Elsevier would like to acknowledge the Traditional Custodians of the lands and waters on which we live and work. We acknowledge that Aboriginal and Torres Strait Islander peoples have continuously passed on knowledge for millennia, using resources from the land and waters to nurture and promote healthy communities, and we pay our respects to Elders past and present.

Elsevier would like to acknowledge the traditional Custodians of the lands and waters on which we live and work. We acknowledge that Aboriginal and Torres Strait Islander peoples have continuously passed on knowledge for millennia, using resources from the land and waters to nurture and promote healthy communities and we pay our respects to Elders past and present.

HAVARD'S NURSING GUIDE TO DRUGS

ADRIANA TIZIANI,
RN, BSC(MON), DIP ED(MELB), MEDST(MON)

MARY BUSHELL, BPHARM (HONS),
PHD, GCTLHE, MPS CRED PHARM (MMR)

KOBI SCHUTZ, RN, MPH

SHAUNAGH DARROCH,
BSC, GRADCERTACAPRAC, MPHARM

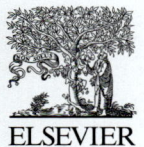
ELSEVIER

12e

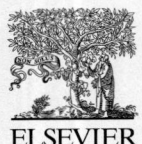

Elsevier Australia. ACN 001 002 357
(a division of Reed International Books Australia Pty Ltd)
Tower 1, 475 Victoria Avenue, Chatswood, NSW 2067

Copyright © 2026 Elsevier Australia. All rights are reserved, including those for text and data mining, AI training, and similar technologies.

Books and Journals published by Elsevier comply with applicable product safety requirements. For any product safety concerns or queries, please contact our authorised representative, Elsevier B.V., at productsafety@elsevier.com.

Publisher's note: Elsevier takes a neutral position with respect to territorial disputes or jurisdictional claims in its published content, including in maps and institutional affiliations.

No part of this publication may be reproduced or transmitted in any form or by any means, electronic or mechanical, including photocopying, recording, or any information storage and retrieval system, without permission in writing from the publisher. Details on how to seek permission, further information about the Publisher's permissions policies and our arrangements with organisations such as the Copyright Clearance Center and the Copyright Licensing Agency, can be found at our website: www.elsevier.com/permissions.

This book and the individual contributions contained in it are protected under copyright by the Publisher (other than as may be noted herein).

ISBN 978-0-7295-9923-8

Notice

Practitioners and researchers must always rely on their own experience and knowledge in evaluating and using any information, methods, compounds or experiments described herein. Because of rapid advances in the medical sciences, in particular, independent verification of diagnoses and drug dosages should be made. To the fullest extent of the law, no responsibility is assumed by Elsevier, authors, editors or contributors for any injury and/or damage to persons or property as a matter of product liability, negligence or otherwise, or from any use or operation of any methods, products, instructions or ideas contained in the material herein.

National Library of Australia Cataloguing-in-Publication Data

A catalogue record for this book is available from the National Library of Australia

---

Senior Content Strategist: Melinda McEvoy
Content Project Manager: Shruti Raj
Edited by Chris Wyard
Proofread by Tim Learner
Cover Design by Gopalakrishnan Venkatraman
Typeset by TNQ Tech
Printed in Australia by Ligare Book Printers

CONTENTS BY THERAPEUTIC CLASS

Icons used in this text	xi
Introduction	xii
Guide to text	xxviii
General Patient Education	xxx
Reviewers	xxxvi
Acne treatment	1
Analgesics and non-steroidal anti-inflammatory drugs (NSAIDs)	10
Anorectics and weight-loss agents	35
Anthelmintics	42
AntiAlzheimer's agents	50
Antianginal agents	58
Antianxiety agents	70
Antiarrhythmic agents	79
Antiasthma agents, bronchodilators and respiratory agents	97
Antibacterial agents	147
Anticoagulants and antithrombotic agents	236
Antidepressants	264
Antidiabetic agents	296
Antidiarrhoeal agents	330
Antidotes, antagonists and chelating agents	334
Antiemetic agents	368
Antiepileptics	384
Antifungal agents	428
Antiglaucoma agents	460
Antigout and uricolytic agents	473
Antihistamines	483
Antihypertensive agents	499
Antimalarial agents	555
Antimigraine agents	569
Antimycobacterial agents	584
Antineoplastic agents	595
Antineoplastic therapy support agents	780
Anti-Parkinson's agents	790
Antiplatelet agents	817
Antiprotozoal agents	825
Antipsychotic and mood-stabilising agents	833
Antiulcer agents	871
Antivenoms	889
Antiviral agents	897
Bladder function disorder agents	942
Bone and calcium regulating agents	957
Cardiac glycosides	979
Cholinergic and anticholinergic agents	981
Corticosteroids	991
Cough suppressants and expectorants	1019
Dermatological agents	1024
Disease-modifying antirheumatic drugs (DMARDs)	1038
Diuretics	1079
Drug dependence	1102
Erectile dysfunction agents	1116
Eye, ear, nose and throat agents	1128
Fibrinolytic agents	1151
Gastrointestinal agents (miscellaneous)	1156
General anaesthetics	1172
Haemopoietic agents	1184
Haemostatics	1194
Hypothalamic and pituitary hormones	1216
Immunomodifiers	1237
Laxatives	1285
Lipid regulating agents	1299
Local anaesthetics	1321
Metabolic disorders agents	1336
Movement disorder agents	1368
Muscle relaxants	1402
Neuromuscular blocking agents	1420
Opioid analgesics	1429
Pregnancy, childbirth and breastfeeding	1456
Pulmonary hypertension agents	1490

Sedatives and hypnotics	1502
Sex hormones	1519
Stimulants	1551
Sympathomimetic agents	1565
Thyroid and antithyroid agents	1579
Vaccines and immunoglobulins	1591
Vasodilators	1632
Vitamins, minerals and electrolytes	1636
Miscellaneous agents	1671
Appendix 1: Poisoning and its treatment	1682
Appendix 2: Poisons information centres	1687
Bibliography	1688
Glossary	1700
Index	1707

CONTENTS BY BODY SYSTEM

Cardiac and Vascular Systems

Antianginal agents	58
Antiarrhythmic agents	79
Anticoagulants and antithrombotic agents	236
Antihypertensive agents	499
Antiplatelet agents	818
Cardiac glycosides	979
Diuretics	1079
Fibrinolytic agents	1151
Haemopoietic agents	1184
Haemostatics	1194
Lipid regulating agents	1299
Pulmonary hypertension agents	1490
Sympathomimetic agents	1565
Vasodilators	1632

Central Nervous System

Anti-Alzheimer's agents	50
Antianxiety agents	70
Antidepressants	264
Antiemetic agents	368
Antimigraine agents	569
Anti-Parkinson's agents	790
Antipsychotic and mood-stabilising agents	833
Drug dependence	1102
Antiepileptics	384
General anaesthetics	1172
Local anaesthetics	1321
Movement disorder agents	1368
Muscle relaxants	1402
Opioid analgesics	1429
Sedatives and hypnotics	1502
Stimulants	1551

Peripheral Nervous System

Cholinergic and anticholinergic agents	981
Neuromuscular blocking agents	1420

Respiratory System

Antiasthma agents, bronchodilators and respiratory agents	97
Cough suppressants and expectorants	1019

Alimentary System

Anorectics and weight-loss agents	35
Antidiarrhoeal agents	330
Antiemetic agents	368
Antiulcer agents	871
Gastrointestinal agents (miscellaneous)	1156
Laxatives	1285
Vitamins, minerals and electrolytes	1636

Musculoskeletal System

Analgesics and non-steroidal anti-inflammatory drugs (NSAIDs)	10
Antigout and uricolytic agents	473
Disease-modifying antirheumatic drugs (DMARDs)	1038

Endocrine System

Antidiabetic agents	296
Bone and calcium regulating agents	957
Corticosteroids	991
Hypothalamic and pituitary hormones	1216
Metabolic disorders agents	1336
Thyroid and antithyroid agents	1579

Urinary System

Bladder function disorder agents	942
Diuretics	1079

Reproductive System

Erectile dysfunction agents	1116
Pregnancy, childbirth and breastfeeding	1456
Sex hormones	1519

Integumentary System

Acne treatment	1
Dermatological agents	1024

Immune System

Antihistamines	483
Antineoplastic agents	595
Antineoplastic therapy support agents	780
Antivenoms	889
Corticosteroids	991
Immunomodifiers	1237
Vaccines and immunoglobulins	1591

Special Senses

Antiglaucoma agents	460
Eye, ear, nose and throat agents	1128

Infection and Infestations

Anthelmintics	42
Antibacterial agents	147
Antifungal agents	428
Antimalarial agents	555
Antimycobacterial agents	584
Antiprotozoal agents	825
Antiviral agents	897

Miscellaneous

Antidotes, antagonists and chelating agents	334
Miscellaneous agents	1671

ICONS USED IN THIS TEXT

Icons are used throughout *Havard's Nursing Guide to Drugs* to highlight important safety information and key considerations related to drug administration. They draw attention to circumstances where additional care, monitoring, or clinical judgement may be required, including dose adjustments, contraindications, and considerations for specific populations.

Icons support rapid identification of critical information and should always be read in conjunction with the accompanying text and current clinical guidelines.

 Hepatic/renal function — dose adjustment may be required in hepatic or renal impairment

 Gerontological considerations

 Sports considerations

 Breastfeeding considerations

 Pregnancy considerations

 Do not crush - dosage form must not be crushed, chewed, or broken

 Crushable/dispersible - dosage form may be crushed or dispersed, if required

 Caution - increased vigilance, monitoring, or clinical judgement required

INTRODUCTION

As with the original aim of the book, *Havard's Nursing Guide to Drugs* continues to be a guide only. This book is meant to be a companion guide to pharmacology texts, something smaller and easier to transport around and reference in the clinical setting, given its availability as an eBook as well.

The Nurse's Role in Drug Therapy

The aims of administering medication are to do it in a safe and efficient manner while observing the patient for both desirable and undesirable effects. Therefore, the nurse needs to:
- assess the patient, including medication history
- have an understanding of the legal requirements associated with the administration of drugs
- have pharmacological knowledge of the medication(s)
- be able to safely administer medications.

Assessing the Patient

Patient assessment should be holistic, looking at the patient's condition and personal circumstances as an entirety, rather than simply as a disease to be treated and this should be reflected in the language used by the nurse (e.g. person with diabetes, not the 'diabetic'). It should include:
- all current medical problems
- comorbidities
- relevant past history
- physical assessment
- medication history (including current medications, over-the-counter (OTC) preparations, herbal preparations, vitamin and mineral supplements, or any other 'alternative' therapy)
- alcohol or tobacco use (and, in some cases, illicit drug use).

Medical history, comorbidities and medication history are intertwined, as a person with comorbidities is often prescribed multiple medications concurrently (polypharmacy), which increases the risk of adverse effects and interactions. Sometimes a person sees more than one medical practitioner (e.g. general practitioner (GP) plus specialist/s), which increases the risk of medications not being regularly reviewed.

People may become confused because medications can have more than one brand/trade name for the same generic drug and they can potentially end up taking the same drug twice (e.g. a patient taking Frusemix-M, Uremide or Lasix (trade names for furosemide (frusemide)) may become quickly dehydrated).

Unfortunately, people do not always complete courses of medications, especially antibiotics, and 'keep the rest for next time' with no understanding of the ramifications of doing this (e.g. bacteria becoming resistant to that antibiotic and the agent becoming ineffective in treating that same infection if it recurs). Other reasons for not completing courses of medications (or not getting prescriptions refilled) include adverse effects, costs or failing to see any obvious benefits from the medication.

Some people believe they are allergic to medications. It is important for the

- to change the route of administration or dosage (e.g. from IV or IM to oral administration) if necessary while maintaining adequate serum levels
- to guide withdrawal of therapy (Knights et al 2023).

Drug route

The effectiveness of a drug often depends on the route of administration. A drug may have a systemic or local effect depending on whether it is taken orally, injected or applied topically (see Glossary, pp. 1700–1706 for forms of preparations). Drugs are formulated to meet the requirements for rapid or slow absorption, metabolism or excretion in order to obtain the required therapeutic blood levels. The two most common routes of drug administration are oral and parenteral.

Oral administration

Many oral preparations are given on an empty stomach because food may decrease the absorption; however, if gastric irritation is a problem they may be given with or immediately after food.

It is recommended that a capsule is preceded by a small amount of water and then taken with half a glass of water to prevent it becoming lodged in the oesophagus. A number of medications are known to cause oesophageal ulceration 'including' aspirin, bisphosphonates (e.g. alendronate), doxycycline, iron tablets, potassium chloride and zidovudine (Gowan & Roller 2010). Enteric-coated, slow-release, extended-release, modified-release, sustained-release and controlled-dosage tablets should be swallowed whole, not crushed or chewed, for a number of reasons, which may include the following:

- absorption will be altered (e.g. MS Contin, Keflor CD, Efexor XR, Dilantin)
- the medication may become unstable (e.g. Augmentin Duo, Nimotop)
- they may cause local irritation (e.g. Cartia, Roaccutane)
- they will not reach the site of the intended action (e.g. Creon, Dipentum)
- unacceptable taste (e.g. Neoral, Coloxyl)
- being hazardous (e.g. Imuran, Myleran, Leukeran).

Care must be taken to select the correct formulation of tablets when several different formulations and/or dosages exist (e.g. verapamil is available as 40 mg or 80 mg, immediate-release tablets and also as 180 mg or 240 mg slow-release tablets), because the consequences may be very serious if the wrong formulation is administered (e.g. substituting verapamil 80 mg (3 tablets), which will act immediately compared with verapamil 240 mg, which is a sustained-release preparation and will act over 24 hours). It is important to check whether different formulations are interchangeable or not (e.g. olapatib is available as a tablet or capsule; however, the strengths are different, as are the recommended dosages, and they are therefore not interchangeable).

Crushing or dispersing medications

It is important to check whether the medication can be dispersed or crushed. As previously stated, sustained- or modified-release medications should not be crushed or dispersed. Important considerations include:

- assessing whether the patient has any swallowing difficulties or is 'at risk' of aspiration. If there are any concerns, referral to a speech pathologist is recommended to determine appropriate fluids or soft foods (e.g. apple purée, yoghurt) that can be used to

administer crushed or dispersed medication
- checking whether the medication is available in a different formulation which is easier to administer (e.g. syrup or solution rather than tablet form)
- preparing only one medication at a time (i.e. only one tablet should be crushed and prepared at a time, not the patient's entire medications)
- any fluid restriction when dispersing medication (e.g. how much fluid should be used to disperse the medication, which should be considered in the patient's overall fluid intake)
- using a closed tablet crusher for medications which are hazardous, cytotoxic or teratogenic
- use of safety glasses, mask and gloves for handling of medications which are hazardous, cytotoxic or teratogenic
- reducing pregnant staff contact with medications that are hazardous, cytotoxic or teratogenic
- ensuring mortar and pestle/tablet crusher are cleaned between medications and between patients (Advanced Pharmacy Australia 2025).

Parenteral administration

Parenteral medications are given either as injections or by infusion. The most common routes are intramuscular (IM), subcutaneous (SC) and intravenous (IV).

Intramuscular

The three main muscles used for intramuscular injections are:
- the lateral aspect of the thigh (the middle third when the thigh is divided into three)
- the upper outer quadrant of the dorsogluteal
- the deltoid.

No more than 5 mL should be administered by intramuscular injection, and less into the deltoid muscle. If a volume > 5 mL is required, the dose should be divided and given into different sites. Furthermore, the deltoid muscle is not recommended for intramuscular injection in children.

Subcutaneous

Subcutaneous injection sites include:
- the upper outer aspect (middle third) of the upper arm
- the upper anterior thigh
- the abdomen below the costal margins to the iliac crests (avoiding the area around the navel by about 5 cm).

When frequent administration is required (e.g. insulin administration in a patient with diabetes mellitus, daily heparin injections), administration sites should be rotated and documented on the medication chart to prevent atrophy of the subcutaneous tissue, increased risk of infection and pain.

Intravenous

A drug may be given by direct IV injection as a bolus in a volume of 20 mL or less in under 1 minute, or by slow IV injection over 5—15 minutes. It is important to check and adhere to the manufacturer's information regarding the required administration time, because administering some drugs too quickly can cause pain and damage the blood vessel, as well as other adverse effects, such as flushing, hyper- or hypotension, syncope, arrhythmias, feelings of warmth or anxiety, depending on the drug administered. IV injection (bolus or slow injection) is used when an immediate effect is required or the drug becomes unstable on reconstitution or dilution. The intermittent infusion method is used when a drug is diluted, when interval dosing is desired and when slow administration is required. The drug is diluted in 50–250 mL and infused over 15 minutes to 2 hours. This minimises stability and incompatibility problems and gives the 'peak' and 'trough' effect in antibiotic therapy. One of the advantages of intermittent IV administration is that the patient can have an intermittent venous access port, which increases client mobility, comfort and safety, as well as providing a cost benefit from not having continuous IV therapy; also the nurse does not have to continuously monitor flow rates.

When a drug must be highly diluted and a steady-state blood level is to be maintained, the continuous infusion method is used, in which the drug is diluted in 500–1000 mL and infused over 4–24 hours (e.g. potassium chloride requires a high dilution and constant blood levels to prevent depression of cardiac function).

The IV flow rate may be controlled by using an infusion pump, a microdrip set or a burette. When a drug is added to the burette during intermittent infusion, details of the additive are indicated on a label that is attached to the burette. Any IV drug admixture must be prepared aseptically, mixed thoroughly and labelled with the name and amount of the additive, the name of the person adding the agent, the name of the person checking the addition and the time of starting the infusion. National recommendations for user-applied labelling of injectable medicines, fluids and lines now exist and it is imperative that nurses understand and comply with these, as consequences of non-labelling can result in a potentially life-threatening situation for the patient. These recommendations include colour coding the route of administration (e.g. red for intra-arterial, blue for intravenous, yellow for epidural or intrathecal and beige for subcutaneous), the process for medicine and label preparation (including label placement), when to discard containers of injectable medicines and special circumstances (ACSQHC 2016a). While these labelling recommendations do not apply to enteral, topical or inhalation routes, the general principles still apply as a way of improving practice and decreasing the risk of errors occurring.

An IV admixture should not be administered if there are signs of physical incompatibility such as a colour change, loss of clarity or precipitate formation. Chemical and physical compatibility and stability of admixtures should be checked *before* administration. If in any doubt, the nurse should consult a pharmacist, textbooks, the manufacturer's information or a drug information centre.

Other administration routes

Drugs generally should not be mixed with blood or blood products.

Other methods of administering medications include the following:

- *Transdermal patches*, which deliver drugs through the skin at a steady concentration, avoiding first-pass metabolism in the liver and any gastric side-effects. Several types of drugs, including glyceryl trinitrate, fentanyl, hormones and nicotine, are available as transdermal patches. Advantages include ease of application and frequency of application (once daily or longer), but the disadvantages include some skin reactions and the low number of drugs available via this route.
- *Intradermal implants*, which are surgically implanted subcutaneously.

dependent on a number of factors, including fetal gestational age on exposure (i.e. the fetus is most at risk during the first trimester, when cells are rapidly proliferating and organs, muscles, CNS, arms, legs, toes and fingers are developing), duration of therapy (including dose, frequency and length of therapy), as well as any other medication taken concurrently (Knights et al 2023). Animal studies have shown considerable differences in species' response with regard to the teratogenic effects of drugs and it may not be possible to extrapolate this data to humans. Fetal abnormalities include missing digits, excessive development or duplication of parts, splitting of parts abnormally, non-splitting of parts, fusion failure or over-fusion of some parts, openings failing to close or open adequately and abnormal placement of parts.

If possible, medications should be avoided during pregnancy. However, this is not always possible or practicable. The woman who is pregnant (or considering pregnancy) should work in partnership with her medical practitioner to develop a medication regimen that balances the benefits to the mother against the potential risks to the fetus. For example, a woman with epilepsy may need to consider the potentially life-threatening risks associated with uncontrolled epilepsy versus the benefits of controlling epilepsy with an agent that has an increased risk of causing fetal abnormalities.

Breastfeeding

Most drugs taken by a mother who is breastfeeding will be excreted to some extent in the breastmilk; however, the amount ingested by the infant will generally be extremely small, and dependent on the age of the infant and the amount of breastmilk consumed (Hotham & Hotham 2015). Some drugs are concentrated in breastmilk relative to the maternal plasma concentration because of their chemical properties, including fat solubility, and may be toxic to the infant because of immaturity of the liver and kidney detoxification systems. Drugs contraindicated during breastfeeding include amiodarone, antineoplastic agents, gold salts, iodine, lithium, oral retinoids and radiopharmaceuticals. Further contraindications during breastfeeding include those very toxic agents where even very small amounts will affect the infant, if the drug has highly allergenic potential, if the maternal renal function is compromised (as this may lead to higher levels being excreted into breastmilk) and the mother having a medical condition requiring prolonged administration of a drug (e.g. cancer) (Hotham & Hotham 2015; Knights et al 2023).

Administering the drug when or immediately after the infant feeds will result in the lowest amount of drug being in the milk at subsequent feedings. If a drug is essential for the mother but of uncertain effect on the infant, it may be necessary to temporarily discontinue breastfeeding and remove contaminated breastmilk (via a breast pump), which should be discarded (Knights et al 2023).

If medication is taken during breastfeeding, the infant should always be closely observed for any side-effects, including poor feeding, listlessness, withdrawal symptoms and other abnormal behaviours, which should be reported if they occur.

Renal and Liver Impairment

Dose reduction is often required in those with any type of kidney and/or liver impairment because these organs are the main sites of drug metabolism and excretion. Monitoring of kidney and liver function throughout any drug therapy may be recommended to ensure that there is no further deterioration caused by the therapy. Furthermore, some medications may damage the liver or kidneys (e.g. large doses of paracetamol are hepatotoxic; non-steroidal anti-inflammatory drugs (NSAIDs) may be nephrotoxic). If potentially nephrotoxic or hepatotoxic agents are given to those with renal or liver impairment, the risk of further damage is greatly increased. Included in this edition are cautions and contraindications specifically related to liver and/or renal impairment.

Legal Requirements

Before a drug can be administered safely, the nurse needs to be aware of the legal aspects of drug administration. This includes knowledge of the laws governing the possession, use and dispensation of drugs and of the directives of the nurse's registering body on the administration of medications to clients. It also means observing the employing health care facility's occupational health and safety (OHS) regulations, which are designed to promote safe storage, handling and use of drugs.

The Nursing and Midwifery Board of Australia (NMBA) is one of the national boards of the Australian Health Practitioner Regulation Agency (Ahpra). With the changes to registration of nurses by Ahpra from 2010, it was decided that enrolled nurses no longer required endorsement for medication administration. The NMBA's goal is for all enrolled nurses (EN) to undertake relevant units of study that will enable them to administer medicines safely as part of their education program. However, for enrolled nurses who have not completed the required units, a notation reading 'Does not hold Board-approved qualifi-cations in administration of medicines' will appear on the national nursing reg-ister against that nurse's name (NMBA Ahpra 2023). Furthermore, ENs with a notation stating 'may only practice in the area of mothercraft nursing' are also unable to administer medications. Jurisdictional legislation and policy specify the routes and schedules of medicines that the enrolled nurse is able to administer and it is therefore of paramount importance that the nurse and employer understand and comply with the drugs and poisons legislation and policy. Furthermore, to administer intravenous medication, the enrolled nurse (Division 2) is required to have completed a separate NMBA-approved unit on the administration and moni-toring of intravenous medications (NMBA Ahpra 2023).

Legal Acts concerning poisons and the poisons regulatory bodies in New Zealand and each state and territory in Australia deal with the control of all drugs, from prescription medication through to agricultural poisons and research drugs. The Standard for the Uniform Scheduling of Medicines and Poisons (SUSMP) applies to sale, supply, containers, disposal, record keeping, storage, labelling, possession, use and advertising. The drugs and poisons contained in the schedules are divided into groups according to their mode of action, therapeutic use, potency, potential for abuse and addiction, and safety.

In Australia, there are currently 10 schedules, with most medications being listed in Schedules 2, 3, 4 or 8 (Therapeutic Goods Administration 2023). Unscheduled substances (i.e. those not contained in these 10 schedules) are not considered a poison by definition and can be supplied to the public; these include laxatives, sunscreens, baby formula, herbal remedies and vitamins (Knights et al 2023). It should be noted, however, that many of these unscheduled substances interact with prescription medications.

While medical practitioners are the main health professionals who advise and prescribe medications, there are members of other health disciplines who have limited prescribing rights. Nurse practitioners, as defined by the *Nurses Act 1993*, are those whose registration has been endorsed as being qualified to obtain and have in their possession and to use, sell or supply Schedule 2, 3, 4 or 8 poisons, as described under the *Drugs, Poisons and Controlled Substances Act 1981* (Version No. 142, 12/11/2025). The approved list of medications (scheduled poisons) is dependent on the nurse practitioner's scope of practice (e.g. an acute care nurse practitioner list will be different to that of a paediatric care nurse practitioner). After completing approved postgraduate education, designated registered nurse prescribers are able to work in partnership with an authorised health practitioner under a prescribing agreement and are able to prescribe Schedule 2, 3, 4 and 8 medicines similar to a nurse practitioner. The major difference between these two roles is that the nurse practitioner practices autonomously whereas the designated registered nurse prescriber must work with an authorised health practitioner (NMBA 2025a, 2025b). In a similar way, midwifes can also be endorsed to prescribe specific Schedule 2, 3, 4 and 8 medicines related to midwifery practice (NMBA 2017).

Dentists are able to prescribe drugs related to their practice (e.g. antibiotics, analgesics); podiatrists with endorsement may prescribe a limited range of Schedule 4 drugs related to podiatry practice (e.g. antibiotics, analgesics); optometrists (in some states, with extra training) are also able to prescribe a limited range of optometry-related Schedule 4 drugs (e.g. eye drops, drugs to treat glaucoma) (Knights et al 2023).

Storage

All medications in a ward or department should be kept in a locked cupboard, medication trolley or some other type of locked container, the key of which is kept by a nurse at all times. Victoria's Drugs, Poisons and Controlled Substances Regulations 2017 are very specific about the storage requirements for Schedule 8 or Schedule 9 poisons (e.g. constructed of steel 10 millimetres thick; fitted with a 6-lever lock; able to resist attack by hand tools for 30 minutes or power tools for 5 minutes) (Victorian Government 2017 (authorised version with amendments November 2025)), with other states having similar requirements. Furthermore, electronic storage and recording equipment can be used to store Schedule 8 poisons if security is equivalent to that previously described, and has features to record and report access, attempted access and discrepancies, as well as visual, electronic or audible alerts if left open, damaged or disconnected from power, and will generate a report that identifies any breaches or attempted breaches to security (Victorian Government 2017 (authorised version with amendments November 2025)).

Drugs or preparations for external use should be stored apart from those intended for internal use, so that errors in administration do not occur. Suppositories, pessaries, insulins, antisera, vaccines, some blood products, some intravenous solutions and some antibiotics (particularly if reconstituted) should be stored in the refrigerator. Nothing else should be stored in the refrigerator (e.g. food) and it should also be kept locked.

The trend towards single-dose units being dispensed contributes to accuracy in dosage, better economy and less risk of product contamination. Many institutions have policies that discourage the use of multidose vials because of the risk of cross-contamination between patients.

Drug Orders

In 2004, Australian health ministers advised that *'to reduce the harm to patients from medication errors, by June 2006, all public hospitals will be using a common medication chart. This means that the same chart will be used wherever a doctor or nurse works and wherever the patient is within a hospital'* (ACSQHC 2019). The result was the National Inpatient Medication Chart (NIMC). Since then, additional national charts have been developed, including the National Residential Medication Chart (NRMC), National Subcutaneous Insulin Chart, Paediatric National Inpatient Medication Chart, Clozapine Titration Chart, NIMC (acute), NIMC (long stay), NIMC (day surgery) and NIMC (day surgery, private hospital). Further work has resulted in the development of electronic medication charts. The introduction and use of electronic medication management (EMM) should enable healthcare services to improve their care by decreasing the number of preventable adverse events, including medication prescribing and dispensing errors (ACSQHC 2025a).

The law in all states requires that a legal drug order must be written either in the prescriber's own handwriting or in a manner approved (by the Public Health and Well Being Act 2008), is written in a legible and durable form, is dated and signed by the prescriber and must include the patient's name and identification number (if applicable), name and strength of the drug, the dose, route of administration, frequency of administration and duration of administration (if applicable). For a Schedule 8 medication, the maximum time it may be supplied must be written in words and numbers. For a Schedule 4 medication, this is required only if required more than once. If there is any doubt about the meaning of the order, the medical officer should be contacted immediately for clarification before administration. Furthermore, since 2021 active ingredient prescribing has been adopted with or without brand names, with prescribers having the option to allow (or not) brand substitution. Prescribers may also prescribe by brand name (rather than active ingredient) if the medication contains four or more active ingredients, or if inclusion of active ingredients is impractical (e.g. ocular lubricants), is for non-medical items (e.g. dressing products, vitamin supplements) or is for vaccines containing various strains (ACSQHC 2021).

Legal Responsibility

Following a medical officer's order was once thought by many to absolve the nurse from all responsibility. However, legal judgments have shown that this is not always the case. The question that is often asked in situations of a drug error occurring is, 'What would the *reasonable* nurse do in this situation?'

Given that administering drugs is an everyday part of the role of most nurses, it is therefore not an unfair expectation that they will have some knowledge of the drugs they are administering. This includes the class of drug, why it is prescribed (purpose), how it works (action), recommended or usual dose range, how it is administered, contraindications, side-effects, potential for causing allergic reactions, any interactions with foods or other drugs and compatibility (especially when multiple intravenous drugs are to be administered).

It is not necessary for the nurse to memorise all this information; however, what is important is that the nurse has ready access to information and knows where or how to readily do so *before* administration. Information on any drug or preparation may be obtained from a pharmacist, textbooks or *reliable* internet sources. Once in possession of this knowledge, the nurse can question an unclear order, assess what skills are required to carry out the order and will understand what to observe in the patient in terms of beneficial and adverse effects.

Drug Incidents (Errors)

Drug incidents (or errors) are any preventable events involving medications that may result in harm and are related to the prescribing, dispensing or administering stages of the process (Jokanovic et al 2019). 'Medication error resulting in serious harm or death' is one of Australia's 10 sentinel events and is considered to be 'wholly preventable' and requires mandatory reporting if it occurs (ACSQHC 2025b). Within the acute care sector, the most common medication errors include mistakes when rewriting drug orders (by doctors) and administration errors (by nurses); however, dispensing errors (by pharmacists) also occur.

Administration incidents (errors) occur when:

- the wrong drug is administered, including the administration of the wrong intravenous fluid (e.g. drugs with similar names; use of abbreviations for names)
- the wrong dose is given (e.g. misreading dosage or units; misinterpreting abbreviations used for units, such as micrograms)
- the drug is given via the wrong route (e.g. an oral drug given intravenously)
- the drug is given to the wrong patient
- the drug is given at the wrong time or frequency, including omission, and/or
- an intravenous infusion is administered at the wrong rate.

Since 2008, standard prescribing terminology, abbreviations and symbols have been introduced in an attempt to reduce the number of associated errors. Abbreviations are used when referring to strength of medications, such as grams (g) and milligrams (mg). For example, the abbreviation for micrograms using the Greek letter μ (mu), that is, μg, is not recommended, nor is mcg, as these may lead to errors; microg is the preferred and recommended abbreviation, or the

INTRODUCTION

whole word (microgram) should be used. Other error-prone abbreviations and symbols that should be avoided include IU (international units — can be mistaken for IV), IVI (intravenous injection — mistaken for IV 1) and qd (every day — mistaken as qid (4 times daily)) (ACSQHC 2023).

The use of 'dose administration aids' (DAAs), commonly found in the community and some residential aged care facilities, may not necessarily reduce the number of administration errors. A 2006 study found that DAAs contained a significant number of errors (incident rate 4.3% of packs and 12% of residents), which included missing medications, the wrong medication or wrong strength of medication dispensed, incorrect dosage instructions supplied or medications being supplied that had been ceased by a doctor (Carruthers et al 2008). A study by Gilmartin and colleagues found similar results, with a proportion of inspected DAAs having additional medications added to them, medications missing and incorrect or inappropriate division of tablets amongst identified errors. Furthermore, while the majority of errors were classified as minor or insignificant, there were also a number of potential major or catastrophic errors (Gilmartin et al 2016). Although on the surface this would appear to be a dispensing- and pharmacy-related problem, it is also the responsibility of the nurse administering the medications to have some idea of what medication a patient has been prescribed (or no longer prescribed), and what the medication(s) actually looks like. DAAs are not suitable for all patients and require careful patient selection (e.g. community-based patients should be motivated and willing to take the medication, and have adequate vision, dexterity and cognition) and awareness of the limitations of the aid selected (e.g. increase in cost, including set-up costs; doses missed if medication is spilled during administration and no back-up available; if home delivered, no opportunity for pharmacist review and counselling; many medicines cannot be packed into a dosing aid; and do not address intentional non-adherence, poor motivation or forgetfulness) (Elliott 2014).

An administration error may or may not have an adverse effect. The seriousness of the outcome (e.g. the adverse effect or lack of effect) does not absolve the nurse from the mistake that was made. It is important to clearly document the error and outcome. Some institutions may also have policies regarding further documentation requirements when an error has occurred (e.g. a 'drug incident' form).

It is important for nurses to practise within their own limitations and within the policies and protocols of the institution. If this is not done and an error occurs (especially a serious one), the nurse may find that the institution (and its insurers) may abrogate any responsibility because the nurse did not follow its policies. The nurse may also be liable under common law.

A Little Pharmacology

For extensive pharmacokinetics and pharmacology, refer to pharmacology texts. Here are some basic concepts that nurses need to understand.

Drug dosage

Dosage depends on the age, weight, sex, renal and liver function and general condition of the patient, and can be based on age, body weight or body

xxi

surface area. As children usually require smaller doses than adults, various rules are used to estimate the fraction of the adult dose (see inside front cover).

Dose interval is important (e.g. anti-infective agents are given at regular intervals, 4-, 6- or 8-hourly, to maintain adequate blood levels, while hormones are given at the same time each day for uniform effect). The time of day must be suitable to the individual's lifestyle. For example, diuretics may be ordered twice daily and normal convention would see them administered at regular intervals (e.g. 8—10-hourly during the day); however, for an older person it may be more practicable to administer the diuretic in the morning and at lunchtime, so that sleep is not disturbed by frequent micturition, increasing the risk of falls.

Drug half-life

The half-life of a drug is a function of both distribution and elimination. In general terms, it is the time required for half of the amount of drug in the body to be eliminated. It is of practical use in calculating the frequency with which multiple doses of a drug can be administered to keep the blood level between the minimum effective concentration and the threshold for toxicity (e.g. a drug with a very short half-life may need to be administered intravenously to maintain levels, while another drug with a long half-life may be suitable for once-daily administration). Furthermore, a drug with a very long half-life may require patient monitoring for some time after the drug has been discontinued or may require a 'washout' period to allow the drug to be removed from the system before the introduction of another agent.

Therapeutic drug monitoring

Some drugs have a narrow therapeutic range (i.e. the difference between overdosing and underdosing). Therapeutic drug monitoring involves measuring drug concentration in the blood. Information accompanying a request form should include the time the blood sample was taken, the time the last dose of the drug was given and its route of administration. The main aim of therapeutic drug monitoring is to optimise drug therapy by achieving adequate drug levels while minimising toxicity. It is especially important in those at the extremes of age (i.e. babies and the elderly).

Why measure drug levels?

Drug levels are measured for a number of reasons, which include:
- to individualise the dose (e.g. lithium, phenytoin, warfarin, levothyroxine)
- to assess the adequacy of loading dose (e.g. phenytoin) or to check levels after dose adjustment
- to avoid or diagnose toxicity (e.g. digoxin, vancomycin)
- to ensure effective blood levels (e.g. prophylactic antiepileptics, gentamicin)
- to check adherence to regimen (e.g. antipsychotic agents)
- to check that comorbidities that may alter drug metabolism and elimination (e.g. renal impairment, hepatic failure, shock, sepsis) are not affecting blood levels
- to ensure that concurrent drug administration is not affecting blood levels
- to diagnose subtherapeutic or failed therapy (to distinguish between ineffective drug treatment, non-adherence and adverse effects that mimic underlying disease)

INTRODUCTION

- to change the route of administration or dosage (e.g. from IV or IM to oral administration) if necessary while maintaining adequate serum levels
- to guide withdrawal of therapy (Knights et al 2023).

Drug route

The effectiveness of a drug often depends on the route of administration. A drug may have a systemic or local effect depending on whether it is taken orally, injected or applied topically (see Glossary, pp. 1700–1706 for forms of preparations). Drugs are formulated to meet the requirements for rapid or slow absorption, metabolism or excretion in order to obtain the required therapeutic blood levels. The two most common routes of drug administration are oral and parenteral.

Oral administration

Many oral preparations are given on an empty stomach because food may decrease the absorption; however, if gastric irritation is a problem they may be given with or immediately after food.

It is recommended that a capsule is preceded by a small amount of water and then taken with half a glass of water to prevent it becoming lodged in the oesophagus. A number of medications are known to cause oesophageal ulceration 'including' aspirin, bisphosphonates (e.g. alendronate), doxycycline, iron tablets, potassium chloride and zidovudine (Gowan & Roller 2010). Enteric-coated, slow-release, extended-release, modified-release, sustained-release and controlled-dosage tablets should be swallowed whole, not crushed or chewed, for a number of reasons, which may include the following:

- absorption will be altered (e.g. MS Contin, Keflor CD, Efexor XR, Dilantin)
- the medication may become unstable (e.g. Augmentin Duo, Nimotop)
- they may cause local irritation (e.g. Cartia, Roaccutane)
- they will not reach the site of the intended action (e.g. Creon, Dipentum)
- unacceptable taste (e.g. Neoral, Coloxyl)
- being hazardous (e.g. Imuran, Myleran, Leukeran).

Care must be taken to select the correct formulation of tablets when several different formulations and/or dosages exist (e.g. verapamil is available as 40 mg or 80 mg, immediate-release tablets and also as 180 mg or 240 mg slow-release tablets), because the consequences may be very serious if the wrong formulation is administered (e.g. substituting verapamil 80 mg (3 tablets), which will act immediately compared with verapamil 240 mg, which is a sustained-release preparation and will act over 24 hours). It is important to check whether different formulations are interchangeable or not (e.g. olapatib is available as a tablet or capsule; however, the strengths are different, as are the recommended dosages, and they are therefore not interchangeable).

Crushing or dispersing medications

It is important to check whether the medication can be dispersed or crushed. As previously stated, sustained- or modified-release medications should not be crushed or dispersed. Important considerations include:

- assessing whether the patient has any swallowing difficulties or is 'at risk' of aspiration. If there are any concerns, referral to a speech pathologist is recommended to determine appropriate fluids or soft foods (e.g. apple purée, yoghurt) that can be used to

- administer crushed or dispersed medication
- checking whether the medication is available in a different formulation which is easier to administer (e.g. syrup or solution rather than tablet form)
- preparing only one medication at a time (i.e. only one tablet should be crushed and prepared at a time, not the patient's entire medications)
- any fluid restriction when dispersing medication (e.g. how much fluid should be used to disperse the medication, which should be considered in the patient's overall fluid intake)
- using a closed tablet crusher for medications which are hazardous, cytotoxic or teratogenic
- use of safety glasses, mask and gloves for handling of medications which are hazardous, cytotoxic or teratogenic
- reducing pregnant staff contact with medications that are hazardous, cytotoxic or teratogenic
- ensuring mortar and pestle/tablet crusher are cleaned between medications and between patients (Advanced Pharmacy Australia 2025).

Parenteral administration

Parenteral medications are given either as injections or by infusion. The most common routes are intramuscular (IM), subcutaneous (SC) and intravenous (IV).

Intramuscular

The three main muscles used for intramuscular injections are:
- the lateral aspect of the thigh (the middle third when the thigh is divided into three)
- the upper outer quadrant of the dorsogluteal
- the deltoid.

No more than 5 mL should be administered by intramuscular injection, and less into the deltoid muscle. If a volume > 5 mL is required, the dose should be divided and given into different sites. Furthermore, the deltoid muscle is not recommended for intramuscular injection in children.

Subcutaneous

Subcutaneous injection sites include:
- the upper outer aspect (middle third) of the upper arm
- the upper anterior thigh
- the abdomen below the costal margins to the iliac crests (avoiding the area around the navel by about 5 cm).

When frequent administration is required (e.g. insulin administration in a patient with diabetes mellitus, daily heparin injections), administration sites should be rotated and documented on the medication chart to prevent atrophy of the subcutaneous tissue, increased risk of infection and pain.

Intravenous

A drug may be given by direct IV injection as a bolus in a volume of 20 mL or less in under 1 minute, or by slow IV injection over 5–15 minutes. It is important to check and adhere to the manufacturer's information regarding the required administration time, because administering some drugs too quickly can cause pain and damage the blood vessel, as well as other adverse effects, such as flushing, hyper- or hypotension, syncope, arrhythmias, feelings of warmth or anxiety, depending on the drug administered. IV injection (bolus or slow injection) is used when an immediate effect is required or the drug becomes unstable on reconstitution or dilution. The intermittent infusion method is used when a drug is diluted, when interval dosing is desired and when slow administration is required. The drug is diluted in 50–250 mL and infused over 15 minutes to 2 hours. This minimises stability and incompatibility problems and gives the 'peak' and 'trough' effect in antibiotic therapy. One of the advantages of intermittent IV administration is that the patient can have an intermittent venous access port, which increases client mobility, comfort and safety, as well as providing a cost benefit from not having continuous IV therapy; also the nurse does not have to continuously monitor flow rates.

When a drug must be highly diluted and a steady-state blood level is to be maintained, the continuous infusion method is used, in which the drug is diluted in 500–1000 mL and infused over 4–24 hours (e.g. potassium chloride requires a high dilution and constant blood levels to prevent depression of cardiac function).

The IV flow rate may be controlled by using an infusion pump, a microdrip set or a burette. When a drug is added to the burette during intermittent infusion, details of the additive are indicated on a label that is attached to the burette. Any IV drug admixture must be prepared aseptically, mixed thoroughly and labelled with the name and amount of the additive, the name of the person adding the agent, the name of the person checking the addition and the time of starting the infusion. National recommendations for user-applied labelling of injectable medicines, fluids and lines now exist and it is imperative that nurses understand and comply with these, as consequences of non-labelling can result in a potentially life-threatening situation for the patient. These recommendations include colour coding the route of administration (e.g. red for intra-arterial, blue for intravenous, yellow for epidural or intrathecal and beige for subcutaneous), the process for medicine and label preparation (including label placement), when to discard containers of injectable medicines and special circumstances (ACSQHC 2016a). While these labelling recommendations do not apply to enteral, topical or inhalation routes, the general principles still apply as a way of improving practice and decreasing the risk of errors occurring.

An IV admixture should not be administered if there are signs of physical incompatibility such as a colour change, loss of clarity or precipitate formation. Chemical and physical compatibility and stability of admixtures should be checked *before* administration. If in any doubt, the nurse should consult a pharmacist, textbooks, the manufacturer's information or a drug information centre.

Other administration routes

Drugs generally should not be mixed with blood or blood products.

Other methods of administering medications include the following:

- *Transdermal patches*, which deliver drugs through the skin at a steady concentration, avoiding first-pass metabolism in the liver and any gastric side-effects. Several types of drugs, including glyceryl trinitrate, fentanyl, hormones and nicotine, are available as transdermal patches. Advantages include ease of application and frequency of application (once daily or longer), but the disadvantages include some skin reactions and the low number of drugs available via this route.
- *Intradermal implants*, which are surgically implanted subcutaneously.

Advantages include the frequency of administration (some may be implanted for 6–8 weeks or longer); however, they require surgical implanting and removal (e.g. etonogestrel (long-term contraception) is left in situ for 3 years before replacement).

Guide for Safe Administration

Some drugs, such as Schedule 8, require double-checking; however, it is important that the double-checking procedure is an independent cognitive task (i.e. the nurse independently calculates the amount required as opposed to checking or glancing at someone else's calculations), rather than it being a superficial routine task. While double-checking is time consuming, it is central to patient safety and reducing drug errors (Ramasamy et al 2013).

Check the order
- Check that the information on the drug name, dose, route, frequency, time due and when the drug was last given are all legible (if any doubt exists, withhold the drug and check with the medical officer) and that the order is signed by the medical officer.
- Check that patient details are correct, including any known allergies (it is important to discuss any allergy/sensitivity history with the patient as cross-sensitivity between products does occur).

Check the drug
- Check the container label against the medication order when selecting the preparation, before measuring out and when replacing the preparation.
- Check the expiry date of the drug.
- Complete the drug calculation and then check the answer with another registered nurse, a pharmacist or a medical officer (ask the second person to do the calculation independently, then compare answers, remembering that it is rare to give less than half a tablet or more than 2 tablets or 1 ampoule at a time).
- Mix liquid contents thoroughly, however rotate or swirl protein preparations gently to prevent denaturation and frothing. If the reconstituted solution containing protein is further diluted, it should be gently inverted (not shaken) to ensure even mixing.
- Note any discolouration, precipitate or foreign bodies (and do not administer if they are present).

Check the patient
- Check the patient's identity carefully (check the wrist identity band, verbally or scan wrist band as well as verbally), taking extra care if there are patients with the same or similar names, or if the patient is unknown to the nurse, especially in situations where the patient may be confused or non-English speaking. An observational study of nurses administering medications found that 79% did not check the patient's identity before administration (Westbrook et al 2015). Where electronic medication management (EMM) is in place, patient identification will involve scanning the person's wristband and the medication to be administered.
- Check if the patient has any known allergies.
- Check that the patient knows the reason for the medication and discuss

INTRODUCTION

any query with the medical officer before giving it.
- Give only medications that you, the nurse, have prepared or seen a pharmacist prepare (i.e. do not administer an IV drug that was drawn up by someone else without you present).
- Give the correct drug and dose.
- Give to the correct patient.
- Give at the correct time.
- Give medication by the prescribed route.
- Do not handle tablets.
- Wait until oral medications are swallowed (never leave medications on bedside tables, lockers or dinner trays).

Documentation
- Ensure that the drug administration sheet is signed after administration.
- Document any discrepancies (e.g. a patient unable or refusing to take medication, a patient absent, medication not available).
- If Schedule 8 drugs are involved, ensure that the drug register is correctly filled in (with date, time, patient, drug (form, strength, amount to be administered), persons administering drug, balance of drug remaining, any drug discarded).
- Observe the patient and document in the patient's history.
- Note beneficial effects and/or report and chart any adverse effects (see the brief discussion below).

Disposal
- Correctly and safely dispose of equipment used (e.g. do not recap syringes, dispose of them safely in a sharps container and return unused medications to pharmacy).

Drug effects
A drug may produce more than one effect, which may be beneficial or not.
- *The desired action* is the physiological response the drug is expected to cause (e.g. antihypertensive medications are expected to lower blood pressure).
- *Adverse effects* refer to an unwanted effect which may or may not be dose related and is usually via a different mechanism to its pharmacological action.
- *Toxic effects* develop after prolonged administration of high doses of medication, or when a drug accumulates in the blood because of impaired metabolism or excretion. Some drugs, such as digoxin and lithium, have a very narrow safety margin and toxicity can occur at recommended or therapeutic doses.
- *Allergic reactions* are unpredictable responses to a drug that acts as an antigen, triggering the release of antibodies. Allergic reactions may be mild (such as urticaria (hives) and pruritus (itching)), or they may be severe (e.g. severe wheezing and respiratory distress) or life threatening (e.g. anaphylactic reaction). Some reactions occur within minutes of the drug being given (e.g. penicillin, streptomycin, radiological contrast media), while other allergic reactions may be delayed for hours or days (e.g. contact sensitivity to local anaesthetic cream).
- *Idiosyncratic reactions* are those where the patient's body either overreacts or underreacts to a drug, or when the reaction is unusual and there is no known cause (e.g. the antihistamine promethazine (Phenergan) is sometimes used for sedation; however, in some people

- (especially children) it can cause insomnia and agitation).
- *Pharmacogenetic reactions* occur because a person may have a genetic trait which leads to abnormal re-actions to drugs (e.g. those with glucose-6-phosphate dehydrogenase (G6PD) deficiency may experience haemolysis if given dapsone, nitrofurantoin, primaquine or sulfamethoxazole) (Knights et al 2023).
- *Drug tolerance* may also occur where a person has a decreased response to a drug over time, necessitating an increase in dosage to achieve the required response (Knights et al 2023).
- *Drug interactions* occur when one drug modifies the action of another drug (e.g. a drug may either increase or decrease the action of other drugs). A drug interaction may be *synergistic* (enhances the effects of another drug) (e.g. probenecid may be given orally before IM procaine penicillin to increase and prolong the serum level of penicillin), *antagonistic* (opposes the effects of another drug) (e.g. protamine sulphate can be given to neutralise the anticoagulant effects of heparin) or *additive* (where the two drug actions are added together (e.g. when alcohol is consumed by a person on heparin, the risk of bleeding is significantly increased)).

Summary

Administering medication is one of the nurse's most important responsibilities and should be treated with the due care it demands. It is not a task merely to be completed, but rather an opportunity for nurses to increase their own knowledge, to ensure that patients have been educated regarding their medications and to observe patients for both expected and unexpected responses — part of holistic nursing care. The right patient has a right to receive the right dose of the right medication in the right form at the right time by the right route for the right duration of therapy. If any doubt exists, the medication should be withheld; remember: WHEN IN DOUBT, DON'T!!

GUIDE TO TEXT

Trade names

This lists the available trade names for the medication.

Available Forms

This section outlines the various formulations for the medication, including the strength/s available.

Action

Because this is not a pharmacology text, only a brief description of the action of each agent is included. For more detailed information, a pharmacology text should be consulted.

Use

The most common uses of drugs (including both hospital and community uses).

Dose

Dosages listed in this book are those for the *average adult* (unless otherwise stated). Occasionally a paediatric dose may be included if that particular agent is used predominantly in children (e.g. growth hormone, agents used to treat attention deficit hyperactivity disorder (ADHD)).

Adverse effects

Adverse effects are generally unwanted effects, some of which are predictable and often dose related. Other adverse effects may be unpredictable and occur less frequently (e.g. anaphylaxis, anaphylactoid reaction). Very common adverse effects are considered to be those that occur in 10% or more of study participants. Common adverse effects are found in 1–10%, uncommon in 1–0.1%, and rare adverse effects in less than 0.1%. The adverse effects listed in this book are generally those that are common or very common, and rare or less common adverse effects are listed when they require some action to be taken. For example, thrombocytopenia may be a rare adverse effect, but there is a requirement for regular monitoring of blood counts.

Interactions

Interactions occur when one drug alters the action of the second drug, or both agents mutually affect each other. As with the adverse effects, the interactions listed are those that occur commonly or are the most dangerous. It should be noted, however, that interactions between any agents are always possible and caution should be taken when multiple agents are given. For detailed explanations of how and why interactions occur, a pharmacological text should be consulted.

Nursing considerations/ Cautions

The points in this section are those most directly applicable to nurses and include:
- IV administration rate
- monitoring advice
- reconstitution and dilution requirements
- incompatibilities
- any specific storage requirements (e.g. refrigeration)
- cautions (e.g. particular patient groups that may need extra monitoring) and contraindications.

Patient education

Included in this section is important information that the patient should receive about their medication and includes:
- taking with food or fluids
- dividing of tablets
- grapefruit juice incompatibility
- driving warning
- when to seek medical advice (see following section for detailed patient education)
- advice regarding contraception if medication causes problems during pregnancy (e.g. teratogenic causing fetal malformations; use of effective contraception during and for some time after last dose).

It is assumed that the nurse will:
- use an aseptic technique when reconstituting medication
- inspect the solution for any particulate matter or cloudiness
- not use the medication if either particulates or cloudiness are present
- administer the medication using a safe, aseptic and correct technique
- dispose of sharps in a safe and responsible manner.

These points *are not* made for every parenteral agent in the text.
- 'Cautions' are the equivalent of amber traffic lights — go slow and take care. For example, a person with renal impairment may not excrete the medication at the same rate as someone with normal renal function, thus increasing the risk of adverse effects and toxicity. Therefore, a reduced dose may be required and/or close monitoring of renal function and drug excretion, as well as monitoring for adverse effects.
- 'Contraindications' are the equivalent of red traffic lights — no go!
  - hypersensitivity to the agent itself is not listed for every agent as it is assumed that this will be checked routinely before administration (i.e. the patient will be asked 'Have you had this medication before? Did you have any problems with it?'). Although cautions and contraindications are often more relevant to the person prescribing the medication, it is important that the nurse is also aware of these factors.

GENERAL PATIENT EDUCATION

Patient education regarding medications is an essential part of care, which often involves the nurse, in addition to the pharmacist, doctor and/or other members of a multidisciplinary team. If possible, take the time to build a rapport with the patient (and their significant other/carer/family member, if appropriate). It is easier to learn from and ask questions of someone you are comfortable with. Also, given the extent of this educational task, it should start on admission rather than a few days before (or on the day of) discharge.

There are a number of factors which may impact on a person's ability to learn (Roach 2005), including the following:
- *Environment and available time:* It may be difficult to teach and/or learn in an area where there are constant distractions or interruptions. Consider using a small room where the door can be closed and at a time when the nurse knows there will not be any interruptions (e.g. not during meal breaks or at other times of reduced staffing or during visiting hours). Although accessing a small room may not be possible, pulling the curtain around the person's bed may alert others that something is taking place, even if it doesn't really afford privacy (curtains are not soundproof). The nurse should also consider how much time they have available to conduct the session. A short session crammed with too much information may cause confusion for the patient, as well as potentially leading to important information being overlooked.
- *Pain and/or discomfort:* Are you able to concentrate if you are tired, in pain, need to go to the toilet, are hungry or thirsty? All of these impact on a person's capacity to concentrate and should be eliminated or minimised before starting a teaching session.
- *Sensory deficits:* Does the patient have a hearing impairment? Do they have

INTRODUCTION

a hearing aid? Do they have it in (and is it turned on)? Can the person read the label on the medication bottle or graduations on a syringe? Is the person dexterous enough to open medication bottles or operate an injector pen or glucometer? Does the person have sufficient coordination to use an inhaler or is a spacer device required?
- *Anxiety/stress/fear:* These are similar to pain and discomfort and should be minimised or alleviated before starting a teaching session.
- *Learning styles:* Not everyone learns in the same manner. Some people learn by reading, others require demonstration, while others may require both (e.g. to demonstrate an injection or puffer technique get the patient to practise, as well as leaving literature for them to read). Consider your own learning style(s) — how do you prefer to learn about a new piece of equipment: play with it until you work out how it works, have it demonstrated to you, read the instruction manual from cover to cover, or a combination of two or more methods? We often teach others in the manner we like to learn; therefore we should also consider teaching using the other, less comfortable ways. Allowing the patient to practise the skills (e.g. injection technique, blood glucose monitoring, puffer technique) gives the nurse an opportunity to observe and anticipate any problems (e.g. the patient may require follow-up by a district nurse on discharge to ensure the technique is correct).
- *Literacy:* Information should be presented at a level that takes into account the patient's education and reading level.
- *Language and culture:* Is an interpreter required? Does consideration need to be given to the nature of the material (e.g. contraception) and the genders of the teacher and patient? It is very difficult to give important information to someone who does not speak the same language as yourself, or who may be able to understand but not able to ask questions. Furthermore, it is important to use a professional interpreter if possible, as using family members (especially children or adults of the opposite sex) can put them into situations where they are not comfortable (e.g. a teenage son interpreting for his mother who is taking medication for gynaecological problems). There are also issues of privacy and patient confidentiality to consider, as well as possible misinterpretation, giving incorrect drug and dosing information, or family members withholding information. It is also necessary to remember these issues of language and culture if giving the patient written information.

Before starting any teaching session, it is important to lay down the 'ground rules' (e.g. how long the session will last, what is going to be discussed, follow-up). Factors which can be alleviated or minimised should be attended to before starting the session. Other general considerations may include the following:
- *Use of appropriate language:* Nurses (and medical professionals in general) often use jargon (e.g. doing 'obs' or the 'meds'), which can be confusing (and daunting or overwhelming) for non-medical people or those people from non-English speaking backgrounds.

- *Speed of conversation:* It is important to consider how quickly the information is delivered (i.e. how quickly does the nurse/doctor/pharmacist/allied health professional talk?) as this can lead to misunderstandings, especially if the patient is elderly, has a hearing impairment or is from a non-English-speaking background (e.g. a patient may be too embarrassed to say they have not understood information because the person is speaking too quickly). Furthermore, when the health professional is feeling rushed, they may also speak faster.
- *Previous knowledge and skills of the person:* Even if the patient has been prescribed the medication before, assessing knowledge and any misunderstandings can be important as this may improve the patient's motivation to take the medication, thereby improving adherence with the regimen. If the medication is new, it is important to determine whether the information and/or skill (such as using an inhaler or administration of insulin) requires more than one session, making discharge planning essential. This extra time gives the patient time not only to practise skills (supervised and/or unsupervised), but also to ask questions and seek clarification on anything that they have not understood (Roach 2005).
- It is important to return at an agreed time to review information and follow up on any other questions the person may have.

Consideration should be given to including the following as part of patient education:

- Why is the person taking the medication (including the benefits)? If the person has any concerns about taking the medication, they should be encouraged to discuss these with their doctor before starting.
- Provide a simplified explanation of how the medication works (however, it is important not to be condescending).
- The importance of telling other health professionals (e.g. dentist, specialist, surgeon, anaesthetist) that they are taking medications (e.g. it may be necessary to discontinue some medications before a procedure). This should also include the patient reminding the health professional of any allergies (including to food(s) or latex) or other medical conditions (past or present) (such as kidney impairment, asthma, tuberculosis, hepatitis B, heart failure, cancer, blood disorders, gastric ulcer or bleeding, diabetes, high blood pressure), and whether they smoke or regularly drink alcohol.
- The importance of telling the doctor if the patient is pregnant, planning to become pregnant, breastfeeding or planning to breastfeed, as many medications cross the placental barrier and/or are excreted in breastmilk.
- Ensuring prescriptions are filled in a timely manner so that the medication does not run out, especially if the person is planning to take a vacation.
- A recommendation that the patient carries a list of current medications (with exact names) in their wallet/purse so that they can ensure that any other health professional knows what is being taken rather than a general description (e.g. 'small blue pill for my heart'). This may also be important in the event of an emergency.

Dosage

- Name and strength of the medication (including information about differing strengths and trade names).
- What the medication looks like (e.g. capsules, tablets, liquid, injection).
- Dose — this may be straightforward (e.g. patient is ordered 10 mg and tablets are supplied as 10 mg) or not (e.g. patient is ordered 15 mg and tablets are supplied as 10 mg, which means splitting one tablet. Depending on the dexterity of the person or the size of the tablet, this may not be a simple task. Is a pill splitter required?)
- When to take (e.g. morning, evening, same time every day, in relation to food or other tablets, once per week, once per month). It can be useful to specify a day. This can make adherence to the regimen simpler.
- Not increasing, decreasing or stopping medication without seeking advice from the doctor.

How to Take

- Swallow whole with glass of water (or other fluids as recommended). Some fluids may interfere with the medication and it is important to know which ones to avoid.
- Importance of taking with or without food. Some medications need to be taken on an empty stomach, so instructions will include an hour before or 2 hours after food.
- Tablets/capsules should generally not be chewed (unless the tablets are chewable), broken, opened or crushed (however, this is dependent on specific medication).
- Techniques (such as inhalation using a puffer or injection) will need to be demonstrated and taught. If the patient is unable to manage, consideration should be given to teaching a carer/family member/significant other, involving a community-based service (e.g. district nursing service) or discussing with a doctor the appropriateness of the medication and the risk of non-adherence with the regimen.
- What to do if a dose is forgotten, omitted or vomiting occurs soon after an oral medication (e.g. seeking advice from a pharmacist or doctor; not taking a double dose to 'catch up').
- What to do if too much medication is taken (e.g. contacting doctor, pharmacist or Poisons Information Centre (131 126 in Australia or 0800 764 766 in New Zealand), going to the nearest Accident and Emergency Department).
- Length of time that the medication will be required (including emphasis on completing the course and not stopping the medication abruptly or without seeking medical advice).
- Whether there is anything that should be avoided while taking the medication (e.g. certain foods or fluids to be avoided, concurrent alcohol use, standing up quickly, not lying down after taking medication).

Adverse Effects

- All medications cause some side/adverse effects. Some of these may be common, mild and transient in nature, while others are more serious (and even life threatening). It is important for the patient to be made aware of any potential side/adverse effects that may require immediate medical attention. Caution should be taken explaining side-effects (e.g.

some patients may become anxious or frightened by potential side-effects and not take medications at all). It may be safer and simpler to suggest seeing a doctor immediately if anything unusual occurs. However, sometimes it is important to give specific directions, such as 'report to your doctor immediately if you develop any yellowing of the skin or whites of the eyes, your urine looks darker than usual, or you develop nausea, vomiting or abdominal pain'.
- Life-threatening side-effects (such as an allergic reaction, including development of wheezing, shortness of breath, rash, skin blistering, difficulty swallowing) should be emphasised as requiring urgent and immediate medical attention (e.g. call an ambulance rather than going to a medical centre).

Storage

- All medications should be kept out of reach of children.
- Medications should be correctly stored. If there are special storage requirements (such as refrigeration), these should be emphasised (e.g. not using if left out of the fridge for 12 hours or more).
- Medications should not be stored in a bathroom, near a sink, on a windowsill or in the car, as heat and dampness may destroy them.
- Most medications should not be frozen.
- Medications should be kept in the original containers/packets with labels intact. Medication should not be taken if the packaging/container is torn or has signs of being tampered with.
- If the medication changes colour, becomes cloudy, has foreign particles present or develops an odour, it should not be used and a pharmacist should be consulted immediately.
- Medications have a 'use by' (or expiry) date and should not be used after this date. It is important to show the patient where this information is located (it can be difficult to see on some containers). Some medications, such as eye drops, ointments and oral suspensions/mixtures, may have a very short life and deteriorate chemically with time, so it is important to write the date opened so that the person knows when to dispose of them.
- Expired medications or medications that are no longer needed should not be disposed of in general waste or sewerage, as they end up in landfill and may be damaging to the environment by ending up in waterways or may be found by children or animals. The Australian Government has established a National Return and Disposal of Unwanted Medicines (NatRUM) program, which collects medicines returned to pharmacies and incinerates them according to Environmental Protection Authority (EPA) requirements (Australian Government, Department of Health, Disability and Ageing, 2023).

Other Issues

These include the following:
- Follow all instructions on the package/container (e.g. 'shake well before use', 'keep refrigerated', 'take 1 hour before meals').
- Seek advice from a doctor if symptoms do not improve or worsen.

- Attend doctor's appointments as requested, including the need for regular blood or other tests to monitor drug levels (e.g. some medications, such as warfarin, require regular monitoring of the therapeutic blood level and the dosage may need to be adjusted accordingly).
- The importance of having a current prescription and getting it filled/refilled before the medication runs out (especially if planning to take a holiday).
- Medications should not be given to others with similar conditions, nor kept for next time the condition recurs (e.g. antibiotics used to treat respiratory infection).
- OTC medications (such as simple analgesics, antacids, laxatives, cold and flu preparations) and herbal preparations or vitamins/minerals may interact with prescribed medications. It is important to consult with the doctor or pharmacist before taking any of these preparations (including those bought from the supermarket or health food stores).
- Consideration should be given to wearing a MedicAlert pendant or bracelet, or some other form of identification for some conditions/medications (e.g. diabetes, anticoagulants, corticosteroids, insulin) in case of an emergency.
- Is the patient able to manage the medications alone (e.g. it may be appropriate to suggest using a dose administration aid (DAA) (e.g. Dosette box)? (See discussion on p. xxi regarding the suitability of patients for administration aids.) Involve a carer in any discussions or refer the patient to a community-based agency (such as the district nursing service) for monitoring). This may also include the ability to open containers or split tablets if needed. Most pharmacies will provide a unit-dose packing service on request at a cost.
- Warn the patient against driving or operating machinery until they know how the medication will affect them. This is particularly important if the medication has known side-effects that affect vision, balance, coordination or reaction time or increases the effects of alcohol. If this is a known occurrence, extra labels will be attached to containers/packages (e.g. 'this medication may cause drowsiness and may increase the effects of alcohol. If affected, do not drive a motor vehicle or operate machinery').
- Other medication-specific considerations are discussed under patient education in each section.

REVIEWERS

Monica O'Halloran
Registered Nurse
Bachelor of Nursing
Master of Nursing (Education)

Claire Stewart
Registered Nurse
Bachelor of Nursing
Graduate Diploma of Advanced Clinical Nursing (Paediatric)
Masters in Adult Vocational Education

Kym Davey
Registered Midwife/Registered Nurse
Bachelor of Nursing
Master of Advanced Midwifery
Fellow of the Higher Education Academy (FHEA)

Technical reviewers

Jerry Perkins
BPharm, BSc

Lynne Margaret Perkins
BPharm, BVA

ACNE TREATMENT

Although a small number of adults (often women) continue to experience acne vulgaris, it is commonly a disorder of teenagers and young adults. After puberty there is an increased sebum production, and blocked follicles result in small cysts (comedones) containing sebum and keratinous material. *Propionibacterium acnes* acts on the sebum leading to release of free fatty acids, which results in inflammation and cyst rupture (Lawley et al 2025).

There are a number of types of lesions that appear in acne vulgaris, including comedones (closed — whiteheads, open — blackheads), papules, pustules, nodules, cysts and scars. Distribution follows the areas of the body with the greatest number of pilosebaceous glands, namely face, neck, chest and back. Comedones are most common on the forehead and cheeks. Papules may evolve quickly over a few hours, are often itchy or painful and become pustules which resolve over a few days (Lawley et al 2021). Nodules and cysts, however, are a sign of deeper inflammation, are more uncomfortable and take longer to resolve. Scarring is a common result, especially if the lesions are scratched, picked or squeezed. For the person experiencing acne, the number or severity of the lesions may not be in proportion to the emotional impact it has on them. It has been found that the severity of the acne tends to be underestimated by the doctor and overestimated by the patient, and a few 'zits/spots' are likely to cause as much angst as many lesions in a teenager. Regardless of the severity of the acne, patients are at greater risk of anxiety and depression compared with those with no acne (Lawley et al 2021).

A number of medications can cause eruptions or worsen pre-existing acne. These include glucocorticoids (topical and systemic), phenytoin, lithium, isoniazid, oral contraceptive pills and androgenic steroids. Genetic factors and polycystic disease may also play a role in the development of secondary acne. Other factors known to aggravate acne include friction and trauma to the area (e.g. chin straps, headbands), some topical preparations (e.g. cosmetics, hair preparations) or exposure to certain industrial compounds (Lawley et al 2021).

Management of acne should always commence with face hygiene using a soap-free face wash and use of oil-free moisturisers, especially after topical treatments (Harris & Cooper 2017).

Treatment of mild-to-moderate acne is usually topical (e.g. topical retinoids, benzoyl peroxide, azelaic acid or salicylic acid), while topical antibacterial agents (e.g. erythromycin, clindamycin) are used as adjuncts. Moderate-to-severe acne is managed with systemic therapy (e.g. minocycline, doxycycline), while oral retinoids are used to manage severe nodulocystic acne that is unresponsive to other therapies. Therapy can be one agent alone (monotherapy) or a combination, with combination therapy being recommended for most patients with acne, as a number of aspects of the disease process are treated simultaneously (Lawley et al 2021). Other therapies for acne management include chemical peels, light, laser and radio frequency; however, there is little long-term research or evidence in these areas to support the use of these treatments. There is some evidence to suggest light therapy is both safe and effective in acne treatment (Lawley et al 2021).

RETINOIDS

General Actions of retinoids
- analogues of vitamin A
- cause epidermal hyperplasia, decreased hyperkeratosis, inhibit sebum production and decrease size of sebaceous glands
- (Acne) assist in the extrusion of fatty substance from comedones and prevent reblocking and formation of new lesions
- some anti-inflammatory action

General Adverse effects of oral retinoids
- pruritus, rash, skin thinning and scaling (especially palms, soles), dermatitis, sticky skin, dry skin, erythema, skin fragility, bullous eruptions
- eye irritation, decreased night vision, conjunctivitis, dry eyes, blurred vision, contact lens intolerance, xerophthalmia
- headache, depression, fatigue, somnolence, anxiety, mood swings
- cheilitis, dry mouth and/or lips, taste disturbance, cracked corners of mouth and lips
- nausea, vomiting, abdominal pain, inflammatory bowel disease, diarrhoea, stomatitis, gingivitis
- flushing
- paronychia, nail fragility
- tinnitus, hearing impairment
- arthralgia, arthritis, myalgia (with or without elevated creatinine phosphokinase (CPK)), joint and bone pain
- drying of mucous membranes, leading to epistaxis or rhinitis
- reversible alopecia, abnormal hair texture
- increased serum cholesterol and triglycerides, raised liver enzymes
- alteration to blood glucose levels
- (Uncommon) photosensitivity
- (Rare, high dose) corneal opacities, erosions or ulceration
- (Rare) benign intracranial hypertension (pseudotumour celebri), skeletal hyperostosis, allergy, suicide, suicidal ideation, pancreatitis, gynaecomastia
- (Overdose, hypervitaminosis A) transient headache, vomiting, facial flushing, dizziness, cheilosis, abdominal pain, ataxia

General Interactions of oral retinoids
- contraindicated with tetracyclines because of risk of benign intracranial hypertension
- contraindicated with other retinoids or vitamin A because of increased risk of hypervitaminosis A
- not recommended with alcohol (especially in women of childbearing potential)
- may reduce efficacy of progestogen-only oral contraceptives

General Nursing considerations/ Cautions for retinoids
- before starting therapy, patient should be assessed for any family history of lipid disorders or obesity, alcohol abuse, diabetes or smoking

ACNE TREATMENT

- liver function should be monitored before starting therapy, weekly during the first 2 months and then at 3-monthly intervals during therapy
- blood lipids (triglycerides and cholesterol) should be monitored before starting and then 1–2 weekly until lipid response is determined (usually 4–8 weeks), then regularly throughout therapy (especially if there is a predisposition to lipid disorders, including family history, diabetes mellitus, obesity or increased alcohol intake)
- exacerbation of cystic acne or psoriasis may occur during initial stages of treatment
- (Long-term therapy) patient should have regular X-rays during therapy to monitor for signs of new, or changes in, bony abnormalities of the spine
- if used in those under 18 years, bone growth and development should be regularly monitored by X-ray and measurement
- caution if used in those with diabetes as glucose tolerance may be affected. Blood glucose levels should be closely monitored, especially at the start of therapy, as they may be elevated
- caution if used in those who have been previously exposed to topical retinoids as this increases the risk of allergic reactions (purpura, allergic vasculitis)
- caution if used in those who have not reached puberty as retinoids may cause premature closure of epiphyseal plates
- caution if used in those with pre-existing or history of depression, psychosis or intestinal disorders
- contraindicated in those with hypersensitivity to any retinoid products, severe liver or kidney impairment, chronically elevated blood lipids or pre-existing hypervitaminosis A

General Patient education for retinoids

Topical therapy
- warn the patient that condition may initially appear worse
- advise the patient to avoid excess sunlight or sunlamps and wear protective clothing and sunscreen with high protective factor (SPF 30+) when going outdoors
- the patient should be advised to avoid extremes of weather/temperature (e.g. wind, extreme cold) during therapy
- if the patient becomes sunburnt, therapy should be discontinued until the skin has completely recovered
- the patient should be warned to wash hands before and after applying gel/cream
- instruct the patient to use moisturising cream/lotion on skin and use lip balm, lubricating eye ointment or tear replacement therapy to overcome some drying of skin, lips and eyes caused by the retinoid therapy
- advise the patient to first wash skin with mild soap and dry before applying gel or cream as per directions, but avoid excessive application
- moisturisers and emollients may be used with retinoid cream, but should be allowed to dry before applying second cream
- avoid application of gel or cream to mucous membranes, eyes, mouth, corners of nose or broken skin. If contact occurs, area should be thoroughly rinsed with water
- to avoid risk of dermatitis, scarring or epidermal stripping, wax epilation should be avoided during and for 5–6 months after stopping therapy
- dermabrasion and laser therapy should be avoided during and for 5–6 months after stopping therapy, because there is an increased risk of hypertrophic scarring and/or skin pigmentation changes
- warn patient not to apply gel/cream more frequently or in greater quantity than prescribed, as this may cause redness, stinging and discomfort and does not increase effect
- if other topical acne products (e.g. benzoyl peroxide) are also used, they should be applied at different times (e.g. retinoid gel/cream in the evening, other therapy in the morning)

- if severe redness, peeling or discomfort occurs, the patient should be advised to decrease frequency of application or use cream/gel of lower strength (if available)

Oral therapy
- warn the patient that condition may initially appear worse
- the patient should be instructed to swallow capsule whole. If capsule is opened, absorption will be altered
- instruct the patient to immediately report any:
  - abdominal pain, rectal bleeding or severe diarrhoea (especially containing blood)
  - visual disturbances, such as blurred vision, decreased night vision or eye irritation
  - hearing loss or ringing in ears
  - skin reactions
  - headache, nausea, vomiting or visual disturbances (if they occur, patient should be screened for papilloedema)
  - sadness, crying, sleeping too much or not being able to fall asleep, change in appetite, trouble with concentration, withdrawal from family, friends and/or previously pleasurable activities, lack of energy and/or thoughts of self-harm
- the patient should be advised to avoid driving or operating machinery if vision (especially night vision) is affected
- instruct the patient not to take vitamin A supplements (or other vitamin supplements containing vitamin A) during therapy
- patients wearing contact lenses should be warned of decreased tolerance during initial therapy
- the patient should be instructed not to donate blood during and for 1 month (isotretinoin) or 3 years (acitretin) after stopping therapy
- patients with diabetes mellitus may find their glucose tolerance is affected and therefore regular monitoring of blood glucose is suggested
- the patient should be advised to avoid alcohol (as a drink or in food or medicine) during and for 2 months after stopping therapy, because alcohol slows the elimination of retinoids
- male patients should be reminded to not share medications, especially with women of childbearing potential or if pregnant
- <u>all</u> women (including those who are not sexually active or have amenorrhoea) should be counselled regarding the importance of using effective contraception
- women of childbearing potential should be given both oral and written information regarding the teratogenic and embryotoxic potential of retinoids. The woman needs to agree to use effective contraception (preferably two different complementary methods, such as oral contraceptive plus condom/diaphragm), starting 1 month before commencement, during and for 3 years following therapy. A negative serum or urine pregnancy test should be completed within 1 week of starting therapy. Monthly pregnancy testing is recommended throughout therapy and for 1–3 months after stopping. Therapy should be started on day 2 or 3 of the menstrual period. Women should also be advised that taking acitretin with alcohol produces etretinate, which is teratogenic, and therefore alcohol should be avoided during therapy and for 2 weeks after stopping. If pregnancy occurs, patient should be counselled regarding continuation or termination given the possible teratogenic effects on the fetus

 Pregnant patients should be warned to avoid opening capsules and making contact with powder. Contraindicated during pregnancy and breastfeeding.

ACITRETIN
Trade name
Neotigason, Zetin

Available forms
Capsules: 10 mg, 25 mg

Action
- metabolite is teratogenic
- half-life 50 hours
- see also General Actions of retinoids (p. 2)

Use
- psoriasis
- severe keratinisation disorders

Dose
- (Psoriasis) initially 25–30 mg orally once daily with food for 2–4 weeks, followed by 25–50 mg daily for 6–8 weeks **OR**
- (Keratinisation disorders) 20 mg orally daily, adjusting dose according to clinical response (daily maximum 50 mg)

Adverse effects
- peripheral oedema
- see also General Adverse effects of oral retinoids (p. 2)

Interactions
- contraindicated with methotrexate because of increased risk of hepatitis
- not recommended with minocycline or doxycycline because of risk of additive toxicity
- see also General Interactions of oral retinoids (p. 2)

Nursing considerations/Cautions
- (Psoriasis) therapy should be stopped when lesions have resolved and any relapses treated as previously
- see also General Nursing considerations/Cautions for retinoids (p. 2)

Patient education
- patients should be advised to take capsules with milk or food
- (Psoriasis) patient should be warned that psoriasis may appear worse during early treatment
- avoid direct sunlight and protect skin with protective clothing
- see also General Patient education for retinoids (oral therapy) (p. 3)

 Contraindicated; do not use in pregnancy as teratogenic.

 Contraindicated; do not use when breastfeeding.

 Contraindicated in severe hepatic impairment.

 If opening capsules for patients with dysphagia, wear a mask and gloves to avoid contact or inhalation of medication.

ISOTRETINOIN
Trade name
Dermatane, Oratane, Roaccutane, Rocta, APO-Isotretinoin, Isotretinoin GX, Isotretinoin Lupin, Isotretinoin-WGR

Available forms
Capsules 10 mg, 20 mg, 40 mg:

Action
- see General Actions of retinoids (p. 2)
- half-life 10–20 hours (half-life of major metabolite 11–50 hours)

Use
- severe cystic acne (unresponsive to conventional therapy including systemic antibiotics)

Dose
- (Severe cystic acne) initially up to 0.5 mg/kg orally daily as a single or 2 divided doses with food for 2–4 weeks, then dose adjusted according to clinical response (for total of 16 weeks)

Adverse effects
- (Rare) inflammatory bowel disease
- see also General Adverse effects of oral retinoids (p. 2)

Interactions
- see General Interactions of oral retinoids (p. 2)

Nursing considerations/Cautions

- (Cystic acne) second course of treatment should not be within 8 weeks of first course
- see also General Nursing considerations/Cautions for retinoids (p. 2)

Patient education

- capsules contain soy, so caution should be used in those with soy or peanut allergy
- see also General Patient education for retinoids (p. 3)

TRETINOIN
Trade name
ReTrieve Cream, Vesanoid

Available forms
Cream: 0.5 mg/g, 1 mg/g;
Capsules: 10 mg

Action
- see General Actions of retinoids (p. 2)

Use
- acne vulgaris where comedones, papules and/or pustules predominate
- dry skin due to photoageing
- acute promyelocytic leukaemia (Vesanoid only)

Dose
- (dry skin due to photoageing) wash and dry skin, then:
  - night 1: apply cream to skin and leave for 5 minutes, then wash off
  - night 2: apply to skin and leave for 10 minutes, then wash off
  - nights 3—6: increasing time by 30 minutes per night until left on for 120 minutes. If no redness or irritation occurs next day, cream can be left on overnight and washed off in the morning. If skin reaction occurs, apply every second night until skin tolerance increases (ReTrieve Cream)

Adverse effects
- transient stinging, feeling of warmth, peeling, erythema, temporary changes to skin pigmentation
- photosensitivity
- reversible elevation of liver enzymes and bilirubin
- (rare) allergy, contact dermatitis

Interactions
- not recommended with other topical medication, especially peeling agents such as resorcinol, benzoyl peroxide, sulfur or salicylic acid
- caution if used with other agents known to cause photosensitivity (e.g. thiazides, phenothiazines, sulfonamides) or those containing high concentrations of alcohol, menthol, lime or spices

Nursing considerations/Cautions

- not recommended as monotherapy for deep cystic nodular acne or severe pustular acne
- caution if applied to neck or other sensitive areas
- not recommended for eczematous skin
- not recommended in those with personal or family history of skin cancer
- see also General Nursing considerations/Cautions for retinoids (p. 2)

Patient education

- advise patient that it may take more than 6 weeks for effects to be seen and treatment should be continued for at least 12 weeks
- see also General Patient education for retinoids (topical therapy) (p. 3)

Note
- Vesanoid is used as an antineoplastic agent (p. 684), not as a general dermatological agent
- contained in Acnatac with clindamycin

TOPICAL AGENTS USED IN ACNE MANAGEMENT

ADAPALENE
Trade name
Differin Topical Cream, Differin Topical Gel

Available forms
Cream: 0.1%;
Gel: 0.1%

ACNE TREATMENT

Action
- retinoid-like properties
- modulates cellular differentiation, keratinisation and inflammatory processes
- normalises differentiation of follicular epithelial cells, resulting in decreased microcomedone formation

Use
- acne vulgaris (with comedones, papules and pustules) of face, chest and back

Dose
- apply thin film to affected areas at night

Adverse effects
- redness, dry skin, burning sensation, scaling, skin irritation, pruritus, sunburn
- (Uncommon) contact dermatitis, flu-like syndrome, headache

Interactions
- not recommended with abrasive cleansers, astringents, strong drying agents or irritants or other topical retinoids, as there may be increased skin irritation

Nursing considerations/Cautions
- not recommended for those with eczema or seborrheic dermatitis

Patient education
- advise patient to wash and dry affected area(s) thoroughly before applying cream/gel
- patient should be warned to avoid contact with eyes, lips and mucous membranes and, if contact occurs, area should be washed immediately with copious amounts of water
- warn patients that preparation should not be applied to broken skin, reddened areas or sunburnt sites, or on skin with eczema or seborrhoeic dermatitis, or if acne covers a large body area
- instruct patient to stop therapy if severe skin reaction occurs
- patient should be warned to use only oil-free moisturisers to manage dry facial skin
- advise patient to avoid excess sunlight or sunlamps and wear protective clothing and sunscreen with high protective factor (SPF 30+) when going outdoors

Available in combination with
- adapalene 0.1% + benzoyl peroxide 2.5% (Epiduo Gel)
- adapalene 0.3% + benzoyl peroxide 2.5% (Epiduo Forte Gel)

AZELAIC ACID
Trade name
Azclear Medicated Lotion, Finacea

Available forms
Gel: 15%;
Lotion: 20%

Action
- antibacterial action that acts on *Propionibacterium acnes*, reducing number of bacteria, as well as reducing free fatty acids in the skin surface lipids
- penetrates damaged skin more rapidly than intact skin
- unknown action in rosacea, although thought to be anti-inflammatory

Use
- mild-to-moderate acne vulgaris
- papulopustular rosacea

Dose
- apply sparingly to affected area twice daily (morning and night) and massage into skin until it vanishes

Adverse effects
- skin burning, pruritus, stinging, tingling, erythema, irritation, dry skin, scaling, rash
- skin discolouration/depigmentation (especially in darker skin)
- (Uncommon) contact dermatitis, folliculitis, skin disorder, acne
- (Rare) allergic reaction

Nursing considerations/Cautions
- duration of therapy depends on the severity of disorder, but improvement is commonly seen in 4–8 weeks

- contraindicated in those with hypersensitivity to propylene glycol
- not to be used under occlusive dressings

Patient education

- instruct patient to wash skin thoroughly with water before applying gel or lotion
- warn patients that adverse effects usually occur at the start of therapy. If adverse effects are severe, therapy should be stopped and the number of applications per day reduced
- advise patient to avoid contact with eyes and if this occurs eyes should be immediately rinsed with copious amounts of water
- patient should be warned that any skin discolouration or depigmentation is temporary

BENZOYL PEROXIDE

Trade name
Benzac, Benzac AC Wash, Oxy Cream, Oxy Vanishing Cream

Available forms
Gel: 2.5%, 5%, 10%;
Cream: 50 mg/g, 100 mg/g

Action
- action not totally understood
- antibacterial action against *Propionibacterium acnes*
- reduces lipids and fatty acids with mild drying and peeling action

Use
- acne vulgaris

Dose
- (Days 1–3) wash and dry affected areas, apply gel once daily and leave on skin for 2 hours, then wash gel off
- (Days 4–6) if no discomfort occurs, apply gel and leave overnight
- if no discomfort occurs and acne is resisting treatment, apply twice daily, once in the morning (and leave on all day), then wash the affected area and reapply at night (and leave overnight) OR (Benzac AC Wash) apply twice daily to affected area using the following instructions. Wet area to be treated and preparation applied to hands; wash affected area with solution, allowing skin contact for 30 seconds, followed by thoroughly rinsing area with water and drying

Adverse effects
- skin dryness, erythema, peeling, pruritus
- allergic contact dermatitis

Interactions
- not recommended with tretinoin, isotretinoin or tazarotene, as these may cause increased irritation and decrease retinoid efficacy
- caution if used with topical sulfonamide, as skin or facial hair may turn orange/yellow temporarily

Patient education

- patient should be warned to wash hands before and after applying gel/cream
- advise patient that mild burning sensation occurs on application of gel/cream and moderate skin reddening and peeling will occur within a few days. Increased peeling and reddening will occur in the first week and then subside within 1–2 days
- warn fair-haired patients that they may be more prone to skin irritation
- if severe irritation occurs, advise patient to stop therapy until it clears and then restart at a decreased frequency
- warn patient to avoid contact with coloured material (e.g. material, hair), as bleaching or discolouration may occur
- cool compresses should be recommended to help reduce irritation
- if used with retinoid gel/cream, advise patient to apply at different times (e.g. benzoyl peroxide in the morning, retinoid in the evening)
- advise patient to avoid contact with eyes, mouth, sensitive neck areas, mucous membranes and angles of nose; if contact occurs, area should be washed thoroughly with water

ACNE TREATMENT

- warn patient that preparation should be applied only to intact skin
- advise patient to avoid excess sunlight or sunlamps and wear protective clothing and sunscreen with high protective factor (SPF 30+) when going outdoors
- if patient becomes sunburnt, therapy should be discontinued until the skin has completely recovered
- warn patient that use with other topical acne preparations is not recommended owing to added skin irritation

Available in combination with
- benzoyl peroxide 2.5% + adapalene 0.1% (Epiduo Gel)
- benzoyl peroxide 2.5% + adapalene 0.3% (Epiduo Forte Gel)
- benzoyl peroxide 5.0% + clindamycin 1.0% (Duac Once Daily Gel)

CLASCOTERONE
Trade name
Winlevi

Available forms
Cream: 10 mg/g

Action
- androgen receptor inhibitor which is structurally similar to non-androgen corticosteroids
- exact mechanism of action unknown
- main metabolite is an intermediate in glucocorticoid synthesis and has weak glucocorticoid properties

Use
- treatment of acne vulgaris (in patients 12 years or older)

Dose
- thin layer applied to acne-prone area twice daily (morning and evening)

Adverse effects
- local irritation (oedema, redness, pruritus, scaling, dry skin, skin atrophy, stinging/burning, striae rubra, telangiectasia)
- nasopharyngitis
- headache

Interactions
- not recommended with other topical preparations that have a strong drying effect (e.g. medicated or abrasive soaps and cleansers, soaps, cosmetics) or with high concentration of alcohol or astringents

Nursing considerations/Cautions
- ensure the patient receives adequate instruction on correct use of cream

Patient education
- the patient should be instructed to:
  - cleanse area to be treated and gently dry
  - cream should be applied in a thin uniform layer
  - wash hands before and after applying cream
  - take care not to transfer cream to eyes, lips, mouth, corners of nose or other mucous membrane. If contact occurs, area should be rinsed well with water
  - do not apply if area has any cuts, abrasions, eczema or sunburn
  - if a dose is missed, cream should be applied when next dose is due (should not double dose)
  - store cream at room temperature (below 25°C) and do not freeze
  - discard any unused cream 6 months after opening
- for best effect, advise the patient that the area should not be spot treated when acne occurs
- ensure the patient understands the cream is for external use only and should not be applied to eyes, vagina or mouth

 Not recommended during pregnancy because of a lack of data for use in pregnancy.

 Benefits to mother versus any possible adverse effects on breastfed child should be evaluated before use.

ANALGESICS AND NON-STEROIDAL ANTI-INFLAMMATORY DRUGS (NSAIDs)

The NSAIDs are a diverse group of compounds, often chemically unrelated, that share some therapeutic actions and side-effects because of their non-selective inhibition of cyclo-oxygenase (COX). Not all drugs in this class possess the anti-inflammatory, antipyretic and analgesic characteristics to the same degree. For example, paracetamol has antipyretic and analgesic properties, but is not useful as an anti-inflammatory. When used as analgesics, these drugs are usually effective against low-to-moderate intensity pain only. As anti-inflammatory agents, they are used in treating musculoskeletal disorders, providing symptomatic relief from pain and inflammation, but leaving the progression of the disease course unchanged. As antipyretics, they are thought to inhibit hypothalamic prostaglandins that act on the thermoregulatory centre in the hypothalamus. The COX-2 inhibitors are a class of agents with similar properties to those of other NSAIDs without having the same side-effects (especially gastrointestinal (GI)) because of their selective inhibition (Grosser et al 2018).

Most NSAIDs are taken orally, while some are applied topically to relieve muscular and/or rheumatic pain. Some are used in ophthalmic preparations to reduce ocular inflammation. A systematic review of the literature found that topical NSAIDs provide a good level of pain relief in acute conditions such as sprains, strains and overuse injuries, with gel preparations providing the best effects with minimal adverse effects (Derry et al 2019).

Simple analgesics are those that contain only one compound (e.g. 500 mg paracetamol), while compound analgesics combine two or more preparations. While this might be an advantage to the patient because only one tablet is taken, it can have its disadvantages, as it is difficult for the clinician to titrate the dose or interval, may be more expensive and/or produce more adverse effects than the individual compounds (Knights et al 2023).

In 2018, the Department of Therapeutic Goods Administration (TGA) amended previously Schedule 2 (Pharmacy Only) and Schedule 3 (Pharmacist Only) preparations containing codeine (e.g. Panadeine = paracetamol plus codeine) to become prescription-only (Schedule 4) (Therapeutic Goods Administration [TGA] 2018). This has resulted in a number of these codeine-containing products no longer being produced by some manufacturers.

General Actions of NSAIDs (not paracetamol)

During the inflammatory response, arachidonic acid is converted by the enzyme cyclo-oxygenase (COX) to prostaglandins and thromboxane A2, and by the enzyme lipoxygenase to leukotrienes, which produce the pain, swelling, redness and heat associated with inflammation (Brenner & Stevens 2017). COX is present in two forms that have distinct properties. Cyclo-oxygenase 1 (COX-1) is found in the stomach, intestines, kidneys and platelets, and appears to be responsible for functions involving prostaglandins, such as renal function, platelet aggregation and cytoprotection of the stomach. NSAIDs inhibit COX-1 non-selectively, resulting in the common side-effects of gastric ulceration and, to a lesser extent, renal toxicity and increased risk of bleeding. Cyclo-oxygenase 2 (COX-2) is found in fewer tissues (including the brain, renal glomeruli and vasculature) at low levels; however, during inflammation, pro-inflammatory substances lead to an increase in COX-2 levels. Selectively inhibiting COX-2 decreases the signs and symptoms of inflammation and pain with less likelihood of causing gastric or renal problems (Grosser et al 2018).

General Adverse effects of NSAIDs (not paracetamol)

- epigastric pain, anorexia, nausea, vomiting, diarrhoea, abdominal pain/cramps, heartburn, dyspepsia, flatulence, constipation, gastritis
- rash, pruritus, erythema, urticaria, dermatitis, sweating, photosensitivity
- tinnitus, temporary deafness
- headache, dizziness, vertigo, fatigue, drowsiness, insomnia
- prolonged bleeding time, increased risk of bruising and bleeding
- fluid retention, peripheral oedema
- hypertension (new, or worsening of existing), palpitations, premature closure of ductus arteriosis
- increased risk of cardiovascular thrombotic events (COX-2 inhibitors)
- elevated liver enzymes (alanine aminotransferase (ALT), aspartate aminotransferase (AST)), decreased serum urea, hyperkalaemia
- blood dyscrasias, iron-deficiency anaemia
- may mask signs and symptoms of infection
- (Females) may impair fertility by delaying or preventing rupture of ovarian follicles
- inhibition of labour, prolongation of gestation
- increased risk of myocardial infarction and stroke
- (Prolonged therapy, high dose) visual disturbances (including blurred vision), acute interstitial nephritis with haematuria, proteinuria, nephrotic syndrome
- (Rare) anaphylactoid reactions, angioedema, serious skin reactions, hypersensitivity reactions (especially in those with asthma or family history), aseptic meningitis
- (Rare) GI bleeding and/or ulceration
- (Rare) renal papillary necrosis, jaundice, hepatitis, liver toxicity

General Interactions of NSAIDs (not paracetamol)

- may increase blood lithium or digoxin levels (except ketoprofen), thereby increasing the risk of toxicity; lithium or digoxin levels should be closely monitored, especially when starting or stopping therapy with NSAIDs

- use with aspirin or other NSAIDs is not recommended because of an increased risk of GI side-effects
- use caution and close monitoring if warfarin is given with NSAIDs because of an increased risk of haemorrhage
- an increased risk of nephrotoxicity if tenofovir, ciclosporin or tacrolimus are given with NSAIDs
- methotrexate toxicity may occur if NSAIDs are given within 24 hours of methotrexate therapy
- use of quinolone antibiotics and NSAIDs may lead to convulsions (not celecoxib)
- the risk of gastric ulceration is increased if aspirin or NSAIDs are taken with alcohol and/or corticosteroids
- not recommended with alendronate or nicorandil because of an increased risk of gastric ulceration
- an increased risk of bleeding if given with selective serotonin reuptake inhibitors (SSRIs), zidovudine, fibrinolytic or antiplatelet agents
- use of antacids may reduce absorption of aspirin or NSAIDs (except ketoprofen, ketorolac trometamol, sulindac and piroxicam)
- may decrease the excretion of aminoglycoside antibiotics, increasing the risk of toxicity
- avoid use with other nephrotoxic agents
- plasma levels may be increased if given with probenecid
- may increase serum potassium levels if given with potassium-sparing diuretics, increasing the risk of nephrotoxicity. Renal function, potassium serum levels and blood pressure should be closely monitored if used together
- may decrease diuretic, natriuretic and antihypertensive effects of loop, potassium-sparing and thiazide diuretics by inhibiting the synthesis of renal prostaglandin
- may potentiate effects of sulfonylureas; therefore blood glucose levels should be closely monitored during therapy to prevent hypoglycaemia
- may reduce antihypertensive effects of beta adrenergic blocking agents, angiotensin converting enzyme (ACE) inhibitors and angiotensin II antagonists
- risk of renal impairment is increased if NSAIDs, thiazide diuretics and ACE inhibitors/angiotensin II antagonists are given together, especially in the elderly or those with pre-existing renal impairment
- may decrease the efficacy of an intrauterine device (IUD)
- not recommended within 8–10 days of mifepristone
- increased elimination if given with colestyramine
- increased risk of bleeding if given with *Ginkgo biloba*

General Nursing considerations/Cautions for NSAIDs (not paracetamol)

- before starting therapy, the patient should be assessed for:
  - any allergic reactions after prior aspirin or other NSAID therapy, as cross-sensitivity occurs
  - any history of asthma (it may induce asthma attack in susceptible individuals) or gastric ulceration/bleeding (because of an increased risk of both) should be assessed before starting therapy
  - cardiovascular risk factors (such as hypertension, hyperlipidaemia, smoking, diabetes)
- if administered preoperatively, the patient should be carefully

ANALGESICS AND NON-STEROIDAL ANTI-INFLAMMATORY DRUGS (NSAIDs)

- monitored for any signs of bleeding intra- or postoperatively
- signs of infection such as fever can be masked by NSAID therapy
- regular ophthalmological examination and haematological and liver enzyme monitoring should all be performed during prolonged therapy
- in patients with concurrent hypertension managed with antihypertensive agents (beta adrenergic blocking agents, ACE inhibitors and angiotensin II antagonists), regular measurement of BP is recommended before starting therapy and then at regular intervals
- caution if used in those with pre-existing oedema because of an increased potential for fluid retention, peripheral oedema and increased blood pressure
- caution if given to those with pre-existing renal disease, uraemia or bleeding disorders
- caution if used in those with inflammatory bowel disease (IBD), as NSAIDs have been associated with exacerbation of IBD-associated spondyloarthropathies
- not recommended in those with uncontrolled hypertension, congestive cardiac failure, ischaemic heart disease or peripheral arterial disease
- contraindicated in those with a history of peptic or GI ulceration or bleeding
- contraindicated in those with bleeding disorders (e.g. haemophilia, von Willebrand disease)
- contraindicated in those with severe liver or kidney insufficiency or severe cardiac failure
- contraindicated in those with salicylate hypersensitivity (as cross-sensitivity between aspirin and other NSAIDs exists)
- contraindicated in those with 'aspirin triad' (a person with asthma who experiences rhinitis with/without nasal polyps, or experiences severe bronchospasm after taking aspirin or NSAIDs)
- contraindicated post coronary artery bypass graft (CABG) surgery

General Patient education for NSAIDs (not paracetamol)

- instruct the patient to take NSAIDs with food or milk (e.g. after meals) to reduce gastric irritation
- warn the patient to avoid alcohol during therapy with NSAIDs to reduce the risk of GI adverse effects
- the patient should be warned to immediately report to their doctor any:
  - changes in hearing or visual disturbances
  - nausea, tiredness, lack of appetite, lethargy, itching, yellowing of skin, eyes, pale bowel motions and dark urine, flu-like symptoms or abdominal tenderness (in the upper outer right quadrant) (as these are signs of impending liver toxicity)
  - breathlessness, difficulty breathing when lying down, any swelling in feet or legs (signs of cardiac failure)
  - sudden and oppressive chest pain (may be a sign of heart attack)
  - severe stomach or throat pain, vomiting blood or black vomit, bleeding from rectum, sticky bowel motions
  - skin rash, hives, blistering or peeling skin, mouth ulcers or swelling of face, lips, mouth, tongue or throat, or wheezing/difficulty breathing

- changes to the amount or colour of urine passed, any blood in urine
- caution patients not to drive or operate machinery if dizziness, drowsiness or visual disturbances occur
- warn patients with diabetes using oral hypoglycaemic agents to monitor blood glucose levels carefully during therapy to prevent hypoglycaemia
- advise a female patient that, if she is having a problem becoming pregnant, NSAID therapy should be stopped
- counsel female patients not to take NSAIDs during pregnancy, especially during the third trimester. If the patient becomes pregnant, she should be advised to tell her doctor immediately

Topical gel/solution
- advise the patient to avoid excess sunlight or sunlamps and wear protective clothing and sunscreen with high protective factor (SPF 30+) when going outdoors, as some topical gels can increase skin sensitivity and therefore the risk of burning
- instruct the patient to wash hands before and after applying gel and avoid contact with eyes or mouth
- warn the patient to avoid contact with eyes, mouth, mucous membrane, angles of the nose or skin which is broken, abraded or infected, or has eczema. If contact occurs, the area should be washed with copious amounts of water
- advise the patient not to use gel under an occlusive dressing or on a large area

Eye drops
- should not be instilled if soft or gas-permeable contact lenses are in situ, as many eye drops contain benzalkonium chloride as a preservative, which may cause discolouration of soft contact lenses. Lenses should be removed before instillation and reinserted after at least a 15-minute interval
- advise the patient not to use drops if they are cloudy or change colour
- instruct the patient in the correct technique for instilling eye drops, including:
  - not allowing the tip of the dispensing container to touch the eye, as it may cause injury and/or contaminate the eye drops
  - if the container is new, remove the protective seal, otherwise check the expiry date
  - wash hands thoroughly with soap and water
  - remove the lid/cap and hold the container upside down in one hand between the thumb and forefinger or index finger
  - using the other hand, gently pull down on the lower eyelid to form a pouch/pocket and tilt the head back, looking up
  - place the tip of the container close to the lower eyelid (taking care not to make contact between tip and eye). Squeezing the bottle gently, release one drop into pouch/pocket formed between eye and eyelid
  - gently close the eye, but do not blink or rub it
  - while the eye is closed, place the index finger against the inside corner of eye and press against the nose for about 2 minutes (this stops medicine from draining through the tear duct into nose and throat)

ANALGESICS AND NON-STEROIDAL ANTI-INFLAMMATORY DRUGS (NSAIDs)

- replace lid/cap tightly
- wash hands again to remove any residue
- warn the patient that vision may be blurred for a few minutes after eye drops have been instilled and it is therefore advisable not to drive or use machinery during this time
- the patient should be advised to write expiry date on eye drops when opened and not to use beyond this date (usually 28 days)

Suppositories
- instruct the adult patient in the correct technique for suppository insertion, including:
  - the need to empty the bowel if possible before suppository insertion
  - wash the hands with soap and water
  - if the suppository feels soft, place it (unwrapped) in the fridge or hold it under cold water to firm it up
  - put on disposable glove if wanted
  - remove the wrapper from the suppository and moisten slightly by dipping it in cool water
  - lie on one side with knees raised to chest
  - push the suppository (blunt end first) gently into the rectum, taking care not to break the suppository
  - remain lying down for a few minutes to allow the suppository to dissolve
  - wash the hands thoroughly after insertion
- advise the patient not to use their bowels for at least 1 hour (if possible) after suppository insertion

Use of these agents during the latter stages of pregnancy may cause closure of the fetal ductus arteriosus, fetal renal impairment and inhibition of platelet aggregation and may delay labour and birth. Therefore, continuous treatment with these agents during the third trimester of pregnancy is generally contraindicated.

Not recommended during labour or delivery.

Not recommended during breastfeeding, as some NSAIDs and/or their metabolites are excreted in breastmilk and their actions on the newborn may be unknown.

ASPIRIN
Trade names
Alka-Seltzer Effervescent, APOHealth Cardio Aspirin, Mayne Pharma Aspirin, Pharmacy Action Low Dose Aspirin, Trust Aspirin EC 100, Aspro Clear, Aspro Clear Extra Strength, Astrix, Cardasa, Cardiprin 100, Cartia, Disprin preparations, Solprin, Spren

Available forms
Capsules: 100 mg;
Tablets: 100 mg, 300 mg, 320 mg, 500 mg;
Tablets (enteric-coated) 100 mg;
Tablets (effervescent): 300 mg, 500 mg

Action
- aspirin is converted to salicylic acid mainly in the GI tract
- absorption is dependent on formulation (e.g. soluble formulation increases rate of absorption)
- irreversibly inhibits cyclo-oxygenase (COX) platelet activity (needed for thromboxane synthesis), resulting in prolonged action. It may take 8–12 days (platelet turnover time) after therapy is stopped to fully recover
- half-life of aspirin is about 20–60 minutes, half-life of salicylate acid is about 6 hours
- see also General Actions of NSAIDs (p. 11)

Use
- relief of mild-to-moderate non-visceral pain
- headache, migraine
- acute febrile illnesses (not for children or teenagers)
- dysmenorrhoea
- rheumatic pain, including juvenile rheumatoid arthritis
- inflammation associated with back or muscular pain/strain
- cold and flu symptoms
- toothache
- antiplatelet therapy (only on medical advice) for prophylaxis against myocardial infarction, unstable angina, transient ischaemic attacks (TIAs) and stroke

Dose
- (Analgesic, antipyretic) 300—1000 mg orally with food 4—6-hourly as required (up to 4 g/day) **OR**
- (Effervescent tablets) 300—1000 mg orally dissolved in 1/2 glass of water 4-hourly as required (up to 4 g/day) **OR**
- (Antiplatelet) 100 mg daily

Adverse effects
- increase in respiratory rate
- (Very high salicylate level) depresses respiration
- (Prolonged therapy, high dose) hypoprothrombinaemia
- see also General Adverse effects of NSAIDs (p. 11)

Interactions
- may increase blood levels of sodium valproate and methotrexate, increasing risk of toxicity and/or adverse effects
- caution if used with anticoagulants because of the increased risk of bleeding
- action of probenecid may be reduced if given with aspirin
- hypoglycaemic action of sulfonylureas may be increased if given with high-dose aspirin; therefore blood glucose levels should be closely monitored
- excretion is increased if given with urinary alkalinisers
- rate and extent of absorption is increased by caffeine
- hydrocortisone may increase metabolism and/or clearance of aspirin. Further, when hydrocortisone is ceased, blood levels of aspirin may rise significantly, increasing the risk of adverse effects and/or toxicity
- increased risk of gastrointestinal bleeding if aspirin is given with high-dose corticosteroids
- may interfere with a number of laboratory tests including measurement of heparin activity and urinary glucose oxidase test in the presence of glycosuria

Nursing considerations/Cautions
- soluble, effervescent, buffered and enteric-coated salicylate preparations reduce gastric irritation
- enteric-coated and sustained-action preparations have delayed absorption, which is useful for regular long-term therapy
- elderly patients are at greater risk of adverse effects, including tinnitus, nausea, anorexia and gastric irritation
- tinnitus (with normal hearing) is a reliable index of therapeutic plasma level, but may not be detected in patients with hearing loss
- therapy should be stopped 1 week before scheduled surgery
- symptoms of salicylism (chronic salicylate intoxication) are hyperventilation, tremor, papilloedema, agitation, paranoia, bizarre behaviour, memory deficits, confusion and stupor, and, rarely, pulmonary oedema, seizures and renal failure
- symptoms of acute salicylate poisoning include nausea, vomiting, tinnitus, hearing loss, sweating and hyperventilation, followed by mixed acid—base disturbance of respiratory alkalosis and metabolic acidosis. Uncommonly, fever, neurological dysfunction, renal failure, acute lung injury (non-cardiogenic pulmonary oedema), cardiac dysrhythmias and hypoglycaemia may occur. Rarely, other complications include rhabdomyolysis, gastric perforation and GI haemorrhage

ANALGESICS AND NON-STEROIDAL ANTI-INFLAMMATORY DRUGS (NSAIDs)

- there is no specific antidote for salicylate toxicity. Treatment of acute salicylate poisoning involves stabilisation of airway, breathing and circulation, correction of volume depletion and metabolic disturbance, GI decontamination and reduction in levels of salicylate. This involves:
  - gastric lavage, followed by single dose of activated charcoal/sorbitol (whole bowel irrigation may be necessary if overdose involves large amounts of enteric-coated or modified-release tablets)
  - assessment of patient's volume and electrolytes. Volume replacement is usually with normal saline with potassium supplementation, as hypokalaemia is common
  - urine alkalisation with IV sodium bicarbonate is more effective than forced diuresis or forced alkaline diuresis
  - urine output should be 1—2 mL/kg/hour
  - serum salicylate and electrolytes should be monitored 1—2-hourly
  - if condition worsens, haemodialysis, peritoneal dialysis or exchange transfusion may be necessary
- not recommended in infants, children and adolescents, including for the treatment of fever and/or muscle pain associated with febrile, viral illness because of the association with Reye's syndrome (see Glossary)
- see also General Nursing considerations/Cautions for NSAIDs (p. 12)

Patient education
- stopping aspirin for any reason (e.g. donation of blood) should be discussed with doctor before discontinuing therapy
- effervescent and soluble preparations should be dissolved in 1/2—1 glass of water for more rapid absorption
- warn patients that sustained-release and enteric-coated preparations should be swallowed whole and not crushed or broken
- advise patient to avoid aspirin within 30 minutes of alcohol
- instruct patient to discuss the need to stop before any surgical procedure with the surgeon
- blood donors should be advised not to take aspirin in the week preceding the donation
- if patient is on a low-sodium diet, they should be cautioned that effervescent preparations contain sodium
- see also General Patient education for NSAIDs (p. 13)

Available in combination with
- aspirin 100 mg + clopidogrel 75 mg tablets (APX-Clopidogrel/Aspirin 75/100, Clopidogrel Winthrop Plus Aspirin, Duo-Cover, DuoPlidogrel, Piax Plus Aspirin);
- aspirin 300 mg + codeine phosphate 8 mg tablets (Aspalgin)

BENZYDAMINE
Trade names
Difflam Anti-inflammatory Gel, Difflam Sore Throat Gargle and Mouth Solution, Difflam Sore Throat Spray, Difflam Sore Throat Spray Forte

Available forms
Throat spray: 1.5 mg/mL, 3 mg/mL;
Gel: 3%, 5%;
Solution: 22.5 mg/15 mL

Action
- analgesic, anti-inflammatory
- chemically unrelated to other NSAIDs

Use
- relief of inflammatory conditions of the mouth and throat (e.g. tonsillitis, radiation mucositis)
- (Topically) inflammatory disorders (e.g. sprains, strains, acute phases of myalgia and bursitis)

Dose
- (Inflammatory disorders) 3% or 5% gel massaged into affected area 3—6 times daily (maximum 6 times daily in severe conditions) for up to 14 days **OR**
- (Throat spray) 4—8 sprays or 2—4 sprays (forte solution) on inflamed area and swallowed gently 1.5—3-hourly for up to 7 days **OR**

HAVARD'S NURSING GUIDE TO DRUGS

- 15 mL (undiluted solution) gargled or swirled in mouth for 30 seconds 1.5–3-hourly for up to 7 days

Adverse effects
- (Gel) erythema, rash, photosensitivity
- (Throat spray, solution) numbness, stinging, tingling, burning, thirst, dryness, altered taste sensation, warm feeling in mouth

Nursing considerations/Cautions
- if sore throat is due to bacterial infection, antibacterial therapy should also be considered
- (Throat spray) not recommended for children under 12 years

Patient education
- advise the patient that oral solution should be used as a rinse or gargled and not swallowed
- if stinging occurs while rinsing or gargling, oral solution can be diluted with water for gargling
- (Throat spray) instruct the patient to prime spray before first use or after a period of non-use. Spray nozzle should be cleaned after each use to prevent clogging
- see also topical gel application advice (p. 14)

Available in combination with
- benzydamine + cetylpyridinium mouth gel and lozenges (Difflam Mouth Gel, Difflam Sore Throat (various flavours))
- benzydamine + lidocaine + dichlorobenzyl alcholol lozenges and throat spray (Difflam Plus Anaesthetic Sore Throat)
- benzydamine + chlorhexidine solution (Difflam PLUS Sore Throat & Mouth Antiseptic + Antiinflammatory Ready to Use)

CELECOXIB
Trade names
Celaxib, Celebrex, Celexi, APX-Celecoxib, Blooms Celecoxib, Celebrex Relief, Celecoxib GH, Celecoxib Sandoz, Celecoxib-WGR, Noumed Celecoxib

Available forms
Capsules: 100 mg, 200 mg

Action
- COX-2 inhibitor preventing prostaglandin synthesis with actions similar to other NSAIDs, with analgesic, antipyretic and anti-inflammatory activity
- half-life 4–15 hours

Use
- osteoarthritis, rheumatoid arthritis, ankylosing spondylitis
- primary dysmenorrhoea
- (Short-term) pain management post-surgery or musculoskeletal/soft tissue injury

Dose
- (Osteoarthritis, ankylosing spondylitis) 200 mg orally daily as single dose or 2 divided doses **OR**
- (Rheumatoid arthritis) 200 mg orally daily in 2 divided doses, increasing to 400 mg daily for short-term management of disease flares/exacerbations **OR**
- (Primary dysmenorrhoea) 400 mg orally daily as single dose or 2 divided doses (first day), then 200 mg daily on following days for up to 5 days maximum **OR**
- (Acute postsurgical pain, musculoskeletal and/or soft tissue injury) initially 400 mg orally daily, then 200 mg 1–2 times daily on following days for up to 5 days maximum

Adverse effects
- pharyngitis, rhinitis, sinusitis
- back pain
- (Rare) increased risk of cardiac and thrombotic events, serious skin reactions
- see also General Adverse effects of NSAIDs (p. 11); however, GI adverse effects occur less frequently

Interactions
- increased plasma levels may occur if given with fluconazole
- increased risk of renal impairment if given with ACE inhibitor/angiotensin receptor antagonist and thiazide diuretic at same time (especially in the elderly)
- may decrease antihypertensive effects of ACE inhibitor, angiotensin receptor antagonist, thiazide diuretics and beta adrenoceptor blocking agents

ANALGESICS AND NON-STEROIDAL ANTI-INFLAMMATORY DRUGS (NSAIDs)

- may decrease natriuretic effect of furosemide (frusemide) and thiazide diuretics because of renal prostaglandin synthesis inhibition
- increased risk of GI adverse effects if given with oral glucocorticoids, especially in the elderly
- increased risk of GI adverse effects if given with aspirin
- increased risk of nephrotoxicity if given with ciclosporin
- may increase plasma levels of digoxin, lithium and warfarin, thereby increasing risk of toxicity; digoxin, lithium and warfarin levels should be closely monitored, especially when starting, stopping or altering doses of celecoxib
- may increase plasma levels of metoprolol and dextromethorphan
- decreased plasma levels may occur if given with aluminium- or magnesium-containing antacids, rifampicin, carbamazepine or barbiturates
- contraindicated with other NSAIDs

Nursing considerations/Cautions

- any dehydration should be corrected before starting therapy
- blood pressure should be regularly monitored during therapy
- any skin reactions usually occur within 4 weeks of starting therapy
- to lessen the risk of cardiovascular events, the lowest effective dose should be used for the shortest possible duration
- (Long-term treatment) haemoglobin or haematocrit levels should be regularly monitored for signs of anaemia
- caution if used in those with high risk of cardiovascular disease or multiple risk factors such as diabetes, hypertension, smoking, cardiac failure or hypercholesterolaemia
- contraindicated in those with sensitivity to sulfonamides
- contraindicated in the treatment of pain in those undergoing coronary artery bypass graft (CABG) surgery
- contraindicated in those with unstable or significant ischaemic heart disease, peripheral arterial disease and/or cerebrovascular disease, congestive heart failure, severe liver or kidney impairment or creatinine clearance < 30 mL/min
- see also General Nursing considerations/Cautions for NSAIDs (p. 13)

Patient education

- advise patient to take antacids 2 hours before or after celecoxib
- warn patient to seek medical advice immediately if the following occurs:
    - fainting, collapse, shortness of breath, tiredness, chest pain or irregular heart beat
    - skin reactions
- see also General Patient education for NSAIDs (p. 13)

Capsules can be opened and dispersed in water, or mixed with spoonful of yoghurt or apple puree.

See General Patient education for NSAIDs (p. 13).

See General Patient education for NSAIDs (p. 13).

Contraindicated in patients with renal disease if CrCl < 30 mL/min.

Contraindicated in patients with severe hepatic impairment.

CHOLINE SALICYLATE
Trade names
Bonjela Mouth Ulcer Gel, Bonjela Teething Gel, Seda-Gel

Available form
Oral gel: 87 mg/g

Action
- local analgesic

Use
- painful oral irritation (e.g. teething)
- lesions of the mouth

Dose
- (Adult) massage 1 cm gel into painful area 3-hourly **OR**
- (Infant > 4 months) massage 0.5 cm gel into painful area 3-hourly if required (up to 6 applications/24 hours)

HAVARD'S NURSING GUIDE TO DRUGS

Adverse effects
- transient stinging on application

Nursing considerations/Cautions
- not recommended in those with salicylate hypersensitivity
- contraindicated in babies less than 4 months old or children under 12 in combination with aspirin-containing products (to avoid excessive salicylate levels)

Patient education
- advise the patient to wash hands before and after applying gel
- warn the patient that gel should not be applied directly to dentures
- (Mouth ulcers) advise the patient to wipe mucus from ulcer surface before applying gel

DICLOFENAC DIETHYLAMINE (DICLOFENAC DIETHYLAMMONIUM)
Trade names
Voltaren Emulgel, Voltaren Osteo Gel 12-hourly

DICLOFENAC POTASSIUM
Trade names
Voltaren Rapid, Cambia, Inflamax Liquid Caps, APOHealth Anti-Inflammatory Pain Relief Rapid 25, Chemists' Own Anti-Inflammatory Pain Relief, Pharmacy Action Diclofenac Rapid 25

DICLOFENAC SODIUM
Trade names
Clonac, Dencorub Anti-Inflammatory Gel, Difenac, Fenac EC, Solaraze 3% Gel, Viclofen, Voltaren, Inflamax Spray, Blooms the Chemist Anti-inflammatory Pain Relief, Chemists' Own Anti-inflammatory Pain Relief, Pharmacy Action Diclofenac 25, Wagner Health Diclofenac

Available forms
Gel: 1%, 2.3%, 3%;
Tablets (enteric-coated): 25 mg, 50 mg;
Tablets (rapid-release): 12.5 mg, 25 mg, 50 mg;
Capsules (liquid, rapid-release): 12.5 mg;
Suppositories: 12.5 mg, 25 mg, 50 mg, 100 mg;
Powder (for oral solution): 50 mg;
Spray: 4%: 30 mL

Action
- selectively inhibits COX-2 at therapeutic doses
- more potent analgesic, antipyretic and anti-inflammatory than aspirin
- see also General Actions of NSAIDs (p. 11)

Use
- rheumatoid arthritis, osteoarthritis
- acute or chronic pain with inflammatory conditions
- primary dysmenorrhoea
- acute migraine, headache
- cold and flu symptoms
- dental pain, back ache, muscle pain
- postoperative pain management in children (suppositories)
- management of actinic keratosis (where other treatment is inappropriate)
- postoperative inflammation following eye surgery

Dose
- (Primary dysmenorrhoea) initially 50–100 mg orally daily, starting with onset of symptoms, followed by 50 mg orally 3 times daily for 3 days **OR**
- (Arthritis, inflammatory conditions) initially 75–150 mg orally daily in 2–3 divided doses, reducing to 75–100 mg orally in divided doses for long-term therapy (enteric-coated tablets, rapid-release tablets) **OR**
- (Arthritis, inflammatory conditions, dental pain, backache) initially 25 mg orally, followed by 12.5–25 mg orally 4–6-hourly if needed (daily maximum 75 mg) (12.5 mg rapid-release tablets) **OR**
- (Acute migraine) 50 mg orally at first sign of migraine, followed by 50 mg 2 hours later if pain is not relieved. If needed, a

ANALGESICS AND NON-STEROIDAL ANTI-INFLAMMATORY DRUGS (NSAIDs)

further 50 mg can be taken at 4—6-hourly intervals (daily maximum 200 mg) **OR**
- (Postoperative pain management in children aged 12 months and above) initially 1—2 mg/kg, followed by 1 mg/kg 3 times daily for up to 3 days if needed (daily maximum 3 mg/kg) (suppositories) **OR**
- (Local pain, soft tissue injury, soft tissue rheumatism) apply gel or spray to affected area and rub gently 3—4 times daily for up to 14 days **OR**
- (Pain, inflammation) apply cherry-size amount of gel, or 4 to 5 sprays, to affected area and rub gently twice daily for up to 21 days (12-hourly gel) **OR**
- (Actinic keratosis) apply to skin twice daily for 30—90 days (daily maximum 8 g) (Solaraze 3% Gel) **OR**
- (Cataract surgery) up to 5 drops to affected eye(s) 3 hours preoperatively, then 1 drop 3 times on day of surgery, then 1 drop 3—5 times daily for 2—4 weeks **OR**
- (Inflamax spray) Adults, children > 15 yrs: 4—5 sprays 3 times daily as necessary; rub in gently; max 15 sprays a day

Adverse effects
- (Suppositories) discomfort, worsening of haemorrhoids
- (Gel, rare) itching, reddened or scaly skin, photosensitivity
- (Gel) contact dermatitis, redness, peeling, skin dryness, numbness, itching, rash, eczema, paraesthesia, hyperaesthesia
- (Eye drops) eye irritation, keratitis, increase in intraocular pressure, blurred vision, delayed corneal healing
- see also General Adverse effects of NSAIDs (p. 11)

Interactions
- (Eye drops) not recommended with topical corticosteroids in patients with corneal inflammation because of the increased risk of delayed healing
- increased plasma levels may occur if given with voriconazole
- decreased plasma levels may occur if given with rifampicin
- see also General Interactions of NSAIDs (p. 11)

Nursing considerations/Cautions
- care should be taken when selecting tablets as rapid-release and slow-release forms are available
- effects may not be seen for up to 30 days after therapy has been stopped
- (Gel) 0.5 g gel (size of pea) is sufficient to cover area 5 cm × 5 cm
- (Gel) duration of treatment varies with condition (14 days for soft tissue injuries, 21 days for osteoarthritis)
- (Gel) not recommended for treatment of bruises
- tablets contain lactose and are therefore not recommended in galactose intolerance, severe Lapp lactase deficiency or glucose—galactose malabsorption
- (100 mg suppositories) should not be used for children or teenagers
- (Suppositories) not recommended in infants under 12 months
- (Suppositories) contraindicated in those with proctitis
- (Gel) contraindicated in those with hypersensitivity to diclofenac, propylene glycol or isopropyl alcohol
- see also General Nursing considerations/Cautions for NSAIDs (p. 12)

Patient education
- instruct the patient that enteric-coated tablets should be swallowed whole (not divided or chewed) with fluids, preferably before food for better absorption and efficacy, but can be taken with food if stomach is upset
- advise the patient that diclofenac should not be used to prevent migraine (prophylaxis), only for management, and should be taken at first sign of headache

- patients who experience night pain and/or morning stiffness should be advised to take oral treatment during the day and suppositories at bedtime for better control of symptoms (daily maximum 150 mg)
- see also suppository insertion advice (p. 15)
- see also eye drop instillation advice (p. 14)
- see also General Patient education for NSAIDs (p. 13)

Rapid-release tablets can be crushed and mixed with water or spoonful of yoghurt or apple puree.

Enteric-coated tablets should not be crushed and should be swallowed whole.

See General Patient education for NSAIDs (p. 13).

See General Patient education for NSAIDs (p. 13).

ETORICOXIB
Trade name
Arcoxia

Available forms
Tablets: 30 mg, 60 mg, 120 mg

Action
- COX-2 inhibitor preventing prostaglandin synthesis, with actions similar to other NSAIDs
- no effect on platelet function
- half-life 22 hours

Use
- osteoarthritis
- acute gouty arthritis
- primary dysmenorrhoea
- minor dental pain

Dose
- (Osteoarthritis) initially 30 mg orally daily, increasing to 60 mg orally daily if needed (daily maximum 60 mg) **OR**
- (Acute gouty arthritis, primary dysmenorrhoea, dental pain) 120 mg orally daily (maximum 8 days) **OR**
- (Dental pain) 90 mg orally daily (up to 8 days maximum)

Adverse effects
- dizziness, headache
- dyspepsia, upper abdominal pain, diarrhoea, nausea, altered taste
- nasopharyngitis, upper respiratory tract infection
- dyspnoea
- urinary tract infection
- peripheral oedema, fluid retention
- hypertension
- increased risk of myocardial infarction and stroke, new or worsened congestive cardiac failure
- (Rare) jaundice, renal injury, serious skin reactions, breast malignant neoplasm

Interactions
- may increase levels of ethinyloestradiol, resulting in an increased risk of adverse effects, such as venous thromboembolic events in at-risk women
- may decrease antihypertensive effects of ACE inhibitor or angiotensin receptor antagonist
- increased risk of renal injury if given with ACE inhibitor or angiotensin receptor antagonist, especially in the elderly and if treated with diuretics
- caution if given with warfarin, especially when starting or stopping therapy. INR should be closely monitored
- may decrease natriuretic effect of furosemide (frusemide) and thiazide diuretics because of renal prostaglandin synthesis inhibition
- contraindicated with aspirin or other NSAIDs
- increased risk of GI adverse effects if given with aspirin
- may reduce clearance of lithium, increasing plasma levels and risk of

toxicity; therefore monitoring during therapy is recommended
- decreased levels (and therefore decreased analgesic effect) may occur if given with rifampicin
- caution if given with methotrexate at doses ≥ 90 mg; therefore monitoring of methotrexate levels is recommended

Nursing considerations/Cautions

- any dehydration should be corrected before starting therapy
- hypertension should be controlled before starting therapy. BP should be monitored every 2 weeks throughout therapy and stopped if there is a significant increase
- to lessen the risk of cardiovascular events, the lowest effective dose should be used for the shortest possible duration
- caution if used in those with increased risk factors for cerebrovascular events (diabetes, hypertension, hypercholesterolaemia, family history of ischaemic heart disease, cardiac failure, left ventricular dysfunction and/or smokers) or pre-existing oedema
- contraindicated in those who have recently undergone coronary artery bypass graft (CABG) surgery or angioplasty
- contraindicated in those with unstable or significant ischaemic heart disease, peripheral arterial disease and/or cerebrovascular disease; hypertension which is not adequately controlled (above 140/90 mmHg); congestive heart failure; severe liver or kidney impairment or creatinine clearance < 30 mL/min; active peptic ulceration or GI bleeding; history of asthma, urticaria or other allergic reaction after taking aspirin or NSAIDs
- see also General Nursing considerations/Cautions for NSAIDs (p. 12)

Patient education

- advise the patient against driving or operating machinery if dizziness occurs
- see also General Patient education for NSAIDs (p. 13)

 See General Patient education for NSAIDs (p. 13).

 See General Patient education for NSAIDs (p. 13).

 Contraindicated in patients with severe renal impairment (CrCl < 30 mL/min).

In patients with mild hepatic impairment (Child—Pugh score 5—6), the maximum dose should be 60 mg daily. In moderate hepatic impairment (Child—Pugh score 7—9), the maximum dose is 60 mg on alternate days (or 30 mg once daily).

FLURBIPROFEN
Trade names
Strepfen Intensive Lozenges, Strepfen Throat Spray

Available forms
Lozenges: 8.75 mg;
Throat spray: 8.75 mg/3 sprays

Action
- anti-inflammatory

Use
- pain, swelling, inflammation associated with severe sore throat

Dose
- 3 sprays to back of throat every 3—6 hours for 3 days maximum (daily maximum 15 sprays) **OR**
- 1 lozenge allowed to dissolve slowly, 3—6-hourly (maximum 8 lozenges/day)

Adverse effects
- (Lozenge) warm sensation/tingling in mouth, taste alteration and, rarely, nausea, vomiting, diarrhoea, dyspepsia, abdominal pain
- (Rare) allergic reaction, hypersensitivity

Interactions
- not recommended with other NSAIDs

Nursing considerations/Cautions
- not recommended in those with heart failure
- not recommended in children < 12 years
- (Throat spray) not recommended in those < 18 years

Patient education
- advise the patient to seek medical advice if symptoms persist
- (Throat spray) instruct the patient to:
  - prime pump with four or more sprays before first use, and one spray if unused recently, until a fine mist is produced
  - depress pump fully with each spray
  - hold the breath during administration
  - do not eat or drink immediately after using the spray
  - discard the pump 6 months after opening (write opening date on pump)

Should be used in the first and second trimesters of pregnancy only on medical advice. Not recommended during the third trimester.

IBUPROFEN
Trade names
Advil, Brufen, Bugesic, FenPaed, Nurofen preparations, AFT Pharmaceuticals Ibuprofen, Chemists' Own Ibuprofen, Pedea Solution for Infusion, Pharmacy Action Ibuprofen, Rafen, WGR-Ibuprofen 400, Zenifen, Caldolor

Available forms
Capsules (liquid): 200 mg;
Caplets: 200 mg, 342 mg;
Tablets: 200 mg, 400 mg;
Tablets (controlled release): 300 mg;
Tablets (chewable): 100 mg;
Syrup/Suspension: 40 mg/mL, 100 mg/5 mL, 200 mg/5 mL;
Gel: 5%;
Vial: 800 mg/8 mL

Action
- analgesic, antipyretic and anti-inflammatory properties similar to those of other NSAIDs
- half-life about 2 hours
- see also General Actions of NSAIDs (p. 11)

Use
- rheumatoid arthritis, including juvenile rheumatoid arthritis, osteoarthritis
- primary dysmenorrhoea
- headache
- migraine
- acute/chronic pain with inflammatory component, including muscle, dental and sinus pain
- fever reduction
- (IV) acute mild-to-moderate postoperative pain, or moderate-to-severe postoperative pain as an adjunct to morphine
- (Topical gel) sprains, strains, sports injuries

Dose
- (Rheumatoid arthritis, osteoarthritis (acute exacerbation)) initially 1200–2400 mg orally daily in 3–4 divided doses with food, reducing to 1600 mg when symptoms stabilise **OR**
- (Primary dysmenorrhoea) 400–800 mg orally with food at the first sign of pain or menstrual bleeding, then 400 mg 4–6-hourly (maximum daily dose 1.6 g) **OR**
- (Minor aches and pains, dental pain, headache) 684 mg (2 caplets) with food initially, then 342–684 mg 4–6-hourly as needed (daily maximum 6 caplets) (342 mg caplets) **OR**
- (Minor aches and pains, dental pain, headache) 200–400 mg orally 4–6-hourly as needed (daily maximum 1.2 g) **OR**

- (Analgesia) 400—600 mg by IV infusion over 30 minutes 6-hourly, as needed (daily maximum 3.2 g for ≤ 2 days) **OR**
- (Fever) initially 400 mg by IV infusion over 30 minutes, then 400 mg IV 4—6-hourly as needed (daily maximum 3.2 g) **OR**
- (Topical gel) apply 4—10 cm of gel 4-hourly (as needed) to affected area and rub gently (maximum 4 applications daily)

Adverse effects
- (Rare) aseptic meningitis with fever and coma
- see also General Adverse effects of NSAIDs (p. 11)

Interactions
- colestyramine may decrease absorption of ibuprofen
- see also General Interactions of NSAIDs (p. 11)

Nursing considerations/Cautions
- (IV) the patient must be well hydrated before IV ibuprofen is used to decrease risk of kidney damage
- (IV) must be diluted with sodium chloride 0.9% or glucose 5% to a concentration of 4 mg/mL before administration
- (Nurofen QuikZorb) each caplet contains 342 mg ibuprofen lysine, which is the equivalent of 200 mg ibuprofen
- chewable tablets contain aspartame and are therefore not recommended in those with phenylketonuria
- caution if used in patients undergoing spinal or epidural analgesia
- caution if used in patients with SLE because of the risk of aseptic meningitis
- see also General Nursing considerations/Cautions for NSAIDs (p. 12)

Patient education
- (Oral solution) advise the patient to shake well before use, and syringe/measuring spoon should be used to measure dose
- (Chewable tablet) instruct the patient to chew tablet, not swallow whole
- see also topical gel administration advice (p. 14)
- see also General Patient education for NSAIDs (p. 13)

 Liquid preparation and chewable tablets are available.

 Liquid-filled capsules and slow-release tablets should not be opened or crushed.

 See General Nursing considerations/Cautions for NSAIDs (p. 12).

 Considered safe for breastfeeding women.

Available in combination with
- ibuprofen 300 mg + paracetamol 1000 mg/100 mL solution for infusion (Maxigesic IV Solution)
- ibuprofen 200 mg + paracetamol 500 mg, tablets/capsules (APOHealth Ibuprofen Plus Paracetamol, Blooms the Chemist Ibuprofen Plus Paracetamol, Chemists' Own Ibuprofen + Paracetamol Duo, Maxigesic, Maxofen, Mersynofen, Nuromol Dual Action Pain Relief, Pharmacy Action Paracetamol & Ibuprofen)
- ibuprofen 200 mg + codeine 12.8 mg, tablets (Amcal Ibuprofen Plus Codeine, Brufen Plus 200/12.8, Ibudeine, Ibuprofen/Codeine-TIH 200/12.8, Ibuprofen/Codeine-WGR 200/12.8, Nurofen Plus, Sandoz Ibuprofen Plus Codeine, Trust Ibuprofen Plus Codeine)
- ibuprofen 200 mg + pseudoephedrine 30 mg tablets (Nurofen Cold & Flu with Decongestant, Sudafed Sinus + Anti-inflammatory Pain Relief)
- ibuprofen 200 mg + phenylephrine 5 mg tablets (Nurofen Cold & Flu, Nurofen Sinus Pain PE)

INDOMETACIN (INDOMETHACIN)

Trade names
Arthrexin, Indocid

Available forms
Capsules: 25 mg;
Suppositories: 100 mg

Action
- more potent analgesic, antipyretic and anti-inflammatory properties than aspirin
- (Oral) half-life about 4.5 hours
- see also General Actions of NSAIDs (p. 11)

Use
- rheumatoid arthritis, osteoarthritis, ankylosing spondylitis
- degenerative hip disease
- gout
- bursitis, capsulitis, tenosynovitis, tendonitis
- sprains and strains
- low back pain (lumbago)
- inflammation, pain and oedema following orthopaedic surgery or reduction, and immobilisation of fractures and dislocations
- primary dysmenorrhoea

Dose
- 50—200 mg orally daily with food in divided doses (daily maximum 200 mg) **OR**
- 100 mg rectal suppository once or twice daily if oral therapy not tolerated **OR**
- in combination (e.g. 25 mg orally 2—4 times daily and 100 mg rectal suppository at night (to a total of 200 mg)) **OR**
- (Acute gouty arthritis) 150—200 mg orally daily with food in divided doses until symptoms subside **OR**
- (Primary dysmenorrhoea) 25 mg orally 3 times daily with food at the first sign of pain or menstrual bleeding, and continuing for as long as the symptoms usually last

Adverse effects
- (Oral) headache, may aggravate pre-existing psychiatric disturbances, epilepsy or Parkinsonism
- (Prolonged therapy) corneal deposits, retinal disturbances
- (Suppository) burning, pain, discomfort, rectal bleeding, proctitis, tenesmus
- see also General Adverse effects of NSAIDs (p. 11)

Interactions
- may cause false negative in dexamethasone suppression test
- see also General Interactions of NSAIDs (p. 11)

Nursing considerations/Cautions
- (Rheumatic conditions) loading dose not required
- capsules contain lactose; therefore are not recommended in those with hereditary galactose intolerance, Lapp lactase deficiency or glucose—galactose malabsorption
- caution if used in those with psychiatric disturbances, epilepsy or Parkinsonism as condition may be aggravated
- (Suppository) contraindicated in those with proctitis or recent rectal bleeding
- see also General Nursing considerations/Cautions for NSAIDs (p. 12)

Patient education
- patients who experience night pain and/or morning stiffness should be advised to take oral treatment during the day and suppositories at bedtime for better control of symptoms
- warn patient that headache may occur early in treatment. If severe, dose can be decreased or therapy stopped if headache persists
- instruct patient to seek medical advice if vision becomes blurred or disturbed
- see also General Patient education for NSAIDs (p. 13)

ANALGESICS AND NON-STEROIDAL ANTI-INFLAMMATORY DRUGS (NSAIDs)

 Capsules can be opened and contents dispersed in water, or mixed with spoonful of yoghurt or apple puree.

 See General Patient education for NSAIDs (p. 13).

 See General Patient education for NSAIDs (p. 13).

KETOPROFEN

Trade name
Oruvail SR

Available form
Capsules (sustained-release): 200 mg

Action
- half-life less than 2 hours
- see also General Actions of NSAIDs (p. 11)

Use
- rheumatoid arthritis, osteoarthritis

Dose
- 200 mg orally in 2—4 divided doses daily with food

Adverse effects
- non-bacterial cystitis (bladder pain, dysuria, haematuria, increased micturition and frequency)
- see also General Adverse effects of NSAIDs (p. 11)

Interactions
- may reduce efficacy of gemeprost and intrauterine contraceptive devices, increasing risk of pregnancy
- increased risk of bleeding if given with pentoxifylline (oxpentifylline)
- see also General Interactions of NSAIDs (p. 11)

Nursing considerations/Cautions
- see General Nursing considerations/Cautions for NSAIDs (p. 12)

Patient education
- recommend that slow-release capsules should not be broken, crushed or chewed but swallowed whole
- warn patient about symptoms of non-bacterial urinary tract infection symptoms, including change in colour, amount or frequency of urine, blood in urine or burning feeling when passing urine
- see also General Patient education for NSAIDs (p. 13)

 Capsules or contents (sustained-release pellets) should not be crushed or chewed. Pellets can be mixed with spoonful of yoghurt or apple puree but must not be chewed.

KETOROLAC

Trade names
Acular Eye Drops, Ketorolac Solution for Injection, Toradol

Available forms
Tablets: 10 mg;
Ampoule: 10 mg/mL, 30 mg/mL;
Eye drops: 5 mg/mL

Action
- inhibits prostaglandin synthesis by inhibiting COX
- potent peripherally acting analgesic with poor anti-inflammatory properties
- half-life 5—6 hours
- platelet inhibition reverses 24—48 hours after stopping

Use
- moderate-to-severe postoperative pain (short term not exceeding 5 days)
- seasonal allergic conjunctivitis (short term); prophylaxis and reduction of inflammation after cataract surgery

Dose
- (Under 65 years) initially 10—30 mg IM, followed by 10—30 mg 4—6-hourly (maximum 90 mg daily) **OR**

- (65 years and over, less than 50 kg or less severe pain) initially 10—15 mg IM, followed by 10—15 mg 4—6-hourly (maximum 60 mg daily) **OR**
- (Under 65 years) 10 mg orally 4—6-hourly (maximum 40 mg daily) **OR**
- (65 years and over) 10 mg orally 6—8-hourly (maximum 30—40 mg daily) **OR**
- (Seasonal allergic conjunctivitis) 1 drop 4 times daily for up to 4 weeks **OR**
- (Prophylaxis and postoperative inflammation) 1—2 drops 4 times daily, starting 24 hours before surgery and for up to 2—4 weeks

Adverse effects
- (Injection site) pain, ecchymosis, bruising, tingling and, rarely, haematoma
- (Rare, but fatal) haemorrhage
- (Eye drops) transient stinging, burning, itching, erythema, keratitis, scratching, foreign body sensation
- see also General Adverse effects of NSAIDs (p. 11)

Interactions
- increased risk of seizure activity if given with antiepileptic agents (e.g. phenytoin, carbamazepine)
- may be used with opioid analgesics to achieve optimal analgesia or when the sedative or anxiolytic effect of the opioid is wanted
- increased risk of hallucinations if given with fluoxetine
- contraindicated with aspirin, NSAIDs, pentoxifylline (oxpentifylline), lithium or probenecid
- (Eye drops) increased risk of delayed corneal healing if given with topical corticosteroids
- see also General Interactions of NSAIDs (p. 11)

Nursing considerations/Cautions
- any hypovolaemia should be corrected before administration of ketorolac trometamol
- IM injection should be given deeply and slowly into large muscle
- pressure should be applied to injection site for 15—30 seconds to decrease local effects
- total duration of use should not exceed 5 days because the risk of adverse effects increases with prolonged use
- conversion from parenteral to oral route should occur as soon as practicable and total combined dose (IM, oral) should not exceed 90 mg (or 60 mg in those aged 65 years and over)
- (Eye drops) contain benzalkonium chloride (preservative), which may discolour soft contact lenses
- contraindicated via epidural or intrathecal route
- contraindicated in those with dehydration, hypovolaemia, moderate/severe kidney impairment, coagulation disorders or on anticoagulant therapy, in surgical procedures with high risk of bleeding, or history of bleeding (GI or intracranial)
- see also General Nursing considerations/Cautions for NSAIDs (p. 12)

Patient education
- (Eye drops) see eye drop instillation advice (p. 486)
- see also General Patient education for NSAIDs (p. 13)

Tablet can be crushed and mixed with water, spoonful of yoghurt or apple puree.

See General Patient education for NSAIDs (p. 13).

See General Patient education for NSAIDs (p. 13).

MEFENAMIC ACID
Trade names
Femin, Ponstan

Available form
Capsules: 250 mg

Action
- half-life 2 hours
- see also General Actions of NSAIDs (p. 11)

ANALGESICS AND NON-STEROIDAL ANTI-INFLAMMATORY DRUGS (NSAIDs)

Use
- primary dysmenorrhoea
- primary menorrhagia
- mild-to-moderate pain (e.g. dental and soft tissue pain)

Dose
- (Primary dysmenorrhoea) 500 mg orally 3 times daily with food from onset of pain for usual duration of pain **OR**
- (Primary menorrhagia) 500 mg orally 3 times daily with food from onset of menses and continued according to doctor's advice, not exceeding 7 days (except on doctor's advice) **OR**
- (Other indications) 500 mg orally 3 times daily with food

Adverse effects
- see General Adverse effects of NSAIDs (p. 11), particularly severe diarrhoea

Interactions
- may cause false positive reaction for urinary bile. Other diagnostic procedures for bilirubinuria are recommended
- see also General Interactions of NSAIDs (p. 11)

Nursing considerations/Cautions
- contraindicated in those who have previously experienced mefenamic acid-induced diarrhoea
- see also General Nursing considerations/Cautions for NSAIDs (p. 12)

Patient education
- advise patient that diarrhoea is dose dependent and disappears when medication is stopped
- see also General Patient education for NSAIDs (p. 13)

MELOXICAM
Trade names
Melobic, Meloxibell, Mobic, Moxicam, APO-Meloxicam, APX-Meloxicam, Cipla Meloxicam, Meloxicam Sandoz, Meloxicam Viatris, Meloxicam-WRG, Pharmcor Meloxicam

Available forms
Tablets: 7.5 mg, 15 mg;
Capsules: 7.5 mg, 15 mg

Action
- selective COX-2 inhibitor
- half-life 20 hours
- see also General Actions of NSAIDs (p. 11)

Use
- osteoarthritis, rheumatoid arthritis

Dose
- (Osteoarthritis) 7.5 mg orally daily with food, increasing to 15 mg daily if needed (daily maximum 15 mg) **OR**
- (Rheumatoid arthritis) 15 mg orally daily with food, decreasing to 7.5 mg daily if condition allows

Adverse effects
- see General Adverse effects of NSAIDs (p. 11)

Interactions
- caution if given with itraconazole, erythromycin, ciclosporin or amiodarone
- not recommended with pemetrexed. If creatinine clearance is 45–79 mL/min, meloxicam should be stopped for 5 days before, on day of and 2 days after pemetrexed administration
- see also General Interactions of NSAIDs (p. 11)

Nursing considerations/Cautions
- contains lactose, therefore is contraindicated in those with hereditary galactose intolerance, Lapp lactase deficiency or glucose–galactose malabsorption
- see also General Nursing considerations/Cautions for NSAIDs (p. 12)

Patient education
- see General Patient education for NSAIDs (p. 13)

 Tablets can be crushed or capsules can be opened and contents dispersed in water, or mixed with spoonful of yoghurt or apple puree.

METHYL SALICYLATE

Trade names
Methyl Salicylate Liniment, Cream and Ointment

Available forms
Cream, Liniment and Ointment:

Action
- salicylate
- topical analgesic properties

Use
- relief of pain and inflammation associated with rheumatic conditions, lumbago, musculoskeletal disorders, sprains and strains

Dose
- massage a small amount into affected area 2—3 times daily

Adverse effects
- acute poisoning can occur if taken orally
- mild skin irritation, erythema

Interactions
- excessive use may increase risk of bleeding in those taking warfarin or other anticoagulants

Nursing considerations/Cautions
- wash hands after use and avoid contact with eyes or mucous membranes

Patient education
- ensure the patient understands the preparation is for external use only
- warn the patient to avoid vigorous rubbing
- instruct the patient not to bandage the area tightly or apply heating pads while the preparation is on skin
- caution the patient to keep medication away from an open flame
- see also topical gel/solution application advice (p. 14)

Available in combination with
- (methyl salicylate + multiple ingredients) Bosisto's Eucalyptus Rub, Deep Heat, Dencorub Extra Strength Heat Gel, Dencorub Pain Relieving Cream, Goanna Heat Cream, Metsal Heat Rub Cream

NAPROXEN

Trade names
Inza, Naprosyn, Naprosyn SR, Phebra, Naproxen Suspension, Proxen SR, Pediapharm Naproxen Oral Suspension USP

NAPROXEN SODIUM

Trade names
Aleve, Anaprox, Crysanal, Naprogesic, APOHealth Period Pain Relief, Chemists' Own Period Pain Relief, Pharmacy Action Period Pain Relief

Available forms
Tablets: 220 mg, 250 mg, 275 mg, 500 mg, 550 mg
Tablets (sustained-release): 660 mg, 750 mg, 1000 mg;
Suspension: 125 mg/5 mL

Action
- half-life 14 hours
- see also General Actions of NSAIDs (p. 11)

Use
- rheumatoid arthritis, osteoarthritis, ankylosing spondylitis, gout
- acute/chronic inflammatory pain
- acute migraine
- primary dysmenorrhoea

Dose
- (Arthritis, spondylitis) initially 500—1100 mg orally daily in 2 divided doses with food, then 375—1000 mg daily (maintenance) **OR**
- (Arthritis, spondylitis) 750—1000 mg orally once daily (SR) (daily maximum 1000 mg) **OR**
- (Primary dysmenorrhoea) 500—550 mg orally with food at the first sign of pain or bleeding, then 250—275 mg 6—8-hourly as required (daily maximum 1250—1375 mg) **OR**
- (Migraine) initially 750—825 mg orally at first sign of impending headache, then 250—550 mg throughout day, but not

before 1 hour of initial dose (daily maximum 1250—1375 mg) **OR**
- (Acute inflammatory pain) initially 500—550 mg orally with food, then 250—275 mg 6—8-hourly (daily maximum 1375 mg)
- (Migraine, 550 mg tablets) 825 mg orally at first sign of impending headache, then 275—550 mg at least 1 hour after initial dose (daily maximum 1375 mg)

Adverse effects
- see General Adverse effects of NSAIDs (p. 11)

Interactions
- may increase serum levels of zidovudine
- may interfere with some tests for 7-ketogenic steroids and some urinary assays for 5-hydroxy-indoleacetic acid
- see also General Interactions of NSAIDs (p. 11)

Nursing considerations/Cautions
- sustained-release preparations should not be used for acute conditions
- suspension contains 8 mg sodium per mL and tablets (Anaprox, Crysanal) contain 50 mg of sodium per 550 mg tablet, which should be considered if patient requires sodium restriction
- see also General Nursing considerations/Cautions for NSAIDs (p. 12)

Patient education
- instruct the patient to discontinue medication 72 hours before adrenal function tests
- advise the patient that sustained-release tablets should be taken whole, not crushed or chewed
- warn the patient that slow-release (SR) tablets are not recommended for acute conditions such as migraine
- the patient should be instructed to shake suspension well before use
- see also General Patient education for NSAIDs (p. 13)

Sustained-release tablets should not be crushed; however, it is available as an oral suspension. Some formulations are very difficult to crush and/or do not disperse easily in water.

PARACETAMOL
Trade names
Dymadon Suspension, Febridol, Lemsip Cold & Flu, Lemsip Max, Osteomol, Panadol preparations, Panamax, Paracetamol preparations, Paracetamol Solution for Infusion, Paradyn, Paralgin, Paramyl Osteo, Parapane, Tylenol

Available forms
Tablets: 500 mg;
Tablets/caplets (modified-release): 665 mg;
Tablets (soluble): 250 mg, 500 mg;
Tablets (chewable): 120 mg;
Caplets: 500 mg;
Suppositories: 125 mg, 250 mg, 500 mg;
Sachets (powder): 500 mg, 1 g;
Syrup/Suspension/Elixir: 120 mg/5 mL, 240 mg/5 mL, 50 mg/mL, 250 mg/5 mL;
Drops: 50 mg/mL, 100 mg/mL;
IV solution: 10 mg/mL

Action
- known as acetaminophen in the USA
- analgesic, antipyretic but has no useful anti-inflammatory properties
- analgesic and antipyretic actions are thought to be related to prostaglandin synthesis inhibition in the CNS
- half-life 1—3 hours

Use
- mild-to-moderate pain
- headache, migraine, tension headache, sinus pain
- muscle ache
- osteoarthritis
- toothache, dental pain post-procedure
- cold and flu symptoms
- fever
- (IV) mild-to-moderate pain when IV route is clinically indicated

- suitable alternative for those with aspirin allergy (including those with asthma), dyspepsia or peptic ulceration, or children with fever caused by viral illness

Dose
- 0.5—1 g orally 4—6-hourly as required (up to 4 g/day) **OR**
- 1330 mg (2 tablets) orally 3 times daily as required (up to 4 g/day (6 tablets)) (modified-release tablets) **OR**
- 0.5—1 g rectal suppository 4—6-hourly as required (up to 4 g/day) **OR**
- (Patient weight > 50 kg) 1 g IV 4-hourly, up to 4 g/day **OR**
- (Patient weight > 33 kg but ≤ 50 kg) 15 mg/kg IV 4-hourly, up to 3 g/day **OR**
- (Patient weight > 10 kg but ≤ 33 kg) 15 mg/kg IV 6-hourly, up to 2 g/day

Adverse effects
- (Rarely) nausea, dyspepsia, allergic or haematological reaction, hypersensitivity, serious skin reactions
- (10—15 g or more) hepatic necrosis, renal dysfunction
- (IV) nausea, vomiting, diarrhoea, dyspepsia, headache, dizziness, increase in liver enzymes, injection site pain and pruritus

Interactions
- (Immediate-release preparations) absorption rate may be increased by metoclopramide but decreased for sustained-release preparations
- prolonged use may require reduction in anticoagulant dose; therefore INR should be closely monitored during therapy and 7 days after stopping therapy
- large or chronic doses of paracetamol increase the likelihood of hepatotoxicity if given with concurrent use of alcohol, other hepatotoxic agents or antiepileptic drugs
- may decrease clearance of busulfan
- increased risk of hepatotoxicity and decreased effectiveness if given with phenytoin
- products containing paracetamol should not be given together (e.g. oral and IV) to avoid risk of overdose and hepatic damage. All routes should be considered when calculating total daily dose
- probenecid reduces clearance
- (IV) metabolism may be increased (therefore increasing level of hepatotoxic metabolites) by barbiturates, anticoagulants, isoniazid, zidovudine, amoxicillin with clavulanic acid or carbamazepine
- absorption may be decreased by agents that decrease gastric emptying (e.g. opioids, propantheline, antidepressants with anticholinergic properties)

Nursing considerations/Cautions
- when estimating total daily dose, all routes (e.g. oral, IV, PR), prescribed and over-the-counter paracetamol-containing products should be considered. Total daily dose should not exceed 4 g (patient weight ≥ 50 kg), 60 mg/kg up to 3 g for patient weight < 50 kg to ≥ 33 kg, and 60 mg/kg for patient weight < 33 kg to ≥ 10 kg
- IV infusion given over 15 minutes
- IV solution has slight yellow colour
- IV administration should be changed to oral administration as soon as practicable
- early overdose symptoms include sweating, pallor, anorexia, nausea, vomiting, abdominal pain or cramping and/or diarrhoea occurring 6—14 hours after ingestion, and lasting about 24 hours
- late overdose symptoms include tenderness or pain in abdominal area, indicating liver necrosis/failure (jaundice, hypoglycaemia, metabolic acidosis) and confusion
- symptoms of overdose in first 48 hours may not reflect potential seriousness, as symptoms of liver failure may not manifest for at least 72 hours. Absorption of SR formulations will be prolonged in overdose
- overdose management: after taking blood for paracetamol assay, overdose should be treated promptly (within 10 hours) with activated charcoal and sorbitol or gastric lavage to reduce gastric absorption and with IV acetylcysteine to

protect against liver damage (see Antidotes, antagonists and chelating agents, p. 334) if 10—15 g or more of paracetamol has been ingested. Liver tests are recommended at the start of overdose management, then daily
- (Febridol tablets) contain sodium metabisulfite, which may cause a hypersensitivity reaction in sensitive individuals
- (Panadol Soluble) may contain sorbitol, which is not recommended in those with fructose intolerance
- (Soluble/effervescent preparations) contain sodium, which should be considered in sodium-restricted diets
- (Soluble/effervescent preparations) contain aspartame and should not be used in those with glucose-6-phosphate dehydrogenase (G6PD) deficiency, as haemolytic anaemia may result
- (IV) if patient has liver disease, daily dose should not exceed 3 g
- (IV) caution if used in those with dehydration, hypovolaemia, chronic malnutrition (including anorexia, bulimia or cachexia) or chronic alcoholism (> 3 drinks/day)
- not recommended for infants under 1 month of age
- caution if used in those with liver or kidney dysfunction
- contraindicated in those with severe liver disease/failure

Patient education

- instruct patient to dissolve effervescent and soluble preparations in 1/2—1 glass of water for more rapid absorption
- warn patient to avoid alcohol during therapy
- advise patient to swallow modified-release tablets whole, not chewed or crushed
- patient should be cautioned regarding risk of overdose if taking multiple paracetamol-containing preparations
- (Powder) instruct patient to pour sachet into mug, fill with hot (not boiling) water and stir until dissolved. May be sweetened with sugar or honey if required
- (Drops/suspension) can be administered to infant mixed with water or fruit juice
- advise patient to seek medical advice if skin reaction occurs
- see also suppository insertion advice (p. 15)

 Modified-release tablets/caplets must be swallowed whole.

 Considered safe to use when pregnant.

 Considered safe to use when breastfeeding.

 Patients with hepatic impairment require a dose reduction of prolonged intervals because of the increased risk of liver damage.

Contraindicated in those with liver failure, decompensated active liver disease or hepatocellular insufficiency. Caution if used in those with severe renal insufficiency (CrCl < 30 mL/min).

Available in combination with
- paracetamol 325 mg + tramadol 37.5 mg (Zaldair)
- paracetamol 500 mg + codeine phosphate 8 mg tablet (Cipla Pain Relief Paracetamol and Codeine 8, Panamax Co)
- paracetamol 500 mg + codeine phosphate 30 mg tablet (APX-Paracetamol/Codeine, Codalgin Forte, Codapane Forte 500/30, Comfarol, Panadeine Forte, Paracetamol/Codeine GH 500/30, Prodeine Forte)
- paracetamol 500 mg + codeine phosphate 15 mg tablet (Amcal Strong Pain Relief Extra 500/15, Codasig, Mydol 15, Paracetamol/Codeine GH 500/15, Prodeineextra)
- paracetamol 500 mg + codeine phosphate 10 mg tablets (Chemists' Own Pain, Chemists' Own Pain Captab)
- paracetamol 450 mg + orphenadrine citrate 35 mg tablets (Norgesic)

HAVARD'S NURSING GUIDE TO DRUGS

- paracetamol 500 mg + codeine phosphate 10 mg + doxylamine succinate 5.1 mg tablets (Dolased Mersyndol, Trust Analgesic Calmative)
- paracetamol 450 mg + codeine phosphate 30 mg + doxylamine succinate 5 mg tablets (Dolased Forte, Mersyndol Forte, Mervadol)
- paracetamol 500 mg + metoclopramide 5 mg (Anagraine, Metomax)
- paracetamol + ibuprofen (see ibuprofen p. 24 in this chapter)
- paracetamol 500 mg + diphenhydramine 25 mg tablets (APOHealth Night Pain Relief, Chemists' Own Night Pain Relief, Panadol Night, Comboleive Day & Night, MersynoNight Night Time Pain Relief)
- paracetamol 500 mg + chlorphenamine 2 mg tablets (APOHealth Cold Relief)
- paracetamol 500 mg + pseudoephedrine 30 mg tablets (APOHelath Sinus & Pain Relief, Chemists' Own Cold & Flu Relief, Codral Original Cold & Flu, Dimetapp Cold & Flu Relief, Lemsip Max Decongestant Cold & Flu Hot Drink, Sudafed Sinus + Pain Relief)
- paracetamol 500 mg + caffeine 65 mg (Chemists' Own Paracetamol Extra)
- paracetemol 500 mg+ phenylephedrine 5 mg tablets (Codral Cold & Flu, Panadol Cold & Flu + Decongestant, Panadol Sinus Relief Original, Pharmacy Action Cold & Flu PSE, Sudafed PE Sinus + Pain Relief)
- paracetamol is also available in multiple ingredient preparations for cough, cold and flu (Sudafed Sinus preparations, Sudafed PE preparations, Lemsip Max preparations, Lemsip Multi-Symptom Relief, Dimetapp preparations, Demazin Cold + Flu preparations, Codral preparations, Chemists' Own Cough, Cold & Flu preparations)

PIROXICAM

Trade names
Feldene D, Feldene Gel, Mobilis, APO-Piroxicam, Mobilis D

Available forms
Capsules: 10 mg, 20 mg;
Tablets (dispersible): 10 mg, 20 mg;
Gel: 5 mg/g

Action
- half-life 36—45 hours
- see also General Actions of NSAIDs (p. 11)

Use
- rheumatoid arthritis, osteoarthritis, ankylosing spondylitis
- acute soft tissue injuries (e.g. sprains, strains, tendonitis)

Dose
- initially 10 mg orally daily, increasing to 20 mg if needed **OR**
- 1 g (3 cm of gel) to affected area 3—4 times daily for up to 2 weeks

Adverse effects
- (Gel) mild skin irritation (erythema, rash, pruritus), transient skin discolouration, photosensitivity, contact dermatitis, eczema
- see also General Adverse effects of NSAIDs (p. 11)

Interactions
- see General Interactions of NSAIDs (p. 11)

Nursing considerations/Cautions
- (Oral) once-daily dose required because of long plasma half-life
- see also General Nursing considerations/Cautions for NSAIDs (p. 12)

Patient education
- advise the patient that gel should be completely rubbed in to prevent skin discolouration or staining of clothes
- see also topical gel administration advice (p. 14)
- see also General Patient education for NSAIDs (p. 13)

 Available as dispersible tablets, or capsule can be opened and contents mixed with spoonful of yoghurt or apple puree.

ANORECTICS AND WEIGHT-LOSS AGENTS

National survey figures in 2022 showed that more than 65% of Australian adults aged 18 years and over were either overweight (34%) or obese (31.7%), 31.6% were normal weight and about 1.7% were underweight (ABS 2022a).

A thorough patient assessment should include an obesity-focused history (e.g. factors contributing to obesity, impact on health, patient goals, expectations and barriers to weight management, motivation), physical examination to determine degree and type of obesity, assessment of comorbid conditions and the patient's willingness to engage in lifestyle changes (Kushner 2022).

To evaluate the degree of obesity, height, weight and waist circumference should be measured (Kushner 2022). Body mass index (BMI) is calculated by dividing the person's weight (kg) by the person's height (in metres squared (m^2)) and is an estimate of body fat, which is related to risk of disease. It should be noted, however, that BMI is a less useful measure in the elderly and those who are fit and muscular (Kushner 2022). A person is classified as obese if their BMI is equal to or greater than 30, while 25–29.9 is considered to be overweight. Waist circumference is a good indicator of visceral fat and is associated with an increased risk of cardiovascular disease and diabetes (Kushner 2022).

The overall goal of therapy is to reduce weight in order to reduce the risk of related comorbidities including cardiovascular disease, type 2 diabetes mellitus, cancer, bone and joint disease, reproductive disorder and increased mortality (Kushner 2022). Management should always start with lifestyle management (diet, physical activity, behaviour modification).

Anorectic and weight-loss agents are considered adjunctive in the management of obesity where other regimens (lifestyle management) have not been successful in achieving an adequate response (e.g. greater than 5% weight loss within 3 months) (Kushner 2022). Sometimes a person who is classified as overweight with a BMI of 27 may be prescribed anorectic and weight-loss agents if they have other obesity-related risk factors such as hypertension, diabetes or dyslipidaemia. Bariatric surgery, such as laparoscopic sleeve gastrectomy or laparoscopic adjustable gastric banding, may be recommended for those with comorbidities and a BMI of 35 kg/m^2 or greater or those with severe obesity ($\geq$ 40 kg/m^2) (Kushner 2022).

The use of anorectic and weight-loss agents should be limited because tolerance and habituation are known to develop. They should be used in conjunction with a well-balanced, calorie-modified diet, appropriate exercise regimen and behaviour modification (Kushner 2022). Secondary causes of obesity should be eliminated before commencing on any weight-loss agent.

LIRAGLUTIDE
Trade name
Saxenda, Victoza

Available form
Prefilled pen: 6 mg/mL 3mL

Action
- glucagon-like peptide-1 (GLP-1) analogue
- protracted release is due to self-association (resulting in slow absorption), binding to albumin and enzymatic stability, resulting in long plasma half-life
- physiological regulator of appetite and calorie intake, as GLP-1 receptors are present in the brain in areas involved in appetite regulation, as well as being present in the intestine
- increases satiety and decreases hunger signals
- peak effect 8–12 hours, duration of action 24 hours, half-life about 13 hours

Use
- type 2 diabetes, chronic weight management in those with BMI $\geq$ 30 kg/m^2 (obese) or $\geq$ 27 kg/m^2 and $<$ 30 kg/m^2 (overweight) with $\geq$ 1 weight-related co-morbidity (e.g. dyslipidaemia, hypertension, obstructive sleep apnoea) (adjunct to reduced calorie diet and increased physical activity) (see Antidiabetic agents, p. 296)

NALTREXONE HYDROCHLORIDE and BUPROPION HYDROCHLORIDE
Trade name
Contrave 8/90

Available form
Tablets (naltrexone hydrochloride 8 mg and bupropion hydrochloride 90 mg) (modified-release)

Action
- naltrexone hydrochloride is a mu-opioid antagonist used as part of alcohol dependence programs and as an adjunct in maintaining abstinence from opioids (see Drugs for alcohol dependence, p. 1108 and Drugs for opioid dependence, p. 1108)
- bupropion hydrochloride selectively inhibits neuronal reuptake of dopamine and noradenaline (norepinephrine) and is used as an adjunct to counselling in management of nicotine dependence (see Drugs for nicotine dependence, p. 1104)
- the exact mode of action of this combination medication on appetite suppression is not totally understood, although it is thought to increase the firing rate of hypothalamic pro-opiomelancortin neurons involved in appetite regulation. Furthermore, in animal studies, a reduced food intake was observed when injected directly into the ventral tegmental area of the mesolimbic circuit, which is associated with reward pathway regulation
- the action of the combinated two agents is thought to be greater than either single agent alone in reducing food intake
- elimination half-life is about 5 hours for naltrexone hydrochloride and 21 hours for bupropion hydrochloride

Use
- as an adjunct in weight management in adults ($\geq$ 18 years) with an initial BMI $\geq$ 30 kg/m^2 (obese) or $\geq$ 27 kg/m^2 to $<$ 30 kg/m^2 (overweight with one or more related co-morbidities including

ANORECTICS AND WEIGHT-LOSS AGENTS

type 2 diabetes, dyslipidaemia or controlled hypertension), along with a reduced calorie diet and increased exercise program

Dose
- (Week 1) 1 tablet orally daily mane
- (Week 2) 1 tablet orally mane and nocte
- (Week 3) 2 tablets orally mane, 1 table orally nocte
- (Week 4 and onwards) 2 tablets orally mane and nocte

Adverse effects
- nausea, vomiting, constipation, upper abdominal pain, altered taste
- dry mouth, toothache
- dizziness, headache, insomnia, feeling jittery, tremor, lethargy, attention disturbance
- palpitations
- tinnitus, vertigo
- hot flush, pruritus, excessive sweating
- alopecia
- (Rare) seizures, angioedema

Interactions
- contraindicated with or within 14 days of stopping MAOIs
- contraindicated with other treatments using naltrexone hydrochloride or bupropion hydrochloride
- caution if used with agents that may lower seizure threshold, including antipsychotics, antidepressants, antimalarials, tramadol, theophylline, systemic corticosteroids, quinolones and sedating antihistamine
- may increase levels of antiarrhythmics, antidepressants, TCAs, SSRIs, antipsychotics and beta adrenergic blocking agents, increasing the risk of adverse effects
- concentration may be increased if given with ticlopidine or clopidogrel
- if patient is undergoing intermittent opioid treatment, therapy should be stopped temporarily or the dose of opioid reduced
- efficacy may be reduced if given with ritonavir, lopinavir or efavirenz
- caution if given with metformin
- CNS toxicity may result if given with levodopa or amantadine
- may produce a false positive in urinary screening test for amphetamines. Further testing is required to differentiate between bupropion and amphetamines
- not recommended with alcohol

Nursing considerations/Cautions
- blood pressure and pulse should be measured before starting and regularly throughout therapy
- therapy should be reviewed after 16 weeks and then annually. If patient has not lost at least 5% of the initial body weight after 16 weeks, therapy should be discontinued
- blood glucose levels should be closely monitored in those with type 2 diabetes at the start of therapy
- if patient experiences seizure, therapy should be stopped and not restarted
- caution if used in those with diabetes as blood glucose levels may be affected, increasing risk of hypoglycaemia and seizure
- caution if used in those with controlled hypertension
- caution if used in those with risk of seizure, including head trauma history, excessive alcohol use and addiction to cocaine or stimulants
- caution if used in those with a history of depression, suicide attempt or suicide ideation
- caution if used in those over 65 years and not recommended in those over 75 years
- not recommended in those with history of myocardial infarction, unstable heart disease or congestive heart failure
- contraindicated in those with severe liver impairment or end-stage kidney failure
- contraindicated in those with uncontrolled hypertension, seizure disorder or history of seizures, known presence of central nervous system tumour, history of bipolar disorder, current or

- past history of an eating disorder or mania
- contraindicated in those with current dependency on opioids or opioid antagonists (e.g. methadone) or currently withdrawing from opioids
- contraindicated in those with rare hereditary problems of galactose intolerance, Lapp lactase deficiency or glucose−galactose malabsorption
- contraindicated in those with hypersensitivity to naltrexone hydrochloride or bupropion hydrochloride

Patient education

- counsel the patient to avoid or minimise intake of alcohol during therapy
- the patient should be advised that adverse effects generally resolve within 4 weeks of starting therapy
- advise the patient to take tablets whole (should not be cut, chewed or crushed)
- patients with type 2 diabetes mellitus should be warned that they may be more likely to experience gastrointestinal adverse effects, including nausea, vomiting and diarrhoea. They should also be advised to closely monitor blood glucose levels at the start of therapy to prevent hypoglycaemia
- instruct the patient to immediately report any:
  - sadness, crying, sleeping too much or not being able to fall asleep, change in appetite, trouble with concentration, withdrawal from family, friends and/or previously pleasurable activities, lack of energy and/or thoughts of self-harm
  - rash, hives, itching, shortness of breath, chest pain, swelling (oedema) (signs of anaphylactic/anaphylactoid reaction)
  - fever, rash, muscle pain, bone pain (signs of delayed hypersensitive reaction)
  - unusual tiredness, persistent loss of appetite, upper abdominal pain, yellowing of eyes or skin, dark urine (signs of hepatitis)
- carers and/or family members should be alerted to the need to monitor the patient's mood or any unusual behaviours in relation to depression or suicidal ideation
- warn the patient that they may be more sensitive to opioids (even low doses) when therapy is stopped, increasing the risk of overdose
- encourage the patient to participate in regular exercise, such as swimming or walking (approved by doctor), in addition to medication for sustained weight loss

 Tablets should not be crushed, cut or chewed.

 Contraindicated during pregnancy.

 Not recommended for use when breastfeeding.

ORLISTAT

Trade name
Prolistat, Xenical

Available form
Capsules: 120 mg

Action
- peripherally acting agent that specifically and reversibly inhibits lipase in the gut by approximately 30%, resulting in weight loss

Use
- management of obesity (BMI $\geq$ 30) or overweight (BMI $\geq$ 27 with other risk factors, such as hypertension or high cholesterol) in conjunction with a mild hypocaloric diet

ANORECTICS AND WEIGHT-LOSS AGENTS

Dose
- 120 mg orally 3 times daily with meals

Adverse effects
- fatty/oily stools, loose stools, faecal urgency, flatulence, oily spotting from rectum, increased frequency of defecation, faecal incontinence
- abdominal pain, nausea, dyspepsia
- headache, asthenia
- (Rare) hepatitis, liver failure, pancreatitis, hypersensitivity skin reaction

Interactions
- because vitamin K absorption may be altered, warfarin plasma levels may also be altered and therefore INR should be closely monitored
- may decrease ciclosporin plasma levels, necessitating monitoring of ciclosporin levels
- may decrease effect of amiodarone
- a decreased oral hypoglycaemic dose may be required with weight loss
- decreases absorption of fat-soluble vitamins A, D, E and beta carotene
- caution if used with antiepileptic agents
- not recommended with acarbose
- not recommended with other anorectic or weight-loss agents

Nursing considerations/Cautions
- effects become obvious within 1–2 days of starting therapy because fatty stools start to appear. Stools return to normal within 48–72 hours of stopping therapy
- those with epilepsy should be monitored for any changes in frequency and/or severity of seizures
- caution if used in those with active peptic ulcer disease, symptomatic cholelithiasis, postsurgical adhesions, eating disorders, psychiatric or neurological disorders, nephrolithiasis, deficiency of fat-soluble vitamins (A, D, E, K), or in those with significant cardiac, liver, kidney, gastrointestinal or endocrine disorders
- contraindicated in those with cholestasis, chronic malabsorption syndrome, chronic pancreatic enzyme deficiency, chronic pancreatitis or after major gastrointestinal surgery

Patient education
- advise the patient that weight loss is usually seen within 2 weeks of starting and continues for 6–12 months during therapy
- instruct the patient that capsules should be swallowed whole and taken with meals or up to 1 hour after meals. If a meal is missed or contains no fat, capsules may be omitted. Daily intake of fat should be spread over 3 main meals rather than concentrated in 1 meal
- advise the patient that the risk of gastrointestinal adverse effects is greater if the meal contains a high fat content
- explain to the patient that some symptoms (e.g. increased wind, abdominal pain, urgent need to open bowels or fatty, oily or liquid stools) will decrease as therapy continues; however, if a meal containing high fat is eaten, symptoms will return
- counsel the patient regarding the benefits of undertaking a nutritionally balanced, calorie-reduced diet and exercise program for continued weight loss. The diet should be nutritionally balanced and rich in fruit and vegetables, with fat making up 30% of the calorie value ($\leq$ 67 g fat/day) and adequate intake of fat-soluble vitamins. Patient should also be counselled to avoid fat-containing foods such as biscuits and chocolate as between-meal snacks
- encourage the patient to read food labels to determine fat content of food
- multivitamin supplement may be needed and should be taken 2 hours before or after medication
- encourage the patient to participate in regular exercise such as swimming or walking (approved by doctor) in addition to medication for sustained weight loss

- advise the patient with type 2 diabetes mellitus that weight loss may require adjustment to oral hypoglycaemic agent in order to maintain stable blood glucose levels and prevent hypoglycaemia

Capsule can be opened and contents dispersed in water or fruit juice, or given with spoonful of yoghurt.

Not recommended for use during pregnancy.

Not recommended for use when breastfeeding owing to limited available data.

PHENTERMINE

Trade name
Alenami, Duromine, Metermine, Phentodur, Supremine ER

Available forms
Capsules, Extended/modified-release capsules: 15 mg, 30 mg, 40 mg;
Tablets, Extended-release: 15 mg, 30 mg, 40 mg

Action
- sympathomimetic agent thought to suppress appetite through action on the hypothalamus
- has effects on the dopaminergic and noradrenergic nervous systems
- long half-life (about 25 hours)

Use
- short-term management of obesity (BMI $\geq$ 30) or overweight (BMI $\geq$ 25—29.9) with other risk factors (such as hypertension or high cholesterol) in conjunction with a mild hypocaloric diet and exercise program

Dose
- initially 30—40 mg orally daily, then 15—40 mg as maintenance

Adverse effects
- insomnia, restlessness, tremor, headache, nervousness, dizziness
- dry mouth, diarrhoea/constipation, nausea, vomiting, unpleasant taste, abdominal cramps
- palpitations, hypertension, tachycardia, praecordial pain
- impotence, disturbed micturition, changes in libido
- rash
- facial oedema
- (Rare) valvular heart disease, primary pulmonary hypertension

Interactions
- contraindicated with MAOIs or within 14 days of stopping MAOI therapy
- may antagonise clonidine and methyldopa sesquihydrate, reducing their antihypertensive actions
- may cause effects of insulin and oral hypoglycaemic agents to vary; therefore blood glucose levels should be closely monitored in those with diabetes
- use cautiously with other sympathomimetics or psychotropic agents, including sedatives
- should not be used with any other anorectic or weight-loss agents
- concurrent use with thyroid agents may cause CNS stimulation
- alcohol may increase CNS effects (e.g. dizziness, confusion)
- not recommended with SSRIs, ergot-related agents or clomipramine

Nursing considerations/Cautions
- cause of obesity should be determined before start of therapy to exclude any organic cause
- blood pressure should be monitored regularly throughout therapy (especially at the start) in those with mild hypertension
- course of treatment should be continued for 12 weeks and then reviewed by doctor
- caution if used in those with mild hypertension, diabetes, epilepsy (may increase frequency/severity of seizure) or if receiving antihypertensive therapy
- not recommended in the elderly

ANORECTICS AND WEIGHT-LOSS AGENTS

- contraindicated in those with glaucoma, moderate-to-severe or uncontrolled hypertension, pulmonary artery hypertension, hyperthyroidism, advanced arteriosclerosis, heart valve abnormalities or heart murmurs, cerebrovascular disease, severe cardiac disease, history of drug/alcohol abuse/dependence or psychiatric illness (including depression or eating disorders)
- contraindicated in those with hypersensitivity to sympathomimetic agents

Patient education

- instruct patients to swallow capsule whole with a glass of water. Capsules should not be chewed or opened
- warn patients to avoid alcohol during therapy
- advise patients not to drive or use machinery if they experience dizziness, tremor or confusion
- to avoid any sleep disturbances at night, suggest taking medication in morning rather than later in the day

- caution patients with diabetes that blood glucose levels should be monitored more frequently as weight loss may necessitate a reduction in dose of insulin and/or oral hypoglycaemic agents, increasing the risk of hypoglycaemia

 Capsules should not be opened or crushed.

 Not recommended during pregnancy.

 Not recommended when breastfeeding.

 In patients with renal impairment, consider a lower dose.

 Not recommended in the elderly.

 Banned in sport.

ANTHELMINTICS

The term 'helminth' is derived from the Greek word 'helmins' meaning worm. Helminths can be subdivided into nematodes (roundworms, hookworms, threadworms, whipworms and filariae), trematodes (flukes) and cestodes (tapeworms) (Keiser et al 2018). Helminth infections can lead to a range of health problems, depending on the type of worm and the organs affected.

Helminth infestations are thought to be present in more than 1.5 billion people worldwide (24% of the world's population). Prevalence is higher in tropical and subtropical areas (World Health Organization [WHO] 2019d) and where there is poor faecal sanitation and limited access to clean water. Adult worms live in human intestines and produce thousands of eggs daily, which are passed in faeces contaminating the soil. Transmission can occur via vegetables grown in contaminated soil that are not adequately washed, from water sources or from playing in contaminated soil and not washing the hands. Transmission is not person to person or via fresh faeces, as the eggs require about 3 weeks to mature and become infective in the soil. Furthermore, hookworm eggs can hatch in soil, and mature larvae can penetrate the skin when a person walks barefoot on contaminated soil (WHO 2019d).

These helminths not only cause ill health, but also have major economic and social consequences in areas where these infestations are endemic. Children in developing countries are particularly at risk of helminth infestation (often mixed), which may lead to impaired growth and physical development, malnutrition, vitamin deficiency, diarrhoea, anaemia and pneumonia (WHO 2019d).

Anthelmintics are drugs used to treat worm infestation. Their actions are selective, by taking advantage of the differences between the worm and host (e.g. different transmitter substances at the neuromuscular junction). These drugs must first be able to penetrate the cuticle of the worm, or its alimentary tract, to be effective. This heterogeneous group works in a variety of ways, including damaging or killing the worm directly, causing the worm to become paralysed and thus expelled in the faeces, damaging the worm in such a way that the host defences then take over, or interfering with the worm's metabolism (Keiser et al 2018).

General Patient education for helminth infestation

- as parasites generally enter the body by the mouth, hygiene is a very important issue for control. Other affected members of a household may require concurrent treatment to prevent reinfection, even if they appear asymptomatic
- eggs are very small and stick to whatever they come into contact with
- everyone in the household should be advised to wear shoes to prevent infestation or reinfestation by eggs
- fingernails should be cut short to avoid scratching the anal area and causing reinfestation (see point below about not shaking bed linen)
- shower or bathe daily
- underwear should be changed daily
- hands and fingernails should be washed thoroughly with soap and water after using the toilet and especially before preparing food or eating
- toilet seats should be thoroughly cleaned after use
- after treatment, bed linen, bedclothes and towels should be washed thoroughly. It is important not to shake bed clothes, bed linen or towels as eggs floating in the air may be swallowed, causing infestation or reinfestation
- bedroom floor should be vacuumed or damp-mopped (not swept) for 3 days post treatment

ALBENDAZOLE
Trade name
Eskazole, Zentel

Available forms
Tablets (chewable): 200 mg, 400 mg

Action
- benzimidazole
- disrupts metabolism, immobilising and killing the worm
- ovicidal (kills eggs), larvicidal (kills larvae) and vermicidal (kills worms)
- poorly absorbed and remains in the gastrointestinal (GI) tract
- active metabolite (albendazole sulfoxide) has a half-life of 8.5 hours

Use
- hydatid disease caused by the tapeworm *Echinococcus granulosus* (where surgery is not possible, multiple cysts are present or as an adjunct pre- or post-surgery)
- cysticercosis (especially with neurological involvement (neurocysticercosis))
- capillariasis (*Capillaria philippinensis*)
- pinworm/threadworm (*Enterobius vermicularis*), roundworm (*Ascaris lumbricoides*), hookworm (*Ancylostoma duodenale, Necator americanus*), whipworm (*Trichuris trichiura*), strongyloides, liver flukes (*Opisthorchis viverrini, Clonorchis sinensis*)
- cutaneous larva migrans
- tapeworm (*Hymenolepis nana* or *Taenia* spp. with other species also present)

Dose
Hydatid disease
- 400 mg orally twice daily with food (for 28 days), which may be repeated for 3 cycles with a 14-day drug-free break between cycles **OR**
- (Under 60 kg) 15 mg/kg/day in divided doses with food (for 28 days), which may be repeated for 3 cycles with a 14-day drug-free break between cycles **OR**
- (Preoperatively) 2 × 28-day cycles as above **OR**
- (Postoperatively) 2 × 28-day cycles as above (if preoperative dose was given less than 14 days, operation was in emergency theatre or if cysts were viable after preoperative treatment) **OR**
- (Inoperable or multiple cysts) 400 mg orally twice daily with food (for 28 days) repeated for 3 cycles with a 14-day drug-free break between cycles

Neurocysticercosis
- 400 mg orally twice daily with food for 3—7 days, which may be repeated for 1 cycle with a 14-day drug-free break between cycles **OR**
- (Under 60 kg) 15 mg/kg/day in divided doses with food, as above

Capillariasis
- 400 mg orally daily with food for 10 days

Pinworm, threadworm, roundworm, hookworm, whipworm
- 400 mg orally on an empty stomach as a single dose

Strongyloides
- 400 mg orally daily on an empty stomach for 3 consecutive days

Cutaneous larva migrans
- 400 mg orally daily with food for 1—3 days

Mixed worm infestation (including liver flukes)
- 400 mg orally twice daily with food for 3 days

Tape worm
- 400 mg orally daily on an empty stomach for 3 days. If ineffective after 21 days, course can be repeated

Adverse effects
- abdominal pain, nausea, vomiting
- dizziness, headache, visual changes
- leucopenia
- rash, pruritus, urticaria
- reversible alopecia (hair thinning and moderate hair loss)
- fever
- transient elevation of liver enzymes
- (Rare) bone pain, proteinuria, hepatitis, pancytopenia, thrombocytopenia
- (Neurocysticercosis) headache, nausea, visual changes, neurological events (including increased intracranial pressure and convulsions) (due to death of parasite)

Interactions
- plasma levels of active metabolite may be increased by praziquantel and dexamethasone
- plasma levels of active metabolite may be decreased by ritonavir, phenytoin, carbamazepine and phenobarbital (phenobarbitone), resulting in decreased efficacy

Nursing considerations/Cautions
- patients should be followed up after 14 days to ensure infestation has been eradicated
- (Neurocysticercosis) oral/IV corticosteroids will prevent increased intracranial pressure if given during the week of treatment. Also recommended are appropriate antihistamines and/or anti-epileptics to prevent hypersensitivity reaction
- (Neurocysticercosis) second course is recommended after a 14-day drug-free interval if no response to the first course
- (Hydatid cyst) if there are no signs of cyst shrinkage (X-ray, ultrasound or CT) within 3 cycles, further improvement of cysts in the liver, lung or peritoneum are unlikely with repeated treatment; bone or brain cysts may require more prolonged treatment
- (Hydatid cyst) blood counts and liver function should be monitored before start of treatment and then 2-weekly during the 28-day cycle
- (Tapeworm) if tapeworm is due to *Hymenolepis nana* infestation, retreatment in 10—21 days is recommended
- therapy should be stopped if liver enzymes reach twice normal level. Therapy can be restarted when levels return to normal, but liver function must be regularly monitored during repeat therapy
- patients with hydatid disease should be monitored for 2 years to detect recurrent cysts
- symptoms of neurocysticercosis may be exacerbated, or neurological symptoms, such as headaches, nausea, convulsions and visual disturbances, may be precipitated

ANTHELMINTICS

- not recommended in children under 6 years of age
- caution if given to those with liver disease as there will be an increased risk of bone marrow depression
- caution if used in those with abnormal liver function
- contraindicated in those with hypersensitivity to albendazole or other benzimadizoles

Patient education

- chewable tablets can be crushed, chewed or swallowed whole
- tablets are better absorbed if taken with a fatty meal
- fever may occur in the first few days of therapy
- patients should be advised not to drive or operate machinery if they experience dizziness
- (Neurocysticercosis) patients should be warned that neurological disturbances, such as headache, nausea, visual disturbances and seizures, may occur or initially become worse
- women of childbearing years should be counselled to use adequate contraception while taking albendazole and for 4 weeks after finishing therapy to prevent pregnancy occurring. If pregnancy is suspected, patient should be advised to consult doctor immediately. Breastfeeding should also be avoided
- see also General Patient education for helminth infestation (p. 43)

Tablets are chewable and can be crushed.

Contraindicated during pregnancy. Women of childbearing age should use effective contraception while taking albendazole and for 4 weeks after treatment to prevent pregnancy. If pregnancy is suspected, consult a doctor immediately.

Breastfeeding is not advised during or within 1 month of stopping treatment.

IVERMECTIN
Trade name
Soolantra, Stromectol

Available forms
Tablets: 3 mg;
Cream: 10 mg/g (1%)

Action
- a broad spectrum avermectin antihelminthic
- inhibits signal transmission in nematodes by stimulating the release of the inhibitory neurotransmitter GABA, without affecting mammalian neurotransmission
- half-life of 12 hours, with an active metabolite half-life of 3 days
- when used topically, it is thought to have anti-inflammatory action

Use
- onchocerciasis (*Onchocerca volvulus*) (also known as river blindness)
- intestinal strongyloidiasis (*Strongyloides stercoralis*)
- crusted scabies (with topical therapy)
- human sarcoptic scabies (where topical treatment is contraindicated or has been ineffective)
- rosacea (papulopustular) in adults > 18 years

Dose
- (Strongyloidiasis) 200 microgram/kg orally as a single dose **OR**
- (Onchocerciasis) 150 microgram/kg orally as a single dose (with repeated dose after 6–12 months) **OR**
- (Sarcoptic scabies, mild crusted scabies) 200 microgram/kg orally given once on day 1 and repeated (second dose) between days 8 and 15 **OR**
- (Moderate-to-severe crusted scabies) as above with third dose **OR**
- (Rosacea) apply thin layer as 5 pea-sized amounts on forehead, chin, nose and each cheek (less than 1 g total) daily for up to 16 weeks

Adverse effects
Strongyloidiasis
- asthenia, fatigue

- anorexia, constipation, diarrhoea, nausea, vomiting, abdominal pain
- dizziness, somnolence, vertigo, tremor
- pruritus, rash, urticaria
- elevated liver enzymes, decreased leucocyte count

Onchocerciasis

- adverse effects of ivermectin in treating onchocerciasis (river blindness) are more frequent and severe owing to allergic or inflammatory responses to the parasite's death, known as the Mazzotti reaction. This occurs in at least one-third of patients, is most severe in those with a high microfilariae count and lessens with repeated courses. Symptoms include pruritus, rash, urticaria, fever, oedema, lymph node enlargement and tenderness, arthralgia and synovitis

Scabies

- exacerbation of pruritus
- headache, lethargy, listlessness, dizziness
- arthralgia
- anorexia, abdominal discomfort

Rosacea

- skin-burning sensation, skin irritation, pruritus, dry skin

Interaction

- (Oral) caution if given with warfarin as INR may be increased

Nursing considerations/Cautions

- dose interval 6–12 months depending on prevalence and/or density of skin microfilariae
- (Scabies) pregnant female mite burrows under stratum corneum, laying eggs that mature in 14 days and emerge as adults, which can then reinvade the same host or the other host. Transmission is via intimate contact with infected person or via contaminated objects. Signs of infestation include blisters, lumps and intense pruritus. Common sites include between fingers, wrists, under arms, female breasts (particularly nipples), stomach, penis, scrotum and buttocks. In children, common sites are face, scalp, palms and soles of the feet
- (Scabies) therapy should be started only when a definitive diagnosis has been made and not based solely on presence of pruritus
- (Crusted scabies) scaling (harbouring mites) can be reduced by using keratolytics (e.g. 6% salicylic acid) when not treated with topical scarbicide (e.g. permethrin) (Lyclear)
- (Rosacea) if no improvement is seen in 12 weeks, therapy should be discontinued
- (Rosacea) course can be repeated if needed
- (Cream) contains cetyl alcohol, stearyl alcohol, methyl hydroxybenzoate and propyl hydroxybenzoate, which can all cause local skin or allergic reactions
- (Cream) caution if used in those with liver or kidney impairment
- caution if used in those with liver impairment
- not recommended in children under 5 years or under 15 kg
- (Rosacea) recommended only for papulopustular rosacea and not other forms of rosacea or facial dermatoses
- (Onchocerciasis) contraindicated in African regions where *O. volvulus* is co-endemic with *Loa loa* owing to the risk of severe post-therapy encephalopathy

Patient education

- patients should be warned against driving or operating machinery if dizziness, sleepiness, fatigue, tremor or vertigo occur
- women of childbearing years should be counselled to use adequate contraception while taking ivermectin to prevent pregnancy occurring, as animal studies have shown fetal damage. If pregnancy is suspected, patient should be advised to consult doctor immediately. Breast-feeding should also be avoided
- see also General Patient education for helminth infestation (p. 43)

ANTHELMINTICS

Scabies
- personal garments, towels and bedclothes should be washed in hot water and dried in a tumble dryer for 30 minutes on hot setting
- blankets should be drycleaned or placed in tumble dryer for 30 minutes on hot setting
- shoes and non-washable items should be placed in a tightly sealed plastic bag for 3 days
- the patient should be warned that itch (pruritus) may continue for 1–2 weeks (sometimes months) after treatment has been completed and mites eliminated

Rosacea
- avoid eyes, eyelids, mouth and lips
- apply a pea-sized amount evenly to the forehead, chin, nose, and cheeks
- after it dries, use SPF 50+ sunscreen on treated areas; cosmetics can be applied afterwards
- wash hands thoroughly after application

Tablets can be dispersed in water or crushed and mixed with water, or given with a spoonful of yoghurt or apple puree.

Safety during pregnancy has not been established; animal studies have shown some fetal damage.

Recommended only if the benefits outweigh the risks. If the mother intends to breastfeed, treatment should be delayed until at least 1 week after delivery.

MEBENDAZOLE
Trade name
Combantrin-1 with Mebendazole, Combantrin-1 with Mebendazole Chocolate Squares, DeWorm, Vermox

Available forms
Tablets (chewable): 100 mg;
Chocolate squares: 100 mg/square;
Suspension: 100 mg/5 mL

Action
- thought to interfere with glucose uptake by worm cells during metabolism, resulting in death of worm

Use
- whipworm, roundworm and/or threadworm infestation, including mixed infestations
- hookworm (under medical supervision)

Dose (adults and children over 2 years)
Threadworm
- 100 mg orally (tablet or suspension) as single dose, repeated in 2–4 weeks to prevent reinfestation

Hookworm, roundworm, whipworm or mixed infestations
- 100 mg orally twice daily for 3 consecutive days. A second course may be necessary after 3 weeks, **OR**
- single 500 mg oral dose

Adverse effects
- nausea, abdominal pain, diarrhoea, vomiting (in those with large numbers of parasites)
- dizziness

Nursing considerations/Cautions
- course can be repeated after 2–4 weeks if infestation recurs
- caution if used in those with Crohn's disease or ulcerative colitis, as absorption may be increased
- caution also in those with liver impairment, as half-life may be prolonged
- contraindicated in children under 2 years

Patient education
- tablets may be chewed or swallowed whole
- shake suspension before use
- advise patient that it can take up to 3 days for dead worms to pass through body

47

- patients should be warned against driving or operating machinery if dizziness or drowsiness occurs
- women of childbearing years should be counselled to use adequate contraception while taking mebendazole. If pregnancy is suspected, patient should be advised to consult doctor immediately. Breastfeeding should also be avoided
- see also General Patient education for helminth infestation (p. 43)

 Tablets can be crushed and chewed.

 Avoid during first trimester. Safety during pregnancy has not been established and mebendazole is therefore best avoided, especially during the first trimester. Animal studies have found it to be embryotoxic and teratogenic.

 May be used; low oral absorption and unlikely excretion in milk.

PRAZIQUANTEL
Trade name
Biltricide

Available form
Tablets: 600 mg

Action
- increases permeability of worm cell membrane to calcium, resulting in paralysis and detachment
- effect is greater in adult than in immature worms
- treatment during acute phase of infection may not prevent progression to chronic phase

Use
- schistosoma infection (flukes)

Dose
- 20 mg/kg orally after food every 4 hours for 3 doses

Adverse effects
- headache, dizziness, drowsiness, somnolence, vertigo
- nausea, vomiting, abdominal pain, anorexia, diarrhoea
- malaise, asthenia, fever, fatigue
- myalgia
- urticaria, rash
- (Rare) cardiac arrhythmias, seizures, bloody diarrhoea, mild increases in liver enzymes

Interactions
- plasma levels may be increased by erythromycin and itraconazole
- plasma levels may be decreased by dexamethasone, antiepileptic agents and hydroxychloroquine
- not recommended with rifampicin
- not recommended with grapefruit juice

Nursing considerations/Cautions
- the patient may show clinical deterioration if treatment is given during acute phase of schistosomiasis when adult worms begin to produce eggs. This deterioration can include paradoxical reactions, serum sickness and Jarisch—Herxheimer-like reaction and may be life threatening
- adverse effects may occur earlier and more frequently if infestation is severe. Adverse effects are also dependent on the species present, extent and duration of infestation and location of parasites
- if the patient has cardiac irregularities, cardiac monitoring is recommended during therapy as cardiac arrhythmias may occur (although rarely)
- extra care and monitoring should occur if there is a potential for the patient to have undiagnosed neurocysticosis
- patients with known neurocysticosis should be treated in hospital setting
- tablets are triple scored to allow precise amounts to be given ($1/4$ tablet = 150 mg)
- caution if used in those with impaired kidney or liver function
- not recommended in those with epilepsy

ANTHELMINTICS

- contraindicated in those with ocular cysticosis as destruction of parasite may result in permanent damage

Patient education

- give with or immediately after food
- the tablet has an extremely bitter taste and may cause gagging or vomiting
- tablets are triple scored to allow precise amounts to be given ($^1/_4$ tablet = 150 mg) and aid in swallowing
- tablets should be swallowed whole
- may cause dizziness/drowsiness; warn patient against driving or operating machinery on day of treatment and the following 24 hours
- see also General Patient education for helminth infestation (p. 43)

Tablet may be cut into halves or quarters, but do not chew.

Safety during pregnancy has not been established.

Minimal excretion in breastmilk. It may be safe to use; however, current advice is women should not nurse on the day of treatment and during the subsequent 72 hours.

PYRANTEL

Trade name
Anthel, Combantrin Chocolate Squares, Early Bird Chocolate Squares

Available forms
Tablets: 125 mg, 250 mg;
Chocolate squares: 100 mg/square

Action

- acts at the neuromuscular junction, resulting in paralysis and immobilisation of the worm, which is then excreted in the faeces

Use

- threadworm, roundworm or hookworm infestation (ineffective against whipworm)

Dose

- 10 mg pyrantel base/kg for adults and children given in a single oral dose as tablets or chocolate squares (e.g. 70 kg adult = 7 squares)

Adverse effects

- nausea, vomiting, abdominal cramps, diarrhoea, anorexia
- dizziness, drowsiness, insomnia, headache, fatigue
- rash
- (Occasionally) elevated liver enzyme levels

Nursing considerations/Cautions

- all family or group members should be treated, even if asymptomatic
- retreatment may be required in 7–10 days if infestation recurs after initial treatment
- (Chocolate squares) dose for children and adults is based on age and weight, with 1 square = 10 kg
- contraindicated in those with acute liver disease or in children under 12 months

Patient education

- all family or group members should be treated even if asymptomatic
- may be given at any time of day, with or without food and without the need for purging
- tablets may be crushed and mixed with honey or jam for administration to young children if necessary
- see also General Patient education for helminth infestation (p. 43)

Tablets may be crushed and mixed with honey or jam for administration to young children if necessary.

Avoid during pregnancy if possible, although animal studies have not shown teratogenic effects.

Safety during breastfeeding has not been established.

ANTIALZHEIMER'S AGENTS

In 1906, Alois Alzheimer first described the brain changes that would become known as Alzheimer's disease (AD). Dementia is an umbrella term that describes a number of conditions that result in a decline in brain functioning and includes impact on memory, speech, cognition, personality, behaviour and mobility (AIHW 2024). In 2023, it was estimated that 15 people in 1000 Australians had dementia, with 63% of those being women. AD is the most common type of dementia, accounting for 50 to 75% of all dementia cases (Alzheimer's Research Australia 2024). It appears that the cholinergic system in the cortex and limbic systems (especially the hippocampus, amygdala and basal forebrain) are damaged and destroyed by structural changes, such as atrophy, neurofibrillary tangles and beta amyloid protein plaques (Rabinovici et al 2022). Risk factors for the development of AD include age (prevalence increases with each decade of adult life), female gender and a positive family history. A history of head trauma with concussion also appears to increase the risk of AD; however, the exact cause remains unknown (Rabinovici et al 2022).

AD generally progresses in three stages. During the first stage, there is an accumulation of protein plaques and tangles and it is usually asymptomatic. During the second stage, cognitive changes start to be noticeable, although not sufficient to impair daily functioning. These changes can include repeated questions, misplacing items and memory loss. In these early stages it is often put down to 'old age'. However, once these changes become noticeable and are evident on a standardised memory test, this is considered mild cognitive impairment or early symptomatic AD. With time the disease progresses to interfere with daily activities, driving, shopping and environmental changes (such as travel, hospitalisation), making these activities problematic. Language becomes impaired over time, and the person may become easily lost and confused; performing tasks that require a sequential order, solving simple puzzles or copying diagrams becomes increasing difficult. In the late stages, some people wander aimlessly, lose their ability to reason and, for some, delusions, disinhibition and belligerent behaviour become increasingly common. End stage results in the person becoming bedridden, rigid, mute, incontinent and requiring full care (Rabinovici et al 2022).

Typical duration of symptomatic AD is 8—10 years, but can range from 1 to 25 years. Death is usually related to complications related to immobility, such as pneumonia (Rabinovici et al 2022).

A number of drugs prevent the symptoms from worsening for a period of time, but to date there is no treatment that will prevent the progress of AD.

General Actions of anti-Alzheimer's agents

- loss of cholinergic neurons in the central nervous system (CNS) (especially those that input from basal forebrain to hippocampus and cerebral cortex) appear to be related to impaired memory and learning, associated with AD. Centrally acting reversible anticholinesterases (cholinesterase inhibitors) increase and prolong acetylcholine levels in the brain, thereby improving cognitive function and slowing decline in function in some (but not all) patients.

General Adverse effects of anti-Alzheimer's agents

- headache, fatigue, malaise
- bradycardia, hypertension, SA/AV heart block, syncope
- nausea, diarrhoea, vomiting, abdominal disturbance, decreased appetite, constipation
- weight loss
- urinary incontinence/frequency, nocturia
- muscle cramps, muscle weakness
- increased sweating
- insomnia, dizziness, depression, somnolence, abnormal dreams, tremor
- confusion, anxiety, agitation, aggression, hallucination
- (Rare) exacerbation or induction of extrapyramidal symptoms (especially in those with existing Parkinson's disease), seizures

General Interactions of anti-Alzheimer's agents

- caution if used with agents known to prolong QTc interval, including disopyramide, amiodarone, sotalol, citalopram, escitalopram, amitriptyline, phenothiazines, ziprasidone, clarithromycin, erythromycin, moxifloxacin, or electrolyte disturbance (hypokalaemia, hypomagnesaemia)
- may increase or prolong muscle relaxation if given with suxamethonium
- may antagonise action of anticholinergic agents
- not recommended with other cholinesterase inhibitors or cholinomimetic agents
- may increase risk of gastric bleeding or ulceration if given with NSAIDs
- caution if given with digoxin or beta adrenoreceptor blocking agents, as heart rate may be further decreased

General Nursing considerations/Cautions for anti-Alzheimer's agents

- therapy should be supervised by a doctor who is experienced in diagnosing and caring for patients with AD
- patient requires a caregiver to supervise medication administration
- any electrolyte disorder should be corrected before starting therapy

- patient should be reassessed after 4 weeks of therapy to determine its effectiveness
- if patient is taking digoxin and/or beta adrenoreceptor blocking agents concurrently, the pulse should be monitored to detect any decrease in heart rate
- not recommended in those recovering from GI surgery or with GI obstruction because cholinesterase inhibitors increase gastric acid secretion
- not recommended in those recovering from bladder surgery or with urinary outflow obstruction because of urinary tract adverse effects, including urinary frequency, nocturia and increased risk of urinary tract infection and incontinence
- caution if used in the immediate post-myocardial infarction period or in those with newly diagnosed atrial fibrillation, heart block (second degree or greater), unstable angina, congestive cardiac failure, sick sinus syndrome or supraventricular cardiac conduction disorders
- caution if used in those with gastric ulcers (or history of ulcer disease), severe asthma, seizures, active pneumonia or chronic obstructive lung disease
- AD rarely occurs during childbearing years; therefore pregnancy and breastfeeding advice has been omitted from this section

General Patient/Carer education for anti-Alzheimer's agents

- carer should be included in patient education, as the person with AD may not remember the information
- patient should be advised not to drive or operate machinery if fatigue, dizziness or somnolence occur. AD may already compromise a person's ability to drive or operate machinery safely
- carer should be advised of the high incidence of loss of appetite, nausea and vomiting at the start of therapy (usually resolves in less than a week). Carer should be advised of the importance of close monitoring of weight during therapy, and reporting any symptoms that persist. Antiemetics may be needed
- carer/patient should be instructed to ensure adequate fluid intake during therapy, especially if nausea and vomiting are problematic
- patient should be monitored for any fainting (syncope) or bradycardia (slow heart rate) as cardiac arrhythmias may occur
- advise patient (and carer) to report any:
    - severe and persistent vomiting or diarrhoea
    - weight loss
    - difficulty passing urine or more frequent urination
    - heartburn, indigestion or stomach pain
    - new or worsening agitation or aggressive behaviour or hallucinations
    - seizures
    - slowed heart rate

DONEPEZIL HYDROCHLORIDE

Trade name
APO-Donepezil, Arazil, Aricept, Aridon APN, Donepezil Sandoz, Donepezil-GH, Donepezil-WGR, Noumed Donepezil

Available forms
Tablets: 5 mg, 10 mg

Action
- reversible specific cholinesterase inhibitor
- active metabolites

ANTIALZHEIMER'S AGENTS

- very long half-life (about 70 hours)
- see also General Actions of anti-Alzheimer's agents (p. 51)

Use
- mild, moderate and severe Alzheimer's disease (AD)

Dose
- initially 5 mg orally nightly before retiring for 4 weeks, then, after at least 4 weeks, increased to 10 mg orally at night if needed (daily maximum 10 mg)

Adverse effects
- (Very rare) neuroleptic malignant syndrome (NMS)
- see also General Adverse effects of anti-Alzheimer's agents (p. 51)

Interactions
- elimination may be increased by phenytoin, phenobarbital (phenobarbitone), rifampicin, dexamethasone or carbamazepine
- may increase the effects of neuromuscular blocking agents or beta adrenoceptor blocking agents that affect cardiac conduction
- see also General Interactions of anti-Alzheimer's agents (anticholinesterases) (p. 51)

Nursing considerations/Cautions
- caution if used in those with risk of aggression as this may worsen during therapy, especially in those with severe AD
- contraindicated in those with a hypersensitivity to piperidine products
- see also General Nursing considerations/Cautions for anti-Alzheimer's agents (p. 52)

Patient/Carer education
- the patient/carer should be advised to immediately report any unexpected high fever, muscle rigidity or altered consciousness (which may be signs of NMS)
- see also General Patient/Carer education for anti-Alzheimer's agents (p. 52)

Tablet can be dispersed in water, or crushed and mixed with water or spoonful of yoghurt or apple puree.

GALANTAMINE
Trade name
APO-Galantamine MR , Galantyl, Gamine XR, Reminyl

Available forms
Capsules (prolonged/modified-release): 8 mg, 16 mg, 24 mg

Action
- reversible cholinesterase inhibitor
- also enhances acetylcholine action on nicotinic receptors (stimulation of nicotinic receptors is thought to improve cognitive function and be neuroprotective against amyloid-induced neurotoxicity)
- active metabolites
- half-life 7—8 hours
- see also General Actions of anti-Alzheimer's agents (p. 51)

Use
- mild-to-moderately severe Alzheimer's disease (AD)

Dose
- initially 8 mg orally daily with meals for 4 weeks, increasing to 16 mg daily for at least 4 weeks, increasing further to 24 mg daily if needed

Adverse effects
- (Rare) serious skin reaction
- see also General Adverse effects of anti-Alzheimer's agents (p. 51)

Interactions
- bioavailability may increase if given with erythromycin, paroxetine, fluoxetine or fluvoxamine, increasing risk of cholinergic side-effects, including nausea and vomiting

- see also General Interactions of anti-Alzheimer's agents (p. 51)

Nursing considerations/Cautions

- use for other types of dementia or memory impairment has not been proven
- if therapy is stopped for more than 2 days, it should be restarted at lowest dose and gradually increased
- increasing dose slowly should decrease side-effects
- contraindicated in those with severe liver or kidney impairment
- see also General Nursing considerations/Cautions for anti-Alzheimer's agents (p. 52)

Patient/Carer education

- prolonged-release capsules should be swallowed whole, not crushed or chewed. Capsules should not be opened
- advise the patient/carer to immediately report any skin rash
- see also General Patient/Carer education for anti-Alzheimer's agents (p. 52)

Prolonged-release capsules should be swallowed whole, not crushed or chewed. Capsules should not be opened.

For those with moderate liver impairment, initial dose should be 8 mg orally every second day for at least 7 days, then dose increased to 8 mg orally daily for at least 4 weeks (daily maximum 16 mg). Contraindicated in those with severe liver impairment (Child—Pugh score > 9) or severe kidney impairment CrCl < 9 mL/min).

MEMANTINE HYDROCHLORIDE
Trade name
APO-Memantine, Ebixa, Memantine Generichealth, Memanxa

Available forms
Tablets: 10 mg, 20 mg

Action
- *N*-methyl-D-aspartate (NMDA) receptor antagonist (it is thought that malfunctioning glutamatergic neurotransmission and especially NMDA receptors may be responsible for neuronal degeneration in dementia)
- protects against chronically raised levels of glutamate in the brain
- metabolites are not active
- half-life 60—100 hours

Use
- moderately severe-to-severe Alzheimer's disease (AD)

Dose
- initially 5 mg orally daily for 1 week, then 10 mg daily for 1 week, then 15 mg daily (given as a 10 mg and 5 mg dose) for 1 week, then 20 mg daily as maintenance

Adverse effects
- peripheral oedema
- constipation, faecal incontinence
- abnormal gait, increased falls risk
- conjunctivitis
- coughing, bronchitis, pneumonia
- urinary incontinence, urinary tract infection
- (rare) cataract formation
- see also General Adverse effects for anti-Alzheimer's agents (p. 51)

Interactions
- not recommended with other NMDA receptor antagonists (e.g. ketamine, amantadine, dextromethorphan)
- may potentiate effects of levodopa, bromocriptine, amantadine or anticholinergics
- caution if given with barbiturates, antipsychotics, antiepileptics, dantrolene or baclofen
- increased levels may occur if given with cimetidine, ranitidine, quinine and nicotine

ANTIALZHEIMER'S AGENTS

Nursing considerations/Cautions

- caution if used in those with recent myocardial infarction, congestive heart failure or uncontrolled hypertension
- caution if used in those with predisposing factors for seizures or epilepsy
- not recommended in those with severe liver impairment
- 10 mg tablets contain lactose and are therefore not recommended in those with rare hereditary problems of galactose intolerance, Lapp lactase deficiency or glucose/galactose malabsorption
- contraindicated in those with epilepsy (or other seizure disorders)
- see also General Nursing considerations/Cautions for anti-Alzheimer's agents (p. 52)

Patient/Carer education

- patients/caregiver should be advised about factors that may increase urinary pH and therefore affect the elimination of memantine (e.g. change to vegetarian diet, severe urinary tract infection)
- instruct patient/carer that the tablet should be taken at the same time every day
- see also General Patient/Carer education for anti-Alzheimer's agents (p. 52)

Tablet can be dispersed in water or crushed and mixed with water or spoonful of yoghurt or apple puree

For those with moderate kidney impairment (CrCl 30—49 mL/min), dose should be 10 mg daily, and after at least 7 days, if tolerated, dose increased to 20 mg daily, titrating slowly as per dosing schedule above. If kidney impairment is severe (5—29 mL/min) dose recommended is 10 mg daily.
Not recommended in those with severe liver impairment

RIVASTIGMINE
Trade name
Exelon, Exelon Patch

Available forms
Capsules: 1.5 mg, 3 mg, 4.5 mg, 6 mg; Transdermal patch: 5 (releases 4.6 mg/24 hours), 10 (releases 9.5 mg/24 hours), 15 (releases 13.3 mg/24 hours)

Action
- 'pseudo-reversible' selective cholinesterase inhibitor
- half-life about 1 hour, duration of action 9 hours
- see also General Actions of anti-Alzheimer's agents (p. 51)

Use
- mild-to-moderately severe Alzheimer's disease (AD)

Dose
- initially 1.5 mg orally twice daily with food, increasing dose gradually every 2—4 weeks to a maximum of 6 mg twice daily if necessary, then 1.5—6 mg orally twice daily as maintenance **OR**
- initially 4.6 mg/24-hour patch applied daily for minimum of 4 weeks. If tolerated, dose is increased to 9.5 mg/24-hour patch. In moderate-to-severe AD, if well tolerated after a minimum of 4 weeks, dose can be increased to 13.3 mg/24-hour patch (transdermal patch)

Adverse effects
- (Transdermal patch) erythema, pruritus, urticaria, blister formation, (rare) allergic contact dermatitis
- see also General Adverse effects of anti-Alzheimer's agents (p. 51)

Interactions
- clearance may be increased by smoking
- not recommended with metoclopramide because of increased risk of extrapyramidal symptoms

- see also General Interactions of anti-Alzheimer's agents (p. 51)

Nursing considerations/Cautions

- if therapy is stopped for more than 3 days, it should be restarted at the lowest dose
- if adverse effects such as nausea, vomiting and abdominal pain persist, dose should be reduced to previously tolerated level
- (Switching from capsules to transdermal patch) total oral daily dose 3—6 mg, switch to 4.6 mg/24-hour patch. If well tolerated after 4 weeks, dose can be increased to 9.5 mg/24-hour patch daily. If daily oral dose is 9—12 mg, switch to 9.5 mg/24-hour patch daily. If daily oral dose is 9 mg but not well tolerated, switch to 4.6 mg/24-hour patch daily and increase to 9.5 mg/24-hour patch if well tolerated after 4 weeks. First patch should be applied the day following the last oral dose
- if allergic contact dermatitis is suspected, allergy testing is recommended and patient not switched to oral formulation unless allergy testing is negative. Some patients may become sensitive to rivastigmine, resulting in them being unable to take rivastigmine in any form
- caution if used in those with very low body weight, as adverse effects may be more pronounced
- contraindicated in those with severe liver disease or with hypersensitivity to carbamates
- (Transdermal patch) contraindicated if allergic contact dermatitis has previously occurred
- see also General Nursing considerations/Cautions for anti-Alzheimer's agents (p. 52)

Patient/Carer education

- if therapy is interrupted for 3 days or more, advice should be sought from doctor before giving next dose
- capsules should be swallowed whole
- ensure the patient (and carer) understands application instructions regarding transdermal patches, including:
  - ensuring previous day's patch has been removed before applying new one (to avoid overdose)
  - only one patch should be worn at a time; it is advisable to date patch
  - if a patch falls off, a new patch should be applied to same site for the remainder of 24-hour period
  - should be applied once daily to dry, clean, intact, hairless skin
  - any reddened, irritated or broken skin areas should be avoided
  - application sites include upper and lower back, upper arm and chest, and should be rotated
  - areas that may be rubbed by tight clothing should be avoided
  - press transdermal patch firmly onto skin for at least 30 seconds until sides stick well
  - bathing normally
  - patch should not be cut into pieces
  - it is important to safely dispose of used patches (fold adhesive sides together)
- the patient (and carer) should be advised to immediately report any increasing redness at the patch application site, especially if it extends beyond the patch size, if there is any swelling, papules or vesicles present, or if there is no improvement in skin condition 48 hours after patch removal
- if switching from oral to patch, the first patch should be applied on the day following the last oral dose

ANTIALZHEIMER'S AGENTS

- (Patch) if skin reaction extends beyond patch size, with increasing redness, swelling and vesicle formation, patch should be removed and medical advice sought if symptoms do not improve within 48 hours of patch removal
- see also General Patient/Carer education for anti-Alzheimer's agents (p. 52)

 Capsule can be opened and contents dispersed in water, or sprinkled on spoonful of yoghurt or apple puree.

ANTIANGINAL AGENTS

Coronary artery disease is caused by an imbalance in the heart between myocardial oxygen demand and supply. Atherosclerosis causes a narrowing of the arteries due to an accumulation of plaques in the arteries, resulting in blood-flow obstruction, which is particularly evident when there is an increased demand during activity, resulting in myocardial ischaemia. Angina pectoris is a condition where myocardial blood flow is temporarily reduced, resulting in transient myocardial ischaemia. It is characterised by chest pain or discomfort described as heaviness, pressure, choking or squeezing and rarely flank pain. It can radiate to either shoulders, both arms, jaw, neck, teeth and epigastrium. However, symptoms may be atypical in women or those with diabetes (Antman & Loscalzo 2019; Knights et al 2023).

Angina may be subdivided into stable angina, unstable angina and variant (Prinzmetal's) angina. *Chronic stable angina* is precipitated by a known cause (e.g. exercise, heavy meal, exposure to the cold, emotional stress) and eased by rest and nitrate treatment. *Unstable angina* has symptoms that are intermediate, between those of stable angina and myocardial infarction; that is, previously stable angina occurs more frequently, lasts longer, is of greater intensity and/or nitrate treatment is no longer as effective. The coronary artery/arteries have become so occluded that they can no longer meet the heart's oxygen demand, increasing the person's risk of myocardial infarction especially if angina occurs at rest. *Variant* (*Prinzmetal's* or *vasospastic*) *angina* is caused by coronary artery spasm, which may or may not be related to atherosclerosis. This type of angina often occurs at rest and usually during the night or in the early hours of the day with chest discomfort that is more severe than with stable angina. In some people, it is related to the atherosclerotic lesion being near the site of the spasm. Prolonged vasospasm may lead to heart block, ventricular arrhythmias or death (Jameson et al 2020; Katzung 2018).

The main aims of antianginal treatment are to manage the acute pain and prevent further attacks by improving perfusion (by relaxing the smooth muscle of the coronary artery) or by reducing the metabolic demand on the heart, or both (Knights et al 2023). However, the antianginal agents treat the symptoms not the cause of the problem. The main pharmacological agents used to treat angina include the organic nitrates (glyceryl trinitrate, isosorbide dinitrate and isosorbide mononitrate) and calcium-channel blockers (verapamil, diltiazem and amlodipine) (see Antihypertensive agents, p. 499).

General Patient education for anti-anginal agents

- understand the importance of lifestyle modifications (e.g. diet, exercise, weight reduction and smoking cessation), managing risk factors like BP, cholesterol and diabetes control, as well as treating sleep apnoea, are crucial for controlling chronic stable angina
- tell your healthcare professional if angina attacks continue or become more frequent despite taking your medication as prescribed
- avoid driving or operating machinery if you experience dizziness or lightheadedness
- instruct patient to take care when first taking medication, not to overdo physical activities and to be especially careful when standing up or getting out of bed, as dizziness, lightheadedness or fainting can occur
- understand the difference between medications for acute angina attacks and those designed to reduce attack frequency
- generally avoid alcohol, as it can increase dizziness and faintness
- ensure you have a sufficient supply of your medication, especially over weekends or during holidays

NITRATES

GLYCERYL TRINITRATE (GTN)
Trade names
DBL Glyceryl Trinitrate Concentrate Injection, Minitran, Nitrolingual Pump Spray, Nitrostat, Transiderm-Nitro

Available forms
Metered dose pump spray: 400 microgram/dose;
Transdermal patch: 5 mg/24 hours, 10 mg/24 hours, 15 mg/24 hours;
Ampoules: 1 mg/mL, 5 mg/mL;
Sublingual tablets: 300 microgram

Action
- organic nitrate relaxes smooth muscle, including vascular muscle, causing vasodilation of peripheral arteries and veins. At low doses the effect is venodilation, whereas arterial dilation occurs at higher doses
- decreases cardiac output and arterial pressure, which results in decreased oxygen demand on the myocardium
- also dilates normal coronary and coronary collateral vessels, increasing perfusion and oxygen delivery to ensure efficient distribution to ischaemic areas of the heart
- does not change contractility or heart rate
- may relieve variant angina by relaxing coronary arteries that are in spasm
- (Sublingual spray and sublingual tablets) onset of action 2–4 minutes, duration less than 60 minutes
- sublingual spray and tablets are absorbed rapidly from the oral mucosa, bypassing the liver to reach the vascular system
- (Transdermal) onset of action greater than 4 hours, duration 8–24 hours
- transdermally, the drug is continuously absorbed through the skin and reaches target organs before being inactivated by the liver
- (IV) onset of action 1–2 minutes, duration 3–5 minutes (although this is dependent on duration of infusion)

Use
- prophylaxis and treatment of angina pectoris (symptom preventer (transdermal patch) and reliever (sublingual tablets and spray, IV))
- (IV) angina pectoris refractory to other treatments, left ventricular failure or congestive heart failure associated with acute myocardial infarction, or control of perioperative hypertension associated with surgical procedures, to produce controlled hypotension during neurosurgery and orthopaedic surgery

Dose
Treatment of acute attack
- (Sublingual spray) (therapeutic) 1 spray (400 micrograms) under the tongue from a metered dose aerosol at the first sign of an attack, followed by a second spray if pain is not relieved within 5 minutes **OR**
- (IV infusion) initially 5 microgram/min (if using a non-adsorbing set), increasing by 5 microgram/min every 3—5 minutes until response is noted; maintain adequate systemic BP and coronary perfusion pressure. If no response at 20 microgram/min, increases of 10 microgram/min can be made. Once a partial BP response is seen, the dose should be decreased and the interval between doses lengthened

Prophylaxis
- (Sublingual spray) (prophylactic) 1—2 sprays (400—800 micrograms) under the tongue from a metered dose aerosol before engaging in activities known to cause an attack **OR**
- (Transdermal patch) initially patch releasing 5 mg/24 hours is applied once daily and left in situ for 12 hours (dose can then be titrated according to clinical response)

Adverse effects
- throbbing headache (requires dose reduction)
- flushing of the face and neck
- tachycardia, dizziness, restlessness
- orthostatic hypotension, syncope
- nausea, vomiting
- (Rare) bradycardia, rash, blurred vision, dry mouth, severe/prolonged headache, methaemoglobinaemia
- tolerance, cross-tolerance to other nitrates/nitrites
- (Abrupt withdrawal) angina, exacerbation of Raynaud's disease/syndrome (in susceptible people) (see Glossary)
- (Transdermal patch/pad) skin irritation, erythema, pruritus, burning sensation, sensitisation phenomena
- (IV) bradycardia, hypotension retrosternal discomfort, abdominal pain, apprehension, restlessness, muscle twitching, alcohol intoxication, hyperosmolarity, nausea, vomiting, dizziness

Interactions
- contraindicated with phosphodiesterase-5 (PDE-5) inhibitors (sildenafil or tadalafil)
- increased risk of orthostatic hypotension and syncope if used with alcohol, calcium-channel blockers, antihypertensive agents, hydralazine, levodopa, opioid analgesics, phenothiazines, prazosin, minoxidil, antipsychotics or TCAs
- effect may be decreased if given with aspirin and other NSAIDs, levodopa, opioid analgesics or hydralazine
- ergot alkaloids may antagonise effects leading to coronary vasoconstriction
- antianginal effects may be reduced by sympathomimetic agents
- hypotension may occur if given with sympathomimetic agents
- may potentiate anticholinergic effects of TCAs
- may decrease effects of heparin
- (IV) may slow morphine metabolism, increasing the risk of overdose and respiratory depression
- may decrease the effect of noradrenaline (norepinephrine)
- (IV) increases neuromuscular blockade induced by pancuronium

ANTIANGINAL AGENTS

- may cause false result on serum cholesterol test (Zlatkis Zak colour reaction)
- may give falsely elevated serum triglyceride results

Nursing considerations/Cautions

- any hypovolaemia should be corrected before starting therapy to decrease risk of hypotension
- tolerance may occur, although less likely with intermittent therapy
- withdrawal should be gradual, reducing dose over 4–6 weeks to prevent withdrawal reaction
- patient may sit or lie down for 10–20 minutes after taking tablets to avoid dizziness
- (Transdermal patch) if there are any signs of hypotension or collapse, remove the transdermal patch and place the patient in a recumbent position with legs raised
- (Transdermal patch) should be removed before cardioversion, DC defibrillation or diathermy to prevent burning
- (IV) continuously monitor heart rate, blood pressure, pulmonary capillary wedge pressure and chest pain, especially at the start of infusion and after a dose increase
- (IV) significant amounts of glyceryl trinitrate are adsorbed by PVC plastics, so dilute and store in glass parenteral solution bottles only and avoid using filters
- (IV) greatest adsorption by PVC occurs when the concentration of glyceryl trinitrate is high, the rate is low and the tubing is long
- (IV) if using a peristaltic action pump, follow the manufacturer's instructions closely, especially if non-adsorbing (non-PVC) tubing is used, as it is less pliable
- (IV) check the administration set for compatibility with the IV infusion solution and that it is recommended for use
- (IV) line should be flushed or replaced if the concentration of solution is altered
- (IV) dosage must be carefully titrated to prevent profound fall in BP
- (IV) must be further diluted before infusing by adding 50 mg (10 mL) ampoule to 490 mL of either glucose 5% or sodium chloride 0.9% to make a concentration of 100 microgram/mL; invert prepared solution several times for uniform dilution
- (IV) administer alone
- (IV) solution diluted with sodium chloride 0.9% or dextrose 5% is stable
- (IV) not given by direct IV injection
- caution if used in industrial workers who may have had long-term high-dose exposure to organic nitrates as tolerance may occur
- cross-tolerance with organic nitrates or nitrites may occur
- increased risk of methaemoglobinaemia if used in those with impaired liver function or if given in high doses
- abrupt withdrawal may precipitate angina and also Raynaud's phenomenon in those who are susceptible
- caution if used in those with increased intraocular pressure (glaucoma), impaired liver function, recent head trauma, lung disease, cor pulmonale, anaemia, hyperthyroidism, hypothyroidism, hypothermia, hypoxaemia, ventilation perfusion imbalance, malnutrition, cerebral vascular disease or severe coronary atherosclerosis
- not recommended within 24 hours of myocardial infarction as severe arterial hypotension with bradycardia may occur
- contraindicated in severe hypotension (systolic BP < 90 mmHg), marked anaemia, uncorrected hypovolaemia, hypertrophic obstructive cardiomyopathy, cardiogenic shock, arterial hypoxaemia, cerebral haemorrhage or raised intracranial pressure caused by head trauma, constrictive pericarditis and pericardial tamponade, cardiogenic shock, primary pulmonary hypertension, obstructive myocardial failure (including aortic or mitral valve stenosis), acute

- circulatory failure or hypersensitivity to nitrates
- (Transdermal patch) contraindicated in those with allergy to adhesive

Patient education

- see General Patient education for anti-anginal agents (p. 59)

Sublingual spray

- priming the spray pump:
  - press the nozzle 5 times before first use
  - prime with 1 spray if unused for 7 days
  - prime with up to 5 sprays if unused for 4 months or longer, until even spray
- using the spray pump:
  - at the onset of an angina attack, spray under the tongue (sublingual) while preferably sitting down
  - hold the canister vertical with the nozzle uppermost and close to your mouth
  - the spray should be applied under your tongue or onto the oral mucosa, and close your mouth immediately after each dose
  - do not inhale the spray
  - avoid swallowing immediately after spraying to ensure the medication is absorbed effectively
- replace plastic cap after use
- if the pain persists after 2 doses, call an ambulance immediately
- store the canister in a cool, dry place below 20°C
- if you experience side effects such as headaches or dizziness, sit or lie down until they pass

Transdermal patch

- GTN patches are for long-term management, not for immediate relief of angina attacks
- (Nitrate-free period) allow a 12-hour patch-free period daily (usually at night) to prevent tolerance. Be aware that some patients may experience nocturnal angina
- patch application:
  - remove old patch before applying a new one. Temporary redness or warmth is normal
  - clean and dry skin thoroughly before applying the patch; avoid creams, lotions and oils
  - apply to hairless areas like the chest or inner arm; avoid scars, irritated skin and areas prone to movement or sweating
  - do not cut or trim the patch
  - if the patch loosens or falls off, apply a new one
- apply once daily. If forgotten, apply as soon as you remember, but don't use two patches simultaneously
- you can bathe or shower with the patch on
- rotate application sites to prevent skin irritation
- handling:
  - wash hands before and after applying
  - dispose of used patches properly, as they still contain medication
  - keep patches out of reach of children
  - storage: store in a cool, dry place, avoiding extreme temperatures. Do not refrigerate

Limited data in pregnancy, but it is generally considered safe. GTN has been used for uterine relaxation in some cases. Recommended during pregnancy if benefits are thought to outweigh risks.

No human data available.

Note

- glyceryl trinitrate is also available as a topical rectal agent (Rectogesic) used for treatment of anal fissure and post-haemorrhoidectomy

ISOSORBIDE DINITRATE

Trade name
Isordil

Available form
Tablet: 5 mg (sublingual)

Action
- exogenous source of nitric oxide
- see also isosorbide mononitrate (p. 63)

Use
- prevent and treat angina and myocardial ischaemia by improving blood flow and reducing myocardial oxygen demand
- manage acute and chronic left ventricular failure by reducing preload and afterload, which improves cardiac performance and stabilises patients, especially in congestive heart failure (rarely used for this indication)

Dose
- (Treatment of acute angina; rapid relief of chest pain) sublingual, 5—10 mg
- (Prophylaxis; prevention of acute angina before activity) sublingual, 5—10 mg taken 10 minutes before activity expected to cause angina

Adverse effects/Interactions/Nursing considerations/Cautions/Patient education
- see Isosorbide mononitrate adverse effects/interactions/Nursing consideration/Cautions/Patient education

Safety of isosorbide dinitrate during pregnancy has not been established. It should be used only if the clinical benefits outweigh the potential risks.

Unknown if excreted in breastmilk; not recommended for nursing mothers unless benefits outweigh risks.

ISOSORBIDE MONONITRATE

Trade names
APO-Isosorbide Mononitrate, Duride, Imdur, Isobide MR, Isosorbide MR-WGR, Monodur

Available forms
Tablets (sustained-release): 60 mg, 120 mg

Action
- organic nitrate; exogenous source of nitric oxide
- see isosorbide mononitrate
- isosorbide mononitrate is an active metabolite of isosorbide dinitrate
- relaxes vascular smooth muscle, producing arterial dilation and vasodilation
- may redistribute coronary blood flow, selectively dilating coronary or coronary collateral vessels, increasing perfusion and oxygen delivery, ensuring efficient distribution to ischaemic areas of heart
- reduces myocardial oxygen demand
- slower onset of action but longer duration than glyceryl trinitrate
- (Controlled-release tablets) onset of action within 1—2 hours, duration up to 24 hours
- half-life is biphasic (first phase 1.1 hours, second phase 7.7 hours)

Use
- prophylaxis of angina

Dose

Prophylactic treatment of angina pectoris, myocardial ischaemia
- initially 30—60 mg orally daily increasing to 120 mg if needed (sustained-release tablets)

Adverse effects
- headache, flushing of face
- vertigo, fainting
- dizziness
- postural hypotension, tachycardia, peripheral oedema
- nausea, vomiting, diarrhoea, dyspepsia, poor appetite, gastrointestinal disturbance,
- sleep disturbances, tiredness
- rash, pruritus
- (Abrupt withdrawal) increased frequency of angina tolerance
- (Uncommon) haemolytic anaemia (in those with glucose-6-phosphate dehydrogenase (G6PD))

Interactions
- contraindicated with phosphodiesterase type 5 (PDE-5) inhibitors (sildenafil or tadalafil)

- increased risk of hypotension if given with TCAs, anticholinergics, phenothiazines or antihypertensive agents, including calcium-channel blocker
- alcohol may increase vasodilation, leading to hypotension
- effect may be decreased if given with aspirin and other NSAIDs, levodopa, opioid analgesics or hydralazine
- (Sustained-release) action may be enhanced if given with methionine, captopril or acetylcysteine, including risk of hypotension
- caution if used with propranolol in those with cirrhosis and portal hypertension
- improved left ventricular function may occur if the SR preparation is given with verapamil-like calcium-channel blockers

Nursing considerations/Cautions

- any hypovolaemia should be corrected before starting therapy
- sustained-release (SR) preparations are recommended only for stable chronic angina (not variant angina or management of acute angina)
- ensure that the correct tablet is administered via the correct route (i.e. some brands have formulations that are sublingual, immediate-release or sustained-release)
- if headache occurs, dose may be reduced
- caution if used in industrial workers who may have had long-term high-dose exposure to organic nitrates as tolerance may occur
- cross-tolerance between organic nitrates or nitrites may occur
- tolerance may be prevented by having a 10–12-hour nitrate-free period in every 24 hours
- withdrawal should be gradual over 2 weeks to prevent increase in the frequency of angina
- (Cardiac failure) pulmonary capillary pressure should not be allowed to fall below 15 mmHg or systolic BP below physiological range for normal or hypertensive patients. If a patient has pre-existing hypotension, range should be 90–100 mmHg
- caution if used in those with G6PD as haemolytic anaemia may occur
- caution if used in patients with hypoxia
- caution if used in those with kidney impairment as accumulation of active metabolite may occur
- caution if given to those with severe coronary or cerebral arteriosclerosis, or pronounced mitral stenosis
- not recommended in those with acute myocardial infarction or congestive cardiac failure
- contraindicated in those with hypersensitivity to nitrates, cardiogenic shock, hypotension, obstructive hypertrophic cardiomyopathy, constrictive pericardial tamponade or pericarditis, isolated right ventricular failure, uncorrected hypovolaemia, severe anaemia, intracranial hypertension or arterial hypoxaemia

Patient education

- may cause dizziness when standing. To minimise this effect, rise gradually from sitting or lying positions. Sit or lie down if you feel dizzy
- isosorbide mononitrate is not suitable for treating acute angina attacks because of its slow onset of action
- take your medication at the time of day when angina is most frequent (e.g. at night for nocturnal angina or in the morning for daytime angina)
- twice-daily dosing is not recommended owing to the risk of developing tolerance from the lack of a nitrate-free interval
- sustained-release tablets should not be crushed, broken or chewed; however, 60 mg SR preparations (but NOT 120 mg SR preparations) are scored and may be halved without altering properties if not crushed during the splitting process
- see also General Patient education for antianginal agents (p. 59)

ANTIANGINAL AGENTS

 Sustained-release tablets should not be crushed; swallow whole.

 Safety during pregnancy has not been established, so not recommended unless the expected benefit outweighs any potential risk.

 Safety has not been established, so not recommended unless the expected benefit outweighs any potential risk.

OTHER ANTIANGINAL DRUGS

IVABRADINE
Trade names
APO-Ivabradine, Coralan, Ivabradine-WGR

Available forms
Tablets: 5 mg, 7.5 mg

Action
- selective I_f channel inhibitor that slows heart rate (by about 10 beats/min) by selectively inhibiting cardiac pacemaker in the sinus node, reducing cardiac workload and therefore myocardial oxygen consumption
- may also interact with retinal current I_h which resembles cardiac I_f resulting in visual adverse effects
- no effect on intra-atrial, AV or intraventricular conduction times, myocardial contractility or ventricular repolarisation
- half-life about 11 hours

Use
- chronic stable angina (in those with normal sinus rhythm who cannot take beta adrenergic blocking agents such as atenolol when heart rate is $\geq$ 70 beats/min but angina is not controlled)
- chronic heart failure (with left ventricular injection fraction $\leq$ 35%, sinus rhythm and HR $\geq$ 77 beats/min)

Dose
- (Angina) initially 5 mg orally twice daily with meals, increasing after 3—4 weeks depending on HR and response (alone or with atenolol 50 mg) **OR**
- (Chronic heart failure) initially 5 mg orally twice daily with meals, increasing/decreasing dose after 2 weeks (depending on HR)

Adverse effects
- blurred vision, transient luminous phenomena (transient enhanced brightness in a limited area of the visual field triggered by sudden variations in light intensity, halo, stroboscopic effects, coloured bright lights, multiple images)
- bradycardia, ventricular extrasystole, tachycardia, AV first-degree block, unstable or aggravated angina, cardiac failure, atrial fibrillation, inadequate BP control
- headache, dizziness
- (Uncommon) prolonged QT interval

Interactions
- contraindicated with itraconazole, clarithromycin, macrolide antibiotics, ciclosporin, gestodene and antiretroviral agents
- contraindicated with calcium-channel blockers such as diltiazem or verapamil, as further heart rate lowering may occur
- not recommended with agents that prolong QT interval (e.g. disopyramide, sotalol, amiodarone, TCAs, antipsychotic agents, IV erythromycin, pentamidine, mefloquine) or agents that cause hypokalaemia (e.g. diuretics, stimulant laxatives, corticosteroids, amphotericin B (amphotericin))
- should not be taken with grapefruit or grapefruit juice as increased serum levels may occur
- metabolism may be increased if given with rifampicin, barbiturates, phenytoin or St John's wort requiring a dose adjustment
- bioavailability may be reduced if given with carbamazepine

Nursing considerations/Cautions
- any heart failure should be stabilised before starting therapy

- serial HR, ECG or ambulatory BP monitoring is recommended before starting or titrating therapy
- therapy should not be started if resting HR < 70 beats/min
- dose titration is according to resting HR:
  - if persistently ≥ 60 beats/min (still symptomatic, initial dose well tolerated), dose should be increased to 7.5 mg
  - if 50–60 beats/min, dose should be maintained
  - if < 50 beats/min rest or patient has symptoms of bradycardia (e.g. dizziness, fatigue, hypotension), dose should be reduced (minimum daily dose 2.5 mg). If bradycardia or heart rate continues below 50 bpm, therapy should be stopped
- transient luminous phenomena usually occur in the first 8 weeks of therapy and last about 12 weeks
- (Angina) if there is no response and angina continues after 12 weeks, therapy should be stopped
- caution in those with aortic stenosis, second-degree heart block, hypertrophic cardiomyopathy, mild-to-moderate hypotension, heart failure, asymptomatic left ventricular dysfunction, end-stage renal failure, moderate liver impairment or retinitis pigmentosa
- not recommended in those with atrial fibrillation or other cardiac arrhythmias that interfere with sinus node function, immediately after stroke or surgery (cardiac or non-cardiac) or QT prolongation (if used, cardiac monitoring is strongly recommended)
- contraindicated in those with galactose intolerance, Lapp lactase deficiency or glucose–galactose malabsorption as tablets contain lactose
- contraindicated in those with artificial pacemaker or sick sinus syndrome, third-degree AV block, unstable or acute heart failure, resting heart rate less than 70 beats/min, severe hypotension (less than 90/50), unstable angina, cardiogenic shock, acute myocardial infarction, sinoatrial block, severe liver impairment or hypertrophic cardiomyopathy (unless co-existing coronary artery disease is proven)

Patient education

- this medication is not to be used in the event of an acute angina attack
- best absorbed with food
- let your health professional know immediately if you experience:
  - fatigue or dizziness (signs of bradycardia)
  - sudden changes in vision, including blurred vision, halo, coloured flashes, multiple/distorted images or bright spots of light (especially when moving quickly between dim and bright light)
  - palpitations or abnormal heartbeat
- blurry vision and seeing bright areas, especially with sudden changes in light, may occur, mostly in the first two months. If affected, avoid driving, particularly at night
- avoid grapefruit and grapefruit juice during therapy
- see also General Patient education for antianginal agents (p. 59)

Tablet does not disperse easily, but can be crushed to fine powder and mixed with spoonful of yoghurt or apple puree.

Contraindicated in pregnancy; limited human data, teratogenic in animal studies; female patients of childbearing potential should be counselled to use adequate contraception during therapy to avoid pregnancy.

Contraindicated during breastfeeding; no available human data

NICORANDIL
Trade names
APO-Nicorandil, Ikotab

Available forms
Tablets: 10 mg, 20 mg

ANTIANGINAL AGENTS

Action
- nitrate properties
- opens ATP-dependent potassium channels in blood vessels, leading to arterial dilation and reduced myocardial afterload
- relaxes vascular smooth muscle, improves blood flow and oxygenation
- reduces coronary artery spasm
- rapidly absorbed with biphasic half-life (first phase about 1 hour, second phase 8—24 hours)

Use
- prevention and treatment of stable angina

Dose
- initially 5—10 mg orally twice daily, increasing to 10—20 mg twice daily if needed

Adverse effects
- headache, dizziness, vertigo, weakness, lethargy
- infection
- vasodilation/flush, palpitations, hypertension, chest pain, angina
- dyspepsia, nausea, vomiting, abdominal pain, weight loss
- myalgia, back pain
- dyspnoea, bronchitis, respiratory disorder
- hyperkalaemia
- (Uncommon) ulceration (skin, gastrointestinal, mucosal, corneal, conjunctival)
- (Rare) gastrointestinal bleeding, tinnitus, hepatitis, jaundice
- (High dose) hypotension

Interactions
- contraindicated with PDE-5 inhibitors (sildenafil, avanafil or tadalafil)
- increased risk of gastric ulceration or gastrointestinal perforation if given with corticosteroids, NSAIDs or aspirin
- caution if given with nitrates owing to risk of additive hypotension occurring
- caution if given with other agents causing hyperkalaemia
- caution if given with antihypertensive agents
- caution if given with tricyclic antidepressants (TCAs)

Nursing considerations/Cautions
- risk of headache may be decreased by starting at a low dose; or if headache is severe the dosage is reduced
- caution in patients with low blood volume, low systolic BP (below 100 mmHg) or liver impairment
- caution if used in those with diverticular disease owing to increased risk of fistula formation or bowel perforation
- contraindicated in those with cardiogenic shock, hypotension, acute myocardial infarction with left ventricular failure (with low filling pressure and hypovolaemia) or hypersensitivity to nicotinamide or nicotinic acid

Patient education
- may cause dizziness; avoid driving or operating machinery if affected
- headaches are common when starting nicorandil but usually improve with continued use; if the headache persists or worsens, seek medical advice
- report immediately if you experience any of the following:
  - skin ulcers or ulcers in the mouth, genital, or anal areas
  - ringing in the ears
  - dark or bloody stools, or bloody diarrhoea
- nicorandil is not for treating acute angina attacks. Always have your emergency angina medication available for sudden chest pain
- see also General Patient education for antianginal agents (p. 59)

Tablet can be dispersed in water (6 minutes), or crushed and mixed with spoonful of yoghurt or apple puree.

Safety during pregnancy has not been established, therefore not recommended unless the expected benefit outweighs any potential risk.

Safety during breastfeeding has not been established, therefore not recommended unless the expected benefit outweighs any potential risk.

PERHEXILINE
Trade names
Pexsig

Available form
Tablets: 100 mg

Action
- non-selective calcium-channel blocker
- appears to increase glucose utilisation, thereby decreasing oxygen demand and increasing myocardial efficiency
- reduces exercise-induced tachycardia, but does not affect resting heart rate
- mild diuretic properties
- half-life 2—6 days, but is variable (up to 30 days)
- narrow therapeutic index

Use
- reduce frequency of moderate-to-severe angina attacks resistant to conventional treatment and not suitable for coronary bypass surgery

Dose
- initially 100 mg orally daily, then adjust dose up or down at 2—4-week intervals depending on response and plasma levels (daily maximum 300—400 mg)
- therapeutic range 0.15—0.6 mg/L (0.5—2 micromol/L); concentration monitoring required.

Adverse effects
Short term (within 24 hours)
- anorexia, nausea, vomiting, weight loss
- transient dizziness, headache, gait disorders, unsteadiness, drunken sensation
- hypoglycaemia (patients with diabetes)

Long term (≥ 12 weeks of continuous therapy)
- cirrhosis, hepatotoxicity (severe and occasionally fatal), elevated liver enzymes, bilirubin, total lipids and triglycerides
- peripheral neuropathy, muscle weakness, ataxia
- extrapyramidal dysfunction
- alterations to ECG

Interactions
- hypoglycaemia may occur if given with hypoglycaemic agents such as insulin or sulfonylureas or beta adrenoceptor blocking agents
- concurrent use with doxorubicin may lead to doxorubicin toxicity
- increased risk of perhexiline toxicity if given with SSRIs
- increased serum transaminases may occur if given with warfarin
- perhexiline is a CYP2D6 substrate (i.e. metabolised by the CYP2D6 enzyme)
- drugs that affect CYP2D6 can alter perhexiline concentrations, either increasing the risk of toxicity or reducing its efficacy. CYP2D6 inhibitors (e.g. SSRIs, bupropion, celecoxib) may raise perhexiline levels, while CYP2D6 inducers (e.g. rifampicin) can lower its levels
- may interfere with ECG, with a slight depression of the T wave and prolonged QT interval

Nursing considerations/Cautions
- measure serum liver enzymes before starting therapy and monitor monthly thereafter
- monitor plasma perhexiline level: at the end of the first week, then monthly, maintaining levels between 0.15 and 0.6 microgram/mL
- patient should be carefully monitored and therapy stopped if any of the following occur:
  - peripheral neuropathy (numbness/tingling in feet/hands, muscle weakness, paraesthesia)
  - hepatic toxicity (weakness, appetite loss, weight loss, persistent elevated liver enzymes)
  - persistent or marked hypoglycaemia
  - excessive weight loss

ANTIANGINAL AGENTS

- papilloedema
- dosing adjustments: dose should only be increased if plasma levels are subtherapeutic after 2—4 weeks of therapy
- doses > 100 mg daily are administered as a divided dose
- use cautiously in patients with ventricular conduction disturbances post myocardial infarction and those with diabetes mellitus.
- (Contraindications) patients with porphyria, renal or hepatic impairment, or if plasma level monitoring is unavailable

Patient education

- ensure the patient understands the importance of regular blood test/monitoring to prevent toxicity.
- seek medical advice immediately if the following symptoms occur:
  - muscle weakness, numbness or tingling in hands or feet, or difficulty walking
  - loss of appetite, nausea, yellowing of eyes/skin, dark urine or upper abdominal pain
- excessive weight loss

- patients with diabetes, especially those on insulin or sulfonylureas, should closely monitor their blood glucose levels for hypoglycaemia, particularly in the first 3 days of therapy
- ensure the patient understands that perhexiline is not for use during an acute angina attack
- see also General Patient education for antianginal agents (p. 59)

 Tablet can be crushed and mixed with water or spoonful of yoghurt or apple puree.

 Not recommended during pregnancy unless the expected benefit outweighs any potential risk.

 No data available on the use of perhexiline during breastfeeding. Not recommended unless the expected benefit outweighs any potential risk.

 Perhexiline is primarily metabolised by the liver, but it can accumulate in patients with renal impairment, especially with prolonged use. Manufacturer contraindicates use in both renal and hepatic impairment.

ANTIANXIETY AGENTS

Mental health is defined as the state of mental well being that allows people to cope with the stresses of life, realise their abilities, learn and work well, and contribute to their community (WHO 2023d) and is integral to a person's overall well-being. A mental disorder is one that impacts significantly on a person's cognition, behaviour and emotions (ABS 2023), with nearly 43% of Australians (8.5 million) reporting a mental disorder (ABS 2023). Anxiety is one of the most common mental disorders reported. In 2020–22, more than 3.4 million Australians (17.2% of the population) aged 16 to 85 years reported an anxiety disorder, up from 2.6 million in 2014–15. Women reported anxiety-related conditions more commonly than males (21.1% compared with 13%), with younger women (15–24 years) reporting anxiety at a rate of 40% (ABS 2023). Females were more likely to consult a health professional than males, with general practitioners (GPs) and psychologists being the most common health professionals consulted (ABS 2023).

Anxiety is a normal human response to a personally threatening situation, such as a threat to one's health, loved ones, job or lifestyle (e.g. performance in exams, moving house, changing job, illness), and can in some instances improve a person's performance because of the increased alertness (e.g. exams, sport, job interview). However, in some instances high levels of anxiety can decrease a person's ability to think clearly, plan or carry out complex tasks, leading to distress and disability (Shelton & Anand 2025).

Anxiety disorders include generalised anxiety disorder, obsessive–compulsive disorder (OCD), panic disorder, social anxiety disorder, specific phobias, separation anxiety, post-traumatic stress disorder (PTSD) and acute stress. Anxiety can also be experienced as part of other psychiatric or mental disorders such as depression (Shelton & Anand 2025).

Management can be either pharmacological with antianxiety (or anxiolytic) agents and/or non-pharmacological, including counselling, stress management, relaxation techniques, graded exposure (e.g. to the cause of the specific phobia) and cognitive behaviour therapy (Shelton & Anand 2025). The choice of pharmacological agent is dependent on the specific anxiety disorder. For example,

ANTIANXIETY AGENTS

benzodiazepines are prescribed for acute (rather than chronic) situations in the treatment of generalised anxiety disorder, to control symptoms and allow the person to return to normal functioning, and should then be discontinued gradually.

It should be noted that antianxiety agents are not recommended for the management of everyday stress or tension.

General Actions of antianxiety agents

- main sites of action of benzodiazepines appear to be the limbic system, thalamus and spinal cord
- suppression of the limbic system is thought to prevent stimulation of the reticular activating centre, resulting in drowsiness
- agents bind to specific receptors in the central nervous system (CNS), either by potentiating gamma aminobutyric acid (GABA)-mediated inhibition or by directly affecting action potential
- agents produce muscle relaxation, sedative–hypnotic effect, antegrade amnesia, anticonvulsant properties and decreased anxiety

General Adverse effects of antianxiety agents

- (Most common) drowsiness, sedation, fatigue, dizziness, lightheadedness, muscle weakness/spasm, ataxia, nervousness, irritability
- headache, tremor, confusion, transient amnesia, insomnia, slurred speech, blurred vision, diplopia, reduced alertness, decreased coordination, slowed reaction time, difficulty concentrating
- depression, irritability, disturbed dreams, altered mood
- nausea, vomiting, anorexia, diarrhoea, dry mouth
- urinary retention/incontinence
- altered libido, sexual dysfunction
- menstrual irregularities
- rash, dermatitis, pruritus
- risk of dependence (physical and psychological) and tolerance (with chronic use)
- (Rare) hypotension, respiratory depression, paradoxical reaction (e.g. excitation, stimulation, acute rage, agitation, increased anxiety), increased intraocular pressure
- (Very rare) blood dyscrasias, jaundice, abnormal liver function

General Interactions of antianxiety agents

- may increase CNS depression if given with alcohol (acute intake), opioid analgesics, some antihistamines, antidepressants (tricyclic, non-selective monoamine oxidase inhibitors (MAOIs)), muscle relaxants, antipsychotics, anaesthetic agents, barbiturates, sedatives and hypnotics, other antianxiety agents or phenothiazines
- increased plasma level may result if given with amiodarone, azole antifungals, calcium-blocking agents (e.g. verapamil, nifedipine), ciclosporin, diltiazem, disulfiram, fluvoxamine, HIV protease inhibitors (e.g. ritonavir), isoniazid, macrolide antibiotics (e.g. erythromycin), grapefruit juice, oestrogens or oral contraceptives
- benzodiazepines may increase the anticholinergic effects of atropine or atropine-like agents, antihistamines or antidepressants
- serum levels of both benzodiazepine and antiepileptic agents may be altered if given together; therefore serum levels of antiepileptic agents should be closely monitored

- may increase euphoria if given with opioid analgesics, increasing the risk of psychological dependence

General Nursing considerations/Cautions for antianxiety agents

- regular reassessment of anxiety level is recommended
- ambulant patients should be started on the lowest possible dose to decrease the risk of falls
- benzodiazepines should be prescribed for only 2–4 weeks (unless used for management of panic disorders, where therapy is usually prolonged); physical and psychological dependence on benzodiazepines may occur after 4–6 weeks and generally results in withdrawal symptoms if they are stopped abruptly
- tolerance of the sedating effect may develop
- withdrawal from benzodiazepines should be gradual (over 4–16 weeks depending on the indication for use) to prevent withdrawal symptoms
- withdrawal symptoms may occur if the patient has developed a physical dependence from taking excessive doses of the benzodiazepine agent over a prolonged period; symptoms may include insomnia, rebound anxiety, palpitations, panic attacks, vertigo, dysphoria, akinesia, myoclonus, metallic taste, hypersensitivity to light, sound and/or touch, delusions, confusion, delirium, abdominal and muscle cramps, tremor, vomiting, sweating, hallucinations, hyperthermia, psychosis and convulsions
- sudden withdrawal of benzodiazepines may result in a temporary increase in the frequency and severity of seizures in patients with epilepsy, or an increase in sleep disturbance in other patients
- 'rebound phenomena' refers to a return to the original presenting symptoms (e.g. anxiety, panic attacks, insomnia) combined with withdrawal symptoms when the benzodiazepine is stopped
- blood counts and liver function tests are advisable during prolonged administration, especially in those with pre-existing kidney or liver impairment
- note and report paradoxical reactions, such as excitement, muscle spasticity, sleep disturbance or acute rage; the benzodiazepine should be stopped if any of these occur
- overdosage is treated with activated charcoal (oral or nasogastric) and flumazenil (see Antidotes, antagonists and chelating agents, p. 348), as well as general supportive measures as appropriate
- not recommended as primary treatment in those with depression or psychosis, as benzodiazepines may increase depression, unmask suicidal tendencies or contribute to deterioration of severe schizophrenia
- caution if used in those with epilepsy, as an increase in frequency and/or severity of seizures may occur, requiring an increase in dosage of antiepileptic agent. Risk of seizure is increased if withdrawal is abrupt and should therefore be avoided
- caution if used in those where decreased blood pressure may lead to cardiac or cerebral complications
- caution should be taken if giving benzodiazepines to patients with narrow-angle glaucoma, pre-existing muscle weakness or spinal/cerebellar ataxia, respiratory depression or impaired liver or kidney function

- contraindicated in those with myasthenia gravis, sleep apnoea, chronic obstructive airways disease with incipient respiratory failure, severe liver impairment, a personal or family history of alcohol or drug dependence, or hypersensitivity to other benzodiazepines

General Patient education for anti-anxiety agents

- warn patient against driving a vehicle or operating machinery if drowsy, dizzy or fatigued
- warn patient about the reduced tolerance to alcohol or other CNS depressants and advise against large intakes of alcohol
- advise patient to avoid grapefruit and grapefruit juice during therapy
- patient should be informed that adverse effects are often seen at the beginning of therapy but usually disappear with continued use or a decrease in dosage
- patient should be warned not to stop benzodiazepines abruptly or alter the prescribed dose
- instruct patient to immediately seek medical advice if any of the following occurs:
  - aggressive behaviour, hostility, anger, violence, hallucinations or sudden anxiety
  - involuntary movements, tremor, shakiness, muscle weakness
  - unexplained nausea, vomiting, abdominal pain, yellowing of skin or eyes, dark urine
- women should be counselled to use adequate contraception to avoid pregnancy

 Benzodiazepines cross the placenta. If taken during the first trimester they may result in congenital abnormalities. If taken late in third trimester or during labour they may cause hypotonia (floppy baby), respiratory depression, difficult drinking or sucking and hypothermia in the newborn. Withdrawal symptoms have been reported in the newborn.

 Benzodiazepines are secreted in breastmilk and may cause hypotonia (floppy baby) and problems with sucking and drinking; therefore they are not recommended while breastfeeding.

 Risk of accumulation of active metabolites exists in the elderly because of age-related changes to the renal and hepatic systems that alter drug metabolism and excretion. Extreme caution should be taken when using benzodiazepines in the elderly because of an associated increased risk of hypotension, falls, confusion, drowsiness and over-sedation. Short-acting benzodiazepines with no active metabolites are the safest option for the elderly.

ALPRAZOLAM

Trade name
Alprax, Kalma

Available forms
Tablets: 0.25 mg, 0.5 mg, 1 mg, 2 mg

Action
- short-acting benzodiazepine with active metabolite
- half-life 11—16 hours; half-life of active metabolite 10—15 hours
- see also General Actions of antianxiety agents (p. 71)

Use
- anxiety disorder
- panic disorders

Dose
- (Anxiety) 0.5—4 mg/day orally daily in 2—3 divided doses **OR**
- (Anxiety with depressive symptoms) 1.5—4.5 mg orally daily in divided doses **OR**

- (Panic disorder) initially 0.5—1 mg orally at bedtime, increasing by 0.25—1 mg every 3 days until adequate response is achieved (daily maximum 10 mg)

Adverse effects
- see General Adverse effects of antianxiety agents (p. 71)

Interactions
- may increase plasma levels of imipramine
- concentration reduced by smoking
- see also General Interactions of antianxiety agents (p. 71)

Nursing considerations/Cautions/Patient education
- half-life is prolonged in Asians and decreased in smokers
- see also General Nursing considerations/Cautions for antianxiety agents (p. 72) and General Patient education for antianxiety agents (p. 73)

Tablets can be dispersed in water, placed under the tongue and allowed to dissolve, or crushed and mixed with spoonful of yoghurt or apple puree.

BROMAZEPAM
Trade name
Lexotan

Available forms
Tablets: 3 mg, 6 mg

Action
- medium-acting benzodiazepine with active metabolite
- half-life 12—24 hours; half-life of active metabolite 20 hours
- see also General Actions of antianxiety agents (p. 71)

Use
- tension, anxiety and agitation

Dose
- (Ambulant patients) 3 mg orally 2—3 times daily before food (daily maximum 60 mg) **OR**
- (Severe hospitalised patients) 6—12 mg orally 2—3 times daily before food

Adverse effects/Interactions
- see General Adverse effects/General Interactions of antianxiety agents (p. 71)

Nursing considerations/Cautions
- tablets contain lactose and therefore are not recommended in those with galactose intolerance, Lapp lactase deficiency or glucose—galactose malabsorption
- it may be an advantage to divide the dosage in such a way as to give a larger dose in the evening or, if the dosage is small (3—6 mg), give as a single dose in the evening
- see also General Nursing considerations/Cautions for antianxiety agents (p. 72)

Patient education
- advise patient to take tablets before meals
- see also General Patient education for antianxiety agents (p. 73)

Tablets can be dispersed in water, or crushed and mixed with spoonful of yoghurt or apple puree.

Lowest dose is recommended in those with mild-to-moderate liver impairment.

Dose reduction is recommended in those aged 50 years and over.

CLOBAZAM
Trade name
Frisium, Pharmcor Clobazam

Available form
Tablets: 10 mg

Action
- anxiolytic agent, chemically distinguishable from other benzodiazepines with some characteristics similar to diazepam

ANTIANXIETY AGENTS

- long-acting benzodiazepine with active metabolite
- does not produce muscle relaxation at normal dosage
- long half-life (18—48 hours); active metabolite long half-life (2—5 days)

Use
- short-term (1 month) treatment of anxiety or sleep disturbances associated with anxiety
- epilepsy (adjunct therapy for partial refractory epilepsy or Lennox—Gastaut epilepsy not stabilised on current antiepileptic therapy in children over 4 years)

Dose
- (Anxiety) 10—30 mg orally daily in 1—2 divided doses **OR**
- (Epilepsy) initially 5 mg orally daily, then 0.3—1.0 mg/kg (maintenance)

Adverse effects
- serious skin reactions (Stevens—Johnson syndrome, toxic epidermal necrolysis)
- see also General Adverse effects of antianxiety agents (p. 71)

Interactions
- increased conversion to metabolite may occur if given with carbamazepine or phenytoin
- see also General Interactions of antianxiety agents (p. 71)

Nursing considerations/Cautions
- the patient should be carefully monitored for skin signs and symptoms, especially in the first 8 weeks of therapy
- (epilepsy) the patient should be reassessed after 4 weeks of therapy for improvement in seizure control
- if dose is divided, a higher proportion should be given at night. Doses of up to 30 mg can be given as a single nightly dose
- see also General Nursing considerations/Cautions for antianxiety agents (p. 72)

Patient education
- advise the patient/carer to seek medical advice immediately if severe blisters and/or bleeding of lips, eyes, mouth, nose and/or genitals occurs
- see also General Patient education for antianxiety agents (p. 73)

 Tablet can be dispersed in water or crushed and mixed with spoonful of yoghurt or apple puree.

DIAZEPAM
Trade name
Antenex, APX-Diazepam, DBL Diazepam Solution, Diazepam WGR, Noumed Diazepam, Orion Diazepam 10 mg/10 mL Elixir, Valium, Valpam

Available forms
Tablets: 2 mg, 5 mg;
Ampoule: 10 mg/2 mL;
Elixir: 10 mg/10 mL

Action
- long-acting benzodiazepine
- long duration of action because of active metabolites (desmethyldiazepam (half-life 20—70 hours) and temazepam (half-life 30—100 hours)), which are then finally metabolised to oxazepam (half-life 5—15 hours)
- crosses the blood—brain and placental barriers
- half-life increases with age and liver or kidney disease
- (IM) onset of action is variable depending on muscle mass
- see also General Actions of antianxiety agents (p. 71)

Use
- anxiety disorders (short-term management)
- allay anxiety before surgery (premedication), cardioversion, endoscopy, and orthopaedic or dental procedures

- relieve acute alcohol withdrawal symptoms
- status epilepticus (IV)
- tetanus spasm (IV)
- muscle spasm, spasticity

Dose

- (Ambulant patient) 2 mg orally 3 times daily **OR**
- (Ambulant patient) 2 mg orally 1—2 times daily plus 5 mg in the evening **OR**
- (Muscle spasm) 10—30 mg orally daily **OR**
- (Hospitalised patient, acute tension, excitation or motor unrest) 10—15 mg orally 3 times daily until acute symptoms subside **OR**
- (Premedication) 10—20 mg orally at least 30 minutes before procedure **OR**
- (Endoscopic procedures) 10—20 mg by slow IV (immediately before) or 5—10 mg IM (30 minutes before procedure) (if IV route is not available) **OR**
- (Status epilepticus, convulsive seizure) initially 5—10 mg by slow IV, repeated in 10—15 minutes if necessary (to a maximum of 30 mg) **OR**
- (Cardioversion) 5—15 mg by slow IV 5—10 minutes before procedure

Adverse effects

- (IV) cardiovascular and respiratory depression (due to propylene glycol)
- (Rapid IV) phlebitis, local irritation, swelling, venous thrombosis, pain, syncope, hypotension, bradycardia, cardiac/respiratory arrest
- (IM) tenderness, local pain, erythema
- see also General Adverse effects of antianxiety agents (p. 71)

Interactions

- plasma levels may be increased if given with isoniazid
- plasma levels may be decreased if given with rifampicin
- may reduce the effects of levodopa, decreasing control of Parkinsonian symptoms (reversible)
- decrease dose of ketamine required if given with diazepam
- absorption increased if given with IV metoclopramide (not oral)
- decreased sedation and anxiolytic effects may result if given with theophylline or caffeine
- metabolism may be inhibited by omeprazole and esomeprazole (but not pantoprazole or lansoprazole), increasing risk of adverse effects
- elimination may be prolonged if given with modafinil and armodafinil
- primary metabolite of idelalisib may increase elimination of diazepam
- can inhibit binding of levothyroxine and liothyronine, resulting in false thyroid function test results
- see also General Interactions of antianxiety agents (p. 71)

Nursing considerations/Cautions

- (Oral) to offset some of the adverse effects, doctor may order most of the daily dose 2/3 at night and the other 1/3 in the morning
- (Acute alcohol withdrawal) dose may be readministered over next 2—7 days if withdrawal symptoms return
- injectable diazepam forms an incompatible precipitate when mixed with other drugs and therefore should be administered alone
- (IV) monitor vital signs, noting hypotension, bradycardia, respiratory depression/apnoea, syncope or muscle weakness
- resuscitation equipment should be available during IV administration
- (IV/IM) maximum dose in 8 hours should not be greater than 30 mg
- if possible, IM administration should be avoided because absorption is erratic
- IV injection administered slowly (5 mg/min) should be into a blood vessel with a large lumen, taking care to avoid extravasation and accidental IA administration. Small vessels should not be used
- hangover effect may occur (mainly in the elderly) as a result of the accumulation of diazepam and its metabolites

- (Tablets) contain lactose and are therefore not recommended for those with rare hereditary problems of galactose intolerance, including Lapp lactase deficiency or glucose—galactose malabsorption
- (Elixir) not recommended for control of status epilepticus or other acute conditions
- (IV) contraindicated in those in shock or coma, acute alcohol intoxication with depressed vital signs or those with respiratory or cardiac insufficiency
- see also General Nursing considerations/ Cautions for antianxiety agents (p. 72)

Patient education
- advise patient that elixir should be stored below 25°C, protected from light and discarded 90 days after opening
- see also General Patient education for antianxiety agents (p. 73)

Elixir is available. Tablets can be dispersed in water, or crushed and mixed with spoonful of yoghurt or apple puree.

LORAZEPAM
Trade name
APO Lorazepam, Ativan, Loraze, Lorazepam Lupin, Lorazepam SXP Solution, Lorazepam Viatris, Lorazepam-WGR

Available forms
Tablets: 1 mg, 2.5 mg

Action
- medium-acting benzodiazepine with no active metabolites
- half-life 10—20 hours
- see also General Actions of antianxiety agents (p. 71)

Use
- anxiety disorders
- premedication (night before or 1—2 hours before procedure)

Dose
- (Anxiety) 2—3 mg orally daily in divided doses (range 1—10 mg) **OR**

ANTIANXIETY AGENTS

- (Insomnia because of anxiety or stress) 1—2 mg orally at bedtime **OR**
- (Premedication) 2—4 mg orally the night before surgery and/or 1—2 hours before surgery

Adverse effects/Interactions/ Nursing considerations/Cautions/ Patient education
- see General Adverse effects/ Interactions/Nursing considerations/ Cautions/Patient education of antianxiety agents (p. 71)

Tablets can be dispersed in water, or placed under the tongue and allowed to dissolve, or crushed and mixed with spoonful of yoghurt or apple puree.

OXAZEPAM
Trade name
Alepam, APO-Oxazepam, Murelax, Oxazepam-WGR, Serepax

Available forms
Tablets: 15 mg, 30 mg

Action
- short-acting benzodiazepine with no active metabolites
- half-life 5—15 hours
- see also General Actions of antianxiety agents (p. 71)

Use
- anxiety disorders
- alcohol withdrawal

Dose
- (Mild-to-moderate anxiety) 7.5—15 mg orally 3—4 times daily **OR**
- (Severe anxiety) 15—30 mg orally 3—4 times daily **OR**
- (Alcohol withdrawal) 15—30 mg orally 3—4 times daily

Adverse effects/Interactions/ Nursing considerations/Cautions/ Patient education
- should not be given if person undergoing alcohol withdrawal is acutely inebriated

HAVARD'S NURSING GUIDE TO DRUGS

* see also General Adverse effects/ Interactions/Nursing considerations/ Cautions/Patient education of antianxiety agents (p. 71)

Tablets can be dispersed in water (although Serepax formulation does not disperse easily).
Tablets can be crushed and mixed with spoonful of yoghurt or apple puree.

ANTIARRHYTHMIC AGENTS

If the conducting system of the heart becomes disrupted, the effect on the electrical activity results in a rhythm disorder, which can be classified as a bradyarrhythmia (HR < 60 bpm) or tachyarrhythmia (HR > 100 bpm). Bradyarrhythmias include sinus bradycardia and atrioventricular (AV) blocks, while tachyarrhythmias include both atrial (e.g. supraventricular tachycardia, atrial fibrillation, atrial flutter) and ventricular tachycardias (e.g. ventricular tachycardia, premature ventricular ectopics, torsades de pointes). Tachyarrhythmias can be classified according to rhythm regularity, site of the rhythm's origin (atrium or ventricle), duration of QRS complex (narrow or wide) and the mechanism involved in the arrhythmia. Bradyarrhythmias are generally managed by reversing the cause of the bradycardia or pacemaker implantation, while tachyarrhythmias are treated by reversing the cause if possible, with medications (e.g. antiarrhythmic agents) or ablation (Banga & Chalfoun 2018).

Antiarrhythmic drugs are divided into four classes according to their mode of action and effect on the cardiac action potential. They may be broadly divided into agents that act mainly on supraventricular arrhythmias, those that act mainly on ventricular arrhythmias and those that act on both. Class I agents are further subdivided by their effect on the duration of the action potential (Knights et al 2023). Some drugs have multiple actions and so belong in more than one class. Adenosine is unique as it is not classified under this system.

CLASS I

- inhibit the fast inward sodium channels responsible for phase 0 of the action potential (sodium channel blockade) and slow membrane repolarisation
- bind to the sodium channel when open or in the refractory phase; therefore the greater the frequency of sodium channels being open, the greater the degree of block by Class I agents
- in slowing conduction speed, may promote tachycardias via re-entry mechanisms
- minor differences are discussed under specific subclasses (Ia, Ib, Ic)

CLASS IA

DISOPYRAMIDE
Trade name
Rythmodan

Available forms
Capsules: 100 mg, 150 mg
(this drug is not marketed in Australia but may be available through the Special Access Scheme (SAS))

Action
* depresses myocardial excitability, prolongs cardiac muscle refractory period of atria and ventricles, prolongs the action potential and refractory period, decreases conduction velocity
* decreases cardiac output, increases peripheral resistance
* slight, transient myocardial depression
* AV node conduction unchanged
* significant anticholinergic effects
* onset of action 3 minutes to 3 hours
* half-life 4—10 hours

Use
* management of life-threatening ventricular arrhythmias

Dose
* initially 800—600 mg orally daily in 3 divided doses, reducing to 300—400 mg orally in 3 divided doses
* for patients with CrCl < 40 mL/min, loading dose: 100—200 mg; maintenance dose: CrCl 30—40 mL/min: 100 mg every 8 hours. CrCl 15—30 mL/min: 100 mg every 12 hours. CrCl < 15 mL/min: 100 mg every 24 hours (adjust according to plasma disopyramide concentrations and clinical response)

Therapeutic drug monitoring
* Therapeutic range 2—4 mg/L (6—12 micromol/L).

Adverse effects
* (Anticholinergic effects) urinary retention, dry mouth, blurred vision, constipation, dizziness
* anorexia, nausea, indigestion, vomiting, diarrhoea, flatulence, bad taste in mouth
* dizziness, fatigue, vertigo, drowsiness
* hypotension, prolongation of QT interval, widening of QRS interval, bradycardia, AV block, severe cardiac failure, disturbance of cardiac conduction, chest pain, oedema, cyanosis, dyspnoea, cardiac arrest, worsening or provocation of ventricular arrhythmias
* rash, pruritus, urticaria, photosensitivity
* profuse sweating
* elevated aspartate aminotransferase (AST) levels
* hypoglycaemia
* aggravation of pre-existing congestive cardiac failure

Interactions
* contraindicated with other antiarrhythmic agents (e.g. flecainide), erythromycin, tricyclic antidepressants (TCAs), tetracyclic antidepressants or pentamidine because of the risk of prolongation of QT interval and 'torsades de pointes' (see Glossary)
* not recommended with stimulant laxatives, amphotericin B (amphotericin), tetracosactide (tetracosactrin), glucocorticoids, mineralocorticoids or diuretics because of the risk of potassium imbalance
* not recommended with phosphodiesterase-5 (PDE-5) inhibitors (sildenafil or tadalafil) used for erectile dysfunction because of the risk of QT interval prolongation
* use with extreme caution with atropine, phenothiazines and other anticholinergic (antimuscarinic) agents owing to increased anticholinergic effects
* serum levels may be decreased by rifampicin, phenytoin, primidone or

carbamazepine and should not be given together
- not recommended with macrolide or azole antifungal agents and roxithromycin because it may increase disopyramide serum levels, therefore increasing the risk of adverse effects
- may increase serum levels of theophylline, human immunodeficiency virus (HIV) protease inhibitors, warfarin and ciclosporin, therefore increasing the risk of adverse effects and/or toxicity

Nursing considerations/Cautions

- proarrhythmic effect: It may worsen arrhythmias; monitor for signs of new or worsening arrhythmias
- contraindicated in those with cardiogenic shock, second/third-degree A-V block (without pacemaker), bundle branch block, double block, pre-existing QT interval prolongation, sinus node dysfunction, cardiac insufficiency or those taking medication that might provoke ventricular arrhythmias or prolong QT interval
- measure serum potassium before starting therapy and regularly during treatment. Correct any potassium imbalance before initiating therapy
- frequent monitoring of ECG (especially for prolongation of PR or QT intervals or QRS widening) is recommended
- regularly check blood pressure
- if cardioversion is planned, start disopyramide 1–2 days beforehand
- monitor blood glucose levels regularly, especially in elderly patients, and those with pre-existing diabetes or kidney insufficiency
- measure intraocular pressure before starting therapy if there is a family history of glaucoma
- monitor closely for hypotension and congestive cardiac failure
- not recommended in those who have had a recent myocardial infarction (within 2 years), structural heart disease and associated heart failure (unless treated and able to be closely monitored during therapy), uncompensated heart failure or hypotension
- not recommended in those with chronic closed-angle glaucoma, urinary retention, benign prostatic hypertrophy or prostatic adenoma because of anticholinergic effects
- caution if used in those with kidney or liver impairment, family history of glaucoma or myasthenia gravis (may precipitate a myasthenic crisis)
- exercise caution in elderly, malnourished patients and those with diabetes mellitus or kidney insufficiency because of the increased risk of hypoglycaemia

Patient education

- advise the patient to seek immediate medical advice and report these symptoms immediately: difficulty urinating, fast or irregular heartbeat, ongoing dizziness or lightheadedness, signs of low blood sugar such as chills, cold sweat, confusion, cool/pale skin, drowsiness, headache, excessive hunger, nausea, shakiness, unusual weakness or tiredness
- advise patients with diabetes to monitor blood glucose levels more frequently because of the risk of hypoglycaemia (low blood sugar).
- advise the patient not to drive or operate heavy machinery if they feel dizzy or light-headed
- advise the patient that, if they open capsules for ease of swallowing, to rinse their mouth carefully afterwards, as the powder can cause mouth ulcers
- warn the patient that dry mouth and throat commonly occur at the start of therapy and may be alleviated by melting chips of ice in the mouth

 Capsules can be opened and contents dispersed in water, or given with a spoonful of apple puree or yoghurt.

Not recommended during pregnancy unless the benefits outweigh the risks, as it can stimulate the uterus and cross into the fetal circulation, potentially leading to preterm labour or impact on fetal development. If used, it requires careful monitoring of both the mother and fetus.

Not recommended during breastfeeding owing to possible anticholinergic or cardiac adverse effects in the infant. If used, the infant should be closely monitored.

Reduce the dose according to the severity of renal impairment. Monitor ECG and plasma disopyramide concentrations regularly to ensure safe and effective dosing.

CLASS IB

- shorten action potential duration (which usually shortens repolarisation)
- increases effective refractory period

LIDOCAINE (LIGNOCAINE)
Trade names
Lignocaine, Xylocard

Available forms
Ampoule: 50 mg/5 mL (1%), 100 mg/5 mL (2%), 200 mg/20 mL (1%), 400 mg/20 mL (2%), 500 mg/5 mL (10%); Prefilled syringe: 20 mg/mL (2%); Vial: 200 mg/20 mL (1%), 400 mg/20 mL (2%)

Action
- amide
- depresses electrical activity reversibly in nerve, muscle and secretory cell membranes
- decreases slow spontaneous depolarisation
- decreases action potential duration and effective refractory period of Purkinje and ventricular cells
- little effect on conduction speed, membrane responsiveness or cardiac output
- less active metabolites
- onset of action 1 minute (IV) or 3—15 minutes (IM)
- half-life 1.6 hours

Use
- treatment or prophylaxis of ventricular arrhythmias and tachycardias associated with acute myocardial infarction, digoxin toxicity, cardiac surgery and after cardiac arrest
- local anaesthetic (see Local anaesthetics, p. 1326)

Dose
- 1 mg/kg slowly IV over 1—2 minutes initially, repeated at 10—20-minute intervals if necessary. No more than 200—300 mg should be administered in a 1-hour period. Infusion should be commenced within 10 minutes
- maintenance, IV infusion drip rate 2—4 mg/min

Therapeutic drug monitoring
- therapeutic range 5—20 micromol/L (1.5—6 microgram/mL)

Adverse effects
- lightheadedness, apprehension, euphoria, nervousness, dizziness, tremors, twitching, drowsiness, agitation, confusion, disorientation, paraesthesia, numbness
- blurred vision, double vision
- dyspnoea
- slurred speech
- tinnitus
- sensations of heat or cold
- anorexia, nausea, vomiting, swallowing difficulties
- (Less common) bradycardia, hypotension, convulsions, psychoses, arrhythmias, methaemoglobinaemia, respiratory and/or cardiac arrest

Interactions
- serum levels may increase if given with fluvoxamine, propranolol and metoprolol, increasing the risk of lidocaine (lignocaine) toxicity

ANTIARRHYTHMIC AGENTS

- lidocaine (lignocaine) and phenytoin have synergistic cardiac effects
- cardiac effects may be potentiated if given with other antiarrhythmic agents
- caution if given with amiodarone, as it may decrease lidocaine (lignocaine) clearance
- caution if given with muscle relaxants (e.g. suxamethonium) because excessive neuromuscular blockade may occur
- may decrease serum levels of inhalational anaesthetics (e.g. nitrous oxide)
- metabolism may be increased by phenytoin, phenobarbital (phenobarbitone), primidone or carbamazepine
- prolonged half-life may occur if given during acute, severe alcohol intoxication
- caution if used with other amide-type local anaesthetics
- may interfere with measurement of creatinine level using enzymatic methods

Nursing considerations/Cautions

- correct hypokalaemia, hypoxia and any acid–base imbalance before starting treatment
- administration advice for lidocaine (lignocaine): (IV injection) use undiluted for IV bolus injections; (IV infusion): lidocaine (lignocaine) is compatible with glucose 5%, glucose/sodium chloride, and sodium chloride 0.9% solutions for IV infusion; ensure appropriate dosage adjustments and continuous monitoring during administration
- continuous ECG monitoring is essential to ensure effectiveness and detect any adverse effects, such as bradycardia or new arrhythmias
- monitor heart rate, blood pressure, plasma lidocaine (lignocaine) levels (especially for those in shock, on prolonged infusion (> 24 hours) or with liver or cardiac failure) and ECG throughout IV administration
- IV infusion should be stopped as soon as cardiac rhythm stabilises or if signs of toxicity appear, including drowsiness, as this may be an early sign of high blood lidocaine (lignocaine) levels
- monitor IV infusion rate closely using an infusion pump
- IV dose should not exceed 100 mg in a single dose or 200–300 mg in a 1-hour period
- IV infusion should be started within 10 minutes of initial IV injection
- IV infusion duration is normally 2 or more days. Usually discontinued 24 hours after last signs of arrhythmia or at first signs of toxicity
- an oral antiarrhythmic agent should replace IV therapy as soon as possible for maintenance
- have available diazepam (for convulsions), isoprenaline and atropine (for reversing bradycardia, hypotension), and facilities for cardiac monitoring, defibrillation and resuscitation (including oxygen therapy)
- caution if given to those with epilepsy, renal or liver failure, congestive cardiac failure, recent myocardial infarction, impaired cardiac conduction, severe digoxin toxicity, hypoxia or respiratory depression, hypovolaemia, severe shock, heart block or severe bradycardia, cardiac decompensation and hypotension, posterior diaphragmal infarction, acute porphyria, cardiac impairment or genetic predisposition to malignant hyperthermia
- contraindicated in those with Stokes–Adams syndrome, myasthenia gravis, severe shock, supraventricular arrhythmias, severe SA, AV or intraventricular block (without pacemaker) or in those with known hypersensitivity to amide-type local anaesthetics

 In renal impairment, active metabolites may accumulate with prolonged treatment. Reduce the dose if treatment exceeds 24 hours or involves repeated IV doses to prevent toxicity.

> In hepatic impairment or reduced blood flow to the liver (e.g. heart failure), lidocaine (lignocaine) may accumulate. Reduce the dose by half for infusions lasting over 24 hours or with repeated IV doses to prevent accumulation.

CLASS IC
- decrease rate of depolarisation and AV conduction time
- decrease contractility

FLECAINIDE
Trade names
APO-Flecainide, Flecainide Sandoz, Flecatab, Tambocor

Available forms
Tablets: 50 mg, 100 mg;
Ampoules: 10 mg/mL

Action
- structurally related to lidocaine (lignocaine)
- increases PR interval, QT interval and QRS duration
- does not alter HR, some increase in systolic and diastolic BP
- slight negative inotropic effect
- some local anaesthetic activity
- (Oral) long half-life 12–27 hours that is slowed by alkaline urine
- therapeutic range 0.2–0.9 mg/L

Use
- suppression and prevention of supraventricular arrhythmias
- life-threatening ventricular arrhythmias (not controlled by other agents)

Dose
- (Sustained ventricular tachycardia) 100 mg orally 12-hourly initially, increasing by 50 mg twice daily every 4 days (maximum 400 mg daily) **OR**
- (Supraventricular arrhythmias) 50 mg orally 12-hourly initially, increasing by 50 mg twice daily every 4 days (maximum 300 mg daily) **OR**
- 2 mg/kg slowly IV over 10–15 minutes, or diluted with glucose 5% and given as a mini-infusion (maximum 150 mg)

Therapeutic drug monitoring
- concentration monitoring: therapeutic range for flecainide: 0.2–0.9 mg/L.

Adverse effects
- may worsen arrhythmias (proarrhythmic effect)
- dizziness, lightheadedness, headache, fatigue, nervousness, tremor, paraesthesia, hypoaesthesia, asthenia
- ataxia
- blurred vision, diplopia, photophobia, visual field defects
- insomnia, somnolence
- nausea, vomiting, anorexia, diarrhoea, constipation, abdominal pain, dry mouth
- urinary retention and frequency, polyuria, dysuria
- increased sweating, flushing, fever
- palpitations, chest pain, congestive heart failure (new or worsening), (serious) ventricular arrhythmias (new or exacerbated), second/third-degree AV block, bradycardia, sinus pause, sinus arrest, angina, conduction disorders, tachycardia, oedema
- dyspnoea, coughing
- rash, pruritus
- tinnitus
- arthralgia, myalgia
- (Rare) blood dyscrasias, pulmonary fibrosis, pneumonitis, interstitial lung disease

Interactions
- alkaline urine decreases elimination
- not recommended with other antiarrhythmic agents
- may increase serum levels of digoxin

Nursing considerations/Cautions
- dilute with glucose 5% only
- any electrolyte imbalance (especially potassium) should be corrected before starting therapy

- IV therapy should be conducted only where cardiac monitoring and defibrillation are readily available
- have available isoprenaline, dopamine or dobutamine, mechanical ventilator and facilities for cardiac monitoring and defibrillation
- IV infusion should not continue for more than 24 hours
- once arrhythmia is controlled, the dose should be reduced to lessen the risk of adverse effects
- (Tablets) dose adjustments should not occur more frequently than every 4 days because of the long half-life
- if changing from another antiarrhythmic agent, at least 2 half-lives should be allowed to elapse before starting flecainide. If withdrawal of antiarrhythmic agent is likely to produce a life-threatening arrhythmia, hospitalisation of the patient is strongly recommended
- caution if used in those with recent myocardial infarction, severe cardiomyopathy, congestive heart failure, sinus node disease, sick sinus syndrome, electrolyte imbalance, alkaline urine, kidney impairment or permanent pacemaker or temporary pacing electrodes in situ
- extreme caution if used in those with structural heart disease, especially if left ventricular ejection fraction ≤ 40%
- not recommended in those with chronic atrial fibrillation or arrhythmias caused by digoxin toxicity
- contraindicated in those with severe liver or kidney impairment
- contraindicated in those with second/third-degree AV block (without pacemaker), right bundle branch block (without pacemaker), cardiogenic shock, severe renal/hepatic impairment, asymptomatic premature ventricular contractions, advanced sinus node disease, non-programmable pacemaker (unless pacing rescue is available) or asymptomatic non-sustained ventricular tachycardia with a history of myocardial infarction

Patient education

- advise the patient not to drive or operate heavy machinery if they experience dizziness, lightheadedness or visual disturbances
- advise the patient to be aware that dry mouth and/or taste disturbance may occur
- advise the patient to report immediately if they experience:
  - rapid or irregular heartbeat
  - chest pain
  - difficulty breathing

 Tablet can be dispersed in 10–20 mL of water, or crushed and given with a spoonful of yoghurt or apple puree.

 Not used in pregnancy unless the expected benefit outweighs any potential risk.

 Not recommended during breastfeeding. Minimal excretion in breastmilk; likely safe, but monitor the nursing infant.

 Renal/hepatic impairment: reduce dose based on plasma concentration.

CLASS II

- inhibit effects of the sympathetic nervous system (beta adrenergic blockade, e.g. atenolol, metoprolol); therefore are effective for arrhythmias induced by excessive sympathetic stimulation
- slow conduction at atria and AV node, increasing the refractory period
- shown to reduce mortality post myocardial infarction
- see also beta adrenoceptor blocking agents in Antihypertensive agents (p. 521)

CLASS III

- prolong the duration of the action potential (increase refractory period)
- decrease AV conduction

AMIODARONE
Trade names
Amiodarone Juno, Amdarone, Amiodarone Sandoz, Aratac, Cordarone X, Amiodarone-GH

Available forms
Tablets: 100 mg, 200 mg;
Ampoule: 150 mg/3 mL

Action
- prolongs action potential duration and hence refractory period of atrial, nodal and ventricular tissues
- increases coronary blood flow by vasodilation
- blocks sodium, calcium and potassium channels
- reduces cardiac oxygen requirement
- suppresses 'ectopic pacemakers'
- onset of action is 3—7 hours; half-life is about 14—59 days (with chronic dosing)
- active metabolite has longer half-life (60—90 days) (chronic dosing) than parent compound
- therapeutic range 1—2.5 mg/L (1.6—4 micromol/L)

Use
- ventricular fibrillation
- atrial flutter and fibrillation
- supraventricular, nodal and ventricular tachycardia refractory to other antiarrhythmic drugs
- severe cardiac arrhythmias (e.g. Wolf—Parkinson—White syndrome)

Dose
- 200 mg orally 3 times daily for 1 week, then reduce to 200 mg orally twice daily for 1 week, then reduce to 200 mg daily or less (maintenance) **OR**
- (IV infusion) 5 mg/kg IV diluted in 250 mL glucose 5% and given over 20 minutes to 2 hours at a rate less than 30 mg/min and repeated if needed (daily maximum 1.2 g) **OR**
- (Emergency; IV injection) 150—300 mg in 10—20 mL glucose 5% IV over 1 to 2 minutes

Therapeutic drug monitoring
- therapeutic range 1—2.5 mg/L (1.6—4 micromol/L)

Adverse effects
- serious adverse effects, including the potential to worsen arrhythmias. These effects can be slow to resolve after stopping the medication owing to its very long half life
- severe bradycardia, atypical ventricular arrhythmia, exacerbation of cardiac failure, cardiac arrest
- reversible benign yellowish-brown corneal micro-deposits
- skin photosensitivity and, rarely, discolouration of exposed areas such as face (slate grey/purple)
- peripheral neuropathy (long-term high dosage above 400 mg/day), myopathy
- insomnia, sleep disorders, vivid dreams and nightmares
- headache, tremor, dizziness, fatigue, vertigo, anxiety
- liver dysfunction, including elevated liver enzymes
- hyperthyroidism, hypothyroidism, weight gain/loss
- gait abnormalities, paraesthesia, muscle weakness, ataxia
- nausea, and, rarely, anorexia; constipation; salty, metallic taste; vomiting
- hair loss, rash, facial flushing
- fever
- (IV, rapid) severe hypotension, transient hot flushes, sweating, nausea
- pneumonitis, pulmonary fibrosis (rare and usually reversible, but potentially fatal), cough
- (Injection site) inflammation, pain, erythema, urticaria, oedema, induration, phlebitis, cellulitis, pigmentation changes, extravasation, necrosis
- (Rare) optic neuritis, optic neuropathy, cardiac failure, cardiac arrest

Interactions
- contraindicated with monoamine oxidase inhibitors (MAOIs)

ANTIARRHYTHMIC AGENTS

- contraindicated when given concurrently with other drugs that may prolong QT interval or induce 'torsades de pointes' (see Glossary), including disopyramide, flecainide, tricyclic antidepressants (TCAs), antihistamines, fluoroquinolones (e.g. moxifloxacin), antipsychotic agents, sotalol, erythromycin IV, pentamidine IV, or agents that may cause hypokalaemia or hypomagnesaemia, such as diuretics, stimulant laxatives, amphotericin B (amphotericin), corticosteroids
- increased risk of life-threatening bradycardia and heart block if given with antiviral agents such as sofosbuvir
- may increase serum levels of digoxin, phenytoin, flecainide and ciclosporin, increasing the toxicity risk; therefore serum levels should be closely monitored
- may increase serum levels of warfarin significantly, increasing the risk of bleeding; therefore INR time should be closely monitored, especially when starting or stopping therapy
- not recommended with calcium channel blockers or beta adrenoceptor blocking agents because of increased bradycardia and risk of conduction disorders
- give cautiously with general anaesthetics and oxygen therapy
- may increase the effects of fentanyl, increasing the risk of toxicity
- increased risk of bleeding if given with dabigatran
- increased serum levels may occur if given with grapefruit juice
- increased risk of myopathy and rhabdomyolysis if given with statins (simvastatin, atorvastatin)
- may alter results of thyroid function tests

Nursing considerations/Cautions

- initial treatment is closely monitored in the hospital
- IV injection is given only in a unit where facilities for monitoring and treating serious arrhythmias are available
- any electrolyte imbalance (especially potassium) should be corrected before starting therapy
- repeated or prolonged IV infusions are preferably given via a central venous catheter (CVC) to avoid thrombophlebitis
- before starting treatment, patients should have a thyroid function test (ultrasensitive thyroid-stimulating hormone (TSH)), serum potassium level measurement and an ECG
- Liver and thyroid function tests, chest X-ray, ophthalmological examination and ECG should be monitored regularly throughout therapy and for several months after stopping therapy
- any hypersensitivity to iodine should be established before starting therapy because amiodarone structurally contains iodine molecules
- oral therapy should replace IV infusion as soon as possible (with up to 2-day overlap to maintain plasma levels)
- functioning of pacemakers or implantable defibrillators should be checked before starting, and regularly during therapy
- should be diluted only in glucose 5%, as amiodarone is incompatible with sodium chloride 0.9%
- administer alone
- IV injections are not recommended as there is a high risk of hypotension, circulatory collapse and thrombophlebitis and therefore recommended only in extreme emergency situations with the patient monitored continuously in a setting such as ICU
- IV injection should not be repeated within 15 minutes of initial injection
- should be infused using a volumetric pump
- (IV) not compatible with heparin or aminophylline
- prepare the infusion solution immediately before use in either a glass or a rigid PVC container and use within 12 hours to reduce adsorption into PVC infusion bags and administration sets

- if surgery is planned, the anaesthetist should be made aware of therapy with amiodarone
- caution if used in those with liver disease/dysfunction or heart failure, as it may be exacerbated
- contraindicated in patients with or a history of thyroid dysfunction, sinus bradycardia, sino-atrial heart block, AV block, sick sinus syndrome (risk of sinus arrest), severe AV conduction disorders (without pacemaker or pacing), cardiomyopathy, circulatory collapse, heart failure, hypotension, severe arterial hypotension and respiratory failure, or in those with iodine hypersensitivity
- (IV) contraindicated in neonates owing to benzyl alcohol content

Patient education

- warn the patient to avoid sun exposure: wear protective clothing, a hat and sunscreen (SPF 30+)
- advise the patient on hepatitis C antiviral medications to seek medical advice if they experience slow heart rate, shortness of breath, lightheadedness, fainting or palpitations
- advise the patient to avoid driving/machinery if they feel dizzy or have vertigo
- advise the patient to avoid grapefruit juice
- advise the patient to report immediately if they experience:
  - blurred or decreased vision
  - blue tinge to skin on exposed areas (face)
  - numbness or tingling in hands/feet
  - nausea, vomiting, yellowing of skin/eyes or dark urine
  - breathing issues or persistent cough
  - skin rashes with blisters
  - symptoms of overactive thyroid (weight loss, sweating, tremor, rapid heartbeat) or underactive thyroid (weight gain, cold intolerance, hair loss)

 Tablets may be crushed and given with water, or a spoonful of yoghurt or apple puree.

 Contraindicated in pregnancy and for 3 months before. If exposure is unavoidable, thyroid function of the newborn infant should be assessed immediately.

 Contraindicated during breastfeeding.

 Use with caution in hepatic impairment because of reduced metabolism, risk of accumulation and potential hepatotoxicity.

SOTALOL
Trade names
APX-Sotalol, Cardol, Sotalol-WGR, Solavert, Sotalol Sandoz, Sotacor

Available forms
Tablets: 80 mg, 160 mg

Action
- non-selective beta adrenergic receptor blocker
- prolongs atrial, ventricular and accessory pathway refractory periods and QT interval
- decreases heart rate; reduces cardiac work and myocardial oxygen demand
- inhibits renin release (at rest and during exercise)
- does not undergo any first-pass metabolism in the liver; therefore bioavailability is 100%. However, this is reduced if given with food, especially milk
- onset of action 2–3 hours, half-life 12–14 hours

Use
- prevention and treatment of supraventricular and ventricular arrhythmias

Dose
- initially 80 mg orally twice daily 1–2 hours before food, increasing at 2–3-

ANTIARRHYTHMIC AGENTS

day intervals to 240—320 mg daily as needed. Renal impairment: adjust dose.

Adverse effects
- cardiac arrhythmias (including 'torsades de pointes' (see Glossary) and serious ventricular arrhythmias), bradycardia, hypotension, chest pain, palpitations, exacerbation of Prinzmetal's (variant) angina
- cold extremities
- oedema
- fatigue, asthenia, dizziness, headache, drowsiness, lightheadedness, sleep disturbance, weakness, tiredness, lethargy, vertigo
- paraesthesia
- anxiety, depression, mood changes
- fever
- dyspnoea
- muscle cramps
- changes in plasma lipid levels
- rash, worsening of pre-existing psoriasis
- diarrhoea, nausea, vomiting, flatulence, dyspepsia, abdominal pain, taste disturbance
- eye irritation, blurred vision, photophobia, eyesight deterioration
- hearing disturbance
- sexual dysfunction

Interactions
- contraindicated with concurrent use of other drugs that may prolong QT interval and induce 'torsades de pointes' (see Glossary), including disopyramide, tricyclic antidepressants (TCAs), calcium-channel blockers, clonidine, amiodarone, erythromycin IV or pentamidine IV, some quinolone antibiotics or agents which cause hypokalaemia or hypomagnesaemia, such as diuretics, stimulant laxatives, corticosteroids and amphotericin B (amphotericin)
- not recommended with clonidine, calcium-channel blockers or other beta adrenoceptor agents
- contraindicated with anaesthetic agents (e.g. methoxyflurane), as myocardial depression may occur
- clearance may be decreased by alcohol
- may prolong hypoglycaemic action of insulin and/or oral hypoglycaemic agents
- may require increased doses of beta receptor stimulants (e.g. isoprenaline, salbutamol, terbutaline)

Nursing considerations/Cautions
- administer 1—2 hours before food to maximise absorption
- should not be withdrawn preoperatively unless there is a clear indication to do so
- serum electrolytes should be measured before and during therapy and any imbalance (especially potassium) corrected
- pulse rate, haemodynamic and ECG monitoring is recommended (especially during initial therapy and with dose increases as arrhythmias may occur)
- dose adjustments should be gradual, allowing 2—3 days to reach a steady state
- medication withdrawal should be gradual over 8—14 days, especially in those with coronary artery disease
- atropine can be used to correct any excessive bradycardia (without/with hypotension)
- those with phaeochromocytoma should be pre-treated with phenoxybenzamine to avoid exacerbation of hypertension
- caution if used in those with congestive heart failure, psoriasis or hyperthyroidism
- caution if used in those with peripheral vascular disease, as symptoms may be worsened
- caution if used in those with diabetes, as signs of hypoglycaemia (e.g. tachycardia) may be masked
- caution if used in those with history of anaphylactic reaction because of an increased risk of reaction
- caution if used in those with hyperthyroidism already managed with beta adrenergic blocking agents. Abrupt withdrawal should be avoided to prevent exacerbation of symptoms including thyroid storm

HAVARD'S NURSING GUIDE TO DRUGS

- not recommended in those with recent myocardial infarction with left ventricular fraction ≤ 40%
- not recommended if QT interval > 450 milliseconds
- not recommended in those with Prinzmetal's (variant) angina because of the risk of exacerbated coronary artery spasm
- contraindicated in those with bronchial asthma, chronic obstructive airways disease, allergies (suggestive of bronchospasm), right ventricular failure (secondary to pulmonary hypertension), right ventricular hypertrophy, bradycardia (< 45–50 beats/min), second/third-degree AV block, sick sinus syndrome (without pacemaker), cardiogenic or hypovolaemic shock, uncontrolled congestive heart failure, kidney impairment (creatinine clearance < 10 mL/min) or congenital/acquired long QT syndrome

Patient education

- warn the patient not to drive or operate machinery if they feel dizzy, fatigued, lightheaded, drowsy or experience visual disturbances
- advise the patient to avoid alcohol while taking sotalol
- advise the patient to take sotalol 1–2 hours before food to improve absorption
- advise patients with diabetes to monitor blood glucose levels closely, as sotalol may prolong the effects of insulin or oral hypoglycaemic medicines
- warn the patient not to stop taking sotalol suddenly and to consult their health professional before making any changes
- advise the patient to seek immediate medical advice if they experience:
  - a very slow heartbeat
  - a very fast or irregular heartbeat, or chest pain
  - or shortness of breath

Tablet can be crushed and mixed with water, or given with a spoonful of yoghurt or apple puree.

Crosses the placental barrier and can cause bradycardia in the fetus and newborn. It should be used during pregnancy, especially in the late stages, only after carefully weighing the mother's needs against the risks to the fetus or newborn. Use with caution and observe the fetus and newborn for signs of beta blockade.

Excreted in breastmilk; therefore not recommended during breastfeeding.

Excretion is reduced in renal impairment; dose adjustment is needed. Sotalol is contraindicated in severe renal impairment (CrCl < 10 mL/min).

Permitted in sport subject to certain restrictions, route or urinary thresholds, or prohibited in some sports but not others.

CLASS IV

- decrease action potential duration
- decrease AV conduction
- decrease contractility
- see also calcium-channel blockers in Antihypertensive agents (p. 532)

ATYPICAL ANTIARRHYTHMIC AGENTS

ADENOSINE
Trade names
Adenocor, Adenosine Viatris, Adenoscan, Adenosine Juno Solution, Adsine

Vial: 6 mg/2 mL (therapeutic), 30 mg/10 mL (for cardiac scanning)

Action
- adenosine is a naturally occurring molecule that results from breakdown of adenosine triphosphate (ATP)
- a number of adenosine receptors (A_1, A_2A, A_2B, A_3) exist throughout the CNS

ANTIARRHYTHMIC AGENTS

- and peripheral tissue, including heart, liver, kidney, GI tract, adipose tissue, lung and blood vessels
- in the heart, binds to A_1 receptors, opening potassium channels leading to hyperpolarisation, inhibiting calcium entry into cells
- at SA node, inhibits pacemaker activity, decreasing spontaneous firing rate
- slows conduction through the AV node and re-establishes normal sinus rhythm
- no systemic haemodynamic effects
- produces peripheral vasodilation by A_2-receptor agonism
- very short half-life (10 seconds)

Use
- rapid conversion to a normal sinus rhythm of paroxysmal supraventricular tachycardias (including those associated with accessory pathways such as Wolff—Parkinson—White syndrome)
- (Diagnostic adjunct) diagnosis of broad and narrow QRS supraventricular tachycardias (Adenoscan)

Dose
- (Intravenous bolus) initially 3 mg rapid IV bolus over 2 seconds; if ineffective within 1—2 minutes, 6 mg may be given and, if necessary, 12 mg after a further 1—2 minutes (flush each dose with 20 mL 0.9% sodium chloride) **OR**
- (Diagnostic adjunct) 140 microgram/kg/min IV over 6 minutes via infusion pump, total dose 0.84 mg/kg, followed by injection of radionuclide after 3 minutes

Adverse effects
- flushing of face, head and body, heat sensation, burning sensation
- headache, lightheadedness, dizziness, apprehension
- paraesthesia
- nausea
- chest pressure/pain/discomfort, severe bradycardia, ventricular excitability, transient increase or decrease in BP, sinus pause, skipped beats, atrial extrasystole, AV block, hypotension
- dyspnoea or urge to breathe deeply
- (Diagnostic adjunct) abdominal discomfort, dry mouth
- (Rare) injection site reaction, bronchospasm

Interactions
- may be antagonised by caffeine, aminophylline and theophylline, and these should therefore be stopped for 24 hours before administration
- contraindicated with dipyridamole
- heart block may be potentiated if given with carbamazepine

Nursing considerations/Cautions
- given by rapid IV injection over 2 seconds, followed by rapid sodium chloride 0.9%
- do not refrigerate, protect from light
- adenosine administration requires close monitoring owing to its rapid effects on heart rhythm
- have cardiorespiratory resuscitation equipment available for immediate use
- ineffective when given as an infusion rather than as a rapid IV bolus
- dipyridamole should be stopped for 24 hours before administration
- coffee, cola, chocolate and other caffeine-containing drinks/food should be stopped for 12 hours before administration
- repeat doses should not be given if patient develops second- or third-degree AV block during administration
- (Diagnostic adjunct) administered undiluted
- (Diagnostic adjunct) HR and BP recorded at 1-minute intervals with continuous ECG monitoring. BP should be measured in opposite arm to infusion
- caution if used in those with a history of seizures
- caution if used in those with prolonged atrial fibrillation or flutter (with accessory pathway), recent heart transplantation (within 12 months), left main coronary stenosis, uncorrected hypovolaemia, left-to-right shunt,

pericarditis, pericardial effusion, autonomic dysfunction, stenotic carotid artery disease with cerebrovascular insufficiency, recent myocardial infarction, heart failure, first-degree AV block, bundle branch block
- contraindicated in those with chronic obstructive lung disease (including asthma), sick sinus syndrome (without pacemaker) or with second/third-degree AV block (without pacemaker), long QT syndrome, severe hypotension and decompensated heart failure

Patient education
- the patient should be warned of 'feeling of impending doom', which occurs transiently after injection

Limited human data. Likely safe because of its short duration and half-life, but should be used in pregnancy only if benefits outweigh risks.

Avoid use, as limited human data.

CARDIAC GLYCOSIDE

DIGOXIN
Trade names
Lanoxin, Sigmaxin

Available forms
Tablets: 62.5 microgram, 250 microgram;
Elixir (paediatric): 50 microgram/mL;
IV solution: 500 microgram/2 mL;
IV solution (paediatric): 50 microgram/2 mL

Action
- cardiac glycoside
- positive inotropic action: increases the force of myocardial contraction by inhibiting the sodium—potassium pump in cardiac myocytes
- negative chronotropic action: slows conduction through the AV node by increasing vagal activity, prolonging refractory periods and reducing ventricular rate
- effects in heart failure:
  - increases vascular resistance and venous tone
  - decreases plasma renin activity and serum aldosterone
  - improves kidney function through enhanced perfusion, promoting diuresis
- (IV administration): onset: 5—30 minutes; peak activity: 1—5 hours (undigitalised patient)
- (Oral administration): onset: 30 minutes to 2 hours; maximal effect: 2—6 hours (undigitalised patient)
- half-life: 36—48 hours (increases to ≥4.5 days in patients with kidney failure)
- steady-state: achieved in 5—7 days
- duration of action: may persist for 3—4 days after withdrawal in digitalised patients
- narrow therapeutic index: requires close monitoring of drug levels
- adult therapeutic range: 0.5—2 nanogram/L

Use
- congestive heart failure
- atrial fibrillation and atrial flutter
- paroxysmal atrial tachycardia

Dose

Digitalising loading dose
- 0.75—1.5 mg (10—20 microgram/kg) orally as a single dose or 3—4 divided doses 4—6 hourly **OR**
- (Elderly) 500—750 micrograms orally as a single dose or 3—4 divided doses 4—6 hourly **OR**
- (Adults, children >10 years) 0.5—1 mg slowly IV over at least 5 minutes as a single dose or in divided doses of 0.25—0.5 mg 4—6-hourly **OR**
- (Elderly) 250—500 micrograms slowly IV over at least 5 minutes as a single dose or in divided doses of 125—250 micrograms every 4—6-hourly

ANTIARRHYTHMIC AGENTS

Maintenance dose
- (Normal renal function) 250 micrograms orally once or twice daily **OR**
- (Elderly or impaired renal function) 125 micrograms orally daily or in 2 divided doses

Adverse effects
- anorexia, nausea, vomiting, diarrhoea, abdominal pain
- rash, urticaria
- blurred vision, visual disturbances (including yellow/green/white vision or coloured haloes)
- dizziness, headache, drowsiness, CNS disturbances
- arrhythmias, bradycardia, bigeminy (coupled beats), trigeminy, PR-prolongation, conduction disturbances
- (Uncommon) depression
- (Rare) intestinal ischaemia, thrombocytopenia, allergic reaction (rash, eosinophilia), gynaecomastia (long-term therapy)
- (Digoxin toxicity) dysrhythmias, decreased appetite, nausea, vomiting, fatigue, malaise, muscle weakness, blurred vision or visual disturbances (such as yellow or green haloes), headache, drowsiness, dizziness, confusion, disorientation, seizures and, rarely, hallucinations and psychosis

Interactions
- the risk of digoxin toxicity is increased by hypokalaemia, which may result from the associated administration of alcohol, amphotericin B (amphotericin), beta2 adrenergic bronchodilators, corticosteroids, corticotrophin, diuretics, edetate disodium, insulin, laxatives, lithium salts, potassium-losing diuretics, sodium polystyrene sulfonate hydrogen or sodium bicarbonate; therefore potassium levels should be closely monitored if given together
- effects of digoxin are enhanced by hypokalaemia, hypomagnesaemia and hypoxia, increasing the risk of digoxin toxicity
- an increased risk of digoxin-induced arrhythmias if given to those with hypercalcaemia or hyperkalaemia. Hyperkalaemia may result from administration of medication that increases serum potassium levels, such as angiotensin converting enzyme (ACE) inhibitors, amiloride, ciclosporin, indometacin, potassium supplements, spironolactone, suxamethonium, tacrolimus and high doses of potassium-containing penicillins; therefore potassium levels should be closely monitored if given together
- ineffective if given when the patient is hypocalcaemic; therefore calcium levels should be rectified before therapy is started
- the risk of toxicity is increased with agents that lower extracellular potassium, such as glucagon, large doses of glucose and glucose—insulin infusions; therefore potassium levels should be closely monitored if given together
- serum digoxin levels may be increased by ACE inhibitors, alprazolam, amiodarone, atorvastatin, IV calcium salts, captopril, ciclosporin, diazepam, diltiazem, diphenoxylate with atropine, erythromycin, felodipine, flecainide, gentamicin, indometacin, itraconazole, nifedipine, prazosin, propantheline, quinine, spironolactone, tetracyclines, trimethoprim or verapamil
- serum digoxin levels are reduced by acarbose, adrenaline (epinephrine), metoclopramide, penicillamine, phenytoin, rifampicin, salbutamol, St John's wort and some bulk-forming laxatives
- absorption of digoxin is reduced by some antacids, colestyramine, kaolin—pectin, neomycin, rifampicin and sulfasalazine
- beta adrenoceptor blocking agents may potentiate bradycardia and heart block. ECG and serum digoxin levels should be carefully monitored during therapy
- may increase the risk of arrhythmias when given with adrenaline (epinephrine), calcium salts (IV), ephedrine,

pancuronium, pseudoephedrine or suxamethonium. ECG monitoring is recommended if given together
- the risk of toxicity increases with hypoxia
- excessive bradycardia may occur if given with verapamil or diltiazem; therefore ECG is recommended if the combination is given
- extreme caution if given with IV magnesium salts, as heart block may occur

Nursing considerations/Cautions

- dosage is highly individualised and toxicity can occur at or close to the therapeutic range in some people
- consideration should be given to whether a digitalising loading dose is required or not. If there is no emergency or urgency, the maintenance dose may be started as the initial dose, but the optimal effect will take 5–7 days to occur
- distribution into body fat is poor, so the dose should be based on ideal lean body weight rather than total body weight
- therapeutic serum digoxin level is close to the toxic concentration, leaving only a narrow margin of safety, so serum levels should be monitored in premature infants, the elderly and patients with impaired kidney or thyroid function or electrolyte imbalance
- symptoms of toxicity commonly occur at serum levels > 2 nanogram/mL
- a blood sample for establishing serum digoxin levels should be taken 6–8 hours after the last dose or immediately before the next dose is due
- serum electrolytes and kidney function (serum creatinine) should be monitored regularly during therapy
- predisposing factors to toxicity include hypercalcaemia, hypokalaemia, hypomagnesaemia and/or co-existing conditions such as renal factors; therefore these conditions should be treated before starting therapy with digoxin if possible. Caution if used in those with hypercalcaemia or hyperkalaemia, as there is an increased risk of primary heart block and/or digitalis-induced arrhythmias
- hypokalaemia sensitises the heart to digoxin and so may induce toxicity. Hypokalaemia can be caused by malnutrition, diarrhoea, dialysis, long-standing heart failure, increased age, prolonged vomiting and some drugs (e.g. corticosteroids, diuretics such as frusemide (furosemide) and thiazides). The patient should be closely monitored if any of these occur
- severe vitamin B_1 deficiency (beriberi) should be corrected before starting therapy
- note any improvement, such as return of heart rate to within normal limits, reduced cyanosis, easier breathing, reduced oedema, reduced pulse deficit and increased urinary output
- select the correct preparation, noting especially when the weaker formulations of digoxin are prescribed: Lanoxin PG (paediatric–geriatric), Lanoxin Paediatric Elixir (50 microgram/mL) or Lanoxin Paediatric Injection (50 microgram/2 mL)
- for a dose of 0.125 mg, give 2 tablets of 62.5 micrograms, not half a 0.25 mg tablet
- IM or SC is not recommended, as digoxin absorption may be unpredictable and cause prolonged intense pain and muscle necrosis
- may be added to sodium chloride 0.9%, glucose 5% or glucose 4% plus sodium chloride 0.18% and given slowly IV over at least 5 minutes, avoiding extravasation
- rapid IV administration should be avoided because it may cause vasoconstriction and hypertension and/or reduced coronary flow
- not given by continuous IV infusion
- anorexia, nausea and vomiting may occur in the absence of digoxin toxicity

- because of gastric irritation and stimulation of the vomiting centre by the drug itself or because of the congestive heart failure
- patients receiving both digoxin and diuretics should have electrolytes measured regularly
- digoxin should be withdrawn 1–2 days before cardiac surgery or cardioversion. In emergency situations, such as cardiac arrest, the lowest possible energy should be applied
- patients with digoxin toxicity are at greater risk of arrhythmias when cardioverted
- digoxin-specific immune antigen binding fragment — f(Ab) — is used for overdosage (see p. 345). It may be several days before a reduction in digoxin dose is reflected in a new serum concentration; however, neurological and visual symptoms may continue after other signs of toxicity have resolved
- digoxin is tissue bound; therefore it is not removed by peritoneal dialysis or haemodialysis
- have facilities available for cardiac monitoring, defibrillation and resuscitation
- patients with malabsorption syndrome or GI reconstruction may require a higher dose to achieve the clinical effect
- caution if used in those with kidney impairment or failure
- caution if used in those with thyroid disease, as hyperthyroidism will make the person less sensitive and hypothyroidism will make the person more sensitive to the effects of digoxin. Half-life is prolonged in hypothyroidism and decreased in hyperthyroidism
- caution if used in those with carotid sinus hypersensitivity, acute glomerulonephritis with cardiac failure, idiopathic hypertrophic subaortic stenosis, hypoxia or sick sinus syndrome
- caution if used in those with ischaemic heart disease, the acute phase of post-myocardial infarction, myxoedema or severe pulmonary/respiratory disease because of an increased risk of digitalis-induced arrhythmias
- not recommended in those with constrictive pericarditis, heart failure associated with cardiac amyloidosis or myocarditis
- contraindicated in those with intermittent complete heart block, second-degree AV block (especially if Stokes–Adams attacks have previously occurred), ventricular tachycardia, ventricular fibrillation, arrhythmias due to digoxin toxicity, supraventricular arrhythmia with accessory AV pathway (e.g. Wolff–Parkinson–White syndrome), hypertrophic obstructive cardiomyopathy or hypersensitivity to other digitalis glycosides

Patient education

- advise the patient to seek medical advice immediately if any of the following occur:
  - loss of appetite, nausea, vomiting or diarrhoea
  - slow heart rate
  - unusual tiredness or extreme weakness
  - blurred vision or coloured haloes around objects
- discuss with the patient the importance of not taking vitamin or potassium supplements, or taking any medications (including herbal preparations or OTC preparations) without first discussing these with the doctor or pharmacist
- warn the patient against driving or operating machinery if dizziness or blurred vision occurs
- if elixir is used, the calibrated dropper should be used to administer the dose
- if the patient is female and of childbearing capacity, counsel them regarding the importance of not becoming

pregnant or immediately seeking medical advice if she becomes pregnant

Tablets do not disperse easily in water. Tablet can be crushed and given with a spoonful of yoghurt or apple puree.

Dose adjustment may be necessary during pregnancy.

Digoxin levels in breastmilk are low and unlikely to cause harm to the infant. To reduce exposure further, avoid breast-feeding for 2 hours after intravenous doses.

Predominantly renally cleared (~50–70%); reduce the dose in renal impairment; when CrCl is < 60 mL/min, the dose should be halved to prevent accumulation and toxicity.

Elderly patients may have reduced renal clearance and increased sensitivity to digoxin. To avoid toxicity, the dose should be reduced, and digoxin concentrations should be closely monitored. Regular monitoring of renal function is also essential in this population.

ANTIASTHMA AGENTS, BRONCHODILATORS AND RESPIRATORY AGENTS

Asthma prevalence in Australia is approximately 11%, equating to just over 2.8 million people, with Australian First Nations people having the higher burden of disease (AIHW 2024). Health expenditure on asthma accounts for approximately 0.6% of the total health care budget (about AU$851 million) in 2020–21. Furthermore, asthma accounted for 467 deaths in 2022, with those aged 5–34 being at the greatest risk (AIHW 2024).

In susceptible people, asthma may be triggered by a number of allergens; however, the common cold is the most likely trigger. Some triggers are avoidable (e.g. cigarette smoke), whereas others are not. Asthma triggers include animal allergens (e.g. pets, animals in workplace), house dust mites, pollen, moulds, airborne or environmental irritants (e.g. cold or dry air, household aerosols, industrial or traffic pollution, perfumes/scents, smoke (e.g. bushfire, indoor wood fires) and more recently thunderstorms). In addition, some medications can trigger asthma, including aspirin, non-steroidal NSAIDs and beta adrenoceptor blocking agents (beta blockers), as well as dietary triggers (e.g. food chemicals or additives, if the person is intolerant) and thermal effects (e.g. cold drinks). Other triggers include physiological exertion (e.g. exercise), and psychological changes (e.g. extreme emotions), hormonal changes (including pregnancy, sexual activity) and comorbid medical conditions (e.g. obesity, allergic rhinitis, nasal polyposis) (National Asthma Council Australia 2022).

During an asthma attack, bronchospasm causes wheezing, coughing, breathing difficulties, mucosal oedema and the formation of mucus. The asthma process is thought to be caused in part by IgE antibodies attaching to mast cells, causing degranulation and the production and release of inflammatory mediators (histamine, leukotrienes, cytokines, eosinophil and neutrophil chemotactic factors) and leading to hyperresponsiveness of the bronchioles. Antihistamines are not useful in asthma management, which suggests that histamine plays only a minor role (Knights et al 2023).

The goal of asthma management is to relieve and control symptoms, prevent acute asthma and death, and maintain best lung function and quality of life for the person with asthma. It therefore involves the use of both symptomatic and prophylactic treatment. Antiasthma drugs can be divided into symptom relievers, symptom controllers and symptom preventers.

Symptom relievers (bronchodilators)
- short-acting beta2 adrenoceptor agonists (e.g. salbutamol, terbutaline)
- anticholinergic (antimuscarinic) agents (e.g. ipratropium)
- xanthines (e.g. theophylline)

Symptom controllers (bronchodilators)
- longer-acting beta2 adrenoceptor agonists (e.g. salmeterol, formoterol (eformoterol))

Symptom preventers (prophylactic and anti-inflammatory drugs)
- mast cell stabilisers (e.g. sodium cromoglycate, nedocromil sodium)
- inhaled corticosteroids (anti-inflammatory) (e.g. budesonide, fluticasone)
- leukotriene-receptor antagonists (anti-inflammatory) (e.g. montelukast)
- oral or parenteral corticosteroids (anti-inflammatory)

The patient should develop a written *asthma action plan* in collaboration with a GP or respiratory doctor. The plan should outline the usual asthma (and allergy) medications, instructions on how to change medications if needed (e.g. if asthma worsens) and when and how to get medical care (especially in the event of an emergency); it should include the name of the person preparing the plan with a date. This plan should be updated regularly (AIHW 2024). In 2020–21, 34% of people across all age groups had a written asthma plan, and 69% of children (14 years and under) had written plans (AIHW 2024).

A study by Roman-Rodriguez and colleagues (2019) found that poor asthma control and exacerbations could, in part, be related to poor inhaler technique resulting in no or insufficient medication reaching the lungs. Given that many of the agents used to manage asthma (both preventers and relievers) are delivered via some sort of inhaler device, it would appear to be of critical importance to optimise inhaler technique. The authors identified a number of issues including poor coordination between actuation and inhalation of the medication when using a metered dose inhaler, incomplete inspiration or failing to hold breath adequately, after inspiration and being prescribed multiple inhaled medications, leading to confusion. The authors concluded that two critical points in improving asthma control were correct device selection and sufficient education (including practice using the device) (Roman-Rodriguez et al 2019).

General Patient education for anti-asthma agents and bronchodilators

- before instructing any patient on correct techniques for monitoring and management of their asthma, it is important to ascertain that the person understands what asthma is (including its seriousness) and identify any avoidable triggers
- instruct patient in the correct technique for:
  - regularly monitoring peak flow using a peak flow meter
  - using metered dose aerosol inhalers, nebulisers, accuhalers, spacers or other inhalation devices (there are a number of 'how to' videos on correct inhaler technique available from

- the importance of carrying a short-acting beta2 agonist (e.g. salbutamol) for use when acute symptom relief is necessary
- long-acting bronchodilators are for maintenance, not acute episodes, and should be used regularly to keep asthma controlled
- ensure that patient is aware of their triggers and knows how to avoid or manage them (e.g. using medication before known exposure)
- advise patient to wear a MedicAlert bracelet or pendant in case of respiratory emergencies, especially if using inhaled or oral corticosteroids
- advise patient to seek medical advice promptly if symptoms worsen or medication does not provide its normal relief, as asthma can be a life-threatening condition
- advise patient against overuse of inhalers containing propellants, as both propellant and active substance can be hazardous in large quantities
- warn patient against driving or operating machinery if dizziness, fatigue, blurred vision or other visual problems occur
- asthma control is important for both maternal and fetal health

Spacer device

- a spacer device may be useful for those with poor inhalation technique or to decrease adverse effects related to the amount of powder directly reaching the mouth and throat
- the patient should be informed that changing brands of spacer device may alter the amount of medication delivered to the lungs
- instruct patient in the correct technique for using their inhaler in conjunction with a spacer device. The inhaler is actuated into the spacer; the patient should then breathe in slowly and as far as possible. Breath is then held for as long as possible before breathing out slowly. If multiple inhalations are required, time in between should be minimised
- the spacer device should be washed with warm water and detergent before first use and then at least monthly. It should be allowed to air dry. A cloth should not be used to dry the spacer device as this produces static electricity, which causes the medication to stick to the sides of the device, thereby reducing the amount available to reach the lungs
- it is important to note that some medication is lost in the spacer because of electrostatic attraction between the plastic spacer device and the medication

Nebuliser

- no substances other than the prescribed diluent should be added to the nebuliser solution (sodium chloride 0.9% or distilled water or propylene glycol spray diluent)
- nebuliser solution may be delivered undiluted, but is usually diluted to allow efficient operation of the nebuliser
- most nebulisers deliver 1 mL of solution over 3 minutes and 2 mL over 8–10 minutes. If given using medical oxygen or medical air rather than via compression pump, the rate should be > 6 L/min
- a small compressed air pump can be used at home to provide pressure for nebulisation
- any solution remaining in the nebuliser after therapy should be discarded. The chamber and mask

should be rinsed after use and allowed to air dry to prevent build-up of medication
- any solution remaining after the stock bottle has been opened for 3 months should be discarded

Aerolizer
- ensure the patient knows the manufacturer's instruction leaflet is in the Aerolizer packet
- instruct patient in the correct use of the Aerolizer, including:
  1. pull cap off inhalation device
  2. to open device, hold base and turn mouthpiece in the direction of the arrow
  3. ensuring fingers/hands are dry, remove capsule from foil pack immediately before use
  4. place capsule in capsule-shaped slot, ensuring that it is on the bottom and lying flat
  5. twist mouthpiece until a 'click' is heard. The mouthpiece is now closed
  6. hold the Aerolizer upright; firmly squeeze the two blue buttons at the same time and then release. This will pierce the capsule — only do this once (piercing more often may release gelatin from the capsule shell, which can then be inhaled into the mouth or throat)
  7. while holding the Aerolizer upright, open the mouthpiece and ensure the capsule is loose so that it can spin on inhalation; close the mouthpiece
  8. breathe out as far as possible
  9. place the mouthpiece well into the mouth, with the lips closed firmly around it and the head tilted back slightly. Breathe in quickly and evenly and as deeply as possible (a whirring sound should be heard as the capsule spins)
  10. hold the breath for as long as possible. Remove the Aerolizer and breathe out through nose
  11. check Aerolizer to see if any powder is left. If there is, repeat steps 8 to 10
  12. remove the empty capsule and wipe the mouthpiece and capsule slot with a dry cloth. Do not use water to clean the Aerolizer
  13. close the mouthpiece and put the cap on

BRONCHODILATORS (BETA2 ADRENOCEPTOR AGONISTS (ALSO CALLED BETA2 AGONISTS))

General Adverse effects of beta2 adrenoceptor agonists

Common effects
- fine skeletal muscle tremor (due to beta effects), especially in the hands, palpitations, increased heart rate/tachycardia (beta effects), nervousness, headache

Less common
- dizziness, insomnia
- anxiety, agitation
- bad taste
- muscle cramps, myalgia
- (Inhalation) cough, mouth and throat irritation, hoarse voice, dry mouth, increase in asthma symptoms, dyspnoea
- (Rare) hyperglycaemia, paradoxical bronchospasm, hypokalaemia, rash, arrhythmias, exacerbation of existing arrhythmias, hypersensitivity reaction
- (Rare, high dose) cardionecrosis, lactic acidosis

ANTIASTHMA AGENTS, BRONCHODILATORS AND RESPIRATORY AGENTS

General Interactions of beta2 adrenoceptor agonists
- theophylline, other xanthines, corticosteroids and potassium-losing diuretics, and hypoxia may increase the risk of hypokalaemia if given with beta2 adrenoreceptor agonists
- hypoxia may aggravate effect of hypokalaemia on cardiac rhythm, increasing the risk of arrhythmia
- increased risk of cardiac arrhythmias if given to those with hypokalaemia induced by salbutamol or another beta2 agonist
- not recommended with sympathomimetic agents
- caution if given with anaesthetic agents, as these may sensitise the myocardium to catecholamines
- increased risk of hypokalaemia and hyperglycaemia when given with glucocorticoids (corticosteroids)
- bronchodilator effect may be inhibited by beta adrenoceptor blocking agents (including ophthalmic preparations), which are therefore not recommended together
- increased risk of arrhythmias if given with digoxin or other cardiac glycosides because of salbutamol or other beta2 agonist-induced hypokalaemia

FORMOTEROL (EFORMOTEROL)
Trade names
Foradile, Oxis Turbuhaler

Available forms
Capsules: 12 microgram (for Aerolizer device);
Metered dose Turbuhaler: 6 microgram/inhalation, 12 microgram/inhalation

Action
- potent, long-acting selective beta2 adrenoceptor agonist
- inhibits histamine and leukotriene release
- some anti-inflammatory properties
- onset 1—3 minutes, peak effect 1—2 hours, duration 12 hours
- symptom controller for maintenance

Use
- long-term regular treatment of reversible airway obstruction associated with asthma in patients having concurrent corticosteroid therapy, including exercise-induced asthma, nocturnal asthma
- prophylaxis and treatment of bronchoconstriction associated with reversible/irreversible chronic obstructive pulmonary disease (COPD)

Dose
- (Asthma) 1—2 inhalations (12—24 micrograms) twice daily (daily maximum 48 micrograms) (Foradile) **OR**
- (Asthma) 6—12 micrograms twice daily, up to 24 micrograms twice daily if necessary (daily maximum 48 micrograms) (Oxis) **OR**
- (COPD) 1 inhalation (12 micrograms) twice daily (Foradile)

Adverse effects
- exacerbation of asthma
- (Rare) prolongation of QT interval
- see also General Adverse effects of beta2 adrenoceptor agonists (p. 100)

Interactions
- increased risk of prolonged QT interval and arrhythmias if given with other agents known to prolong QT interval such as monoamine oxidase inhibitors (MAOIs), tricyclic antidepressants (TCAs), erythromycin, disopyramide, phenothiazines or antihistamines
- not recommended with other long-acting beta2 adrenoceptor agonists
- see also General Interactions of beta2 adrenoceptor agonists

Nursing considerations/Cautions
- should be used only as an adjunct to inhaled corticosteroid therapy in those with asthma
- therapy should not be started in those with unstable or acutely deteriorating asthma
- once symptoms are controlled, consideration should be given to reducing dose

- not recommended in those under 5 years
- not recommended in those whose asthma can be managed with short-acting beta2 agonists
- can increase blood glucose levels; therefore use with caution in those with diabetes mellitus
- use with caution in those with ischaemic heart disease, arrhythmias or severe heart failure as they are more likely to experience cardiovascular side-effects
- use with caution in those with idiopathic subvalvular aortic stenosis, hypertrophic obstructive cardiomyopathy, acquired/congenital QT interval prolongation, thyrotoxicosis or inadequately controlled hyperthyroidism, severe hypertension, phaeochromocytoma, aneurysm or severe cardiac decompensation
- contraindicated in those with rare hereditary galactose intolerance, Lapp lactase deficiency or glucose—galactose malabsorption, as capsules contain lactose

Patient education

- ensure the patient understands that this medication is not recommended for use during an acute asthma episode
- the patient should be advised to continue concurrent corticosteroid therapy, even if symptoms are improved
- warn the patient that tremor and palpitations may be experienced
- those with diabetes should be instructed to monitor blood glucose levels, especially when starting therapy
- if the patient has underlying heart disease, advise them to seek medical advice immediately if chest pain or signs of worsening heart disease, including shortness of breath, occur during therapy
- ensure that the patient understands capsules are for use with the Aerolizer, and not to be taken orally
- instruct the patient on the correct use of the Aerolizer (p. 100) or Turbuhaler (p. 110)

- see also General Patient education for antiasthma agents and bronchodilators (p. 98)

Limited data available, but considered safe when breastfeeding.

Prohibited in and out of competition orally or via nebuliser. Conditional use in and out of competition via metered dose inhaler (maximum dose 54 micrograms in 24 hours)

Available in combination with

- aclidinium 340 microgram/actuation + formoterol fumarate dihydrate 12 microgram/actuation powder for inhalation
- beclometasone dipropionate + formeterol fumarate dihydrate combination (see beclometasone p. 123)
- beclometasone dipropionate + formeterol fumarate dihydrate + glycopyrronium combination (see beclometasone p. 123)
- budesonide + formoterol fumarate dihydrate combinations (see budesonide p. 124)
- fluticasone propionate + formoterol fumarate dihydrate combinations (see fluticasone propionate p. 130)

INDACATEROL
Trade name
Onbrez Breezhaler

Available form
Powder for inhalation: 150 microgram, 300 microgram

Action
- ultra-long-acting beta2 adrenergic agonist
- rapid onset within 5 minutes, peak effect 2—4 hours, long duration of action

Use
- treatment of airflow limitation in those with chronic obstructive pulmonary disease (COPD)

Dose
- 150 micrograms once daily by inhalation via Breezhaler, increasing to 300 micrograms if needed

Adverse effects
- nasopharyngitis, cough, upper respiratory tract infection, sinusitis, oropharyngeal pain, rhinorrhoea
- headache
- muscle spasm, myalgia
- dry mouth
- hypokalaemia
- hyperglycaemia
- peripheral oedema, chest pain
- (Rare) hypersensitivity (breathing or swallowing difficulties, swelling of tongue, lips or face, urticaria, rash), paradoxical bronchospasm, prolongation of QT interval

Interactions
- increased risk of prolonged QT interval and arrhythmias if given with other agents known to prolong QT interval, such as monoamine oxidase inhibitors (MAOIs), tricyclic antidepressants (TCAs), erythromycin, disopyramide, phenothiazines or antihistamines
- not recommended with other beta2 adrenoceptor agonists
- see also General Interactions of beta2 adrenoceptor agonists (p. 101)

Nursing considerations/Cautions
- should not be used in those with asthma or mixed airways disease, which should be excluded before starting therapy
- not recommended for initial treatment of acute symptomatic COPD exacerbations
- if COPD worsens despite treatment, the patient should be re-evaluated
- not recommended in those < 18 years
- beta2 adrenoceptor agonists can increase blood glucose levels; therefore use with caution in those with diabetes mellitus
- use with caution in those with coronary artery disease, acute myocardial infarction, cardiac arrhythmia, hypertension, epilepsy or thyrotoxicosis, or if the patient is known to be unresponsive to beta2 adrenergic agonist therapy
- contraindicated in those with rare hereditary galactose intolerance, Lapp lactase deficiency or glucose—galactose malabsorption, as capsules contain lactose

Patient education
- advise the patient to continue long-term inhaled corticosteroids with indacaterol therapy
- instruct the patient to seek medical advice if they have difficulty breathing or swallowing, or swelling of the tongue, lips or face occurs
- ensure the patient understands that indacaterol should not be used to relieve an acute attack of breathlessness or wheezing
- if the patient has underlying heart disease, advise them to seek medical advice immediately if chest pain or signs of worsening heart disease, including shortness of breath, occur during therapy
- those with diabetes should be instructed to monitor blood glucose levels, especially when starting therapy
- instruct patient that:
  1. capsules are for use with the Breezhaler only and should not be taken orally
  2. it should be administered at the same time each day
  3. capsules should be stored in the blister pack and only removed just before use
  4. the correct use of the Breezhaler (inhalation device supplied) is important to ensure the whole dose is administered, including:
  5. remove the cap and open the mouthpiece

6. after removing the capsule from the blister pack, place in the chamber and close the mouthpiece (until a click is heard)
7. do not shake, but press the side buttons in once and then release
8. breathe out gently (away from the inhaler) and then place the mouth over the mouthpiece (without biting) to form a good seal
9. breathe in quickly and steadily (the capsule should vibrate)
10. hold the breath for as long as is comfortable (or at least 5 seconds)
11. while holding the breath, remove the inhaler from the mouth and breathe out gently (away from the inhaler)
12. open the mouthpiece and remove the used capsule
13. if other doses are required, repeat steps 3—8
14. close the mouthpiece and cap
- see also General Patient education for antiasthma agents and bronchodilators (p. 98)

Limited human data available, but considered safe when breastfeeding.

Prohibited in sport and requires approval in the form of a therapeutic use exemption.

Available in combination with
- indacaterol 110 microgram + glycopyrronium 50 microgram powder for inhalation (Ultibro Breezhaler 110/50)
- indacaterol 114 microgram + glycopyrronium 46 microgram + mometasone furoate 68 microgram powder for inhalation (Enerzair Breezhaler 114/46/68)
- indacaterol 114 microgram + glycopyrronium 46 microgram + mometasone furoate 136 microgram powder for inhalation (Enerzair Breezhaler 114/46/136)
- indacaterol 125 microgram + mometasone furoate 62.5 microgram powder for inhalation (Atectura Breezhaler 125/127.5)
- indacaterol 125 microgram + mometasone furoate 127.5 microgram powder for inhalation (Atectura Breezhaler 125/127.5)
- indacaterol 125 microgram + mometasone furoate 260 microgram powder for inhalation (Atectura Breezhaler 125/260)

SALBUTAMOL (known as albuterol in the USA)
Trade names
Airomir Autohaler and Inhaler, Asmol CFC-free Inhaler, Ventolin preparations, Ventolin Obstetric Injection, Zempreon CFC-Free Inhaler

Available forms
Inhaler/Autohaler: 100 microgram/metered dose;
Nebules/Sterinebs/Ampoules (for inhalation): 2.5 mg/2.5 mL, 5 mg/2.5 mL;
Syrup (sugar free): 2 mg/5 mL;
Rotacap capsules: 200 microgram;
Injection: 500 microgram/mL, 1 mg/mL

Action
- selective beta2 adrenoreceptor stimulant causing bronchodilation, mainly by stimulating pulmonary receptors
- relaxes uterine and blood vessel smooth muscle
- some cardiac stimulation
- onset of action 5—15 minutes, duration of action 3—6 hours
- symptom reliever

Use
- prevention of relief-reversible bronchospasm in asthma or chronic obstructive pulmonary disease (COPD)
- acute prophylaxis against exercise-induced asthma (or other known triggers)
- management of uncomplicated premature labour (24—33 weeks' gestation) (see Pregnancy, childbirth and breastfeeding, p. 1475)

ANTIASTHMA AGENTS, BRONCHODILATORS AND RESPIRATORY AGENTS

Dose
- 2—4 mg (5—10 mL) orally 3—4 times daily **OR**
- 5 mg via nebuliser 4- to 6-hourly **OR**
- 1—2 inhalations (100—200 micrograms) 4-hourly as required (if 2 inhalations are required, allow a 1-minute interval) (daily maximum 16 inhalations (8 treatments) (metered dose aerosol inhaler / Autohaler) **OR**
- 500 micrograms SC or IM 3—4-hourly **OR**
- 200—300 micrograms over 1 minute IV, repeated after 15 minutes if required **OR**
- 200 micrograms IV over 1 minute (loading dose), then 5—20 microgram/min as IV infusion

Adverse effects
- (IM, SC, IM) stinging, pain
- see also General Adverse effects of beta2 adrenoreceptor agonists (p. 100)

Interactions
- combination of nebulised salbutamol and ipratropium may result in closed-angle glaucoma
- see also General Interactions of beta2 adrenoceptor agonists (p. 101)

Nursing considerations/Cautions
- monitor vital signs, noting that an elevation of heart rate may be a side-effect and a reduced heart rate a sign of improvement
- before increasing dose, patient inhaler techniques should be checked
- symptoms of overdose are eased by rest and reassurance
- note and report any cardiac arrhythmias, especially in patients receiving digoxin, as these may result from salbutamol-induced hypokalaemia
- patient may also be prescribed an inhaled corticosteroid (e.g. fluticasone), in which case it is taken about 10 minutes after the salbutamol. Salbutamol promotes bronchodilation, maximising inhalation of the corticosteroid
- excessive inhalation of the aerosol should be avoided to prevent overdose of the active therapeutic agent and reduce the risk of hazards from the propellant and of worsening hypoxaemia
- parenteral salbutamol (IM, IV) is used only in cases of severe bronchospasm or status asthmaticus, in conjunction with glucocorticoids and oxygen therapy
- adverse effects are more common when salbutamol is given IV or IM
- if used IV in those with diabetes mellitus, solution should be diluted using sodium chloride 0.9% only
- if given by injection, IM is the route of choice
- (Nebuliser) most nebulisers deliver 1 mL over 3 minutes or 2 mL over 8—10 minutes
- (Nebuliser) fresh dilution should be prepared for each inhalation, any residue discarded and nebuliser cleaned
- can increase blood glucose levels; therefore use with caution in those with diabetes mellitus
- use with caution in those with liver or kidney dysfunction as lower doses may be required
- use with caution in those who have hypertension, coronary artery disease, congestive cardiac failure, phaeochromocytoma, diabetes mellitus, recent myocardial infarction, hyperthyroidism or thyrotoxicosis
- (Dry powder inhaler formulation) is contraindicated in patients with severe milk protein allergy

Patient education
- instruct the patient that exercise-induced bronchospasm may be prevented by 2 inhalations (200 micrograms) 15 minutes before exertion
- advise the patient of the benefit of a small dose early in an attack before bronchospasm becomes too severe

- counsel patient that, in an emergency, 6 puffs are taken immediately then 1 puff every 5 minutes while seeking medical attention
- warn patient against overuse of inhaled salbutamol as it may lead to worsening of hypoxaemia
- overdose may be avoided by instructing the patient thoroughly in the correct use of the metered dose aerosol inhaler, other inhaler devices and nebuliser, and ensuring that the inhaler is not used if the patient is receiving salbutamol by another means
- warn patient that tremor and palpitations are commonly experienced
- instruct patient to seek medical advice immediately if not obtaining adequate relief (i.e. if effect of each dose lasts for less than 3 hours)
- warn patient to avoid mist contacting eyes (e.g. ensuring nebulising mask fits correctly), especially if person is predisposed to glaucoma
- patient with diabetes should be advised to closely monitor blood glucose levels during therapy
- instruct patient that oral syrup may be diluted with purified water only. Diluted mixture should be used within 28 days and protected from light
- patients should be advised not to drive or operate machinery if they experience adverse effects
- if patient has underlying heart disease, advise them to seek medical advice immediately if experiencing chest pain or signs of worsening heart disease, including shortness of breath, occur during therapy
- see also General Patient education for antiasthma agents and bronchodilators (p. 98)

Metered dose aerosol inhaler
- advise patient that the manufacturer's instruction leaflet is in the inhaler packet and should be referred to
- instruct patient in the correct technique for a metered dose aerosol inhaler:
  - load inhaler with salbutamol canister
  - remove the mouthpiece cap and shake the inhaler well
  - prime the inhaler by activating the aerosol 2 or 3 times into the air to ensure the spray is even
  - hold the inhaler vertically with the mouthpiece at the bottom and breathe out slowly and fully
  - place the mouthpiece well into the mouth, with lips closed firmly around it and the head tilted back slightly
  - inhale rapidly and deeply through the mouthpiece, at the same time administering a metered dose by pressing the canister downwards
  - release pressure on the canister and remove the inhaler while holding the breath for as long as possible (10 seconds)
  - breathe out slowly through the mouth and replace the mouthpiece cap
- if two inhalations are required, allow a 5-minute interval before taking the second to enable better assessment of the first inhalation and deeper penetration of the second inhalation
- the patient can practise with a placebo inhaler (contains air)
- warn patient that the pressurised container should be kept intact and away from heat
- the canister is about 1/4 full if it floats at about 45 degrees on the surface of a bowl of water (i.e. the patient needs to obtain new canister)
- children can usually manage a metered dose aerosol inhaler from about 7 years of age, but should be supervised by a responsible adult until competent
- a CFC-free inhaler needs to be primed before first use or if unused for 5 days or more
- canisters should be protected from frost, as cold temperatures may decrease therapeutic effect
- the inhaler should be cleaned at least once a week by removing the metal canister from the plastic casing as well as

ANTIASTHMA AGENTS, BRONCHODILATORS AND RESPIRATORY AGENTS

the mouthpiece cover. The actuator should be rinsed under warm running water and then dried inside and out. The metal canister and mouthpiece cover should then be replaced. The metal canister should not be put into water

Rotahaler

- the Rotahaler is a breath-actuated device that breaks the Rotacap in half, while the airflow through the device during inspiration disperses the powder in the inspired air
- suitable for children aged from 3 to 6 years and others unable to coordinate the use of the metered dose aerosol inhaler, and in severe asthma with low inspiratory flow rate
- ensure the patient understands that Rotacaps are not for oral use
- instruct the patient in the correct technique for the Rotahaler:
  1. remove the Rotahaler from the container and hold it vertically by the dark blue mouthpiece with the light blue body uppermost
  2. turn the light blue body of the Rotahaler as far as it will go in either direction
  3. push the Rotacap, clear end first, firmly into the square hole, forcing any previously used Rotacap shell into the Rotahaler
  4. holding the Rotahaler horizontally to prevent its contents from falling out, turn the light blue body as far as it will go in the opposite direction to open the Rotacap
  5. breathe out slowly and, keeping the Rotahaler completely level, grip the mouthpiece between the teeth, with the lips closed firmly around it and head tilted back slightly
  6. inhale rapidly and deeply through the mouthpiece
  7. remove the Rotahaler, hold the breath as long as possible, then breathe out slowly through the mouth
  8. after each use, pull the two halves of the Rotahaler apart and remove loose Rotacap shells
  9. reassemble and store in the container
- the Rotahaler may be cleaned once every 2 weeks by rinsing both halves in warm water and drying thoroughly (removing empty shells first)
- protect the Rotahaler from heat and from dirt and damage by keeping it in its container
- Rotacaps are designed to be used with the Rotahaler for patients unable to satisfactorily use a metered dose aerosol inhaler, including children. Children's use should be supervised by a responsible adult

Autohaler

- advise the patient that the manufacturer's instruction leaflet is in the Autohaler packet
- instruct the patient in the correct technique for the Autohaler:
  1. if the Autohaler is new or unused for 2 weeks, release 4 puffs into the air (away from the face)
  2. remove the mouthpiece cover by unclipping it from the back. Check that it is clean
  3. hold the Autohaler upright and shake vigorously
  4. continue holding the Autohaler upright (without blocking the vents in the base) and push the lever up
  5. breathe out as far as possible and close the lips around the mouthpiece
  6. breathe in slowly and deeply, and continue to do so when you hear a click and feel the puff in mouth
  7. hold the breath for as long as comfortable (or at least 10 seconds) and then breathe out slowly
  8. after each puff, return the lever to the down position while keeping the Autohaler upright
  9. push the lever up before each puff and gently back down afterwards,

keeping the Autohaler upright. The lever should be left down between treatments
10. if more than 1 dose is required, steps 4—8 should be repeated
- the Autohaler should be cleaned weekly by wiping the mouthpiece only with a clean dry cloth. Other parts of the Autohaler should not be cleaned
- to check if the Autohaler is empty, remove the mouthpiece cover by unclipping it from the back. Shake the Autohaler and, holding it upright with the mouthpiece away from you, push the lever up and release a puff by pushing the dose-release slide on the bottom of the Autohaler in the direction of the arrow. To release a second puff, first return the lever to the down position and repeat. Repeat this 4 times in total. If the Autohaler is empty, you will not feel or hear a puff being discharged
- the dose-release slide is for testing the Autohaler ONLY; it should not be used to deliver medication

Salbutamol metered dose aerosol inhalers are considered safe to use in pregnancy.

Salbutamol is considered safe when breastfeeding.

(IV, oral) banned in sport.

(Inhalers, nebulising solution) use in sport subject to conditions.

SALMETEROL
Trade name
Serevent

Available form
Accuhaler: 50 microgram/blister

Action
- selective long-acting beta2 adrenoceptor agonist
- onset of action within 10—30 minutes, peak effect 3—4 hours, duration 12 hours
- symptom controller

Use
- long-term management of reversible airways obstruction in asthma or chronic obstructive pulmonary disease (COPD) (with concurrent corticosteroid therapy)

Dose
- 50—100 micrograms (1—2 blisters) twice daily via Accuhaler

Adverse effects
- see General Adverse effects of beta2 adrenoreceptor agonists (p. 100)

Interactions
- not recommended with itraconazole, clarithromycin, ritonavir, saquinavir, nelfinavir or atazanavir
- see also General Interactions of beta2 adrenoceptor agonists (p. 101)

Nursing considerations/Cautions
- therapy should not be started if asthma is unstable or significantly deteriorating
- has slow onset of action; therefore a faster-acting beta2 agonist should be used if rapid bronchodilation is needed
- can increase blood glucose levels; therefore caution is required if used in those with diabetes mellitus
- use with caution in those with pre-existing cardiovascular disease or predisposition to low serum potassium levels

Patient education
- the patient should be advised not to stop or reduce the dose of corticosteroids without medical advice
- ensure the patient understands that salmeterol is long acting and should not be used in the event of an acute asthma episode
- instruct the patient that use before exercise is not appropriate because of the slow onset of action (10—30 minutes) and the full effect requires repeated doses

ANTIASTHMA AGENTS, BRONCHODILATORS AND RESPIRATORY AGENTS

- instruct the patient on the correct technique for using the Accuhaler (p. 132)
- see also General Patient education for antiasthma agents and bronchodilators (p. 98)

 Consider use, as limited data available.

 Considered safe to use when breastfeeding.

 Is permitted in sport subject to certain restrictions

Available in combination with
- fluticasone propionate 100 microgram/actuation + salmeterol 50 microgram/actuation powder for inhalation Pavtide Accuhaler 100/50, Seretide Accuhaler (100/50))
- fluticasone propionate 250 microgram/actuation + salmeterol 50 microgram/actuation powder for inhalation (Fluticasone Salmeterol Ciphaler 250/50, Pavtide Accuhaler 250/50, Salflumix Easyhaler 250/50, SalplusF DPI 250/50, Seretide Accuhaler)
- fluticasone propionate 500 microgram/actuation + salmeterol 50 microgram/actuation powder for inhalation (Fluticasone Salmeterol Ciphaler 500/50, Pavtide Accuhaler 500/50, Salflumix Easyhaler 500/50, SalplusF DPI 500/50, Seretide Accuhaler (500/50))
- fluticasone propionate 125 microgram/actuation + salmeterol 25 microgram/actuation inhalation metered dose inhaler (Evocair MDI 125/50, Fluticaone + Salmeterol Cipla 125/25, Pavtide MDI 125.25, SalplusF 125/25, Seretide MDI (125/25))
- fluticasone propionate 250 microgram/actuation + salmeterol 25 microgram/actuation inhalation metered dose inhaler (Evocair MDI 250/25, Fluticasone + Salmeterol Cipla 250/25, Pavtide MDI 250/25, SalplusF 250/25, Seretide MDI (250/25))
- fluticasone propionate 50 microgram/actuation + salmeterol 25 microgram/actuation inhalation metered dose inhaler (Pavtide 50/25, Seretide MDI (50/25))

TERBUTALINE
Trade name
Bricanyl

Available forms
Injection: 0.5 mg/mL;
Turbuhaler: 500 microgram/inhalation

Action
- direct-acting sympathomimetic agent with some selective beta2 adrenoreceptor stimulant activity in the lungs
- also improves mucociliary clearance
- onset of action 30 minutes (SC), 1 hour (inhalation), duration 4—5 hours
- symptom reliever

Use
- relief of bronchospasm associated with asthma and chronic obstructive pulmonary disease (COPD)
- prophylaxis of exercise-induced asthma or other bronchospasm-inducing situation

Dose
- 1 inhalation (500 micrograms) 4—6 hourly as required (may require up to 3 inhalations in severe cases, but should not exceed 12 inhalations in 24 hours) **OR**
- 250 micrograms SC 6-hourly as required

Adverse effects
- nausea, vomiting, diarrhoea
- sweating
- rash, urticaria
- see also General Adverse effects of beta2 adrenoreceptor agonists (p. 100)

Interactions
- see General Interactions of beta2 adrenoreceptor agonists (p. 101)

Nursing considerations/Cautions
- SC administration is for acute management only

109

HAVARD'S NURSING GUIDE TO DRUGS

- caution if used in those with thyrotoxicosis, hypertension, coronary artery disease, arrhythmias or diabetes mellitus
- contraindicated in those with hypersensitivity to other sympathomimetic agents

Patient education

- ensure patient understands that this should not be used in emergency or acute situations
- advise patient to continue oral or inhaled corticosteroids or leukotriene antagonists
- patients with diabetes should be advised to monitor blood glucose levels closely during therapy
- if patient has underlying heart disease, advise them to seek medical advice immediately if experiencing chest pain, or signs of worsening heart disease, including shortness of breath, occur during therapy
- see also General Patient education for antiasthma agents and bronchodilators (p. 98)

Turbuhaler
- advise the patient that the manufacturer's instruction leaflet is in the packet
- the Turbuhaler is a breath-actuated multiple dose inhaler device that allows dispersion of the very fine propellant-free powder in the inspired air
- suitable for children aged from 3—4 years and others unable to coordinate the use of the metered dose aerosol inhaler, in severe asthma with low inspiratory flow rate and in patients sensitive to freon propellants
- instruct patient in the correct Turbuhaler technique:
    1. unscrew the cap and lift it off
    2. hold the Turbuhaler upright and twist the coloured base to the right as far as it will go, then twist it back to the left until it clicks
    3. breathe out slowly, put the mouthpiece fully between the lips and inhale deeply through the mouth without covering the air vents
    4. remove the Turbuhaler, hold the breath as long as possible, then breathe out slowly through the mouth
    5. the Turbuhaler has a dose indicator window in which a red mark appears when there are 20 doses remaining
    6. the Turbuhaler should be cleaned 2—3 times per week by removing the mouthpiece and gently wiping away any particles that have collected inside the mouthpiece with a dry tissue or cloth (do not wash the mouthpiece with water)

 Considered safe to use in pregnancy.

 Considered safe to use when breastfeeding.

 Banned in sport; can be used only with a therapeutic use exemption.

ANTICHOLINERGIC AGENTS

General Adverse effects of anticholinergic agents

- (Local) irritated throat, cough, dry mouth, hoarseness
- dry mouth, dysphagia, thirst, constipation, nausea, vomiting, taste alteration, dyspepsia
- headache, nervousness, insomnia, confusion, drowsiness, dizziness
- urinary urgency, difficulty and retention
- impotence
- flushing and dryness of skin, decreased sweating
- tachycardia, palpitations, arrhythmias
- mydriasis, photophobia, cycloplegia, blurred vision, eye pain
- (Less common) raised intraocular pressure, glaucoma, angina, heat intolerance, hypersensitivity, hyperpyrexia
- (Rare) paradoxical bronchoconstriction

General Nursing considerations/ Cautions for anticholinergic agents

- caution if used in those with unstable angina, myocardial infarction (in last 6 months), newly diagnosed arrhythmia

ANTIASTHMA AGENTS, BRONCHODILATORS AND RESPIRATORY AGENTS

(in last 3 months), or hospitalised for heart failure (class III or IV) (last 12 months)
- caution if used in those with symptomatic prostatic hyperplasia, bladder neck obstruction or narrow-angle glaucoma
- contraindicated in those with hypersensitivity to atropine and related substances

General Patient education for anticholinergic agents

- advise the patient not to drive or operate machinery if dizziness, drowsiness, confusion or blurred vision occurs
- warn the patient that persistent dry mouth can lead to dental caries; therefore it is important to maintain good mouth and dental hygiene
- if the patient has poor metered dose inhaler technique, suggest using a spacer device (p. 99)
- instruct the patient to seek medical advice if any of the following occur:
  - difficulty passing urine, painful urination
  - any eye pain/discomfort, blurred vision, visual halos, coloured images and/or red eyes
  - rapid or irregular heartbeat

ACLIDINIUM
Trade name
Bretaris Genuair

Available form
Powder for inhalation: 322 microgram/dose

Action
- anticholinergic (antimuscarinic agent) that acts on M3 receptors in airway smooth muscle to induce bronchodilation
- onset of action within 5—15 minutes, half-life 2—3 hours

Use
- long-term bronchodilator maintenance treatment for chronic obstructive pulmonary disease (COPD)

Dose
- 322 micrograms (1 inhalation) twice daily

Adverse effects
- diarrhoea, toothache, abdominal discomfort
- nasopharyngitis, sinusitis, rhinitis
- see also General Adverse effects of anticholinergic agents (p. 110)

Interaction
- not recommended with other anticholinergic agents owing to additive effects

Nursing considerations/Cautions

- not recommended in those with asthma
- not recommended in those under 18 years
- contains lactose and is therefore contraindicated in those with rare hereditary problems of galactose intolerance, Lapp lactase deficiency or glucose—galactose malabsorption
- see also General Nursing considerations/Cautions for anticholinergic agents (p. 110)

Patient education

- advise patient that aclidinium should not be used for acute episodes of bronchospasm
- instruct patient in the correct use of the Genuair inhaler device:
  1. check the dose counter (taking care not to shake the device)
  2. remove the green protective cap by squeezing the arrows on each side and pulling outwards
  3. hold with the green button facing upwards (not tilted)
  4. press and release the green button while breathing out completely away from the inhaler (do not continue to hold green button down)
  5. make sure the control window is showing green. If window shows red, repeat the above steps

6. place your lips tightly around the mouthpiece and breathe in strongly and deeply through the inhaler (you should hear a click; continue to breathe in after this has occurred)
7. remove the inhaler from your mouth and hold the breath for as long as comfortable, then breathe out slowly through your nose
8. the control window should return to red (to show dose has been administered). If the control window is still green, continue inhaling through the mouthpiece
9. replace the green protective cap after use
10. when red stripes appear in the dose indicator window, a new prescription should be obtained

- see also General Patient education for antiasthma agents and bronchodilators (p. 98) and General Patient education for anticholinergic agents (p. 111)

Considered safe to use when breastfeeding.

Available in combination with
- aclidinium 340 microgram/actuation + formoterol fumarate dihydrate 12 microgram/actuation powder for inhalation (Brimica Genuair 340/12)

GLYCOPYRRONIUM (GLYCOPYRROLATE)
Trade name
Seebri Breezhaler

Available form
Inhalation powder capsules: 50 microgram
Action
- long-acting anticholinergic (antimuscarinic) agent
- onset of action 5 minutes, half-life 33—57 hours (inhalation)

Use
- long-term bronchodilator maintenance treatment for chronic obstructive pulmonary disease (COPD)

Dose
- 50 micrograms via Breezhaler once daily

Adverse effects
- gastroenteritis, dyspepsia
- (Uncommon) musculoskeletal pain, pain in extremity, rash, fatigue, asthenia, productive cough, congested sinus, throat irritation, blood nose, rhinitis
- see also General Adverse effects of anticholinergic agents (p. 110)

Interactions
- not recommended with other anticholinergic agents owing to additive effects

Nursing considerations/Cautions
- caution if used in those with severe kidney impairment
- contains lactose and is therefore contraindicated in those with rare hereditary problems of galactose intolerance, Lapp lactase deficiency or glucose—galactose malabsorption
- see also General Nursing considerations/Cautions for anticholinergic agents (p. 110)

Patient education
- advise the patient that glycopyrronium should not be used for acute episodes of bronchospasm
- ensure the patient understands that capsules are not to be taken orally and are for use only with inhaler device
- instruct patient in correct use of the Breezhaler, including:
  1. remove the cap and flip the mouthpiece to open
  2. remove the capsule from the blister pack and insert into the chamber
  3. close the mouthpiece (a click should be heard)
  4. press the side buttons in once and then release (taking care not to shake the device)
  5. breathe out gently (away from the device), then place the mouthpiece between the teeth and close the lips to form a tight seal

ANTIASTHMA AGENTS, BRONCHODILATORS AND RESPIRATORY AGENTS

6. breathe in quickly and steadily (capsule should vibrate) and then hold the breath for 5 seconds, or as long as comfortable
7. while holding the breath, remove the device from the mouth
8. breathe out gently (away from the device)
9. open the device to remove the capsule and repeat process if more than 1 dose is required
10. close the mouthpiece and cap

- see also General Patient education for antiasthma agents and bronchodilators (p. 98) and General Patient education for anticholinergic agents (p. 111)

 Considered safe to use when breastfeeding.

Available in combination with
- glycopyrronium + beclometasone dipropionate + formoterol fumarate dihydrate combination (see beclometasone dipropionate p. 123)
- glycopyrronium 50 microgram powder for inhalation + indacaterol 110 microgram, capsules (Ultibro Breezhaler 110/50)
- glycopyrronium + indacaterol + mometasone furoate combination (see indacaterol p. 102)

IPRATROPIUM
Trade names
Cipla Ipratropium, Atrovent preparations

Available forms
Metered dose aerosol: 21 microgram/inhalation;
Nebuliser solution: 250 microgram/mL, 500 microgram/mL;
Nasal spray: 22 microgram/dose, 44 microgram/dose

Action
- anticholinergic (antimuscarinic) agent
- causes bronchodilation by blocking vagal reflexes
- (Nasal spray) inhibits secretions from serous and seromucous glands lining nasal mucosa without altering any physiological nasal functions such as smell
- (Inhalation) onset of action 3—5 minutes, peak response at 1.5—2 hours, duration of 4—6 hours, half-life 1.5—4 hours
- (Asthma) symptom reliever

Use
- chronic asthma, moderate asthma attack, chronic obstructive bronchitis with bronchospasm
- bronchospasm during/after surgery, during ventilation with respirator
- rhinorrhoea associated with allergic or non-allergic rhinitis and common cold (nasal spray)

Dose
- 42—84 micrograms (2—4 puffs) 3—4 times daily (metered dose aerosol) **OR**
- 250—500 micrograms (1—2 mL) diluted to 2—3 mL with sodium chloride 0.9% and given 6-hourly via nebuliser until entire volume is inhaled (may be repeated after 2 hours as required) (daily maximum 2 mg) **OR**
- (Rhinorrhoea associated with allergic/non-allergic rhinitis) 44—88 micrograms into each nostril 2—3 times daily, decreasing dose/frequency when rhinorrhoea improves (nasal spray) **OR**
- (Rhinorrhoea associated with cold) 88 micrograms into each nostril 3—4 times daily decreasing dose when rhinorrhoea improves (for up to 4 days) (nasal spray)

Adverse effects
- (Local, nasal spray) nose bleed, nasal discomfort, irritation and dryness, headache, blood-tinged mucus, pharyngitis, nausea
- mild, reversible visual disturbances (blurred vision, eye pain, halo vision) if it accidentally enters eyes
- hypersensitivity (skin rash, angioedema of tongue, lips and face, urticaria, laryngospasm)

- see also General Adverse effects of anticholinergic agents (p. 110)

Interactions
- not recommended with other anticholinergic agents owing to additive effects
- bronchodilation may be enhanced if used with xanthines and beta2 adrenoceptor agonists
- increased risk of glaucoma (in those with history of narrow-angle glaucoma) if given simultaneously with beta2 adrenoceptor agonists

Nursing considerations/Cautions
- (Asthma) may be used alone or in combination with other bronchodilator agents and corticosteroids
- (Common cold, nasal spray) treatment should be limited to 4 days
- if using wall oxygen/air with nebuliser, 6–8 L/min is the recommended flow rate
- (Nasal spray) contains benzalkonium chloride, which may cause irritation of nasal mucosa
- caution if used in those with cystic fibrosis, as they have an increased risk of gastrointestinal motility disturbance
- see also General Nursing considerations/Cautions for anticholinergic agents (p. 111)

Patient education
- instruct patient on correct use of the metered dose aerosol inhaler (p. 101)
- warn patient to avoid mist contacting eyes (e.g. ensuring nebulising mask fits correctly), especially if person is predisposed to glaucoma
- instruct patient in correct use of nasal spray, including:
  - when taking nasal spray from foil pouch for first time, write expiry date (4 months) on space provided on nasal spray bottle. This should be checked each time nasal spray is used. Discard after this date
  - do not spray near or in eyes
  - do not attempt to pierce or enlarge hole in nozzle
  - do not shake pump spray
- before first use, prime spray pump by activating spray 5–7 times until an even spray is released. If pump is unused for 24 hours, it should be re-primed by spraying once or until a fine mist appears
- blow nose before nasal administration
- insert spray adapter into nostril and administer spray while breathing gently through nose. Repeat for required number of sprays. Repeat in other nostril if required
- replace protective cap and store upright
- if nasal tip becomes clogged, run under warm running water for about 60 seconds, then dry tip and re-prime before replacing protective cap
- see also General Patient education for antiasthma agents and bronchodilators (p. 98) and General Patient education for anticholinergic agents (p. 111)

 Limited data available; use with caution during first trimester of pregnancy.

 Considered safe to use when breastfeeding.

TIOTROPIUM
Trade names
Braltus, Spiriva, Spiriva Respimat, Tiotropium Lupin

Available forms
Capsule (for inhalation device): 13 microgram, 18 microgram;
Solution for inhalation: 2.5 microgram/actuation

Action
- long-acting anticholinergic (antimuscarinic) agent
- relaxes bronchial smooth muscle by inhibiting muscarinic receptors (M3)
- long duration of action (about 24 hours), allowing once-daily administration

ANTIASTHMA AGENTS, BRONCHODILATORS AND RESPIRATORY AGENTS

Use
- prophylaxis and maintenance treatment of bronchospasm and dyspnoea associated with chronic obstructive pulmonary disease (COPD)
- maintenance treatment for moderate-to-severe asthma

Dose
- (COPD) 13 micrograms (1 capsule) via inhalation once daily via Zonda device OR
- (COPD) 18 micrograms (1 capsule) via inhalation once daily via HandiHaler **OR**
- (COPD, asthma) 5 micrograms (2 puffs) daily via Respimat inhalation device

Adverse effects
- hypersensitivity reaction
- see also General Adverse effects of anticholinergic agents (p. 110)

Interactions
- not recommended with other anticholinergic agents owing to additive effects

Nursing considerations/Cautions
- not first-line treatment in asthma management
- (Capsules) contains 5.5 mg lactose/capsule; therefore use with caution; not recommended in those with rare hereditary problems of galactose intolerance, Lapp lactase deficiency or glucose—galactose malabsorption
- caution if used in those with moderate-to-severe kidney impairment (creatinine clearance ≤ 50 mL/min)
- see also General Nursing considerations/Cautions for anticholinergic agents (p. 110)

Patient education
- ensure the patient understands that tiotropium should not be used for treatment of acute episodes of bronchospasm or relief of acute symptoms. A rapid beta2 agonist is recommended to treat an acute attack
- avoid contact with eyes, especially if the person is predisposed to glaucoma
- ensure the patient understands that capsules should not be taken orally and are for use only in an inhaler device
- instruct the patient in the correct technique for the Respimat inhaler, HandiHaler and Zonda devices (instructions below)
- see also General Patient education for antiasthma agents and bronchodilators (p. 98) and General Patient education for anticholinergic agents (p. 111)

HandiHaler
- advise the patient that the manufacturer's instruction leaflet is in the packet
- instruct the patient in the correct technique for the HandiHaler, including:
  1. open the dust cap by pulling upwards and then open the mouthpiece
  2. remove the capsule gently from the blister pack immediately before use
  3. place the capsule in the centre chamber and close the mouthpiece firmly until a click is heard (leaving the dust cap open)
  4. hold the device with the mouthpiece upwards; press the green button completely (once) and release (this pierces the capsule, releasing powder for inhalation)
  5. breathe out fully away from the inhaler
  6. close the lips tightly around the mouthpiece and breathe in slowly and deeply, at a rate that causes the capsule to vibrate
  7. hold the breath for as long as comfortable, remove the device from mouth and resume normal breathing
  8. repeat steps 5 to 7
  9. open the mouthpiece and remove the used capsule
- to clean the HandiHaler, open the dust cap and mouthpiece. Then open the base by lifting the piercing button, rinse with warm water and allow to air dry (this may take 24 hours)
- capsules should be used within 5 days of opening the blister strip

Zonda device

- advise the patient that the manufacturer's instruction leaflet is in the packet
- instruct the patient in the correct technique for the Zonda device, including:
  1. pull the cap upwards
  2. firmly hold the base of inhaler and pull the mouthpiece upwards to open
  3. remove the Braltus capsule from the bottle and place it in the capsule-shaped compartment at the bottom of inhaler (ensure the lid of bottle is closed tightly after the capsule is removed)
  4. close the mouthpiece (a click should be heard) leaving the cap open
  5. hold the inhaler with the mouthpiece upwards, press piercing the button once only and release the button
  6. breathe out fully (away from the inhaler)
  7. place the mouthpiece in the mouth closing the lips around it to form a tight seal then breathe in deeply and steadily (the capsule should vibrate)
  8. hold the breath for as long as possible, then breathe out normally
  9. repeat the last two steps to ensure the capsule is empty
  10. empty the capsule from the mouthpiece
  11. the Zonda device should be discarded after 30 uses

Respimat inhalation device

- advise the patient that the manufacturer's instruction leaflet is in the packet
- instruct the patient in the correct technique for the Respimat device, including:
  1. keep cap closed
  2. remove clear base: press safety catch while firmly pulling off base with other hand
  3. insert cartridge into inhaler
  4. place inhaler on a firm surface and push down firmly until it clicks into place
  5. put clear base back into place until it clicks
  6. turn clear base in direction of arrows on label until it clicks (half a turn)
  7. open cap fully, point towards the ground and press dose-release button
  8. close cap
  9. repeat steps 7–10 until a cloud is visible and then repeat 7–10 3 more times directions for use
  10. hold inhaler upright with cap closed
  11. turn base in direction of arrows on label until it clicks (half a turn)
  12. open cap fully
  13. breathe out gently
  14. place mouthpiece in mouth and close lips to form a good seal
  15. breathe in slowly and deeply through the mouth and, at the same time, press the dose-release button
  16. continue to breathe in slowly and deeply
  17. hold breath for 5 seconds or as long as comfortable
  18. while holding breath, remove inhaler from mouth
  19. breathe out gently
  20. close cap

 Limited data available; consider before use.

 Considered safe to use when breastfeeding.

 Consider use with patients with impaired renal function, as tiotropium is renally cleared. There is an increased risk of anticholinergic adverse effects in patients with CrCl < 50 mL/min.

ANTIASTHMA AGENTS, BRONCHODILATORS AND RESPIRATORY AGENTS

Available in combination with
- tiotropium 2.5 microgram/actuation + olodaterol 2.5 microgram/actuation inhalation solution (Spiolto Respimat)

UMECLIDINIUM

Trade name
Incruse Ellipta

Available form
Powder for inhalation: 62.5 microgram/dose

Action
- long-acting anticholinergic (antimuscarinic) agent
- onset of action 15 minutes, duration of action 24 hours, half-life 19 hours

Use
- long-term bronchodilator maintenance treatment for chronic obstructive pulmonary disease (COPD)

Dose
- 62.5 micrograms once daily via inhaler

Adverse effects
- upper respiratory tract infection, sinusitis, nasopharyngitis
- urinary tract infection
- arthralgia
- see also General Adverse effects of anticholinergic agents (p. 110)

Interactions
- not recommended with other anticholinergic agents owing to additive effects

Nursing considerations/Cautions
- therapy should not be started in those with acutely deteriorating COPD
- not recommended in those with asthma
- contains lactose and is therefore contraindicated in those with rare hereditary problems of galactose intolerance, Lapp lactase deficiency or glucose–galactose malabsorption
- contraindicated in those with severe milk protein allergy
- see also General Nursing considerations/Cautions for anticholinergic agents (p. 110)

Patient education
- warn the patient that umeclidinium is not for use if symptoms are acute
- advise the patient to use inhaler only once per day
- instruct the patient in the correct use of the Ellipta inhaler, including:
    - the inhaler should not be removed from the sealed container/tray until the patient is ready to inhale medication
    - ensure the inhaler is in the 'closed' position. If the cover is opened and then closed without inhaling, the dose will be lost and held inside the device
    - do not shake the inhaler at any time
    - slide the cover down until you hear a click (the dose counter should also count down). If there is no click, the device may be faulty and needs to be returned to the pharmacy
    - holding the inhaler away from the mouth, breathe out as far as is comfortable and then put the mouthpiece between the lips. Close the lips firmly around the mouthpiece, taking care not to block air vents with fingers
    - take a long steady deep breath in and hold for 3–4 seconds (or as long as is comfortable)
    - remove the inhaler from the mouth and breathe out slowly (away from the mouthpiece)
    - you may or may not taste or feel medication when inhaling
    - the mouthpiece can be cleaned using dry tissue, then close the cover
    - when less than 10 doses remain in the inhaler, half of the dose counter will show red. The inhaler is empty when 0 appears on the dose counter, which will appear red
    - the inhaler should be discarded 6 weeks after opening the container/tray
- see also General Patient education for antiasthma agents and bronchodilators (p. 98) and General Patient education for anticholinergic agents (p. 111)

Considered safe to use when breastfeeding.

Available in combination with
- umeclidinium 62.5 microgram/actuation + vilanterol 25 microgram/actuation powder for inhalation (Anoro Ellipta)
- fluticasone furoate 100 microgram/actuation + umeclidinium 62.5 microgram/actuation + vilanterol 25 microgram/actuation powder for inhalation (Trelegy Ellipta 100 mcg/62.5 mcg/25 mcg)
- fluticasone furoate 200 microgram/actuation + umeclidinium 62.5 microgram/actuation + vilanterol 25 microgram/actuation powder for inhalation (Trelegy Ellipta 200 mcg/62.5 mcg/25 mcg)

XANTHINES

AMINOPHYLLINE
Trade names
DBL Aminophylline Injection

Available form
Ampoule: 250 mg/10 mL

Action
- aminophylline dissociates to theophylline in biological tissue (1 mg aminophylline = 0.8 mg theophylline)
- narrow therapeutic index
- symptom reliever
- see also Action of theophylline (p. 121)

Use
- reversible bronchospasm associated with chronic bronchitis, emphysema, bronchial asthma and chronic obstructive pulmonary disease (COPD)
- paroxysmal dyspnoea associated with left-sided heart failure

Dose
- (Bronchospasm not currently undergoing theophylline therapy, cor pulmonale or congestive heart failure) 6 mg/kg IV over 20–30 minutes (loading dose), then 0.5–1.2 mg/kg/hour IV infusion for 12 hours, then reduced to 0.1–1 mg/kg/hour IV infusion **OR**
- (Currently undergoing theophylline therapy and unable to obtain serum concentration) 3 mg/kg IV over 20–30 minutes (loading dose), then 0.5–1.2 mg/kg/hour IV infusion for 12 hours, then reduced to 0.1–1 mg/kg/hour IV infusion

Adverse effects
- (Rapid administration) anxiety, headache, nausea, vomiting, severe hypotension, profound bradycardia, flushing, faintness, praecordial pain
- see also Adverse effects of theophylline (p. 121)

Interactions
- contraindicated with other xanthines owing to risk of additive toxicity
- aminophylline should be withheld for 36 hours before myocardial perfusion studies, as it reverses the effects of dipyridamole
- inhibition of bronchodilatory effect may occur if given with beta adrenoceptor blocking agents (beta blockers), including ophthalmic preparations
- cardiotoxicity and hypoglycaemia may occur if given with beta adrenergic agonists
- may reduce or reverse sedative effects of benzodiazepines
- may antagonise non-depolarising neuromuscular blocking agents
- may cause toxicity if given with cardiac glycosides
- may produce false positive on serum uric acid test (using Bittner or colorimetric methods)
- see also Interactions of theophylline (p. 121)

Nursing considerations/Cautions
- dosage is calculated on lean body mass and highly individualised, preferably on the basis of serum theophylline monitoring, to achieve a therapeutic

- concentration of 5–20 microgram/mL (27.5–110 micromol/L)
- coagulation time should be monitored regularly during therapy
- maintenance dose is dependent on patient's age, heart, liver or lung function, and/or smoking status
- if patient is already taking theophylline, dose may depend on serum theophylline concentration (aminophylline is converted to theophylline in the body)
- monitor vital signs during IV administration, which should be at a rate not greater than 20–25 mg/min. Rapid administration should be avoided, as it may result in anxiety, headache, nausea, vomiting, severe hypotension, dizziness, faintness, lightheadedness, palpitations, syncope, flushing, bradycardia or cardiac arrest
- IV therapy should be replaced by oral theophylline as soon as possible
- if it is necessary to prepare an IV admixture, consult a compatibility chart, manufacturer's literature, a pharmacist or drug information centre, because aminophylline is chemically or physically incompatible with an extensive list of drugs
- precipitates in acidic solutions (see previous comment about compatibility)
- not given IM because of intense pain and tissue sloughing
- not used if solution contains crystals
- chronic overdose symptoms and toxicity can occur at lower serum concentration (40 microgram/mL) than acute overdosage (90 microgram/mL). Management of overdose should be symptomatic and supportive
- caution if used in those with epilepsy, as seizure threshold may be lowered
- caution if used in the elderly or those with decreased liver or kidney function, congestive cardiac failure, cor pulmonale, chronic alcohol use, chronic obstructive pulmonary disease (COPD), acute pulmonary oedema, hypothyroidism, acute febrile state and viral infection (including pneumonia, influenza or influenza immunisation), as clearance may be decreased thus increasing the risk of toxicity
- caution if used in those with compromised cardiac or circulatory function, hypertension, tachyarrhythmias, angina or acute myocardial injury where cardiac effects may be harmful
- caution if used in those with hyperthyroidism, diabetes mellitus, or glaucoma, as there may be an exacerbation of the conditions
- caution if used in those with gastric ulceration or gastro-oesophageal reflux disease (GORD) because of an increase in gastric acid secretion
- contraindicated in those with hypersensitivity to xanthines or ethylenediamine, or with coronary artery disease or bronchiolitis

Patient education

- warn the patient not to take other xanthine derivatives or excessive amounts of caffeine-containing beverages such as coffee, tea, cola or energy drinks (e.g. Red Bull) concurrently

Not to be used during pregnancy unless the expected benefit outweighs any potential risk. It crosses placental barrier, therefore if given near delivery the neonate should be closely monitored for any adverse effects.

Consider before use, theophylline is excreted in breastmilk; therefore, minimise dosage to the mother to avoid irritability and restlessness in the infant.

Consider reduction in dose for patients with renal impairment.

Reduce dose in the elderly, as theophylline clearance is reduced.

CAFFEINE CITRATE
Trade name
Cafnea

Available forms
Vial: 40 mg/2 mL;
Oral solution: 25 mg/5 mL

Action
- methylxanthine related to theophylline and aminophylline
- centrally acting respiratory stimulant that increases respiratory rate significantly in premature infants, as well as decreasing apnoea attacks
- direct effect on myocardium, increasing the heart rate
- reduces pulmonary resistance and increases lung compliance, with a reduction in amount of inspired oxygen required
- may also increase cerebral blood flow (but this has not been conclusively proven)
- poorly metabolised in preterm infants
- half-life in neonates is 65—102 hours, prolonged to 80—120 hours in preterm infants (28—32 weeks)

Use
- short-term management of apnoea in premature infants (gestational age 28 — < 33 weeks)

Dose
- 20 mg/kg IV over 30 minutes using a syringe infusion pump (loading dose), followed by 5 mg/kg daily IV over 10 minutes or orally, and further increased to 10 mg/kg once daily if apnoea persists (maintenance)

Adverse effects
- injection site reaction
- irritability, restlessness, jitteriness
- tachycardia, increased left ventricular output, increased stroke volume
- feeding intolerance, increased gastric aspirate
- vomiting, constipation, gastro-oesophageal reflux, dilated loops of bowel
- hypoglycaemia, hyperglycaemia
- anaemia
- hyponatraemia, increased calcium excretion, increased urine flow, increased creatinine clearance
- rash
- necrotising enterocolitis

Interactions
- increased serum levels may occur if given with artemisinin, fluvoxamine, fluconazole or verapamil
- decreased serum levels may occur if given with phenytoin
- may antagonise effects of benzodiazepines
- increases levels of both endogenous and oral melatonin
- increases serum levels of clozapine
- may reduce bioavailability of fluvoxamine
- half-life increased and clearance decreased by ciprofloxacin and norfloxacin
- not recommended with aminophylline or theophylline

Nursing considerations/Cautions
- other causes of apnoea (e.g. CNS disorders, primary lung disease, anaemia, sepsis, metabolic or cardiovascular disturbances, obstructive apnoea) should be evaluated and/or treated before starting therapy
- baseline serum caffeine levels should be measured if mothers have consumed caffeine-containing fluids before delivery (caffeine crosses the placenta)
- the maintenance dose should be adjusted weekly according to changes in body weight
- the maintenance dose begins 24 hours after the loading dose and may be given IV over 10 minutes or orally if the infant is tolerating full enteral feeds
- if the mother shows signs of caffeine toxicity (e.g. tachycardia, tachypnoea, jitteriness, tremors, unexplained seizures and vomiting), the dose can be reduced or withheld

ANTIASTHMA AGENTS, BRONCHODILATORS AND RESPIRATORY AGENTS

- therapy should be stopped when apnoea ceases or therapy is no longer required
- the infant should be closely monitored for any signs of necrotising enterocolitis, which occurs commonly in preterm or low birthweight babies. Symptoms include abdominal distension, tenderness, blood in stool, bilious vomiting/drainage from enteral feeding tube, unstable temperature, apnoea, bradycardia, hypotension, acidosis and lethargy
- caution if used in infants with cardiovascular disease, as caffeine may increase heart rate, left ventricular output and stroke volume
- caution if used in infants with seizure disorders or impaired kidney or liver function
- contraindicated in those with known sensitivity to caffeine or citrate

THEOPHYLLINE
Trade names
Nuelin Syrup, Nuelin SR

Available forms
Tablets (sustained-release): 200 mg, 250 mg, 300 mg;
Syrup: 133.3 mg/25 mL

Action
- smooth muscle relaxation, especially bronchial muscle and pulmonary blood vessels
- stimulant effect on myocardium (increasing heart rate and contractility), CNS and respiration (via medullary respiratory centre)
- decreases peripheral resistance by increasing pulmonary vasodilation
- diuresis (transient)
- increases gastric secretion
- active metabolite (less activity than theophylline)
- narrow therapeutic range
- therapeutic level 10—20 microgram/mL (doses above linked to adverse effects)
- half-life (3—12 hours) and clearance are affected by age, heart, liver and lung disease, viral infection, fever, some medications and smoking
- symptom reliever

Use
- relief and prophylaxis of reversible bronchospasm in asthma, chronic bronchitis, emphysema and related conditions

Dose
- 25 mL (133.3 mg) orally 6-hourly before meals (syrup) **OR**
- 200—300 mg orally 12-hourly, gradually increasing/decreasing dose by 100—150 mg if needed to achieve desired effects with minimal side-effects (sustained-release tablets)

Adverse effects
- anorexia, nausea, vomiting, epigastric pain, diarrhoea, abdominal cramps
- insomnia, headache, tremor, nervousness, restlessness, dizziness, anxiety, lightheadedness
- palpitations, tachycardia, hypotension, cardiac arrhythmias
- tachypnoea
- increased urination, albuminuria, haematuria
- hyperglycaemia, hypokalaemia
- flushing
- rash
- alopecia
- reactivation of peptic ulcer or gastrooesophageal reflux disease (GORD), haematemesis
- (High dose) inappropriate antidiuretic hormone (ADH) secretion
- (Early signs of toxicity) nausea, anorexia, vomiting, headache, irritability, agitation, anxiety, insomnia, hypotension, tachycardia, palpitations
- (Late signs of toxicity) delirium, extreme thirst, sensory disturbance, confusion, delirium, hyperthermia, ventricular arrhythmias, convulsions

Interactions
- not recommended with other xanthine derivatives or concurrent excessive amounts of caffeine-containing products

such as coffee, tea, cola and some energy drinks
- clearance may be decreased, increasing serum levels and risk of adverse effects and toxicity by alcohol, allopurinol (high dose > 600 mg/day), beta adrenergic blocking agents, ciprofloxacin, clarithromycin, diltiazem, disulfiram, erythromycin, methotrexate, norfloxacin, oral contraceptives, propranolol, recombinant alpha interferons, thyroid hormones, ticlopidine, verapamil
- clearance may be increased, decreasing serum levels by barbiturates, carbamazepine, isoprenaline, phenytoin, phenobarbital (phenobarbitone), primidone, rifampicin, St John's wort, tobacco or marijuana smoking
- additive effect (e.g. increased nausea, insomnia, nervousness) when given with sympathomimetic agents; therefore caution if given together
- may decrease seizure threshold if given with ketamine
- may antagonise cardiovascular effects of adenosine
- may increase excretion of lithium, causing decreased serum concentrations; therefore serum levels should be closely monitored

Nursing considerations/Cautions

- dosage should be highly individualised, preferably on the basis of serum theophylline concentration monitoring
- monitor serum concentrations by sampling blood immediately before morning dose (trough level), then 1–2 hours after dose (5–10 hours if SR) for peak concentration, provided that therapy has been established for 48 hours and no excess drug has been given or doses missed
- serum concentrations should be regularly monitored if daily dose is greater than 1 g in adults (or 24 mg/kg in children)
- xanthine/caffeine-containing beverages (e.g. tea, coffee, cola, cocoa, energy drinks) may interfere with the theophylline assay
- caution if used in those with decreased liver function, congestive cardiac failure, chronic obstructive pulmonary disease (COPD), acute pulmonary oedema, severe hypoxia, decreased thyroid function, acute febrile state and viral infection (including pneumonia, influenza or influenza immunisation), as clearance may be decreased, increasing the risk of toxicity
- caution if used in those with arrhythmias, coronary artery disease, unstable angina, cardiomyopathy or severe hypertension where cardiac effects may be harmful
- caution if used in those with gastric ulceration or GORD because of an increase in gastric acid secretion
- contraindicated in those with hypersensitivity to xanthines

Patient education

- SR tablets may be broken along score line, but are not to be crushed or chewed
- the patient should be advised that SR theophylline should not be used in acute asthma
- warn the patient not to take other xanthine derivatives or excessive amounts of caffeine-containing products, such as coffee, tea, cola or energy drinks
- advise the patient not to drive or operate machinery if dizziness persists
- serum concentrations are affected by smoking, therefore the patient should be instructed to advise a doctor if starting/stopping smoking
- theophylline has interactions with many other medications. The patient should be instructed to discuss taking any other medications with a doctor or pharmacist
- (Syrup) advise the patient to take syrup 1 hour before meals with glass of water; however, if GI irritation is a problem, it may be taken with or just after food

ANTIASTHMA AGENTS, BRONCHODILATORS AND RESPIRATORY AGENTS

 Available as a syrup. Sustained-release tablets should not be crushed or chewed.

 Not to be used during pregnancy unless the expected benefit outweighs any potential risk. Crosses the placental barrier; therefore if given near delivery the neonate should be closely monitored for any adverse effects.

 Consider before use, theophylline is excreted in breastmilk; therefore, minimise dosage to the mother to avoid irritability and restlessness in the infant.

 Consider reduction in dose for patients with renal impairment.

 Reduce dose in the elderly as theophylline clearance is reduced.

CORTICOSTEROIDS

BECLOMETASONE (BECLOMETHASONE)
Trade names
Beconase Allergy & Hayfever, Qvar

Available forms
Metered dose inhaler: 50 microgram/inhalation, 100 microgram/inhalation;
Autohaler: 50 microgram/inhalation, 100 microgram/inhalation;
Nasal spray: 50 microgram/inhalation

Action
- inhibits inflammatory cells and prevents release of inflammatory mediators
- has an active metabolite, resulting in some systemic activity
- (Asthma) symptom preventer

Use
- prophylaxis of symptoms of asthma (Qvar)
- prophylaxis and treatment of allergic rhinitis for up to 6 months (Beconase)

Dose
- (Mild-to-moderate asthma) 50–200 micrograms twice daily (daily maximum 800 micrograms) (metered dose inhaler) **OR**
- (Severe asthma) up to 400 micrograms twice daily (daily maximum 800 micrograms) (metered dose inhaler) **OR**
- (Allergic rhinitis) initially 100 micrograms (2 sprays) twice daily to each nostril, then reducing to 50 micrograms (1 spray) twice daily to each nostril when symptoms are controlled (maximum 400 micrograms (8 sprays/day)) (nasal spray)

Adverse effects
- hoarseness, pharyngitis
- taste sensation
- (Nasal spray) stinging sensation, sneezing, bleeding, unpleasant taste and smell, dryness/irritation to nose and throat
- (Rare) oral candidiasis, paradoxical bronchospasm, Cushing's syndrome, Cushingoid features, anxiety, sleeping disorders, hypersensitivity, cataract formation, elevated intraocular pressure, visual disturbances

Nursing considerations/Cautions
- not recommended for acute asthma episode or status asthmaticus
- asthma should be stable before adding inhaled corticosteroid to usual asthma maintenance regimen
- discontinuation of oral corticosteroids may cause exacerbation of pre-existing allergic diseases such as atopic eczema, which can be treated symptomatically
- if the patient experiences any visual disturbances, referral to an ophthalmologist is recommended
- if the patient has been on oral corticosteroids, these may need to be restarted rapidly in times of stress or when there is airway obstruction or mucus that compromises inhaled route
- (Nasal spray) if therapy is prolonged, twice-yearly examination of nasal mucosa is recommended

- Autohaler is breath actuated and automatically releases medication during inhalation; therefore it is suitable for those with poor inhaler technique
- the canister does not require shaking before use, test firing if unused for a period of time or waiting between actuations
- (Allergic rhinitis) any respiratory, nasal passage or paranasal sinus infection should be treated promptly with antibiotics
- (Nasal spray) if used for several months, nasal mucosa should be examined regularly for any signs of mucosal damage
- (Qvar) contains propellant hydrofluoroalkane (norflurane)
- caution if used in those with active or latent tuberculosis (TB)
- (Nasal spray) not recommended in those with nasal septal ulcers or recent nasal injury or surgery until healing has occurred
- (Nasal spray) contraindicated if severe nasal infection is present or if patient has bleeding disorder or history of recurrent nasal bleeding

Patient education

- the patient should be advised not to exceed the recommended dose
- instruct the patient to rinse mouth with water after using a metered dose inhaler
- (Allergic rhinitis) warn the patient that benefits of therapy may take at least a week to become apparent, and therapy should be continued as prescribed
- advise the patient to report any blurred vision or other visual disturbances
- instruct the patient in the correct technique for using a metered dose inhaler (p. 106), Autohaler (p. 102) and nasal spray (p. 114)
- see also General Patient education for antiasthma agents and bronchodilators (p. 98)

Considered safe to use in pregnancy.

Considered safe to use when breastfeeding.

Available in combination with

- beclometasone dipropionate 100 microgram/actuation + formoterol fumarate dihydrate 6 microgram/actuation inhalation metered dose inhaler (Fostair 100/6)
- beclometasone dipropionate 200 microgram/actuation + formoterol fumarate dihydrate 6 microgram/actuation inhalation metered dose inhaler (Fostair 200/6)
- beclometasone dipropionate 100 microgram/actuation + formoterol fumarate dihydrate 6 microgram/actuation + glycopyrronium 10 microgram/actuation inhalation metered dose inhaler (Trimbow 100/6/10)
- beclometasone dipropionate 200 microgram/actuation + formoterol fumarate dihydrate 6 microgram/actuation + glycopyrronium 10 microgram/actuation inhalation metered dose inhaler (Trimbow 200/6/10)

BUDESONIDE

Trade names
Budamax, Budenofalk, Budenofalk Foam, Cortiment, Entocort, Jorveza, Pulmicort, Rhinocort, Rhinocort Hayfever & Allergy

Available forms
Nebulising solution (respules): 0.5 mg/2 mL, 1 mg/2 mL;
Turbuhaler: 100 microgram/inhalation, 200 microgram/inhalation, 400 microgram/inhalation;
Nasal spray: 32 microgram/dose, 64 microgram/dose;
Capsules: 3 mg;
Enema: 2 mg;
Tablet (prolonged-release): 9 mg;
Orally disintegrating tablet 0.5 mg, 1 mg

Action
- glucocorticoid is related to hydroxyprednisolone, with fewer systemic

ANTIASTHMA AGENTS, BRONCHODILATORS AND RESPIRATORY AGENTS

- effects than beclometasone, although twice as potent
- lower influence on hypothalamo-pituitary-adrenal axis
- (Crohn's) anti-inflammatory with local action on intestinal mucosa
- (Oral) half-life 3—4 hours
- (Asthma) symptom preventer

Use
- treatment and prophylaxis of asthma (Pulmicort)
- laryngotracheobronchitis (croup) (Pulmicort)
- treatment and prophylaxis of allergic rhinitis (seasonal, perennial), nasal polyps (Budamax, Rhinocort)
- crohn's disease (Budenofalk, Entocort)
- ulcerative colitis (active rectal and rectosigmoid disease) (Budenofalk Foam Enema)
- induction of remission in mild-to-moderate ulcerative colitis where mesalazine was insufficient or not tolerated (Cortiment)
- eosinophilic oesophagitis (Jorveza)

Dose
- (Mild asthma) 400—800 micrograms daily in divided doses (Turbuhaler) **OR**
- (When starting therapy, during severe asthma or reducing oral corticosteroid dose) 400—2400 micrograms daily in 2—4 divided doses, reducing to lowest dose (100—400 micrograms daily) to maintain the patient symptom free (Turbuhaler) **OR**
- (When starting therapy, during severe asthma or reducing oral corticosteroid dose) 1—2 mg twice daily, reducing to 0.5—1 mg twice daily via nebuliser **OR**
- (Acute laryngotracheobronchitis) 2 mg via nebuliser **OR**
- (Allergic rhinitis) initially 128 micrograms in each nostril daily (morning) **OR**
- (Allergic rhinitis) initially 64 micrograms twice daily in each nostril morning and evening **OR**
- (Allergic rhinitis, maintenance) reducing to 32—64 micrograms in each nostril daily **OR**
- (Nasal polyps) 64 micrograms twice daily into each nostril morning and evening **OR**
- (Acute Crohn's disease) 9 mg orally 30 minutes before food in the morning, for up to 12 weeks, with dose being tapered over the last 2—4 weeks (sustained-release capsules) **OR**
- (Acute Crohn's disease) 3 mg orally 30 minutes before food 3 times daily (morning, noon, evening) for no more than 8 weeks **OR**
- (Active ulcerative colitis) 2 mg enema once daily (morning or evening) for 6—8 weeks **OR**
- (Induction of remission of ulcerative colitis) 9 mg orally daily (morning) for up to 8 weeks **OR**
- (Eosinophilic oesophagitis) Induction: 1 mg twice daily for 6—12 weeks. Maintenance: 0.5 to 1 mg twice daily.

Adverse effects
- (Oral) nausea, abdominal pain, dyspepsia, dry mouth, loose stools, diarrhoea, muscle/joint pain, headache, fatigue, insomnia, altered mood, depression, irritability, euphoria
- (Inhalation) hoarseness, sore throat, cough, dry mouth, irritation of throat, tongue and mouth, oral candidiasis (thrush)
- (Enema) rectal burning sensation and pain, headache, abdominal pain, diarrhoea, acne, depression, irritability, euphoria, muscle/joint pain, muscle weakness, osteoporosis
- (Nasal spray) stinging, sneezing, dry/irritated nose, larynx and throat, unpleasant or strong smell and taste, dry mouth, nasal crust, increased sputum, sinusitis, epistaxis, headache, dizziness, tiredness, cough, dyspnoea, rhinitis, fever, rash
- (High dose, prolonged therapy) corticosteroid systemic effects (see Corticosteroids, p. 123), including increased risk of infection
- (Nasal spray, prolonged use) nasal atrophy and perforation
- (Inhalation, rare) paradoxical bronchospasm with wheezing

- (Rare) hypersensitivity reaction, visual disturbances, cataract formation

Interactions
- (Oral) increased serum levels may occur if given with itraconazole, ritonavir, clarithromycin and grapefruit juice
- (Oral) decreased serum levels may occur if given with carbamazepine and rifampicin
- (Oral) not recommended with live attenuated virus vaccines
- (Oral) absorption may be decreased if given with colestyramine or antacids
- (Oral) may cause increased potassium excretion, which may potentiate effects of digoxin
- (Oral) may cause false results on adrenocorticotrophic hormone (ACTH) stimulation test for diagnosing pituitary or adrenal insufficiency

Nursing considerations/Cautions
- (Asthma, non-oral corticosteroid dependent) if the patient has large amounts of mucus, a short course (2 weeks) of oral corticosteroids may be recommended in addition to inhaled corticosteroid
- (Asthma) therapy should be started when the patient's asthma is stable
- (Ulcerative colitis) therapy is for active rectal or rectosigmoid disease only, not maintenance
- (Ulcerative colitis, Cortiment) prolonged release formulation may result in lower corticosteroid levels than conventional (immediate release formulation) oral glucocorticoid therapy. Signs of adrenocortical suppression may be seen when the patient is transferred from immediate-release formulations with higher systemic effects
- (Oral) discontinuation should be tapered
- if the patient experiences any visual disturbances, referral to an ophthalmologist is recommended
- (Nasal spray) if the patient has severe nasal obstruction/congestion, treatment with local decongestant can be used for 2—3 days
- (Nasal spray) if therapy is prolonged, twice-yearly examination of nasal mucosa is recommended
- (Allergic rhinitis, nasal polyposis) any respiratory, nasal passage or paranasal sinus infection should be treated promptly with antibiotics
- long-term use in children is not recommended because of potential growth suppression
- (Asthma) caution if used in those transferring from oral to inhaled steroid therapy, as there is an increased risk of adrenal impairment
- caution if given to those with active/latent tuberculosis, respiratory tract infection or severe liver impairment
- use with caution in those with hypertension, diabetes mellitus (or family history of), osteoporosis, peptic ulceration, glaucoma (or family history of) or cataracts where corticosteroid therapy may have undesired effects
- (Crohn's disease) enteric-coated capsules are not recommended in those with upper GI Crohn's disease or extraintestinal symptoms (e.g. skin, eyes, joints), as therapy appears to be ineffective
- (Enteric-coated capsules) contain lactose and sucrose and are therefore not recommended in those with rare hereditary problems of galactose or fructose intolerance, glucose—galactose malabsorption, sucrose isomaltase insufficiency, Lapp lactase deficiency or congenital lactase deficiency
- (Inhaled therapy) not recommended for bronchospasm relief or as sole therapy for acute asthma episodes or status asthmaticus
- (Nasal spray) not recommended in those with nasal septal ulcers or recent nasal injury or surgery until healing has occurred
- (Nasal spray) contraindicated if severe nasal infection is present or if the patient has bleeding disorder or a history of recurrent nasal bleeding

ANTIASTHMA AGENTS, BRONCHODILATORS AND RESPIRATORY AGENTS

- (Prolonged-release tablets) contraindicated in those with rare hereditary galactose intolerance, Lapp lactase deficiency or glucose—galactose malabsorption, as capsules contain lactose. Tablets also contain lecithin (of soya origin) and are therefore contraindicated in those with known lecithin sensitivity
- contraindicated in those with cirrhosis of the liver

Patient education

- warn the patient not to drive or operate machinery if visual disturbances or dizziness occur
- the patient should be advised to seek medical advice if blurred vision or other visual disturbances occur

Asthma

- the patient should have full understanding of effects (i.e. it is not suitable for rapid relief of bronchospasm during acute asthma attack and is taken prophylactically regularly and should be continued even when the patient is asymptomatic)
- the patient should be instructed in correct use of metered dose inhalers (p. 106)
- the patient using nebulised solution should be encouraged to wash the face after use to reduce risk of facial irritation
- incidence of oral candidiasis and hoarseness may be reduced by encouraging the patient to rinse the mouth with water after each inhalation
- if the patient requires 400 micrograms or less for asthma treatment, it may be given as a single daily dose (either morning or evening)
- if the patient is also on bronchodilators, they should be taken several minutes before the budesonide to allow adequate penetration into the bronchial tree and bronchial dilation
- Turbuhaler is breath actuated, therefore it is suitable for those with poor inhaler technique
- advise the patient that nebulised solution may be diluted to 2 mL if necessary
- warn the patient that the pressurised container should be kept intact and away from heat
- canisters should be protected from frost, as cold temperatures may decrease therapeutic effect
- see also General Patient education for antiasthma agents and bronchodilators (p. 98)

Allergic rhinitis

- (Allergic rhinitis) warn the patient that full effects may not be seen for 2—3 days (and rarely, up to 2 weeks)
- (Allergic rhinitis) advise the patient to start therapy before exposure to allergen
- (Nasal spray) if using decongestant for severe nasal congestion, it should be used 2—3 minutes before the nasal spray

Crohn's disease, ulcerative colitis

- (Oral) instruct the patient to avoid grapefruit juice during therapy
- (Oral) the patient should be advised to seek medical advice if any of the following occurs:
  - feeling unwell in a non-specific way (e.g. muscle or joint pain)
  - tiredness, headache, nausea and vomiting (may be signs of insufficient corticosteroid effect)
- (Crohn's disease, ulcerative colitis) advise the patient to avoid close personal contact with chicken pox, herpes zoster and measles as minor illness can be fatal in those who are immunocompromised. If contact occurs, instruct the patient to seek medical advice immediately
- (Oral, sustained-release capsules) advise the patient to swallow capsules whole, not chewed, crushed or broken. However, if the patient has problems swallowing, capsules may be opened and the contents swallowed whole (not chewed or crushed) with water
- (Oral, prolonged-release tablets) instruct the patient to swallow tablets whole, not broken, crushed or chewed

- (Oral) if the patient is also taking antacids and/or colestyramine, they should be separated by at least 2 hours from budesonide capsules
- (Foam enema) instruct the patient in the correct use of foam enema, including:
  - ensure enema is at room temperature before use
  - warn the patient that burning sensation or pain on using enema is normal feeling
  - empty the bowel (if possible) before insertion of enema
  - wash hands with soap and water
  - fit the applicator onto the spray can spout and shake for 15 seconds to mix contents
  - remove the safety tab under the pump dome and twist dome until the semicircular gap is in line with the nozzle
  - place a finger on top of the pump dome and turn the spray can upside down (must be pointing down)
  - insert the applicator into the rectum (as far as comfortable) and push the pump dome fully once, holding for 5 seconds and release. Wait for 15 seconds for foam to be delivered and withdraw the applicator from the rectum
  - remove the applicator from the spray can and dispose of safely
  - wash hands with soap and water
  - try not to open the bowels for as long as possible (despite a feeling of urgency to empty bowel — this is normal)
- (Foam enema) instruct the patient that the enema should not be used after 4 weeks of opening container

Capsule/tablet should not be crushed.

Considered safe to use in pregnancy.

Considered safe to use when breastfeeding.

Oral and rectal preparations are banned in competition. Inhaled route is not prohibited.

Available in combination with
- budesonide 100 microgram/actuation + formoterol fumarate dihydrate 3 microgram/actuation inhalation (Rilast Rapihaler 100/3, Symbicort 100/3)
- budesonide 200 microgram/actuation + formoterol fumarate dihydrate 6 microgram/actuation inhalation (Bufomix Easyhaler 200/6, DuoResp Spiromax 200/6, Rilast Rapihaler 200/6, Symbicort Rapihaler 200/6, Symbicort Turbuhaler 200/6)
- budesonide 100 microgram/actuation + formoterol fumarate dihydrate 6 microgram/actuation powder for inhalation (Symbicort Turbuler 100/6)
- budesonide 400 microgram/actuation + formoterol fumarate dihydrate 12 microgram/actuation powder for inhalation (Bufomix Easyhaler 400/12, DuoResp Spiromax 400/12, Rilast Turbuhaler, Symbicort Turbuhaler 400/12)

CICLESONIDE
Trade names
Alvesco, Omnaris Nasal Spray

Available forms
Metered dose inhaler: 80 microgram/inhalation, 160 microgram/inhalation;
Metered dose nasal spray: 50 microgram/spray

Action
- non-halogenated glucocorticosteroid that acts on the lungs without significant systemic effects
- prodrug, converted to active metabolite in the lung
- half-life about 1 hour (and 2.8 hours for metabolite)
- (Asthma) symptom preventer

Use
- prophylactic management of asthma (metered dose inhaler)

ANTIASTHMA AGENTS, BRONCHODILATORS AND RESPIRATORY AGENTS

- treatment of seasonal or perennial allergic rhinitis (nasal spray)

Dose
- (Asthma) 80—320 micrograms via metered dose inhaler daily (dose dependent on severity of asthma) **OR**
- (Allergic rhinitis) 100 micrograms (2 sprays) per nostril daily (daily total 200 micrograms)

Adverse effects
- (Metered dose inhaler) hoarseness, cough, pharyngeal pain, headache, bronchitis, nasopharyngitis, influenza, sinusitis, upper respiratory tract infection, back pain
- (Nasal spray) stinging, sneezing, dry/irritated nose and throat, unpleasant taste, dry mouth, dyspepsia, headache, epistaxis, nasopharyngitis, pharyngolaryngeal pain, ear pain
- (Nasal spray, prolonged use) nasal atrophy and nasal septum perforation
- (Rare) hypersensitivity reactions, paradoxical bronchospasm, visual disturbances

Interactions
- not recommended with itraconazole, ritonavir or nelfinavir

Nursing considerations/Cautions
- (Asthma) for mild asthma, dose should start at 160 microgram, moderate asthma 160—320 microgram, severe asthma 320 micrograms
- if paradoxical bronchospasm with wheezing occurs after dose is given, an inhaled short-acting bronchodilator should be used. If ineffective and large number of inhalations are needed, medical advice should be sought
- if changing from oral corticosteroid to inhaled ciclesonide, patient should be stable. High doses of ciclesonide should be given with oral corticosteroid for about 10 days, then gradually reduce oral corticosteroid to the lowest dose possible
- higher dosage may be required if the patient was previously on an inhaled corticosteroid
- if the patient experiences any visual disturbances, referral to an ophthalmologist is recommended
- when transferring from oral corticosteroids, pre-existing allergic conditions (e.g. allergic rhinitis, eczema) may be unmasked
- (Nasal spray) not recommended in those with nasal septal ulcers or recent nasal injury or surgery until healing has occurred
- caution if given to those with active/latent tuberculosis or respiratory tract infection or liver impairment

Patient education
- (Asthma) the patient should have full understanding of effects (i.e. it is not suitable for rapid relief of bronchospasm during acute asthma attack and is taken prophylactically regularly, and should be continued even when patient is asymptomatic)
- advise the patient to seek medical advice if any blurred vision or visual disturbances occur
- the patient should be warned not to drive or operate machinery if any blurred vision or visual disturbances occur
- (Asthma) the patient should be advised not to stop therapy suddenly
- (Asthma) instruct the patient in correct use of metered dose inhaler (p. 106)
- instruct the patient in the correct technique for using nasal spray (p. 114), with the following exceptions:
    - shake the bottle gently before removing the cap
    - re-priming is required only if the nasal spray has not been used for 4 days
- see also General Patient education for antiasthma agents and bronchodilators (p. 98)

Considered safe to use in pregnancy.

Considered safe to use when breastfeeding.

FLUTICASONE PROPIONATE
Trade names
Axotide, Flixonase Allergy & Hayfever 24 hr, Flixonase Nasule Drops, Flixotide, Flixotide Nebules, Fluair Inhaler

Available in combination with
- fluticasone propionate 50 microgram/actuation + formoterol fumarate dihydrate 5 microgram/actuation inhalation, 120 actuations
- fluticasone propionate 125 microgram/actuation + formoterol fumarate dihydrate 5 microgram/actuation inhalation, 120 actuations
- fluticasone propionate 250 microgram/actuation + formoterol fumarate dihydrate 10 microgram/actuation inhalation, 120 actuations
- fluticasone propionate + salmeterol combinations (see salmeterol p. 108)
- fluticasone propionate 50 micrograms + azelastine (HCl) 125 micrograms per spray nasal spray (APOHealth Allergy and Hayfever Relief, Chemists' Own Allermist, Dymista 125/50, Dymista Allergy, Misty-Duo Allergy)

FLUTICASONE FUROATE
Trade names
Arnuity Ellipta, Avamys

Available forms
Accuhaler blister: 100 microgram/inhalation, 250 microgram/inhalation, 500 microgram/inhalation;
Ellipta inhaler: 100 microgram/inhalation, 200 microgram/inhalation;
Metered dose inhaler (CFC free): 50 microgram/inhalation, 125 microgram/inhalation, 250 microgram/inhalation;
Nasal spray: 27.5 microgram/spray, 50 microgram/spray;
Nasal suspension (drops): 400 microgram/400 microlitre;
Nebuliser solution (nebules): 0.5 mg/2 mL, 2 mg/2 mL

Action
- corticosteroid that acts on the lungs without significant systemic effects
- (Asthma) symptom preventer

Use
- prophylactic management of asthma
- mild-to-moderate nasal polyps
- allergic rhinitis (seasonal, perennial) (short-term treatment, 3—6 months)

Dose
- (Asthma) 100—200 micrograms via inhalation once daily (Arnuity Ellipta) **OR**
- (Mild asthma) 100—250 micrograms via inhalation twice daily, then reducing to lowest dose to control symptoms (Flixotide) **OR**
- (Moderate asthma) 250—500 micrograms via inhalation twice daily, then reducing to lowest dose to control symptoms (Flixotide) **OR**
- (Severe asthma) 500—1000 micrograms via inhalation twice daily, then reducing to lowest dose to control symptoms (Flixotide) **OR**
- (Severe asthma) 2 mg via nebuliser twice daily (Flixotide Nebules) **OR**
- (Allergic rhinitis) initially 2 sprays (55 micrograms) per nostril daily, decreasing to 1 spray (27.5 micrograms) per nostril daily (nasal spray) (Avamys) **OR**
- (Allergic rhinitis) initially 2 sprays (100 micrograms) per nostril daily, decreasing to 1 spray (50 micrograms) per nostril daily (nasal spray) (Flixonase) **OR**
- (Nasal polyps) 400 micrograms 1—2 times daily divided evenly between two nostrils (nasal drops) (Flixonase Nasule Drops)

Adverse effects
- (Nasal spray/drops) stinging, sneezing, dry/irritated nose and throat, unpleasant or strong smell and taste, dry mouth, nasal crust, headache, nosebleed, nasal ulceration

ANTIASTHMA AGENTS, BRONCHODILATORS AND RESPIRATORY AGENTS

- (Inhalation) mouth or throat candidiasis, lower/upper respiratory tract infection, influenza, hoarseness, bronchitis, nasopharyngitis, pharyngitis, sinusitis, headache, toothache, oropharyngeal pain, cough, back pain
- (Inhalation, rare) paradoxical bronchospasm
- (Rare, nasal spray, prolonged use) nasal atrophy and nasal septal perforation
- (Rare) hypersensitivity reaction, impaired wound healing, glaucoma, increased intraocular pressure, cataract formation
- (Long-term use) decreased bone mineral density

Interactions
- not recommended with ritonavir
- caution if used with itraconazole
- (Nasal spray) caution if used with other formulations of corticosteroids because of the increased risk of adverse effects

Nursing considerations/Cautions
- the Accuhaler is breath actuated and is suitable for anyone with difficulties using a metered dose aerosol inhaler
- (Allergic rhinitis) if prophylaxis is required, nasal spray should be administered before exposure to allergen
- (Nasal spray) if therapy is prolonged, twice-yearly examination of nasal mucosa is recommended
- if the patient experiences any visual disturbances, referral to an ophthalmologist is recommended
- (Nebules) can be diluted with sodium chloride if needed
- (Nasal spray) caution if used in children as growth may be retarded
- caution if used in those with risk factors for reduced body mass (e.g. prolonged immobilisation, family history of osteoporosis or chronic use of agents that decrease body mass)
- (Inhalation) caution if used in those with liver impairment. For those with moderate-to-severe liver impairment, a maximum daily dose of 100 micrograms is recommended
- (Nasal spray) not recommended in those with nasal septal ulcers or recent nasal injury or surgery until healing has occurred
- (Arnuity Ellipta) contraindicated in those with severe milk-protein allergy or hypersensitivity to lactose
- contraindicated in those with hypersensitivity to other corticosteroids

Patient education
- the patient should be advised that fluticasone is not recommended for acute asthma episodes or status asthmaticus
- warn the patient not to drive or operate machinery if blurred vision or visual disturbance occurs
- (Arnuity Ellipta) instruct the patient that inhalation should be used at the same time every day (either morning or night)
- if using the nebuliser with a mask, advise the patient to wash face thoroughly after therapy
- ensure that the patient is aware of detailed instructions for using the metered dose aerosol inhaler (p. 106), Ellipta inhaler and Accuhaler (see p.132). Extension tubes (spacers) are designed for attachment to the mouthpiece to increase lung deposition of inhaled drug if the patient is unable to master the inhaler technique
- (Allergic rhinitis) warn the patient that it may take several days for the full effect to be evident
- (Allergic rhinitis) instruct the patient to seek medical advice if there is no improvement in symptoms in 7 days
- (Nasal drops) instruct the patient in the correct use of nasal drops, including:
  1. gently blow the nose to clear both nostrils before using drops
  2. one nasule is sufficient for both nostrils
  3. flick/shake container several times to ensure solution is well mixed
  4. hold the top of the container and flick downwards in one quick

HAVARD'S NURSING GUIDE TO DRUGS

  motion to remove any solution from the neck of the container
5. twist and remove the top
6. to instil drops, the patient should lie on their back with head supported
7. squeeze the container to insert 6 drops (half container/dose) into one nostril, then repeat in the other nostril
8. keep the head in position for at least 1 minute
9. avoid contact with eyes; however, if contact occurs, rinse eyes well with water
10. drops should be protected from light and not frozen

- (Accuhaler) instruct the patient in correct use of the Accuhaler device, including:
  1. before starting, check the dose counter and then open the cover using a thumb grip
  2. hold the device horizontally and load the dose by sliding the lever until a click is heard
  3. breathe out gently (away from the inhaler) and place the mouth around the mouthpiece (closing lips to form a good seal and keeping the device horizontal)
  4. breathe in deeply and steadily, and then hold the breath for as long as comfortable (at least 5 seconds)
  5. remove the inhaler from the mouth (while still holding the breath)
  6. breathe out gently (away from the inhaler)
  7. if another dose is needed, repeat steps 3—6
  8. close the cover and click shut
  9. rinse mouth with water after use
- (Ellipta inhaler) instruct the patient in the correct use of the Ellipta device, including:
  1. opening and closing the device cover without inhaling medication results in loss of dose
  2. check the dose counter. A new device will show 30 doses. When fewer than 10 doses are left, half the dose cover will be red. When the last dose has been used, the dose counter will show 0
  3. do not shake the device but slide the cover down until a click is heard
  4. breathe out gently (away from the inhaler), then place the mouth over the mouthpiece to form a good seal, but taking care not to cover the air vent
  5. breathe in deeply and steadily and then hold the breath for as long as comfortable (or at least 5 seconds) and remove the inhaler
  6. breathe out gently (away from the inhaler)
  7. slide the cover upwards as far as it will go to cover the mouthpiece
  8. rinse the mouth with water after use
- (Nasal spray) instruct the patient in the correct use of nasal spray (see p. 114) with the following exceptions:
  - shake the bottle well before use
  - when finished, clean the nozzle carefully with tissue and replace cap
  - therapy can be continued for up to 6 months
  - nasal spray should be discarded 12 weeks from first use or after expiry date
- see also General Patient education for antiasthma agents and bronchodilators (p. 98)

 Should be used when breastfeeding only if benefits outweigh risks as no data are available.

Available in combination with
- fluticasone furoate 100 microgram/actuation + umeclidinium 62.5 microgram/actuation + vilanterol 25 microgram/actuation powder for inhalation (Anoro Ellipta)
- fluticasone furoate + umeclidinium + vilanterol combinations (see umeclidinium p. 117)
- fluticasone furoate 100 microgram/actuation + vilanterol 25 microgram/

ANTIASTHMA AGENTS, BRONCHODILATORS AND RESPIRATORY AGENTS

- actuation powder for inhalation, (BreoEllipta 100/25)
- fluticasone furoate 200 microgram/actuation + vilanterol 25 microgram/actuation powder for inhalation, (BreoEllipta 200/25)

OTHER RESPIRATORY AGENTS

BENRALIZUMAB
Trade name
Fasenra

Available form
Prefilled pen: 30 mg/mL

Action
- antibody that binds to interleukin-5 receptor (IL-5R) (IL-5 receptor is expressed on surface of eosinophils and basophils)
- reduces eosinophilic inflammation, which is an important component in asthma pathogenesis

Use
- severe eosinophilic asthma (eosinophil count ≥ 300 cells/microlitre or ≥ 150 cells/microlitre if on oral corticosteroid therapy)

Dose
- 30 mg SC every 4 weeks for 3 doses, then every 8 weeks

Adverse effects
- headache
- pharyngitis, cough
- arthralgia
- fever
- injection site reaction
- hypersensitivity

Nursing considerations/Cautions
- before starting therapy, treatment with high-dose inhaled corticosteroids and long-acting beta agonists should be optimised
- any helminth infection should be treated before starting therapy. If infestation occurs during therapy and does not respond to antihelminth therapy, benralizumab should be stopped until infestation is treated successfully
- corticosteroid therapy can be gradually decreased if appropriate, but should not be stopped abruptly
- patient should be closely monitored for hypersensitivity reaction, which can occur within hours of administration (but can also be delayed)
- patient can be instructed in SC administration

Patient education
- ensure the patient understands that benralizumab should not be used to treat acute asthma exacerbation
- the patient should be instructed to seek medical advice immediately if:
  - asthma remains uncontrolled or worsens after starting therapy
  - any signs of delayed hypersensitivity (e.g. urticaria, rash) occur
- ensure the patient understands administration instructions (see Mepolizumab Patient education, p. 141)

 Not recommended during pregnancy unless benefits outweigh risks, as there are limited data in humans.

 Not recommended when breastfeeding unless benefits outweigh risks, as there are no data in humans.

BERACTANT
Trade name
Survanta

Available form
Vial: 25 mg/mL

Action
- pulmonary surfactant that lowers surface tension on alveolar surfaces during respiration and stabilises alveoli against collapse at resting transpulmonary pressures
- deficiency of surfactant causes respiratory distress syndrome (hyaline membrane disease) in premature infants

133

Use
- prevention of respiratory distress syndrome (RDS) in premature infants weighing less than 1250 g or with evidence of surfactant deficiency (preferably within 15 minutes of birth)
- treatment of confirmed RDS in infants requiring mechanical ventilation (as soon as possible, preferably within 8 hours of birth)

Dose
- 100 mg/kg (4 mL/kg) via intratracheal administration 4 times in first 48 hours of life, administered no more frequently than 6-hourly

Adverse effects
- transient bradycardia, hypotension, hypertension
- oxygen desaturation, hypercarbia, hypocarbia, apnoea
- endotracheal tube reflux, endotracheal blockage
- pallor, vasoconstriction
- increased risk of post-treatment nosocomial sepsis

Nursing considerations/Cautions
- should be used only in neonatal intensive care settings where infants can be frequently monitored with arterial or transcutaneous measurement of systemic oxygen and carbon dioxide
- oxygenation may improve markedly within minutes of administration; therefore the infant should be frequently observed and monitored
- if transient bradycardia and desaturation occurs, the procedure should be stopped and symptoms treated accordingly
- endotracheal suctioning is generally not required after administration unless airway obstruction occurs. Rales and moist breath sounds occur transiently after administration
- for intratracheal administration only
- the solution is off-white to light brown in colour
- if the solution has settled during storage, it should be swirled gently (not shaken) to redisperse
- allow to warm to room temperature for at least 20 minutes before administration. Alternatively, it can be warmed in the hand for at least 8 minutes
- artificial warming methods should not be used
- there are three different methods of administration involving end-hole catheter and disconnection of ventilator, instillation through the secondary lumen of the double lumen of an endotracheal tube with no disconnection from the ventilator, and a third method being a combination of both. Consult the manufacturer's instructions or institutional policies for administration details
- repeat doses are administered according to the infant's birthweight and are determined by ongoing respiratory distress
- repeat doses should not be given within 6 hours of the previous dose
- if given for prophylaxis, repeat doses should be given only after X-ray confirmation of RDS
- manual hand-bag ventilation should not be used to administer repeat doses. Ventilator settings may be changed to maintain appropriate oxygenation and ventilation
- unopened, unused vials that have been warmed to room temperature can be returned to the refrigerator within 8 hours; however, this should only occur once
- not recommended in infants weighing $<$ 600 g or $>$ 1750 g

DORNASE ALFA
Trade name
Pulmozyme

Available form
Inhalation solution: 1 mg/mL

Action
- mucolytic
- produced by genetically modified Chinese hamster ovary cells containing DNA that codes for DNase. Recombinant DNase is similar to the human enzyme that hydrolyses DNA in accumulated neutrophils in sputum, reducing viscosity of purulent lung secretions
- those with cystic fibrosis produce infected sputum that contains large amounts of mucus glycoproteins and extracellular DNA
- half-life 3–4 hours

Use
- respiratory complications in those with cystic fibrosis

Dose
- 2.5 mg nebulised once daily (may increase to twice daily if needed in those > 21 years)

Adverse effects
- pharyngitis, hoarse voice, laryngitis, rhinitis, dyspnoea, decreased lung function
- rash, urticaria
- dyspepsia
- fever
- conjunctivitis
- non-cardiac chest pain

Nursing considerations/Cautions
- therapy continuation should be based on clinical response and lung function tests (if possible)
- ultrasonic nebulisers should not be used for administration
- (Children < 5 years) administration should be via tight-fitting mask
- contraindicated in those with hypersensitivity to Chinese hamster ovary cell products

Patient education
- advise the patient of the following:
  - nebulise using compressed air at 6–8 L/minute
  - do not dilute or mix with other drugs
- may be used safely in conjunction with other standard treatments for cystic fibrosis
- unused portion of opened ampoules should be discarded
- should not be used if solution is cloudy or discoloured
- normal chest physiotherapy should continue as normal
- patient should be advised not to stop medication suddenly

Not recommended during pregnancy because no human data are available.

Not recommended when breastfeeding because no human data are available.

IVACAFTOR
Trade name
Kalydeco

Available forms
Tablet: 150 mg;
Granules: 25 mg, 50 mg, 75 mg

Action
- selective potentiator of cystic fibrosis (CF) transmembrane conductance regulator (CFTR) protein, thought to enhance chloride transport; however, the exact mechanism of action is not completely understood
- active metabolite
- half-life about 12 hours

Use
- treatment of CF in those ≥ 4 months who have G551D or other gating (class III) mutation in the CFTR gene

Dose
- (≥ 25 kg) 150 mg orally twice daily (tablet) **OR**
- (> 14 kg – < 25 kg) 75 mg orally twice daily (granules) **OR**
- (≥ 7 kg – < 14 kg) 50 mg orally twice daily (granules) **OR**
- (≥ 5 kg) 25 mg orally twice daily (granules)

Adverse effects

- dizziness, headache
- abdominal pain, diarrhoea, nausea, vomiting
- rash
- fever
- productive cough, upper respiratory tract infection, nasal congestion, pharyngeal erythema, oropharyngeal pain, rhinitis, sinus congestion, nasopharyngitis
- ear pain, ear discomfort, tinnitus, vestibular disorder, ear congestion
- bacteria in sputum
- (Uncommon) elevated liver enzymes
- (Rare) congenital lens opacities (cataract) (without vision impact)

Interactions

- serum levels may be increased by itraconazole, posaconazole, voriconazole, clarithromycin, fluconazole and erythromycin
- serum levels may be decreased by grapefruit juice, Seville oranges, rifampicin, rifabutin, dexamethasone, prednisolone (high dose), phenobarbital (phenobarbitone), carbamazepine, phenytoin and St John's wort
- may increase serum levels of midazolam, alprazolam, and diazepam, increasing the risk of adverse effects
- may increase serum levels of digoxin, ciclosporin and tacrolimus, increasing risk of adverse effects; therefore serum levels should be monitored during therapy
- caution if given with warfarin; therefore INR should be closely monitored, especially when starting or stopping therapy

Nursing considerations/Cautions

- the patient should receive therapy only if accurate and validated genotyping has been performed to confirm presence of gating (class III) mutation in at least one allele of the CFTR gene
- baseline and regular ophthalmological examinations are recommended
- liver function tests are recommended before starting, 3-monthly during first year, then yearly during therapy. Therapy should be interrupted if AST or ALT levels are greater than 5 times the upper normal limit
- contains lactose and are therefore not recommended in those with rare hereditary problems of galactose intolerance, Lapp lactase deficiency or glucose—galactose malabsorption
- caution if used in those with severe kidney impairment (creatinine clearance $\leq$ 30 mL/minute) or end-stage kidney disease
- not recommended in those with severe liver impairment
- not recommended in transplant patients
- not recommended in those with CF who are homozygous for the F508del mutation in the CFTR gene

Patient education

- instruct the patient to swallow tablets whole, not crushed, chewed, broken or dissolved
- the patient should be advised to take medication with fat-containing snack or meal, including those prepared with oil or butter, containing eggs, cheeses, nuts, avocado, whole milk, full-fat yoghurt or meats
- advise the patient to avoid food containing grapefruit juice or Seville oranges during therapy
- warn the patient to avoid driving or operating machinery if dizziness occurs
- (Granules) sachet should be mixed with teaspoon (5 mL) of age-appropriate soft food/liquid (e.g. pureed fruits/vegetables, milk, yoghurt, water, juice) and should be ingested within 1 hour of mixing
- (Granules) food/liquid should be at room temperature or lower when mixing with granules

Granules can be dispersed in 5 mL of water, milk or juice or mixed with spoonful of pureed fruit or vegetables.

 Tablets should be swallowed whole.

 Not recommended in pregnancy, as limited data are available.

 Consider use carefully when breastfeeding owing to limited clear data. If used, consider monitoring the infant's bilirubin and liver enzymes.

 Caution if used in those with severe renal impairment (CrCl<30 mL/min) or end stage renal disease (ESRD).
Not recommended in those 6 years and older with severe liver impairment (Child-Pugh Class C) and dose reduction in those with moderate liver impairment (Child-Pugh Class B).
In infants 4-6 months, not recommended in those with any level of liver impairment unless benefits outweigh risks. If given, dose reduction (25 mg granules daily) or less frequent dosing is recommended.
In infants 1-4 months with liver impairment, therapy is not recommended.

Available in combination with
- ivacaftor 37.5 mg + elexacaftor 50 mg + tezacaftor 25 mg tablet and ivacaftor 75 mg tablet (Trikafta 50 mg/25 mg/37.5 mg + 75 mg Tablets composite pack)
- ivacaftor 75 mg + elexacaftor 100 mg + tezacaftor 50 mg tablet and ivacaftor 150 mg tablet (Trikafta 100 mg/50 mg/75 mg + 150 mg Tablets composite pack)
- ivacaftor 60 mg + elexacaftor 80 mg + tezacaftor 40 mg granules and ivacaftor 59.5 mg granules (Trikafta 80 mg/40 mg 60 mg + 59.5 mg Granules composite pack)
- ivacaftor 75 mg + elexacaftor 100 mg + tezacaftor 50 mg granules & ivacaftor 75 mg granules (Trikafta 100 mg/50 mg/75 mg + 75 mg Granules composite pack)
- ivacaftor 125 mg + lumacaftor 100 mg tablet/granules (Orkambi 100/125)
- ivacaftor 125 mg + lumacaftor 200 mg (Orkambi 200/125)
- ivacaftor 94 mg + lumacaftor 75 mg granules (Orkami 75/94 Granules)
- ivacaftor 188 mg + lumacaftor 150 mg granules (Okambi 150/188)
- ivacaftor 75 mg + tezacaftor 50 mg tablet & ivacaftor 75 mg tablet (Symdeko 50 mg/75 mg + 75 mg Tablets composite pack)
- ivacaftor 150 mg + tezacaftor 100 mg tablet & ivacaftor 150 mg tablet (Symdeko 100 mg/150 mg + 150 mg Tablets composite pack)

MANNITOL
Trade names
Aridol, Bronchitol

Available forms
Powder for inhalation: 40 mg;
Diagnostic kit containing capsules (0 mg, 5 mg, 10 mg, 20 mg, 40 mg) and inhalation device:

Action
- when inhaled, increases osmolarity in airways in a similar way to other bronchial provocation tests causing a release of mediators from airway inflammatory cells that result in bronchoconstriction
- (Diagnostic) response is greater in patient with asthma or exercise-induced asthma
- airway response is measured using forced expiratory volume in 1 second (FEV_1)
- (Treatment) mannitol is spray-dried and delivered to lungs using a specific inhaler device to improve lung hygiene by correcting impaired mucociliary clearance
- (Treatment) thought to change viscoelastic properties of mucus, but exact action is unknown

HAVARD'S NURSING GUIDE TO DRUGS

Use
* treatment of cystic fibrosis, either as adjunctive therapy with dornase alfa (p. 134) or in those intolerant to or with inadequate response to dornase alfa (Bronchitol)
* identifying bronchial hyper-responsiveness to help in diagnosis of asthma (Aridol)

Dose
* cumulative dose of 635 mg given (or until positive response is achieved) (Aridol) **OR**
* 400 mg via inhaler device twice daily (morning and 2−3 hours before bedtime) (after initiation dose assessment has been completed) (Bronchitol)

Adverse effects
* bronchospasm (chest tightness, cough or wheezing)
* cough, pharyngolaryngeal pain, rhinorrhea, haemoptysis, dyspnoea, nasopharyngitis, sinusitis
* eye pruritus
* nausea, vomiting, diarrhoea, upper abdominal pain, decreased appetite
* back pain, arthralgia, musculoskeletal pain
* headache, dizziness, fatigue, insomnia, sinus headache
* chest discomfort/tightness
* throat irritation, tonsillitis
* epistaxis
* flu-like illness
* rash
* fever

Interactions
* inhaled corticosteroids will reduce response and should be withheld before procedure

Nursing considerations/Cautions
* given by inhalation only

Diagnostic procedure
* the patient must be supervised at all times during the procedure
* medication to treat severe bronchospasm, bronchodilators and oxygen must be present in the testing area
* spirometry should be performed before challenge, to determine resting FEV_1
* seat the patient comfortably and encourage them to maintain good posture during the procedure to achieve effective delivery into the lungs
* apply the nose clip and direct the patient to breathe through mouth
* place the capsule (0 mg) in the inhalation device and puncture it by depressing buttons on the side of the device slowly (capsule should only be punctured once, to prevent fragmenting occurring)
* advise the patient to exhale completely, then inhale from the device in a controlled, rapid, deep inspiration. A 60-second timer should be set and the patient asked to hold the breath for 5 seconds, then exhale and remove the nose clip. At the end of 60 seconds, FEV_1 should be measured twice (this is the baseline). The procedure is then repeated using 5 mg, 10 mg, 20 mg, 40 mg, etc. until a cumulative dose of 635 mg has been given or the patient has a positive response
* a positive response is achieved when FEV_1 is 15% less than baseline (0 mg dose) or there is 10% incremental fall in FEV_1 between doses. A beta2 agonist may be given to accelerate recovery and patients should be monitored until FEV_1 is within 5% of baseline levels
* there should be minimal delay between FEV_1 measurement and next dose
* at least 2 repeatable FEV_1 measurements should be obtained after each dose
* 80 mg and 160 mg doses are given in multiples of 40 mg capsules (e.g. 2 × 40 mg) with no interval between doses (i.e. one capsule should be followed immediately by the next capsule until the total dose has been inhaled)
* a new inhalation device should be used for each test (not cleaned during test)

- a number of agents may interfere with response and should be withheld, including:
  - smoking (at least 6 hours)
  - vigorous exercise (not performed on day of testing)
  - significant amounts of coffee, tea and other caffeine-containing foods and drinks (day of testing)
  - inhaled non-steroidal anti-inflammatory agents (6—8 hours)
  - short-acting beta2 agonists (e.g. salbutamol) (8 hours)
  - inhaled corticosteroids or anticholinergic bronchodilatore (e.g ipratropium) ipratropium (12 hours)
  - long-acting beta2 agonists (e.g. salmeterol) and xanthines (e.g. theophyliine) (24 hours)
  - inhaled corticosteroids plus long-acting beta2 agonists (24 hours)
  - long-acting anticholinergics (e.g. tiotropium bromide)
  - tiotropium bromide, antihistamines (72 hours)
  - leukotriene receptor antagonists (4 days)
- if 0 mg capsule induces a FEV_1 fall > 10% or the patient experiences spirometry-induced asthma, further testing should not be done and the patient should be administered a bronchodilator
- pharyngolaryngeal pain may be reduced by rinsing the mouth after testing
- caution if the patient has ventilatory impairment (resting FEV_1 < 70% normal predicted value or an absolute value of 1.5 L in adults), spirometry-induced bronchoconstriction, haemoptysis (of unknown origin), pneumothorax, recent abdominal, thoracic or eye surgery, unstable angina, inability to perform spirometry of suitable quality or respiratory tract infection (upper or lower) in previous 2 weeks
- contraindicated in those where conditions may be compromised by induced bronchospasm or repeated blowing manoeuvres (e.g. aortic or cerebral aneurysms, myocardial infarction, uncontrolled hypertension or stroke in previous 6 months)

Treatment
- an initiation dose assessment for bronchial hyperresponsiveness should be conducted under supervision before staring therapy. Assessment requires measurement of oxygen saturation (SpO_2) and performing spirometry. Drugs and equipment for management of acute bronchospasm should be readily available in the event of an emergency
- initiation dose assessment:
  - the patient should be instructed in the correct inhaler technique
  - baseline FEV_1 and SpO_2 are measured
  - the patient is premedicated with bronchodilator 5—15 minutes before dose
  - all subsequent FEV_1 and SpO_2 measurements should be performed 1 minute after dose
  - the patient inhales 40 mg, then SpO_2 is monitored
  - the patient inhales 80 mg, then SpO_2 is monitored
  - the patient inhales 120 mg, then FEV_1 is measured, SpO_2 is monitored
  - the patient inhales 160 mg, then FEV_1 is measured, SpO_2 is monitored
  - FEV_1 is measured 15 minutes after last dose
- the patient is considered hyperresponsive if:
  - SpO_2 falls $\geq$ 10% at any stage of the assessment
  - FEV_1 fall $\geq$ 20% at the cumulative 240 mg dose
  - FEV_1 fall $\geq$ 20% (from baseline) at the end of assessment and does not return to within $\leq$ 20% of baseline within 15 minutes
  - FEV_1 fall $\geq$ 50% (from baseline) at the end of assessment
- the patient should be closely monitored to ensure FEV_1 returns to baseline level after assessment is complete

- the patient should be monitored carefully for any signs of significant haemoptysis and therapy stopped if massive/severe haemoptysis (> 240 mL/ 24 hours or recurrent bleeding ≥ 100 mL over several days) occurs
- the patient should be reviewed after 6 weeks of therapy for any signs of drug-induced bronchospasm. If any uncertainty exists, the initiation assessment should be repeated
- caution if used in those with history of asthma
- not recommended in those who are unable to complete spirometry or complete the initiation dose assessment
- not recommended in those with history of significant haemoptysis (> 60 mL) in previous 12 weeks, impaired lung function (FEV_1 < 30%), liver or kidney impairment or non-cystic fibrosis bronchiectasis
- contraindicated in those with hypersensitivity or with bronchial hyper-responsiveness to mannitol (either pre-existing or determined by initiation dose assessment)

Patient education

- (Bronchitol) instruct the patient:
  - in the correct inhaler technique (each capsule is loaded separately into the device, capsules are inhaled using the inhaler device with one or two breaths, then the empty capsule discarded before inserting the next capsule into device)
  - to replace the inhaler device weekly
- if needed, the inhaler device can be washed with warm water and allowed to completely dry before re-use
- use a bronchodilator 5—15 minutes before mannitol
- normal physiotherapy and dornase alfa therapy (if used) should be completed as normal after mannitol
- the patient should be advised to report any persistent cough when using mannitol therapy

 Considered safe to use in pregnancy if benefits outweigh the risk owing to an increased chance of mannitol-induced bronchospasm.

 Considered safe to use when breastfeeding.

 Banned in sport.

Note
- also available as Osmitrol Intravenous Infusion for use as an osmotic diuretic (see p. 1098)

MEPOLIZUMAB
Trade name
Nucala

Available forms
Vial: 100 mg;
Prefilled syringe/pen: 100 mg/mL

Action
- humanised monoclonal antibody (IgG_1 kappa) that targets human interleukin-5 (IL-5) responsible for growth, differentiation, recruitment, activation and survival of eosinophils
- half-life 16—22 days

Use
- adjunctive therapy for severe refractory eosinophilic asthma (EA)
- relapsed or refractory eosinophilic granulomatosis with polyangiitis (EGPA)

Dose
- (Severe EA) 100 mg SC once every 4 weeks **OR**
- (Relapsed or refractory EGPA) 300 mg SC every 4 weeks

Adverse effects
- headache, fatigue
- pruritus, eczema
- abdominal pain, nausea, vomiting, diarrhoea

ANTIASTHMA AGENTS, BRONCHODILATORS AND RESPIRATORY AGENTS

- back pain, muscle spasm, arthralgia
- dyspnoea, nasal congestion, nasopharyngitis, pharyngitis
- bronchitis, allergic rhinitis, exacerbation of asthma, viral respiratory infection, sinusitis, upper respiratory tract infection
- herpes zoster, influenza, urinary tract infection
- hypersensitivity (urticaria, angioedema, rash, bronchospasm, hypotension)
- development of neutralising antibodies
- (Injection site) pain, redness, swelling, itching, burning sensation

Nursing considerations/Cautions

- patient should be monitored for any signs of hypersensitivity after SC administration
- any helminth infection should be treated before starting therapy. If helminth infection occurs during therapy, the patient should be treated. However, if the patient is unresponsive to helminth therapy, mepolizumab therapy should be interrupted
- rotate SC administration sites (upper arm, thigh or abdomen)
- the patient may be taught to self-administer using prefilled syringe/pen
- to reconstitute the vial, add 1.2 mL water for injections vertically onto the centre of the powder and gently swirl in circular motion for 10 seconds, then allow the vial to rest for further 5 seconds until the powder is dissolved, avoiding any foaming or frothing
- reconstituted solution may be colourless to pale yellow or pale brown in colour
- do not shake reconstituted solution before administration to prevent foaming or precipitation
- caution if used in patients with pre-existing helminth infestation
- not recommended in children < 12 years

Patient education

- advise the patient that this should not be used for management of acute asthma episodes
- the patient should be instructed to seek medical advice immediately if asthma remains uncontrolled or symptoms worsen after starting therapy
- advise the patient to continue with corticosteroid therapy and not to stop this abruptly
- warn the patient that hypersensitivity reaction (urticaria, angioedema, rash, bronchospasm, hypotension) may be delayed and occur days after starting therapy. If this occurs, the patient should seek medical advice immediately
- ensure the patient understands administration using a prefilled syringe/pen, including:
  - the pen/syringe should not be shaken or used if it is damaged or has been dropped on a hard surface
  - the needle cap should not be removed until ready to use
  - the pen/syringe should be removed from fridge, the pack opened and allowed to stand at room temperature for 30 minutes before administration (should not be warmed using hot water, direct sunlight or microwave)
  - check expiry date and solution (not cloudy or containing particles), which should be colourless to pale yellow to pale brown
  - choose injection site (abdomen or, if carer is administering injection, upper arm) and allow 5 cm between injection sites if more than one injection is needed. Injection site should be at least 5 cm from navel
  - the injection site should be free of scarring, bruising, redness or tenderness
  - hands should be washed with soap and water
  - the injection site should be cleaned with alcohol wipe and area allowed to dry

Pen instructions

- remove the cap from the pen but do not touch the yellow needle guard
- place the pen on the injection site with the yellow needle guard against skin.

Push pen down at a 90-degree angle until the first click is heard (injection started). Pen should be kept in place until a second click is heard. Continue holding pen against skin while counting to 5 and then lift pen from skin (this ensures full dose is given)

Syringe instructions
- remove the needle cap (pulling firmly away from needle)
- do not touch the needle or plunger or expel any air bubbles from syringe
- skin at the injection site should be pinched up and the needle inserted into pinched skin at a 45-degree angle
- slowly push the plunger down to inject the full dose (using thumb on plunger) until the stopper reaches the bottom of the syringe
- lift the thumb slowly to allow the plunger to come up and the needle to retract into the syringe
- release pinched skin
- the needle should not be recapped
  - if small drop of blood appears at injection site, press a cotton wool ball or gauze against site for a few seconds
  - the injection site should not be rubbed
  - used pen/syringe should be disposed of appropriately and safely in a sharps container
  - the prefilled pen/syringe can be removed from the fridge and kept in unopened pack for up to 7 days at room temperature (below 30°C and protected from light)
  - should be administered within 8 hours of opening the pack
  - discard if more than 8 hours has passed after opening the pack
  - the prefilled pen/syringe should be stored in fridge at 2—8°C but not frozen

Should be used during pregnancy only if benefits outweigh risks owing to limited data available.

Should be used when breastfeeding only if benefits outweigh risks owing to limited data available.

MONTELUKAST
Trade names
Lukair, Montelair, Singulair

Available forms
Tablets (chewable): 4 mg, 5 mg;
Tablets: 10 mg

Action
- selective leukotriene receptor antagonist that specifically inhibits the leukotrienes LTC4, LTD4 and LTE4 that are potent pro-asthmatic mediators (leukotrienes mediate bronchoconstriction, mucus secretion, vascular permeability and eosinophil recruitment)
- symptom preventer
- bronchodilation within 2 hours

Use
- prophylaxis and treatment of chronic asthma
- symptomatic treatment of seasonal allergic rhinitis

Dose
- 10 mg orally (at night for asthma, individualised time for allergic rhinitis)

Adverse effects
- fever
- headache, dizziness, fatigue, asthenia
- agitation, anxiety, aggression, insomnia, abnormal dreams, sleep walking, depression, tremor, hallucinations, disorientation, hostility
- dyspepsia, abdominal pain, diarrhoea
- dental pain
- cough, nasal congestion
- rash
- elevated liver enzymes
- (Rare) vasculitis, vasculitic rash, eosinophilia, eosinophilic granulomatosis with polyangiitis (EGPA, Churg—Strauss syndrome), suicidal ideation, worsening lung condition

ANTIASTHMA AGENTS, BRONCHODILATORS AND RESPIRATORY AGENTS

Nursing considerations/Cautions
- not used for relief of acute asthma attack
- chewable tablets (4 and 5 mg) contain aspartame therefore caution if used in those with phenylketonuria

Patient education
- the patient should be warned not to drive or operate machinery if dizziness or fatigue are ongoing
- advise the patient to keep taking medication regardless of their asthma status (i.e. whether stable or during an acute attack)
- can be given with inhaled corticosteroids. Corticosteroid dose may be reduced during therapy, but the patient should understand that montelukast is not an inhaled steroid therapy substitute
- instruct the patient (or carer) to seek medical advice if any of the following occur:
  - insomnia, sleep disturbance, sleep walking, abnormal dreams, hostility, aggression, restlessness, irritability, depression, tremor or hallucinations
  - any thoughts of self-harm, depressed mood or suicidal thoughts
- see also General Patient education for antiasthma agents and bronchodilators (p. 98)

 Chewable and plain tablets can be crushed and mixed with spoonful of yoghurt or apple puree.

 Considered safe to use when breastfeeding.

OMALIZUMAB
Trade names
Xolair, Omlyclo

Available forms
Vial: 150 mg;
Prefilled syringe: 75 mg/0.5 mL, 150 mg/mL

Action
- recombinant monoclonal antibody that selectively binds to IgE, which is thought to be responsible for degranulation of mast cells releasing histamines, leukotrienes, cytokines and other mediators

Use
- moderate-to-severe asthma (in those who have raised IgE concentrations (> 30 IU/mL) and concurrent inhaled steroid therapy)
- chronic spontaneous urticaria (CSU) as an adjunct to antihistamine therapy where symptoms are not controlled
- chronic rhinosinusitis with nasal polyps (CRSwNP)

Dose
- (Allergic asthma (patients greater than or equal to 6 yrs), CRSwNP (adults)) 75-600 mg SC every 4 weeks OR 225-375 mg SC every 2 weeks based on bodyweight, baseline serum IgE (max 750 mg/4 weeks).
- (CSU) 150—300 mg SC every 4 weeks (with antihistamine therapy)

Adverse effects
- (Injection site) pain, swelling, itching, redness
- headache, fatigue and, less commonly, dizziness and somnolence
- fever
- weight gain, nausea, upper abdominal pain, diarrhoea
- urticaria, rash
- cough, pharyngitis, nasopharyngitis, sinusitis, upper respiratory tract infection (viral)
- myalgia, arthralgia, back pain
- decreased platelet count (asymptomatic)
- allergic reactions (immediate or delayed)
- (Rare) arterial thromboembolic events, eosinophilic granulomatosis with polyangiitis (EGPA), Churg—Strauss syndrome), hypereosinophilic syndrome, development of antibodies

Interactions
- may interfere with skin prick test, patch testing and RAST testing for hypersensitivity to potential allergens; therefore caution is recommended when interpreting test results

Nursing considerations/Cautions
- allergic reactions can occur after first and subsequent dose, often within the first 2 hours (but sometimes delayed); adrenaline (epinephrine) and resuscitation equipment should be readily available
- dose and frequency are determined by body weight and IgE concentrations and given every 2 or 4 weeks
- doses greater than 750 mg are not recommended
- if patient gains weight, dose will need to be adjusted
- IgE concentrations are usually measured only before starting therapy and if therapy has been stopped for 12 months or more. If therapy is stopped for less than 1 year, the dose should be based on IgE level before the initial dose. IgE remains elevated for up to 12 months after therapy is stopped
- platelet count is recommended before starting and then regularly during therapy
- the patient's response to therapy should be assessed after 16 weeks. If the patient's asthma is well controlled, withdrawal of inhaled corticosteroids may be attempted (with medical supervision)
- administered SC only
- SC sites should be rotated
- (Vial) add 1.4 mL water for injections to the vial (held upright) and swirl contents for 1 minute to wet the powder, but do not shake. Continue swirling for 5–10 seconds every 5 minutes to dissolve the powder (process usually requires 15–30 minutes). Invert the vial for 15 seconds to allow solution to drain towards the stopper. Using a new 3 mL syringe and large-bore needle (18 gauge), insert the needle tip into the vial (bottom of solution) and withdraw solution. Replace the needle with 25 gauge for SC administration
- (Vial) reconstituted solution should be clear and slightly opaque to pale brown-yellow in colour with no gel-like particles present. There may be small bubbles or foam around vial edge
- (Vial) reconstituted solution is viscous in nature; therefore care should be taken that entire dose is retrieved when withdrawing solution from vial
- (Vial) because of viscosity of solution, it may take 5–10 seconds to administer
- (Prefilled syringe) the patient may be taught to self-administer, but the first 3 doses should be given under supervision
- (Prefilled syringe) doses greater than 150 mg should be given into more than one site
- (Prefilled syringe) contains latex and should not be handled by those with latex sensitivity
- (Prefilled syringe) allow to come to room temperature for about 20 minutes before administration. Syringe should not be kept at room temperature for longer than 4 hours
- caution if used in those with (or a history of) thrombocytopenia
- caution if used in those with liver or kidney impairment
- caution if used in those with history of anaphylaxis, as they are at increased risk of allergic reaction

Patient education
- as allergic reactions can be delayed (1–5 days after injection or more), advise the patient to seek medical attention immediately if an allergic reaction occurs (including rash, fever, swollen glands, joint pain, stiffness)
- warn the patient against driving or operating machinery if fatigue, dizziness or somnolence are problematic
- (Prefilled syringe) instruct the patient in correct administration technique, including importance of rotation of SC

ANTIASTHMA AGENTS, BRONCHODILATORS AND RESPIRATORY AGENTS

sites, injection techniques, correct storage and disposal of used syringes

Caution if used during pregnancy owing to limited data available.

Caution if used when breastfeeding owing to limited data available.

PORACTANT ALFA
Trade names
Curosurf

Available forms
Vial: 120 mg/1.5 mL, 240 mg/3 mL

Action
- pulmonary surfactant that reduces surface tension at air—liquid interface on the alveoli during ventilation
- stabilises alveoli against collapse at resting transpulmonary pressures
- lack of surfactant in preterm infants results in respiratory distress syndrome (RDS) with poor lung expansion, inadequate gas exchange and gradual lung collapse (atelectasis)

Use
- treatment for RDS in preterm infants
- prophylaxis for infants at risk of RDS

Dose
- (Treatment for RDS) 200 mg/kg (2.5 mL/kg) intratracheal as soon as RDS is diagnosed, followed by up to 2 further doses of 100 mg/kg (1.25 mL/kg) at 12-hour intervals if needed (maximum total dose (400 mg/kg) 5 mL/kg) **OR**
- (Prophylaxis of RDS) 100—200 mg/kg as a single dose within 15 minutes of birth, with further doses of 100 mg/kg given 6—12 hours after initial dose, then 12 hours later in babies who have persistent symptoms of RDS and are ventilator dependent (maximum total dose 300—400 mg/kg)

Adverse effects
- bradycardia, hypotension
- endotracheal tube blockage
- oxygen desaturation

Nursing considerations/Cautions
- should be administered only in a neonatal intensive care setting
- any acidosis, hypotension, anaemia, hypoglycaemia or hypothermia should be treated before starting therapy
- infants receiving therapy should be frequently monitored, as medication can affect oxygenation and lung compliance, rapidly requiring modification to oxygen and ventilator support
- if transient adverse effects occur (e.g. bradycardia, hypotension, endotracheal tube blockage, oxygen desaturation), therapy should be stopped and adverse effects treated
- for intratracheal administration only
- administered via a 5 French end-hole catheter while briefly disconnecting the endotracheal tube from the ventilator or via the secondary lumen of a dual lumen endotracheal tube without interrupting mechanical ventilation
- before instillation, proper position and patency of the endotracheal tube should be established. If needed, the endotracheal tube may be suctioned, but the infant should be allowed to stabilise before instillation of therapy
- for endotracheal tube instillation with 5 French end-hole catheter: contents of the vial should be withdrawn into a 3 or 5 mL syringe through a large gauge ($\geq$ 20 gauge) needle and then a syringe attached to a precut 8 cm 5 end-hole French catheter. The catheter should be filled with solution and then excess solution discarded (through the catheter), leaving the exact dose in the syringe. Before administration, change the infant's ventilator settings to 40—60 breaths/minute, inspiratory time 0.5 seconds and supplemental oxygen

sufficient to maintain oxygen saturation (SaO$_2$) > 92%. With the infant in neutral position (head and body aligned with no inclination), disconnect the endotracheal tube from the ventilator. The precut 5 French catheter should be inserted into the endotracheal tube and 1.25 mL/kg instilled, and the infant positioned on either the right or left side. Remove the catheter and manually ventilate the infant with 100% oxygen for 1 minute at 40–60 breaths/minute. When the infant is stable, repeat the procedure on the other side with the remaining solution. Suctioning should not occur within 1 hour of instillation unless significant airway obstruction occurs. Ventilator management should return to pre-instillation settings

- for instillation via the secondary lumen of a dual lumen endotracheal tube: withdraw the contents into a 3 or 5 mL syringe through a large gauge ($\geq$ 20 gauge) needle. The infant should be in neutral position (with head and body aligned and no inclination). Administer solution via the secondary lumen as a single dose without interrupting ventilation. After dosing, some transient increase in ventilatory management may be required
- the solution should be white to creamy white and allowed to come to room temperature slowly before administration
- the vial should be slowly inverted (but not shaken) to ensure uniform distribution of solution
- unopened, unused vials that have been warmed to room temperature can be returned to the fridge within 24 hours for storage; however, this should not occur more than once

ANTIBACTERIAL AGENTS

Organisms which can produce infection in humans include bacteria, mycoplasma, spirochaetes, fungi and viruses. Agents used to treat bacterial infections (antibacterial agents) will be discussed in this section, while antiviral agents, antifungal agents and antimycobacterial agents are discussed in other sections.

The 'ideal' antibacterial drug harms the invading organism without harming the host (known as 'selective' toxicity) (Knights et al 2023). Antibacterial agents exploit the differences between the host and the invading organism and generally act in one of the following general ways:
- inhibiting bacterial cell wall synthesis (e.g. penicillins, cephalosporins, monobactams and carbapenems, glycopeptides)
- inhibiting bacterial protein synthesis (e.g. aminoglycosides, tetracyclines, chloramphenicol, macrolides, lincosamides, oxazolidinones, streptogramins)
- inhibiting synthesis of bacterial DNA (e.g. quinolones)
- disrupting bacterial cell membrane (e.g. colistimethate)
- interfering with metabolic processes such as bacterial nucleic acid synthesis or folate metabolism (e.g. sulfonamides, trimethoprim) (Knights et al 2023)

Bactericidal drugs kill susceptible microorganisms, whereas *bacteriostatic* drugs inhibit their growth but do not kill the organisms. Whether a drug is bacteriostatic or bactericidal may be dependent on the dose given and the concentration achieved at the site of action. Because bacteriostatic drugs slow the growth of the organisms, they give the body's immune system time to become activated and rid itself of the invading organisms. Whether or not an antibacterial agent is successful in destroying or suppressing bacterial growth is dependent on factors such as bacterial load (concentration of bacteria present), phase of bacterial growth, ability to achieve an adequate drug concentration at the site of the infection and the minimum inhibitory concentration of the antibacterial agent (this is the lowest amount of drug needed to prevent visible bacterial growth, and this is dependent on the antibacterial agent, the organism and the person being affected) (Knights et al 2023).

Antibacterial agents are often overused for many reasons, including doctors prescribing multiple antibiotics when one is sufficient, prescribing long courses unnecessarily, prescribing for self-limiting illnesses that don't require antibiotics, overuse as prophylaxis before surgery, over-the-counter (OTC) sales in some countries (encouraging inappropriate and/or indiscriminate use), and use in animal feeds to promote growth and prevent infection (Levison 2014). One outcome of this overuse is the development of resistance, resulting in fewer agents being effective in treating infection. Some organisms have innate (or intrinsic) resistance to some antimicrobial agents (i.e. they have always been resistant to them), while others have acquired resistance (i.e. the organism changes its genetic make-up or acquires new DNA) (Knights et al 2023). Antibacterial resistance has developed through the following processes:

- the antibacterial agent is unable to reach the target site because some organisms may form a protective membrane (e.g. glycocalyx or biofilm) that stops the antibacterial agent from reaching the bacterial cell wall. Gram-negative bacteria produce porins (outer membrane proteins) which allow diffusion of molecules (including antibacterials) into cytoplasm; however, mutations to porins impede antibacterial access (e.g. tobramycin-resistant *Pseudomonas aeruginosa*)
- developing enzymes that inactivate the drug (e.g. beta lactamase is an enzyme produced by staphylococci that inactivates the penicillins and many of the cephalosporins). Extended-spectrum beta lactamases have developed, which have led to bacteria having cross-resistance to penicillin and cephalosporins, as well as being resistant to other classes of antibacterial agents
- the antibacterial target site is altered so the drug can no longer bind to the site. Penicillin-binding proteins (PBP) are membrane-associated enzymes present in the cell wall of peptidoglycan-containing organisms. Changes to PBP can result in resistance occurring (e.g. *Staphylococcus aureus* resistance to beta-lactam antibiotics results from the development of highly resistant PBP)
- the antibacterial agent is pumped out by an efflux pump found in both Gram-positive and Gram-negative organisms (e.g. tetracycline-resistant *S. aureus*); development of bypass pathways that compensate for loss of function due to antibacterial agents (e.g. resistance to sulfonamides) (Brenner & Stevens 2017; Knights et al 2023).

Many resistant strains of bacteria exist in Australia, including methicillin-resistant *S. aureus* (MRSA) and vancomycin-resistant *Enterococcus faecium* (VRE). Other issues include the emergence of multi-drug-resistant HIV and *Mycobacterium tuberculosis* (Knights et al 2023). From a clinical perspective, it is this acquired resistance that has become a serious problem as it has reduced the number of drugs available to treat infection, potentially resulting in increased hospitalisation, longer lengths of stay in hospital and increased mortality (Knights et al 2023).

Many programs are in place that attempt to combat this drug resistance, including limiting the availability of some antibacterial agents (e.g. vancomycin, teicoplanin, imipenem) unless they are specifically required, using combinations rather than single agents in certain circumstances (e.g. mixed infections), or using them in rotation, as well as ensuring that the lowest effective dose is used (Knights et al 2023). It is therefore important that antibacterial agents are used only to treat bacterial infections (not viral or other types of infections), and that the organism is identified, along with its susceptibility or resistance (however, if the infection is life threatening, treatment should be started immediately) (Knights et al 2023). Use a dose that is high enough to be efficacious with minimal toxicity but has the narrowest spectrum of that organism and is used for the shortest duration possible (unless evidence suggests that longer is possible/advantageous) (Knights et al 2023).

General Nursing considerations/ Cautions for antibacterial agents

- appropriate culture and sensitivity testing should be done to isolate and identify the organism(s) and determine susceptibility to antibacterial agents
- mild- to life-threatening antibiotic-associated pseudomembranous colitis (caused by *Clostridioides difficile* toxin; see Glossary) may occur weeks after finishing a course of antibiotics. The condition may be worsened or prolonged if peristalsis-delaying drugs are given (e.g. opioid analgesics)
- monitor for signs of *C. difficile*: diarrhoea, abdominal pain and cramping, fever, nausea, loss of appetite, dehydration, pseudomembranous colitis, blood or pus in stools, elevated white blood cell count (leukocytosis)
- careful routine history is taken to exclude previous reactions to antibacterial agents (e.g. penicillin, cephalosporin), other allergens or severe asthma in order to avoid anaphylaxis
- all relevant medical staff must be informed of any antibiotic allergy, and medical history, medication chart and patient suitably labelled (e.g. patient identification label) (as per workplace guidelines)
- after administration of drugs (especially penicillins and cephalosporins), observe patient closely for bronchospasm, urticarial rash, signs of cardiovascular collapse or angioneurotic oedema (anaphylactoid reactions can occur with the first dose)
- ensure hand-washing occurs after patient contact by all staff to prevent cross-infection with organisms
- note and report signs of superinfection, such as stomatitis, 'black tongue', vaginal and/or oral moniliasis. Superinfection occurs because of an overgrowth by non-susceptible microorganisms (e.g. *Candida albicans*) during therapy
- ensure administration at regular (and prescribed) intervals to maintain adequate plasma drug levels
- lidocaine (lignocaine) toxicity may occur in patients with hepatic disease if lidocaine (lignocaine) is used repeatedly as a diluent to reduce the pain of IM injection. Lidocaine (lignocaine) should not be used for IV administration and is contraindicated in anyone with a known hypersensitivity to lidocaine (lignocaine) or other amide-type local anaesthetics, or in those with non-paced heart block, severe heart failure or infants less than 30 months

- IM injections should be given into large muscle mass, ensuring that injection sites are rotated
- when giving IM, avoid intravascular injection by aspirating syringe plunger prior to administration and checking for blood
- ensure that IV drugs are handled carefully to avoid spillage and spraying into the air during reconstitution and/or administration
- reconstitute drugs according to the manufacturer's instructions. Dry powders are generally reconstituted with water for injections (and then diluted with appropriate and compatible infusion fluid (e.g. sodium chloride 0.9%) if necessary). It is especially important to consult the manufacturer's product information if the antibacterial agent can be given both IM and IV, as the amount of diluent required may vary according to the route of administration
- if the recommended method of administration is by slow infusion, dilute the reconstituted drug in 50—100 mL of compatible infusion fluid and infuse over 30—60 minutes via a burette (some drugs are infused over 1—6 hours)
- if a slow bolus injection is necessary, the drug should be reconstituted with or diluted in 10—20 mL water for injections and injected over 1—10 minutes into side arm (injection port) of flowing administration set or through three-way tap, followed by flush with sodium chloride 0.9%. Slow bolus means **slow** — this prevents irritation to the vein and reduces pain and some adverse reactions related to administration
- maintain asepsis during administration of IV antibacterial agents
- maintain activity of drug by correct storage conditions (especially if not administered immediately)
- have adrenaline (epinephrine), IV corticosteroids, oxygen and resuscitation equipment available in the event of anaphylaxis

General Patient education for antibacterial agents

- the patient should be advised to obtain a MedicAlert bracelet or pendant if they have an allergy to antibacterial agent (or other drugs, foods, dyes or preservatives)
- instruct the patient to inform any medical or nursing personnel of allergy, especially when antibacterial agent is being administered
- emphasise the importance of completing the entire course of the prescribed antibacterial agent, even if the patient feels better quickly. Discourage keeping any antibacterial agents and self-medicating if symptoms recur
- instruct the patient to immediately seek medical advice if any of the following occurs:
  - diarrhoea (especially if severe, watery or bloody), severe stomach cramps and/or fever during therapy or up to several weeks after stopping antibacterial agents
  - it is essential to stress the importance of not taking any medication to stop the diarrhoea, as this may worsen the condition
  - skin rash or hives, blistering or peeling of skin, swelling to face, lips, mouth or throat making it difficult to breathe or swallow or any breathing difficulty, including wheezing

- advise patient to seek medical advice (but not an emergency) if vaginal itching or discharge (vaginal thrush) or white, sore, furry tongue and mouth (oral thrush) occurs
- ensure patient understands when to take oral preparations in relation to food (e.g. before or after meals) and other medications such as antacids
- instruct patient to keep any antibacterial mixtures/suspensions/syrups in the refrigerator (not freezer) and discard as advised by pharmacist
- advise patient not to drive or operate machinery if they experience dizziness, lethargy, tiredness, blurred vision or other similar side-effects which may impair judgement or driving ability
- as many antibacterial agents have been implicated in reducing the effectiveness of oral contraceptives, women are advised to check with the prescriber to ascertain whether additional contraceptive precautions (e.g. barrier method) are required during therapy
- with female patients of childbearing potential, the importance of seeking medical advice if they become pregnant or plan to breastfeed during therapy must be discussed

INHIBITORS OF BACTERIAL CELL WALL SYNTHESIS

Penicillins, cephalosporins, monobactams and carbapenems all contain a beta-lactam ring, which relates them structurally. It is this ring that is essential for antibacterial activity. Many bacteria produce beta lactamase (penicillinase), an enzyme that breaks the beta-lactam ring, thereby rendering the antibacterial agent ineffective against that bacterial strain. It is now possible to add beta-lactamase inhibitors to penicillins, making them active against previously resistant strains; however, this does increase the cost (Knights et al 2023). These inhibitors include clavulanic acid and tazobactam. Furthermore, some Gram-negative organisms have a phospholipid membrane that prevents some of the penicillins from entering the cell, making those organisms resistant to penicillin.

PENICILLINS

General Actions of penicillins
- selectively inhibit formation of a rigid bacterial cell wall
- bactericidal
- Gram-negative bacilli are generally resistant to penicillins
- classified as:
    - narrow spectrum (e.g. benzylpenicillin, phenoxymethylpenicillin)
    - narrow spectrum, penicillinase resistant (e.g. dicloxacillin)
    - moderate spectrum beta-lactamase-sensitive aminopenicillins (e.g. amoxicillin, ampicillin)
    - broad and extended spectrum (e.g. piperacillin, ticarcillin)

General Uses of penicillins
- infections where the organisms are not resistant to penicillins, including:
    - upper and lower respiratory tract infections
    - skin and skin structure infections
    - bone and joint infections
    - urinary tract infections
    - gynaecological infections
    - septicaemia, bacteraemia
    - intra-abdominal infections
    - sexually transmitted infections (e.g. gonorrhoea, syphilis, yaws, bejel, pinta)
    - scarlet fever
    - meningitis
    - fusospirochaetosis (Vincent's gingivitis and pharyngitis)
    - Group A streptococci infection without bacteraemia

- surgical (including obstetric and colorectal) prophylaxis (where there is significant risk of postoperative infection)
- prophylaxis of rheumatic fever, rheumatic heart disease and acute glomerulonephritis
- prophylaxis of subacute bacterial endocarditis (SBE)

General Adverse effects of penicillins

- hypersensitivity reaction, including urticaria, exfoliative dermatitis, maculopapular rash, rash, pruritus
- anaemia, leucopenia, thrombocytopenia, agranulocytosis, purpura and, rarely, prolongation of bleeding time and prothrombin time
- headache
- glossitis, stomatitis, black hairy tongue
- diarrhoea, nausea, vomiting, abdominal pain, taste/smell disturbance
- fever
- superinfection (vaginal and/or oral moniliasis), pseudomembranous colitis, serum sickness-like reaction (chills, fever, oedema, arthralgia), allergic reaction
- (High doses, rare) interstitial nephropathy
- (Rare) hepatitis, cholestatic jaundice
- (Rare, high doses) convulsions, dizziness, confusion, encephalopathy
- (Rare) anaphylactic shock, anaphylactoid reaction, severe skin reactions
- (Rapid IV) convulsions
- (IV) phlebitis, pain, burning, erythema, swelling
- (IM) pain
- (Rare, repeated IM injection) quadriceps femoris fibrosis and atrophy

General Interactions of penicillins

- aminoglycosides and penicillins are physically and/or chemically incompatible
- increased risk of aminoglycoside-associated nephrotoxicity if aminoglycosides and penicillins are given together, especially in those with renal impairment. If given together, renal function should be closely monitored
- penicillins may affect the stability of anticoagulant control, therefore prothrombin time should be carefully monitored, especially when starting and stopping therapy
- increased risk of bleeding if given in high-dose IV with antiplatelet agents. If given together, patient should be closely monitored for any signs of bleeding
- probenecid increases and prolongs serum penicillin levels
- effect of penicillins may be reduced by the bacteriostatic agents chloramphenicol, erythromycin and tetracycline, therefore therapeutic response should be closely monitored
- some penicillins may cause failure of combined oral contraceptives, which may be due to increased oestrogen metabolism or decreased oestrogen reabsorption in the gut
- may decrease clearance of methotrexate, potentially resulting in methotrexate toxicity. If given together, methotrexate levels should be closely monitored
- lidocaine (lignocaine) toxicity may occur in patients with liver disease or reduced liver blood flow if lidocaine (lignocaine) is used repeatedly as a diluent to reduce the pain of IM injection
- increased risk of pseudomembranous colitis if given with peristalsis-delaying agents such as opioid analgesics or atropine/diphenoxylate combination
- absorption may be decreased by antacids
- may cause false positive result on urine glucose testing with some reagents

General Nursing considerations/ Cautions for penicillins

- (Meningitis) blood—brain barrier permeability is increased with inflammation, leading to an increased risk of

ANTIBACTERIAL AGENTS

- encephalopathy occurring at a lower dose, therefore patients should be closely monitored
- probenecid 1 g may be given orally 30 minutes before injection to increase and prolong the serum penicillin level
- penicillin should be handled carefully by staff to prevent self-sensitisation
- when only part of a vial's contents is required (e.g. 750 mg from a 1 g vial), reconstitution should be according to dilution table found in the manufacturer's information; discard any remaining solution
- needle blockage is less likely if a small-bore syringe and 20-gauge needle are used
- if giving IM with lidocaine (lignocaine) (without adrenaline (epinephrine)), it is important to ensure patient does not have a hypersensitivity to lidocaine (lignocaine)
- treatment should continue 48—72 hours after symptoms have abated
- treatment should generally not exceed 14 days
- if treatment is prolonged, blood counts and liver and renal function should be monitored
- IV injection should be given over at least 3—5 minutes to prevent pain and convulsions
- if single-dose therapy is used for urinary tract infection, urine should be cultured post therapy — if organisms are still present, a longer or higher dose treatment regimen is recommended
- if treating streptococcal disease, cultures should be taken at the end of therapy to ensure total eradication of organism
- all patients with gonorrhoea should also have serological testing for syphilis at time of diagnosis and then monthly for at least 4 months
- electrolyte monitoring is recommended if given in high doses and/or for prolonged therapy in some patients (e.g. those with heart or renal disease) for whom sodium intake may have an impact
- care should be taken if the person is on a salt-restricted diet as many parenteral preparations have a high sodium content that may worsen cardiac failure
- oxygen, adrenaline, IV corticosteroids and intubation equipment should be readily available in the case of a severe hypersensitivity reaction occurring
- caution if used in those with a history of GI diseases (especially colitis), mononucleosis, bleeding disorders, cardiac disease, cystic fibrosis, impaired renal or liver function
- caution if used in those with allergic tendencies
- contraindicated in those with known hypersensitivity to beta-lactam antibiotics (penicillins and cephalosporins)
- (With lidocaine (lignocaine)) contraindicated in those with amide-type local anaesthetic hypersensitivity
- see also General Nursing considerations/Cautions for antibacterial agents (p. 149)

General Patient education for penicillins

- some penicillins should be taken on an empty stomach, while others may be taken with food.
- if antacids are used, patient should be instructed to separate by at least 2 hours from oral penicillins
- warn patient to avoid taking oral preparations with acidic fruit juices or liquids because these may accelerate drug decomposition
- advise patient to seek medical advice immediately if any of the following occur:
  - severe skin reaction
  - yellowing of skin or eyes, loss of appetite, nausea, upper abdominal pain, itchy skin, dark urine, pale stools (even if these occur weeks after stopping therapy)

- see also General Patient education for antibacterial agents (p. 150)

Penicillins are considered safe to use during pregnancy.

Generally considered safe, but penicillins may cause loose bowel movements in the breastfeeding infant and, though rare, could sensitize them, leading to allergic reactions. Risks and benefits should be assessed before use during breastfeeding.

Most penicillins are excreted by the kidneys through glomerular filtration and tubular secretion. Dose adjustments may be necessary in patients with impaired renal function to avoid toxicity.

AMOXICILLIN

Trade names
Alphamox, Amiloxyn, Amoxicillin-WGR, Amoxil, Amoxycillin Generichealth, APO-Amoxycillin, Fisamox, Ibiamox, Maxamox, Noumed Amoxicillin

Available forms
Capsules: 250 mg, 500 mg;
Tablets: 1 g;
Vial: 500 mg, 1 g;
Syrup/suspension: 125 mg/5 mL, 250 mg/5 mL, 500 mg/5 mL;
Paediatric drops: 100 mg/mL

Action
- broad spectrum, acid-stable aminopenicillin that is not penicillinase resistant
- activity spectrum is the same as for ampicillin
- active against broader range of Gram-negative organisms than benzylpenicillin but not Gram-positive organisms
- half-life about 1 hour
- see also General Actions of penicillins (p. 151)

Use
- see General Uses of penicillins (p. 151)

Dose
- (Upper respiratory tract infection, genitourinary tract infection, skin and soft tissue infections) 250 mg IM, by IV infusion over 30—60 minutes or IV bolus over 3—4 minutes 6—8-hourly **OR**
- (Upper respiratory tract infection, genitourinary tract infection, skin and soft tissue infections) 250 mg orally 8-hourly **OR**
- (Lower respiratory tract infections) 500 mg orally, IM, by IV infusion over 30—60 minutes or IV bolus over 3—4 minutes 8-hourly **OR**
- (Acute uncomplicated urinary tract infection, urethritis, gonorrhoea) 3 g as single oral dose **OR**
- (Bacterial septicaemia) 1 g 6-hourly by slow IV injection over 3—4 minutes or IV infusion over 30—60 minutes **OR**
- (Prophylaxis — subacute bacterial endocarditis (SBE) after dental procedures, no anaesthetic and no penicillin taken in the past month) 3 g orally 1 hour before the procedure, followed by 3 g 6 hours later if necessary **OR**
- (Prophylaxis — SBE, no penicillin taken in the past month, dental procedures with a general anaesthetic, oral antibiotics are not appropriate) 1 g IM immediately before induction, followed by 500 mg orally 6 hours later **OR**
- (Prophylaxis — SBE after dental procedure; patient has taken penicillin in the past month and the patient needs general anaesthetic or has prosthetic valve replacements and needs general anaesthetic or has had one or more attacks of SBE) 1 g IM with 120 mg gentamicin IM immediately before induction or 15 minutes before dental procedure, followed by 500 mg orally 6 hours later **OR**
- (Prophylaxis — SBE for genitourinary surgery/procedure under general anaesthesia) 1 g IM with 120 mg gentamicin IM immediately before induction, followed by 500 mg orally or IM 6 hours later **OR**
- (Prophylaxis — SBE for genitourinary surgery/procedure under general anaesthesia) 1 g IM with 120 mg

ANTIBACTERIAL AGENTS

- gentamicin IM immediately before induction, followed by 500 mg orally or IM 6 hours later **OR**
- (Prophylaxis — SBE for obstetric and gynaecological procedures or GI procedures with prosthetic valve replacement) 1 g IM with 120 mg gentamicin IM immediately before induction, followed by 500 mg IM 6 hours later **OR**
- (Prophylaxis — SBE for upper respiratory tract surgery/procedure in patient without prosthetic valve replacement) 1 g IM immediately before induction, followed by 500 mg IM 6 hours later

Adverse effects
- (Rare) crystalluria, superficial tooth discolouration in children
- see also General Adverse effects of penicillins (p. 152)

Interactions
- increased risk of skin rashes if given with allopurinol; therefore not recommended together. If given together, patient should be monitored for appearance of any rash
- see also General Interactions of penicillins (p. 152)

Nursing considerations/Cautions
- doses greater than 500 mg not given as single IM injection
- ensure patient is adequately hydrated to maintain high urinary output during therapy with amoxicillin
- if patient has IDC in situ, regularly monitor for any crystalluria as high levels of amoxicillin may precipitate out at room temperature
- (SBE) dental procedures include tooth extraction, scaling or surgery involving gingival tissue
- (SBE) if given with gentamicin, should not be mixed in same syringe
- (Acute lower urinary tract infection) urine should be cultured after single dose is given. If culture is positive, longer or larger course may be required
- may be given by IV infusion run over 30—40 minutes or slow IV injection over 3—5 minutes (to prevent convulsions)
- harmless, transient pink colouration or slight cloudiness may appear during reconstitution of IM or IV solution may be diluted with lidocaine (lignocaine) 1% or procaine 0.5% to reduce pain IM
- parenteral solution contains 2.6—3.3 mmol sodium per 1 g amoxicillin, which may be a consideration in those with a sodium restriction
- (Syrup/paediatric drops) contain aspartame and therefore not recommended in those with phenylketonuria
- (Syrup/paediatric drops) contain benzoates; therefore may cause reaction in those with hypersensitivity
- not recommended for sore throat or pharyngitis because of increased risk of skin rash if amoxicillin is given to those with infectious mononucleosis (glandular fever)
- increased risk of rash if given to those with lymphatic leukaemia;, therefore should be given with caution and patient closely monitored
- see also General Nursing considerations/Cautions for penicillins (p. 152)

Patient education
- if parent is going to administer paediatric syrup to child, the following instructions should be given:
  - shake bottle well before use
  - use syringe adapter (provided to withdraw required dose)
  - rinse syringe well after use
  - refrigerate but do not freeze
  - discard 14 days after opening
- see also General Patient education for penicillins (p. 153)

 Syrup/suspension is available. Tablet can be crushed or capsule opened and mixed with water or spoonful of yoghurt or apple puree.

Safe to use.

 Safe to use; however, it may cause loose bowel movements in the infant. Use when the benefit outweighs the risk.

 In patients with renal impairment, high parenteral doses and/or prolonged treatment may lead to electrolyte disturbances (due to sodium content) and neurotoxicity (from penicillin accumulation, such as seizures or coma). The risk of neutropenia may also be increased.

Available in combination with
- amoxicillin 125 mg/5 mL + clavulanic acid 31.25 mg/5 mL powder for oral suspension (Augmentin 400, Augmentin, Curam 125/31.25)
- amoxicillin 500 mg + clavulanic acid 125 mg tablet (Alphaclav Duo Viatris 500/125, Amoxicillin/Clavulanic Acid Viatris 500/125, Amoxicillin Clavulanic Acid WGR-500/125, APO-Amoxy/Clav 500/125, APX-Amoxicillin/Clavulanic Acid 500/125, Augmentin Duo, Curam Duo 500/125)
- amoxicillin 875 mg + clavulanic acid 125 mg tablet (Alphaclav Duo Forte Viatris 875/125, Amoxicillin/Clavulanic Acid-WGR 875/125, AmoxyClav Generihealth 875/125, APO-AmoxyClav 875/125, APX-Amoxicillin/Clavulanic Acid 500/125, Augmentin Duo Forte, Blooms the Chemist Amoxicillin/Clavulanic Acid 875/125, Curam Duo Forte 875/125)
- amoxicillin 400 mg/5 mL + clavulanic acid 57 mg/5 mL powder for oral suspension (Curam Duo 400/57)
- (Combination pack) amoxicillin 500 mg capsule + esomeprazole 20 mg enteric tablet + clarithromycin 500 mg tablet for the eradication of *Helicobacter pylori* (Esomeprazole Sandoz Hp7, Nexium Hp7)
- amoxicillin 1000 mg + clavulanic acid 200 mg powder for injection (Amoxiclav Juno 1000/200, Curam 1000/200)
- amoxicillin 2000 mg + clavulanic acid 200 mg powder for injection (Amoxiclav Juno 2000/200, Curam 2000/200)
- amoxicillin 500 mg + clavulanic acid 100 mg powder for injection (Amoxiclav Juno 500/100, Curam 500/100)

AMOXICILLIN WITH CLAVULANIC ACID
Trade names
Alphaclav Duo Forte Viatris, Amoxicillin/Clavulanic Acid Viatris, Amoxicillin/Clavulanic Acid-WGR, Amoxiclav Juno. APO-Amoxy/Clav, Augmentin Duo, Blooms The Chemist Amoxicillin/Clavulanic Acid 875/125, Curam, Curam Duo, Curam Duo Forte 875/125

Available forms
Vial: 500 mg amoxicillin/100 mg clavulanic acid, 1000 mg amoxicillin/200 mg clavulanic acid, 2000 mg amoxicillin/200 mg clavulanic acid;
Tablets: 500 mg amoxicillin/125 mg clavulanic acid, 875 mg amoxicillin/125 mg clavulanic acid;
Syrup/suspension: 125 mg amoxicillin/31.25 mg clavulanic acid/5 mL, 400 mg amoxicillin/57 mg clavulanic acid/5 mL

Action
- clavulanic acid is a potent inhibitor of beta lactamase (penicillinase) and is added to some penicillins to enhance their activity against many previously resistant strains
- clavulanic acid is a beta-lactamase inhibitor that irreversibly binds to beta-lactamase enzymes produced by certain bacteria. Beta lactamase is an enzyme bacteria produced to break down beta-lactam antibiotics (like penicillins), rendering them ineffective. Clavulanic acid inhibits this enzyme, protecting the penicillin from degradation and allowing the antibiotic to maintain its antibacterial activity
- this broadens the spectrum of penicillins to include beta-lactamase producing previously resistant strains of bacteria
- active against a range of Gram-positive and Gram-negative aerobic organisms
- see also General Actions of penicillins (p. 151)

Use
- see General Uses of penicillins (p. 151)

Dose
- 1000 mg amoxicillin/200 mg clavulanic acid by slow IV over 3–4 minutes or IV infusion over 30–40 minutes 6- to 8-hourly **OR**
- (Serious infection) 2000 mg amoxicillin/200 mg clavulanic acid by slow IV over 3–4 minutes or IV infusion over 30–40 minutes 6- to 8-hourly **OR**
- (Surgical prophylaxis) 1000 mg amoxicillin/200 mg clavulanic acid – 2000 mg amoxicillin/200 mg clavulanic acid by slow IV over 3–4 minutes at induction, then repeated after 2 hours if needed **OR**
- 500 mg amoxicillin/125 mg clavulanic acid 12-hourly orally immediately before food or with first mouthful **OR**
- (Severe infections) 875 mg amoxicillin/125 mg clavulanic acid orally 12-hourly immediately before food or with first mouthful **OR**
- (Syrup) 250 mg amoxicillin/62.5 mg clavulanic acid – 500 mg amoxicillin/125 mg clavulanic acid (5–10 mL) 8-hourly immediately before food or with first mouthful

Adverse effects
- see General Adverse effects of penicillins (p. 152)

Interactions
- amoxicillin increases risk of skin rashes if given with allopurinol; therefore not recommended together
- see also General Interactions of penicillins (p. 152)

Nursing considerations/Cautions
- (Parenteral) not given IM
- (Parenteral) reconstitute using 10 mL water for injections for 600 mg vial or 20 mL for 1.2 or 2.2 mg vial and then further dilute using 50–100 mL for IV infusion
- (Tablets) each preparation is different and the dose is based on the amoxicillin content, and therefore correct preparation should be selected (clavulanic acid content is the same in tablet preparation (125 mg) but varies in the syrup/suspension)
- 400 mg amoxicillin/57 mg clavulanic acid oral suspension/syrup is intended for paediatric use and dose is based on child's weight. If child weighs ≥ 40 kg, dose should be according to adult guidelines
- (Suspension) contains aspartame and is therefore not recommended in those with phenylketonuria
- (Parenteral) vials contain 31.4–125.9 mg sodium, which may need to be considered if patient has salt restriction
- (Parenteral) vials contain 19.6–39.3 mg potassium, which may need to be considered if patient has reduced kidney function or requires potassium-controlled diet
- (Parenteral) less stable in solutions containing glucose, dextran or bicarbonate
- (Parenteral) should not be mixed with blood products, protein hydrolysates or IV lipid emulsions
- not recommended in those with moderate-to-severe kidney impairment (creatinine clearance ≤ 30 mL/min)
- contraindicated in those with previous history of amoxicillin/clavulanic acid-associated jaundice or liver dysfunction
- see also Nursing considerations/Cautions for amoxicillin (p. 154)

Patient education
- take it with food. Food helps improve absorption and may reduce gastrointestinal side effects (e.g. nausea)
- advise patient/parent/carer to check discarding information carefully as some oral suspensions should be discarded 14 days after opening, while others after 7 days
- instruct patient not to substitute tablets (e.g. 2 Augmentin for Augmentin Duo Forte, as they are not equivalent)
- see also Patient education for amoxicillin (p. 153)

Tablets can be crushed and mixed with water, a spoonful of yoghurt, or apple puree.

Amoxicillin/clavulanic acid is generally considered safe for use during pregnancy. However, some studies have raised concerns about an increased risk of necrotising enterocolitis in preterm infants when the drug is used, particularly close to delivery. Use when benefits outweigh risks.

Amoxicillin/clavulanic acid is generally considered safe to use during breastfeeding. However, it can be excreted in small amounts into breastmilk, which may cause loose bowel movements in the nursing infant. Use when benefits outweigh risks.

Amoxicillin is primarily renally cleared, with about 50—70% of the drug excreted unchanged in the urine. For clavulanic acid, around 25—40% is renally excreted. Due to significant renal clearance, dose adjustments are typically required in patients with impaired renal function to avoid drug accumulation and associated toxicity, especially with high doses or prolonged use.

AMPICILLIN

Trade names
Ampicyn, Austrapen, Ibimycin

Available form
Vial: 500 mg, 1 g

Action
- moderate spectrum, acid-stable aminopenicillin
- not penicillinase resistant, i.e. can be broken down by beta-lactamase enzymes (penicillinases) produced by certain bacteria
- similar to benzylpenicillin, but more active against some Gram-negative bacilli and some *Enterobacteriaceae*
- half-life 1 hour (prolonged up to 20 hours in those with kidney impairment)
- see also General Actions of penicillins (p. 151)

Use
- see General Uses of penicillins (p. 151)

Dose
- (Respiratory tract infection) 250—500 mg IM, IV injection over 3—5 minutes or IV infusion over 30—40 minutes 6-hourly **OR**
- (Chronic bronchitis) 0.5—1 g IM, IV injection over 3—5 minutes or IV infusion over 30—40 minutes 6-hourly **OR**
- (Urinary tract infection) 500 mg IM, IV injection over 3—5 minutes or IV infusion over 30—40 minutes 6-hourly **OR**
- (GI infections) 500—750 mg IM, IV injection over 3—5 minutes or IV infusion over 30—40 minutes 6-hourly **OR**
- (Bacterial meningitis, septicaemia) 200 mg/kg daily IV in divided doses 4—6-hourly (daily maximum 12 g)

Adverse effects
- (Rare) crystalluria. May cause the formation of crystals in the urine, which can lead to kidney damage, urinary obstruction or even acute kidney injury, especially in patients receiving high doses or those who are dehydrated
- see also General Adverse effects of penicillins (p. 151)

Interactions
- increased risk of skin rashes if given with allopurinol
- see also General Interactions of penicillins (p. 152)

Nursing considerations/Cautions/Patient education
- ensure patient is adequately hydrated to maintain high urinary output during therapy with ampicyllin
- if patient has IDC in situ, regular monitoring for crystalluria is recommended as high levels of ampicillin may precipitate out at room temperature
- may be given IM, by IV infusion run over 30—40 minutes or by slow IV injection over 3—5 minutes (to prevent convulsions)
- should be administered immediately after being reconstituted with diluents
- may also be given by intraperitoneal, intrapleural or intra-articular injection

ANTIBACTERIAL AGENTS

- contains 2.7 mmol sodium per gram ampicillin, which may need to be considered if patient has salt restriction
- not recommended intrathecally
- not recommended for sore throat or pharyngitis because of increased risk of skin rash if ampicillin is given to those with infectious mononucleosis (glandular fever)
- increased risk of rash if given to those with lymphatic leukaemia
- see also General Nursing considerations/Cautions for penicillins (p. 152) and General Patient education for penicillins (p. 153)

Generally considered safe to use during pregnancy.

Generally considered safe to use while breastfeeding. However, it may cause loose bowel movements or mild gastrointestinal disturbances in the breastfeeding infant. The benefits of continuing breastfeeding usually outweigh these mild effects.

If CrCl < 10 mL/min, the dose of ampicillin should be reduced to avoid accumulation and potential toxicity.

BENZATHINE BENZYLPENICILLIN

Trade names
Bicillin L-A

Available forms
Prefilled syringe: 600,000 units/1.17 mL, 1,200,000 units/2.3 mL

Action
- slowly absorbed and converted to benzylpenicillin, resulting in lower but more prolonged blood levels than other parenteral penicillins
- see also General Actions of penicillins (p. 151)

Use
- see General Uses of penicillins (p. 151)

Dose
- (Venereal disease — primary, secondary and latent syphilis) 2,400,000 units as single IM injection **OR**
- (Venereal disease — tertiary syphilis with neurosyphilis) 2,400,000 units IM weekly for 3 weeks (total 3 doses) **OR**
- (Venereal disease — yaws, bejel, pinta) 1,200,000 units as single IM injection **OR**
- (Rheumatic fever, glomerulonephritis acute attack) 1,200,000 units IM monthly, adult/child > 20 kg, IM 1.2 million units as a single dose; child < 20 kg, IM 600,000 units as a single dose **OR**
- (Rheumatic fever, glomerulonephritis) adult, child > 20 kg, IM 1.2 million units every 3–4 weeks; child < 20 kg, IM 600,000 units every 3–4 weeks **OR**
- (Streptococcal (group A) upper respiratory tract infection) single IMI of 1,200,000 units for adults; a single injection of 900,000 units for older children; a single injection of 300,000 to 600,000 units for infants and children under 27 kg

Adverse effects
- (Syphilis) Jarisch–Herxheimer reaction (malaise, fever, chills, sore throat, myalgia, headache, tachycardia)
- severe agitation, confusion, visual/auditory hallucinations, fear of impending death
- see also General Adverse effects of penicillins (p. 152)

Interactions/Nursing considerations/Cautions/Patient education
- benzathine benzylpenicillin and benzylpenicillin are not therapeutically interchangeable
- given as deep IM injection
- accidental IV administration may cause severe neurovascular damage and CNS effects such as anxiety, agitation, fear of death and hallucinations, usually resolving in 15–30 minutes but may last up to 24 hours
- NEVER give IV
- administer alone
- before administration, the syringe should be rolled between the palms of the hands to resuspend contents
- administer at a slow and steady rate to prevent needle blockage

- contains hydroxybenzoates, which may cause allergic reaction in hypersensitive individuals
- benzathine benzylpenicillin products contain soy lecithin
- see also General Nursing considerations/Cautions for penicillins (p. 152)

Generally considered safe to use during pregnancy.

Generally considered safe to use while breastfeeding. However, it may cause loose bowel movements or mild gastrointestinal disturbances in the breastfeeding infant. The benefits of continuing breastfeeding usually outweigh these mild effects.

For patients with renal impairment, dose adjustment may be required to avoid risks like electrolyte disturbances, neurotoxicity (seizures, coma), and neutropenia, especially with high doses or prolonged treatment.

BENZYLPENICILLIN (crystalline penicillin, penicillin G)

Trade names
BenPen

Available forms
Vial: 600 mg, 1.2 g, 3 g

Action
- narrow-spectrum penicillin
- active against most Gram-positive organisms (e.g. streptococci, pneumococci, non-beta-lactamase-producing staphylococci, clostridia) and some Gram-negative organisms (e.g. gonococci and meningococci, and also some spirochaetes)
- reaches high blood levels quickly, which prevents resistance
- drug of choice for streptococcal pneumonia
- see also General Actions of penicillins (p. 151)

Use
- see General Uses of penicillins (p. 151)

Dose
- 300 mg IM or IV 6-hourly (increasing dose/frequency in more serious infections) **OR**
- (Severe infections) 4—24 g/24 hours in 4—6 divided doses IM or IV **OR**
- (Prophylaxis — surgery) 600 mg IV immediately before surgery, then 4—8-hourly for duration of procedure if necessary **OR**
- (Treatment of SBE) not less than 1.2 g IV daily in divided doses for 4—6 weeks **OR**
- (Treatment of SBE *Streptococci viridans*) 6—12 g IV daily in divided doses for 4—6 weeks **OR**
- (Clostridial infection) 1.2 g IV 6-hourly for 48 hours **OR**
- (Meningococcal meningitis (children)) initially 600 mg IM, then 300 mg IM 4—6-hourly **OR**
- (Pneumococcal meningitis (children)) at least 300 mg IM 4-hourly for 2 weeks, then 6-hourly for 7 days

Adverse effects
- (Syphilis) Jarisch—Herxheimer reaction (malaise, fever, chills, sore throat, myalgia, headache, tachycardia)
- see also General Adverse effects of penicillins (p. 152)

Interactions
- actions antagonised by chloramphenicol, erythromycin and tetracyclines
- see also General Interactions of penicillins (p. 152)

Nursing considerations and Cautions/Patient education
- do not add to IV infusions, as benzylpenicillin is unstable at room temperature
- incompatible with some antihistamines, other antibacterial agents, noradrenaline (norepinephrine), metaraminol, thiopentone and phenytoin
- must be used immediately after reconstitution with water for injections
- for IM doses of 600 mg, reconstitute with 1.6 mL water for injections. For doses

greater than 600 mg, refer to the manufacturer's reconstitution table
- for IV administration, the recommended concentration is 60 mg/mL
- contains 3.0 mmol sodium per 1 g of benzylpenicillin. Electrolyte monitoring is recommended for high doses, prolonged therapy or in patients with heart failure
- see also General Nursing considerations/Cautions for penicillins (p. 152) and General Patient education for penicillins (p. 153)

Safe to use.

Safe to use; however, it may cause loose bowel movements in the infant. Use when the benefit outweighs the risk.

Primarily renally cleared, and dose adjustments are required in patients with reduced renal function to prevent accumulation and toxicity. For adults with renal impairment and CrCl < 10 mL/min, the maximum recommended dose of benzylpenicillin is 6 g daily.

DICLOXACILLIN
Trade names
Distaph, Dicloxacillin Viatris

Available form
Capsules: 250 mg, 500 mg

Action
- narrow-spectrum antibiotic active against *Streptococcus pyogenes*, *S. viridans*, *S. pneumoniae* and penicillinase-producing staphylococci
- see also General Actions of penicillins (p. 151)

Use
- see General Uses of penicillins (p. 151)

Dose
- 250–500 mg orally 6-hourly 1–2 hours before food

Adverse effects
- (over 55 years, prolonged therapy) hepatitis, cholestatic jaundice
- (Rare) oesophageal burning, oesophagitis, oesophageal ulceration
- see also General Adverse effects of penicillins (p. 152)

Interactions
- may decrease phenytoin and warfarin levels; therefore levels should be carefully monitored during therapy
- see also General Interactions of penicillins (p. 152)

Nursing considerations/Cautions
- white blood cell count and differential cell count should be measured before starting therapy, and then weekly during therapy. Urinalysis, serum urea, creatinine and liver enzymes should also be monitored
- not recommended in patients over 55 years unless clearly indicated because of the risk of cholestatic hepatitis
- can be used as an alternative to flucloxacillin
- monitor hepatic function if treatment continues for more than 2 weeks, especially if risk factors are present
- see also General Nursing considerations/Cautions for penicillins (p. 152)
- dicloxacillin is contraindicated in patients with a history of cholestatic hepatitis related to dicloxacillin or flucloxacillin

Patient education
- take capsules with a large glass of water and avoid lying down immediately after to prevent irritation of the oesophagus. Do not take at bedtime
- take on an empty stomach (one hour before food or 2 hours after food)
- immediately report any yellowing of the eyes or skin or darkening of urine, especially in patients over 55, during therapy or weeks after therapy has stopped
- see also General Patient education for penicillins (p. 153)

The capsule can be opened and dispersed in water, or mixed with a spoonful of yoghurt or apple puree.

 Safe to use.

 Safe to use; it is excreted in low amounts into breastmilk, and adverse effects in breastfed infants are unlikely. However, it may cause loose bowel movements in the infant. Use when the benefit outweighs the risk.

 Primarily renally cleared with some hepatic metabolism. Dose adjustments are generally not needed in mild to moderate renal impairment. However, in severe renal impairment (CrCl < 10 mL/min), the dose should be adjusted to 250–500 mg orally every 6–8 hours, with a maximum of 4 g daily. Renal function should be monitored throughout treatment to prevent drug accumulation.

FLUCLOXACILLIN

Trade names
Flucil, Flubiclox, Flucloxacillin Kabi, Flopen Viatris, Staphylex

Available forms
Vial: 500 mg, 1 g;
Capsules: 250 mg, 500 mg;
Syrup: 125 mg/5 mL, 250 mg/5 mL

Action
- acid stable and penicillinase resistant
- narrow-spectrum antibiotic active against *S. pyogenes* or *S. pneumoniae,* and beta-lactamase producing and penicillin-sensitive *Staphylococcus aureus*
- not active against Gram-negative bacilli, *Streptococcus faecalis* or MRSA
- see also General Actions of penicillins (p. 151)

Use
- see General Uses of penicillins (p. 151)

Dose
- 250 mg orally 6-hourly 30–60 minutes before meals **OR**
- 250 mg IM 6-hourly **OR**
- 250–1000 mg 6-hourly by IV bolus or infusion over 3–4 minutes

Adverse effects
- (Over 55 years or prolonged therapy) severe hepatitis, cholestatic jaundice
- see also General Adverse effects of penicillins (p. 152)

Interactions
- increased risk of metabolic acidosis if given with paracetamol
- see also General Interactions of penicillins (p. 152)

Nursing considerations/Cautions
- IV bolus may cause pain and irritation at injection site
- may also be given by intrapleural or intra-articular injection
- (IV) reconstitute 1 g in 20 mL water for injections
- (IM) reconstitute 1 g in 2.5 mL water for injections
- (Parenteral) contains 2 mmol sodium per 1 g flucloxacillin
- (IV) should not be mixed with blood or protein-containing products
- (IV) incompatible with aminoglycosides, amiodarone, atropine, buprenorphine, calcium gluconate, chlorpromazine, ciprofloxacin, diazepam, dobutamine, erythromycin, metoclopramide, morphine, pethidine, prochlorperazine and verapamil
- (Syrup) contains benzoates, which may cause hypersensitivity reaction in sensitive individuals
- not recommended for those over 55 years because of increased risk of severe hepatitis and cholestatic jaundice
- contraindicated in those with flucloxacillin-associated jaundice or liver dysfunction, or for use in the eye (locally or conjunctivally)
- see also General Nursing considerations/Cautions for penicillins (p. 152)

Patient education
- advise patient (especially if over 55 years) to immediately report any

- yellowing of eyes or skin, or darkening of urine, during therapy or weeks after therapy has stopped
- (Syrup) instruct patient to shake bottle well before use and discard 14 days after opening
- see also General Patient education for penicillins (p. 153)

Available as syrup/suspension. Capsules can be opened and mixed with water, yoghurt, or apple puree for easier administration, especially for children or those with swallowing difficulties.

Safe to use.

Safe to use; however, it may cause loose bowel movements in the infant. Use only when the benefit outweighs the risk.

Flucloxacillin should be reduced if creatinine clearance (CrCl) < 10 mL/min to avoid drug accumulation and potential toxicity. Monitoring of renal function is recommended throughout treatment to adjust dosing appropriately.

PHENOXYMETHYLPENICILLIN
Trade names
Aspecillin VK, Cilicaine V, Cilicaine VK, LPV, Phenoxymethylpenicillin-AFT

Available forms
Tablets: 250 mg, 500 mg;
Capsules: 250 mg, 500 mg;
Suspension: 125 mg/5 mL, 150 mg/5 mL, 250 mg/5 mL

Action
- narrow-spectrum penicillin, less active than benzylpenicillin
- mainly effective against Gram-positive bacteria like *Streptococcus* species and penicillin-sensitive *Staphylococcus aureus*
- limited activity against Gram-negative bacteria
- it is not effective against beta-lactamase producing bacteria
- see also General Actions of penicillins (p. 151)

Use
- common uses include upper respiratory infections, rheumatic fever prophylaxis and dental infections
- see also General Uses of penicillins (p. 151)

Dose
- (Mild-to-moderately severe streptococcal infections, including scarlet fever) 125—250 mg orally 6—8-hourly 1 hour before meals for 10 days **OR**
- (Mild-to-moderately severe pneumococcal infections, otitis media) 250—500 mg orally 4—6-hourly 1 hour before meals until patient has been afebrile for 2 days **OR**
- (Mild-to-moderately severe fusospirochaetosis of oropharynx) 250—500 mg orally 6—8-hourly 1 hour before meals **OR**
- (Prevent recurrence of rheumatic fever and/or chorea) 125—250 mg orally twice daily 1 hour before meals **OR**
- (Prophylaxis — SBE) 2 g orally 30 minutes before procedure, then 500 mg orally 1 hour before meals 6-hourly for 8 doses

Adverse effects/Interactions
- see General Adverse effects and Interactions of penicillins (p. 152)

Nursing considerations/Cautions/Patient education
- (Streptococcal infection) therapy should be continued for at least 10 days
- (Suspension) contains hydroxybenzoates, which may cause hypersensitivity reaction in sensitive individuals
- not recommended for severe pneumonia, empyema, bacteraemia, pericarditis or arthritis during acute phase of illness
- see also General Nursing considerations/Cautions for penicillins (p. 152)

and General Patient education for penicillins (p. 153)

Available as syrup/suspension. Tablets can be crushed, or capsules opened and mixed with water, yoghurt, or apple puree for easier administration, especially for children or those with swallowing difficulties.

Safe to use.

Safe to use; however, it may cause loose bowel movements in the infant. Use when the benefit outweighs the risk.

In renal impairment, high parenteral doses or prolonged treatment may require dose adjustments because of the risk of electrolyte disturbances (from sodium content), neurotoxicity (e.g. seizures, coma) and increased risk of neutropenia. Monitoring is advised, especially in severe impairment (CrCl < 10 mL/min).

PIPERACILLIN WITH TAZOBACTAM

Trade names
PiperTaz, PipTaz, Tazopip

Available form
Vial: 4 g piperacillin/0.5 g tazobactam

Action
- piperacillin is broad spectrum
- tazobactam is a beta-lactamase inhibitor (that helps protect piperacillin from being broken down by beta-lactamase enzymes produced by certain bacteria)
- active against a broad spectrum of both Gram-negative and Gram-positive beta-lactamase and non-beta-lactamase producing organisms
- half-life 0.7–1.2 hours
- see also General Actions of penicillins (p. 151)

Use
- see General Uses of penicillins (p. 151)

Dose
- 4 g piperacillin/0.5 g tazobactam by slow IV infusion over 20–30 min, 6–8-hourly

Adverse effects
- transient increases in liver enzymes (ALT, AST)
- increased blood urea nitrogen (BUN) and serum creatinine levels (indicative of kidney dysfunction)
- (Rare) electrolyte disturbances (e.g. hypokalaemia)
- see also General Adverse effects of penicillins (p. 152)

Interactions
- may prolong neuromuscular blockade of vecuronium; therefore caution if given with neuromuscular blocking agents
- increased risk of hypokalaemia if given in high doses with diuretics or cytotoxic therapy
- increased risk of kidney damage if given with vancomycin
- see also General Interactions of penicillins (p. 152)

Nursing considerations/Cautions/Patient education
- liver and renal function and blood counts should be monitored if therapy extends beyond 21 days or if the patient has pre-existing liver or kidney impairment
- serum potassium should be monitored during treatment for patients at risk of developing hypokalaemia, as this combination can cause or exacerbate low potassium levels
- treatment should last a minimum of 5 days and be continued for 48 hours after the fever or symptoms resolve (with a maximum of 14 days)
- administer alone
- reconstitute with 20 mL water for injections, and it can be further diluted with 50 mL sodium chloride 0.9% or glucose 5%

ANTIBACTERIAL AGENTS

- it is not recommended to mix with blood products (including albumin) or solutions with a basic pH, such as lactated Ringer's solution, sodium bicarbonate, or other solutions
- contains 56 mg of sodium per gram of piperacillin. Use with caution in patients with heart failure or those on sodium-restricted diets
- piperacillin/tazobactam is often used in combination with an aminoglycoside (e.g. in febrile neutropenia). However, in febrile neutropenia, adding an aminoglycoside may not enhance efficacy but increases the risk of adverse effects, particularly nephrotoxicity. Renal function should be closely monitored owing to the increased risk of renal impairment when combining these drugs
- patients with cystic fibrosis are at an increased risk of developing a rash or fever
- it is not recommended for use in meningitis or brain infections
- see also General Nursing considerations/Cautions for penicillins (p. 152)

Safe to use.

Safe to use; however, it may cause loose bowel movements in the infant. Use when the benefit outweighs the risk.

Piperacillin with tazobactam is primarily eliminated by the kidneys, so in patients with impaired renal function, dosage adjustments are needed to avoid accumulation and toxicity. Reduce dose if CrCl < 40 mL/min.

PROCAINE BENZYLPENICILLIN (PROCAINE PENICILLIN)
Trade names
Cilicaine Syringe

Available form
Syringe: 1.5 g

Action
- penicillin antibiotic

- as for benzylpenicillin, but for moderately severe infections
- procaine salt has low solubility; therefore particles dissolve slowly allowing administration 1—2 times daily only
- see also General Actions of penicillins (p. 151)

Use
- see General Uses of penicillins (p. 151)

Dose
- 1.5 g IM daily for 2—5 days **OR**
- (Gonorrhoea) 4.8 g as single IM dose with oral probenecid **OR**
- (Gonorrhoea) 1 g IM daily for 7—14 days **OR**
- (Syphilis) 1 g IM daily for 10—14 days

Adverse effects
- (Syphilis) Jarisch—Herxheimer reaction (malaise, fever, chills, sore throat, myalgia, headache, tachycardia)
- extreme anxiety, sensation of impending death (thought to be caused by procaine; self-limiting and generally subsides after 15—30 minutes)
- see also General Adverse effects of penicillins (p. 152)

Interactions
- see General Interactions of penicillins (p. 152)

Nursing considerations/Cautions/Patient education
- only given IM
- NEVER given IV as neurovascular damage may occur
- may cause permanent neurological damage if given into or near nerves
- slowly absorbed and maintains antibacterial blood levels for up to 24 hours, but concentration achieved is lower than for benzylpenicillin
- not recommended in those with Brugada syndrome (because of procaine content) (potentially life-threatening cardiac rhythm disorder) or known cardiac conduction abnormalities
- contraindicated in those with known hypersensitivity to procaine

- see also General Nursing considerations/Cautions for penicillins (p. 152) and General Patient education for penicillins (p. 153)

Should be used during pregnancy only if clearly necessary. Animal studies show no harm, but adequate and well-controlled studies in pregnant women are lacking, and potential risks to the fetus cannot be fully excluded.

Excreted in human milk; use with caution.

Dose adjustments may be necessary for patients with renal impairment, especially for those with severe impairment, as penicillin is primarily excreted via the kidneys.

CEPHALOSPORINS

General Actions of cephalosporins
- selectively interfere with bacterial cell wall synthesis, as with penicillin
- bactericidal
- broad spectrum, often second line of treatment in many infections
- divided into first, second, third and fourth generation
- some of the newer generation of cephalosporins resist the action of beta lactamase (penicillinase)
- *Staphylococcus aureus* (MRSA), *Clostridium difficile*, *Pseudomonas aeruginosa* and *Enterococcus faecalis* are resistant to the cephalosporins

General Uses of cephalosporins
- infections where the organisms are not resistant to cephalosporins, including:
  - upper and lower respiratory tract infections
  - skin and skin structure infections
  - bone and joint infections
  - urinary tract infection (complicated or uncomplicated)
  - intra-abdominal infections, including biliary tract infections
  - gynaecological infections
  - septicaemia, endocarditis
  - febrile neutropenia
  - meningitis
  - gonorrhoea
  - ear, nose and throat infections
  - surgical prophylaxis

General Adverse effects of cephalosporins
- nausea, vomiting, dyspepsia, bad taste, abdominal pain/cramps, diarrhoea
- rash, urticaria, fever, pruritus
- dizziness, headache, insomnia, somnolence, malaise
- hypoprothrombinaemia
- superinfection (oral and/or vaginal moniliasis)
- granulocytopenia, leucopenia, neutropenia, eosinophilia
- anaphylactic shock, anaphylactoid reaction (rare), serum sickness-like reaction (rash, arthritis/arthralgia, fever), hypersensitivity
- (Transient) elevation in liver enzymes and, rarely, hepatitis, cholestatic jaundice
- (High dose) reversible encephalopathy, neurotoxicity, seizures
- (Rare) reversible nephritis, elevated serum creatinine and blood urea nitrogen levels, interstitial nephritis
- (Rare) haemolytic anaemia, agranulocytosis
- (Rare) severe skin reactions
- (Rare but often fatal) pseudomembranous colitis (see Glossary)
- (IM) pain, induration, tenderness
- (IV) pain, inflammation, phlebitis, thrombophlebitis

General Interactions of cephalosporins
- cephalosporins may affect stability of warfarin; therefore prothrombin time should be closely monitored especially when starting and stopping therapy
- probenecid increases and prolongs serum levels of most cephalosporins by inhibiting excretion (not ceftriaxone or ceftazidime)

ANTIBACTERIAL AGENTS

- increased risk of renal damage if used with other potentially nephrotoxic agents such as colistin, gentamicin, tobramycin, etacrynic acid (large doses) and furosemide (frusemide) (large doses) and therefore renal function should be monitored regularly
- absorption decreased by aluminium- and magnesium-containing antacids and therefore administration should be spaced 2 hours apart
- physical/chemical incompatibility with aminoglycosides
- lidocaine (lignocaine) toxicity may occur in those with liver disease if lidocaine (lignocaine) is used repeatedly as diluent to reduce pain of IM injection
- increased risk of GI ulceration and bleeding if given with NSAIDs, salicylates or sulfinpyrazone
- increased risk of hypoprothrombinaemia if given in high doses with high doses of salicylates
- if active against *Salmonella typhi* organisms, may interfere with live typhoid vaccine if given within 24 hours of last dose
- increased risk of pseudomembranous colitis if given with peristalsis-delaying agents such as opioid analgesics or atropine/diphenoxylate combination
- may cause false positive Coombs' test and false positive glucose test (urine)
- false high creatinine levels may occur using Jaffe technique; therefore blood samples for creatinine levels should not be drawn within 2 hours of drug administration

General Nursing considerations/ Cautions for cephalosporins

- penicillin is the usual drug of choice for treatment and prophylaxis of streptococcal infections including rheumatic fever prevention
- serum sickness-like reaction often occurs after second (or subsequent) dose and occurs more frequently in children than in adults
- white blood cell monitoring is recommended if therapy > 7 days
- liver and/or renal function monitoring is recommended if liver or renal insufficiency exists
- all patients with gonorrhoea should also have serological testing for syphilis at time of diagnosis and then 3 months later
- therapy should be continued for 2 days after signs and symptoms have resolved unless treating a group A beta-haemolytic streptococci infection. Therapy should be given for at least 10 days to decrease risk of rheumatic fever or glomerulonephritis
- when reconstituting powders for injection, it is important to note the amount of diluent required for the specific route (e.g. IM cefepime 500 mg requires 1.5 mL of diluent, whereas IV it needs 5 mL of diluent to give the required level)
- reconstituted solution may darken on storage, but efficacy is not affected
- do not mix with other drugs in the same syringe or IV infusion container as a precipitate will form
- if cephalosporins are being administered by a Y-line infusion method, the primary or main infusion is stopped to avoid incompatibility
- incompatible with aminoglycosides and vancomycin as precipitation will occur if given together. Lines should be flushed between administration if given one after the other
- the amount of sodium should be noted as this may be important for those with cardiac disease or if a sodium restriction is required
- caution if used in those with allergic tendencies including asthma
- caution if given to those with a history of GI diseases (especially colitis or enteritis), impaired kidney or liver function or those with impaired or low vitamin K synthesis because of the increased risk of bleeding

167

- caution if used in those with history of bleeding disorders
- caution if used in those with pre-existing seizure disorders
- contraindicated in those with a history of anaphylaxis to penicillins, penicillin derivatives, penicillamine or cephalosporin-related bleeding disorder
- (with lidocaine (lignocaine)) contraindicated in those with amide-type local anaesthetic hypersensitivity
- see also General Nursing considerations/Cautions for antibacterial agents (p. 149)

General Patient education for cephalosporins

- instruct patient to seek medical advice immediately if any of the following occurs:
  - signs of frequent infection including fever, sore throat, swollen glands or mouth ulcers
  - unusual bleeding or bruising under skin
  - tiredness, headache, dizziness, paleness, shortness of breath
  - yellowing of skin or eyes
- see also General Patient education for antibacterial agents (p. 150)

Cephalosporins are generally considered safe in pregnancy. However, there is limited human data for ceftaroline, ceftolozane, or ceftazidime with avibactam. Use these drugs during pregnancy only when the benefits outweigh the risks.

While cephalosporins are generally considered safe during breastfeeding (generally low excretion rate in breastmilk), they may occasionally cause diarrhoea or gastrointestinal disturbances in breastfed infants. Use only when the benefits outweigh the risks. Monitor the infant for such side effects.

Most cephalosporins are primarily renally cleared, meaning that dose adjustments are often required in patients with renal impairment to prevent drug accumulation and reduce the risk of adverse effects, such as neurotoxicity (e.g. seizures). Regular monitoring of renal function (e.g. creatinine clearance) is recommended.

CEFACLOR

Trade names
Ceclor, Ceclor CD, Cefaclor SUN, Keflor, Keflor CD

Available forms
Tablets (sustained-release): 375 mg;
Suspension: 125 mg/5 mL, 250 mg/5 mL

Action
- *Pseudomonas* spp., *Acinetobacter calcoaceticus,* enterococci, *Enterobacter* spp., indole-positive *Proteus* and *Serratia* spp. are resistant to cefaclor
- second generation cephalosporin
- half-life 40—60 minutes (increased to 2.3—2.8 hours in those with anuria)
- see also General Actions of cephalosporins (p. 166)

Use
- see General Uses of cephalosporins (p. 166)

Dose
- (Bronchitis, pneumonia) 250 mg orally 8-hourly (daily maximum 2 g) **OR**
- (Severe infection) 500 mg orally 8-hourly (daily maximum 2 g) **OR**
- (Skin or skin structure infection) 250 mg orally 8—12-hourly (daily maximum 2 g) **OR**
- 375 mg orally twice daily with food (SR preparation) **OR**
- (Pneumonia, acute bacterial sinusitis) 750 mg orally twice daily with food (SR preparation) **OR**
- (Lower urinary tract infection) 500 mg orally daily with food (SR preparation)

Adverse effects/Interactions
- see General Adverse effects for cephalosporins (p. 166) and General Interactions for cephalosporins (p. 166)

ANTIBACTERIAL AGENTS

Nursing considerations/Cautions
- therapy should be continued for 10 days for acute bacterial sinusitis
- daily dose of 2 g should not be exceeded
- see also General Nursing considerations/ Cautions for cephalosporins (p. 167)

Patient education
- advise patient that tablets (sustained-release) should be swallowed whole and not chewed or crushed and taken with food to improve absorption
- if taking suspension, instruct patient to shake bottle well before use and discard 14 days after opening
- see also General Patient education for cephalosporins (p. 168)

 Sustained-release (SR) tablets should not be crushed. Cefaclor suspension can be used if the patient has difficulty swallowing.

CEFALEXIN
Trade names
Cephalex, Cephalexin, Ibilex, Keflex

Available forms
Capsules: 250 mg, 500 mg;
Suspension: 125 mg/5 mL, 250 mg/5 mL

Action
- not active against most strains of enterococci, some strains of staphylococci, most strains of *Enterobacter* spp., *Morganella morganii, Proteus vulgaris, Pseudomonas* spp., *Acinetobacter calcoaceticus*
- first generation cephalosporin
- see also General Actions of cephalosporins (p. 166)

Use
- see General Uses of cephalosporins (p. 166)

Dose
- 1—4 g orally in divided doses **OR**
- (Streptococcal pharyngitis, tonsillitis, skin or skin structure infection) 500 mg orally twice daily
- (Uncomplicated UTI) Adult: oral 500 mg every 12 hours for 5 days for women, and 7 days for men; Child: oral 12.5 mg/kg (maximum 500 mg) every 6 hours for 3 days

Adverse effects
- see General Adverse effects of cephalosporins (p. 166)

Interactions
- may decrease clearance of metformin
- see also General Interactions of cephalosporins (p. 166)

Nursing considerations/Cautions
- if daily dose is greater than 4 g, parenteral cephalosporin therapy should be considered
- twice daily dosing is not recommended when doses are greater than 1 g daily
- not recommended for bacterial infections of brain or spinal column
- see also General Nursing considerations/ Cautions for cephalosporins (p. 167)

Patient education
- (Suspension) advise patient to shake suspension well before use, refrigerate solution and discard 14 days after opening
- see also General Patient education for cephalosporins (p. 168)

 Syrup/suspension is available. Capsule can be opened and contents mixed with water or spoonful of yoghurt or apple puree. Patient should be warned of bitter taste.

CEFAZOLIN
Trade names
Cefazolin-AFT, Cefazolin Viatris, Kefzol

Available form
Vial: 500 mg, 1 g, 2 g

Action
- not active against many strains of enterococci, *Enterobacter cloacae*,

indole-producing *Proteus* spp., *Serratia* spp., *Pseudomonas* spp., methicillin-resistant staphylococci and *Acinetobacter calcoaceticus*
- see also General Actions of cephalosporins (p. 166)

Use
- see General Uses of cephalosporins (p. 166)

Dose
- (Mild infections) 250–500 mg IM or by IV bolus over 3–5 minutes or IV infusion 8-hourly **OR**
- (Moderate-to-severe infections) 0.5–1 g IM or by IV bolus over 3–5 minutes or IV infusion 6- to 8-hourly **OR**
- (Serious infection (e.g. endocarditis)) 6 g IM or by IV bolus over 3–5 minutes or IV infusion daily in divided doses

Adverse effects/Interactions
- see General Adverse effects of cephalosporins (p. 166) and General Interactions of cephalosporins (p. 166)

Nursing considerations/Cautions/Patient education
- must not be given intrathecally, as convulsions may occur
- (IM) reconstitute using sodium chloride 0.9% or water for injections
- (IV) reconstitute using water for injections
- not recommended via intraventricular route
- contains 43.3 mg sodium per 1 g cefazolin sodium
- see also General Nursing considerations/Cautions for cephalosporins (p. 167) and General Patient education for cephalosporins (p. 168)

CEFEPIME
Trade names
Cefepime-AFT, Cefepime Kabi

Available form
Vial: 1 g, 2 g

Action
- bactericidal
- inhibits cell wall synthesis, leading to bacterial cell death
- not active against *Clostridium difficile*, *Stenotrophomonas* spp., most strains of enterococci and some strains of *Enterobacter*
- fourth generation cephalosporin
- see also General Actions of cephalosporins (p. 166)

Use
- see General Uses of cephalosporins (p. 166)

Dose
- (Mild-to-moderate urinary tract infection) 0.5–1 g IM or by IV bolus over 3–5 minutes or IV infusion over 30 minutes 12-hourly **OR**
- (Mild-to-moderate infections) 1 g IM or by IV bolus over 3–5 minutes or IV infusion over 30 minutes 12-hourly **OR**
- (Severe infections) 2 g by IV bolus over 3–5 minutes or IV infusion over 30 minutes 12-hourly **OR**
- (Very severe or life-threatening infections) 2 g by IV bolus over 3–5 minutes or IV infusion over 30 minutes 8-hourly **OR**
- (Prophylaxis – surgery) 2 g stat by IV infusion over 30 minutes, given 60 minutes before first surgical incision (with metronidazole 500 mg IV when cefepime infusion is finished). If surgical procedure lasts for longer than 12 hours, a second dose of cefepime and metronidazole should be given 12 hours after the initial dose

Adverse effects/Interactions
- see General Adverse effects of cephalosporins (p. 166) and General Interactions of cephalosporins (p. 166)

Nursing considerations/Cautions/Patient education
- reserved for treating infections caused by multi-resistant organisms, such as *Pseudomonas aeruginosa*, and is commonly used in the empirical treatment of sepsis in patients with neutropenia

ANTIBACTERIAL AGENTS

- reconstitute carefully according to manufacturer's instructions as the amount of diluent required varies with the size of the vial and the administration route
- when given for surgical prophylaxis with metronidazole, ensure line is flushed in between cefepime and metronidazole to prevent precipitation occurring
- not compatible with gentamicin, metronidazole, vancomycin or tobramycin
- contraindicated in those with hypersensitivity to L-arginine
- see also General Nursing considerations/Cautions for cephalosporins (p. 167) and General Patient education for cephalosporins (p. 168)

Dose reduction is needed in renal impairment owing to increased risk of neurotoxicity (seizures, coma) at high doses. There is also an increased risk of neutropenia with prolonged use. Renal impairment.

CEFOTAXIME

Trade names
DBL Cefotaxime Sodium for Injection

Available form
Vial: 1 g

Action
- not active against methicillin-resistant staphylococci, *Clostridium perfringens*, *Enterococcus faecalis* and *Enterobacter cloacae*
- third generation cephalosporin
- see also General Actions of cephalosporins (p. 166)

Use
- see General Uses of cephalosporins (p. 166)

Dose
- (Urinary tract infection) 1 g IM or IV bolus over 3—5 minutes or IV infusion over 30 minutes 12-hourly **OR**
- (Other infections) 1 g IM or IV bolus over 3—5 minutes or IV infusion over 30 minutes 12-hourly, increasing to 3, 4 or 6 g daily if necessary **OR**
- (Gonorrhoea — non-beta-lactamase producing organism) 1 g as a single IM dose **OR**
- (Gonorrhoea — beta-lactamase producing organism) 0.5 g as single IM dose plus probenecid, 1 g orally, taken 1 hour earlier **OR**
- (Prophylaxis — biliary surgery) 1 g as IV bolus over 3—5 minutes or IV infusion over 30 minutes at induction **OR**
- (Prophylaxis — caesarean section) 1 g IV bolus over 3—5 minutes or IV infusion over 30 minutes after umbilical cord is clamped, followed by 1 g at 6 and 12 hours from first dose (total 3 doses) **OR**
- (Prophylaxis — vaginal or abdominal hysterectomy) 1 g IM 30—60 minutes before incision, 1 g on completion of surgery, then 1 g 8-hourly for a total of 24 hours

Adverse effects
- (Rare, rapid IV via CVC line) arrhythmias
- Jarisch—Herxheimer reaction (malaise, fever, chills, sore throat, myalgia, headache, tachycardia)
- see also General Adverse effects of cephalosporins (p. 166)

Interactions
- not recommended with tetracycline, erythromycin or chloramphenicol
- concurrent use with aminoglycosides (e.g. gentamicin) increases the risk of nephrotoxicity
- see also General Interactions of cephalosporins (p. 166)

Nursing considerations/Cautions
- if patient is treated for more than 7 days, WBC count monitoring is recommended
- incompatible with sodium bicarbonate and aminoglycosides
- 0.5% lidocaine (lignocaine) (without adrenaline (epinephrine)) may be added to reduce pain at IM site

HAVARD'S NURSING GUIDE TO DRUGS

- not more than 4 mL given into single IM injection site
- if daily dose > 2 g or if frequency is more than twice daily, IV route is preferred
- contains 48.2 mg sodium per 1 g cefotaxime
- contraindicated in those with severe heart failure or non-paced heart block or infants less than 30 months
- see also General Nursing considerations/Cautions for cephalosporins (p. 167)

Patient education
- see General Patient education for cephalosporins (p. 168)

Generally considered safe to use during pregnancy; may be used when the benefits outweigh the risks, particularly in serious infections.

Generally considered safe during breastfeeding. It can be used when the benefits outweigh the risks. Small amounts pass into breastmilk; it may occasionally cause loose stools or gastrointestinal upset in the infant. Monitor infant.

Dose reduction is needed in renal impairment (CrCl < 5 mL/min, halve the dose). Increased risk of neurotoxicity (seizures, coma) with high doses in renal impairment. Risk of neutropenia with prolonged use.

CEFOXITIN
Trade names
Cefoxitin Juno Powder for Injection

Available form
Vial: 1 g

Action
- not active against *Pseudomonas* spp., most strains of enterococci, methicillin-resistant staphylococci and many strains of *Enterobacter cloacae*
- second generation cephalosporin
- see also General Actions of cephalosporins (p. 166)

Use
- see General Uses of cephalosporins (p. 166)

Dose
- (Uncomplicated infection) 1 g IM or by IV bolus over 3–5 minutes or IV infusion 6–8-hourly **OR**
- (Moderate to severe infection) 2 g IM or by IV bolus over 3–5 minutes or IV infusion 6–8-hourly **OR**
- (Severe infections) 2–3 g IM or by IV bolus over 3–5 minutes or IV infusion 4–6-hourly (daily maximum 12 g) **OR**
- (Gonorrhoea) 2 g as a single IM dose plus probenecid, 1 g orally, taken immediately or 1 hour earlier **OR**
- (Prophylaxis — surgery) 2 g IM 1 hour before surgery or by IV bolus over 3–5 minutes or IV infusion just before surgery, then 2 g IM or IV at 6 and 12 hours after first dose **OR**
- (Prophylaxis — caesarean section) 2 g after umbilical cord is clamped, then 2 g IM or by IV bolus over 3–5 minutes or IV infusion at 4 and 8 hours after first dose

Adverse effects
- see General Adverse effects of cephalosporins (p. 166)

Interactions
- may interfere with measurement of urine corticosteroids
- see also General Interactions of cephalosporins (p. 166)

Nursing considerations/Cautions/Patient education
- contains 51.2 mg sodium per 1 g cefoxitin
- 0.5% or 1% lidocaine (lignocaine) without adrenaline (epinephrine) may be added to reduce pain at IM site
- not recommended for treatment of meningitis or brain abscesses
- see also General Nursing considerations/Cautions for cephalosporins

ANTIBACTERIAL AGENTS

(p. 167) and General Patient education for cephalosporins (p. 168)

Generally considered safe, but use only when benefits outweigh risks.

Generally considered safe during breastfeeding, though it may cause mild gastrointestinal disturbances, such as loose stools in the infant. Use only when benefits outweigh risks, and observe the infant for any adverse effects.

Dose reduction may be needed in renal impairment, as impaired renal function can lead to drug accumulation. Renal impairment increases the risk of neurotoxicity (such as seizures or coma) at high doses, particularly in patients with severe renal dysfunction.

CEFTAROLINE
Trade names
Zinforo

Available form
Vial: 600 mg

Action
- ceftaroline fosamil is a prodrug converted to active ceftaroline
- active against Gram-positive and Gram-negative bacteria including methicillin-resistant *Staphylococcus aureus* (MRSA) and penicillin non-susceptible *Streptococcus pneumoniae*
- half-life 2.5 hours
- see also General Actions of cephalosporins (p. 166)

Use
- see General Uses of cephalosporins (p. 166)

Dose
- 600 mg by IV infusion over 60 minutes twice daily

Adverse effects
- see General Adverse effects of cephalosporins (p. 166)

Nursing considerations/Cautions/Patient education
- (Complicated skin and soft tissue infection) duration 5—14 days
- (Community-acquired pneumonia) duration 5—7 days
- reconstitute using 20 mL water for injections and then dilute further for IV infusion
- caution if used in those with epilepsy or moderate-to-severe kidney impairment
- contraindicated in those with hypersensitivity to L-arginine
- see also General Nursing considerations/Cautions for cephalosporins (p. 167) and General Patient education for cephalosporins (p. 168)

Limited data on the use of ceftaroline in pregnancy. Generally not recommended. Use only if the potential benefit outweighs the risk.

Limited data on use in breastfeeding. Generally not recommended. Use only if the potential benefit outweighs the risk.

Reduce dose when CrCl < 50 mL/min to prevent drug accumulation and reduce the risk of toxicity. Close monitoring of renal function is recommended; adjust dosing appropriately.

CEFTAZIDIME
Trade names
Ceftazidime Powder for Injection

Available form
Vial: 1 g, 2 g

Action
- not active against *Enterococcus faecalis*, many other enterococci, methicillin-resistant staphylococci, *Listeria monocytogenes*, *Campylobacter* spp. or *Clostridium difficile*
- third generation cephalosporin with antipseudomonal activity

- see also General Actions of cephalosporins (p. 166)

Use
- see General Uses of cephalosporins (p. 166)

Dose
- (Urinary tract or less serious infections) 0.5—1 g IM, by IV bolus over 3—5 minutes or IV infusion over 30 minutes 12-hourly **OR**
- (Other infections) 1—2 g IM, by IV bolus over 3—5 minutes or IV infusion over 30 minutes 8—12-hourly **OR**
- (Serious infections) 2 g by IV bolus over 3—5 minutes or IV infusion over 30 minutes 8—12-hourly

Adverse effects
- see General Adverse effects of cephalosporins (p. 166)

Interactions
- not recommended with chloramphenicol
- see also General Interactions of cephalosporins (p. 166)

Nursing considerations/Cautions/Patient education
- doses greater than 1 g should be given IV
- vials supplied are under reduced pressure and, as the product dissolves, carbon dioxide is released, causing effervescence and a positive pressure develops
- amount of diluent required depends on dose and route of administration (e.g. 1 g IM requires 3 mL whereas 2 g IV requires 10 mL). Manufacturer's instructions should be consulted
- colour of solution may vary from pale yellow to amber
- to preserve sterility, a gas relief needle should not be inserted until product has completely dissolved
- 0.5% lidocaine (lignocaine) (without adrenaline (epinephrine)) may be added to reduce pain at the IM site, but stable for only half the time compared with addition of water for injections
- solution contains 52 mg sodium per 1 g ceftazidime
- not recommended to treat CNS infections such as meningitis or brain abscess
- see also General Nursing considerations/Cautions for cephalosporins (p. 167) and General Patient education for cephalosporins (p. 168)

Insufficient data on the effects in pregnancy. Avoid use. Use only if the benefits clearly outweigh the risks.

Insufficient data on the effects in breastfeeding. Avoid use. Use only if the benefits clearly outweigh the risks.

CEFTAZIDIME WITH AVIBACTAM
Trade names
Zavicefta

Available form
Vial: 2 g ceftazidime/0.5 g avibactam

Action
- cephalosporin with avibactam (beta-lactamase inhibitor)
- ceftazidime has little or no activity against most Gram-positive organisms or anaerobes
- avibactam does not inhibit class B enzymes (metallo-beta lactamases) or class D enzymes
- half-life of both ceftazidime and avibactam is about 2 hours
- see also General Actions of cephalosporins (p. 166)

Use
- complicated intra-abdominal infection (with metronidazole)
- complicated urinary tract infection, including pyelonephritis
- hospital-acquired pneumonia, including ventilator-associated pneumonia

Dose
- (Complicated intra-abdominal infection) 2 g ceftazidime/0.5 g avibactam by IV infusion over 2 hours 8-hourly for 5—14 days (with metronidazole) **OR**
- (Complicated urinary tract infection, pyelonephritis) 2 g ceftazidime/0.5 g

ANTIBACTERIAL AGENTS

avibactam by IV infusion over 2 hours 8-hourly for 5—10 days **OR**
* (Hospital-acquired pneumonia) 2 g ceftazidime/0.5 g avibactam by IV infusion over 2 hours 8-hourly for 7—14 days

Adverse effects
* hypokalaemia
* tachycardia, hypotension, hypertension
* pleural effusion, dyspnoea, cough
* peripheral oedema
* see also General Adverse effects of cephalosporins (p. 166)

Interactions
* caution if given with other nephrotoxic agents or potent diuretics owing to risk of nephrotoxicity
* not recommended with probenecid
* not recommended with chloramphenicol
* may cause false positive Coombs' test

Nursing considerations/Cautions
* (Complicated urinary tract infection, pyelonephritis) if patient has bacteraemia, therapy can be extended to 14 days
* reconstitute powder using 10 mL water for injections, shake vial to dissolve powder then further dilute for IV infusion
* to preserve product sterility, gas relief needle should not be inserted before product is dissolved
* vial contains 148 mg sodium
* reconstituted solution is clear and colourless to yellow solution
* contraindicated in those with hypersensitivity to cephalosporins, other beta-lactam antibacterial agents or avibactam
* see also General Nursing considerations/Cautions for cephalosporins (p. 167)

Patient education
* see General Patient education for cephalosporins (p. 168)

Insufficient data available on its use during pregnancy. Generally not recommended. Use only if the benefits clearly outweigh the risks.

Insufficient data available on its use during breastfeeding. Generally not recommended. Use only if the benefits clearly outweigh the risks.

In reduced renal function, dose adjustment is required to prevent drug accumulation and reduce the risk of toxicity. Close monitoring of renal function (e.g. serum creatinine, creatinine clearance) is essential.

CEFTOLOZANE WITH TAZOBACTAM
Trade names
Zerbaxa

Available form
Vial: 1 g ceftolozane/0.5 g tazobactam

Action
* cephalosporin with tazobactam (beta-lactamase inhibitor)
* half-life of ceftolozane 3 hours, tazobactam 1 hour
* see also General Actions of cephalosporins (p. 166)

Use
* see General Uses of cephalosporins (p. 166)

Dose
* (Complicated intra-abdominal infection) 1 g ceftolozane/0.5 g tazobactam by IV infusion over 60 minutes 8-hourly for 4—14 days (with metronidazole 500 mg IV 8-hourly) **OR**
* (Complicated urinary tract infections including pyelonephritis) 1 g ceftolozane/0.5 g tazobactam by IV infusion over 60 minutes 8-hourly for 7 days
* (Nosocomial pneumonia including ventilator associated pneumonia) 2 g ceftolozane/1 g tazobactam by IV infusion over 60 minutes 8-hourly for 8 to 14 days

Adverse effects
* hypokalaemia
* atrial fibrillation, hypotensions
* see also General Adverse effects of cephalosporins (p. 166)

Interactions
- increased serum levels may occur if given with probenecid, diclofenac or cimetidine

Nursing considerations/Cautions/Patient education
- reconstitute using 10 mL water for injections or sodium chloride 0.9%, shaking gently to dissolve
- reconstituted solution is clear to slightly yellow
- for IV infusion, reconstituted solution should be added to 100 mL sodium chloride 0.9% or glucose 5% and infused over 60 minutes
- administer alone
- caution if used in those who are severely immunocompromised, receiving immunosuppressive therapy or with severe neutropenia
- contraindicated in those with hypersensitivity to tazobactam or piperacillin/tazobactam
- see also General Nursing considerations/Cautions for cephalosporins (p. 167) and General Patient education for cephalosporins (p. 168)

Insufficient data available on its use during pregnancy. Generally not recommended.

Limited human data exist on the use of ceftolozane during breastfeeding. It is generally not recommended. Use with caution and only when the benefits outweigh the risks. Monitor the infant for any adverse reactions.

In patients with reduced renal function, dose adjustment is required to prevent drug accumulation and reduce the risk of toxicity. Close monitoring of renal function (e.g. serum creatinine, creatinine clearance) is essential.

CEFTRIAXONE
Trade names
Ceftriaxone Powder for Injection

Available form
Vial: 500 mg, 1 g, 2 g

Action
- active against some species of *Pseudomonas aeruginosa* but other *Pseudomonas* spp. are resistant. Most species of group D streptococci, including *Enterococcus faecalis* and *E. faecium*, are resistant
- third generation cephalosporin
- half-life 5.8—8.7 hours
- see also General Actions of cephalosporins (p. 166)

Use
- see General Uses of cephalosporins (p. 166)

Dose
- 1—2 g IM or by IV bolus over 2—4 minutes, or by IV infusion over 30 minutes daily, or in equally divided doses 12-hourly **OR**
- (Uncomplicated gonorrhoea) 250 mg as single IM dose **OR**
- (Prophylaxis — surgery) 1 g IM or IV 0.5—2 hours before surgery

Adverse effects
- (Rare) pancreatitis, precipitations in gallbladder (not gallstones)
- (Rare, neonates) lung and kidney precipitates (if given with calcium-containing solutions)
- see also General Adverse effects of cephalosporins (p. 166)

Interactions
- probenecid does not alter elimination of ceftriaxone
- (Neonates) not recommended with or within 48 hours of calcium-containing solutions

Nursing considerations/Cautions/Patient education
- contains 83 mg sodium per g
- incompatible with vancomycin, fluconazole, aminoglycosides or calcium-containing fluids (e.g. Hartmann's solution, Ringer's solution)
- 1% lidocaine (lignocaine) (without adrenaline (epinephrine)) may be added to reduce pain at IM site

ANTIBACTERIAL AGENTS

- no more than 1 g injected IM into one site
- reconstituted solutions have a harmless yellowish tinge and may have a slight cloudiness
- caution if used in those with risk factors for biliary stasis or biliary sludge as this increases the risk of pancreatitis
- see also General Nursing considerations/Cautions for cephalosporins (p. 167) and General Patient education for cephalosporins (p. 168)

Generally considered safe, but use only when benefits outweigh risks.

Safe to use during breastfeeding, though it may cause loose stools in the child. Use only when benefits outweigh risks, and monitor the infant for any side effects.

Ceftriaxone is primarily excreted via the biliary system, with partial renal excretion. While dose adjustment is generally not required in mild-to-moderate renal impairment, caution should be exercised in patients with severe renal impairment (CrCl < 10 mL/min) or in those with concomitant hepatic impairment. In such cases, accumulation may occur, and monitoring for adverse effects, such as biliary sludge or neurotoxicity, is recommended.

CEFUROXIME
Trade names
Cefuroxime SXP, Pharmacor Cefuroxime, Zinnat, Zinnat Suspension

Available forms
Tablets: 250 mg;
Powder for injection: 750 mg;
Suspension: 125 mg/5 mL

Action
- prodrug which is hydrolysed to active cefuroxime
- not active against *Clostridium difficile*, *Pseudomonas* spp., *Campylobacter* spp., *Acinetobacter calcoaceticus*, *Proteus vulgaris*, *Morganella morganii*, *Serratia* spp., *Listeria monocytogenes*, *Bacteroides fragilis*, *Enterococcus faecalis*, *Enterobacter* spp., methicillin-resistant staphylococci or *Citrobacter* spp.
- second generation cephalosporin
- see also General Actions of cephalosporins (p. 166)

Use
- see General Uses of cephalosporins (p. 166)

Dose
- (Acute or chronic bronchitis) 250—500 mg twice daily after a light meal (for 5—7 days) **OR**
- (Uncomplicated gonorrhoea) 1 g as single oral dose after a light meal **OR**
- (Other infections) 250 mg twice daily after a light meal (for 7—10 days) **OR**
- (Orthopaedic surgery prophylaxis) 1.5 g IV with induction of anaesthesia **OR**
- (Cardiac surgery prophylaxis) 1.5 g IV with induction of anaesthesia followed by 750 mg 8-hourly for two more doses

Adverse effects
- see General Adverse effects of cephalosporins (p. 166)

Interactions
- bioavailability may be decreased if given with ranitidine
- may decrease efficacy of oral contraceptives containing oestrogen
- see also General Interactions of cephalosporins (p. 166)

Nursing considerations/Cautions
- tablets and suspension are not bioequivalent and should not be substituted
- food increases absorption. Give with or soon after food for the best absorption
- suspension is recommended for paediatric use
- daily dose should not exceed 500 mg in those with kidney impairment
- (Suspension) contains aspartame and is therefore not recommended in those with phenylketonuria
- (Suspension) contains 3 g sucrose per dose (125 mg/5 mL), which may need to

- be considered if patient has diabetes mellitus
- see also General Nursing considerations/Cautions for cephalosporins (p. 167)

Patient education

- (Suspension) advise parent/carer to shake bottle well before administering dose to child
- (Suspension) instruct parent/carer to store bottle in fridge and discard 10 days after opening
- may cause dry mouth
- see also General Patient education for cephalosporins (p. 168)

Syrup/suspension is available. Tablet can be dispersed in 40–60 mL orange, grape or apple juice or chocolate milk, or tablet can be crushed and mixed with water or spoonful of yoghurt, apple puree or ice-cream.

Generally considered safe, but use only when benefits outweigh risks.

Safe to use during breastfeeding, though it may cause loose stools in the child. Use only when benefits outweigh risks, and monitor the infant for any side effects.

Dose adjustment is required in renal impairment to prevent drug accumulation. Monitor renal function regularly and adjust doses accordingly.

MONOBACTAMS AND CARBAPENEMS

General Uses of monobactams and carbapenems

- monobactams (aztreonam) and carbapenems (imipenem, meropenem and ertapenem) are both classes of beta-lactam antibiotics, but they differ in their structure, spectrum of activity and clinical use
- moderate-to-serious infections of the lower respiratory tract, intra-abdominal infections, gynaecological infection, bacterial septicaemia, endocarditis, skin, bone and joint infections, including multi-bacterial infections
- diabetic foot infections (in those unable to tolerate other antibiotics or with resistant organisms)
- Gram-negative infections (e.g. gonorrhoea, urinary tract)
- meningitis (*Haemophilus influenzae, Neisseria meningitidis*) with other antibacterial agents
- *Pseudomonas* spp. infections (with aminoglycosides)

General Adverse effects of monobactams and carbapenems

- nausea, vomiting, altered taste, diarrhoea, abdominal pain/cramps, mouth ulcers
- increase in liver enzymes
- rash, urticaria, pruritus, fever, flushing, sweating
- headache, dizziness
- encephalopathy (confusion, impaired consciousness, seizures, movement disorders)
- superinfection
- pseudomembranous colitis
- hypersensitivity, anaphylaxis, anaphylactoid reaction
- haematological disorders (eosinophilia, neutropenia, thrombocytopenia), positive direct or indirect Coombs' test
- (Rare) convulsions, severe skin reactions, jaundice, liver failure
- (IV site) phlebitis, thrombophlebitis, pain/discomfort, erythema, induration
- (IM) pain

General Interactions for monobactams and carbapenems

- increased serum levels may occur if given with probenecid
- increased risk of pseudomembranous colitis if given with peristalsis-delaying

ANTIBACTERIAL AGENTS

agents, such as opioid analgesics or diphenoxylate/atropine combination

General Nursing considerations/Cautions for monobactams and carbapenems

- cross-sensitivity can exist between penicillins, cephalosporins, imipenem, aztreonam and meropenem, so patients sensitive to one of these agents may also be sensitive to the others
- renal, liver and haematological function should be monitored regularly with prolonged therapy
- administer alone, ensuring IV line is adequately flushed before and after administration
- amount of diluent required for reconstitution is dependent on route of administration (IM or IV), therefore manufacturer's instructions should be consulted before reconstitution
- adrenaline (epinephrine), IV corticosteroids, oxygen and resuscitation equipment should be available in the event of anaphylaxis
- caution if used in those with kidney impairment
- caution if used in those with liver impairment. If used, liver function should be closely monitored during therapy
- contraindicated in those with hypersensitivity to monobactams, carbapenems or beta lactams
- see also General Nursing considerations/Cautions for antibacterial agents (p. 149)

General Patient education for monobactams and carbapenems

- warn patient against driving or operating heavy machinery if dizziness, somnolence or seizure occurs
- see also General Patient education for antibacterial agents (p. 150)

Both monobactams (aztreonam) and carbapenems (limipenem, meropenem and ertapenem) should be used with caution in patients with kidney impairment, as these drugs are primarily excreted by the kidneys. Dose adjustments are often required to prevent drug accumulation, which can increase the risk of toxicity, particularly neurotoxicity. Monitoring of kidney function (serum creatinine and creatinine clearance) should be conducted regularly during treatment.

AZTREONAM
Trade name
Azactam

Available form
Vial: 1 g

Action
- synthetic monocyclic beta lactam (monobactam) that binds to penicillin-binding proteins resulting in bacterial cell wall synthesis inhibition
- bactericidal against most aerobic Gram-negative bacteria
- resists the action of beta lactamase (penicillinase, cephalosporinase)
- not well absorbed orally
- half-life 1.4—2.2 hours (normal renal function)

Use
- reserved for Gram-negative infections where other antibacterial agents are inappropriate or contraindicated

Dose
- (Moderately severe infections) 1—2 g 8—12-hourly IM, by slow IV injection over 3—5 minutes or IV infusion over 30 minutes (daily maximum 8 g) **OR**
- (Severe infections) 2 g 6—8-hourly by slow IV injection over 3—5 minutes or IV infusion over 30 minutes (daily maximum 8 g) **OR**
- (Urinary tract infection) 0.5—1 g 8—12-hourly IM, by slow IV injection over 3—5 minutes or IV infusion over 30 minutes (daily maximum 8 g) **OR**

- (Uncomplicated gonorrhoea, acute cystitis) 1 g as a single deep IM dose

Adverse effects
- see General Adverse effects of monobactams and carbapenems (p. 178)

Interactions
- increased serum levels may occur if given with furosemide (frusemide)
- see also General Interactions of monobactams and carbapenems (p. 178)

Nursing considerations/Cautions
- not used as monotherapy for management of meningitis
- (Meningitis) therapy should be continued for 7—10 days (*Neisseria meningitidis*) and 10—14 days (*Haemophilus influenzae*)
- IV route is recommended for single doses over 1 g or in those with septicaemia, intra-abdominal abscess, peritonitis or severe systemic/life-threatening infections
- (IV infusion) reconstitute the powder with water for injections or sodium chloride 0.9% and shake contents immediately and vigorously, then dilute further for IV infusion with at least 50 mL compatible fluid per gram aztreonam
- (IV bolus) reconstitute with 6—10 mL water for injections
- (IM) reconstitute with at least 3 mL water for injections per gram of aztreonam
- colour of reconstituted IV solution may vary from colourless to pale yellow with a slight pink tint on standing
- IM injection is usually well tolerated and local anaesthetic is not required
- not recommended for gynaecological infections or other sites where aerobic Gram-negative organisms are not common
- see also General Nursing considerations/Cautions for monobactams and carbapenems (p. 179)

Patient education
- see General Patient education for monobactams and carbapenems (p. 179)

 Crosses placenta and enters fetal circulation; therefore should be used during pregnancy only if clearly needed.

 Can be used during breastfeeding when the benefits outweigh the risks. While generally safe, it may occasionally cause loose stools in the infant. Monitoring for side effects is advised.

 Reduce dose if CrCl < 30 mL/min.

ERTAPENEM
Trade names
Invanz

Available form
Vial: 1 g

Action
- bactericidal antibiotic
- beta-lactam antibiotic
- carbapenem, which inhibits bacterial wall synthesis
- wide activity against Gram-positive and Gram-negative aerobic and some anaerobic organisms
- half-life of about 4 hours

Use
- see General Uses of monobactams and carbapenems (p. 178)

Dose
- (Moderate-to-severe infections, diabetic foot infections) 1 g daily IM or by IV infusion over 30 minutes for 3—14 days

Adverse effects
- see General Adverse effects of monobactams and carbapenems (p. 178)

Interactions
- may decrease serum levels of valproic acid (sodium valproate) reducing

seizure control; therefore levels should be monitored throughout therapy
- see also General Interactions of monobactams and carbapenems (p. 178)

Nursing considerations/Cautions/Patient education
- as with other broad-spectrum antibiotics, prolonged use of ertapenem may lead to superinfections, including *Clostridioides difficile*-associated diarrhoea. Monitor for signs of secondary infections like diarrhoea, oral thrush or vaginal yeast infections.
- not recommended with glucose-containing diluents
- reconstitute using 10 mL water for injections or sodium chloride 0.9%, then dilute to 50 mL using sodium chloride 0.9% for IV infusion
- for IM use, may be diluted using 3.2 mL lidocaine (lignocaine) (without adrenaline (epinephrine)) to reduce pain
- caution if used in those with CNS disorders (e.g. brain abscess, epilepsy, history of seizures) and/or liver impairment owing to increased risk of seizures
- not recommended for meningitis or other CNS infections in children owing to increased risk of seizures
- contraindicated in those with hypersensitivity to lidocaine (lignocaine) or amide-type local anaesthetics, or with severe shock or heart block (if diluted using lidocaine (lignocaine))
- see also General Nursing considerations/Cautions for monobactams and carbapenems (p. 179) and General Patient education for monobactams and carbapenems (p. 179)

Not recommended during pregnancy unless benefits outweigh risks.

Generally considered safe while breastfeeding and can be used when the benefit outweighs the risk. It may occasionally cause loose stools in the infant, so monitor for any side effects.

Assess renal function prior to starting ertapenem, especially in elderly or renally impaired patients. Dosage adjustments may be necessary based on creatinine clearance to avoid toxicity.

IMIPENEM (with cilastatin)
Trade names
Primaxin

Available form
Vial: imipenem 500 mg/cilastatin 500 mg

Action
- imipenem is a carbapenem resistant to beta lactamases, but is inactivated by a renal dihydropeptidase; therefore it is formulated in combination with cilastatin sodium, the specific inhibitor of the renal enzyme
- bactericidal against most aerobic and anaerobic Gram-negative and Gram-positive microorganisms
- carbapenems are related to beta-lactam antibiotics (penicillins, cephalosporins), but are structurally different

Use
- see General Uses of monobactams and carbapenems (p. 178)

Dose
- 0.5—1 g 6—8-hourly by IV infusion over 20—60 minutes (daily maximum 4 g or 50 mg/kg)

Adverse effects
- hypotension, somnolence
- (Uncommon/rare) tremor, confusion, vertigo
- see also General Adverse effects of monobactams and carbapenems (p. 178)

Interactions
- may decrease serum levels of valproic acid (sodium valproate), reducing seizure control; therefore levels should be monitored throughout therapy
- increased risk of seizures if given with ganciclovir; therefore these agents are not recommended together

- probenecid can inhibit the renal excretion of imipenem, leading to increased levels of imipenem in the blood, which may enhance both its efficacy and its toxicity. Concurrent use is generally avoided
- see also General Interactions of monobactams and carbapenems (p. 178)

Nursing considerations/Cautions/Patient education

- dosages greater than 2 g per day are associated with increased risk of CNS-adverse effects (especially in those with renal impairment)
- for doses of less than or equal to 500 mg, infusion should be over 20—30 minutes; for 1 g dose, infusion over 40—60 minutes is recommended
- if patient develops nausea, slow the rate of IV infusion
- do not mix with other drugs in the same syringe or IV container
- reconstitute with 10 mL water for injections and dilute to 100 mL with compatible infusion fluid, mixing solution well until clear, then infuse over 30 minutes via burette (1 g infused over 40—60 minutes; 500 mg infused over 20—30 minutes)
- harmless pale yellow colour may occur
- contains 37.5 mg sodium per 500 mg imipenem, which may need to be considered if patient is on a salt restriction diet
- incompatible with lactate
- not recommended for meningitis because of increased risk of seizures
- see also General Nursing considerations/Cautions for monobactams and carbapenems (p. 179) and General Patient education for monobactams and carbapenems (p. 179)

Limited data on its safety in human pregnancy. Use during pregnancy only if benefits outweigh risks.

Generally considered safe while breast-feeding and can be used when the benefit outweighs the risk. It may occasionally cause loose stools in the infant, so monitor for any side effects.

Use with caution in patients with renal impairment. Reduced renal function increases the risk of drug accumulation; dose reduction is necessary. Accumulation can lead to an increased risk of neurotoxicity, including seizures.

MEROPENEM

Trade names
Meropenem

Available forms
Vial: 500 mg, 1 g

Action
- carbapenem active against Gram-positive aerobes, Gram-negative aerobes and some anaerobic bacteria
- *Enterococcus faecium, Stenotrophomonas maltophilia* and methicillin-resistant *Staphylococcus aureus* (MRSA) are resistant to meropenem
- carbapenems are related to beta-lactam antibiotics (penicillins, cephalosporins), but are structurally different
- half-life about 1 hour

Use
- see General Uses of monobactams and carbapenems (p. 178)

Dose
- 0.5—1 g by IV bolus over 5 minutes or IV infusion over 15—30 minutes 8-hourly **OR**
- (Febrile neutropenia) 1 g by IV bolus over 5 minutes or IV infusion over 15—30 minutes 8-hourly **OR**
- (Meningitis) 2 g by IV bolus over 5 minutes or IV infusion over 15—30 minutes 8-hourly

Adverse effects
- see General Adverse effects of monobactams and carbapenems (p. 178)

Interactions
- may decrease serum sodium valproate levels, reducing seizure control; therefore serum levels should be monitored
- see also General Interactions of monobactams and carbapenems (p. 178)

Nursing considerations/Cautions/Patient education
- administer alone
- reconstitute using water for injections (10 mL/500 mg meropenem) and then further dilute to 50–200 mL for IV infusion
- reconstituted solution may be clear to pale yellow
- see also General Nursing considerations/Cautions/Patient education for monobactams and carbapenems (p. 179)

Use during pregnancy only if benefits outweigh risks.

Generally considered safe while breastfeeding and can be used when the benefit outweighs the risk. It may occasionally cause loose stools in the infant, so monitor for any side effects.

GLYCOPEPTIDES

General Actions of glycopeptides
- inhibit bacterial wall synthesis, but at a different site from beta-lactam antibacterial agents
- generally bactericidal
- primarily active against Gram-positive organisms
- growing resistance, particularly with vancomycin-resistant enterococci (VRE) and some strains of *Staphylococcus aureus*

General Adverse effects of glycopeptides
- nausea, vomiting, diarrhoea
- hearing loss, tinnitus, vertigo, vestibular disorders
- dizziness, headache
- eosinophilia, leucopenia, neutropenia, thrombocytopenia and, rarely, agranulocytosis
- increase in liver enzymes
- increased creatinine and urea, kidney failure
- 'red man' syndrome is caused by rapid infusion of glycopeptides, particularly vancomycin. It is not an allergic reaction, but symptoms are related to histamine release. Symptoms include fever, chills, erythema and a rash on the face and upper torso, which can progress to hypotension, angioedema and itching. Managed with antihistamines (e.g. promethazine)
- (IV site) redness, pain, phlebitis, abscess formation, thrombophlebitis
- (Rapid IV infusion) 'red neck' or 'red man' syndrome (pruritus, and flushing to face, neck, upper body, back and arms)
- superinfection, pseudomembranous colitis
- (Rare) hypersensitivity reactions, anaphylactoid reaction (hypotension, palpitations, substernal pressure, tachycardia), severe cutaneous reactions
- (Rare) ototoxicity

General Nursing considerations/Cautions for glycopeptides
- serial audiograms are recommended with prolonged therapy (especially in those over 60 years, if renal impairment is present or if given with other ototoxic agents such as aminoglycosides)
- blood tests, renal and liver function studies should be carried out regularly during prolonged therapy or in patients with renal insufficiency
- slowing or stopping infusion may stop 'red man' syndrome; it usually resolves within 20 minutes but may last several hours
- patient should be closely monitored for any signs of rash with blisters or oral

- lesions and therapy stopped if they occur
- contraindicated in those with glycopeptide hypersensitivity, deafness, hearing loss or kidney disease
- see also General Nursing considerations/Cautions for antibacterial agents (p. 149)

General Patient education for glycopeptides

- patients should be advised to seek medical advice immediately if any of the following occur:
  - ringing in the ears or changes to hearing
  - blistering or peeling of skin
- warn patient to avoid driving or operating machinery if dizziness or vertigo occurs
- see also General Patient education for antibacterial agents (p. 150)

Limited data available; use only if benefits outweigh risks. Recommended only for severe infections with no safer alternatives. Monitor mother and fetus closely.

Glycopeptides, such as vancomycin and teicoplanin, are generally considered safe during breastfeeding, as only small amounts pass into breastmilk. Monitor the infant for gastrointestinal disturbances such as diarrhoea. Use only when the benefit outweighs the risk.

In patients with reduced renal function, dose adjustments are necessary to prevent drug accumulation and reduce the risk of nephrotoxicity and ototoxicity. Regular monitoring of renal function is essential, especially during prolonged or high-dose treatments. Close observation is also required for elderly patients, as they are more susceptible to renal impairment.

TEICOPLANIN

Trade names
Targocid, Teicoplanin Medsurge, Teicoplanin Sandoz

Available form
Vial: 400 mg

Action
- very long elimination half-life (70—100 hours)
- cross-sensitivity is possible between vancomycin and teicoplanin
- no cross-resistance with beta lactams, macrolides, aminoglycosides, tetracycline, rifampicin or chloramphenicol
- see also General Actions of glycopeptides (p. 183)

Use
- staphylococcal or streptococcal infection that cannot be treated using other antibiotics
- osteomyelitis, septic arthritis, septicaemia, non-cardiac bacteraemia

Dose
- (Septicaemia/bacteraemia, acute/chronic osteomyelitis) initially 6—12 mg/kg as an IV bolus over 5 minutes or IV infusion over 30 minutes 12-hourly for 3 doses, then 6 mg/kg IM or IV daily for 2—4 weeks (bacteraemia) or 3—6 weeks (osteomyelitis) **OR**
- (Septic arthritis) initially 12 mg/kg as an IV bolus over 5 minutes or IV infusion over 30 minutes 12-hourly for 3 doses, then 12 mg/kg IM or IV daily for 3—6 weeks

Adverse effects
- fever, rigors
- rash, pruritus
- see also General Adverse effects of glycopeptides (p. 183)

Interactions
- use with caution if given with other nephrotoxic or ototoxic drugs (e.g. amphotericin B (amphotericin), aminoglycosides, furosemide (frusemide), ciclosporin). If given together, blood, liver and kidney function should be closely monitored

Nursing considerations/Cautions
- teicoplanin is well tolerated when administered by IV infusion
- (IM) should not exceed 400 mg (3 mL) at a single site

ANTIBACTERIAL AGENTS

- loading dose of 12 mg/mL at 12-hourly intervals is given to achieve rapid steady state plasma levels. Creatinine levels should be closely monitored in addition to blood, liver and kidney function
- reconstitute by adding all of the supplied diluent slowly down the side of the vial, gently rolling between the palms of the hands until the powder is dissolved, taking care to avoid foaming. The vial should not be shaken. If foamy, allow to stand for 15 minutes until foam subsides. May be further diluted for IV infusion with sodium chloride 0.9%, glucose 5%, sodium chloride 0.18% or lactated Ringer's solution
- incompatible with aminoglycosides as precipitate will form
- caution if used in those with known hypersensitivity to vancomycin (however, history of 'red man' syndrome is not a contraindication in itself)
- see also General Nursing considerations/Cautions for glycopeptides (p. 183)

Patient education
- see General Patient education for glycopeptides (p. 184)

VANCOMYCIN
Trade names
Vancocin, Vancocin CP, Vancomycin Powder for Infusion

Available forms
Capsules: 125 mg, 250 mg;
Vial: 500 mg, 1 g

Action
- alters bacterial wall permeability and RNA synthesis
- elimination half-life 4—6 hours
- cross-sensitivity is possible between vancomycin and teicoplanin
- active against Gram-positive organisms, with Gram-negative organisms, mycobacteria and fungi resistant
- poorly absorbed orally
- not removed by haemodialysis or peritoneal dialysis
- resistance emerging; therefore recommendations/guidelines have been developed regarding usage and should be followed closely
- see also General Actions of glycopeptides (p. 183)

Use
- life-threatening infections caused by beta-lactam-resistant Gram-positive organisms or in patients who have serious allergies to beta-lactam antibacterial agents
- prophylaxis for endocarditis before some procedures in those at high risk of endocarditis
- surgical prophylaxis for major procedures involving prostheses or device implantation where risk of MRSA or MRSE is high
- life-threatening *Clostridium difficile*-associated disease (relapse or unresponsive to metronidazole)
- (Oral route) recommended only for treatment of staphylococcal enterocolitis or antibiotic-induced pseudomembranous colitis

Dose
- 500 mg IV 6-hourly or 1 g IV 12-hourly by infusion over at least 60 minutes **OR**
- (antibiotic-associated pseudomembranous colitis) 0.5—2 g orally daily in 3—4 divided doses for 7—10 days **OR**
- (antibiotic-associated pseudomembranous colitis) 250 mg orally 6-hourly for 5—10 days

Adverse effects
- (Rapid IV infusion) rash, generalised pruritus, chills, fever, severe hypotension and (rarely) cardiac arrest
- chills
- (Oral) nausea, vomiting, diarrhoea, indigestion, stomach ache
- see also General Adverse effects of glycopeptides (p. 183)

Interactions

- concurrent or sequential use of vancomycin and other neurotoxic and/or nephrotoxic agents (e.g. amphotericin B (amphotericin), aminoglycosides, colistin, cisplatin) is not recommended and should be very carefully monitored
- serum levels may be altered if given with furosemide (frusemide); therefore close monitoring is recommended especially when starting or stopping therapy
- increased risk of infusion-related events (e.g. hypotension, flushing, pruritus, urticaria) if given with anaesthetic agents; therefore vancomycin infusion should be completed before anaesthetic induction
- caution if given with other agents known to cause neutropenia
- not recommended with other agents known to cause ototoxicity
- may increase neuromuscular blockage if given with vecuronium or suxamethonium
- (Oral) absorption decreased by colestyramine

Nursing considerations/Cautions

- given by slow IV infusion (500 mg over 1 hour, 1 g over 2 hours) to decrease risk of hypersensitivity reaction and severe hypotension
- should be used for 48—72 hours after fever and symptoms have resolved
- avoid extravasation and never administer intramuscularly (risk of tissue irritation/necrosis)
- for IV infusion, reconstitute drug with 10 mL water for injections for 500 mg, or 20 mL for 1 g, then dilute with 100 mL of fluid for 500 mg, or 200 mL for 1 g. This should minimise risk of thrombophlebitis
- incompatible with beta lactams (penicillins, cephalosporins), as precipitation may occur. IV lines should be carefully flushed before and after administration
- poorly absorbed orally, but is used in the treatment of antibiotic-associated pseudomembranous colitis
- for oral (or nasogastric) administration, 500 mg is reconstituted with 30 mL distilled or deionised water and then flavoured to improve taste (extremely unpalatable); however, capsules may eliminate the need to do this
- renal function monitoring is recommended if given with aminoglycosides
- adrenaline (epinephrine), IV corticosteroids and oxygen should be available to treat anaphylactic/anaphylactoid reaction
- (Oral) caution if given to those with GI inflammatory disorders, which may increase absorption and the risk of systemic adverse effects
- caution if used in those with known hypersensitivity to teicoplanin
- caution if used in those with kidney impairment. If used, dose and/or dose intervals should be adjusted and kidney function carefully monitored
- see also General Nursing considerations/Cautions for glycopeptides (p. 183)

Patient education

- advise patient to swallow capsules whole with full glass of water
- (Oral) if taking colestyramine as well, instruct patient to separate by at least 2 hours from vancomycin
- see also General Patient education for glycopeptides (p. 184)

 Capsules should not be opened.

INHIBITORS OF BACTERIAL PROTEIN SYNTHESIS

AMINOGLYCOSIDES

General Actions of aminoglycosides

- interfere with bacterial protein synthesis by binding irreversibly to ribosomal (30S) subunits of susceptible organisms
- bactericidal
- inhibit a wide range of Gram-negative and some Gram-positive organisms

ANTIBACTERIAL AGENTS

- *Streptococcus pneumoniae* and the aerobic organisms *Bacteroides* and *Clostridium* spp. have shown resistance to aminoglycosides
- poorly absorbed from GI tract

General Uses of aminoglycosides
- serious or life-threatening infection where other antibacterial agents are contraindicated or ineffective

General Adverse effects of aminoglycosides
- ototoxicity (auditory and vestibular, including tinnitus, vertigo, dizziness) (hearing loss may be permanent)
- nephrotoxicity, increased or decreased urinary frequency, decreased creatinine clearance, azotaemia, increase in serum urea
- neurotoxicity (including ataxia, dizziness, peripheral neuritis, paraesthesia, tremor)
- nausea, vomiting, diarrhoea
- rash, pruritus, urticaria
- superinfection, pseudomembranous colitis
- drug fever
- (Rare) blood dyscrasias
- (IM) pain
- (IV) thrombophlebitis

General Interactions of aminoglycosides
- nephrotoxicity and ototoxicity of aminoglycosides are increased when given with furosemide (frusemide) or other potent diuretics
- not recommended concurrently or sequentially with other neurotoxic or nephrotoxic agents (e.g. other aminoglycosides, amphotericin B (amphotericin), bacitracin, colistin, cisplatin, clindamycin, vancomycin)
- inactivated by solutions containing beta-lactam antibiotics (penicillins and cephalosporins)
- enhanced neuromuscular blockade (including respiratory paralysis) may occur intraoperatively or postoperatively if given with anaesthetics, neuromuscular blocking agents, other medications with neuromuscular activity or massive transfusions with citrated, anticoagulated blood
- increased risk of nephrotoxicity and enhanced neuromuscular blockade if given with methoxyflurane
- increased serum level may occur if given with NSAIDs (as NSAIDs may decrease renal function). If given together, drug level and renal function should be closely monitored

General Nursing considerations/ Cautions for aminoglycosides
- baseline renal function should be measured before starting therapy and then regularly throughout course of treatment, especially in those with known or suspected renal impairment
- once-daily administration has proven to be as efficacious as, safe as and less costly than divided dose administration and is recommended in those with normal renal function
- urine should be monitored for specific gravity, protein, cells and casts to monitor for renal irritation
- if possible, serial audiograms are recommended before starting and throughout therapy, especially in those with renal impairment
- blood urea nitrogen, serum creatinine, calcium, magnesium and sodium and creatinine clearance should be monitored regularly throughout therapy
- note and report oliguria as therapy may need to be stopped if urine output decreases
- patients should be well hydrated during therapy to avoid nephrotoxicity, and hydration should be increased if any signs of renal irritation occur
- monitoring for blood levels is not required if duration of therapy is < 48 hours. If therapy duration is > 48 hours, blood level monitoring is recommended in addition to other testing previously

discussed. Blood for trough level is sampled immediately before the next IM or IV dose; blood for peak level is obtained approximately 1 hour after IM or IV injection and 30 minutes after completion of a 30-minute IV infusion or at the completion of a 1-hour IV infusion; levels should be remeasured every 72 hours. The goal is to avoid excessive peak and/or trough level as this increases risk of ototoxicity and nephrotoxicity
- do not mix with other drugs in the same syringe or IV infusion container
- dilute and give by IV infusion according to manufacturer's instructions
- IV injection to be given very slowly over 2–3 minutes
- caution if used in those with muscular disorders, such as Parkinsonism, as muscle weakness may be aggravated
- caution if used in those with extensive burns, as serum levels may be lowered. Serum levels should be monitored closely to ensure adequate concentrations are reached
- caution if used in those with known hearing impairment, fever, low haematocrit, advanced age or renal damage/impairment, as risk of ototoxicity is increased
- caution if used in the elderly, as there may be pre-existing kidney and/or hearing impairments present
- contraindicated in those with myasthenia gravis
- contraindicated in those with known hypersensitivity to aminoglycosides or with subclinical renal or eighth nerve damage caused by nephrotoxic or ototoxic agents
- see also General Nursing considerations/Cautions for antibacterial agents (p. 49)

General Patient education for aminoglycosides

- patient should be advised to immediately seek medical advice if any of the following occur:
  - headache, dizziness, nausea, vomiting, ataxia, nystagmus, vertigo, tinnitus (buzzing or ringing in the ears), hearing loss or roaring in the ears (signs of ototoxicity)
  - numbness, skin tingling, muscle twitching or convulsions (signs of neurotoxicity), even after therapy has stopped, as damage can occur after drug has been discontinued
- female patients of childbearing potential should be counselled to use adequate contraception during therapy to avoid pregnancy
- see also General Patient education for antibacterial agents (p. 149)

 Contraindicated during pregnancy. Aminoglycosides cross the placenta and may damage the eighth cranial nerve in the developing fetus. All aminoglycosides should be considered potentially nephrotoxic and ototoxic to the fetus regardless of maternal therapeutic blood levels.

 Aminoglycosides (amikacin, gentamicin and tobramycin) are generally considered safe during breastfeeding owing to their poor oral absorption. This means that very little of the drug passes into breastmilk or is absorbed by the infant's gastrointestinal tract. However, it is important to use these medications only when the benefits outweigh the risks and to monitor the infant for any signs of gastrointestinal upset, such as diarrhoea.

 Aminoglycosides are predominantly renally cleared. Renal impairment increases risk of toxicity due to higher plasma concentrations.

AMIKACIN
Trade names
Amikacin Medsurge, Amikacin SXP, Amikacin Wockhardt, DBL Amikacin

Available form
Ampoules: 500 mg/2 mL

Action
- derivative of kanamycin used for treatment of many Gram-negative organisms

ANTIBACTERIAL AGENTS

that are resistant to gentamicin or tobramycin
- half-life 2–3 hours (but greatly prolonged in severe renal failure to 30–86 hours)
- desirable serum levels: peak 15–30 microgram/mL and trough 5–10 microgram/mL
- see also General Actions of aminoglycosides (p. 186)

Use
- second-line treatment of serious staphylococcal infections or neonatal sepsis not responsive to other aminoglycosides
- see also General Uses of aminoglycosides (p. 187)

Dose
- 15 mg/kg/day IM or by IV infusion over 30–60 minutes in 2–3 divided doses **OR**
- (Non-pseudomonal urinary tract infections) 250 mg IM or by IV infusion over 30–60 minutes 12-hourly

Adverse effects
- (Rare) increased liver enzymes, hepatotoxicity, hepatomegaly
- see also General Adverse effects of aminoglycosides (p. 187)

Interactions
- see General Interactions of aminoglycosides (p. 187)

Nursing considerations/Cautions
- some response to treatment should be seen in 24–48 hours. If no clinical response is seen in 72–120 hours, bacterial sensitivities should be rechecked
- treatment should be limited to 10 days. If treatment is greater than 10 days, daily renal and auditory function monitoring is recommended
- IM is the preferred route of administration, with IV used if IM is unavailable or infection is life threatening
- prolonged peak serum levels > 30–35 microgram/mL increases risk of toxicity
- total treatment dose > 15 g increases risk of nephrotoxicity and ototoxicity
- contains sodium bisulfite, which may cause allergy reactions in susceptible people (e.g. those with asthma)
- see also General Nursing considerations/Cautions for aminoglycosides (p. 187)

Patient education
- see General Patient education for aminoglycosides (p. 188)

FRAMYCETIN
Trade names
Soframycin Ear, Soframycin Eye Drops

Available forms
Ear drops: 5 mg/mL (0.5%);
Eye drops: 5 mg/mL (0.5%)

Action
- aminoglycoside used to treat Gram-positive and Gram-negative infections

Use
- otitis externa
- infected corneal ulcer (bacterial keratitis), bacterial conjunctivitis, post removal of foreign bodies, blepharitic corneal abrasions and burns

Dose
- (Ear infection) 2–3 drops into the affected ear(s) 3 times daily **OR**
- (Eye infection) 2 drops into the affected eye(s) 1–2-hourly, then 2–3 drops 3 times daily

Adverse effects
- (Eye drops) redness, discharge, irritation, pain, oedema
- (Rare) hypersensitivity (eyelid swelling and irritation)

Nursing considerations/Cautions
- (Ear drops) may also be applied to a wick and inserted into external auditory meatus
- caution if used in those with known hypersensitivity to neomycin because cross-sensitivity may exist
- (Ear drops) contraindicated if there is perforation of the tympanic membrane

Patient education

Eye drops
- ensure patient has instructions on correct instillation of eye drops (see p. 1128)

Ear drops
- instruct patient in correct instillation technique for ear drops, including:
  - check expiry date
  - if the ear drops are new, break safety cap and open
  - wash hands thoroughly with soap and water
  - hold bottle upside down in one hand (between thumb and middle finger)
  - tilt head to one side with affected ear facing up (it may be easier in sitting or lying position)
  - place dropper tip close to (but not touching) ear and gently tap or press base of container to release drops
  - continue holding head in same position for 1 minute to allow drops to reach deeper into the ear
  - repeat for other ear if needed
  - replace cap on bottle and close tightly
  - wash hands to remove any residue
- warn patient that feeling of drops flowing deeper into ear may be unpleasant
- advise patient that a bad taste in the mouth may occur after using ear drops
- patient should be advised to note opening date and discard after that date (e.g. 28 days)

Available in combination with
- framycetin sulfate 0.5% + gramicidin 0.005% + dexamethasone 0.05% ear drops (Otodex, Sofradex)

GENTAMICIN

Trade names
DBL Gentamicin Solution for Injection BP, Gentamicin Noriderm Solution for Injection, Pfizer (Australia) Gentamicin Injection BP

Available form
Ampoules: 80 mg/2 mL

Action
- aminoglycoside antibiotic which is active against *Pseudomonas aeruginosa*, and *Proteus, Salmonella, Shigella, Klebsiella, Enterobacter, Serratia* and *Staphylococcus* spp.
- not active against anaerobic organisms
- half-life about 2 hours
- see also General Actions of aminoglycosides (p. 186)

Use
- first-line treatment for Gram-negative sepsis
- see also General Uses of aminoglycosides (p. 187)

Dose
- (Severe infections) 3 mg/kg/day IM or by IV infusion over at least 30 minutes in 3 divided doses 8-hourly for 7–10 days **OR**
- (Life-threatening infections) initially 5 mg/kg/day IM or by IV infusion over at least 30 minutes in 3–4 divided doses 6–8 hourly, reducing to 3 mg/kg/day as soon as possible for total of 7–10 days

Adverse effects
- nephrotoxicity, ototoxicity, neuromuscular blockade
- see also General Adverse effects of aminoglycosides (p. 187)

Interactions
- may inhibit actions of IV vitamin K
- added nephrotoxicity and ototoxicity may occur if given with cisplatin
- see also General Interactions of aminoglycosides (p. 187)

Nursing considerations/Cautions
- (IV) dose should never exceed 5 mg/kg/day without serum levels being closely monitored
- IM is the preferred route, with IV being used if IM route is not available or infection is life threatening
- peak levels above 12 microgram/mL or trough levels above 2 microgram/mL should be avoided
- (IV) administer alone

ANTIBACTERIAL AGENTS

- (IV) treatment should not exceed 10—14 days
- (IV) dilute in 100—200 mL sodium chloride 0.9% or glucose 5% and then infuse over at least 30 minutes at a rate not exceeding 1 mg/mL
- when given as an IV bolus, serum levels initially rise into the toxic range but rapidly fall. However, the safety of this administration method has not been established
- (Bone infection) wire chain should be removed after 10—14 days (short-term management of chronic recurrent osteomyelitis) or after 3 months (long-term management of chronic recurrent osteomyelitis where bone grafting is intended)
- (Soft tissue infection) wire chain should be removed after 7—10 days
- see also General Nursing considerations/Cautions for aminoglycosides (p. 187)

Patient education

- if the patient is receiving gentamicin for more than 7—10 days, there is a risk that their kidneys may not function as well, but this typically improves once the drug is stopped
- in some cases, hearing and balance can be affected, and permanent hearing loss is possible. If hearing worsens, the patient should let their health professional know immediately
- it is important for the patient to inform their health professional if they feel unsteady, dizzy or off-balance, especially when they sit up, stand up or walk
- see also General Patient education for aminoglycosides (p. 188)

 Renally cleared. Before starting gentamicin treatment, calculate the patient's creatinine clearance (CrCl) to assess renal function.

For patients on gentamicin with renal impairment, there is an increased risk of toxicity due to reduced drug clearance. Dosing should be adjusted based on renal function and drug levels.

If treatment lasts more than 48 hours, monitor both drug concentration and serum creatinine levels to adjust dosing and avoid toxicity.

TOBRAMYCIN SULFATE

Trade names
DBL Tobramycin, Tobi, Tobi Podhaler, Tobra-Day, Tobramycin Injection, Tobramycin PF, Tobramycin SUN, Tobramycin Viatris, Tobramycin WKT, Tobrex

Available forms
Ampoules: 80 mg/2 mL, 500 mg/5 mL;
Eye drops: 0.3%;
Eye ointment: 0.3%;
Solution for inhalation: 300 mg/5 mL;
Powder for inhalation: 28 mg

Action
- aminoglycoside active against *Pseudomonas aeruginosa*, *Escherichia coli*, and *Proteus*, *Salmonella*, *Shigella*, *Klebsiella*, *Enterobacter*, *Serratia*, *Citrobacter*, *Providencia* and *Staphylococcus* spp., and with low-order activity against Gram-positive organisms
- half-life 2—3 hours (prolongs to 5—70 hours in those with kidney impairment)
- see also General Actions of aminoglycosides (p. 186)

Use
- acute lung exacerbation including *P. aeruginosa* infection in cystic fibrosis
- eye infection
- see also General Uses of aminoglycosides (p. 187)

Dose
- (Mild-to-moderate urinary tract infection) 2—3 mg/kg/day IM or by IV infusion over 20—60 minutes in 2—3 divided doses 8—12-hourly for 7—10 days **OR**
- (Severe infections) 3 mg/kg/day IM or by IV infusion over 20—60 minutes in 3 equal divided doses 8-hourly **OR**
- (Life-threatening infections) up to 5 mg/kg/day IM or by IV infusion over

20—60 minutes in 3—4 divided doses, reducing to 3 mg/kg/day as soon as possible **OR**
- (Cystic fibrosis) initially 10 mg/kg/day by IV infusion over 30—60 minutes, adjusting dose according to serum levels, renal function and patient response, for 10—14 days (500 mg/5 mL) **OR**
- (Cystic fibrosis) 300 mg via nebuliser over 10—15 minutes twice daily for 28 days, repeated after drug-free 28-day interval **OR**
- (Cystic fibrosis) 112 mg (4 capsules) twice daily by inhalation via Tobi Podhaler **OR**
- (Eye infection) 1—2 drops into affected eye(s) 4-hourly or 2 drops hourly (if severe) until improvement **OR**
- (Eye infection) 1—1.5 cm ointment 2—3 times daily or 3—4-hourly (if severe) until improvement

Adverse effects
- (Rare) neurotoxicity
- (Inhalation) bronchospasm, cough, haemoptysis, voice alteration, tinnitus (transient), dizziness, pharyngitis, dyspnoea, oropharyngeal pain, increased serum creatinine
- see also General Adverse effects of aminoglycosides (p. 187)

Interactions
- (IV) activity may be decreased by calcium and magnesium ions
- see also General Interactions of aminoglycosides (p. 187)

Nursing considerations/Cautions
- monitor renal function (serum creatinine, creatinine clearance) regularly
- assess serum tobramycin levels to ensure therapeutic dosing and prevent toxicity
- observe for signs of nephrotoxicity (e.g. decreased urine output, elevated creatinine) and ototoxicity (e.g. tinnitus, hearing loss)
- ensure adequate hydration to support renal clearance
- adjust dosage or frequency in patients with impaired renal function
- (IV) if duration of treatment is > 10 days, renal and auditory monitoring is recommended. IV therapy should not exceed 10—14 days
- serum potassium, calcium, sodium, magnesium and urea levels should be monitored throughout therapy
- IV vial should be diluted with 50—100 mL sodium chloride 0.9% or glucose 5% and infused over 20—60 minutes
- (Inhalation) first dose should be given under supervision with FEV_1 measured before and after inhalation administration to detect bronchospasm. Bronchodilator therapy may be required
- (Inhalation) caution if concurrent tobramycin therapy is given (e.g. IV and inhalation) as there is a risk of cumulative toxicity
- (Podhaler) children 10 years and under should be supervised using Podhaler to ensure correct use
- (IV) contains sodium metabisulfite; therefore should be given with caution in susceptible people (e.g. those with asthma)
- caution if used in those with malignant disease as complex metabolic syndrome (hypocalcaemia, hypomagnesaemia, hypokalaemia, hypoalbuminaemia, hypophosphataemia, hypouricaemia) may occur 2—8 weeks after finishing therapy
- see also General Nursing considerations/Cautions for aminoglycosides (p. 187)

Patient education
- immediately report any signs of nephrotoxicity (reduced urine output, swelling, fatigue) or ototoxicity (ringing in the ears, hearing loss, balance issues)
- be aware that dizziness or balance problems may occur owing to the drug's effects on the inner ear

ANTIBACTERIAL AGENTS

- maintain adequate hydration to help your kidneys clear the drug, especially if the medication is taken intravenously or orally
- see also General Patient education for aminoglycosides (p. 188)

Inhaled therapy
- advise patient that inhalation therapy should be 12 hours apart if possible, but not less than 6-hour interval
- if patient is taking multiple inhaled medications, tobramycin inhalation should be taken last
- patient should know that therapy is a 28-day drug cycle followed by a 28-day drug-free interval
- if using nebuliser solution, patient should be aware that it should not be mixed with other medications in the nebuliser
- ensure that patient knows that Tobi Podhaler capsules are for use in the Podhaler only and should not be taken orally
- ensure patient has instructions on correct use of Podhaler, including:
  - remove Podhaler from case holding base and twisting top off case (counter-clockwise direction)
  - holding body of inhaler, unscrew and remove mouthpiece (set mouthpiece aside)
  - peel back foil from capsule card to reveal capsule and remove
  - insert capsule into inhaler chamber and replace mouthpiece, screwing on firmly until it stops (but don't over-tighten)
  - to puncture capsule, hold inhaler with mouthpiece down, press button firmly with thumb (as far as it goes) and release
  - exhale fully, and place inhaler mouth over mouthpiece to make tight seal
  - inhale fully with a single continuous inhalation
  - remove inhaler and hold breath for about 5 seconds, then exhale normally after a few normal breaths, perform second inhalation from same capsule
  - unscrew mouthpiece, remove capsule and inspect used capsule to ensure it is punctured and empty
  - if capsule is punctured but is not empty, replace in chamber (with punctured side inserted first), replace mouthpiece and take 2 more inhalations, then reinspect capsule
  - if capsule is unpunctured, place back in chamber, replace mouthpiece and press button firmly (as far as it goes) and take 2 more inhalations. If capsule remains full, replace inhaler device and repeat steps 4–10
  - repeat for 3 remaining capsules to administer full dose
  - replace mouthpiece and screw it firmly until it stops
  - when 4 capsules have been administered, wipe mouthpiece with a clean dry cloth
  - store inhaler in storage case
  - inhaler should not be washed with water
  - Podhaler should be discarded after 7 days and a new Podhaler used for subsequent inhalations
- rinse your mouth after each inhalation to prevent throat irritation

Eye infections
- ensure patient has instructions on correct instillation of eye drops (see p. 1128)
- ensure patient has instructions on correct instillation of eye ointment, including:
  - check expiry date
  - wash hands thoroughly before applying eye ointment
  - tilt head back gently and gently pull lower eyelid down
  - squeeze 1.5 cm of eye ointment inside lower eyelid (however, not allowing tip of tube to touch eye, eyelid or lashes)
  - release eyelid slowly and close eyes gently for 1–2 minutes or blink a few times to help spread the ointment over the eye

- blot any excessive ointment from around the eye with a tissue
- wash hands thoroughly after finishing applying eye ointment

Tobramycin is primarily cleared by the kidneys through glomerular filtration. Renal impairment can significantly reduce its clearance, leading to drug accumulation and increased risk of nephrotoxicity and ototoxicity.

TETRACYCLINES

General Actions of tetracyclines
- interfere with bacterial protein synthesis by blocking 30S ribosomal subunit
- bacteriostatic
- broad spectrum
- bind strongly to calcium ions and concentrate in developing teeth and bone
- not the drug of choice in staphylococcal infections
- oral tetracyclines are well absorbed and distributed in most body fluids

General Uses of tetracyclines
- infections due to susceptible strains of *E. coli*, *Enterobacter* spp., *H. influenzae*, *Klebsiella* spp., *Proteus* spp., *S. pyogenes*, *S. faecalis*

General Adverse effects of tetracyclines
- anorexia, dysphagia, nausea, vomiting, dyspepsia, diarrhoea, abdominal pain, glossitis, black hairy tongue, inflammatory lesions of the anogenital region
- photosensitivity
- (Rare) oesophagitis, oesophageal ulceration
- dizziness, headache, tinnitus, vertigo, lightheadedness, asthenia
- increase in serum urea, elevated liver enzymes
- tooth and nail discolouration (if given during pregnancy or to children under 8 years), tooth discolouration in adults
- urticaria, rash
- benign intracranial hypertension (pseudotumour cerebri) (symptoms include headache and blurred vision), bulging fontanelles in infants
- enterocolitis, pseudomembranous colitis, superinfection
- (Prolonged therapy) microscopic discolouration (black/brown) of thyroid gland (but thyroid function not affected)
- (Rare) blood dyscrasias, acute renal failure, aggravated pre-existing kidney failure
- (Rare) cholestatic hepatitis, fatty liver degeneration, severe skin reactions, hypersensitivity
- (IV) phlebitis

General Interactions of tetracyclines
- contraindicated with methoxyflurane because it increases the risk of fatal renal toxicity
- increased intracranial pressure (benign) may occur if given with oral retinoids (acitretin, isotretinoin) or vitamin A and is therefore contraindicated
- absorption may be reduced by milk, food, sodium bicarbonate, colestipol, colestyramine, oral iron, calcium, magnesium and aluminium salts (and any supplements or antacids containing these), sucralfate
- may reduce the activity of penicillins; therefore should not be given together
- may affect the stability of oral anticoagulant control; therefore prothrombin time should be closely monitored, especially when starting and stopping therapy
- may cause failure of oral oestrogen-containing contraceptives
- increased risk of pseudomembranous colitis if given with agents that delay peristalsis, such as opioid analgesics and diphenoxylate/atropine combination
- anti-anabolic action and increased serum urea levels may occur if given with diuretics
- may give false positive result on urinary catecholamine assay

ANTIBACTERIAL AGENTS

General Nursing considerations/Cautions for tetracyclines

- therapy should be continued for 24—48 hours after fever and symptoms have resolved. If treating group A beta haemolytic streptococcal infection, therapy should continue for 10 days
- if patient has prolonged therapy with tetracyclines, blood counts and renal and liver function should be monitored regularly
- all patients with gonorrhoea should also have serological testing for syphilis at time of diagnosis and monthly for at least 4 months
- see manufacturer's instructions for information about reconstituting solutions and stability
- avoid using out-of-date or deteriorated tetracyclines because degraded products cause reversible Fanconi's syndrome
- not recommended in those with renal impairment (except doxycycline)
- contraindicated in those with known hypersensitivity to tetracyclines, severe renal impairment or SLE
- see also General Nursing considerations/Cautions for antibacterial agents (p. 149)

General Patient education for tetracyclines

- warn patient to avoid sunlamps or sunbeds or direct exposure to sunlight and if this cannot be avoided, they should wear protective clothing and sunscreen with high sun protection factor (SPF 30+) owing to increased risk of photosensitivity. Reaction may be immediate or up to 3 days after sun exposure
- instruct patient not to take oral preparations while lying down (especially doxycycline). Tablets/capsules should be taken with at least 100 mL of fluid and the patient advised to remain upright for 30 minutes after ingestion to reduce risk of oesophageal ulceration
- patient should be advised to seek medical advice immediately if any of the following occur:
  - headache with any of the following: nausea, vomiting, dizziness and/or blurred vision
  - severe sunburn (redness, itching, swelling, blistering) occurring more quickly than usual
  - any diarrhoea or colitis (even if the antibacterial agent was ceased some weeks ago)
- warn patient to avoid driving or using heavy machinery if dizziness, headache, tinnitus, visual disturbances or lightheadedness are ongoing problems
- advise patient to separate tetracycline administration from antacids or iron supplements by at least 2 hours to achieve maximum effect
- female patients should be counselled to use barrier method contraception in addition to oral contraceptives during therapy with tetracyclines and for 7 days after completion of course to avoid unwanted pregnancy
- see also General Patient education for antibacterial agents (p. 150)

Not recommended during pregnancy (after 18 weeks), breastfeeding or in the first 8 years of life because tetracyclines accumulate in the growing skeleton and may induce hypoplasia of enamel and permanent discolouration of teeth.

DOXYCYCLINE

Trade names
APX-Doxycycline, Doryx, Doxsig, Doxycycline Sandoz, Doxycycline-WGR, Doxylin, Mayne Pharma Doxycycline

Available forms
Tablets: 50 mg, 100 mg;
Capsules: 50 mg, 100 mg

Action
- long half-life (10—24 hours), which enables once-daily administration

- available in two different salts of the same drug: doxycycline hyclate (water-soluble salt form) and doxycycline monohydrate (less water-soluble salt form)
- doxycycline monohydrate = Doxycycline Sandoz
- doxycycline hyclate = APX-Doxycycline, Doryx, Doxsig, Doxylin, Doxycycline-WGR, Mayne Pharma Doxycycline.
- see also General Actions of tetracyclines (p. 194)

Use
- acne
- rosacea
- chlamydial infection
- non-gonococcal genital infection
- malaria prophylaxis
- treatment of uncomplicated malaria (with quinine)
- see also General Uses of tetracyclines (p. 194)

Dose
- 100 mg orally 12-hourly on the first day, then 100 mg as a single daily dose or 50 mg (or 100 mg for severe infections) 12-hourly **OR**
- (Treatment for louse-borne or scrub typhus) 100–200 mg orally as a single dose **OR**
- (Prevention of scrub typhus) 200 mg orally as single dose **OR**
- (Gonococcal infection) 100 mg orally twice daily for 5–7 days **OR**
- (Syphilis) 150 mg orally twice daily for at least 10 days **OR**
- (Malaria prophylaxis) 100 mg orally daily starting 2 days before entering a malarial area, continued while in the area and 2 weeks after departure **OR**
- (Severe acne) 50 mg orally daily for 12 weeks

Adverse effects
- see General Adverse effects of tetracyclines (p. 194)

Interactions
- plasma levels may be reduced by alcohol, barbiturates, phenytoin, carbamazepine, sodium bicarbonate, sodium lactate and acetazolamide
- increased risk of ergot toxicity if given with ergometrine or methysergide
- see also General Interactions of tetracyclines (p. 194)

Nursing considerations/Cautions
- may cause oesophageal irritation and ulceration. Take a single daily dose in the morning rather than at night
- give with a glass of water and ensure the person remains upright for one hour
- food and milk do not markedly affect absorption. May be given with meals and a glass of water or milk to reduce gastric irritation
- (Malaria prophylaxis) maximum 100 mg daily for 8 weeks is recommended
- not recommended late at night due to increased risk of oesophageal ulceration
- see also General Nursing considerations/Cautions for tetracyclines (p. 195)

Patient education
- instruct patient that tablets/capsules may be given with meals and a glass of water or milk to reduce gastric irritation
- see also General Patient education for tetracyclines (p. 195)

Tablet should be softened in 20 mL water, then crushed and mixed with milk, apple juice, chocolate pudding, yoghurt or apple puree.
Capsules can be opened and contents given with yoghurt or apple puree but pellets must not be chewed.

Use in pregnancy (16 weeks post conception) is contraindicated. After 18 weeks of pregnancy, doxycycline can cause discolouration of the developing baby's teeth.

Doxycycline should not be used in breast-feeding women; however, with specialist advice, a single 7–10-day course of doxycycline may be considered safe during breastfeeding. Prolonged use is contraindicated as it may harm the breastfeeding baby.

ANTIBACTERIAL AGENTS

Doxycycline should generally be handled with caution by health professionals who are pregnant. While handling intact tablets or capsules is typically considered low risk, crushing or splitting the tablets can release powder that could be inhaled or absorbed through the skin, potentially posing a risk to the developing fetus.

MINOCYCLINE
Trade names
Akamin, Minomycin

Available form
Tablets: 50 mg

Action
- semisynthetic derivative of tetracycline
- active against *Staphylococcus aureus* organisms
- half-life about 13 hours
- see also General Actions of tetracyclines (p. 194)

Use
- may be used for tetracycline-resistant acne
- see also General Uses of tetracyclines (p. 194)

Dose
- initially 200 mg orally, then 100 mg 12-hourly (continued for 24—48 hours after fever and symptoms have resolved) **OR**
- (Tetracycline-resistant acne) 50 mg orally twice daily (for up to 12 weeks)

Adverse effects
- blue-black cutaneous and mucous membrane hyperpigmentation (especially with prolonged use)
- decreased hearing
- (Rare) hepatoxicity
- see also General Adverse effects of tetracyclines (p. 194)

Interactions
- caution if used with hepatotoxic agents
- see also General Interactions of tetracyclines (p. 194)

Nursing considerations/Cautions
- food and milk do not influence absorption so may be taken at any time
- acne usually resolves in 12 weeks
- caution if used in those with acne vulgaris, rheumatoid arthritis, pemphigus or pemphigoid as risk of blue-black hyperpigmentation is increased
- caution if used in those with liver dysfunction
- see also General Nursing considerations/Cautions for tetracyclines (p. 195)

Patient education
- advise patient that blue-black discolouration usually resolves when minocycline is stopped; however, it may take months to years to resolve completely
- see also Patient education for tetracyclines (p. 195)

Tablet can be crushed and mixed with water or spoonful of yoghurt or apple puree. Follow the dose with a glass of water or thickened fluid to help ensure the dose is swallowed completely and to prevent any irritation to the throat or oesophagus.

Use in pregnancy (16 weeks post-conception) is contraindicated. After 18 weeks of pregnancy, doxycycline can cause discolouration of the developing baby's teeth.

Should not be used in breastfeeding women; however, with specialist advice, a single 7—10 day course of doxycycline may be considered safe during breastfeeding. Prolonged use is contraindicated as it may harm the breastfeeding baby.

Although it can generally be used without dose adjustment in mild-to-moderate renal impairment, the manufacturer contraindicates its use in patients with severe renal impairment because of the risk of accumulation and potential toxicity.

> Hepatotoxicity is more likely to occur in patients with hepatic impairment, particularly with higher doses. Avoid high doses.

> Should generally be handled with caution by health professionals who are pregnant. While handling intact tablets is typically considered low risk, crushing or splitting the tablets can release powder that could be inhaled or absorbed through the skin, potentially posing a risk to the developing fetus.

TIGECYCLINE

Trade names
Tygecycline Juno, Tygacil

Available form
Vial: 50 mg

Action
- glycylcycline tetracycline structurally related to minocycline but with expanded spectrum of activity against tetracycline-resistant organisms (e.g. penicillin-resistant *Streptococcus pneumonieae,* methicillin-resistant *Staphylococcus aureus* (MRSA), methicillin-resistant *Staphylococcus epidermidis* (MRSE), vancomycin-resistant *Enterococcus* (VRE))
- some resistance documented
- see also General Actions of tetracyclines (p. 194)

Use
- see General Uses of tetracyclines (p. 194)

Dose
- initially 100 mg by IV infusion over 30—60 minutes, then 50 mg 12-hourly for 5—14 days

Adverse effects
- (IV site) phlebitis, pain, inflammation, swelling
- increased bilirubin, hypoproteinaemia
- (Uncommon) pancreatitis
- see also General Adverse effects of tetracyclines (p. 194)

Interactions
- see General Interactions of tetracyclines (p. 194)

Nursing considerations/Cautions
- bolus IV administration is not recommended
- reconstitute using 5.3 mL of sodium chloride 0.9% or glucose 5%, swirl gently to dissolve powder, further dilute according to manufacturer's instructions and administer over 30—60 minutes
- reconstituted solution should be yellow to orange. If this does not occur, solution should be discarded
- administer alone
- incompatible with amphotericin B (amphotericin), chlorpromazine, diazepam, esomeprazole, methylprednisolone, omeprazole and voriconazole
- caution if used to treat complicated intra-abdominal infections secondary to intestinal perforation
- caution if used in those with liver impairment
- not recommended for hospital- or community-acquired pneumonia or diabetic foot infections
- see also Nursing considerations/Cautions for tetracyclines (p. 195)

Patient education
- advise patient to seek medical advice immediately if any signs of pancreatitis occur including nausea, vomiting, tender abdomen, abdominal pain that radiates to the back, upper abdominal pain, abdominal pain that is worse after eating, or rapid pulse and fever
- see also General Patient education for tetracyclines (p. 195)

> Avoid. No human data. Animal studies indicate risks, including bone discoloration in rats, increased fetal loss in rabbits, and decreased fetal weight and delayed bone ossification in both species.

> Avoid. Excretion in human breastmilk unknown.

ANTIBACTERIAL AGENTS

Reduced hepatic function: no dosage adjustment is necessary for mild-to-moderate hepatic impairment (Child Pugh A and B). In patients with severe hepatic impairment (Child Pugh C), reduce the dose to 100 mg initially, followed by 25 mg every 12 hours. Patients with severe hepatic impairment should be monitored closely for treatment response.

MACROLIDES

General Actions of macrolides
- contain a common macrocyclic lactone ring with attached sugars
- bind to bacterial ribosomal subunit 50S, inhibiting RNA-dependent protein synthesis
- bacteriostatic
- bactericidal in high levels (selected organisms)
- wide spectrum of action against Gram-positive and Gram-negative aerobic organisms and some anaerobes
- most strains of methicillin-resistant *Staphylococcus aureus* (MRSA), Enterobacteriaceae, and *Pseudomonas* and *Acinetobacter* spp. show resistance to macrolides, and *Streptococcus pneumoniae* is showing increasing resistance
- cross-resistance may exist between clarithromycin, erythromycin and other macrolides, as well as lincomycin and clindamycin

General Uses of macrolides
- community-acquired pneumonia, upper and lower respiratory tract infections (including Legionnaire's disease and pharyngitis)
- uncomplicated skin or skin structure infections
- disseminated or localised mycobacterial infection (including prevention of *Mycobacterium avium* complex (MAC) infections in HIV-infected adults with other antimycobacterial agents)
- sinusitis, otitis media
- diphtheria (adjunct to antitoxin)
- non-gonococcal urethritis
- chlamydial infections, gonorrhoea, syphilis, acute pelvic inflammation (due to *Neisseria gonorrhoeae*)
- prophylaxis of SBE in penicillin-resistant patients
- combination therapy for peptic ulcer treatment associated with *Helicobacter pylori* infection

General Adverse effects of macrolides
- decreased appetite, nausea, vomiting, diarrhoea, abdominal pain, dyspepsia, constipation
- dizziness, headache, asthenia
- fever
- rash, pruritus, urticaria
- reversible hearing loss (high dose, prolonged therapy)
- dyspnoea
- altered liver enzymes, cholestatic jaundice, hepatic dysfunction
- pseudomembranous colitis, superinfection
- (Uncommon) taste alteration, flatulence, depression, flushing, increased prothrombin time, photophobia
- (Rare) hypersensitivity, angioedema, anaphylaxis, photosensitivity, tongue discolouration, severe skin reactions
- (Rare) cardiac arrhythmia, prolongation of QT interval, palpitations, chest pain
- (Rapid IV) arrhythmias, hypotension
- (IV site) pain, inflammation

General Interactions of macrolides
- contraindicated with statins (HMG-CoA reductase inhibitors) owing to risk of myopathy and/or rhabdomyolysis
- may cause peripheral vasospasm and dysaesthesia (ergot toxicity) if given with ergot alkaloids such as ergotamine or dihydroergotamine; therefore contraindicated with these agents
- caution if given with agents known to prolong QT interval such as class IA and

III antiarrhythmic agents, antipsychotics, antidepressants, antifungals, fluoroquinolones or agents that cause electrolyte disturbance (e.g. diuretics) especially hypokalaemia and hypomagnesaemia
- may enhance effects of alprazolam and midazolam, causing increased and prolonged sedation, so should be used with caution (and avoid altogether with erythromycin)
- may increase serum digoxin levels increasing the risk of toxicity; therefore digoxin serum levels should be monitored carefully during therapy
- increased risk of neurotoxicity if given with carbamazepine (not azithromycin)
- caution if given with agents that delay peristalsis, such as opioid analgesics or diphenoxylate/atropine combination, because of the increased risk of antibiotic-associated pseudomembranous colitis
- may increase serum levels of phosphodiesterase inhibitors (sildenafil, tadalafil), increasing risk of adverse effects and toxicity
- may increase serum levels of alprazolam, carbamazepine, cilostazol, ciclosporin, disopyramide, ibrutinib, midazolam, methylprednisolone, phenytoin, quetiapine, rifabutin, sildenafil, sodium valproate, tacrolimus, tadalafil, theophylline, triazolam, vinblastine and warfarin, thereby increasing the risk of toxicity; serum levels should be closely monitored during therapy
- effects may be increased by protease inhibitors such as ritonavir
- increased risk of nephrotoxicity and/or neurotoxicity if given with ciclosporin or tacrolimus
- may increase the anticoagulant effects of warfarin, therefore INR should be closely monitored, especially when starting or stopping therapy

General Nursing considerations/Cautions for macrolides

- any electrolyte imbalance (especially hypokalaemia or hypomagnesaemia) should be corrected before starting therapy
- sensitivity checking is recommended for community-acquired pneumonia or moderate-to-severe skin and soft tissue infections owing to emerging resistance to macrolides
- 5–10 days of treatment for streptococcal throat infection or 20 days for non-gonococcal genital infections
- caution if used in those with myasthenia gravis, as disease exacerbation may occur
- caution or not recommended in those with predisposition to prolongation of the QT interval, bradycardia, cardiac arrhythmias or cardiac insufficiency
- caution if used in those with severe liver impairment
- contraindicated in those with known hypersensitivity to other macrolides
- see also General Nursing considerations/Cautions for antibacterial agents (p. 149)

General Patient education for macrolides

- patient should be advised to avoid driving or operating machinery if dizziness occurs
- warn patient to seek medical advice immediately if any of the following occur:
    - unexplained muscle pain or weakness
    - hearing difficulties
    - severe skin reactions, including blistering and peeling
    - yellowing of skin or eyes, loss of appetite, nausea, upper abdominal pain, itchy skin, dark urine, pale stools (even if these occur weeks after stopping therapy)
    - rapid or irregular heart beat
- see also General Patient education for antibacterial agents (p. 150)

 Macrolides can be considered during pregnancy, but should be used only if the

> benefits outweigh the potential risks and no safer alternative is available.
>
> While generally safe for breastfeeding, macrolides should be used cautiously, as they may cause loose stools in the infant. Use only when the benefits outweigh the risks.

AZITHROMYCIN

Trade names
APO-Azithromycin, Azith, Azithromycin-AFT, Azithromycin Medsurge, Azithromycin Mylan, Azithromycin Sandoz, Azithromycin Viatris, Azithromycin-WGR, Zedd, Zithro, Zithromax, Zithromax IV

Available forms
Tablets: 500 mg, 600 mg;
Oral suspension: 200 mg/5 mL;
Vial: 500 mg

Action
- shows cross-resistance with erythromycin-resistant Gram-positive organisms and Gram-negative *P. aeruginosa*
- long half-life (68 hours)
- see also General Actions of macrolides (p. 199)

Use
- see General Uses of macrolides (p. 199)

Dose
- (Chlamydial infections) 1 g orally as single dose 1 hour before or 2 hours after food **OR**
- (Chlamydial infections) 500 mg orally daily 1 hour before or 2 hours after food for 3 days **OR**
- (Other infections) initially 500 mg orally daily (day 1) 1 hour before or 2 hours after food, then 250 mg daily (days 2—5) **OR**
- (Other infections) 500 mg orally daily 1 hour before or 2 hours after food for 3 days **OR**
- (Conjunctivitis due to *Chlamydia trachomatis*) 1 g orally 1 hour before or 2 hours after food as either a single dose or weekly for up to 3 weeks **OR**
- (Prevention of disseminated *Mycobacterium avium* complex (MAC)) 1.2 g orally 1 hour before or 2 hours after food weekly alone or with rifabutin **OR**
- (Community-acquired pneumonia) 500 mg daily as IV infusion over 60 minutes for 2 days, followed by 500 mg orally 1 hour before or 2 hours after food daily (total course 7—10 days)

Adverse effects
- see General Adverse effects of macrolides (p. 199)

Interactions
- should not be given with magnesium or aluminium-containing antacids
- see also General Interactions of macrolides (p. 199)

Nursing considerations/Cautions
- because of long half-life, allergic symptoms may continue after therapy has been ceased
- should not be given IM or as an IV bolus
- IV infusion rate should not exceed 2 mg/mL (administered over 1 hour) to avoid local site reactions
- reconstitute using 4.8 mL water for injections, then dilute further and infuse over 60 minutes
- administer alone IV
- (Suspension) contains 3.87 g sucrose/5 mL and is therefore not recommended in those with fructose intolerance, glucose—galactose malabsorption or sucrase—isomaltase deficiency and should be used with caution in those with diabetes
- see also General Nursing considerations/Cautions for macrolides (p. 200)

Patient education
- see General Patient education for macrolides (p. 200)
- advise patient to separate tablet or oral suspension by at least 2 hours from magnesium- or aluminium-containing antacids

- instruct patient that tablets should be taken 1 hour before or 2 hours after meals but oral suspension can be taken with meals
- advise patient to discard suspension 10 days after opening
- if patient taking suspension has diabetes mellitus, they should be warned of the sucrose content

Tablet can be crushed and mixed with water or spoonful of yoghurt or apple puree. Syrup/suspension is available.

Generally considered safe to use during pregnancy if it is the treatment of choice. Animal studies have not demonstrated a risk to the fetus, and there are no adequate studies in pregnant women, but it is commonly used when necessary.

Generally considered safe to use while breastfeeding, but it may cause loose bowel movements in the nursing infant, which is a common and typically mild side effect. Use when the benefit outweighs the risk.

Undergoes hepatic metabolism and is excreted mainly via bile into the faeces. Only a small proportion (about 6—12%) is excreted unchanged in the urine. Therefore, it does not usually require dose adjustment in patients with impaired renal function, but caution is advised, and dose reduction may be needed in those with severe hepatic impairment.

CLARITHROMYCIN

Trade names
Clarithro, Clarithromycin Sandoz, Kalixocin, Klacid, Noumed Clarithromycin

Available forms
Tablets: 250 mg, 500 mg;
Oral suspension: 250 mg/5 mL

Action
- not active against *Pseudomonas* spp., Enterobacteriaceae or *Mycobacterium tuberculosis*
- more potent than erythromycin against atypical mycobacteria
- metabolite has antibacterial properties
- half-life about 7 hours
- see also General Actions of macrolides (p. 199)

Use
- see General Uses of macrolides (p. 199)

Dose
- (Non-mycobacterial infections) 250—500 mg orally twice daily for 7—14 days **OR**
- (Legionnaire's disease) 500 mg orally twice daily for 4 weeks **OR**
- (Treatment of mycobacterial infection) 500 mg orally twice daily **OR**
- (Prophylaxis of mycobacterial infection (MAC) in HIV-infected adults) 500 mg orally twice daily **OR**
- (*Helicobacter pylori* eradication) 500 mg orally twice daily for 7—10 days (with amoxicillin 1 g twice daily and omeprazole 20 mg daily)

Adverse effects
- (Immunocompromised patient) rash, dyspnoea, altered taste
- see also General Adverse effects of macrolides (p. 199)

Interactions
- colchicine, domperidone, ergometrine, oral midazolam, simvastatin and ticagrelor are contraindicated when using clarithromycin owing to the risk of serious drug interactions that may lead to increased toxicity or adverse effects
- clarithromycin is a strong inhibitor of CYP3A4, an enzyme responsible for metabolising many drugs. Common examples of medications metabolised by CYP3A4 include some statins (atorvastatin, fluvastatin, simvastatin), antiepileptics like carbamazepine, and anticoagulants such as warfarin and rivaroxaban. It also affects immunosuppressants like ciclosporin and tacrolimus, calcium channel blockers (felodipine, lercanidipine, nifedipine, nimodipine and verapamil) and sildenafil, which are used for erectile dysfunction. Due to these

ANTIBACTERIAL AGENTS

- interactions, clarithromycin can significantly increase the serum levels of these drugs, leading to a higher risk of adverse effects. Therefore, it is important to exercise caution and closely monitor patients when clarithromycin is prescribed alongside CYP3A4 substrates
- not recommended in daily doses > 1 g with HIV protease inhibitors
- simultaneous administration of clarithromycin tablets and zidovudine in patients with HIV infection may lead to decreased absorption of zidovudine
- serum levels may be decreased by carbamazepine, efavirenz, etravirine, nevirapine, phenytoin, phenobarbital (phenobarbitone), St John's wort, tolterodine, rifabutin and rifampicin
- may increase serum levels of rifabutin, tolterodine and colchicine
- increased risk of hypotension, lactic acidosis and bradyarrhythmias if given with verapamil
- if given with itraconazole, serum levels of both agents may be raised, increasing risk of toxicity
- caution if given with calcium-channel blocker because of the risk of acute kidney injury and hypotension
- significant hypoglycaemia may occur if given with insulin and/or oral hypoglycaemic agents
- caution if used with ototoxic agents such as aminoglycosides. Vestibular and auditory function should be monitored during and after therapy if given together
- see also General Interactions of macrolides (p. 199)

Nursing considerations/Cautions

- (MAC prophylaxis) some authorities recommend delaying therapy until CD4 cell count < 50 cells/mm
- (Suspension) contains sucrose; therefore not recommended in those with rare hereditary problems of fructose intolerance, glucose—galactose malabsorption or sucrase—isomaltase insufficiency, and should be taken into consideration if patient has diabetes mellitus
- caution if used in those with severe kidney impairment
- see also General Nursing considerations/Cautions for macrolides (p. 200)

Patient education

- this medicine interacts with many drugs. Advise patient to inform their prescriber and pharmacist that they are taking this medicine before starting or stopping any other medications, including herbal remedies and over-the-counter products
- advise patient that oral doses of clarithromycin should be separated from zidovudine by at least 2 hours to prevent decreased absorption of zidovudine
- if patient taking suspension has diabetes mellitus, they should be advised to monitor blood glucose levels owing to sucrose levels
- see also General Patient education for macrolides (p. 200)

 Syrup/suspension is available. Tablet can be dispersed in 20 mL water or crushed and mixed with spoonful of yoghurt or apple puree.

 Considered safe to use during pregnancy if it is the treatment of choice.

 Safe to use; however, it may cause loose bowel movements in the infant. Use when the benefit outweighs the risk.

 Approximately 20—30% of clarithromycin is excreted unchanged via the kidneys. Because of this renal clearance, dose adjustments are recommended in patients with significant renal impairment, particularly when creatinine clearance is less than 30 mL/min.

Available in combination with

- contained in combination pack for eradication of *H. pylori*
  - clarithromycin 500 mg tablet + esomeprazole 20 mg enteric tablet +

amoxicillin 500 mg capsule (Esomeprazole Sandoz Hp7, Nexium Hp7)

ERYTHROMYCIN ETHYL SUCCINATE
Trade names
EMycin Mayne Pharma Erythromycin

ERYTHOMYCIN LACTOBIONATE
Trade names
Erythrocin IV Erythromycin SKX

Available forms
Tablets: 400 mg;
Capsules: 250 mg;
Oral suspension: 200 mg/5 mL, 400 mg/5 mL;
Vial: 1 g

Action/Use
- not active against strains of *Haemophilus influenzae* and staphylococci
- half-life 1.4 hours (prolonged in anuric patient to 6 hours)
- see also General Actions and General Uses of macrolides (p. 199)

Dose
- 250—400 mg orally 6-hourly 1 hour before meals, or 500—800 mg 12-hourly 1 hour before meals (daily maximum 4 g) **OR**
- (Severe infections) 15—20 mg/kg/day IV in divided doses (up to 4 g/day) **OR**
- (Legionnaire's disease) 0.8—1.6 g orally 6-hourly 1 hour before meals for 14 days **OR**
- (Legionnaire's disease) 1—4 g IV daily in divided doses **OR**
- (Chlamydial or mycoplasma infection) 500 mg orally 8-hourly 1 hour before meals for 10 days, 800 mg orally 6-hourly for 7 days, or 400 mg 6-hourly for 14 days **OR**
- (Primary syphilis) total dose of 30—64 g orally given over 10—15 days in divided doses 1 hour before meals **OR**
- (Streptococcal prophylaxis) 250—400 mg orally 1 hour before meals twice daily for 10 days **OR**
- (Prophylaxis — endocarditis prophylaxis) 1—1.6 g orally 90 minutes—2 hours before dental or surgical procedure, then 500—800 mg 6-hourly 1 hour before meals for 6—8 doses **OR**
- (Acute pelvic inflammatory disease) 500 mg IV 6-hourly for 3 days, then 250—400 mg orally 6-hourly 1 hour before meals for 7 days **OR**
- (Acne vulgaris) 250—400 mg orally 1 hour before meals 4 times daily for 2 weeks, continued for 3 months, adjusting dose 4—6-weekly as necessary

Adverse effects
- visual impairment
- (Rare) infantile hypertrophic pyloric stenosis
- see also General Adverse effects of macrolides (p. 199)

Interactions
- may decrease the clearance of zopiclone, increasing its sedative/hypnotic effects
- may antagonise the effects of clindamycin, lincomycin, chloramphenicol, streptomycin, tetracyclines, colistin, penicillins and cephalosporins
- may interfere with urinary catecholamine determination
- see also General Interactions of macrolides (p. 199)

Nursing considerations/Cautions
- transfer from IV route to oral as soon as possible
- (IV) reconstitute with 20 mL water for injections only, then dilute further with sodium chloride 0.9% or lactated Ringer's solution for IV administration at a rate of 1—5 mg/mL over 60 minutes
- administer alone
- should not be given as IV bolus to prevent high serum levels and risk of QT prolongation
- see also General Nursing considerations/Cautions for macrolides (p. 200)

Patient education
- instruct patient that most oral preparations are taken 1 hour before or 2 hours after food to improve absorption;

ANTIBACTERIAL AGENTS

however, some preparations can be given before or with food, so pharmacist should be consulted
- instruct patient to seek medical advice immediately if any changes to vision occur
- (Suspension) instruct patient to discard suspension 10 days after opening
- see also General Patient education for macrolides (p. 200)

 Syrup/suspension is available. Tablet can be crushed, or capsule opened and mixed with water or spoonful of yoghurt or apple puree; however, contents of capsule must not be chewed.

 Safe. However, observational studies have reported cardiovascular malformations in infants exposed to erythromycin during early pregnancy. Erythromycin crosses the placenta but with generally low fetal levels. Use erythromycin during pregnancy only if necessary.

 Caution. Concentrated in breastmilk, and adverse effects such as gastrointestinal disturbances, pyloric stenosis or sensitisation can occur in breastfed infants.

 Reduced renal function: Erythromycin clearance is reduced in severe renal impairment, potentially requiring dose adjustment. Half-life may increase to 6 hours in anuric patients. No adjustment is needed for mild to moderate impairment.

Reduced hepatic function: Caution. Primarily excreted by the liver. Contraindicated in severe hepatic impairment owing to risk of hepatitis, jaundice and abnormal liver function.

 Elderly patients may be more susceptible to drug-associated effects on the QT interval. Erythromycin should be used with caution in elderly patients with pre-existing cardiac conditions, coronary artery disease, or electrolyte imbalances, as they may be at increased risk of QT prolongation and arrhythmias.

ROXITHROMYCIN

Trade names
APX-Roxithromycin, Roxithromycin-WGR, Roxar, Roxithromycin Sandoz

Available forms
Tablets: 150 mg, 300 mg;
Tablets (for suspension): 50 mg

Action
- shows activity against *Haemophilus influenzae* and *Staphylococcus aureus* (not methicillin resistant)
- long half-life (12 hours) (prolonged in the elderly or those with liver or kidney impairment)
- see also General Actions of macrolides (p. 199)

Use
- see General Uses of macrolides (p. 199)

Dose
- 300 mg orally daily 1 hour before or 3 hours after food for 5–10 days **OR**
- (Atypical pneumonia) 150 mg orally twice daily 1 hour before or 3 hours after food for 5–10 days

Adverse effects
- see General Adverse effects of macrolides (p. 199)

Interactions
- may increase serum levels of disopyramide; therefore ECG monitoring is recommended
- see also General Interactions of macrolides (p. 199)

Nursing considerations/Cautions
- contraindicated in those with severe liver impairment
- see also General Nursing considerations/Cautions for macrolides (p. 200)

Patient education
- advise patient that tablets should be swallowed whole with fluid

- see also General Patient education for macrolides (p. 200)

Tablets can be crushed and mixed with spoonful of yoghurt or apple puree. Crushing roxithromycin tablets can alter the drug's absorption, potentially leading to higher serum concentrations compared with taking whole tablets. This can increase the risk of adverse effects owing to faster or greater absorption of the drug.

Considered safe to use during pregnancy if it is the treatment of choice.

Safe to use; however, it may cause loose bowel movements in the infant. Use when the benefit outweighs the risk.

Roxithromycin is primarily cleared through the liver. It undergoes hepatic metabolism and is excreted mainly in the bile and faeces. A smaller portion is excreted unchanged in the urine. Because of its hepatic clearance, dose adjustments are generally not needed in patients with renal impairment but may be necessary in those with significant liver impairment.

LINCOSAMIDES

General Actions of lincosamides
- bind to bacterial ribosomal subunit 50S, inhibiting protein synthesis
- bacteriostatic but bactericidal at high doses with selected organisms

General Uses of lincosamides
- serious infections caused by streptococci, staphylococci, pneumococci and anaerobic bacteria, including infections of the bone and joints, pelvis, intra-abdominal area, skin and soft tissue, pneumonia, septicaemia
- reserved for infections where penicillin is inappropriate

General Adverse effects of lincosamides
- nausea, vomiting, diarrhoea, abdominal discomfort
- rash, urticaria, pruritus
- abnormal liver function
- eosinophilia
- pseudomembranous colitis
- superinfection
- (Rare) anaphylactoid reaction, thrombocytopenia, agranulocytosis, polyarthritis, jaundice, severe skin reactions
- (Rapid IV administration) cardiac arrest, hypotension
- (IM site) pain, sterile abscess, induration, irritation
- (IV site) thrombophlebitis

General Interactions of lincosamides
- may enhance the action of neuromuscular blocking agents and therefore should not be given together
- use with erythromycin or chloramphenicol is not recommended
- increased risk of pseudomembranous colitis if given with peristalsis-delaying agents such as opioid analgesics and diphenoxylate/atropine combination

General Nursing considerations/Cautions for lincosamides
- cross-resistance exists between clindamycin, erythromycin and lincomycin; therefore a careful history is taken on admission to ascertain any previous allergic reactions
- blood counts, kidney and liver function should be monitored during prolonged therapy
- not to be given as an IV bolus because hypotension and cardiac arrest may occur
- not recommended for treatment of meningitis or non-bacterial infections
- caution if used in those with GI diseases (especially colitis, ulcerative colitis or regional enteritis) or severe kidney or liver impairment
- contraindicated in those with known hypersensitivity to lincomycin or clindamycin
- see also General Nursing considerations/Cautions for antibacterial agents (p. 150)

General Patient education for lincosamides

- warn patient to seek medical advice immediately if any of the following occur:
  - unusual tiredness or weakness, bleeding or bruising easily
  - joint pains
  - severe skin reactions, including blistering and peeling
  - yellowing of skin or eyes, loss of appetite, nausea, upper abdominal pain, itchy skin, dark urine, pale stools (even if these occur weeks after stopping therapy)
- see also General Patient education for antibacterial agents (p. 150)

 Considered safe in pregnancy when the benefits outweighs the risks.

 Generally considered safe to use during breastfeeding, but may cause loose stools or gastrointestinal disturbances in the infant. Monitor the infant for adverse effects. Use only when benefit outweighs the risk.

 Dose adjustments may be needed in renal and hepatic impairment.

CLINDAMYCIN HYDROCHLORIDE
Trade names
APO-Clindamycin, Calindamin, Clindamycin Lu, Clindamycin-WGR, Clindamyk, ClindaTech, Dalacin C Capsules

CLINDAMYCIN PHOSPHATE
Trade names
Clindamycin Viatris, Dalacin C Phosphate Injection, Dalacin T Topical Lotion, Dalacin V Cream 2%

Available forms
Ampoules: 300 mg/2 mL, 600 mg/4 mL;
Capsules: 150 mg;
Topical solution: 10 mg/mL (1%);
Vaginal cream: 20 mg/1 g (2%)

Action
- semisynthetic derivative of lincomycin; therefore some cross-resistance between clindamycin and lincomycin but more effective
- clindamycin phosphate is hydrolysed in the skin to active clindamycin
- resistance to *Propionibacterium acnes* has emerged
- half-life 2–3 hours
- see also General Actions of lincosamides (p. 206)

Use
- acne vulgaris (where comedomes, papules and pustules predominate)
- bacterial vaginosis
- see also General Uses of lincosamides (p. 206)

Dose
- 150–450 mg orally 6-hourly **OR**
- (Serious or complicated infections, intra-abdominal or female pelvic infection) 1.2–2.7 g IM in 2, 3 or 4 equally divided daily doses **OR**
- (Serious or complicated infections, intra-abdominal or female pelvic infection) 1.2–2.7 g in 2, 3 or 4 equally divided daily doses infused IV at a rate not exceeding 30 mg/min (over 10–60 minutes) **OR**
- (Uncomplicated infections) 600–1200 mg IM or IV in 3–4 equally divided daily doses
- (Bacterial vaginosis) 1 applicator-full (5 g) intravaginally nightly for 7 consecutive days **OR**
- (Acne) apply thin film (using applicator if supplied) 1–2 times daily

Adverse effects
- (Topical lotion) irritation, dry skin, peeling, pruritus, erythema, warm sensation, burning, dermatitis, diarrhoea
- (Vaginal cream) irritation, itching, discharge
- eye irritation
- see also General Adverse effects of lincosamides (p. 206)

Interactions
- decreased serum levels may occur if given with rifampicin
- see also General Interactions of lincosamides (p. 207)

Nursing considerations/Cautions
- for beta-haemolytic streptococcal infections, treatment can be continued for 10 days minimum
- not more than 600 mg is given at a single IM site or not more than 1.2 g in a single 1-hour infusion
- (IV) should be diluted to concentration not greater than 12 mg/mL and infused at a rate not exceeding 30 mg/min
- (Acne) therapy should be reviewed after 6–8 weeks for effectiveness
- (IV) incompatible with ampicillin, clindamycin, phenytoin, barbiturates, aminophylline, calcium gluconate, magnesium sulfate, ceftriaxone and ciprofloxacin
- caution if used in atopic individuals
- (Topical) not recommended with other topical anti-acne preparations or topical preparations containing alcohol
- not recommended for meningitis as it does not diffuse adequately into CSF
- not recommended for severe and deep nodulocystic acne
- see also General Nursing considerations/Cautions for lincosamides (p. 206)

Patient education
- capsules should be given with a full glass of water to prevent oesophageal ulceration
- (Acne) patient should be given the following instructions:
  - avoid contact with eyes, eyelids, mucous membranes, nasal folds or abraded skin or near mouth owing to unpleasant taste
  - wash face with warm water and pH neutral soap, rinse and pat dry, ensuring all cosmetics are removed. Shave if necessary
  - after washing and shaving, wait 15 minutes before applying lotion
  - shake bottle well before use
  - apply lotion to face (using applicator if provided)
  - do not use lotion more than 1–2 times daily (as per instructions). Greater use does not improve outcome and causes skin drying
  - wash hands well after application
  - acne may initially worsen when starting treatment and take 8–12 weeks before full improvement is seen. Advise patient to seek medical advice if there is no improvement in 6 weeks
- patient should be instructed in the correct technique for insertion of intravaginal cream, including:
  - wash hands before and after application
  - remove cap from cream and screw applicator to tube; squeeze cream from base of tube to force cream into applicator
  - choose comfortable position for insertion, remembering that cream should be inserted as high as possible into vagina
  - part lips of vagina with finger of one hand and grasp applicator between thumb and middle finger of other hand. Insert (open end first) into vagina as deeply as possible
  - slowly push plunger in until it stops and then carefully withdraw applicator
  - use new applicator (disposable) for each dose
- (Vaginal cream) counsel patient not to use condom or vaginal contraceptive device with or within 72 hours of finishing therapy because cream may weaken latex or rubber
- (Vaginosis) advise patient to avoid vaginal intercourse or use vaginal products (such as tampons) during therapy
- see also General Patient education for lincosamides (p. 207)

Available in combination with
- clindamycin 1% + benzoyl peroxide (5%) (Duac Once Daily Gel)
- clindamycin 1% + tretinoin 0.025% (Acnatac)

LINCOMYCIN
Trade names
Lincocin, Lincomycin SXP

Available form
Ampoules: 300 mg/mL

Action
- not active against most strains of *Enterococcus faecalis, Neisseria gonorrhoeae, N. meningitides, Haemophilus influenza* or other Gram-negative organisms
- half-life 4.4–6.4 hours
- see also General Actions of lincosamides (p. 206)

Use
- see General Uses of lincosamides (p. 206)

Dose
- 600 mg IM daily (or 12-hourly for more serious infections) **OR**
- 600 mg–1 g by IV infusion over at least 1 hour 8–12-hourly

Adverse effects/Interactions/Nursing considerations/Cautions/Patient education
- maximum recommended daily dose 8 g
- for beta haemolytic streptococcal infections, therapy should be continued for at least 10 days to decrease risk of subsequent rheumatic fever or glomerulonephritis
- (IV) diluted with 100–400 mL or more of glucose 5% or sodium chloride 0.9% and infuse over 1–4 hours (depending on dose)
- incompatible with erythromycin and phenytoin
- contains benzyl alcohol; therefore contraindicated in newborns
- see also General Adverse effects/Interaction/Nursing considerations/Cautions/Patient education for lincosamides (p. 206)

OTHER MISCELLANEOUS INHIBITORS OF BACTERIAL PROTEIN SYNTHESIS

CHLORAMPHENICOL
Trade names
Cholfen APOHealth Chloramphenicol Eye Drops,Chemists' Own Clorah Eye Drops, Chloromycetin Succinate, Chlorsig, Minims Chloramphenicol 0.5% Eye Drops

Available forms
Vial: 1 g;
Eye drops: 0.5%;
Eye ointment: 1%

Action
- potent inhibitor of protein synthesis by binding to bacterial 50S ribosomal subunit
- bacteriostatic
- broad-spectrum antibacterial and antirickettsial antibiotic
- chloramphenicol succinate is hydrolysed to active chloramphenicol in the liver
- half-life 1.6–3.3 hours
- development of resistance appears to be low

Use
- serious infections (e.g. bacterial meningitis, typhoid fever, rickettsial infections, septicaemia)
- intraocular infections, bacterial conjunctivitis

Dose
- (Serious infections) 50 mg/kg/day IV or IM divided into 6-hourly doses, increasing to 100 mg/kg/day for septicaemia, meningitis or infections due to resistant organisms **OR**
- (Intraocular infections, bacterial conjunctivitis) 1–2 drops to affected eye(s) 2–6-hourly for 2–3 days **OR**
- (Intraocular infections, bacterial conjunctivitis) 1.5 cm ointment to affected eye(s) 3-hourly, or 1.5 cm nightly if used concurrently with drops

Adverse effects
- bone marrow depression, blood dyscrasias, aplastic anaemia
- fever
- delirium, confusion, depression
- nausea, vomiting, glossitis, stomatitis, diarrhoea
- rash, urticaria, angioedema
- peripheral neuritis, optic neuritis
- pseudomembranous colitis, superinfection
- (Eye drops, ointment) redness, itching, swelling, burning sensation, delayed corneal ulcer healing

Interactions
- not recommended during active immunisation
- not recommended with other agents that cause bone marrow depression or aplastic anaemia
- not recommended with agents that delay peristalsis because of the risk of pseudomembranous colitis
- caution if used with erythromycin, lincomycin or clindamycin
- may decrease clearance and prolong duration of action of alfentanil if chloramphenicol is used preoperatively or perioperatively
- may reduce efficacy of oral contraceptive containing oestrogen
- metabolism may be increased by rifampicin and phenobarbital (phenobarbitone)
- may increase serum level of tacrolimus, increasing risk of toxicity

Nursing considerations/Cautions
- blood counts should be measured before starting and regularly throughout therapy
- plasma chloramphenicol levels should be monitored in those with severe kidney impairment or premature/full-term neonates with immature metabolic processes
- (IV) not recommended for prophylaxis
- (IV) to reconstitute, add 2.5–10 mL of water for injections, sodium chloride 0.9% or glucose 5% (see manufacturer's instructions) to vial and swirl gently to dissolve
- (IV) prolonged use may cause haemolytic anaemia in those with glucose-6-phosphate dehydrogenase (G6PD) deficiency and should be used only with great caution
- eye drops should be continued for 2 days after symptoms resolve, but therapy duration should not be longer than 5 days
- caution if used in those with pre-existing haematological disorders
- (Eye preparations) not recommended in those with photophobia, severe eye pain or swelling, decreased or blurred vision, restricted eye movement, cloudy cornea, copious purulent discharge, eye injury (including after recent welding without eye protection), abnormal pupils, eye surgery or laser treatment in last 6 months, glaucoma, dry eyes or suspected foreign body present. Patient should be advised to see doctor or ophthalmologist
- not recommended in neonates because of risk of 'grey baby syndrome' (see Glossary)
- contraindicated if hypersensitivity to chloramphenicol exists

Patient education
- patient should be advised to immediately seek medical advice if any of the following occur:
  - diarrhoea
  - unusual tiredness, weakness, bleeding or bruising more easily than normal
  - eye pain, blurred vision or blind spots
  - numbness, tingling or weakness in the extremities
- instruct patient to discard eye drops and ointment 4 weeks after opening

ANTIBACTERIAL AGENTS

- ensure patient has instructions on correct technique for instilling eye drops (p. 1128 or eye ointment p. 1129)
- (Eye infection) advise patient to seek medical advice immediately if symptoms worsen or if symptoms have not improved in 48 hours, and not to use drops for longer than 5 days
- (Eye infection) if patient wears contact lenses, advise patient to not insert lenses during or for 24 hours after stopping therapy
- female patients of childbearing potential should be warned that oral contraceptives containing oestrogen may lose their efficacy during therapy with chloramphenicol, and another form of contraception should be used to prevent pregnancy
- see also General Patient education for antibacterial agents (p. 50)

(Injection) not recommended in the week before birth because of the risk of 'grey baby syndrome', which includes hypothermia and cyanosis (see Glossary).

(Injection) avoid during breastfeeding, as adverse reactions like vomiting, excessive intestinal gas and drowsiness in breastfed infants have been reported.

SODIUM FUSIDATE
Trade names
Fucidin, Fucidin Topical

Available forms
Tablets: 250 mg;
Topical ointment: 2%

Action
- inhibits protein synthesis by preventing translocation on ribosome
- bactericidal
- no activity against Gram-negative organisms or fungi

Use
- staphylococcal infections, including skin lesions (e.g. boils, impetigo, folliculitis)
- osteomyelitis

Dose
- (Adult) 250–500 mg orally 2–3 times daily for 5–10 days **OR**
- (Child 5–12 years) 250 mg every 8 hours **OR**
- (Osteomyelitis, septic arthritis due to MRSA) (adult) 500 mg orally every 8–12 hours, with oral rifampicin **OR**
- (Skin lesions) apply thin film 2–3 times daily (without dressing) or daily if covered with protective dressing for 7 days

Adverse effects
- nausea, vomiting, dyspepsia, diarrhoea, flatulence, abdominal pain
- headache, lethargy, fatigue, asthenia
- urticaria
- (Uncommon) elevated liver enzymes
- (Topical) mild irritation, burning sensation, rash, urticaria, pruritus, redness
- (Rare) jaundice, hypersensitivity, rash, pruritus, blood dyscrasias, serious skin reactions

Interactions
- contraindicated with or within 7 days of statins (lipid-lowering agents) because of increased risk of rhabdomyolysis, muscle weakness and pain
- caution if given with saquinavir, ritonavir or other HIV protease inhibitors because of risk of hepatoxicity

Nursing considerations/Cautions
- regular liver function tests are recommended for prolonged or high-dose therapy, or in patients with pre-existing liver disease
- caution if used in those with liver impairment or biliary disease/obstruction
- tablets contain lactose; therefore are not recommended in those with rare hereditary problems of galactose intolerance, Lapp lactase deficiency or glucose–galactose malabsorption
- see also General Nursing considerations/Cautions for antibacterial agents (p. 149)

Patient education

- advise patient to take on an empty stomach (1 hour before or 2 hours after food) for best absorption. If it upsets their stomach, they can take it with or shortly after food
- (Topical) warn patient to avoid contact with eyes
- see also General Patient education for antibacterial agents (p. 150)

If the person is unable to swallow the tablet whole, it can be crushed and mixed with water. If the person cannot swallow thin fluids, crush the tablet and mix with a spoonful of yoghurt or apple puree.

No human data. Avoid use particularly in the last month because of theoretical risk of kernicterus.

Secreted in breastmilk;, therefore should be used with great caution during breastfeeding.

Use cautiously in hepatic impairment; dose reduction may be needed.

LINEZOLID

Trade names
Linevox, Zyvox, Linezolid Kabi, Pharmcor Linezolid

Available forms
Infusion solution: 2 mg/mL;
Tablets: 600 mg;
Oral suspension: 20 mg/mL

Action
- oxazolidinone antibacterial which selectively inhibits bacterial protein synthesis by binding to a different ribosomal subunit (proximal to 50S subunit) than other antibacterial agents. Because site of action is different to other antibacterial agents, likelihood of cross-resistance is decreased
- active against Gram-positive aerobic and some anaerobic organisms, and some Gram-negative organisms
- not active against *Haemophilus influenzae*, *Neisseria* spp., Enterobacteriaceae or *Pseudomonas aeruginosa*
- combination therapy may be necessary if there is a concurrent Gram-negative organism
- well absorbed orally
- half-life 5—7 hours

Use
- serious infections due to Gram-positive organisms where other antibacterial agents are contraindicated or not appropriate because of resistance

Dose
- (Community-acquired pneumonia, nosocomial pneumonia) 600 mg orally or IV infusion twice daily for 10—14 days **OR**
- (Skin and soft tissue infections) 400—600 mg orally or 600 mg IV infusion twice daily for 10—14 days **OR**
- (Enterococcal infections) 600 mg IV infusion or orally twice daily for 14—28 days

Adverse effects
- headache
- diarrhoea, nausea, vomiting, altered taste
- abnormal liver function
- myelosuppression, including thrombocytopenia, anaemia, leucopenia, neutropenia, eosinophilia
- superinfection
- pseudomembranous colitis
- (Rare) peripheral and optic neuropathy, convulsions, lactic acidosis, tongue and/or tooth discolouration

Interactions
- contraindicated with or within 2 weeks of MAO inhibitors A or B
- caution if given with other myelosuppressive agents
- increased risk of pseudomembranous colitis if given with peristalsis-delaying agents, such as opioid analgesics or diphenoxylate/atropine combination
- not recommended with directly or indirectly acting sympathomimetic agents

ANTIBACTERIAL AGENTS

(e.g. pseudoephedrine), vasopressor agents (e.g. adrenaline (epinephrine), noradrenaline (norepinephrine)) or dopaminergic agents (e.g. dopamine, dobutamine)
- not recommended with serotonergic agents (e.g. SSRIs, TCAs, pethidine, 5HT1 receptor agonists) because of risk of serotonin syndrome

Nursing considerations/Cautions

- blood pressure should be monitored regularly throughout therapy
- visual function (e.g. visual acuity, colour vision, visual field) should be monitored if therapy is prolonged (greater than 12 weeks)
- monitoring of blood counts weekly is recommended if therapy extends beyond 14 days (especially in those with pre-existing myelosuppression, taking other myelosuppressive agents or with chronic previously treated infection)
- therapy duration should not exceed 28 days
- (IV) administer alone
- IV infusion over 30–120 minutes
- infusion should be kept in foil wrapping and carton until just before use
- discoloured or hazy solution should be discarded
- reconstituted oral suspension should be stored in outer container and gently inverted (not shaken) before use
- IV solution is incompatible with amphotericin B (amphotericin), chlorpromazine, sulfamethoxazole/trimethoprim, pentamidine, diazepam, erythromycin, phenytoin and ceftriaxone
- not recommended for treatment of central venous catheter-related bloodstream infections
- not recommended in those with uncontrolled hypertension, phaeochromocytoma or thyrotoxicosis unless blood pressure can be carefully monitored during therapy
- caution if given to those with pre-existing myelosuppression, GI disorders (especially colitis), epilepsy, kidney and liver insufficiency
- see also General Nursing considerations/Cautions for antibacterial agents (p. 149)

Patient education

- instruct patient to seek medical advice immediately if any of the following occurs:
    - any visual impairment, such as blurred vision or changes to colour vision
    - recurrent nausea and vomiting (may be first signs of lactic acidosis)
    - tiredness, paleness, headache, shortness of breath on exercising
    - fever, chills, sore throat, mouth ulcers
    - unusual bleeding or bruising
    - numbness, weakness or tingling in extremities
    - extreme fever, shivering, lack of co-ordination, dizziness, confusion
    - changes to colour of teeth or tongue
- (Oral suspension) instruct patient not to shake bottle. To mix suspension before use, advise patient to invert bottle gently several times
- see also General Patient education for antibacterial agents (p. 150)

A syrup/suspension is available, and the tablet can be crushed and mixed with water, yoghurt or apple puree for easier consumption.

Limited human data. Avoid use.

Avoid use. Appears in breastmilk, but no published safety data is available.

Linezolid's metabolites accumulate in patients with creatinine clearance (CrCl) < 30 mL/min, though the clinical significance of this accumulation remains unknown.

MUPIROCIN

Trade names
Bactroban, Bactroban Nasal Ointment, Supirocin

Available forms
Cream: 20 mg/g;
Ointment: 20 mg/g;
Nasal ointment: 20 mg/g

Action
- inhibits bacterial protein synthesis by binding to bacterial transfer RNA synthetase
- mainly active against Gram-positive aerobes, including *Staphylococcus* spp. and *Streptococcus* spp.
- no cross-resistance with other antibacterial agents

Use
- topical treatment of mild impetigo (ointment) and infected skin lesions (cream)
- elimination of nasal carriage of *Staphylococcus*, including MRSA

Dose
- apply to affected area 3 times daily (cover with gauze dressing if desired) for up to 10 days **OR**
- apply to inside of each nostril 2–3 times daily for no more than 5–7 days

Adverse effects
- (Nasal) irritation, tingling, burning, itching, rhinitis, stinging, soreness, pain over the maxilla, postnasal drip, sinusitis, conjunctivitis
- itching, burning, erythema, stinging, pain, swelling, dryness
- nausea, headache, diarrhoea
- (Rare) superinfection, anaphylaxis, hypersensitivity

Interaction
- not recommended with other topical preparations

Nursing considerations/Cautions
- not suitable for application to cannulation site
- not suitable for eyes or other mucous membranes
- (Bactroban) not recommended for application to large surface areas because of polyethylene glycol (preservative) content (especially in those with moderate-to-severe kidney impairment)

Patient education
- avoid contact with eyes and mucous membranes. Wash area well with water if contact occurs
- use only the specially formulated nasal ointment in the nose
- apply a match-head-sized amount of nasal ointment to a swab or finger. Spread it inside each nostril by pressing the sides of the nose together
- avoid prolonged treatment to reduce the risk of developing resistance
- children with impetigo should be kept home until appropriate treatment is started. Cover sores on exposed surfaces with a watertight dressing when the child returns to school or during child care

Safe to use.

Safe to use. If used on cracked nipples during breastfeeding, nipples should be washed well before breastfeeding.

INHIBITORS OF DNA SYNTHESIS

QUINOLONES (ALSO KNOWN AS FLUOROQUINOLONES)

General Actions of quinolones
- inhibit bacterial DNA synthesis by interfering with enzymes involved in supercoiling DNA needed for duplication, transcription and repair of bacterial DNA
- bactericidal
- increasing bacterial resistance with cross-resistance existing between quinolones

ANTIBACTERIAL AGENTS

General Uses of quinolones
- respiratory tract infections, including mild-to-moderate community-acquired pneumonia, acute exacerbation of chronic bronchitis, acute sinusitis, Legionnaire's disease
- severe complicated skin and skin structure infections, bone and joint infections
- complicated urinary tract infections, gonorrhoeal urethritis and cervicitis, chronic bacterial prostatitis, epididymo-orchitis
- shigellosis, traveller's diarrhoea, gastro-enteritis
- septicaemia
- post-exposure inhalation anthrax

General Adverse effects of quinolones
- nausea, vomiting, diarrhoea, bad taste, dyspepsia, gastric irritation, abdominal pain, flatulence, dry mouth
- headache, dizziness, weakness, fatigue, drowsiness, nervousness, tremor, restlessness, lightheadedness, agitation, insomnia, somnolence, depression
- rash, pruritus, urticaria
- fever
- photosensitivity
- eosinophilia
- pain, inflammation or rupture of tendon
- transient increase in liver enzymes, increased bilirubin
- crystalluria
- visual disturbances
- (IV) thrombophlebitis, burning pain, pruritus, erythema
- (Rare) pseudomembranous colitis, hypersensitivity, superinfection, anaphylaxis, anaphylactoid reaction
- (Rare) hallucinations, confusion, seizures, psychoses, suicidal ideation
- (Rare) interstitial nephritis, blood dyscrasias, haemolytic anaemia, QT prolongation, peripheral neuropathy

General Interactions of quinolones
- caution if given with agents known to prolong QT interval, such as class IA and III antiarrhythmic agents, antipsychotics, antidepressants, antifungals, fluoroquinolones or agents that cause electrolyte disturbance (e.g. diuretics), especially hypokalaemia and hypomagnesaemia
- may increase theophylline levels, thereby increasing risk of theophylline toxicity
- renal clearance may be decreased if given with probenecid
- may prolong half-life of caffeine
- may enhance effects of warfarin, therefore INR should be closely monitored especially when starting or stopping therapy
- metoclopramide may accelerate absorption of quinolones
- quinolones (high dose) and some NSAIDs (not aspirin) may increase risk of CNS stimulation and seizures if given together
- iron, sucralfate, highly buffered drugs (e.g. antiretroviral agents) and antacids containing magnesium, aluminium or calcium interfere with quinolone absorption
- increased risk of pseudomembranous colitis if given with peristaltic-delaying agents such as opioid analgesics and diphenoxylate/atropine combination
- increased risk of tendon rupture if given with corticosteroids
- if given with ciclosporin, may cause a transient increase in serum creatinine

General Nursing considerations/Cautions for quinolones
- before starting therapy, a careful history should be taken to exclude hypokalaemia or any family history of QT prolongation
- patient should be well hydrated and have good urine output throughout therapy to prevent crystalluria
- blood counts, renal and liver function should be monitored during prolonged therapy
- anaphylactoid reactions have occurred with quinolones (sometimes after the first dose), therefore patients should be closely observed, even if there is no known history of allergy
- all patients with gonorrhoea should also have serological testing for syphilis at

- time of diagnosis and then monthly for 4 months
- IV solution should be administered alone
- caution if used in those with epilepsy (as seizure threshold may be lowered), reduced brain flow, altered brain structure or stroke
- used with great caution in patients with myasthenia gravis because symptoms may be exacerbated
- caution if used in those with positive family history of aneurysm disease, or those with pre-existing aortic aneurysms and/or dissection, or with risk factors for aortic aneurysm and dissection
- caution if used in those with glucose-6-phosphate dehydrogenase (G6PD) deficiency because of increased risk of haemolytic anaemia
- caution if used in those with liver or renal impairment
- caution if used in those who have experienced quinolone-associated tendon rupture, are over 60 years of age and/or taking corticosteroids concurrently as there is an increased risk of tendon rupture. Young athletes undertaking extensive training are also at increased risk
- contraindicated in those with known hypersensitivity to quinolones
- see also General Nursing considerations/cautions for antibacterial agents (p. 149)

General Patient education for quinolones

- advise patient to take oral doses 2 hours before or 2 hours after dietary supplements containing zinc, magnesium or iron, 2 hours before or 4 hours after antacids containing calcium, aluminium or magnesium
- advise patient to drink plenty of fluids to maintain adequate hydration and urinary output to prevent crystalluria
- advise patient to avoid direct sunlight, wear protective clothing when outdoors and use a suitable sunscreen
- advise patient to avoid driving, operating machinery, or engaging in activities requiring mental alertness and coordination if you experience adverse effects like dizziness, drowsiness, or confusion
- patient should be advised to seek medical advice if any of the following occur:
  - pain, inflammation or suspected rupture of a tendon may occur within 48 hours of starting or up to 6 months after stopping therapy.
  - patient should also be advised to rest, refrain from exercising and stop therapy
  - pain, weakness, burning, tingling or numbness
  - rapid or irregular heart rate
  - fitting
  - depression, changes in mood, self-harming behaviours
- see also General Patient education for antibacterial agents (p. 150)

CIPROFLOXACIN HYDROCHLORIDE
Trade names
CFlox, CiloQuin, Ciloxan, Ciloxan Ear Drops, Ciprofloxacin Sandoz, Ciprofloxacin-WGR, Ciprol, APO-Ciprofloxacin, Noumed Ciprofloxacin

CIPROFLOXACIN LACTATE
Trade names
Aspen Ciprofloxacin Injection for Intravenous Infusion

Available forms
Infusion solution: 100 mg/50 mL, 200 mg/100 mL;
Tablets: 250 mg, 500 mg, 750 mg;
Eye/ear drops: 0.3% (3 mg/mL)

ANTIBACTERIAL AGENTS

Action
- Gram-negative organisms are more sensitive to ciprofloxacin than are Gram-positive organisms
- resistance to ciprofloxacin occurs in a significant number of those with cystic fibrosis who have *Pseudomonas aeruginosa* infections. This can occur after a single course
- metabolites have some antibacterial activity
- half-life about 4 hours
- see also General Actions of quinolones (p. 214)

Use
- infected corneal ulcer (bacterial keratitis), bacterial conjunctivitis
- chronic suppurative otitis media
- see also General Uses of quinolones (p. 215)

Dose
- (Severe or complicated urinary tract, moderate lower respiratory tract infection) 200 mg by IV infusion over 60 minutes 12-hourly **OR**
- (Severe lower respiratory tract infection; skin, skin structure, blood, bone or joint infection) 300 mg by IV infusion over 60 minutes 12-hourly **OR**
- (Post-exposure to inhalation of anthrax) 400 mg by IV infusion over 60 minutes 12-hourly for 60 days, starting as soon as possible after exposure **OR**
- (Post-exposure to inhalation of anthrax) 500 mg orally 12-hourly for 60 days, starting as soon as possible after exposure **OR**
- (Bronchial, skin, bone or joint infection) 500–750 mg orally 12-hourly **OR**
- (Chronic bacterial prostatitis) 250–500 mg orally 12-hourly for 14–28 days **OR**
- (Urinary tract infection) 250–500 mg orally 12-hourly **OR**
- (Acute uncomplicated gonorrhoeal urethritis) 250 mg as single oral dose **OR**
- (Gastroenteritis) 500 mg orally 12-hourly for 5 days **OR**
- (Corneal ulcers) 2 drops to affected eye(s) every 15 minutes for 6 hours, then 2 drops every 30 minutes for remainder of day 1, then 2 drops hourly for day 2, then 2 drops 4-hourly days 3—14 **OR**
- (Bacterial conjunctivitis) 1 drop into conjunctival sac(s) 2-hourly for 2 days (while awake), then 1 drop 4-hourly for next 5 days **OR**
- 5 drops to affected ear(s) twice daily for 9 days

Adverse effects
- (Ear drops) ear pain, stinging, ear pruritus, bitter taste, transient dizziness, headache, vertigo
- (Eye drops) discomfort, foreign body sensation, white precipitate, itching, redness, bitter taste
- see also General Adverse effects of quinolones (p. 215)

Interactions
- hypoglycaemia may occur when given with sulfonylureas (e.g. glibenclamide)
- serum levels may be decreased by omeprazole
- may increase or decrease serum levels of phenytoin; therefore levels should be monitored during therapy with ciprofloxacin
- may increase serum levels of methotrexate, increasing risk of toxicity; therefore close monitoring is recommended
- may increase serum levels of sildenafil, leading to adverse effects
- may increase serum levels of agomelatine and zolpidem and they are therefore not recommended together
- may decrease clearance of lidocaine (lignocaine)
- may increase serum levels of duloxetine, clozapine, olanzapine and ropinirole
- may interfere with *Mycobacterium* spp. culture, causing false negative result
- see also General Interactions of quinolones (p. 215)

Nursing considerations/Cautions
- ensure the patient is well hydrated before starting IV therapy, and avoid

- alkaline urine to reduce the risk of crystalluria
- treatment typically lasts 7—14 days, continued for 2 days after fever and symptoms resolve. Bone/joint infections may require 4—6 weeks of treatment, and chronic bacterial prostatitis may need 14—28 days. The IV route should be used only when the oral route is contraindicated. Switch to oral therapy as soon as possible to avoid toxicity
- avoid positioning the IV cannula in small veins of the hand to prevent local site reactions
- IV solutions are incompatible with alkaline solutions, penicillins and heparin
- IV solution will precipitate at cool temperatures and should not be refrigerated. Precipitate dissolves at room temperature
- Aspen Ciprofloxacin Injection contains 55 mg glucose/mL, which may affect blood glucose levels in patients with diabetes mellitus
- not recommended for pneumococcal infections
- not recommended for prepubertal children (except for post-exposure to inhaled anthrax) due to the risk of musculoskeletal effects
- see also General Nursing considerations/Cautions for quinolones (p. 215)

Patient education

- instruct patient on correct technique for insertion of ear drops (p. 1143)
- (Ear drops) if ear drops are cold, advise patient to warm in hands for 1—2 minutes before instillation
- instruct patient on correct technique for insertion of eye drops (p. 1128)
- (Eye drops) advise patient to discard eye drops 14 days after opening
- (Eye drops) if patient wears soft contact lenses, warn him/her not to insert lenses during therapy as eye drops contain benzalkonium chloride (preservative) which discolour soft contact lenses and can cause eye reaction
- see also General Patient education for quinolones (p. 216)

Ciprofloxacin tablets can be crushed and mixed with water or a spoonful of apple puree, but they should not be given with yoghurt or other milk-based products because calcium in these products can bind to the drug. This reduces its absorption and effectiveness by forming insoluble complexes, which decrease the amount of ciprofloxacin available in the bloodstream.

Not recommended during pregnancy because of potential risks to fetal cartilage development. While available data do not conclusively show an increased risk of abnormalities, ciprofloxacin should be used only in severe or life-threatening infections when no safer alternatives are available.

Generally considered safe to use; however, it may cause loose bowel movements in the infant. Use when the benefit outweighs the risk.

Reduce the dose of ciprofloxacin if CrCl < 30 mL/min to prevent drug accumulation and potential toxicity.

Available in combination with
- ciprofloxacin 2 mg + hydrocortisone 10 mg/mL (Ciproxin HC Ear Drops)

MOXIFLOXACIN
Trade names
Avelox, Moxifloxacin APO, Moxifloxacin Kabi, Moximed

Available forms
Tablets: 400 mg;
IV solution: 400 mg/250 mL

Action
- see General Actions of quinolones (p. 214)

ANTIBACTERIAL AGENTS

Use
- see General Uses of quinolones (p. 215)

Dose
- (Acute sinusitis) 400 mg orally daily for 10 days **OR**
- (Acute bacterial exacerbation of chronic bronchitis) 400 mg orally or IV infusion over 60 minutes for 5 days **OR**
- (Community-acquired pneumonia) 400 mg orally or IV infusion over 60 minutes for 10 days (oral) or 7—14 days (sequential IV and oral therapy) **OR**
- (Major skin or skin structure infection) 400 mg (sequential IV and oral therapy) for 7—21 days

Adverse effects
- see General Adverse effects of quinolones (p. 215)

Interactions
- see General Interactions of quinolones (p. 215)

Nursing considerations/Cautions
- IV infusion should be given over 60 minutes and NEVER as a bolus injection
- administer alone
- do not refrigerate IV solution, as precipitate will occur
- because of sodium content (34 mmol sodium per 250 mL), caution if used in those where sodium load may be important (e.g. congestive cardiac failure, renal failure)
- no dose adjustment is necessary when changing from IV to oral
- incompatible with sodium chloride 10% or 20%, or sodium hydrogen carbonate 4.2% or 8.4%
- see also General Nursing considerations/Cautions for quinolones (p. 215)

Patient education
- swallow tablets whole; do not crush or chew
- antacids, or iron or zinc supplements, may reduce absorption. Do not take them within 2 hours of a moxifloxacin dose
- notify your doctor if you experience palpitations, fainting spells, weakness, yellow skin, dark urine or a severe rash while taking moxifloxacin
- see also General Patient education for quinolones (p. 216)

 Swallow tablets whole; do not crush or chew.

 Not recommended during pregnancy because of potential risks to fetal cartilage development. While available data do not conclusively show an increased risk of abnormalities, moxifloxacin should be used only in severe or life-threatening infections when no safer alternatives are available.

 Generally considered safe to use; however, it may cause loose bowel movements in the infant. Use only when the benefit outweighs the risk.

NORFLOXACIN

Trade name
APO-Norfloxacin

Available form
Tablets: 400 mg

Action
- broad spectrum
- active metabolites have less antibacterial activity than norfloxacin
- half-life 3—4 hours
- see also General Actions of quinolones (p. 214)

Use
- see General Uses of quinolones (p. 215)

Dose
- (Urinary tract infection) 400 mg orally twice daily 1 hour before or 2 hours after food for 7—10 days or 3 days (uncomplicated urinary tract infection) **OR**
- (Suppression of chronic recurrent urinary tract infection) 400 mg orally twice daily 1 hour before or 2 hours after food for 4—12 weeks **OR**

- (Shigellosis, traveller's diarrhoea) 400 mg orally twice daily 1 hour before or 2 hours after food for 5 days

Interactions
- antibacterial action may be antagonised by nitrofurantoin and therefore should not be given together

Adverse effects/Nursing considerations/Cautions/Patient education
- take norfloxacin 1 hour before or 2 hours after meals for best absorption, and drink plenty of fluids while taking it
- if treating shigellosis or traveller's diarrhoea, you can take it with or without food
- avoid dairy products, antacids, iron, zinc or calcium supplements within 2 hours of a norfloxacin dose as they can reduce absorption
- norfloxacin may increase the effects of caffeine; you may need to reduce your caffeine intake
- avoid sun exposure, and wear protective clothing and sunscreen while taking norfloxacin, as it may increase sensitivity to sunlight
- see also General Adverse effects/General Nursing considerations/Cautions/General Patient education for quinolones (p. 214)

Tablet can be crushed (very bitter taste) and mixed with water or apple puree. Should not be given with yoghurt or milk-based products.

Not recommended during pregnancy because of potential risks to fetal cartilage development. While available data do not conclusively show an increased risk of abnormalities, norfloxacin should be used only in severe or life-threatening infections when no safer alternatives are available.

Generally considered safe to use; however, it may cause loose bowel movements in the infant. Use only when the benefit outweighs the risk.

For patients with CrCl < 30 mL/min, the recommended dose of norfloxacin is 400 mg orally once daily to prevent drug accumulation and reduce the risk of toxicity.

OFLOXACIN
Trade name
Ocuflox

Available form
Eye drops: 3 mg/mL (0.3%)

Action
- see General Actions of quinolones (p. 215)

Use
- infected corneal ulcer (bacterial keratitis), severe bacterial conjunctivitis

Dose
- (Corneal ulcers) 1–2 drops to affected eye(s) every 30 minutes while awake and 1–2 drops 4 hours after going to bed and again 2 hours later (days 1–2), 1–2 drops hourly while awake (days 3–7) and then 1–2 drops 4 times daily until ulcer has healed (usually 21 days) **OR**
- (Bacterial conjunctivitis) 1 drop 4-hourly to affected eye(s) for 2 days, then 1 drop 6-hourly for up to 8 days

Adverse effects
- corneal precipitates and perforation (in those with pre-existing corneal ulcer or defect)
- burning, stinging, tearing, itching, foreign body sensation, photophobia, blurred vision, eye pain, dry eyes, eye/periorbital/facial oedema
- nausea
- dizziness

Nursing considerations/Cautions/Patient education
- instruct patient on correct technique for insertion of eye drops (p. 1128)
- (Eye drops) advise patient to discard eye drops 28 days after opening

ANTIBACTERIAL AGENTS

- (Eye drops) if patient wears soft contact lenses, warn them not to insert lenses during therapy, as eye drops contain benzalkonium chloride (preservative), which discolour soft contact lenses and can cause eye reaction

No human studies. Generally considered as safe to use as systemic absorption is minimal.

Ofloxacin eye drops are generally considered safe to use during breastfeeding because the systemic absorption is minimal when used topically in the eyes.

To further reduce any potential risk, apply pressure to the tear duct (punctal occlusion) for a minute or two after administering the drops to limit systemic absorption.

DISRUPTING BACTERIAL CELL MEMBRANE

COLISTIN (AS COLISTIMETHATE SODIUM)
Trade name
Tadim

Available form
Powder (for nebulisation): 1 million IU

Action
- polypeptide that attaches to the bacterial cell membranes, altering its permeability causing disruption and lysis
- bactericidal
- not recommended for infections due to *Proteus* spp. or *Neisseria* spp.
- half-life 1.5 hours (IV), prolonged to 2–4.8 hours in those with cystic fibrosis
- 1 million IU = 80 mg

Use
- colonisation and lung infection due to *P. aeruginosa* in those with cystic fibrosis

Dose
- (Cystic fibrosis – initial colonisation) 2 million IU via nebuliser twice daily for 3 weeks (with oral/parental antibiotics) **OR**
- (Cystic fibrosis – frequent, recurrent infections) up to 2 million IU via nebuliser 3 times daily for up to 12 weeks (with oral/parental antibiotics) **OR**
- (Cystic fibrosis – chronic colonisation) 1–2 million IU via nebuliser twice daily (with oral/parental antibiotics for acute exacerbations)

Adverse effects
- (Nebulisation) coughing, bronchospasm, chest tightness, sore mouth and/or throat
- (Rare) hypersensitivity, superinfection

Interactions
- neuromuscular blockade may be potentiated if given with non-depolarising muscle relaxants and should be used with extreme caution
- caution if used with other nephrotoxic or neurotoxic agents
- increased risk of nephrotoxicity if given with cefalotin

Nursing considerations/Cautions
- (Cystic fibrosis) sputum cultures to confirm colonisation with sensitive *P. aeruginosa* is recommended before starting therapy
- (Cystic fibrosis) first dose should be administered via nebuliser under medical supervision, observing for bronchospasm or bronchial hyperactivity by measuring FEV_1 before and after dose
- (Cystic fibrosis) I-neb AAD system is recommended for efficient nebulisation
- (Cystic fibrosis) pre-dosing with bronchodilator is recommended
- (Cystic fibrosis) if used with other therapies, should be used after physiotherapy and any other inhaled therapies

- (Nebulisation) reconstitute powder with water for injections
- caution if used in those with impaired renal function or porphyria
- not recommended in those with myasthenia gravis

Patient education

- (Cystic fibrosis) instruct patient to complete chest physiotherapy and/or inhaled therapy before using colistimethate
- see also General Patient education for antibacterial agents (p. 150)

No human safety during pregnancy has been established; therefore not recommended during pregnancy unless benefits outweigh risks.

Not recommended during breastfeeding unless benefits outweigh risks.

OTHER ANTIBACTERIAL AGENTS

CO-TRIMOXAZOLE (TRIMETHOPRIM WITH SULFAMETHOXAZOLE)

Trade names
Bactrim 400/80 Infusion Concentrate, Bactrim DS, DBL Sulfamethoxazole 400 mg and Trimethoprim 80 mg, Resprim, Resprim Forte, Septrin Forte, Septrin Sugar Free Oral Suspension

Available forms
Ampoules: 400 mg sulfamethoxazole/ 80 mg trimethoprim/5 mL;
Tablets (DS/Forte): 800 mg sulfamethoxazole/160 mg trimethoprim;
Tablets: 400 mg sulfamethoxazole/80 mg trimethoprim;
Oral suspension: 200 mg sulfamethoxazole/ 40 mg trimethoprim/5 mL

Action
- combination is bactericidal because it blocks two consecutive steps in bacterial folate metabolism, resulting in an inability to synthesise nucleic acids
- sulfamethoxazole and other sulfonamides block the conversion of para-aminobenzoic acid (PABA) to the coenzyme dihydrofolic acid, whereas trimethoprim inhibits the enzyme dihydrofolate reductase, which converts dihydrofolic acid to tetrahydrofolic acid
- combination should not be used if organism is sensitive to trimethoprim but not sensitive to sulfamethoxazole
- trimethoprim has an active metabolite
- half-life 10 hours (trimethoprim) and 11 hours (sulfamethaxole)

Use
- respiratory tract infections (upper and lower), renal and urinary tract infections, genital tract infections, GI infections, skin and wound infections, septicaemia

Dose
- (800 mg sulfamethoxazole/160 mg trimethoprim) 1/2—1 1/2 tablets orally twice daily after meals for 5 days or until symptom free for 48 hours (DS or Forte tablets) **OR**
- (400 mg sulfamethoxazole/80 mg trimethoprim) 2 tablets orally twice daily, increasing to 3 tablets twice daily for severe infections after meals for 5 days or until symptom free for 48 hours **OR**
- (*Pneumocystis carinii* pneumonitis) trimethoprim 20 mg/kg and sulfamethoxazole 100 mg/kg/day orally or by IV infusion in 4 divided doses for 14 days **OR**
- 800 mg sulfamethoxazole/160 mg trimethoprim (10 mL) by IV infusion twice daily **OR**
- (Severe infection) 1200 mg sulfamethoxazole/240 mg trimethoprim (15 mL) by IV infusion twice daily

Adverse effects
- nausea, vomiting, anorexia
- rash, pruritus, urticaria
- photosensitivity reactions
- arthralgia, myalgia

ANTIBACTERIAL AGENTS

- fever, symptoms resembling serum sickness
- crystalluria, oliguria, anuria, impaired kidney function
- aplastic anaemia, agranulocytosis, thrombocytopenia, leucopenia, bone marrow depression
- ataxia, convulsions, confusion, depression, apathy, hallucinations, nervousness
- vertigo, tinnitus
- peripheral and optic neuropathy
- headache, fatigue, insomnia
- hyperkalaemia, hyponatraemia
- increased liver enzymes and bilirubin, hepatitis
- hypersensitivity, allergic reactions
- pseudomembranous colitis, superinfection
- Stevens—Johnson syndrome (rare but possibly fatal) (see Glossary)
- (Rare) diuresis, hypoglycaemia, haemolytic anaemia (associated with glucose-6-phosphate dehydrogenase (G6PD) deficiency), aseptic meningitis, rhabdomyolysis
- (IV) pain, inflammation, thrombophlebitis

Interactions

- may decrease effectiveness of tricyclic antidepressants (TCAs)
- not recommended with amiodarone, paclitaxel and clozapine
- increased risk of delirium and myoclonus if given with amantadine or memantine
- increased risk of haematological adverse effects if given with azathioprine, zidovudine or mercaptopurine; therefore blood counts should be closely monitored if given together
- increased antibacterial activity may occur if given with polymyxin
- may increase serum levels of digoxin, increasing risk of toxicity
- may increase serum levels of methotrexate, increasing the risk of bone marrow depression
- may increase serum levels of phenytoin, thereby increasing their risk of toxicity; therefore levels should be closely monitored, especially when starting or stopping therapy
- may enhance the effect of sulfonylurea hypoglycaemic agents; therefore blood glucose levels should be closely monitored
- increased risk of pseudomembranous colitis if given with peristalsis-delaying agents such as opioid analgesics and diphenoxylate/atropine combination
- not recommended with local anaesthetics (PABA derivatives such as procaine) as antibacterial activity may be antagonised
- increased risk of thrombocytopenia if given with thiazide diuretics in the elderly
- may decrease serum levels of ciclosporin
- caution if given with other agents that may cause hyperkalaemia
- increased risk of methaemoglobinaemia if given with dapsone
- may potentiate effects of warfarin; therefore INR should be closely monitored, especially when starting or stopping therapy
- rifampicin may decrease half-life of trimethoprim
- caution if given with ACE inhibitors or angiotensin receptor blockers
- may interfere with a number of laboratory tests including *Lactobacillus casei* serum folate assay and *Lactobacillus leishmania* serum cyanocobalamin (57Co) (vitamin B_{12}) assay

Nursing considerations/Cautions

- blood cell counts should be monitored during prolonged therapy (greater than 14 days), especially in those with predisposition to folate deficiency, or in those with malnutrition or treatment with antiepileptic agents
- urinalysis (with microscopic examination), renal function tests and serum potassium and sodium are recommended during prolonged therapy greater than 14 days

- patient should be well hydrated and have an adequate fluid intake during therapy
- urinary output should be monitored and kept above 1500 mL/day to reduce crystalluria and stone formation
- alkalinisation may be necessary to increase solubility of some sulfonamides and reduce the risk of crystalluria
- therapy should be discontinued if rash appears
- patients with AIDS who are being treated for PCP (*Pneumocystis jirovecii*, previously called *Pneumocystis carinii*) may show a higher incidence of rash, fever and leucopenia and should be carefully monitored during therapy
- cross-sensitivity may occur with other sulfonamides such as some antithyroid drugs, acetazolamide, thiazide diuretics and oral hypoglycaemic agents
- IV route is recommended only when oral route is unavailable
- (High dose) serum potassium and kidney function should be closely monitored during therapy
- (Oral) therapy should continue for at least 5 days or until patient has been symptom free for 48 hours
- should not be given undiluted or as an IV bolus
- dilute ampoule before administration according to manufacturer's instructions in 125–500 mL of IV fluid and mix well
- IV infusion should be completed within 90 minutes
- IV therapy should be limited to 3 days or less
- IV ampoule solution may precipitate if stored at low temperatures. If this occurs, solution should be discarded
- (IV) contains sodium metabisulfite, which may cause allergic reaction in sensitive individuals
- (Suspension) contains hydroxybenzoates, polysorbate and sorbitol
- caution if used in those with liver or kidney impairment, urinary obstruction, blood dyscrasias, asthma, allergies, porphyria or thyroid dysfunction
- not recommended in those with serious haematological disorders
- caution if used in those with folate deficiency, hypoglycaemia and electrolyte imbalance (especially hyperkalaemia)
- caution if used in those with malnutrition because of increased risk of crystalluria
- caution if used in the elderly because of increased risk of adverse effects
- caution if used in those with oedema of cardiac origin, as sulfonamides may induce diuresis
- not recommended in those with G6PD deficiency because of risk of haemolytic anaemia
- not recommended in patients receiving peritoneal dialysis
- not recommended in infants under 12 weeks
- contraindicated in newborns during first 6 weeks of life or premature infants
- contraindicated for streptococcal pharyngitis
- contraindicated in those with known hypersensitivity to sulfonamides or trimethoprim, or blood dyscrasias, bone marrow depression, parenchymal liver damage or severe renal impairment (creatinine clearance < 15 mL/min)
- see also Nursing considerations/Cautions for antibacterial agents (p. 149)

Patient education

- patients with diabetes taking sulfonylurea hypoglycaemics should be advised that blood glucose control may be altered during therapy
- warn patient to avoid sunlamps or sunbeds or direct exposure to sunlight and, if this cannot be avoided, should wear protective clothing and sunscreen with high sun protection factor (SPF 30+)

ANTIBACTERIAL AGENTS

- instruct patient to seek medical advice immediately if any of the following occur:
  - rash, sore throat, fever, bleeding, painful joints
  - cough, shortness of breath, pallor
  - bleeding under skin
  - yellowing of skin or whites of the eyes
- patient should be advised to avoid driving or operating machinery if dizziness, drowsiness, confusion, insomnia, vertigo or fatigue are ongoing problems
- advise patient to increase fluid intake by drinking extra glasses of water during the day unless told not to do so by doctor
- advise patient to shake suspension well before use
- see also General Patient education for antibacterial agents (p. 150)

Syrup/suspension is available. Tablet can be crushed and mixed with water or spoonful of yoghurt or apple puree.

Sulfonamides should not be given to women before delivery because they may cause jaundice and/or haemolytic anaemia in the newborn and are contraindicated in late pregnancy. Animal studies have shown trimethoprim causes birth defects because of interference to folic acid metabolism, and therefore folic acid supplements should be given if trimethoprim or trimethoprimesulfonamide combination must be used during pregnancy.

Sulfonamides are contraindicated during breastfeeding of infants under 2 months or if infant has G6PD deficiency. Trimethoprim is not recommended during breastfeeding.

Caution if used in those with renal impairment, a reduced or less frequent dose is recommended to avoid accumulation of trimethoprim in the blood. Close monitoring for signs of toxicity is recommended if used in those with severe renal impairment.

DAPTOMYCIN
Trade names
Cipla Daptomycin, Daptomycin Dr.Reddy's, Daptomycin Juno, Daptomycin Lupin

Available forms
Vial: 350 mg, 500 mg

Action
- cyclic lipopeptide
- binds to bacterial membrane, causing depolarisation of membrane potential in growing and stationary phase cells, inhibition of protein, DNA and RNA synthesis
- active against Gram-positive organisms only

Use
- complicated skin and skin structure infections (where other antibacterial agents are ineffective or inappropriate)
- bacteraemia (due to *Staphylococcus aureus*), including right-sided valve infective endocarditis

Dose
- (Complicated skin and skin structure infection) 4 mg/kg daily as IV bolus over 2 minutes, or infusion over 30 minutes for 7–14 days or until infection has resolved **OR**
- (Bacteraemia, right-sided endocarditis) 6 mg/kg daily as IV bolus over 2 minutes, or infusion over 30 minutes for 2–6 weeks

Adverse effects
- fungal infection, urinary tract infection
- anaemia
- anxiety, insomnia
- dizziness, headache
- hypertension, hypotension
- GI/abdominal pain, diarrhoea, nausea, vomiting, flatulence, bloating, distension, constipation
- rash, pruritus
- fever, asthenia
- increased creatine phosphokinase (CPK), muscle pain, (uncommon) weakness, rhabdomyolysis

HAVARD'S NURSING GUIDE TO DRUGS

- abnormal liver function
- eosinophilic pneumonia (fever, dyspnoea, hypoxic respiratory insufficiency, diffuse pulmonary infiltrates)
- hypersensitivity, pseudomembranous colitis, superinfection
- peripheral neuropathy
- (IV site) infusion site reaction

Interactions
- caution if used with other agents associated with myopathy and rhabdomyolysis (e.g. statins (HMG CoA reductase inhibitors), fibrates, ciclosporin)
- may cause false prolongation of prothrombin time and elevation of INR

Nursing considerations/Cautions
- plasma CPK should be measured before starting therapy and then weekly during therapy
- kidney function and plasma CPK should be measured regularly (> once per week) in anyone with pre-existing kidney impairment
- closely monitor patients for any muscle pain or weakness (especially in extremities)
- if infection persists or relapses, repeat blood cultures are recommended. Appropriate surgical intervention, such as debridement or removal of prosthetic devices, should also be considered
- add 7 mL sodium chloride 0.9% to 350 mg vial (or 10 mL to 500 mg vial) and gently rotate, taking care to avoid foaming. The vial should not be shaken. Allow vial to stand for 10 minutes and then swirl gently for several minutes to ensure powder is reconstituted
- if administering as an IV infusion over 30 minutes, further dilution with sodium chloride 0.9% is required
- not compatible with glucose-containing diluents or solutions
- administer alone
- not indicated for pneumonia or left-sided endocarditis
- caution if used in those with kidney impairment. If creatine clearance is < 30 mL/min, dosing interval should be lengthened to 48 hours and kidney function closely monitored
- not recommended in children < 12 months
- see also General Nursing considerations/Cautions for antibacterial agents (p. 149)

Patient education
- advise patient to seek medical advice if any of the following occur:
  - tender or aching muscles, muscle weakness
  - unusual tingling or numbness in feet or hands, loss of feeling, difficulty moving
  - new or worsening fever, cough or difficulty breathing
- see also General Patient education for antibacterial agents (p. 150)

 No human data. Used during pregnancy only if benefits outweigh the risks.

 While small amounts may pass into breastmilk, the effects on a breastfed infant are unknown. Given its poor oral absorption, the risk to the nursing infant is likely low.

 Primarily eliminated by the kidneys. A dosage adjustment is recommended for adult patients with creatinine clearance (CrCl) < 30 mL/min, including those receiving hemodialysis or continuous ambulatory peritoneal dialysis.

FIDAXOMICIN

Trade name
Dificid

Available form
Tablets: 200 mg

Action
- macrocyclic antibacterial
- inhibits RNA synthesis by RNA polymerases at a site different from the rifamycins
- active metabolite

ANTIBACTERIAL AGENTS

- half-life 7—16 hours
- bactericidal against *Clostridium difficile*

Use
- confirmed infection with *C. difficile*-associated disease

Dose
- 200 mg orally twice daily for 10 days

Adverse effects
- nausea, constipation, vomiting, abdominal pain, diarrhoea
- headache, dizziness, fatigue, insomnia
- pruritus
- fever, chills
- peripheral oedema
- hypotension
- dyspnoea
- increased liver enzymes
- urinary tract infection, pneumonia
- hypokalaemia, hyperkalaemia, hypomagnesaemia
- anaemia
- back pain
- (Rare) hypersensitivity

Nursing considerations/Cautions
- caution if used in those with severe kidney or liver insufficiency
- not recommended for systemic infections
- caution if used in those with known hypersensitivity to macrolides
- see also General Nursing considerations/Cautions for antibacterial agents (p. 149)

Patient education
- see General Patient education for antibacterial agents (p. 150)

Tablet can be crushed and mixed with water or spoonful of apple puree.

No human data. Used during pregnancy only if needed and benefits outweigh the risks.

No data available.

FOSFOMYCIN
Trade name
Monurol

Available form
Granules: 3 g/sachet

Actions
- inhibits first stage of bacterial wall synthesis
- bactericidal
- also reduces bacterial adhesion to bladder mucosa
- not metabolised and is excreted unchanged via kidneys
- half-life 4 hours

Use
- treatment of uncomplicated lower urinary tract infections (acute cystitis) in females due to Enterobacteriaceae spp. (including *Escherichia coli*) and *Enterococcus faecalis*

Dose
- (Females > 12 years) 3 g orally as single dose on empty stomach or 2—3 hours after meals, preferably before bedtime

Adverse effects
- vulvovaginitis
- headache, dizziness
- diarrhoea, nausea, dyspepsia
- hypersensitivity, pseudomembranous colitis

Interactions
- may increase or decrease prothrombin time; therefore close monitoring of INR is recommended if patient is taking warfarin
- not recommended with metoclopramide, as decreased serum levels of fosfomycin may occur
- not recommended with urinary alkalinisers

Nursing considerations/Cautions
- culture and susceptibility studies should be performed to identify causative organism and sensitivity. Therapy can be started before results are known
- only one dose should be used per single episode of acute cystitis. Repeated

doses are not recommended as clinical outcomes are not improved, but risk of adverse events increases
- contains sucrose; therefore not recommended in those with hereditary problems of fructose intolerance, glucose–galactose malabsorption or sucrase–isomaltase insufficiency
- not recommended for treatment of pyelonephritis or perinephric abscess, or if resistance is likely (as indicated by previous treatment failure)
- not recommended in male patients
- contraindicated in those with severe kidney insufficiency (creatinine clearance < 10 mL/min) or undergoing haemofiltration, haemodialysis or peritoneal dialysis
- see also General Nursing considerations/Cautions for antibacterial agents (p. 149)

Patient education

- works best when taken before bedtime, after emptying the bladder, to allow for maximum drug concentration in the urinary tract
- advise patient to:
  - take on an empty stomach or at least 2–3 hours after meals, preferably before bedtime after emptying bladder
  - dissolve granules in glass of water and take immediately
  - hot water should not be used to dissolve granules
  - dry granules should not be ingested
- instruct patient that medicines such as sodium bicarbonate, Ural® or Citravescent® can reduce the effectiveness of fosfomycin for treating urinary tract infections and therefore should not be taken together.
- see also General Patient education for antibacterial agents (p. 150)

Granules can be dispersed in 120–150 mL water, or dissolved in 5 mL water and then mixed with spoonful of yoghurt or apple puree.

Not recommended during pregnancy, as evidence suggests that a single dose of fosfomycin does not increase the risk of congenital malformations. However, it should be used during pregnancy only when other treatment options are unsuitable.

Not recommended during breastfeeding, as no human data. Small amounts of fosfomycin pass into breastmilk. A single oral dose is likely to be safe, though it may cause loose bowel movements in the baby. Use only when benefit outweighs the risk.

Predominantly renally cleared and is not recommended for use in patients with a CrCl < 10 mL/min owing to reduced drug clearance and potential for toxicity.

METHENAMINE (HEXAMINE) HIPPURATE

Trade names
APOHealth Urinary Tract Antibacterial, Chemists' Own Urinary Tract Antibacterial, Hiprex, Uramet

Available form
Tablets: 1 g

Action
- broad-spectrum antibacterial agent that is active against both Gram-negative and Gram-positive organisms
- antibacterial action occurs when it is excreted in the urine, where it dissociates to hippuric acid (bacteriostatic) and methenamine (which is further hydrolysed to ammonia and formaldehyde (bacteriostatic))
- takes 30 minutes to 2 hours to reach peak urinary formaldehyde level

Use
- long-term treatment of chronic or recurrent urinary tract infections

Dose
- 1 g orally twice daily

Adverse effects
- (Occasionally) nausea, upset stomach, rash, dysuria, stomatitis

Interactions
- crystalluria may occur if administered with sulfonamides

Nursing considerations/Cautions/Patient education
- ensure patient is adequately hydrated before starting therapy
- only active if urinary pH is less than 5.5; therefore check pH frequently and do not alkalinise urine
- avoid taking medications like sodium bicarbonate, Ural® or Citravescent® as they make methenamine less effective
- restrict alkalinising foods (e.g. vegetarian diet)
- additional urine acidification may be achieved by administration of ascorbic acid 2 g daily in divided doses
- contraindicated in those with kidney or liver insufficiency, metabolic acidosis, severe dehydration or parenchymal infection (as monotherapy)
- see also General Nursing considerations/Cautions for antibacterial agents (p. 149) and General Patient education for antibacterial agents (p. 150)

The tablet can be halved to make it easier to swallow, or it can be crushed and mixed with water, milk, or fruit juice for easier administration.

Safe to use.

Safe to use.

It is ineffective in patients with renal impairment owing to inadequate concentrations in the renal tubules, which limit its efficacy. Additionally, there is a risk of hippurate crystalluria in cases of severe renal impairment.

It is contraindicated in patients with severe hepatic impairment because stomach acid hydrolyses methenamine, leading to the production of ammonia, which can exacerbate hepatic encephalopathy.

NITROFURANTOIN
Trade names
APX-Nitrofurantoin, Macrodantin, Nitrofurantoin BNM

Available forms
Capsules: 50 mg, 100 mg

Action
- inhibits bacterial protein, DNA, RNA and cell wall synthesis, disrupting multiple essential processes within the bacterial cell. This broad mechanism of action makes nitrofurantoin effective against a range of urinary tract pathogens
- bacteriostatic in low levels, bactericidal in high levels
- active against both Gram-positive and Gram-negative urinary tract pathogens
- half-life 20 minutes

Use
- treatment of urinary tract infections (UTIs), such as cystitis and pyelitis, caused by susceptible pathogens
- effective against common UTI-causing bacteria, including *Escherichia coli*, and is typically prescribed for uncomplicated infections

Dose
- (Acute UTI treatment, adult) 50—100 mg orally 4 times daily with or after food for 7 days then continue until urine sterile for 3 days (daily maximum 400 mg) **OR**
- (Acute UTI treatment, child > 1 month) 0.75—1.75 mg/kg (maximum 100 mg) orally 4 times daily for 5—7 days

- (UTI prophylaxis, adult) 50–100 mg orally at bedtime
- (UTI prophylaxis, child > 1 month) 1–2 mg/kg (maximum 100 mg) orally at bedtime.

Adverse effects
- anorexia, nausea, vomiting, diarrhoea, abdominal pain, dyspepsia, flatulence, constipation
- headache, drowsiness, dizziness, nystagmus, vertigo, depression, asthenia, confusion, amblyopia
- peripheral neuropathy, including optic neuritis
- eosinophilia, anaemia
- elevated liver enzymes
- rash, urticaria, pruritus, dermatitis, transient alopecia
- superinfection, hypersensitivity
- (Rare) pulmonary hypersensitivity (acute, allergic pneumonitis, chronic interstitial pulmonary fibrosis), hepatitis, pseudomembranous colitis, psychosis, benign intracranial hypertension, blood dyscrasias including haemolytic anaemia, severe skin reactions

Interactions
- action may be inhibited by phenobarbital (phenobarbitone)
- excretion is decreased by acidifying drugs and increased by alkalising drugs
- antacids reduce effectiveness
- increased serum levels may result if given with probenecid or sulfinpyrazone, increasing the risk of toxicity
- increased risk of pseudomembranous colitis if given with peristalsis-delaying agents such as opioid analgesics and diphenoxylate/atropine combination
- interferes with some laboratory tests (e.g. serum bilirubin, urinary glucose, urine creatinine, serum urea)

Nursing considerations/Cautions
- pulmonary function (including X-ray examination) should be monitored 6-monthly during prolonged therapy
- liver function should be monitored regularly during prolonged therapy
- treatment should be continued for at least 3 days after clear urine culture has been obtained
- note and report muscle weakness, numbness and tingling (peripheral neuritis) because this necessitates ceasing therapy
- caution if used in those with glucose-6-phosphate dehydrogenase (G6PD) deficiency
- caution if used in those with GI disorders, especially colitis, because of increased risk of developing pseudomembranous colitis
- increased risk of peripheral neuropathy if given to those with renal impairment, anaemia, diabetes mellitus, electrolyte imbalance or vitamin B deficiency
- risk of pulmonary hypersensitivity is increased with prolonged therapy > 6 months
- caution if used in those with kidney impairment or acidosis. If therapy is prolonged, blood pH, CO_2 content, urea nitrogen and non-protein nitrogen should be monitored
- contraindicated in those with hypersensitivity to furan derivatives or with renal impairment (creatinine clearance (CrCl) < 60 mL/min or elevated serum creatinine), anuria or oliguria
- see also General Nursing considerations/Cautions for antibacterial agents (p. 149)

Patient education
- warn patient that urine may become harmless brown colour
- instruct patient that GI side-effects can be lessened if given with food or milk

ANTIBACTERIAL AGENTS

- patient should be advised to seek medical advice immediately if any of the following occur:
  - fever, chills, cough, chest pain, rash or shortness of breath (as these may indicate acute pneumonitis)
  - malaise, shortness of breath on exertion, cough, blue tinge to lips or fingernails (chronic interstitial pulmonary fibrosis)
  - yellowing of eyes or skin, loss of appetite, nausea, upper abdominal pain, dark urine (jaundice/hepatitis)
  - numbness or tingling of feet or hands (peripheral neuropathy)
- advise patient to take antacids 2 hours apart from nitrofurantoin
- patient should be warned to avoid driving or operating machinery if dizziness, drowsiness or vertigo are ongoing problems
- male patients should be counselled regarding decreased sperm count that may occur during therapy
- see also General Patient education for antibacterial agents (p. 150)

Capsule can be opened and mixed with water or spoonful of yoghurt or apple puree.

Generally safe during pregnancy, except in the last trimester, because of a theoretical risk of haemolytic anaemia in the neonate. It may cause haemolytic anaemia in newborns with G6PD deficiency and is therefore contraindicated during labour or delivery if labour is imminent.

Use with caution; avoid use if the baby is under 4 weeks old or has G6PD deficiency, as it may cause haemolysis.

Contraindicated by the manufacturer if CrCl < 60 mL/min because of concerns about adverse effects and decreased effectiveness.

RIFAXIMIN
Trade name
Xifaxan

Available form
Tablet: 550 mg

Action
- non-aminoglycoside, semisynthetic, non-systemic antibiotic derived from rifamycin
- binds to beta subunit of bacterial DNA-dependent RNA polymerase, resulting in inhibition of bacterial RNA synthesis
- broad spectrum
- active against Gram-positive, Gram-negative, aerobic and anaerobic organisms causing intestinal infection
- (Recurrent hepatic encephalopathy) thought to affect GI flora

Use
- prevention of hepatic encephalopathy (HE) (where other treatment is inappropriate)

Dose
- (Hepatic encephalopathy) 550 mg orally twice daily

Adverse effects
- nausea, vomiting, flatulence, abdominal pain, constipation, rectal tenesmus, defecation urgency
- fever
- headache
- (HE) anaemia, peripheral oedema, muscle spasm, back pain, dizziness, rash, pruritus, dyspnoea
- (Rare) hypersensitivity, pseudomembranous colitis

Interactions
- charcoal may decrease absorption
- caution if given with ciclosporin
- may increase or decrease INR, therefore caution if given with warfarin. INR should be closely monitored especially when starting or stopping therapy

Nursing considerations/Cautions
- (HE) caution if used in those with severe liver impairment
- not recommended in children under 12 years
- contraindicated in those with intestinal obstruction or with hypersensitivity to rifamycins
- see also General Nursing considerations/Cautions for antibacterial agents (p. 149)

Patient education
- see General Patient education for antibacterial agents (p. 150)

Generally not recommended to be crushed, as crushing could alter the drug's release and absorption characteristics, even though it is poorly absorbed systemically. If crushing is necessary because of patient difficulty in swallowing, some pharmacies can make a suspension from crushed tablets.

Limited human data. Rifaximin has minimal absorption and acts locally in the gastrointestinal tract. While unlikely to significantly affect the fetus, use only when the benefits outweigh the risks.

Limited human data. As it is poorly absorbed from the gastrointestinal tract, it is considered unlikely to pass into breastmilk in significant amounts or cause harm to a breastfeeding infant. Use only when the benefits outweigh the risks.

Use with caution in severe hepatic impairment (Child—Pugh class C) as systemic concentrations of rifaximin may be increased.

Patients with Model for End-stage Liver Disease (MELD) scores > 25 were excluded from clinical trials, so safety and efficacy in this population are not well-established. Monitor such patients closely if treatment is necessary.

SILVER SULFADIAZINE
Trade name
Flamazine

Available form
Cream: 1%

Action
- sulfonamide combined with silver
- structurally similar to para-amino benzoic acid (PABA) and blocks conversion of PABA to dihydrofolic acid (reduced form of folic acid); therefore bacteria are deprived of folic acid because of incomplete synthesis and so cease to multiply
- active against both Gram-negative and Gram-positive organisms
- silver is reported to have some antibacterial properties of its own

Use
- prevention and treatment of infection in severe burns
- treatment of infections in leg ulcers and pressure injuries
- conservative management of fingertip injuries (where pulp, nail loss and/or partial loss of distal phalanx have occurred)

Dose
- applied with a sterile spatula or gloved hand in a layer 3—5 mm thick and changed at least daily

Adverse effects
- systemic effects (in those with more than 20% burns), including nausea and vomiting
- (Local reactions) pain, burning, itching, rash, contact dermatitis/eczema, pruritus
- (Rare) skin discolouration (argyria) (due to silver), systemic absorption, transient leucopenia

Interactions
- may inactivate enzymatic debriding agents

ANTIBACTERIAL AGENTS

- (Large burns) caution if given with phenytoin or oral hypoglycaemic agents

Nursing considerations/Cautions/Patient education

- avoid contact with eyes
- (Burns) assess the burn wound regularly for signs of infection, healing progress and potential adverse reactions to treatment. Prolonged use of silver sulfadiazine can delay healing in superficial or partial-thickness burns, so careful observation is required
- limit the use of silver sulfadiazine to the first 3 days after a burn for infection prevention, as extended use can inhibit the healing process in superficial or partial-thickness burns
- (Long-term therapy) blood count monitoring is recommended
- (Extensive burns) kidney function and serum sulfonamide levels should be monitored. Urine should also be checked for sulfonamide crystals
- may alter appearance of burn wound and/or delay separation of burn eschar
- non-ulcerated areas should be avoided to prevent skin maceration
- each jar or tube is for single patient use only; any remaining cream should be discarded after completion of treatment
- (Fingertip injury) after haemostasis has been achieved, finger dressing can be applied over cream and changed every 2–3 days
- (Leg ulcers/pressure injuries) cream should fill ulcer cavity, then be covered with absorbent pad/dressing and covered with compression bandaging (leg ulcers) if needed
- (Hand burn) after applying cream, whole hand can be enclosed in glove or clear plastic bag, then closed at the wrist. Patient should be encouraged to move fingers and hand
- not recommended for leg ulcers or pressure injuries with high levels of exudate
- contraindicated in those with known hypersensitivity to sulfonamides, silver, cetyl alcohol or propylene glycol

Avoid use during the last month of pregnancy if possible because of the theoretical risk of kernicterus, jaundice and haemolytic anaemia in the neonate.

Use with caution in patients with impaired renal function, especially those undergoing prolonged treatment for extensive burns, as systemic absorption of the drug may occur. Monitor use.

TRIMETHOPRIM

Trade names
Alprim, Trimethoprim Viatris, Trimethoprim WGR, Triprim

Available form
Tablets: 300 mg

Action
- selectively interferes with bacterial synthesis of nucleic acids and proteins by binding to bacterial dihydrofolate reductase enzyme
- half-life 8–12 hours
- not active against *Pseudomonas* spp.

Use
- treatment of acute urinary tract infection (not caused by *Pseudomonas* spp.)
- prostatitis
- prophylaxis of urinary tract infection

Dose
- (Acute, uncomplicated UTI women) 300 mg orally nightly with food for 3 days (preferably before bedtime to maximise urinary concentration)
- (Acute, uncomplicated UTI men) 300 mg orally nightly with food for 7 days (preferably before bedtime to maximise urinary concentration)
- (Acute, uncomplicated UTI child) 3–4 mg/kg orally (maximum 150 mg) twice daily for 3 days.
- (Recurrent UTI) 300 mg orally nightly with food for 10–14 days (preferably before bedtime to maximise urinary concentration)
- (Prophylaxis UTI adult) 150 mg orally nightly

- (Prophylaxis UTI child) 2 mg/kg orally (maximum 150 mg) nightly
- (Prostatitis) 300 mg orally nightly with food for 14 days (preferably before bedtime to maximise urinary concentration) (4 weeks for chronic)

Adverse effects
- rash, pruritus, exfoliative dermatitis
- nausea, vomiting, epigastric pain, glossitis
- blood dyscrasias
- fever
- elevated liver enzymes, bilirubin and serum creatinine
- hyperkalaemia, hyponatraemia
- (Rare) severe skin reactions, hypersensitivity

Interactions
- may potentiate anticoagulant action of warfarin; therefore INR should be closely monitored, especially when starting or stopping therapy
- folate supplements may be required if given with other antifolate drugs such as methotrexate
- serum levels may be decreased by rifampicin
- increased risk of nephrotoxicity if given with ciclosporin
- hyponatraemia may occur if given with diuretics
- increased risk of myelosuppression and megaloblastic anaemia if given with methotrexate or pyrimethamine
- may increase serum level of dapsone while having own serum level increased by dapsone
- increased risk of severe hyperkalaemia if given with ACE inhibitors, prednisolone or potassium-sparing diuretics
- may increase serum levels of phenytoin and digoxin
- may decrease excretion and therefore increase serum levels of zidovudine and lamivudine, increasing risk of haematological toxicity
- may interfere with assay for creatinine (produces overestimation) and serum methotrexate assay

Nursing considerations/Cautions
- any folate deficiency should be corrected before starting therapy with trimethoprim
- monthly blood counts are recommended if trimethoprim therapy is long term
- serum potassium should be monitored during therapy (especially in those with kidney insufficiency or taking agents that increase potassium levels)
- therapy should be stopped if any rash appears
- caution if used in the elderly or in those with blood dyscrasias, actual/potential folate deficiency or impaired liver or kidney function
- not recommended in those with porphyria
- contraindicated in those with severe kidney impairment (creatinine clearance (CrCl) < 10 mL/min unless plasma trimethoprim levels can be monitored regularly during therapy), severe haematological disorders or megaloblastic anaemia due to folate deficiency, or trimethoprim hypersensitivity
- see also General Nursing considerations/Cautions for antibacterial agents (p. 149)

Patient education
- patient should be advised to immediately seek medical advice if any of the following occur:
    - rash (especially if there is any blistering or peeling)
    - sore throat, mouth ulcers, fever, chills
- advise patient to take tablets with food to minimise gastric irritation

ANTIBACTERIAL AGENTS

- see also General Patient education for antibacterial agents (p. 150)

 Tablet can be dispersed in water, or crushed and mixed with spoonful of yoghurt or apple puree.

 Avoid use in the first trimester because of the risk of congenital anomalies (e.g. cardiovascular and neural tube defects, oral clefts) and miscarriage. Short courses in the second and third trimesters may be safe, but should be used only when the benefits outweigh the risks.

 Generally considered safe to use; however, observe the infant for potential adverse effects such as vomiting, diarrhoea or rash. May be used when the benefits outweigh the risks.

 Use with caution in patients with renal impairment, as it can lead to elevated serum creatinine and an increased risk of hyperkalaemia, requiring careful dose adjustment or avoidance in severe cases to prevent toxicity. It is contraindicated if CrCl < 10 mL/min, and the dose should be reduced if CrCl is 10−30 mL/min (the manufacturer does not recommend its use if CrCl < 15 mL/min).

Available in combination with
- see trimethoprim + sulfamthoxazole combination (p. 222)

ANTICOAGULANTS AND ANTITHROMBOTIC AGENTS

Normally, blood vessels are kept free of thrombi by maintaining a balance between deposition of fibrinogen and its breakdown (fibrinolysis). When this balance is shifted towards fibrinogen deposition, the result is the formation of a blood clot (thrombus), which may then threaten to occlude the vessel. Arterial thrombi usually form as a result of damage to the endothelial layer of the vessel wall, whereas venous thrombi are caused by venous stasis, which allows platelets and fibrin to build up. Arterial thrombi are composed mainly of platelets with little fibrin, so antiplatelet agents (p. 817) are more appropriate treatments because they are able to prevent platelet aggregation and clot formation. Venous thrombi are mainly composed of fibrin and red blood cells, with fewer platelets. This composition makes them particularly responsive to treatment with anticoagulants (Hogg & Weitz 2018; Knights et al 2023).

Anticoagulants are used in the prophylaxis and treatment of thromboembolic disorders, including the prevention of fibrin deposition and extension of existing thrombus. However, they do not dissolve existing clots or restore tissue ischaemic injury caused by clot occlusion of blood vessel. Anticoagulant agents are divided into:
- heparin and the low molecular weight heparins (e.g. dalteparin, enoxaparin, danaparoid, nadroparin) (these are the drugs of choice for rapid anticoagulation)
- vitamin K antagonists (e.g. warfarin)
- agents that directly inhibit thrombin (e.g. bivalirudin, dabigatran, argatroban)
- direct inhibitors of factor Xa (e.g. rivaroxaban, apixaban) (Knights et al 2023).

The main side-effect of anticoagulants is bleeding, which can range from mild to severe. Administering and maintaining the correct dosage within the therapeutic range is achieved by regular monitoring of blood concentrations. These blood tests use plasma in which clotting has been prevented by a calcium-sequestering agent (citrate or oxalate). Calcium and an activating agent are then added to the blood, and the time for clot formation is measured (Knights et al 2023). Several tests measure different parts of the clotting cascade, including:

ANTICOAGULANTS AND ANTITHROMBOTIC AGENTS

- *prothrombin time* (PT) measures factor VII and the common pathway in the clotting cascade. Thromboplastin is used as the activating agent. Because the thromboplastin reagent varies in sensitivity with each new batch, the standard way to report PT is as a ratio of patient PT to control PT, raised to the power of the International Sensitivity Index (ISI), which is established for each new batch of thromboplastin. This ratio is called the International Normalised Ratio (INR) and is used to regulate warfarin dosage
- *activated partial thromboplastin time* (aPTT) measures the extent to which heparin inhibits thrombin, factor Xa and factor IXa. aPTT is used to monitor heparin therapy, although low-dose heparin therapy does not require monitoring (Knights et al 2023).

General Patient education for anticoagulants

- patient should be advised to seek medical advice immediately if there is:
  - any unexplained/prolonged bleeding, bruising or swelling
  - bleeding from gums when brushing teeth
  - unusual nosebleeds
  - oozing from wounds
  - coughing or vomiting blood
  - blood in urine or stool
  - unusual pain (especially in back or stomach)
- patient should be advised of the importance of wearing a MedicAlert or other medical alert-type bracelet or pendant informing others of the anticoagulant therapy (especially if the person is unconscious or unable to speak). This information can also be included on the patient's mobile phone under 'medical ID'
- advise patient to inform dentist of anticoagulant therapy if any dental procedure is planned because of the risk of local bleeding
- warn patient not to drive or operate machinery if dizziness occurs
- patient should be instructed to seek advice from doctor or pharmacist before taking OTC analgesics (including aspirin)

HEPARIN and LOW MOLECULAR WEIGHT HEPARINS (LMWHs)

HEPARIN
Trade names
DBL Heparin Sodium Injection, Heparin Sodium Injection, Heparinised Saline Injection

Available forms
Ampoules: 1000 IU/1 mL, 5000 IU/0.2 mL, 5000 IU/1 mL, 5000 IU/5 mL, 25,000 IU/5 mL

Action
- complex proteoglycan consisting of protein core with repeating disaccharide units attached, varying in molecular weight from 5000 to 40,000
- combines with antithrombin III (heparin co-factor), inactivating factor X and inhibiting the conversion of prothrombin to thrombin
- if thrombus exists, heparin inhibits further coagulation by inactivating thrombin, preventing conversion of fibrinogen to fibrin

- prevents stable clot formation by inhibiting activation of fibrin-stabilising factor
- sourced from pig mucosa
- onset of action is immediate (IV) or 20—60 minutes (SC); acts for 3—6 hours and trebles blood-clotting time to 15—30 minutes
- half-life is dose dependent and generally 1—6 hours
- not absorbed from the GI tract; therefore ineffective if given orally
- prevents further clotting but does not affect existing clot
- does not cross the placenta or enter breastmilk
- prolonged aPTT in those over 60 years

Use
- prophylaxis and treatment of thromboembolic disorders (e.g. deep vein thrombosis (DVT), pulmonary embolus (PE) or thrombophlebitis)
- prophylaxis of thromboembolic complications arising from heart and vascular surgery
- anticoagulant in blood collected for transfusion or laboratory tests
- extracorporeal circulation (heart/lung and renal dialysis machines)
- patency of IV devices (heparinised saline)

Dose
- (DVT prophylaxis postoperatively) 5000 units by SC injection 2 hours before surgery, then 8—12 hourly for 7—10 days or until patient is fully mobile **OR**
- (DVT/PE treatment) initially 5000 units by IV bolus, then 20,000—40,000 units in sodium chloride 0.9% 1 L over 24 hours by continuous IV infusion **OR**
- (DVT/PE treatment) initially 10,000 units IV bolus followed by 5000—10,000 units 4—6-hourly (intermittent IV injection) **OR**
- (DVT/PE treatment) 5000 units IV, then 10,000 units by deep SC injection 8-hourly or 15,000 units by deep SC injection 12-hourly **OR**
- (Heart and blood vessel surgery) initially not less than 150 units/kg (300 units/kg may be used for surgery duration < 60 minutes or 400 units/kg > 60 minutes) **OR**
- (IV device patency) 10—50 units 4-hourly

Adverse effects
- haemorrhage (ranging from mild ecchymosis to severe bleeding)
- thrombocytopenia
- osteoporosis (4—12 weeks after prolonged, high-dose heparin therapy)
- hyperkalaemia
- elevated liver enzymes
- (SC injection site) local irritation, erythema, mild pain, haematoma, ulceration
- (High dose, prolonged therapy) suppression of kidney function
- hypoaldosteronism (rare), rebound hyperlipidaemia (when heparin is stopped), reversible hypereosinophilia
- (Rare) skin necrosis at the injection site, alopecia (delayed, transient), priapism, heparin-induced thrombocytopenia (HIT), heparin-induced thrombocytopenia and thrombosis (HITT) (also called white clot syndrome), delayed HIT, delayed HITT, allergic reactions (e.g. pruritus, urticaria, chills, fever, headache)

Interactions
- decreased anticoagulant effect when given with antihistamines, digoxin, ascorbic acid (vitamin C), nicotine or tetracyclines
- decreased prothrombin time may occur if given simultaneously with IV glyceryl trinitrate; therefore should be given with caution, especially when starting or stopping therapy
- increased risk of hypoprothrombinaemia if given with large doses of aspirin
- increased anticoagulant effect and risk of bleeding when given with abciximab, alcohol (heavy use), alprostadil, alteplase, antiplatelet agents, asparaginase (colaspase), aspirin, clopidogrel, contrast media (some), corticosteroids (systemic), dextran, dipyridamole, epoprostenol, etacrynic acid, hydroxychloroquine,

ANTICOAGULANTS AND ANTITHROMBOTIC AGENTS

ibuprofen, indomethacin, NSAIDs, penicillins (high dose), probenecid, propylthiouracil, reteplase, rivaroxaban, sodium valproate, tenecteplase, ticlopidine, tirofiban, warfarin or vitamin K antagonists
* hyperkalaemia may occur if given with ACE inhibitors, potassium-sparing diuretics or potassium supplements; therefore potassium levels should be monitored regularly, especially in those who are at risk of hyperkalaemia
* may antagonise effects of insulin, corticosteroids and ACTH
* may interfere with aminotransferase determination of myocardial infarction, pulmonary embolus or liver disease; therefore results should be interpreted with caution

Nursing considerations/Cautions

Subcutaneous injection technique
* use care with SC administration to avoid local haematoma formation and ensure uniform absorption
* use a tuberculin syringe and a short-gauge (25—26-gauge) needle
* injection site is the subcutaneous fat of the anterior abdominal wall or anterior thighs, given at an angle perpendicular to the skin surface
* inject slowly at the rate of 1 mL/minute to prevent pain
* do not rub site of injection
* rotate and document the injection sites regularly

General
* heparin sodium may be given IV or SC
* to prevent painful haematoma formation, avoid giving IM
* all unnecessary procedures that might cause vascular damage (except IV injections) should be avoided if possible
* patient should be closely monitored for signs of spinal haematoma (e.g. midline back pain, numbness, weakness, lower limb paralysis, bowel/bladder dysfunction) if they have a spinal puncture or insertion/removal of epidural/spinal needle/catheter. Risk of haematoma formation is increased if the patient is taking NSAIDs, antiplatelet agents or other anticoagulants, or if the procedure is repeated or traumatic
* be alert to the early signs of overdose by looking for bruising and testing the urine daily for blood (therapeutic dose only)
* platelet counts, haematocrit and occult blood test should be measured before starting and regularly throughout therapy
* if platelet count $< 100,000$ mm^3 or recurrent thrombosis occurs, therapy should be stopped and an alternative anticoagulant considered
* heparin dose is adjusted to keep the aPTT at 1.5—2 times the control value (or whole blood-clotting time 2.5—3 times control value)
* oral anticoagulants may be started 3—5 days before gradually reducing and then discontinuing heparin
* when given with warfarin, and prothrombin time is required, at least 5 hours from last IV dose or 24 hours from last SC heparin dose should elapse before blood is drawn
* there are two types of thrombocytopenia which can result from heparin therapy:
  * an acute mild form occurring within 1—4 days of starting heparin, which usually resolves without stopping therapy
  * a more serious delayed onset form that occurs within 7—11 days of starting heparin and necessitates ceasing therapy
* heparin-induced thrombocytopenia (HIT) and thrombosis (HITT) (also referred to as 'white clot syndrome') starts as a heparin-induced antibody-mediated reaction resulting from irreversible aggregation of platelets and progressing to new thrombus formation with thrombocytopenia induced. It may lead to thromboembolic complications such as skin necrosis, gangrene, DVT and

- pulmonary embolism. HIT and HITT can occur as a delayed reaction several weeks after heparin is stopped
- (Heparinised saline) IV device should be flushed with sodium chloride 0.9% before and after administration of heparinised saline
- when preparing infusion bags, it is important to invert the bag at least 6 times to ensure even distribution of heparin throughout IV fluid
- monitor IV infusion rate closely using an infusion pump
- heparin infusion should be administered alone as there are many incompatibilities
- heparin therapy should be continued for several days after therapeutic aPTT level has been reached and then stopped (without tapering)
- dose should be reduced or stopped if the person is having an oral surgical (dental) procedure
- heparin overdose resulting in severe bleeding should be treated with protamine sulfate (a small basic protein that counteracts the anticoagulant effect of heparin by neutralising its acidic charge) (see Antidotes, antagonists and chelating agents, p. 359). Minor bleeding can be managed by stopping heparin
- derived from animal source; therefore should be used with caution in those with a history of allergy or asthma
- caution if used in those with diabetes mellitus or renal insufficiency owing to increased risk of hyperkalaemia occurring
- caution if used in those with fever, thrombosis, thrombophlebitis, infection (with thrombosing tendencies), myocardial infarction, cancer, antithrombin III deficiency or post surgery as there is an increased risk of heparin resistance occurring
- caution if used in those with continuous tube drainage of stomach/small intestine, mild-to-moderate liver/kidney disease, hypertension, history of ulcers (gastric or duodenal), retinal vascular disease, hereditary antithrombin III deficiency or if over the age of 60 years (particularly women)
- (Heparinised saline) not recommended in neonates
- contraindicated in those with active or potential bleeding or bleeding disorders (e.g. haemophilia, vitamin C deficiency, bleeding haemorrhoids), threatened abortion, immediately postpartum, subacute/acute bacterial endocarditis, severe hypertension, GI ulcerative disorders (at risk of bleeding), advanced kidney/liver disease, during or immediately post-surgery/injury (especially to brain, eye or spinal cord and also including spinal puncture and spinal/epidural anaesthesia), shock, severe thrombocytopenia, previous heparin-induced thrombocytopenia or haemorrhagic stroke, or if there are inadequate laboratory facilities to monitor blood clotting regularly
- heparin is commonly sourced from pig mucosa, which can cause allergic reactions in individuals sensitive to pork products

Patient education

- see General Patient education for anticoagulants (p. 237)

 Although heparin does not cause fetal malformations, there is an increased risk of fetal loss and prematurity associated with maternal haemorrhage if given in last trimester of pregnancy or the immediate postpartum period

 Caution and dose reduction required if used in those with liver or renal impairment

 Dose reduction and careful monitoring required in those over 60 years (especially women)

LOW MOLECULAR WEIGHT HEPARINS

DALTEPARIN
Trade names
Fragmin

Available forms
Fixed single dose syringe: 2500 IU/0.2 mL, 5000 IU/0.2 mL, 12,500 IU/0.5 mL, 15,000 IU/0.6 mL, 18,000 IU/0.72 mL;
Graduated single-dose syringe: 10, 000 IU/1 mL

Action
- low molecular weight heparin (LMWH, a smaller fragment of heparin prepared from unfractionated heparin using enzymatic or chemical methods, with a molecular weight about a third of heparin)
- increases neutralisation rate of factor Xa mainly, but also factor XIIa and kallikrein by antithrombin
- little effect on platelet function and adhesion compared with heparin
- some antithrombotic properties may be caused by an action on the vessel wall or fibrinolytic system
- half-life is 2 hours (IV) or 3–4 hours (SC)

Use
- prophylactically against thrombotic complications of haemodialysis
- treatment of acute deep vein thrombosis (DVT)
- treatment of symptomatic venous thromboembolism (VTE) or to reduce recurrence in those with solid tumour cancers
- treatment of unstable coronary artery disease (CAD) (e.g. unstable angina and non-Q wave myocardial infarction (also called non-ST elevation myocardial infarction (NSTEMI))
- prophylactically against thromboembolic complications during the perioperative and postoperative periods

Dose
Acute DVT treatment
- initially 100 IU/kg twice daily SC, or 100 IU/kg over 12 hours by continuous IV infusion, and then adjusted according to serum levels of prothrombin complex factors (factors II, VII, IX and X), usually about 5 days

Treatment of symptomatic VTE in those with solid tumour cancers
- 200 IU/kg SC daily (month 1), then 150 IU/kg SC daily (months 2—6) (daily maximum 18,000 IU)

Anticoagulation for haemodialysis
- (Haemodialysis > 4 hours, chronic renal failure, no bleeding risk) 30—40 IU/kg IV bolus followed by 10—15 IU/kg/hour IV infusion **OR**
- (Haemodialysis of 4 hours maximum, chronic renal failure) as above, or 5000 IU IV bolus only **OR**
- (Haemodialysis, acute renal failure, high bleeding risk) 5—10 IU/kg IV bolus followed by 4—5 IU/kg/hour IV infusion

Thromboprophylaxis (surgery)
- 2500 IU SC 1—2 hours before surgery, followed by 2500 IU SC 12 hours later then daily for 5—7 days until patient is mobile

Thromboprophylaxis (general surgery associated with high thrombosis risk)
- 5000 IU SC the evening before surgery, followed by 5000 IU SC the following evenings for 5—7 days until patient is mobile **OR**
- 2500 IU SC 1—2 hours before surgery, followed by 2500 IU SC 12 hours later, then 5000 IU SC each morning for 5—7 days until patient is mobile

Thromboprophylaxis (orthopaedic surgery e.g. hip replacement)
- 5000 IU SC the evening before surgery, followed by 5000 IU SC the following evenings for 5 weeks **OR**
- 2500 IU SC 1—2 hours before surgery, followed by 2500 IU SC 8—12 hours later,

then 5000 IU SC each morning for 5 weeks

Unstable CAD
- 120 IU/kg SC twice daily for 6 days (maximum 10,000 IU/12 hours) with low-dose aspirin

Adverse effects
- bleeding tendency (especially at high doses), mild thrombocytopenia
- transient elevation of liver transaminases
- hyperkalaemia
- (Uncommon) allergic reactions, rash, urticaria, pruritus
- (Long term) osteoporosis
- (Injection site) subcutaneous haemorrhage or haematoma, pain

Interactions
- anticoagulant effect increased by aspirin, cytostatic agents, dextran, dipyridamole, etacrynic acid, fibrinolytic agents, NSAIDs, probenecid, vitamin K antagonists
- anticoagulant effect decreased by antihistamines, digoxin, tetracyclines and ascorbic acid
- increased risk of hyperkalaemia if given with potassium-sparing agents, potassium supplements or angiotensin converting enzyme (ACE) inhibitors; therefore potassium levels should be monitored during therapy

Nursing considerations/Cautions
- not interchangeable with heparin or other LMWHs
- should not be given IM
- doses above 5000 IU increase bleeding tendency
- new patients undergoing haemodialysis should have anti-Xa concentrations monitored during first few weeks
- routine monitoring of anti-Xa is not required (unless the patient has cancer, kidney or liver failure, is very thin/morbidly obese, pregnant or is at increased risk of bleeding), but platelet concentrations should be measured before starting therapy and regularly throughout, for the early detection of thrombocytopenia
- the patient should be closely monitored for signs of spinal haematoma (e.g. midline back pain, numbness, weakness, lower limb paralysis, bowel/bladder dysfunction) if they have a spinal puncture or insertion/removal of epidural/spinal needle/catheter. Risk of haematoma formation is increased if the patient is taking NSAIDs, antiplatelet agents or other anticoagulants, or if the procedure is repeated or traumatic. Insertion/removal of an epidural or spinal catheter should be delayed 10–24 hours (depending on dose) after last administration
- overdose treated with protamine sulfate at a dose of 1 mg protamine for 100 anti-Xa IU dalteparin. If aPTT remains prolonged 2–4 hours after first protamine infusion, a second infusion (0.5 mg protamine/100 anti-Xa IU dalteparin) can be given
- (High dose) caution if used in those who have undergone recent surgery
- caution if used in those with a history of osteoporosis or spontaneous fractures
- caution if used in those with uncontrolled hypertension, hypertensive or diabetic retinopathy, primary or metastatic brain tumours, severe liver/kidney insufficiency, osteoporosis or spontaneous fractures, recent surgery, patients with cancer, high risk of bleeding, platelet disorder, thrombocytopenia or hereditary antithrombin III deficiency
- caution if used in those with diabetes mellitus, chronic renal failure or pre-existing metabolic acidosis owing to an increased risk of hyperkalaemia
- not recommended for prosthetic heart valve prophylaxis
- contraindicated in those with hypersensitivity to heparin or other LMWHs, or pork products
- contraindicated in those with a history of heparin-induced thrombocytopenia,

ANTICOAGULANTS AND ANTITHROMBOTIC AGENTS

cerebral haemorrhage, GI ulceration, ulcerative colitis, severe coagulation disorder, acute/subacute bacterial endocarditis, sympathetic block, spinal/epidural puncture (not contraindicated in doses less than 5000 IU), surgery (brain, spinal cord, eyes, ears), haemorrhagic stroke or severe hypertension

Patient education
- see General Patient education for anticoagulants (p. 37)

Considered safe, it does not cross the placenta.

While dalteparin is safe for the developing fetus, there is an increased risk of complications such as fetal loss and prematurity, which can arise from maternal haemorrhage. This risk is a concern with all anticoagulants, as they increase the likelihood of bleeding.

Considered safe. LMWHs, due to their large molecular size and properties, are minimally transferred into breastmilk.

Use cautiously if renal function is impaired, as they are primarily eliminated by the kidneys and can accumulate, increasing the risk of bleeding. Check anti-factor Xa levels to ensure therapeutic levels are maintained without reaching toxic levels.

DANAPAROID
Trade name
Orgaran

Available form
Ampoule: 750 antifactor Xa units/0.6 mL

Action
- heparinoids (not a low molecular weight heparin (LMWH))
- inhibits thrombus formation
- little effect on platelet function and adhesion
- peak activity 4—5 hours, half-life 25 hours (SC) or 7 hours (IV)

Use
- prophylaxis of venous thromboembolism (VTE) after surgery (general or orthopaedic)

Dose
- 750 anti-Xa units SC twice daily for 7—10 days

Adverse effects
- bleeding
- hypersensitivity (occasionally)
- (Rare) thrombocytopenia, changes in liver enzymes
- (Injection site) bruising and/or pain

Interactions
- caution when used with other anticoagulants, antiplatelet agents, NSAIDs or corticosteroids
- prolonged bleeding time may occur if given with aspirin
- may cause unreliable results if blood is taken within 5 hours of administration for prothrombin monitoring

Nursing considerations/Cautions
- LMWHs and danaparoid are not interchangeable
- should not be given IM
- rotate SC injection sites
- routine clotting assays are not suitable if anticoagulant monitoring is required
- if given preoperatively, last dose should be 1—4 hours before procedure
- the patient should be closely monitored for signs of spinal haematoma (e.g. midline back pain, numbness, weakness, lower limb paralysis, bowel/bladder dysfunction) if they have a spinal puncture or insertion/removal of an epidural/spinal needle/catheter. Risk of haematoma formation is increased if the patient is taking NSAIDs, antiplatelet agents or other anticoagulants, or if the procedure is repeated or traumatic
- platelet count should be monitored before starting and during therapy for the early detection of thrombocytopenia

- caution if used in those with moderate kidney or liver impairment (with impaired haemostasis), GI tract lesions or other organs/sites at risk of bleeding
- contains sulfite, therefore is contraindicated in those with known hypersensitivity to sulfites
- contraindicated in those with diabetic retinopathy, acute/subacute bacterial endocarditis, severe hypertension, severe kidney or liver insufficiency, history of heparin-induced thrombocytopenia, uncontrolled active bleeding, severe gastric or duodenal ulceration (unless this is the reason for surgery), haemophilia or other bleeding disorders

Patient education

- see General Patient education for anticoagulants (p. 237)

Considered safe.

Considered safe.

Use cautiously if CrCl is < 30 mL/min. Regularly check anti-factor Xa levels. Adjust dosage based on monitoring results.

ENOXAPARIN
Trade names
Clexane, Clexane Forte, Exarane, Exarane Forte

Available forms
Prefilled syringe: 20 mg/0.2 mL, 40 mg/0.4 mL, 60 mg/0.6 mL, 80 mg/0.8 mL, 100 mg/mL, 120 mg/0.8 mL, 150 mg/mL

Action
- low molecular weight heparin (LMWH, a smaller fragment of heparin prepared from unfractionated heparin using enzymatic or chemical methods, with a molecular weight about a third of heparin)
- binds to and accelerates antithrombin III action
- inactivates factor Xa and factor IIa (thrombin), leading to decreased thrombin formation, preventing fibrin clot formation
- has four times the effect on factor Xa compared with factor IIa
- minimal effect on bleeding

Use
- prophylaxis of venous thromboembolism (VTE) after surgery (general, orthopaedic) or bedridden acutely ill patients
- prevention of thrombosis in extracorporeal circulation during haemodialysis
- treatment of established deep vein thrombosis (DVT)
- unstable angina and non-Q wave myocardial infarction (with aspirin)
- treatment of acute ST segment elevation myocardial infarction (STEMI) (adjunct with fibrinolytics)

Dose
- (Prophylaxis of venous thrombosis — high risk) 40 mg SC once daily for 7–10 days, initial dose 12 hours before surgery **OR**
- (Prophylaxis of venous thrombosis — medium risk) 20 mg SC once daily for 7–10 days, initial dose 2 hours before surgery **OR**
- (Prophylaxis of venous thrombosis — medical patient) 40 mg SC once daily for 6–14 days or until patient is fully mobile **OR**
- (Prolonged thromboembolic prophylaxis, e.g. total hip replacement) 40 mg SC once daily for 30 days postoperatively **OR**
- (Treatment of DVT) 1 mg/kg SC twice daily or 1.5 mg/kg SC once daily for at least 5 days **OR**
- (Haemodialysis) 1 mg/kg into the arterial line of the dialysis unit at start of session, with 0.5–1 mg/kg fresh addition if fibrin rings form and depending on time before end of dialysis **OR**
- (Haemodialysis, high risk of haemorrhage) 0.5 mg/kg (double vascular

ANTICOAGULANTS AND ANTITHROMBOTIC AGENTS

access) or 0.75 mg/kg (single vascular access) **OR**
- (Unstable angina and non-Q wave myocardial infarction) 1 mg/kg SC 12-hourly (with aspirin 100–325 mg daily) for 2–8 days **OR**
- (Treatment of STEMI) 30 mg as IV bolus along with 1 mg/kg SC, then 1 mg/kg SC 12-hourly (with fibrinolytic therapy) for 8 days or until hospital discharge

Adverse effects
- haemorrhage, anaemia, mild transient thrombocytopenia
- nausea, diarrhoea
- fever
- peripheral oedema
- urticaria, pruritus, erythema
- elevated liver enzymes
- confusion, headache
- (Uncommon) allergic reaction
- (Injection site) haematoma, pain, swelling, bleeding
- (Rare) hyperkalaemia, alopecia
- (Prolonged therapy) osteoporosis

Interactions
- other drugs (e.g. anticoagulants, fibrinolytics, NSAIDs, aspirin, aspirin-containing preparations, ticlopidine, dextran, antiplatelet agents, clopidogrel, corticosteroids) affecting haemostasis should be withdrawn before starting therapy
- increased risk of hyperkalaemia if given with potassium-sparing agents, potassium supplements or angiotensin-converting enzyme (ACE) inhibitors; therefore potassium levels should be monitored during therapy

Nursing considerations/Cautions
- LMWHs are not interchangeable
- should not be given IM
- (IV) administer alone, ensuring IV lines are well flushed with sodium chloride 0.9% or dextrose 5% before and after administration
- if a patient has percutaneous coronary revascularisation procedure, 0.3 mg/kg IV bolus should be given if last enoxaparin dose was > 8 hours before balloon inflation. If a closure device is used, the sheath should be removed immediately. If manual compression is used to achieve haemostasis, the sheath should be removed 6 hours after last dose. Enoxaparin should not be administered within 6–8 hours of sheath removal. Site should be closely monitored for any signs of bleeding or haematoma formation
- (Acute STEMI treatment) enoxaparin should be given between 15 minutes before and 30 minutes after the start of fibrinolytic therapy. Aspirin (100–300 mg) should also be started (unless contraindicated)
- therapy should be ceased for 12–24 hours (depending on dose) before the insertion/removal of epidural/spinal needle/catheter and next dose given at least 4 hours after the procedure. If blood was present during needle/catheter placement, the next dose should be delayed by 24 hours. Site should be closely monitored for any signs of spinal haematoma. The patient should be advised to immediately report any numbness/weakness of lower limbs, back pain or bowel/bladder dysfunction
- the patient should be closely monitored for signs of spinal haematoma (e.g. midline back pain, numbness, weakness, lower limb paralysis, bowel/bladder dysfunction) if they have a spinal puncture or insertion/removal of epidural/spinal needle/catheter. Risk of haematoma formation is increased if the patient is taking NSAIDs, antiplatelet agents or other anticoagulants, or if the procedure is repeated or traumatic
- (DVT treatment) therapy with warfarin should be started within 72 hours of commencing enoxaparin and continued for at least 5 days and until INR is 2.0–3.0
- should not be mixed with other injections or infusions

- platelet count should be monitored before starting and throughout therapy. If counts fall to 30—50% of pre-therapy level or below 100,000/mm^3, the drug should be withdrawn
- when therapy is for DVT, warfarin is usually started 72 hours after enoxaparin and the two continued until the INR is 2.0—3.0
- routine monitoring of blood clotting is generally not required
- SC injection sites should be rotated
- SC injection site should not be rubbed after administration
- the entire length of needle should be injected at 90 degrees to the skin, which has been gently pinched between thumb and finger and held throughout injection
- prefilled syringe needles are coated with silicone to enhance ease of skin penetration. Needles should not be wiped or enoxaparin allowed to crystallise as this will damage the silicone coating
- air bubble should not be expelled from prefilled syringe before injection
- if overdosage occurs, it may be neutralised using protamine sulfate as IV infusion (1 mg protamine sulfate will neutralise 1 mg enoxaparin) if enoxaparin was given in the previous 8 hours. If > 8 hours, 0.5 mg protamine sulfate is used for each 1 mg enoxaparin. If > 12 hours, protamine may not be necessary (depending on clinical circumstances)
- close monitoring for thromboembolism is recommended if patient has BMI > 30 kg/m^2
- caution if used in women weighing less than 45 kg or men weighing less than 57 kg because of the increased risk of bleeding
- caution if used in those with diabetes, chronic kidney failure or pre-existing metabolic acidosis because of the increased risk of hyperkalaemia
- caution if used in those with bacterial endocarditis, congenital/acquired bleeding disorders, active ulceration, GI disease, haemorrhagic stroke, recent surgery (brain, eye, spine), uncontrolled hypertension, bleeding disorders, liver impairment, diabetic retinopathy, recent ischaemic stroke or impaired haemostasis
- caution if used in those with kidney impairment, as clearance is decreased resulting in increased risk of bleeding
- not recommended for thromboembolism prophylaxis in those with prosthetic heart valves
- contraindicated in those with hypersensitivity to heparin or other LMWHs
- contraindicated in those with a history of heparin-induced thrombocytopenia (within last 10 years or with antibodies present), thrombocytopenia (with antibodies), cerebral haemorrhage, gastric ulcer, ulcerative colitis, severe coagulation/bleeding disorders, acute/subacute bacterial endocarditis, spinal/epidural puncture, surgery (brain, spinal cord, eyes, ears), conditions with bleeding tendencies, haemorrhagic stroke or severe hypertension

Patient education

- instruct the patient in self-administration. This should include information on injection technique (under the skin and not into muscle), rotation of injection sites, not rubbing site after injection, correct storage and disposal of used syringes
- see also General Patient education for anticoagulants (p. 237)

Considered safe, it does not cross the placenta. While safe for the developing fetus, there is an increased risk of complications such as fetal loss and prematurity, which can arise from maternal haemorrhage. This risk is a concern with all anticoagulants, as they increase the likelihood of bleeding.

Considered safe. LMWHs, due to their large molecular size and properties, are minimally transferred into breastmilk.

 Use cautiously if renal function is impaired, as they are primarily eliminated by the kidneys and can accumulate, increasing the risk of bleeding. Check anti-factor Xa levels to ensure therapeutic levels are maintained without reaching toxic levels.

NADROPARIN CALCIUM

Trade names
Fraxiparine, Fraxiparine Forte

Available forms
Ungraduated prefilled syringe: 2850 IU anti-Xa/0.3 mL, 3800 IU anti-Xa/0.4 mL;
Graduated prefilled syringe: 5700 IU anti-Xa/0.6 mL, 7600 IU anti-Xa/0.8 mL, 9500 IU anti-Xa/mL, 11, 400 IU anti-Xa/0.6 mL, 15,200 IU anti-Xa/0.8 mL, 19, 000 anti-Xa/mL

Action
- low molecular weight heparin (LMWH) with a high ratio of anti-Xa activity to anti-IIa compared with unfractionated heparin
- has both immediate and prolonged antithrombotic actions
- high affinity for antithrombin III, leading to a rapid inhibition of factor Xa (and also factor IIa to a lesser extent) contributing to antithrombotic activity
- also activates fibrinolysis via release of tissue plasminogen activator, decreases blood viscosity and increases platelet and granulocyte membrane fluidity

Use
- prophylaxis and treatment of deep vein thrombosis (DVT) associated with general and orthopaedic surgery
- prophylaxis of venous thromboembolism (VTE) in at-risk medical patients
- prevention of clotting during haemodialysis

Dose
- (DVT treatment) dose is weight dependent and based on 171 anti-Xa IU/kg SC once daily for 10 days (Fraxiparine Forte) **OR**
- (DVT prophylaxis — general surgery) 2850 anti-Xa IU/0.3 mL SC 2—4 hours before surgery, then daily on subsequent days for at least 7 days until patient is ambulant (Fraxiparine) **OR**
- (DVT prophylaxis — orthopaedic surgery) dose is weight dependent and based on 38 anti-Xa IU/kg SC starting 12 hours before and after surgery, then once daily to third postoperative day, then increasing dose by 50% from fourth postoperative day for at least 10 days and until patient is ambulant (Fraxiparine) **OR**
- (DVT treatment) dose is weight dependent and based on 86 anti-Xa IU/kg SC twice daily for 10 days (Fraxiparine) **OR**
- (Prevention of clotting during haemodialysis) 2850 anti-Xa IU/0.3 mL (weight < 50 kg), 3800 anti-Xa IU/0.4 mL (weight 50—69 kg) or 5700 anti-Xa IU/0.6 mL (weight ≥ 70 kg) injected into arterial line at start of dialysis (for sessions up to 4 hours). If session > 4 hours, an additional smaller dose may be given (Fraxiparine) **OR**
- (Thromboembolism prophylaxis in medical patients) 3800 anti-Xa IU/0.4 mL (weight ≤ 70 kg) or 5700 anti-Xa IU/0.6 mL (weight > 70 kg) started within 12—24 hours of admission and continued for up to 28 days

Adverse effects
- bleeding, anaemia
- transient elevated transaminases
- (Rare) thrombocytopenia, rash, urticaria, erythema, pruritus
- (Very rare) cutaneous necrosis (preceded by purpura and painful erythematous blotches), reversible hyperkalaemia, hypersensitivity
- (Injection site) haematoma, reaction

Interactions

- not recommended with aspirin, other salicylates, NSAIDs, ticlopidine or other antiplatelet agents owing to an increased risk of bleeding
- caution if given with dextrans or systemic corticosteroids
- if used with warfarin, nadroparin calcium should be continued until INR is stabilised at target level
- increased risk of hyperkalaemia if given with potassium-sparing agents, potassium supplements or angiotensin-converting enzyme (ACE) inhibitors; therefore potassium levels should be monitored during therapy

Nursing considerations/Cautions

- LMWHs are not interchangeable
- should not be given IM
- platelet count should be monitored before starting and throughout therapy
- (Medical patients) therapy should be started only if immobility/bed rest is expected to last longer than 3 days
- (DVT treatment) oral anticoagulant should be started as soon as possible (unless contraindicated), but nadroparin calcium should not be stopped until INR target level is reached and stabilised
- SC injection sites should be rotated (abdomen and thigh are recommended sites)
- (Fraxiparine ungraduated syringe) entire dose is injected
- (Fraxiparine ungraduated syringe) air bubble in syringe does not have to be removed before administration
- (Fraxiparine, Fraxiparine Forte graduated syringe) hold vertically with the needle uppermost and air bubble at the top of the syringe. Plunger should be advanced to the volume/dose required, expelling the air bubble and any excess
- the SC injection site should not be rubbed after administration
- a prefilled syringe may contain dry natural latex rubber, which can cause allergic reactions in those with latex hypersensitivity
- the patient should be closely monitored for signs of spinal haematoma (e.g. midline back pain, numbness, weakness, lower limb paralysis, bowel/bladder dysfunction) if they have a spinal puncture or insertion/removal of epidural/spinal needle/catheter. The risk of haematoma formation is increased if the patient is taking NSAIDs, antiplatelet agents or other anticoagulants, or if the procedure is repeated or traumatic. A minimum of 12—24 hours (depending on dose) should elapse before insertion/removal of the spinal/epidural catheter
- there is an increased risk of hyperkalaemia if used in those with pre-existing raised plasma potassium, diabetes mellitus, chronic renal failure or pre-existing metabolic acidosis or taking agents that cause hyperkalaemia (e.g. ACE inhibitors, NSAIDs). Potassium levels should be closely monitored
- in the event of serious overdosage, protamine sulfate can be given by slow IV injection (6 mg protamine sulfate neutralises about 950 IU anti-Xa (about 0.1 mL)), taking into account the time elapsed from the nadroparin injection. Fresh frozen plasma can be used if transfusion is needed
- caution if used in those at increased risk of bleeding, including kidney impairment, liver insufficiency, liver failure, severe arterial hypertension, history of peptic ulceration or other lesion likely to bleed, vascular disorder of chorio-retina, or postoperatively after brain, eye or spinal cord surgery
- caution if used in those with history of heparin-induced thrombocytopenia and should be used only if necessary. If used, the patient should be carefully monitored including daily platelet count assessment, as there is an increased risk of thrombocytopenia occurring

ANTICOAGULANTS AND ANTITHROMBOTIC AGENTS

- not recommended in those under 18 years
- contraindicated in those with a history of nadroparin-induced thrombocytopenia, increased risk of haemorrhage (including bleeding disorders), active bleeding or organic lesions likely to bleed (e.g. active peptic ulceration), infective endocarditis, haemorrhagic cerebrovascular accident or with severe kidney failure (creatinine clearance < 30 mL/min) receiving treatment for DVT

Patient education
- see General Patient education for anticoagulants (p. 237)

Limited human data. Not recommended unless benefits outweigh risks.

Limited human data. Avoid use.

Dosage adjustments may be needed in patients with reduced renal function.

VITAMIN K ANTAGONISTS

WARFARIN SODIUM
Trade names
Coumadin, Marevan

Available forms
Tablets: 1 mg, 2 mg, 3 mg, 5 mg

Action
- long-acting coumarin derivative
- interferes with vitamin K-dependent synthesis of prothrombin (factor II) and factors VII, IX and X in the liver, preventing the extension of established clot or the formation of new clot(s)
- also decreases synthesis of proteins C and S (vitamin K-dependent anticoagulant proteins)
- onset of action 24—48 hours, duration of action 2—5 days
- half-life 25—60 hours (average 40 hours)
- narrow therapeutic index
- some genetic variation in response and some patients may have a hereditary resistance to warfarin
- anticoagulant effect influenced by diet, drugs and disease states

Use
- prevention and management of venous thrombosis (e.g. deep vein thrombosis (DVT), pulmonary embolism (PE))
- prevention and management of thromboembolism in atrial fibrillation (AF), myocardial infarction or those with prosthetic heart valves
- adjunct in treatment of coronary occlusion

Dose
- initially 10 mg orally daily for 2—4 days, then maintenance dose of 2—10 mg daily based on INR

Adverse effects
- haemorrhage (mild, severe or life threatening, affecting any tissue or organ)
- nausea, vomiting, diarrhoea, flatulence/bloating, taste alteration, abdominal pain
- pruritus, rash, urticaria
- fatigue, lethargy, malaise, asthenia
- headache, dizziness
- alopecia
- elevated liver enzymes, hepatitis
- fever, chills, cold intolerance, paraesthesia
- (Rare) systemic cholesterol microemboli, purple toe syndrome (see Glossary), skin (or tissue) necrosis, hypersensitivity reaction, calciphylaxis
- (Long-term therapy, rare) tracheal or tracheo-bronchial calcification

Interactions
- alcohol (acute intoxication), allopurinol, alteplase, amiodarone, amoxicillin, aspirin, azithromycin, bivalirudin, cefazolin, cefoxitin, ceftriaxone, celecoxib, chloramphenicol, ciprofloxacin,

clarithromycin, clopidogrel, danazol, dextran, diazoxide, diclofenac, diflunisal, disopyramide, disulfiram, doxycycline, efavirenz, erythromycin, fenofibrate, fluconazole, fluorouracil, fluvastatin, gefitinib, gemcitabine, glucagon (high dose), heparin, ibuprofen, ifosfamide, indometacin, influenza virus vaccine, interferons, isoniazid, itraconazole, ketorolac, ketoprofen, levothyroxine, liothyronine, mefenamic acid, mefloquine, mesterolone, methylprednisolone, methyl salicylate ointment (topical), metronidazole, miconazole, nadroparin, nandrolone, naproxen, norfloxacin, olsalazine, omeprazole, oxandrolone, pentoxifylline (oxpentifylline), paracetamol, piroxicam, posaconazole, prednisolone, prednisone, propranolol, quinine, ranitidine, rosuvastatin, roxithromycin, simvastatin, sodium valproate, sulfamethoxazole, sulindac, tamoxifen, testosterone, tetracyclines, ticlopidine, tramadol, trimethoprim/sulfamethoxazole, vitamin E and voriconazole enhance the activity of oral anticoagulants, which may lead to bleeding episodes
- activity reduced by chronic abuse of alcohol, aminoglutamide, aprepitant, ascorbic acid (vitamin C) (high dose), azathioprine, bosentan, carbamazepine, carbimazole, colestyramine, dicloxacillin, flucloxacillin, griseofulvin, isotretinoin, mercaptopurine, pheno barbital (phenobarbitone), primidone, propylthiouracil, ribavirin, rifabutin, rifampicin, spironolactone, sucralfate, vitamin K, vitamin K-rich diet
- extra caution if used with aspirin or NSAIDs, as inhibition of platelet aggregation will occur in addition to the increased risk of GI bleeding, peptic ulceration and/or perforation
- may enhance hypoglycaemic effects of hypoglycaemic agents
- increased risk of bleeding if given with selective serotonin reuptake inhibitors (SSRIs) and serotonin and noradrenaline (norepinephrine) reuptake inhibitors (SNRIs)
- if given with phenytoin, there may be a transient increase in anticoagulant effect, followed by a decrease in anticoagulant effect
- may increase serum levels of phenytoin
- caution if given with ciclosporin, cyclophosphamide, oestrogens, mesalazine or corticotrophin, as effects are unpredictable
- increased activity if given with glucosamine
- increased anticoagulant effect may occur if used with garlic, ginkgo or curcumin
- warfarin metabolism may be increased by St John's wort, ginseng or co-enzyme Q10, leading to decreased INR

Nursing considerations/Cautions

- Coumadin and Marevan should not be interchanged, as bioequivalence has not been established
- large loading doses (e.g. 30 mg) are not recommended because of the increased risk of bleeding and complications
- patient should be assessed for any risk factors for bleeding, including INR > 4.0. age ≥ 75 years, highly variable INRs and long duration of warfarin therapy
- bleeding can occur within the therapeutic range and may be due to the unmasking of a lesion such as a tumour
- if large daily doses are required to maintain INR within the normal therapeutic range, acquired or inherited warfarin resistance should be considered as a cause
- signs of bleeding are dependent on location and extent of bleeding
- avoid IM injections, and any SC injection sites should be observed for haematoma
- if IM injections cannot be avoided, they should be restricted to upper extremities where manual compression, application of pressure bandage and easy observation of site are possible

ANTICOAGULANTS AND ANTITHROMBOTIC AGENTS

- observe for early signs of overdose such as bleeding, especially from the gums
- urine is not routinely tested daily for blood
- oral therapy is usually initiated at the same time or soon after starting heparin or low molecular weight heparins (LMWHs); heparin/LMWH is stopped gradually once the effect of oral anticoagulant is apparent, usually in 36—48 hours
- when heparin and warfarin are given together, blood for prothrombin activity is taken 5 hours after last IV heparin bolus dose, 4 hours after stopping IV heparin infusion or 24 hours after the last SC heparin injection
- the optimal dose is highly individual and the dose is adjusted by monitoring the prothrombin activity of the blood, usually measured as INR (see p. 237); however, after dose adjustment, response is usually not apparent for 2—3 days
- baseline INR should be measured before starting therapy, then daily for first 5 days. When there are two consecutive INRs in the target range, the INR monitoring interval can be increased
- additional monitoring is recommended when other medications are started, stopped or dosages are changed, if the patient's medical condition alters (e.g. alcohol intake, dehydration, diarrhoea, oedema, poor nutrition), and/or if there are changes to other conditions such as diet and environment
- INR is maintained at 2.0—2.5 (prophylaxis of DVT), 2.0—3.0 (treatment of DVT, PE and AF), 2.5—3.5 (recurrent DVT and PE, myocardial infarction, arterial grafts, cardiac prosthetic valves and grafts)
- duration of therapy is dependent on reason for use (e.g. DVT or PE prophylaxis — usually at least 3 months, mitral stenosis — indefinite, rheumatic mitral valve disease — long term)
- (AF non-valvular) treatment is usually continued for at least 1 month after normal sinus rhythm has been established (unless contraindicated)
- oral anticoagulants are withdrawn gradually over 3—4 weeks
- therapy should be stopped 5 days before procedures with moderate-to-high risk of bleeding to allow the INR to normalise. If the patient is at high risk of thrombosis (e.g. prosthetic heart valve) LMWH can be used for 12—24 hours before procedure
- the patient should be educated before discharge (see Patient education (p. 252) for a list of teaching considerations)
- treatment of overdose is dependent on the extent of the bleeding. Severe life-threatening bleeding should be managed by stopping warfarin therapy, and administration of phytomenadione (vitamin K) IV 5—10 mg over 30 seconds with fresh frozen plasma or prothrombin complex concentrate. Prothrombin time should be measured 3 hours later and a further dose given if response is inadequate
- caution if used in those over 70 years as there is an increased risk of bleeding, especially for females
- caution if used in those with congenital/acquired protein S or protein C deficiency because of an increased risk of skin necrosis
- caution if given to those with severe-to-moderate liver/kidney insufficiency, moderate-to-severe hypertension, infectious diseases, disturbance to GI flora (including antibacterial therapy), trauma which may result in internal bleeding, surgery/trauma resulting in extensive wounds, indwelling catheters, bacterial endocarditis, pericarditis, pericardial effusion, cerebral aneurysm, dissecting aorta, known/suspected deficiency or protein C mediated anticoagulation response, warfarin resistance (inherited or acquired), polycythaemia vera, vasculitis or severe diabetes
- caution if used in those with congestive cardiac failure, as a greater response may be seen, requiring more frequent INR monitoring

contraindicated in those with active bleeding or bleeding tendency (with or without active ulceration), blood dyscrasias, threatened abortion, eclampsia or pre-eclampsia, alcoholism, psychosis, spinal puncture or regional lumbar block anaesthesia, malignant hypertension, recent (or planned) surgery of the CNS or eyes or resulting in extensive surgical wounds, or lack of patient cooperation (including those with dementia with no supervision) or if there are inadequate laboratory facilities available

Patient education

- emphasise the importance of carrying the Anticoagulant handbook/booklet because it includes laboratory test results and daily anticoagulant dose
- advise the patient of the importance of attending doctor's visits and having regular blood tests, as these determine the dose to be taken
- advise the patient that tablets are to be taken whole, not chewed or crushed, and taken at the same time every day (in the evening). The patient should be further instructed not to take a 'make up' dose (e.g. double dose) if the dose is missed and to seek advice from doctor or pharmacist if this occurs
- instruct the patient to seek medical advice immediately if any of the following occur:
  - unusual or prolonged bleeding or bruising
  - increased menstrual flow or vaginal bleeding
  - unusual nosebleeds
  - bleeding gums when brushing teeth
  - vomiting or coughing up blood
  - red or dark brown urine
  - tarry (black or dark brown) or red stools
  - well-demarcated red skin lesions (thighs, buttocks, toes, breast) occurring 2–5 days after starting therapy where the centre of the lesion becomes necrotic
  - blackness in tissue at extremities such as fingers, toes or penis
  - toes that become dark purple or mottled in colour, blanching with moderate pressing and fade with elevation, painful or tender (usually occurring 3–10 weeks after starting therapy)
  - intense pain in a leg, foot or toes
  - new foot ulcers or severe skin wounds
  - abdominal, joint, chest, back or flank pain
  - fever, headache, dizziness or weakness
  - painful swelling or discomfort
  - swollen ankles
  - persistent diarrhoea
- instruct the patient to avoid any activity that could result in traumatic injury
- advise the patient of the importance of seeking medical advice immediately if any serious fall or injury occurs
- warn the patient to avoid alcohol during therapy
- emphasise the importance of notifying others (e.g. dentist or surgeon) of the anticoagulant therapy before any procedure
- warn the patient that effects last for 2–5 days after warfarin has been stopped
- the patient should not stop warfarin therapy abruptly or stop/start any other medication (including OTC medications such as aspirin and other analgesics, herbal or vitamin preparations) without first seeking medical advice (doctor, pharmacist), as *many* preparations interact with warfarin
- discuss the importance of maintaining a balanced diet and avoid large increases in vegetables containing vitamin K (e.g. green leafy vegetables)
- seek medical advice if travel is planned or if person becomes unwell (e.g. prolonged diarrhoea), which might also result in dietary change or exposure to prolonged hot weather (i.e. possibility of dehydration), as these are all factors that

- can affect the individual's response to warfarin
- women of childbearing years should be counselled to use effective contraception to avoid pregnancy while taking warfarin and should seek medical advice if pregnancy should occur
- see also General Patient education for anticoagulants (p. 237)

Marevan tablets will disperse in 5 minutes; however, Coumadin tablets do not disperse easily. Marevan and Coumadin tablets can be crushed and mixed with a spoonful of yoghurt or apple puree.

Warfarin is contraindicated during pregnancy as it crosses the placenta and fetal blood concentrations are similar to those of mother. Warfarin use has been associated with fetal haemorrhage, birth malformations, increased risk of spontaneous abortion and perinatal bleeding.

Safe to use.

ANTITHROMBIN III-DEPENDENT ANTICOAGULANTS

FONDAPARINUX
Trade names
Arixtra

Available form
Prefilled syringe: 2.5 mg/0.5 mL

Action
- synthetically produced selective inhibitor of factor Xa
- inhibits both thrombin formation and development of thrombus
- has no effect on platelet aggregation or thrombin
- not neutralised by protamine sulfate
- half-life is about 17 hours (prolonged to about 20 hours in the elderly)

Use
- prevention of venous thromboembolism associated with major orthopaedic (hip, knee) or abdominal surgery
- treatment of acute deep vein thrombosis (DVT) or pulmonary embolus (PE)
- treatment of unstable angina or non-ST segment elevation myocardial infarction (UA/NSTEMI) in patients where urgent invasive management is not indicated
- treatment of ST-segment elevation myocardial infarction (STEMI) in patients managed without any initial reperfusion therapy

Dose
- (Prophylaxis of venous thromboembolism, < 75 years, no kidney or liver impairment, mild kidney impairment) 2.5 mg SC daily, starting 6 hours after surgical closure, for 5—9 days or as long as thromboembolic risk exists (maximum 31 days) **OR**
- (Treatment of acute DVT or PE) 7.5 mg (5 mg if patient weight < 50 kg, 10 mg if patient weight >100 kg) SC daily for at least 5 days and until INR range is within 2—3 (until oral anticoagulant therapy is established) **OR**
- (UA/NSTEMI treatment) 2.5 mg SC once daily for up to 8 days or hospital discharge if earlier **OR**
- (STEMI treatment) initially 2.5 mg IV, then 2.5 mg SC once daily for up to 8 days or hospital discharge if earlier

Adverse effects
- bleeding, anaemia, purpura
- hypokalaemia
- insomnia, headache, dizziness, confusion
- hypotension, hypertension
- nausea, vomiting, diarrhoea, dyspepsia, constipation
- increase in liver enzymes
- rash, bullous eruption
- urinary retention, urinary tract infection
- fever
- oedema
- cough, pneumonia
- increased wound drainage

HAVARD'S NURSING GUIDE TO DRUGS

- pain, back pain
- (Rare) angioedema, allergic reaction

Interactions
- agents increasing risk of bleeding should be stopped before starting fondaparinux. If this is not possible, closely monitor for bleeding

Nursing considerations/Cautions
- first dose should be given no earlier than 6 hours post surgical closure and achievement of haemostasis
- should not be given IM
- platelet count should be monitored at the start and end of therapy
- (Orthopaedic patients) kidney function should be monitored regularly throughout therapy
- (STEMI, UA/NSTEMI) therapy should be stopped 24 hours before coronary artery bypass graft surgery and restarted after 48 hours
- if the patient is to undergo percutaneous coronary intervention, therapy should not be restarted earlier than at least 2 hours (UA/NSTEMI) or 3 hours (STEMI) after sheath removal
- (IV, first dose, STEMI patients only) may be given as IV injection through existing line or via sodium chloride 0.9% mini bag (25–50 mL) and given over 1–2 minutes. IV line should be well flushed with sodium chloride 0.9% after administration
- SC injection sites should be rotated and documented
- to use the prefilled syringe the following instructions should be followed:
  - the safety syringe is made up of a needle guard, plunger, finger grip and security sleeve
  - the needle guard should be removed by twisting and pulling it straight off and then discarding the shield
  - the air bubble should not be expelled before use
  - the full length of needle should be inserted at 90 degrees into a skin fold
  - after SC injection, the needle will automatically withdraw into the security sleeve to lock permanently
  - discard the used prefilled syringe into a sharps disposal container
- the patient should be closely monitored for signs of spinal haematoma (e.g. midline back pain, numbness, weakness, lower limb paralysis, bowel/bladder dysfunction) if they have a spinal puncture or insertion/removal of epidural/spinal needle/catheter. Risk of haematoma formation is increased if the patient is taking NSAIDs, antiplatelet agents or other anticoagulants, or if the procedure is repeated or traumatic
- for orthopaedic surgery where risk of venous thromboembolism persists, therapy may continue for up to 31 days
- the patient can be taught self-administration
- (Treatment of acute DVT or PE) oral anticoagulant should be started within 72 hours
- if switching to heparin or another low molecular weight heparin (LMWH), therapy should start 1 day after last fondaparinux injection
- the needle guard may contain latex rubber, which may cause allergic reaction in those with latex allergy
- caution if used in patients with a history of heparin-induced thrombocytopenia
- caution if used in those weighing less than 50 kg, over 75 years of age, or with renal impairment (creatinine clearance < 50 mL/min) or severe liver impairment
- caution if used in those at increased risk of bleeding, or with congenital/acquired bleeding disorders, active GI ulceration, recent surgery (brain, spinal, eye) or recent intracranial haemorrhage
- contraindicated in those with severe kidney impairment (creatinine clearance < 30 mL/min), acute bacterial endocarditis or major bleeding

ANTICOAGULANTS AND ANTITHROMBOTIC AGENTS

Patient education
- instruct the patient in self-administration. This should include information on the injection technique (under the skin and not into muscle), rotation of injection sites, not rubbing the site after injection, correct storage and disposal of used syringes
- advise patients to wear a medical alert bracelet or necklace that indicates they are on anticoagulant medication. This can be crucial in emergency situations where they may not be able to communicate their medical status
- see also General Patient education for anticoagulants (p. 237)

Limited human data.

Heparin or LMWH is the preferred treatment for VTE during pregnancy.

Generally not recommended owing to insufficient data on safety during breastfeeding.

Reduced clearance in renal impairment leads to prolonged anticoagulant effect.

Contraindicated: CrCl < 30 mL/min owing to high bleeding risk.

Use with caution: CrCl 30–50 mL/min; consider dose reduction.

DIRECT THROMBIN INHIBITORS

BIVALIRUDIN
Trade names
Bivalirudin ARX

Available form
Vial: 250 mg

Action
- synthetic analogue of hirudin (anticoagulant found in leech saliva)
- reversible and specific thrombin inhibitor
- half-life 25 minutes

Use
- percutaneous coronary intervention (PCI) (with aspirin)
- treatment of moderate-to-high risk acute coronary syndrome (ACS) (e.g. unstable angina/non-ST segment elevation myocardial infarction (non-STEMI)) undergoing early invasive management

Dose
- (PCI) initially 0.75 mg/kg IV bolus, then 1.75 mg/kg/hour IV infusion for remainder of procedure or up to 4 hours post-procedure as needed (with 300–325 mg aspirin) **OR**
- (ACS) initially 0.1 mg/kg IV bolus, then 0.25 mg/kg/hour IV infusion for up to 72 hours (with aspirin 300–325 mg orally). If patient then has PCI, additional 0.5 mg/kg IV bolus should be given at the start of the procedure, then 1.75 mg/kg/hour IV infusion for remainder of procedure. When procedure is complete, IV infusion is decreased to 0.25 mg/kg/hour for 4–12 hours as needed

Adverse effects
- bleeding
- nausea, vomiting
- fever
- atrial fibrillation, hypotension, hypertension, angina, bradycardia
- back pain, chest pain
- headache, insomnia
- (IV site) pain, bleeding, haematoma
- (Uncommon) hypersensitivity

Interactions
- heparin should be discontinued for 30 minutes before starting bivalirudin
- low molecular weight heparins (LMWHs) should be discontinued for 8 hours before starting bivalirudin
- increased risk of bleeding if given with other anticoagulant or antiplatelet agents; should therefore be given with caution

Nursing considerations/Cautions

- not given IM
- (PCI) patient should be closely monitored for signs and symptoms of myocardial infarction throughout infusion
- (PCI) patient should be closely observed for at least 24 hours post procedure, as STEMI patients are at increased risk of acute stent thrombosis (especially in first 4 hours after procedure)
- therapy should be commenced just prior to PCI
- reconstitute using 5 mL water for injections, swirl gently until dissolved then dilute using sodium chloride 0.9% or glucose 5% for a total volume of 50 mL and concentration of 5 mg/mL
- incompatible with alteplase, amiodarone, amphotericin B (amphotericin), chlorpromazine, diazepam, prochlorperazine, reteplase and vancomycin as precipitation may occur. Other incompatibilities include dobutamine (4 mg/mL), haloperidol (0.2 mg/mL) and promethazine (2 mg/mL)
- not recommended during gamma brachytherapy (radiation therapy where the radiation source is placed in direct contact with the tumour)
- caution if used in patients who are at risk of bleeding
- contraindicated in those with increased risk of active bleeding, irreversible coagulation disorders, severe uncontrolled hypertension, subacute bacterial endocarditis or severe kidney impairment (creatinine clearance < 30 mL/min) or in dialysis-dependent patients

Patient education

- see General Patient education for anticoagulants (p. 237)

Limited human data. Not recommended during pregnancy unless potential benefits outweigh risks.

Limited human data. Caution if used during breastfeeding.

Adjustments and monitoring are essential for patients with reduced renal function to ensure safe and effective use during procedures like PCI.

Monitor activated clotting time (ACT) closely in patients with renal impairment.

Lower infusion rate if CrCl < 30 mL/min during PCI.

Some manufacturers contraindicate use with CrCl < 30 mL/min.

DABIGATRAN ETEXILATE

Trade names
APX-Dabigatran, Dabigatran Sandoz, Pharmacor Dabigatran, Pradaxa

Available forms
Capsules: 75 mg, 110 mg, 150 mg

Action
- dabigatran etexilate is a prodrug which is converted to the active metabolite dabigatran
- direct thrombin inhibitor
- dabigatran inhibits both free and clot-bound thrombin by binding specifically to the thrombin's active site
- half-life 8—10 hours (single dose) or 14—17 hours (multiple doses)

Use
- prophylaxis of venous thromboembolic event (VTE) after major orthopaedic surgery (total hip, knee replacement)
- treatment of deep vein thrombosis (DVT) or pulmonary embolism (PE) and prevention of recurrent DVT or PE
- prophylaxis of stroke and systemic embolism in those with non-valvular atrial fibrillation and at least one additional risk factor for stroke

Dose
- (Prophylaxis of VTE after major orthopaedic surgery) initially 110 mg orally

ANTICOAGULANTS AND ANTITHROMBOTIC AGENTS

- 1—4 hours after completed surgery, then 220 mg orally once daily for 10 days (knee replacement) or 28—35 days (hip replacement) **OR**
- (Prophylaxis of stroke and systemic embolism in those with non-valvular atrial fibrillation) 150 mg orally twice daily **OR**
- (Treatment or prevention of recurrent DVT or PE) 150 mg orally twice daily

Adverse effects

- bleeding, anaemia
- nausea, vomiting, dyspepsia, diarrhoea, constipation
- dizziness, headache, insomnia
- fever
- increased wound discharge/complication
- arthralgia, muscle spasm, extremity pain
- hypotension, syncope, atrial fibrillation, hypertension
- urinary tract infection, urinary retention
- rash, pruritus, erythema, blistering
- peripheral oedema
- hypokalaemia
- abnormal liver enzymes

Interactions

- contraindicated with verapamil (either starting verapamil and dabigatran simultaneously or adding verapamil to stable dabigatran therapy)
- contraindicated with glecaprevir/pibrentasvir combination
- not recommended with heparin, low molecular weight heparins (LMWHs), aspirin, antiplatelet agents, fondaparinux, fibrinolytic agents, ticagrelor, dextran or warfarin
- not recommended with itraconazole, tacrolimus, ciclosporin, ritonavir, nelfinavir
- increased risk of bleeding if given with selective serotonin reuptake inhibitors (SSRIs) or serotonin and noradrenaline (norepinephrine) reuptake inhibitors (SNRIs)
- not recommended with P glycoprotein inducers such as carbamazepine, rifampicin, phenytoin and St John's wort, as decreased serum level may occur
- increased serum levels may occur if given with P glycoprotein inhibitors such as amiodarone, clarithromycin, ritonavir and glecaprevir; should therefore be used with caution if at all
- increased risk of bleeding if given with NSAIDs (with half-life > 12 hours)
- may cause false positive INR elevation

Nursing considerations/Cautions

- liver and kidney function should be assessed before starting therapy
- (DVT/PE) treatment should be started with parenteral anticoagulant for at least 5 days before starting oral therapy with dabigatran
- dabigatran should be stopped 1—5 days preoperatively or pre-procedure to decrease risk of bleeding. The exact length of time is dependent on patient's risk of bleeding (high or standard), surgery type (e.g. major) and kidney function. If an acute intervention is required, it should be delayed at least 12 hours after the last dose to lessen risk of bleeding if possible
- (Prophylaxis of VTE after major orthopaedic surgery) if treatment is not started on day of surgery, it should be started with a 220 mg dose
- if switching from dabigatran etexilate to parenteral anticoagulant, 12—24 hours should be allowed to elapse from the last oral dose to starting parenteral anticoagulant
- if switching from parenteral anticoagulant to dabigatran etexilate, the dabigatran etexilate dose should be given up to 2 hours before the next dose is due, or, if parenteral anticoagulant is being administered by continuous IV, dabigatran etexilate should be started when the infusion is stopped
- if switching from dabigatran etexilate to warfarin, the starting time of warfarin

- should be based on creatinine clearance (CrCl):
  - CrCl > 50 mL/min, warfarin should be started 3 days before stopping dabigatran etexilate
  - CrCl 31–50 mL/min, warfarin should be started 2 days before stopping dabigatran etexilate
  - CrCl 15–30 mL/min, warfarin should be started 1 day before stopping dabigatran etexilate
- if switching from warfarin to dabigatran etexilate, warfarin should be stopped and dabigatran etexilate started when INR < 2.0
- the patient should be closely monitored for signs of spinal haematoma (e.g. midline back pain, numbness, weakness, lower limb paralysis, bowel/bladder dysfunction) if they have a spinal puncture or insertion/removal of epidural/spinal needle/catheter. Risk of haematoma formation is increased if the patient is taking NSAIDs, antiplatelet agents or other anticoagulants, or if the procedure is repeated or traumatic
- INR should not be used for anticoagulation monitoring as it is unreliable and may produce false positive results
- if rapid reversal is required for emergency surgery/procedures or in the case of life-threatening bleeding, IV idarucizumab (see p. 352) can be used as it immediately reverses anticoagulant effects. A second dose may be required, as dabigatran's anticoagulant actions may re-emerge up to 24 hours after first infusion
- dosage should be reduced in those aged ≥ 75 years or with moderate kidney impairment (CrCl 30–50 mL/min)
- capsules contain sunset yellow (FCF C/15985 (E110)), which is known to cause allergic reactions in some people
- not recommended in patients undergoing hip surgery, those with a PE and who are haemodynamically unstable, or who are eligible for fibrinolytic therapy or pulmonary embolectomy
- not recommended in those under 18 years
- caution if used in patients who are at risk of bleeding (including those with aPTT > 80 seconds), aged 75 years or older, congenital or acquired coagulation disorders, thrombocytopenia, functional platelet defect, recent biopsy, major trauma, recent intracranial haemorrhage, bacterial endocarditis or kidney impairment (creatinine clearance 30–50 mL/min)
- not recommended in those with a history of thrombosis and antiphospholipid syndrome
- contraindicated in those with kidney impairment (creatinine clearance < 30 mL/min), increased risk of active bleeding, haemorrhagic stroke (within the last 6 months), active peptic ulcer disease with recent bleeding, liver impairment/disease, history of intracranial, intraocular, spinal, retroperitoneal or atraumatic intra-articular bleeding, within 12 months of GI bleeding (unless permanently treated) or prosthetic heart valves, or within 2 hours of removal of an indwelling spinal/epidural catheter, bleeding disorders, lesions or tumours at risk of bleeding, recent brain or spinal injury, recent brain or spinal surgery or injury, recent eye surgery, known or suspected oesophageal varices, arteriovenous malformations, vascular aneurysm, or major intraspinal or intracerebral vascular abnormalities

Patient education

- advise patient to swallow capsules whole, not chewed, broken or opened
- see also General Patient education for anticoagulants (p. 237)

Capsules should not be opened or crushed.

Limited human data.

Heparin or LMWH is the preferred treatment for VTE during pregnancy.

ANTICOAGULANTS AND ANTITHROMBOTIC AGENTS

Generally not recommended owing to insufficient data on safety during breastfeeding.

(Renal) contraindicated: if CrCl < 30 mL/min

Reduced dosage: for patients with a CrCl 30—50 mL/min

(Hepatic) use is contraindicated if liver enzymes are more than two times the ULN, or if there is hepatic disease that could impact survival.

Dose should be reduced in those aged 75 and over.

DIRECT FACTOR XA INHIBITORS

General Action of direct factor Xa inhibitors
- highly selective and reversible inhibitor of Factor Xa
- by inhibiting Factor Xa, the conversion of prothrombin to thrombin is prevented. Thrombin is essential for converting fibrinogen to fibrin, the main protein involved in clot formation
- does not require cofactor antithrombin III for its activity (which is required by indirect inhibitors like heparins)

APIXABAN
Trade names
Eliquis

Available forms
Tablet: 2.5 mg, 5 mg

Action
- inhibits both free and clot-bound factor Xa and prothrombinase activity
- no direct effect on platelet aggregation
- half-life about 12 hours
- see also General Action of direct factor Xa inhibitors above

Use
- prophylaxis of venous thromboembolism (VTE) after knee or hip replacement
- prophylaxis of stroke and systemic embolism in those with non-valvular atrial fibrillation with at least one other stroke risk factor
- treatment and prophylaxis of deep vein thrombosis (DVT)
- treatment and prophylaxis of pulmonary embolus (PE)

Dose
- (VTE prophylaxis after knee or hip surgery) 2.5 mg orally twice daily, starting 12—24 hours after surgery **OR**
- (Prophylaxis of stroke and systemic embolism) 5 mg orally twice daily **OR**
- (Treatment of DVT and PE) initially 10 mg orally twice daily for 7 days, then 5 mg orally twice daily **OR**
- (Prophylaxis of DVT or PE) 2.5 mg orally twice daily after at least 6 months of treatment for DVT or PE (see above)

Adverse effects
- nasopharyngitis
- hypokalaemia

Interactions
- strong combined inhibitors of CYP3A4 and P-GP: oral ketoconazole, itraconazole, voriconazole, posaconazole, HIV-protease inhibitors
- inducers such as rifampicin, phenytoin, phenobarbital, St John's wort, carbamazepine

Nursing considerations/Cautions
- duration of therapy depends on type of orthopaedic surgery: knee replacement 10—14 days, hip replacement 32—38 days
- epidural catheter should not be removed within 20—30 hours of administration of apixaban, and apixaban should not be started within 5 hours of epidural catheter removal
- (Stroke prophylaxis) dose should be decreased to 2.5 mg twice daily in patients with at least two of the following characteristics if body weight ≤60kg, serum creatinine ≥133 micromol/L or over 80 years of age
- if switching to or from parenteral anticoagulants, this should be done at next dose

- if switching from warfarin, warfarin should be stopped and apixaban started when INR < 2.0
- if switching to warfarin, apixaban should be continued for 48 hours. After the first dose of warfarin, INR should be measured and both continued until INR ≥ 2.0
- can be started or continued during cardioversion procedure
- if the patient has not previously received anticoagulant therapy, at least 5 doses of 5 mg apixaban (or 2.5 mg twice daily) should be given before procedure
- if the procedure is required before 5 doses can be given, a loading dose of 10 mg should be given at least 2 hours before the procedure
- not recommended for haemodynamically significant rheumatic heart disease or mitral stenosis
- contraindicated in those with significant active bleeding, lesions at increased risk of bleeding, bleeding disorders or moderate-to-severe liver impairment (especially those associated with coagulopathy and risk of bleeding), recent surgery (brain, spinal, eyes), recent intracranial haemorrhage, known/suspected oesophageal varices, AV malformation, vascular aneurysm, major intraspinal/intracerebral vascular abnormalities, recent brain/spinal injury or severe kidney impairment (creatinine clearance < 25 mL/min)

Patient education
- see General Patient education for anticoagulants (p. 237)

Tablet can be crushed and mixed with water, apple juice, apple puree or glucose 5%.

Limited human data.

Heparin or LMWH is the preferred treatment for VTE during pregnancy.

Generally not recommended owing to insufficient data on safety during breastfeeding.

In patients with reduced renal function, it is important to note that data are limited and recommendations can vary.

Apixaban is contraindicated in patients with renal impairment creatinine clearance <25 mL/min

RIVAROXABAN
Trade names
Ixarola, Rivoxa, Xarelto, APO-Rivaroxaban, ARX-Rivaroxaban, Relaban, Riveralto, Rivaroxaban Dr. Reddy's Tablets, Rivaroxaban Lupin, Rivaroxaban Sandoz, Rivaroxaban-Teva, Rivaxib,

Available forms
Tablet: 2.5 mg, 10 mg, 15 mg, 20 mg

Action
- half-life 5–9 hours (prolonged to 11–13 hours in the elderly)

Use
- prophylaxis of venous thromboembolism (VTE) after knee or hip replacement
- prophylaxis of stroke and systemic embolism in those with non-valvular atrial fibrillation (AF) with at least one other stroke factor
- treatment of deep vein thrombosis (DVT) and prophylaxis of recurrent DVT and pulmonary embolus (PE)
- prophylaxis of cardiovascular events in patients with coronary artery disease (CAD) and/or peripheral arterial disease (PAD) (with aspirin)

Dose
- (VTE prophylaxis for knee/hip surgery) 10 mg orally daily, starting 6–10 hours after surgery (when haemostasis has been established) **OR**

ANTICOAGULANTS AND ANTITHROMBOTIC AGENTS

- (Stroke and systemic embolism prophylaxis) 20 mg orally once daily. For patients with severe and moderate renal impairment (Creatinine clearance: 15–49 mL/min), one 15 mg tablet should be taken once daily. Due to limited clinical data caution should be taken in patients with severe renal impairment (Creatinine clearance (CrCl) 15–29 mL/min) **OR**
- (Treatment of DVT and prophylaxis of recurrent DVT and PE) initially 15 mg orally twice daily for 3 weeks, then 20 mg orally daily (while risk of VTE exists) **OR**
- prophylaxis of cardiovascular events in patients with CAD and/or PAD) 2.5 mg orally twice daily (with aspirin 100 mg orally daily)

Interactions
- contraindicated with HIV protease inhibitors and azole antifungal agents (except fluconazole)
- caution if given with fluconazole

Nursing considerations/Cautions
- duration of therapy depends on type of orthopaedic surgery: knee replacement 2 weeks, hip replacement 5 weeks
- epidural catheter should not be removed within 18 hours of rivaroxaban or longer if the puncture was traumatic, and rivaroxaban should be started within 6 hours of epidural catheter removal
- therapy can be started or continued with cardioversion procedure. Therapy should be started at least 4 hours before procedure in patients not previously receiving anticoagulant therapy
- if switching from parenteral anticoagulant, rivaroxaban should be given up to 2 hours before the next parenteral dose is due or when continuous IV therapy is stopped
- if switching from warfarin, warfarin should be stopped and rivaroxaban started when INR $\leq$ 3.0 (for stroke/systemic embolism prophylaxis) or INR $\leq$ 2.5 (for DVT treatment or prophylaxis of recurrent DVT/PE)
- (Recurrent DVT/PE prophylaxis) risk of recurrent DVT or PE should be reassessed after 6–12 months of therapy. Dose reduction to 10 mg daily may be considered
- (Prophylaxis of cardiovascular event in those with CAD and/or PAD) caution if used in those > 75 years because of increased risk of bleeding
- caution if used in those at risk of ulcerative GI disease. Prophylactic therapy is recommended
- (Prophylaxis of cardiovascular event in those with CAD and/or PAD) not recommended in those who are within 4 weeks of experiencing an ischaemic, non-lacunar stroke
- not recommended for hip fracture surgery or prosthetic heart valves
- tablets contain lactose and are not recommended in those with galactose intolerance, Lapp lactase deficiency or glucose–galactose malabsorption
- caution in those with bronchiectasis or history of pulmonary bleeding
- contraindicated in those with significant active bleeding, lesions at increased risk of bleeding, bleeding disorders or moderate-to-severe liver impairment associated with coagulopathy, undergoing dialysis or severe kidney impairment (creatinine clearance (CrCl) < 15 mL/min)

Patient education
- advise patient that 15 mg or 20 mg tablets should be taken with food
- women of childbearing years should be counselled to use adequate contraception during therapy to prevent pregnancy

 Tablet can be crushed and mixed with water or a spoonful of apple puree.

Limited human data. Use contraindicated. Use heparin or low molecular weight heparin for VTE treatment during pregnancy.

Limited human data. Use contraindicated.

Primarily cleared by the kidneys, dosage adjustments are necessary in patients with reduced renal function.

CrCl < 15 mL/min: contraindicated owing to high risk of bleeding.

CrCl 15—50 mL/min: AF patients: reduce dose.

Limited data <30 mL/min: extra caution needed; data are insufficient.

OTHER THROMBOTIC AGENTS

PROTEIN C
Trade names
Ceprotin

Available forms
Vial: 500 IU, 1000 IU

Action
- normally synthesised in the liver as a vitamin K-dependent plasma protein which is converted by thrombin—thrombomodulin complex on endothelial surface to activated protein C, which is a protease with anticoagulant activity, especially with co-factor protein S
- activated protein C inhibits activated forms of factors V and VIII, resulting in decreased thrombin formation
- half-life 4.4—15.8 hours, but is shortened in conditions with acute thrombosis such as purpura fulminans and skin necrosis

Use
- purpura fulminans (intravascular thrombosis and haemorrhagic skin infarction)
- coumarin-induced skin necrosis in those with severe congenital protein C deficiency

Dose
- initially 60—80 IU/kg IV (to achieve protein C activity level of 100%), then adjusting dose based on protein C activity (maintained at above 25%)

Adverse effects
- (Injection site) reaction, burning, stinging
- dizziness, restlessness, headache
- nausea, vomiting
- chest tightness, wheezing
- fever, sweating
- bleeding, thrombosis
- hypotension, tachycardia, cardiac arrhythmias, chest pain
- rash, urticaria, pruritus, skin ulceration
- bleeding, thrombosis
- hypersensitivity reaction, heparin-induced thrombocytopenia, protein C antibody development

Interactions
- transient hypercoagulable state may occur if given with vitamin K antagonist anticoagulants (e.g. warfarin) before anticoagulant effect becomes evident

Nursing considerations/Cautions
- should be administered only where protein C monitoring is available
- protein C activity should be estimated using protein C-specific chromogenic substrates and measured before starting therapy, every 6 hours until patient is stabilised, then twice daily and always before next injection
- patient being treated during acute phase of disease may display lower increase in protein C activity
- resuscitation should be readily available in the case of acute allergic-type hypersensitivity occurring
- if patient is switched to permanent oral anticoagulant prophylaxis, protein C

should be stopped only when anti-coagulation has stabilised. Anti-coagulation should be started at low dose and slowly increased
- reconstitute using water for injections, gently rotating vial to dissolve powder. Reconstituted solution should then be withdrawn using sterile filter needle and then administered immediately via IV route. A separate sterile filter needle should be used for each individual vial used
- administration rate should not exceed 2 mL/min (except for children under 10 kg, where the rate should not be greater than 0.2 mL/kg/min)
- derived from human plasma; therefore carries a risk of transmission of infectious diseases. Vaccination against hepatitis A and B should be considered if patient is likely to receive regular or repeated doses
- may contain a trace amount of heparin, which may cause heparin-induced allergic reactions including heparin-induced thrombocytopenia (HIT). HIT starts as a heparin-induced antibody-mediated reaction resulting from irreversible aggregation of platelets and progressing to new thrombus formation with thrombocytopenia induced. If HIT is suspected, the platelet count should be determined and therapy stopped if needed
- contains sodium and the daily dose may exceed 200 mg, which may be of importance in those on a sodium-controlled diet
- not recommended in those with combined severe congenital protein C deficiency and activated protein C resistance
- contraindicated in those with hypersensitivity to mouse protein or heparin (except in life-threatening thrombotic complications) including any previous heparin-induced thrombocytopenia

Patient education

- instruct patient to immediately report any signs of allergy including hives, tightness in chest or wheezing

Limited human data. Should be used during pregnancy only if benefits are thought to outweigh risks.

Safety during breastfeeding has not been established.

ANTIDEPRESSANTS

In 2020–22, 8.5 million Australians (or 43% of the population) aged 16–85 years reported experiencing a mental illness at some time in their life. Of these, 1 in 7 (16%) reported depression and 17.2% (3.4 million) reported anxiety, with females reporting feelings of depression and anxiety at a higher rate than males (ABS 2023). Depression occurs throughout the life span, peaking in youth, early adulthood and early old age, with an average age of onset being the mid 20s, but 40% have had their first episode by the time they are 20 (Mahli et al 2021).

There are a number of risk factors for depression, including family history (e.g. high risk in families with history of depression or alcoholism), life events (e.g. recent negative experiences such as death, relationship break-up, health changes), childhood experiences (e.g. significant loss or disruptive/hostile environment), postpartum, personality traits (e.g. insecure, introverted, stress-sensitive, obsessive) or lack of social networks (Mahli et al 2021). Causes of depression can include some medications, substances of abuse (including alcohol), neurological diseases (e.g. dementias, Huntington's disease, multiple sclerosis), infectious diseases (e.g. HIV, tuberculosis, infectious hepatitis), cancers, metabolic and endocrine disorders (e.g. diabetes, thyroid disorders), collagen-vascular conditions (e.g. rheumatoid arthritis), cardiovascular disease (e.g. post myocardial infarction, chronic heart disease) and postpartum (Gao 2024).

Symptoms of depression can vary from person to person and can be quite subtle, meaning that people often don't seek help until they become more marked. Symptoms include depressed or irritable/angry mood, lack of interest in activities that would normally please or decreased ability to feel pleasure (anhedonia), problems with memory and concentration, indecisiveness, anxiety, restlessness, agitation, thoughts involving helplessness or hopelessness, changes in weight or appetite, insomnia or hypersomnia, low energy/fatigue, feelings of worthlessness or guilt and/or suicidal ideation (Gao 2024). Treatment should be tailored to the individual and the type of depression (psychotic, manic, melancholic, reactive). Major depressive disorder is the most common presentation in the community, with the aims of treatment being complete remission of symptoms with full recovery to premorbid functioning, reduction of associated morbidity, and limiting disability and risk of self-harm or fatality while focusing on the person's strengths in order to develop skills and resilience to prevent recurrence (Mahli et al 2024).

Pharmacotherapy is only one part of a treatment plan. Management of depression should also include sleep restoration, regular exercise, diet modification, addressing smoking, alcohol and substance misuse, and psychological therapies (e.g. cognitive behaviour therapy, interpersonal psychotherapy, mindfulness-based cognitive therapy) and general psychosocial interventions (e.g. self-help literature, drug and alcohol support groups, family or couples counselling) (Gao 2024; Mahli et al 2021). Other therapies are sometimes considered when the depression fails to respond and may include electroconvulsive therapy (ECT), light therapy and transcranial magnetic stimulation (Mahli et al 2021).

The decision to use antidepressants is very much based on clinical judgement of the doctor in collaboration with the patient. The first antidepressant (imipramine) became available in the 1950s and the range of agents used to treat depression has expanded since then to include:

- tricyclic antidepressants (tricyclics, TCAs) and related agents
- monoamine oxidase inhibitors (MAO inhibitors or MAOIs)
- reversible inhibitors of monoamine oxidase (RIMAs)
- selective serotonin reuptake inhibitors (SSRIs)
- serotonin and noradrenaline (norepinephrine) reuptake inhibitors (SNRIs)
- atypical antidepressants.

Antidepressants should be trialled for a minimum of 3 weeks at therapeutic dose in order to determine clinical response. It can take 2–4 weeks to determine effectiveness; therefore regular follow-up is necessary, to determine not only clinical response, but also adverse effects, including the potential of some antidepressants to produce suicidal thoughts and behaviours (especially in young adults or adolescents) (Mahli et al 2021).

Serotonin syndrome occurs when there is excessive serotonin acting on the CNS, resulting in effects that range from mild to life threatening. It is often the result of a drug interaction, commonly involving SSRIs. Other drugs implicated in serotonin syndrome are lithium, St John's wort, amphetamines (including recreational drugs), cocaine, anorectics, LSD, tramadol, pethidine, MAOIs, moclobemide, atypical antidepressants, TCAs, sumatriptan and tryptophan. They act by blocking serotonin reuptake, inhibiting its metabolism or being a serotonin agonist, precursor or releaser. Clinical symptoms of serotonin syndrome include agitation, confusion, hypomania, hyperactivity, restlessness, hyperthermia, sweating, tachycardia, hypertension, flushing, shivering, clonus, hyperreflexia, hypertonia, ataxia and tremor. Hyperreflexia and clonus are the main diagnostic symptoms of serotonin syndrome. Treatment should include ceasing the drug, ensuring adequate hydration and urine output, and monitoring of vital signs, and may involve aggressive measures to treat hyperthermia. Serotonin antagonists such as cyproheptadine may also be useful.

General Nursing considerations/ Cautions for antidepressants

- patients should be screened carefully before starting therapy to determine the risk for bipolar disorders, including detailed psychiatric history and family history of depression, suicide and bipolar disorder
- all patients should be carefully monitored during initial stages of therapy or when the dosage is changed, because the risk of suicide remains high. Family members/carers should be alerted to this possibility. Prescriptions are usually written for the smallest quantity to decrease the risk of overdose
- observe for a beneficial elevation in mood (although this may take weeks to become apparent)
- maintenance therapy should continue for at least 6—12 months after depressive symptoms have abated to avoid relapse
- observe for mania, hypomania, hallucinations, delusions and suicidal tendencies, which will necessitate discontinuation of therapy (especially those with pre-existing schizophrenia, bipolar disorder or paranoid delusions)
- when stopping therapy, the dose should be slowly tapered to prevent withdrawal symptoms, which include dizziness, paraesthesia, tremor, anxiety, nausea and palpitations. The risk of withdrawal symptoms is dependent on dose, duration of therapy and the slowness of the tapering regimen
- a washout period may be necessary when switching from one antidepressant to another and is based on the drug's half-life — the longer the half-life, the longer the washout period
- caution if used in those with unstable epilepsy or history of seizures because of the risk of increased seizure activity
- caution if used to treat depression in those with schizophrenia as psychotic symptoms may be intensified; in manic depression there may be a shift towards mania, and paranoid delusion may be aggravated
- caution if used in those with kidney or liver impairment. Liver and kidney function should be monitored regularly during therapy

General Patient education for antidepressants

- the patient should be advised that antidepressant effects are usually seen after 7—10 days and progress over 2—4 weeks, whereas a sedative effect is seen almost immediately and disappears with time
- the patient (or carer) should be advised to seek medical advice immediately if any of the following occur:
  - thoughts/talk about self-harm, harm to others, suicide or death or recent attempts at self-harm or increase in aggression or hostility
  - change in mood, abnormal thinking or hallucinations
  - worsening of depression
- warn the patient against driving a vehicle or operating machinery if dizziness, drowsiness, visual disturbances or concentration is impaired, especially during the initial period of treatment when sedation is common, and if the dose is being increased

- advise the patient that dizziness, lightheadedness and/or fainting (due to hypotension) can be avoided by moving gradually to a sitting or standing position, especially after sleep. Warn the patient that postural hypotension is made worse by prolonged standing, hot baths or showers, hot weather, physical exertion, large meals and drinking alcohol
- warn the patient to avoid alcohol during therapy
- advise the patient against abruptly stopping therapy

TRICYCLIC AND RELATED ANTIDEPRESSANTS (TCAs)

General Actions of TCAs
- prevent reuptake of noradrenaline (norepinephrine) and serotonin (5HT), prolonging their actions at the receptors
- histamine (H_1) receptor antagonist
- marked anticholinergic and sedative effects
- not used as first-line treatment because of potentially serious adverse effects

General Adverse effects of TCAs
- nausea, vomiting, anorexia, peculiar taste, diarrhoea, epigastric distress, black tongue, changes in appetite, weight gain, thirst, dry mouth
- dental caries
- elevated liver enzymes
- tinnitus
- slurred speech
- yawning
- hot flushes, increased sweating
- dizziness, headache, fatigue, drowsiness
- numbness, tingling and paraesthesia of extremities, ataxia
- disturbed concentration/attention and memory, tremor, delirium, weakness, sedation, somnolence, insomnia, nightmares, confusion, anxiety, agitation, disorientation, hallucinations, excitement, restlessness, aggression
- tachycardia, palpitations, postural hypotension, occasionally hypertension, altered conduction, arrhythmias, heart block and non-specific ECG changes
- (anticholinergic effects) dry mouth, blurred vision, constipation, urinary retention/difficulty with micturition, sweating, hyperpyrexia, increased intraocular pressure, paralytic ileus
- testicular swelling, gynaecomastia, impotence, erectile dysfunction, changes to libido (males)
- breast enlargement, galactorrhoea, changes to libido (females)
- allergic reaction (oedema of face/tongue, rash, urticaria, photosensitivity)
- withdrawal syndrome (nausea, headache, malaise, vomiting, diarrhoea, abdominal pain, anxiety, dizziness, sleep and dream disturbance, restlessness, nervousness, irritability)
- (Rare) blood dyscrasias, hepatitis, syndrome of inappropriate antidiuretic hormone secretion (SIADH), hyponatraemia, glaucoma, paralytic ileus, peripheral neuropathy, neuroleptic malignant syndrome, serotonin syndrome (see p. 265), suicidal ideation, seizures, glaucoma, alopecia, altered blood glucose levels
- (Overdose) initially urinary retention, dry mucous membranes, decreased bowel motility, then temporary confusion, disturbed concentration, transient visual hallucinations, agitation, hyperactive reflexes, muscle rigidity, vomiting, drowsiness, hypothermia, tachycardia and other arrhythmias, dilated pupils, metabolic acidosis, hypokalaemia, hyponatraemia, convulsions, severe hypotension, stupor, coma

General Interactions of TCAs
- contraindicated with or within 14 days of monoamine oxidase inhibitors (MAOIs) because this combination may cause coma, hyperpyrexia, convulsions and death

- when substituting a TCA for an MAOI, allow 14 days to elapse after discontinuing MAOI therapy
- serotonin toxicity may occur if given with moclobemide (reversible MAOI), which is therefore contraindicated with TCAs
- increased risk of agranulocytosis if given with carbimazole or propylthiouracil
- (ECT) hazards may be increased when ECT and TCAs are used together
- increased risk of toxicity (including cardiac arrhythmias) and increases therapeutic effects of both agents if TCAs and thyroid hormones are given together
- high doses may cause conduction defects and arrhythmias; therefore contraindicated with agents known to prolong QT interval such as antiarrhythmic agents and SSRIs
- may potentiate cardiovascular effects of sympathomimetic agents such as adrenaline (epinephrine), noradrenaline (norepinephrine) or amphetamines
- if given with phenothiazines, serum levels of both agents may be increased, increasing the risk of seizures and neuroleptic malignant syndrome
- CNS depressant effects may be enhanced by alcohol, barbiturates, benzodiazepines or general anaesthetic agents
- may precipitate hyperpyrexia, delirium and/or paralytic ileus if given with antihistamines, antiparkinsonian (anticholinergic) drugs, atropine, phenothiazines (with anticholinergic effects) or anticholinergic drugs
- hyperpyrexia may occur if given with antipsychotic (neuroleptic) drugs, especially during hot weather
- increased risk of convulsions if given with tramadol
- delirium may occur if TCAs are given with disulfiram
- serum levels may be decreased by barbiturates, carbamazepine, colestyramine, colestipol, phenobarbital (phenobarbitone), phenytoin, St John's wort, rifampicin or nicotine (including smoking)
- serum levels may be increased by alprazolam, cimetidine, disulfiram, methylphenidate, phenothiazines, fluoxetine, fluvoxamine, paroxetine, sertraline or sodium valproate
- serotonin syndrome may occur if TCAs are given with serotonin-enhancing agents such as SSRIs (e.g. citalopram, fluoxetine, fluvoxamine, paroxetine, sertraline), SNRIs or lithium and are therefore not recommended together
- not recommended within 14–21 days of fluoxetine (as washout period is required)
- TCAs decrease hypotensive effects of clonidine and methyldopa
- hypokalaemia (or use of potassium-losing diuretics) may increase risk of prolonged QT interval and associated arrhythmias and they are therefore not recommended together
- may potentiate effects of oral anticoagulants; therefore INR should be carefully monitored throughout therapy, especially when starting or stopping therapy
- TCAs may increase serum levels of phenytoin or carbamazepine, increasing risk of toxicity
- increased risk of bone fracture if given with SSRIs in those over 50 years

General Nursing considerations/Cautions for TCAs

- blood pressure should be measured before starting therapy
- any hypokalaemia should be corrected before starting therapy
- blood counts and ECG should be regularly monitored during therapy
- liver enzymes and renal function should be regularly monitored during therapy in those with pre-existing liver and kidney disease
- dosage should be started at a low level and increased gradually; however, higher doses may be used in severely depressed, hospitalised patients

ANTIDEPRESSANTS

- entire daily dose may be given in the morning, at night, or in divided doses, depending on requirements
- should be withdrawn before surgery as TCAs may increase the risk of arrhythmias if given with general anaesthetics
- caution if used in those with narrow angle glaucoma, raised intraocular pressure, urinary retention, chronic constipation and prostatic hyperplasia because symptoms may be exacerbated by anticholinergic actions of TCAs
- caution if used in those with hyperthyroidism, tumours of the adrenal medulla (may provoke hypertensive crisis), liver or kidney impairment, or cardiovascular disorders (including tachycardia, conduction disorders, arrhythmias and cardiac insufficiency)
- (Depression) not recommended in those under 18 years
- contraindicated in those with or recovering from myocardial infarction, congenital long QT syndrome, epilepsy or with low seizure threshold (e.g. due to brain damage) or liver failure
- contraindicated in those with known hypersensitivity to other TCAs as cross-sensitivity is possible
- see also General Nursing considerations/Cautions for all antidepressant agents (p. 266)

General Patient education for TCAs

- the patient (or carer) should be advised to seek medical advice immediately if any of the following occur:
  - difficulty passing urine
  - increase in breast size, changes in libido (in both men and women)
  - numbness or tingling in feet or hands
  - fever, chills, mouth ulcers, unusual tiredness or sore throat, swollen glands
  - ringing in the ears
  - fast or irregular heart beat
  - unusual bruising or bleeding
- the patient should have regular dental checks and maintain good dental hygiene throughout therapy as TCAs are known to increase the incidence of dental caries
- contact lens wearers should be warned about the potential for damage to the corneal epithelium from decreased lacrimation and accumulation of mucoid secretions
- regular ophthalmological examination is recommended for all patients
- warn the patient to avoid alcohol and over-the-counter drugs that contain pseudoephedrine or phenylephrine (especially cough and cold preparations, antihistamines and weight-reduction tablets) during and for 2 weeks after stopping therapy
- if insomnia is a troublesome symptom, dose may be divided so that a higher amount is taken as the evening dose
- if the patient is a smoker, they should be warned not to suddenly stop smoking, as serum levels of TCA will be altered. Patient should stop smoking under medical supervision
- instruct the patient that constipation may be treated with increased fluid intake, added dietary roughage or a laxative
- the patient should be warned to avoid exposing skin to direct sunlight. When outdoors, patient should wear protective clothing, hat and sunscreen (with SPF 30+ or greater)
- see also General Patient education for all antidepressant agents (p. 266)

 If used during pregnancy, benefits to the mother should be weighed against potential risks to the newborn infant, as some have shown withdrawal symptoms when mothers have had prolonged therapy with TCAs. Gradual withdrawal before delivery date is recommended.

 Many TCAs are excreted in breastmilk; therefore therapy may need to be stopped or breastfeeding discontinued.

 Lower doses are generally recommended in those over 65 years.

AMITRIPTYLINE HYDROCHLORIDE

Trade name
Amitriptyline -WGR, APX-Amitriptyline, Amitriptyline Lupin, Amitriptyline Viatris, Endep, Entrip

Available forms
Tablets: 10 mg, 25 mg, 50 mg

Action
- active metabolite (nortriptyline) (half-life 26 hours)
- half-life about 22 hours
- see also General Actions of TCAs (p. 267)

Use
- major depression
- nocturnal enuresis (after organic causes have been excluded)

Dose
Depression
- (Outpatient) initially 75 mg orally daily in divided doses, increasing gradually to a daily total of 150 mg if needed **OR**
- (Outpatient) initially 50—100 mg orally at night, increasing by 25—50 mg to a daily total of 150 mg if needed **OR**
- (Hospitalised patients) initially 100 mg orally daily, increasing gradually to 200—300 mg daily if needed **OR**
- (Maintenance) 50—100 mg orally daily

Enuresis
- (11—16 years) 25—50 mg orally at night **OR**
- (6—10 years) 10—20 mg orally at night **OR**
- (Less than 6 years) 10 mg orally at night

Adverse effects
- (Enuresis) (common) drowsiness, anticholinergic effects (but less frequent than for depression)
- see also General Adverse effects/Interactions of TCAs (p. 267)

Interactions
- see General Interactions of TCAs (p. 267)

Nursing considerations/Cautions
- 50 mg tablets are recommended for maintenance therapy only. Should not be used in those who are acutely ill and/or at risk of suicide
- (Enuresis) any organic pathology (e.g. urinary tract infection) should be excluded before starting therapy
- (Enuresis) response is usually seen within a few days but continued treatment is required
- should not be used for children in the management of depression
- see also General Nursing considerations/Cautions for TCAs (p. 268)

Patient education
- tablets are not scored and the patient should be advised to use a pill cutter for a smaller dose (to ensure the tablet is evenly divided)
- warn the patient that the crushed tablet has a bitter/burning taste and may cause numbness to the mouth. The patient should be advised to rinse mouth well and avoid hot drinks and food immediately after to avoid the possibility of burning mouth
- see also General Patient education for TCAs (p. 269)

 Tablets can be crushed and mixed with spoonful of yoghurt or apple puree.

CLOMIPRAMINE HYDROCHLORIDE

Trade name
Anafranil, APO-Clomipramine, Clomipramine-WGR, Placil

Available form
Tablets: 25 mg

Action
- derivative of imipramine
- active metabolite (half-life 13—25 hours)
- half-life 12—36 hours
- see also General Actions of TCAs (p. 267)

ANTIDEPRESSANTS

Use
- major depression
- cataplexy associated with narcolepsy
- obsessive compulsive disorder (OCD)
- phobias

Dose
- (OCD, phobias, depression) initially 25 mg orally 2–3 times daily, increasing by 25 mg every 3–4 days to 100–150 mg daily in 2–3 divided doses, then 50–100 mg daily maintenance in 2–3 divided doses **OR**
- (Catalepsy) 25–75 mg daily orally

Adverse effects
- see General Adverse effects of TCAs (p. 267)

Interactions
- serum levels may be increased by grapefruit, grapefruit juice or cranberry juice
- see also General Interactions of TCAs (p. 267)

Nursing considerations/Cautions
- tablets contain lactose and sucrose, and therefore should not be used in those with galactose intolerance, fructose intolerance, sucrase–isomaltase insufficiency or glucose–galactose malabsorption
- nocturnal medication should be given only in cases where clomipramine does not exacerbate insomnia (cataplexy associated with narcolepsy)
- see also General Nursing considerations/Cautions for TCAs (p. 268)

Patient education
- advise the patient to avoid grapefruit, grapefruit juice or cranberry juice during therapy
- patients with panic disorders should be advised that intensified anxiety may occur at the start of therapy, but subsides within 2 weeks
- see also General Patient education for TCAs (p. 269)

 Tablet can be dispersed in 10–20 mL of water, or crushed (sugar coating may be hard to crush) and then mixed with water or spoonful of yoghurt or apple puree.

DOSULEPIN (DOTHIEPIN) HYDROCHLORIDE
Trade name
Dolsulepin Viatris, Dothep

Available forms
Capsules: 25 mg; Tablets: 75 mg

Action
- equivalent to amitriptyline but less potent than imipramine
- active metabolite
- biphasic elimination: phase one 15–18 hours, whole-body elimination 51 hours
- narrow therapeutic range, with onset of toxicity within 4–6 hours
- see also General Actions of TCAs (p. 267)

Use
- major depression

Dose
- (Depression) initially 25 mg orally 3 times daily for 7–14 days, then increasing daily dose by 25–50 mg after 1–2 weeks if needed (daily maximum 200 mg) (up to 150 mg of daily dose may be given as single nightly dose)

Adverse effects/Interactions/ Nursing considerations/Cautions/ Patient education
- 75 mg tablets are recommended for maintenance therapy only
- should not be used in those who are acutely ill and/or at risk of suicide
- see also General Adverse effects/ Interactions/Nursing considerations/ Cautions/Patient education for TCAs (p. 267)

Capsules can be opened or tablets crushed and contents dispersed in water, or mixed with spoonful of yoghurt or apple puree. Powder/crushed tablet may lead to mouth numbness; therefore care should be taken to rinse mouth and avoid hot drinks or food immediately after administration.

Reduced dose is recommended in those with kidney or liver impairment.

DOXEPIN
Trade name
Deptran

Available forms
Capsules: 10 mg, 25 mg;
Tablets: 50 mg

Action
- active metabolite (half-life is longer than parent compound)
- half-life 8–24 hours, extended in overdose
- see also General Actions of TCAs (p. 267)

Use
- major depression

Dose
- (Mild depression) initially 30 mg orally daily in 3 divided doses, increasing to 50 mg daily if needed **OR**
- (Moderate–severe depression) initially 75 mg orally daily in 3 divided doses, increasing up to 300 mg daily if necessary; dose may be reduced once a satisfactory therapeutic response has been achieved

Adverse effects/Interactions/Nursing considerations/Cautions
- initial dose is dependent on severity of presenting symptoms
- 50 mg tablets are recommended for maintenance therapy only
- if insomnia is a problem, up to 150 mg of the dose can be given in the evening
- see also General Adverse effects/Interactions/Nursing considerations/Cautions for TCAs (p. 267)

Patient education
- warn the patient that mouth numbing may occur if capsules are opened or tablets crushed. The patient should be advised to rinse the mouth well after dose and avoid hot drinks or food immediately after dose to prevent burning mouth
- see also General Patient education for TCAs (p. 269)

Capsules can be opened and contents dispersed in water, or mixed with spoonful of yoghurt or apple puree. Tablets can be crushed and mixed with water, or spoonful of yoghurt or apple puree.

IMIPRAMINE HYDROCHLORIDE
Trade name
Imipramine Hydrochloride Tablets USP, Tofranil

Available forms
Tablets: 10 mg, 25 mg

Action
- active metabolite (desmethylimipramine)
- half-life 20 hours
- see also General Actions of TCAs (p. 267)

Use
- major depression
- nocturnal enuresis (after organic causes have been excluded)

Dose
Depression
- (Ambulant patient) initially 25 mg orally 3 times daily, increasing gradually to 150–200 mg by the end of the first week and maintained until there is improvement in condition, then reduced to 50–100 mg daily as maintenance **OR**
- (Hospitalised patient) initially 25 mg orally 3 times daily increasing by 25 mg increments to 200 mg until condition

improves, then reduced to 100 mg daily as maintenance

Enuresis
- (Over 12 years) 25—75 mg orally at night
OR
- (9—12 years) 25—50 mg orally at night
OR
- (5—8 years) 20—30 mg orally at night

Interactions
- serum levels may be increased by verapamil, diltiazem, labetalol and propranolol
- see also General Interactions of TCAs (p. 267)

Adverse effects/Nursing considerations/Cautions
- tablets contain lactose and sucrose, and therefore should not be used in those with galactose intolerance, fructose intolerance, severe lactase insufficiency, sucrase—isomaltase insufficiency or glucose—galactose malabsorption
- see also General Adverse effects/Nursing considerations/Cautions for TCAs (p. 267)

Patient education
- warn the patient that mouth numbing may occur if tablets are crushed. The patient should be advised to rinse the mouth well after dose and avoid hot drinks or food immediately after dose to prevent burning the mouth
- see also General Patient education for TCAs (p. 269)

 Tablets can be crushed and mixed with water or spoonful of yoghurt or apple puree.

NORTRIPTYLINE
Trade name
Allegron, NortriTABS

Available forms
Tablets: 10 mg, 25 mg

Action
- see General Actions of TCAs (p. 267)

Use
- major depression

Dose
- (Depression) 25 mg orally 3—4 times daily increasing gradually if needed (daily maximum 100 mg)

Adverse effects/Interactions/Nursing considerations/Cautions/Patient education
- see General Adverse effects/Interactions/Nursing considerations/Cautions/Patient education for TCAs (p. 267)

 Tablets can be dispersed in water, or crushed and mixed with spoonful of yoghurt or apple puree.

MONOAMINE OXIDASE INHIBITORS (MAOIs)

General Actions of MAOIs
- monoamine oxidase (MAO) is a mitochondrial enzyme that inactivates the biogenic amines (adrenaline (epinephrine), noradrenaline (norepinephrine), dopamine and serotonin). By inhibiting this enzyme, the level of the biogenic amines is allowed to increase
- two types of MAO enzymes exist in the body. MAO-A is located throughout the body and metabolises adrenaline (epinephrine), noradrenaline (norepinephrine), dopamine and serotonin, producing diverse effects. MAO-B is found in human platelets
- long delay in mood improvement
- metabolism is via acetylation; therefore rate is dependent on whether the person is a slow or rapid acetylator
- when therapy is stopped, MAO activity usually recovers in 3—5 days, but may take up to 2 weeks
- considered second- or third-line treatment of depression if other antidepressants have been ineffective or inappropriate

General Uses of MAOIs
- major depression (not first-line treatment because of adverse effects and dietary restrictions where other antidepressants have been ineffective or inappropriate)

General Adverse effects of MAOIs
- insomnia, disturbed sleep
- drowsiness, dizziness, weakness, fatigue, headache, tremors, twitching/muscle spasm, hyperreflexia, myoclonic movements
- postural hypotension, oedema
- palpitations, tachycardia
- impotence, ejaculation disorders
- dry mouth, constipation, weight gain, nausea, diarrhoea, abdominal pain, anorexia
- elevated liver enzymes
- withdrawal symptoms
- (Uncommon) urinary retention, blurred vision, glaucoma, pruritus, rash, sweating, chills, tinnitus
- (Rare) blood dyscrasias, hypomania and agitation (high dose, prolonged therapy), hepatitis, suicidal ideation, syndrome of inappropriate antidiuretic hormone secretion (SIADH), syncope, hallucinations (especially in the elderly)
- (Severe, possibly fatal) hypertensive crisis
- (High dose) tolerance and dependence (in those with pre-existing drug dependence)

General Interactions of MAOIs
- contraindicated with pethidine (or related opioids) (because of the risk of respiratory depression) and dextromethorphan (risk of psychosis)
- contraindicated with other MAOIs
- should not be given within 10 days of stopping therapy with another MAOI or other antidepressants
- contraindicated with, or within 21 days of, tricyclic antidepressants (TCAs) as combination may cause hyperpyrexia, diffuse intravascular coagulation and status epilepticus
- contraindicated with, or within 14 days of, selective serotonin reuptake inhibitors (SSRIs) or serotonin and noradrenaline (norepinephrine) reuptake inhibitors (SNRIs)
- contraindicated with carbamazepine because of the risk of hyperpyrexia, hypertensive crises and/or convulsions. MAOI should be stopped for at least 2 weeks before starting carbamazepine
- contraindicated with sympathomimetic agents, local anaesthetics or cocaine with added adrenaline (epinephrine), amphetamines, dopamine, fenfluramine, methylphenidate, adrenaline (epinephrine), noradrenaline (norepinephrine), ephedrine and phenylephrine (including over-the-counter (OTC) cold, flu and hay fever preparations), levodopa, l-tyrosine, methyldopa, phenylalanine or tryptophan
- contraindicated with tyramine-containing foods and drinks as they cause a 'cheese reaction' (see Glossary)
- contraindicated with, or within 14 days of, bupropion
- not recommended with high doses of caffeine or caffeine-containing drinks or food
- not recommended with or within 14 days of buprenorphine because of the risk of serotonin syndrome
- effects may be potentiated/prolonged if given with barbiturates. Barbiturates should be given at a reduced dose
- exaggerated hypotension may occur if given with antihypertensive agents
- increased hypotension and CNS depression may occur if given with inhalation anaesthetics
- increased risk of serotonin syndrome if sumatriptan is given with or within 14 days of MAOIs; therefore this should be avoided
- may cause profuse sweating, tremors and hyperpyrexia if given with anti-Parkinson's agents
- may potentiate hypoglycaemic agents or alter glucose metabolism

- may lower convulsive threshold by antagonising antiepileptic agents
- see also General Nursing considerations/Cautions for antidepressant agents (p. 266)

General Nursing considerations/Cautions for MAOIs

- blood pressure should be measured before starting and regularly throughout therapy
- may suppress anginal pain, which acts as a warning of myocardial ischaemia
- may cause excessive stimulation in schizophrenic patients or swing from depression to mania in those with bipolar disorder
- observe for hypoglycaemia in patients with diabetes
- TCAs and SSRIs generally should not be given within 10–14 days of MAOIs (allow 5 weeks if giving with fluoxetine)
- should be discontinued at least 10–14 days before elective surgery or other procedures requiring general anaesthetic or local anaesthestic containing adrenaline (epinephrine)
- treatment of hypertensive crisis includes discontinuing MAOI, giving phentolamine 5 mg slowly IV (to lower blood pressure) and treating hyperpyrexia/fever symptomatically with external cooling (such as a fan). Acute symptoms usually subside within 24 hours
- caution if used in those with epilepsy, diabetes, hyperthyroidism, impaired kidney function or angina
- caution if used in those with pre-existing drug dependence issues as tolerance and dependence may occur
- not recommended in those under 18 years for management of depression or other psychiatric disorders
- contraindicated in those over 60 years
- contraindicated in those with phaeochromocytoma, porphyria, liver disease (or with abnormal liver function), congestive cardiac failure, cerebrovascular disease, cardiovascular disease, hypertension, recurrent/frequent headaches or blood dyscrasias

General Patient education for MAOIs

- the patient must seek medical advice before taking any other preparations with MAOIs (including OTC preparations)
- warn the patient to avoid alcohol and OTC products (including cough and cold preparations with dextromethorphan, nasal decongestants (tablets, drops, sprays), hay fever/sinus preparations, asthma inhalants, antiappetite/weight-reduction preparations or tryptophan-containing products) during and for 2 weeks after stopping therapy, unless advised by the doctor
- the patient should be instructed to avoid tyramine-containing foods and drinks because these may cause a severe hypertensive crisis (including nausea, severe headache, neck stiffness/soreness, palpitations, substernal pain, sweating, pallor, tachycardia/bradycardia and fainting). Foods include cheeses (especially matured/aged such as blue, brie, parmesan, stilton, gruyere), aged, cured and pickled meats and fish (e.g. game, caviar, herring, sausages (kabana, pepperoni, salami, hot-dogs), corned beef, bacon), vegetables (e.g. over-ripe avocado, broad beans, pickled vegetables (e.g. sauerkraut), soy products (e.g. soy sauce), fruits (e.g. over-ripe figs, bananas, raisins or pineapples), meat or yeast extracts (e.g. Bonox, Vegemite, stock cubes, packet soups) and alcoholic beverages (e.g. red wine (especially Chianti), sherry, beer, liqueurs). These foods should also be avoided for 14 days after stopping therapy with MAOIs. Medical advice should be sought immediately if patient eats tyramine-containing food
- if the patient stops taking MAOI (under medical supervision), a normal diet (with

- tyramine-containing foods and drink) should not be resumed for 2 weeks after discontinuation
- advise the patient about the need to continue therapy and to keep follow-up appointments
- the patient should be warned to avoid large intakes of caffeine (including tea, coffee, cola and chocolate) during therapy
- instruct the patient to immediately report any headache (which may radiate frontally), rapid or slowed heart rate, nausea, vomiting, neck stiffness or soreness, photophobia, dilated pupils, sweating (sometimes with fever and cold/clammy skin) and constricting chest pain
- if insomnia is a problem, the patient can be advised to take last dose before 3 pm
- if the patient has diabetes, they should be instructed to monitor blood glucose levels closely during therapy
- see also General Patient education for antidepressant agents (p. 266)

Safety in pregnancy has not been established. If given during third trimester, may result in withdrawal symptoms in newborn.

Secreted in breastmilk; therefore should be used with caution during breastfeeding.

Contraindicated in those over 60 years.

PHENELZINE
Trade name
Nardil

Available form
Tablets: 15 mg

Action
- two metabolites, although it is unknown if they are clinically active
- short half-life (1.2 hours)
- see also General Actions of MAOIs (p. 273)

Dose
- (Depression) initially 15 mg orally 3 times daily, increasing to 60—90 mg daily for at least 4 weeks, then reduced slowly to as low as 15 mg daily or every second day (maintenance)

Action/Use/Adverse effects/ Interactions/Nursing considerations/ Cautions/Patient education
- see General Uses/Adverse effects/ Interactions/Nursing considerations/Cautions/Patient education for MAOIs (p. 274)

Tablet can be crushed and mixed with water or spoonful of yoghurt or apple puree.

TRANYLCYPROMINE
Trade name
Parnate

Available form
Tablets: 10 mg

Dose
- (Depression) initially 20 mg orally daily (given as 10 mg morning and 10 mg evening); if ineffective after 2 weeks, add a further 10 mg at midday; when response is established, dose may be reduced to 10—20 mg daily (daily maximum 30 mg) **OR**
- (Treatment in combination with ECT) 10 mg orally twice daily during ECT therapy, then 10 mg daily

Interactions
- contraindicated with, or within 14 days of, moclobemide
- see also General Interactions of MAOIs (p. 274)

Action/Use/Adverse effects/Nursing considerations/Cautions/Patient education
- tablets contain sucrose and are therefore not recommended in those with rare hereditary problem of fructose intolerance, glucose—galactose malabsorption or sucrase—isomaltase insufficiency

ANTIDEPRESSANTS

- see also General Actions/Uses/Adverse effects/Nursing considerations/Cautions/Patient education for MAOIs (p. 273)

 Tablet can be crushed and mixed with water or spoonful of yoghurt or apple puree.

REVERSIBLE INHIBITORS OF MONOAMINE OXIDASE TYPE A (RIMAs)

MOCLOBEMIDE
Trade name
Amira, APO-Moclobemide, Aurorix, Clobemix, Moclobenide-WRG, Moclobenide Sandoz

Available forms
Tablets: 150 mg, 300 mg

Action
- selectively inhibits monoamine oxidase A (MAO A) over MAO B in a ratio of 4:1
- causes an increase in extracellular levels of noradrenaline (norepinephrine), dopamine and serotonin, which results in an increase in mood and psychomotor activity, relieving symptoms such as dysphoria, poor concentration, exhaustion and lack of drive
- MAO activity is restored within 1—2 days of stopping therapy
- increases total sleep time while not impairing alertness or reaction time
- half-life 2 hours

Use
- major depression

Dose
- initially 300—450 mg orally daily in 2 divided doses after meals, increasing after at least a week if needed to 300—600 mg in 2 divided doses (maintenance)

Adverse effects
- nausea, diarrhoea, constipation, dry mouth
- dizziness, headache
- restlessness, anxiety, agitation, irritability
- insomnia
- paraesthesia
- hypotension
- rash
- (rare) confusion, suicidal ideation, serotonin syndrome (see p. 265)

Interactions
- contraindicated with TCAs, SSRIs or irreversible MAOIs because of the increased risk of serotonin syndrome
- contraindicated with selegiline, clomipramine, pethidine, tramadol, triptans, bupropion, linezolid or dextromethorphan
- may increase pressor effect if given with sympathomimetic agents at high doses
- may increase effects of opioids and therefore should be used with caution
- may increase serum levels of proton pump inhibitors
- not recommended with dextropropoxyphene
- not recommended with St John's wort because of the increased risk of serotonin syndrome
- caution if used with venlafaxine
- caution if used with buprenorphine because of the risk of serotonin syndrome

Nursing considerations/Cautions
- allow the correct amount of time to elapse between stopping SSRIs and starting moclobemide (5 weeks after stopping fluoxetine; 2 weeks after stopping paroxetine; 1 week after stopping citalopram or fluvoxamine)
- may theoretically precipitate hypertensive crisis in patients with thyrotoxicosis or phaeochromocytoma; therefore caution if used
- caution if used in those with liver or kidney impairment
- not recommended in those with rare hereditary problems of galactose intolerance, Lapp lactase deficiency or glucose—galactose malabsorption

- not recommended in those under 18 years for the treatment of depression
- contraindicated in those with acute confusion
- see also General Nursing considerations/Cautions for antidepressant agents (p. 266)

Patient education
- advise patient to take tablets after meals
- restriction of tyramine-rich foods is not as stringent as for MAOIs; however, some people may be sensitive to tyramine and therefore ingesting large amounts of tyramine-rich food should be discouraged ('cheese reaction', see Glossary)
- hypertensive patients should be advised to avoid tyramine-rich foods
- warn patient to avoid alcohol and OTC products (including cough and cold preparations with dextromethorphan)
- see also General Patient education for antidepressant agents (p. 266)

 Tablet can be crushed and mixed with water, or spoonful of yoghurt or apple puree.

 Safety in pregnancy has not been established; therefore it should be used only if benefits outweigh risks to fetus.

 Very small amount secreted in breastmilk; therefore should be used with caution during breastfeeding.

 Dose should be reduced by one-half or one-third in those with severe liver impairment.

SELECTIVE SEROTONIN REUPTAKE INHIBITORS (SSRIs)

General Actions of SSRIs
- selectively inhibit reuptake of serotonin (5-hydroxytryptamine, 5HT), prolonging serotonin action
- anxiolytic action
- increases prolactin levels
- suppresses rapid eye movement (REM) sleep and increases deep slow-wave sleep

General Adverse effects of SSRIs
- palpitations, tachycardia, hypotension (including postural hypotension)
- dizziness, tremor, headache, migraine, asthenia, twitching, amnesia, apathy, anxiety, nervousness, aggravated depression, fatigue, agitation, paraesthesia, impaired concentration, confusion
- anorexia, nausea, vomiting, abdominal pain, diarrhoea, altered taste, dry mouth, flatulence, increased appetite, increased/decreased weight, dyspepsia, increased saliva, constipation
- hot flushes, increased sweating, chills, fever
- insomnia, somnolence, abnormal dreams
- yawning
- decreased libido/impotence, ejaculation disorders
- bone fractures
- amenorrhoea, menstrual disorders
- myalgia, arthralgia, back pain
- cough, pharyngitis, rhinitis, sinusitis
- rash, pruritus, urticaria
- polyuria, urinary frequency
- blurred vision, mydriasis
- tinnitus
- bleeding disorders (purpura, ecchymosis, haematoma, epistaxis, GI and vaginal bleeding, postpartum haemorrhage)
- (Rare) hyponatraemia, syndrome of inappropriate antidiuretic hormone secretion (SIADH), akathisia/psychomotor restlessness, increased risk of bone fractures, seizures, suicidal ideation, suicidal behaviours, mania, serotonin syndrome (see p. 265), prolongation of QT interval
- withdrawal symptoms (nausea, vomiting, diarrhoea, headache, dizziness, paraesthesia, insomnia, nightmares, disturbed dreams, visual disturbances, palpitations, emotional instability,

ANTIDEPRESSANTS

anxiety, agitation, tremor, confusion, sweating)

General Interactions of SSRIs

- contraindicated with, or within 14 days of, stopping MAOIs or linezolid because of the increased risk of serotonin syndrome
- contraindicated with, or within 1 day of, stopping moclobemide
- moclobemide should not be started within 14 days of stopping SSRIs
- not recommended with 5HT agonists (serotonergic agents) (e.g. sumatriptan, tramadol, tryptophan, fentanyl, lithium, St John's wort) as the risk of serotonin syndrome is increased
- use with alcohol should be avoided
- not recommended with SNRIs because of the risk of serotonin syndrome and increased serum levels and toxicity of SNRIs
- not recommended with TCAs or antipsychotic agents
- not recommended with other agents known to prolong QT interval
- prothrombin time should be carefully monitored if given with warfarin (not citalopram)
- caution if given with agents that lower seizure threshold, such as other SSRIs, TCAs, antipsychotic agents, tramadol, bupropion or mefloquine
- caution if given with other centrally acting agents
- caution if used with ECT
- may prolong action of neuromuscular blocking agents such as suxamethonium and mivacurium
- increased effects may occur if given with tryptophan
- increased serum levels may result if given with omeprazole
- caution if given with lithium
- increased risk of bleeding if given with aspirin, NSAIDs, antiplatelet agents, anticoagulants, TCAs, atypical antipsychotics, phenothiazines or other agents affecting coagulation
- glycaemic control may be affected; therefore blood glucose levels should be closely monitored and antidiabetic agent dose adjusted accordingly
- may increase serum levels (and therefore associated adverse effects/toxicity) of phenytoin, carbamazepine, flecainide, metoprolol (when used for cardiac failure), clomipramine, nortriptyline, imipramine, risperidone, theophylline, methadone, clozapine, ciclosporin, tacrine or haloperidol

General Nursing considerations/ Cautions for SSRIs

- any hypokalaemia and/or hypomagnesaemia should be corrected before starting, and potassium and magnesium levels should be monitored regularly throughout therapy
- treatment should be over at least 6 months to prevent relapse
- electrolytes should be monitored at the start of therapy in the elderly because of the increased risk of hyponatraemia
- ECG monitoring is recommended for patients with any risk factors for QT interval prolongation
- sexual dysfunction may continue after therapy is stopped
- not recommended in those with unstable heart disease or recent history of myocardial infarction
- not recommended in those under 18 years for the treatment of major depression
- caution if used in those with a history of bleeding disorders or taking drugs affecting platelet function, epilepsy or history of seizures, impaired kidney or liver function, diabetes, acute narrow-angle glaucoma or raised intraocular pressure
- caution if used in those at risk of QT interval prolongation such as congestive cardiac failure, bradyarrhythmias or predisposition to hypokalaemia or hypomagnesaemia

HAVARD'S NURSING GUIDE TO DRUGS

- contraindicated in those with congenital long QT syndrome
- see also General Nursing considerations/Cautions for antidepressant agents (p. 266)

General Patient education for SSRIs

- if patient has diabetes, instruct them to carefully monitor blood glucose levels as glucose tolerance may be disrupted
- advise patients that nausea usually decreases within first 2 weeks of therapy
- patients should be advised to seek medical advice immediately if any of the following occur:
  - unusual bleeding or bruising
  - change in heart rate (fast, irregular) and/or fainting
  - unpleasant or distressing restlessness, inability to sit or stand still
- see also General Patient education for antidepressant agents (p. 266)

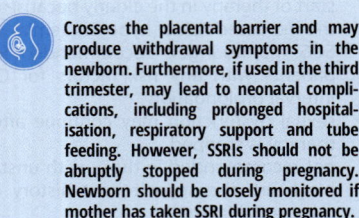

Crosses the placental barrier and may produce withdrawal symptoms in the newborn. Furthermore, if used in the third trimester, may lead to neonatal complications, including prolonged hospitalisation, respiratory support and tube feeding. However, SSRIs should not be abruptly stopped during pregnancy. Newborn should be closely monitored if mother has taken SSRI during pregnancy.

Excreted in breastmilk; therefore breastfeeding is not recommended or contraindicated.

CITALOPRAM

Trade name
A-Citalopram, APO-Citalopram, APX-Citalopram, Auro-Citalopram, Celapram, Cipramil, Citalopram Sandoz, Citalopram-GA, Citalopram WGR, Noumed Citalopram, Pharmcor Citalo, Talam

Available forms
Tablets: 10 mg, 20 mg, 40 mg

Action
- active metabolites have SSRI properties but less than citalopram itself
- long half-life 36 hours
- see also General Actions of SSRIs (p. 278)

Use
- major depression

Dose
- initially 20 mg orally daily, increasing by 10 mg at 2—3-weekly intervals to 40 mg daily maximum if necessary

Adverse effects/Interactions/ Nursing considerations/Cautions/ Patient education

- tablets contain lactose and therefore should not be used in those with galactose intolerance, Lapp lactase insufficiency or glucose—galactose malabsorption
- see also General Adverse effects, Interactions/Nursing considerations/ Cautions/Patient education for SSRIs (p. 278)

Tablets can be dispersed in water (stir for 5—10 minutes), or crushed and given with spoonful of yoghurt or apple puree.

Recommended starting dose for those with mild-to-moderate liver impairment is 10 mg. Dose may be increased after 2—3 weeks to 20 mg (maximum dose).

Recommended starting dose is 10 mg daily for those 65 years and over. Dose may be increased after 2—3 weeks to 20 mg (maximum dose).

ESCITALOPRAM

Trade name
APO-Escitalopram, APX-Escitalopram, Blooms Escitalopram, Blooms the Chemist Escitalopram, Cilopam-S, Escitalopram-GH, Escitalopram Sandoz, Escitalopram-TIH, Esipram, Lexapro, Loxalate, Noumed Escitalopram

Available forms
Tablets: 10 mg, 20 mg;

ANTIDEPRESSANTS

Oral solution: 20 mg/mL

Action
- long half-life (30 hours) (extended in those with mild-to-moderate liver impairment or over 65 years)
- see also General Actions of SSRIs (p. 278)

Use
- major depression
- social anxiety disorder (social phobia), generalised anxiety disorder
- obsessive compulsive disorder (OCD)

Dose
- (Major depression, social or generalised anxiety disorder, OCD) initially 10 mg orally daily, increasing gradually to a daily maximum of 20 mg

Adverse effects/Interactions/ Nursing considerations/Cautions
- contraindicated in those with hypersensitivity to citalopram
- see also General Adverse effects/ Interactions/Nursing considerations/ Cautions for SSRIs (p. 278)

Patient education
- warn patient that crushed tablet has bitter taste

Oral solution
- instruct patient to turn bottle upside down completely. If no drops come out, tap bottle lightly to start flow
- advise patient that 10 mg = 10 drops of the 20 mg/mL solution
- drops should be added to drink (water, apple or orange juice but no other fluids), stirred and drunk
- oral solution should be stored below 25°C and discarded 2 months after opening
- see also General Patient education for SSRIs (p. 280)

Oral solution is available. Tablet can be dispersed in water (some brands are slow to disperse), or crushed and mixed with spoonful of yoghurt or apple puree.

Maintenance dose should not exceed 10 mg in those 65 years and over.

Recommended dose for those with liver impairment is 5 mg. May be increased to 10 mg after to 2 weeks if needed with caution.

FLUOXETINE
Trade name
APO-Fluoxetine, Blooms the Chemist Fluoxetine, Fluotex, Fluoxetine Generichealth, Fluoxetine Sandoz, Nuomed Fluoxetine, Prozac, Zactin

Available forms
Capsules: 20 mg;
Tablets (dispersible): 20 mg

Action
- active metabolite norfluoxetine (long half-life 4—16 days)
- half-life is 1—3 days (acute administration), which is extended to 4—6 days with chronic administration
- slow elimination and long half-life means that, even after therapy is stopped, drug/metabolite will persist for weeks
- see also General Actions of SSRIs (p. 278)

Use
- major depression
- obsessive—compulsive disorder (OCD)
- premenstrual dysphoric disorder (PMDD)

Dose
- (Depression, OCD) initially 20 mg orally morning, increasing to twice-daily dosage (morning, noon) after several weeks if no clinical improvement is noted (daily maximum 80 mg) **OR**
- (PMDD) 20 mg orally daily **OR**
- (PMDD) 20 mg orally daily starting 14 days before anticipated onset of menstruation, continuing until first day of menses, repeating for each menstrual cycle

Adverse effects
- (Common) rash, urticaria
- (Rare) allergy, anaphylactic events

- see also General Adverse effects of SSRIs (p. 278)

Interactions
- may increase serum levels of diazepam, alprazolam and imipramine
- may decrease efficacy of tamoxifen
- may alter lithium levels
- see also General Interactions of SSRIs (p. 279)

Nursing considerations/Cautions/Patient education
- patient should be advised to immediately seek medical advice if any rash or hives occur
- advise patient to swallow capsule whole or dissolve tablets in 100 mL water
- see also General Nursing considerations/Cautions/Patient education for SSRIs (p. 279)

Dispersible tablets available. Capsule can be opened and contents mixed with yoghurt or apple puree.

A lower or less frequent dose is recommended in those with liver impairment owing to prolonged elimination.

FLUVOXAMINE MALEATE
Trade name
APO-Fluvoxamine, Faverin, Fluvoxamine-WGR, Luvox, Movox

Available form
Tablets: 50 mg, 100 mg

Action
- half-life is 12–13 hours (single dose) or 22 hours (repeated dosing)
- metabolite has similar half-life
- see also General Actions of SSRIs (p. 278)

Use
- major depression
- obsessive–compulsive disorder (OCD)

Dose
- (Depression) initially 50 mg orally at night for 7 days, increasing gradually by 50 mg/week if needed (daily maximum 300 mg) **OR**
- (OCD) initially 50 mg orally daily for 3–4 days, then increasing by 50 mg every 4–6 days until effective (daily maximum 300 mg)

Interactions
- may increase serum levels of caffeine, propranolol, midazolam, haloperidol, ropinirole, alprazolam and diazepam
- serum levels may be decreased by smoking
- see also General Interactions of SSRIs (p. 279)

Adverse effects/Nursing considerations/Cautions
- doses greater than 150 mg should be given in 2–3 doses
- see also General Adverse effects/Nursing considerations/Cautions for SSRIs (p. 278)

Patient education
- instruct patient that tablets should be swallowed whole
- warn patient not to suddenly stop smoking without first seeking medical advice
- see also General Patient education for SSRIs (p. 280)

Tablet is difficult to crush and does not disperse. If crushed, crush finely and mix with spoonful of yoghurt or apple puree.

Starting at low dose and careful monitoring is recommended in those with kidney or liver impairment.

PAROXETINE
Trade name
APX-Paroxetine, Aropax, Blooms the Chemist Paroxetine, Extine, Noumed Paroxetine, Paroxetine GH, Paroxetine Sandoz, Paroxetine-WGR, Paxtine, Roxtine 20

Available form
Tablets: 20 mg

ANTIDEPRESSANTS

Action
- half-life about 24 hours
- see also General Actions of SSRIs (p. 278)

Use
- major depression
- obsessive—compulsive disorder (OCD)
- social anxiety disorder (social phobia), generalised anxiety disorder
- post-traumatic stress disorder (PTSD)

Dose
- (Depression) initially 20 mg orally daily, increasing by 10 mg at weekly intervals if needed (daily maximum 50 mg) **OR**
- (OCD) initially 20 mg orally daily, increasing by 10 mg at weekly intervals if needed (daily maximum 60 mg) **OR**
- (Panic disorder) initially 10 mg orally daily, increasing by 10 mg at weekly intervals if needed (daily maximum 60 mg) **OR**
- (Social anxiety disorder/social disorder, anxiety, PTSD) initially 20 mg orally daily, increasing by 10 mg at weekly intervals if needed (daily maximum 50 mg)

Interactions
- decreased serum levels may occur if given with ritonavir/fosamprenavir
- may decrease efficacy of tamoxifen
- see also General Interactions of SSRIs (p. 279)

Adverse effects/Nursing considerations/Cautions/Patient education
- (Panic disorder) low starting dose and slow increase in dosage is recommended to decrease the risk of associated anxiety early in the management of this disorder
- advise patient that tablets should be swallowed whole, not chewed
- see also General Actions/Adverse effects/Nursing considerations/Cautions/Patient education for SSRIs (p. 278)

 Tablet does not disperse in water, but can be crushed and mixed with spoonful of yoghurt or apple puree.

 Doses at lower end of range are recommended for those with kidney or liver impairment.

 Daily maximum dose should not exceed 40 mg in those > 65 years.

SERTRALINE
Trade name
APO-Sertraline, Blooms the Chemist Sertraline, Eleva, Noumed Sertraline, Sertra, Sertraline Generichealth, Sertraline Sandoz, Sertraline TIH, Sertraline-WGR, Setrona, Zoloft

Available forms
Tablets: 50 mg, 100 mg

Action
- half-life about 24 hours
- metabolite has less activity but longer half-life
- see also General Actions of SSRIs (p. 278)

Use
- major depression
- obsessive—compulsive disorder (OCD)
- panic disorder
- premenstrual dysphoric disorder (PMDD)
- social anxiety disorder (social phobia), generalised anxiety disorder

Dose
- (Major depression) initially 50 mg orally daily, increasing at weekly intervals if needed (daily maximum 200 mg) **OR**
- (Panic disorder, social phobia) initially 25 mg orally daily, increasing to 50 mg daily after 1 week **OR**
- (PMDD) 50 mg orally daily, increasing by 50 mg per menstrual cycle if needed (daily maximum 150 mg) **OR**
- (PMDD) 50 mg orally daily for 14 days before anticipated menstruation continued until first day of menses, repeated each menstrual cycle. Dose can be increased by 50 mg per menstrual cycle if needed (daily maximum 100 mg)

- (OCD, 6—12 years) initially 25 mg orally daily for 7 days, then increase to 50 mg **OR**
- (OCD, 13—18 years) initially 50 mg orally daily **OR**
- (OCD, adult) initially 50 mg orally daily, increasing at weekly intervals if needed (daily maximum 200 mg)

Adverse effects/Interactions/ Nursing considerations/Cautions/ Patient education

- increases serum levels of diazepam
- should not be used in those under 18 years for management of major depression
- see also General Adverse effects/ Interactions/Nursing considerations/ Cautions/Patient education for SSRIs (p. 278)

 Tablet can be dispersed in water or crushed and mixed with spoonful of yoghurt or apple puree.

SEROTONIN AND NORADRENALINE (NOREPINEPHRINE) REUPTAKE INHIBITORS (SNRIs)

General Actions of SNRIs

- selective serotonin and noradrenaline (norepinephrine) reuptake inhibitor that prolongs action of serotonin and noradrenaline (norepinephrine) at receptor sites

General Adverse effects of SNRIs

- nausea, vomiting, diarrhoea, constipation, dry mouth, anorexia, decreased/increased weight, dyspepsia, abdominal pain, altered taste
- headache, fatigue, asthenia, dizziness, somnolence, insomnia, disturbed dreams, tremor, paraesthesia, anxiety, altered concentration, irritability, agitation, feeling jittery, nervousness
- ecchymosis, haematoma, epistaxis, petechiae, GI bleeding, postpartum haemorrhage
- yawning
- tinnitus, vertigo
- sweating, hot flushes
- pruritus, rash
- palpitations, tachycardia, increased BP, postural hypotension, syncope
- (Males) abnormal ejaculation, erectile dysfunction, impotence, decreased libido, testicular pain
- (Females) abnormal orgasm, menorrhagia
- dysuria, urinary retention, urinary hesitancy, proteinuria
- blurred vision, mydriasis
- chills
- increased serum cholesterol and triglycerides, elevated liver enzymes, altered glycaemic control
- withdrawal symptoms (nausea, vomiting, fatigue, dizziness, headache, lethargy, agitation, anxiety, confusion, irritability, vertigo, somnolence, insomnia, vivid nightmares, sweating, paraesthesia, seizures)
- (Rare) hyponatraemia, suicide ideation, seizures, syndrome of inappropriate antidiuretic hormone secretion (SIADH), akathisia/psychomotor restlessness, hypomania/mania, serotonin syndrome (see p. 265), neuroleptic malignant syndrome

General Interactions of SNRIs

- contraindicated with, or within 14 days of stopping, MAOIs
- should be stopped for at least 7 days before starting an MAOI
- contraindicated with reversible MAOIs (RIMAs) (e.g. moclobemide, linezolid, IV methylene blue)
- increased risk of serotonin syndrome if given with SSRIs, other SNRIs, TCAs, amphetamine, lithium, sibutramine, fentanyl, methadone, St John's wort, triptans, tramadol, pethidine or tryptophan
- caution if used with other CNS active agents

ANTIDEPRESSANTS

- SNRIs may inhibit metabolism of TCAs, increasing serum levels and anticholinergic effects
- INR should be monitored if given with warfarin, especially when starting, stopping or adjusting dose
- not recommended with tryptophan supplements
- not recommended with alcohol
- increases risk of bleeding if given with NSAIDs, aspirin, warfarin or other agents
- increased risk of hyponatraemia if given with diuretics (especially in the elderly)

General Nursing considerations/Cautions for SNRIs

- any dehydration, hypovolaemia or pre-existing hypertension should be corrected before starting therapy
- BP monitoring is recommended (especially in those with hypertension or cardiac disease). If BP remains elevated, the dose should be reduced or therapy stopped
- liver function (including serum lipids and cholesterol) should be monitored regularly during therapy
- sexual dysfunction may continue for some time after stopping therapy
- those at risk of narrow angle glaucoma should be closely monitored throughout therapy
- caution if used in those with pre-existing or uncontrolled hypertension, history of bleeding disorders, unstable heart disease, hyperthyroidism, heart failure, recent myocardial infarction, cerebrovascular disease, raised serum cholesterol or triglycerides, dehydration, hypovolaemia, history of seizures or mania, raised intraocular pressure, at risk of narrow-angle glaucoma, urinary retention, prostatic hypertrophy or those over 65 years with hypertension and/or other cardiac disease
- see also General Nursing considerations/Cautions for antidepressant agents (p. 266)

General Patient education for SNRIs

- patients with diabetes should be instructed to monitor blood glucose levels closely during therapy
- advise the patient to seek medical advice if any of the following occur:
  - rash or hives (allergy)
  - unpleasant or distressing restlessness, inability to sit or stand still (akathisia/psychomotor restlessness)
  - headache, difficulty concentrating, impaired memory, confusion, weakness, unsteadiness (hyponatraemia)
- women should be advised to discuss pregnancy with their doctor and are recommended to use adequate contraception throughout therapy
- see also General Patient education for antidepressant agents (p. 266)

Should be used during pregnancy only if benefits outweigh potential risks to the fetus. Increased risk of postpartum haemorrhage if taken during last month of pregnancy. Increased risk of pre-eclampsia if given in mid to late pregnancy. Withdrawal symptoms or other adverse effects may occur in the newborn if given during third trimester.

May be excreted in breastmilk: therefore not recommended during breastfeeding. If used, infant should be closely observed.

DESVENLAFAXINE

Trade name
APO-Desvenlafaxine MR, BTC Desvenlafaxine, Desfax, Desvenlafaxine Amneal, Desvenlafaxine GH XR, Desvenlafaxine Sandoz, Deesvenlafaxine-WGR XR, Medven, Pristiq

Available forms
Tablets (extended/modified-release): 50 mg, 100 mg

Action
- active metabolite of venlafaxine

- half-life 11 hours (prolonged in those with kidney impairment)
- see also General Actions of SNRIs (p. 284)

Use
- major depression

Dose
- initially 50 mg orally daily, increasing dose gradually at 1-week intervals if needed (daily maximum 200 mg)

Interactions
- not recommended with venlafaxine
- caution if used with midazolam because of the risk of increased sedation
- may cause false positive results on urine immunoassay screening for amphetamine and phencyclidine (PCP) for up to several days after therapy is stopped
- see also General Interactions of SNRIs (p. 284)

Adverse effects/Nursing considerations/Cautions
- contraindicated in those with hypersensitivity to venlafaxine
- see also General Adverse effects/Nursing considerations/Cautions for SNRIs (p. 284)

Patient education
- patient should be advised to take tablets whole, not crushed or chewed
- warn patient that inert tablet matrix/shell may be noticed when defecating or via colostomy. Active medication has already been absorbed
- see also General Patient education for SNRIs (p. 285)

Tablets should not be dispersed, crushed or chewed.

For those with end-stage kidney disease or severe kidney impairment, recommended dose is 50 mg every second day.

DULOXETINE
Trade name
APO-Duloxetine, Cymbalta, Depreta, Duloxecor, Duloxetine Sandoz, Dytrex, Tixol

Available forms
Capsules (enteric-coated): 30 mg, 60 mg

Action
- half-life is about 12 hours with no difference between males and females
- see also General Actions of SNRIs (p. 284)

Use
- major depression
- generalised anxiety disorder
- diabetic neuropathic pain

Dose
- (Depression, diabetic neuropathic pain) 60 mg orally daily **OR**
- (Generalised anxiety disorder) initially 30 mg orally daily, increasing at 30 mg increments if needed (daily maximum 120 mg)

Interactions
- contraindicated with fluvoxamine
- may decrease efficacy of tamoxifen
- may increase serum levels of flecainide and risperidone
- clearance may be decreased by paroxetine or other SSRIs increasing serum levels and risk of adverse effects
- caution if used with agents which may slow motility or increase gastric pH
- see also General Interactions of SNRIs (p. 284)

Adverse effects/Nursing considerations/Cautions/Patient education
- not recommended in those with acute or chronic liver disease (including those who consume large amounts of alcohol)
- not recommended for those aged 18 years or under
- contraindicated in those with liver impairment

ANTIDEPRESSANTS

- see also General Adverse effects/Nursing considerations/Cautions/Patient education for SNRIs (p. 284)

Capsules should not be crushed. Capsules can be opened and pellets dispersed in apple juice or sprinkled on apple juice. Pellets should not be chewed.

If CrCl < 30 mL/min, the recommended dose is 30 mg orally daily.

REBOXETINE
Trade name
Edronax

Available form
Tablets: 4 mg

Action
- weakly inhibits serotonin uptake
- half-life is about 12 hours
- see also General Actions of SNRIs (p. 284)

Use
- major depression (including prevention of relapse)

Dose
- initially 4 mg orally twice daily, increasing after 3 weeks up to 10 mg daily if needed

Adverse effects
- see General Adverse effects of SNRIs (p. 284)

Interactions
- contraindicated with or within 14 days of MAOIs
- serum levels may be decreased by carbamazepine or phenobarbital (phenobarbitone)
- caution if used with antihypertensive agents, as orthostatic hypotension may be exacerbated
- use with ergot alkaloids may increase hypertension; therefore BP should be closely monitored during therapy
- increased serum levels may occur if given with azole antifungal agents, macrolide antibiotics (e.g. erythromycin) and fluvoxamine
- caution if given with lithium

Nursing considerations/Cautions/Patient education
- see General Nursing considerations/Cautions/Patient education for SNRIs (p. 285)

Tablets can be dispersed in water or crushed and given with spoonful of yoghurt or apple puree.

Recommended starting dose for those with kidney or moderate-to-severe liver impairment is 2 mg orally twice daily.

Recommended starting dose for those > 65 years is 2 mg orally twice daily, increasing up to 6 mg daily after 3 weeks if needed.

VENLAFAXINE HYDROCHLORIDE
Trade name
APO-Venlafaxine XR, Blooms the Chemist Venlafaxine XR, Efexor XR, Elaxine SR, Enlafax-XR, Sandoz Venlafaxine XR, Venlafaxine Generichealth, Venlafaxine XR-WRG

Available forms
Capsules (modified-release): 37.5 mg, 75 mg, 150 mg

Action
- half-life 8—11 hours
- active metabolite (half-life 9—13 hours)
- see also General Actions of SNRIs (p. 284)

Use
- major depression
- generalised anxiety disorder, social anxiety disorder
- panic disorder

Dose
- (Panic disorder) initially 37.5 mg orally daily with food for 4—7 days, then increasing to 75 mg daily. If needed, dose can be increased at 2-week intervals by 75-mg increments (daily maximum 225 mg) **OR**
- (Depression, generalised or social anxiety disorder) initially 75 mg orally daily with food, increasing after 2 weeks to

150 mg daily, then gradually at 2-week intervals to 225 mg if necessary

Adverse effects
- sustained hypertension
- (Uncommon) rash, pruritus
- (Rare) prolongation of QTc interval, stress cardiomyopathy
- see also General Adverse effects of SNRIs (p. 284)

Interactions
- may increase serum levels of clozapine, haloperidol, lithium or risperidone with its associated toxicity/adverse effects
- increased serum levels may occur if given with erythromycin, fluconazole or grapefruit juice
- caution if given with metoprolol, as antihypertensive effect may be reduced
- caution if given with other agents that prolong QTc interval
- may decrease serum levels of indinavir
- see also General Interactions of SNRIs (p. 284)

Nursing considerations/Cautions
- caution if used in those at risk of QTc prolongation
- not recommended in those under 18 years
- see also General Nursing considerations/Cautions for SNRIs (p. 285)

Patient education
- patient should be advised to seek medical advice if any of the following occur:
  - rash, hives or other skin condition develops
  - heart rate becomes rapid or irregular
- advise patient that tablets should be swallowed whole and not chewed or crushed
- instruct patient to avoid grapefruit juice during therapy
- see also General Patient education for SNRIs (p. 285)

Capsules and contents should not crushed. Efexor XR (only) — capsules can be opened and contents given with spoonful of apple puree.

Dose reduction by 25—50% is recommended in those with kidney impairment (GFR 10—70 mL/min).
Dose reduction of 50% is recommended in those with moderate-to-severe liver impairment or receiving haemodialysis.

ATYPICAL ANTIDEPRESSANT AGENTS

AGOMELATINE
Trade name
Agomelatine Lupin, Agomelatine Sandoz, Domion, Valdoxan, Agomelatine-WGR

Available form
Tablets: 25 mg

Action
- melatonin receptor (MT_1 and MT_2) agonist and $5HT_{2C}$ receptor antagonist
- increases noradrenaline (norepinephrine) and dopamine in prefrontal cortex specifically, thereby decreasing GI, sexual function and cardiovascular adverse effects
- improves sleep
- rapid half-life (1—2 hours)

Use
- major depression (including prevention of relapse)
- generalised anxiety disorder

Dose
- initially 25 mg orally at night (bedtime) for 2 weeks (for depression) or 4 weeks (for generalised anxiety disorder), increasing to 50 mg orally if needed

Adverse effects
- elevated liver enzymes
- nausea, vomiting, dry mouth, diarrhoea, abdominal pain, dyspepsia, constipation
- increased weight

ANTIDEPRESSANTS

- headache, migraine, dizziness, tremor, anxiety, fatigue, irritability
- insomnia, somnolence, abnormal dreams, sedation
- sweating
- back pain, arthralgia
- (Rare) hepatitis, suicidal ideation, urinary retention

Interactions

- contraindicated with fluvoxamine and ciprofloxacin
- caution if given with oestrogens (oral contraceptives), propranolol and rifampicin
- caution if used with other antidepressants
- not recommended with alcohol

Nursing considerations/Cautions

- before starting therapy, patient should be assessed for any risk factors for liver injury including alcohol use, substantial alcohol intake, non-alcoholic fatty liver disease, diabetes, being overweight or obese
- liver function tests are recommended before starting therapy, at 3, 6, 12 and 24 weeks and then regularly or if increasing dose to 50 mg
- therapy should not be started if liver enzymes are more than 3 times the upper limit of normal
- if liver enzymes become elevated, liver function test should be repeated within 48 hours
- if liver transaminases are more than 3 times normal upper limits or if patient has signs of liver injury, therapy should be stopped
- dose does not need to be tapered when discontinuing therapy
- therapy should be continued for at least 6 months after response to ensure symptoms do not recur
- if switching from SSRI or SNRI, agomelatine can be started immediately while tapering the dose of SSRI/SNRI. Tapering should be gradual to prevent discontinuation symptoms
- tablets contain lactose and therefore should not be used in those with galactose intolerance, Lapp lactase insufficiency or glucose–galactose malabsorption
- caution if used in those with elevated liver enzymes or at risk of liver impairment (e.g. obese, overweight, non-alcoholic fatty liver, substantial alcohol use, concurrent use of hepatotoxic medications)
- not recommended for those under 18 years
- not recommended for major depression in patients with dementia
- contraindicated in those with liver impairment including cirrhosis and active liver disease, or with liver transaminases more than 3 times upper normal limit
- see also General Nursing considerations/Cautions for antidepressant agents (p. 266)

Patient education

- advise patient to immediately report any abdominal pain, tiredness, yellowing of skin or eyes or dark urine
- see also General Patient education for antidepressant agents (p. 266)

 Tablets can be crushed and mixed with water or spoonful of yoghurt or apple puree.

 Safety has not been established in pregnancy and therefore is not recommended.

 Not recommended during breastfeeding unless benefits to mother outweigh risks to newborn.

 Not recommended to treat depression in those 75 years or over or to treat generalised anxiety disorder in those over 65 years.

ESKETAMINE
Trade name
Spravato

Available form
Nasal spray: 28 mg

Action
* enantiomer of ketamine
* non-selective, non-competitive antagonist of *N*-methyl-D-aspartate (NMDA) receptor
* diverse from other antidepressant actions as does not involve monoamine, GABA or opioid receptors
* rapidly absorbed by nasal mucosa
* half-life 7–12 hours

Use
* treatment-resistant depression (where there has been no adequate response to at least 2 different antidepressants at adequate dose and treatment duration) in conjunction with a newly started oral antidepressant

Dose
* Induction phase (weeks 1–4) < 65 years: 56 mg intranasally (first dose), then 56 or 84 mg twice weekly
* Maintenance phase (evidence of therapeutic benefit established) weeks 5–8 < 65 years: 56 or 84 mg weekly week 9 onward 56 or 84 mg every two weeks or once weekly (lowest dosing frequency to maintain response)

Adverse effects
* somnolence, sedation
* dissociation, perception disturbances, anxiety, euphoria, mental impairment, tremor, lethargy, slowed speech, feeling abnormal or drunk, confusion, asthenia
* dizziness, vertigo, headache
* abnormal taste, nausea, vomiting, dry mouth
* tachycardia, elevated blood pressure
* nasal discomfort
* throat irritation, oropharyngeal pain
* sweating
* urinary frequency and urgency, dysuria
* (Rare) respiratory depression

Interactions
* increased risk of sedation if given with CNS depressants including benzodiazepines, opioids and alcohol
* increased BP may result if given with amphetamine, methylphenidate, modafinil or armodafinil
* use with MAOI, including tranylcypromine, selegiline or phenelzine, may result in increased BP
* should be separated by at least a 1-hour interval from other nasal preparations

Nursing considerations/Cautions
* the patient should be assessed for any cardiovascular or cerebrovascular conditions before starting therapy. Patient should be stable and free of any cardiac symptoms if there is a history of myocardial infarction
* administration is under direct supervision of doctor/health care professional
* 28 mg = 1 device, 56 mg = 2 devices, 84 mg = 3 devices
* BP must be measured before administration and not administered if elevated (> 140 mmHg systolic, > 90 mmHg diastolic)
* BP should be monitored for at least 40 minutes post administration
* device should NOT be primed before use
* doctor/health professional will instruct patient in self-administration
* a 5-minute interval should be allowed between administration when more than one device is required
* the patient should also be monitored for sedation and dissociation symptoms post administration until clinically stable
* caution if used in those with history of drug abuse or dependence, as there is a risk for misuse or abuse (although this is lessened as administration is under direct supervision of doctor/health professional)
* caution if used in those with unstable or poorly controlled hypertension, within 6 weeks of myocardial infarction, within

ANTIDEPRESSANTS

- 6 months of ischaemic stroke or transient ischaemic attack, significant valvular heart disease (e.g. mitral regurgitation, aortic stenosis, aortic regurgitation), or heart failure (NYHA Class III or IV) (regardless of aetiology)
- caution if used in those with or with a history of psychoses, mania, bipolar mania, insufficiently treated hyperthyroidism, uncontrolled bradyarrhythmias or tachyarrhythmias leading to haemodynamic instability, history of brain injury, hypertensive encephalopathy, intrathecal therapy with ventricular shunts or other conditions associated with raised intracranial pressure
- not recommended in those with severe liver impairment
- contraindicated in those in whom an increase in BP or intracranial pressure may pose a serious risk, or in those with known intracranial, thoracic or abdominal aortic aneurysm or history of intracerebral haemorrhage
- contraindicated in those with known hypersensitivity to ketamine or esketamine

Patient education

- the patient should be instructed not to eat for 2 hours before administration or drink liquids at least 30 minutes before administration
- if the patient uses a nasal decongestant or nasal corticosteroid, advise them to not use these within 1 hour of administration
- the patient should be warned that their blood pressure will be monitored before and after administration
- warn the patient not to drive or operate machinery until next day after a good night's sleep
- self-administration instructions should include:
  - blowing nose before administration
  - device is NOT primed before use
  - reclining head at a 45-degree angle for administration
  - inserting tip of device into nostril with nose rest, touch skin between nostrils
  - close opposite nostril
  - breathe in while pushing plunger all the way until it stops
  - sniff gently to keep medication inside nostril
  - move device to other nostril and repeat to deliver second spray
  - doctor/health professional will check device to ensure all medication has been administered
  - rest for 5 minutes in semireclined position taking care not to blow nose
  - if another dose is required, the steps are repeated
- women of childbearing potential should be advised to use adequate contraception during therapy and for 6 weeks after stopping therapy to avoid pregnancy occurring

Animal studies with ketamine have shown developmental neurotoxicity; therefore not recommended during pregnancy.

Thought to be excreted in breastmilk; therefore not recommended during breastfeeding.

Dose reduction is recommended for those 65 years and over, with starting dose of 28 mg intranasally, then increasing to 56 mg or 84 mg in 28-mg increments depending on patient tolerance and response.

MIANSERIN HYDROCHLORIDE
Trade name
Lumin

Available forms
Tablets: 10 mg, 20 mg

Action
- tetracyclic antidepressant (chemically unrelated to tricyclic antidepressants (TCAs)) that blocks noradrenaline (norepinephrine) uptake
- also acts on serotonin (5HT) receptors on CNS
- anxiolytic, promotes sleep
- long half-life (21–61 hours)

Use
- major depression

Dose
- initially 30 mg orally daily as 3 divided doses or single at night (bedtime) dose, slowly increasing at weekly intervals to a maintenance dose of 30–90 mg daily if needed (daily maximum 120 mg)

Adverse effects
- tiredness, lethargy, drowsiness, sedation, headache, tremor, dizziness, faintness, weakness, vertigo
- dry mouth, constipation
- (Rare) altered glucose tolerance, hypotension
- (Very rare) convulsions, bone marrow depression (neutropenia, thrombocytopenia, agranulocytosis), jaundice, hypomania, bradycardia, QT prolongation, cardiac arrest

Interactions
- contraindicated with or within 2 weeks of monoamine oxidase inhibitors (MAOIs)
- MAOIs should not be commenced within 2 weeks of stopping mianserin
- may have unpredictable effects on warfarin serum levels; therefore INR levels should be closely monitored, especially when starting or stopping therapy, or adjusting dose
- CNS depressant effects enhanced by alcohol, barbiturates and benzodiazepines
- not recommended with alcohol
- BP monitoring is recommended if given with antihypertensive agents
- caution if given with other agents that prolong QTc interval
- serum levels may be decreased by phenytoin and carbamazepine

Nursing considerations/Cautions
- any hypokalaemia or hypomagnesaemia should be corrected before starting therapy
- blood glucose levels should be carefully monitored in those with diabetes because glucose tolerance may be altered
- full blood count is recommended if patient complains of sore throat, malaise, mouth ulcers, flu-like symptoms or infection
- caution if used in elderly with a history of white cell disorders, or those with narrow-angle glaucoma, diabetes, prostatic hypertrophy, epilepsy, liver/renal impairment, who are female or aged 65 years and over
- caution if used in those with cardiac impairment (including recent myocardial infarction, heart block and unstable heart disease), structural heart disease, left ventricular dysfunction or those at risk of QT prolongation including long QT syndrome
- not recommended in those under 18 years
- contraindicated in those with mania or severe liver disease
- see also General Nursing considerations/Cautions for antidepressant agents (p. 266)

Patient education
- advise the patient to swallow tablet whole between meals
- if the patient has diabetes, instruct them to carefully monitor blood glucose levels, as glucose tolerance may be disrupted
- instruct the patient that the daily dose should be divided or may be taken as a single dose at night
- the patient should be advised to seek medical advice immediately if any of the following occur:
  - sore throat, fever, chills, mouth ulcers, malaise, flu-like symptoms or signs of infection
  - unusual bleeding or bruising
  - change in heart rate (fast, irregular) and/or fainting
- see also General Patient education for antidepressant agents (p. 266)

 Tablet can be dispersed in water (2–5 minutes), or crushed and given with spoonful of yoghurt or apple puree.

ANTIDEPRESSANTS

Should be used during pregnancy only if benefits outweigh risks.

Not recommended during breastfeeding.

Contraindicated in those with severe liver disease

MIRTAZAPINE
Trade name
APX-Mirtazapine, Avanza, Axit, Blooms the Chemist Mirtazapine, Mirtanza, Mirtazapine Sandoz, Mirtazapine-WGR, Noumed Mirtazapine, Mirtanza ODT

Available forms
Tablets: 15 mg, 30 mg, 45 mg;
Tablets (dissolvable): 15 mg, 30 mg, 45 mg

Action
- tetracyclic antidepressant (TCA) that is an analogue of mianserin but unrelated to TCAs, selective serotonin reuptake inhibitors (SSRIs) or monoamine oxidase inhibitors (MAOIs)
- increases release of noradrenaline (norepinephrine) and serotonin (5HT)
- blocks $5HT_2$ and $5HT_3$ receptors, allowing serotonin to act on $5HT_1$ receptors
- weak anticholinergic properties
- sedative properties
- half-life (20—40 hours), with shorter half-life noted in young men

Use
- major depression

Dose
- initially 15 mg orally at night, increasing gradually to 30—45 mg if no response in 2—4 weeks (daily maximum 60 mg)

Adverse effects
- drowsiness, sedation (during first weeks of treatment)
- oedema (local or generalised)
- increased appetite, weight gain
- (Uncommon) dizziness, headache, severe skin reaction
- (Rare) bone marrow depression, postural hypotension, hyponatraemia, seizures, serotonin syndrome (see p. 265), suicidal ideation, akathisia/psychomotor restlessness

Interactions
- contraindicated with or within 2 weeks of MAOIs
- caution if given with agents that prolong QTc interval
- INR should be closely monitored if given with warfarin, especially when stopping or starting therapy, or adjusting dose
- may potentiate effects of alcohol, antipsychotics, antihistamines, opioids, sedatives or benzodiazepines
- risk of serotonin syndrome is increased if given with other serotonergic agents, including SSRIs, lithium, tramadol, linezolid, triptans, L-tryptophan, St John's wort, serotonin and noradrenaline (norepinephrine) reuptake inhibitors (SNRIs) and methylene blue
- serum levels may be decreased if given with carbamazepine, rifampicin or phenytoin
- caution if used with azole antifungal agents, HIV protease inhibitors or erythromycin as serum levels may be increased
- not recommended with alcohol

Nursing considerations/Cautions
- any dehydration, hypovolaemia or electrolyte imbalance should be corrected before starting therapy
- liver function and blood counts should be measured before starting therapy and regularly throughout
- not recommended in those under 18 years
- (Dissolvable tablets) contain aspartame and are therefore not recommended in those with phenylketonuria

- tablets contain lactose/sucrose and therefore should not be used in those with galactose intolerance, Lapp lactase insufficiency, fructose intolerance or glucose—galactose malabsorption
- caution if used in those with epilepsy, organic brain syndrome, liver/kidney impairment, hypotension, dehydration, hypovolaemia, prostate hypertrophy, raised intraocular pressure, narrow-angle glaucoma, recent myocardial infarction, angina or diabetes mellitus
- see also General Nursing considerations/Cautions for antidepressant agents (p. 266)

Patient education

- advise the patient that tablets should be swallowed whole, without chewing
- instruct the patient that dose may be divided into morning and evening doses
- if the patient has diabetes, instruct them to carefully monitor blood glucose levels as glucose tolerance may be disrupted
- if the patient is taking dissolvable tablets, the following instructions should be given:
  - take care not to crush tablets when removing from foil
  - carefully peel off foil lid starting at corner indicated by arrow
  - ensure hands/fingers are dry
  - place dissolvable tablet on tongue, then swallow when dissolved (with or without water)
- the patient should be advised to seek medical advice immediately if any of the following occur:
  - sore throat, fever, chills, mouth ulcers, malaise, flu-like symptoms or signs of infection
  - seizures (fits)
  - feeling sick, weak, confused, exhausted, muscle weakness or cramping (signs of low sodium level)
  - unpleasant or distressing restlessness, inability to sit or stand still
  - skin reaction
- see also General Patient education for antidepressant agents (p. 266)

 Available as an orally dissolving tablet which can be dissolved on the tongue with or without water. Tablet can be crushed and given with spoonful of apple puree or yoghurt.

 Should be used during pregnancy only if benefits clearly outweigh potential risks to the fetus.

 Not recommended during breastfeeding.

VORTIOXETINE
Trade name
Brintellix

Available forms
Tablets: 5 mg, 10 mg, 15 mg, 20 mg

Action
- serotonin receptor activity modulator, 5HT transporter reuptake inhibitor
- long half-life 66 hours

Use
- major depression (including prevention of relapse)

Dose
- initially 10 mg orally daily, increasing to 20 mg or decreasing to 5 mg daily if needed

Adverse effects
- headache, dizziness, somnolence, sedation, fatigue, asthenia
- insomnia
- sweating, pruritus
- decreased appetite, nausea, vomiting, dry mouth, dyspepsia, abdominal discomfort
- back pain, arthralgia
- nasopharyngitis, flu-syndrome
- sexual dysfunction
- (Rare) seizure, serotonin syndrome (see p. 265), neuroleptic malignant syndrome, abnormal bleeding (ecchymoses, purpura and GI haemorrhage), hyponatraemia, mania/hypomania

ANTIDEPRESSANTS

Interactions
- contraindicated with or within 2 weeks of monoamine oxidase inhibitors (MAOIs), including irreversible nonselective MAOI (e.g. selegiline, rasagiline), reversible MAO-A (e.g. moclobemide), reversible nonselective MAOI (e.g. linezolid)
- increased risk of serotonin syndrome if given with serotonergic agents (e.g. tramadol, lithium, selective serotonin reuptake inhibitors (SSRIs), sumatriptan and other triptans)
- increased risk of adverse effects and serotonin syndrome if given with St John's wort
- increased risk of seizures if given with agents that lower seizure threshold such as SSRIs, serotonin and noradrenaline (norepinephrine) reuptake inhibitors (SNRIs), phenothiazines, thioxanthenes, butyrophenones, mefloquine, bupropion and tramadol
- decreased serum levels may occur if given with rifampicin
- increased serum levels and therefore risk of adverse effects may occur if given with bupropion
- may increase serum levels of tricyclic antidepressants (TCAs), increasing the risk of toxicity and serotonin syndrome
- caution if given with anticoagulants or other agents that affect platelet function because of the risk of bleeding
- caution if used with other agents that cause hyponatraemia
- caution if used with ECT
- may cause a false positive urine drug screen for methadone

Nursing considerations/Cautions
- unlike many other antidepressants, may be stopped without gradual reduction
- not recommended in those under 18 years
- see also General Nursing considerations/Cautions for antidepressants (p. 266)

Patient education
- see General Patient education for antidepressants (p. 266)

 Tablet can be crushed and mixed with water or spoonful of yoghurt or apple puree.

 Used during pregnancy only if benefits outweigh risks.

 Not recommended during breastfeeding.

 Dose should be started at 5 mg in those 65 years and over.

ANTIDIABETIC AGENTS

Diabetes mellitus is classified according to the process that leads to hyperglycaemia. Earlier classification used criteria such as age of onset (e.g. juvenile onset diabetes) or type of therapy (e.g. insulin dependent, non-insulin dependent). However, both of these are now outdated as it is now recognised that diabetes can develop at any age and those who start as non-insulin dependent may become insulin dependent as the disease progresses. The two main categories of diabetes are type 1 and type 2, but there are other forms of diabetes that share characteristics of type 1 and/or type 2 (Powers, Niswender & Evans-Mollina 2022).

Worldwide, the prevalence of diabetes was estimated at 537 million in 2021 (1 in 10 adults) and is thought to increase to 643 million (1 in 9 adults) by 2030 if the current rates continue (IDF 2021). Australian data for 2021 showed 1.3 million people (1 in 20) (or 5% of Australian adults) had diabetes, this having increased from 460,000 people in 2000. In the same time period (2021—22), 10% of all hospitalisations were associated with diabetes and contributed to 11% of all deaths (AIHW 2024). The rate of diabetes prevalence, hospitalisation, mortality and burden of disease is almost three times higher for Aboriginal and Torres Strait Islander people than for non-indigenous Australians (AIHW 2024).

Normally, beta cells in the islets of Langerhans in the pancreas release *insulin* to regulate blood glucose levels (BGLs), keeping them between 4.0 and 7.8 mmol/L. Insulin is made up of 51 amino acids arranged in A and B chains joined by disulfide bonds. It has a short half-life (3—5 minutes) and is mainly metabolised in the liver, but also in the kidney and muscles. After a meal and when BGLs are >3.9 mmol/L, insulin release is stimulated and enters the portal venous system (Powers, Niswender & Evans-Mollina 2022). Insulin has a number of functions, including:

- stimulating the storage of glucose in the liver as glycogen and in adipose tissue as triglycerides
- stimulating the storage of amino acids in muscle as protein
- inhibiting the breakdown of triglycerides, glycogen and protein and conversion of amino acids to glucose (Powers, Niswender & Evans-Mollina 2022).

Types of diabetes include:
- *type 1*, which accounts for about 15% of diabetes overall and results from complete or near-complete insulin deficiency and can occur at any age, although commonly before 20 years of age. The insulin deficiency is due to autoimmune destruction of the pancreatic beta cells, while other pancreatic cells (e.g. alpha, delta) remain intact and function normally. Although the exact cause is unknown, the autoimmune response may be triggered by an environment factor such as viral infection. Family history is also thought to play a role (IDF 2021).
- *type 2*, a heterogeneous group of disorders characterised by degrees of insulin resistance, impaired insulin secretion and increased glucose production. Risk factors for developing type 2 diabetes include family history, obesity (especially central and visceral fat), physical inactivity, race/ethnicity, history of gestational diabetes mellitus, hypertension, elevated HDL cholesterol and triglycerides, polycystic ovary syndrome and history of cardiovascular disease. Those with pre-diabetes or at risk of diabetes may be able to prevent or delay the onset of diabetes by addressing some of the related lifestyle factors such as weight management, increased exercise and control of blood pressure and lipids (Powers, Niswender & Evans-Mollina 2022).
- *gestational diabetes mellitus*, which occurs in some women during the second or third trimester of pregnancy when glucose intolerance develops. Blood glucose levels generally return to normal after delivery; however, these women have a substantial risk (35—60%) of developing type 2 diabetes in later life. In 2021—22, one in six pregnant women in Australia developed gestational diabetes. The incidence of gestational diabetes doubled from 2012—13 to 2021—22, and was thought to be related to increased maternal age, higher rates of maternal overweight and obesity, and growing proportions of higher risk ethnic groups in the population, but most importantly to an introduction of new diagnostic guidelines between 2011 and 2013 (AIHW 2024).

Monitoring BGLs is an important part of diabetes management in order to decrease microvascular complications such as neuropathy, retinopathy and nephropathy, and other cardiovascular complications. BGLs can be monitored using a drop of blood from a finger prick or by a continuous glucose monitoring (CGM) device that is worn by the person continuously. There are two types of CGM available: one that produces real time monitoring every 1 to 5 minutes, or the intermittently scanned data that stores BGL data when the sensor is scanned by a device or smartphone app (Sly & Taylor 2023). Both of these systems provide real time BGLs. Glycated haemoglobin (HbA1c) is a blood test that looks at the long-term diabetes management. HbA1c measures the average blood glucose level over the previous 3 months, but doesn't reflect any variations that may have occurred during that time (e.g. highs and/or lows). Persistently elevated blood glucose levels correlate with diabetes-related complications (Powers, Niswender & Evans-Mollina 2022).

Patient education is an important part of the management plan and the newly diagnosed person should receive education about nutrition, exercise, care of diabetes during illness, how and when to monitor blood glucose levels, medication (how and when to administer), how to look after themselves generally to prevent complications (e.g. the importance of correct footwear, regular inspection of feet, ophthalmology review and podiatry visits), as well as managing associated conditions such as dyslipidaemia, hypertension, cardiovascular disease and obesity (Powers, Fowler & Rickels 2022). It is important that regular reviews are scheduled and attended. Education should not be a once-off occurrence, but should be ongoing, especially if there are any changes or problems (e.g. changing from an oral hypoglycaemic agent to insulin; hypoglycaemia occurring frequently; eyesight problems changing a person's ability to manage their own insulin injection; a change from one type of device to another, such as from a syringe to an insulin prefilled pen). Many of these issues are considered below in more detail.

INSULINS

Early insulin preparations were from beef (bovine) or pork (porcine) pancreas. Currently, insulin with an amino acid sequence identical to that of human insulin is obtained by either enzymatic modification of purified pork insulin (emp) (semisynthetic) or recombinant DNA techniques using bacteria (crb, prb) or yeast (pyr) (biosynthetic). Human insulins are less likely to cause antigen reactions than are beef insulins, which are no longer commonly used in Australia.

Insulins are classified according to onset, peak and duration of action (e.g. ultra-short, short, intermediate and long acting). Insulins are also available in a premixed combination (e.g. short acting plus intermediate, or ultra-short plus long acting).

Available forms
Vial, prefilled/cartridge pens 100 U/mL, 300 U/mL

- formulations include ultra-short-acting, short-acting, intermediate-acting and long-acting insulins (see Table, p. 303)
- premixed (or biphasic) insulins — include both short-acting and long-acting insulins in the same formulation

General Actions of insulins
- duration of action is dependent on dose, formulation, site of injection, blood supply to the area, temperature and physical activity
- see also introduction (p. 296)

General Use of insulins
- type 1 diabetes
- type 2 diabetes not adequately controlled by diet and/or oral hypoglycaemic agents, or at times of increased or unusual stress such as pregnancy, infection, illness, trauma or surgery
- gestational diabetes mellitus
- emergency management of diabetic ketoacidosis (regular insulin)
- hyperglycaemic (hyperosmolar), non-ketotic coma

Dose
- no standard dose
- dose is individual and determined in consultation with the medical practitioner, and is dependent on BGLs, as well as the person's weight, diet, lifestyle, exercise levels, stress, illness, pregnancy, type of insulin and regimen in order to avoid fluctuation in BGLs and hypo- or hyperglycaemia
- generally given SC

General Adverse effects of insulins
- hypoglycaemia (timing is dependent on action profile of particular insulin; signs and symptoms include cold sweats, cool pale skin, tremor, nervousness, anxiety, tiredness, weakness, confusion, altered concentration, drowsiness, excessive hunger, visual disturbance, headache, nausea and palpitations; severe hypoglycaemia can lead to unconsciousness, brain impairment and death). Some patient groups (e.g. elderly people, those

ANTIDIABETIC AGENTS

- with long-standing diabetes or markedly improved glycaemic control or on concurrent medications which interact with insulin) may not experience the typical early warning symptoms of a hypoglycaemic reaction
- hyperglycaemia (due to inadequate dosing or stopping therapy, especially in those with type 1 diabetes)
- (Initially) sodium retention, oedema, visual impairment, including refraction anomalies, acute reversible painful neuropathy
- (Injection site reaction) erythema, pain, swelling, hives or itching
- nasopharyngitis, sinusitis, rhinitis
- nausea, upper abdominal pain, gastroenteritis
- back pain, arthralgia
- fatigue, dizziness, headache
- (Local allergic reaction) pruritus, rash, redness, induration
- (Uncommon) lipodystrophy (lipoatrophy or lipohypertrophy) at injection site, which disappears slowly if site is changed. Lipodystrophy will delay insulin absorption from that site
- (Rare) (systemic allergic reaction) urticaria, pruritus, angioedema, bronchospasm, shortness of breath, sweating, fast pulse, hypotension, generalised skin reaction
- (Rare) insulin resistance (requiring a change to purified porcine or human insulin), antibody development

General Interactions of insulins

- alcohol, clonidine, lithium, isoniazid, interferons, oestrogen-containing oral contraceptives and beta adrenoceptor blocking agents can produce variable effects (either increasing or decreasing actions of insulin)
- insulin requirements may be increased if given with beta2 stimulants (e.g. salbutamol), clozapine, corticosteroids, danazol, diazoxide, glucagon, growth hormone, lanreotide, octreotide, olanzapine, oxymetholone, phenothiazines, progestogens, somatotrophin, sympathomimetic agents, thiazide diuretics and thyroid hormones
- insulin requirements may be decreased if given with angiotensin-converting enzyme (ACE) inhibitors (captopril, enalapril), alcohol, alpha adrenoceptor blocking agents (e.g. prazosin), beta adrenoceptor blocking agents (non-selective), anabolic steroids (except danazol and oxymetholone), fibrates, fluoxetine, monoamine oxidase inhibitors (MAOIs), octreotide, pentoxifylline (oxpentifylline), oral hypoglycaemic agents, perhexiline, quinine, salicylates and sulfonamides
- increased risk of hypoglycaemia if given with oral hypoglycaemic agents
- caution if given with protease inhibitors, as hyperglycaemia may occur
- extreme caution if given with disopyramide because of the additive hypoglycaemia risk (especially in the elderly or those with malnutrition, kidney or cardiac impairment)
- if given with pentamidine, there is an increased risk of hypoglycaemia, which may be followed by hyperglycaemia
- beta adrenoceptor blocking agents may mask the symptoms and delay recovery from hypoglycaemia by blocking gluconeogenesis
- increased risk of congestive cardiac failure if given with thiazolidinediones (pioglitazone)

General Nursing considerations/Cautions for insulins

- it is important to review patient education and injection technique regularly, especially if the person has an increase in the frequency of hypo- or hyperglycaemic episodes or uncontrolled BGLs
- hypoglycaemia is likely if BGL is less than 3 mmol/L; convulsions may occur if it is less than 2 mmol/L

- changes between types, brand or species of insulin should be done with caution and careful monitoring
- have available 50% glucose and glucagon (glucagon is injected to increase the BGL temporarily to treat any severe hypoglycaemic reaction when the person cannot or will not swallow or is unconscious; see Antidotes, antagonists and chelating agents, p. 350). Glucagon can be given IM or SC, but glucose must be given IV by a medical professional if the person has not responded to glucagon in 10—15 minutes
- if using an insulin-infusion pump, it is important to check if the insulin is recommended for use in the pump (as there are some that are not)
- (Lantus) should not be diluted or mixed with other insulins or solutions
- (Fiasp) must not be diluted or mixed with other products except infusion fluids (glucose 5% or sodium chloride 0.9%)
- caution in those using protamine-containing insulin if protamine is used to reverse heparinisation after cardiac catheterisation, as a severe anaphylactic-type reaction is possible
- caution if used in those who have had recent surgery or trauma or who have liver or kidney impairment, fever, severe infection, hyperthyroidism, adrenal or pituitary disorders (not adequately controlled), diarrhoea, intestinal obstruction or vomiting
- insulin is contraindicated in those with hypoglycaemia or with hypersensitivity to insulin preparations

Short-acting insulin
- includes very short-acting (aspart, lispro, glulisine) and short-acting (neutral) preparations
- clear solution, usually given SC, but may be given IV or IM in emergencies such as diabetic ketoacidosis, pre-coma and coma
- when given IM, onset of action is more rapid than SC but duration is shorter
- usually given 15—30 minutes before meals
- cloudy solutions should be discarded
- injection should be followed by carbohydrate-containing snack/meal within 15—30 minutes (depending on the very short-acting or short-acting insulin)

Long-acting insulin
- appears white and cloudy
- contains zinc or protamine, allowing slow release of insulin, so prolonging the duration of action
- used in people with stabilised insulin-sensitive diabetes
- given SC, never IM or IV or in an emergency
- should be gently shaken or agitated by rolling in the palms of the hands to evenly distribute insulin throughout solution before using (should not be vigorously shaken)
- newer formulations (e.g. insulin detemir, insulin glargine) should not be mixed

Storage
- store unopened insulin (vials/cartridges/prefilled pens) at 2—8°C, but do not freeze and do not store next to freezer compartment or freezer packs
- before first use, insulin should be allowed to come to room temperature for 1—2 hours as injecting cold insulin is painful
- insulin in use can be stored at room temperature provided that the room temperature does not exceed 25°C; mark date of opening on label and discard after 28 days
- avoid overexposure to light or heat
- insulin should be discarded if it has been frozen or exposed to high temperatures (as the protein becomes denatured), if discoloured or if any lumps or flakes are present
- do not store cartridge pens (that are in use) in the refrigerator

ANTIDIABETIC AGENTS

Preparation
- select correct preparation
- porcine insulin should not be given to those of Islamic or Jewish faith
- not mixed with other drugs
- keep insulin at room temperature for at least 1–2 hours before use to reduce pain
- check expiry date
- suspensions are rotated gently (not vigorously shaken) and inverted several times to ensure full dispersion and prevent frothing
- insulin of one brand should not be mixed with insulin of another brand
- model and brand of syringe or needle should not be changed without consulting the doctor
- when mixing insulins, use the same procedure every time for accuracy and constant effect
- short-acting insulin is drawn up first to prevent its contamination in the vial by the long-acting insulin (containing zinc or protamine), which binds soluble insulin, thereby reducing the amount of soluble insulin available for immediate effect. The mixture should be injected immediately after mixing
- the majority of insulins are available in 100 units/mL vials, together with a standard insulin syringe marked in units for U100 insulin (dose ranges from 10 to 100 or more units, depending on the severity of the diabetes, and is adjusted according to blood glucose level). The exception to this is glargine insulin (Toujeo), which is available as 300 units/mL
- incompatible with agents containing thiols or sulfites

Administration
- ineffective if given orally
- usually given SC; avoid IV injection by withdrawing syringe plunger before injecting
- the area should not be massaged after injection because this may speed up absorption
- given usually 30 minutes before breakfast (however, some of the ultra-rapid insulins can be given just before or with a meal) or, if twice daily, give a second injection before the evening meal
- injection sites include the upper arms, thighs and abdomen; however, because absorption rates vary so much it is advisable to rotate injection sites within the same anatomical location, preferably the abdomen, which has the most rapid absorption rate
- injection sites are rotated so that the same site is not injected more than once per month to prevent thickening and dimpling of the site (lipodystrophy), which may result in decreased insulin absorption
- instructions enclosed with the injection pen and cartridge vial must be followed carefully to ensure correct dose is administered

General Patient education for insulins

After diagnosis, patient education should begin at least several days before hospital discharge in order to give the person the opportunity to ask questions and practise skills such as blood sugar monitoring and injection techniques. Education needs to be ongoing and life long.
- emphasise the importance of exercise, maintaining a healthy weight range and correct diet (referral to a dietitian may be necessary)
- advise the patient about the temporary changes to vision that can occur at the start of treatment with insulin, which can impact on ability to drive or operate machinery
- type of insulin to be used (e.g. short-acting, long-acting) and an understanding of why it is being used
- monitoring of BGLs, including technique, when to monitor, recording of information

- understanding how to manage BGL if fasting for diagnostic or surgical procedures
- choice of appropriate insulin devices, depending on:
  - the person's vision and ability to see the dose (e.g. some devices have an audible click when insulin doses are dialled up and this may maintain a visually impaired person's independence)
  - fine motor skills (e.g. some devices require the person to load a cartridge and dial up the dose, while others are preloaded)
  - ability to manage the actual device itself, including loading cartridges, performing safety test (if needed), cleaning, knowing when the device has malfunctioned and what to do if there is a problem
- emphasise the importance of checking insulin label (on cartridge, reusable pen or vial) before each injection to ensure correct insulin is being used. This is especially important if the person uses more than one formulation type. Insulin should also be checked for any cloudiness or particles, and not used if they are present and the insulin solution is not clear
- injection technique (with opportunity to practise skills), including not massaging area after injection
- importance of rotating injection sites (e.g. not using the same site more than once per month) including abdomen, thigh, buttock and upper arm
- if injection pen is damaged or not working, it should not be used
- disposal of sharps into a sharps container, including not reusing needles and not sharing needles or devices with others
- correct storage of insulin (both unopened and opened; with or without needles attached)
- importance of following injection with carbohydrate-containing meal or snack
- significance of carrying some form of oral glucose at all times (e.g. jelly-beans, barley sugar) to prevent hypoglycaemia
- if using an infusion pump, understanding the importance of having an alternative delivery device in case of pump failure (e.g. SC therapy) and understanding pump use and changing of infusion set. The person should understand that pump malfunction may lead to fast onset of hypoglycaemia and ketosis and what to do if any of these occur
- recognising symptoms of hypoglycaemia (e.g. cool pale skin, fatigue, drowsiness, unusual tiredness, sweating, shaking, anxiety, crying, vomiting, headache, excessive hunger, visual changes, palpitations and confusion). However, it is important to emphasise that symptoms vary between people, with some experiencing only a few symptoms and others many. It is essential that the person knows what their individual symptoms are and acts immediately
- anticipating when hypoglycaemia is likely to occur (e.g. increased exercise) and working out a snack or meal pattern to prevent or overcome it
- understanding that hypoglycaemia causes slower reaction time (important when driving or operating machinery)
- recognising symptoms of hyperglycaemia including loss of appetite, drowsiness, flushed dry skin, dry mouth, increased thirst, blurred vision, passing large amounts of urine and 'fruity' breath
- the patient/carer needs to understand that hyperglycaemia is a potentially life-threatening situation
- the benefits of obtaining and wearing a MedicAlert bracelet or pendant (especially in the event of confusion or loss of consciousness)
- the need for extra food requirements before or during increased activity such as sport or, alternatively, that the insulin dose may require adjustment. If the patient exercises regularly, a doctor should be consulted regarding food intake and insulin requirements to ensure that hypoglycaemia is prevented
- the patient should be instructed to seek advice from a doctor/diabetes educator when travelling overseas and crossing

ANTIDIABETIC AGENTS

CHARACTERISTICS OF DIFFERENT INSULIN PREPARATIONS

Preparation	Examples	Onset	Peak	Duration
Ultra short-acting (rapid)				
Insulin glulisine	Apidra	15 minutes	1 hour	
Insulin lispro	Humalog	15 minutes	1–3 hours	3–5 hours
Insulin aspart	Fiasp NovoRapid	15 minutes	1–3 hours	3–5 hours
Short-acting				
Neutral (regular, soluble) insulin	Actrapid Humulin R	30 minutes	2–5 hours	6–8 hours
Intermediate-acting				
Isophane insulin (with protamine)	Humulin NPH Protaphane	1–2.5 hours	4–10 hours	16–24 hours
Long-acting (basal)				
Insulin glargine	Lantus Toujeo Optisulin	1–2 hours	Steady state	24 hours (does not peak)
Insulin detemir	Levemir	3–4 hours	3–14 hours	12–24 hours
Biphasic/combination				
30/70 or 50/50 mixtures of short-acting plus intermediate-acting insulin; or ultra-short-acting plus long-acting insulin	Humalog Mix (insulin lispro + insulin lispro protamine); Humulin 30/70 (insulin isophane human + insulin neutral human) Mixtard (insulin isophane human + insulin neutral human)	0.5–1 hour	2–12 hours	16–24 hours
	NovoMix (insulin aspart +insulin aspart protamine)			
	Ryzodeg 70/30 (insulin aspart + insulin degludec)			

303

time zones, as these may affect administration times of insulin, increasing the risk of unstable BGLs. It is also important for the person to carry a letter from the doctor explaining why he/she has injecting pens and needles
- advise the patient that if feeling ill (including cold and flu, or vomiting), they should continue to use insulin, take food in liquid form as replacement and consult a doctor if unable to eat a normal diet or if blood or urine tests become positive for glucose and/or ketones. Infection and fever often increase insulin requirements
- changes in insulin strength, brand, type and/or species should be done under medical supervision as requirements may change. Early warning symptoms of hypoglycaemia may also be altered when changing from an animal source insulin to another type
- a relative, friend, colleague or teacher should be alerted that the person has diabetes and instructed on how to identify and deal with hypoglycaemia or hyperglycaemia, including recognising symptoms and what to do if the person loses consciousness (e.g. place on side, get medical assistance, do not give the person who is unconscious anything to eat or drink as they may choke; they may be instructed in injecting glucagon if the person has hypoglycaemia)
- if the person wears glasses and is currently experiencing uncontrolled BGLs, they should be advised to postpone obtaining new corrective lenses until BGLs have stabilised for 3—6 weeks, as it can take this length of time for visual disturbances to stabilise
- warn the patient of the dangers of drinking alcohol (especially excessive amounts), as it can affect the actions of insulin and may lead to hypoglycaemia occurring. Alcohol may also predispose the person to hyperglycaemia on the morning following alcohol intake
- female patients should be advised to inform the doctor if they become pregnant or are planning pregnancy
- advise the patient about organisations such as Diabetes Australia and Diabetes New Zealand, which are able to provide further information about diabetes and management

Insulin requirements usually fall in the first trimester and increase during the second and third trimesters of pregnancy. Insulin requirements fall to pre-pregnancy levels within 6 weeks of delivery. BGLs should be monitored closely post-delivery to prevent hypoglycaemia from occurring as insulin requirements may decrease 24—72 hours after delivery.

If breastfeeding, insulin requirements, diet or both may need to be adjusted.

Insulin requirements may be reduced in those with liver or kidney impairment. Close monitoring of BGLs is recommended.

Insulin preparations are banned in sport.

ORAL HYPOGLYCAEMIC AGENTS

- sulfonylureas (e.g. glibenclamide)
- biguanides (e.g. metformin hydrochloride)
- alpha glucosidase inhibitors (e.g. acarbose)
- thiazolidinediones (e.g. pioglitazone)
- dipeptidyl peptidase 4 (DPP-4) inhibitors (e.g. linagliptin)
- glucagon-like peptide-1 (GLP-1) analogues (e.g. exenatide)
- sodium—glucose cotransporter 2 inhibitors (SGLT2 inhibitors) (e.g. canagliflozin)

ANTIDIABETIC AGENTS

General Nursing considerations/Cautions for oral hypoglycaemic agents

- caution if using these agents in those who are elderly, malnourished and/or debilitated
- contraindicated in those with type 1 diabetes mellitus, diabetic ketoacidosis, diabetic coma or pre-coma or severe kidney/liver impairment/dysfunction

General Patient education for oral hypoglycaemic agents

- it is important that the patient understands and adheres to managing their diet and weight, personal hygiene and physical exercise, as well as identifying and managing any cardiovascular risk factors, including hypertension and dyslipidaemia
- ensure the patient understands the need to avoid infection and report to the doctor if any signs of illness occur
- instruct the patient how oral hypoglycaemic agents work and the importance of not stopping medication if blood glucose levels (BGLs) appear stable
- the patient should be educated on:
  - how to monitor BGLs and the importance of regular medical checks, especially if blood glucose control is not optimal or if they are changing antidiabetic agents
  - not increasing the dose if a dose is missed. It is important to discuss what to do if a dose or meal is missed and understand the consequences of skipping a meal after the oral hypoglycaemic agent has been taken
  - identification of the symptoms of hypoglycaemia, which include weakness, listlessness, sweating, hunger, nausea, vomiting, trembling/shaking, restlessness, sleep disturbance, impaired concentration, alertness and/or reactions, lightheadedness, irritability, numbness around lips/tongue, headache, palpitations and confusion. This list is not extensive and varies from person to person
  - how to treat hypoglycaemia and the importance of having carbohydrates readily available. For example, eating 5–7 jelly beans, 3 teaspoons of sugar/honey, drinking 1/2 can of non-diet soft drink, 2–3 glucose tablets or a tube of glucose gel, followed up by extra carbohydrates such as plain biscuits, fruit or milk if the next meal is not within the next 10 to 15 minutes
  - anticipate when hypoglycaemia is likely to occur and work out a snack or meal pattern to prevent or overcome it. Risk factors for hypoglycaemia include not understanding directions for medication use (e.g. taking too much), the need to monitor BGLs, malnutrition, irregular meal intake (including skipping meals or fasting), dietary changes, imbalance between exercise and carbohydrate intake and physical problems (e.g. kidney or liver impairment)
  - identification of the symptoms of hyperglycaemia, including nausea, vomiting, drowsiness, dry mouth, flushed dry skin, polyuria, polydipsia, decreased appetite and acetone ('fruity') breath
- warn the patient to take care when driving or operating machinery, because hypoglycaemia causes slow reaction time, or decreased alertness
- hypoglycaemia may occur during the first month of therapy because sulfonylureas also cause insulin to be released from the pancreas
- warn the patient that hyperglycaemia is a potentially life-threatening situation
- the patient should be closely monitored during times of unusual stress, such as infection, fever, surgery and trauma, as this predisposes them to hyperglycaemia and ketosis; the patient may require insulin during this time. Other

causes of hyperglycaemia include eating more carbohydrates than usual, too little hypoglycaemic agent, too little exercise (depending on usual level) and other medications
* ensure that the patient understands there is a reduced tolerance to alcohol, which may also affect blood levels of oral hypoglycaemic agents, and therefore it is best to be avoided altogether. If alcohol is consumed, it is important to warn the patient to immediately report any flushing, headache, problems with breathing, rapid heart rate, stomach pain, feeling nauseous and/or vomiting (possible disulfiram-like reaction) (see Glossary)
* a relative, friend, colleague or teacher needs to know how to identify and deal with hypoglycaemia and hyperglycaemia
* advise the patient to wear a MedicAlert bracelet or pendant
* instruct the patient to immediately tell the doctor of the return of any symptoms, such as lethargy, tiredness, headache, thirst, blurred vision or passing large amounts of urine, or if BGLs are unstable/fluctuating, as this may indicate the particular oral hypoglycaemic agent is no longer effective at lowering BGLs

SULFONYLUREAS

General Actions of sulfonylureas

* orally active sulfonylurea (sulfonamide derivative) agents that stimulate insulin release from functioning pancreatic cells
* improve sensitivity of beta cells of the pancreas to glucose stimulus, leading to insulin secretion
* enhance peripheral sensitivity to insulin
* reduce basal glucose production by the liver
* decreases both fasting and postprandial (after meals) glucose levels

General Uses of sulfonylureas

* type 2 diabetes (unresponsive to diet alone and in whom other antidiabetic agents have been ineffective)

General Adverse effects of sulfonylureas

* hypoglycaemia and, rarely, severe or prolonged and fatal hypoglycaemia
* anorexia, nausea, vomiting, epigastric fullness/pressure, abdominal pain, constipation, diarrhoea, dyspepsia, heartburn
* weight gain
* rash, pruritus, erythema, urticaria, photosensitivity
* blurred vision, changes to accommodation, diplopia (transient, at start of therapy)
* abnormal liver enzymes and function, (rare) cholestatic jaundice, hepatitis, pancreatitis
* (Rare) hyponatraemia, syndrome of inappropriate antidiuretic hormone secretion (SIADH)
* (Rare) anaemia, leucopenia, thrombocytopenia, agranulocytosis

General Interactions of sulfonylureas

* hypoglycaemic action enhanced by alcohol (acute intake), anabolic steroids, angiotensin converting enzyme (ACE) inhibitors, antidiabetic agents (oral), aspirin, beta adrenoceptor blocking agents, biguanides, chloramphenicol, clarithromycin, clonidine, cyclophosphamide, disopyramide, fibrates, fluconazole, fluoxetine, gemfibrozil, heparin, ifosfamide, insulin, miconazole, monoamine oxidase inhibitors (MAOIs), NSAIDs, pentoxifylline (oxpentifylline) (high dose, IV), phosphamides, probenecid, fluoroquinolone antibacterial agents, ranitidine, salicylates, sulfonamides, testosterone, tetracyclines and voriconazole, which may result in loss of blood glucose control
* hypoglycaemic effects reduced by acetazolamide, barbiturates, chronic

ANTIDIABETIC AGENTS

alcohol use, calcium-channel blockers, clonidine, corticosteroids, diazoxide, furosemide (frusemide), glucagon, isoniazid, laxatives (prolonged use), nicotinic acid (high dose), oral contraceptives, oestrogens, phenothiazines, phenytoin, progestogens, rifampicin, sympathomimetics, thiazide diuretics or thyroid hormones
- may either increase or decrease warfarin effects; therefore should be given with caution and INR closely monitored
- may increase serum levels of ciclosporin, increasing the risk of toxicity; therefore levels should be closely monitored, especially if starting or stopping sulfonylureas
- (Rare) when combined with alcohol, may cause a disulfiram-like reaction (see Glossary)
- beta adrenoceptor blocking agents, clonidine, H_2-receptor antagonists (e.g. cimetidine) may prolong or mask the symptoms of hypoglycaemia
- increased hypoglycaemia may occur if given to those with acute alcohol intoxication
- decreased duration of action may occur in those who ingest alcohol chronically

General Nursing considerations/Cautions for sulfonylureas

- when first starting therapy, clinical status should be checked after 4–8 weeks and then regularly to ascertain that the dosage is correct to maintain blood glucose levels (BGLs) within normal range
- patient should be closely monitored if changing from one sulfonylurea to another sulfonylurea/other hypoglycaemic agent
- sulfonylureas are not oral insulins, but are capable of increasing circulating insulin in a person with a functioning pancreas
- any hypersensitivity reaction requires prompt discontinuation
- caution if used in those with alcoholism, insulinoma, or adrenal, thyroid or pituitary insufficiency because they may have increased sensitivity to sulfonylureas
- caution if used in those with porphyria, as the condition may be exacerbated
- there is an increased risk of hypoglycaemia if the person is undertaking intense or prolonged exercise (especially if there is an imbalance between exercise and carbohydrate intake), drinks alcohol, has a decreased food intake (e.g. dietary changes, periods of fasting) or irregular meal times, is taking multiple antidiabetic agents, has severe endocrine disorders or adrenal/pituitary insufficiency, or the person is elderly, debilitated, malnourished or has liver or kidney impairment
- not recommended in those with glucose-6-phosphate dehydrogenase (G6PD) deficiency, as haemolytic anaemia may occur
- contraindicated in those with type 1 diabetes, diabetes complicated with ketosis, diabetic ketoacidosis, serious metabolic decompensation with acidosis (especially pre-coma or coma), or severe kidney or liver dysfunction or impairment
- contraindicated if given to those with sensitivity to another sulfonamide or thiazide diuretic because cross-sensitivity may be possible
- see also General Nursing considerations/Cautions for oral hypoglycaemic agents (p. 307)

General Patient education for sulfonylureas

- the patient should be instructed to protect skin by using protective clothing and sunscreen with high protective factor (SPF 30+) as skin may be more sensitive to sunlight
- advise the patient to ensure meal has adequate amount of carbohydrates to prevent hypoglycaemia occurring

- advise the patient to seek medical advice immediately if any of the following occur:
  - yellowing of skin and/or eyes, tiredness, loss of appetite, nausea, vomiting, upper abdominal pain, dark urine, pale stools
  - unexplained bleeding or bruising
  - pale appearance, tiredness, shortness of breath during exercise or exertion
  - rash, hives, skin redness, itching
- see also General Patient education for oral hypoglycaemic agents (p. 307)

Animal studies have shown sulfonylureas to be embryotoxic and cause fetal abnormalities, and are therefore contraindicated during pregnancy. May also cause neonatal hypoglycaemia. Oral hypoglycaemics should be replaced with insulin during pregnancy.

Contraindicated during breastfeeding.

GLIBENCLAMIDE
Trade name
Daonil

Available form
Tablets: 5 mg

Action/Use
- inhibits glucagon-producing alpha cells and increases release of somatostatin from delta cells in the pancreas
- has a mild diuretic action
- metabolite has weak hypoglycaemic activity
- peak effect 2–6 hours, half-life 2–10 hours
- see also General Actions of sulfonylureas and General Uses of sulfonylureas (p. 306)

Dose
- initially 2.5 mg orally daily before breakfast, increasing by 2.5 mg at 7-day intervals if needed (daily maximum 20 mg)

Adverse effects
- see General Adverse effects of sulfonylureas (p. 306)

Interactions
- contraindicated with bosentan because of the increased risk of hepatotoxicity. In addition, serum levels of both agents can be significantly decreased if given together
- see also General Interactions of sulfonylureas (p. 306)

Nursing considerations/Cautions/Patient education
- if the patient has only a light breakfast, the first dose should be delayed until lunchtime
- if the patient is changed from insulin to glibenclamide, test urine for ketones and glucose 3 times daily during changeover period. For patients receiving up to 40 units/day, insulin can be stopped gradually and glibenclamide started (2.5 mg for < 20 units or 5 mg for 20–40 unit). Dose can be increased in increments of 1.25–2.5 mg/day at intervals of 2–10 days, depending on patient response and tolerance
- if changing from another oral antidiabetic agent, dose should be started at 2.5–5 mg. Depending on the characteristics of the previous antidiabetic agent (e.g. length of half-life), transition period may require a drug-free period to prevent overlapping effects of the two agents resulting in hypoglycaemia
- doses up to 10 mg can be given as a single daily dose before breakfast. Amounts in excess of 10 mg can be given with the evening meal
- caution if used in those with coronary artery disease because of the increased risk of cardiovascular mortality
- see also Nursing considerations/Cautions for sulfonylureas and Patient education for sulfonylureas (p. 307)

ANTIDIABETIC AGENTS

Available in combination with
- glibenclamide 2.5 mg + metformin hydrochloride 500 mg (Glucovance 500/2.5)
- glibenclamide 5 mg + metformin hydrochloride 500 mg (Glucovance 500/5)

GLICLAZIDE
Trade names
APO-Gliclazide MR, APX-Gliclazide, Ardix Gliclazide 60 mg MR, Diamicron 60 mg MR, Gliclazide Lupin MR, Gliclazide MR Viatris, Nidem, Pharmcor Gliclazide MR

Available forms
Tablets: 80 mg;
Tablets (modified-release): 30 mg, 60 mg

Action/Use
- reduces platelet adhesiveness and aggregation, increases vascular endothelial fibrinolytic activity and has some antioxidant properties
- peak effect 4—6 hours, half-life 12—16 hours
- see also General Actions of sulfonylureas and General Uses of sulfonylureas (p. 306)

Dose
- initially 40 mg daily, increasing up to 320 mg if necessary **OR**
- initially 30 mg daily, increasing by 30 mg every 14 days if needed (up to 120 mg daily) (modified-release tablets)

Adverse effects
- see General Adverse effects of sulfonylureas (p. 306)

Interactions
- caution if used with fluoroquinolones as blood glucose levels may become disturbed
- efficacy may be decreased if given with St John's wort
- caution if given with chlorpromazine (high dose)
- contraindicated with miconazole
- not recommended with danazol
- see also General Interactions of sulfonylureas (p. 306)

Nursing considerations/Cautions
- (Tablets) up to 160 mg as a single dose at the same time every morning; amounts in excess of 160 mg should be taken in divided doses morning and evening
- modified-release tablets are scored and can be divided
- transferring from insulin is not recommended
- tablets contain lactose and therefore are not recommended in those with galactose intolerance, glucose—galactose malabsorption or Lapp lactose deficiency
- see also General Nursing considerations/Cautions for sulfonylureas (p. 307)

Patient education
- suggest to patient that dose should be taken at breakfast
- (Modified-release tablets) patient should be advised to swallow tablets whole, not chewed or crushed; however, tablet is scored and can be broken in half if a half-dose is required
- see also General Patient education for sulfonylureas (p. 307)

 Immediate-release (80 mg) tablets can be dispersed in 10—20 mL water, or crushed and mixed with spoonful of yoghurt or apple puree.

 Modified-release (30 mg, 60 mg) tablets should not be crushed.

GLIMEPIRIDE
Trade names
Amaryl, ARX-Glimepiride, Glimepiride Sandoz, Glimepiride-WGR

Available forms
Tablets: 1 mg, 2 mg, 3 mg, 4 mg

Action/Use
- active metabolite
- peak effect 2.5 hours, half-life 5—8 hours, duration of action 24 hours

- see also General Actions of sulfonylureas and General Uses of sulfonylureas (p. 306)

Dose
- initially 1 mg orally daily before breakfast. If needed, may be increased by 1 mg at 1–2 week intervals according to response, then 1–4 mg daily (maintenance)

Adverse effects/Interactions/Nursing considerations/Cautions/Patient education
- if the patient has only a light breakfast, the first dose should be delayed until lunchtime
- see also General Adverse effects/Interactions/Nursing considerations/Cautions/Patient education for sulfonylureas (p. 306)

 Tablet can be dispersed in water (1–3 minutes), or crushed and mixed with spoonful of yoghurt or apple puree.

GLIPIZIDE
Trade name
Minidiab

Available form
Tablets: 5 mg

Action/Use
- peak action 1–3 hours, half-life 2–4 hours
- see also General Actions of sulfonylureas and General Uses of sulfonylureas (p. 306)

Dose
- initially 5 mg orally daily 30 minutes before breakfast, increasing gradually after several days in increments of 2.5–5 mg if needed (maximum total daily dose is 40 mg)

Adverse effects
- dizziness, drowsiness, vertigo, headache
- see also General Adverse effects of sulfonylureas (p. 306)

Interactions/Nursing considerations/Cautions/Patient education
- amounts in excess of 15 mg should be divided and given before meals
- if single dose is not effective, dosage may be divided and given twice daily
- contraindicated in those with severe thyroid dysfunction, severe trauma, infections, febrile conditions, major surgical procedures or gangrene
- see also General Interactions/Nursing considerations/Cautions/Patient education for sulfonylureas (p. 306)

 Tablet can be dispersed in water or crushed and mixed with spoonful of yoghurt or apple puree.

 Recommended initial dose in those with liver disease is 2.5 mg orally.

 Recommended initial dose in the elderly is 2.5 mg orally.

BIGUANIDES

METFORMIN HYDROCHLORIDE
Trade names
APO-Metformin, APO-Metformin XR, APX Metformin, Blooms the Chemist Metformin, Blooms the Chemist Metformin XR, Diabex, Diabex XR, Diaformin Alphapharrm XR, Diaformin Viatrix, Formet, Glucobete, Metex XR, Metformin GH, Metformin Mylan, Metformin XR Mylan, Metformin WGR, Metformin WGR XR, Metformin Sandoz, Pharmcor Metformin XR, TIH-Metformin

Available forms
Tablets: 500 mg, 850 mg, 1000 mg; Tablets (extended-release): 500 mg, 1000 mg

Action
- orally active biguanide derivative
- lowers both basal and postprandial glucose

ANTIDIABETIC AGENTS

- does not stimulate insulin release, but does require insulin to be present to be effective
- inhibits gluconeogenesis in the liver and glucose absorption from the GI tract, and increases peripheral uptake and utilisation in muscle by increasing insulin sensitivity
- increases insulin sensitivity via increasing number of receptors and affinity for receptors
- decreases risk of diabetes-related complications or mortality
- affects lipid metabolism by reducing total cholesterol, low-density lipoprotein cholesterol and triglycerides
- considered first-line treatment for type 2 diabetes mellitus
- peak effect 2–3 hours, half-life 3 hours

Use
- type 2 diabetes (unresponsive to diet and exercise alone as monotherapy, with insulin or with other oral hypoglycaemic agents)

Dose
- initially 500 mg orally 1–2 times daily with meals, increasing slowly to 1 g 3 times daily if needed (daily maximum 2 g) **OR**
- initially 500–750 mg orally with evening meal, increasing dose by 500–750 mg every 10–15 days if needed (daily maximum 2 g) (extended-release tablets)

Adverse effects
- (Mild, transient) diarrhoea, nausea, vomiting, metallic taste, anorexia, abdominal pain
- (Very rare) mild erythema, pruritus, urticaria
- decreased vitamin B_{12} absorption, decreased vitamin B_{12} levels
- (Very rare) serious and often fatal lactic acidosis (nausea, vomiting, abdominal pain, diarrhoea, malaise, myalgia, somnolence, hyperventilation, decreased blood pH), liver function abnormalities, hepatitis

Interactions
- contraindicated with contrast media (containing iodine) used for radiological examination owing to risk of altered kidney function and lactic acidosis. Must be discontinued for 48 hours before examination
- risk of lactic acidosis may be increased if given with alcohol or diuretics (especially loop diuretics), acetazolamide, topiramate or zonisamide, in cases of renal impairment or with doses greater than 2 g per day
- alcohol may delay and/or mask the symptoms of hypoglycaemia and also increase the risk of lactic acidosis and therefore not recommended together
- angiotensin converting enzyme (ACE) inhibitors and calcium-channel blockers may affect blood glucose control; therefore should be given with caution, and dose adjustment of metformin may be required according to blood glucose levels (BGLs)
- beta adrenoceptor blocking agents may mask signs of hypoglycaemia (e.g. tachycardia) as well as potentiating the hyperglycaemic action
- increased plasma levels may occur if given with nifedipine
- may increase elimination time of vitamin K antagonists; therefore prothrombin time should be monitored when starting, stopping or changing doses
- clearance may be decreased if given with dolutegravir, triamterene or trimethoprim
- if given with agents that intrinsically elevate BGLs (e.g. glucocorticoids, tetracosactides, danazol, chlorpromazine (doses > 100 mg/day), thyroid hormones and diuretics) more frequent monitoring of BGLs is recommended, especially when starting or stopping therapy or adjusting doses of either agent
- caution if used with other agents which may impair kidney function (e.g. NSAIDs, thiazide diuretics, antihypertensive agents)

- efficacy may be decreased if given with verapamil
- efficacy and GI absorption may be increased if given with rifampicin

Nursing considerations/Cautions

- creatinine clearance (CrCl) and/or serum creatinine should be assessed before starting therapy and then yearly (if patient has normal kidney function) or 2—4 times yearly (if patient is elderly or has serum creatinine levels at the upper side of normal levels)
- regular monitoring of liver and cardiovascular function is also recommended, especially if patient has pre-existing heart failure
- vitamin B_{12} levels should be measured before starting therapy, at 6 months then yearly if therapy is continuous
- should be stopped before and for at least 48 hours after radiological examination using IV iodinated contrast medium or surgery. Should be restarted only after renal function is evaluated and found to be normal
- does not normally cause hypoglycaemia when given as monotherapy
- may be used with insulin
- switching to extended-release tablets is not recommended in patients managed on immediate-release metformin dose > 2000 mg/day
- switching to extended-release tablets, the starting dose should be the same as the daily dose (immediate release) given as a single dose in the evening
- if switching from another antidiabetic agent, stop the other agent and commence with 500 mg orally (modified-release tablet) in the evening and then titrate as needed
- caution if given to the elderly, those with kidney impairment or in doses over 2 g/day because of an increased risk of life-threatening lactic acidosis
- contraindicated in those with type 1 diabetes mellitus, diabetes mellitus (controlled by diet alone), during/after surgery where insulin is needed, diabetic ketoacidosis, lactic acidosis, diabetic precoma, kidney dysfunction/failure (CrC < 60 mL/min), other conditions that could affect kidney function (e.g. shock, dehydration, severe infection, IV administration of iodinated contrast agents), severe liver insufficiency, alcoholism, acute alcohol intoxication, acute/chronic disease causing tissue hypoxia (e.g. recent myocardial infarction, cardiac/respiratory failure, sepsis), pulmonary embolism, gangrene or pancreatitis
- see also General Nursing considerations/Cautions for oral hypoglycaemic agents (p. 305)

Patient education

- patient should be advised to avoid alcohol during therapy
- caution patient against taking NSAIDs without first discussing with doctor
- instruct patient that GI adverse effects may be avoided if metformin is taken with food and dose is increased slowly
- advise the patient to swallow extended-release tablets whole, not broken, crushed or chewed
- warn patient that tablet shell may appear in the faeces (and this is normal)
- patient should be advised that BGL control usually takes about 2 weeks to achieve
- ensure that patient understands that lactic acidosis is a medical emergency and can be life threatening. The patient should be therefore advised to immediately report any of the following:
  - abdominal cramps
  - muscle pain or cramping
  - nausea, vomiting, loss of appetite, diarrhoea
  - feeling generally unwell, unusually tired or sleepy
  - weakness
  - shivering, feeling extremely cold
  - fast, shallow breathing
- see also General Patient education for oral hypoglycaemic agents (p. 305)

ANTIDIABETIC AGENTS

 Immediate-release tablets can be crushed and mixed with water or spoonful of yoghurt or apple puree.

 Modified-release and extended-release tablets should not be crushed.

 Oral hypoglycaemics should be replaced with insulin during pregnancy.

 Contraindicated if used during breast-feeding, as animal studies have shown metformin to be secreted in breastmilk.

 Initial and maintenance dose should be conservative in the elderly, malnourished or debilitated patients. Kidney function should be closely monitored to reduce risk of lactic acidosis.

Available in combination with

- metformin 500 mg + alogliptin 12.5 mg (NesinaMet 12.5/500)
- metformin 850 mg + alogliptin 12.5 mg (NesinaMet 12.5/850)
- metformin 1000 mg + alogliptin 12.5 mg (NesinaMet 12.5/1000)
- metformin 500 mg + dapagliflozin 10 mg (XigduoXR 10/500)
- metformin 1000 mg + dapagliflozin 5 mg (XigduoXR 5/1000)
- metformin 1000 mg + dapagliflozin 10 mg (XigduoXR 10/1000)
- metformin 500 mg + empagliflozin 5 mg (Jardiamet 5/500)
- metformin 500 mg + empagliflozin 12.5 mg (Jardiamet 12.5/500)
- metformin 1000 mg + empagliflozin 5 mg (Jardiamet 5/1000)
- metformin 1000 mg + empagliflozin 12.5 mg (Jardiamet 12.5/1000)
- metformin 500 mg + glibenclamide 2.5 mg (Glucovance 500/2.5 mg)
- metformin 500 mg + glibenclamide 5 mg (Glucovance 500/5 mg)
- metformin 500 mg + linagliptin 2.5 mg (Trajentamet 2.5/500)
- metformin 850 mg + linagliptin 2.5 mg (Trajentamet 2.5/850)
- metformin 1000 mg + linagliptin 2.5 mg (Trajentamet 2.5/1000)
- metformin 500 mg + saxagliptin 5 mg (KombiglyzeXR 5/500)
- metformin 1000 mg + saxagliptin 2.5 mg (KombiglyzeXR 2.5/1000)
- metformin 1000 mg + saxagliptin 5 mg (KombiglyzeXR 5/1000)
- metformin 500 mg + sitagliptin 50 mg (Janumet 50/500)
- metformin 850 mg + sitagliptin 50 mg (Janumet 50/850)
- metformin 1000 mg + sitagliptin 50 mg (Janumet 50/1000)
- metformin 1000 mg + sitagliptin 50 mg (Janumet XR 50/1000)
- metformin 1000 mg + sitagliptin 100 mg (Janumet XR 100/1000)
- metformin 500 mg + sitagliptin 50 mg (Sitagliptin/Metformin Mylan 50/500)
- metformin 850 mg + sitagliptin 50 mg (Sitagliptin/Metformin Mylan 50/850)
- metformin 1000 mg + sitagliptin 50 mg (Sitagliptin/Metformin Mylan 50/1000)
- metformin 500 mg + sitagliptin 50 mg (Sitagliptin/Metformin Sandoz 50/500)
- metformin 850 mg + sitagliptin 50 mg (Sitagliptin/Metformin Sandoz 50/850)
- metformin 1000 mg + sitagliptin 50 mg (Sitagliptin/Metformin Sandoz 50/1000)
- metformin 1000 mg + sitagliptin 50 mg (Sitagliptin/Metformin Sandoz XR 50/1000)
- metformin 1000 mg + sitagliptin 100 mg (Sitagliptin/Metformin Sandoz XR 100/1000)
- metformin 500 mg + sitagliptin 50 mg (Velmetia 50/500)
- metformin 850 mg + sitagliptin 50 mg (Velmetia 50/850)
- metformin 1000 mg + sitagliptin 50 mg (Velmetia 50/1000)
- metformin 500 mg + vildagliptin 50 mg (Galvumet 50/500)
- metformin 850 mg + vildagliptin 50 mg (Galvumet 50/850)
- metformin 1000 mg + vildagliptin 50 mg (Galvumet 50/1000)

ALPHA GLUCOSIDASE INHIBITORS

ACARBOSE
Trade names
Acarbose Viatris, Glybosay

Available forms
Tablets: 50 mg, 100 mg

Action
- complex oligosaccharide with action on GI tract
- inhibits intestinal alpha glucosidase involved in the breakdown of disaccharides, oligosaccharides and polysaccharides, but not monosaccharides, leading to delayed digestion
- monosaccharides are absorbed more slowly into the blood, reducing the fluctuation in blood glucose levels (BGLs) throughout the day related to food ingestion
- does not induce hypoglycaemia
- has no effect on the pancreas
- active metabolite
- half-life about 2 hours

Use
- type 2 diabetes (when diet alone or diet and other oral hypoglycaemic agents have been ineffective)

Dose
- initially 50 mg orally daily for the first week, increasing to 50 mg orally twice daily in the second week, 50 mg orally 3 times daily in the third week, increasing further after 4–8 weeks if necessary (daily maximum 600 mg)

Adverse effects
- (Very common) flatulence
- (Common) diarrhoea, abdominal pain
- (Uncommon) nausea, vomiting, dyspepsia, distension, bloating, increased serum transaminases (transient, reversible)
- (Rare) hepatitis, jaundice, oedema

Interactions
- use with thiazide diuretics, furosemide (frusemide), corticosteroids, phenothiazines, oestrogens, oral contraceptives, thyroid hormones, phenytoin, nicotinic acid, sympathomimetics or isoniazid may result in loss of blood glucose control
- if given concurrently with colestyramine, effects may be increased
- use with digoxin may require dose adjustment of digoxin
- use with charcoal or enzyme preparations is not recommended
- if hypoglycaemia occurs when given with sulfonylureas or metformin, dose of both agents should be reduced

Nursing considerations/Cautions
- hypoglycaemia does not occur when acarbose is given alone, but may occur if given with insulin, metformin or sulfonylureas
- hypoglycaemia should be treated using glucose. Cane sugar/sucrose should not be given to patients treated with acarbose alone or in combination with another hypoglycaemic agent because the breakdown of sucrose will be slowed and hypoglycaemia will persist
- if diarrhoea persists, the patient should be closely monitored and the dose decreased
- starting at a low dose helps to alleviate some of the adverse intestinal effects
- liver enzymes should be monitored monthly for the first 6–12 months and, if changes occur, the dose reduced or withdrawn and enzymes monitored weekly until normal
- contraindicated in those with severe renal impairment (creatinine clearance < 25 mL/min), malabsorption disorders, ulcerative colitis, Crohn's disease, predisposition to intestinal obstruction or ileus, partial bowel obstruction or conditions aggravated by intestinal gas formation or under 18 years of age

ANTIDIABETIC AGENTS

- see also General Nursing considerations/Cautions for oral hypoglycaemic agents (p. 305)

Patient education
- advise the patient to swallow tablets whole before meals or chew with the first mouthful of the meal
- the patient should be advised to avoid cane sugar (sucrose) or products containing cane sugar as they may cause stomach pains/discomfort and possibly diarrhoea
- warn the patient that it is common for side-effects (flatulence/wind, stomach rumbling, feeling full, sometimes stomach cramps) to occur in the first few days of therapy, especially if foods containing sugar are eaten. If symptoms persist for longer than 2—3 days or are severe, the patient should seek medical advice
- if hypoglycaemia occurs, cane sugar/sucrose should not be given in patients treated with acarbose alone or in combination with another hypoglycaemic agent because the breakdown of sucrose will be slowed and hypoglycaemia will persist. Glucose should be used
- instruct the patient to not use antacids to treat indigestion as they will be ineffective
- see also General Patient education for oral hypoglycaemic agents (p. 305)

Tablet can be chewed with first mouthful of food, or can be crushed and mixed with spoonful of yoghurt.

Contraindicated during pregnancy.

Contraindicated during breastfeeding.

THIAZOLIDINEDIONES

PIOGLITAZONE
Trade names
Actos, ARX-Pioglitazone, Noumed Pioglitazone, Pioglitazone Sandoz, Vexazone

Available forms
Tablets: 15 mg, 30 mg, 45 mg

Action
- thiazolidinedione that depends on insulin to be present to be effective
- improves insulin sensitivity in the liver, skeletal muscle and adipose tissue
- inhibits gluconeogenesis in the liver
- decreases insulin resistance
- decreases circulating free fatty acid level
- may take several weeks for full effect to become noticeable
- 3 active metabolites
- peak effect 2—4 hours, half-life 5—23 hours (parent and metabolites)

Use
- type 2 diabetes inadequately controlled by diet and exercise alone (as monotherapy, or with metformin, insulin or sulfonylurea)

Dose
- (Monotherapy) initially 15—30 mg orally daily, increasing after 4 weeks to 45 mg daily if necessary (daily maximum 45 mg) **OR**
- (Double therapy) 15—30 mg orally daily (with insulin, metformin or sulfonylurea) **OR**
- (Triple therapy) 30 mg orally daily, increasing to 45 mg if needed (with metformin and sulfonylureas)

Adverse effects
- increased incidence of bone fractures (upper arm, hand, foot) (women)
- hypoglycaemia (if given with insulin, metformin or sulfonylureas)
- peripheral oedema, fluid retention, new or worsening cardiac failure

- weight gain
- fatigue, headache
- back pain
- decreased haemoglobin (anaemia) and haematocrit
- upper respiratory tract infection, pharyngitis, sinusitis
- abnormal liver function test results, transient increase in creatine phosphokinase (CPK) levels
- asthenia, malaise
- myalgia, leg cramps
- upper abdominal pain, diarrhoea
- tooth disorder
- abnormal vision
- urinary tract infection
- (Female) increased risk of oedema, resumption of ovulation
- (Rare) bladder cancer with prolonged use
- (Very rare) new/worsening diabetic macular oedema, decreased visual acuity

Interactions
- may decrease effectiveness of oral contraceptives
- increased serum levels if given with gemfibrozil
- decreased serum levels may occur if given with rifampicin
- increased risk of hypoglycaemia if given with insulin and/or oral antidiabetic agent

Nursing considerations/Cautions
- (Female patient) dose should be started at 15 mg and increased gradually, monitoring for any oedema
- (Double therapy) if patient is using insulin, pioglitazone should be started at 15 mg once daily
- liver function tests should be monitored every second month for the first year, and regularly thereafter
- blood tests (haemoglobin and haematocrit) should be monitored regularly throughout therapy
- patients should be closely monitored for any signs of cardiac failure during therapy, including excessive rapid weight gain, dyspnoea and/or oedema
- caution if used in those with pre-existing oedema
- caution if used in those with class I heart failure (New York Heart Association (NYHA) classification). Close monitoring is recommended
- not recommended in those with current or history of bladder cancer, active liver disease or liver transaminases > 2.5 times the upper normal limit
- contraindicated in those with class II, III or IV heart failure (NYHA classification), type 1 diabetes mellitus or for the treatment of diabetic ketoacidosis
- see also General Nursing considerations/Cautions for oral hypoglycaemic agents (p. 305)

Patient education
- warn the patient to seek medical advice if there is blood, pain and burning when passing urine (as these could be symptoms of bladder cancer)
- warn the patient that weight gain is a common side-effect
- the patient should be advised to seek medical advice immediately if any of the following occur:
  - loss of appetite, nausea, vomiting, upper abdominal pain, dark urine, pale stools, fatigue or yellowing of skin and/or eyes
  - excessive rapid weight gain, difficulty breathing, swelling of ankles, feet and hands
  - eye problems, including blurred or double vision
  - urinary urgency or blood in urine
- female patients should be counselled regarding the need to use additional contraceptive methods to protect against unwanted pregnancy, as therapy may result in resumption of ovulation, increasing the risk of pregnancy in anovulatory premenopausal women with insulin resistance (e.g. polycystic ovary syndrome)

ANTIDIABETIC AGENTS

- female patients should be warned that pioglitazone may decrease effectiveness of oral contraceptive
- see also General Patient education for oral hypoglycaemic agents (p. 305)

 Tablets can be crushed and mixed with water or spoonful of yoghurt or apple puree.

 Use during pregnancy only if benefits to mother outweigh risks to fetus.

 Not recommended during breastfeeding.

 Dose should be started at 15 mg orally daily in those with liver impairment, and dose increased cautiously if needed. Therapy should not be started if liver enzyme (alanine aminotransferase) is 2.5 times above upper limit of normal.

DIPEPTIDYL PEPTIDASE-4 (DPP-4) INHIBITORS

General Actions of DPP-4 inhibitors
- dipeptidyl peptidase 4 (DPP-4) enzyme inhibitor that enhances levels of incretin hormones (glucagon-like peptide 1 (GLP1) and glucose-dependent insulinotropic polypeptide (GIP)), which are released by the intestine in response to a meal and are involved in the regulation of glucose homeostasis
- improves pancreatic beta cell responsiveness to glucose, as well as increasing insulin synthesis and release
- reduces glucagon secretion from pancreatic alpha cells, decreasing liver glucose

General Uses of DPP-4 inhibitors
- type 2 diabetes (inadequately controlled by diet and exercise alone) as monotherapy or in combination with metformin, sulfonylurea, insulin or other hypoglycaemic agents

General Adverse effects of DPP-4 inhibitors
- nasopharyngitis, sinusitis, upper respiratory tract infection
- headache
- rash
- pancreatitis
- hypoglycaemia (when combined with sulfonylurea)
- hypersensitivity (urticaria, angioedema, localised skin reaction, bronchial hyperreactivity)
- (Rare) arthralgia, bullous pemphigoid

General Nursing considerations/Cautions for DPP-4 inhibitors
- not recommended in those under 18 years
- not recommended in those with type 1 diabetes or for treatment of diabetic ketoacidosis
- contraindicated in those with hypersensitivity to DPP-4 inhibitors
- see also General Nursing considerations/Cautions for oral hypoglycaemic agents (p. 305)

General Patient education for DPP-4 inhibitors
- advise the patient to seek medical advice immediately if any of the following occur:
  - any allergic reactions such as shortness of breath, wheezing, difficulty breathing, face/lips/tongue swelling, skin rash, itching or hives
  - any persistent abdominal pain, especially if associated with nausea and/or vomiting (as these may be signs of pancreatitis)
  - new or exacerbation of joint pain
  - rash, skin blistering or ulceration
- ensure the patient is aware of the increased risk of hypoglycaemia if they are taking a DPP-4 inhibitor as part of combination therapy

Not recommended during pregnancy.

 Not recommended during breastfeeding.

ALOGLIPTIN
Trade name
Nesina

Available forms
Tablets: 6.25 mg, 12.5 mg, 25 mg

Action/Use
- peak activity 1—2 hours, half-life 21 hours
- see also General Actions of DPP-4 inhibitors and General Uses of DPP-4 inhibitors (p. 317)

Dose
- 25 mg orally daily

Adverse effects
- abdominal pain, gastro-oesophageal reflux disease
- rash, pruritus
- (Rare) liver damage
- see also General Adverse effects of DPP-4 inhibitors (p. 317)

Nursing considerations/Cautions
- if patient has any signs of liver injury, liver function tests should be conducted immediately
- dose should be reduced if given with insulin or sulfonylurea to decrease risk of hypoglycaemia
- caution if used in those with congestive cardiac failure
- not recommended for those with severe liver impairment
- see also General Nursing considerations/Cautions for DPP-4 inhibitors (p. 317)

Patient education
- advise patient to seek medical advice immediately if any of the following occur:
  - yellowing of eyes/skin, loss of appetite, nausea, vomiting, upper abdominal pain, dark urine or pale stools (signs of liver impairment)
- see also General Patient education for DPP-4 inhibitors (p. 317)

 Tablets can be crushed and mixed with water or spoonful of yoghurt or apple puree.

 For those with moderate kidney impairment, recommended daily dose is 12.5 mg. If patient has severe kidney impairment or is on dialysis, recommended daily dose is 6.25 mg (regardless of the timing of dialysis).

Available in combination with
- alogliptin 12.5 mg + metformin 500 mg (NesinaMet 12.5/500)
- alogliptin 12.5 mg + metformin 850 mg (NesinaMet 12.5/850)
- alogliptin 12.5 mg + metformin 1000 mg (NesinaMet 12.5/1000)

LINAGLIPTIN
Trade name
Trajenta

Available form
Tablets: 5 mg

Action/Use
- peak effect 1.5 hours, triphasic half-life
- see also General Actions of DPP-4 inhibitors and General Uses of DPP-4 inhibitors (p. 317)

Dose
- 5 mg orally daily

Adverse effects
- increased uric acid levels
- (Uncommon) cough, constipation
- see also General Adverse effects of DPP-4 inhibitors (p. 317)

ANTIDIABETIC AGENTS

Nursing considerations/Cautions/Patient education
- see General Nursing considerations/Cautions/Patient education for DPP-4 inhibitors (p. 317)

Tablets can be crushed and mixed with water or a spoonful of yoghurt and apple puree.

Available in combination with
- linagliptin 5 mg + empagliflozin 10 mg (Glyxambi 10/5)
- linagliptin 5 mg + empagliflozin 25 mg (Glyxambi 25/5)
- linagliptin 2.5 mg and metformin 500 mg (Trajentamet 2.5/500)
- linagliptin 2.5 mg and metformin 850 mg (Trajentamet 2.5/850)
- linagliptin 2.5 mg and metformin 1000 mg (Trajentamet 2.5/1000)

SAXAGLIPTIN
Trade name
Onglyza

Available forms
Tablets: 2.5 mg, 5 mg

Action/Use
- active metabolite (half as potent as saxagliptin) (half-life 3.1 hours)
- peak effect 2 hours, duration of action 24 hours, half-life 2.5 hours
- see also General Actions of DPP-4 inhibitors and General Uses of DPP-4 inhibitors (p. 317)

Dose
- 5 mg orally daily

Adverse effects
- urinary tract infection
- heart failure
- see also General Adverse effects of DPP-4 inhibitors (p. 317)

Nursing considerations/Cautions
- kidney function should be assessed before starting therapy and then monitored regularly during therapy
- dose should be decreased if given with sulfonylurea to decrease risk of hypoglycaemia
- caution if used in those with moderate-to-severe kidney impairment or cardiac failure
- not recommended in those with end-stage kidney disease on haemodialysis
- see also General Nursing considerations/Cautions for DPP-4 inhibitors (p. 317)

Patient education
- see General Patient education for DPP-4 inhibitors (p. 317)

Tablets can be crushed and mixed with water or spoonful of yoghurt or apple puree; however, they do not disperse readily in water and tablets are hard to crush.

Kombiglyze XR tablets (combination saxagliptin and metformin) should not be crushed.

Dose should be reduced to 2.5 mg orally daily in those with moderate-to-severe kidney impairment.

Available in combination with
- saxagliptin 5 mg + dapagliflozin 10 mg (Qtern 5/10)
- saxagliptin 2.5 mg + metformin 1000 mg (Kombiglyze XR 2.5/1000)
- saxagliptin 5 mg + metformin 500 mg (Kombiglyze XR 5/500)
- saxagliptin 5 mg + metformin 1000 mg (Kombiglyze XR 5/1000)

SITAGLIPTIN
Trade names
Januvia, Sitagliptin Mylan, Sitagliptin Sandoz, Sitagliptin Sun, Sitaglo, Xelevia

Available forms
Tablets: 25 mg, 50 mg, 100 mg

Action/Use
- peak effect 1–4 hours, half-life 12.4 hours
- see also General Actions of DPP-4 enzyme inhibitors and General Uses of DPP-4 enzyme inhibitors (p. 317)

Dose
- 100 mg orally daily (as monotherapy or in combination with other hypoglycaemic agents)

Adverse effects
- diarrhoea, constipation
- hypertension
- back ache, osteoarthritis, pain in extremities
- see also General Adverse effects of DPP-4 inhibitors (p. 317)

Nursing considerations/Cautions/ Patient education
- kidney function should be monitored before starting and regularly throughout therapy
- see also General Nursing considerations/Cautions/ Patient education for DPP-4 inhibitors (p. 317)

Tablets can be crushed and mixed with water or spoonful of yoghurt or apple puree; however, tablets do not disperse readily in water and are difficult to crush.

Janumet XR (sitagliptin and metformin) is an extended-release tablet and should not be crushed, chewed or broken.

In those with moderate kidney impairment, dose should be reduced to 50 mg daily; for those with severe kidney impairment or on dialysis, dose should be reduced to 25 mg daily.

Available in combination with
- sitagliptin + metformin combination (see Metformin p. 313)

VILDAGLIPTIN

Trade name
Galvus

Available form
Tablets: 50 mg

Action/Use
- peak effect 1.75 hours, half-life 2—3 hours
- see also General Actions of DPP-4 inhibitors and General Uses of DPP-4 inhibitors (p. 317)

Dose
- (Combination therapy) 50 mg orally once or twice daily **OR**
- (Monotherapy) 50 mg orally twice daily

Adverse effects
- peripheral oedema
- headache, dizziness
- constipation
- (Rare) changes in liver enzymes, liver dysfunction, hepatitis
- see also General Adverse effects of DPP-4 inhibitors (p. 317)

Nursing considerations/Cautions
- liver and kidney function should be assessed before starting therapy and then monitored 3-monthly during therapy
- tablets contain lactose and therefore are not recommended in those with galactose intolerance, glucose—galactose malabsorption or Lapp lactose deficiency
- not recommended in those with moderate-to-severe kidney impairment, end-stage kidney disease on haemodialysis or those with liver impairment (alanine aminotransferase (ALT) or aspartate aminotransferase (AST) 2.5 times > upper normal limit) or cardiac failure (NYHA functional class IV)
- see also General Nursing considerations/Cautions for DPP-4 inhibitors (p. 317)

Patient education
- advise the patient to seek medical advice if any loss of appetite, nausea, vomiting, upper abdominal pain, lethargy, dark urine or pale stools occurs
- warn the patient not to drive or operate machinery if dizziness is an ongoing problem
- see also General Patient education for DPP-4 inhibitors (p. 317)

ANTIDIABETIC AGENTS

Tablets can be crushed and mixed with water, or a spoonful of yoghurt or apple puree.

In those with moderate, severe or end-stage kidney disease, daily dose should be reduced to 50 mg.

Available in combination with
- vildagliptin + metformin combination (see Metformin p. 313)

GLUCAGON-LIKE PEPTIDE-1 (GLP-1) ANALOGUES

General Actions of GLP-1 analogues
- binds to and activates glucagon-like peptide-1 (GLP-1) receptors mimicking incretin, leading to increase in synthesis and secretion of insulin by the pancreas
- suppresses glucagon secretion in those with type 2 diabetes, leading to decreased glucose output by the liver
- does not impair normal glucagon response to hypoglycaemia
- slows gastric emptying

General Uses of GLP-1 analogues
- type 2 diabetes (as either monotherapy or combination therapy with other hypoglycaemic agents where glycaemic control has not been achieved)

General Adverse effects of GLP-1 analogues
- nausea, vomiting, decreased appetite, anorexia, diarrhoea, constipation, dyspepsia, abdominal pain and distension, GI reflux disease, belching
- headache
- fatigue, asthenia, malaise
- upper respiratory tract infection
- hypoglycaemia (if given with sulfonylurea)
- risk of pulmonary aspiration
- (Injection site) pruritus, redness, pain, haematoma, induration and, rarely, abscess formation, cellulitis, ulceration, necrosis
- (Rare) acute renal failure, pancreatitis, kidney impairment, worsening of chronic kidney failure, antibody production

General Interactions of GLP-1 analogues
- caution if given with agents that require rapid GI absorption (e.g. bisphosphonates) because of the delay in GI emptying, or those that can cause GI irritation (e.g. tetracyclines)
- increased risk of hypoglycaemia if given with sulfonylureas (in those with type 2 diabetes)

General Nursing considerations/Cautions for GLP-1 analogues
- not given IV or IM
- dose of sulfonylurea may be reduced to lessen risk of hypoglycaemia if given as combination therapy
- administer alone
- caution if used in patients undergoing general anaesthesia or deep sedation because of the risk of pulmonary aspiration, as GLP-1 analogues delay gastric emptying
- caution if used in those with history of pancreatitis, gallstones, alcoholism or severe hypertriglyceridaemia
- caution if used in those with congestive cardiac failure
- not recommended in those with diabetes mellitus type 1, treatment of diabetic ketoacidosis or those with history of pancreatitis
- contraindicated in those with history of GLP-1 analogue-associated pancreatitis
- see also General Nursing considerations/Cautions for oral hypoglycaemic agents (p. 305)

General Patient education for GLP-1 analogues
- the patient should be educated:
  - in the correct use of pen for self administration (see also General Patient education for insulins (p. 301))

- on the importance of rotating injection sites to include upper arms, thighs and abdomen
- to inject into skin (not into veins or muscle)
- not to use solution if cloudy, coloured or if it contains particles, or if expiry date has passed
- to store pen in fridge, but should not be frozen. Pen should be discarded if it becomes frozen
- safe disposal of used pens/syringe
- that if dose is missed and there is less than 3 days before next dose, dose should not be given, but administered on next scheduled day
- the patient should be instructed to seek medical advice immediately if any of the following occur:
  - any persistent severe abdominal pain, especially if accompanied by diarrhoea, nausea and/or vomiting
  - vomiting, upset stomach, rapid pulse, fever, abdominal pain or tenderness (signs of pancreatitis)
- see also General Patient education for oral hypoglycaemic agents (p. 305)

Not recommended during pregnancy unless benefits outweigh risks to fetus. Insulin is recommended during pregnancy.

Not recommended during breastfeeding unless benefits to mother outweigh risks to infant.

DULAGLUTIDE
Trade name
Trulicity

Available form
Prefilled pen: 1.5 mg/0.5 mL

Action/Use
- half-life 4.7 days (making it suitable for once-weekly administration)
- see also General Actions of GLP-1 analogues and General Uses of GLP-1 analogues (p. 321)

Dose
- 1.5 mg weekly SC

Adverse effects
- fatigue
- sinus tachycardia
- elevated pancreatic enzymes
- hypersensitivity
- see also General Adverse effects of GLP-1 analogues (p. 321)

Interactions
- see General Interactions of GLP-1 analogues (p. 321)

Nursing considerations/Cautions
- not recommended in those with end-stage kidney disease
- see also General Nursing considerations/Cautions for GLP-1 analogues (p. 321)

Patient education
- advise patient that gastrointestinal adverse effects usually peak in first 2 weeks and then decline over next 4 weeks
- see also General Patient education for GLP-1 analogues (p. 321)

LIRAGUTIDE
Trade names
Saxenda, Victoza

Available form
Prefilled pen: 6 mg/mL

Action
- protracted release is due to self-association (resulting in slow absorption), binding to albumin and enzymatic stability, resulting in long plasma half-life
- physiological regulator of appetite and calorie intake as glucagon-like peptide 1 (GLP-1) receptors are present in the brain in areas involved in appetite regulation, as well as being present in the intestine
- increases fullness and satiety and decreases hunger signals

ANTIDIABETIC AGENTS

- decreases plasma triglycerides, total cholesterol, low-density lipoprotein (LDL) and very-low-density lipoprotein (VLDL) while increasing high-density lipoprotein (HDL), but does not reduce size of any existing plaques
- peak effect 8–12 hours, duration of action 24 hours, half-life about 13 hours
- see also General Actions of GLP-1 analogues (p. 321)

Use
- reduces risk of cardiovascular events as an adjunct to standard care
- chronic weight management in those with BMI $\geq$ 30 kg/m^2 (obese) or $\geq$ 27 kg/m^2 and $<$ 30 kg/m^2 (overweight) with $\geq$ one weight-related co-morbidity (e.g. dyslipidaemia, hypertension, obstructive sleep apnoea) (adjunct to reduced calorie diet and increased physical activity) (Saxeda)
- see also General Uses of GLP-1 analogues (p. 321)

Dose
- (Type 2 diabetes) initially 0.6 mg SC once daily, then increasing to 1.2 mg after 7 or more days, increasing to 1.8 mg after a further 7 days if needed (maximum daily dose 1.8 mg) (Victoza) **OR**
- (Weight management) initially 0.6 mg SC once daily, increasing by 0.6 mg increments at 7-day intervals to 3 mg (as maintenance) (Saxenda)

Adverse effects
- gastritis, flatulence, altered taste, dry mouth, belching
- increased heart rate, hypotension
- insomnia (especially in first 12 weeks of therapy), fatigue, asthenia
- dizziness
- (Uncommon) rash, urticaria, pruritus
- cholelithiasis, cholecystitis, elevated liver enzymes
- (Uncommon) dehydration
- (Rare) increased blood calcitonin, goitre, thyroid adenomas/carcinomas, allergic reactions, depression, suicidal ideation
- injection site reactions
- see also General Adverse effects of GLP-1 analogues (p. 321)

Interactions
- (Saxenda) caution if used with other agents that increase heart rate such as sympathomimetic agents
- not recommended with other agents containing GLP-1 analogues
- (Saxenda) not recommended with other weight loss products (including over-the-counter or complementary/herbal medicines)
- see also General Interactions of GLP-1 analogues (p. 321)

Nursing considerations/Cautions
- (Weight management) if there has not been a weight loss of at least 5% of initial body weight on 3 mg daily dose after 12 weeks, therapy should be stopped
- (Weight management) heart rate should be monitored regularly during therapy
- should not be used as substitute for insulin
- (Weight management) intervals of at least 7 days are needed to improve GI tolerability. If increasing dose to next level is not tolerated for 2 consecutive weeks, stopping treatment should be considered
- (Weight management) therapy should be reviewed each time prescription is written and at least annually
- caution if used in those with pre-existing thyroid disease
- (Weight management) not recommended in those with obesity secondary to endocrinological issues or eating disorders
- (Saxenda) not recommended in those with liver insufficiency or kidney impairment
- (Saxenda) not recommended for type 2 diabetes management
- (Saxenda) not recommended in those with inflammatory bowel disease or diabetic gastroparesis
- (Saxenda) increased risk of GI adverse effects in those $>$ 65 years
- (Saxenda) not recommended in those $>$ 75 years

- not recommended in those with end-stage kidney disease or heart failure (NYHA class IV)
- (Saxenda) not recommended in those with history of major depression or other psychiatric illnesses
- see also General Nursing considerations/Cautions for GLP-1 analogues (p. 321)

Patient education

- the patient should be advised to avoid dehydration during therapy, especially if nausea, vomiting and/or diarrhoea occur
- warn the patient that severe diarrhoea can impact on absorption of oral medications
- warn the patient not to drive or operate machinery if dizziness is ongoing
- advise the patient to seek medical advice if any of the following occur:
  - palpitations, feelings of racing heartbeat while at rest
  - upper right-sided abdominal pain, yellowing of eyes or skin
  - lump or swelling in neck, hoarseness, difficulty swallowing, shortness of breath
  - sadness, depression, change in mood, ideas of self-harm
- see also General Patient education for GLP-1 analogues (p. 321)

SODIUM–GLUCOSE COTRANSPORTER 2 INHIBITORS (SGLT2 INHIBITORS)

General Actions of SGLT2 inhibitors

- reversibly inhibit sodium–glucose cotransporter 2 (SGLT2) in the proximal renal tubules. Normally SGLT2 is responsible for most of the reabsorption of filtered glucose from renal tubular lumen. Those with diabetes have raised renal glucose reabsorption, which adds to persistently elevated blood glucose levels (BGLs). SGLT2 is inhibited, reducing reabsorption of filtered glucose, lowering the renal glucose threshold and increasing glucose excretion, resulting in decreased blood glucose levels (BGLs)
- blood glucose excretion leads to osmotic diuresis (and therefore decreased fluid load), caloric loss and subsequent weight reduction
- improve both fasting and postprandial plasma glucose level
- do not depend on insulin secretion or sensitivity

General Uses of SGLT2 inhibitors

- type 2 diabetes mellitus with diet and exercise (as monotherapy when metformin is not tolerated or inappropriate, or as combination therapy with other antidiabetic agents)
- heart failure
- chronic kidney disease

General Adverse effects of SGLT2 Inhibitors

- hypotension, dehydration, hypovolaemia
- thirst
- polyuria, renal impairment, decreased creatinine clearance
- urinary tract infection, genital infection (vulvovaginal, balanitis)
- constipation
- back pain
- (Uncommon) pyelonephritis, urosepsis
- hypoglycaemia (when given with insulin or sulfonylurea)
- ketoacidosis
- (Rare) Fournier's gangrene

General Nursing considerations/Cautions for SGLT2 inhibitors

- any volume deficit should be corrected before starting therapy. Volume status should be assessed using physical examination, BP measurements and laboratory tests (including haematocrit)
- the patient should be assessed for any risk factors predisposing to ketoacidosis such as insulin deficiency (e.g. insulin pump failure, pancreatic surgery, history of pancreatitis), decreased insulin dose, increased insulin requirements, reduced

ANTIDIABETIC AGENTS

- caloric intake (such as low-carbohydrate diet), surgery, acute illness, dehydration, alcohol abuse or previous ketoacidosis
- kidney function should be monitored before starting and yearly during therapy. If any medications are added that impair kidney function, the test should be conducted again and, if the patient has moderate kidney impairment, kidney function tests should be 2—4 times yearly
- lower doses of insulin or sulfonylurea may be needed if used as combination therapy to decrease risk of hypoglycaemia
- the patient should be monitored for any signs and symptoms of urinary tract infection during therapy
- therapy should be interrupted if the patient develops pyelonephritis or urosepsis
- therapy should be interrupted temporarily:
  - prior to major surgery, and restarted when patient's condition has stabilised and oral intake is normal
  - if patient develops condition leading to volume depletion such as acute illness, severe infection, heat stress or gastrointestinal illness
- caution if used in those with cardiovascular disease, taking antihypertensive agents, a history of hypotension or in the elderly where a fall in blood pressure could pose a risk
- not recommended in those with diabetes mellitus type 1 or treatment for diabetic ketoacidosis
- not recommended in patients receiving loop diuretics, who are volume depleted or have a history of hypotension or dehydration when receiving diuretics
- contraindicated in those with moderate-to-severe kidney or liver impairment

General Patient education for SGLT2 inhibitors

- the patient should be instructed to seek medical advice immediately if any of the following occurs:
  - feeling dizzy or lightheaded
  - vomiting or diarrhoea, severe thirst, urinating less than normal
  - increased urination, urgent need to urinate, cloudy urine, strong odour, burning sensation on urination, passing frequent small amounts of urine
  - pain, tenderness, rash, redness or swelling in genital/perineal area, fever or malaise
  - nausea, vomiting, abdominal pain, malaise, shortness of breath (signs of ketoacidosis)
- advise the patient to take care in going from lying or sitting position to standing as lightheadedness, dizziness or fainting may occur
- instruct the patient to take adequate fluids to avoid dehydration, especially during infection or illness (especially GI with vomiting and/or diarrhoea) or in hot conditions
- see also General Patient education for oral hypoglycaemic agents (p. 305)

 Contraindicated during pregnancy.

 Contraindicated during breastfeeding.

DAPAGLIFLOZIN
Trade name
Forxiga

Available form
Tablets: 10 mg

Action/Use
- peak activity within 2 hours, half-life 13 hours
- see also General Actions/Uses of SGLT2 inhibitors (p. 324)

Dose
- (Type 2 diabetes) 10 mg orally once daily (as mono or combination therapy) **OR**
- (Heart failure, chronic kidney disease) 10 mg orally once daily

Adverse effects
- see General Adverse effects of SGLT2 inhibitors (p. 324)

Interactions
- not recommended with pioglitazone because of an increased risk of bladder cancer
- may increase clearance of lithium, requiring a dose adjustment

Nursing considerations/Cautions
- not recommended in those > 75 years or with severe liver impairment (eGFR < 25 mL/min/1.75 m^2)
- see also General Nursing considerations/Cautions for SGLT2 inhibitors (p. 324)

Patient education
- see General Patient education for SGLT2 inhibitors (p. 325)

Tablet can be crushed and mixed with water, or spoonful of yoghurt or apple puree.

Xigduo XR (dapagliflozin and metformin) tablets are extended release and should not be crushed, chewed or broken.

Available in combination with
- dapagliflozin + metformin combination (see Metformin p. 313)
- dapagliflozin 10 mg + saxagliptin 5 mg (Qtern 5/10)
- dapagliflozin 10 mg + sitagliptin 100 mg (Sidapvia 10/100)

EMPAGLIFLOZIN
Trade name
Jardiance

Available forms
Tablets: 10 mg, 25 mg

Action/Use
- peak activity 1.5 hours, half-life 12.4 hours
- see also General Actions of SGLT2 inhibitors and General Uses of SGLT2 inhibitors (p. 324)

Dose
- (Type 2 diabetes) initially 10 mg orally once daily, increasing to 25 mg if additional glycaemic control is needed
- (Heart failure, chronic kidney disease) 10 mg orally once daily

Adverse effects
- see General Adverse effects of SGLT2 inhibitors (p. 324)

Interactions
- not recommended with glucagon-like peptide 1 (GLP-1) analogues
- may cause positive glucose result on urine test
- increased risk of dehydration and hypotension if given with thiazide and loop diuretics
- may increase lithium clearance, requiring dose adjustment
- increase risk of hypoglycaemia if given with insulin or sulfonylureas

Nursing considerations/Cautions
- tablets contain lactose and are therefore not recommended in those with galactose intolerance, Lapp lactase deficiency or glucose–galactose malabsorption
- contraindicated in those with severe kidney impairment, including those on dialysis (creatinine clearance < 30 mL/min)
- see also General Nursing considerations/Cautions for SGLT2 inhibitors (p. 324)

Patient education
- see General Patient education for SGLT2 inhibitors (p. 325)

Available in combination with
- empagliflozin 10 mg + linagliptin 5 mg (Glyxambi 10/5)
- empagliflozin 25 mg + linagliptin 5 mg (Glyxambi 25/5)
- empagliflozin + metformin combination (see Metformin p. 313)

SEMAGLUTIDE

Trade names
Ozempic, Wegovy, Rybelsus

Available forms
Prefilled Pen: 0.25 mg, 0.5 mg, 1 mg, 2 mg;
Tablet: 3 mg, 7 mg, 14 mg

Action
- see General Actions of GLP-1 analogues (p. 321)

Use
- chronic weight management in those with BMI $\geq$ 30 kg/m^2 (obese) or $\geq$ 27 kg/m^2 and with $\geq$ 1 weight-related co-morbidity (e.g. dyslipidaemia, hypertension, obstructive sleep apnoea) (adjunct to reduced calorie diet and increased physical activity)
- see also General Uses of GLP-1 analogues (p. 321)

Dose
- (Type 2 diabetes) initially 0.25 mg SC weekly for 4 weeks, increasing to 0.5 mg SC weeks for 4 weeks, increasing to 1 mg weekly if needed (Ozempic) **OR**
- (Weight management) initially 0.25 mg SC weekly (weeks 1—4), then 0.5 mg SC weekly (weeks 5—9), 1 mg SC weekly (weeks 10—14), 1.7 mg SC weekly (weeks 15—19), then 2.4 mg SC weekly (maintenance dose) (maximum dose 2.4 mg) (Wegovy) **OR**
- (Type 2 diabetes) initially 3 mg orally daily for 1 month, increasing to 7 mg orally daily for 1 month, then, if needed, increasing to 14 mg orally daily (maximum daily dose 14 mg) (Rybelsus)

Adverse effects
- see General Adverse effects of GLP-1 analogues (p. 321)

Nursing considerations/Cautions
- (Weight management) if patient does not tolerate 2.4 mg, dose can be decreased to 1.7 mg as maintenance. If tolerated, dose should be increased to 2.4 mg
- not recommended for patients with severe liver impairment or end-stage renal disease
- not recommended in those with uncontrolled or unstable diabetic retinopathy
- see also General Nursing considerations/Cautions for GLP-1 analogues (p. 321)

Patient education
- the patient should be advised to prevent dehydration during therapy, especially if they experience gastrointestinal adverse effects
- if the patient has diabetic retinopathy, they should be warned that it might temporarily worsen as glucose control improves
- see also General Patient education for GLP-1 analogues (p. 321)

TIRZEPATIDE

Trade names
Mounjaro, Mounjaro KwikPen

Available forms
Vial: 2.5 mg/0.5 mL, 5 mg/0.5 mL, 7.5 mg/0.5 mL, 10 mg/0.5 mL, 12.5 mg/0.5 mL, 15 mg/0.5 mL;
Prefilled pen (KwikPen): 4.17 mg/mL, 8.33 mg/mL, 12.5 mg/mL, 16.67 mg/mL, 20.83 mg/mL, 25 mg/mL

Actions
- protracted release is due to self-association (resulting in slow absorption), binding to albumin and enzymatic stability, resulting in long plasma half-life
- physiological regulator of appetite and calorie intake, as glucagon-like peptide 1 (GLP-1) receptors are present in the brain in areas involved in appetite regulation, as well as being present in the intestine
- increases fullness and satiety and decreases hunger signals
- decreases plasma triglycerides, total cholesterol, low-density lipoprotein (LDL) and very-low-density lipoprotein

(VLDL) while increasing high-density lipoprotein (HDL), but does not reduce size of any existing plaques
* half-life 5 days (allowing weekly administration)
* see also General Actions of GLP-1 analogues (p. 321)

Use
* chronic weight management in those with BMI $\geq$ 30 kg/m^2 (obese) or $\geq$ 27 kg/m^2 and < 30 kg/m^2 (overweight) with $\geq$ 1 weight-related co-morbidity (e.g. dyslipidaemia, hypertension, obstructive sleep apnoea) (adjunct to reduced calorie diet and increased physical activity)
* see also General Uses of GLP-1 analogues (p. 321)

Dose
* (Type 2 diabetes, weight management) initially 2.5 mg SC weekly, increasing to 5 mg SC after 4 weeks, and, if needed, increasing by 2.5 mg increments at 4-weekly intervals (maximum weekly dose 15 mg)

Adverse effects
* nausea, vomiting, diarrhoea, dehydration, constipation, abdominal pain/discomfort, belching, flatulence, dyspepsia, gastro-oesophageal reflux, decreased appetite, metallic/bitter taste
* headache, fatigue, dizziness
* injection site reaction
* hair loss
* hypotension
* (Uncommon) cholelithiasis, pancreatitis, hypersensitivity, malnutrition, acute renal failure, depression, suicidal ideation
* hypoglycaemia (if given with insulin or sulfonylurea)

Interactions
* see General Interactions of GLP-1 analogues (p. 321)

Nursing considerations/Cautions
* the patient should be assessed for risk of malnutrition and nutritional support considered
* if the patient experiences severe gastrointestinal adverse effects, dose adjustment or stopping therapy should be considered
* caution if the patient is undergoing general anaesthesia or deep sedation because of the increased risk of pulmonary aspiration resulting from delayed gastric emptying
* caution if used in those with diabetic macular oedema, proliferative diabetic retinopathy or non-proliferative diabetic retinopathy requiring acute therapy
* caution if used in those at risk of malnutrition including those with low body weight, vitamin and mineral deficiency or protein deficiency
* not recommended in those with end-stage kidney disease or liver impairment
* not recommended in those with a history of major depression or other psychiatric illnesses
* not recommended in those with inflammatory bowel disease or diabetic gastroparesis, type 1 diabetes or ketoacidosis
* see also General Nursing considerations/Cautions for GLP-1 analogues (p. 321)

Patient education
* instruct the patient that the day of the weekly dose can be changed as long as there is a minimum of 72 hours between injections
* the patient should be advised to avoid dehydration during therapy, especially if nausea, vomiting and/or diarrhoea occur
* if the patient has diabetic retinopathy, they should be warned that condition may temporarily worsen at the start of therapy
* ensure the patient is instructed in correct self-administration including use of a KwikPen, which is a multi-dose device drawing-up technique using vial (see General Patient education for GLP-1

ANTIDIABETIC AGENTS

analogues (p. 321) for SC injection technique, storage and safe disposal)
- advise the patient to seek medical advice if any of the following occur:
  - sadness, depression, change in mood, ideas of self-harm
  - vomiting, stomach upset, rapid pulse, fever, abdominal tenderness or pain, or abdominal pain that radiates to back (signs of pancreatitis)
- see also General Patient education for GLP-1 analogues (p. 321)

ANTIDIARRHOEAL AGENTS

Diarrhoea can be defined as frequent passage of loose (liquid or unformed) stools and may be acute (lasting < 2 weeks), persistent (2–4 weeks) or chronic (lasting > 4 weeks). For most people, diarrhoea is self-limiting and does not require any intervention; however, acute infectious diarrhoea is still one of the most common causes of mortality (especially in infants) in developing countries (Camilleri & Murray 2026).

Acute diarrhoea is primarily caused by infectious agents and often accompanied by vomiting, fever and abdominal pain, while a smaller proportion may be due to medication (e.g. antibiotics, non-steroidal NSAIDs, some antidepressants), ischaemia, toxins, food-related and other conditions. Those most at risk of developing acute diarrhoea include travellers (especially to Asia, Africa and Latin America), immunodeficient individuals, those in institutions such as hospitals and long-term care facilities, children attending day care and their family members, and consumers of some foods (e.g. *Listeria* from uncooked foods or soft cheeses, *Salmonella* from eggs, seafood, cream, mayonnaise) (Camilleri & Murray 2022).

Management of severe acute diarrhoea should include:

- investigating the underlying cause (e.g. a stool sample may be collected to isolate an organism), recommended if the patient has diarrhoea that is profuse with dehydration, grossly bloody stools, fever $\geq 38.5°C$, lasting longer than 48 hours without improvement, recent antibiotic use, associated with abdominal pain (especially if over 70 years), immunocompromised or if there is a current community outbreak (Camilleri & Murray 2022). Caution should be used if diarrhoea is thought to be a result of antibiotic-induced colitis or pseudomembranous colitis
- preventing/treating fluid and electrolyte imbalance, especially in the elderly and very young, because dehydration can occur very quickly
- use of antibacterial agents (if appropriate), which may reduce the severity and duration of the diarrhoea depending on the causative organism
- antimotility and antisecretory agents (e.g. loperamide) can be useful in

controlling symptoms in moderately severe non-febrile and non-bloody diarrhoea (Camilleri & Murray 2022).

Chronic diarrhoea is generally non-infectious and should be investigated to rule out serious underlying pathology. Causes of chronic diarrhoea include chronic alcohol intake, decreased absorption due to bowel resection, disease or fistula, lactase deficiency, gluten intolerance, idiopathic inflammatory bowel disease (e.g. Crohn's disease, ulcerative colitis), irritable bowel syndrome, eating disorders (with laxative abuse), ileal resection and radiation enterocolitis. Management of chronic diarrhoea is dependent on identification and management of the underlying cause if possible, as this will result in control of the diarrhoea (Camilleri & Murray 2022).

General Nursing considerations/ Cautions for antidiarrhoeal agents

- agents that delay or inhibit intestinal motility may induce toxic megacolon in patients with Crohn's disease or ulcerative colitis and therefore should be stopped at the first signs of abdominal distension or other untoward symptoms
- it may not always be appropriate to slow the motility of the bowel (e.g. if the cause is infectious), because this may allow time for the organism to replicate further or the toxin to accumulate

General Patient education for antidiarrhoeal agents

- the patient should be warned against driving or operating machinery if drowsiness, dizziness or confusion occur
- advise the patient to avoid alcohol while taking medication
- instruct the patient to stop taking the medication when bowel motions return to normal
- advise the patient to seek medical advice if diarrhoea persists for more than 2 days or if there is blood present in the diarrhoea
- instruct the patient to drink plenty of liquids (such as rehydration solution) to prevent becoming dehydrated. Milk, dairy products, fatty or fried foods, chocolate, fruit, acidic vegetables and alcohol should be avoided as these may make the diarrhoea worse. Food intake should be restricted during first few days to unbuttered toast, plain crackers, boiled potatoes, rice and pasta. Normal diet can be restarted when the diarrhoea stops

DIPHENOXYLATE

Trade names
Lofenoxal, Lomotil

Available form
Tablets: 2.5 mg

Action
- pethidine-related drug that reduces peristalsis and allows increased fluid absorption
- contains atropine
- half-life is 2.5 hours
- active metabolite

Dose
- recommended starting dose in adults is dose is 5 mg (two tablets) three or four times daily
- reduce to meet requirements of individual patients

Use
- treatment of acute and chronic diarrhoea (adjunctive therapy)

Adverse effects
- drowsiness, sedation, headache, confusion, dizziness, restlessness, euphoria, malaise, lethargy
- numbness of extremities
- anorexia, nausea, vomiting, abdominal discomfort
- anaphylaxis, urticaria, rash, pruritus
- gum swelling
- paralytic ileus, toxic megacolon
- (Atropine) tachycardia, dry mouth and skin, flushing, hyperthermia, urinary retention
- (High dose) addiction/dependency

Interactions
- may precipitate hypertensive crisis if given with monoamine oxidase inhibitors (MAOIs)
- may have additive effect when given with alcohol and other CNS depressants

Nursing considerations/Cautions
- the patient should be assessed for cause of diarrhoea
- the patient should be closely monitored for any signs of fluid and/or electrolyte imbalance, and treated if it occurs
- combined with small amount of atropine to discourage excessive self-medication and misuse
- may induce toxic megacolon if given to patients with ulcerative colitis
- respiratory depression may occur up to 30 hours after overdose, therefore patients should be monitored for at least 48 hours if overdose does occur. Respiratory depression should be treated with naloxone (IV) initially, then given SC or IM for more prolonged effect if respiratory depression does not improve. Repeated doses may be required, as naloxone has a short duration of action
- caution if used in those with abnormal liver function or hepatorenal disease, as hepatic coma can occur
- caution if used in those with a history of drug addiction or currently taking drugs that may be addictive, as diphenoxylate hydrochloride has the potential to be addictive
- caution (because of atropine content) if used in those with Down syndrome
- contraindicated in those with jaundice, bacterial/amoebic colitis, diarrhoea associated with pseudomembranous enterocolitis or inflammatory bowel disease (e.g. Crohn's disease, ulcerative colitis) and in children under 12 years (accidental overdosage may result in severe, even fatal, respiratory depression)
- see also General Nursing considerations/Cautions for antidiarrhoeal agents (p. 331)

Patient education
- warn the patient not to take more than 8 tablets per 24 hours
- see also General Patient education for antidiarrhoeal agents (p. 331)

 Tablets can be crushed and mixed with water (do not readily disperse), or given with a spoonful of yoghurt or apple puree.

 Chemically related to pethidine and may cause respiratory depression in the newborn; therefore should not be given at or near term.

 Not recommended during breastfeeding owing to limited data available.

Available in combination with
- diphenoxylate hydrochloride 2.5 mg + atropine sulfate monohydrate 25 microgram tablet (Lofenoxil; Lomotil)

LOPERAMIDE HYDROCHLORIDE
Trade names
Chemists' Own Diarrhoea Relief, Diareze, Gastrex, Gastro-Stop, Harmonise, Imodium, Pharmacy Action Diarrhoea Relief, Stop-It

Available forms
Tablets: 2 mg;
Capsules: 2 mg;
Dissolvable tablets (melts): 2 mg

ANTIDIARRHOEAL AGENTS

Action
- binds to opiate receptors in the gut wall, reducing peristalsis by suppressing intestinal motility through direct action on circular and longitudinal muscles of the intestinal wall
- may also increase anal sphincter tone, decreasing urgency and incontinence
- no analgesic properties
- more potent as an antidiarrhoeal agent than diphenoxylate hydrochloride (3 times) and codeine phosphate (25 times)
- onset of action (symptomatic improvement) in 1—3 hours, half-life 9—14 hours

Use
- relief of acute non-specific diarrhoea
- to reduce the volume of discharge in patients with ileostomies and colostomies, chronic diarrhoea

Dose
- (Acute diarrhoea) initially 4 mg orally, then 2 mg after each unformed stool, up to 16 mg/day **OR**
- (Chronic diarrhoea or to reduce volume of ileostomy/colostomy discharge) initially 4 mg orally, then 2 mg after each unformed stool, then maintained on 4—8 mg daily as a single or divided dose

Adverse effects
- nausea, abdominal pain/cramps, constipation, flatulence, abdominal distension
- (Very rare) dizziness, drowsiness
- (Melts) burning, prickling sensation on tongue

Interactions
- caution if used with alcohol
- increased plasma levels may occur if given with ritonavir
- action may be potentiated by monoamine oxidase inhibitors (MAOIs)

Nursing considerations/Cautions
- the patient should be carefully assessed for the cause of diarrhoea
- the patient should be closely monitored for any signs of fluid and/or electrolyte imbalance, and treated if they occur
- improvement is usually seen in 48 hours
- therapy should be stopped if constipation, abdominal distension or ileus develops
- sublingual tablets (melts) are recommended for those with swallowing difficulties
- may induce toxic megacolon if given to patients with ulcerative colitis or Crohn's disease
- caution if used in those with AIDS because of the risk of toxic megacolon
- caution if used in those with urinary retention, glaucoma, pyloric obstruction, gastric retention or intestinal stasis
- caution if used in those with liver dysfunction, as CNS toxicity may occur
- contraindicated in those with constipation, conditions where constipation should be avoided, high fever, blood in stools of unknown origin, acute dysentery, inflammatory bowel disease, bacterial enterocolitis, antibiotic-induced pseudomembranous colitis, megacolon or toxic megacolon, or in children under 12 years
- loperamide may be misused: serious cardiac adverse events (QT interval prolongation, torsades de pointes, ventricular arrhythmias, cardiac arrest) and death have been reported with high doses (e.g. 40 mg—300 mg daily)
- see also General Nursing considerations/Cautions for antidiarrhoeal agents (p. 331)

Patient education
- (Melt tablets) advise the patient to place tablet on tongue and allow to melt, then swallow with saliva
- see also General Patient education for antidiarrhoeal agents (p. 331)

 Capsules can be opened and contents dispersed in water, or sprinkled on apple puree. Tablets can be crushed and mixed with water or a spoonful of apple puree.

 Not recommended during pregnancy or breastfeeding unless the expected benefit outweighs any potential risk.

ANTIDOTES, ANTAGONISTS AND CHELATING AGENTS

Antidotes, chelating agents and antagonists play a crucial role in counteracting the toxic effects of various substances within the body, whether these substances are introduced externally (exogenous) or produced within the body (endogenous).

ACETYLCYSTEINE
Trade names
Acetadote Concentrated Injection,
Acetylcysteine-Link Injection Concentrate,
DBL Acetylcysteine Injection Concentrate

Available forms
Ampoules: 200 mg/mL, 6 g/30 mL

Action
- Normal metabolism of paracetamol:
  - The liver metabolises paracetamol mainly through glucuronidation and sulfation pathways, producing non-toxic metabolites
  - A small amount of paracetamol is metabolised by the CYP2E1 enzyme to form a toxic intermediate metabolite called N-acetyl-p-benzoquinone imine (NAPQI)
  - NAPQI is usually detoxified by conjugation with glutathione, forming non-toxic compounds that are excreted by the kidneys
- Paracetamol overdose:
  - In overdose situations, glutathione stores in the liver are rapidly depleted. Without sufficient glutathione, excess NAPQI binds to liver proteins and lipids, leading to oxidative stress, hepatocellular damage and hepatic necrosis. Hepatic necrosis can be seen at 6 g and death at 15 g of paracetamol
  - IV administration of acetylcysteine, a sulfhydryl donor, within 10 hours of paracetamol ingestion prevents severe liver damage, primarily by restoring glutathione levels

Use
- antidote for paracetamol poisoning
- prevents hepatotoxicity following paracetamol overdose by replenishing glutathione stores in the liver and enhancing the detoxification of the toxic metabolite, NAPQI

Dose
- initially 150 mg/kg IV in 200 mL glucose 5% over 15–60 minutes (loading dose), followed by continuous infusion of 50 mg/kg in 500 mL over 4 hours, followed by 100 mg/kg in 1 L over 16 hours (total dose 300 mg/kg in 20 hours)

Adverse effects
- rash, urticaria, flushing, sweating
- fever

ANTIDOTES, ANTAGONISTS AND CHELATING AGENTS

- blurred vision, eye pain
- cyanosis
- facial pain, facial and periorbital oedema
- arthralgia
- hypokalaemia, acidosis, decreased liver function
- nausea, vomiting
- hypotension/hypertension, tachycardia, bradycardia, chest pain, ECG changes
- anxiety, malaise, rigors
- bronchospasm, coughing, stridor, dyspnoea, angioedema
- injection site reaction
- (Rare) anaphylactoid reaction, seizures, thrombocytopenia

Interactions

- hepatoxicity may occur at lower paracetamol doses if taken with rifampicin, isoniazid, phenytoin, carbamazepine, primidone, phenobarbital (phenobarbitone) or sodium valproate, or with chronic alcohol intake
- false positive for urinary ketones may occur with dipstick testing

Nursing considerations/Cautions

- urea, electrolytes (including potassium to monitor for hypokalaemia), Hb, WBC count, platelets, blood glucose, urea and bilirubin, liver function, ECG, blood gases and prothrombin should be monitored on admission and then daily for coagulation disorders, hepatic encephalopathy, renal failure and cardiac toxicity
- general management for paracetamol overdose should include tests as above, airway management, cardiac monitoring and then infusion of acetylcysteine
- if the patient is conscious and within 1 hour of paracetamol ingestion, activated charcoal (1–2 g/kg (maximum 50 g)) should be given
- liver damage may not be apparent (biochemically) for 24–48 hours and the patient may appear well, but hepatic necrosis is preventable if treatment can be instituted within 10–12 hours of ingestion
- obtain urgent serum paracetamol levels (but no earlier than 4 hours after ingestion as they may be unreliable) and ascertain the degree of potential liver damage from the semilogarithmic graph of serum paracetamol levels plotted against hours since ingestion (for single ingestion). The graph may not be useful in determining acetylcysteine requirements if there was multiple or chronic ingestion or if sustained preparations were taken
- the decision to give acetylcysteine is made on the basis of the amount of paracetamol ingested and should not be delayed pending laboratory results. If the time of ingestion is unknown, paracetamol levels should be measured immediately
- may be used 15 hours after paracetamol overdose, but this should be discussed first with doctors experienced in the treatment of paracetamol poisoning for use in high-risk patients, as effectiveness has not been proven
- dose/volume may need to be adjusted if the patient weighs less than 40 kg or if on a fluid restriction to decrease risk of hyponatraemia and seizures
- anaphylactic-like reactions (bronchospasm, dyspnoea, hypotension, tachycardia, shock, urticaria) occur most commonly during or after loading dose has been administered. The patient should be closely monitored during this time
- dilute in glucose 5% or sodium chloride 0.9% before administration
- slight colour change (pink/purple) may occur when the stopper is punctured; however, this does not indicate any loss of activity
- not compatible with rubber and some metals (iron, copper, nickel)
- caution if used in those with asthma or bronchospasm, or oesophageal varices

or peptic ulceration (because of an increased risk of bleeding with associated vomiting) or in those with known liver/kidney impairment
- caution if used in those with a history of chronic alcohol use or taking medications such as antiepileptics, isoniazid or rifampicin as there is an increased risk of hepatotoxicity due to paracetamol overdose

Benefits can be assumed to outweigh potential risks. Limited clinical experience has not shown adverse effects on the fetus.

Safe to use. Due to its minimal oral bioavailability, it is unlikely to affect the breastfed infant when administered to the mother.

CALCIUM FOLINATE
Trade names
Leucovorin Calcium Injection and Tablets

Available forms
Tablets: 15 mg;
Vial: 50 mg/5 mL, 300 mg/30 mL

Action
- also known as folinic acid, which is the active form of folic acid
- member of the water-soluble vitamin B group
- neutralises folic acid antagonists
- active metabolite

Use
- administered a few hours after folic acid antagonists (e.g. methotrexate) to 'rescue' the normal cells of the host preferentially, after the drug has been bound within tumour cells
- impaired elimination or overdose of methotrexate
- megaloblastic anaemia (not vitamin B_{12} deficiency)
- pyrimethamine overdose

Dose
- (Folinic acid rescue) 15 mg IV, IM or orally 6-hourly starting 24 hours after beginning methotrexate administration for 10 doses or until methotrexate serum level decreases and then dose and interval altered accordingly **OR**
- (Impaired methotrexate elimination or overdose) 10 mg/m^2 IV, IM or orally 6-hourly until methotrexate serum levels are less than 10^{-8} M. Dose may be increased to 100 mg/m^2 IV 3-hourly if creatinine is 50% over baseline or methotrexate level is 5×10^{-6} M (at 24 hours) or 9×10^{-7} M or greater (at 48 hours) **OR**
- (Megaloblastic anaemia) up to 1 mg IM daily **OR**
- (Megaloblastic anaemia) 5—15 mg orally daily **OR**
- (Pyrimethamine overdose) 3—9 mg/day IM for 3 days or until platelet and leucocyte counts have returned to acceptable limits

Adverse effects
- fever, rash, pruritus
- leukocytosis, thrombocytopenia
- (High dose) nausea, vomiting and rarely, insomnia, agitation, depression
- (Rare) seizures, syncope, urticaria, allergic reaction, severe skin reaction

Interactions
- high doses may counteract antiepileptic action of phenytoin, primidone and phenobarbital (phenobarbitone)
- high doses may reduce efficacy of intrathecal methotrexate or other folic acid antagonists if given together
- may enhance toxicity (enterocolitis, diarrhoea, dehydration) of fluorouracil
- incompatible with droperidol and foscarnet

Nursing considerations/Cautions
- should be administered as soon as possible after methotrexate overdose to ensure effectiveness
- serum methotrexate and creatinine are monitored daily to determine dose and duration of therapy. Blood leucocyte and thrombocyte counts and serum

ANTIDOTES, ANTAGONISTS AND CHELATING AGENTS

- electrolytes should also be closely monitored
- parenteral route is recommended for doses greater than 25 mg, or if the patient is vomiting or at risk of not absorbing oral dose
- not administered intrathecally
- may be diluted to 1 L with sodium chloride 0.9% or glucose 5% for IV administration
- injection rate should be no greater than 160 mg/min (because of calcium content)
- (Folinic acid rescue) hydration (3 L/day), urinary alkalisation (pH $\geq$7) and therapy with calcium folinate should be continued until methotrexate level is less than 5×10^{-8} M
- caution if used in those with CNS metastases because of an increased risk of seizures and/or syncope
- contraindicated in those with pernicious anaemia or vitamin B_{12} deficiency anaemias

Patient education

- instruct the patient to take oral doses on an empty stomach
- advise the patient to seek medical advice immediately if any of the following occur:
  - fitting
  - fever, rash, itching, hives, swelling (face, lips, tongue, other body parts), shortness of breath or difficulty breathing

Tablets can be dispersed in water, or crushed and mixed with a spoonful of yoghurt or apple sauce.

Safe to use.

Safe to use.

CHARCOAL, ACTIVATED
Trade name
Carbosorb X

Available form
Oral suspension: 0.2 g/mL

Action
- physically adsorbs drugs and toxic agents onto its surface (including aspirin, barbiturates, phenytoin, tricyclic antidepressants (TCAs), digoxin, quinine, amphetamine, morphine, cocaine, paracetamol and phenothiazines) in the gastrointestinal tract (GIT), thereby reducing or preventing systemic absorption

Use
- poisoning and drug overdose by oral ingestion

Dose
- 1 g/kg orally or via nasogastric/orogastric tube as soon as possible after ingestion or suspected ingestion of the potential poison, or after induced emesis or stomach washout (may be repeated 2–6-hourly until first black stool has been passed (maximum dose 50 g))

Adverse effects
- vomiting, constipation, black-coloured faeces
- (Multiple doses) electrolyte imbalance, intestinal obstruction
- (Rare) aspiration pneumonia

Interactions
- not recommended with agents that reduce gut motility (including supportive agents such as atropine and verapamil), as this may result in repeated doses of activated charcoal being given, increasing the risk of intestinal obstruction
- not recommended at same time as emetics
- should not be given with specific oral antidotes because they may become inactivated

Nursing considerations/Cautions

- should be given within 1 hour of ingestion to absorb maximum amount of poison/drug from the GIT
- patient should be closely monitored for any signs of vomiting because of the risk of aspiration pneumonia
- if a specific antidote is available, it should be given in preference to activated charcoal
- for nasogastric/orogastric administration, it should be diluted with water (ratio 0.25 parts water to 1 part activated charcoal) and administered via nasogastric tube
- shake container well before administration
- given after emptying stomach contents by emesis or washout. However, if the patient is drowsy (or likely to become drowsy within 30 minutes of receiving emetic), unconscious or fitting, induced emesis is not recommended because of the risk of aspiration
- other medication should preferably be given parenterally
- monitor for fluid and electrolyte changes (especially if multiple doses are administered in children) because activated charcoal can absorb vitamins, minerals and amino acids from the GIT
- contains sucrose (0.33 g/mL) and should be used with care in those with diabetes mellitus
- use with great caution if the person has diminished or no bowel sounds, has taken a large quantity of agent that reduces gut motility (such as opioid) or is at risk of GI haemorrhage or perforation
- contraindicated if poisoning is caused by strong acids or alkalis or iron salts, cyanides, sulfonylureas, malathion, lithium, ethanol, methanol, ethylene glycol or hydrocarbons, as adsorptive capacity is too low
- contraindicated if the patient has an unprotected airway (due to risk of aspiration) or the GIT is not intact (e.g. recent surgery)

Note

- the potency of activated charcoal is enhanced when combined with the osmotic laxative sorbitol (in Carbosorb XS); however, it is contraindicated in children < 1 year
- also used in tablet and capsule form as a GI adsorbent to reduce symptoms of bloating and flatulence from intestinal gas (Charcocaps, Charcotabs)
- Charcotrace is used in addition to stereotactic or ultrasonic localisation of small impalpable breast lesions for later surgical incision
- may be used locally as a deodorant in ostomy pouches, wounds and ulcers

DEFERASIROX

Trade names
Deferasirox, Eferas, Jadenua, Pharmacor Deferasirox

Available forms
Tablets: 90 mg, 180 mg, 360 mg;
Dispersible tablets: 500 mg

Action
- chelates iron and promotes excretion, mainly in the faeces
- low affinity for zinc and copper
- half-life 8–16 hours

Use
- chronic iron overload due to blood transfusion (transfusion haemosiderosis)
- chronic iron overload in children 2–5 years (when desferrioxamine is inappropriate or ineffective)
- chronic iron overload in those with non-transfusion-dependent thalassaemia syndrome

Dose

Chronic iron overload due to blood transfusion
- (Adult, receiving > 4 units of blood/month) 21 mg/kg body weight orally daily **OR**
- (Adult, receiving < 2 units of blood/month) 7 mg/kg body weight orally daily **OR**

- initially ⅓ dose of desferrioxamine orally daily 30 minutes before food **OR**
- (Maintenance) 3.5—7 mg/kg/day, adjusting dose at 3—6-month intervals according to serum ferritin levels (up to 28 mg/kg/day)

Non-transfusion-dependent thalassaemia syndrome
- initially 7 mg/kg orally daily, then adjusted every 3—6 months if needed, by increments of 3.5—7 mg/kg (up to 14 mg/kg)

Adverse effects
- nausea, vomiting, diarrhoea, abdominal pain/distension, dyspepsia, constipation
- headache, fatigue
- fever, flu-like syndrome
- cough, pharyngitis, nasopharyngitis, nasopharyngeal pain
- arthralgia
- increased serum creatinine, elevated liver enzymes
- proteinuria
- rash, pruritus
- (Uncommon) loss of hearing, lens opacities, cataract formation, increased intraocular pressure, retinal disorders
- (Uncommon) GI ulceration and/or haemorrhage
- (Rare) neutropenia, thrombocytopenia, hypersensitivity, severe skin reaction

Interactions
- not recommended with other iron-chelating agent or aluminium-containing antacids
- increased risk of GI ulceration/haemorrhage if given with other ulcerogenic agents (e.g. NSAIDs, corticosteroids, oral bisphosphonates) and therefore not recommended together
- may decrease serum levels of midazolam, ciclosporin, simvastatin, colestyramine and oral contraceptives
- decreased serum levels may occur if given with rifampicin, phenytoin, ritonavir and phenobarbital (phenobarbitone)
- may increase serum levels of theophylline, clozapine, imipramine, haloperidol, fluvoxamine, naproxen, olanzapine and zolmitriptan, increasing risk of toxicity and are therefore not recommended together
- caution if given with busulfan. Busulfan levels should be closely monitored if given together
- blood glucose levels should be closely monitored if given with repaglinide

Nursing considerations/Cautions
- therapy should be started after about 20 units of blood have been transfused (100 mL/kg) or when serum ferritin > 1000 microgram/L
- dose should be rounded to nearest whole tablet size
- ensure the patient is adequately hydrated before starting therapy (especially if diarrhoea or vomiting occurs)
- serum ferritin should be measured monthly and the dose adjusted every 3—6 months if needed on that basis. If level falls consistently below 500 microgram/L, therapy interruption may be considered
- serum creatinine and/or creatinine clearance should be measured before starting therapy and then monthly (weekly monitoring for the first month is recommended in those with kidney impairment or if taking medication which may depress kidney function)
- blood counts and urine (for protein) should be monitored monthly
- liver function should be measured before starting therapy, every second week for 4 weeks, then monthly. If liver enzymes increase due to therapy (other causes ruled out), therapy should be stopped until they return to normal and then restarted slowly at a lower dose
- vision and hearing should be checked before starting, then yearly during treatment (disturbances of vision or hearing are reversible if the drug is stopped early)

- (Non-transfusion-dependent thalassaemia syndrome) therapy should be started when the liver iron concentration (LIC) ≥ 5 mg iron/g dry weight or serum ferritin is consistently > 800 microgram/L
- (Non-transfusion-dependent thalassaemia syndrome) doses > 14 mg/kg are not recommended
- (Non-transfusion-dependent thalassaemia syndrome) if LIC is not assessed and serum ferritin ≤ 2000 microgram/L, dose should not be greater than 7 mg/kg
- (Non-transfusion-dependent thalassaemia syndrome) once LIC is satisfactory (< 3 mg/g dry weight or serum ferritin < 300 microgram/L), therapy should be interrupted and resumed if chronic iron overload recurs
- body weight and longitudinal growth should be measured regularly in children
- caution if used in the elderly who are at increased risk of adverse effects, those with pre-existing kidney conditions or using agents that suppress renal function, or if creatinine clearance (CrCl) is between 40 and 90 mL/min
- dispersible tablets contain lactose and therefore are not recommended in those with galactose intolerance, Lapp lactase deficiency or glucose—galactose malabsorption
- not recommended in those with severe liver impairment, and dose should be reduced in those with moderate liver impairment
- contraindicated in those with CrCl < 40 mL/min, serum creatinine more than twice age-appropriate upper normal limit or if platelet count is less than 50 × 10^9/L, in those at high risk of myelodysplastic syndrome or other haematological/non-haematological disorders where chelation therapy would not be beneficial

Patient education

- instruct the patient to take tablets on empty stomach or with a light meal (not high fat content)
- the patient should be advised to seek medical advice if any of the following occur:
  - hearing difficulties
  - blurry or loss of vision
  - vomiting with blood and/or black stools
  - upper abdominal pain, yellowing of skin or eyes, dark urine and drowsiness (liver problem)
  - reduced urine output (kidney problem)
  - frequent heartburn or stomach pain, especially when taking medication or after eating
  - rash, severe skin reaction
- female patients should be counselled regarding the possibility of oral contraceptive failure and the need to use a non-hormonal contraceptive device (e.g. condom, diaphragm) to prevent an unwanted pregnancy from occurring

Tablets can be crushed and sprinkled on yoghurt or apple puree and taken immediately.

Limited human data. No abnormalities have been observed in reports of exposure up to 22 weeks of gestation. Should be used during pregnancy only if benefits outweigh risks.

No human data; not recommended during breastfeeding.

Reduce the starting dose if CrCl < 60 mL/min. Avoid use when CrCl < 40 mL/min or serum creatinine > twice the upper limit of normal (ULN) (contraindicated by the manufacturer).

Hepatic impairment increases deferasirox concentration. Use cautiously and

ANTIDOTES, ANTAGONISTS AND CHELATING AGENTS

reduce the starting dose in moderate hepatic impairment (Child—Pugh class B). Avoid use in severe hepatic impairment (Child—Pugh class C).

DEFERIPRONE
Trade name
Ferriprox

Available forms
Tablets: 500 mg, 1 g;
Oral solution: 100 mg/mL

Action
- chelates iron in a ratio of 3:1
- half-life 2—3 hours

Use
- iron overload in thalassaemia major (when desferrioxamine is inappropriate or ineffective)

Dose
- 25—33 mg/kg orally 3 times daily (daily total 75—100 mg/kg body weight)

Adverse effects
- abdominal pain/discomfort, nausea, vomiting, increased appetite, increased weight, dyspepsia, diarrhoea, anorexia
- headache
- arthralgia, back pain, joint swelling, pain in extremities
- neutropenia, agranulocytosis, thrombocytopenia
- increased liver enzymes, liver fibrosis
- red/brown urine
- peripheral oedema
- (Rare) QT prolongation

Interactions
- not recommended with aluminium-based antacids
- not recommended with other agents known to cause neutropenia or agranulocytosis
- caution if used with vitamin C
- caution if used with agents known to prolong QT interval or cause electrolyte imbalance (e.g. diuretics)

Nursing considerations/Cautions
- neutrophil count should be measured before starting therapy, and therapy not commenced if the patient is found to be neutropenic
- monitoring neutrophil count weekly is recommended. If the patient develops neutropenia, therapy should be stopped and the patient advised to avoid any potential risk of infection. Blood counts (including WBC, neutrophil and platelet counts) should be monitored daily until neutrophil count returns to normal, then weekly for 3 weeks to ensure complete recovery
- liver function tests are recommended in patients with hepatitis C
- therapy should be interrupted if the patient develops infection. Neutrophil should be monitored more frequently. If neutropenia occurs, daily blood counts are recommended until the neutrophil count recovers, then weekly for 3 consecutive weeks to ensure full recovery has occurred
- serum ferritin and plasma zinc levels should be monitored every 2—3 months during therapy; zinc supplementation may be required
- dose adjustment is dependent on serum ferritin levels and therapy interrupted if levels fall below 500 microgram/L
- daily doses greater than 100 mg/kg not recommended
- dose should be calculated to nearest half tablet or 2.5 mL
- (Oral solution) contains yellow colouring agent (sunset yellow (E110)), which may cause an allergic reaction in sensitive individuals
- caution if used in those with liver or kidney impairment
- caution if used in those at risk of QT prolongation, including those with bradycardia, congestive heart failure or cardiac hypertrophy, or if taking agents that may cause electrolyte imbalance, especially hypokalaemia or hypomagnesaemia

HAVARD'S NURSING GUIDE TO DRUGS

- not recommended in immunocompromised patients, such as those with HIV
- contraindicated in those with recurrent neutropenia or history of agranulocytosis

Patient education

- the patient should be advised to seek medical advice immediately if any of the following occur:
  - any fever, sore throat or flu-like symptoms
  - palpitations, irregular heartbeat, dizziness, lightheadedness, fainting
- warn the patient that urine discolouration (reddish/brown) is normal
- instruct the patient to separate medication by 2 hours from aluminium-based antacids and not to take vitamin C
- oral solution should be refrigerated and used within 35 days of opening
- women of childbearing years should be advised to use adequate contraception during therapy and to tell the doctor if she plans to become or becomes pregnant

Available as an oral solution. If crushing tablets, mask and gloves should be worn. Mix with a spoonful of yoghurt or apple puree.

Contraindicated during pregnancy because it is embryotoxic and teratogenic, meaning it can cause harm to the developing fetus.

Contraindicated during breastfeeding because of the potential risk of harm to the nursing infant.

DESFERRIOXAMINE

Trade name
DBL Desferrioxamine Mesylate for Injection BP

Available form
Vial: 500 mg, 2 g

Action
- chelating agent that forms ferrioxamine, a non-toxic stable complex (chelate) with iron
- parenteral desferrioxamine removes iron from various iron-containing proteins (ferritin, haemosiderin), but not from haemoglobin or iron-containing enzymes; the water-soluble chelate is excreted rapidly in urine and some in bile
- does not remove iron deposits from lungs
- chelates copper, aluminium, calcium and zinc
- suppresses lymphocytes
- neurotoxic (possibly due to chelation of copper or zinc)
- causes release of histamine (causing acute hypotension) with rapid IV administration
- 1 g desferrioxamine binds 85 mg ferric iron (500 mL transfusion of whole blood adds 250 mg iron to body); however, iron excretion is non-linear; therefore there is reduced efficiency when given at high doses

Use
- transfusion haemosiderosis (chronic iron overload from repeated transfusions in thalassaemia and other chronic anaemias)
- acute iron poisoning (as an adjunct to other measures)
- diagnosis of iron storage disease

ANTIDOTES, ANTAGONISTS AND CHELATING AGENTS

Dose
Chronic iron overload
- 20–40 mg/kg SC or IV 3–7 times weekly (frequency depending on the extent of the iron overload) (daily maximum 80 mg/kg)

Acute iron poisoning (as adjunct to standard measures)
- (Normotensive patient) 2 g deeply IM stat **OR**
- (Hypotensive patient) 15 mg/kg/hour IV, reduced after 4–6 hours to a daily maximum of 80 mg/kg

Diagnostic desferrioxamine test
- 500 mg IM then collect urine for 6 hours to measure iron content

Treatment in terminal renal failure
- 1–4 g IM or IV weekly (patient on haemodialysis or haemofiltration)

Adverse effects
- (Rapid IV or high dose) pain, induration, swelling, pruritus, erythema, weal formation
- (Prolonged SC infusion, IV, IM) local irritation
- (Rapid IV) flushing, urticaria, hypotension, shock
- nausea, vomiting, abdominal pain, black stools
- hypotension, tachycardia, shock
- fever
- transient bone pain, leg cramps
- dysuria, urine discolouration ('vin rose'), kidney failure, aggravation of pyelonephritis
- hypocalcaemia (transient), hyperparathyroidism
- growth retardation, bone changes (especially if given in first 3 years of life)
- headache, dizziness, reversible aphasia, convulsion
- (Prolonged therapy, high dose) disturbances of vision and hearing (may be irreversible), pulmonary toxicity
- liver impairment
- (Rare) rash, fever, oedema, anaphylactic shock
- (Very rare) blood dyscrasias, fungal infection
- (Dialysis patients) aluminium toxicity ('dialysis dementia'), renal impairment, aggravation of pyelonephritis

Interactions
- use with prochlorperazine may result in temporary but severe change in consciousness and are therefore not recommended together
- use with phenothiazines or methyldopa sesquihydrate may potentiate neuro-ophthalmic toxicity
- increased risk of cataract formation and impaired cardiac function if given long term with vitamin C (ascorbic acid)
- addition of oral vitamin C (ascorbic acid) (up to 200 mg) may increase excretion of formed iron complex (but should not be started until desferrioxamine therapy has been in progress for at least 1 week)

Nursing considerations/Cautions
- therapy should be started after 10–20 units of blood have been transfused or when serum ferritin = 1000 microgram/L
- dose should be estimated according to iron levels to prevent toxic effects. Expected iron excretion rate is 10–20 mg/day
- normal serum ferritin is less than 300 microgram/L
- patients with heavy iron load may require treatment 5–7 times weekly to prevent iron toxicity occurring. Regular doses > 50 mg/kg/day are not recommended unless intense chelation is required
- vision and hearing should be checked before starting, then at 3-monthly intervals during treatment (disturbances of vision or hearing are reversible if the drug is stopped early)
- urine output should be carefully measured and, if oliguria or anuria occurs, peritoneal dialysis or haemodialysis may be necessary

343

- urinary iron is initially measured daily and dose adjusted by increments of 0.5 g daily until excretion reaches a plateau
- vitamin C (ascorbic acid) (150—250 mg daily) may be given as adjunctive therapy after initial 4 weeks of chelation therapy because it increases urinary excretion of iron and it should be given on same day as desferrioxamine 1—2 hours after IV infusion has started
- cardiac function should be monitored if given with vitamin C (ascorbic acid)
- (Children) height and weight should be measured 3-monthly and doses should be kept to a minimum
- IM administration is less effective than SC or IV. May also be added to dialysis fluid and given via intraperitoneal route
- if given IM, reconstitute using $\geq$ 1.5 mL water for injections, diluted to a volume of at least 3 mL and then administered using more than one site (0.5—1.5 g per site) (per treatment) to reduce pain and ensure adequate dilution and distribution
- addition of 1—2 mg hydrocortisone and dilution reduces local reaction at IM site
- monitor IV infusion rate closely by using a burette or infusion pump and do not exceed 15 mg/kg/hour
- not given by IV bolus, as rapid IV infusion may result in hypotension, flushing, tachycardia, urticaria and/or collapse
- caution if flushing IV line, as this is the same as giving an IV bolus (see above point)
- continuous IV infusion is recommended in those unable to continue SC infusion or if patient has a cardiac problem related to iron overload
- (IV) reconstitute by adding water for injections (not sodium chloride) (5 mL for 500 mg vial, 20 mL for 2 g vial), making a 10% solution, which may then be further diluted with glucose 5%, sodium chloride 0.9% or Ringer's solution
- incompatible with heparin because precipitation or cloudiness may occur
- IV infusion can be administered at the same time as blood transfusion via Y-adapter
- SC needle should not be inserted too close to the skin
- continuous SC infusion is controlled by battery-operated syringe pump and can be given over 8—12 hours 5—6 nights/week (or 3—5 nights/week if iron load is low)
- (Prolonged therapy, high dose, IV) the patient should be closely monitored in first 32—72 hours for any signs of respiratory distress
- (Acute poisoning) gastric lavage, emesis, control of shock and correction of any acid—base imbalance
- (Acute poisoning) plasma/serum iron levels should be measured 3—4 hours after ingestion of iron products. After 4 hours, results may be an underestimate because iron may have bound to ferritin or been distributed into tissues
- (Acute poisoning) if slow-release/enteric-coated tablets have been ingested, levels should be repeated 6—8 hours later as absorption may be erratic
- (Acute poisoning) if serum iron is between 62 and 90 micromol/L, brief chelation therapy is indicated; 90—180 micromol/L, vigorous support and chelation therapy; greater than 180 micromol/L, vigorous support, chelation and possible transfusion and haemo/peritoneal dialysis is recommended
- (Acute poisoning) if oliguria or anuria develops, peritoneal or haemodialysis may be needed
- (Acute poisoning) end point of treatment is when 'vin rose'-coloured urine disappears, when serum iron is less than 54 micromol/L or when symptoms have disappeared
- (Desferrioxamine test) excretion of 1—1.5 mg over 6 hours is suggestive of iron overload; > 1.5 mg is considered pathological (if kidney function is normal)

ANTIDOTES, ANTAGONISTS AND CHELATING AGENTS

- if used in those on haemodialysis without iron overload, may cause increase in plasma aluminium levels
- caution if used in those with severe kidney failure or pyelonephritis
- not recommended in those with primary haemochromatosis
- contraindicated if iron overload has not been proven

Patient education

- the patient should be advised to seek medical advice if any of the following occur:
    - high fever, painful inflamed sore throat, abdominal pain and/or severe diarrhoea
    - blurred vision or other problems with sight
    - hearing problems, ringing in ears
- reassure the patient that reddish discolouration ('vin rose') in the urine is normal and indicates the iron is being removed from the body
- warn the patient not to drive or operate machinery if dizziness or vision problems occur
- instruct patients (and carers) in the reconstitution of medication, insertion of SC needles, rotation of sites and operation and care of the SC pump, as well as correct storage of medication vials and disposal of used needles

Appears to be safe for use during pregnancy. In cases of acute iron poisoning, the benefits to the mother are expected to outweigh any potential risks to the fetus.

Should not be used during breastfeeding unless the expected benefit outweighs any potential risks. While oral bioavailability is low, making it unlikely that desferrioxamine will be absorbed by the nursing child, caution should still be exercised.

Use with caution in patients with severe renal impairment. For patients undergoing dialysis, the usual dose can be used, as deferoxamine is removed by dialysis.

DIGOXIN-SPECIFIC IMMUNE ANTIGEN BINDING FRAGMENT (FAB)

Trade name
DigiFab

Available form
Vial: 40 mg

Action
- digoxin binding antibody derived from immunised sheep that binds free (unbound) digoxin
- Fab fragment—digoxin complex is excreted from the kidneys, alleviating symptoms within 30 minutes of administration
- 38/40 mg digoxin immune Fab binds approximately 0.5 mg digoxin
- half-life 15—20 hours (normal kidney function)

Use
- digoxin overdose (life threatening)

Dose
- dose is dependent on the number of digoxin tablets ingested and is administered IV over 30 minutes. Half the estimated dose is given, and the response monitored for 6—12 hours. Remainder may be given within 2 hours if no clinical response is evident or if toxicity recurs

Adverse effects
- (IV site) phlebitis
- hypokalaemia, hyperkalaemia
- headache, confusion, fatigue
- nausea, vomiting, diarrhoea, constipation, abdominal distension
- flu-like illness
- kidney failure
- exacerbation of cardiac failure, chest pain, hypotension, orthostatic hypotension
- hypersensitivity reaction (urticaria, pruritus, erythema, angioedema, bron-

chospasm with cough or stridor, laryngeal oedema, hypotension)

Interactions
- will interfere with digoxin immunoassay measurements; therefore the standard serum digoxin concentration may be misleading until Fab is eliminated (several days to a week depending on kidney function)

Nursing considerations/Cautions
- if the overdose is intentional, toxic effects of other drugs or poisons should be considered if no response is seen
- serum digoxin levels should be established before starting therapy if possible, but at least 5–6 hours after ingestion
- any electrolyte or acid–base imbalance or hypoxia should be corrected and any cardiac arrhythmias treated
- serum potassium levels should be frequently monitored throughout therapy and treatment given with great caution (because potassium shifts in and out of cells leading to hyper- and hypokalaemia). Serum potassium may fall rapidly when therapy is discontinued
- temperature, BP and ECG (for deterioration of cardiac function) should be monitored during and after therapy and the patient should be closely observed for any signs of hypersensitivity
- bolus injection is possible if cardiac arrest is imminent
- redigitalisation should not occur until antibodies have been eliminated from the body (several days), or longer if the patient has kidney impairment
- skin testing has not proven to be useful in predicting allergic response
- for reconstitution, gently add 4 mL water for injections to give a concentration of 9.5–10 mg/mL. May be further diluted with sodium chloride 0.9% and should be infused through a membrane filter (0.22 micrometre)
- not recommended in those with known allergy to sheep protein or papaya extracts, or who have been previously treated with digoxin immune Fab

The benefit of using Fab products during pregnancy is expected to outweigh the risk.

Multiple studies suggest that Fab drugs may be actively secreted into breastmilk. Caution is advised, although the risk of harmful effects to the infant is considered small, as any fragments ingested through breastmilk would probably be digested in the infant's stomach.

DISODIUM EDETATE
Trade names
Biological Therapies Disodium Edetate

Available form
Vial: 3 g/100 mL

Action
- disodium salt of EDTA (ethylenediamine tetra-acetic acid) dehydrate, which is a chelating agent that incorporates a heavy metal ion into the ring structure
- also removes iron, zinc, calcium, cadmium and lead
- sodium ascorbate is added as it acts synergistically as a weak chelating agent as well as having antioxidant activity, which is protective during metal mobilisation
- 3 g disodium edetate can remove about 324 mg of calcium ions, which can cause a rapid drop in serum calcium levels if given too rapidly IV
- lead poisoning can occur by ingestion or inhalation of lead dust or fumes. Signs and symptoms of poisoning include metallic taste, anorexia, irritability, apathy, abdominal colic, vomiting, diarrhoea, constipation, headache, leg cramps, black stools, oliguria, stupor, convulsions and coma
- chronic lead poisoning may involve the central nervous system, blood-forming organs and gastrointestinal tract
- diagnosis of lead poisoning includes blood lead levels, hair analysis, urine

testing, 12-hour urine collection and X-rays of long bones and abdomen
- there are no recognised safe limits for lead poisoning

Use
- low-level lead accumulation and lead poisoning (with or without hypercalcaemia)
- temporary reduction of serum calcium levels in hypercalcaemia
- management of severe digitalis arrhythmias where rapid response is needed
- elimination of some radioactive metals (e.g. calcium, strontium, radium, cobalt and plutonium)

Dose
- (Removal of lead, lead poisoning, elimination of radioactive metals) 50 mg disodium edetate/kg IV over 3—4 hours daily (daily maximum 3 g disodium edetate) for 5 days, followed by 2-day drug-free interval. Cycle is repeated twice more **OR**
- (Digitalis arrhythmia) 15 mg/kg/hour IV up to max 60 mg/kg/day

Adverse effects
- nausea, vomiting, diarrhoea
- transient paraesthesia, numbness, headache
- transient drop in both diastolic and systolic BP
- febrile reaction
- hyperuricaemia
- anaemia
- exfoliating dermatitis, skin and mucous membrane reactions
- nephrotoxicity
- (Excessive dose) damage to reticuloendothelial system with haemorrhagic tendency
- thrombophlebitis

Interactions
- not recommended with other chelating agents
- may interfere with oxalate method of measuring serum calcium; therefore other methods should be used for accurate measurement

Nursing considerations/Cautions
- not recommended IM
- creatinine clearance should be measured at each infusion and therapy not given if there is a decreased creatinine clearance or elevated serum creatinine
- urine should be checked with each course of treatment for proteinuria and haematuria to monitor for any kidney damage; however, severe acute lead poisoning can also produce proteinuria and haematuria. If proteinuria worsens, or there are large renal epithelial cells or an increasing number of red blood cells in the urine, therapy should be stopped
- urine flow should be established before administration of first dose using IV fluids if not clinically contraindicated. This is especially necessary if the patient has been vomiting and is dehydrated. If urine flow stops, therapy should be stopped
- because minerals are chelated during therapy, it is recommended that:
  - the patient is monitored for any signs of hypocalcaemic tetany, convulsions and respiratory arrest
  - zinc supplementation should be considered after each treatment (as it is more prone to removal by edentates)
- ECG, BP and pulse should be monitored during therapy
- plasma calcium levels should be closely examined
- potassium may be added to IV solution if hypokalaemia is present
- magnesium may be added to infusion to reduce pain and venous wall spasm
- heparin (2000 U) may be added (if not contraindicated) to reduce clotting at the injection site

- local anaesthetic (procaine hydrochloride) may be used to reduce injection site pain
- pH of solution should be between 7 and 7.4. If needed, sodium bicarbonate 8.4% may be added
- any additions to the IV solution (e.g. magnesium, potassium) should be added individually and mixed well before addition of next ingredient
- (Removal of lead, lead poisoning) initial test dose of 20 mg disodium edetate/kg may be given to check patient sensitivity
- (Lead encephalopathy) any acute increase in intracranial pressure (ICP) should be treated before starting therapy
- must be further diluted before administration in 500 mL of sodium chloride 0.45% or glucose 5%
- ensure the solution is isotonic before administration
- caution if used in those with congestive cardiac failure, history or seizures/epilepsy or on anticoagulant therapy
- caution if used in those with hypertension and/or a previous history of kidney disease. If given, the dose should be adjusted
- contraindicated in those with inadequate kidney function, active liver disease, a history of tuberculosis or hypocalcaemia

 Recommended during pregnancy only if benefits outweigh risks.

Available in combination with
- Disodium Edetate 3 g+Sodium Ascorbate 5 g in 50 mL Solution

FLUMAZENIL
Trade names
Anexate, Flumazenil-Baxter, Flumazenil Kabi

Available form
Ampoules: 0.5 mg/5 mL
Action
- benzodiazepine antagonist that acts competitively at CNS benzodiazepine receptors, reversing sedative effects
- has some weak antiepileptic action
- hypnotic/sedative effects reversed after 1–2 minutes (IV), but may return (depending on the half-life of the benzodiazepine)
- half-life 53 minutes, prolonged in those with moderate-to-severe liver impairment

Use
- reverses acute benzodiazepine effects (in hospitalised patients)

Dose
- (Reversal of benzodiazepine effects at therapeutic doses) 200 micrograms IV over 15 seconds, followed at 1-minute intervals by further doses of 100 micrograms if necessary (up to a total dose of 1 mg) **OR**
- (Known or suspected overdose of benzodiazepines) 300 micrograms IV over 15 seconds followed at 1-minute intervals by further doses of 300 micrograms until the patient wakes up or up to a total dose of 2 mg; if drowsiness recurs, an IV infusion of 100–400 microgram/hour may be commenced

Adverse effects
- nausea, vomiting
- withdrawal symptoms (agitation, anxiety, emotional lability, mild confusion, sensory distortion)
- panic attacks (in patients with panic disturbances)
- seizures (in patients with epilepsy or liver impairment)
- convulsions, cardiac arrhythmias (mixed drug overdose including tricyclic antidepressants (TCAs))
- (Infrequent) dizziness, vertigo, anxiety, fearfulness, depression, tearfulness, agitation, palpitations
- (Rare) hypersensitivity

Interactions
- (Anaesthesia) should not be used until neuromuscular blocking agent effects have been reversed
- withdrawal may precipitate convulsions or withdrawal symptoms
- antagonises non-benzodiazepines (e.g. zopiclone)

ANTIDOTES, ANTAGONISTS AND CHELATING AGENTS

Nursing considerations/Cautions
- may be diluted with glucose 5% or sodium chloride 0.9%
- administered by an anaesthetist or experienced doctor
- the patient should be closely monitored for signs of respiratory depression or resedation or withdrawal symptoms (e.g. agitation, anxiety, mild confusion, sensory distortion and/or emotional lability)
- should not be used to treat benzodiazepine dependence
- not recommended in those with epilepsy, especially in those treated with benzodiazepines for a prolonged time
- caution should be taken when used in mixed drug overdose (because some of the toxic effects of other drugs may emerge with the benzodiazepine reversal), or in those with benzodiazepine dependence, or if large doses have been taken recently (before overdose), as withdrawal symptoms or convulsions may be provoked
- caution if used in those with head injuries as it may cause raised intracranial pressure and/or altered cerebral blood flow
- caution if used in those with liver impairment or panic disorders
- contraindicated if benzodiazepine has been used to control status epilepticus or intracranial pressure, or in mixed drug overdose containing tricyclic antidepressants (TCAs)

Patient education
- warn the patient against driving a vehicle or operating machinery within 24 hours of reversal, as sedation and dizziness may occur

Should be used during pregnancy only if the benefits are considered to outweigh the risks. It should be avoided in benzodiazepine-dependent women because of the risk of precipitating withdrawal symptoms in the fetus.

No human studies, adnd therefore should be used with caution during breastfeeding.

Caution if used in those with liver impairment as delayed benzodiazepine effects may occur.

FOMEPIZOLE
Trade name
Antizol Concentrated Injection

Available form
Vial: 1 g/mL

Action
- competitive inhibitor of alcohol dehydrogenase (which catalyses oxidation of ethanol to acetaldehyde, as well as the initial steps in ethylene glycol and methanol metabolism to toxic metabolites)
- ethylene glycol (main component of antifreeze and coolant) is metabolised to glycolaldehyde and oxalate, which are responsible for metabolic acidosis and kidney damage in poisoning (a lethal dose of ethylene glycol is 1.4 mL/kg)
- methanol (the main component of windshield wiper fluid) is slowly metabolised via alcohol dehydrogenase to formic acids, which is responsible for metabolic acidosis and visual disturbances in methanol poisoning (a lethal dose of methanol is about 1−2 mL/kg)
- lack of treatment leads to accumulation of toxic metabolites
- half-life varies with dose

Use
- treatment of ethylene glycol or methanol poisoning

Dose
- 15 mg/kg IV over 30 minutes (loading dose), followed by 10 mg/kg 12-hourly for 4 doses, then 15 mg/kg 12-hourly until the concentration of ethylene glycol or methanol is either undetectable or reduced below 20 mg/dL and the patient is asymptomatic with normal pH

Adverse effects
- fever
- facial flushing
- headache, feeling drunk, agitation, seizures, anxiety, drowsiness, toxic encephalopathy, dizziness, lightheadedness
- abdominal pain or tenderness, vomiting, nausea, haematemesis, diarrhoea, metallic/bad taste
- abnormal smell
- transient blurred vision
- hypotension, bradycardia, hypertension, collapse
- back ache
- anuria, worsening acute kidney failure
- anaemia, lymphangitis, disseminated intravascular coagulation (DIC), eosinophilia
- hypocalcaemia
- pulmonary oedema, pharyngitis, sinusitis, rhinitis
- (IV site) bleeding, burning/tingling
- (Rare) allergic reaction (major and minor)

Interactions
- ineffective in the treatment of ethanol intoxication and would prolong intoxication if given together
- ethanol decreases the rate of elimination

Nursing considerations/Cautions
- therapy should be started on suspicion of ethylene glycol or methanol poisoning, based on patient history, anion gap metabolic acidosis, increased osmolar gap, visual disturbances or oxalate crystals in urine or documented levels of ethylene glycol or methanol > 20 mg/dL
- the patient should be managed for metabolic acidosis, acute kidney failure (ethylene glycol), adult respiratory syndrome, visual disturbances (methanol) and hypocalcaemia. Supportive therapy should include fluids and sodium bicarbonate, in addition to oxygen, and potassium and calcium supplements. If the patient is anuric or has severe metabolic acidosis or azotaemia, haemodialysis is recommended
- ECG, liver enzymes, WBC, blood gases, pH, serum electrolytes, creatinine and urea, and urinalysis should be monitored regularly
- should not be given undiluted or by bolus injection
- if the solution has solidified in the vial, it can be liquefied by running the vial under warm water or holding it in the hand. This does not affect stability
- to dilute, add the calculated dose from the vial to 100 mL sodium chloride 0.9% or glucose 5% and mix well. Administer by infusion over 30 minutes
- the patient should be closely monitored for signs of allergic reaction
- contraindicated in patients with ethanol intoxication, other poisons alone or in combination with ethylene glycol or methanol
- contraindicated in those with hypersensitivity to other pyrazoles

 Not recommended during pregnancy unless the benefit outweighs the risk.

 Caution if used during breastfeeding.

GLUCAGON HYDROCHLORIDE
Trade name
GlucaGen HypoKit

Available form
Vial: 1 mg

Action
- polypeptide hormone, synthesised from yeast cells, which is identical to human hormone
- increases blood glucose level by mobilising liver glycogen (but not muscle glycogen)
- stimulates secretion of insulin from beta cells in the pancreas, as well as catecholamines
- reduces the tone and motility of the gastrointestinal tract (GIT)

ANTIDOTES, ANTAGONISTS AND CHELATING AGENTS

- onset of action is 5—15 minutes (IM) or 1 minute (IV), duration of action is 10—40 minutes (IM) or 5—20 minutes (IV)
- when treating hypoglycaemia, the action on blood glucose is within 10 minutes
- short half-life (3—6 minutes)

Use
- treatment of severe hypoglycaemia
- as an aid in radiological examination of the GIT to inhibit motility

Dose
- (Hypoglycaemia) 0.5—1 mg SC, IM or IV **OR**
- (Endoscopy and radiography) 0.2—2 mg IM or IV

Adverse effects
- nausea, vomiting, abdominal pain
- secondary hypoglycaemia
- (Diagnostic procedure, fasting) nausea, hypoglycaemia, BP changes

Interactions
- may increase effects of warfarin when given in high doses
- has positive inotropic effects, which can reverse cardiac depression caused by beta blockade; therefore should be given with caution in those taking beta adrenoceptor blocking agents
- antagonises insulin
- unpredictable effects if given with indometacin

Nursing considerations/Cautions
- no effect will be seen if patient is fasting, has chronic hypoglycaemia, adrenal insufficiency or alcohol-induced hypoglycaemia
- not given as IV infusion
- reconstitute with accompanying diluent (in prefilled syringe) and use immediately
- when the patient responds (usually within 10 minutes), or at the end of a diagnostic procedure (especially if patient has been fasting), supplemental oral carbohydrate should be given to prevent secondary hypoglycaemia by restoring liver glycogen
- IV glucose must be given if a patient with hypoglycaemia fails to respond to glucagon. IV glucose is preferred if hypoglycaemia has been induced by sulfonylureas. If glucagon is used alone, secondary hypoglycaemia may occur. Blood glucose levels should be closely monitored
- (Diagnostic procedure) onset of action if given IV is within 1 minute, with a duration of 5—20 minutes (depending on the organ being examined). If given IM, onset is 5—15 minutes, with a duration of 10—40 minutes (depending on the organ being examined)
- (Diagnostic procedure) caution if used in the elderly with cardiac disease, or in patients with diabetes undergoing radiological procedures using glucagon
- contraindicated in those with insulinoma, glucagonoma or phaeochromocytoma (as an acute hypertensive crisis may be provoked)

Patient/Carer education
- although glucagon is an emergency drug, patients, relatives, friends, colleagues or teachers can be educated on its proper use. During a hypoglycaemic emergency, glucagon can be administered subcutaneously or intramuscularly in the thigh, buttock or upper arm
- if the patient does not regain consciousness within 10 minutes of glucagon administration, it is critical to seek immediate medical assistance
- after using glucagon, it is essential to inform your health professional, as it may affect further treatment and management of hypoglycaemia
- patients should be advised not to drive after undergoing a diagnostic procedure where glucagon is used until they have eaten carbohydrate-containing food to prevent potential hypoglycaemia

IDARUCIZUMAB

Trade name
Praxbind

Available form
Vial: 50 mg/mL

Action
- monoclonal antibody fragment that binds to dabigatran and its metabolites with high affinity, neutralising anticoagulant effect
- degraded to smaller molecules such as peptides and amino acids, which are then reabsorbed and used for protein synthesis
- does not reverse effects of other anticoagulants

Use
- specific reversal agent for dabigatran when rapid anticoagulant reversal is needed (e.g. emergency surgery, urgent procedures, life-threatening or uncontrolled bleeding)

Dose
- 5 g IV as either bolus dose or 2 consecutive infusions (2 × 2.5 g/50 mL) over 5–10 minutes each

Adverse effects
- headache
- nasopharyngitis
- diarrhoea
- back pain, musculoskeletal stiffness
- skin irritation
- transient proteinuria (not indicative of renal damage)
- pain at catheter site
- (Uncommon) recurrence of elevated coagulation parameters up to 24 hours after administration
- thrombotic events
- hypersensitivity

Nursing considerations/Cautions
- anticoagulant therapy should be resumed as soon as medically appropriate to reduce the risk of thromboembolic events. Anticoagulation therapy with dabigatran can be started after 24 hours of administration of idarucizumab
- a second dose may be required if there is a recurrence of clinically relevant bleeding with prolonged clotting times, or if the patient requires second emergency surgery or urgent procedure and has prolonged clotting times
- administer alone
- flushing IV line with sodium chloride 0.9% before and after administration is recommended
- contains sorbitol (4 g); therefore benefits versus risks should be considered if emergency situation arises in a patient with hereditary fructose intolerance
- contains 50 mg sodium per dose, which may need to be considered if the patient is on a controlled sodium diet

 No human data; use only if the benefit outweighs the risk.

 No human data.

 In patients with renal impairment, the elimination of idarucizumab is delayed, which may lead to a prolonged effect of the drug. Careful monitoring is required in such patients to ensure appropriate management of its extended action.

LANTHANUM

Trade name
Fosrenol

Available form
Tablets (chewable): 500 mg, 750 mg, 1000 mg

Action
- dietary phosphate binder that forms insoluble complex that is then excreted

Use
- hyperphosphataemia (in those with chronic renal failure on haemodialysis or peritoneal dialysis)

Dose
- (Serum phosphate 1.8–2.4 mmol/L) initially 250 mg orally 3 times daily with food **OR**
- (Serum phosphate 2.4–2.9 mmol/L) initially 500 mg orally 3 times daily with food **OR**
- (Serum phosphate > 2.9 mmol/L) initially 750 mg orally 3 times daily with food **OR**
- (Maintenance) dose adjusted every 2–3 weeks depending on serum phosphate levels

Adverse effects
- nausea, vomiting, diarrhoea, abdominal pain, dyspepsia, flatulence, constipation, taste alteration
- bronchitis, rhinitis
- headache, dizziness, vertigo
- hypocalcaemia, hypercalcaemia
- hypotension
- dialysis graft occlusion/complication

Interactions
- activity may be affected by agents which alter gastric pH (e.g. proton pump inhibitors)
- may increase gastric pH and affect absorption of hydroxychloroquine, thyroid hormones and fluoroquinolone antibiotics
- may impact on results of abdominal X-rays, causing a radio-opaque appearance

Nursing considerations/Cautions
- serum phosphate and calcium should be monitored regularly throughout therapy. Calcium supplements may be required
- liver function monitoring is recommended in those with reduction in bile flow
- caution if used in those with biliary atresia or other causes of reduced bile flow, as this may result in higher serum levels and deposition in tissue
- caution if used in those with predisposition to bowel obstruction (such as GI surgery, diverticular disease, GI cancer or ulceration, Crohn's disease or ulcerative colitis) or hypomotility disorders (e.g. constipation, diabetic gastroparesis)
- caution if used in those with renal insufficiency, as hypocalcaemia may occur
- contraindicated in those with hypophosphataemia

Patient education
- the patient should be advised to immediately report any abdominal distension or constipation
- instruct the patient to continue recommended diet to control phosphate and fluids
- advise the patient to chew tablets completely, and not swallow them whole
- if the patient has dentures and is unable to chew tablets, they should be advised to crush tablets
- instruct the patient to separate lanthanum by 2 hours from hydroxychloroquine, thyroid hormones and some antibiotics (e.g. tetracyclines)
- if the patient is also prescribed norfloxacin or ciprofloxacin, they should be instructed to take it either 2 hours before or 4 hours after lanthanum
- warn the patient against driving or operating machinery if dizziness or vertigo occurs

Thoroughly chew the tablets before swallowing to help minimise the risk of serious gastrointestinal side-effects. If chewing is difficult, crush the tablets and mix with water or spoonful of yoghurt or apple puree.

No human data. therefore should not be used during pregnancy unless benefits outweigh risks.

May be excreted in breastmilk; therefore not recommended during breastfeeding.

METHYLENE BLUE TRIHYDRATE
Trade names
Methylene Blue Injection, Proveblue Solution

Available forms
Ampoule: 50 mg/10 mL;
Vial: 50 mg/5 mL

Action
- thiazide dye able to stain tissue
- in methaemoglobinaemia, methylene blue lowers levels in RBCs by activating a normally dormant reductase enzyme system which reduces methylene blue to leucomethylene blue, which then reduces methaemoglobin to haemoglobin
- monoamine oxidase inhibitor properties
- weak antiseptic and bacteriological staining properties
- binds irreversibly to viral nucleic acid, causing disruption of virus molecule on light exposure

Use
- treatment of drug-induced or idiopathic methaemoglobinaemia
- bacteriological stain
- diagnostic stain (e.g. to detect fistula)
- delineation of some body tissues during surgery

Dose
- (Methaemoglobinaemia) 1–2 mg/kg by IV injection over 5 minutes, may be repeated after 1 hour if needed (maximum dose 7 mg/kg) **OR**
- (Parathyroid gland staining) 5 mg/kg diluted in 500 mL glucose 5% and given as IV infusion over 60 minutes **OR**
- 5–10 mL diluted in 100–200 mL water for injections and taken orally immediately after dilution

Adverse effects
- nausea, vomiting, abdominal pain, unusual or metallic taste
- headache, dizziness, anxiety, tremor, fever, aphasia, confusion, agitation, paraesthesia
- hypertension, hypotension, arrhythmias, chest pain, tachycardia
- dyspnoea, tachypnoea, hypoxia
- pain in extremities
- mydriasis
- profuse sweating, photosensitivity
- rash (blue macules, severe burning pain)
- skin, urine, faeces and saliva coloured blue
- (High dose) haemolysis, methaemoglobinaemia, thrombophlebitis
- (Injection site) pain
- anaphylaxis

Interactions
- not recommended with selective serotonin reuptake inhibitors (SSRIs), serotonin and noradrenaline (norepinephrine) reuptake inhibitors (SNRIs), monoamine oxidase inhibitors (MAOIs) or other serotonergic agents to reduce risk of serotonin toxicity
- may cause false positive result on phenolsulfonphthalein excretion test or interfere with the bispectral index (BIS)
- may cause underestimation of oxygen saturation using pulse oximetry

Nursing considerations/Cautions
- IV route is recommended for management of methaemoglobinaemia
- serotonin toxicity has occurred when used, monitor for signs
- blood pressure and ECG monitoring is recommended during therapy to monitor for hypotension and/or arrhythmias
- full blood count (including reticulocyte count, haemoglobin and methaemoglobin levels) should be monitored throughout therapy to ensure anaemia or haemolysis has not occurred
- slow injection rate is recommended to prevent high concentration, as necrotic abscess may result if extravasation occurs
- should not be diluted with sodium chloride 0.9% as precipitation will occur

ANTIDOTES, ANTAGONISTS AND CHELATING AGENTS

- ensure solution is adequately diluted (not more than 350 mg methylene blue in 500 mL) to prevent thrombophlebitis
- any skin discolouration can be removed with hypochlorite solution
- incompatible with caustic alkalis, iodides and dichromates, and oxidising and reducing substances
- cumulative dose of 4 mg/kg should not be exceeded in those with dapsone-induced methaemoglobinaemia
- caution if used in those with mild-to-moderate kidney impairment
- caution if used in those with hyperglycaemia or diabetes mellitus if diluting using glucose 5%
- caution if used to treat aniline-induced methaemoglobinaemia, as Heinz body formation and haemolytic anaemia may be exacerbated. Lower doses are recommended
- not recommended in infants < 4 months
- contraindicated SC or by intrathecal administration
- contraindicated in those with known hypersensitivity of other thiazide dyes, severe kidney impairment or if methaemoglobinaemia is due to chlorate or cyanide poisoning
- contraindicated in those with G6PD deficiency, as there is a reduced capacity to convert methylene blue to leucomethylene blue, as well as being susceptible to haemolytic anaemia induced by methylene blue

Patient education

- inform patient that methylene blue may cause blue-green discolouration of saliva, skin, urine and faeces
- advise patient to avoid strong light sources, such as direct sunlight and intense indoor lighting, and to use protective measures, such as wearing protective clothing, applying sunblock and limiting exposure to strong lights

Avoid use. It can cross the placenta and has been associated with ileal abnormalities, including fetal intestinal atresia. It should be used only if needed and the potential benefits outweigh the risks to the fetus.

Methylene blue is excreted into breastmilk and may cause harm to the breastfed infant. It is generally advised that breastfeeding be discontinued while the mother is receiving methylene blue treatment. If methylene blue is considered necessary, the risks and benefits should be carefully weighed.

NALOXONE HYDROCHLORIDE

Trade names
DBL Naloxone Hydrochloride Injection, Naloxone Juno, Naloxone SXP, Narcan, Nyxoid, Prenoxad

Available forms
Ampoule: 400 microgram/mL, 1 mg/mL; Nasal spray: 1.8 mg/100 microlitre

Action
- antagonises effects of opioids (narcotics) by competing for the same receptor sites
- acts on mu, kappa and sigma opioid receptors in the CNS
- prevents or reverses opioid effects, including respiratory depression, sedation and hypotension
- also reverses effects of partial agonists or mixed agonist/antagonists but requires higher doses and may be incomplete
- reverses analgesic effects of opioids
- no pharmacological effect in the absence of opioids or opioid agonists
- does not reverse respiratory depression caused by non-opioid agents
- onset of action 1–2 minutes (IV), duration 1–4 hours, half-life 60–90 minutes

Use
- reversal of opioid-induced depression, including respiratory depression, sedation and hypotension

- (Nasal spray) reversal of opioid-induced depression, including respiratory depression, sedation and hypotension in home or other non-medical settings
- diagnosis and treatment of suspected acute opioid overdose

Dose
- (Postoperative opioid-induced depression) 0.1–0.2 mg IV over 1 minute repeated every 2–3 minutes depending on response. Additional doses may be needed at 1–2-hour intervals **OR**
- (Opioid overdose — known or suspected) 0.4–2 mg IV over 1 minute repeated every 2–3 minutes up to 10 mg (if no response at 10 mg, question diagnosis) **OR**
- (Opioid overdose) 1 spray into nostril. If no response after 2–3 minutes or if respiratory depression relapse occurs, readminister to other nostril using new container

Adverse effects
- nausea, vomiting
- headache, dizziness
- tachycardia, hypotension, hypertension
- (Opioid overdose reversal) nausea, vomiting, sweating, tachycardia, hypertension, tremulousness, seizures, ventricular tachycardia and fibrillation, pulmonary oedema, cardiac arrest
- withdrawal syndrome

Interactions
- antagonises analgesic and respiratory depressant effects of opioids and opioid agonists
- caution if used with agents with cardiovascular effects such as hypotension, ventricular tachycardia or fibrillation or pulmonary oedema

Nursing considerations/Cautions
- IV administration is recommended in emergencies, but can be given SC or IM if the IV route is not available
- when used to reverse opioid-induced depression or opioid overdose, the patient can wake up violently, in extreme pain or angry
- may be diluted with glucose 5% or sodium chloride 0.9% (2 mg in 500 mL) to give a solution of 4 microgram/mL and given IV
- cardiopulmonary resuscitative measures may be required, so resuscitation equipment including vasopressors should be readily available
- observe respiration, heart rate and BP, and for signs of reversal of analgesia such as nausea, vomiting, sweating, tachycardia or raised BP and also any recurrence of respiratory depression (if opioid is long acting)
- (Nasal spray) nasal spray device should not be tested before use as this device is then no longer usable
- administer with caution if there is known or suspected physical dependence on opioids, or if large doses of opioids have been taken, as acute withdrawal syndrome may be precipitated
- signs and symptoms of withdrawal include nausea, vomiting, diarrhoea, abdominal cramps, sneezing, yawning, sweating, tearing, stuffy or runny nose, dysphoria, disrupted sleep, irritability, pupil dilation, weakness, nervousness, restlessness, inability to concentrate or focus, piloerection (goose bumps), anxiety, shivering, feeling of skin crawling, fasciculations, fever, hypertension, tachycardia and muscle aches or cramps
- repeated doses may be necessary because the duration of action (short or long acting) of some opioids may exceed that of the antagonist
- (Narcan) contains 17.7 mg sodium/2 mg dose (5 mL), which may need to be taken into consideration in a sodium-restricted diet
- incompatible with preparations that contain sulfite or metasulfite, are alkaline or contain long chain or high molecular weight anions
- caution if used in those with cardiovascular disease (including those taking

ANTIDOTES, ANTAGONISTS AND CHELATING AGENTS

medications with cardiovascular effects), liver or kidney impairment
- caution if used in those with pre-existing lung disease, as sudden worsening of disease may occur

Patient education

- advise the patient not to drive, operate machinery or engage in physically or mentally exerting activities for at least 24 hours after opioid reversal, as opioid effect may recur, especially if a long-acting opioid was used
- (Nasal spray) the following instructions should be given to the person using the nasal spray device:
  - know the signs of overdose (breathing problems, severe sleepiness, not responding to loud noise or touch)
  - call an ambulance before administering the nasal spray
  - the person should be lying on their back with their head allowed to tilt back supporting the neck
  - ensure the nose is clear if possible
  - remove the nasal spray device from the blister pack
  - do not prime or test the device before use (this will make it unusable)
  - place the thumb on the bottom of plunger with the first and middle fingers on either side of the nozzle
  - the nozzle should be gently inserted into one nostril
  - press the plunger firmly until it clicks to administer the dose
  - remove from the nostril
  - place the person in the recovery position on one side with mouth open pointing towards the ground
  - continue to observe the person for improvement in breathing, alertness and response to noise and touch until the ambulance arrives. If the person starts breathing normally, no further dose is needed
  - if there is no improvement in 2–3 minutes and an ambulance has not arrived, a second dose can be given into the other nostril using a new device

 Can be used during pregnancy when the benefits to the mother outweigh potential risks to the fetus. In cases of opioid overdose, naloxone may be lifesaving for both mother and baby.

 Poorly absorbed when taken orally, which means that even if a small amount of the drug passes into breastmilk, it is unlikely to be absorbed by the infant if ingested. In the case of an opioid overdose, the immediate concern is the health of the mother. Naloxone can be life saving, and its benefits in such situations far outweigh any theoretical risks associated with breastfeeding.

Available in combination with

- Buprenorphine (for use in drug dependence)
  - naloxone 500 micrograms + buprenorphine 2 mg sublingual film (Suboxone 2 mg/0.5 mg film)
  - naloxone 2 mg + buprenorphine 8 mg sublingual film (Suboxone 8 mg/2 mg film)

- Oxycodone (as an analgesic)
  - naloxone hydrochloride 1.25 mg + oxycodone hydrochloride 2.5 mg modified-release tabletadd (ARX-Oxycodone/Naloxone 2.5/1.25)
  - naloxone hydrochloride 2.5 mg + oxycodone hydrochloride 5 mg modified-release tablet (ARX - Oxycodone/Naloxone 10/5 mg)
  - naloxone hydrochloride 5 mg + oxycodone hydrochloride 10 mg modified-release tablet (ARX-Oxycodone/Naloxone 10/5 mg, Targin 10/5 mg)

- naloxone hydrochloride 7.5 mg + oxycodone hydrochloride 15 mg modified-release tablet (ARX-Oxycodone/Naloxone 15/7.5 mg, Targin 15/7.5 mg)
- naloxone hydrochloride 10 mg + oxycodone hydrochloride 20 mg modified-release tablet (ARX-Oxycodone/Naloxone 20/10 mg, Targin 20/10 mg)
- naloxone hydrochloride 15 mg + oxycodone hydrochloride 30 mg modified-release tablet (ARX-Oxycodone/Naloxone 30/15 mg, Targin 30/15 mg)
- naloxone hydrochloride 20 mg + oxycodone hydrochloride 40 mg modified-release tablet (ARX-Oxycodone/Naloxone 40/20 mg, Targin 40/20 mg)
- naloxone hydrochloride 30 mg + oxycodone hydrochloride 60 mg modified-release tablet (ARX-Oxycodone/Naloxone 60/30 mg, Targin 60/30 mg)
- naloxone hydrochloride 40 mg + oxycodone hydrochloride 80 mg modified-release tablet (ARX-Oxycodone/Naloxone 80/40 mg, Targin 80/40 mg0)

PATIROMER

Trade name
Veltassa

Available forms
Powder for oral suspension: 8.4 g, 16.8 g

Action
- a non-absorbed cation exchange polymer containing a calcium-sorbitol complex (as a counter-ion)
- increased faecal potassium excretion through potassium binding in GI tract lumen reducing concentration of free potassium, thereby reducing serum potassium levels
- onset of action 4—7 hours after administration
- potassium levels may return to pre-treatment levels within 2 days of stopping therapy

Use
- treatment of hyperkalaemia in adults

Dose
- initially 8.4 g orally once daily, adjusting daily dose at weekly intervals of 8.4 g increments according to serum potassium levels (daily maximum 25.2 g)

Adverse effects
- hypomagnesaemia, hypokalaemia
- constipation, diarrhoea, abdominal pain, flatulence, nausea, vomiting

Interactions
- should be separated by at least 3 hours from oral medications, as it may decrease GI absorption and efficacy
- may reduce bioavailability of ciprofloxacin, levothyroxine and metformin
- caution if given with thiamine
- if given with agents with narrow therapeutic index, close monitoring is recommended

Nursing considerations/Cautions
- reversible causes of hyperkalaemia should be excluded before starting therapy
- serum potassium levels should be monitored throughout therapy including after any changes to other agents affecting serum potassium or when dose is titrated
- serum magnesium should be monitored for at least 4 weeks after starting therapy and continued if there is a decrease in magnesium levels. If low magnesium levels occur, supplementation should be considered
- serum calcium levels should be monitored in those at risk of hypercalcaemia. Calcium is part of the counter-ion complex and is partially released, which may lead to absorption
- when therapy is stopped, potassium levels return to pre-treatment levels. Therapy should not be stopped without consulting doctor
- should not be used as the sole emergency treatment of hyperkalaemia

- caution if used in those at risk of hypercalcaemia
- caution if used in those with a history of bowel obstruction or major GI surgery, severe GI disorders or swallowing problems because of the increased risk of GI ischaemia, necrosis and/or intestinal perforation (reported with other potassium binders)

Patient education
- ensure the patient understands the following:
  - powder should initially be mixed with 40 mL of water and then stirred. Another 40 mL of water is then added and the solution mixed thoroughly
  - if the powder does not dissolve and the solution looks cloudy, more water can be added
  - the mixture should be drunk immediately. If powder remains in the glass, water should be added, stirred and drunk. This should be repeated until no powder remains in the glass
  - apple juice or cranberry juice can be used instead of water
  - other fluids containing high levels of potassium should not be used (e.g. juices from oranges, tomatoes, prunes, apricots or grapefruit)
  - the solution should not be heated or added to hot food or liquids
  - the dry form should not be taken
  - the solution should be taken after food at the same time every day
  - the solution should be taken at least 3 hours apart from any other oral medications
  - therapy should not be stopped suddenly without first consulting a doctor

No human data. Not absorbed systemically; maternal use is not anticipated to cause harm.

No human data. Not absorbed systemically; not anticipated to cause harm.

PROTAMINE SULFATE
Trade names
Fisons Protamine Sulphate Injection BP

Available form
Ampoules: 10 mg/mL

Action
- basic protein that combines with acidic heparin to form a stable inactive complex

Use
- neutralises anticoagulant action of heparin (e.g. before surgery, if excessive bleeding occurs after overdose)

Dose
- based on 1 mg neutralising approximately 100 units of mucous heparin or 80 mg of lung heparin; given slowly by IV injection over 10 minutes and repeated depending on the whole blood clotting time or plasma activated partial thromboplastin time (aPTT)

Adverse effects
- sudden drop in BP, bradycardia, pulmonary/systemic hypertension
- nausea, vomiting
- weakness, exhaustion
- dyspnoea, non-cardiogenic pulmonary oedema
- transitory flushing, feeling of warmth
- back pain
- (Rapid administration) severe hypotension, anaphylactoid reaction, hypersensitivity
- (Rare) thrombocytopenia, antibody formation

Nursing considerations/Cautions
- should not be administered rapidly, as anaphylaxis and/or hypotension may occur
- resuscitation equipment should be readily available
- dose reduction is required if heparin was administered more than 15 minutes earlier
- vital signs should be monitored closely

HAVARD'S NURSING GUIDE TO DRUGS

- no more than 50 mg to be given at any one time
- if used in excess or in the absence of heparin, it has an anticoagulant action
- ineffective in overdose of oral anticoagulants
- caution if used in those who may have an increased risk of allergic reaction (e.g. known allergy to fish, use of protamine insulin, previous exposure to protamine during procedures such as coronary angioplasty or cardiopulmonary bypass, infertile men or men having had a vasectomy who may have protamine antibodies)
- caution if repeated doses are given, as rebound bleeding may occur (up to 18 hours)

Avoid use. No human data. Should be used only if the potential benefit outweighs the potential risk to the fetus.

Avoid use. No human data.

SEVELAMER
Trade names
APX-Sevelamer, Renagel, Sevelamer Lupin

Available form
Tablets: 800 mg

Action
- phosphate binder that lowers serum phosphate concentration (those with end-stage kidney disease retain phosphorus)
- also lowers low-density lipoprotein (LDL) and total serum cholesterol
- does not contain calcium; therefore decreased risk of hypercalcaemia compared with other phosphate-binding agents

Use
- hyperphosphataemia (stage 4/5 chronic renal disease)

Dose
- (No previous phosphate binder, serum phosphorus 1.78–2.42 mmol/L) initially 800 mg orally 3 times daily with food **OR**
- (No previous phosphate binder, serum phosphorus 2.42–2.91 mmol/L) initially 1600 mg orally 3 times daily with food **OR**
- (No previous phosphate binder, serum phosphorus > 2.91 mmol/L) initially 1600 mg orally 3 times daily with food **OR**
- (Previous calcium-based phosphate binder) initial equivalent dose orally daily **OR**
- (Maintenance) dose adjusted at 2-week intervals depending on serum phosphorus levels

Adverse effects
- headache
- fever
- pain in limb, arthralgia, back pain
- hypertension
- nausea, vomiting, dyspepsia, diarrhoea, flatulence, abdominal pain, constipation
- cough, dyspnoea, nasopharyngitis, bronchitis, upper respiratory tract infection
- pruritus
- (Rare) intestinal obstruction

Interactions
- may decrease bioavailability of ciprofloxacin
- caution if given with levothyroxine; therefore thyroid-stimulating hormone levels should be monitored if given together
- caution if given with antiepileptic agents or antiarrhythmic agents
- if given with ciclosporin, mycophenolate mofetil or tacrolimus, serum levels should be monitored, especially when stopping therapy
- may increase phosphate levels if given with proton pump inhibitors

Nursing considerations/Cautions
- serum phosphorus is measured regularly and the dose adjusted accordingly
- serum calcium, bicarbonate, chloride, vitamin A, D, E and K should be monitored throughout therapy and supplementation given if needed

ANTIDOTES, ANTAGONISTS AND CHELATING AGENTS

- an increased risk of hypocalcaemia or hypercalcaemia in those with renal insufficiency
- caution in those with GI disorders, swallowing problems, severe constipation, motility disorders or major GI surgery
- not recommended in those under 18 years or pre-dialysis patients
- contraindicated in those with hypophosphataemia or bowel obstruction

Patient education

- patients should be advised to swallow tablets whole with water and not crushed, broken or chewed
- instruct patient to report any constipation as it may precede intestinal obstruction

Tablets should not be crushed, broken or dispersed in water.

Limited human data. In animal studies, some adverse effects were observed at high doses. Use during pregnancy is recommended only if the potential benefit outweighs the risk to the fetus.

No human data. Use only if the potential benefit outweighs the risk.

SODIUM NITRITE

Trade names
Hope Pharmaceuticals Sodium Nitrite Solution

Available form
Vial: 300 mg/10 mL

Action
- cyanide poisoning is rapidly fatal in high doses. Low doses cause toxicity within minutes
- cyanide has affinity for ferric ions, reacting with ferric ion in mitochondrial cytochrome oxidase
- reacts with haemoglobin to form methaemoglobin, to which cyanide will preferentially bind, thereby restoring cytochrome oxidase activity. Cyanide dissociates and is converted to thiocyanate (non-toxic)
- vasodilatory activity on smooth muscle
- peak effect within 30–70 minutes (IV)

Use
- antidote to cyanide poisoning (with sodium thiosulfate)

Dose
- 300 mg IV at 75–150 mg/min (followed by sodium thiosulfate)

Adverse effects
- hypotension, syncope, tachycardia, methaemoglobinaemia
- headache, dizziness
- nausea, vomiting, abdominal pain
- cyanosis, dyspnoea, tachypnoea

Nursing considerations/Cautions

- should be used only in severe poisoning (e.g. loss of consciousness, decreasing vital signs)
- methaemoglobin levels should be monitored throughout therapy and not allowed to exceed 40%
- BP should be monitored throughout therapy and the IV rate decreased if hypotension occurs
- if symptoms recur, a half dose of sodium nitrite and sodium thiosulfate can be given after 30 minutes
- rapid administration should be avoided because hypotension may occur
- a characteristic bitter almond smell usually occurs with cyanide poisoning; however, not everyone is able to detect its presence
- should be administered alone because it has a large number of incompatibilities
- incompatible with caffeine, citrate, chlorates, iodides, mercury salts, morphine, oxidising agents, permanganate, phenazone, sulfites and tannic acid
- caution if used in those with congenital/acquired methaemoglobinaemia (because the condition may be exacerbated) or with

glucose-6-phosphate dehydrogenase (G6PD) (because of the risk of haemolysis)
- contraindicated in those who have asymptomatic poisoning or combined smoke inhalation, or combined carbon monoxide and cyanide poisoning (unless treated at the same time with hyperbaric oxygen)

No human data. Animal studies suggest that some sodium nitrite crosses the placenta and may cause fetal methaemoglobinaemia. However, in life-threatening cyanide poisoning, the risk to the mother and fetus from untreated poisoning may outweigh the potential risk of sodium nitrite use.

It is unknown if sodium nitrite is excreted into breastmilk. However, in cases of life-threatening cyanide poisoning, the potential benefit of treating the mother is likely to outweigh any potential risk.

SODIUM POLYSTYRENE SULFONATE HYDROGEN (POLYSTYRENE SULFONATE)

Trade names
Resonium A

Available form
Powder: 999.3 mg/g

Action
- cation exchange resin
- removes potassium ions from the body by exchanging sodium ions for potassium ions in the large intestine
- not selective for potassium and may remove other cations (e.g. magnesium, calcium)
- potassium exchange can be variable (about 1 mmol/g)

Use
- hyperkalaemia

Dose
- 15 g orally with sufficient water/syrup to make solution of 3–4 mL/g of resin 3–4 times daily **OR**
- 30–50 g mixed with glucose 10% and/or water up to 150 mL as a retention enema daily

Adverse effects
- anorexia, nausea, vomiting, gastric irritation and, occasionally, diarrhoea
- (Large dose, elderly patients) constipation, faecal impaction
- sodium retention, hypokalaemia, hypocalcaemia and, sometimes, hypomagnesaemia
- (Rare) aspiration pneumonia, ischaemic colitis, intestinal obstruction, gastrointestinal stenosis

Interactions
- may increase the risk of toxicity if given with digoxin (if hypokalaemia develops)
- may decrease the absorption of lithium or levothyroxine
- increased risk of alkalosis if given with magnesium hydroxide
- not recommended with sorbitol because intestinal necrosis may occur
- should be separated by a 3-hour interval from oral medications
- may cause intestinal obstruction if given with aluminium hydroxide

Nursing considerations/Cautions
- if a rapid decrease in serum potassium is required, may be administered both orally and rectally. Dialysis may be required because therapy with sodium polystyrene sulfonate hydrogen may take hours to days to be effective
- in extreme hyperkalaemia, serum potassium level can be decreased temporarily by IV glucose and insulin or IV sodium bicarbonate
- electrolytes (especially potassium, magnesium and calcium) should be monitored daily during therapy. Serum potassium levels should be measured more frequently if patient is taking digoxin. Therapy should be stopped in all patients if the potassium level falls below 5 mmol/L
- small amounts of magnesium and calcium ions can be lost during therapy together with potassium ions;

therefore observe for features of electrolyte imbalance including anorexia, nausea, vomiting, dry mouth, thirst, excessive diuresis, oliguria, weakness, lethargy, hypotension and tachycardia
- not given in fruit juices, as many have a high potassium content
- mild laxative relieves constipation and avoids faecal impaction. If severe constipation occurs, therapy should be stopped and should be restarted only when normal bowel habits return
- magnesium-containing laxatives should be avoided
- rectal administration should be used if the patient is vomiting or has paralytic ileus
- the patient should be encouraged to retain the enema for at least 9 hours, followed by colonic irrigation to remove resin
- caution if used in those affected by increased sodium levels (even small amounts) (e.g. congestive cardiac failure, severe hypertension, severe oedema or kidney damage)
- contraindicated in those with obstructive bowel disease or if potassium levels are less than 5 mmol/L

Patient education
- instruct the patient to use the spoon provided to measure 15 g accurately and to mix with water or syrup, but not fruit juices (as these contain potassium)
- warn the patient to avoid inhaling powder
- the patient should be advised to report any constipation (especially if patient is elderly), as bowel obstruction may occur
- advise the patient to separate administration by at least 3 hours from oral medications
- if the patient has gastroparesis, advise them to separate administration by at least 6 hours from oral medications

 No human data. Use only if the expected benefit outweighs the potential risk.

 No human data. Use only if the expected benefit outweighs the potential risk.

Note
- calcium polystyrene sulfonate hydrogen (Calcium Resonium) can be used at the same dosages with similar effects

SODIUM THIOSULFATE
Trade names
DBL Sodium Thiosulfate Solution, Hope Pharmaceuticals Sodium Thiosulfate Solution

Available forms
Vial: 2.5 g/10 mL, 12.5 g/50 mL

Action
- combines with cyanide ions from cyanohaemoglobin to form the relatively harmless thiocyanate, which is excreted in the urine
- cytochrome oxidase is protected from the cyanide ions by an initial injection of sodium nitrite, which oxidises haemoglobin to methaemoglobin, with which the cyanide ions combine preferentially, forming cyanohaemoglobin
- poorly absorbed orally

Use
- cyanide poisoning (in combination with sodium nitrite)
- prevention of sodium nitroprusside-induced cyanide toxicity

Dose
- (Cyanide poisoning) 12.5 g slowly IV over 10 minutes at a rate of 5 mL/minute **OR**
- (Prevention of sodium nitroprusside-induced cyanide toxicity) 5–10 times dose rate of sodium nitroprusside IV (with sodium nitroprusside)

Adverse effects
- hypotension
- headache, agitation, disorientation, delusions, hallucination
- diarrhoea, nausea, vomiting
- arthralgia, hyperreflexia, muscle cramps
- blurred vision, tinnitus

- diuresis, osmotic disturbances

Nursing considerations/Cautions

- if signs of toxicity are still present 0.5–2 hours after infusion, may be repeated at half dose (with sodium nitrite)
- if given with sodium nitrite, should be administered immediately after sodium nitrite infusion has been completed
- caution if used in those with hypertension, congestive cardiac failure, liver cirrhosis, renal impairment or toxaemia of pregnancy because symptoms may be exacerbated

No human data. In life-threatening cyanide poisoning, the risk to the mother and fetus from untreated poisoning may outweigh the potential risk of sodium thiosulfate use.

Unknown if excreted in breastmilk, but use if the benefit outweighs potential risks.

SUCROFERRIC OXYHYDROXIDE
Trade name
Velphoro

Available form
Tablets (chewable): 2.5 g (equivalent 500 mg iron)

Action
- phosphate binder

Use
- control of serum phosphate in patients with chronic kidney disease on dialysis

Dose
- initially 3 tablets orally daily with meals, then titrating up or down in increments of 1 tablet, at 2–4-week intervals until serum phosphorus levels are acceptable (daily maximum 3 g iron = 6 tablets)

Adverse effects
- diarrhoea, discoloured faeces, nausea, vomiting, constipation, dyspepsia, abdominal pain, flatulence, abnormal taste, temporary discolouration of tongue and/or teeth
- hyperphosphataemia, hypophosphataemia, hyperkalaemia, hypocalcaemia, hypercalcaemia
- hypertension, hypotension
- dyspnoea
- nasopharyngitis
- fever
- muscle spasm
- headache
- anaemia

Interactions
- if used with agents known to interact with iron (e.g. alendronate, doxycycline, levothyronine), it should be separated and given 1 hour before or 2 hours later

Nursing considerations/Cautions

- serum phosphate levels should be closely monitored during therapy
- contains sucrose (750 mg), starches and iron
- caution if used within 3 months of peritonitis, significant gastric or liver disorders or major GI surgery
- not recommended in those with rare hereditary problems of fructose intolerance, glucose–galactose malabsorption or sucrase–isomaltase insufficiency
- contraindicated in those with haemochromatosis and other iron accumulation disorders

Patient education

- advise the patient that tablets should be chewed, not swallowed whole and may be crushed if needed
- if taken with other agents that interact with iron (e.g. alendronate, cefalexin, doxycycline, thyroid hormone), instruct the patient that tablets should be taken 1 hour before or 2 hours after other medications
- warn the patient that discolouration of tongue and/or teeth is temporary and that faeces is coloured black

ANTIDOTES, ANTAGONISTS AND CHELATING AGENTS

 Tablets are chewable, or can be crushed and mixed with spoonful of yoghurt or apple puree.

 Limited human data. Should be used during pregnancy and breastfeeding only if benefits outweigh risks.

SUGAMMADEX
Trade names
Sugammadex Accord, Sugammadex ARX, Sugammadex Dr. Reddy, Sugammadex Juno, Sugammadex Lupin, Sugammadex Sandoz, Sugammadex Viatris, Sugammadex-Teva

Available forms
Vial: 200 mg/2 mL, 500 mg/5 mL

Action
- modified gamma cyclodextrin
- selective relaxant binding agent that forms a complex with neuromuscular blocking agents (vecuronium, rocuronium), reducing the amount available to bind with receptors at neuromuscular junctions
- result is reversal of neuromuscular blockade induced by vecuronium or rocuronium

Use
- reversal of neuromuscular blockade induced by vecuronium or rocuronium

Dose
- (Routine reversal, rocuronium or vecuronium) 4.0 mg/kg IV if recovery has reached 1–2 post-tetanic counts (recovery time approx. 3 minutes) **OR**
- (Routine reversal, rocuronium or vecuronium) 2.0 mg/kg IV if recovery is spontaneous (recovery time approx. 2 minutes) **OR**
- (Immediate reversal of rocuronium) 16 mg/kg IV administered 3 minutes after bolus dose of rocuronium (1.2 mg/kg) (recovery time approx. 1.5 minutes)

Adverse effects
- procedural pain, anaesthetic complication (e.g. limb movement, coughing, grimacing, sucking endotracheal tube during surgery/anaesthetic procedure)
- nausea, vomiting, constipation, abdominal pain, diarrhoea
- hypotension, hypertension
- cough, oropharyngeal pain
- headache, dizziness, hypoaesthesia, insomnia
- fever, chills
- back pain, generalised pain
- prolonged activated partial thromboplastin time (aPTT) and prothrombin time (PT) (INR)
- peripheral oedema
- recurrence of blockade (suboptimal dose)
- (Rare) marked bradycardia, hypersensitivity

Interactions
- recovery time may be delayed if given with toremifene (on the same day as operation/anaesthetic procedure) or fusidic acid
- may decrease efficacy of oral contraceptives
- may interfere with serum progesterone assay

Nursing considerations/Cautions
- all patients require ventilator support and respiratory function monitoring until spontaneous respiration is restored. Haemodynamic monitoring is also required during and after reversal of neuromuscular blockage
- coagulation (APTT, PT and INR) should be assessed before and after treatment
- suboptimal doses (< 2 mg/kg) are not recommended
- recurrence of neuromuscular blockade is possible (especially if suboptimal doses are administered)
- given rapidly as IV bolus over 10 seconds directly into vein or IV line
- if readministration is required after immediate reversal, a 24-hour interval should be allowed between doses
- not compatible with verapamil, ondansetron and ranitidine

- not recommended in patients with severe kidney impairment (creatinine clearance < 30 mL/min) or severe liver impairment (with or without coagulopathy)
- not recommended for reversal of other neuromuscular blocking agents other than rocuronium or vecuronium
- caution if used in those who are older, or have cardiovascular disease, pre-existing coagulation disorders or oedema, as longer recovery times may occur

Patient education

- can reduce the effectiveness of hormonal contraception; female patients should be counselled to use a non-hormonal contraceptive (e.g. condom) in addition to hormonal contraceptive for next 7 days to avoid unwanted pregnancy

No human data are available. Should be used during pregnancy only if benefits are thought to outweigh risks.

No human data are available. Should be used only if benefits are thought to outweigh risks.

Limited data in reduced renal function. The manufacturer advises against use when CrCl is < 30 mL/min.

VITAMIN K (PHYTOMENADIONE) (VITAMIN K₁)

Trade names
Konakion, Konakion MM Paediatric

Available forms
Ampoules (adult): 10 mg/mL; (paediatric): 2 mg/0.2 mL

Action
- promotes hepatic biosynthesis of prothrombin (factor II) and coagulation factors VII, IX and X and coagulation inhibitors protein C and protein S
- antagonises the effects of indirect, orally acting anticoagulants

Use
- prothrombin deficiency
- prophylaxis and treatment of vitamin K deficiency bleeding in infants
- hypovitaminosis K
- reverse of oral anticoagulant overdose

Dose

Adults
- (Severe life-threatening haemorrhage) 5—10 mg IV over 30 seconds with fresh frozen plasma (FFP) and prothrombin complex concentrate (PCC) **OR**
- (INR 5—9, with or without mild haemorrhage) 0.5—1 mg IV over 30 seconds, or 1—2.5 mg orally **OR**
- (INR > 9, with or without mild haemorrhage) 1 mg IV over 30 seconds, or 2.5—5.0 mg orally

Paediatrics
- (Prophylaxis, healthy neonate) 1 mg IM at birth **OR**
- (Prophylaxis, healthy neonate) 2 mg orally at birth, at 3—5 days and at 4 weeks **OR**
- (Neonate with special risk factor) 1 mg IM at birth **OR**
- (Neonate with special risk factors weighing < 1.5 kg) 0.5 mg IM at birth **OR**
- (Treatment of vitamin K deficiency bleeding) initially 1 mg IV, with further doses based on coagulation status (with whole blood or coagulation factor transfusion)

Adverse effects
- facial flushing, sweating, unusual taste
- (IV site) local pain, phlebitis or irritation
- (IV rare) anaphylactoid reaction, thromboembolism

Interactions
- antagonises coumarin-type anticoagulants
- action may be impaired by antiepileptic agents
- effects inhibited by some cephalosporin antibiotics

ANTIDOTES, ANTAGONISTS AND CHELATING AGENTS

Nursing considerations/Cautions

- (Reversal of anticoagulant overdose) oral anticoagulant should be stopped
- should not be given IM
- ineffective in heparin or heparin-like (e.g. low molecular weight heparin) overdose
- prothrombin time should be estimated 3 hours after IV administration and may be repeated if necessary. Blood transfusion may also be necessary
- administer alone
- should not be diluted
- vitamin K is contained in many multivitamin preparations in varying quantities, which may undermine control of warfarin
- (Adult oral administration) withdraw required amount from vial, remove needle and administer directly into the patient's mouth, followed by fluid to wash it down
- elderly patients are more sensitive to reversal of anticoagulation and should be prescribed lower doses
- (Paediatric) if the newborn is not breastfed (i.e. formula is used), the last oral dose can be omitted
- (Paediatric) special risk factors for decreased dose include prematurity, birth asphyxia, delay in establishing oral feeding, maternal use of anticoagulants, antiepileptic, antibiotic or antimycobacterial agents, prolonged use of antibiotics, liver dysfunction with obstructive jaundice and malabsorption
- (Paediatric) dispenser delivers 2 mg at the mark and should be placed directly into the infant's mouth
- (Paediatric) if the infant spits the oral dose out, vomits or has diarrhoea within 24 hours of administration, a repeat dose is recommended
- caution if used in those with severe liver impairment (INR should be monitored), biliary atresia, fat malabsorption syndromes or pancreatic insufficiency
- contraindicated in those with severe allergic predisposition

Limited human data. Does not readily cross the placental barrier.

Used in women with hypovitaminosis K due to anticoagulation therapy or those on liver enzyme-inducing antiepileptics (carbamazepine, phenytoin)

Poorly excreted in breastmilk. There is no clear evidence of harm to breastfed infants, making it generally safe to use while breastfeeding. However, it is not recommended for prophylactic use to prevent neonatal bleeding in breastfed infants.

Lower doses are recommended in those over 65, as they may be more sensitive to anticoagulation.

ANTIEMETIC AGENTS

The emetic centre (in the medulla) receives input from a number of other areas, including the chemoreceptor trigger zone (CTZ, located in the fourth ventricle), the vestibular apparatus, higher brain centres (relaying sensory input, such as pain, smell and sight), and organs such as the heart and parts of the gastrointestinal tract (GIT). All of these areas have different densities of receptors (e.g. dopamine, serotonin, histamine, muscarinic, neurokinin-1 (NK_1). For example, the CTZ has high concentrations of dopamine D2 receptors, opioid receptors and possibly serotonin ($5HT_3$) receptors and NK1 receptors, while the vestibular apparatus is rich with muscarinic (M1) and histamine (H1) receptors (Fantry 2024; Knights et al 2023).

Because the CTZ sits outside the blood–brain barrier, it can be stimulated by blood-borne emetics (e.g. chemical and bacterial toxins, drugs), cerebrospinal fluid-borne emetics and 5-hydroxytryptamine (5HT, serotonin) released from the stomach and small intestine. The vomiting or emetic centre is activated by a number of triggers, including smells, strong or unpleasant emotions, severe pain, increased intracranial pressure, labyrinthine disturbances (motion sickness and inner ear disturbances), endocrine and metabolic disturbances (including pregnancy), toxic reactions to drugs, GIT disease (including obstruction and ischaemia), GIT inflammatory diseases, infection, radiation treatment and chemotherapy. The emetic centre sends messages via a number of pathways and neurotransmitters to the upper GIT, diaphragm and abdominal muscles, causing contraction, which results in vomiting (emesis). Neurotransmitters involved in the process include 5HT (serotonin), acetylcholine, dopamine, histamine and substance P (Fantry 2024; Knights et al 2023).

Management of nausea and vomiting should include symptom control (usually with antiemetic agents), prevention or management of dehydration, resumption of normal oral intake and prevention of abnormal blood glucose levels, especially in those with diabetes (Hasler 2022).

Antiemetics act by blocking transmission of neurotransmitters. For example, dopamine antagonists (e.g. domperidone, metoclopramide, prochlorperazine) act to block dopamine receptors (D2) in the stomach and CTZ; $5HT_3$ receptor antagonists (e.g. granisetron, ondansetron, tropisetron) block $5HT_3$ receptors in the GIT, CTZ and vomiting centre; anticholinergics (e.g. hyoscine) block muscarinic receptors; and neurokinin-1 (NK_1) receptor antagonists (e.g. apreprant, fosaprepitant) block NK_1 receptors located in the CNS (Fantry 2024; Hasler 2022; Knights et al 2022).

Note
- highly emetogenic chemotherapy includes cisplatin
- less emetogenic chemotherapy includes carboplatin, cyclophosphamide, doxorubicin

$5HT_3$ RECEPTOR ANTAGONISTS

General Adverse effects of $5HT_3$ receptor antagonists
- headache, dizziness, fatigue
- diarrhoea, constipation, abdominal pain
- fever
- changes in liver enzymes
- insomnia, somnolence, drowsiness
- (Uncommon) bradycardia, arrhythmias, hypotension, angina, ECG changes
- (Rare) prolongs QT interval, torsades de pointes (see Glossary)
- (Rare) seizures, extrapyramidal reactions, hypersensitivity reactions, serotonin syndrome (see Glossary)

General Interactions of $5HT_3$ receptor antagonists
- caution if given with other agents known to prolong QT interval, cause arrhythmias or cause electrolyte imbalances
- serotonin syndrome may occur if given with other serotonergic agents such as selective serotonin reuptake inhibitors (SSRIs)

General Nursing considerations/Cautions for $5HT_3$ receptor antagonists
- any electrolyte imbalance such as hypo- or hyperkalaemia should be corrected before starting therapy
- pulse and ECG should be monitored during therapy
- the patient should be monitored for any signs of subacute intestinal obstruction
- the patient should be carefully observed for any signs of serotonin syndrome if given with other serotonergic agents. Clinical symptoms of serotonin syndrome include agitation, confusion, hypomania, hyperactivity, restlessness, hyperthermia, sweating, tachycardia, hypertension, flushing, shivering, clonus, hyperreflexia, hypertonia, ataxia and tremor
- not recommended in those with congenital QT syndrome
- caution in those who have or may develop QT prolongation, cardiac rhythm or conduction disturbances, with electrolyte disturbance or receiving cardiotoxic chemotherapy
- caution if used in those with subacute intestinal obstruction as stimulation of gastric motility may be dangerous
- caution if used in those with hypersensitivity to other $5HT_3$ antagonists, as cross-sensitisation may occur

General Patient education for $5HT_3$ receptor antagonists
- the patient should be advised not to drive or operate machinery if dizziness, fatigue or insomnia occur
- instruct the patient to seek medical advice if any chest pain or changes to

heart rate (such as palpitations or pounding heart) are felt

Not used during pregnancy unless the expected benefit outweighs any potential risk.

Not recommended during breastfeeding.

GRANISETRON
Trade names
Granisetron-AFT, Granisetron Kabi, Kytril

Available forms
Tablets: 2 mg;
Ampoules: 1 mg/1 mL, 3 mg/3 mL

Action
- selective serotonin (5HT$_3$) receptor antagonist
- (Oral) half-life 9 hours

Use
- prevention of nausea and vomiting associated with chemotherapy, radiotherapy
- postoperative nausea and vomiting

Dose
- (Prophylaxis of nausea and vomiting associated with chemotherapy) 2 mg orally daily up to 6 days following chemotherapy, with first dose given 1 hour before the start of chemotherapy **OR**
- (Prophylaxis of nausea and vomiting associated with chemotherapy) 3 mg by IV infusion over 5 minutes, starting 30 minutes before and completed just prior to chemotherapy **OR**
- (Treatment of established nausea and vomiting after chemotherapy) 1 mg by IV infusion over 5 minutes, repeated at 10-minute intervals if needed (daily maximum 9 mg) **OR**
- (Prophylaxis of nausea and vomiting associated with radiotherapy) 3 mg by IV infusion over 5 minutes before start of radiotherapy, or oral 2 mg once daily 1 hour before radiotherapy; **OR**
- (Prophylaxis of postoperative nausea and vomiting) 1 mg IV over 30 seconds before induction of anaesthesia or radiotherapy **OR**
- (Treatment of established postoperative nausea and vomiting) 1 mg IV over 30 seconds as a single dose

Adverse effects
- constipation, headache, dizziness, transient rise in hepatic aminotransferases
- asthenia
- agitation, anxiety, CNS stimulation
- alopecia
- anaemia, thrombocytopenia, leucopenia
- hypertension
- anorexia, altered taste
- see also General Adverse effects of 5HT$_3$ antagonists (p. 369)

Interactions
- see General Interactions of 5HT$_3$ receptor antagonists (p. 369)

Nursing considerations/Cautions
- do not give IM
- efficacy is increased by adding a corticosteroid (e.g. dexamethasone 8–20 mg IV) just before chemotherapy
- solution should be diluted with 20–50 mL of infusion fluid before IV administration
- dilution fluids include glucose 5%, sodium chloride 0.9%, mannitol 10%, Hartmann's solution, sodium chloride 0.18%/glucose 4% and compound sodium lactate
- should be administered alone, but may be mixed with dexamethasone
- (Postoperative nausea and vomiting) give IV over 30 seconds
- tablets not recommended in those with hereditary problems of galactose intolerance, Lapp lactase deficiency or glucose–galactose malabsorption

ANTIEMETIC AGENTS

- see also General Nursing considerations/Cautions for 5HT₃ receptor antagonists (p. 369)

Patient education
- see General Patient education for 5HT₃ receptor antagonists (p. 369)

Tablets can be crushed and mixed with water, or a spoonful of yoghurt or apple puree.

May be used for nausea and vomiting if other drugs are inadequate. If used, ondansetron is preferred because of greater experience; limited data for granisetron (human data lacking for tropisetron and palonosetron).

ONDANSETRON
Trade names
APX-Ondansetron, Ondansetron Injection, Ondansetron Viatris, Ondansetron Tablets, Zofran, Zotren

Available forms
Tablets: 4 mg, 8 mg;
Wafers: 4 mg, 8 mg;
Oral liquid: 4 mg/5 mL;
Ampoules: 4 mg/2 mL (IM or IV), 8 mg/4 mL (IV)

Action
- serotonin antagonist highly selective against selective serotonin (5HT₃) receptors

Use
- prevention and treatment of nausea and vomiting induced by radiotherapy or chemotherapy
- prevention and treatment of postoperative nausea and vomiting

Dose
Highly emetogenic chemotherapy
- 8–12 mg by slow IV injection or IV infusion over 15 minutes immediately before chemotherapy, followed by further IV doses if necessary (daily maximum 16 mg; maximum 8 mg if age >75 years) **OR**
- orally 16–24 mg 1–2 hours before chemotherapy

Radiotherapy or less emetogenic chemotherapy
- 8–12 mg by slow IV injection or IV infusion over 15 minutes immediately before chemotherapy or radiotherapy (8 mg if age >75 years), then 8 mg orally 12-hourly **OR**
- 8 mg orally 2 hours before chemotherapy or radiotherapy, then 8 mg orally 12-hourly or 16 mg PR daily for up to 5 days

Postoperative nausea and vomiting
- (Prevention) 4 mg IM or slow IV at induction of anaesthesia or oral 16 mg 1 hour before anaesthesia **OR**
- (Treatment) 4–8 mg IM or slow IV 4 mg single dose. Doses up to 8 mg have been used

Adverse effects
- sensation of flushing or warmth
- anxiety
- dry mouth
- (Uncommon) hiccups
- (IV) local reaction, shivering
- (Rapid IV administration) transient visual disturbances (including blurred vision or blindness), dizziness
- see also General Adverse effects of 5HT₃ receptor antagonists (p. 369)

Interactions
- may decrease the analgesic effect of tramadol
- increased clearance and decreased antiemetic effect may occur if given with phenytoin, carbamazepine or rifampicin
- contraindicated with apomorphine
- see also General Interactions of 5HT₃ receptor antagonists (p. 369)

Nursing considerations/Cautions
- do not administer any other drug in the same syringe or infusion

- see manufacturer's instructions for dilution and compatibility with other drugs
- diluted solutions that are hazy, discoloured or contain visible particulate matter must be discarded
- IV doses over 8 mg should be given as an IV infusion over 15 minutes
- should not be given rapidly, as visual disturbances may occur. Transient blindness should resolve within 20 minutes
- a single dose of IV dexamethasone (20 mg) administered before the first ondansetron dose will potentiate the antiemetic effect in patients receiving highly emetogenic chemotherapy
- wafers contain aspartame and should be used with caution in those with phenylketonuria
- wafers should be placed on the tongue, allowed to dissolve and then swallowed
- see also General Nursing considerations/Cautions for $5HT_3$ receptor antagonists (p. 369)

Patient education

- advise the patient to place wafer on tongue and allow to dissolve before swallowing
- see also General Patient education for $5HT_3$ receptor antagonists (p. 369)

There is conflicting data about the association of ondansetron, used in the first trimester, with a small increased risk of malformations, e.g. orofacial clefts.

Reduce dose in severe hepatic impairment.

Wafers should be used if the patient has swallowing difficulties

In breastfeeding avoid (long half-life); ondansetron is preferred.

PALONOSETRON HYDROCHLORIDE

Trade names
Aloxi, Palonosetron Medsurge, Palonosetron Dr. Reddy's

Available form
Vial: 250 microgram/5 mL

Action
- selective serotonin ($5HT_3$) receptor antagonist
- half-life about 40 hours

Use
- prevention of nausea and vomiting induced by cytotoxic therapy
- prevention of nausea and vomiting postoperatively for up to 24 hours

Dose
- 250 micrograms IV over 30 seconds given 30 minutes before start of cytotoxic therapy **OR**
- (Postoperatively) 75 micrograms IV as a single dose before induction of anaesthesia

Adverse effects
- weakness, asthenia, anxiety
- hyperkalaemia
- (IV site) burning, pain, discomfort, induration
- see also General Adverse effects of $5HT_3$ receptor antagonists (p. 369)

Interactions
- see General Interactions of $5HT_3$ receptor antagonists (p. 369)

Nursing considerations/Cautions
- IV line should be flushed with 0.9% sodium chloride before and after administration of palonosetron
- administer alone

- see also General Nursing considerations/Cautions for 5HT$_3$ receptor antagonists (p. 369)

Patient education
- the patient should be advised not to drive or operate machinery if dizziness, fatigue or insomnia are ongoing

 Avoid in breastfeeding (long half-life); ondansetron is preferred.

Available in combination with
- contained in Akynzeo with netupitant (a substance P neurokinin-1 receptor antagonist) and Akynzeo IV intravenous infusion (Fosnetupitant, Palonosetron)

TROPISETRON
Trade names
Tropisetron-AFT, Tropisetron MYX

Available forms
Ampoules: 2 mg/2 mL, 5 mg/5 mL

Action
- selective serotonin (5HT$_3$) receptor antagonist
- long duration of action (24 hours)

Use
- prevention of nausea and vomiting induced by cytotoxic therapy (5 mg/5 mL ampoule only)
- treatment and prevention of postoperative nausea and vomiting (2 mg/2 mL ampoule only)

Dose

Prevention of nausea and vomiting induced by cytotoxic therapy
- 5 mg IV infusion over 15 minutes or slow IV injection over at least 60 seconds immediately before chemotherapy (day 1), then
- days 2—6: 5 mg orally in the morning 1 hour before food

Postoperative nausea and vomiting
- 2 mg by slow IV injection over at least 30 seconds or infusion just before induction of anaesthesia

Adverse effects
- (Rare) collapse, syncope
- see also General Adverse effects of 5HT$_3$ receptor antagonists (p. 369)

Interactions
- rifampicin and phenobarbital (phenobarbitone) may reduce serum levels of tropisetron
- see also General Interactions of 5HT$_3$ receptor antagonists (p. 369)

Nursing considerations/Cautions
- for IV use, ampoule may be diluted to 100 mL with sodium chloride 0.9%, glucose 5%, mannitol 10% or Ringer's solution
- should be avoided in doses of 10 mg or greater in patients with uncontrolled hypertension
- the antiemetic effect may be enhanced if given with dexamethasone
- see also General Nursing considerations/Cautions for 5HT$_3$ receptor antagonists (p. 369)

Patient education
- see General Patient education for 5HT$_3$ receptor antagonists (p. 369)

 Contraindicated during pregnancy. Ondansetron preferred.

 Contraindicated during breastfeeding. Ondansetron preferred. Human data are lacking.

 Prolonged QT interval or risk factors for prolonged QT interval — use with caution, as QT prolongation (usually transient and clinically insignificant) has been reported, mainly with IV administration.

NEUROKININ-1 (NK₁) RECEPTOR ANTAGONISTS

APREPITANT
Trade names
Aprepitant ARX, Aprepitant Lupin

Available forms
Capsules: 40 mg, 80 mg, 125 mg, 165 mg

Action
- neurokinin-1 (NK1) receptor antagonist which blocks substance P
- half-life 9—13 hours

Use
- prevention of acute and delayed nausea and vomiting associated with moderately or highly emetogenic chemotherapy (e.g. cisplatin) (with ondansetron and dexamethasone)
- prevention of postoperative nausea and vomiting

Dose

Chemotherapy-induced nausea and vomiting (highly emetogenic)
- 165 mg orally 1 hour before chemotherapy (with dexamethasone 12 mg orally and ondansetron 32 mg IV 30 minutes before chemotherapy) (day 1), followed by dexamethasone 8 mg orally mane (day 2), then dexamethasone 8 mg orally BD (days 3 and 4) **OR**
- 125 mg orally 1 hour before chemotherapy (with dexamethasone 12 mg orally and ondansetron 32 mg IV 30 minutes before chemotherapy) (day 1), then 80 mg orally mane (with dexamethasone 8 mg orally) (days 2 and 3), then dexamethasone 8 mg orally mane (day 4)

Chemotherapy-induced nausea and vomiting (moderately emetogenic)
- 165 mg orally 1 hour before chemotherapy (with dexamethasone 12 mg orally and ondansetron 32 mg IV 30 minutes before chemotherapy) **OR**
- 125 mg orally 1 hour before chemotherapy (with dexamethasone 12 mg orally and ondansetron 32 mg IV 30 minutes before chemotherapy) (day 1), then 80 mg orally mane (days 2 and 3)

Prevention of postoperative nausea and vomiting
- 40 mg orally within 3 hours of anaesthetic induction

Adverse effects
- asthenia, fatigue, dizziness, insomnia, somnolence, anxiety
- fever
- anorexia, nausea, burping, abdominal pain, flatulence, constipation or diarrhoea, dyspepsia, reflux
- headache
- anaemia, febrile neutropenia
- hiccups
- increase in liver enzymes
- pruritus, rash, urticaria
- hypotension, bradycardia

Interactions
- may result in decreased prothrombin time if given with warfarin; therefore INR should be closely monitored for 14 days following therapy
- may decrease efficacy of oral contraceptives during and for 28 days following therapy
- caution if given with ciclosporin, tacrolimus or sirolimus
- may decrease serum levels of phenytoin and warfarin
- may increase serum levels of dexamethasone, methylprednisolone, midazolam, alprazolam
- decreased plasma levels may result if given with rifampicin and paroxetine
- not recommended with St John's wort
- caution if given with ifosfamide, as neurotoxicity may occur

Patient education
- patient should be advised not to drive or operate machinery if they experience fatigue or dizziness

ANTIEMETIC AGENTS

- female patients using hormonal contraceptives should be instructed to use alternative or extra contraception methods during therapy and for 1 month after last dose
- (165 mg capsule) advise the patient to take either with a light meal or on an empty stomach

Capsules can be opened and contents dispersed in water or sprinkled on a spoonful of yoghurt or apple puree.

Not recommended during pregnancy unless benefits outweigh potential risks.

Not recommended during pregnancy or breastfeeding unless benefits outweigh potential risks.

FOSAPREPITANT

Trade names
Emend IV, Medsurge, Fosaprepitant MSN, Fosaprepitant-AFT

Available form
Vial: 150 mg powder

Action
- prodrug of aprepitant (neurokinin-1 (NK_1) receptor antagonist which blocks substance P)
- conversion to aprepitant occurs within 30 minutes of IV infusion being completed

Use
- prevention of acute and delayed nausea and vomiting associated with moderate to highly emetogenic chemotherapy (e.g. cisplatin) (with ondansetron and dexamethasone)

Dose
- (Highly emetogenic chemotherapy) 150 mg IV over 20—30 minutes, 30 minutes before chemotherapy (dexamethasone 12 mg orally and ondansetron 30 minutes before chemotherapy) (day 1), then dexamethasone 8 mg orally mane (day 2), then dexamethasone 8 mg orally twice daily (days 3 and 4) **OR**
- (Moderately emetogenic chemotherapy) 150 mg IV over 20—30 minutes, 30 minutes before chemotherapy (dexamethasone 12 mg orally and ondansetron 30 minutes before chemotherapy)

Adverse effects
- IV site reaction
- (High dose) thrombosis
- (Rare) hypersensitivity reaction
- see also Adverse effects for Aprepitant (p. 374)

Interactions
- see Interactions for Aprepitant (p. 374)

Nursing considerations/Cautions
- should not be given as bolus injection or IM or SC
- to reconstitute the powder, inject sodium chloride 5 mL gently into the vial and swirl gently to avoid foaming
- inject the reconstituted solution into the sodium chloride infusion bag (for 150 mg IV infusion, volume of infusion bag should be 145 mL; for 115 mg IV infusion, volume of infusion bag should be 110 mL (extra sodium chloride will need to be added to infusion bags to make up the correct volume))
- invert the infusion bag gently 2—3 times to ensure even mixing
- IV infusion given over 20—30 minutes
- administer alone
- incompatible with solutions containing divalent cations (e.g. Mg^{2+}, Ca^{2+}), including Hartmann's solution and lactated Ringer's solution
- contraindicated in those with hypersensitivity to aprepitant or polysorbate 80
- see also Nursing considerations/Cautions for Aprepitant (p. 374)

Patient education
- see Patient education for Aprepitant (p. 374)

Possible adverse effects of aprepitant on nursing infants — a decision should be made whether to discontinue nursing or to discontinue the drug.

DOPAMINE ANTAGONISTS

DOMPERIDONE
Trade names
Motilium, APO-Domperidone

Available form
Tablets: 10 mg

Action
- prokinetic agent
- dopamine antagonist that seldom causes extrapyramidal reactions because it does not cross the blood—brain barrier
- antiemetic action thought to be caused by peripheral effects, as well as antagonism of central dopamine receptors in the chemoreceptor trigger zone (CTZ)
- half-life 7—9 hours

Use
- intractable nausea and vomiting
- treatment (short term) of diabetic gastroparesis symptoms

Dose
- 10 mg orally, 3 times daily 15—30 minutes before meals and before retiring if needed (daily maximum 30 mg)

Adverse effects
- mild abdominal cramps, diarrhoea, dry mouth
- headache, somnolence, akathisia, asthenia, depression, anxiety
- endocrine disturbance (including breast enlargement, breast tenderness or pain, irregular menstruation, amenorrhoea), decreased libido
- (Uncommon) increase in prolactin levels, thirst, nervousness, insomnia, dizziness, lethargy, irritability
- (Rare) extrapyramidal symptoms, QT prolongation, arrhythmias, sudden cardiac death

Interactions
- contraindicated with erythromycin, fluconazole, voriconazole, clarithromycin and amiodarone because of QT interval prolongation
- antacids and antisecretory drugs (e.g. ranitidine) reduce bioavailability of domperidone and block absorption
- effects decreased if given with anticholinergic agents. If given before atropine, may decrease relaxation of lower oesophageal sphincter
- plasma levels may be increased by azole antifungal agents, macrolide antibiotics, HIV protease inhibitors, calcium-channel blockers, amiodarone or aprepitant; therefore not recommended together
- may affect the absorption of enteric-coated or sustained-release preparations
- caution if used with agents that cause electrolyte disturbance, as it may increase risk of QT prolongation

Nursing considerations/Cautions
- any electrolyte disturbance should be corrected before starting therapy
- (Acute nausea and vomiting) therapy should be continued for more than 7 days
- contains lactose and therefore is not recommended in those with lactose intolerance, galactosaemia or glucose—galactose malabsorption
- (Diabetic gastroparesis) once diabetic control has been established (either by diet or insulin or both), domperidone should be stopped
- may lead to increased serum prolactin levels with prolonged use; therefore it should be used with caution in those with a history of breast cancer, as some are prolactin dependent
- caution if used in those over 60 years or in patients with diabetes or cardiac

ANTIEMETIC AGENTS

disease because of the increased risk of cardiac death
- not recommended in children or if the patient weighs < 35 kg
- not recommended in those with liver or kidney impairment
- contraindicated in those with moderate-to-severe liver impairment, or with prolactin-releasing pituitary tumours (prolactinoma), where stimulation of gastric motility may be dangerous such as GIT haemorrhage or obstruction, or in those with QT prolongation, cardiac disease or significant electrolyte disturbance

Patient education
- advise the patient to take domperidone 2 hours apart from any antacid or antisecretory preparation
- warn the patient not to drive or operate machinery if any dizziness or somnolence occurs
- instruct the patient to seek medical advice immediately if any of the following occur:
  - uncontrollable face, leg or arm movements, excessive trembling, unusual muscle stiffness or spasm
  - fast or irregular heart rate
  - swelling of hands, ankles or feet
  - unusual milk secretion from breast, breast enlargement, breast tenderness or pain, irregular or absent menstruation, decreased sex drive

> Tablets can be dispersed in water, or crushed and mixed with water or a spoonful of yoghurt or apple puree.

> Not to be used during pregnancy unless the expected benefit outweighs any potential risk.

> Not to be used during breastfeeding unless the expected benefit outweighs any potential risk.

> Patients with severe renal impairment on prolonged therapy should be reviewed regularly.

> Domperidone is contraindicated for patients with moderate-to-severe hepatic impairment.

METOCLOPRAMIDE HYDROCHLORIDE

Trade names
Emexlon, Maxolon, Metoclopramide Injection, Pramin

Available forms
Tablets: 10 mg;
Ampoules: 10 mg/2 mL

Action
- prokinetic agent with dopamine antagonistic actions
- stimulates the motility of the upper GIT without affecting gastric, biliary or pancreatic secretions
- increases rate of gastric emptying by enhancing peristalsis, thereby accelerating intestinal transit time
- increases resting tone of lower oesophageal sphincter
- little or no effect on colon or gallbladder activity
- increases prolactin secretion and circulating aldosterone levels (transient)
- effective within 1–3 minutes (IV), 10–15 minutes (IM) or 30–60 minutes (oral); duration 1–2 hours, half-life 2.5–5 hours (increased to about 15 hours in those with kidney impairment)

Use
- controls nausea and vomiting in most cases, except for motion sickness or other labyrinth disturbances
- adjunct to radiological examination of stomach and duodenum
- facilitates and accelerates introduction of tubes or biopsy capsules into small intestine

- enhances absorption of a range of drugs, including aspirin in a migraine attack (given IM 10 minutes before aspirin)
- after gastric surgery for gastric retention
- assists with intestinal intubation
- mild-to-moderate diabetic gastroparesis

Dose
- (Nausea/vomiting) 10 mg orally, slow IV over 1–2 minutes or IM 1–3 times daily **OR**
- (Diagnostic purpose) 10–20 mg slow IV over 1–2 minutes or IM 5–10 minutes before examination
- Total daily dose should not exceed 0.5 mg/kg or 30 mg (whichever is less).

Adverse effects
- restlessness, drowsiness, lassitude, fatigue, insomnia, headache, dizziness
- nausea, constipation or diarrhoea
- extrapyramidal reactions (e.g. dystonic type, such as facial muscle spasm, trismus, oculogyric crises, increase in muscle tone, hyperextension/spasticity of head, neck and back) (dystonic reactions are more common in children and young adults)
- tardive dyskinesia (especially in the elderly on long-term therapy)
- hypertensive crisis (if the patient has phaeochromocytoma)
- raised prolactin levels, galactorrhoea, breast enlargement
- (Rare) Parkinsonian symptoms (new or exacerbated, including tremor, rigidity, akinesia, bradykinesia), methaemoglobinaemia
- (Very rare) neuroleptic malignant syndrome, acute depression, hypersensitivity, bradycardia, heart block
- (Rapid IV) anxiety, agitation, restlessness, drowsiness

Interactions
- contraindicated or use with great caution with other agents known to cause extrapyramidal reactions such as phenothiazines
- not recommended with monoamine oxidase inhibitors (MAOIs)
- may prolong recovery time if given with suxamethonium
- may increase absorption of paracetamol, tetracyclines, alcohol, levodopa or controlled-release preparations of morphine
- may decrease absorption of digoxin, bromocriptine or penicillin
- may potentiate action of other CNS depressants, such as alcohol, barbiturates, anaesthetics, sedatives, hypnotics, opioid analgesics and tranquillisers
- effects on GI motility are antagonised by anticholinergic agents and opioid analgesics
- may increase bioavailability of ciclosporin; therefore ciclosporin blood levels should be closely monitored to prevent toxicity
- increased risk of neuroleptic malignant syndrome and extrapyramidal symptoms if given with phenothiazines
- increased risk of neurotoxicity if given with lithium
- may increase plasma levels of diazepam
- diabetic control may be affected because the rate of food absorption will be altered, necessitating an adjustment in dose and/or time of insulin

Nursing considerations/Cautions
- the cause of vomiting should be identified before treatment. If vomiting persists despite therapy, the patient should be reassessed to exclude underlying causes, such as cerebral irritation
- treatment should be no longer than 5 days
- should be withheld for 3–4 days post GI surgery (e.g. pyloroplasty, anastomosis), as wound healing may be inhibited by vigorous muscular contraction
- extrapyramidal reaction (see Glossary) may not develop if the drug is stopped when the early sign of fine vermicular

ANTIEMETIC AGENTS

- (worm-like) movements of the tongue occurs
- extrapyramidal reactions usually occur within 36 hours of starting and cease within 24 hours of stopping therapy. The patient should be closely observed if this occurs
- acute dystonic reactions may occur after a single dose, especially in children and young adults
- tardive dyskinesia may occur after therapy has been stopped; the risk is greatest in elderly females on high-dose therapy
- compatible with morphine or pethidine when mixed in the same syringe, if the resultant solution is used within 15 minutes and there is no precipitation
- see the manufacturer's instructions for compatibility with cytotoxic and other agents
- slow IV administration over 1—2 minutes is advised to prevent intense feelings of anxiety, restlessness and drowsiness (transient)
- if given as IV infusion, should be diluted in 50 mL and administered over 15 minutes. Suitable fluids include glucose 5%, sodium chloride 0.9%, Hartmann's solution and Ringer's solution
- discard any ampoules showing yellow discolouration
- caution if used in those with a prior history of depression, breast cancer, impaired kidney or liver function or Parkinson's disease
- caution if used in those with hypertension
- not recommended in those under 20 (because of the increased risk of dystonic reactions), except for severe intractable vomiting of known cause, to aid with GI intubation or vomiting associated with radiotherapy and intolerance to cytotoxic agents
- contraindicated in those with phaeochromocytoma (because of the risk of hypertensive crisis), where increase in GI motility may be dangerous (e.g. obstructed or perforated bowel), in those with epilepsy or porphyria, or in those with known sensitivity to procaine owing to possible cross-sensitivity

Patient education

- warn the patient against driving a vehicle or operating machinery if drowsy or dizzy
- the patient should be instructed to seek medical advice promptly if any of the following occur:
  - nausea and vomiting persist despite therapy
  - fast heartbeat
  - uncontrolled or repeated movements (such as darting tongue, chewing movement, uncontrolled movement of legs or arms), muscle spasm, upturned eyes, locked jaw or shuffling walk
  - sudden increase in body temperature
- advise the patient to avoid using alcohol during therapy

 Tablets can be crushed and mixed with water, or spoonful of yoghurt or apple puree.

 Not recommended during pregnancy unless the expected benefit outweighs any potential risk.

 Not recommended during breastfeeding unless the expected benefit outweighs any potential risk.

Available in combination with

- metoclopramide hydrochloride 5 mg + paracetamol 500 mg tablets (Anagraine, Metomax)

PROCHLORPERAZINE MALEATE
Trade names
Nausetil, APO-Prochlorperazine, Procalm, APOHealth Nausea Relief, Chemists' Own Procalm, Nausrelief

PROCHLORPERAZINE MESILATE
Trade names
Stemetil Solution for Injection

Available forms
Tablets: 5 mg;
Ampoules: 12.5 mg/mL

Action
- centrally acting phenothiazine that has antidopamine actions, antagonises alpha adrenoreceptors, blocks noradrenaline (norepinephrine) reuptake and has weak anticholinergic, antihistamine and antiserotonin actions
- has an effect on temperature control and blocks conditioned avoidance response
- less sedating than chlorpromazine
- half-life about 24 hours

Use
- nausea and vomiting
- vertigo, labyrinthitis

Dose
- 5–10 mg orally 2–3 times daily if required **OR**
- (Nausea and vomiting) 5–10 mg orally 2–3 times daily **OR**
- (Acute nausea) 20 mg orally, followed by 10 mg 2 hours later if necessary **OR**
- (Vertigo) 5–10 mg orally 3–4 times daily, reduced gradually over several weeks to 5–10 mg daily

Adverse effects
- constipation, dry mouth
- drowsiness, akathisia, extrapyramidal reactions (Parkinsonian type), blurred vision, tardive dyskinesia
- urinary retention/hesitancy
- endocrine disturbances (including breast enlargement, breast tenderness or pain, irregular menstruation, amenorrhoea), decreased libido
- very serious acute dystonic reactions in children
- (IV) hypotension
- (IM) postural hypotension with tachycardia, local pain, nodule formation
- (Rare) neuroleptic malignant syndrome, prolongation of QT interval, ECG changes, photosensitivity, hyperglycaemia, blood dyscrasias

Interactions
- caution if used with other agents known to prolong QT interval, induce bradycardia or cause hypokalaemia
- may increase hypotensive effects of most antihypertensive agents, especially alpha adrenergic blocking agents
- high dose may decrease response to hypoglycaemic agents
- may increase serum levels of amitriptyline, increasing the risk of adverse effects
- may lower convulsive threshold; therefore the antiepileptic dose may need adjustment
- use with propranolol may result in increased serum levels of both drugs
- may induce transient metabolic encephalopathy (loss of consciousness for 48–72 hours) when given simultaneously with desferrioxamine
- thiazide diuretics may accentuate orthostatic hypotension
- not recommended with levodopa, clonidine, adrenaline (epinephrine) or neuroleptic agents
- CNS depressant effects are enhanced by alcohol and other depressant drugs
- may potentiate anticholinergic effects of tricyclic antidepressants (TCAs) and atropine-like drugs
- use with procarbazine may result in the potentiation of extrapyramidal side-effects
- may result in increased and/or impaired phenytoin metabolism if given together; therefore phenytoin levels should be closely monitored during therapy

ANTIEMETIC AGENTS

- may diminish effects of oral anticoagulants; therefore INR should be closely monitored
- caution if used with other antipsychotic agents
- absorption may be decreased if given with lithium, anti-Parkinson's agents or antacids
- increased risk of neurotoxicity if given with lithium
- increased risk of agranulocytosis if given with carbamazepine or myelosuppressive agents

Nursing considerations/Cautions

- blood counts should be monitored regularly during prolonged therapy
- acute dystonic reactions should be managed with benztropine IM immediately
- extrapyramidal reaction (see Glossary) may not develop if drug is stopped when the early sign of fine vermicular (worm-like) movements of the tongue occurs
- should be stopped immediately if tardive dyskinesia symptoms occur
- do not use darkened solution (more than pale yellow)
- not normally mixed in the same syringe with other drugs, but is compatible with morphine or pethidine when mixed in the same syringe, if the resultant solution is used within 15 minutes and there is no precipitation
- (Solution) avoid contact with skin to prevent sensitisation occurring
- response may be delayed in those with schizophrenia
- do not use oral forms in children and adolescents under 18 years of age.
- caution if used in the elderly because of the risk of hypotension, sedation and/or extrapyramidal reactions
- caution if used with spinal anaesthesia because hypotension may occur
- caution if used in those with liver impairment, epilepsy or a history of seizures, urinary dysfunction, constipation or acute narrow-angle glaucoma
- caution if used in those with hypoparathyroidism because of the increased risk of dystonic reactions
- caution if used in those with congenital or acquired prolongation of QT interval
- caution if used in those with risk factors for stroke or thromboembolism
- not recommended in those with a history of agranulocytosis or narrow-angle glaucoma
- not recommended in those with kidney impairment, hypothyroidism, Parkinson's disease, dementia, phaeochromocytoma, prostatic hypertrophy, cardiac failure or myasthenia gravis
- contraindicated in those with CNS depression (e.g. coma, drug intoxication), circulatory collapse, bone marrow depression or previous hypersensitivity to other phenothiazines owing to the possibility of cross-sensitivity

Patient education

- advise the patient to take antacids 2 hours apart from therapy
- warn the patient against driving a vehicle or operating machinery if blurred vision, drowsiness, dizziness or lightheadedness occurs
- if the patient has diabetes mellitus, careful monitoring of blood glucose levels should be suggested, as they may become erratic
- advise the patient to avoid alcohol during therapy, as dizziness or lightheadedness may worsen
- instruct the patient to avoid exposure to sun or wear long-sleeved garments and SPF 30+ sunscreen during therapy, as skin may be more sensitive to sun
- warn the patient to keep cool in hot weather and warm in cool weather, and avoid swimming in cold water as temperature regulation may be affected
- instruct patient in the correct suppository insertion technique (see General Patient education for NSAIDs, p. 13)

HAVARD'S NURSING GUIDE TO DRUGS

- advise the patient to immediately seek medical advice if any of the following occur:
  - muscle spasm or unusual trembling, uncontrolled movements of tongue, face, mouth and jaw, rigid posture, twitching or restlessness
  - sudden increase in body temperature
  - unexplained fever or infection
  - fitting (seizures)
  - unusual milk secretion from the breast, breast enlargement, breast tenderness or pain, irregular or absent menstruation, decreased libido

Tablets can be dispersed in water, or crushed and mixed with water or a spoonful of yoghurt or apple puree.

High doses of phenothiazines used late in pregnancy may cause jaundice, hyperreflexia, hyporeflexia or prolonged extrapyramidal symptoms in the newborn, therefore not used during pregnancy or breastfeeding unless the expected benefit outweighs any potential risk.

If unavoidable to use prochlorperazine for a child, the dosage is 250 micrograms/kg bodyweight 2 or 3 times a day.

Do not use orally in children and adolescents under 18 years of age.

It should not be given to children by the intramuscular route.

When treating children, it is recommended that the 5 mg tablets are used.

CYCLIZINE HYDROCHLORIDE
Trade name
Nausicalm

CYCLIZINE LACTATE
Trade names
Valoid, Cyclizine Juno Solution

Available forms
Ampoule: 50 mg/mL;
Tablets: 50 mg

Action
- piperazine antihistamine (H_1 receptor antagonist) with anticholinergic and antiemetic actions
- half-life about 14 hours

Use
- postoperative nausea and vomiting
- prevention and treatment of motion sickness

Dose
- (Treatment of postoperative nausea and vomiting) 50 mg IV up to 3 times daily (for up to 48 hours) **OR**
- (Prevention of postoperative nausea and vomiting) 50 mg IV 20 minutes before end of surgery **OR**
- (Prevention and treatment of motion sickness) 50 mg orally 6—8-hourly starting 1—2 hours before anticipated travel (daily maximum 150 mg)

Adverse effects
- (Anticholinergic side-effects) dry mouth, nose and throat, constipation, urinary retention, blurred vision, tachycardia, asthenia, somnolence, headache, drowsiness, oculogyric crisis
- extrapyramidal symptoms
- (IV site) erythema, pain, thrombophlebitis and (rarely) chills, pruritus, heavy sensation
- (Rare) transient paralysis, decreased consciousness, blood dyscrasias, liver dysfunction, jaundice

Interactions
- may increase effects of alcohol and CNS depressants such as hypnotics, opioid analgesics, anaesthetics and tranquillisers
- may enhance side-effects of other anticholinergic agents if given together
- antiemetic effect may be decreased if given with atropine
- caution if given with aminoglycosides because of the risk of masking ototoxicity

Nursing considerations/Cautions
- should be given within 24 hours of surgery for best effect. For prophylaxis, the

ANTIMETIC AGENTS

first dose should be given 20 minutes before the anticipated end of surgery
- the patient should be carefully observed for any signs of limb paralysis, which may occur within minutes of administration and usually resolves within hours of stopping medication
- (Motion sickness) not recommended for longer than 48 hours
- (Motion sickness) not recommended in children under 12 years
- caution if used in those with neuromuscular disorders, asthma, chronic obstructive pulmonary disease, urinary retention or obstruction, prostatic hypertrophy, closed-angle glaucoma, untreated intraocular hypertension, uncontrolled open-angle glaucoma, GI obstructive disorder, phaeochromocytoma, liver disease, hypertension or epilepsy
- not recommended in those with porphyria
- contraindicated in those with sensitivity to other piperazines or with severe heart failure, acute myocardial infarction or acute alcohol intoxication

Patient education

- advise the patient to avoid alcohol during therapy
- the patient should be advised to be careful when getting out of bed or going from bed to chair to prevent dizziness occurring
- the patient should be warned not to drive or operate machinery if somnolence or drowsiness occur
- (Motion sickness) the patient should be advised to take tablet 1–2 hours before anticipated travel

 Tablet is difficult to crush and does not disperse in water. If crushed, can be given with a spoonful of yoghurt or apple puree.

 Not recommended during pregnancy.

 Not recommended during breastfeeding.

ANTIEPILEPTICS

Epilepsy is one of the most common neurological conditions with about 151,000 (0.6%) of Australians having a diagnosis. Epilepsy accounted for about 31,400 hospitalisations in 2018–2019 and over 20,600 emergency department presentations in the same time period. Furthermore, in 2019, there were about 1100 deaths attributed to epilepsy (AIHW 2022). This demonstrates the enormous impact that epilepsy can have not only on the individual but also the broader health care system.

A *seizure* is a 'transient alteration of behaviour due to the disordered synchronous and rhythmic firing of populations of brain neurons', while *epilepsy* is considered to be a condition in which a person has recurrent seizures due to a chronic underlying aetiology, suggesting that a single seizure or recurrent seizures due to correctable causes (e.g. induced by medication or biochemical abnormalities) does not mean the person has epilepsy (Rao & Lowenstein 2022; Ropper et al 2023).

Seizures are classified as:
- *generalised*, and include absence (either typical or atypical), tonic–clonic (grand mal), clonic, tonic, atonic or myoclonic seizures. Generalised seizures involve both hemispheres and may result from cellular, biochemical or structural abnormalities of the brain (Ropper et al 2023).
- *focal* (previously known as partial) seizures start at a particular focus and do not spread beyond one hemisphere and may be associated with structural brain abnormalities. Focal seizures can further be described as having intact or impaired awareness, motor or non-motor onset and can develop into a generalised seizure (Ropper et al 2023).
- *unclassifiable* or *unknown onset* seizures are those that cannot easily be classified as generalised or focal (Ropper et al 2023).
- *status epilepticus* is a life-threatening medical emergency in which there is no regaining of consciousness between seizures (i.e. the seizures are continuous for at least 30 minutes) and may be caused by nonadherence with antiepileptic medications, cerebral irritation, CNS tumours or infection, trauma, hypoglycaemia or low blood levels of calcium. First-line treatment is usually fast-acting benzodiazepines (e.g. diazepam, clonazepam, midazolam)

generally given IM or IV, followed by a long-acting antiepileptic (e.g. phenytoin, phenobarbital (phenobarbitone), sodium valproate) (Ropper et al 2023).

Antiepileptics (also known as anticonvulsants) are required to control primary recurrent seizures. The ideal antiepileptic agent is one that is highly effective, with low toxicity; is inexpensive; controls a number of seizure types without adverse effects, such as sedation; does not interact with other medications; is long acting and does not result in the development of tolerance. Unfortunately, such an agent does not exist, with current antiepileptic agents failing to control seizures completely or having adverse effects that range from unwanted (e.g. drowsiness, nausea) to severe (e.g. liver failure, blood dyscrasias) (Ropper et al 2023).

Selection of a particular antiepileptic medication is generally determined by the type of seizure. For example, phenytoin and carbamazepine are considered first-line drugs for generalised tonic–clonic seizures, whereas sodium valproate is used for myoclonic seizures. Other factors which may need to be considered in choosing an epileptic agent include age, sex, other medications, other medical or psychiatric conditions, and kidney and liver function (Rao & Lowenstein 2022; Ropper et al 2023). Therapy usually commences as a single drug (monotherapy) starting at a low dose, which is then increased gradually until seizure activity is controlled or adverse reactions become unacceptable to the patient. Combination therapy (consisting of two or more antiepileptic drugs) is required in people who are refractory to treatment or who have two or more types of seizures (Rao & Lowenstein 2022; Ropper et al 2023). It is important that plasma drug concentrations are measured at the start of therapy, when doses are adjusted, if therapeutic effect is not achieved or toxic adverse effects appear, or if multiple drug therapy is initiated (Ropper et al 2023).

Antiepileptic therapy is usually continued until a person has been seizure free for 2–3 years; however, some patients continue to have seizures despite treatment because of pharmacoresistance (defined as failure to control seizure despite adequate doses of two antiepileptic agents). In some patients, seizures may recur after ceasing antiepileptic agents. Risk factors for recurrence include age of seizure onset (i.e. after 12 years of age), family history, abnormal EEG despite therapy, total number of seizures, taking 2–6 years to achieve seizure control, or presence of mental retardation or organic neurological disorder/s (Ropper et al 2023).

General Adverse effects of antiepileptics
- drowsiness, dizziness, headache, fatigue, somnolence, insomnia, asthenia, vertigo
- ataxia, gait or balance disturbance (and associated falls), muscle weakness
- nausea, vomiting
- rash
- diplopia, blurred vision, nystagmus
- confusion, hostility, irritation, nervousness, anxiety, tremor, aggressiveness, hyperactivity, inability to concentrate, memory impairment,

- depression, sleep disturbances including night terrors, disorientation, transient amnesia
- increased seizure activity
- (Rare) suicidal behaviours and ideation

General Nursing considerations/ Cautions for antiepileptics

- changing from one antiepileptic agent to another should be done gradually because sudden withdrawal may precipitate seizures
- some antiepileptic agents require regular monitoring of blood levels. This is especially recommended if there is any increase in seizure activity, during pregnancy, in children or adolescents, if there is a suspected malabsorption disorder, or if the patient's adherence to therapy is questionable
- many antiepileptics increase the risk of suicidal thoughts or behaviours, and patients should therefore be closely monitored for any signs of depression, suicidal thoughts or behaviour, or any changes in mood or behaviour
- tolerance, physical and psychological dependence may occur with barbiturates
- drug withdrawal should be gradual to prevent provoking withdrawal seizure, and patients should be cautioned about abruptly stopping medication
- patients may be discontinued from antiepileptics if they have been seizure free for 2—3 years
- long-term antiepileptic therapy has been associated with decreased folate levels; therefore folic acid supplements (5 mg daily) are recommended 4 weeks before and for the first 12 weeks of pregnancy to decrease the risk of spina bifida in the fetus

General Patient education for antiepileptics

- instruct the patient to immediately report any changes in seizure activity (either frequency or severity). Encourage patient to keep a diary documenting seizure activity, including triggers and medication
- the patient should be advised to be aware of and try to avoid (if possible) seizure triggers, such as poor nutrition, lack of sleep, excess alcohol, fever, stress, bright lights (especially flashing and strobe), or changes in levels of fluids, electrolytes and hormones. Some drugs are also known to provoke seizures or reduce the seizure threshold
- many antiepileptic agents cause drowsiness, dizziness, vertigo, blurred or double vision and impaired concentration. Patients should therefore be advised of the dangers of driving or operating machinery while these adverse effects are occurring. Many of these adverse effects are transient and occur at the start of therapy
- advise the patient that fatigue, amnesia and muscle weakness are transient and generally disappear with ongoing therapy
- warn the patient about reduced tolerance to alcohol. Alcohol intake can also result in increased/ decreased serum antiepileptic agent levels (depending on acute or chronic intake) and should therefore be avoided during therapy
- many antiepileptic agents interact with other medications (prescription and non-prescription); therefore it is

- important that the patient is advised not to start or stop any medication without first consulting their doctor
- instruct the patient to continue therapy and not stop medication abruptly (as this may provoke withdrawal symptoms, including increased seizure activity). Non-adherence to medications may be a particular issue with adolescent patients who may be struggling with having a chronic condition requiring ongoing medications (and wanting to appear normal in the eyes of their peers)
- ensure the patient understands the importance of keeping follow-up appointments, blood tests and any other examinations required during therapy
- it is important that the person discusses driving with their doctor so that they have a full understanding of the requirements to hold a driver's licence, including the need for an annual medical review. Requirements vary depending on the type of seizure/epilepsy the person has and whether the person requires a private or commercial licence. For example, for a conditional commercial licence to be granted to someone with epilepsy, the person must provide an EEG that is clear of any epileptiform activity (Austroads 2022)
- other safety issues for consideration could include swimming (e.g. not swimming alone), operation of unguarded machinery and climbing ladders. If the person participates in sporting or leisure activities, ensure peers know what to do if a seizure occurs
- emphasise the importance of seeking medical advice if any of the following occur:
    - rash or skin reactions
    - changes in mood or behaviour, including aggression, hostility, anger, anxiety or nervousness
    - sleep disturbances
    - signs of depression, thoughts of self-harm or harm to others, or thoughts of suicide. This should also be discussed with family members, carers or significant others
- many antiepileptic agents interact with hormonal contraceptives. Female patients should be warned that breakthrough bleeding can occur and an alternative method of contraception should be used
- advise female patients that seizure activity may increase during menstruation
- women of childbearing potential should be counselled regarding the risks of using antiepileptic agents when pregnant versus the risks to the fetus of uncontrolled epilepsy. This pregnancy counselling and planning should occur on diagnosis (in an adult). Uncontrolled epilepsy is a greater danger to both mother and fetus than is the risk of having an abnormal child as a result of taking antiepileptic agents. The risk of fetal abnormalities in a mother taking antiepileptics is about three times that of the general population (Ropper et al 2023). Taking more than one antiepileptic agent increases the risk of fetal abnormalities; therefore monotherapy at the lowest dose to control seizure activity is recommended. Fetal malformations due to the older antiepileptic agents, such as phenytoin, carbamazepine and sodium valproate, are well documented. However, long-term studies involving the newer agents have not been

carried out and therefore the longer term risks are not well known (e.g. those adverse effects which might emerge in childhood) (Ropper et al 2023)
- supplementation with folic acid is advised if a woman is planning pregnancy, with 5 mg daily recommended 4—12 weeks before conception and for first 12 weeks of pregnancy to reduce the risk of spina bifida

Some antiepileptic agents have been associated with coagulation defects, with haemorrhage risk in the fetus and newborn, which may be prevented by giving vitamin K prophylactically to the mother before delivery.

Most antiepileptic agents are excreted in breastmilk in varying amounts. Those excreted in high concentration include phenobarbital (phenobarbitone), primidone, ethosuximide, zonisamide and benzodiazepines.

ACETAZOLAMIDE
Trade names
Acetazolamide Powder for Injection, Diamox, Glaumox Powder for Injection

Available forms
Tablets: 250 mg;
Vial: 500 mg

Action
- non-bacterial sulfonamide derivative that inhibits the action of carbonic anhydrase
- appears to retard abnormal, paroxysmal excessive discharge from CNS neurons
- decreases secretion of aqueous humour, thereby reducing intraocular pressure
- increases bicarbonate excretion in the renal tubules and consequently sodium, potassium and water excretion, resulting in an alkaline diuresis

Use
- some types of epilepsy (absence (petit mal) and unlocalised seizures)
- adjunctive treatment in chronic simple (open-angle) glaucoma, secondary glaucoma and preoperatively in acute closed-angle glaucoma (see Antiglaucoma agents, p. 462)
- cardiac and drug-induced oedema, oedema associated with altitude sickness (see Diuretics, p. 1081)

Dose
- (Epilepsy) 250—1000 mg orally or IV daily in divided doses (alone or with other antiepileptic agents)

Adverse effects
- (IV site) pain
- see also Adverse effects of acetazolamide in Diuretics (p. 1081)

Interactions
- not recommended with other carbonic anhydrase inhibitors
- see also Interactions of acetazolamide in Diuretics (p. 1081)

Nursing considerations/Cautions
- if used with other antiepileptic agents, the dose should be started at 250 mg daily and increased slowly
- reconstitute powder using at least 5 mL of water for injections and administer IV
- IV route should be used only short term until oral route is available
- see also Nursing considerations/Cautions for acetazolamide in Diuretics (p. 1081)

Patient education
- see General Patient education for antiepileptics (p. 386)

ANTIEPILEPTICS

 Tablet can be crushed and mixed with water or spoonful of yoghurt or apple puree. Chocolate syrup can be used to mask the bitter taste.

 Teratogenic in animal studies; therefore not recommended during pregnancy, especially during first trimester.

 Caution if used during breastfeeding.

 Banned in sport.

BRIVARACETAM
Trade name
Brivact

Available forms
Vial: 50 mg/5 mL;
Tablets: 25 mg, 50 mg, 75 mg, 100 mg;
Oral solution: 10 mg/mL

Action
- antiepileptic action unclear, but thought to be related to selective affinity for synaptic vesicle protein 2A in the brain
- half-life 9 hours

Use
- as adjunctive therapy of partial-onset seizures (with or without secondary generalisation) in those aged 4 years and over

Dose
- initially 50 mg orally or IV twice daily, increasing in increments of 50 mg per day every 2 weeks if needed (dose range 50–200 mg daily)

Adverse effects
- diarrhoea, constipation, upper abdominal pain, toothache, decreased appetite, weight increase/decrease
- hyponatraemia
- myalgia, back pain, pain in extremities
- nasopharyngitis, upper respiratory tract infection, flu-like symptoms, cough, dyspnoea
- paraesthesia
- pruritus, eczema
- (IV) infusion site pain
- (Rare) hypersensitivity (bronchospasm and angioedema)
- see also General Adverse effects of antiepileptic agents (p. 386)

Interactions
- serum levels may be decreased if given with rifampicin
- may increase serum levels of carbamazepine epoxide (active metabolite of carbamazepine)
- may decrease serum levels of carbamazepine, phenobarbital (phenobarbitone) and phenytoin
- may increase effects of alcohol; therefore not recommended together

Nursing considerations/Cautions
- (IV) may be administered as an IV bolus undiluted, or diluted with sodium chloride 0.9% or glucose 5% and given over 15 minutes
- not recommended in those with end-stage kidney disease undergoing dialysis
- see also General Nursing considerations/ Cautions for antiepileptics (p. 386)

Patient education
- (IV) warn the patient that a bitter taste may be experienced after IV administration
- (Oral solution) ensure the patient understands how to use adaptor/syringe for oral solution, including:
  - press the cap down and turn it clockwise to open the bottle
  - separate the adapter from the syringe (both provided with oral solution)
  - the adaptor should be inserted into the neck of the bottle, ensuring it is well fitted

- insert the syringe into the adaptor opening and turn the bottle upside down
- fill the syringe with a small amount of solution by pulling the piston down, then push it upwards to remove any air bubbles
- pull the piston down to the graduation mark that corresponds to dose in mL (as prescribed by doctor)
- turn the bottle the right way up and remove syringe from adaptor
- empty the contents of the syringe into a glass of water and drink immediately
- close solution bottle with the cap
- wash the syringe with water only
- store at less than 30°C
• advise the patient to seek medical advice if any of the following occur:
  - wheezing or difficulty breathing
  - swelling of face, lips, tongue or other body parts
  - rash, itching or hives on the skin
• see also General Patient education for antiepileptics (p. 386)

Oral solution available. Tablet can be crushed and mixed with water or spoonful of yoghurt or apple puree.

Not recommended during pregnancy unless benefit outweighs risk.

Caution if used in those with liver impairment. Daily dose should not exceed 150 mg in two divided doses.

- for moderate liver impairment, initial dose should be started at 1.25 mg/kg orally twice daily, increasing to 2.5 mg/kg twice daily after 7 days (daily maximum 10 mg/kg)
- for severe liver impairment, initial dose should be started at 0.5 mg/kg orally twice daily, increasing to 1 mg/kg twice daily after 7 days (daily maximum 4 mg/kg)

CANNABIDIOL
Trade name
Epidyolex

Available form
Oral solution: 100 mg/mL

Action
- reduces neuronal hyperexcitability
- half-life 56—61 hours

Use
- adjunctive therapy in the management of seizures associated with Lennox—Gestaut syndrome or Dravet syndrome in those over 2 years

Dose
- initially 2.5 mg/kg orally twice daily for 7 days, then increasing to 5 mg/kg twice daily (maximum 20 mg/kg/day)

Adverse effects
- changes in appetite (increased or decreased), weight decrease
- cough, pneumonia, bronchitis, nasopharyngitis, urinary tract infection
- irritability, agitation, aggression, abnormal behaviour, lethargy, tremor, fatigue
- diarrhoea, vomiting,
- elevated liver transaminases and bilirubin, abnormal liver function
- rash
- fever
- sedation, somnolence, insomnia,
- (Rare) increased seizure activity, suicidal ideation and behaviour

Interactions
- serum levels decreased if given with rifampicin, carbamazepine or St John's wort
- increase sedation and somnolence may occur if given with clobazam. Dose of clobazam should be reduced if given together
- increased incidence of diarrhoea and loss of appetite may occur if given with sodium valproate
- caution if given with phenytoin

ANTIEPILEPTICS

- may increase serum levels of lamotrigine, everolimus, sirolimus, tacrolimus and ciclosporin
- monitoring is recommended if given with digoxin
- caution if given with warfarin and rapaglinide
- may increase serum levels of omeprazole or those with a narrow therapeutic index

Nursing considerations/Cautions

- before starting therapy, serum transaminases (alanine aminotransferase (ALT) and aspartate aminotransferase (AST)) and total bilirubin levels should be measured, then at 2 weeks, 1 month, 2 months, 3 months, 6 months and then as clinically needed
- calculated dose should be rounded to closest graduation for syringe
- if discontinued, dose should be decreased gradually by about 10% per day for 10 days
- if one or two doses are missed, they should not be caught up. If not administered for 7 or more days, titration should be restarted from initial dose
- food impacts serum levels and therefore administration should be consistent (i.e. either with or without food)
- oral solution contains alcohol
- contraindicated if transaminases are 3 times or more above upper normal level and bilirubin levels are 2 times or more above upper normal level
- contraindicated in those with hypersensitivity to sesame oil

Patient education

- the patient/carer should be advised to take/administer medication consistently either with or without food
- the patient/carer should be instructed on correct administration including:
    - understanding that the 1 mL syringe is for administration of 100 mg or less and 5 mL syringe is for doses between 100 and 500 mg. For doses > 500 mg, the 5 mL syringe will be used more than once
    - ensure the correct syringe is chosen
    - check the expiry date
    - removing the child-proof cap and insert the bottle adapter firmly in bottle neck
    - insert correct syringe into bottle adapter, and turn bottle upside down
    - slowly pull syringe plunger back to draw solution into syringe to line plunger up with required volume
    - turn bottle right side up and remove syringe from adapter
    - place tip of syringe inside cheek and gently push plunger to release medication into cheek
    - medication should not be directed to back of mouth or throat
    - replace lid (bottle adapter does not need to be removed)
    - oral syringe should be washed by drawing water in and out of syringe using the plunger. Plunger should be removed from barrel and both parts should be rinsed under running water
    - syringe should be allowed to air dry until next use
    - syringe should not be washed in dishwasher
    - if syringe is not completely dry, it will cause solution to become cloudy, however this does not change the efficacy of the solution
    - date solution bottle when opened and discard after 8 weeks
    - store below 25°C
- the patient should be advised not to drive or operate machinery if sedation or somnolence occurs. They should also be aware that, since this is a cannabis-based medication, driving when using this medication may have legal implications depending on state laws
- the patient/carer should be advised to immediately report:
    - unexplained nausea, vomiting, loss of appetite, right upper quadrant abdominal pain, fatigue, darkening

urine, yellowing of skin or whites of eyes

Not recommended during pregnancy unless benefits outweigh risks to fetus.

Not recommended during breastfeeding.

CARBAMAZEPINE
Trade names
Avloire, Carbamazepine Sandoz, Tegretol

Available forms
Tablets: 100 mg, 200 mg;
Tablets (controlled-release): 200 mg, 400 mg;
Suspension: 100 mg/5 mL

Action
* antiepileptic, neurotrophic, psychotropic
* stabilises hyperexcited nerve membranes
* inhibits repetitive neuronal discharge
* reduces propagation of excitatory impulse
* anticholinergic, antidiuretic activity
* decreases turnover of dopamine and noradrenaline (norepinephrine) (psychotropic (antimania) effects)
* active metabolite (carbamazepine-epoxide) (half-life 6 hours)
* half-life 16—24 hours (with repeated dosing)

Use
* generalised tonic—clonic (grand mal) epilepsy
* partial seizures (complex or simple) (with or without generalisation)
* mixed seizures (tonic—clonic and partial)
* trigeminal neuralgia, glossopharyngeal neuralgia
* mania, bipolar disorder (see Antipsychotic and mood stabilising agents, p. 842)

Dose
* (Epilepsy, adults and children >15 years) initially 100—200 mg orally once or twice daily with or after food, increasing gradually until optimal response is achieved (usually 400 mg 2—3 times daily) **OR**
* (Neuralgia) initially 100—200 mg orally twice daily with or after food, increasing gradually for several days until pain is controlled, then reduced to a minimum effective level (maximum daily dose 1200 mg)

Adverse effects
* dry mouth
* urticaria, allergic dermatitis
* leucopenia, thrombocytopenia, eosinophilia
* elevated liver enzymes
* oedema, fluid retention, increased weight, hyponatraemia, decreased blood osmolarity
* (Rare) lens opacities, conjunctivitis, urinary frequency and retention, cholestatic hepatitis, folate deficiency
* (Very rare) serious dermatological reactions, blood dyscrasias, hypersensitivity
* see also General Adverse effects of antiepileptics (p. 385)

Interactions
* contraindicated with or within 2 weeks of stopping monoamine oxidase inhibitors (MAOIs)
* if given with aripiprazole, haloperidol, lithium or metoclopramide may lead to neurotoxicity (even at therapeutic serum concentrations)
* may reduce tolerance to alcohol
* may decrease serum levels of albendazole, amitriptyline, apixaban, aprepitant, atorvastatin, buprenorphine, bupropion, citalopram, clobazam, clomipramine, clonazepam, clozapine, cyclophosphamide, ciclosporin, dabigatran, dexamethasone, digoxin, doxycycline, ethosuximide, everolimus, felodipine, haloperidol, imatinib, imipramine, indinavir, itraconazole, ivabradine, lapatinib, lamotrigine, levothyroxine, lovastatin, methadone, mianserin, midazolam, nortriptyline, olanzapine, oral contraceptives, oxcarbazepine,

ANTIEPILEPTICS

- paliperidone, paracetamol, phenytoin, praziquantel, prednisolone, primidone, progesterone-containing products, quetiapine, rifabutin, risperidone, ritonavir, sertraline, simvastatin, sirolimus, sodium valproate, tacrolimus, tadalafil, theophylline, tiagabine, topiramate, tramadol, voriconazole, warfarin and ziprasidone
- serum levels may be increased by acetazolamide, antiviral protease inhibitors, clarithromycin, ciprofloxacin, dantrolene, danazol, diltiazem, erythromycin, fluconazole, fluoxetine, fluvoxamine, grapefruit juice, ibuprofen, isoniazid, itraconazole, loratadine, nicotinamide (high dose), olanzapine, omeprazole, oxybutynin, paroxetine, primidone, quetiapine, ritonavir, sodium valproate, ticlopidine, TCAs, verapamil, vigabatrin and voriconazole, resulting in adverse reactions
- serum levels may be decreased by aminophylline, barbiturates, cisplatin, clonazepam, doxorubicin, isotretinoin, oxcarbazepine, phenobarbital (phenobarbitone), phenytoin, primidone, rifampicin, sodium valproate, St John's wort and theophylline
- use with lamotrigine may result in carbamazepine toxicity, as well as decreasing serum levels of lamotrigine
- increased risk of toxicity if given with levetiracetam
- may decrease serum levels of hormonal contraceptives, increasing the risk of bleeding
- hepatotoxicity may occur if given with isoniazid
- may increase metabolism of paracetamol, reducing its analgesic effects as well as increasing risk of hepatotoxicity due to an increase in levels of hepatoxic metabolite
- may reduce serum levels of isotretinoin and other retinoids by increasing clearance
- in those with hypothyroidism, serum levels of thyroid hormones may be reduced, requiring an increase in dosage. Thyroid function should be closely monitored
- may antagonise non-depolarising muscle relaxants (e.g. pancuronium)
- hyponatraemia may result if given with furosemide (frusemide) or hydrochlorothiazide. If given together, serum sodium levels should be measured before starting, after 2 weeks and monthly for 12 weeks during therapy
- may decrease serum levels of apixaban, rivaroxaban and dabigatran, increasing the risk of thrombus formation
- may cause serotonin syndrome (see Glossary) if given with selective serotonin reuptake inhibitor (SSRI) antidepressants
- may interfere with some serological tests

Nursing considerations/Cautions

- elderly patients may become confused or agitated and so will require close supervision
- full blood count (including serum iron) is recommended before starting therapy, then weekly for the first month, then monthly for the first year
- baseline and regular ophthalmological and liver function tests (especially in the elderly or those with liver impairment), complete urinalysis and blood urea nitrogen (BUN) are recommended
- absorption of oral suspension is faster than for tablets
- if changed from immediate-release tablets to suspension, dose should remain the same, but frequency should be increased
- if switching from immediate release to controlled release tablets, dose may need to be increased
- (Epilepsy, oral solution) daily maximum is 1200 mg
- (Neuralgia) large doses should be given as 3—4 divided doses
- (Neuralgia) attempts to discontinue should be at intervals not more than 12 weeks, as there may be periods of remission from the neuralgia

- caution if used in the elderly or others at risk of confusion, agitation or psychosis
- caution if used in those with pre-existing kidney conditions associated with low sodium or in those treated with sodium-lowering medications (e.g. diuretics). Sodium levels should be measured before starting therapy, after 2 weeks, then monthly for 3 months
- caution if used in those with glaucoma, urinary retention or prostatism (because of anticholinergic adverse effects)
- caution if used in those with mixed seizures, as seizure activity may be exacerbated
- caution if used in those with history of cardiac, liver or kidney damage, previous interrupted course of carbamazepine or those who have had previous haematological reactions to other drugs
- caution if used in those with hypothyroidism, as thyroid replacement therapy may need to be increased. Regular thyroid function monitoring is also recommended
- caution if used in those with genetic risk of severe dermatological reactions, including those from Japan, Southern India or Asia (Philippines, Thailand, Malaysia, Hong Kong, Taiwan, North China), or Indigenous Americans or those of Hispanic or Arabic descent. Genetic testing for specific gene is recommended (if available) and not recommended in those with the HLA-A*3101 or HLA-B*1502 allele positive
- suspension contains para-hydroxybenzoates, which can cause allergic reactions, and also sorbitol, and therefore should not be given to those with hereditary fructose intolerance
- cross-hypersensitivity can occur with primidone, phenobarbital (phenobarbitone), phenytoin, oxcarbazepine and carbamazepine
- contraindicated in those with AV block, systemic lupus erythematosus (SLE), porphyrias, bone marrow depression or liver failure
- see also General Nursing considerations/Cautions for antiepileptics (p. 386)

Patient education

- sustained/controlled-release tablets should be swallowed whole (not crushed or chewed), but those which are scored may be halved
- remind the patient to shake the suspension well before administration
- the patient should be warned to avoid grapefruit and grapefruit juice during therapy
- advise the patient against taking paracetamol for a prolonged period during therapy
- the patient should be advised to seek medical advice immediately if any of the following occur:
  - flu-like symptoms (e.g. fever, sore throat, swollen glands, aching joints, lack of energy)
  - frequent infections including fever, chills, sore throat or mouth ulcers
  - persistent nausea and vomiting, loss of appetite, generally feeling unwell
  - darkened urine, yellowing of skin or whites of the eyes
  - easy bruising or bleeding
  - lethargy, vomiting, headache, confusion
  - rash or other skin lesions
- the patient should be advised to have regular ophthalmological examinations
- see also General Patient education for antiepileptics (p. 386)

Oral liquid is available. A plain tablet can be dispersed in water or crushed and mixed with flavoured syrup.

Controlled-release tablets should not be crushed, chewed or broken.

Associated with spina bifida, hypospadias, craniofacial defects, cardiovascular malformations, fingernail hypoplasia and developmental disability. May also cause coagulation defects, leading to the risk of

ANTIEPILEPTICS

fetal haemorrhage, which may be prevented by prophylactic administration of vitamin K to the mother before delivery. May also cause neonatal withdrawal syndrome (vomiting, diarrhoea and/or reduced feeding), as well as seizures and/or respiratory depression.

 Secreted in breastmilk; therefore use with great caution and observe the newborn for skin reactions, including jaundice or excessive sleepiness.

CLONAZEPAM

Trade names
Paxam, Rivotril

Available forms
Tablets: 0.5 mg, 2 mg;
Suspension: 2.5 mg/mL;
Ampoule: 1 mg/mL

Action
- benzodiazepine closely related to nitrazepam, with antiepileptic, sedative and muscle-relaxant properties
- long half-life (31—47 hours)
- tolerance may occur after 4—24 weeks, leading to increase in seizure frequency

Use
- status epilepticus (IV)
- generalised epilepsy (myoclonic, akinetic, tonic, tonic—clonic)
- partial epilepsy (including psychomotor seizures)

Dose
- (Adult) initially 0.5 mg orally twice daily, then 4—8 mg in 3—4 divided doses as maintenance (daily maximum 20 mg) **OR**
- (Status epilepticus) 1 mg by slow IV injection over 2—4 minutes or IV infusion at 0.25—0.5 mg/min, repeated IV or IV infusion until status is controlled (maximum 10 mg)

Adverse effects
- ankle/face oedema
- dyspepsia, increased appetite, constipation, dysphagia
- hirsutism
- leucopenia, eosinophilia, anaemia
- dysuria, nocturia, enuresis, urinary retention
- double vision (high-dose or long-term therapy)
- shortness of breath, respiratory depression
- transient amnesia
- hypersalivation (especially in infants and children)
- bronchial hypersecretions
- (IV) respiratory depression, tachycardia, palpitations
- (IV) thrombophlebitis
- dependence, tolerance, withdrawal syndrome on stopping therapy suddenly, abuse potential
- (Rare) paradoxical reactions (agitation, nervousness, hostility, anxiety, sleep and dream disturbance, rage, excitement), hypotension, cardiac failure, thrombocytopenia
- see also General Adverse effects of antiepileptics (p. 385)

Interactions
- CNS depressant effects enhanced by alcohol
- may enhance effects of other CNS depressant drugs such as other antiepileptic agents, barbiturates, antipsychotic agents, anaesthetics, sedatives, hypnotics, lithium, tricyclic antidepressants (TCAs), antihistamines, opioid analgesics, monoamine oxidase inhibitors (MAOIs)
- serum levels may be decreased by phenytoin, phenobarbital (phenobarbitone), sodium valproate, lamotrigine and carbamazepine
- serum levels may be increased by disulfiram
- may decrease serum levels of carbamazepine
- may increase or decrease serum levels of phenytoin
- may increase anticholinergic effects of antihistamines, some antidepressants and atropine-like drugs
- if given with sodium valproate, may produce absence seizures

Nursing considerations/Cautions

- clonazepam can be absorbed by PVC; therefore glass containers should be used or, if PVC infusion bags are used, the mixture should be infused immediately at greater than 60 mL/hour and short tubing used
- BP and respiratory rate should be monitored continually during IV administration
- blood counts and liver function should be monitored if therapy is longer than 4 weeks
- only large vessels should be used for IV administration to avoid thrombophlebitis
- contents of ampoule to be mixed thoroughly with supplied diluent
- IV infusion prepared by diluting 3 mg in 250 mL of sodium chloride 0.9%, glucose 5% or 10% or sodium chloride 0.45% plus glucose 2.5%
- (IV) not compatible with sodium bicarbonate, as precipitation will occur
- regular blood counts and liver function tests are recommended in those with impaired liver or kidney function
- changes in behaviour (e.g. agitation, hostility, anxiety) suggestive of paradoxical reaction may require withdrawal of drug
- tablets contain lactose and are therefore not recommended in those with rare hereditary problems of galactose intolerance, Lapp lactase deficiency or glucose–galactose malabsorption
- ampoules contain benzyl alcohol and may lead to irreversible brain damage in newborn infants, so should be avoided unless no alternative is available
- in the case of overdose, flumazenil should be given with extreme caution, as it may provoke seizures
- suspension contains lactose and therefore not recommended in those with galactose intolerance
- caution if used in the elderly (because of the increased risk of falls) or those with a predisposition to hypotension, glaucoma, myasthenia gravis, respiratory depression, ataxia, blood dyscrasias, kidney impairment or porphyria
- not recommended in those with pre-existing depression, psychosis, schizophrenia, spinal or cerebellar ataxia or sleep apnoea
- contraindicated in those with hypersensitivity to benzodiazepines, alcohol/drug dependency (or history), chronic obstructive pulmonary disease (COPD) (with developing respiratory failure) or severe liver impairment
- see also General Nursing considerations/Cautions for antiepileptics (p. 386)

Patient education

- advise the patient that tablet is scored if half or quarter tablet is required
- (Suspension) suspension is recommended for infants
- suspension is delivered via dropper (1 drop = 0.1 mg clonazepam). Instruct the patient (or carer) to use the supplied dropper to measure dose and deliver onto a spoon (not directly into mouth)
- oral suspension is compatible with fruit juice, water or tea
- see also General Patient education for antiepileptics (p. 386)

Suspension available. Tablet can be dispersed in 5–20 mL water, or crushed and mixed with a spoonful of apple puree.

Clonazepam is a benzodiazepine and if given during pregnancy may result in hypotonia, respiratory depression and hypothermia of the newborn. The newborn may also display signs of withdrawal symptoms.

Not recommended during breastfeeding as it may cause drowsiness and feeding difficulties.

Caution if used in those with mild-to-moderate liver impairment. Lowest dose possible should be prescribed.

ANTIEPILEPTICS

 Caution if used in the elderly because of the increased risk of falls. Lowest dose possible is recommended.

ETHOSUXIMIDE
Trade names
Ethosuximide Essential Generics, Zarontin

Available forms
Capsules: 250 mg;
Suspension: 250 mg/5 mL

Action
- succinimide that may depress the motor cortex and elevate convulsive threshold, reducing the frequency of seizures

Use
- simple partial (petit mal) epilepsy

Dose
- initially 20–30 mg/kg orally given in 2 divided doses, increasing by 250 mg every 4–7 days until control is achieved with minimal side-effects (daily maximum 1.5 g)

Adverse effects
- anorexia, cramps, diarrhoea, epigastric pain, upper abdominal pain, weight loss, gum hypertrophy, tongue swelling
- hiccups
- urticaria
- blood dyscrasias
- (Rare) SLE, myopia, vaginal bleeding, hirsutism, hypersensitivity, serious skin reactions, haematuria, psychosis, increased libido, liver and kidney impairment
- see also General Adverse effects of antiepileptics (p. 385)

Interactions
- serum levels may be altered if given with sodium valproate
- may increase phenytoin serum levels

Nursing considerations/Cautions
- doses greater than 1.5 g/ day in divided doses only, administered under strict medical supervision
- be aware of the possibility of increased frequency of tonic—clonic (grand mal) seizures when ethosuximide is used alone in mixed types of epilepsy
- full blood count weekly for the first month, then monthly for the first year
- regular urinalysis and liver function tests are recommended during therapy
- caution if used in those with blood dyscrasias, liver or kidney impairment
- contraindicated in those with hypersensitivity to succinimides
- see also General Nursing considerations/Cautions for antiepileptics (p. 386)

Patient education
- advise the patient to seek medical advice immediately if any of the following occurs:
  - rash, blistering, fever, swollen glands (especially in first 28 days of therapy)
  - flu-like symptoms (e.g. fever, sore throat, swollen glands, aching joints, lack of energy)
  - frequent infections, including fever, chills, sore throat or mouth ulcers
  - easy bruising or bleeding
- see also General Patient education for antiepileptics (p. 386)

 Oral suspension is available. Contents of capsule cannot be extracted easily.

 Not recommended during pregnancy, as birth defects may occur.

 Excreted in high concentration in breast-milk; therefore not recommended during breastfeeding unless benefits outweigh risks to the fetus.

GABAPENTIN

Trade names
APX-Gabapentin, Gabacor, Gabapentin Sandoz, Gabapentin-WGR, Gapentin, Neurontin, Nupentin, Pharmacor Gabapentin, WP-Gabapentin

Available forms
Tablets: 600 mg, 800 mg;
Capsules: 100 mg, 300 mg, 400 mg

Action
* structurally related to the neurotransmitter GABA, but its exact antiepileptic action is unknown, although it is not thought to interact with the sodium channels
* half-life 5–7 hours

Use
* as adjunct therapy for partial seizures, including generalised tonic–clonic seizures in patients who have not achieved control with standard antiepileptic drugs
* neuropathic pain

Dose
* (Epilepsy) 300 mg on day 1 (at night to minimise adverse effects), 300 mg twice daily (day 2), and 300 mg 3 times daily (day 3), increasing dose further if needed (up to 2.4 g) **OR**
* (Neuropathic pain) initially 300 mg orally 3 times daily, increasing if necessary (daily maximum 3.6 g)

Adverse effects
* abdominal pain, increased appetite, weight increase, dyspepsia, dry mouth, constipation, diarrhoea, dental abnormalities
* impotence
* rhinitis, pharyngitis, coughing
* pruritus, acne
* myalgia, back pain
* peripheral oedema
* leucopenia
* fever
* (Rare) drug rash with eosinophilia and systemic symptoms (DRESS), anaphylaxis, abuse and dependence, respiratory depression
* see also General Adverse effects of antiepileptics (p. 385)

Interactions
* bioavailability may be decreased by antacids and therefore should be separated by a 2-hour interval
* increased risk of CNS depression if given with morphine
* may produce false positive reading on urinary protein test

Nursing considerations/Cautions
* the patient should be be carefully assessed for any current or past history of abuse or dependence on opioids or benzodiazepines, as abuse and dependence can lead to overdose and/or death if used with opioids and other CNS depressants
* caution in those with mixed epilepsy that includes absence seizures, because gabapentin may exacerbate absence seizures
* caution if used in those with kidney insufficiency or on dialysis
* caution if used in those with a current or past history of abuse or dependence on opioids and/or benzodiazepines
* see also General Nursing considerations/Cautions for antiepileptics (p. 386)

Patient education
* the patient should be advised not to allow more than 12 hours between doses. If a dose is missed by less than 4 hours, it may be taken. If more than 4 hours, the dose should be missed and the next dose taken at the usual time
* may be taken with or without food
* advise the patient not to take antacids for heartburn or reflux within 2 hours of gabapentin
* instruct the patient to seek medical advice immediately if any of the following occur:

ANTIEPILEPTICS

- fever, swollen glands or rash
- breathing difficulty, swelling of lips, throat or tongue, feeling light-headed
- see also General Patient education for antiepileptics (p. 386)

Capsules can be opened and contents dispersed in water or orange juice. Tablet can be crushed and mixed with water or orange juice, or a spoonful of apple puree or chocolate pudding. (Note: tablet is very hard to crush.)

Use during pregnancy only if benefits outweigh risks to the fetus.

Use during breastfeeding only if benefits outweigh risks.

Dose reduction is required for those with kidney impairment, with dose and frequency determined by patient kidney function (creatinine clearance).

LACOSAMIDE
Trade names
Lacoress, Lacosam, Lacosamide ARX, Lacosamide Lupin, Lacosamide Sandoz, Vimcosa, Vimpat

Available forms
Tablets: 50 mg, 100 mg, 150 mg, 200 mg;
Oral liquid: 10 mg/mL;
Ampoule: 200 mg/20 mL

Action
- appears to selectively enhance slow inactivation of voltage-gated sodium channels, reducing hyperexcitability of neuronal membranes
- half-life about 13 hours

Use
- therapy for partial seizures, with or without secondary generalisation (in patients over 16 years) as monotherapy or adjunct therapy

Dose
- (Monotherapy) 200 mg orally or IV infusion over 15–60 minutes (loading dose), then 50 mg twice daily, increasing dose at weekly intervals if needed to maximum daily dose 600 mg **OR**
- (Adjunctive therapy) 200 mg orally or IV infusion over 15–60 minutes (loading dose), then 50 mg twice daily, increasing dose at weekly intervals if needed to maximum daily dose 400 mg

Adverse effects
- tinnitus
- muscle spasm
- constipation, flatulence, dry mouth, dyspepsia, diarrhoea
- pruritus
- nasopharyngitis
- (Rare) PR interval prolongation, elevated liver enzymes, hepatitis
- (IV) pain, discomfort, irritation, erythema
- see also General Adverse effects of antiepileptics (p. 385)

Interaction
- caution if used with other agents known to prolong PR interval or class I antiarrhythmic agents

Nursing considerations/Cautions
- IV route is recommended where oral route is not feasible
- if a loading dose is not required, dose should be started at 50 mg twice daily
- (IV) can be given undiluted, or as diluted solution with sodium chloride 0.9%, glucose 5% or lactated Ringer's solution
- IV infusion should be given over 15–60 minutes
- conversion from IV to oral dosage can be done without titrations
- if converting to monotherapy from other antiepileptic agents, other agents should be withdrawn over at least 6 weeks
- ECG is recommended before starting therapy
- when discontinuing therapy, gradual withdrawal at a rate of 200 mg per week is recommended

- dose reduction is recommended in those with severe kidney impairment
- caution if used in those with severe liver impairment
- caution if used in those with known conduction problems (e.g. sick sinus syndrome without pacemaker, marked first degree AV block), severe cardiovascular disease, diabetic neuropathy
- contraindicated in those with second or third degree AV block
- see also General Nursing considerations/Cautions for antiepileptics (p. 386)

Patient education

- advise the patient that oral solution can be diluted in water if needed
- instruct the patient to discard oral solution 2 months after opening and stored below 30°C but not frozen or refrigerated
- the patient should be advised to seek medical advice immediately if any of the following occur:
    - lightheadedness and/or fainting
    - slow or irregular pulse
    - shortness of breath or palpitations
- see also General Patient education for antiepileptics (p. 386)

Oral solution available. Tablet can be dispersed in water or crushed and mixed with spoonful of yoghurt or apple puree.

Recommended during pregnancy only if benefits to mother clearly outweigh risks to fetus.

Maximum daily dose of 250 mg is recommended for those with severe kidney impairment.

Maximum daily dose of 300 mg is recommended for those with mild-to-moderate liver impairment, and administered to those with severe liver impairment only if the benefits outweigh the risks.

LAMOTRIGINE

Trade names
APX-Lamotrigine, Lamictal, Lamitan, Lamotrigine GH, Lamotrigine-WGR, Lamotrust, Logem, Noumed Lamotrigine, Reedos, Sandoz Lamotrigine, Torlemo DT

Available forms
Tablets (dispersible/chewable): 2 mg, 5 mg, 25 mg, 50 mg, 100 mg, 200 mg

Action
- phenyltriazine compound
- exact mechanism of action unknown, but thought to inhibit voltage-gated sodium channels and decrease release of glutamate and aspartate (excitatory amino acids)
- half-life 29 hours

Use
- partial and generalised seizures, as both monotherapy and adjunct therapy
- prevention of depressive episodes in patients with bipolar disorder

Dose
- (Epilepsy, monotherapy) initially 25 mg orally daily for 2 weeks, increased to 50 mg (weeks 3 and 4), then increasing by 50—100 mg every 1—2 weeks until optimum dose is achieved, and then maintained on 100—200 mg orally daily or in 2 divided doses **OR**
- (Epilepsy, with sodium valproate) initially 25 mg orally on alternate days for 2 weeks, increased to 25 mg daily (weeks 3 and 4), then increasing by 25—50 mg every 1—2 weeks until optimum dose is achieved, and then maintained on 100—200 mg daily or in 2 divided doses **OR**
- (Epilepsy, with other antiepileptic agents) initially 25—50 mg orally for 2 weeks, then increased by 50—100 mg every 1—2 weeks, and then maintained on 100—400 mg daily in divided doses **OR**
- (Bipolar disorder, adjunct therapy) initially 25 mg orally on alternate days

ANTIEPILEPTICS

for 2 weeks, then 25 mg orally daily (weeks 3 and 4), then 50 orally (as either single daily or divided dose) (week 5), increasing to 100 mg (as either single daily or divided dose) (daily maximum 200 mg)

Adverse effects
- maculopapular rash, Stevens—Johnson syndrome (see Glossary), toxic epidermal necrolysis
- pharyngitis
- elevated liver enzymes, diarrhoea
- (Bipolar disorder) worsening of symptoms or appearance of new symptoms of bipolar disorder
- (Uncommon) transient haematological abnormalities, hypersensitivity
- (Rare) liver dysfunction, aseptic meningitis, worsening of parkinsonian symptoms, haemophagocytic lymphohistiocytosis, arrhythmias, Brugada-type ECG
- see also General Adverse effects of antiepileptics (p. 385)

Interactions
- metabolism may be increased by phenytoin, carbamazepine, phenobarbital (phenobarbitone), primidone, rifampicin, ritonavir and combined oral contraceptives
- serum levels may be increased by sodium valproate, increasing the risk of severe rash
- serum levels may be decreased by oral contraceptives; therefore caution when starting or stopping therapy, as dose of lamotrigine may need to be adjusted
- CNS adverse effects may be increased by carbamazepine
- not recommended with other sodium channel blocking agents owing to the risk of arrhythmias
- may interfere with some rapid urine drug screen leading to false positive for phencyclidine (PCP)

Nursing considerations/Cautions
- skin rash usually appears within 8 weeks of starting therapy and disappears on withdrawal. Stopping therapy is recommended at first sign of rash unless the rash is known to be non-drug related
- if the patient has stopped therapy (not associated with development of rash), was previously on a high dose and requires restarting the therapy again, consideration should be given to restarting at the maintenance dose (rather than the initial dose) to decrease the risk of serious dermatological adverse effects
- if being used as an add-on therapy and discontinuing of the other antiepileptic is required, careful monitoring is needed. Depending on what the other antiepileptic was and whether it impacted on serum levels, the dose of lamotrigine may need to be adjusted
- caution if used in those with Parkinson's disease, or kidney or liver failure
- caution if used in those with a history of allergy or antiepileptic-induced rash, as the risk of severe skin reactions is increased
- caution if used in those with bipolar disorder or a history of suicidal thoughts or behaviours
- (Epilepsy) not recommended as monotherapy in newly diagnosed children
- (Bipolar disorder) not recommended in those under 18 years
- (Epilepsy) not recommended in those with cardiac conduction disorders, cardiac disease or abnormality (e.g. structural heart disease), ventricular arrhythmias or Brugada syndrome
- see also General Nursing considerations/Cautions for antiepileptics (p. 386)

Patient education
- advise the patient that dispersible/chewable tablets can be swallowed whole, chewed or dispersed in a small amount of water
- warn parents that children have a higher risk of serious skin reactions
- the patient/carer should be advised to seek medical advice immediately if any of the following occur:
  - rash or skin reaction

- fever, rash, swollen glands (especially if they occur 8–24 days after starting therapy)
- headache, fever, neck stiffness, photophobia, nausea, vomiting, rash, chills, muscle aches, change in consciousness and sleepiness (which may occur 1-45 days after starting therapy)
- (Bipolar disorder) the patient/carer should be warned to immediately report any change in mood, depression, thoughts of self-harm or suicide
- see also General Patient education for antiepileptics (p. 386)

Tablets can be dispersed in 2.5 mL water and then mixed with spoonful of yoghurt or apple puree.

May cause cleft palate if used during pregnancy; therefore should be avoided unless the benefits outweigh risks to the fetus.

Use during breastfeeding only if the benefits outweigh risks to the newborn.

Caution is recommended if used in those with kidney failure.

Dose should be reduced by 50 to 75% depending on the severity of the liver impairment.

Pregnant staff should not disperse tablets.

LEVETIRACETAM
Trade names
APO-Levetiracetam, Auro-Levetiraceam, Hospira Levetiracetam Concentrate for IV Infusion, Keppra Oral, Kerron, Kevtam, Levactam, Levecetam, Levetiracetam-GH, Levetiracetam IV ARX, Levetiracetam Medsurge, Levetiracetam Sandoz, Levetiracetam SZ, Levetiracetam Viatris, Levetiracetam AFT, Levetiracetam-GH, Levetiracetam-WGR, Levi, Levitam, Noumed Levetiracetam

Available forms
Vial: 500 mg/5 mL;
Tablets: 250 mg, 500 mg, 1000 mg; Suspension: 100 mg/mL

Action
- unknown antiepileptic action, although thought to interact with specific binding site in CNS
- active metabolite
- half-life about 6–8 hours

Use
- as monotherapy or adjunct therapy in partial seizures (with or without secondary generalisation), myoclonic seizures in those with juvenile myoclonic epilepsy, or primary generalised tonic–clonic seizures in those with idiopathic generalised epilepsy

Dose
- (Monotherapy) initially 250 mg orally or by IV infusion twice daily for 2 weeks, then increasing to 500 mg twice daily for 2 weeks; further increases of 250 mg increments twice daily at 2-week intervals may be necessary, depending on clinical response (daily maximum 1500 mg twice daily) **OR**
- (Adjunct therapy) initially 500 mg orally or by IV infusion twice daily, increasing by 500 mg twice-daily increments at 2–4-week intervals if necessary (daily maximum 1500 mg twice daily)

Adverse effects
- upper respiratory tract infection, flu-like syndrome, increased cough, pharyngitis, rhinitis, sinusitis, nasopharyngitis, bronchitis
- fever
- eczema, pruritus
- anorexia, gastroenteritis, gingivitis, tooth disorders, weight gain, abdominal pain
- ecchymosis, thrombocytopenia
- myalgia, back pain
- (Rare) QT interval prolongation, blood dyscrasias
- (Very rare) acute kidney damage

ANTIEPILEPTICS

- see also General Adverse effects of antiepileptics (p. 385)

Interactions
- probenecid inhibits renal clearance of metabolite but not levetiracetam
- caution if used with other agents that prolong QT interval or cause electrolyte disturbance
- may decrease methotrexate clearance increasing serum levels and risk of adverse effects
- increased risk of anorexia if given with topiramate

Nursing considerations/Cautions
- any electrolyte disturbance should be corrected before starting therapy
- IV should be used only when oral administration is not possible
- oral and IV dosages are the same
- should not be given as a direct IV injection or rapid infusion
- dilute IV concentrate with at least 100 mL of sodium chloride 0.9%, glucose 5% or lactated Ringer's solution
- IV infusion given over 15 minutes
- (IV) not compatible with IV phenytoin
- (IV) administer alone
- not suitable for status epilepticus
- (Oral solution) contains hydroxybenzoates, which may cause allergic reactions in susceptible individuals
- (Oral solution) contains glycerol and is not recommended in those with fructose intolerance
- caution if used in those with known QT prolongation, cardiac disease or electrolyte disturbances
- contraindicated in those with hypersensitivity to pyrrolidine derivatives
- see also General Nursing considerations/Cautions for antiepileptics (p. 386)

Patient education
- advise the patient that an oral suspension may be diluted with water
- warn the patient that a bitter taste may be experienced after oral administration
- instruct the patient (or carer) to write the date of opening oral solution on the bottle and discard 7 months after opening. Should be stored below 25°C and protected from light
- see also General Patient education for antiepileptics (p. 386)

 Available as an oral liquid. Tablet can be crushed and mixed with water, or spoonful of yoghurt or apple puree.

 Use during pregnancy only if benefits outweigh risks to fetus.

 Secreted in breastmilk; therefore not recommended during breastfeeding.

 Dose adjustment is required in those with impaired kidney function and should be based on creatinine clearance. 50% maintenance dose reduction is recommended if CrCl < 60 mL/min.

 Dose adjustment is recommended in those > 65 years who have kidney impairment.

OXCARBAZEPINE
Trade name
Trileptal

Available forms
Tablets: 150 mg, 300 mg, 600 mg;
Oral suspension: 60 mg/mL

Action
- analogue of carbamazepine
- inhibits voltage-sensitive sodium channels, stabilising hyperexcited neural membrane, inhibiting repetitive neural firing and decreasing synaptic impulse propagation
- increases potassium conductance and modulates high-voltage-activated calcium channels
- activity due to active metabolite
- half-life 1.3—2.3 hours, metabolite half-life 7.5—11 hours

Use
- partial or generalised tonic—clonic seizures in adults or children as either monotherapy or adjunctive therapy

Dose
- (Adult) initially 300 mg orally twice daily, increasing by 600 mg per day at weekly intervals if required (maximum daily dose 2400 mg)

Adverse effects
- abdominal pain, constipation, diarrhoea, weight increase
- asymptomatic hyponatraemia
- alopecia, acne
- (Rare) hypersensitivity, anaphylaxis, angioedema, multi-organ hypersensitivity
- (Very rare) Stevens—Johnson syndrome (see Glossary), toxic epidermal necrolysis, erythema multiforme, hypothyroidism, blood dyscrasias
- see also General Adverse effects of antiepileptics (p. 385)

Interactions
- caution if used with St John's wort
- serum levels may be increased by phenobarbital (phenobarbitone)
- may increase serum levels of amitriptyline, citalopram, clomipramine, cyclophosphamide, diazepam, imipramine, lansoprazole, omeprazole, pantoprazole, phenobarbital (phenobarbitone), phenytoin, progesterone, proguanil, propranolol and sodium valproate
- serum levels may be lowered by phenytoin
- serum levels may be increased by ciclosporin
- may increase hyponatraemic effects of drugs that lower serum sodium levels
- may decrease serum levels of felodipine and carbamazepine
- may decrease effectiveness of combined oral contraceptives containing progestogens
- may increase sedative effects of alcohol
- active metabolite levels may be decreased if given with rifampicin, carbamazepine, phenytoin or phenobarbital (phenobarbitone)

Nursing considerations/Cautions
- doses of oral suspension and tablets are bioequivalent
- regular weight measurement is recommended in those with cardiac insufficiency/failure to detect any fluid retention. Serum sodium levels should be measured if fluid retention occurs
- serum sodium levels should be measured before starting, after 2 weeks then monthly throughout therapy, especially in those who have low sodium levels (due to either medical conditions or sodium-lowering agents or in the elderly)
- thyroid function should be monitored in children starting therapy
- (Oral suspension) contains parabens, which can cause an allergic reaction in susceptible individuals
- (Oral suspension) contains sorbitol, which is converted to fructose and may be problematic for those with fructose intolerance
- caution if used in those with a genetic risk of severe dermatological reactions, including those from Japan, Southern India, Asia (Philippines, Thailand, Malaysia, Hong Kong, Taiwan, North China), in Indigenous Americans, or of Hispanic or Arabic descent. Genetic testing for specific gene is recommended (if available) and not recommended in those with the HLA-A*3101 or HLA-B*1502 allele positive
- cross-hypersensitivity can occur with phenytoin, oxcarbazepine and carbamazepine
- caution if used in those with AV block, arrhythmias or other conduction disorders
- caution in those with liver or kidney impairment
- see also General Nursing considerations/Cautions for antiepileptics (p. 386)

ANTIEPILEPTICS

Patient education
- the patient should be advised to seek medical advice immediately if any of the following occur:
  - rash or skin reactions
  - headache, lethargy, dizziness, nausea, vomiting or confusion (may be signs of hyponatraemia)
  - any swelling of eyelids, lips, mouth or throat
- the patient should be advised to shake the suspension well before administration
- the patient should be advised to use the supplied dosing syringe for administration of oral suspension
- the oral suspension may be taken directly from syringe or mixed with water and taken immediately
- female patients should be warned of a potential decrease in effectiveness of oral contraceptives during therapy and advised to use a non-hormonal or barrier form of contraception
- see also General Patient education for antiepileptics (p. 386)

An oral suspension is available. Tablet can be crushed and mixed with water, or spoonful of yoghurt or apple puree. Tablet is hard to crush and should be crushed in a closed tablet crusher.

Not recommended during pregnancy. Related to carbamazepine, which is teratogenic.

Oxcarbazepine and active metabolite are excreted in breastmilk; therefore are not recommended during breastfeeding.

In those with kidney impairment, if creatinine clearance is < 30 mL/min, the starting dose should be halved (300 mg daily) and increased slowly to achieve the clinical result.

Dose reduction is recommended in those > 65 years if creatinine clearance is < 30 mL/min.

Staff should wear gown and gloves if crushing tablets.

PERAMPANEL
Trade name
Fycompa

Available form
Tablets: 2 mg, 4 mg, 6 mg, 8 mg, 10 mg, 12 mg;

Action
- alpha-amino-3-hydroxy-5-methyl-4-isoxazolepropionic acid (AMPA) glutamate receptor antagonist (glutamate is a CNS excitatory neurotransmitter thought to be involved in neurological disorders involving neuronal overexcitation)
- half-life 25 hours
- decreased clearance in females

Use
- adjunctive treatment of partial-onset seizures (with or without generalised seizures) in patients over 12 years
- adjunctive treatment of primary generalised tonic–clonic seizures in adults and those over 12 years with idiopathic generalised epilepsy

Dose
- initially 2 mg orally at night, increasing in increments of 2 mg/day at 1–2-weekly intervals to a daily maintenance of 4–8 mg (depending on response and tolerance to a daily maximum 12 mg)

Adverse effects
- arthralgia, myalgia, musculoskeletal pain, back pain
- constipation, weight gain
- cough

- (Rare) multiorgan hypersensitivity, hepatotoxicity
- see also General Adverse effects of antiepileptics (p. 385)

Interactions
- may decrease efficacy of combined oral contraceptives
- decreased plasma levels may occur if given with carbamazepine, phenytoin, oxcarbazepine, rifampicin or St John's wort
- caution if given with alcohol or other CNS depressants

Nursing considerations/Cautions
- tablets contain lactose and should not be used in those with rare hereditary problems of galactose intolerance, Lapp lactase deficiency or glucose—galactose malabsorption
- caution if used in the elderly because of the increased risk of dizziness and falls
- caution if used in those with a history of substance abuse
- not recommended in children under 4 years
- not recommended in those with moderate-to-severe kidney failure, on haemodialysis or with severe liver impairment
- not recommended as monotherapy
- see also General Nursing considerations/Cautions for antiepileptics (p. 386)

Patient education
- women of childbearing potential taking combined oral contraceptives should be counselled to use additional non-hormonal contraceptive methods (e.g. condom, intrauterine advice) during therapy to avoid the risk of pregnancy
- see also General Patient education for antiepileptics (p. 386)

 Tablets can be dispersed in water, or crushed and mixed with spoonful of yoghurt or apple puree.

 Not recommended during pregnancy unless the benefits are thought to outweigh the risks to the fetus.

 Not recommended during breastfeeding.

 Dose should not exceed 8 mg in those with mild-to-moderate liver impairment.

PHENOBARBITAL (PHENOBARBITONE)

Trade names
Orion Phenobarbital Elixir, Phenobarbital Injection, Phenobarb

Available forms
Tablets: 30 mg;
Ampoules: 200 mg/mL;
Suspension: 15 mg/5 mL

Action
- long-acting barbiturate with sedative, hypnotic and antiepileptic properties
- thought to mimic or enhance actions of gamma aminobutyric acid (GABA)
- depresses synaptic transmission and increases threshold for electrical stimulation in the motor cortex
- long half-life (90—100 hours)
- therapeutic serum level 15—40 microgram/mL (65—170 microM/L)

Use
- epilepsy (grand mal and psychomotor)
- status epilepticus
- sedation

Dose
- (Epilepsy) 60—240 mg orally in 2—3 divided doses daily **OR**
- (Epilepsy) 100—300 mg IM, repeated if necessary (daily maximum 600 mg) **OR**
- (Status epilepticus) 10—20 mg/kg IM or slow IV injection, repeated after 20 minutes if necessary (maximum daily total 1—2 g) **OR**

ANTIEPILEPTICS

- (Sedative) 30–120 mg orally daily in 2–3 divided doses **OR**
- (Sedative) 30–120 mg IM daily in 2–3 divided doses

Adverse effects
- sedation, disorientation, dizziness, depression, drowsiness, lethargy, hangover effect, confusion, restlessness, irritability, excitement, memory impairment, mood changes
- rash, bullae (skin blisters)
- dependence (physical and psychological), tolerance, withdrawal syndrome (including status epilepticus) if abruptly stopped
- (Uncommon) folate deficiency, hypocalcaemia, megaloblastic anaemia, injection site reactions, nausea, vomiting, diarrhoea, vitamin D deficiency
- (Rare) rickets, osteomalacia, exacerbated hyperthyroid symptoms, fibromas, Dupuytren's contracture, frozen shoulder, joint pain
- (IV extravasation) tissue necrosis

Interactions
- CNS depressant effects may be increased by other CNS depressants, including alcohol, monoamine oxidase inhibitors (MAOIs), benzodiazepines, antihistamines, phenothiazines, anaesthetics and opioid analgesics
- hypotension, respiratory depression and prolonged recovery time may occur if given with ketamine
- not recommended with MAOI tranylcypromine owing to increased CNS depressant effects
- may impair the absorption of griseofulvin
- may decrease the effects of warfarin by increasing metabolism; therefore prothrombin time should be closely monitored, especially when starting, stopping and changing doses
- may increase the metabolism of paracetamol, increasing the level of toxic metabolite and risk of hepatotoxicity
- absorption may be decreased by amphetamines
- effects may be reduced by folic acid (high dose) or alkalinising the urine
- serum levels may be decreased by St John's wort. Serum levels should be monitored when starting or stopping therapy
- serum levels may be increased by sodium valproate, disulfiram, methylphenidate, flu vaccine or chloramphenicol
- may decrease the effectiveness of oral contraceptives by increasing metabolism of both oestrogen and progestogen components
- increased risk of hepatotoxicity if given with halothane or enflurane
- may increase the metabolism of opioid analgesics, leading to withdrawal symptoms
- may potentiate hepatotoxicity of sodium valproate
- may alter levels (unpredictable) of phenytoin; therefore serum levels should be closely monitored
- phenytoin may alter serum levels of phenobarbital (phenobarbitone); therefore serum levels should be closely monitored
- may increase the metabolism (and therefore decrease the serum levels and effectiveness) of antiarrhythmics, carbamazepine, chloramphenicol, chlorpromazine, corticosteroids, corticotrophin, ciclosporin, digoxin, disopyramide, doxycycline, etoposide, haloperidol, itraconazole, lamotrigine, metronidazole, nifedipine, paracetamol, phenothiazines, propranolol, ritonavir, tacrolimus, theophylline, selective serotonin reuptake inhibitors (SSRIs) and tricyclic antidepressants (TCAs). Serum level monitoring is recommended

- increased risk of hypothermia if given with other hypothermia-producing agents
- increased risk of nephrotoxicity if given with methoxyflurane (even several weeks after phenobarbital (phenobarbitone) has been stopped)
- increased risk of respiratory depression may occur if given with TCAs
- increased risk of osteopenia if given with carbonic anhydrase inhibitors such as acetazolamide
- may decrease the effects of vitamin D by increasing metabolism, increasing the risk of osteomalacia with long-term therapy
- may interfere with a number of laboratory tests

Nursing considerations/Cautions

- blood counts should be monitored at the start and regularly throughout long-term therapy
- therapeutic serum levels should be monitored regularly if therapy is ongoing
- calcium and vitamin D supplements are recommended during long-term therapy
- regular bone mineral density monitoring is recommended with long-term therapy
- physical dependency and tolerance may develop; therefore therapy should not be discontinued suddenly to prevent withdrawal symptoms occurring
- hypotension and vasodilation may occur if given by rapid IV administration
- highly alkaline; may cause tissue necrosis if extravasation occurs
- not given SC or intra-arterially because of the risk of tissue necrosis
- (IV) dilute solution 1 in 10 with water for injections and administer at a rate less than 60 mg/min to decrease the risk of respiratory depression and circulatory collapse
- oxygen, vasopressor agents and resuscitation equipment should be readily available when given IV because of the risk of overdose and CNS depression (including respiratory depression) occurring
- injection given deep IM (not greater than 5 mL per site)
- tablets not recommended in those with rare hereditary problems of galactose intolerance, total lactase deficiency or glucose–galactose malabsorption
- caution if used in the elderly (as confusion, depression or excitement may occur) or in those with asthma, urticaria, angioedema, hypotension, hypoadrenalism, hyperthyroidism, history of haematological disorders, cardiovascular or respiratory disease, or kidney or liver dysfunction
- contraindicated if used in those with acute or chronic pain (especially if uncontrolled), as paradoxical excitement may occur or other symptoms may be masked
- contraindicated in those with hypersensitivity to barbiturates, severe folate-deficiency anaemia, porphyria, severe depression, suicidal tendencies, severe respiratory, kidney or liver impairment, sleep apnoea, acute intoxication to sedatives/hypnotics or alcohol, a history of drug abuse or dependence, nephritis, premonitory signs of hepatic coma, severe uncontrolled asthma, diabetes mellitus, or in the elderly if nocturnal confusion/restlessness from sedatives or hypnotics has occurred
- see also General Nursing considerations/ Cautions for antiepileptics (p. 386)

Patient education

- the patient should be advised to seek medical advice if any of the following occur:
  - sore throat, fever, bruising or bleeding, bloody nose (sign of blood dyscrasias)
  - signs of infection
  - rash or other skin reactions, severe itching
- encourage the patient to have adequate sunlight exposure (or take

ANTIEPILEPTICS

- vitamin D supplement) and regular weightbearing exercise
- advise the female patient using oral contraceptives that additional forms of contraception are required to prevent pregnancy occurring
- see also General Patient education for antiepileptics (p. 386)

Available as oral liquid. Tablets can be crushed and mixed with water or fruit juice, or a spoonful of yoghurt or apple puree.

Barbiturates distribute throughout fetal tissue, especially liver and brain, and may be associated with minor craniofacial defects, fingernail hypoplasia, developmental disability and brain tumours. Barbiturate withdrawal may be seen in newborns up to 2 weeks after birth.

CNS depression and withdrawal symptoms may be seen in breastfed babies. Infant serum levels should be closely monitored.

Dose reduction is recommended in those with kidney or liver dysfunction.

Caution if used in the elderly (as confusion, depression or excitement may occur); therefore dose reduction is recommended.

Do not crush tablets if pregnant.

PHENYTOIN, PHENYTOIN SODIUM

Trade names
Dilantin, DBL Phenytoin Injection BP, Phenytoin Juno

Available forms
Tablets (chewable): 50 mg;
Capsules: 30 mg, 100 mg;
Ampoules: 100 mg/2 mL, 250 mg/5 mL;
Suspension: 30 mg/5 mL

Action
- hydantoin
- acts by preventing the spread of seizure activity across the motor cortex (promotes efflux of sodium ions from neurons), stabilises excitability threshold
- antiarrhythmic actions (positive inotropic effect and enhances AV conduction, decreases automaticity, shortens refractory period, shortens QT interval and duration of action potential)
- not effective for absence (petit mal) seizures
- (Oral) absorption is slow and variable, especially in neonates
- onset of action 30—60 minutes (IV), duration of action up to 24 hours
- half-life 7—42 hours (average 24 hours); however, this is dependent on dose and serum levels

Use
- psychomotor seizures
- tonic—clonic (grand mal) epilepsy
- status epilepticus
- prophylactic control of seizures during and after neurosurgery or after severe head trauma
- arrhythmias not responding to other antiarrhythmic agents or cardioversion

Dose
- (Epilepsy) initially 4—5 mg/kg orally daily in 2—3 divided doses, adjusting dose at 2-week intervals according to plasma levels (daily maximum 600 mg) **OR**
- (Status epilepticus) 10—15 mg/kg slowly IV (loading dose), then 100 mg IV or orally 6—8-hourly given with a short-acting IV benzodiazepine to control seizure rapidly **OR**
- (Neurosurgery prophylaxis) 250 mg slowly IV 6—12-hourly until oral administration is possible **OR**
- (Cardiac arrhythmias) 3—5 mg/kg slow IV injection initially, at a rate not exceeding 50 mg/min and repeated if necessary

Adverse effects
- constipation, altered taste, epigastric pain, weight loss
- hyperplasia of gums and gum bleeding, lip enlargement
- coarsened facial features
- acne
- abnormal thyroid function
- lymphadenopathy, anaemia, thrombocytopenia, agranulocytosis, megaloblastic anaemia, leucopenia, pancytopenia
- hirsutism, hypertrichosis
- (Rapid IV infusion) hypotension, cardiac arrhythmias, impaired cardiac conduction, CNS depression, respiratory depression
- (Long-term therapy > 10 years) vitamin D deficiency, osteomalacia, bone fractures
- (IV) irritation, thrombophlebitis, inflammation, pain, tissue necrosis, purple glove syndrome (oedema, pain and discolouration distal to the injection site)
- (Rare) hypersensitivity, toxic hepatitis, liver damage, phenytoin-induced dyskinesia, anticonvulsant hypersensitivity syndrome, angioedema, hyperglycaemia (patients with diabetes)
- (Phenytoin toxicity) lateral gaze/nystagmus, ataxia, dysarthria, followed by tremor, hyperreflexia, dizziness, somnolence, drowsiness, lethargy, slurred speech, blurred or double vision, hypotension, confusion, hallucinations, clumsiness, nausea and vomiting, and, in severe poisoning or overdose, respiratory depression, bradycardia and heart block
- see also General Adverse effects of antiepileptics (p. 385)

Interactions
- serum levels may be increased or decreased (unpredictable effect) by benzodiazepines, carbamazepine, ciprofloxacin, phenobarbital (phenobarbitone), phenothiazines, primidone, sodium valproate and theophylline; therefore serum levels should be closely monitored
- serum levels may be increased by acute alcohol intake, amiodarone, amphotericin B (amphotericin), capecitabine, chloramphenicol, clopidogrel, diazepam, diltiazem, disulfiram, erythromycin, ethosuximide, fluconazole, fluorouracil (5FU), fluvastatin, fluvoxamine, fluoxetine, gabapentin, halothane, isoniazid, itraconazole, methylphenidate, miconazole, nifedipine, oestrogens, omeprazole, oxcarbazepine, phenothiazines, ranitidine, salicylates, sertraline, selective serotonin reuptake inhibitors (SSRIs), sodium valproate, sulfonamides, tacrolimus, ticlopidine, topiramate, voriconazole and warfarin
- serum levels may be decreased by chronic alcohol abuse, aminophylline, bleomycin, calcium folinate, carboplatin, carmustine, ciprofloxacin, cisplatin, diazoxide, folic acid, HIV protease inhibitors, methotrexate, oral contraceptives, rifabutin, rifampicin, sucralfate, St John's wort, theophylline, vigabatrin and vinblastine
- absorption is interfered with by calcium ions; therefore administration of antacids containing calcium should be staggered
- tricyclic antidepressants (TCAs), haloperidol, tramadol, antipsychotic agents and monoamine oxidase inhibitors (MAOIs) may precipitate seizures in susceptible patients by lowering convulsive threshold
- reduces the efficacy of aminophylline, amiodarone, amlodipine, azole antifungal agents, carbamazepine, clozapine, corticosteroids, ciclosporin, digoxin, doxycycline, felodipine, furosemide (frusemide), ivabradine, lamotrigine, lercanidipine, methadone, nifedipine, nimodipine, oestrogens, combined oral contraceptives, perampanel, praziquantel, progestogens, teniposide, theophylline, verapamil and vinca alkaloids

ANTIEPILEPTICS

- caution if given with other highly protein-bound drugs such as nifedepine and verapamil
- may decrease serum levels of topiramate and increase serum levels of phenytoin if given together
- large doses may increase serum glucose levels, increasing insulin and/or oral hypoglycaemic agent requirements
- caution if given with warfarin, as effects may be unpredictable; therefore drug levels and INR should be monitored during therapy
- food and enteral feeding may affect phenytoin absorption
- seizure control may be decreased if given with folic acid because of increased phenytoin metabolism
- may increase metabolism of vitamin D, increasing the risk of osteoporosis and bone fractures
- if combined with cranial irradiation and gradual decreasing doses of corticosteroids, may result in severe skin reactions
- caution if used with pancuronium, as recovery time from neuromuscular blockade may be faster
- chronic phenytoin therapy may result in resistance to vecuronium-induced neuromuscular blockage, requiring higher dose
- an increased risk of hyperammonaemia if given with sodium valproate
- (IV) additive cardiac depressive effects may occur if given with lidocaine (lignocaine) or beta adrenergic blocking agents
- (IV) bradycardia and hypotension may occur if given with dopamine
- may interfere with thyroid function, folic acid, calcium, dexamethasone and metyrapone tests

Nursing considerations/Cautions

- any hypoalbuminaemia should be corrected immediately because it may lead to toxicity (due to increased levels of unbound phenytoin)
- serum levels should be measured 7–10 days after starting therapy, if dose is altered, if adding or subtracting another antiepileptic agent or when switching from one formulation to another, or at first signs of toxicity, as prolonged high phenytoin levels may lead to encephalopathy and/or confusional state
- recommended serum level is between 10 and 20 microgram/mL
- regular blood count monitoring is recommended for long-term therapy
- long-term therapy requires adequate vitamin D and folic acid intake in diet or supplements. Bone density should also be measured regularly
- (Status epilepticus) short-acting IV benzodiazepine is usually administered first for rapid control of the seizure, followed by slow administration of IV phenytoin
- IV administration should not exceed 50 mg/min to prevent cardiac arrhythmias and/or hypotension. The patient requires constant heart rate, blood pressure and ECG monitoring and observation for respiratory depression
- injectable solutions are strongly alkaline, so avoid mixing with other drugs or IV solutions, as crystallisation/precipitation may occur
- (IV) risk of purple glove syndrome (pain, oedema and discolouration distal to the IV site)
- SC or IM administration is not recommended. IM absorption is also slow and erratic
- (IV) contains propylene glycol, which can cause toxicity if used for a prolonged period, which may occur several days after IV administration. Toxicity includes CNS depression, hyperosmolarity, lactic acidosis and renal insufficiency
- (IV) not for dilution
- IV lines should be flushed with sodium chloride 0.9% before and after administration of phenytoin
- (IV) if solution is refrigerated, precipitate may form. This will dissolve at room

HAVARD'S NURSING GUIDE TO DRUGS

- temperature with no adverse effects on solution
- (IV) avoid extravasation as tissue necrosis may occur
- (suspension) it is suggested that phenytoin should not be administered with continuous enteral feeds. Phenytoin should be administered 2 hours after an intermittent feed and a 2-hour interval allowed before the next feed is commenced
- suspension should be diluted before administration via feeding tube. Tube should be flushed well after administration
- not effective in the management of seizures due to hypoglycaemia or other metabolic causes
- caution if used in the elderly or those with porphyria, liver or kidney impairment, (IV) hypotension or severe myocardial insufficiency or diabetes (as hyperglycaemia may be increased)
- caution if used in those who have experienced or have a family history of anticonvulsant hypersensitivity syndrome previously (to phenytoin or other antiepileptic agents) or are immunosuppressed
- caution if used in those of Chinese heritage, as there is an increased risk of severe skin reactions
- extreme caution if combined with cranial irradiation, as gradually decreasing doses of corticosteroids may result in severe skin reactions
- contraindicated in those with hypersensitivity to hydantoins, sinus bradycardia, SA block, second/third degree AV block or Stokes—Adams syndrome
- see also General Nursing considerations/Cautions for antiepileptics (p. 385)

Patient education

- advise the patient to take tablets with at least half a glass of water before meals, but if there is a tendency to nausea then take with or after food (always taken in the same relation to food for consistent absorption)
- if gastric irritation is a problem, splitting the dose into 3 is recommended
- advise the patient (or carer) to shake the suspension well before use
- instruct the patient to seek medical advice immediately if any of the following occur:
  - fever or sore throat (early signs of bone marrow depression)
  - any rash or skin reaction including blisters or itching
  - joint or muscle pain, fever, chills, yellowing of skin or eyes, fatigue, itching, nausea, vomiting, loss of appetite, abdominal pain
- advise about good oral hygiene (e.g. frequent brushing, gum massage) to reduce gingival (gum) hyperplasia especially during first 6 months of therapy
- if the patient has diabetes, they should be advised to monitor blood glucose more frequently because of the risk of hyperglycaemia
- (IV) the patient should be advised to report any pain, swelling or discolouration away from the IV site towards the hand
- see also General Patient education for antiepileptics (p. 386)

Oral suspension available. Capsules can be opened and contents dispersed in water. Tablets can be crushed and mixed with water.

Has been associated with fetal hydantoin syndrome (craniofacial defects, fingernail hypoplasia, developmental disability, growth retardation and, less often, oral clefts and cardiac anomalies). May also cause coagulation defects, with a haemorrhage risk in the fetus and newborn, which may be prevented by giving vitamin K prophylactically to the mother before delivery.

Not recommended during breastfeeding.

ANTIEPILEPTICS

Lower or less frequent dosing may be required in those > 65 years.

(Status epilepticus) IV rate should not exceed 25 mg/min.

If opening capsules or crushing tablets, mask and gloves should be worn. Pregnant staff should not open capsules or crush tablets.

PREGABALIN

Trade names
APO-Pregabalin, BTC-Pregabalin, Cipla-Pregabalin, Lyrica, Lyzalon, Neuroccord Pregabalin, Noumed Pregabalin, Prebalin, Pregabalin Lupin, Pregabalin Sandoz, Pregabalin-DRLA, Pregabalin-WGR

Available forms
Capsules: 25 mg, 50 mg, 75 mg, 100 mg, 150 mg, 200 mg, 225 mg, 300 mg

Action
- analogue of gamma aminobutyric acid (GABA) with analgesic and antiepileptic properties
- binds to protein subunit of voltage-gated calcium channels in CNS
- reduces release of glutamate, noradrenaline and substance P, although the significance of this is currently unknown
- half-life 6.3 hours

Use
- adjunct therapy in partial seizures with or without secondary generalisation
- neuropathic pain

Dose
- (Epilepsy, neuropathic pain) initially 75 mg orally twice daily, increasing to 150 mg twice daily after 3—7 days. After a further 7-day interval, this can be increased to 300 mg twice daily if needed

Adverse effects
- flatulence, dry mouth, diarrhoea, bloating, increased appetite, weight gain
- peripheral oedema, generalised oedema
- blurred vision
- decreased libido and, uncommonly, erectile dysfunction, sexual dysfunction, dysmenorrhoea
- muscle cramp, back pain, arthralgia, limb pain
- nasopharyngitis
- elevated creatine kinase levels
- (Rare) myopathy, rhabdomyolysis, hypersensitivity, skin reaction, kidney failure, respiratory depression
- see also General Adverse effects of antiepileptics (p. 385)

Interactions
- may enhance the effects of alcohol, oxycodone and lorazepam
- increased risk of respiratory depression, severe sedation, coma and death if used with opioid analgesics; therefore are not recommended together, or if given together the dose should be adjusted and the patient should be carefully monitored
- increased risk of constipation, paralytic ileus and bowel obstruction if given with opioid analgesics or other agents that slow intestinal time leading to constipation

Nursing considerations/Cautions
- therapy should be stopped if creatine kinase levels are markedly elevated or if there are any signs of myopathy
- the patient should be assessed for any current or past history of opioid and/or benzodiazepines, as pregabalin has the potential for abuse or misuse and dependence
- high risk of overdose and death if used with opioids and/or benzodiazepines
- if the patient has diabetes, kidney function should be measured before starting therapy and the dose adjusted if needed
- (Neuropathic pain) if pain is not adequately controlled in 12 weeks, risk versus benefit to the patient should be assessed before continuing therapy

- (Epilepsy) not recommended as monotherapy
- caution if used in those with congestive cardiac failure, respiratory impairment, respiratory or neurological disease, or kidney impairment
- not recommended in those with hereditary problems of galactose intolerance, lactase deficiency or glucose–galactose malabsorption
- see also General Nursing considerations/Cautions for antiepileptics (p. 386)

Patient education

- the patient should be advised of weight gain and counselled regarding healthy eating options, especially if the person also has diabetes; added weight may require dose adjustment of hypoglycaemic agents
- the patient should be warned that dizziness and somnolence may persist throughout therapy;, however, blurred vision usually resolves with continued therapy
- warn the patient to immediately seek medical advice if any of the following occurs:
  - swelling of face, lips or upper airway
  - skin reaction, especially any blistering
- see also General Patient education for antiepileptics (p. 386)

 Capsules can be opened and the contents dispersed in 120 mL water, or mixed with a spoonful of yoghurt or apple puree.

 Not recommended during pregnancy unless benefits are thought to outweigh risks to fetus.

 Dose adjustment needed in those with kidney impairment is dependent on creatinine clearance (CrCl). If the patient is receiving haemodialysis, the daily dose should be based on CrCl, followed by a supplementary dose given immediately after a 4-hour dialysis treatment (also based on CrCl)

 Increased risk of dizziness and somnolence if given to those > 65 years.

PRIMIDONE
Trade name
Mysoline

Available form
Tablets: 250 mg

Action
- barbiturate
- reduces sensitivity to stimuli that might provoke seizure activity
- active metabolites include phenobarbital (phenobarbitone) and phenylethylmalonamide

Use
- tonic–clonic (grand mal) epilepsy
- temporal lobe (psychomotor) epilepsy
- partial (focal) epileptic seizures
- myoclonic jerks, akinetic attacks

Dose
- initially 125 mg orally at night, gradually increasing by increments of 125 mg every 3 days until 500 mg is reached, then increasing by increments of 250 mg every 3 days until control is achieved (750–1500 mg daily in 2 divided doses, morning and evening)

Adverse effects
- severe skin eruptions
- tolerance, dependence, withdrawal syndrome
- (Rare) megaloblastic anaemia, Dupuytren's contracture, arthralgia, osteomalacia
- see also General Adverse effects of antiepileptics (p. 385)

Interactions
- may alter serum levels of other antiepileptic agents
- if given with warfarin, INR should be closely monitored
- may reduce effectiveness of oral contraceptives
- may enhance effects of alcohol and other CNS depressants

ANTIEPILEPTICS

- affects metabolism of vitamin D
- decreased serum levels may occur if given with mianserin, sertraline, oxycodone, tyrosine kinase inhibitors, ifosfamide, antiviral agent, azole antifungals, anticoagulant agents, bosentan, nimodipine, alcohol and St John's wort; therefore not recommended together

Nursing considerations/Cautions

- it is advisable to give the larger part of the dose when the seizures are known to be more frequent (e.g. if the seizures are nocturnal, most of the dose is given in the evening)
- bone mineral density should be measured regularly with long-term use
- vitamin D supplements are recommended with long-term therapy
- contraindicated in those with porphyria
- see also General Nursing considerations/Cautions for antiepileptics (p. 386)

Patient education

- female patients should be counselled to use other methods of contraception to avoid pregnancy occurring, as oral contraceptives may be ineffective during therapy
- warn the patient to report any skin reaction, especially blistering (particularly in the first 10 weeks of therapy)
- see also General Patient education for antiepileptics (p. 386)

 Tablet can be dispersed in water, or crushed and mixed with a spoonful of yoghurt or apple puree.

 Barbiturates distribute throughout fetal tissue, especially liver and brain, and may be associated with minor craniofacial defects, fingernail hypoplasia, developmental disability and brain tumours. Barbiturate withdrawal may be seen in newborns up to 2 weeks after birth.

 CNS depression and withdrawal symptoms may be seen in breastfed babies.

Infant serum levels should be closely monitored.

 A reduced dose is recommended in those with kidney or liver impairment.

 Caution if used in those > 65 years.

 Pregnant staff should not crush tablets.

RUFINAMIDE
Trade name
Inovelon

Available form
Tablets: 100 mg, 200 mg, 400 mg

Action
- modulates sodium channel activity, prolonging an inactive state
- half-life 6—10 hours

Use
- adjunct therapy to seizures associated with Lennox—Gastaut syndrome in patients 4 years and older. (Lennox—Gastaut syndrome is a rare, complex and severe epilepsy which starts in childhood (usually between 3 and 5 years), and can persist into adulthood. It is characterised by multiple and concurrent seizure types.)

Dose
- (Adults, adolescents and children > 4 years and > 30 kg, not receiving sodium valproate) initially 200 mg orally twice daily, increasing by increments of 400 mg daily if needed (daily maximum 1.8 g—3.2 g depending on patient weight) **OR**
- (Adults, adolescents and children > 4 years and > 30 kg, receiving sodium valproate) initially 200 mg orally twice daily, increasing by increments of 400 mg daily if needed (daily maximum 1.2 g—2.2 g depending on patient weight) **OR**

- (Children > 4 years and < 30 kg, not receiving sodium valproate) initially 100 mg orally twice daily, increasing at 3-day intervals of 200 mg daily increments if needed (daily maximum 600 mg) **OR**
- (Children > 4 years and < 30 kg, receiving sodium valproate) initially 100 mg orally twice daily, increasing at 2-day intervals of 200 mg daily increments if needed (daily maximum 1 g)

Adverse effects
- pneumonia, flu-like symptoms, nasopharyngitis, sinusitis, rhinitis
- ear infection
- back pain
- oligomenorrhoea
- decreased appetite, anorexia, upper abdominal pain, constipation, dyspepsia, diarrhoea, weight change
- (Rare) hypersensitivity reaction, increased liver enzymes, decrease in QTc interval
- see also General Adverse effects of antiepileptics (p. 385)

Interactions
- serum levels increased by sodium valproate
- decreased serum levels may occur if given with primidone, phenobarbital (phenobarbitone), carbamazepine or vigabatrin
- may decrease efficacy of oral contraceptives
- caution if given with triazolam
- caution if used with amiodarone, aprepitant, atorvastatin, carbamazepine, ciclosporin, felodipine, hydrocortisone, HIV protease inhibitors, simvastatin, tacrolimus, tyrosine kinase inhibitors (e.g. axitinib), verapamil, zolpidem. Patients should be closely monitored for 2 weeks at the start, end or dose adjustment if given with rufinamide
- caution if given with warfarin or digoxin. Serum levels should be closely monitored if given together

Nursing considerations/Cautions
- treatment should be started by a paediatrician or neurologist specialised in the management of epilepsy
- caution if used in those with, or a family history of, congenital short QT syndrome
- caution if used in patients with mild-to-moderate liver impairment. Careful dose titration is recommended
- not recommended in patients with severe liver impairment
- tablets contain lactose and are therefore not recommended in those with rare hereditary problems of galactose intolerance, Lapp lactase deficiency or glucose—galactose malabsorption
- see also General Nursing considerations/Cautions for antiepileptics (p. 386)

Patient education
- see General Patient education for antiepileptics (p. 386)

 Tablet can be crushed and mixed with water.

 Not recommended during pregnancy unless the benefits are thought to outweigh risks to the fetus.

 Thought to be excreted in breastmilk; therefore not recommended during breastfeeding.

SODIUM VALPROATE
Trade names
APO-Sodium Valproate, Epilim, Epilim IV, Sodium Valproate Juno, Sodium Valproate Sandoz, Sodium Valproate Wockhardt, Valpro EC, Valproate Winthrop, Valproate SXP Solution

Available forms
Tablets (sustained-release): 200 mg, 500 mg;
Tablets (crushable): 100 mg;
Sugar free liquid: 200 mg/5 mL;
Syrup: 200 mg/5 mL;
Vial: 400 mg

ANTIEPILEPTICS

Action
- anticonvulsant, antipsychotic
- thought to raise brain levels of the inhibitory synaptic transmitter gamma aminobutyric acid (GABA), as well as blocking voltage-dependent sodium channels
- half-life 8—12 hours

Use
- simple partial (petit mal) epilepsy
- tonic—clonic (grand mal) epilepsy
- myoclonic epilepsy
- mono or adjuvant therapy in partial (focal) epilepsy
- mania (see Antipsychotics and mood stabilising agents, p. 867) (where other agents are inadequate or inappropriate)

Dose
- initially 600 mg orally daily with or after food, increasing by 200 mg daily at 3-day intervals until control is reached (1000—2000 mg). If control is not reached after 2 weeks, dosage may be increased to a maximum of 2500 mg daily or another antiepileptic agent may be added **OR**
- initially 400—800 mg (up to 10 mg/kg) IV over 3—5 minutes or by IV infusion, then 1—2 mg/kg/hour (daily maximum 2.5 g or another antiepileptic agent may be added)

Adverse effects
- anorexia, diarrhoea, abdominal cramps, increased appetite, weight gain
- transient hair loss, nail/nailbed disorder
- gingival hyperplasia
- elevated liver enzymes, hyponatraemia
- dysmenorrhoea
- urinary incontinence
- prolonged bleeding time (reversible), thrombocytopenia
- (Rare) liver damage/failure, pancreatitis, vasculitis, hyperammonaemia (with or without symptoms, including lethargy, coma, vomiting, ataxia, clouded consciousness), hypersensitivity, severe skin reaction
- (IV) pain, discomfort, erythema, inflammation
- see also General Adverse effects of antiepileptics (p. 385)

Interactions
- not recommended with carbapenem antibiotics
- increased risk of liver damage if given with salicylates, including aspirin
- increased risk of neutropenia/leucopenia if given with quetiapine
- use with clozapine may result in increased serum levels of either clozapine or sodium valproate
- may increase serum levels of midazolam, primidone, nimodipine and zidovudine, increasing the risk of adverse effects
- may decrease renal clearance of lorazepam
- may inhibit metabolism of tricyclic antidepressants (TCAs); therefore serum levels should be monitored
- may increase serum levels of diazepam and inhibit its metabolism, increasing the risk of sedation
- use with clonazepam may result in absence seizures
- use with aspirin may result in increased sodium valproate serum levels by displacement from receptor site, as well as inhibiting its metabolism
- may increase or decrease serum phenytoin levels; therefore close monitoring of serum levels is recommended
- may inhibit metabolism of carbamazepine (and its metabolite), lamotrigine, phenobarbital (phenobarbitone) and ethosuximide, increasing the risk of toxicity; therefore monitoring of serum levels is recommended
- may decrease serum levels of olanzapine and propofol
- increased risk of encephalopathy and/or hyperammonaemia if given with topiramate or acetazolamide
- use with antidepressants may decrease seizure threshold in patients whose seizures have not been stabilised
- may potentiate CNS effects of alcohol, antidepressants, antipsychotics,

417

- benzodiazepines, phenobarbital (phenobarbitone) and monoamine oxidase inhibitors (MAOIs)
- serum levels are decreased by phenytoin, phenobarbital (phenobarbitone), carbamazepine, colestyramine, protease inhibitors (e.g. ritonavir), imipenem, rifampicin or meropenem
- serum levels are increased by erythromycin, fluoxetine, chlorpromazine, felbamate, MAOIs, TCAs or selective serotonin reuptake inhibitors (SSRIs)
- seizures may occur if given with mefloquine
- caution if given with warfarin, as serum levels of warfarin may be increased; therefore the INR should be closely monitored especially when starting or stopping therapy
- may give false positive results to ketone bodies in urine testing in those with diabetes (ketone bodies are produced from elimination of sodium valproate by the kidneys). May also alter thyroid function tests

Nursing considerations/Cautions

- may take 2–6 weeks for optimal seizure control to be achieved
- risk of urea cycle disorders should be evaluated before starting therapy (including those with unexplained encephalopathy or coma, encephalopathy associated with protein, pregnancy or postpartum, cyclical vomiting and lethargy, extreme irritability, ataxia, low blood nitrogen urea (BUN) or protein avoidance)
- liver function is assessed before starting therapy, then monitored monthly for 6 months, then less frequently
- blood counts (including prothrombin time, serum fibrinogen and albumin) and platelet counts should be monitored before and regularly throughout therapy and especially before surgery (because bleeding time may be prolonged)
- pregnancy should be excluded before starting therapy
- enteric-coated tablets are recommended for those requiring higher doses
- not recommended IM because of the risk of tissue necrosis
- (IV) administer alone
- (IV) reconstitute using 4 mL of provided diluent
- (IV) administer by slow IV injection or infusion
- (IV) the patient should be transferred to oral therapy as soon as practicable
- if the patient requires surgery, platelet function should be closely monitored
- increased risk of rhabdomyolysis if given to those with carnitine palmitoyltransferase (CPT) type II deficiency
- caution if used in those with ornithine transcarbamylase deficiency because of the risk of hyperammonaemia
- caution if used in those with pancreatitis, impaired kidney or liver function or systemic lupus erythematosus (SLE)
- contraindicated in those with liver dysfunction (including a family history of hepatitis), porphyria or known urea cycle disorders, or some mitochondrial disorders
- see also General Nursing considerations/Cautions for antiepileptics (p. 386)

Patient education

- the patient should be advised to take the dose with or after food to reduce gastrointestinal (GI) adverse effects, but avoid taking with carbonated water
- warn the patient that GI symptoms are usually transient at the start of therapy and usually disappear within a few days
- the patient should be warned about hair loss as a common adverse effect. Hair usually grows back but may be curly
- instruct the patient to take the regular dose at least 3 times daily to avoid excessive fluctuations in serum and brain drug levels
- advise the patient to take with milk to avoid an unpleasant taste
- warn the patient not to remove tablets from foil until ready to ingest as they absorb water

- care should be taken when using Epilim syrup in patients with diabetes because it contains 3.6 g sucrose/5 mL. Sugar free liquid is available as an alternative
- syrup should be shaken well before use
- normal syrup may be diluted but used within 14 days; sugar free liquid should not be diluted
- the patient should be advised to seek medical advice immediately if any of the following occur:
  - sudden bruising or bleeding (signs of blood dyscrasias)
  - nausea, vomiting, anorexia and/or abdominal pain (signs of pancreatitis)
  - ongoing lethargy, vomiting or changes in mental state (hyperammonaemia)
  - signs of liver dysfunction (malaise, weakness, lethargy, facial oedema, anorexia, vomiting, abdominal pain, drowsiness, yellowing of skin or eye whites, darkened urine)
  - skin reaction especially any blistering
- warn the patient against using aspirin for pain or as an antipyretic
- counsel the patient about possible weight gain and a suitable diet
- female patients of childbearing age should be counselled regarding the need to use two reliable forms of contraception (including a barrier method) during therapy and the need to seek medical advice if pregnancy occurs
- male patients should be counselled not to donate sperm during or for 3 months after stopping therapy and the need to seek medical advice if they plan to father a child. Contraception should be used during and for 3 months after stopping therapy
- see also General Patient education for antiepileptics (p. 386)

 Available as a syrup or crushable tablet. Crushable tablets can be crushed and mixed with water, or a spoonful of yoghurt or apple puree.

 Contraindicated during pregnancy because of the increased risk of neural tube defects if taken during the first trimester. Pregnant women taking sodium valproate should be encouraged to consider ultrasound and amniocentesis for diagnosis of possible abnormalities. A haemorrhagic syndrome related to hypofibrinaemia in neonates has also been seen (decreased coagulation factors). It is recommended that fibrinogen serum levels, platelet count and coagulation should be monitored carefully in the neonate.

 Secreted in breastmilk; therefore mothers are advised against breastfeeding.

 Lower doses are required in those with kidney impairment.

 Pregnant staff should not disperse or crush tablets.

STIRIPENTOL
Trade name
Diacomit

Available forms
Capsules: 250 mg, 500 mg;
Sachets: 250 mg, 500 mg

Action
- potentiates gamma aminobutyric acid (GABA) transmission both presynaptically (increasing GABA release from nerve terminals) and postsynaptically (increasing brain levels of GABA)
- half-life 4–13 hours (dose dependent)

Use
- adjunctive therapy in treatment of generalised tonic–clonic seizures associated with severe myoclonic epilepsy in infancy (known as Dravet syndrome) in those not adequately controlled with a benzodiazepine (usually clobazam) and sodium valproate

Dose
- dose is calculated on mg/kg of body weight and then divided into 2 or 3 daily doses

- initially 20 mg/kg/day (for first week), then increasing to 30 mg/kg/day (for second week), then increasing according to the child's age (recommended daily dose is 50 mg/kg/day)

Adverse effects
- anorexia, loss of appetite, weight loss, nausea, vomiting
- insomnia, aggressiveness, irritability, behaviour disorders, opposing behaviour, hyperexcitability, sleep disorders
- drowsiness, ataxia, hypotonia, dystonia, hyperactivity, inability to concentrate
- neutropenia
- elevated liver enzymes
- (Uncommon) photosensitivity, rash, urticaria
- (Rare) thrombocytopenia

Interactions
- not recommended with carbamazepine, phenytoin or phenobarbital (phenobarbitone)
- clobazam or sodium valproate dose should be reduced if given with stiripentol
- increased risk of neutropenia if given with clobazam or sodium valproate
- not recommended with tacrolimus, ciclosporin or sirolimus, as serum levels and the risk of adverse effects and toxicity are increased
- increased risk of adverse effects such as rhabdomyolysis if given with statins; therefore not recommended together
- caution if used with macrolide antibacterial agents or azole antifungals
- caution if used with citalopram, omeprazole, HIV protease inhibitors, antihistamines, calcium-channel blockers, statins, codeine and oral contraceptives. Plasma levels should be monitored if given together
- not recommended with caffeine or theophylline, or agents with narrow therapeutic index
- increased action if given with other agents that enhance GABA activity such as benzodiazepines, barbiturates and bromides

Nursing considerations/Cautions
- starting therapy should be done slowly, with dose escalation depending on child's age. During the third week:
  - (child < 6 years) an additional 20 mg/kg/day (to a recommended dose of 50 mg/kg/day)
  - (child > 6 years but < 12 years) an additional 10 mg/kg/day each week, achieving a recommended daily dose of 50 mg/kg/day in 4 weeks
  - (child > 12 years, adolescent) an additional 5 mg/kg/day each week until optimum dose is achieved
- formulations are not bioequivalent; therefore switching from one formulation to the other should be done under medical supervision
- blood count and liver function tests are recommended before starting therapy and then 6-monthly
- growth rate in children should be closely monitored during therapy (especially if the combination therapy causes gastrointestinal side-effects including anorexia, loss of appetite, nausea and vomiting)
- safety in children under 3 years has not been established
- not recommended in those with any liver or kidney impairment
- contraindicated in those with a history of psychoses or delirium

Patient education
- parents/carers should be instructed not to switch formulations without seeking medical advice
- advise the patient/parent/carer that capsules should be swallowed whole with a glass of water during a meal. If using a sachet, powder should be mixed in glass of water and taken with the meal
- instruct the patient/parent/carer that medication should not be taken with milk or dairy products (including yoghurt, ice cream, soft cream cheese), carbonated drinks, fruit juice or foods/

ANTIEPILEPTICS

drinks which contain caffeine (e.g. cola drinks, energy drinks) or theophylline (e.g. chocolate)
- advise the patient/parent/carer to seek medical advice if any of the following occur:
  - drowsiness or excessive sleepiness
  - depressed mood, self-harming behaviours, suicidal thoughts

 Capsule can be opened, or sachet contents can be mixed with spoonful of honey or jam.

SULTHIAME
Trade name
Ospolot

Available form
Tablets: 50 mg, 200 mg

Action
- sulfonamide derivative with no antibacterial actions
- carbonic anhydrase inhibitor

Use
- temporal lobe epilepsy
- myoclonic seizures
- tonic—clonic (grand mal) epilepsy
- partial motor (Jacksonian) seizures
- hyperkinetic behaviour

Dose
- initially 100 mg orally twice daily with fluids after meals, increasing gradually to 200 mg 3 times daily (maintenance)
OR
- initially 50 mg orally 3 times daily with fluids after meals, increasing gradually to 200 mg 3 times daily (maintenance)

Adverse effects
- paraesthesia of face and extremities
- hyperpnoea, dyspnoea, tachypnoea
- anorexia, weight loss
- angina
- hiccups
- (Rare) calcium and vitamin D metabolism disturbance
- see also General Adverse effects of antiepileptics (p. 385)

Interactions
- use with primidone may lead to severe adverse effects, including psychosis
- increased serum levels of phenytoin may occur when added to established phenytoin therapy; therefore phenytoin serum levels should be closely monitored
- may lead to increased lamotrigine, phenobarbital (phenobarbitone) and carbamazepine serum levels
- use with alcohol is not recommended because of the risk of disulfiram reaction occurring
- caution if used with carbonic anhydrase inhibitors such as topiramate and acetazolamide
- may interfere with barbiturate estimation test

Nursing considerations/Cautions
- kidney function should be closely monitored during therapy
- caution if used in those with kidney or liver impairment
- not recommended in those with psychiatric history
- not recommended in those with rare hereditary problems of galactose intolerance, lactase deficiency or glucose—galactose malabsorption
- contraindicated in those with hypersensitivity to sulfonamides, acute porphyria, hyperthyroidism or arterial hypertension
- see also General Nursing considerations/Cautions for antiepileptics (p. 386)

Patient education
- the patient should be advised to report any shortness of breath, or rapid or difficulty breathing
- ensure the patient understands the importance of not consuming alcohol

during therapy because of the risk of a severe reaction, including severe flushing, pulsating headache, decreased breathing, nausea, vomiting, low BP and racing heart
- see also General Patient education for antiepileptics (p. 386)

 Tablets can be dispersed in water, or crushed and mixed with a spoonful of yoghurt or apple puree.

 Not recommended during pregnancy.

 Not recommended during breastfeeding.

 Pregnant staff should not disperse or crush tablets.

TIAGABINE HYDROCHLORIDE
Trade name
Gabitril

Available form
Tablets: 5 mg, 10 mg, 15 mg

Action
- selectively inhibits uptake of gamma aminobutyric acid (GABA) in neurons and glial cells
- half-life 7—9 hours

Use
- partial seizures (as adjunct therapy where epilepsy is not controlled by other antiepileptics)

Dose
- initially 2.5—5 mg orally 3 times daily with food, increasing at weekly intervals by 5—15 mg weekly until an optimal response is achieved, 30—50 mg daily (maintenance) (daily maximum 70 mg)

Adverse effects
- diarrhoea, abdominal pain
- pharyngitis, rhinitis, flu syndrome
- (Rare) visual field defects, bleeding, serious skin reactions
- see also General Adverse effects of antiepileptics (p. 385)

Interactions
- contraindicated with St John's wort
- metabolism enhanced by phenytoin, carbamazepine, phenobarbital (phenobarbitone) and primidone; therefore serum levels should be closely monitored

Nursing considerations/Cautions
- if visual symptoms occur, the patient should be referred to an ophthalmologist
- caution if used in those with a history of behavioural problems including anxiety and depression or mild-to-moderate liver impairment
- not recommended in those under 12 years
- contraindicated in those with severe liver impairment
- see also General Nursing considerations/Cautions for antiepileptics (p. 386)

Patient education
- instruct the patient to seek medical advice immediately if any of the following occur:
  - bruising or bleeding
  - visual changes
  - rash or blistering
- warn the patient that tablets should not be refrigerated
- see also General Patient education for antiepileptics (p. 386)

 Tablet can be crushed and mixed with water or a spoonful of yoghurt or apple puree.

 Caution if used during pregnancy, as animal studies have demonstrated some fetal abnormalities.

 Should be used during breastfeeding only if benefits are thought to outweigh risks to newborn.

ANTIEPILEPTICS

TOPIRAMATE

Trade names
APO-Topiramate, Epiramax, Noumed Topiramate, RBX Topiramate, Tamate, Topamax, Topiramate Sandoz, Topiramate-WGR

Available forms
Tablets: 25 mg, 50 mg, 100 mg, 200 mg; Sprinkle capsules: 15 mg, 25 mg, 50 mg

Action
- reduces the frequency of neuronal action potential generation
- enhances the activity of GABA by an action different to that of barbiturates
- antagonises the ability of kainate to activate glutamate receptors
- has weak carbonic anhydrase inhibitor activity (less than acetazolamide)
- antimigraine action is unknown
- half-life 21 hours

Use
- newly diagnosed epilepsy (monotherapy)
- primary generalised tonic—clonic seizures
- partial seizures with or without secondary generalised seizures (adjunct therapy)
- drop attacks associated with Lennox—Gastaut syndrome
- migraine prophylaxis

Dose
- (Epilepsy — monotherapy) initially 25 mg orally at night for 7 days or longer, increasing by 25—50 mg daily at weekly or longer intervals until a clinical response is achieved (daily maximum 500—1000 mg) **OR**
- (Epilepsy — add-on therapy) initially 25—50 mg orally at night or in divided doses for 7 days or longer, increasing by 25—100 mg daily at weekly or longer intervals until a clinical response is achieved (daily maximum 1000 mg) **OR**
- (Migraine prophylaxis) initially 25 mg orally at night for 7 days, increasing by 25 mg per day at weekly intervals to 100 mg daily in 2 divided doses

Adverse effects
- myalgia, muscle spasm, arthralgia
- anorexia, weight loss, alteration to taste, dyspepsia, dry mouth, diarrhoea, abdominal pain
- leucopenia, bleeding (mild to severe), anaemia
- paraesthesia, hypoaesthesia
- ear pain, tinnitus
- dyspnoea
- (Rare) renal calculi, oligohidrosis, hyperthermia, eye pain, dry eyes, acute myopia, decreased visual acuity, redness, increased intraocular pressure, decreased serum sodium bicarbonate, metabolic acidosis, hyperammonaemia, dysuria, nephrolithiasis, serious skin reaction
- see also General Adverse effects of antiepileptics (p. 385)

Interactions
- may increase serum levels of phenytoin and lithium, increasing the risk of toxicity
- may decrease digoxin serum levels; therefore levels should be closely monitored especially when starting or stopping therapy
- not recommended with alcohol or other CNS-depressant drugs
- may decrease efficacy of combined oral contraceptives
- serum levels may be decreased by phenytoin and carbamazepine
- serum levels may be increased by hydrochlorothiazide
- increased risk of hypokalaemia if given with hydrochlorothiazide
- may alter serum levels of metformin, glibenclamide and pioglitazone; therefore blood glucose levels should be closely monitored
- caution if used with carbonic anhydrase inhibitors, as these may increase the risk of oligohidrosis and hyperthermia

- the risk of nephrolithiasis is increased if given with other agents that predispose to it
- increased risk of hyperammonaemia (with or without encephalopathy) if given with sodium valproate
- caution if given with warfarin;. INR should be closely monitored during therapy

Nursing considerations/Cautions

- any dehydration should be corrected before starting therapy
- the patient should be closely monitored for any decreased sweating and/or increase in body temperature
- sodium bicarbonate levels should be monitored during therapy
- caution if used in those with psychiatric history, kidney or liver impairment or prior kidney stone formation or hypercalciuria
- see also General Nursing considerations/Cautions for antiepileptics (p. 386)

Patient education

- the patient should be advised to maintain good hydration throughout therapy (especially if exercising or exposed to warm conditions) to decrease the risk of renal calculi formation
- instruct patients (especially children) to avoid exposure to high temperatures and maintain hydration in order to avoid heat stroke, as medication can decrease sweating and raise body temperature
- advise the patient to seek medical advice immediately if any of the following occur:
  - eye pain or changes in vision
  - fatigue, anorexia or hyperventilation
  - numbness or tingling of hands or feet
  - decreased sweating
  - kidney or flank pain
  - changes to consciousness, lethargy, confusion
  - serious skin reaction
  - changes to mental status, vomiting, unexplained lethargy
- women taking oral contraceptives should be counselled to report any changes in bleeding patterns and use alternative contraceptive methods (e.g. barrier) to avoid pregnancy occurring during therapy
- warn the patient that, if sprinkle capsules are used in food, the food should not be stored
- (Migraine prophylaxis) advise the patient that medication should not be used for an acute attack
- see also General Patient education for antiepileptics (p. 386)

 Capsules can be opened and mixed with yoghurt or apple puree. Tablet can be dispersed in water (has bitter taste) or mixed with a spoonful of yoghurt or apple puree.

 Increased risk of cleft palate, hypospadias and body anomalies if given during pregnancy; therefore use only if benefits outweigh risks. Folic acid supplementation is recommended to decrease the risk of spina bifida.

 Not recommended during breastfeeding, as diarrhoea and somnolence may occur in the newborn if breastfed.

 Half the starting and maintenance dose is recommended in those with moderate-to-severe kidney impairment. If the patient is undergoing haemodialysis, a supplemental dose (half of the daily dose) is recommended on the days of dialysis, given in divided doses at the start and end of dialysis.

 Pregnant staff should not open capsules or crush or disperse tablets.

VIGABATRIN
Trade name
Sabril

Available forms
Tablets: 500 mg;

ANTIEPILEPTICS

Powder: 500 mg

Action
- inhibitor of gamma aminobutyric acid (GABA) breakdown, leading to an increase in GABA levels, which leads to reduced neuronal activity
- half-life 5–8 hours

Use
- epilepsy (unresponsive to other drugs)

Dose
- initially 2 g orally daily in 1–2 doses, increasing or decreasing as necessary at weekly (or more) increments of 1 g (daily maximum 4 g)

Adverse effects
- weight gain
- abdominal pain
- oedema
- alopecia
- anaemia
- arthralgia
- visual field defects, blurred vision, double vision, and rarely, optic neuritis, optic atrophy
- (Rare) encephalopathy
- see also General Adverse effects of antiepileptics (p. 5)

Interactions
- may decrease serum levels of phenytoin
- contraindicated with retinotoxic agents
- caution if used with clonazepam because of increased sedation
- liver function tests may be unreliable in those taking vigabatrin. May also result in false positive test for some rare genetic metabolic disorders because of an increased level of amino acids in urine

Nursing considerations/Cautions
- visual fields (including visual acuity) should be measured before starting and then monitored every 6 months throughout therapy
- therapy is usually started as add-on therapy to other antiepileptic agents
- not recommended in those with pre-existing significant visual field defects
- caution if used in those with a history of depression, psychosis or behavioural problems, or kidney impairment (creatinine clearance (CrCl) < 60 mL/min)
- see also General Nursing considerations/Cautions for antiepileptics (p. 386)

Patient education
- the patient should be advised to seek medical advice immediately if any changes to vision occur
- advise the patient that granules should be dissolved in water or soft drink just before administration
- see also General Patient education for antiepileptics (p. 386)

 Powder can be dissolved in 100 mL water or soft drink. Tablet can be dispersed in water, or crushed and mixed with a spoonful of yoghurt or apple puree.

 Not recommended during pregnancy unless benefits outweigh risks to the fetus.

 Dose reduction is recommended in those with CrCl < 60 mL/min.

 If CrCl is < 60 mL/min, a low starting dose is recommended in those > 65 years.

 Pregnant staff should not prepare oral solutions or crush or disperse tablets.

ZONISAMIDE
Trade name
Zonegran

Available form
Capsules: 25 mg, 50 mg, 100 mg

Action
- benzisoxazole unrelated to other antiepileptic agents that preferentially acts on seizures coming from the cortex
- acts on sodium and calcium channels

425

- enables dopaminergic and serotonergic neurotransmission
- effective against tonic (not clonic) seizure types
- raises generalised seizure threshold
- shortens seizure duration
- inhibits carbonic anhydrase
- half-life about 60 hours

Use
- (Monotherapy) adults with partial seizures (with or without secondary generalisation) (newly diagnosed, intolerant to other agents or where other agents are contraindicated)
- (Adjunctive therapy) adults with partial seizures (with or without secondary generalisation)

Dose
- (Monotherapy) 100 mg orally daily (weeks 1 and 2), increasing to 200 mg orally daily (weeks 3 and 4), increasing to 300 mg orally (weeks 5 and 6), then 300 mg orally daily as maintenance. If a higher dose is needed, the dose can be increased at 100 mg increments at 2-weekly intervals to a maximum of 500 mg **OR**
- (Adjunctive therapy with carbamazepine, phenytoin, phenobarbital (phenobarbitone)) 25 mg orally twice daily (week 1), increasing to 50 mg orally twice daily (week 2), then increasing at weekly intervals of 100 mg (weeks 3 to 5), with maintenance of 300–500 mg (once daily or in divided doses) **OR**
- (Adjunctive therapy, or in those with renal/liver impairment) 25 mg orally twice daily (weeks 1 and 2), increasing to 50 mg orally twice daily (weeks 3 and 4), then increasing at 2-weekly intervals of up to 100 mg (weeks 5 to 10), with maintenance of 300–500 mg (once daily or in divided dose)

Adverse effects
- abdominal pain, anorexia, constipation, diarrhoea, dry mouth, dyspepsia, altered taste, weight loss
- ecchymosis, leucopenia
- arthralgia, myasthenia
- otitis media, tinnitus
- urinary tract infection, nephrolithiasis
- metabolic acidosis, decreased bicarbonate, osteomalacia, osteoporosis, decreased serum phosphorus
- acne, oligohidrosis, hyperthermia
- increased cough, pharyngitis, rhinitis, sinusitis
- pancreatitis
- (Rare) allergic reaction, flu-like syndrome, hypersensitivity, serious skin reaction, acute myopia and secondary angle-closure glaucoma, hyperammonaemia and encephalopathy
- see also General Adverse effects of antiepileptics (p. 385)

Interactions
- not recommended with carbonic anhydrase inhibitors (e.g. topiramate) because of the increased risk of metabolic acidosis and nephrolithiasis
- caution if given with bicarbonate-lowering drugs such acetazolamide because of the increased risk of metabolic acidosis
- increased risk of kidney stone development if given with other agents that cause urolithiasis
- caution if given with phenytoin, carbamazepine, phenobarbital (phenobarbitone) and rifampicin
- increased risk of hyperammonaemia and encephalopathy if given with topiramate and sodium valproate
- caution if used with other agents with anticholinergic activity or carbonic anhydrase inhibitors, as these predispose to heat disorders (e.g. heat stroke)

Nursing considerations/Cautions
- the patient should be monitored for signs of metabolic acidosis, which can occur at any dose, although more commonly at high doses and early in treatment. If metabolic acidosis occurs, the dose should be decreased or the drug discontinued

ANTIEPILEPTICS

- monitor the patient for any signs of muscle weakness or muscle pain. If they occur, creatine phosphokinase should be measured
- if the patient develops any unexplained changes to mental status, lethargy and/or vomiting, serum ammonia levels should be measured, as these can be signs of hyperammonaemia that can lead to encephalopathy
- serum bicarbonate levels should be measured before starting therapy, when reaching maintenance dose, if doses are increased, if other antiepileptic agents are added to the regimen and then 6-monthly
- 100 mg capsules contain yellow colouring (sunset yellow), which may cause allergic reaction
- caution if used in those with low body weight (< 40 kg)
- caution if used in younger patients, as metabolic acidosis occurs more frequently and more severely
- caution if given to those with a predisposition to metabolic acidosis, such as kidney disease, respiratory disorders, status epilepticus, diarrhoea, surgery, ketogenic diet or if taking bicarbonate-lowering drugs
- caution if used in those with risk factors for nephrolithiasis, including previous kidney stone formation, a family history of nephrolithiasis and hypercalciuria
- caution if used in those with a history of eye disorders because of the risk of acute myopia
- caution if used in those with inborn errors of metabolism or reduced liver mitochondrial activity because of the increased risk of hyperammonaemia and encephalopathy
- not recommended in those under 18 years or with severe liver impairment
- contraindicated in those with hypersensitivity to sulfonamides
- see also General Nursing considerations/Cautions for antiepileptics (p. 386)

Patient education

- advise patients (especially children) to avoid exposure to high temperatures and maintain hydration in order to avoid heat stroke, as medication can decrease sweating and raise body temperature
- the patient should be instructed to increase fluid intake during therapy to decrease the risk of kidney stones forming
- warn the patient to avoid a ketogenic diet during therapy because of the increased risk of metabolic acidosis
- instruct the patient to seek medical advice immediately if any of the following occur:
    - rash or skin blistering
    - significant weight loss
    - loss of appetite, fatigue, rapid breathing
    - nausea, vomiting, fever, chills, abdominal pain radiating to the back, pale fatty stools
    - eye pain, changes to vision
    - kidney or flank pain
    - muscle pain or weakness
    - vomiting, lethargy, unexplained changes in mental status
- women of childbearing potential should be counselled to use reliable contraception during and for 4 weeks after therapy is discontinued
- see also General Patient education for antiepileptics (p. 386)

 Capsules can be opened and the contents dispersed in water, or mixed with a spoonful of yoghurt or apple puree.

 Teratogenic in animal studies; therefore should be used in pregnancy only if the benefits are thought to outweigh risks to the fetus.

 Excreted in breastmilk in similar concentrations to serum; therefore breastfeeding is not recommended during or for 4 weeks after therapy is discontinued.

 Pregnant staff should not open capsules.

ANTIFUNGAL AGENTS

Fungal infections (termed mycoses) are usually caused by:
- moulds (which grow in filamentous forms (hyphae) at room temperature and in invaded tissue, e.g. dermatophytes such as *Tinea* spp., which cause 'athlete's foot', and *Aspergillus*)
- yeasts (rounded, single cells or budding organisms, e.g. *Cryptococcus* (the cause of cryptococcal meningitis), *Candida* spp. (oral and vaginal thrush))
- dimorphic fungus (these grow as yeasts but are filamentous at room temperature in the environment in which they occur, e.g. blastomycosis, histoplasmosis) (Edwards 2018).

Fungal infections can be superficial (e.g. skin, nails) or systemic (e.g. organs, deeper tissue) with deep organ infections causing severe illness and, at times, becoming fatal (Edwards 2018). *Endemic* fungal infections are acquired from environmental sources (and most commonly inhaled), while *opportunistic* fungal infections occur when normally occurring human flora overgrow owing to suppression of the immune system (Edwards 2018). For example, *Candida albicans* is a yeast-like fungus that normally resides in the gastrointestinal tract (GIT) and vagina, and is usually kept under control by the normal bacteria that also reside in those areas. When a person is treated with antibacterial agents, corticosteroids, monoclonal antibodies or antineoplastic agents, the fungus is no longer under control and overgrowth occurs (Edwards 2018).

Antifungal agents are used topically, orally or parenterally to treat infections and have no activity against other organisms such as bacteria or viruses. Classes of antifungal agents include azoles (e.g. fluconazole, isavuconazole, itraconazole, ketoconazole, miconazole, posaconazole, voriconazole), echinocandins (e.g. anidulafungin, caspofungin, micafungin) and other agents which have similar modes of action.

AMOROLFINE
Trade names
Aporyl, Chemists' Own Amer-Fine Nail Lacquer, Loceryl, MycoNail, Pharmacy Action Antifungal Nail Treatment

Available form
Nail lacquer: 5%

Action
- alters fungal cell membrane targeting ergosterol, changing cell permeability and causing leakage of cell contents

ANTIFUNGAL AGENTS

- broad spectrum
- penetrates and diffuses through nail plate effectively

Use
- onychomycoses (fungal nail infections) caused by dermatophytes, yeasts and moulds

Dose
- apply nail lacquer to affected finger(s) or toe(s) 1—2 times weekly

Adverse effects
- itching, pruritus, erythema, periungual scaling
- (Rare) nail discolouration, brittle/broken nails, transient burning sensation, contact dermatitis

Nursing considerations/Cautions
- should not be used in those who have shown previous hypersensitivity reaction

Patient education
- instruct the patient that affected finger/toenails should be cut short to allow better penetration of the antifungal agent
- the patient should be advised to:
  - file and clean nails (using the supplied nail file and cleansing pad) before applying or reapplying the lacquer
  - avoid applying lotion to skin surrounding nail
  - allow nails to dry (3—5 minutes) after the entire surface of affected nail has been coated using the supplied reusable spatula, taking care not to apply lacquer to surrounding healthy tissue
- discard the nail file after use and do not reuse it because of reinfection risk
- clean the neck of bottle and spatula with the supplied cleansing pad after each use
- ensure the bottle is tightly closed immediately after use
- treatment should be continued uninterrupted for 6 months (fingernails) or longer (toenails) until the nail has regrown and the area is cured
- the patient should be advised not to use cosmetic nail polish, artificial nails, other topical medications or occlusive dressings on the nail(s) being treated with amorolfine
- warn the patient to wear impermeable gloves if working with solvents such as paint thinners to protect the nail lacquer

 Not recommended during pregnancy unless benefits outweigh risks. Human data are limited.

 Limited human data.

AMPHOTERICIN B
Trade names
AmBisome, Amphotericin Liposomal SUN, Fungilin

Available forms
Vial: 50 mg;
Lozenges: 10 mg

Action
- binds to ergosterol, leading to membrane permeability and leakage of cell contents, causing potassium loss
- fungistatic or fungicidal (depending on concentration and/or susceptibility of organisms)
- lipid formulations have been developed to overcome nephrotoxicity and infusion reactions. The liposomal vesicles stay intact during prolonged circulation until they selectively bind to the fungal cell membrane and release the amphotericin B (amphotericin)
- not absorbed from GIT
- (IV) elimination half-life 26—32 hours (depending on dose)

Use
- oral and perioral candidiasis

- prophylaxis and treatment of potentially fatal systemic fungal infections (in liver transplant patients)
- presumed fungal infection in those with febrile neutropenia (where fever has not responded to broad-spectrum antibiotics)
- visceral leishmaniasis due to *Leishmania infantum*

Dose

Oral candidiasis
- 10 mg orally (1 lozenge) sucked and allowed to dissolve slowly, 4 times daily after meals and nightly for 7–14 days

Systemic fungal infections
- (Systemic mycoses) initially 3 mg/kg daily by IV infusion over 30–60 minutes, increasing gradually to 5 mg/kg if needed **OR**
- (Prophylaxis of fungal infection in liver transplantation) 1 mg/kg daily by IV infusion over 30–60 minutes for 5 days following transplantation **OR**
- (HIV-associated disseminated cryptococcosis) 3 mg/kg daily by IV infusion over 30–60 minutes for up to 42 days **OR**
- (Visceral leishmaniasis, immunocompromised patient) 1–1.5 mg/kg daily by IV infusion over 30–60 minutes for 21 days **OR**
- (Visceral leishmaniasis, immunocompetent patient) as for immunocompromised patient, or 3.0 mg/kg daily by IV infusion over 30–60 minutes for 10 days **OR**
- (Febrile neutropenia with presumed fungal infection) 1–3 mg/kg by IV infusion over 30–60 minutes, adjusting the dose according to clinical condition

Adverse effects
- (Oral) mild nausea, vomiting, diarrhoea, transient yellowing of teeth
- (Infusion reaction) chills, fever, rigors, back pain (usually within minutes of infusion starting)
- nausea, vomiting, abdominal pain, diarrhoea
- headache, tremor
- back pain
- hypotension, tachycardia, vasodilation, flushing, chest pain
- dyspnoea, cough
- rash, pruritus
- abnormal liver/kidney function, hypokalaemia, hyperglycaemia, hyponatraemia, hypomagnesaemia, hypocalcaemia, hyperbilirubinaemia, increased creatinine and blood urea
- toxic nephropathy
- (Rare) anaphylactoid reactions, anaphylaxis

Interactions
- risk of digitalis toxicity is increased in the presence of amphotericin-induced hypokalaemia when given with digoxin; therefore serum potassium and digoxin levels should be closely monitored
- not recommended with azole antifungal agents owing to an antagonistic effect reducing antifungal activity
- increased risk of pulmonary toxicity if given with or near to leucocyte transfusion, so should be separated for the longest possible time period. Lung function should be monitored
- increased risk of myelotoxicity and nephrotoxicity if given with zidovudine
- effects of skeletal muscle relaxants may be potentiated in the presence of amphotericin-induced hypokalaemia. The patient should be monitored for any enhanced neuromuscular blockade if given together
- increases nephrotoxicity of ciclosporin, nephrotoxic antibiotics (e.g. aminoglycosides), other nephrotoxic agents and parenteral pentamidine; therefore renal function should be closely monitored if given together
- increased risk of nephrotoxicity, bronchospasm and hypotension if given with antineoplastic agents such as cisplatin and nitrogen mustard compounds

ANTIFUNGAL AGENTS

- corticosteroids and corticotrophin may increase amphotericin-induced hypokalaemia, predisposing to cardiac arrhythmias; therefore serum potassium level and cardiac function should be closely monitored if given together
- increased risk of toxicity if given with flucytosine
- caution if used with loop diuretics. If given together, serum potassium and kidney function should be monitored

Nursing considerations/Cautions

- should not be used for superficial infections
- (Lozenge) should not be used to treat systemic infections
- blood counts, serum electrolytes, kidney and liver function should be monitored at least weekly during prolonged therapy (especially if receiving a concurrent nephrotoxic agent). Potassium supplements may be required
- slowing infusion rate may decrease infusion-related reaction symptoms
- resuscitation equipment should be readily available during IV administration
- reconstitute using water for injections only and shake the solution until any yellow sediment has dissolved, withdraw the required amount from vial(s), discard the needle and replace with a 5 micron high-flow filter needle (supplied) and inject into glucose 5% solution
- administer alone using separated IV line or ensure the existing IV line is adequately flushed with glucose 5% before administration
- an in-line filter (1 micron or greater) may be used for IV infusion
- leucocyte transfusion should be separated for the longest possible period to avoid the risk of acute lung toxicity. Lung function should be closely monitored
- if the patient is having renal dialysis, amphotericin B (amphotericin) should not be administered until dialysis is completed. Monitoring of serum potassium and magnesium is recommended
- should not be mixed with solutions containing sodium chloride or potassium
- contains 900 mg sucrose per vial; therefore blood glucose levels should be closely monitored if the patient has diabetes mellitus
- should be used omly after dialysis has been completed in those with kidney impairment

Patient education

- (Lozenge) advise the patient that dentures should be removed while sucking lozenges and then thoroughly cleaned
- (Lozenge) the patient should be warned that any yellowing of teeth is from sucking lozenges and is temporary. It can be removed by brushing teeth
- (Infusion) inform the patient that infusion-related reactions (e.g. fever, chills, rigors, chest pain, or back pain) may occur during the administration. These reactions typically resolve after stopping the infusion and may not occur with future doses. However, the patient should report any reactions immediately
- (Infusion) the patient should be aware of the potential for electrolyte imbalances, such as hypokalaemia (low potassium) and hypomagnesaemia (low magnesium). Supplementation may be required, and symptoms like muscle cramps or weakness should be reported
- (Infusion) regular monitoring of renal function (creatinine levels) and serum electrolytes (especially potassium and magnesium) will be necessary

Should be used during pregnancy only if the potential benefits outweigh the risks.

Breastfeeding should be discontinued during therapy.

Renal Impairment: dosage reduction is unnecessary in patients with renal impairment. However, further

> impairment may occur during treatment, especially with prolonged use.
>
> Co-administration with nephrotoxic drugs (e.g. aminoglycosides, cyclosporin) may increase the likelihood of renal impairment. Avoid combination therapy if possible or ensure close monitoring of renal function when these drugs are used together.

ANIDULAFUNGIN

Trade name
Eraxis

Available form
Vial: 100 mg

Action
- echinocandin that inhibits glucan synthesis in the fungal wall (which is not present in human cells)
- fungicidal for *Candida* species
- fungistatic for *Aspergillus* species
- elimination half-life 20 hours

Use
- invasive candidiasis, including candidaemia

Dose
- (Adults with invasive candidiasis, including candidaemia): initially 200 mg IV over 180 minutes (day 1, loading dose), then 100 mg daily over 90 minutes continued for at least 14 days after last positive culture (but not exceeding 28 days)
- (Children > 1 month): loading dose (day 1): 3 mg/kg (not exceeding 200 mg), maintenance dose (from day 2 onwards): 1.5 mg/kg (not exceeding 100 mg) once daily. Continued for at least 14 days after the last positive culture (but not exceeding 28 days)

Adverse effects
- thrombocytopenia, coagulopathy, decreased platelet count
- hyperkalaemia, hypokalaemia, hypomagnesaemia
- increase in liver enzymes, elevated bilirubin and creatinine
- headache, flushing
- diarrhoea
- rash, pruritus
- seizures
- prolonged QT interval
- (Rare) anaphylactic reaction
- (Infusion reaction) rash, pruritus, flushing, urticaria, dyspnoea, bronchospasm, hypotension

Nursing considerations/Cautions
- fungal culture and histopathology should be performed on specimen to identify species before starting therapy
- liver function, FBC, ECG and electrolytes should be monitored during therapy
- administer intravenously (IV)
- do not administer by bolus injection; only slow IV infusion is recommended
- reconstitute each vial with sterile water for injection, resulting in a concentration of 3.33 mg/mL
- after reconstitution, further dilute with either 9 mg/mL (0.9%) sodium chloride or 50 mg/mL (5%) glucose for infusion. The final concentration should be 0.77 mg/mL
- the rate of infusion should not exceed 1.1 mg/min (or 84 mL/hour). The minimum infusion duration is: 200 mg dose: 180 minutes (3 hours); 100 mg dose: 90 minutes (1.5 hours)
- inspect visually for particulate matter or discolouration before administration. If present, discard the solution
- the final infusion solution should be used within 48 hours if stored at 25°C

Patient education
- advise the patient to seek medical advice if any of the following occur:
  - increased heart rate
  - fever, infection
  - unexplained bleeding or bruising
  - seizures (fitting)

ANTIFUNGAL AGENTS

- female patients of childbearing potential should be counselled to use adequate and effective contraception during therapy and contact doctor if pregnancy occurs during therapy

Not recommended during pregnancy, as human safety data not available. Effective contraception should be used in women of childbearing potential.

Not recommended during breastfeeding unless benefits outweigh risks.

BIFONAZOLE
Trade names
Canesten Bifonazole Once Daily Body, Canesten Once Daily Antifungal Athlete's Foot

Available form
Topical cream: 1% (10 mg/g)

Action
- imidazole antifungal agent that inhibits ergosterol synthesis in fungal cell membrane
- fungicidal against dermatophytes, fungistatic against yeasts

Use
- mycoses of skin caused by dermatophytes and yeasts
- pityriasis versicolor caused by *Malassezia furfur*

Dose
- applied thinly to affected area and rubbed gently into skin once daily before sleeping

Adverse effects
- burning, pruritus, irritation, erythema, scaling
- (Less frequent) contact dermatitis

Nursing considerations/Cautions
- not recommended for fungal infections of the mucous membranes or eyes

Patient education
- the patient should be advised to complete the course of treatment, which may continue for days/weeks after symptoms have resolved. If there is no resolution of the symptoms after the treatment period, the diagnosis should be reassessed or the likelihood of resistance to the agent used should be considered
- warn the patient that superficial fungal infections can be highly contagious
- advise the patient not to share clothing or personal linen (e.g. face washers, towels)
- the patient should be advised to continue treatment uninterrupted for the following times:
  - 3 weeks for tinea pedis, tinea pedis interdigitalis
  - 2–3 weeks for tinea corporis, tinea cruris, tinea manuum
  - 2 weeks for pityriasis versicolor
  - 2–4 weeks for superficial candidiasis of the skin
- the patient being treated for tinea pedis should be encouraged to wash and dry the feet (especially between the toes) carefully each day and apply antifungal powder. They should also be advised to wear shoes or sandals that are well ventilated (if possible), wear waterproof sandals in public showers, change hosiery (preferably cotton socks) daily and dust shoes inside with powder
- instruct the patient not to use cream for fungal infection of other areas of the body, particularly the vagina or mouth

Safety during pregnancy has not been established; animal studies have shown bifonazole to be embryotoxic.

Available in combination with
- bifinazole 100 mg/g + urea 400 mg/g tube (Canesten Fungal Nail Treatment)

CASPOFUNGIN

Trade name
Caspofungin AN

Available forms
Vial: 50 mg, 70 mg

Action
- echinocandin that inhibits glucan synthesis in the fungal wall (which is not present in human cells)
- fungicidal for *Candida*, fungistatic for *Aspergillus*

Use
- invasive candidiasis (including candidaemia)
- oesophageal candidiasis
- invasive aspergillosis (when other treatment was ineffective or inappropriate)
- fungal infection in febrile neutropenia patient (when fever has failed to respond to other treatments)

Dose
- (Invasive candidiasis, invasive aspergillosis, febrile neutropenia) initially 70 mg by slow IV infusion over 1 hour (day 1, loading dose), then 35—50 mg daily IV (maintenance) **OR**
- (Oesophageal candidiasis) 35—50 mg daily by slow IV infusion over 1 hour

Adverse effects
- myalgia
- diarrhoea, nausea, vomiting, abdominal pain
- fever, chills, sweating, flushing
- dyspnoea
- rash, pruritus, erythema
- tremor, insomnia
- headache
- tachycardia, hypertension
- increased liver enzymes, hypokalaemia, hypomagnesaemia, increased creatinine and bilirubin
- (Hypersensitivity reaction) rash, pruritus, facial swelling, bronchospasm, flushing sensation
- (IV site) phlebitis, thrombophlebitis, pain

Interactions
- not recommended with ciclosporin because of the increased risk of liver toxicity. If given together, liver function should be closely monitored
- may decrease serum levels of tacrolimus; therefore blood levels should be monitored
- serum levels decreased if given with rifampicin (if added to already existing rifampicin therapy), efavirenz, nevirapine, phenytoin, dexamethasone or carbamazepine

Nursing considerations/Cautions
- treatment should continue for a minimum of 14 days and at least 28 days after neutropenia and clinical symptoms have resolved
- not compatible with glucose
- administer alone
- allow the vial to come to room temperature, then reconstitute using water for injections or sodium chloride 0.9% (10.5 mL) and mix gently. When the solution clears, inspect for particulate matter or discolouration, then dilute with sodium chloride 0.9% infusion bag (100—250 mL) and infuse over 1 hour
- caution if used in those with moderate liver impairment or with a history of allergic skin reactions

 Caspofungin should be used during pregnancy only if the potential benefits outweigh the potential risks to the fetus.

 Not recommended during breastfeeding.

 Hepatic impairment: moderate hepatic impairment (Child—Pugh score 7—9): there is a more significant increase (~76%) in plasma concentrations, and therefore a reduced daily dose of 35 mg is recommended following a loading dose of 70 mg.

ANTIFUNGAL AGENTS

Severe hepatic impairment (Child—Pugh score > 9): there is no clinical experience with caspofungin use in this population, and therefore its use is not recommended without close monitoring.

Elderly patients (65+ years) experience slightly higher plasma concentrations of caspofungin (~28% increase in AUC), but no dosage adjustment is typically necessary.

CICLOPIROX
Trade name
Rejuvenail

Available form
Solution: 80 mg/g

Action
- pyridone antifungal agent with some anti-inflammatory activity

Use
- treatment of mild-to-moderate fungal nail infections (onychomycosis) caused by dermatophytes, yeasts and moulds

Dose
- applied topically to infected nail(s) at night until healthy nail has regrown
- treatment course can last from 6 months (fingernails) to 9—12 months (toenails), depending on the severity of the infection

Adverse effects
- pain, irritation, redness, burning, tenderness, ingrown nail

Patient education
- the patient should be advised to:
  - wash and dry the infected nail
  - apply a thin layer to within 5 mm of surrounding skin and under the nail if possible
  - allow to dry for 30 seconds
  - the area should not be washed for 6 hours

- fingernails may require up to 6 months of treatment, toenails 9—12 months

Caution if used during pregnancy although systemic absorption is minimal.

Caution if used during breastfeeding owing to lack of safety data.

CLOTRIMAZOLE
Trade names
Apohealth Anti-Fungal, Canesten Clotrimazole Antifungal, Canesten Clotrimazole Athletes Foot, Clonea, Pharmacy Action Anti-Fungal, Clonea Clotrimazole Thrush Treatment 3 Day Cream, Clonea Clotrimazole Thrush Treatment 6 Day Cream, Clozole Topical Cream, Clozole Vaginal Cream

Available forms
Topical cream: 10 mg/g;
Solution: 10 mg/mL (1%);
Vaginal cream: 10 mg/g, 20 mg/g;
Vaginal pessaries: 100 mg, 500 mg

Action
- imidazole antifungal agent that inhibits ergosterol synthesis in fungal cell membrane

Use
- dermatophytes (e.g. tinea pedis, tinea cruris, tinea corporis, pityriasis versicolor)
- onychia, paronychia
- candidiasis, cutaneous candidiasis, vaginal and vulvovaginal candidiasis

Dose

Cutaneous candidiasis, dermatophytes
- gently massage cream into affected and surrounding skin areas 2—3 times daily for at least 2 weeks after symptoms have resolved **OR**
- apply cream or solution 2—3 times daily sparingly to affected areas

Vaginal, vulvovaginal candidiasis

- 5 g (1 applicator full) inserted nightly as deeply as possible into the vagina for 6 successive days (vaginal cream 1%) or 3 doses (vaginal cream 2%) or 1 dose (vaginal cream 10%) **OR**
- 100 mg nightly inserted as deeply as possible into the vagina for 6 successive days (vaginal tablet/pessary) or 2 × 100 mg tablets for 3 doses or 1 × 500 mg (vaginal tablet/pessary) as a single dose

Adverse effects

- (Cream/solution) erythema, oedema, pruritus, urticaria, stinging/burning, blistering, peeling, general irritation of skin
- (Pessaries/vaginal tablets) (uncommon) mild burning, skin rash, lower abdominal pain

Interactions

- vaginal cream may reduce effectiveness of latex products (e.g. condoms, diaphragms)

Nursing considerations/Cautions

- (Skin conditions) treatment time depends on the location of the infection:
  - dermatomycoses: 2–4 weeks
  - onychia and paronychia: 4–8 weeks
  - tinea pedis, corporis: 4 weeks
  - tinea cruris: 2 weeks
  - cutaneous candidiasis: 2 weeks
- if there is no improvement in 4 weeks, the diagnosis should be reviewed
- vaginal cream and pessaries can be used together to manage vulvovaginitis or perianal infection
- caution if used in those with sensitivity to another azole

Patient education

- the patient should be advised to complete the course of treatment, which may continue for days/weeks after symptoms have resolved. If there is no resolution of the symptoms after the treatment period, the diagnosis should be reassessed or the likelihood of resistance to the agent used considered
- warn the patient that superficial fungal infections can be highly contagious
- advise the patient not to share clothing or personal linen (e.g. face washers, towels)
- patients being treated for tinea pedis should be encouraged to wash and dry the feet (especially between toes) carefully each day and apply antifungal powder. They should also be advised to wear shoes or sandals that are well ventilated (if possible), wear waterproof sandals in public showers, change hosiery (preferably cotton socks) daily and dust shoes inside with powder

Vaginal/Vulvovaginal candidiasis

- ensure the patient understands the correct insertion technique for vaginal cream, pessaries and tablets
- advise the patient that a second course of treatment may be required if the first course was unsuccessful
- treatment should be timed to avoid menstruation or to be complete before its onset or should be continued if menstruation occurs
- warn the patient that vaginal cream/pessaries may decrease the effectiveness and safety of condoms and diaphragms
- for prevention of reinfection, the partner(s) should be treated locally at the same time with application of cream to the glans penis
- if the patient is pregnant and in second or third trimester, digital insertion of tablets/pessaries is recommended rather than plastic applicator
- instruct women being treated for vaginal infection that they should refrain from sexual intercourse or encourage the partner to use a condom. Sexual

partner(s) should also be treated to prevent reinfection. Perineal pads (or panty liners) will prevent staining of underwear or clothing when vaginal tablets or creams are used. Wearing cotton underwear and pantyhose with a cotton gusset is also recommended (especially if infection recurs). Use of tampons or douching between doses of vaginal medications is not recommended

 Intravaginal antifungal preparations, such as clotrimazole, are usually not recommended during the first trimester of pregnancy unless the potential benefits outweigh the risks.

Available in combination with
- clotrimazole 1% cream + fluconazole 150 mg tablet (APO Health Thrush Treatment Duo Combination pack, Canesoral Duo Combination pack, Chemists' Own Femazole Duo Combination pack)
- hydocortison 1% + clotrimazole 1% cream (Candacort MiniPak, CandaDerm, Canesten Extra Antifungal Anti-Inflammatory Cream, Canesten Plus Antifungal Anti-Inflammatory Cream, Hydrozole Cream, Trimacorte Cream)

ECONAZOLE
Trade names
Pevaryl Anti-Fungal Cream, Pevaryl Foaming Solution

Available forms
Foaming solution: 1%;
Cream: 1%

Action
- azole antifungal
- imidazole antifungal agent that inhibits ergosterol synthesis in fungal cell membrane

Use
- tinea pedis, tinea cruris, tinea corporis, tinea versicolor (pityriasis versicolor)

Dose
- apply foaming solution to wet body (skin and scalp) after showering nightly. Rub in well for 3–5 minutes and then allow to dry, rinse off the following morning and repeat for 3 consecutive evenings **OR**
- apply cream to affected area 2–3 times daily for up to 14 days until symptoms disappear, to prevent relapse

Adverse effects
- (Foaming solution) tightening of facial skin

Nursing considerations/Cautions
- the course should be repeated after 4 weeks and again at 12 weeks after initial treatment to prevent recurrence
- caution if used in those with sensitivity to another azole

Patient education
- the patient should be advised to complete the course of treatment, which may continue for days/weeks after symptoms have resolved. If there is no resolution of the symptoms after the treatment period, the diagnosis should be reassessed or the likelihood of resistance to the agent used should be considered
- warn the patient that superficial fungal infections can be highly contagious
- advise the patient not to share clothing or personal linen (e.g. face washers, towels)
- the patient should be advised to avoid contact with eyes
- patients being treated for tinea pedis should be encouraged to wash and dry the feet (especially between toes) carefully each day and apply antifungal powder. They should also be advised to wear shoes or sandals that are well ventilated (if possible), wear waterproof sandals in public showers, change hosiery (preferably cotton socks) daily and dust shoes inside with powder

Limited human data. Should be used only if the benefits outweigh potential risks, particularly in the first trimester.

It is unknown whether econazole is excreted in breastmilk. However, due to low systemic absorption following topical or vaginal administration, the risk to a nursing infant is minimal.

FLUCONAZOLE

Trade names
Apo-Fluconazole, ApoHealth Fluconazole One, Aspen Fluconazole Injection for Intravenous Infusion, Canesoral, Chemists' Own Femazole One, Diflucan, Diflucan One, Dizole, Dizole One, Fluconazole Sandoz, Fluconazole-Baxter, Fluconazole-WGR, Flufeme, Fluzole, Ozole, Pharmacy Action Femrelief One

Available forms
Capsules: 50 mg, 100 mg, 150 mg, 200 mg; Powder (for oral suspension): 50 mg/5 mL; Infusion bags: 100 mg/50 mL, 200 mg/100 mL, 400 mg/200 mL

Action
- azole
- triazole (similar to the imidazoles) which shows good penetration into body fluids including ocular fluid and CSF
- inhibits ergosterol synthesis in fungal cell membrane
- (Oral, IV) half-life about 30 hours, prolonged in those with impaired kidney function (98—125 hours)

Use
- treatment and prophylaxis of cryptococcal meningitis (in those unable to tolerate amphotericin B (amphotericin) or prevent relapse in patients with AIDS)
- serious or life-threatening *Candida* infections (in patients unable to tolerate amphotericin B (amphotericin))
- oropharyngeal or oesophageal candidiasis
- vaginal candidiasis (where topical therapy has failed)
- extensive tinea infection (in immunocompromised patients where topical treatment has failed or is not practicable)

Dose
- (Cryptococcal meningitis) 400 mg orally or IV on first day, then 200—400 mg orally or IV daily and continue for 10—12 weeks after CSF becomes culture negative **OR**
- (Prevention of relapse of cryptococcal meningitis in patient with AIDS) 100—200 mg orally or IV daily after full course of primary treatment **OR**
- (Oropharyngeal candidiasis) 100 mg orally or IV on first day, then 50 mg orally or IV daily for 2—3 weeks **OR**
- (Oesophageal candidiasis) 200 mg on first day, then 100 mg daily for 2—3 weeks **OR**
- (Secondary prophylaxis against oropharyngeal candidiasis in HIV patients) 150 mg as a single weekly oral or IV dose **OR**
- (Serious candidiasis where amphotericin B (amphotericin) is unable to be used) 400 mg orally or IV on first day, then 200—400 mg orally or IV daily for a minimum of 4 weeks and at least 2 weeks after symptoms have resolved **OR**
- (Failed topical treatment of vaginal candidiasis) 150 mg as single oral dose **OR**
- (Extensive tinea infection) 150 mg as a single weekly dose for 4 weeks

Adverse effects
- nausea, vomiting, abdominal pain, diarrhoea, dyspepsia
- headache, dizziness
- rash, acne
- elevated liver enzymes
- (Rare) anaphylaxis, prolonged QT interval, hepatotoxicity, serious cutaneous reactions, leucopenia

Interactions
- contraindicated with agents known to prolong QT interval such as erythromycin

ANTIFUNGAL AGENTS

- not recommended with voriconazole
- serum levels may be decreased by rifampicin
- increased risk of uveitis if given with rifabutin
- may enhance anticoagulant effect of warfarin; therefore prothrombin time should be closely monitored during therapy, especially when starting or stopping therapy
- may increase serum levels of alfentanil, amitriptyline, carbamazepine, ciclosporin, calcium-channel blockers (nifedipine, amlodipine, verapamil, felodipine), celecoxib, methadone, midazolam, nortriptyline, NSAIDs, phenytoin, rifabutin, sirolimus, tacrolimus and theophylline, increasing the risk of adverse effects and toxicity. Patients receiving concurrent therapy should be closely observed and serum levels monitored if appropriate
- may increase the serum levels of sulfonylureas and risk of hypoglycaemia
- serum levels may increase when given with hydrochlorothiazide
- may decrease metabolism of zidovudine, leading to increased serum levels increasing the risk of adverse effects
- may decrease antihypertensive effect of losartan
- increased risk of myopathy and rhabdomyolysis if given with 3-hydroxy-3-methylglutaryl coenzyme A (HMG-CoA) reductase inhibitors (statins)
- if given long term with prednisolone, the patient should be monitored for adrenal cortex insufficiency when fluconazole is stopped
- may increase respiratory depression if given with fentanyl
- may increase serum bilirubin and creatinine if given with cyclophosphamide
- increased risk of neurotoxicity if given with vinca alkaloids
- increased risk of CNS adverse effects if given with vitamin A
- not recommended with amphotericin B (amphotericin), as it reduces antifungal activity

Nursing considerations/Cautions

- IV fluconazole should be given only when oral administration is not possible
- monitor liver function frequently during therapy
- (Cryptococcal meningitis) if no response after 60 days, alternative therapy should be considered
- IV rate not to exceed 200 mg/hour
- should not be mixed with other IV drugs
- compatible with Ringer's solution and sodium chloride 0.9%
- IV solution contains 15 mmol sodium chloride/100 mL, which may need to be considered if the patient has a sodium restriction
- development of rash in immunocompromised patients may require withdrawal of the drug
- oral suspension contains sucrose and capsules contain lactose; therefore not recommended in those with rare hereditary problems of galactose intolerance, Lapp lactase deficiency or glucose–galactose malabsorption
- caution if used in those with known cardiac arrhythmias, structural heart disease or electrolyte imbalance, or if given with other agents that are known to prolong the QT interval
- caution if used in patients with HIV or AIDS infection, as there is an increased likelihood of adverse effects occurring
- caution if used in those with kidney impairment
- contraindicated in those with sensitivity to another azole

Patient education

- if the patient has diabetes treated with sulfonylureas, they should be advised to monitor blood glucose levels carefully, as there is a risk of hypoglycaemia occurring

- if the patient has HIV infection or is immunocompromised, they should be instructed to immediately report any rash, as this may require stopping fluconazole
- warn the patient against driving or operating machinery if dizziness occurs
- advise the patient to seek medical advice if any of the following occur:
  - yellowing of eyes or skin, loss of appetite, lethargy or tiredness, upper abdominal pain, dark urine, pale stools
  - fast or irregular heart rate
  - sudden severe itching, hives or rash
- the patient should be advised to swallow capsules whole and take with water
- instruct the patient to shake the oral suspension well before measuring and discard after 14 days
- patients being treated for tinea pedis should be encouraged to wash and dry the feet (especially between toes) carefully each day and apply antifungal powder. They should also be advised to wear shoes or sandals that are well ventilated (if possible), wear waterproof sandals in public showers, change hosiery (preferably cotton socks) daily and dust shoes inside with powder
- women of childbearing potential should be advised to use adequate contraception throughout therapy to avoid pregnancy and for 1 week after finishing therapy

Available as oral solution. Capsules can be opened and contents dispersed in water, or mixed with a spoonful of yoghurt or apple puree.

Not recommended during pregnancy or in women of childbearing potential not using effective contraception owing to the risk of spontaneous abortion or congenital abnormalities (at high doses for prolonged courses of treatment).

Excreted into human breastmilk at concentrations similar to those found in plasma. Not recommended for nursing mothers unless the potential benefits outweigh the risks to the infant.

Available in combination with
- fluconazole 150 mg tablets + clotrimazole 1% cream (Canesoral Duo Combination, Chemists' Own Femazole Duo)

GRISEOFULVIN
Trade name
Grisovin

Available form
Tablets: 125 mg, 500 mg

Action
- derived from *Penicillium* species and inhibits fungal mitosis
- deposited in the keratin precursor cells, mainly in the diseased tissue, causing the new keratin to become highly resistant to fungal invasion, allowing uninfected new growth to replace older infected structures
- has no antibacterial action and is therefore unlikely to upset GI flora
- absorption is variable and incomplete (fatty food will increase rate and extent of absorption)
- half-life 9–21 hours

Use
- fungal infections of skin, scalp, hair and nails (where topical therapy has failed or is inappropriate)

Dose
- 500–1000 mg orally once daily after meals

Adverse effects
- nausea, vomiting, diarrhoea, thirst, flatulence, dyspepsia, GI bleeding, oral thrush

ANTIFUNGAL AGENTS

- headache (sometimes severe), drowsiness, vertigo, fatigue, confusion, insomnia, lethargy, impaired performance
- peripheral neuritis
- rash, urticaria, erythema, photosensitivity
- leucopenia, neutropenia
- albuminuria
- (Rare) systemic lupus erythematosus (SLE)-like syndrome, exacerbation of existing SLE, hepatotoxicity, proteinuria, menstrual irregularities, nephrosis, serum sickness, angioedema

Interactions

- may enhance effects of alcohol
- absorption and effectiveness may be decreased by barbiturates
- reduces the effectiveness of oral contraceptives
- warfarin effects may be reduced; therefore prothrombin time should be closely monitored especially when starting or stopping therapy
- blood levels and effectiveness may be decreased by sedatives and hypnotics

Nursing considerations/Cautions

- administer with food or milk to enhance absorption
- contraindicated for prophylaxis
- treatment may last for at least 4 weeks (hair and skin) and extend to 12 months for some nail infections and should continue for at least 2 weeks after symptoms have disappeared
- monitor blood cell count weekly for 4 weeks and then regularly during therapy. Kidney and liver function should also be monitored periodically (especially if therapy is prolonged)
- contraindicated in those with porphyria, SLE, severe liver failure or hepatocellular failure

Patient education

- instruct patient to take tablets with meals (which include some fat) or milk to help with absorption
- advise the patient to immediately seek medical advice if any of the following occur:
  - menstrual irregularities
  - confusion
  - numbness, tingling, pain or weakness in hands or feet
  - sore throat, fever
  - yellowing of skin or eyes
- warn the patient to avoid skin exposure to direct or intense sunlight (real or artificial) and of the need to wear sunscreen (at least SPF 30+), protective clothing, hat and sunglasses when outside
- advise the patient not to drive or operate machinery if drowsy or dizzy
- the patient should be warned that the effects of alcohol may be enhanced and should be avoided during therapy. If the patient has alcohol, and rapid heartbeat, flushing, redness in the face and/or increased sweating occurs (disulfiram—alcohol reaction) (see Glossary), they should seek medical advice immediately
- oral contraceptives may be less effective while taking griseofulvin; use additional non-hormonal contraceptive methods during treatment and for 1 month after stopping the medication.
- women and men should be advised to use adequate contraception during therapy and for 4 weeks (women) or 24 weeks (men) after ceasing therapy, as griseofulvin can cause birth defects
- patients should be advised to adopt hygienic measures to minimise the risk of reinfection. Items such as footwear and, in the case of scalp infections, headwear and pillows should be treated or replaced to avoid the spread of infection

 Tablet can be crushed and mixed with water or milk, or a spoonful of yoghurt.

 Contraindicated in pregnancy and in women planning to become pregnant during or within 1 month after treatment

because of teratogenic effects. Women should be advised not to become pregnant within 4 weeks of taking griseofulvin.

Men should allow 6 months after treatment before fathering children because griseofulvin may cause abnormal segregation of chromosomes after cell division.

Avoid use. Excretion in human breastmilk unknown.

Hepatic impairment: contraindicated in patients with severe hepatic disease, as it may worsen liver function. Regular monitoring of liver function is advised during treatment owing to the risk of hepatotoxicity.

ISAVUCONAZOLE

Trade name
Cresemba

Available forms
Vial: 200 mg;
Capsules: 100 mg

Action
- azole antifungal
- triazole (subclass)
- inhibits ergosterol synthesis in fungal cell membrane
- isavuconazole sulfate is a prodrug converted to active isavuconazole

Use
- treatment of invasive aspergillosis and mucormycosis in patients where amphotericin B is inappropriate

Dose
- 200 mg orally or IV infusion over 1 hour 8-hourly for 6 doses (loading dose), followed by 200 mg orally or IV infusion over 1 hour once daily

Adverse effects
- elevated liver enzymes
- decreased appetite, nausea, vomiting, abdominal pain, diarrhoea
- dyspnoea, acute respiratory failure
- headache, confusion, delirium, somnolence, fatigue
- chest pain
- rash, pruritus
- hypokalaemia
- kidney failure
- infusion-related reaction
- injection site reaction, thrombophlebitis
- (Rare) severe skin reactions, hypersensitivity

Interactions
- contraindicated with high-dose ritonavir (> 200 mg every 12 hours), rifampicin, rifabutin, carbamazepine, long-acting barbiturates (e.g. phenobarbital (phenobarbitone)), phenytoin, St John's wort, efavirenz and etravirine
- caution if used with agents known to decrease QT interval
- increased plasma levels may occur if given with clarithromycin and other protease inhibitors; therefore should be given with caution
- decreased plasma levels may occur if given with aprepitant or pioglitazone
- caution if given with mycophenolate mofetil, ciclosporin, sirolimus or tacrolimus. If given together, plasma levels should be closely monitored
- not recommended with prednisolone
- may increase plasma levels of midazolam, colchicine, dabigratran, metformin, vincristine, vinblastine, daunorubicin, doxorubicin, irinotecan or topotecan, leading to adverse effects
- may decrease plasma levels of bupropion, cyclophosphamide or nelfinavir
- digoxin plasma levels should be closely monitored if given together

Nursing considerations/Cautions
- liver enzymes should be measured before starting therapy and monitored regularly throughout therapy
- duration of treatment is determined by clinical response; however, if the therapy is longer than 6 months, risk versus benefit should be considered
- IV infusion should be stopped if an infusion-related reaction (hypotension,

dyspnoea, dizziness, paraesthesia, nausea, headache) occurs
- to reconstitute, add 5 mL water for injections to vial, shake well to dissolve, then further dilute by adding to 250 mL infusion bag of either glucose 5% or sodium chloride 0.9% and inverting the bag gently several times to minimise particulate formation. Diluted solution may contain fine white-to-translucent particulates, which can be removed by administration through an in-line filter
- must be administered using an in-line filter (0.2–1.2 micrometre pore size) made of polyether sulfone (PES)
- administer alone
- infuse over at least 1 hour to reduce the risk of infusion-related reactions
- IV infusion should be completed within 6 hours of reconstitution and dilution
- caution if used in patients with hypersensitivity to other azole antifungals
- not recommended in those with severe liver impairment or in those under 18 years
- contraindicated in patient with a family history of short QT syndrome

Patient education

- instruct the patient that capsules should be swallowed whole and not chewed, crushed, opened or dissolved
- advise the patient not to drive or operate machinery if any confusion, dizziness, somnolence or syncope occurs

Capsules should not be opened, crushed or dissolved.

However, in situations where a patient cannot swallow capsules, they may open the capsule and disperse the contents in water.

If the patient cannot swallow thin fluids, the capsule's contents can be mixed with a spoonful of yogurt or apple puree, which are thicker consistencies, to aid ingestion.

Not recommended during pregnancy unless fungal infection is severe or life threatening.

Avoid use, as limited human data. Can be transferred into breastmilk.

Health professionals should not open the capsule if they are pregnant.

ITRACONAZOLE

Trade name
Itracap, Itranox, Lozanoc

Available forms
Capsules: 50 mg, 100 mg

Action
- azole antifungal
- triazole (subclass) which has poor penetration into CSF
- inhibits ergosterol synthesis in the fungal cell membrane
- variable oral absorption, although this improves if taken with food
- metabolite has equal antifungal activity

Use
- oral and oesophageal candidiasis (when other treatment has been ineffective or inappropriate)
- vaginal candidiasis (not responding to topical treatment)
- pityriasis versicolor (tinea versicolor) (not responding to treatment)
- systemic mycoses, aspergillosis, histoplasmosis, sporotrichosis
- fungal keratitis (not responding to treatment, progressing or threatening sight)
- superficial dermatomycosis (tinea corporis, tinea cruris, tinea pedis, tinea manus, tinea unguium) (not responding to topical treatment)
- onychomycosis (caused by dermatomycoses)
- disseminated/chronic histoplasmosis in patient with AIDS (treatment and maintenance)

- non-invasive candidiasis (non-neutropenic patient not responding to other treatments)
- prophylaxis of fungal infection (neutropenic patient)

Dose
- (Superficial dermatomycosis) 100 mg orally daily for 2–4 weeks **OR**
- (Superficial dermatomycosis) 50 mg orally daily for 2–4 weeks (Lozanoc) **OR**
- (Onychomycosis) 200 mg orally daily for 3 months **OR**
- (Onychomycosis) 100 mg orally daily for 3 months (Lozanoc) **OR**
- (Onychomycosis — pulsed) 200 mg orally twice daily for 7 days, followed by drug-free 21 days, repeated for fingernails (2 pulses) or repeated twice more (3 pulses) for toenails **OR**
- (Onychomycosis — pulsed) 100 mg orally twice daily for 7 days, followed by drug-free 21 days, repeated for fingernails (2 pulses) or repeated twice more (3 pulses) for toenails (Lozanoc) **OR**
- (Vulvovaginal candidiasis) 200 mg orally twice daily for 1 day, or 200 mg daily for 3 days **OR**
- (Vulvovaginal candidiasis) 100 mg orally twice daily for 1 day, or 100 mg daily for 3 days (Lozanoc) **OR**
- (Fungal keratitis) 200 mg orally daily for 3 weeks **OR**
- (Fungal keratitis) 100 mg orally daily for 3 weeks (Lozanoc) **OR**
- (Pityriasis versicolor) 200 mg orally daily for 1 week **OR**
- (Pityriasis versicolor) 100 mg orally daily for 1 week (Lozanoc) **OR**
- (Oral candidiasis in immunosuppressed patients) 100–200 mg for 4 weeks **OR**
- (Oral candidiasis in immunosuppressed patients) 50–100 mg for 4 weeks (Lozanoc) **OR**
- (Oesophageal candidiasis) 100 mg (1 measuring cup, i.e. 10 mL) daily for a minimum treatment of three weeks. Treatment should continue for 2 weeks following resolution of symptoms. Doses up to 200 mg (2 measuring cups, i.e. 20 mL) per day may be used based on the clinical response of the patient **OR**
- (Aspergillosis) 200 mg orally daily for 2–5 months (increasing the dose to 200 mg twice daily for invasive or disseminated disease) **OR**
- (Aspergillosis) 100 mg orally daily for 2–5 months (increasing the dose to 100 mg twice daily for invasive or disseminated disease) (Lozanoc) **OR**
- (Candidiasis) 100–200 mg orally daily for 3 weeks to 7 months **OR**
- (Candidiasis) 50–100 mg orally daily for 3 weeks to 7 months (increasing the dose to 100 mg twice daily for invasive or disseminated disease) (Lozanoc) **OR**
- (Histoplasmosis) 200 mg orally daily for 8 months, increasing the dose to 200 mg twice daily if needed **OR**
- (Histoplasmosis) 100 mg orally daily for 8 months, increasing the dose to 100 mg twice daily if needed (Lozanoc) **OR**
- (Sporotrichosis) 100 mg orally daily for 12 weeks, increasing the dose to 200 mg daily if needed **OR**
- (Sporotrichosis) 50 mg orally daily for 12 weeks, increasing the dose to 100 mg daily if needed (Lozanoc)

Adverse effects
- abdominal pain, constipation, diarrhoea, dyspepsia, nausea, vomiting
- dizziness, headache
- increased hepatic enzymes (reversible)
- (Rare) erectile dysfunction, menstrual disorders
- (Rare) pruritus, rash, urticaria, angioedema, hepatitis (with prolonged therapy), hepatotoxicity, peripheral neuropathy, severe congestive cardiac failure, QT prolongation, transient or permanent hearing loss

Interactions
- contraindicated with disopyramide, domperidone, ergot alkaloids, felodipine, 3-hydroxy-3-methylglutaryl coenzyme A (HMG-CoA) reductase inhibitors (statins) (e.g. simvastatin), irinotecan, lercanidipine, methadone, midazolam, ticagrelor

ANTIFUNGAL AGENTS

- contraindicated with colchicine and solifenacin in those with severe kidney impairment or moderate-to-severe liver impairment
- not recommended with apixaban, dabrafenib, darifenacin, sunitinib, or tolvaptan
- may increase serum levels of sulfonylureas, leading to hypoglycaemia
- decreased plasma levels may occur when given with carbamazepine, isoniazid, phenobarbital (phenobarbitone), phenytoin, rifabutin or rifampicin; therefore not recommended together
- increased risk of toxicity when given with busulfan, docetaxel or vinca alkaloids (e.g. vincristine)
- may increase serum levels of alfentanil, alprazolam, atorvastatin, calcium-channel blockers, carbamazepine, ciclosporin, disopyramide, digoxin, eletriptan, fentanyl, glucocorticoids (budesonide, dexamethasone, fluticasone, methylprednisolone), imatinib, midazolam (IV), norethisterone, phenytoin, reboxetine, rifabutin, ritonavir, sildenafil, sirolimus or tacrolimus, increasing the risk of toxicity/adverse effects, so serum levels should be closely monitored
- may increase the activity of warfarin, increasing the risk of bleeding, so prothrombin time should be closely monitored
- absorption decreased by antacids, H_2-receptor antagonists and proton pump inhibitors (e.g. omeprazole); therefore should not be given together
- increased serum levels may occur if given with clarithromycin, erythromycin or ritonavir, increasing the risk of adverse effects
- caution if given with calcium-channel blockers because of the increased risk of oedema and chronic heart failure
- can inhibit metabolism of calcium-channel blockers
- not recommended with amphotericin B (amphotericin), as it reduces antifungal activity. May also affect liver function; therefore liver enzymes should be monitored during therapy

Nursing considerations/Cautions

- (Disseminated mycoses) monitoring of itraconazole serum levels is recommended regularly throughout therapy
- (Systemic candidiasis) sensitivity should be checked before starting therapy
- liver function monitoring is recommended throughout therapy
- oral availability may be decreased in those who are immunocompromised, requiring an increase in dosage
- capsules and oral solution are not interchangeable
- (Lozanoc) capsules have a higher bioavailability than other itraconazole formulations: 50 mg Lozanoc = 100 mg other itraconazole formulations; therefore these are not interchangeable
- not recommended in patients with life-threatening systemic fungal infections
- not recommended for treatment of oral and/or oesophageal candidiasis in severely neutropenic patients
- caution if used in those with known sensitivity to another azole
- caution if used in those with impaired liver or kidney function
- caution if used in those with cystic fibrosis, as therapeutic levels may vary and an alternative therapy may be considered if the response is suboptimal
- contraindicated in those with congestive cardiac failure (or history of) unless the infection is life threatening

Patient education

- the patient should be advised to complete the course of treatment, which may continue for days/weeks after symptoms have resolved. If there is no resolution of the symptoms after the treatment period, the diagnosis should be reassessed or the likelihood of resistance to the agent used considered
- warn the patient that superficial fungal infections can be highly contagious

- advise the patient not to share clothing or personal linen (e.g. face flannels, towels)
- the patient should be advised against driving or operating machinery if dizziness is a problem
- those with diabetes treated with sulfonylureas should be warned to monitor blood glucose levels closely throughout therapy because of the increased risk of hypoglycaemia
- instruct the patient to take capsules with food
- advise the patient to take capsules 2 hours apart from antacids
- if the patient has achlorhydria or is taking H$_2$-receptor antagonists (e.g. ranitidine) or proton pump inhibitors (e.g. omeprazole), advise taking capsules with an acidic drink (e.g. cola) because adequate gastric acidity is required for tablet dissolution
- warn the patient to immediately seek medical advice if any of the following occur:
  - unusual fatigue, loss of appetite, nausea, vomiting, abdominal pain, yellowing of skin/eyes, dark urine or pale stools
  - numbness/tingling or weakness of feet/hands
  - hearing loss
  - skin disorder with peeling or blistering
  - swelling of the hands or feet, shortness of breath, unusual fatigue, unexpected weight gain
- (Vulvovaginal candidiasis) for prevention of reinfection, the partner(s) should be treated locally at the same time, with application of antifungal cream to the glans penis
- counsel women of childbearing years to use adequate contraception during therapy and for one menstrual cycle after completion

Capsules can be opened and contents dispersed in apple juice or cola, or mixed with a spoonful of yoghurt or apple puree.

Contraindicated during pregnancy unless fungal infection is life threatening and benefits outweigh risks to fetus.

Should be used during breastfeeding only if benefits outweigh risks to infant.

KETOCONAZOLE

Trade names
DaktaGOLD cream, Nizoral Cream and Anti-Dandruff Shampoo, Sebizole Shampoo

Available forms
Cream: 20 mg/g;
Shampoo: 10 mg/g (1%), 20 mg/g (2%)

Action
- azole antifungal (imidazole subclass)
- inhibits ergosterol synthesis in the fungal cell membrane
- action in seborrhoeic dermatitis is unknown

Use
- (Shampoo) seborrhoeic dermatitis and dandruff (associated with fungal infection)
- cutaneous candidiasis, dermatophyte infections

Dose
- (Dermatophyte and *Candida* infections) apply cream to the affected area 1–2 times daily for 14 days after symptoms have disappeared **OR**
- (Seborrhoeic dermatitis) apply cream to the affected area twice daily for up to 4 weeks **OR**
- (Seborrhoeic dermatitis, dandruff) shampoo twice weekly for up to 4 weeks

Adverse effects
- (Cream) pruritus, burning sensation, dermatitis
- (Shampoo) burning sensation, itchiness, oiliness/dryness of hair/scalp, rash, erythema and, rarely, discolouration of hair (grey or coloured)

Nursing considerations/Cautions
- has a high affinity for keratin and remains active in the skin for 7–14 days after the last topical application

ANTIFUNGAL AGENTS

- (Seborrhoeic dermatitis) if previously treated with topical corticosteroids, skin should be allowed to recover for at least 2 weeks before using ketoconazole cream to avoid skin sensitisation
- not indicated for nail or hair infections
- more resistant cases should be treated twice daily
- caution if used in those with sensitivity to another azole

Patient education

- the patient should be advised to continue treatment uninterrupted for the following times:
  - 4—6 weeks for tinea pedis
  - 3—4 weeks for tinea corporis
  - 2—4 weeks for tinea cruris
  - 2—3 weeks for pityriasis versicolor
  - 2—3 weeks for superficial candidiasis of the skin
- the patient should be advised to complete the course of treatment, which may continue for days/weeks after symptoms have resolved. If there is no resolution of the symptoms after the treatment period, the diagnosis should be reassessed, or the likelihood of resistance to the agent used should be considered
- warn the patient that superficial fungal infections can be highly contagious
- advise the patient not to share clothing or personal linen (e.g. face washers, towels)
- instruct the patient to wet the hair, add sufficient shampoo to lather, leave for 3—5 minutes and rinse thoroughly with water, avoiding contact with eyes. The eyes should be thoroughly washed with cold water if contact occurs
- the patient should be instructed to allow a 4-week gap between consecutive courses of treatment with shampoo

 Human safety data lacking; therefore use during pregnancy only if benefits outweigh risks.

 Topical ketoconazole is unlikely to be absorbed in significant amounts or excreted into breastmilk in quantities that would affect a breastfeeding infant.

MICAFUNGIN
Trade name
Mycamine

Available form
Vial: 50 mg, 100 mg

Action
- echinocandin that non-competitively inhibits glucan, which is essential in fungal cells but not present in mammalian cells
- fungicidal against most *Candida* species and inhibits *Aspergillus* species
- cross-resistance with other echinocandins possible
- half-life 10—17 hours

Use
- treatment of invasive candidiasis
- treatment of oesophageal candidiasis in those over 16 years
- prophylaxis of *Candida* infection in those undergoing allogenic haematopoietic stem cell transplantation or are expected to have neutropenia (absolute neutrophil count (ANC) < 500 cells/micromol) for 10 or more days

Dose

Invasive candidiasis
- (Body weight > 40 kg) 100 mg daily IV over 1 hour for a minimum of 14 days **OR**
- (Body weight ≤ 40 kg) 2 mg/kg daily IV over 1 hour for a minimum of 14 days

Oesophageal candidiasis
- (Body weight > 40 kg) 150 mg daily IV over 1 hour for a minimum of 7 days after symptoms have resolved **OR**
- (Body weight ≤ 40 kg) 3 mg/kg daily IV over 1 hour for a minimum of 7 days after symptoms have resolved

Candida infection prophylaxis
- (Body weight > 40 kg) 50 mg daily IV over 1 hour for a minimum of 7 days after neutrophil recovery **OR**
- (Body weight ≤ 40 kg) 1 mg/kg daily IV over 1 hour for a minimum of 7 days after neutrophil recovery

Adverse effects
- anorexia, nausea, vomiting, abdominal pain, dyspepsia, diarrhoea, constipation, mucosal inflammation
- fever, rigors
- fatigue, headache, insomnia, anxiety
- peripheral oedema, fluid overload
- back pain, arthralgia
- tachycardia, atrial fibrillation, arrhythmia, hypotension
- hypokalaemia, hypomagnesaemia, hypocalcaemia, hyperglycaemia, hyponatraemia
- elevated liver enzymes
- rash, pruritus
- cough, dyspnoea, epistaxis
- hypotension, hypertension
- thrombocytopenia, neutropenia, anaemia
- bacteraemia, sepsis, pneumonia
- (Rare) hypersensitivity, severe skin reaction, haemolysis, haemolytic anaemia, hepatotoxicity
- (IV site) phlebitis

Interactions
- caution if used with other hepatotoxic agents
- may increase serum levels of sirolimus, nifedipine and itraconazole, increasing the risk of toxicity

Nursing considerations/Cautions
- liver function should be monitored during therapy and stopped if there is any persistent and significant elevation of liver enzymes
- (Invasive candidiasis) therapy should continue for at least 1 week after two sequential negative blood cultures have been obtained and symptoms have resolved
- to reconstitute, add 5 mL sodium chloride 0.9% or glucose 5% slowly to the vial to avoid foaming. Rotate the vial gently (not shaking) to dissolve the powder and then add to 100 mL infusion bag (final concentration between 0.5 mg/mL and 2 mg/mL depending on dose)
- administer alone
- caution if used in those with severe liver impairment, chronic liver disease or congenital enzyme defects
- contraindication in those with hypersensitivity to other echinocandins

Patient education
- advise the patient to immediately report any rash

 Should be used during pregnancy only if the potential benefit justifies the potential risk to the fetus, as it has shown some adverse effects in animal studies.

 Avoid use. It is not known if micafungin is excreted in human breastmilk. Caution is advised when using during breastfeeding because of potential adverse effects.

MICONAZOLE
Trade names
Daktarin (cream, oral gel, powder, spray, tincture), Eulactol Antifungal (spray), Resolve (solution), Resolve Jock Itch (cream), Resolve Tinea (cream), Decozol Oral Gel

Available forms
Oral gel: 20 mg/mL;
Topical cream: 2% (20 mg/g);
Lotion/Solution: 2%;
Powder: 2%;
Spray powder: 2%;
Tincture: 2%;
Spray (liquid): 2%

Action
- imidazole, which inhibits ergosterol synthesis in the fungal cell membrane

ANTIFUNGAL AGENTS

Use
- candidiasis (cutaneous, oral)
- dermatophytosis, pityriasis versicolor
- seborrhoeic dermatitis (scalp)

Dose
- (Dermatophytosis, pityriasis versicolor, cutaneous candidiasis) apply a thin layer and rub well into skin daily (tinea versicolor (pityriasis versicolor)) or twice daily (tinea pedis, cruris or corporis, cutaneous candidiasis) **OR**
- (Powder) apply powder directly to the lesion twice daily and also dust inside articles of clothing in contact with affected areas until the lesion is completely healed **OR**
- (Tincture) apply tincture to the affected nail and surrounding skin twice daily (after cutting very short) for at least 2 months or until new nail has grown **OR**
- (Spray powder) apply spray twice daily to affected area for at least 14 days after symptoms resolve **OR**
- (Oral candidiasis) half of the supplied measuring spoon 4 times daily dropped on tongue and kept in mouth as long as possible before swallowing

Adverse effects
- (Oral) nausea, vomiting, regurgitation of food
- (Topical cream, lotion) stinging, local irritation, pruritus, warmth at application site
- superinfection (prolonged therapy)
- (Rare) anaphylaxis, angioedema, serious skin reactions

Interactions

Oral administration
- may increase serum levels of alfentanil, alprazolam, busulfan, calcium-channel blockers, carbamazepine, ciclosporin, disopyramide, docetaxel, methylprednisolone, midazolam (IV), phenytoin, reboxetine, rifabutin, saquinavir, sildenafil, sirolimus, tacrolimus or vinca alkaloids, increasing the risk of adverse effects
- increased risk of hypoglycaemia if given with sulfonylureas
- contraindicated with midazolam (oral) (owing to prolonged sedation), simvastatin (an increased risk of rhabdomyolysis), ergot alkaloids (risk of ergotism) and any agents known to prolong QT interval
- contraindicated with warfarin, as anticoagulant effects may be enhanced, increasing the risk of bleeding, so prothrombin time should be closely monitored
- antifungal action may be blocked by amphotericin B (amphotericin)

Nursing considerations/Cautions
- if the patient is unresponsive to treatment, check for undiagnosed diabetes
- candida should be treated for not less than 2 weeks and dermatophytes not less than 4 weeks
- contraindicated in those with sensitivity to another azole
- (Oral gel) contraindicated in those with liver impairment or in infants under 6 months

Patient education
- the patient should be advised to complete the course of treatment, which may continue for days/weeks after symptoms have resolved. If there is no resolution of the symptoms after the treatment period, the diagnosis should be reassessed or the likelihood of resistance to the agent used should be considered
- warn the patient that superficial fungal infections can be highly contagious
- advise the patient not to share clothing or personal linen (e.g. face washers, towels)
- patients being treated for tinea pedis should be encouraged to wash and dry the feet (especially between toes) carefully each day and apply antifungal powder. They should also be advised to wear shoes or sandals that are well

ventilated (if possible), wear waterproof sandals in public showers, change hosiery (preferably cotton socks) daily and dust shoes inside with powder

Oral gel

* advise the patient (or carer) that gel should be placed on the tongue and left for as long as possible before swallowing. Gel may be applied to dentures and left overnight. However, it should be washed off before reinsertion of dentures in the morning
* instruct the patient/carer that gel should be measured only with the supplied measuring spoon
* advise the patient/carer to continue for at least 7 days after symptoms have subsided

Spray powder

* advise the patient to shake the can well before use and hold iot about 15 cm from the area to be treated
* warn the patient to avoid contact with eyes

Topical cream

* instruct the patient to cleanse the skin using a soap alternative, as normal soap may cause skin irritation
* warn the patient to avoid contact with eyes

Tincture

* instruct the patient to:
  * cut nails as short as possible before applying tincture. Apply under the nail also if possible
  * continue treatment until the new nail has grown and the area is cured (8 weeks or more)
  * clean the nail using acetone-based nail polish remover before reapplying tincture
* ensure the patient understands that a nail falling off is due to infection, not the treatment, which should not be interrupted
* warn the patient that the tincture contains alcohol and should not be applied to open lesions

Available in combination with

* Miconazole nitrate: 20 mg/g (2% w/w) + hydrocortisone: 5 mg/g (0.5% w/w) (Resolve Plus 0.5 Cream)
* Miconazole nitrate: 20 mg/g (2% w/w) + hydrocortisone: 10 mg/g (1.0% w/w) (Resolve Plus 1.0 Cream)
* Miconazole nitrate: 20 mg/g (2% w/w) + zinc oxide: 150 mg/g (15% w/w) (Daktozin Ointment)

NYSTATIN

Trade names

Chemists' Own Nystatin, Mycostatin, Nilstat Oral, Nilstat Vaginal, Nystatin [Omegapharm], Pharmacy Action Nystatin, Trust Nystatin

Available forms

Tablets: 500,000 units;
Capsules: 500,000 units;
Oral drops: 100,000 units/mL;
Vaginal cream: 100,000 units/5 g

Action

* alters fungal cell membrane, targeting ergosterol, changing cell permeability and causing leakage of cell contents
* not absorbed from the GIT

Use

* prophylaxis and treatment of infections caused by *Candida* spp. (vulvovaginal, cutaneous, oral, intestinal)

Dose

* (Cutaneous candidiasis) apply liberally to affected areas 2—3 times daily (topical cream) **OR**
* (Intestinal candidiasis) 500,000—1,000,000 units (1—2 tablets or capsules) 3 times daily and continued for 48 hours after symptoms resolve **OR**
* (Oral candidiasis) 100,000 units (1 mL) 4 times daily, swirled around mouth as long as possible before swallowing, and continued for 48 hours after symptoms have resolved (oral drops) **OR**
* (Vaginal candidiasis) 1 full applicator (5 g) 1—2 times daily for 14 days (vaginal cream)

ANTIFUNGAL AGENTS

Adverse effects
- (Oral, large doses, uncommon) nausea, vomiting, diarrhoea, oral irritation
- (Rare, oral) urticaria, rash, angioedema
- (Vaginal cream, uncommon) irritation

Nursing considerations/Cautions
- not suitable for systemic fungal infections
- to prevent relapse, oral administration should continue for at least 48 hours after clinical cure
- smears or other diagnostic methods should be used to rule out other causes of infection and repeated if there is no response to therapy
- if symptoms persist or worsen after 14 weeks, alternate therapy should be considered
- (Oral drops) caution if used in those with known hypersensitivity to hydroxybenzoates

Patient education
- the patient should be advised to complete the course of treatment, which may continue for days/weeks after symptoms have resolved. If there is no resolution of the symptoms after the treatment period, the diagnosis should be reassessed or the likelihood of resistance to the agent used should be considered
- warn the patient that superficial fungal infections can be highly contagious
- advise the patient not to share clothing or personal linen (e.g. face flannels, towels)

Vaginal candidiasis
- instruct the patient to continue treatment even if menstruation occurs
- ensure the patient has instructions for correct insertion of vaginal cream and cleaning instructions for the applicator (taking plunger and barrel apart and washing with warm water and mild soap)
- for prevention of reinfection, the partner(s) should be treated locally at the same time with application of cream to the glans penis
- the patient should be advised that vaginal cream may decrease the effectiveness and safety of latex products such as condoms and diaphragms
- instruct women being treated for vaginal infection that they should refrain from sexual intercourse or encourage their partner to use a condom. Sexual partner(s) should also be treated to prevent reinfection. Perineal pads (or panty liners) will prevent staining of underwear or clothing when vaginal tablets or creams are used. Wearing cotton underwear and pantyhose with a cotton gusset is also recommended (especially if infection recurs). Use of tampons or douching between doses of vaginal medications is not recommended

Oral drops
- 1 mL four times daily. The drops should be swirled around the mouth for as long as possible before swallowing. Continue treatment for 48 hours after symptoms resolve.
- instruct the patient to:
  - shake bottle well before use
  - use a graduated dropper to measure correct amount
  - keep drops in the mouth as long as possible before swallowing
  - wash the dropper with hot water after use
  - discard drops after the expiry date
  - avoid food or drink for 1 hour after oral drops

Capsules can be opened and contents dispersed in water, or tablet crushed and mixed with water.

(Oral) use during pregnancy only if clearly needed.

Unknown whether excreted in breastmilk; use with caution.

Available in combination with
- triamcinolone + neomycin + gramicidin + nystatin (Kenacomb ointment, Kenacomb Otic ear ointment, Kenacomb Otic ear drops, Otocomb Otic ear ointment, Otocomb Otic ear drops)

POSACONAZOLE
Trade names
Noxafil, Pharmacor Posaconazole, Posaconazole ARX, Posaconazole Dr. Reddy, Posaconazole Juno, Posaconazole Sandoz, Posaconazole-WGR

Available forms
Vial: 300 mg/16.7 mL;
Oral suspension: 40 mg/mL;
Modified-release tablets: 100 mg

Action
- broad-spectrum triazole that inhibits ergosterol synthesis in fungal cell membrane
- effective against a number of species, including fluconazole-resistant *Candida* spp.
- half-life 20–66 hours (oral suspension) or 27 hours (IV)

Use
- invasive aspergillosis (where other agents are inappropriate or ineffective)
- fusariosis, zygomycosis, coccidioidomycosis, chromoblastomycosis and mycetoma (where other agents are inappropriate or ineffective)
- oropharyngeal candidiasis (in immunocompromised patients or those resistant to itraconazole or fluconazole)
- prophylaxis of invasive fungal infections (in patients at high risk)

Dose
- (Refractory invasive fungal infection) 400 mg orally twice daily with food or nutritional supplement (oral suspension) **OR**
- (Refractory invasive fungal infection) 200 mg orally 4 times daily with food or nutritional supplement (oral suspension) **OR**
- (Refractory invasive fungal infection) 300 mg orally or IV infusion twice daily (day 1) then 300 mg daily (concentrated solution, modified-release tablets) **OR**
- (Oral candidiasis refractory to itraconazole or fluconazole) 400 mg orally twice daily with food or nutritional supplement (oral suspension) **OR**
- (Prophylaxis of invasive fungal infection) 200 mg orally 3 times daily with food or nutritional supplement (oral suspension) **OR**
- (Prophylaxis of invasive fungal infection) 300 mg orally or IV infusion twice daily (day 1), then 300 mg daily (concentrated solution, modified-release tablets) **OR**
- (Oral candidiasis in immunocompromised patient) 200 mg orally daily (day 1) (loading dose), then 100 mg orally daily for 13 days (oral suspension)

Adverse effects
- neutropenia, anaemia, thrombocytopenia
- anorexia, dry mouth, nausea, vomiting, abdominal pain, diarrhoea, dyspepsia, flatulence, constipation, inflamed mucosa
- electrolyte imbalance (e.g. hypokalaemia, hypomagnesaemia), elevated liver function test, elevated liver enzymes and bilirubin
- dizziness, headache, somnolence
- paraesthesia
- rash, peticchiae
- asthenia, fatigue, fever, chills
- peripheral oedema
- hypertension
- cough, dyspnoea, epistaxis
- (Rare) hepatitis, QT prolongation

Interactions
- contraindicated with any agents that prolong QT interval
- contraindicated with ergot alkaloids because of the risk of ergotism
- contraindicated with 3-hydroxy-3-methylglutaryl coenzyme A (HMG-CoA) reductase inhibitors (statins) because of

ANTIFUNGAL AGENTS

- the increased risk of myopathy and rhabdomyolysis
- not recommended with phenytoin, rifabutin, H$_2$-receptor antagonists or efavirenz, as decreased serum levels may occur
- may increase serum levels of atazanavir/ritonavir, calcium-channel blockers, ciclosporin, digoxin, fosamprenavir, rifabutin, sirolimus, tacrolimus or vinca alkaloids
- increased risk of hypoglycaemia if given with sulfonylureas
- not recommended with amphotericin B (amphotericin), as it reduces antifungal activity
- increased risk of prolonged sedation if given with benzodiazepines (e.g. alprazolam, midazolam)
- increased risk of neurotoxicity and other serious adverse effects if given with vinca alkaloids

Nursing considerations/Cautions

- liver function and serum electrolytes should be monitored (especially potassium, magnesium and calcium) before starting and throughout therapy (especially if receiving concentrated solution). Any imbalance should be corrected before starting therapy
- tablets and oral suspension are not interchangeable
- ensure the vial is at room temperature before dilution with 150–283 mL of suitable fluid to give a concentration of 1–2 mg/mL, and infused over 90 minutes via central venous catheter (CVC) or peripherally inserted central catheter (PICC)
- multiple infusions via a peripheral venous line are not well tolerated. If used, the infusion should be over 30 minutes
- should not be administered as an IV bolus
- a concentrated solution should not be diluted with lactated Ringer's solution, 5% dextrose with lactated Ringer's or 4.2% sodium bicarbonate
- caution if used in those with sensitivity to another azole
- caution if used in those with liver impairment, known arrhythmias or at risk of QT prolongation
- (Concentrated injection) not recommended in those with moderate-to-severe kidney impairment. If used, serum creatinine should be closely monitored

Patient education

- if the patient has diabetes and is treated using sulfonylureas, instruct them to monitor blood glucose levels closely, as hypoglycaemia may occur
- instruct the patient to shake an oral suspension well before use and use the measuring spoon provided
- advise the patient to take an oral suspension with food or at least 240 mL of nutritional supplement
- warn the patient that tablets should be swallowed whole, not chewed, crushed or divided
- warn the patient not to drive or operate machinery if dizziness occurs
- the patient should be advised to seek medical advice if any of the following occur:
  - tingling or numbness of hands or feet, muscle weakness
  - fatigue, loss of appetite, any yellowing of eyes or skin, upper abdominal pain, dark urine, pale stools
- women of childbearing potential should be counselled to use adequate contraception throughout and for at least 2 weeks after completing therapy

Modified-release tablets should not be crushed or broken. Oral liquid is available.

Not recommended during pregnancy unless benefits to mother outweigh risks to fetus. Women of childbearing

potential should use effective contraception during treatment and for at least 2 weeks after completing therapy.

Avoid use, as no human studies. Excreted in the milk of lactating rats.

Renal impairment: posaconazole is not significantly renally excreted, so no dose adjustment is required for mild-to-moderate renal impairment. However, in patients with severe renal impairment (eGFR < 20 mL/min), there is high variability in drug exposure, and these patients should be closely monitored for breakthrough fungal infections.

Hepatic impairment: half-life is doubled in severe impairment. Use with caution.

TERBINAFINE
Trade names
APO-Terbinafine, Chemists' Own Tamsil Cream, Lamisil Cream, Lamisil DermGel, Lamisil Once, Lamisil Spray, Lamisil Tablets, Noumed Terbinafine, SolvEasy Tinea Cream, SolvEasy Tinea Gel, SolvEasy Tinea Spray, Tamsil, Terbinafine Sandoz, Terbinafine-DRLA, Terbinafine-WGR, Tinasil, Trust Terbinafine Cream

Available forms
Tablets: 250 mg;
Solution/Gel/Cream/Spray: 10 mg/g (1%)

Action
- allylamine (mainly active against dermatophytes) that prevents ergosterol (lipid) synthesis of the fungal cell membrane, resulting in cell disruption and death
- (Oral) concentrates in superficial tissues, including nails, hair and skin

Use
- (Oral) *Tinea* infection (not responding to topical treatment)
- onychomycosis
- cutaneous candidiasis

Dose
- 250 mg orally daily **OR**
- apply to clean and dry affected area and surrounding skin, and rub lightly daily (solution, cream, spray or gel) **OR**
- apply solution daily in a thin layer to BOTH feet around and between the toes (even if there is no sign of infection), covering the sole and sides of feet (1.5 cm) and allow to dry for 1—2 minutes

Adverse effects
- (Oral) nausea, vomiting, anorexia, dyspepsia, gastritis, belching, diarrhoea, flatulence, abdominal discomfort and cramps, feeling of fullness, taste loss (ageusia)
- (Oral) headache, depression, dizziness, lightheadedness
- (Oral) myalgia, arthralgia
- (Oral) visual impairment
- (Oral) rash, pruritus, urticaria, erythema and, uncommonly, photosensitivity
- (Cream/gel/solution) itching, stinging, redness and, rarely, rash, pruritus, urticaria
- (Oral) (rare) transient increase in liver enzymes, jaundice, blood dyscrasias, serious skin reactions

Interactions
Oral
- plasma clearance may be increased by rifampicin, leading to decreased serum levels
- may cause menstrual abnormalities in women taking oral contraceptives
- may inhibit metabolism of antiarrhythmic agents (class 1A, 1B, 1C), beta adrenoceptor blocking agents, tricyclic antidepressants (TCAs), selective serotonin reuptake inhibitors (SSRIs) and monoamine oxidase inhibitors (MAOIs) (type B)
- may affect prothrombin time if given with warfarin; therefore it should be closely monitored throughout therapy
- may decrease clearance of caffeine and theophylline, leading to increased serum levels

ANTIFUNGAL AGENTS

- may increase clearance of ciclosporin, leading to decreased serum levels
- may increase serum levels of amiodarone and fluconazole
- may increase serum levels of dextromethorphan

Nursing considerations/Cautions

- (Oral) liver function tests are recommended before starting and then every 4—6 weeks during therapy
- if therapy is longer than 6 weeks, blood counts should be monitored
- oral therapy is recommended when topical therapy is ineffective or the site, severity or extent of infection warrants oral therapy
- length of administration depends on cause:
  - tinea pedis, tinea cruris, tinea corporis: oral treatment 2—6 weeks
  - tinea cruris, tinea corporis: oral treatment 2—4 weeks
  - onychomycosis: oral treatment 6 weeks—3 months, cream: 1—4 weeks)
- (Oral) caution if used in those with psoriasis or lupus erythematosus, as conditions may be precipitated and/or exacerbated
- (Oral) not recommended in those with impaired kidney function (creatinine clearance < 50 mL/min or serum creatinine > 300 micromol/L)
- (Oral) contraindicated in those with severe liver disease (chronic or active)

Patient education

- if tablets cause upset stomach, the patient should be instructed to take after a light meal
- the patient should be advised to complete the course of treatment, which may continue for days/weeks after symptoms have resolved. If there is no resolution of the symptoms after the treatment period, the diagnosis should be reassessed or the likelihood of resistance to the agent used should be considered
- warn the patient that superficial fungal infections can be highly contagious
- advise the patient not to share clothing or personal linen (e.g. face flannels, towels)
- advise the patient to immediately seek medical advice if any of the following occur:
  - unusual fatigue or tiredness, loss of appetite, nausea, vomiting, right upper abdominal pain, yellowing of skin/eyes, dark urine or pale stools
  - fever, sore throat, mouth ulcers, chills, tiredness, swollen glands and aching joints
- warn the patient not to drive or operate machinery if dizziness or lightheadedness occurs
- the patient should be advised that loss of taste usually recovers within several weeks of discontinuing oral therapy
- instruct the patient that both feet should be treated even if only one is symptomatic. Feet should be washed and dried before applying solution to one foot at a time. Solution should be applied between and all around toes, soles and 1.5 cm up the sides of feet, and then allowed to dry (not massaged into skin). Feet should not be washed for 24 hours after application of the solution
- advise the patient to their wash hands thoroughly after using the solution and avoid contacting eyes with solution
- for infections which are sub-breast, between the digits, inguinal or intergluteal, gauze may be used to cover cream or gel, especially at night
- (Solution) warn the patient that the solution should not be massaged into skin and that the treated area should not be washed for 24 hours after application

- advise the patient to seek medical advice if there is no improvement in 7 days
- (Oral) female patients taking tablets and oral contraceptives should be warned of the possibility of menstrual disorders

Should be used during pregnancy only if the potential benefits outweigh any potential risks.

Avoid, as excreted in human breastmilk.

Renal impairment: reduce the dose if CrCl is less than 50 mL/min, as terbinafine clearance decreases by about 50%, increasing the risk of drug accumulation and adverse effects.

Hepatic impairment: contraindicated in patients with severe, chronic or active hepatic disease. The drug has been associated with hepatotoxicity even in patients without pre-existing liver disease. Liver function tests should be monitored before initiating treatment, and the drug should be discontinued immediately if liver enzyme elevations occur. Rare cases of liver failure leading to liver transplant or death have been reported.

TOLNAFTATE

Trade name
Tinaderm Powder

Available form
Powder spray: 0.9 mg/g

Action
- fungicidal

Use
- ringworm
- tinea pedis

Dose
- (Ringworm, tinea) sprinkle or spray enough powder to cover affected area 2–3 times daily; powder should also be dusted into footwear **OR**
- (Prevention of tinea) dust footwear and feet regularly

Adverse effects
- mild irritation

Nursing considerations/Cautions
- review diagnosis if there is no improvement after 4 weeks of treatment
- powder/spray powder are recommended as adjunctive treatment with other antifungal treatments

Patient education
- the patient should be advised to complete the course of treatment, which may continue for days/weeks after symptoms have resolved. If there is no resolution of the symptoms after the treatment period, the diagnosis should be reassessed or the likelihood of resistance to the agent used should be considered
- warn the patient that superficial fungal infections can be highly contagious
- advise the patient not to share clothing or personal linen (e.g. face washers, towels)
- warn the patient to avoid contact with eyes or mucous membranes or inhaling powder preparations
- the patient being treated for tinea pedis should be encouraged to wash and dry the feet (especially between toes) carefully each day and apply antifungal powder. They should also be advised to wear shoes or sandals that are well ventilated (if possible), wear waterproof sandals in public showers, change hosiery (preferably cotton socks) daily and dust shoes inside with powder
- (Spray powder, liquid) shake can well before use

Available in combination with
- tolnaftate 10 mg/g + chlorhexidine hydrochloride 2.5 mg/g (Mycil Healthy Feet Dusting Powder)

ANTIFUNGAL AGENTS

VORICONAZOLE

Trade names
Vfend, Voricon, Voriconazole AFT, Voriconazole InterPharma, Voriconazole Sandoz, Voriconazole Wockhardt, Vttack, Vzole

Available forms
Vial: 200 mg;
Tablets: 50 mg, 200 mg;
Powder (for oral suspension): 40 mg/mL

Action
* broad-spectrum triazole that inhibits ergosterol synthesis in fungal cell membrane
* active against *Candida* spp., *Aspergillus*, *Scedosporium* and *Fusarium*
* half-life about 6 hours

Use
* invasive aspergillosis (first-line treatment)
* serious *Candida* infections (including oesophageal and systemic candidiasis)
* serious infections caused by *Scedosporium* and *Fusarium* species
* other fungal infections (when other therapy has been ineffective or inappropriate)
* prophylaxis in high-risk patients

Dose
* initially 6 mg/kg 12-hourly by IV infusion for 24 hours (loading dose), then 3–4 mg/kg 12-hourly (maintenance) **OR**
* 200–400 mg orally either 1 hour before or after food, 12-hourly for 24 hours (loading dose), then 100–200 mg twice daily (maintenance) **OR**
* (Prophylaxis) initially 6 mg/kg 12-hourly by IV infusion for 24 hours (loading dose), then 4 mg/kg 12-hourly (maintenance) **OR**
* (Prophylaxis) 100–200 mg orally either 1 hour before or after food 12-hourly

Adverse effects
* dry mouth, nausea, vomiting, diarrhoea, abdominal pain, dyspepsia, cheilitis, gingivitis
* sinusitis, respiratory distress syndrome, pulmonary oedema
* fever, chills
* headache, dizziness, tremor, paraesthesia, somnolence, fainting
* confusion, depression, hallucinations, anxiety, agitation, insomnia, asthenia
* back pain
* hypotension
* chest pain, tachycardia, bradycardia, arrhythmia
* rash, pruritus, photosensitivity, alopecia, dermatitis, purpura
* oedema (peripheral, facial)
* visual disturbances (including blurred vision, changes in colour perception), photophobia, retinal haemorrhage
* hypokalaemia, hypoglycaemia, hyponatraemia
* elevated liver enzymes, jaundice, cholestatic jaundice
* elevated creatinine, acute kidney failure, haematuria
* agranulocytosis, anaemia, leucopenia, pancytopenia, thrombocytopenia
* (IV site) inflammation, phlebitis, thrombophlebitis, infusion-related reactions (e.g. chest tightness, dyspnoea, flushing, fever, nausea, pruritus, rash, sweating, tachycardia)
* (Rare) optic neuritis, papilloedema, QT prolongation, periostitis, severe skin reactions

Interactions
* contraindicated with any agents that prolong QT interval or cause electrolyte imbalance
* contraindicated with ergot alkaloids (increased risk of ergotism), carbamazepine, rifabutin, rifampicin, sirolimus and long-acting barbiturates (e.g. phenobarbital (phenobarbitone)) (increased risk of toxicity), ritonavir (high dose, 800 mg daily) and efavirenz (daily doses > 400 mg) and St John's wort (decreased efficacy of voriconazole)
* not recommended with everolimus, fluconazole, phenytoin or ritonavir (low dose 200 mg daily)
* may decrease metabolism of 3-hydroxy-3-methylglutaryl coenzyme A (HMG-

457

- CoA) reductase inhibitors (statins), increasing serum levels and risk of rhabdomyolysis
- may increase serum levels of efavirenz, NSAIDs, tacrolimus, oxycodone and other long-acting opioids, and ciclosporin, increasing the risk of adverse effects
- may increase prothrombin time if given with warfarin; therefore closely monitor throughout therapy
- may increase the risk of hypoglycaemia by increasing serum levels of sulfonylureas
- may prolong the sedative effect of midazolam and alprazolam
- increased risk of respiratory depression if given with alfentanil, fentanyl or remifentanil
- increased risk of neurotoxicity if given with vinca alkaloids
- may increase serum levels of methadone, increasing the risk of toxicity and QT interval prolongation
- serum levels may be decreased by phenytoin, rifabutin and HIV protease inhibitors
- if therapy is added to already existing omeprazole, the omeprazole dose should be halved
- increased risk of toxicity if given with HIV protease inhibitors
- may increase adverse effects if given with oral contraceptives containing norethisterone and ethylestradiol
- not recommended with amphotericin B (amphotericin), as it reduces antifungal activity

Nursing considerations/Cautions

- any hypokalaemia, hypomagnesaemia or hypocalcaemia should be corrected before starting therapy
- liver and kidney function (including serum creatinine and bilirubin) should be monitored weekly for the first month and then monthly throughout therapy. Pancreatic function (amylase, lipase) monitoring is also recommended in those at risk of acute pancreatitis (e.g. recent chemotherapy)
- (Long-term therapy) regular dermatological monitoring is recommended to detect any premalignant lesions
- (IV) the patient should be carefully observed at the start of infusion for any infusion-related reaction
- (IV) if the response to 3 mg/kg is inadequate, the dose should be increased to 4 mg/kg; if the patient is intolerant to 4 mg/kg, the dose can be reduced to 3 mg/kg
- reconstitute IV powder using 19 mL water for injections, shake thoroughly and further dilute with a compatible fluid (e.g. sodium chloride 0.9%, glucose 5%, compounded lactate sodium IV infusion, glucose 5% and sodium chloride 0.45%)
- should not be given as an IV bolus
- recommended administration rate is 3 mg/kg/hour over 1—2 hours
- (IV) not compatible with blood products or concentrated electrolyte solutions. If infused with non-concentrated electrolyte solutions or total parenteral nutrition (TPN), the infusion should be via separate lines
- (Vial) contains 217.6 mg sodium, which should be considered if the patient has sodium restriction
- (Tablets) contain lactose and are not recommended in those with galactose intolerance, Lapp lactase deficiency or glucose—galactose malabsorption
- (Oral powder) (used to make up suspension) contains sucrose and is not recommended in those with fructose intolerance, sucrase—isomaltase deficiency or glucose—galactose malabsorption
- if the patient has creatinine clearance < 50 mL/min (including those on dialysis), oral (not IV) therapy is recommended
- caution if used in those with risk factors for pancreatitis (e.g. chemotherapy, stem cell transplantation)

ANTIFUNGAL AGENTS

- use with great caution in patients who are at risk of QT prolongation, including those with existing symptomatic arrhythmias, congenital or acquired QT prolongation, sinus bradycardia, cardiomyopathy or if given with other agents that may prolong the QT interval, induce arrhythmias or cause electrolyte imbalance (e.g. hypokalaemia)
- caution if used in those with sensitivity to another azole
- (IV) not recommended for oesophageal candidiasis

Patient education

- (IV) warn the patient that mild visual disturbances (e.g. blurred vision, colour vision changes, photophobia) occur commonly and usually resolve within 60 minutes of infusion completion
- instruct the patient to avoid direct sunlight during therapy and when outdoors to wear sunscreen (at least SPF 30+), protective clothing, hat and sunglasses
- if the patient is receiving long-term therapy, advise them to have regular skin checks by a dermatologist
- the patient should be advised not to drive or operate machinery if photophobia, visual problems (e.g. blurred vision, colour vision changes), hypotension, dizziness, confusion or hallucinations occur. The patient should be warned against driving at night
- warn the patient to immediately seek medical advice if any of the following occur:
  - any rash or other skin condition such as skin flaking or blistering
  - any ongoing changes to vision or sensitivity to light
  - bone pain
  - any new or changing skin lesions
  - increased or irregular heart rate
  - yellowing of skin or eyes, lethargy, loss of appetite, upper abdominal pain, dark urine, pale stools
  - signs of frequent or worsening infections such as fever, chills, sore throat and/or mouth ulcers
  - face or limb swelling
  - blood in urine
- instruct the patient to take tablets or oral suspension 1 hour before or 1 hour after meals
- the patient should be advised to shake the solution well before using and measured using the supplied syringe and amount slowly squirted into the mouth towards the cheek. Oral suspension should not be mixed with any other medication or water. The syringe should be taken apart and rinsed with warm water each time it is used
- advise the patient to discard the oral suspension 14 days after opening
- female patients of childbearing years should be counselled to use effective contraception during therapy to prevent pregnancy occurring

Oral liquid is available. Tablet can be crushed and mixed with water or a spoonful of yoghurt or apple puree.

Use is not recommended unless the potential benefit to the mother outweighs the risks to the fetus. It should be considered only for severe or life-threatening fungal infections where no safer alternative is available.

Avoid use, as no human studies. Unknown if excreted in breastmilk.

ANTIGLAUCOMA AGENTS

Glaucoma is an eye condition characterised by optic disk cupping and visual field loss, usually associated with a raised intraocular pressure; however, it can occur at normal or near-normal pressure. Although raised intraocular pressure may be symptomless in the early stages, damage to the optic nerve leads to loss of vision and, when severe, is one of the leading causes of preventable blindness worldwide. Risk factors for glaucoma include family history, increasing age, high intraocular pressure, extreme short-sightedness, co-morbidities such as diabetes and hypertension, and some medications such as long-term corticosteroids (Salmon 2018).

The main types of glaucoma are open-angle, closed-angle and secondary glaucoma. Open-angle glaucoma, the most common type, is caused by impaired outflow of aqueous humor due to abnormalities in the drainage system of the anterior chamber. It develops slowly and accounts for about 80% of all glaucoma cases. Closed-angle glaucoma occurs when access to the drainage system is obstructed, leading to a sudden increase in intraocular pressure and requiring immediate medical intervention. Secondary glaucoma arises from other medical conditions, such as diabetes or eye injuries, that contribute to elevated eye pressure. Among these, open-angle glaucoma progresses gradually and often without symptoms in the early stages (Salmon 2018).

Glaucoma management involves reducing intraocular pressure by either decreasing the production of aqueous humor or increasing its outflow, using medical, laser or surgical therapy (Salmon 2018).

Pharmacological management may include the following drugs:

- alpha adrenergic agonists/sympathomimetic agents (apraclonidine, brimonidine)
- beta adrenoceptor blocking agents (betaxolol, timolol) (first-line management)
- carbonic anhydrase inhibitors (acetazolamide, brinzolamide, dorzolamide)
- prostaglandin analogues (bimatoprost, latanoprost, travoprost) (first-line management)
- parasympathomimetic agents (pilocarpine)
- prostamide analogue (bimatoprost)
- hyperosmotic agent (mannitol)

ANTIGLAUCOMA AGENTS

General Actions of antiglaucoma agents
- decrease intraocular pressure (either by increasing aqueous output or reducing production) since sustained intraocular pressure and poor ocular perfusion result in damage to the head of the optic nerve and loss of visual field
- agents may be used alone or in combination to reduce intraocular pressure

General Ocular Adverse effects of antiglaucoma agents
- ocular pruritus, ocular ache or pain
- tearing, burning or stinging, blurring of vision, decreased visual acuity
- discomfort, foreign body sensation, eye irritation
- lid oedema or erythema, eyelid crusting
- ocular hyperaemia
- ocular allergic reaction
- conjunctivitis, conjunctival oedema, conjunctival follicles
- dry eyes
- discharge
- photophobia

General Adverse effects (uncommon) of antiglaucoma agents
- headache, asthenia, malaise, dizziness, nervousness, depression, insomnia, somnolence, fatigue, drowsiness, decreased coordination
- chest pain, palpitations, bradycardia, hypotension
- dry mouth, taste perversion
- dry nose, rhinitis
- dermatitis

General Nursing considerations/Cautions for antiglaucoma agents
- regular intraocular pressure (IOP) monitoring is essential, especially early in treatment, to assess effectiveness and prevent vision loss
- IOP varies throughout the day, so it should be measured at different times for accurate monitoring and therapy adjustments
- some antiglaucoma eye drops contain benzalkonium chloride, which can irritate the eyes and discolour soft contact lenses. Lenses should be removed before use and not replaced for 15 minutes
- drug effectiveness may decrease over time, requiring therapy adjustments

General Patient education for antiglaucoma agents
- encourage adherence to antiglaucoma medications, as non-adherence is common. Only 15% of patients maintain good adherence over 4 years. Up to 30% never fill their first prescription and 50% stop after the first refill. Others struggle with correct eye drop instillation, leading to poor outcomes and glaucoma progression (Newman-Casey & Myers 2019)
- avoid driving or operating machinery if visual disturbances, dizziness, fatigue, or drowsiness occur
- eye drops may cause temporary blurred vision; avoid driving or machinery use until vision clears
- seek immediate medical advice for new eye conditions, reactions to drops, or infections
- be aware that benzalkonium chloride in eye drops may irritate and discolour soft lenses. Do not use eye drops with contact lenses in place; remove lenses and wait at least 15 minutes before reinserting
- attend regular ophthalmologist appointments
- eye preparations are for individual use only. Mark the expiry date on eye drops and discard them after

28 days; do not use if cloudy or discoloured
- do not stop administering drops suddenly
- if using multiple eye drops, wait at least 5 minutes between doses

Instillation of eye drops
- instruct patient in the correct technique for instilling eye drops, including:
    - do not allow the tip of the dispensing container to touch the eye, as it may cause injury and/or contaminate the eye drops
    - if the container is new, remove the protective seal, otherwise, it is important to check the expiry date
    - wash hands thoroughly with soap and water
    - remove the lid/cap and hold the container upside down in one hand between thumb and forefinger or index finger
    - using the other hand, gently pull down on the lower eyelid to form a pouch/pocket and tilt the head back looking up
    - place tip of container close to lower eyelid (taking care not to make contact between tip and eye). Squeezing bottle gently, release one drop into pouch/pocket formed between the eye and the eyelid, taking care not to allow the tip to touch the eye
    - gently close the eye, but do not blink or rub the eye
    - while the eye is closed, place index finger against the inside corner of the eye and press against the nose for about 2 minutes (this stops the medicine from draining through the tear duct into the nose and throat)
    - replace the lid/cap tightly
    - wash hands again to remove any residue

ACETAZOLAMIDE
Trade names
Diamox, Glaumox Powder for Injection, Acetazolamide Powder for Injection (USP)

Available forms
Tablets: 250 mg;
Vial: 500 mg

Action
- non-bacteriostatic sulfonamide derivative
- inhibits the action of carbonic anhydrase in the ciliary process of the eye, inhibiting secretion of aqueous humour, so reducing intraocular pressure
- (Tablets) onset of action 1—1.5 hours, peak effect 2—4 hours, duration of action 8—12 hours
- (IV) onset of action 2 minutes, peak effect 15 minutes, duration of action 4—5 hours

Use
- adjunctive treatment in chronic simple (open-angle) glaucoma, secondary glaucoma and preoperatively in acute closed-angle glaucoma (where delay in surgery is required to lower intraocular pressure)
- for other uses see Antiepileptics (p. 388)

Dose
- (Open-angle glaucoma) Oral dose: 250 mg to 1 g per day (in divided doses if more than 250 mg); IV dose: 250 mg to 1 g per day (in divided doses if more than 250 mg) **OR**
- (Secondary glaucoma and preoperatively in acute closed-angle glaucoma) Oral dose: 250 mg every 4 hours. Alternatively, start with 500 mg, then give 125 mg to 250 mg every 4 hours, depending on the situation **OR**

ANTIGLAUCOMA AGENTS

- (Acute glaucoma) Oral or IV: Start with 500 mg, then continue with 125 to 250 mg every 4 hours.

Adverse effects
- See Adverse effects for acetazolamide in Diuretics, p. 1081

Interactions
- See Interactions for acetazolamide in Diuretics, p. 1081

Nursing considerations/Cautions
- doses should be adjusted according to symptoms and intraocular pressure readings
- doses > 250 mg should be given as divided doses
- daily doses > 2 g show no increased effects
- IV route should be used when rapid relief from raised intraocular pressure is required
- IV administration should be used only when oral route is not available
- avoid combining aspirin and acetazolamide owing to the risk of severe toxicity; metabolic acidosis can occur, even in patients with normal kidneys
- contraindicated in those with hypersensitivity to sulfonamides or related products as long-term therapy in chronic non-congestive angle-closure glaucoma, severe liver or kidney impairment, hyperchloraemic acidosis, hypokalaemia, hyponatraemia or suprarenal failure
- see also General Nursing considerations/Cautions for acetazolamide in Diuretics (p. 1082)

Patient education
- see General Patient education for acetazolamide in Diuretics (p. 1082)

 Not recommended during pregnancy, especially during the first trimester.

 Not recommended during breastfeeding unless benefits to mother outweigh risks to infant.

 Reduced renal function: contraindicated in patients with a GFR <10 mL/min. For GFR >10 mL/min, reduce the dose by half or increase the dosing interval to every 12 hours.

Reduced hepatic function: contraindicated in patients with marked liver disease or impaired liver function, including cirrhosis, because of the risk of hepatic encephalopathy and reduced ammonia clearance.

 Use with caution.

 Banned in sport.

APRACLONIDINE
Trade name
Iopidine

Available form
Eye drops: 5 mg/mL (0.5%)

Action
- alpha2 adrenergic agonist
- onset of action 1 hour, peak effect 3–5 hours

Use
- control of intraocular pressure in patients with glaucoma who are on maximum tolerated therapy

Dose
- 1 drop to affected eye(s) 2–3 times daily

Adverse effects
- corneal changes
- (Uncommon) depression
- see also General Ocular Adverse effects of antiglaucoma agents (p. 461) and General Adverse effects of antiglaucoma agents (p. 461)

Interactions
- contraindicated with MAOIs, TCAs or systemic sympathomimetic agents
- caution if given with beta adrenoceptor blocking agents (systemic or ophthalmic), antihypertensive agents, clonidine or digoxin
- may have additive CNS depressive effects if given with alcohol, barbiturates, opioids, sedatives or anaesthetics

Nursing considerations/Cautions
- if used with cardiovascular agents, heart rate and BP should be closely monitored
- if patient has severe cardiovascular disease, they should be closely monitored at start of therapy for vasovagal attack
- therapy should be limited to 3 months. Any decision to continue therapy beyond this time should be based on continued effectiveness of therapy and ophthalmological examination for any corneal changes
- caution if used in those with coronary or cerebral insufficiency, recent myocardial infarction, severe uncontrolled cardiac disease, Raynaud's disease or thromboangiitis obliterans, chronic renal failure, impaired liver function, hypertension, cerebrovascular disease, postural hypotension, depression or previous history of vasovagal attacks in patients with cardiovascular disease
- contraindicated in those with hypersensitivity to clonidine
- see also General Nursing considerations/Cautions for antiglaucoma agents (p. 461)

Patient education
- advise patient to report any:
  - changes in mood or depression
  - chest pain or irregular heart beat
- see also General Patient education for antiglaucoma agents (p. 461)

No human studies available. Use only if the potential benefits outweigh the risks.

No studies available. Use only if the benefits outweigh the risk.

Caution if used in those with impaired liver function or renal failure.

BETAXOLOL
Trade names
Betoptic, Betoquin

Available forms
Eye drops: 5 mg/mL (0.5%)

Action
- beta1 adrenoceptor blocking agent that decreases production of aqueous humour
- onset of action 30 minutes, peak effect 2 hours, duration of action 12—18 hours

Use
- chronic open-angle glaucoma
- ocular hypertension

Dose
- 1 drop in the affected eye(s) twice daily

Adverse effects
- (Systemic) asthma, bradycardia, bronchospasm, congestive cardiac failure, dyspnoea, heart block, respiratory failure
- see also General Ocular Adverse effects of antiglaucoma agents (p. 461) and General Adverse effects of antiglaucoma agents (p. 461)

Interactions
- not recommended with other beta adrenoceptor blocking agents, calcium-channel blockers or antiarrhythmic agents
- may prolong AV conduction time if given with digoxin and therefore not recommended together
- additive reduction in intraocular pressure may occur if given with IV acetazolamide or topical miotic agents

ANTIGLAUCOMA AGENTS

- caution if used with catecholamine-depleting agents (e.g. adrenergic psychotropic drugs) owing to risk of hypotension and/or bradycardia
- hypotension may occur if given with phenothiazines
- may decrease effectiveness of adrenaline (epinephrine)

Nursing considerations/Cautions

- those with severe cardiac disease should be closely monitored at start of therapy for any cardiac-related adverse effects
- if used to treat angle-closure glaucoma, should be given with miotic agent
- should be stopped gradually 24–48 hours before surgery with a general anaesthetic
- because there may be systemic absorption and effects, caution if used in those with asthma, myasthenia gravis or thyrotoxicosis
- caution if used in those with diabetes mellitus, as signs of hypoglycaemia (tachycardia) may be masked
- caution if used in those with thyrotoxicosis, as thyroid storm may be provoked if withdrawal is abrupt
- caution if used in those with sick sinus syndrome, Prinzmetal's (variant) angina, hypotension, metabolic acidosis, first-degree heart block, hypotension, cerebrovascular insufficiency, phaeochromocytoma (untreated), hyperthyroidism, cardiac failure, severe COPD, asthma, severe peripheral circulatory insufficiency (e.g. Raynaud's disease), severe allergic rhinitis or bronchial hyperreactivity
- contraindicated in those with sinus bradycardia (greater than first-degree block), cardiac failure or cardiogenic shock
- see also General Nursing considerations/Cautions for antiglaucoma agents (p. 461)

Patient education

- see General Patient education for antiglaucoma agents (p. 461)

 Use only if benefits outweigh risks. May cause bradycardia in fetus.

 Caution if used during breastfeeding.

 Generally banned in sport, but may be permitted under certain circumstances or in some sports.

BIMATOPROST

Trade names
Bimprozt, Lumigan Eye Drops, Lumigan PF, Vizo-PF Bimatoprost, Bimatoprost Sandoz, Bimatoprost-WGR

Available form
Eye drops: 0.3 mg/mL (0.03%)

Action
- prostamide analogue that increases outflow of aqueous humour through trabecular meshwork and enhances uveoscleral outflow
- onset of action within 4 hours, peak effect in 8–12 hours, duration of action 24–36 hours

Use
- chronic open-angle glaucoma or ocular hypertension (as monotherapy or adjunctive therapy with beta adrenoceptor blocking agents)

Dose
- 1 drop to affected eye(s) once daily, at night

Adverse effects
- increased iris pigmentation
- pigmentation of periocular and eyelid skin
- eyelash darkening, thickening, lengthening, increased number of lashes and misdirected growth
- macular oedema
- see also General Ocular Adverse effects of antiglaucoma agents (p. 461) and General Adverse effects of antiglaucoma agents (p. 461)

Nursing considerations/Cautions

- caution if used in those with liver or kidney impairment, compromised lung function, aphakia (absence of lens in the eye) or with a torn posterior lens capsule, uncontrolled congestive cardiac failure, heart block (> first degree), predisposition to hypotension or low heart rate or those with risk factors for macular oedema (e.g. diabetic retinopathy, intraocular surgery) or active intraocular inflammation (e.g. uveitis) (as inflammation may be exacerbated)
- see also General Nursing considerations/Cautions for antiglaucoma agents (p. 461)

Patient education

- warn patient that iris colour may darken, eyelashes darken, thicken and lengthen, and eyelid skin and skin around eyes may also darken. If only one eye is being treated, this may cause a noticeable difference between the eyes
- advise patient to avoid allowing solution to run onto cheeks or other skin areas
- see also General Patient education for antiglaucoma agents (p. 461)

 Not recommended during pregnancy owing to lack of adequate human studies.

 Not recommended during breastfeeding.

Available in combination with

- bimatoprost 0.03% + timolol 0.5% in a 3 mL bottle (for multiple uses) (Ganfort 0.3/5)
- bimatoprost 0.03% + timolol 0.5%, but in 0.4 mL single-use vials (for one-time application, typically to reduce the risk of contamination) (Ganfort PG.3/5)

BRIMONIDINE
Trade names
Alphagan Eye Drops, Alphagan P, Enidin

Available forms
Eye drops: 1.5 mg/mL (0.15%), 2 mg/mL (0.2%)

Action
- alpha2 adrenergic agonist that reduces aqueous humour production and increases uveoscleral outflow
- rapid onset of action, peak effect 2 hours, duration of action 8—12 hours

Use
- chronic open-angle glaucoma or ocular hypertension (monotherapy or adjunctive therapy)

Dose
- 1 drop in affected eye(s) twice daily (approximately 12-hourly) (alone or with beta adrenoceptor blocking agent)

Adverse effects
- see General Ocular Adverse effects of antiglaucoma agents (p. 461) and General Adverse effects of antiglaucoma agents (p. 461)

Interactions
- contraindicated with MAOIs, TCAs or systemic sympathomimetic agents
- caution if given with beta adrenoceptor blocking agents (systemic or ophthalmic), antihypertensive agents, clonidine or cardiac glycosides
- may have additive CNS depressive effects if given with alcohol, barbiturates, opioids, sedatives and anaesthetics

Nursing considerations/Cautions

- if used with cardiovascular agents, heart rate and BP should be closely monitored
- if patient has severe cardiovascular disease, they should be closely monitored at start of therapy for vasovagal attack

ANTIGLAUCOMA AGENTS

- therapy should be limited to 3 months. Any decision to continue therapy beyond this time should be based on continued effectiveness of therapy and ophthalmological examination for any corneal changes
- caution if used in those with coronary or cerebral insufficiency, recent myocardial infarction, severe uncontrolled cardiac disease, Raynaud's disease or thromboangiitis obliterans, chronic renal failure, hypertension, cerebrovascular disease, postural hypotension, depression or previous history of vasovagal attacks in patients with cardiovascular disease
- contraindicated in those with hypersensitivity to clonidine
- see also General Nursing considerations/Cautions for antiglaucoma agents (p. 461)

Patient education

- see General Patient education for antiglaucoma agents (p. 461)

No human studies available; crosses placenta in animals. Avoid use.

Not recommended during breastfeeding. Animal studies suggest excretion in breastmilk.

Available in combination with

- brimonidine tartrate 0.2% + timolol 0.5% (eye drops) (Combigan)
- brimonidine tartrate 0.2% + brinzolamide 1% (eye drops) (Simbrinza)

BRINZOLAMIDE

Trade names

Azopt Eye Drops 1%, BrinzoQuin Eye Drops 1%

Available form

Eye drops: 10 mg/mL (1%)

Action

- carbonic anhydrase inhibitor which decreases production of aqueous humour
- duration of action 8–12 hours

Use

- chronic open-angle glaucoma
- ocular hypertension

Dose

- 1 drop in affected eye(s) twice daily

Adverse effects

- see General Ocular Adverse effects of antiglaucoma agents (p. 461) and General Adverse effects of antiglaucoma agents (p. 461)

Interactions

- not recommended with oral carbonic anhydrase inhibitors

Nursing considerations/Cautions

- if changing from another antiglaucoma agent, patient should be advised to use first agent on last day at usual dose, then next day start brinzolamide at recommended dose
- caution if used in those liver impairment, diabetes mellitus or corneal dystrophies
- contraindicated in those with hypersensitivity to sulfonamides, severe kidney impairment or hyperchloraemic acidosis
- see also General Nursing considerations/Cautions for antiglaucoma agents (p. 461)

Patient education

- patients wearing soft contact lenses should remove them before applying eye drops. Wait at least 15 minutes after instillation before reinserting the lenses
- see also General Patient education for antiglaucoma agents (p. 461)

Animal studies show reproductive toxicity and placental transfer of brinzolamide. Avoid use.

Not recommended during breastfeeding unless the benefits to the mother outweigh risks to the infant.

Available in combination with

- brinzolamide 1% + brimonidine 0.2% (eye drops) (Simbrinza)

- brinzolamide 1% + timolol 0.5% (eye drops) (Azarga)

DORZOLAMIDE
Trade names
Trusamide, Trusopt

Available form
Eye drops: 20 mg/mL (2%)

Action
- topical carbonic anhydrase inhibitor that decreases the production of aqueous humour
- non-bacteriostatic sulfonamide
- duration of action 8–12 hours

Use
- chronic open-angle glaucoma or ocular hypertension (monotherapy or adjunctive therapy with beta adrenoceptor blocking agent)

Dose
- (Monotherapy) 1 drop to the affected eye(s) 3 times daily **OR**
- (Adjunct to beta adrenoceptor antiglaucoma agents) 1 drop to affected eye(s) twice daily

Adverse effects
- transient bitter taste
- see also General Ocular Adverse effects of antiglaucoma agents (p. 461) and General Adverse effects of antiglaucoma agents (p. 461)

Interactions
- not recommended with oral carbonic anhydrase inhibitors

Nursing considerations/Cautions
- not recommended in those with severe kidney or liver impairment or with sulfonamide sensitivity
- see also General Nursing considerations/Cautions for antiglaucoma agents (p. 461)

Patient education
- see General Patient education for antiglaucoma agents (p. 461)

 Not recommended during pregnancy, as no human studies available.

 Caution if used during breastfeeding.

Available in combination with
- dorzolamide 2% + timolol 0.5% eye drops (Cosdor, Cosopt, Vizo-PF Dorzalatim)

LATANOPROST
Trade names
APO-Latanoprost, Latanoprost-WGR, Latanoprost Sandoz, Xalaprost, Xalatan

Available form
Eye drops: 50 microgram/mL (0.005%)

Action
- prostaglandin analogue (F_{2alpha})
- prodrug that is hydrolysed to active form in the aqueous humour
- increases outflow by secondary pathway (uveoscleral flow)
- onset of action 3–4 hours, peak action 8–12 hours, duration of action 24–36 hours

Use
- chronic open-angle glaucoma
- ocular hypertension

Dose
- 1 drop to affected eye(s) nightly

Adverse effects
- iris colour change
- pigmentation of periocular and eyelid skin
- eyelash darkening, thickening, lengthening, increased number of lashes and misdirected growth
- (Rare) macular oedema
- see also General Ocular Adverse effects of antiglaucoma agents (p. 461) and General Adverse effects of antiglaucoma agents (p. 461)

ANTIGLAUCOMA AGENTS

Interactions
- precipitation may occur if given with thiomersal containing eye drops; therefore should be separated by at least 5 minutes
- not recommended with other prostaglandin analogues

Nursing considerations/Cautions
- caution if used in those with aphakia (absence of lens in the eye), pseudoaphakia, or those with risk factors for macular oedema (e.g. diabetic retinopathy, intraocular surgery), inflammatory or neovascular glaucoma, inflammatory ocular conditions, congenital glaucoma, during perioperative cataract surgery, recurrent history of herpes simplex keratitis, with risk factors for iritis or uveitis
- see also General Nursing considerations/Cautions for antiglaucoma agents (p. 461)

Patient education
- warn patient of possible change in eye colour, particularly in those with mixed eye colour (e.g. blue–brown, grey–brown), which generally occurs within first 8 months of treatment
- patients should be advised that eyelashes may darken, thicken and lengthen and eyelid skin and skin around eyes may also darken
- contains benzalkonium chloride, which can be absorbed by contact lenses. Remove lenses before applying drops; reinsert after 15 minutes.
- see also General Patient education for antiglaucoma agents (p. 461)

No human studies available. Not recommended during pregnancy.

Use only if benefits outweigh risks.

Available in combination with
- latanoprost 0.005% + timolol 0.5% eye drops (APO-Latanoprost/Timolol 0.05/5, Xalacom, Xalamol 50/5)

PILOCARPINE
Trade name
Isopto Carpine

Available forms
Eye drops: 10 mg/mL (1%), 20 mg/mL (2%), 40 mg/mL (4%)

Action
- parasympathomimetic agent (cholinergic)
- decreases intraocular pressure
- miotic
- action within 30 minutes, peak effect 1–1.25 hours, duration of action 4–12 hours

Use
- chronic open-angle glaucoma
- emergency management of acute narrow-angle glaucoma

Dose
- 1–2 drops to affected eye(s) 3–4 times daily **OR**
- (Emergency management of acute narrow-angle glaucoma) 1 drop to affected eye(s) every 5 minutes until miosis is achieved

Adverse effects
- (Uncommon) retinal tear
- (Rare) retinal detachment, ciliate muscle spasm
- see also General Ocular Adverse effects of antiglaucoma agents (p. 461) and General Adverse effects of antiglaucoma agents (p. 461)

Interactions
- miotic effects may be reduced by belladonna alkaloids

Nursing considerations/Cautions
- available in a range of strengths, so select correct preparation

- may cause bronchospasm in susceptible individuals
- not recommended if there is acute inflammation of anterior chamber
- caution if used in those with cardiac failure, asthma, peptic ulcer, hyperthyroidism, GI spasm, recent myocardial infarction, Parkinson's disease, urinary tract obstruction or hypo/hypertension
- caution if used in those with corneal or conjunctival damage
- contraindicated where pupillary constriction is not desirable (e.g. acute iritis and uveitis, anterior uveitis), previous history of retinal detachment or conditions that predispose to retinal detachment
- see also General Nursing considerations/Cautions for antiglaucoma agents (p. 461)

Patient education

- these drops may cause blurred vision. Avoid driving or operating machinery if affected, and be cautious in low-light conditions
- may cause stinging and eye watering, which could dilute and reduce the effectiveness of other eye drops. If using multiple eye drops, apply pilocarpine last
- see also General Patient education for antiglaucoma agents (p. 461)

 Limited human studies. Avoid use.

 Use during breastfeeding only if benefits outweigh risks.

TIMOLOL
Trade names
Timoptol, Timoptol XE

Available forms
Eye drops: 2.5 mg/mL (0.25%), 5 mg/mL (0.5%)

Action
- non-selective beta adrenoceptor blocking agent which reduces production of aqueous humour
- onset of action 20 minutes, peak effect 1–2 hours, duration of action 24 hours

Use
- chronic open-angle glaucoma
- ocular hypertension

Dose
- 1 drop of 0.25% ophthalmic solution to affected eye(s) 1–2 times daily until intraocular pressure is at satisfactory level, then once daily (0.5% solution may be required if response is inadequate)

Adverse effects
- see General Ocular Adverse effects of antiglaucoma agents (p. 461) and General Adverse effects of antiglaucoma agents (p. 461)

Interactions
- not recommended with methoxyflurane
- increased risk of tachycardia and hypotension if given with anaesthetics
- decreased AV conduction and bradycardia may occur if given with digoxin
- increased risk of rebound hypertension if given with clonidine
- increased risk of hypotension if given with nifedipine
- increased risk of conduction disorders if given with verapamil or diltiazem
- decreased heart rate may occur if given with SSRIs
- may prolong QT interval if given with mefloquine
- caution if given with adrenaline (epinephrine) owing to the risk of bradycardia and/or hypertensive crisis
- increased effect if given with oral beta adrenoceptor blocking agents
- not recommended with other topical beta adrenoceptor blocking agents
- increased serum levels may occur if given with hydralazine
- may mask signs of hypoglycaemia (tachycardia)
- may increase effects of insulin
- caution if given with amiodarone owing to risk of bradycardia
- not recommended with lidocaine (lignocaine)

ANTIGLAUCOMA AGENTS

Nursing considerations/Cautions
- cardiac failure should be controlled before starting therapy
- intraocular pressure should be reassessed 2–4 weeks after starting therapy
- should be stopped gradually 24–48 hours before surgery with a general anaesthetic
- because there may be systemic absorption and effects, caution if used in those with asthma, myasthenia gravis or thyrotoxicosis
- caution if given to those with myasthenia gravis owing to risk of increased muscle weakness
- caution if used in those with diabetes mellitus as signs of hypoglycaemia (tachycardia) may be masked
- caution if used in those with thyrotoxicosis as thyroid storm may be provoked if withdrawal is abrupt
- caution if used in those with metabolic acidosis, severe cardiac disease, cerebrovascular insufficiency or with a history of atopy or anaphylaxis
- caution if used in those with severe peripheral circulatory insufficiency (e.g. Raynaud's disease)
- contraindicated in those with severe COPD, asthma, reactive airway disease, bronchospasm, SA block, sinus bradycardia (greater than first degree), AV block (second- or third-degree block), cardiac failure, cardiogenic shock or hypersensitivity to timolol or other beta adrenoceptor blocking agents
- see also General Nursing considerations/Cautions for antiglaucoma agents (p. 461)

Patient education
- see General Patient education for antiglaucoma agents (p. 461)

Use only if benefits outweigh risks. May cause bradycardia in fetus.

Caution if used during breastfeeding.

Generally banned in sport during competition, but may be permitted under certain circumstances. This also includes combination eyedrops that contain timolol.

Available in combination with
- timolol 0.5% + bimatoprost 0.03% (eye drops) (Ganfort 0.3/5)
- timolol 0.5% + bimatoprost 0.03% eye drops (30 × 0.4 mL ampoules) (eye drops) (Ganfort PF 0.3/5)
- timolol 0.5% + brimonidine tartrate 0.2% (eye drops) (Combigan)
- timolol 0.5% + brinzolamide 1% (eye drops) (Azarga)
- timolol 0.5% + dorzolamide 2% (eye drops) (Cosdor, Cosopt, Vizo-PF Dorzolatim)
- timolol 0.5% + latanoprost 0.005% (eye drops) (APO-Latanoprost/Timolol, Xalacom, Xalamol 50/5)
- timolol 0.5% + travoprost 0.004% (eye drops) (DuoTrav)

TRAVOPROST

Trade name
Travatan Eye Drops

Available form
Eye drops: 40 microgram/mL (0.004%)

Action
- prostaglandin analogue
- prodrug of prostaglandin F_2 alpha analogue which increases aqueous humour outflow
- onset of action 2 hours, peak effect 12 hours, duration of action 24–36 hours

Use
- chronic open-angle glaucoma
- ocular hypertension

Dose
- 1 drop into affected eye(s) daily, in the evening

Adverse effects
- iris colour change
- pigmentation of periocular and eyelid skin
- eyelash darkening, thickening, lengthening, increased number of lashes and misdirected growth
- macular oedema
- see also General Ocular Adverse effects for antiglaucoma agents (p. 461)

Nursing considerations/Cautions
- caution if used in those with aphakia (absence of lens in the eye), pseudoaphakia, or those with risk factors for macular oedema (e.g. diabetic retinopathy, intraocular surgery), acute intraocular inflammation or risk factors for uveitis or iritis
- see also General Nursing considerations/Cautions for antiglaucoma agents (p. 461)

Patient education
- warn patient of possible change in eye colour, particularly in those with mixed eye colour (e.g. blue—brown, grey—brown), which generally occurs within first 8 months of treatment
- patient should be advised that eyelashes may darken, thicken and lengthen, and eyelid skin and skin around eyes may also darken. Advise patient to wipe off any excess solution from the skin to reduce risk of skin darkening
- women of childbearing potential should be counselled to use adequate contraception during therapy
- see also General Patient education for antiglaucoma agents (p. 461)

 Limited human data. Due to the theoretical risk of uterine contractions and its known effects in animal studies (increased post-implantation loss and teratogenic effects), use should be avoided.

 Avoid use, as limited human data.

Available in combination with
- travoprost 0.004% + timolol 0.5% eye drops, 2.5 mL (DuoTrav)

ANTIGOUT AND URICOLYTIC AGENTS

Gout is a metabolic disorder primarily caused by excess uric acid (hyperuricaemia) in the blood, leading to the formation of uric acid crystals in the joints. This can cause severe pain and inflammation, commonly affecting the big toe but also other joints such as the wrists, fingers, elbows, ankles and knees. While the global prevalence of gout varies, it is more common in developed countries. In Australia, around 224,000 people, or approximately 0.9% of the population, were estimated to be living with gout in 2022 (AIHW 2024e). The disease accounted for 0.7% of the total burden from musculoskeletal conditions in 2023 (AIHW 2024e).

Though gout is often seen as a non-serious condition, its impact on quality of life is significant. It not only causes debilitating pain but also affects a person's ability to function and work. In 2021–22, there were 7100 hospitalisations in Australia with a principal diagnosis of gout, equating to 27 per 100,000 people. Gout also contributed to 573 deaths in 2022, or 2.2 deaths per 100,000 people, representing 0.3% of all deaths and 5.5% of deaths from musculoskeletal conditions (AIHW 2024e). Of these, gout was the underlying cause in 34 deaths (5.9%), while it was recorded as an associated cause in the remaining 539 deaths (94%).

Gout is often associated with co-morbidities such as hypertension, diabetes mellitus, ischaemic heart disease, obesity and kidney disease (Capuano et al 2017). Screening for these conditions in patients presenting with gout is essential to manage the broader health risks associated with the disease. Despite the chronic nature of gout and its associated risks, gout mortality rates (including both underlying and associated causes) have remained relatively stable over the past decade, with little change between 2012 and 2022 (1.4 and 1.6 per 100,000 population, respectively).

Uric acid is produced in the body from purines (adenosine, guanine) via a number of steps catalysed by the enzyme xanthine oxidase. It is normally filtered by the kidneys, reabsorbed and then excreted in the urine. Conditions that may cause the uric acid to crystallise (the crystals are known as 'tophi') include an acid environment (such as in the kidney filtrate) or temperatures less than 37°C (such as body extremities). When the uric acid crystallises as urates in the joint spaces (usually toes and/or ankles) an inflammatory response is mediated, resulting in swelling, heat, inflammation and pain. Initially, one joint is affected; however, with subsequent attacks, other joints become involved. In the renal tubules, the crystals can lead to stone formation and impaired renal function, which can proceed to renal failure. Early attacks usually subside without treatment in 3–10 days with no residual symptoms (Schumacher & Chen 2018).

The primary goal of gout therapy is to reduce serum urate levels, aiming to prevent gout flares (acute gouty attacks) and resolve tophi, if present. Urate-lowering therapy should be titrated to a target serum urate concentration of less than 0.36 mmol/L for those without tophi, and less than 0.30 mmol/L for those with tophi, as the presence of tophi indicates a higher urate load. (Robinson & Stamp 2016). While patients should be aware that gout flares may still occur for 12–18 months after serum urate levels reach target concentrations, these flares should become less frequent and eventually cease if the target urate levels are maintained. Lifelong urate-lowering therapy is recommended for all patients with confirmed gout, especially those with tophaceous gout, renal manifestations of gout or chronic gouty arthritis. Acute gout flares are typically managed with NSAIDs or colchicine, while oral corticosteroids may be used in patients who are intolerant or have contraindications to these treatments. NSAIDs and colchicine are also used prophylactically to prevent flares during the initiation of urate-lowering therapy, typically for at least 6 months or 3 months after reaching the target serum urate levels in patients without tophi, or 6 months for those with tophi.

Non-adherence to urate-lowering therapy is a common issue, often due to misconceptions about the medications or a reluctance to start lifelong treatment. Patients must understand that, while gout flares may persist in the short term, the long-term goal is to eliminate these flares by maintaining target serum urate levels. Patient education is critical to improving adherence and understanding the chronic nature of gout. While dietary modifications (low purine) are often discussed, there is limited evidence supporting their effectiveness in managing gout. However, avoiding large intakes of sugar and sweetened soft drinks has been shown to reduce the risk of gout flares (Robinson & Stamp 2016).

First-line urate-lowering therapy generally involves allopurinol or a xanthine oxidase inhibitor (Therapeutic Guidelines 2024). Monitoring serum uric acid concentration monthly during the dose titration phase helps to enable treatment efficacy. Allopurinol is well tolerated, but in rare cases it can lead to severe adverse reactions such as allopurinol hypersensitivity syndrome. In cases where allopurinol is contraindicated or not tolerated, alternative therapies such as febuxostat or probenecid may be considered. It is important to note that starting or increasing urate-lowering therapy carries a high risk of precipitating a gout flare. Starting with a low dose and gradually increasing it, along with flare prophylaxis, can help manage this risk (Therapeutic Guidelines 2024). Additionally, patients should not discontinue or adjust their urate-lowering therapy during an acute attack, as sudden changes in serum uric acid concentrations can worsen or prolong the attack.

Managing gout involves a combination of acute and long-term strategies, patient

ANTIGOUT AND URICOLYTIC AGENTS

education and adherence to therapy. Lifelong management with urate-lowering therapy is key to preventing recurrent flares and complications associated with gout (Therapeutic Guidelines 2024).

XANTHINE OXIDASE INHIBITORS

ALLOPURINOL
Trade names
Allopurinol Alphapharm, Allopurinol-WGR, APO-Allopurinol, Allopurinol Sandoz, Allosig, Noumed Allopurinol, Zyloprim, Progout Viatris

Available forms
Tablets: 100 mg, 300 mg

Action
- reduces uric acid levels in both body fluids and urine by inhibiting xanthine oxidase, which catalyses the conversion of hypoxanthine and xanthine to urate/uric acid
- active metabolite (oxypurinol)
- half-life of allopurinol 1–2 hours, while the active metabolite oxypurinol has a half-life of 15 hours

Use
- chronic gout (gouty arthritis, skin tophi)
- hyperuricaemia resulting from neoplastic disease or myeloproliferative disorders (with high cell turnover), antineoplastic or thiazide diuretic therapy or radiotherapy
- recurrent renal stones (mixed calcium oxalate) with hyperuricaemia (where other forms of management have failed) or enzyme disorders resulting in overproduction of urate

Dose
Gout
- (Mild) 100–200 mg orally daily after food **OR**
- (Moderately severe) 300–600 mg orally daily after food **OR**
- (Severe) 700–900 mg orally daily after food

High urate turnover conditions
- dosage should be started at lower range (see mild gout above)

High urate turnover conditions (with renal impairment)
- initially 100 mg orally daily after food, increasing only if serum and/or urinary urate levels do not respond

Adverse effects
- rash
- nausea, vomiting
- headache, fever, malaise, somnolence, vertigo, asthenia, ataxia
- (Rare) hypersensitivity reaction (fever, arthralgia, eosinophilia, exfoliation), hepatotoxicity, bone marrow depression, ataxia

Interactions
- prolongs the activity of azathioprine and mercaptopurine; therefore lower doses of both agents are recommended
- excretion of active metabolite (oxypurinol) may be increased when given with probenecid or high-dose salicylates
- may increase theophylline or ciclosporin plasma concentrations, requiring more frequent monitoring to decrease the risk of toxicity, especially at start of therapy or when increasing the dose of allopurinol
- may increase the frequency of rash in patients receiving ampicillin or amoxicillin; therefore not recommended together
- may increase the risk of toxicity of ifosamide, pyrazinamide or cyclophosphamide if given with allopurinol
- increased risk of bone marrow depression if given with other agents which also depress bone marrow

Nursing considerations/Cautions
- should not be started until an acute attack has subsided (otherwise further attacks may be precipitated)
- serum urate and urinary urate/uric acid levels should be measured regularly during therapy

- if the dose is greater than 300 mg and gastric symptoms are present, the dose may be divided
- if allopurinol is stopped because of rash, it can be restarted at a lower dose when the rash has totally disappeared and the dose gradually increased. However, if rash recurs the therapy should be stopped immediately and not restarted, as there is an increased risk of hypersensitivity
- the dose is dependent on the severity of gout
- colchicine or NSAIDs may also be given in the early stages of allopurinol therapy as prophylaxis for acute gout attacks
- (High urate turnover conditions) any hyperuricaemia and/or hyperuricosuria should be corrected before starting cytotoxic therapy. Adequate hydration is also required to ensure optimal diuresis to minimise kidney stone formation or deposition in the urinary tract
- (High urate turnover conditions with renal impairment) the dose may be started at less than 100 mg per day or 100 mg at a longer interval (e.g. every second day)
- in those with pre-existing liver disease, regular liver function tests are recommended, especially early in therapy
- allopurinol is removed by renal dialysis; therefore alternate dose (300–400 mg orally immediately after dialysis) should be considered if dialysis is needed 2 to 3 times per week
- caution if used in those with liver or renal impairment, as a lower dose is required
- caution if used in those with hypertension, cardiac insufficiency with renal impairment, haemochromatosis or abnormal iron storage conditions

Patient education

- warn the patient not to take allopurinol during an acute attack of gout
- the patient should be warned that acute gout attacks may occur early in therapy because of mobilisation of urate from tissue and this is managed with NSAIDs or colchicine for at least 4 weeks
- advise the patient to take with food or milk to minimise gastric irritation
- if not contraindicated, fluid intake should be increased to maintain a urinary output of at least 2 L/24 hours and urine made alkaline to minimise kidney stone formation or deposition in the urinary tract
- instruct the patient to report rash, pruritus (itch), anorexia (loss of appetite) or weight loss immediately to the doctor because this indicates the need to stop therapy
- warn the patient against driving a vehicle or operating machinery if drowsy or experiencing vertigo or ataxia
- advise the patient to avoid using aspirin, foods with high purine content such as organ meat (e.g. kidney, liver), sardines, anchovies, mackerel, herring, minced meat, shrimp, broth, consommé, gravies and yeast, and limit the use of alcohol and fructose-containing foods and drinks

 Tablet can be broken in half and dispersed with water, or crushed and mixed with water or a spoonful of yoghurt or apple puree.

 Limited human data. Use in pregnancy only if benefits outweigh potential risks.

 Not recommended during breastfeeding.

 Use a lower starting dose in renal impairement and increase gradually to achieve serum urate < 0.36 mmol/L (< 0.3 mmol/L if tophi).

ANTIGOUT AND URICOLYTIC AGENTS

COLCHICINE
Trade names
Colcine, Colgout, Lengout, Colchicine-WGR

Available form
Tablets: 500 microgram

Action
- inhibits leucocyte migration and phagocytosis in gouty joints, counteracting the inflammatory response to urate crystals
- decreases deposition of urate crystals, although it has no effect on production or excretion of uric acid
- has no analgesic properties, but does have prophylactic, suppressive effects reducing the incidence of acute attacks
- half-life 4.4 hours, which increases to 18.8 hours in kidney dysfunction

Use
- acute gout (where NSAIDs are contraindicated or are ineffective)
- gout flare prophylaxis, including start of urate-lowering therapy
- familial Mediterranean fever (FMF)

Dose
- (Acute gout flare) initially 1 mg orally, then 0.5 mg 1 hour later (maximum 1.5 mg per course). Do not repeat the course within 3 days.
- (Gout flare prophylaxis, including start of urate-lowering therapy (ULT)) 0.5 mg orally once or twice daily, depending on response and gastrointestinal tolerance (maximum 1.5 mg per 3 days)

Adverse effects
- nausea, vomiting, diarrhoea, abdominal pain
- rash, urticaria, purpura, dermatitis
- delayed or impaired corneal wound healing
- reversible azoospermia and oligospermia, decreased sperm motility
- anuria, bladder spasm, oliguria
- increased alkaline phosphatase
- muscle weakness, myopathy
- (Long-term or prolonged therapy or overdose) blood dyscrasias, hair loss (body and scalp), anorexia, myopathy, peripheral neuropathy, rhabdomyolysis, vascular damage, malabsorption syndrome, hypersensitivity
- (Toxic dose) haemorrhagic diarrhoea, dehydration, metabolic acidosis, hypotension, shock, haematuria, oliguria, renal damage

Interactions
- increased risk of myopathy and/or rhabdomyolysis if used with ciclosporin, especially if kidney impairment is also present
- toxicity may occur if given with erythromycin and clarithromycin (especially if liver/kidney impairment exists or in the elderly)
- increased serum levels, and therefore risk of toxicity, may occur if given with clarithromycin, erythromycin, atazanavir, ritonavir or itraconazole
- inhibited by acidifying agents such as ammonium chloride and ascorbic acid
- potentiated by alkalinising agents such as sodium bicarbonate and potassium citrate
- may increase sensitivity to CNS depressants (e.g. opioids, sedatives, hypnotics, alcohol, benzodiazepines)
- increased risk of GI toxicity if given with alcohol
- alcohol increases blood uric acid levels, thereby decreasing prophylactic actions of colchicine
- increased risk of GI bleeding/ulceration if given with NSAIDs
- increased risk of bone marrow depression if given with radiation treatment and/or cytolytic antineoplastic agents
- increased risk of bleeding if given with other agents that impair blood clotting or cause haemorrhage
- may cause reversible malabsorption of vitamin B_{12}
- leucopenic and/or thrombocytopenic effects may be increased if given with myelotoxic agents (i.e. those with bone

HAVARD'S NURSING GUIDE TO DRUGS

- marrow depressing effects or those causing blood dyscrasias)
- action may be decreased if given with antineoplastic agents which cause rapid cell turnover
- may affect a number of laboratory tests

Nursing considerations/Cautions

- treatment is continued during an acute attack until relief, or if nausea and diarrhoea occur (even if an acute attack has not subsided). The patient should be advised to note the cumulative dose at which GI symptoms occurred and remain below this with subsequent treatments
- additional treatment should not occur within 3 days of completing a course
- therapy should be stopped before any eye surgery because of delayed or impaired corneal wound healing
- complete blood counts are recommended if therapy is prolonged or long term
- any dental work should be delayed if leucopenia or thrombocytopenia occur owing to an increased risk of gum bleeding, delayed healing and infection
- overdose symptoms may be delayed 2–12 hours after ingestion; therefore it is recommended the patient is monitored for at least 12 hours after overdose or acute poisoning
- caution if used in the elderly (especially if under 50 kg) or debilitated, or those with heart, kidney or GI disease
- contraindicated in those with kidney and/or liver disease/impairment, severe GI or cardiac disorders and blood dyscrasias

Patient education

- warn the patient to avoid alcohol during therapy
- the patient should be advised to avoid vitamin C preparations because they acidify the urine, leading to the possibility of renal stone formation
- instruct the patient to continue therapy until relief occurs or abdominal pain, diarrhoea, nausea or vomiting appear. These symptoms usually occur within 8–12 hours of starting therapy (especially if a maximum dose is given). The patient should also be asked to take a note of the total dose taken when the symptoms occurred and seek medical advice immediately
- warn the patient to not take colchicine again within 3 days of stopping treatment or abdominal pain, diarrhoea, nausea or vomiting occurring
- advise the patient to avoid using aspirin, and foods with high purine content, such as organ meat (e.g. kidney, liver), sardines, anchovies, mackerel, herring, minced meat, shrimp, broth, consommé, gravies and yeast, and limit the use of alcohol and fructose-containing foods and drinks
- advise the patient to avoid grapefruit juice, as it may increase colchicine levels in the bloodstream and raise the risk of side-effects.
- the patient should be instructed to seek medical advice immediately if any of the following occur:
  - burning sensation in throat or stomach
  - severe stomach pain, nausea or vomiting
  - severe diarrhoea with bloody or black stools
  - difficulty passing urine or urine containing blood
  - muscle weakness
  - numbness in fingers or toes

Tablets can be dispersed in water, or crushed and given with water or a spoonful of yoghurt or apple puree.

Not recommended during pregnancy. Animal studies have shown embryotoxicity and teratogenic effects.

ANTIGOUT AND URICOLYTIC AGENTS

Considered safe during breastfeeding, but it is recommended to take the medication after feeding to minimise the infant's exposure. Regular monitoring of the baby for any side-effects is advised.

Kidney: clearance is reduced in renal impairment, increasing the risk of side-effects. Dose reduction and close monitoring are advised.

Acute gout: increase the interval between doses when CrCl < 30 mL/min; avoid use in CrCl < 80 mL/min if on prophylaxis.

Prophylaxis/FMF/pericarditis: use a lower starting dose if CrCl < 30 mL/min.

Hepatic: reduced clearance raises the risk of adverse effects. Dose adjustments and monitoring are necessary.

Acute gout: extend intervals in severe impairment; avoid if on prophylaxis.

FMF/prophylaxis/pericarditis: start with a lower dose in severe impairment.

Do not crush or disperse the tablets if pregnant.

FEBUXOSTAT
Trade name
Adenuric

Available form
Tablets: 80 mg

Action
- non-purine selective xanthine oxidase inhibitor
- active metabolites
- half-life 5—8 hours

Use
- chronic gout
- gouty arthritis and/or tophus formation

Dose
- (Chronic gout) initially 40 mg orally daily, increasing to 80 mg daily after 2—4 weeks if serum uric acid levels are greater than 357 micromol/L (6 mg/dL); (maximum 120 mg orally daily)

Adverse effects
- gout flares (acute gouty attacks)
- liver function abnormalities
- diarrhoea, nausea
- headache
- rash
- oedema
- (Uncommon) dizziness, somnolence, paraesthesia, blurred vision, altered taste
- (Rare) severe hypersensitivity reaction

Interactions
- not recommended with mercaptopurine or azathioprine owing to increased risk of toxicity
- caution if given with theophylline, as there may be an increase in levels of theophylline's metabolite
- metabolism may be increased by phenytoin. Serum uric acid should be monitored 12 weeks after starting therapy if given together
- may increase serum levels of tacrolimus

Nursing considerations/Cautions
- therapy should not be started until acute gout has subsided
- gout flares (acute gouty attacks) commonly occur soon after start of therapy and during first 6 months of therapy because of the mobilisation of urate from tissue deposits resulting in changing serum uric acid levels. Gout flares can be prevented by concurrent therapy with colchicine or NSAIDs for up to 6 months
- liver function tests are recommended before starting and regularly throughout therapy. If the patient experiences symptoms of liver dysfunction, liver function tests should be completed immediately and therapy stopped if alanine aminotransferase (ALT) is three times greater than normal levels
- the patient should be carefully monitored for signs and symptoms of stroke or myocardial infarction during therapy

- tablets contain lactose and therefore are not recommended in those with hereditary problems of galactose intolerance, Lapp lactase deficiency or glucose–galactose malabsorption
- caution if used in those with thyroid dysfunction, or liver or kidney impairment
- not recommended in those with ischaemic heart disease or congestive heart failure, or organ transplant recipients
- not recommended in those with an increased rate of urate formation such as during treatment for malignancy or those with Lesch–Nyhan syndrome

Patient education

- warn the patient that gout flares may occur more frequently during the first 6 months of therapy because of changes in serum uric acid levels, but will decrease in both frequency and intensity. Febuxostat should be continued during these gout flares
- the patient should be advised not to drive or operate machinery if somnolence, dizziness, blurred vision or numbness occurs
- advise the patient to seek medical advice immediately if any of the following occur:
  - rash, itchiness, breathing difficulties, limb/face swelling
  - skin/eyes yellowing, dark urine, fatigue, loss of appetite, pain in right upper abdomen
  - increase in gout symptoms

Tablet may be crushed and mixed with water or a spoonful of yoghurt or apple puree.

Not recommended during pregnancy owing to limited safety data.

Not recommended during breastfeeding owing to lack of safety data.

Reduced renal function: clearance is reduced. Dose adjustment is required. Avoid use in severe renal impairment (eGFR < 30 mL/min).

Reduced hepatic function: metabolism is reduced. Avoid use in severe hepatic impairment or in patients with both renal and hepatic impairment.

OTHER DRUGS FOR GOUT

PROBENECID

Trade name
Pro-Cid

Available form
Tablets: 500 mg

Action
- promotes uric acid excretion by inhibiting its renal tubular absorption (uricosuric)
- reduces renal tubular excretion of some anti-infective agents, thereby prolonging and increasing their plasma concentrations by 2—4 times
- half-life 6—12 hours

Use
- chronic gout
- adjuvant to therapy with penicillins and most cephalosporins (beta lactam antibacterial agents)

Dose
- (Gout) 250 mg orally twice daily for 1 week, then increased to 500 mg twice daily. If needed, dose may be further increased by 500 mg every 4 weeks (maximum daily dose 2 g) **OR**
- (Beta lactam co-therapy) 500 mg orally 4 times daily **OR**
- (Uncomplicated gonorrhoea) 1 g orally as a single dose taken with a single high dose of oral ampicillin, IM procaine benzylpenicillin (procaine penicillin) or IM cefoxitin sodium

Adverse effects
- headache, dizziness

ANTIGOUT AND URICOLYTIC AGENTS

- flushing, dermatitis, alopecia
- sore gums
- anorexia, nausea, vomiting
- urinary frequency, renal colic, renal stones (with or without haematuria)
- hypersensitivity reaction, including skin reactions
- exacerbation of gout
- anaemia, haemolytic anaemia

Interactions

- contraindicated with aspirin or other salicylates, as they antagonise uricosuric action
- may prolong action of sulfonylureas, increasing risk of hypoglycaemia
- may decrease excretion of sulfonamides
- may increase plasma concentrations of penicillins, dapsone, some cephalosporins, midazolam, nitrazepam, methotrexate, paracetamol, rifampicin, NSAIDs, antiviral agents, lorazepam, ketorolac, ciprofloxacin, famotidine
- increased plasma concentrations of both if given with allopurinol
- may increase plasma concentrations of methotrexate leading to toxicity; therefore plasma concentrations should be closely monitored and dose adjusted as needed
- may potentiate the effects of thiazide diuretics
- may increase and prolong anaesthetic effect of ketamine and thiopental
- may decrease the dose needed for induction using thiopental
- may cause a false positive test for glycosuria using reagent strips containing copper sulfate

Nursing considerations/Cautions

- therapy should not be started until an acute attack has subsided. If acute gout is precipitated, probenecid should be continued with colchicine, indometacin or other agents to control the acute attack
- gastric symptoms (anorexia, nausea and vomiting) may indicate overdose, and the dose may be reduced without losing clinical response
- alkaline urine can be achieved by taking sodium bicarbonate (3–7.5 g/day) or potassium citrate (7.5 g/day) and this should be continued until serum uric acid levels return to normal and tophi have disappeared. Acid–base balance should be closely monitored during this time
- if the patient has been free of acute attacks for 6 months and serum uric acid levels are normal, the dose may be reduced
- blood glucose levels (BGLs) should be monitored frequently in patients with diabetes who are treated concurrently with sulfonylureas and probenecid
- when used in gonorrhoea, oral ampicillin is given at the same time, whereas IM penicillin or cefoxitin should be given 30 minutes after probenecid
- not effective if the patient has chronic renal insufficiency and the glomerular filtration rate is less than 30 mL/min
- caution if used in those with GI disease (e.g. peptic ulcer) or chronic kidney insufficiency
- contraindicated in those with blood dyscrasias or uric acid stones

Patient education

- the patient should be warned not to start therapy until acute attack has settled
- the patient should be advised to take paracetamol instead of aspirin for pain relief
- instruct the patient to report any loss of appetite, nausea and/or vomiting to doctor immediately
- if the patient is involved in elite sport, he/she should be advised that probenecid is banned in sport both in and out of competition
- if the patient has diabetes and is managed using sulfonylureas, he/she should be warned that there is an increased risk of hypoglycaemia occurring
- if the patient has diabetes, they should be advised that false positive test results

may occur if the test involves copper sulfate
- warn the patient against driving a vehicle or operating machinery if experiencing dizziness
- instruct the patient to drink plenty of water while taking probenecid to prevent kidney stones from forming
- advise the patient to seek medical advice if blood appears in the urine, severe/sharp pain occurs in the side or lower back, fever, infection, increased bruising or bleeding, unusual hair loss or painful swollen joints occurs
- advise the patient to avoid aspirin, foods with a high purine content such as organ meat (e.g. kidney, liver), sardines, anchovies, mackerel, herring, minced meat, shrimp, broth, consommé, gravies and yeast, and limit the use of alcohol and fructose-containing foods and drinks

Can be dispersed in water, or crushed and given in water or a spoonful of yoghurt or apple puree.

Crosses the placental barrier and should be used in pregnancy only if benefits outweigh risks.

Avoid use.

Reduced renal function:

Do not use if there's a history of uric acid kidney stones.

CrCl < 50 mL/min: effectiveness may decrease. Monitor serum urate levels.

CrCl < 10 mL/min: avoid, as it is ineffective.

Banned in sport (in and out of competition). Probenecid is considered a masking agent, as it can be used to inhibit the excretion of other substances (such as performance-enhancing drugs) in urine, thereby hiding the use of prohibited substances such as anabolic steroids or stimulants.

RASBURICASE RYS
Trade name
Fasturtec

Available form
Vial: 1.5 mg

Action
- recombinant urate oxidase
- catalyses oxidation of uric acid to allantoin, which is water soluble and therefore more easily excreted by the kidney
- produces hydrogen peroxide as a byproduct
- half-life 19 hours

Use
- prophylaxis and treatment of acute hyperuricaemia (caused by malignancy with high risk of rapid tumour lysis)

Dose
- 0.20 mg/kg/day administered as an IV infusion over 30 minutes once daily for 5–7 days

Adverse effects
- fever
- nausea, vomiting
- rash, urticaria
- (Uncommon) bronchospasm, allergic reaction, antibody formation, haemolytic anaemia, methaemoglobinaemia, headache, diarrhoea, hypotension
- (Rare) anaphylaxis

Nursing considerations/Cautions
- the patient should be carefully monitored during therapy for any signs of allergy including skin reactions and bronchospasm
- if the patient is already hyperuricaemic, chemotherapy should be administered within 48 hours of rasburicase rys
- if the patient is not hyperuricaemic, chemotherapy should be administered within 24 hours of rasburicase rys
- the patient should be monitored for hyperphosphataemia, hyperkalaemia and hypocalcaemia, as these can also arise from rapid tumour lysis

ANTIGOUT AND URICOLYTIC AGENTS

- when reconstituting solution, it should be swirled gently and not shaken
- after reconstitution, solution should be further diluted using sodium chloride 0.9% to make up a total infusion of 50 mL
- reconstituted solution should be inspected for any particulate matter
- an inline filter should not be used
- administer as a 30-minute intravenous infusion
- use a separate line from other chemotherapeutic agents, or flush the line with saline if sharing the same line
- if a separate IV line is not available, IV should be flushed with sodium chloride between chemotherapy and rasburicase rys
- if blood is needed for uric acid concentrations, it should be collected into pre-chilled tubes (with heparin to prevent coagulation), samples placed in ice/water bath, centrifuged in a precooled centrifuge, plasma kept in ice/water bath and analysed within 4 hours of collection
- physically incompatible with glucose
- caution if used in those with a history of atopic allergies because of the increased risk of hypersensitivity reactions
- contraindicated in those with glucose-6-phosphate dehydrogenase (G6PD) deficiency or other metabolic disorders because of the hydrogen peroxide byproduct, which is known to induce haemolytic anaemia in susceptible individuals or those with uricase hypersensitivity

No human data. Animal studies show teratogenicity at high doses. Use only if the benefit to the mother outweighs the risk to the fetus.

Unknown if excreted in human milk. Avoid use during breastfeeding.

483

ANTIHISTAMINES

Histamine is a naturally occurring amine that is stored in mast cells or in circulating basophils and is the major mediator of inflammation, anaphylaxis and gastric acid secretion. Mast cells are found in large numbers in bronchial smooth muscle and small blood vessels, which may account for some of the immediate hypersensitivity and allergic responses. Histamine has also been found stored in the GI mucosa, epidermis and the CNS. It should be noted that some medications act directly, causing mast cells to release histamine, leading to adverse effects (Skidgel 2018).

Antihistamines block the effects of histamine by binding to histamine receptors, particularly H_1-receptors. This prevents histamine from causing itching, swelling, and redness associated with allergies. Broadly, antihistamines can be categorised into sedating and non-sedating types. Sedating antihistamines, also known as first-generation antihistamines, include drugs such as cinnarizine with dimenhydrinate, cyclizine, cyproheptadine, dexchlorpheniramine, diphenhydramine, doxylamine and promethazine. Non-sedating antihistamines are bilastine, cetirizine, desloratadine, fexofenadine, levocetirizine and loratadine. The older style sedating antihistamines (e.g. promethazine, chlorpheniramine) have also been used as mild hypnotic agents because they cross the blood—brain barrier and cause sedation, and also as antiemetics, especially in the treatment of motion sickness (Skidgel 2018).

H_1-receptor antagonists are commonly referred to as 'antihistamines' and are used in the treatment of allergic disorders, including seasonal allergic rhinitis (hay fever), allergic skin reactions, including rash, pruritus and insect stings, and also with adrenaline (epinephrine) in the management of anaphylaxis or severe angioedema.

General Actions of antihistamines
- block main actions of histamine at H_1 receptors

General Adverse effects of antihistamines
Non-sedating antihistamines
- sedation-related effects: sedation, decreased motor skills and coordination, fatigue, dizziness, headache, somnolence, insomnia, confusion, anxiety, hallucinations
- anticholinergic effects: dry eyes, nose and mouth, blurred vision, urinary

ANTIHISTAMINES

hesitancy/retention, constipation, tachycardia
- gastrointestinal effects: nausea, vomiting, diarrhoea, dyspepsia
- other effects: tinnitus, vertigo, pruritus, rash, urticaria, allergic dermatitis
- rare effects: blood dyscrasias
- sedation-related effects (rare): dizziness, headache, fatigue (less common)
- gastrointestinal effects: nausea, dyspepsia
- other side effects: rash, urticaria (less common)

General Interactions of antihistamines
- may enhance CNS depressant effects of alcohol and other CNS depressing agents, such as barbiturates, hypnotics, sedatives, anticholinergics, antipsychotics and opioid analgesics

General Nursing considerations/ Cautions for antihistamines
- should be discontinued 48—72 hours before skin testing for allergies is performed
- caution if used in those with epilepsy (especially in children), liver or kidney impairment
- caution if used in the elderly, as they are more prone to adverse effects, such as confusion, dizziness, sedation and hypotension, which increases the risk of falls
- caution/contraindicated if used in those with cardiovascular disease, hypertension, narrow-angle glaucoma, predisposed to urinary retention (e.g. prostatic hypertrophy, spinal cord lesion), bladder neck obstruction, pyloroduodenal obstruction, stenosing peptic ulcer, thyroid disease or raised intraocular pressure

General Patient education for antihistamines
- counsel the patient to avoid contact with allergen (if possible) and to take antihistamine before start of exposure (e.g. at the beginning of hay fever season)
- ensure the patient understands that antihistamine does not protect against allergic reactions
- (Sedating antihistamine) advise the patient against driving a vehicle or operating machinery if drowsy, dizzy or experiencing any other CNS adverse effects
- (Sedating antihistamine) warn the patient about reduced tolerance to alcohol and the need to avoid it during therapy with antihistamine

Nasal spray instillation
- if using a nasal spray, instruct the patient to:
  1. ensure nasal spray is primed for use, if new, dust cover has been left off or device has been unused for some time (priming instructions vary from nasal spray to nasal spray, but essentially involves vigorously shaking container (with cap on) for 10 seconds and then priming by releasing 6—7 sprays until spray is uniform)
  2. blow nose
  3. insert spray adapter/nozzle into nostril while closing other nostril
  4. tilt head slightly forwards, keeping nasal spray container upright
  5. avoid tilting head back as this will result in bitter smell/taste

6. depress pump while breathing gently and slowly through the nostril
7. repeat procedure in same nostril if second spray per nostril is required
8. remove adapter/nozzle from nostril and repeat in other nostril
9. after prescribed amount has been delivered, remove adapter/nozzle from nostril and wipe with tissue
10. wash spray adapter/nozzle regularly with warm water
11. re-prime with 2 sprays after cleaning
12. if nozzle/adapter becomes blocked, pins or other sharp devices should not be used to unblock device as it may become damaged and not deliver required amount of nasal spray
13. replace dust cap after each use

Eye drop instillation

- instruct the patient in the correct technique for instilling eye drops, including:
  1. removal of contact lenses before using eye drops and not replacing lenses for at least 15 minutes (eye drops contain preservative benzalkonium chloride, which discolours contact lenses)
  2. not allowing tip of dispensing container to touch eye, as it may cause injury and/or contaminate eye drops
  3. if container is new, remove protective seal, otherwise it is important to check expiry date
  4. when opening for first time, container should be dated and discarded 28 days after opening
  5. wash hands thoroughly with soap and water
  6. remove lid/cap and hold container upside down in one hand between thumb and forefinger or index finger
  7. using other hand, gently pull down on lower eyelid to form a pouch/pocket and tilt head back, looking up
  8. place tip of container close to lower eyelid (taking care not to make contact between tip and eye). Squeezing the bottle gently, release 1 drop into pouch/pocket formed between eye and eyelid, taking care not to allow tip to touch eye
  9. gently close eye, but do not blink or rub eye
  10. while eye is closed, place index finger against inside corner of eye and press against nose for about 2 minutes (this stops medicine from draining through tear duct into nose and throat)
  11. blot any excess solution from around the eye with a tissue
  12. replace lid/cap tightly
  13. wash hands again to remove any residue

AZELASTINE

Trade names
Azep Nasal Spray, Eyezep

Available forms
Metered dose nasal spray: 137 microgram/0.137 mL;
Eye drops: 0.5 mg/mL

Action
- active metabolite (half-life 56 hours)
- half-life 22 hours
- (Nasal spray) onset of action 15 minutes, duration up to 12 hours

ANTIHISTAMINES

- see also General Actions of antihistamines (p. 484)

Use
- seasonal or perennial allergic rhinitis, seasonal/non-seasonal (perennial) allergic conjunctivitis

Dose
- (Nasal spray) 1 spray to each nostril twice daily **OR**
- (Eye drops) 1 drop per eye twice daily, increasing to 4 times daily if needed

Adverse effects
- (Nasal spray) nasal stinging, itching, sneezing, rhinitis, bitter taste, nausea, epistaxis, headache
- (Eye drops) mild transient burning or stinging and, uncommonly, bitter taste

Interactions
- see General Interactions of antihistamines (p. 485)

Nursing considerations/Cautions
- (Perennial allergic rhinitis) treatment should not exceed 6 weeks
- (Non-seasonal conjunctivitis) treatment should not exceed 6 months
- (Eye drops) not recommended in those with eye infections
- (Eye drops) contains benzalkonium chloride (preservative), which can cause irritation and discolouration of soft contact lenses
- see also General Nursing considerations/Cautions for antihistamines (p. 485)

Patient education
- (Nasal spray) prime 2—3 times before first use, and again if not used for > 3 days until spray is even
- (Eye drops) if allergen exposure is anticipated, should be instilled before exposure
- see also General Patient education for antihistamines (including instillation instructions for nasal spray and eye drops) (p. 485)

 Not recommended during pregnancy unless benefits are thought to outweigh risks.

 Caution if used during breastfeeding.

Available in combination with
- (Nasal spray) azelastine with fluticasone (Dymista, APOHealth Allergy and Hayfever Relief, Chemists' Own Allermist, Misty-Duo)

BILASTINE
Trade name
Allertine

Available form
Tablet: 20 mg

Action
- non-sedating, long-acting histamine antagonist with a high affinity for peripheral H_1 receptors and no affinity for muscarinic receptors
- binds to the H_1 receptor, stabilising it in an inactive form
- reduces the effects of histamine
- it prevents histamine from causing allergic symptoms like itching, sneezing and swelling
- reaches maximum plasma concentration approximately 1.3 hours after oral administration

Use
- allergic rhinoconjunctivitis (AR), which includes both seasonal allergic rhinitis (SAR) and perennial allergic rhinitis (PAR)
- urticaria (hives), including chronic idiopathic urticaria (CIU).

Dose
- adults and children over 12 years: 20 mg orally once daily

Adverse effects
- abdominal pain, diarrhoea, fatigue, nasopharyngitis, dizziness, headache, somnolence, pharyngolaryngeal pain

Interactions

- food reduces bioavailability: high-fat and standard low-fat meals reduce the oral bioavailability of bilastine by 30% and 25%, respectively. It is recommended to take bilastine 1 hour before or 2 hours after food
- grapefruit juice decreases bilastine bioavailability by 30% because of inhibition of the OATP1A2 transporter, which bilastine is a substrate for
- co-administration with P-glycoprotein inhibitors such as cyclosporin or diltiazem may increase bilastine plasma concentrations, leading to a higher risk of adverse effects like dizziness, headache and nausea
- co-administration with ketoconazole or erythromycin can double bilastine levels, but this doesn't significantly affect its safety

Nursing considerations/Cautions

- administer bilastine at least 1 hour before or 2 hours after food to avoid reducing its bioavailability

Patient education

- take bilastine at least 1 hour before or 2 hours after food to avoid reducing its bioavailability
- avoid grapefruit juice, as it can reduce bilastine's effectiveness by decreasing absorption
- may cause drowsiness in some people; the patient should be advised to avoid driving or operating machinery if they feel sleepy

Avoid use, as there are limited data on the use of bilastine in pregnant women. Animal studies in rabbits have shown skeletal variations at high, maternotoxic doses.

Avoid use, as no human data. Animal studies indicate that bilastine is excreted in milk at levels approximately half of those in maternal plasma. The relevance of these findings for humans is unknown.

CETIRIZINE

Trade names
Alzene, Pharmacy Action Cetrelief, Zyrtec

Available forms
Tablets: 10 mg;
Oral solution: 1 mg/mL;
Oral drops: 10 mg/mL (2.5 mg/5 drops)

Action
- non-sedation antihistamine
- half-life 8 hours
- see also General Actions of antihistamines (p. 484)

Use
- seasonal or perennial allergic rhinitis
- chronic idiopathic urticaria

Dose
- (Adults, children > 12 years) initially 10 mg orally daily, increasing to 20 mg if necessary

Adverse effects
- (Rare) severe skin reactions
- see also General Adverse effects of antihistamines (p. 484)

Interactions
- see General Interactions of antihistamines (p. 485)

Nursing considerations/Cautions

- (Oral drops) not recommended in children < 1 year
- (Oral solution) not recommended in children < 2 years, as sorbitol may cause diarrhoea
- (Tablets) not recommended in children < 6 years
- (Zyrtec) tablets are not recommended in those with galactose intolerance, Lapp lactase deficiency or glucose–galactose malabsorption
- (Oral solution) not recommended in those with fructose intolerance
- contraindicated in those with hypersensitivity to hydroxyzine or piperazine derivatives, or severe kidney impairment (creatinine clearance < 10 mL/min)
- see also General Nursing considerations/Cautions for antihistamines (p. 485)

ANTIHISTAMINES

Patient education
- the patient should be advised to seek medical advice immediately if any pustules with fever occur within the first 2 days of treatment (especially in skin folds, trunk or upper extremity)
- see also General Patient education for antihistamines (p. 485)

Available as oral solution. Tablet can be crushed and mixed with water or a spoonful of yoghurt or apple puree.

Generally considered safe, although there are limited human studies. There is more experience with older sedating antihistamines.

Generally considered safe.

Contraindicated in those with severe liver impairment (CrCl < 10 mL/min).

CYPROHEPTADINE

Trade name
Periactin

Available form
Tablets: 4 mg

Action
- serotonin and histamine antagonist with anticholinergic and sedative actions

Use
- acute and chronic allergies, pruritus
- anaphylactic reaction (with adrenaline (epinephrine) after acute manifestations have subsided)
- prophylaxis and treatment of migraine and vascular headache
- sometimes used in the treatment of serotonin syndrome because of its antagonist activity at serotonin receptors

Dose
- (Allergy, pruritus) initially 4 mg orally 3 times daily, then dose adjusted according to response (not exceeding 32 mg daily) **OR**
- (Prophylaxis and treatment of migraine/headache) initially 4 mg orally, repeated in 30 minutes if necessary, then 4 mg every 4–6 hours if needed (not exceeding 8 mg in any 4–6-hour period)

Adverse effects
- see General Adverse effects of antihistamines (p. 484)

Interactions
- contraindicated with monoamine oxidase inhibitors (MAOIs) because anticholinergic effects may be prolonged and intensified
- may interfere with selective serotonin reuptake inhibitors (SSRIs)
- may cause false positive on urine drug screen for tricyclic antidepressants (TCAs)
- see also General Interactions of antihistamines (p. 485)

Nursing considerations/Cautions
- caution if used in those with hyperthyroidism, cardiovascular disease, hypertension, a history of asthma or raised intraocular pressure because of atropine-like actions
- contraindicated in those with acute asthma attack or lower respiratory tract symptoms
- see also General Nursing considerations/Cautions for antihistamines (p. 485)

Patient education
- see General Patient education for antihistamines (p. 485)

Tablet can be dispersed in 10–20 mL of water and settles quickly, so should be mixed well before use. Tablet can be crushed and mixed with a spoonful of yoghurt or apple puree.

Generally considered safe in pregnancy when clearly needed, as no proven harmful effects have been observed in humans.

It is not known whether cyproheptadine is excreted in human milk but, due to the risk of serious side-effects in nursing infants, its use is contraindicated during breastfeeding.

DESLORATADINE

Trade names
Aerius, Children's ClaratyneDES, Desonex

Available forms
Tablets: 5 mg;
Syrup: 0.5 mg/mL

Action
- long-acting, non-sedating antihistamine
- peak effect 3 hours
- half-life 27 hours
- see also General Actions of antihistamines (p. 484)

Use
- seasonal or perennial allergic rhinitis

Dose
- 5 mg orally daily

Adverse effects/Interactions
- see General Adverse effects/Interactions for antihistamines (p. 484)

Nursing considerations/Cautions
- tablets are not recommended for those under 12 years
- contraindicated in those with hypersensitivity to loratadine
- see also General Nursing considerations/Cautions for antihistamines (p. 485)

Patient education
- see General Patient education for antihistamines (p. 485)

Available as liquid. Tablet can be crushed and mixed with a spoonful of yoghurt or apple puree.

Generally considered safe, although there are limited human studies. There is more experience with older sedating antihistamines.

Generally considered safe. Can be used when the benefit outweighs the risk, as only small amounts pass into breastmilk, and the likelihood of harm to the infant is low.

DEXCHLORPHE NIRAMINE

Trade name
Polaramine

Available forms
Tablets: 2 mg;
Oral suspension: 2 mg/5 mL

Action
- sedating antihistamine with no antiemetic actions
- onset of action 30—60 minutes, peak effect hours, duration of action 4—8 hours
- see also General Actions of antihistamines (p. 484)

Use
- seasonal allergic rhinitis, vasomotor rhinitis, allergic conjunctivitis, mild skin manifestations of urticaria and angioedema
- relief of itch associated with allergic eczema, pruritus ani/vulvae and atopic/contact dermatitis, insect bites and drug reactions

Dose
- 2 mg orally 6-hourly (tablet or syrup)

Adverse effects
- (Children) paradoxical excitation
- photosensitivity
- see also General Adverse effects of antihistamines (p. 484)

Interactions
- contraindicated with monoamine oxidase inhibitors (MAOIs) because anticholinergic effects may be prolonged and intensified
- may decrease effects of anticoagulants
- see also General Interactions of antihistamines (p. 485)

Nursing considerations/Cautions
- (Tablets) not recommended in children < 12 years
- oral suspension contains sorbitol which may cause diarrhoea
- see also General Nursing considerations/Cautions for antihistamines (p. 485)

ANTIHISTAMINES

Patient education
- instruct patient to wear sun protection (sunscreen (SPF 30+ or greater), hat, protective clothing) when outdoors
- see also General Patient education for antihistamines (p. 485)

Suspension is available. Tablets can be crushed and mixed with a spoonful of yoghurt or apple puree.

Safe for use in early pregnancy but avoid in the third trimester because of risks to newborns.

Use with caution; drug passes into breastmilk and may cause sedation in infants.

DIPHENHYDRAMINE
Trade names
Snuzaid Tabs, Unisom Sleepgels

Available forms
Capsules: 50 mg;
Tablets: 50 mg

Action
- crosses the blood—brain barrier causing sedation
- peak effect 1—4 hours, half-life 2.4—9.3 hours
- see also General Actions of antihistamines (p. 484)

Use
- insomnia (short-term management)

Dose
- (Insomnia) 50 mg orally at night, 20—30 minutes before retiring (capsules, tablets)

Adverse effects
- see General Adverse effects of antihistamines (p. 484)

Interactions
- contraindicated with monoamine oxidase inhibitors (MAOIs) and tricyclic antidepressants (TCAs) or with other products containing diphenhydramine hydrochloride (see 'Available in combination with' below)
- see also General Interactions of antihistamines (p. 485)

Nursing considerations/Cautions
- not recommended in children < 12 years
- see also General Nursing considerations/Cautions for antihistamines (p. 485)

Patient education
- the patient should be advised to seek medical advice if insomnia lasts for > 10 days
- see also General Patient education for antihistamines (p. 485)

Tablets can be crushed and mixed with water or a spoonful of yoghurt or apple puree.

Safe: used by a large number of pregnant women without any proven increase in malformations or other harmful effects on the fetus.

Limited human data. Avoid use, as excreted into breastmilk; there is a risk of sedation in the nursing infant.

Available in combination with
- Diphenhydramine 12.5 mg + Phenylephrine 5 mg oral liquid (Paedamin Decongestant and Antihistamine)
- Diphenhydramine 14 mg + Ammonium Chloride 135 mg oral liquid (Benadryl Original)
- Diphenhydramine 14 mg + Ammonium Chloride 135 mg oral liquid (Codral Dry Cough & Cold with Antihistamine)
- Diphenhydramine 14 mg + Ammonium Chloride 135 mg + Sodium Citrate + Menthol oral liquid (Chemists' Own Difenacol)
- Diphenhydramine 25 mg + Paracetamol 500 mg tablet, (Chemists' Own Night Pain Relief)

- Diphenhydramine 25 mg + Paracetamol 500 mg tablet (Apohealth Night Pain Relief)
- Diphenhydramine 25 mg + Paracetamol 500 mg tablet (MersynoNight Night Time Pain Relief)
- Diphenhydramine 25 mg + Paracetamol 500 mg tablet (Panadol Night)

DOXYLAMINE SUCCINATE

Trade names
Dozile, APOhealth Sleep Assist, Restavit

Available form
Tablets: 25 mg

Action
- sedating antihistamine with anticholinergic actions
- peak activity 2—3 hours, half-life 10 hours
- see also General Actions of antihistamines (p. 484)

Use
- temporary insomnia

Dose
- (Insomnia) 25—50 mg orally, 20—30 minutes before bed

Adverse effects
- (High dose) nervousness, tremor, insomnia, agitation, irritability
- see also General Adverse effects of antihistamines (p. 484)

Interactions
- contraindicated with monoamine oxidase inhibitors (MAOIs) and tricyclic antidepressants (TCAs) because of prolonged and intensified anticholinergic and CNS effects
- see also General Interactions of antihistamines (p. 485)

Nursing considerations/Cautions
- not recommended in children < 12 years
- see also General Nursing considerations/Cautions for antihistamines (p. 485)

Patient education
- patient should be advised to seek medical advice if insomnia lasts for >10 days
- see also General Patient education for antihistamines (p. 485)

Tablet can be crushed and mixed with water or a spoonful of yoghurt or apple puree.

Safe: taken by a large number of pregnant women without any proven increase in malformations or other harmful effects on the fetus.

Avoid use, as may be excreted into breastmilk in small amounts and may cause unusual excitement or irritability in infants. It may have anticholinergic effects that could inhibit lactation.

Available in combination with
- Doxylamine 5 mg + Paracetamol 500 mg + Codeine 10 mg tablet (Dolased)
- Doxylamine 5 mg + Paracetamol 500 mg + Codeine 30 mg tablet (Dolased Forte)
- Doxylamine 5 mg + Paracetamol 500 mg + Codeine 9.6 mg tablet (Maxydol)
- Doxylamine 5 mg + Paracetamol 450 mg + Codeine 9.75 mg tablet (Mersyndol)
- Doxylamine 5 mg + Paracetamol 450 mg + Codeine 9.75 mg tablet (Mersyndol Caplet)
- Doxylamine 5 mg + Paracetamol 500 mg + Codeine 30 mg + tablet (Mersyndol Forte)
- Doxylamine 5 mg + Paracetamol 500 mg + Codeine 30 mg tablet (Mevadol Forte)
- Doxylamine 5 mg + Paracetamol 500 mg + Codeine 9.6 mg tablet (Trust Analgesic Calmative)
- Doxylamine 6.25 mg + Paracetamol 500 mg + Dextromethorphan 10 mg

ANTIHISTAMINES

- soft capsule (Dimetapp Cough Cold & Flu Daytime/Nightime)
- Doxylamine 6.25 mg + Paracetamol 500 mg + Pseudoephedrine 30 mg + Dextromethorphan 10 mg soft capsule (Dimetapp PSE Cough Cold & Flu Day & Night)
- Doxylamine 6.25 mg + Paracetamol 500 mg + Pseudoephedrine 30 mg + Dextromethorphan 10 mg mg soft capsule (Dimetapp PSE Cough Cold & Flu Night Relief)

FEXOFENADINE
Trade names
Fexo, Pharmacy Action Fexorelief, Fexotabs, Telfast, Trust Fexit, Xergic

Available forms
Tablets: 60 mg, 120 mg, 180 mg;
Oral suspension: 6 mg/mL

Action
- non-sedating antihistamine with no anticholinergic actions
- half-life 14–15 hours
- see also General Actions of antihistamines (p. 484)

Use
- seasonal allergic rhinitis, urticaria

Dose
- (Allergic rhinitis) 60 mg orally twice daily **OR**
- (Seasonal allergic rhinitis) 120–180 mg orally daily **OR**
- (Urticaria) 180 mg orally daily

Adverse effects
- see General Adverse effects of antihistamines (p. 484)

Interactions
- serum levels may be increased by erythromycin
- bioavailability reduced by magnesium- or aluminium-containing antacids
- see also General Interactions of antihistamines (p. 485)

Nursing considerations/Cautions
- (Oral suspension) children > 6 months
- (Oral suspension) contains hydroxybenzoates, which may cause hypersensitivity reaction in sensitive individuals
- see also General Nursing considerations/Cautions for antihistamines (p. 485)

Patient education
- advise the patient that magnesium- or aluminium-containing antacids should be taken 2 hours before or after fexofenadine
- see also General Patient education for antihistamines (p. 485)

 Available as oral suspension. Tablets can be dispersed in 10–20 mL of water (Telfast). Tablets can be crushed and mixed with a spoonful of yoghurt or apple puree.

 Generally considered safe, although there are limited human studies. There is more experience with older sedating antihistamines.

 Can be used when the benefit outweighs the risk, as only small amounts pass into breastmilk, and the likelihood of harm to the infant is low.

Available in combination with
- fexofenadine 60 mg + 120 mg of pseudoephedrine (Telfast Decongestant)

LEVOCABASTINE
Trade names
Livostin Eye Drops, Livostin Nasal Spray, Zyrtec Eye Drops, Zyrtec Nasal Spray

Available forms
Eye drops: 0.5 mg/mL;
Nasal spray: 0.5 mg/mL

Action
- (Eye drops) immediate action, duration of action several hours
- half-life 33 hours
- see also General Actions of antihistamines (p. 484)

Use
- (Eye drops) allergic conjunctivitis
- (Nasal spray) seasonal or perennial allergic rhinitis

Dose
- (Eye drops) 1 drop to each eye twice daily, may be increased to 3–4 times daily if needed (for up to 8 weeks) **OR**
- (Nasal spray) 2 sprays to each nostril twice daily, increasing to 3–4 times if needed (up to 8 weeks)

Adverse effects
- headache, somnolence, fatigue, dizziness
- (Eye drops) eye irritation
- (Nasal spray) epistaxis, nasal irritation, sinusitis, nausea, pharyngolaryngeal pain, epistaxis, cough

Interactions
- oxymetazoline may transiently decrease absorption of nasal spray

Nursing considerations/Cautions
- (Eye drops) contains benzalkonium chloride (preservative), which can cause irritation and discolouration of soft contact lenses
- use should be limited to 8 weeks
- (Nasal spray) caution if used in those with kidney impairment, especially if therapy is prolonged
- see also General Nursing considerations/Cautions for antihistamines (p. 485)

Patient education
- patient should be advised not to drive or operate machinery if fatigue or somnolence occurs
- see also General Patient education for antihistamines (including instillation instructions for nasal spray and eye drops) (p. 485)

No human data. Animal studies have shown evidence of fetal harm at high doses, including embryolethality and teratogenic effects. Use only if the potential benefit outweighs the risk to the fetus.

May pass into breastmilk. Avoid use during breastfeeding unless necessary.

(Kidney) increased drug exposure in moderate-to-severe kidney impairment. Dose reduction should be considered, particularly with prolonged use of the nasal spray.

LORATADINE
Trade names
Allereze, Children's Claratyne Chewable Tablets, Children's Claratyne Syrup, Claratyne, Claratyne Reditabs, Lorano, Lorapaed

Available forms
Tablets: 10 mg;
Tablets (effervescent/disintegrating): 10 mg;
Tablets (chewable): 5 mg;
Oral suspension/syrup: 1 mg/mL

Action
- long-acting, non-sedating antihistamine
- active metabolite (desloratadine) (half-life 20 hours)
- rapid onset 1 hour, half-life 12 hours
- see also General Actions of antihistamines (p. 484)

Use
- seasonal and perennial allergic rhinitis
- chronic urticaria

Dose
- (Adults and children > 30 kg) 10 mg orally once daily.
- (Children 2–12 years, < 30 kg) 5 mg orally once daily.
- (Severe hepatic impairment) administer the standard dose on alternate days.

ANTIHISTAMINES

Adverse effects/Interactions
- see General Adverse effects/Interactions of antihistamines (p. 484)

Nursing considerations/Cautions
- (Syrup, grape flavoured) contains sorbitol and maltitol, which may cause diarrhoea
- (Chewable tablets) contain phenylalanine and are not recommended in those with phenylketonuria
- contraindicated in those with hypersensitivity to desloratadine or sodium benzoate (oral suspension)
- see also General Nursing considerations/Cautions for antihistamines (p. 485)

Patient education
- advise the patient that effervescent tablets should be dissolved in a glass of water
- instruct the patient (or parent/carer) that chewable tablets for children should be chewed before swallowing
- see also General Patient education for antihistamines (p. 485)

Available as oral liquid, chewable and effervescent tablets.

Generally considered safe, although there are limited human studies. There is more experience with older sedating antihistamines.

Generally considered safe.

Severe hepatic impairment: administer the standard dose on alternate days.

Available in combination with
- loratadine 5 mg + 120 mg pseudoephedrine (should not be crushed) (Claratyne D with Decongestant Repetabs)

OLOPATADINE
Trade names
Paladopt, Patanol

Available form
Eye drops: 1 mg/mL (0.1%)

Action
- antihistamine
- inhibits pro-inflammatory mediator release from conjunctival mast and epithelial cells
- half-life 8—12 hours

Use
- seasonal allergic conjunctivitis

Dose
- 1—2 drops into affected eye(s) twice daily for up to 14 weeks

Adverse effects
- headache, asthenia
- blurred vision
- burning, stinging, dry eye(s), foreign body sensation, lid oedema, hyperaemia
- pharyngitis, rhinitis, sinusitis
- pruritus
- altered taste, nausea
- hypersensitivity

Nursing considerations/Cautions
- not for injection or oral ingestion
- contains benzalkonium chloride (preservative), which can cause irritation and discolouration of soft contact lenses
- see also General Nursing considerations/Cautions for antihistamines (p. 485)

Patient education
- advise patient that blurred vision may occur just after instillation of eye drops and should wait until this has resolved before driving or operating heavy machinery
- see General Patient education for antihistamines (including instillation instructions for eye drops) (p. 485)

Safe to use.

 Safe to use.

Available in combination with
- Olopatadine 665 micrograms + Mometasone 25 micrograms nasal spray (Ryaltris)

PROMETHAZINE
Trade names
Allersoothe, Apohealth Promethazine Allergy Relief, Chemists' Own Antihistamine for Allergy Relief, DBL Promethazine Hydrochloride Injection, Fenezine, Phenergan, Wagner Health Promethazine

Available forms
Tablets: 10 mg, 25 mg;
Ampoules: 50 mg/2 mL;
Oral suspension: 1 mg/mL

Action
- long-acting sedating phenothiazine derivative antihistamine with mild anticholinergic and antiserotonin actions
- other actions due to CNS effects include antiemetic, antivertigo, anti-motion sickness, hypnotic and tranquilliser
- antihistamine action lasts 4—12 hours, sedative effect 2—8 hours, half-life 5—14 hours
- onset of action 3—5 minutes (IV) or 20 minutes (IM)

Use
- motion sickness
- nausea and vomiting, or where avoiding vomiting is essential (e.g. after neuro- or eye surgery)
- allergic conditions (e.g. drug, insect bites and stings, urticaria, contact dermatitis)
- relief from excessive upper respiratory tract secretions (e.g. hay fever, allergic rhinitis)
- sedation (short-term management)
- pre-anaesthetic medication

Dose
- (Allergy) 10—20 mg orally 2—3 times daily **OR**
- (Allergy, sedation) 25—75 mg orally at night **OR**
- (Allergy) 25—50 mg deep IM or slow IV, may be repeated after 2 hours if needed (daily maximum 150 mg) **OR**
- (Motion sickness) 25 mg orally the night before travel and repeated 6—8 hours on following day if needed (for long journey) **OR**
- (Motion sickness) 25 mg orally 1—2 hours before short journey **OR**
- (Nausea and vomiting) 25 mg orally 4—6-hourly (daily maximum 100 mg) **OR**
- (Nausea and vomiting, not related to motion sickness) 12.5—25 mg deep IM or slow IV 4-hourly as needed **OR**
- (Preoperative or postoperative sedation, hypnotic) 25—50 mg deep IM or slow IV 1—2 hours before surgery (usually with pethidine and atropine) **OR**
- (Sedation, hypnotic) 25—50 mg deep IM or slow IV **OR**
- (Obstetric sedation, early labour) 50 mg deep IM **OR**
- (Obstetric sedation, established labour) 25—75 mg deep IM or slow IV (with reduced dose of opioid analgesic), may be repeated 1—2 times at 4-hourly intervals (daily maximum 100 mg)

Adverse effects
- marked irregular respiration
- jaundice
- photosensitisation
- angioneurotic oedema
- oculogyric crisis, seizures, extrapyramidal symptoms, tardive dyskinesia, hysteria, catatonic state
- (Rare) paralytic ileus (if given with anticholinergic agents)
- (Rare) neuroleptic malignant syndrome, cardiac arrhythmias, QT prolongation
- (IV site) venous thrombosis
- (Rapid IV) transient hypotension
- (High dose, IV) extrapyramidal reactions

ANTIHISTAMINES

- see also General Adverse effects of antihistamines (p. 484)

Interactions

- contraindicated after large doses of other CNS depressants, including alcohol
- QT prolongation is possible with phenothiazines; therefore not recommended with other agents known to prolong QT interval
- effects potentiated if given with anticholinergic agents, increasing the risk of adverse effects such as constipation, paralytic ileus and heat stroke
- may lower seizure threshold; therefore the antiepileptic dose may require adjustment during therapy
- if given with propranolol may result in increased plasma levels of both agents, resulting in increased hypotension, irreversible retinopathy, cardiac arrhythmias and tardive dyskinesia
- may increase serum prolactin levels, interfering with effects of bromocriptine
- may block the action of levodopa
- increased severity and frequency of extrapyramidal effects may occur if given with other phenothiazines
- may block the actions of adrenaline (epinephrine), resulting in severe hypotension and tachycardia and should not be used for phenothiazine overdose
- may decrease pressor response to adrenaline (epinephrine) and metaraminol
- may block the effects of centrally acting appetite suppressants and amphetamines
- increased risk of hypotension, extrapyramidal and anticholinergic effects if given with tricyclic antidepressants (TCAs)
- increased risk of hepatotoxicity if given with other hepatotoxic agents
- may increase hypotension caused by antihypertensive agents
- may mask tinnitus and dizziness caused by ototoxic agents such as aminoglycosides
- may enhance the CNS depressant effects of alcohol and other CNS depressing agents, such as barbiturates, hypnotics, sedatives, antipsychotics and opioid analgesics
- not recommended with monoamine oxidase inhibitors (MAOIs) or TCAs because anticholinergic and CNS depressant effects may be prolonged and intensified
- may interfere with pregnancy test and glucose tolerance test

Nursing considerations/Cautions

- (IV) a very long list of incompatibilities and should usually be administered alone
- preferably given by deep IM
- slow IV injection is recommended only if benefits outweigh risks (e.g. emergency situations, where IM route is contraindicated)
- large vessels should be used IV; wrist and hand veins are not recommended
- IV site should be carefully monitored for extravasation and/or any signs of burning, pain, phlebitis, swelling or blistering, as these may be early signs of tissue injury
- contraindicated SC or intra-arterially to avoid tissue damage and necrosis
- (IV) should be diluted 1 in 10 with water for injections or given into the tubing of a free-flowing infusion
- a transient fall in BP and increased risk of tissue damage may occur if given rapidly IV
- IV rate should not exceed 25 mg/min
- caution if used in those with eczema or rheumatoid conditions (increased risk of solar dermatitis) or epilepsy (may increase severity of convulsions)
- caution if used in children because of an increased risk of central and obstructive apnoea and decreased arousal. Excessive doses can cause hallucinations, convulsions and sudden death in children
- caution if used in those with acute or chronic respiratory impairment

HAVARD'S NURSING GUIDE TO DRUGS

- caution if used in those at risk of QT prolongation
- (25 mg tablets) not recommended for children 12 years and under
- not recommended in children or adolescents with signs of Reye's syndrome (see Glossary)
- not recommended in anyone experiencing hypertensive crisis
- (IV, IM) contains sodium metabisulfite, sodium sulfite or sodium benzoate and is therefore contraindicated in those with known hypersensitivity
- contraindicated in those with history of phenothiazine-induced jaundice or hypersensitivity to phenothiazines
- contraindicated in children under 2 years because of the risk of respiratory depression
- contraindicated in comatose patients
- see also General Nursing considerations/Cautions for antihistamines (p. 485)

Patient education

- instruct the patient that tablets should not be taken for more than 10 days. If symptoms persist, the patient should seek medical advice
- warn the patient that, if taken for sedation at bedtime, a 'hangover' effect can exist in the morning, increasing the risk of accidents and/or falls. The patient should be further advised not to drive or operate machinery while this exists
- the patient should be advised to immediately seek medical advice if any of the following occur:
  - any abdominal pain, cramping and/or distension with failure to pass wind or stools
  - high fever, sweating, muscle cramps or stiffness, dizziness, very bad headache, fast heart rate, confusion, agitation, hallucinations
  - irregular heart rate
  - yellowing of eyes or skin
  - fits
  - twitching or jerking movements
- instruct the patient to wear sun protection (sunscreen (SPF 30+ or greater), hat, protective clothing) when outdoors (especially if the patient has eczema or rheumatism, owing to the risk of solar dermatitis)
- see also General Patient education for antihistamines (p. 485)

 Available as suspension. Tablet can be dispersed in water, or crushed and mixed with a spoonful of yoghurt or apple puree.

 Avoid use, as high doses during late pregnancy can cause prolonged neurological disturbances in the newborn. Not recommended during pregnancy unless the potential benefits outweigh the risks.

 Avoid use, as excreted in breastmilk and can cause irritability or excitement in infants.

 Avoid use, as elderly patients are more likely to experience CNS depressive side effects, such as confusion and sedation. They are also more susceptible to anticholinergic effects (urinary retention, constipation and hypotension). Paradoxical excitation may occur in some elderly patients. Less sedating antihistamines are preferred.

Available in combination with

- Promethazine 5 mg + Paracetamol 250 mg + Codeine 5 mg oral liquid (Painstop Night-Time Pain Reliever)

ANTIHYPERTENSIVE AGENTS

Approximately 1 in 10 (11.6%) people in Australia have hypertension. There is a similar prevalence in males and in females (11.7% and 11.6% respectively). These numbers have remained relatively stable over the last 10 years. The proportion of the population with hypertension increases with age, especially over 35 years, with the highest proportion (42.9%) being those aged 75 years and over (ABS 2023).

Normal adult blood pressure (BP) is considered to be 120—129 mmHg systolic and 80—84 mmHg diastolic. Although definitions vary, one definition of mild hypertension is an elevation of systolic BP between 140 and 159 mmHg, diastolic BP above 90—99 mmHg, or both based on measurements taken on several separate occasions (Heart Foundation 2023). Lowering of elevated BP by even 1—2 mmHg reduces absolute cardiovascular disease risk (i.e. risk of having stroke or myocardial infarction). Modifiable risk factors include smoking status, BP, total cholesterol/HDL cholesterol ratio, waist circumference and body mass index (BMI), nutrition, physical activity level and alcohol intake (Heart Foundation 2023). Non-modifiable risk factors include age, sex, family history of premature cardiovascular disease and social history (e.g. cultural identity, ethnicity, socioeconomic status). Related conditions include diabetes, chronic kidney disease (with albuminuria), familial hypercholesterolaemia and/or evidence of atrial fibrillation.

Management of hypertension should begin with modification of lifestyle factors, such as weight and alcohol reduction, smoking cessation, increasing physical daily activity to 30 minutes if possible and limiting salt intake (Knights et al 2023). If lifestyle changes do not lower blood pressure to the target level, antihypertensive medicines should be considered.

Antihypertensive medication is usually recommended in individuals with persistently elevated BP $\geq$ 160/100 mmHg (at least two measurements of seated BP on separate occasions). Ambulatory blood pressure monitoring (ABPM) is a better predictor of outcomes than clinical BP measurement and should be used to monitor BP lowering therapy (Heart Foundation 2023). The decision of which antihypertensive agent to use is based on the patient's age, any comorbidities that may determine target BP (e.g. < 140/90 mmHg for adults with diabetes) and potential drug interactions. Implications for adherence and cost should also be considered (Heart Foundation 2023).

Suitable first-line drugs in the treatment of hypertension include:
- angiotensin converting enzyme (ACE) inhibitors (e.g. captopril)
- angiotensin II receptor antagonists (e.g. irbesartan)
- dihydropyridine calcium-channel blockers (e.g. amlodipine)
- thiazide and thiazide-like diuretics (e.g. indapamide) (may be used as first-line management > 65 years).

The first-line antihypertensive is selected with consideration of patient-specific factors, e.g. comorbidities and potential drug interactions.

Suitable second-line drugs in the treatment of hypertension include:
- beta adrenoceptor blocking agents (e.g. atenolol)
- centrally acting alpha2 agonist agents (e.g. clonidine)
- non-dihydropyridine calcium-channel blockers (e.g. diltiazem)
- potassium-sparing diuretics (e.g. spironolactone)
- direct-acting vasodilators (e.g. hydralazine).

Antihypertensive therapy usually begins with a single drug, starting with a small-to-moderate dose of a first-line drug. If the target is not achieved after 4 to 6 weeks, a second antihypertensive from a different class is usually added to the patient's regimen, rather than increasing the dose of the first agent. Individuals commonly require 2 or more drugs to reach the BP target. If after 3 months, the target is still not reached but the patient is tolerating both drugs, the dose of one agent is usually increased. It is important to assess also any non-adherence issues, possible hypertensive effects of other medications and any undisclosed alcohol or recreational drug use or high salt intake (Heart Foundation 2016).

Some manufacturers have produced 'fixed-dose combination' medications (e.g. ACE inhibitor plus dihydropyridine calcium-channel blocker; angiotensin II receptor antagonists plus a thiazide). These combination products decrease the number of tablets needed, potentially increasing patient adherence.

General Patient education for antihypertensive agents

- ensure the patient understands the risks and benefits of therapy and the risks of not treating hypertension (increased risk of stroke and myocardial infarction)
- postural hypotension can be avoided by moving gradually from a sitting to a standing position. Postural hypotension is made worse by prolonged standing, hot baths or showers, hot weather, physical exertion, large meals or alcohol ingestion. If you feel dizzy or faint, you are advised to sit or lie down
- if drowsiness or dizziness is a problem, do not drive or operate machinery
- avoid alcohol
- do not stop your antihypertensive/s suddenly, as rebound hypertension may occur
- consider lifestyle modification strategies (e.g. smoking cessation, weight loss, physical activity, healthy diet)
- adherence to antihypertensives is low. Studies show that many (50%)

ANTIHYPERTENSIVE AGENTS

patients stop taking antihypertensives after about 2 years, while 19% do not get a second prescription filled

 It should also be noted that those antihypertensive combinations with diuretics are generally banned in sport.

ALPHA ADRENOCEPTOR BLOCKING AGENTS

General Adverse effects of alpha adrenoceptor blocking agents
- 'first-dose' effect (see General Nursing considerations, below)
- postural hypotension, palpitations, tachycardia, syncope, oedema
- headache, drowsiness, dizziness, lightheadedness, asthenia, drowsiness, weakness, fatigue, nervousness, depression
- dyspnoea
- blurred vision, miosis
- nasal congestion
- abnormal ejaculation, impotence, increased frequency, incontinence
- dry mouth, nausea, vomiting, diarrhoea, constipation
- rash, pruritus
- intraoperative floppy iris syndrome (during cataract surgery)
- (Uncommon) angina
- (Rare) priapism

General Nursing considerations/Cautions for alpha adrenoceptor blocking agents
- 'first-dose' effect may occur with the first dose, an increase in dosage or if there is an interruption to the regimen. Symptoms including marked hypotension (especially in the upright position), dizziness and syncope usually occur within 30–90 minutes of the initial dose
- both supine and standing systolic and diastolic BP should be monitored (especially when starting therapy or when adjusting dose) in all patients, regardless of the indication for use
- caution if used in those with ischaemic heart disease, angina (because angina may be exacerbated), cerebral or coronary arteriosclerosis, marked renal impairment or where a fall in BP or tachycardia is not desirable (e.g. recovery period after acute myocardial infarction (AMI))
- not recommended in those with congestive heart failure caused by aortic or mitral valve stenosis, pulmonary embolism or restrictive pericardial disease
- contraindicated in those with any hypersensitivity to alpha adrenoceptor blocking agents

General Patient education for alpha adrenoceptor blocking agents
- advise patient to take the first dose (and any increase in dosage) before sleep, to reduce the 'first-dose' effect
- warn patient to avoid driving or operating machinery or other hazardous activities for 12 hours after initial dose, when the dose is increased or after an interruption to the therapy and the medication is resumed, or if dizziness, drowsiness, blurred vision or lightheadedness continues
- male patient should be instructed to seek medical advice immediately if prolonged (lasting > 4 hours) painful penile erection occurs
- see also General Patient education for antihypertensive agents (p. 500)

 Use during pregnancy or breastfeeding only if benefits outweigh potential risks.

PHENOXYBENZAMINE
Trade name
Dibenyline

Available form
Capsules: 10 mg

Action
- long-acting
- irreversible non-selective alpha1 and alpha2 adrenoceptor antagonists
- blocks uptake of amines, potentiating effects of noradrenaline (norepinephrine) and adrenaline (epinephrine) on beta adrenergic receptors
- non-competitive block of histamine, serotonin and muscarinic (acetylcholine) receptors
- increases blood flow to skin, mucosa and abdominal viscera, lowering both standing and supine BP
- blocks alpha receptors on distal urethral sphincter and smooth muscle of bladder neck, resulting in decreased bladder outflow resistance, improving urinary flow and reducing bladder urine volume
- does not block beta adrenoceptor receptors
- oral absorption variable

Use
- hypertension associated with pheochromocytoma
- urinary retention due to neuropathic bladder

Dose
- (Hypertension associated with pheochromocytoma) initially 10 mg orally twice daily, increasing gradually at 4-day intervals to 20—60 mg in 2 divided doses as required **OR**
- (Urinary retention) 10 mg orally twice daily

Adverse effects
- see General Adverse effects of alpha adrenoceptor blocking agents (p. 501)

Interactions
- may block noradrenaline (norepinephrine)-induced hyperthermia
- not recommended with sympathomimetic agents (e.g. adrenaline (epinephrine)), as exacerbated hypotension and reflex tachycardia will occur

Nursing considerations/Cautions/Patient education
- may require beta adrenoceptor blocking agents to control tachycardia and arrhythmias in pheochromocytoma, with the alpha adrenoceptor blocking agent started first
- (Pheochromocytoma) a 4-day interval should be allowed after each dose increase to observe patient response
- (Urinary retention) if therapy is not effective in 2—3 weeks it should be discontinued
- caution if used in those with respiratory infection as symptoms may be exacerbated
- contraindicated in those where a fall in BP is undesirable (e.g. cerebral vascular accident (CVA), recovery period after acute myocardial infarction (AMI))
- see also General Nursing considerations/Cautions/Patient education for alpha adrenoceptor blocking agents (p. 501) and General Nursing considerations/Cautions/Patient education for antihypertensive agents (p. 500)

 Contents can be dispersed in water, or mixed with spoonful of yoghurt or apple puree.

 Limited human data. Use only if clearly needed, weighing the potential benefits against possible risks.

 Avoid. Potential for serious adverse reactions in infants.

 Elderly patients may be more sensitive to the hypotensive effects of phenoxybenzamine. Start at a low dose and monitor carefully, particularly for postural hypotension.

 If opening capsule, mask and gloves should be worn (do not open capsules if pregnant).

ANTIHYPERTENSIVE AGENTS

PRAZOSIN
Trade name
Minipress

Available forms
Tablets: 1 mg, 2 mg, 5 mg

Action
- quinazoline derivative
- high affinity for alpha1A, alpha1B and alpha1D receptors, with little affinity for alpha2 receptors, resulting in peripheral vasodilation with no reflex tachycardia
- BP is lowered in both supine and standing positions with diastolic effect more pronounced
- no rebound hypertension when therapy is stopped
- blocks alpha receptors on distal urethral sphincter and smooth muscle of bladder neck, resulting in decreased bladder outflow resistance, improving urinary flow and reducing bladder urine volume
- increased plasma renin activity (in those with congestive cardiac failure)
- peak concentration in 1—3 hours, half-life 2.5—3.5 hours (6—8 hours in heart failure)

Use
- hypertension
- congestive heart failure (CCF) (refractory to cardiac glycosides and diuretic therapy)
- Raynaud's disease, Raynaud's phenomenon
- benign prostatic hyperplasia

Dose
- (Hypertension) initially 0.5 mg orally twice daily for 3 days, then increased to 1 mg 2—3 times daily for a further 3 days, then 2 mg 2—3 times daily, then up to 20 mg in divided doses if needed **OR**
- (Congestive heart failure) initially 0.5 mg orally daily, increasing to 4—20 mg daily in 2—3 divided doses **OR**
- (Raynaud's disease/phenomenon) initially 0.5 mg orally twice daily for 3—7 days, increasing to 1—2 mg twice daily if needed **OR**
- (Benign prostatic hyperplasia) 0.5 mg orally twice daily for 3—7 days, increasing to 2—4 mg twice daily if needed

Adverse effects
- see General Adverse effects of alpha adrenoceptor blocking agents (p. 501)

Interactions
- hypotension may be increased if given with beta adrenoceptor blocking agents, diuretics and calcium-channel blockers
- caution if used with phosphodiesterase-5 (PDE-5) inhibitors owing to increased risk of hypotension
- may cause false positive in screening test for pheochromocytoma

Nursing considerations/Cautions/Patient education
- (Hypertension) response should be seen within 14 days, although optimal response may require 6 weeks
- (Raynaud's disease) BP should be monitored during initial administration and dose titrated accordingly
- (Benign prostatic hypertrophy) prostatic carcinoma should be excluded before starting therapy
- if given with other antihypertensive agents, other agent dose should be reduced when starting prazosin
- diuretic may be added to therapy for hypertension to increase efficacy (usually started when patient is at 2 mg dose)
- caution if used in those with liver impairment as dose may need to be reduced
- caution if used in those with ischaemic heart disease as angina may be exacerbated
- contraindicated in those with any hypersensitivity to alpha adrenoceptor blocking agents or quinazolines
- see also General Nursing considerations/Cautions/Patient education for alpha adrenoceptor blocking agents (p. 501) and General Nursing considerations/Cautions for antihypertensive agents (p. 500)

Tablets can be dispersed in water or crushed and mixed with spoonful of yoghurt or apple puree.

 Dose adjustment may be required in those with kidney or liver impairment.

 Caution if used in the elderly (especially those with cerebrovascular disease) because of the risk of hypotension, exacerbation of pre-existing angina, new onset angina and myocardial infarction.

ANGIOTENSIN CONVERTING ENZYME (ACE) INHIBITORS

General Actions of ACE inhibitors
- prevent conversion of angiotensin I to angiotensin II (which is a powerful vasoconstrictor) by inhibiting ACE, resulting in reduced peripheral vascular resistance and therefore decreased BP
- decreases aldosterone production (from the adrenal cortex), thereby reducing sodium and water reabsorption, which also plays a role in BP reduction
- increase plasma renin levels by negative feedback
- inhibit degradation of bradykinin leading to accumulation of both bradykinin and substance P sensitising airways and producing cough
- most ACE inhibitors are prodrugs that are converted in the body to an active form after oral ingestion (except captopril and lisinopril)
- most ACE inhibitors (except captopril) have a long duration of action, allowing once-daily administration

General Adverse effects of ACE inhibitors
- hypotension, palpitations, tachycardia, chest pain
- dizziness, vertigo, fatigue, headache, weakness, asthenia
- abdominal pain, nausea, anorexia, diarrhoea, dry mouth, taste disturbances (including decreased taste or metallic taste)
- persistent, dry, non-productive cough (may require discontinuance of therapy), dyspnoea
- rash (with or without fever/arthralgia), pruritus and, uncommonly, photosensitivity
- elevated potassium levels, hyperkalaemia, hyponatraemia
- hypoglycaemia (in patients with diabetes)
- raised liver enzyme levels
- proteinuria, nephrotic syndrome
- neutropenia, agranulocytosis
- (Rare) angioedema (head and neck) with or without urticaria (may be delayed for weeks to months), intestinal angioedema
- (Rare) anaphylactoid reaction
- (Rare) cholestatic jaundice, hepatitis, renal impairment
- (Rare) loss of libido, impotence, insomnia, somnolence, syndrome of inappropriate antidiuretic hormone (SIADH)

General Interactions of ACE inhibitors
- contraindicated with or within 36 hours of sacubitril (nepilysin inhibitor) because of risk of angioedema
- significant hypotension may occur if given with other antihypertensive agents, diuretics, alpha-adrenoceptor blocking agents, tricyclic antidepressants (TCAs), antipsychotics and some anaesthetic agents
- antihypertensive effect may be decreased if given with sympathomimetic agents
- hyperkalaemia may occur when given potassium-sparing diuretics, potassium supplements or agents that increase potassium levels
- increased risk of hyperkalaemia if given with trimethoprim/sulfamethoxazole combination
- increased risk of hyperkalaemia and decreased hypotensive effect if given with NSAIDs and therefore not recommended together
- increased risk of renal impairment if given concurrently with combination of NSAIDs and thiazide diuretics

ANTIHYPERTENSIVE AGENTS

- may increase serum concentrations of lithium, increasing the risk of lithium toxicity; risk is further increased if there is also a concurrent diuretic. Lithium levels and renal function should be closely monitored if given together
- increased risk of 'first-dose hypotension' if given with loop diuretic (e.g. furosemide (frusemide)) in patient with hypovolaemia or hyponatraemia
- increased risk of hypokalaemia and renal impairment if given with loop diuretic
- may cause facial flushing, nausea, vomiting and hypotension if given with sodium aurothiomalate (gold)
- effects of alcohol may be potentiated
- bioavailability may be decreased if given with antacids; therefore should be given 2 hours apart
- increased risk of hypoglycaemia if given with insulin and oral hypoglycaemic agents
- may decrease absorption of tetracyclines
- increased risk of angioedema if given with mTOR inhibitors (e.g. temsirolimus, sirolimus, everolimus) or DPP-IV inhibitors (e.g. vildagliptin)

General Nursing considerations/ Cautions for ACE inhibitors

- before starting an ACE inhibitor, diuretic therapy should be stopped for at least 3 days to prevent 'first-dose hypotension'. If diuretic cannot be stopped, initial dose of ACE inhibitor should be as low as possible and patient carefully monitored for several hours after administration
- any volume or salt depletion should be corrected before starting therapy
- check for urinary protein before treatment, then monthly for the first 8 months and periodically thereafter in those with renal disease
- BP is recorded every 15 minutes for 1 hour after the initial dose and, if a hypotensive response occurs, the patient placed in a supine position
- medical supervision should be maintained for at least 1 hour after the initial dose
- transient hypotension may be minimised by giving the initial dose at night
- regular monitoring of serum potassium, sodium and urea is recommended (especially if taking diuretics concurrently)
- white blood count (WBC) count monitoring (with differential) is recommended before starting and regularly throughout therapy in those with diseases affecting bone marrow function, collagen diseases, pre-existing neutropenia or if taking medication that is associated with bone marrow depression
- persistent non-productive cough is common. If the cough becomes intolerable, switching to another class of antihypertensive is recommended
- angioedema may be fatal if associated with laryngeal oedema
- (Congestive heart failure) BP and renal function should be monitored before starting and regularly during therapy
- (Myocardial infarction) therapy can be started within 1–3 days of myocardial infarction and usually in combination with aspirin, beta adrenoceptor blocking agent and fibrinolytic (thrombolytic) agent
- anaphylactoid reaction may occur during exposure to the high-flux dialysis/ lipoprotein apheresis membrane
- should be withheld while patient is undergoing desensitisation to hymenoptera (ant, honey bee, wasp) venom
- should be stopped for 24 hours before surgery or anaesthesia to decrease the risk of excessive hypotension
- low-density lipoprotein (LDL) apheresis with dextran or haemodialysis using high-flux polyacrylonitrite (AN 69) membranes is not recommended during ACE therapy, as there is an increased risk of anaphylactoid reactions
- caution if used in those of African origin, as risk of angioedema is higher

- caution if used in those with liver impairment, as most ACE inhibitors are converted to active form in the liver
- caution if used in those with renal failure, aortic stenosis, hypertrophic cardiomyopathy, systemic lupus erythematosus (SLE), scleroderma, bone marrow depression, cerebrovascular or cardiac insufficiency
- contraindicated in those with known hypersensitivity to ACE inhibitors, hyperkalaemia, renal transplant or impairment, severe renal artery stenosis or history of hereditary/idiopathic angioedema or ACE inhibitor-induced angioedema

General Patient education for ACE inhibitors

- patients should be advised to avoid driving or operating machinery or other hazardous activity for 12 hours after initial dose, when the dose is increased or after an interruption to the therapy and the medication is resumed or if dizziness continues
- patient should be advised to seek medical advice immediately if any of the following occur:
  - rash, fever or sore throat (early signs of neutropenia)
  - rash, with or without urticaria (red patches and weals on skin)
  - persistent non-productive cough
  - swelling of the face, lips, tongue, throat, hands or feet (signs of facial angioedema)
  - unusual abdominal pain (with or without nausea or vomiting), especially if accompanied by facial angioedema (as described in previous point)
  - yellowing of eyes or skin, itching, upper abdominal pain, nausea, vomiting, tiredness, dark urine (signs of liver impairment)
- warn patient to avoid dehydration and excessive perspiration as it may lead to a greater fall in BP, increasing the risk of fainting; therefore patient should maintain hydration within prescribed limits (e.g. there may be a fluid restriction for those with cardiac failure). Excessive vomiting or diarrhoea may also cause dehydration and increase the risk of fainting
- instruct patient against taking over-the-counter NSAIDs as these interact with ACE inhibitors
- patient should be advised that loss of taste or metallic taste often occurs with ACE inhibitors and this usually lasts for 2–3 months
- warn patient that rash may occur in first 4 weeks of therapy and often resolves without need for any intervention. However, antihistamines may be used if pruritus (itchiness) exists as well as rash
- advise the patient that brief, mild light-headedness may be experienced after the first few days of therapy. If fainting occurs, this should be reported immediately to a doctor
- instruct the patient that a low-salt diet may be beneficial in reducing BP. However, potassium-containing salt substitutes are not recommended because of the increased risk of hyperkalaemia
- patients with diabetes mellitus should be advised to carefully monitor blood glucose levels during therapy (especially first month)
- women of childbearing potential should be counselled to avoid pregnancy during therapy by using adequate contraception, and if pregnancy occurs to immediately report to a doctor. Pregnancy should be excluded before starting therapy
- see also General Patient education for antihypertensive agents (p. 500)

CAPTOPRIL
Trade name
Zedace

Available forms
Tablets: 25 mg, 50 mg

ANTIHYPERTENSIVE AGENTS

Action
- onset of action 15—60 minutes, duration of effect 6—12 hours
- see also General Actions of ACE inhibitors (p. 504)

Use
- hypertension
- heart failure
- myocardial infarction
- diabetic nephropathy (studies have shown ACE inhibitors decrease the progression of renal impairment)

Dose
- (Hypertension) initially 12.5 mg orally daily 1 hour before meals, then increased to 25 mg twice daily. If satisfactory BP decrease has not occurred in 2—4 weeks then increase to 50 mg twice daily. If BP is still not satisfactory after a further 2 weeks, a thiazide diuretic may be added (daily maximum 50 mg) **OR**
- (Severe refractory hypertension or high-dose diuretics/low-salt diet or dialysis) initially 6.25—12.5 mg orally daily 1 hour before meals, then titrated to 25—50 mg twice daily **OR**
- (Severe hypertension) up to 75 mg twice daily 1 hour before meals **OR**
- (Heart failure) initially 6.25 mg (2.5 mg in sodium-depleted patients or with high doses of diuretics) orally 3 times daily 1 hour before meals, increasing gradually at 2-week intervals to 25—75 mg twice daily (maximum daily dose 150 mg) **OR**
- (Myocardial infarction) initially 6.25 mg orally daily 1 hour before meals, increasing to 25 mg 3 times daily during next 2—3 days, then increasing gradually over several weeks to 50 mg orally 3 times daily **OR**
- (Diabetic nephropathy) 75—100 mg orally daily in 3 divided doses 1 hour before meals

Adverse effects
- see General Adverse effects of ACE inhibitors (p. 504)

Interactions
- glyceryl trinitrate and other nitrates should be discontinued when starting captopril and, if recommenced, should be started at a lower dose
- may cause false positive on acetone urine test
- see also General Interactions of ACE inhibitors (p. 504)

Nursing considerations/Cautions
- may cause neutropenia, especially in patients with renal impairment, collagen vascular disease, or those on immuno-suppressant therapy. Routine white blood cell monitoring is recommended for these patients.
- (Hypertension) if possible, any other antihypertensive agent should be stopped before starting therapy
- if the patient is receiving diuretics or has renal damage, the first dose may cause a precipitous fall in BP, so give a test dose of 6.25 mg
- if patient has renal disease or daily dose > 150 mg, urine protein estimation (using first morning urine sample) is recommended before starting and regularly during therapy
- (Myocardial infarction) usually started 3 days post infarction for best effect
- (Diabetic neuropathy) if patient has microalbuminuria, BP and blood glucose levels should be optimised to prevent progression to proteinuria
- see also General Nursing considerations/Cautions for ACE inhibitors (p. 505)

Patient education
- advise patient that tablets should be taken 1 hour before meals for best effect

HAVARD'S NURSING GUIDE TO DRUGS

- see also General Patient education for ACE inhibitors (p. 6)

Tablet can be dispersed in water, or crushed and mixed with spoonful of yoghurt or apple puree.

Contraindicated. Risks of fetal injury and neonatal complications, including hypotension, skull hypoplasia and irreversible renal damage.

Avoid use. Excreted in breastmilk in low concentrations.

ENALAPRIL

Trade names
Acetec, APO-Enalapril, Enalapril-WGR, Enalapril Sandoz, Malean, Renitec

Available forms
Tablets: 5 mg, 10 mg, 20 mg

Action
- enalapril (prodrug) is converted to active metabolite enalaprilat
- onset of action 60 minutes, duration of effect 24 hours
- see also General Actions of ACE inhibitors (p. 504)

Use
- hypertension
- heart failure with reduced ejection fraction
- asymptomatic left ventricular dysfunction
- diabetic nephropathy
- post myocardial infarction

Dose
- (Essential hypertension) initially 5 mg orally daily, increasing gradually to 10–40 mg orally daily as a single or 2 divided doses **OR**
- (Congestive heart failure) initially 2.5 mg orally daily, increasing gradually at 2–4-week intervals to 10–20 mg as a single or 2 divided doses **OR**
- (Left ventricular dysfunction without heart failure) initially 2.5 mg orally twice daily, then increasing gradually at 2–4-week intervals to 10 mg twice daily

- if the patient has renal failure or if is receiving a diuretic, the initial dose is 2.5 mg as a single dose once daily dose

Adverse effects/Interactions/Nursing considerations/Cautions/Patient education
- see General Adverse effects/Interactions/Nursing considerations/Cautions/Patient education for ACE inhibitors (p. 504)

Tablet can be crushed and mixed with water, or a spoonful of yoghurt or apple puree.

Contraindicated. Risk of fetal toxicity, including renal failure, hypotension and death.

Avoid use. No human data. Present in the milk of lactating rats.

Reduced renal function: Monitor renal function during therapy. Dosage adjustment is necessary in patients with renal impairment.

Elderly patients may be more sensitive to hypotensive effects. Start at 2.5 mg, adjusting based on response. Monitor blood pressure and renal function closely, especially during the first weeks or after dose changes, because of a higher risk of renal impairment or volume depletion.

Available in combination with
- enalapril 20 mg + hydrochlorothiazide 6 mg tablets (Enalapril/HCT Sandoz, Renitec Plus 20/6)(these are banned in sport)
- lercanidipine 10 mg + enalapril 10 mg tablets (Zan-Extra 10/10)
- lercanidipine 10 mg + enalapril 20 mg tablets (Zan-Extra 10/20)

FOSINOPRIL

Trade name
Monopril

Available form
Tablets: 10 mg

ANTIHYPERTENSIVE AGENTS

Action
- fosinopril (prodrug) is converted to active fosinopril diacid
- onset of action less than 60 minutes, duration of action 24 hours
- see also General Actions of ACE inhibitors (p. 504)

Use
- hypertension
- heart failure with reduced ejection fraction
- post myocardial infarction
- diabetic kidney disease

Dose
- (Hypertension, heart failure) initially 10 mg orally daily, increasing gradually to 40 mg daily

Interactions
- decreased absorption may occur if given with antacids; therefore should be separated by 2 hours
- may cause false low serum digoxin levels if charcoal absorption method is used for estimation
- should be discontinued for 2 days before parathyroid function test
- see also General Interactions of ACE inhibitors (p. 504)

Adverse effects/Nursing considerations/Cautions/Patient education
- see General Adverse effects/Nursing considerations/Cautions/Patient education for ACE inhibitors (p. 504)

Tablet can be crushed and mixed with water, or mixed with spoonful of yoghurt or apple puree.

Contraindicated owing to their association with fetal death in utero.

Avoid use.

Reduced renal function: close monitoring is recommended, CrCl < 10 mL/min and initial dose should be reduced to 5 mg.

Tablet should not be crushed or dispersed by pregnant staff.

Available in combination with
- fosinopril 20 mg + hydrochlorothiazide 12.5 mg tablets (Fosetic)

LISINOPRIL
Trade names
APO-Lisinopril, Fibsol, Lisinopril Sandoz, Lisinopril-WGR, Zestril, Zinopril

Available forms
Tablets: 5 mg, 10 mg, 20 mg

Action
- onset of action 60 minutes, duration of action 24 hours
- see also General Actions of ACE inhibitors (p. 504)

Use
- hypertension
- heart failure with reduced ejection fraction
- post myocardial infarction
- diabetic kidney disease

Dose
- (Hypertension) initially 5–10 mg orally daily (2.5 mg for diuretic-treated or salt/volume-depleted patients), increasing gradually at 2–4-week intervals to 10–20 g daily (maximum daily dose 40 mg) **OR**
- (Heart failure) initially 2.5 mg orally daily, increasing gradually at increments ≤ 10 mg at 2-week intervals to 5–20 mg daily **OR**
- (Acute myocardial infarction (AMI), within 24 hours of onset of symptoms) initially 5 mg (2.5 mg if systolic BP is less than 120 mmHg or if within 72 hours of AMI) orally daily, 5 mg 24 hours later, 10 mg after 48 hours, then 10 mg orally daily for 6 weeks

Adverse effects/Interactions/Nursing considerations/Cautions/Patient education
- may be started within 24 hours of symptoms of acute myocardial infarction; however, should not be started until patient is haemodynamically stable. If systolic BP < 90 mmHg for more

than 60 minutes, therapy should be stopped, or if systolic BP ≤ 100 mmHg a maintenance dose of 5 mg is recommended
- if patient with AMI develops heart failure, therapy should be continued beyond 6 weeks
- see also General Adverse effects/Interactions/Nursing considerations/Cautions/Patient education for ACE inhibitors (p. 504)

Tablet can be crushed and mixed with water, or mixed with spoonful of yoghurt or apple puree.

Contraindicated. Transition women to an alternative antihypertensive as soon as possible during the first trimester. Use during the second and third trimesters is associated with fetal renal dysfunction, oligohydramnios and fetal death in utero.

Avoid.

Reduced renal function: patients with CrCl < 30 mL/min may require a lower starting dose and cautious dose titration.

PERINDOPRIL ARGININE
Trade names
APO-Perindopril Arginine, APX-Perindopril Arginine, Coversyl, Perindopril Arginine Sandoz, Perindopril Arginine-WGR, Prexum

Available forms
Tablets: 2.5 mg, 5 mg, 10 mg

PERINDOPRIL ERBUMINE
Trade names
APO-Perindopril Arginine, Idaprex, Indosyl Mono, Oxapace, Perindo, Perindopril-WGR, Perisyl

Available forms
Tablets: 2 mg, 4 mg, 8 mg

Action
- perindopril (prodrug) is converted to active perindoprilat
- less 'first-dose' hypotension when compared with enalapril or captopril in those with congestive cardiac failure
- onset of action 3—6 hours, duration of action 24 hours
- see also General Actions of ACE inhibitors (p. 504)

Use
- hypertension
- heart failure with reduced ejection fraction
- post myocardial infarction
- diabetic kidney disease

Dose
- (Hypertension) initially 4—5 mg orally daily (2—2.5 mg for renovascular hypertension or salt/volume-depleted patients) 1 hour before meals, increasing gradually to daily maximum of 8—10 mg **OR**
- (Heart failure) initially 2—2.5 mg orally daily 1 hour before meals, increasing gradually to 4—5 mg daily **OR**
- (Reduction of risk of cardiovascular event) initially 4—5 mg orally daily 1 hour before meals for 14 days, then increasing to 8—10 mg daily (depending on tolerance and/or renal function)

Adverse effects
- see General Adverse effects of ACE inhibitors (p. 504)

Interactions
- see General Interactions of ACE inhibitors (p. 504)

Nursing considerations/Cautions
- if patient has episode of angina during first 4 weeks of therapy, risk analysis should be conducted to determine benefits of continuing therapy
- see also General Nursing considerations/Cautions for ACE inhibitors (p. 505)

Patient education
- advise patient to take tablets 1 hour before food

ANTIHYPERTENSIVE AGENTS

- see also General Patient education for ACE inhibitors (p. 506)

Tablet can be crushed and mixed with water, or mixed with a spoonful of yoghurt or apple puree.

Use of ACE inhibitors during pregnancy is contraindicated owing to their association with fetal death in utero.

Available in combination with
- perindopril erbumine 4 mg + indapamide 1.25 mg tablet (APO-Perindopril/Indapamide 4/1.35, Perindopril Indapamide-WGR 4/1.25, Perisyl Combi 4/1.25)
- perindopril arginine 10 mg + amlodipine 10 mg tablets (APX-Perindopril Arginine/Amlodipine 10 mg/10 mg, Coveram 10 mg/ 10 mg, Perindopril Arginine/Amlodipine-WGR 10 mg/10 mg, Reaptan 10 mg/10 mg)
- perindopril arginine 10 mg + amlodipine 5 mg tablets (APX-Perindopril Arginine/Amlodipine 10 mg/5 mg, Coveram 10 mg/ 5 mg, Perindopril Arginine/Amlodipine-WGR 10 mg/5 mg, Reaptan 10 mg/5 mg)
- perindopril arginine 5 mg + amlodipine 10 mg tablets (APX-Perindopril Arginine/Amlodipine 5 mg/10 mg, Coveram 5 mg/10 mg, Perindopril Arginine/Amlodipine-WGR 5 mg/10 mg, Reaptan 5 mg/10 mg)
- perindopril arginine 5 mg + amlodipine 5 mg tablets (APX-Perindopril Arginine/Amlodipine 5 mg/5 mg, Coveram 5 mg/5 mg, Perindopril Arginine/Amlodipine-WGR 5 mg/5 mg, Reaptan 5 mg/5 mg)
- perinodpril arginine 5 mg + indapamide 1.25 mg tablets (Coversyl Plus 5/1.25, Prexum Combi 5 mg/1.25 mg)
- perinodpril arginine 2.5 mg + indapamide 0.625 mg tablets (Coversyl Plus 2.5/0.625, Prexum Combi LD 2.5 mg/0.625 mg)

RAMIPRIL
Trade names
APO-Ramipril, Prilace, Ramipril Sandoz, Ramipril Viatris, Ramipril-WGR, Tritace, Tryzan, Vascalace

Available forms
Tablets: 1.25 mg, 2.5 mg, 5 mg, 10 mg; Capsules: 1.25 mg, 2.5 mg, 5 mg, 10 mg

Action
- ramipril (prodrug) is converted to active ramiprilat
- onset of action 1—2 hours, duration of action 24 hours
- see also General Actions of ACE inhibitors (p. 504)

Use
- hypertension
- heart failure with reduced ejection fraction
- post myocardial infarction
- diabetic kidney disease
- prevention of progressive renal failure in patients with persistent proteinuria > 1 g/day

Dose
- (Hypertension) initially 2.5 mg orally daily (1.25 mg for diuretic-treated or salt/volume-depleted patients), increasing gradually at 2—3-week intervals to 5—10 mg daily **OR**
- (After myocardial infarction) initially 1.25—2.5 mg orally twice daily, increasing gradually at 1—3-day intervals to 5 mg twice daily, starting 2—10 days after infarction **OR**
- (Reducing risk of cardiovascular event) initially 2.5 mg orally daily, doubling dose after 1 week, then increasing to 10 mg daily after 3 weeks **OR**
- (Prevention of progressive renal failure in patients with persistent proteinuria > 1 g/day) initially 1.25 mg orally daily, then doubling dose at 2—3-week intervals to 5 mg daily

Adverse effects
- see General Adverse effects of ACE inhibitors (p. 504)

Interactions
- contraindicated with angiotensin II receptor antagonists in patients with diabetic nephropathy and not recommended in other patients taking angiotensin II receptor antagonists
- see also General Interactions of ACE inhibitors (p. 504)

Nursing considerations/Cautions/Patient education
- increased risk of hypotension post myocardial infarction if patient has impaired renal function
- if the patient has a creatinine clearance of 20–50 mL/min, the dose should be started at 1.25 mg daily and increased at 2–3-day intervals as tolerated
- see also General Nursing considerations/Cautions/Patient education for ACE inhibitors (p. 505)

Tablet can be crushed and mixed with water, or mixed with spoonful of yoghurt or apple puree. Capsule can be opened and contents dispersed in water or apple juice, or mixed with spoonful of apple puree.

Contraindicated owing to their association with fetal death in utero.

Avoid use.

Reduced renal function: CrCL 20–50 mL/min, initiate Ramipril at 1.25 mg once daily and titrate carefully based on tolerance. Monitor renal function closely, as further dose adjustments may be necessary based on patient response.

Start at a lower dose (1.25 mg once daily). Careful monitoring of blood pressure, renal function and electrolytes is recommended during treatment. Dose adjustments may be necessary based on individual response.

Available in combination with
- ramipril 5 mg + felodipine 5 mg modified-release tablet (Triasyn 5.0/5.0)(Modified-release tablets should not be crushed or chewed)

TRANDOLAPRIL
Trade names
Dolapril, Gopten, Tranalpha

Available forms
Capsules: 0.5 mg, 1 mg, 2 mg, 4 mg

Action
- prodrug trandolapril is converted to active trandolaprilat
- onset of action 60 minutes, duration of action 48 hours
- see also General Actions of ACE inhibitors (p. 504)

Use
- hypertension
- heart failure with reduced ejection fraction
- post myocardial infarction
- diabetic kidney disease

Dose
- (Hypertension) initially 1 mg orally daily (0.5 mg for diuretic-treated, renally impaired or salt-depleted patients), increasing gradually to 2–4 mg daily **OR**
- (Left ventricular dysfunction after myocardial infarction) after 0.5 mg test dose, 1 mg orally daily for 3 days, then increased to 2 mg for 4 weeks, then further increased to 4 mg daily

ANTIHYPERTENSIVE AGENTS

Adverse effects/Interactions/Nursing considerations/Cautions/Patient education

- patient should be advised to take medication at the same time every day (i.e. 24-hour interval) and as a single (not divided) dose
- response should be seen in 2—4 weeks
- see also General Adverse effects/Interactions/Nursing considerations/Cautions/Patient education for ACE inhibitors (p. 504)

Capsule can be opened and contents mixed with water, or mixed with spoonful of yoghurt or apple puree.

Contraindicated. Transition women to an alternative antihypertensive as soon as possible during the first trimester. Use during the second and third trimesters is associated with fetal renal dysfunction, oligohydramnios and fetal death in utero.

Avoid use; safety unknown. Consider alternatives. If used, monitor infant for hypotension and renal issues.

Reduced renal function: dose adjustment may be required. Use with caution in patients with renal impairment; monitor renal function regularly. Avoid use in severe renal impairment (eGFR < 30 mL/min).

Available in combination with

- trandolapril 2 mg + verapamil hydrochloride 180 mg modified-release tablet (Tarka 2/180)
- trandolapril 4 mg + verapamil hydrochloride 240 mg modified-release tablet (Tarka 4/240) (modified-release tablets should not be crushed or chewed)

ANGIOTENSIN II RECEPTOR ANTAGONISTS

General Actions of angiotensin II receptor antagonists

- also known as 'sartans'
- antagonise angiotensin II receptors (AT1 subtype) on vascular smooth muscle and adrenal cortex (angiotensin II is responsible for vasoconstriction, stimulation of aldosterone, regulation of salt and water homeostasis, and cell growth stimulation)
- increases renal blood flow and maintains/increases glomerular filtration rate while decreasing renal vascular resistance
- no inhibition of angiotensin converting enzyme (ACE), therefore no potentiation of bradykinin and substance P activity (which are thought to be responsible for non-productive cough associated with ACE inhibitors)
- some angiotensin II receptor antagonists are prodrugs, which are converted to active form
- antihypertensive effect may be slightly less in those of African origin

General Adverse effects of angiotensin II receptor antagonists

- hyperkalaemia
- hypotension, palpitations, tachycardia, chest pain
- dizziness, headache, fatigue, asthenia (weakness)
- back pain, myalgia, arthralgia
- nausea, vomiting, abdominal pain, diarrhoea, dyspepsia
- flu-like symptoms, upper respiratory tract infection, rhinitis, pharyngitis, dyspnoea, cough
- urinary tract infection
- hypertriglyceridaemia
- decreased haematocrit, decreased haemoglobin
- raised liver enzymes
- (Rare) angioedema

General Interactions of angiotensin II receptor antagonists

- risk of hyperkalaemia is increased if given with potassium-sparing diuretics or potassium supplements, salt

substitutes containing potassium, other agents that raise potassium levels such as heparin, or trimethoprim/sulfamethoxazole
- not recommended with ACE inhibitors in those with diabetic neuropathy
- may increase serum lithium levels, increasing the risk of toxicity; therefore levels should be closely monitored, especially when starting, stopping or adjusting dose
- while commonly used in combination with other antihypertensive agents, increased hypotension may occur
- increased risk of renal impairment if given in combination with NSAIDs and diuretics (triple whammy)
- efficacy decreased by NSAIDs, especially indometacin

General Nursing considerations/Cautions for angiotensin II receptor antagonists

- any sodium or intravascular volume depletion should be corrected before initiating therapy
- if changing from a beta adrenoceptor blocking agent, dose should be gradually decreased over 8–14 days before starting the angiotensin II receptor antagonist
- serum potassium and creatinine levels should be regularly monitored if used for heart failure or in those also taking ACE inhibitors and/or potassium-sparing diuretics
- thiazide diuretic or another antihypertensive agent may be added to the regimen if BP is not adequately controlled by angiotensin II receptor antagonist alone
- caution if used in patients undergoing haemodialysis
- caution if used during anaesthesia and surgery owing to increased risk of hypotension
- not recommended in those with primary hyperaldosteronism or with heart failure
- caution if used in those with volume/sodium depletion, severe congestive heart failure or renal disease (e.g. renal artery stenosis), aortic or mitral valve stenosis, obstructive hypertrophic cardiomyopathy, mild-to-moderate liver impairment or renal impairment
- contraindicated in those with known hypersensitivity to angiotensin II receptor antagonists or who have haemodynamically significant bilateral renovascular disease or severe stenosis of solitary functioning kidney

General Patient education for angiotensin II receptor antagonists

- patients should be advised to avoid potassium-based salt substitutes
- women of childbearing potential should be counselled to avoid pregnancy during therapy and immediately report pregnancy if it occurs
- see also General Patient education for antihypertensive agents (p. 500)

 Contraindicated during pregnancy because of the association with abnormalities such as renal dysfunction, skull hypoplasia and decreased amniotic fluid, and also because of increased risk of fetal death in utero.

 Generally not recommended/contraindicated during breastfeeding.

 Contraindicated in patients with severe renal impairment (creatinine clearance < 30 mL/min).

Contraindicated in patients with severe hepatic impairment (Child–Pugh score 10–15) or biliary obstruction.

ANTIHYPERTENSIVE AGENTS

CANDESARTAN

Trade names
Adesan, APO-Candesartan, Atacand, BTC Candesartan, CANDESAN, Candesartan GA, Candesartan Sandoz, Candesartan-WGR, Noumed Candesartan

Available forms
Tablets: 4 mg, 8 mg, 16 mg, 32 mg

Action
- prodrug (candesartan cilexetil) is converted to active candesartan in the GI tract
- time to peak effect 6—8 hours, half-life 5—10 hours
- see also General Actions of angiotensin II receptor antagonists (p. 513)

Use
- hypertension
- heart failure with reduced ejection fraction (when ACE inhibitors are not tolerated)

Dose
- (Hypertension) 8—16 mg orally daily, increasing to 32 mg daily if needed **OR**
- (Heart failure) initially 4 mg orally daily, increasing at 2-week intervals to 32 mg

Adverse effects/Interactions/Nursing considerations/Cautions/Patient education
- may take 4 weeks for effective BP control to be achieved
- contraindicated in those with severe liver impairment and/or cholestasis
- see also General Adverse effects/ Interactions/Nursing considerations/ Cautions/Patient education for angiotensin II receptor antagonists (p. 513)

 Tablet can be crushed and mixed with water, or mixed with spoonful of yoghurt or apple puree.

 Contraindicated. Risk of spontaneous abortion, oligohydramnios (low amniotic fluid) and newborn renal dysfunction.

 Not recommended during breastfeeding.

 Reduced renal function: lower doses may be needed if the creatinine clearance (CrCl) is less than 30 mL/min.

Available in combination with
- candesartan 16 mg + hydrochlorothiazide 12.5 mg tablet (Adesan HCT 16/12.5, APO-Candesartan HCTZ 16/12.5, Atacand Plus 16/12.5, BTC-Candesartan HCT 16/12.5, Candesan Combi 16/12.5, Candesartan HCTZ-WGR 16/12.5, Candesartan/HCT Sandoz 16/12.5, Noumed Candesartan HCT 16/12.5)
- candesartan 32 mg + hydrochlorothiazide 12.5 mg tablet (Adesan HCT 32/12.5, APO-Candesartan HCTZ 32/12.5, Atacand Plus 32/12.5, BTC-Candesartan HCT 32/12.5, Candesan Combi 32/12.5, Candesartan HCTZ-WGR 32/12.5, Candesartan HCT Sandoz 32/12.5, Noumed Candesartan HCT 32/12.5)
- candesartan 32 mg + hydrochlorothiazide 25 mg tablet (Adesan HCT 32/25, APO-Candesartan HCTZ 32/25, Atacand Plus 32/25, Auro-Candesartan HCT 32/25, BTC-Candesartan HCT 32/25, Candesan Combi 32/25, Candesartan HCTZ-WGR 32/25, Candesartan HCT Sandoz 32/12.5, Noumed Candesartan HCT 32/25)

IRBESARTAN

Trade names
Abisart, APO-Irbesartan, Avapro, Avsartan, Blooms Irbesartan, Irbesartan Actavis, Irbesartan GH, Irbesartan Sandoz, Irbesartan-WGR, Irprestan, Karvea, Noumed Irbesartan

Available forms
Tablets: 75 mg, 150 mg, 300 mg

Action
- time to peak effect 3—6 hours, half-life 11—15 hours
- see also General Actions of angiotensin II receptor antagonists (p. 513)

Use
- hypertension
- delaying progression of renal disease in those with type 2 diabetes and persistent microalbuminaemia (> 30 mg/day) or urinary protein (> 900 mg/day)

Dose
- (Hypertension) initially 150 mg orally daily (75 mg daily for volume- or salt-depleted patients), increasing to 300 mg if needed **OR**
- (Hypertension and type II diabetic renal disease) 300 mg orally daily

Interactions
- see General Interactions of angiotensin II receptor antagonists (p. 513)

Adverse effects/Nursing considerations/Cautions/Patient education
- see General Adverse effects/Nursing considerations/Cautions/Patient education for angiotensin II receptor antagonists (p. 513)

Tablet can be crushed and mixed with water, or mixed with spoonful of yoghurt or apple puree.

Contraindicated. May cause fetal renal dysfunction and oligohydramnios (decreased amniotic fluid volume for gestational age), which may cause fetal death.

Not recommended during breastfeeding.

Reduced renal function: use with caution in patients with severe renal impairment (CrCl ≤ 30 mL/min).

Elderly patients may be at a higher risk of hypotension, particularly if volume depleted. Close monitoring of renal function and electrolyte levels is recommended.

Teratogen. Do not crush or disperse the tablet if you are pregnant.

Available in combination with
- irbesartan 150 mg + hydrochlorothiazide 12.5 mg (Avapro HCT 150/12.5, Karvezide 150/12.5, Abisart HCTZ 150/12.5, APO-Irbesartan 150/12.5, Avsartan HCT 150/12.5, Irbesartan HCTZ-WGR 150/12.5, Irbesartan/HCT Sandoz 150/12.5)
- irbesartan 300 mg + hydrochlorothiazide 12.5 mg (Avapro HCT 300/12.5, Karvezide 300/12.5, Abisart HCTZ 300/12.5, APO-Irbesartan HCTZ 300/12.5, Avsartan HCT 300/12.5, Irbesartan HCTZ-WGR 300/12.5, Irbesartan/HCT Sandoz 300/12.5)
- irbesartan 300 mg + hydrochlorothiazide 25 mg (Avapro HCT 300/12.5, Karvezide 300/12.5, Abisart HCTZ 300/12.5, APO-Irbesartan HCTZ 300/12.5, Avsartan HCT 300/12.5, Irbesartan HCTZ-WGR 300/12.5, Irbesartan/HCT Sandoz 300/12.5)

LOSARTAN
Trade names
Cozaar, Cozavan

Available forms
Tablets: 25 mg, 50 mg

Action
- active metabolite (half-life 4—9 hours)
- time to peak effect 6 hours, half-life 1.5—2 hours
- see also General Actions of angiotensin II receptor antagonists (p. 513)

Use
- hypertension
- delaying progression of renal disease in those with type II diabetes and persistent microalbuminaemia (> 30 mg/day) or urinary protein (> 900 mg/day)

Dose
- initially 50 mg orally daily (25 mg daily for volume- or salt-depleted patients). If BP is not adequately controlled, then 25 mg orally twice daily, increasing to 100 mg orally daily if necessary

Adverse effects/Interactions/Nursing considerations/Cautions/Patient education
- maximum BP effect in 3—6 weeks after starting therapy
- see also General Nursing considerations/Cautions for angiotensin II receptor antagonists (p. 515)

ANTIHYPERTENSIVE AGENTS

 Tablet can be crushed and mixed with water, or mixed with spoonful of yoghurt or apple puree.

 May cause fetal renal dysfunction and oligohydramnios (decreased amniotic fluid volume for gestational age), which may cause fetal death. Contraindicated by manufacturers.

 Not recommended during breastfeeding.

 Lower doses may be needed in renal impairment.

OLMESARTAN MEDOXOMIL
Trade names
Olmertan, Olmetec, Olsetan

Available forms
Tablets: 10 mg, 20 mg, 40 mg

Action
- olmesartan medoxomil (prodrug) is hydrolysed to active olmesartan in the GI tract
- time to peak effect 1.4–2.8 hours, half-life 12–18 hours
- see also General Actions of angiotensin II receptor antagonists (p. 513)

Use
- hypertension

Dose
- (Hypertension) initially 20 mg orally daily (10 mg for volume-depleted patients or impaired renal function), increasing to 40 mg daily if needed

Adverse effects
- sprue-like enteropathy (severe, chronic diarrhoea with significant weight loss, abdominal pain, fatigue, bloating, nausea, vomiting, and anaemia. It is caused by atrophy of the small intestinal villi and occurs months to years after therapy has started). While a rare adverse effect, It is more common with olmesartan than other sartans. Symptoms resolve gradually, over weeks to months, after ceasing olmesartan.
- see also General Adverse effects of angiotensin II receptor antagonists (p. 513)

Interactions
- bioavailability may be reduced if given with antacids
- see also General Interactions for angiotensin II receptor antagonists (p. 513)

Nursing considerations/Cautions
- see General Nursing considerations/Cautions for angiotensin II receptor antagonists (p. 514)

Patient education
- patient should be advised to seek medical attention if severe chronic diarrhoea with weight loss occurs
- see also General Patient education for angiotensin II receptor antagonists (p. 514)

 Tablet can be crushed and mixed with water, or mixed with spoonful of yoghurt or apple puree.

 May cause fetal renal dysfunction and oligohydramnios (decreased amniotic fluid volume for gestational age), which may cause fetal death. Contraindicated by manufacturers.

 Not recommended during breastfeeding.

 Contraindicated in individuals with severe kidney impairment (creatinine clearance (CrCl) < 30 mL/minute), biliary obstruction or severe liver impairment.

Available in combination with:
- olmesartan 20 mg + hydrochlorothiazide 12.5 mg tablets (APO-Olmesartan/HCTZ 20/12.5, APX-Olmesartan/HCTZ 20/12.5, Olmertan Combi 20/12.5, Olmesartan HCTZ-WGR 20/12.5, Olmesartan/HCT Sandoz 20/12.5, Olmetec Plus 20/12.5, Pharmacor Olmesartan HCTZ 20/12.5)

- olmesartan 40 mg + hydrochlorothiazide 12.5 mg tablets (APO-Olmesartan/HCTZ 40/12.5, APX-Olmesartan/HCTZ 40/12.5, Olmertan Combi 40/12.5, Olmesartan HCTZ-WGR 40/12.5, Olmesartan/HCT Sandoz 40/12.5, Olmetec 40/12.5, Pharmacor Olmesartan HCTZ 40/12.5)
- olmesartan 40 mg + hydrochlorothiazide 25 mg tablets (APO-Olmesartan/HCTZ 40/25, APX-Olmesartan/HCTZ 40/25, Olmertan Combi 40/25, Olmesartan HCTZ-WGR 40/25, Olmesartan/HCT Sandoz 40/25, Olmetec 40/25, Pharmacor Olmesartan HCTZ 40/25)
- olmesartan 20 mg + amlodipine 5 mg tablets (APO-Olmesartan/Amlodipine 20/5, Olmekar 20/5, Olmesartan Amilodipine-WGR 20/5, Olmesartan/Amlodipine Sandoz 20/5, Pharmacor Olmesartan Amilodipine 20/5, Sevikar 20/5)
- olmesartan 40 mg + amlodipine 10 mg tablets (APO-Olmesartan/Amlodipine 40/10, Olmekar 40/10, Olmesartan Amilodipine-WGR 40/10, Olmesartan/Amilodipine Sandoz 40/10, Pharmacor Olmesartan Amilodipine 40/10, Sevikar 40/10)
- olmesartan 40 mg + amlodipine 5 mg tablets (APO-Olmesartan/Amlodipine 40/5, Olmekar 40/5, Olmesartan Amilodipine-WGR 40/5, Olmesartan/Amlodipine Sandoz 40/5, Pharmacor Olmesartan Amilodipine 40/5, Sevikar 40/5)
- olmesartan 20 mg + amlodipine 5 mg + hydrochlorothiazide 12.5 tablets (APO-Olmesartan/Amlodipine HCTZ 20/5/12.5, Olamlo HCT 20/5/12.5, Sevikar HCT 20/5/12.5
- olmesartan 40 mg + amlodipine 10 mg + hydrochlorothiazide 12.5 mg tablets (APO-Olmesartan/Amlodipine HCTZ 40/10/12.5, Olamlo HCT 40/10/12.5, Sevikar HCT 40/10/12.5
- olmesartan 40 mg + amlodipine 10 mg + hydrochlorothiazide 25 mg tablets (APO-Olmesartan/Amlodipine HCTZ 40/10/25, Olamlo HCT 40/10/25, Sevikar HCT 40/10/25
- olmesartan 40 mg + amlodipine 5 mg + hydrochlorothiazide 12.5 mg tablets (APO-Olmesartan/Amlodipine HCTZ 40/5/12.5, Olamlo HCT 40/5/12.5, Sevikar HCT 40/5/12.5
- olmesartan 40 mg + amlodipine 5 mg + hydrochlorothiazide 25 mg tablets (APO-Olmesartan/Amlodipine HCTZ 40/5/25, Olamlo HCT 40/5/25, Sevikar HCT 40/5/25

TELMISARTAN
Trade names
APO Telmisartan, Micardis, Mizart, Noumed Telmisartan, Pharmacor Telmisartan, Telmisartan Sandoz, Teltartan

Available forms
Tablets: 40 mg, 80 mg

Action
- peak effect 0.5–1 hour, half-life 24 hours
- see also General Actions of angiotensin II receptor antagonists (p. 513)

Use
- hypertension
- prevention of cardiovascular morbidity or mortality in those ≥ 55 years, with coronary artery disease, peripheral arterial disease, previous stroke, transient ischaemic attacks, or high-risk diabetes with evidence of end-organ damage

Dose
- (Hypertension) initially 40 mg orally daily, increasing to 80 mg daily if needed
OR
- (Prevention of cardiovascular morbidity/mortality) 80 mg orally daily

Adverse effects
- see General Adverse effects of angiotensin II receptor antagonists (p. 513)

Interactions
- may increase serum levels of digoxin, increasing the risk of toxicity; therefore digoxin levels should be closely monitored, especially when starting or stopping therapy or adjusting dose
- systemic corticosteroids may decrease antihypertensive effects

ANTIHYPERTENSIVE AGENTS

- see also General Interactions of angiotensin II receptor antagonists (p. 513)

Nursing considerations/Cautions

- may take 4—8 weeks for effective BP control to be achieved
- (Prevention of cardiovascular morbidity/mortality) BP should be closely monitored during therapy
- contains sorbitol (338 mg); therefore not recommended in those with hereditary fructose intolerance
- caution if used in those with diabetes owing to risk of undiagnosed cardiac disease
- caution if used in those with mild-to-moderate liver impairment; dose should not exceed 40 mg
- contraindicated in those with biliary obstructive disorder or severe liver impairment
- see also General Nursing considerations/Cautions for angiotensin II receptor antagonists (p. 514)

Patient education

- see General Patient education for angiotensin II receptor antagonists (p. 514)

Tablet can be crushed and mixed with water, or mixed with spoonful of yoghurt or apple puree.

Telmisartan is contraindicated in pregnanacy; it may cause fetal renal dysfunction and oligohydramnios, which can cause fetal death.

Not recommended during breastfeeding.

Available in combination with:

- telmisartan 40 mg + hydrochlorothiazide 12.5 mg tablets (APO-Telmisartan HCTZ 40/12.5, Micardis Plus 40/12.5, Mizart HCT 40/12.5, Telmisartan HCTZ-WGR 40/12.5, Telmisartan HCT Sandoz 40/12.5, Teltartan HCT 40/12.5)
- telmisartan 80 mg + hydrochlorothiazide 12.5 mg tablets (APO-Telmisartan HCTZ 80/12.5, Micardis Plus 80/12.5, Mizart 80/12.5, Telmisartan HCTZ-WGR 80/12.5, Telmisartan HCT Sandoz 80/12.5, Teltartan HCT 80/12.5)
- telmisartan 80 mg + hydrochlorothiazide 25 mg tablets (APO-Telmisartan HCTZ 80/25, Micardis Plus 80/25, Mizart 80/25, Telmisartan HCTZ-WGR 80/25, Telmisartan HCT Sandoz 80/25, Teltartan HCT 80/25)
- telmisartan 40 mg + amlodipine 10 mg tablets (Pritor/Amlodipine 40/10, Twynsta 40/10)
- telmisartan 40 mg + amlodipine 5 mg (Pritor/Amlodipine 40/5, Twynsta 40/5)
- telmisartan 80 mg + amlodipine 5 mg tablets (Pritor/Amlodipine 80/5, Twynsta 80/5)
- telmisartan 80 mg + amlodipine 10 mg tablets (Pritor/Amlodipine 80/10, Twynsta 80/10)

VALSARTAN

Trade names
Dilart, Diovan

Available forms
Tablets: 40 mg, 80 mg, 160 mg, 320 mg

Action
- peak effect in 2 hours, half-life 6—9 hours
- see also General Actions of angiotensin II receptor antagonists (p. 513)

Use
- hypertension
- heart failure (with diuretic and/or digoxin in those intolerant to ACE inhibitors)
- post myocardial infarction

Dose
- (Hypertension) initially 80 mg orally daily, increasing to 160 mg daily after 4 weeks if BP control is not achieved (daily maximum 320 mg) **OR**
- (Heart failure) initially 40 mg orally twice daily, increasing to 80—160 mg twice daily if needed **OR**

- (Post myocardial infarction) initially 20 mg orally twice daily, increasing to 40 mg twice daily, then 80 mg twice daily, to 160 mg twice daily, over a number of weeks as tolerated by the patient

Adverse effects
- neutropenia
- see also General Adverse effects of angiotensin II receptor antagonists (p. 513)

Interactions
- caution if given with rifampicin, ciclosporin and ritonavir
- not recommended with ACE inhibitors
- see also General Interactions of angiotensin II receptor antagonists (p. 513)

Nursing considerations/Cautions/Patient education
- (Hypertension) maximum effect is usually seen after 4 weeks. f further BP reduction is needed, diuretic may be added or dose may be increased to 320 mg daily
- (Myocardial infarction) therapy can be started within 12 hours of myocardial infarction
- (Heart failure, post myocardial infarction) renal function should be monitored regularly during therapy
- (Post myocardial infarction) dose may be reduced if patient becomes hypotensive or if renal function declines
- contraindicated in those with severe liver impairment, biliary cirrhosis and cholestasis
- see also General Nursing considerations/Cautions for angiotensin II receptor antagonists (p. 514)

The tablet can be crushed and mixed with water, or it can be mixed with a spoonful of yogurt or apple puree for administration.

Pregnant women who take valsartan may be at risk of spontaneous abortion, oligohydramnios (low amniotic fluid), and newborn renal dysfunction. Valsartan is contraindicated in pregnant women.

Not recommended during breastfeeding.

For patients with severe renal impairment (creatinine clearance (CrCl) < 30 mL/minute), the maximum daily dose of valsartan should be limited to 80 mg.

Available in combination with:
- sacubitril 24.3 mg + valsartan 25.7 mg tablets (Entresto 25/26, Omtralo 25/26, Pharmacor Sacubitril/Valsartan 25/26, Sacubitril/Valsartan Alphapharm 25/26, Valtresto 25/26)
- sacubitril 48.6 mg + valsartan 51.4 mg tablets (Entresto 49/52, Omtralo 49/52, Pharmacor Sacubitril/Valsartan 49/52, Sacubitril/Valsartan Alphapharm 49/52, Valtresto 49/52)
- sacubitril 97.2 mg + valsartan 102.8 mg tablets (Entresto 97/103, Omtralo 97/103, Pharmacor Sacubitril/Valsartan 97/103, Sacubitril/Valsartan Alphapharm 97/103, Valtresto 97/103)
- amlodipine 10 mg + valsartan 160 mg tablets (Amlodipine/Valsartan Novartis 10/160, Exforge 10/160)
- amlodipine 10 mg + valsartan 320 mg tablets (Amlodipine/Valsartan Novartis 10/320, Exforge 10/320)
- amlodipine 5 mg + valsartan 160 mg tablets (Amlodipine/Valsartan Novartis 5/160, Exforge 5/160)
- amlodipine 5 mg + valsartan 320 mg tablets (Amlodipine/Valsartan Novartis 5/320, Exforge 5/320)
- amlodipine 5 mg + valsartan 80 mg tablets (Amlodipine/Valsartan Novartis 5/80, Exforge 5/80)
- valsartan 160 mg + hydrochlorothiazide 12.5 mg tablets (Co-Diovan 160/12.5, Dilart HCT 160/12.5)
- valsartan 160 mg + hydrochlorothiazide 25 mg tablets (Co-Diovan 160/25, Dilart HCT 160/25)
- valsartan 320 mg + hydrochlorothiazide 12.5 mg tablets (Co-Diovan 320/12.5, Dilart HCT 320/12.5)

- valsartan 320 mg + hydrochlorothiazide 25 mg tablets (Co-Diovan 320/25, Dilart HCT 320/25)
- valsartan 80 mg + hydrochlorothiazide 12.5 mg tablets (Co-Diovan 80/12.5, Dilart HCT 80/12.5)
- amlodipine 10 mg + valsartan 160 mg + hydrochlorthiazide 12.5 mg tablets (Amlodipine/Valsartan/HCT Novartis 10/160/12.5, Exforge HCT 10/160/12.5)
- amlodipine 10 mg + valsartan 160 mg + hydrochlorthiazide 25 mg tablets (Amlodipine/Valsartan/HCT Novartis 10/160/25, Exforge HCT 10/160/25)
- amlodipine 10 mg + valsartan 320 mg+ hydrochlorthiazide 25 mg tablets (Amlodipine/Valsartan/HCT Novartis 10/320/25, Exforge HCT 10/320/25)
- amlodipine 5 mg + valsartan 160 mg + hydrochlorthiazide 12.5 mg tablets (Amlodipine/Valsartan/HCT Novartis 5/160/12.5, Exforge HCT 5/160/12.5)
- amlodipine 5 mg + valsartan 160 mg + hydrochlorthiazide 25 mg tablets (Amlodipine/Valsartan/HCT Novartis 5/160/25, Exforge HCT 5/160/25)

BETA ADRENOCEPTOR BLOCKING AGENTS

General Actions of beta adrenoceptor blocking agents

- also known as 'beta adrenoceptor antagonists', 'beta blockers' or β-blockers
- competitively inhibit beta adrenoceptors (sympathetic nervous system), reducing some of the body's responses to adrenaline (epinephrine), noradrenaline (norepinephrine) and isoprenaline
- beta1 receptors are primarily found in the heart (cardiac nodal tissue, cardiac myocytes and other heart conduction pathway tissues), kidneys and adipose tissue
- beta2 receptors are widely distributed in the respiratory tract, particularly in airway smooth muscle. They are also located in the heart, blood vessel smooth muscle, kidneys, pancreas, uterus, brain and liver
- cardioselective beta blockers (i.e. atenolol, bisoprolol, betaxolol, esmolol, metoprolol, nebivolol) have more affinity for beta1 receptors; this selectivity is reduced with high doses
- non-cardioselective beta blockers (i.e. propranolol, timolol) have equal affinity for both beta1 (heart) and beta2 (lung) receptors.
- some non-cardioselective beta blockers also block alpha1 adrenoceptors (i.e. carvedilol, labetalol)
- reduce rate of impulses through the cardiac conducting system
- reduce cardiac rate and force of contraction
- reduce cardiac output and myocardial oxygen demand
- reduce BP by decreasing cardiac output
- inhibits exercise-induced tachycardia
- precipitate bronchospasm
- inhibition of renin release from the kidneys
- inhibition of catecholamine-induced lipid and carbohydrate metabolism
- decreases melatonin release via blockage of central beta1 adrenoreceptors (possibly contributing to sleep disturbances)
- (Non-selective) increases plasma levels of triglycerides and lowers HDL
- reduction of elevated, as well as normal, intraocular pressure, probably by reducing aqueous humour formation (see Antiglaucoma agents p. 461)

General adverse effects of beta adrenoceptor blocking agents

- bronchospasm (uncommon but serious), dyspnoea on exertion, coughing, wheezing, asthma, nasal congestion (including topical beta blockers), exacerbation of allergic conditions (e.g. allergic rhinitis (hay fever) during pollen season)
- bradycardia, heart block, hypotension, postural hypotension, arrhythmias, development or worsening of heart failure, exacerbation of angina, tachycardia
- nausea, vomiting, diarrhoea, constipation, abdominal pain, indigestion, dry mouth

- cold extremities, exacerbation of Raynaud's phenomenon or other circulation disorders such as intermittent claudication
- fatigue, dizziness, headache, malaise, asthenia
- sleep disturbances, including vivid dreams and nightmares, insomnia
- oedema (generalised, leg and/or dependent)
- impotence, decreased libido
- blurred vision, dry eyes/decreased lacrimation
- rash, pruritus, reversible alopecia, exacerbation of psoriasis
- increase in free thyroxine (T4) levels
- hypoglycaemia, elevated triglyceride levels
- (Uncommon) depression, confusion, mood changes, hallucinations
- (Rarely) thrombocytopenia, purpura, elevated liver enzymes, urea and creatinine levels, hepatic toxicity

General interactions of beta adrenoceptor blocking agents

- may cause bradycardia, hypotension and asystole when given with verapamil (and diltiazem to a lesser degree); it is not recommended to use together
- caution if used with dihydropyridine calcium-channel blockers (e.g. felodipine, amlodipine) because of an increased risk of increased hypotension and deterioration of ventricular pump function
- may enhance the effects of other antihypertensive agents
- careful monitoring is required if given with other beta adrenoceptor blocking agents (including eye drops) and generally not recommended together
- not recommended with Class I antiarrhythmic agents
- caution if given with amiodarone owing to prolongation of AV conduction time
- may cause loss of diabetic control and delayed recovery from hypoglycaemia, requiring adjustment of insulin and/or oral hypoglycaemic agents
- use with clonidine may result in severe withdrawal symptoms (rebound hypertension and arrhythmias) and is not recommended. If used together, the beta adrenoceptor blocking agent should be withdrawn first, at least 3 days before clonidine, which is then gradually stopped
- may cause excessive bradycardia if given with digoxin in the treatment of digoxin toxicity; therefore heart rate should be closely monitored
- hypotensive effect may be decreased if given with prostaglandin-synthesis blocking NSAIDs (e.g. ibuprofen, indometacin)
- increased hypotension may occur if given with phenothiazines, barbiturates or tricyclic antidepressants (TCAs)
- effects may be counteracted if given with sympathomimetic agents (e.g. adrenaline (epinephrine))
- peripheral circulation disturbance may be exacerbated if given with ergot alkaloids
- decreased serum levels may occur if given with rifampicin
- caution if given with amisulpride owing to increased bradycardia
- not recommended with monoamine oxidase inhibitors (MAOIs) because of the increased risk of bradycardia and hypotension and also the risk of hypertensive crisis

General Nursing considerations/ Cautions for beta adrenoceptor blocking agents

- contraindicated in bradycardia (45–50 beats/min), second or third-degree AV block, sick sinus syndrome (without pacemaker), severe hypotension, cardiogenic or hypovolaemic shock, uncontrolled heart failure, right ventricular failure secondary to pulmonary hypertension, significant right ventricular hypertrophy, severe untreated peripheral arterial circulatory disturbance and metabolic acidosis

ANTIHYPERTENSIVE AGENTS

- before giving the drug, note bradycardia (especially if the heart rate is 45–50 beats/min), hypotension, dyspnoea, cyanosis and circulation in the extremities
- not recommended in those with systolic BP < 120 mmHg with first-degree heart block
- during therapy, if heart rate 50–55 beats/min at rest or patient has signs of bradycardia, dose should be decreased or stopped gradually
- (Heart failure) patient should be monitored closely for any signs of bradycardia, vasodilation or worsening heart failure before increasing dose. Any symptoms should be stabilised before increasing dose. Check weight and keep a fluid chart to detect fluid retention
- (Coronary artery disease) should not be stopped abruptly, as exacerbation of angina, myocardial infarction and cardiac arrhythmias may occur. Discontinuation should be over 8–14 days
- not recommended in those with variant (Prinzmetal's) angina, as coronary artery spasm may be exacerbated
- not recommended in Raynaud's disease (reduced blood flow to the fingers and toes when exposed to cold temperatures or stress), as it may exacerbate the condition
- may exacerbate intermittent claudication (lower extremity skeletal muscle pain that occurs during exercise)
- may exacerbate pre-existing psoriasis
- contraindicated in asthma, chronic obstructive pulmonary disease (COPD), bronchospasm or other conditions involving airway obstruction as they can precipitate bronchospasm. Beta1-selective beta blockers (e.g. metoprolol) may be considered for patients with well-controlled asthma (on specialist advice) or COPD.
- caution if used in diabetes mellitus or history of spontaneous hypoglycaemia (early signs of hypoglycaemia such as tachycardia and palpitations may be masked); pain also masked
- (Surgery) anaesthetist must be informed that the patient is taking a beta blocker
- caution if used in those with hyperthyroidism (clinical signs may be masked)
- contraindicated in untreated pheochromocytoma (tumour in the adrenal gland)
- contraindicated in those with known allergy or hypersensitivity to beta blocker agents

General Patient education for beta adrenoceptor blocking agents

- advise patient not to stop the drug abruptly to decrease the risk of angina pectoris, acute myocardial infarction or cardiac arrhythmias
- contact lens users should be advised that dry eye may occur because of decreased lacrimation
- warn patient with diabetes mellitus regarding:
  - masked signs (e.g. tachycardia, palpitations) of hypoglycaemia
  - prolonged recovery from hypoglycaemia
  - need to monitor blood glucose levels vigilantly because of the potential loss of diabetic control, necessitating adjustment of insulin and/or hypoglycaemic agent dose
- advise patient to seek medical advice immediately if any of the following occur:
  - slowed heart rate
  - dizziness, fainting
  - tingling, pins and needles
  - sexual problems
  - skin rash, itchiness
  - dry eyes
  - increase in cramp-like pain in one or both legs when walking
- counsel female patients of childbearing potential to use adequate contraception to avoid pregnancy during therapy
- see also General Patient education for antihypertensive agents (p. 500)

Start treatment at a lower dose because of the increased risk of adverse effects. Monitor closely for side effects like bradycardia, hypotension and fatigue. Adjust dose as needed.

Beta adrenoceptor blocking agents are banned in sport, but may be allowed in some circumstances, or banned in some sports but not others.

ATENOLOL
Trade names
Tenormin, Noten, Tensig, APX-Atenolol, Atenolol-GH, Atenolol Sandoz, Atenolol-AFT Oral Liquid, Atenolol-WGR, Blooms the Chemist Atenolol

Available forms
Tablets: 50 mg;
Oral liquid: 50 mg/10 mL

Action
- cardioselective (block beta1 receptors)
- decreases the size of infarction and incidence of ventricular dysrhythmia; decreases mortality in first 7 days post infarction
- antiarrhythmic action due to anti-sympathetic effect depressing both sinus and AV node function and prolonging atrial refractory period
- slightly less effective in those of Afro-Caribbean origin
- half-life 7–9 hours
- see also General Actions of beta adrenoceptor blocking agents (p. 521)

Use
- hypertension
- angina
- tachyarrhythmia
- myocardial infarction

Dose
- (Hypertension) initially 50 mg orally daily, increasing weekly by 50 mg, then up to 200 mg if necessary **OR**
- (Angina) initially 50 mg orally daily, increasing to 100 mg daily as a single or 2 divided doses if needed **OR**
- (Cardiac arrhythmias) controlled with other IV agents initially, then 50–100 mg orally daily (maintenance) **OR**
- (Myocardial infarction, late intervention with patient presenting 12 hours after onset of chest pain) 50 mg orally daily for 1–3 years

Adverse effects/Interactions/Nursing considerations/Cautions/Patient education
- oral doses of 50–100 mg are given once daily; doses greater than 100 mg should be divided
- (Myocardial infarction) most beneficial if given in first 48 hours post myocardial infarction
- absorption reduced by apple juice
- (Oral liquid) contains hydroxybenzoates and propylene glycol, which may cause hypersensitivity reaction in sensitive individuals
- see also General Nursing considerations/Cautions for beta adrenoceptor blocking agents (p. 523)

Available as oral liquid. Tablet can be crushed and mixed with spoonful of yoghurt (but not apple puree).

Atenolol crosses the placental barrier and may affect fetal growth and development. There is a concern about potential adverse effects on the fetal heart rate and blood circulation.

Not recommended during breastfeeding, as atenolol accumulates in breastmilk potentially causing adverse effects.

BISOPROLOL
Trade names
Bicor, Bicard, Bispro, APO-Bisoprolol, Bisoprolol Dr. Reddy's, Bisoprolol Generihealth, Bisoprolol Sandoz, Bisoprolol-WGR, Noumed Bisoprolol

Available forms
Tablets: 1.25 mg (starter pack), 2.5 mg, 5 mg, 10 mg

ANTIHYPERTENSIVE AGENTS

Action
- cardioselective (block beta1 receptors). Bisoprolol is more cardioselective than metoprolol and atenolol
- compared with non-selective beta blockers, cardioselective beta blockers (like bisoprolol) are preferred in patients with COPD and well-controlled asthma
- half-life 10—12 hours
- see also General Actions of beta adrenoceptor blocking agents (p. 521)

Use
- stable, chronic moderate-to-severe heart failure

Dose
- (Stable chronic moderate-to-severe heart failure) initially 1.25 mg orally daily for 1 week, then (if tolerated) 2.5 mg for 1 week, then 3.75 mg for 1 week, then 5 mg for 4 weeks, then 7.5 mg for 4 weeks, then 10 mg daily (maintenance) (with ACE inhibitor, diuretic +/− digoxin)

Interactions
- AV conduction and risk of bradycardia may be increased if given with cholinergic (parasympathomimetic) agents
- increased risk of bradycardia if given with mefloquine
- may decrease effects of dobutamine or isoprenaline
- slight decrease in half-life if given with rifampicin
- see General Interactions of beta adrenoceptor blocking agents (p. 522)

Adverse effects/Nursing considerations/Cautions/Patient education
- contraindicated in those with acute heart failure
- patient should be in stable condition after heart failure (without any acute failure in the previous 6 weeks) and stabilised on therapy for the previous 2 weeks before starting bisoprolol
- heart rate, BP, ECG and any signs of worsening heart failure should be monitored during dose titration. If heart rate ≤ 50—55 beats/minute, the dose should be decreased gradually
- each increase should be monitored for any signs of intolerance
- transient worsening of heart failure, hypotension and/or bradycardia may occur during titration period
- see also General Nursing considerations/Cautions for beta adrenoceptor blocking agents (p. 522)

 Tablets are film coated they should be swallowed with liquid and should not be chewed.

 Not recommended during pregnancy unless benefits outweigh risk to the fetus including reduced placental perfusion and impaired fetal growth and development.

 Not recommended during breastfeeding.

 Bisoprolol is lipid soluble and eliminated by both the liver and the kidneys. Dose reduction is generally not required; however, caution is advised.

CARVEDILOL
Trade names
Carvidol, Dicarz, Dilatrend, Volirop, APO-Carvedilol, Carvedilol Sandoz, Carvedilol-WGR

Available forms
Tablets: 3.125 mg, 6.25 mg, 12.5 mg, 25 mg

Action
- non-selective (blocks beta1, beta2 and alpha1 receptors)
- half-life 6—10 hours
- see also General Actions of beta adrenoceptor blocking agents (p. 521)

Use
- hypertension
- heart failure

Dose
- (Hypertension) initially 12.5 mg orally daily for 2 days, then increasing at 2-week intervals to 25 mg daily and, if necessary, increasing to 50 mg daily if needed **OR**

525

- (Heart failure) initially 3.125 mg orally twice daily with food for 2 weeks, then doubling of dose at 2-week intervals if tolerated (daily maximum 50 mg (if < 85 kg or with severe heart failure), 100 mg (if > 85 kg) in 2 divided doses)

Adverse effects
- increased sweating
- arthralgia, myalgia, back pain
- see also General Adverse effects of beta adrenoceptor blocking agents (p. 521)

Interactions
- may increase serum levels of ciclosporin and digoxin, increasing the risk of adverse effects; therefore serum levels should be closely monitored during therapy
- caution if given with fluoxetine if patient is clinically unstable
- serum levels may be increased by grapefruit juice
- see also General Interactions of beta adrenoceptor blocking agents (p. 522)

Nursing considerations/Cautions
- contraindicated in people with asthma — can precipitate (cause or trigger) bronchospasm
- contraindicated by the manufacturer in significant liver dysfunction (the main route of carvedilol elimination is the liver)
- (Severe congestive heart failure) patient should be assessed for any signs of peripheral oedema, systolic BP ≥ 85 mmHg and other therapies (digoxin, diuretics, ACE inhibitors) should be stabilised first before introducing carvedilol
- (Congestive heart failure) patient should be monitored for any symptoms of worsening heart failure, vasodilation or bradycardia before each dose increase
- (Congestive heart failure) if pulse rate < 55 beats/min, dose should be reduced
- caution if used in those with labile or secondary hypertension
- see also General Nursing considerations/Cautions for beta adrenoceptor blocking agents (p. 522)

Patient education
- Advise the patient to avoid use of grapefruit juice during therapy
- see also General Patient education for beta adrenoceptor blocking agents (p. 523)

 Tablets can be dispersed in water or crushed and mixed with spoonful of yoghurt or apple puree.

 Not recommended during pregnancy unless benefits outweigh risk to the fetus including reduced placental perfusion and impaired fetal growth and development.

 Carvedilol should not be used during breastfeeding unless the benefits outweigh the potential risks to the nursing infant.

ESMOLOL
Trade name
Brevibloc

Available form
Vial: 100 mg/10 mL

Action
- cardioselective
- rapid onset, short duration of action, half-life 5—23 minutes
- active metabolite (half-life 3.7 hours, which is prolonged tenfold in those with severe kidney disease)
- see also General Actions of beta adrenoceptor blocking agents (p. 521)

Use
- supraventricular tachycardia

Dose
- (Supraventricular tachycardia) initially 500 microgram/kg/min IV over 1 minute (loading dose), then 50 microgram/kg/min for 4 minutes
- if satisfactory response, then 50 microgram/kg/min by IV infusion (maintenance)
- if unsatisfactory response, repeat initial loading dose of 500 microgram/kg/min

ANTIHYPERTENSIVE AGENTS

IV over 1 minute, followed by 100 microgram/kg/min for 4 minutes. This may be repeated, increasing the maintenance dose by 50 microgram/kg/min until response is satisfactory. As satisfactory heart rate or BP is approached, infusion rate should be decreased

Adverse effects
- symptomatic hypotension with sweating and dizziness, asymptomatic hypotension
- dizziness, somnolence, confusion, headache, agitation, fatigue, paraesthesia, asthenia
- nausea, vomiting
- sweating
- (IV site) inflammation, induration, swelling, redness, skin discoloration, thrombophlebitis and, rarely, skin necrosis (from extravasation)

Interactions
- plasma level may be increased by IV morphine
- may prolong suxamethonium's neuromuscular blockade
- not recommended with dopamine, adrenaline (epinephrine) or noradrenaline (norepinephrine) to slow heart rate owing to risk of blocking contraction
- contraindicated within 48 hours of discontinuing verapamil
- increased risk of hypotension if given with nifedipine and amlodipine
- increased serum level may occur if given with warfarin or digoxin
- increased AV conduction time may occur if given with disopyramide or amiodarone
- may decrease serum levels of digoxin
- see also General Interactions of beta adrenoceptor blocking agents (p. 522)

Nursing considerations/Cautions/Patient education
- overdoses of esmolol can cause cardiac arrest
- ECG, heart rate and BP should be monitored continuously during therapy. If pulse falls to less than 50—55 beats/minute with symptoms of bradycardia, dose should be reduced
- therapy should be limited to 24 hours
- infusion into small veins or at levels greater than 10 mg/mL is not recommended
- butterfly needles are not recommended
- intervals may be increased from 5 to 10 minutes if necessary
- avoid extravasation and monitor IV site regularly to prevent venous irritation and/or tissue necrosis
- 100 mg vial is pre-diluted and ready to administer
- incompatible with sodium bicarbonate, furosemide (frusemide), diazepam and thiopentone
- maintenance dose should not exceed 200 microgram/kg/min owing to risk of increased hypotension
- contains about 20% alcohol, and this should be considered if this is administered to young children of those who have suffered from alcoholism
- therapy should be discontinued gradually once arrhythmia has been controlled, patient is stable and alternative antiarrhythmic agent has been started
- caution if used to control ventricular rate
- contraindicated if patient requires inotropic agents and/or vasodilators to maintain systemic BP and cardiac output
- see also General Nursing considerations/Cautions for beta adrenoceptor blocking agents (p. 522)

 When used in late pregnancy (third trimester) and labour, esmolol caused fetal bradycardia that continued even after the drug infusion was stopped.

 Not recommended during breastfeeding.

LABETALOL

Trade names
Labetalol SXP, Presolol

Available forms
Tablets: 100 mg, 200 mg;
Ampoules: (solution for IV injection) 5 mg/mL

Action
- beta blockade is non-selective, blocks beta1, beta2 and alpha1 receptors
- alpha receptor blockade is mainly on peripheral arterioles, resulting in a reduction of peripheral resistance (additional vasodilation)
- beta blockade on the heart causes reflex peripheral vasodilation, reducing BP without cardiac stimulation
- half-life 5.5—8 hours (however, hypotensive effect may last for up to 11 hours after administration)
- see also General Actions of beta adrenoceptor blocking agents (p. 521)

Use
- hypertension
- hypertensive emergency

Dose
- (Hypertension) initially 100—200 mg orally twice daily after meals, increasing at weekly intervals up to 2400 mg daily in 3—4 divided doses if needed
- (Hypertensive emergency) refer to local protocols for specific treatment guidelines. *IV bolus adult:* initially 20 mg IV over about 2 minutes, then 40 mg after 10—20 minutes if needed. Further doses up to 80 mg can be given at 10—20-minute intervals, maximum 300 mg in 24 hours. Consider IV infusion if BP is not controlled by bolus injection. *IV infusion adult:* administer 2 mg per minute IV until desired BP is achieved (usual dose 50—200 mg)
- (Severe hypertension in pregnancy) initially administer 20 mg/hour IV, with the option to increase by 20 mg/hour at 20-minute intervals, up to a maximum rate of 160 mg/hour (maximum dose 300 mg in 24 hours).

Adverse effects/Interactions/Nursing considerations/Cautions/Patient education
- may interfere with some laboratory tests including assays using fluorimetric or photometric methods
- may also produce false positive result using urine screening for amphetamines
- see also General Nursing considerations/Cautions for beta adrenoceptor blocking agents (p. 522)

Tablets can be dispersed in water or crushed and mixed with spoonful of yoghurt or apple puree.

Labetolol is considered safe to use during pregnancy and is often recommended at first-line management for high BP in pregnant women. However it does cross the placental barrier, carrying some potential risks to the fetus.

Labetolol is excreted in breastmilk. While it is preferred in breastfeeding over other beta blockers, it is generally not recommended.

METOPROLOL TARTRATE

Trade names
APX-Metoprolol, Betaloc, Metoprolol Sandoz, Metoprolol IV Viatris, Metoprolol-WGR, Minax, Noumed Metoprolol

METOPROLOL SUCCINATE

Trade names
Metrol-XL, Minax-XL, Toprol-XL, Topreloc-XL

- metoprolol succinate is long acting (controlled release) and taken once daily, while metoprolol tartrate is short acting and typically taken at least twice daily

Available forms
Tablets: 50 mg, 100 mg;
Tablets (controlled-release): 23.75 mg, 47.5 mg, 95 mg, 190 mg;
Ampoules: 5 mg/5 mL

Action
- cardioselective
- half-life 3—5 hours
- see also General Actions of beta adrenoceptor blocking agents (p. 521)

Use
- mild-to-severe hypertension
- angina pectoris prophylaxis
- myocardial infarction (definite or suspected)
- migraine prophylaxis
- cardiac arrhythmias (IV)
- stable chronic heart failure

Dose
- (Mild hypertension) 50—100 mg orally daily **OR**
- (Severe hypertension) 50—100 mg orally twice daily **OR**
- (Angina pectoris) 50—100 mg orally 2—3 times daily **OR**
- (Myocardial infarction) initially 50 mg orally twice daily for 48 hours, then 100 mg twice daily **OR**
- (Migraine prophylaxis) 100—150 mg orally daily in 2 divided doses **OR**
- (Cardiac arrhythmias, particularly supraventricular tachyarrhythmias) 5 mg IV at 1—2 mg/min repeated at 5-minute intervals as required, up to a dose of 15 mg **OR**
- (Heart failure) initially 11.875—23.75 mg (1/2—1 tablet) orally once daily for 2 weeks, then 47.5 mg daily for 2 weeks, then 95 mg daily for 2 weeks, then 190 mg daily or the highest tolerated dose once daily (maintenance) (controlled-release tablets)

Interactions
- plasma levels may be increased by alcohol, diphenhydramine, fluoxetine, hydralazine, sertraline and paroxetine
- caution if given with hydroxychloroquine or diphenhydramine
- caution if given with warfarin as increased anticoagulation may occur. INR should be monitored during therapy
- plasma levels may be decreased by rifampicin
- see also General Interactions of beta adrenoceptor blocking agents (p. 522)

Adverse effects/Nursing considerations/Cautions
- parenteral administration is conducted only in a unit where suitable monitoring and resuscitation equipment is available
- (IV) BP and ECG should be monitored throughout therapy
- (IV) caution if systolic BP < 100 mmHg, as further significant decrease in BP can occur
- no equivalence has been shown between controlled-release tablets and immediate-release formulations
- controlled-release tablets should be used only for chronic heart failure
- if dose ≤ 150 mg, it may be given as a single daily dose
- caution if used in those with liver cirrhosis, as clearance may be decreased, leading to elevated serum levels
- see also General Adverse effects/ Nursing considerations/Cautions for beta adrenoceptor blocking agents (p. 521)

Patient education
- patient should be advised to avoid alcohol during therapy
- advise patient that controlled-release tablets may be halved
- patient should be instructed that controlled-release tablets should be swallowed whole (or halved if tablets are scored), not chewed or crushed
- see also General Patient education for beta adrenoceptor blocking agents (p. 523)

Modified-release tablets should not be chewed or crushed. Tablets that are non-modified release can be dispersed in water, or crushed and mixed with spoonful of yoghurt or apple puree.

Avoid use. May reduce placental perfusion, leading to potential risks such as growth retardation, intrauterine death, preterm birth or miscarriage. May cause bradycardia in the fetus and newborn.

Caution advised. Excreted into breastmilk. Monitor infant for symptoms such as bradycardia.

Reduced hepatic function: metabolised in the liver. Dose adjustments may be necessary. Close monitoring of liver function is recommended.

NEBIVOLOL

Trade names
Nebilet, Nepiten, APO-Nebivolol, Nebaloc, Nebivolol Lupin, Nebivolol Sandoz, Nebivolov Viatris

Available forms
Tablets: 1.25 mg, 5 mg, 10 mg

Action
- cardioselective with very high affinity for beta1 adrenoceptors
- causes vasodilation through release of nitrous oxide in endothelial cells
- active metabolite
- half-life about 10 hours
- see also General Actions of beta adrenoceptor blocking agents (p. 521)

Use
- hypertension (monotherapy or with diuretic)
- stable chronic heart failure (adjunct therapy in those > 70 years with diuretic and/or digoxin and/or angiotensin-converting enzyme (ACE) inhibitor and/or angiotensin II antagonist)

Dose
- (Hypertension) 5 mg orally daily **OR**
- (Heart failure) initially 1.25 mg orally daily increasing at 1—2-week intervals to 2.5 mg daily, then 5 mg daily and up to 10 mg daily

Adverse effects
- paraesthesia, hypoaesthesia
- nervousness
- myalgia, back pain
- increased sweating
- chest pain
- see also General Adverse effects of beta adrenoceptor blocking agents (p. 521)

Interactions
- increased serum levels may occur if given with paroxetine and fluoxetine, increasing the risk of excessive adverse effects including bradycardia
- increased hypotension may occur if given with baclofen or amifostine
- see also General Interactions of beta adrenoceptor blocking agents (p. 522)

Nursing considerations/Cautions
- (Hypertension) effects should be seen in 2 weeks; however, may take 4 weeks in some patients
- (Heart failure) condition should be stable with acute heart failure in the last 6 weeks before starting therapy
- (Heart failure) other standard drug therapy (e.g. diuretic, ACE inhibitor and/or angiotensin II antagonist) should be stabilised in 2 weeks before starting nebivolol
- (Heart failure) therapy should be started under medical supervision over at least 2 hours to monitor BP, heart rate, ECG and signs of worsening heart failure to ensure clinical condition remains stable
- (Heart failure) should not be stopped abruptly to prevent worsening heart failure
- tablets contain lactose and are therefore not recommended in those with rare hereditary problems of galactose intolerance, Lapp lactase deficiency or glucose—galactose malabsorption
- contraindicated in those with liver insufficiency or impairment
- see also General Nursing considerations/Cautions for beta adrenoceptor blocking agents (p. 522)

Patient education
- see General Patient education for beta adrenoceptor blocking agents (p. 523)

ANTIHYPERTENSIVE AGENTS

Tablets can be dispersed in water, or crushed and mixed with spoonful of yoghurt or apple puree.

May cause reduced placental perfusion, which can lead to growth retardation, intrauterine death or premature delivery. It may also cause hypoglycaemia and bradycardia in the fetus or newborn. If used during pregnancy, close monitoring of the uteroplacental blood flow and fetal growth is recommended.

Not recommended during breastfeeding as it may cause bradycardia in the infant.

In patients over 65 years old, the recommended starting dose for hypertension is 2.5 mg daily, which may be increased to 5 mg if necessary.

PROPRANOLOL

Trade names
APO-Propranolol, Deralin, Inderal, Propranolol-WGR

Available forms
Tablets: 10 mg, 40 mg, 160 mg

Action
- non-selective beta blocker (blocks both beta1 and beta2 receptors)
- active metabolite
- half-life 3—6 hours
- see also General Actions of beta adrenoceptor blocking agents (p. 521)

Use
- hypertension
- angina
- myocardial infarction
- essential tremor
- migraine prophylaxis
- preoperatively for pheochromocytoma
- cardiac dysrhythmia (including anxiety tachycardia, drug-induced dysrhythmia)
- Fallot's tetralogy (relief of right ventricular outflow tract shutdown)

Dose
- (Hypertension) initially 40 mg orally twice daily, increasing at weekly intervals according to response to 60—160 mg twice daily (daily maximum 320 mg)
- (Angina) 40 mg orally 2—3 times daily, increasing at weekly intervals according to response up to 60—160 mg twice daily
- (Essential tremor) 40 mg orally 2—3 times daily, increasing at weekly intervals according to response to 40—80 mg twice daily
- (Migraine prophylaxis) 40 mg orally twice daily, increasing to 40—80 mg twice daily
- (Myocardial infarction) initially 40 mg orally 4 times daily for 2—3 days, then 80 mg twice daily
- (Preoperatively for pheochromocytoma) 60 mg orally daily for 3 days in divided doses, then 30 mg daily in divided doses (maintenance) (with alpha receptor blockade)
- (Cardiac dysrhythmias) 10—40 mg orally 3—4 times daily
- (Fallot's tetralogy — children) up to 1 mg/kg orally 3—4 times daily

Adverse effects
- (Rare) hearing loss, tinnitus
- see also General Adverse effects of beta adrenoceptor blocking agents (p. 521)

Interactions
- not recommended with lidocaine (lignocaine) as may increase its serum levels
- may increase serum levels of rizatriptan
- increased serum levels may occur if given with alcohol or hydralazine
- propranolol and chlorpromazine given together may result in increased plasma levels of both drugs
- see also General Interactions of beta adrenoceptor blocking agents (p. 522)

Adverse effects/Nursing considerations/Cautions/Patient education
- advise patient to avoid alcohol during therapy
- (Migraine prophylaxis) response generally seen in 12 weeks. If significant

- reduction in frequency of migraine is seen, therapy may be gradually stopped
- increased risk of hepatic encephalopathy
- caution if used in those with liver impairment including decompensated cirrhosis and portal hypertension
- see also General Adverse effects/Nursing considerations/Cautions/Patient education for beta adrenoceptor blocking agents (p. 522)

 Tablets can be dispersed in water, or crushed and mixed with spoonful of yoghurt or apple puree.

 Avoid use. Can reduce placental perfusion, potentially leading to fetal death, premature deliveries or other complications.

 Not recommended during breastfeeding unless benefits outweigh risks. If used, the infant should be monitored for any potential adverse effects.

 Reduced renal function: half-life may be prolonged, potentially necessitating dose adjustments.

Reduced hepatic function: metabolism is slowed in patients with hepatic impairment, requiring careful dose titration and monitoring for adverse effects.

 Start with lower doses and adjust according to response to minimise side effects like bradycardia and hypotension.

CALCIUM-CHANNEL BLOCKERS (CCBs)

General Actions of calcium-channel blockers

- also known as calcium antagonists
- impede the influx of calcium ions into vascular smooth muscle and cardiac muscle during depolarisation, improving myocardial oxygen supply and cardiac output and reducing myocardial work by reducing afterload
- dilate coronary artery decreasing resistance, improving oxygen supply to ischaemic area, as well as improving blood flow to collateral vessels
- dilate peripheral arteries and arterioles, reducing peripheral vascular resistance and therefore BP
- half-life increased in the elderly (e.g. amlodipine, diltiazem, felodipine, verapamil)
- subdivided into:
  - dihydropyridines (e.g. amlodipine, felodipine, nifedipine, nimodipine, lercanidipine, clevidipine)
    - dihydropyridines act mainly on arteriolar smooth muscle to reduce peripheral vascular resistance (relax blood vessels) and BP. They have minimal effect on myocardial cells
  - non-dihydropyridines: phenylalkylamine type (e.g. verapamil), benzothiazepine type (e.g. diltiazem)
    - act on cardiac and arteriolar smooth muscle. They reduce cardiac contractility (negative ionotropic effect), heart rate (negative chronotropic effect) and conduction, reducing the workload of the heart

General Adverse effects of calcium-channel blockers

- headache, dizziness/vertigo, flushing (feeling of warmth), lightheadedness, fatigue, somnolence, asthenia/weakness, malaise
- nausea, vomiting, dyspepsia, constipation, abdominal pain, flatulence, dry mouth
- gingivitis, gingival hyperplasia
- rash, pruritus, urticaria
- AV block, palpitations, tachycardia, hypotension, exacerbation of angina
- (Rare) elevated liver enzymes, severe skin reactions, hyperglycaemia, impotence, gynaecomastia, bronchospasm, asthma aggravation
- Peripheral oedema: dihydropyridines, due to their vasodilatory effects on the arterioles, commonly cause peripheral

ANTIHYPERTENSIVE AGENTS

oedema because of redistribution of extracellular fluid (rather than fluid retention); this does not respond to treatment with diuretics

General Interactions of calcium-channel blockers
- grapefruit juice may increase CCB serum levels (grapefruit juice contains substances known as furanocoumarins, which inhibit the activity of the CYP3A4 enzyme in the liver and intestines that metabolises CCB)
- great caution if used with beta adrenoceptor blocking agents, as may result in profound (potentially life-threatening) bradycardia, heart block and hypotension
- may enhance hypotensive effect of other antihypertensives and diuretics
- excessive cardiovascular depression may occur if given with inhalation anaesthetics
- increased vasodilation (hypotension and faintness) may occur if given with nitrates

General Nursing considerations/Cautions for calcium-channel blockers
- contraindicated in those with sick sinus syndrome (without pacemaker), second- or third-degree AV block (without pacemaker), severe bradycardia (< 40 beats/min), hypotension (< 90 mmHg systolic), severe uncompensated heart failure, cardiogenic shock, unstable angina, within 4–8 weeks of acute myocardial infarction or left ventricular failure with pulmonary congestion
- contraindicated in those with hypersensitivity to calcium-channel blockers
- gingival enlargement can be avoided or reversed by attention to dental hygiene
- ER (extended-release) or SR (slow- or sustained-release) are not bioequivalent to immediate-release tablets and should not be substituted
- (Sustained-release preparation) caution if used in those with previous history of severe gastrointestinal narrowing or obstruction because of the increased risk of bowel obstruction due to the non-conformable nature of sustained-release formulation
- caution if used in those with short bowel syndrome, Crohn's disease, ulcerative colitis or other conditions with chronic diarrhoea, as transit time is shortened, resulting in inadequate serum levels
- caution if used in those with bronchial hyperreactivity, including asthma, as bronchospasm may occur
- caution if used in those with diabetes mellitus
- caution if used in those with aortic stenosis, heart failure, liver or kidney impairment, bradycardia or first-degree AV block

General Patient education for calcium-channel blockers
- patient should be advised that ER (extended-release) or SR (slow- or sustained-release) tablets should be swallowed whole (not divided, crushed or chewed)
- instruct patient to maintain good dental hygiene (e.g. brush teeth twice daily, floss daily) and to attend regular professional teeth cleaning to decrease gingival hyperplasia
- warn patient to immediately report any
  - skin reaction (e.g. red, painful or itchy spots, blisters, skin peeling) that persists
  - wheezing or difficulty breathing
- advise patient not to stop therapy suddenly, as severe angina may occur
- patient should be warned to avoid grapefruit or grapefruit juice during therapy
- patients with diabetes should be instructed to monitor blood glucose levels closely during therapy
- see also General Patient education for antihypertensive agents (p. 500)

Generally not recommended/contraindicated during pregnancy, as these agents have the potential to produce fetal hypoxia associated with maternal hypotension (nifedipine has an accepted indication of preterm labour).

Passes into human breastmilk. Use with caution if breastfeeding, and consider alternatives if possible. If treatment is necessary, monitor the infant for any potential side effects, such as hypotension or feeding issues.

Reduced hepatic function: use with caution. CCBs are primarily metabolised by the liver. Reduced hepatic function may lead to increased plasma concentrations, increasing the risk of side effects. Dose adjustment may be needed.

Start treatment at a lower dose because of the increased risk of side-effects such as hypotension, bradycardia or dizziness.

AMLODIPINE

Trade names
Amlo, Amlodipine GH, Amlodipine Sandoz, Amlodipine-WGR, APO-Amlodipine, Blooms Amlodipine, Blooms the Chemist Amlodipine, Nordip, Norvasc, Pharmacor Amlodipine

Available forms
Tablets: 5 mg, 10 mg

Action
- dihydropyridine
- peak effect 6—12 hours, half-life 35—50 hours
- see also General Actions of calcium-channel blockers (p. 532)

Use
- hypertension
- chronic stable angina (as monotherapy or with other antianginal agents)

Dose
- (Hypertension, angina) 2.5—5 mg orally daily, increasing at 7—14-day intervals to a daily maximum of 10 mg if needed

Interactions
- increased risk of hypotension if given with clarithromycin
- caution if given with simvastatin
- serum levels may be increased if given with erythromycin, itraconazole or ritonavir
- decreased serum levels may occur if given with rifampicin or St John's wort
- may increase serum levels of tacrolimus

Adverse effects/Nursing considerations/Cautions/Patient education
- dose titration should occur over 7—14 days to assess patient response to dose changes
- 5 mg tablets are scored and can be divided for smaller dose
- see also General Adverse effects/Nursing considerations/Cautions/Patient education for calcium-channel blockers (p. 532), General Patient education for antihypertensive agents (p. 500) and General Patient education for antianginal agents (p. 58)

Tablet can be dispersed in water, or crushed and mixed with spoonful of yoghurt or apple puree. Crushed tablet has a bitter taste.

Not recommended during pregnancy unless benefits outweigh risks. Animal studies have shown adverse effects.

Breastfeeding should be discontinued during therapy.

Reduced hepatic function: amlodipine is extensively metabolised by the liver. A lower starting dose and careful monitoring are recommended because of the risk of worsened liver function.

Available in combination with
- amlodipine + atorvastatin (see Atorvastatin in Lipid regulating agents p. 1302)

ANTIHYPERTENSIVE AGENTS

- amlodipine + valsartan + hydrochlorothiazide (see Valsartan in this chapter p. 519)
- amlodipine + olmesartan (see Olmesartan p. 517)
- amlodipine + olmesartan + hydrochlorothiazide (see Olmesartan p. 517)
- amlodipine + perindopril (see Perindopril p. 510)
- amlodipine + telmisartan (see Telmisartan p. 518)

CLEVIDIPINE
Trade name
Cleviprex

Available form
Vial: 0.5 mg/mL

Action
- dihydropyridine
- see also General Actions of calcium-channel blockers (p. 532)

Use
- short-term hypertension management when oral therapy is not feasible or desirable

Dose
- initially 1–2 mg/hour, doubling dose every 90 seconds until BP is approaching target level, then dose adjustments should be every 5–10 minutes until desired target is reached (maximum 32 mg/hour)

Adverse effects
- atrial fibrillation, tachycardia, ventricular tachycardia, supraventricular extrasystoles
- hypotension
- peripheral oedema
- headache, dizziness
- fever, feeling hot, flushing
- polyuria
- atelectasis, pulmonary oedema, wheezing, dyspnoea, pneumonia
- anxiety, restlessness, disorientation, insomnia
- renal insufficiency, acute renal failure
- nausea, vomiting, constipation
- pruritus
- (Rare) congestive cardiac failure, hypersensitivity, decreased oxygen saturation

Interactions
- beta adrenoceptor blocking agents should not be used to treat any clevidipine-induced tachycardia

Nursing considerations/Cautions
- BP and heart rate should be monitored continuously during therapy until vital signs are stable
- dose should be decreased if hypotension and reflex tachycardia occur with worsening clinical outcome
- when transitioning to an oral antihypertensive agent, clevidipine should be titrated downwards or stopped, and BP should continue to be monitored
- if patient is not being transitioned to oral antihypertensive agent, BP and heart rate should continue to be monitored for at least 8 hours after stopping infusion as rebound hypertension may occur
- no more than 1000 mL or an average of 21 mg/mL is recommended per 24 hours because of lipid content
- vial should be inverted gently before infusion to ensure emulsion is evenly distributed
- should not be diluted
- administer alone
- should be used within 12 hours and any remaining solution discarded after this time
- contains 0.2 g lipid/mL (2.0 kcal), which may need to be considered if patient has lipid load restrictions
- caution if used in elderly patients. Patients should be closely monitored and titration of dose started at low end of dose range
- caution if used in those with heart failure, as negative inotropic effects can exacerbate heart failure. If used, patient should be closely monitored during therapy

- not recommended in children or adolescents
- not recommended in those with defective lipid metabolism (e.g. pathological hyperlipidaemia, lipoid nephrosis, acute pancreatitis with hyperlipidaemic) or severe aortic stenosis
- contraindicated in those with known allergies to soybeans, soy products, eggs or egg products

DILTIAZEM

Trade names
Cardizem, Cardizem CD, Vasocardol, Vasocardol CD

Available forms
Tablets: 60 mg;
Capsules (extended-release): 180 mg, 240 mg, 360 mg

Action
- non-dihydropyridine calcium-channel blocker
- decreases conduction through the sinoatrial (SA) and atrioventricular (AV) nodes.
- inhibits coronary artery spasm
- onset of action 30 minutes (immediate-release), 30–60 minutes (controlled-release)
- peak effect 2–3 hours (immediate-release) or 6–11 hours (controlled-release)
- duration of action 4–8 hours (immediate-release) or 12 hours (controlled-release)
- half-life about 3.5 hours (single or chronic dosing)
- see also General Actions of calcium-channel blockers (p. 532)

Use
- chronic stable angina pectoris
- hypertension
- atrial fibrillation or atrial flutter (ventricular rate control)

Dose
- (Hypertension) initially 180–240 mg orally daily, increasing at 2-week intervals to 240–360 mg daily if needed (extended-release capsules) **OR**
- (Angina) initially 30 mg orally 4 times daily before meals and at night, increasing at 1–2-day intervals until response is achieved (usually 180–240 mg) (daily maximum 360 mg) (immediate-release tablets) **OR**
- (Angina) initially 180 mg orally daily, increasing gradually over 7–14 days if needed to 360 mg daily (extended-release capsules)

Adverse effects
- mood changes, depression
- see also General Adverse effects of calcium-channel blockers (p. 532)

Interactions
- contraindicated with dantrolene and ivabradine
- may decrease clearance of some beta adrenoceptor blocking agents, increasing serum levels
- increased risk of bradycardia if given with amiodarone
- increased hypotension may occur if given with alpha adrenoceptor blocking agents
- avoid grapefruit and grapefruit juice
- not recommended with antiarrhythmic agents
- serum levels may be increased by cimetidine or ranitidine
- may increase serum levels of digoxin, theophylline, ciclosporin, cilostazol, methylprednisolone, midazolam, triazolam, phenytoin or carbamazepine, increasing the risk of toxicity; therefore serum levels should be closely monitored especially when starting or stopping therapy
- serum levels may be decreased by diazepam and rifampicin
- increased risk of neurotoxicity if given with lithium
- caution if given with statins, as there is an increased risk of myalgia and rhabdomyolysis due to increased serum levels

ANTIHYPERTENSIVE AGENTS

- caution if given with aspirin, other salicylates or antiplatelets because of the increased risk of bleeding
- increased risk of depression if given with beta adrenoceptor blocking agents
- caution if given with X-ray contrast media because of the increased risk of hypotension
- see also General Interactions of calcium-channel blockers (p. 532)

Nursing considerations/Cautions
- immediate-release tablets are used only as antianginal agents, not as antihypertensives
- sustained-release preparations are recommended only for chronic stable angina, not variant angina
- see also General Nursing considerations/Cautions for calcium-channel blockers (p. 533)

Patient education
- advise patient to seek medical advice if low mood or depression occurs
- see also General Patient education for antianginal agents (p. 58), General Patient education for calcium-channel blockers (p. 533) and General Patient education for antihypertensive agents (p. 500)

Tablet can be crushed and mixed with a spoonful of yoghurt or apple puree.

Capsules can be opened and pellets mixed with yoghurt. Do not crush the controlled-release capsule or the contents.

Not recommended during pregnancy unless benefits outweigh risks.

Avoid use. Excreted in breastmilk.

Reduced renal function: use cautiously; may increase drug levels. Monitor renal function and adjust dose if needed.

Reduced hepatic function: use cautiously; may increase drug levels. Monitor heart rate and adjust dose accordingly.

Elderly patients may have higher plasma concentrations and increased incidence of adverse reactions such as bradycardia, dizziness and peripheral oedema. Careful titration and monitoring is recommended.

FELODIPINE
Trade names
Felodil XR, Felodur ER, Plendil ER

Available forms
Tablets (extended-release): 2.5 mg, 5 mg, 10 mg

Action
- dihydropyridine
- mild natriuretic and diuretic effect
- no effect of conduction or contractility
- onset of action 120–300 minutes, peak effect 2.5–5 hours, duration of action 24 hours, biphasic half-life (4 hours, 24 hours)
- see also General Actions of calcium-channel blockers (p. 532)

Use
- hypertension

Dose
- (Hypertension) initially 2.5–5.0 mg orally daily, increasing gradually to 5–10 mg orally daily (daily maximum 20 mg) (extended-release tablets)

Interactions
- serum levels may be reduced by carbamazepine, phenobarbital (phenobarbitone), rifampicin, phenytoin and St John's wort
- serum levels may be increased if given with grapefruit juice, itraconazole, cimetidine or erythromycin
- may increase serum levels of tacrolimus, increasing the risk of toxicity
- see also General Interactions of calcium-channel blockers (p. 533)

Adverse effects
- mood changes, depression
- see also General Adverse effects of calcium-channel blockers (p. 532)

Nursing considerations/Cautions/Patient education
- (Felodur ER) contains lactose and is not recommended in those with hereditary galactose intolerance or glucose–galactose malabsorption
- advise patient that extended-release tablets should be swallowed whole, not chewed, broken or divided
- patient should be warned to seek medical advice if low mood or depression occurs
- see also General Nursing considerations/Cautions for calcium-channel blockers (p. 533)

 Extended-release tablets should not be broken, chewed or crushed.

Available in combination with
- felodipine 5 mg + ramipril 5 mg (controlled release) (Triasyn 5.0/5.0)

LERCANIDIPINE
Trade names
APX-Lercanidipine, Lercan, Lercanidipine-WGR, Zanidip, Zircol

Available forms
Tablets: 10 mg, 20 mg

Action
- dihydropyridine
- peak effect 1.5–3 hours, duration of action 24 hours
- see also General Actions of calcium-channel blockers (p. 532)

Use
- hypertension

Dose
- (Hypertension) initially 10 mg orally daily at least 15 minutes before food, increasing after 2 weeks to 20 mg if necessary

Interactions
- not recommended with alcohol because of potentiation of vasodilation
- increased serum levels may occur if given with erythromycin, ritonavir, itraconazole and fluoxetine
- decreased serum levels may occur if given with phenytoin, metoprolol, carbamazepine and rifampicin resulting in decreased hypertensive effect
- caution if given with amiodarone or other antiarrhythmic agents
- may increase serum levels of simvastatin
- contraindicated with ciclosporin
- see also General Interactions of calcium-channel blockers (p. 533)

Nursing considerations/Cautions
- food causes increased absorption; therefore should be administered at least 15 minutes before food
- if given in patients undergoing peritoneal dialysis, peritoneal effluent may become cloudy, which can be mistaken for infection
- contraindicated in those with severe renal (creatinine clearance < 12 mL/min) or liver impairment
- see also General Nursing considerations/Cautions for calcium-channel blockers (p. 533)

Patient education
- patients should be advised to avoid alcohol
- food causes an increase in drug absorption; therefore instruct the patient to take medication at least 15 minutes before food
- if patient is taking simvastatin concurrently, advise taking lercanidipine in the morning and simvastatin in the evening
- see also General Patient education for calcium-channel blockers (p. 532) and General Patient education for antihypertensive agents (p. 530)

ANTIHYPERTENSIVE AGENTS

 Tablet can be crushed and mixed with water or spoonful of yoghurt or apple puree.

 Contraindicated in those with severe renal impairment (CrCl < 12 mL/min) or liver impairment.

Available in combination with
- lercanidipine 10 mg + enalapril 10 mg tablet (Zan-Extra 10 mg/10 mg)
- lercanidipine 10 mg + enalapril 20 mg tablet (Zan-Extra 10 mg/20 mg)

NIFEDIPINE
Trade name
APO-Nifedipine XR

Available forms
Tablets (controlled-/modified-release): 30 mg, 60 mg

Action
- dihydropyridine
- inhibits coronary artery spasm
- decreases myocardial oxygen consumption at rest, during exercise and during episodes of coronary artery spasm
- onset of action 15 minutes, peak effect 0.5—1 hour, duration of action 4—8 hours
- elimination may be decreased in South Asian patients
- see also General Actions of calcium-channel blockers (p. 532)

Use
- angina
- mild-to-moderate hypertension
- (Accepted) preterm labour

Dose
- (Hypertension) initially 30 mg orally daily, increasing (or decreasing) at 7—14-day intervals if necessary to 120 mg daily (controlled-/modified-release tablets). Titration to doses above 120 mg/day is not recommended
OR
- (Chronic stable angina) initially 30 mg orally once daily, increasing gradually to 90 mg if needed (controlled-/modified-release tablets)

Interactions
- nifedipine is metabolised via the cytochrome P450 3A4 (CYP3A4) system. Drugs that are known to inhibit or induce CYP3A4 may, therefore, alter the first pass or the clearance of nifedipine
- contraindicated with rifampicin
- serum levels may be increased if given with sodium valproate, fluoxetine, erythromycin, HIV protease inhibitors (e.g. ritonavir) or diltiazem
- may potentiate the effects of salbutamol and terbutaline
- may increase hypotensive effect of candesartan or irbesartan
- may increase serum levels of digoxin increasing the risk of toxicity
- may alter (increase or decrease) serum levels of theophylline; therefore should be given together with caution
- serum levels may be decreased if given with carbamazepine, phenytoin or phenobarbital (phenobarbitone)
- may increase serum level of tacrolimus, increasing risk of toxicity
- may cause false positive result on barium contrast X-ray
- see also General Interactions of calcium-channel blockers (p. 533)

Adverse effects/Nursing considerations/Cautions
- contraindicated within 8 days of acute myocardial infarction or in those with cardiogenic shock or ileostomy after proctocolectomy (Kock pouch)
- see also General Nursing considerations/Cautions for calcium-channel blockers (p. 533)

Patient education
- instruct the patient to swallow tablets whole (not crushed or chewed)):
- see also General Patient education for antianginal agents (p. 58)
- see also General Patient education for calcium-channel blockers (p. 533)

Extended-release tablets should not be crushed, broken or chewed.

NIMODIPINE
Trade names
Nimodipine Juno, Nimotop

Available forms
Tablets: 30 mg;
Infusion solution: 10 mg/50 mL

Action
- dihydropyridine calcium-channel blocker that preferentially dilates cerebral vessels, increasing cerebral perfusion especially in areas of early damage or restricted circulation
- onset of action 15 minutes, peak effect 1—1.5 hours, half-life 1.2—1.8 hours (IV) or 5—10 hours (oral)

Use
- prophylaxis and treatment of ischaemic neurological deficits caused by cerebral vasospasm after subarachnoid haemorrhage caused by ruptured intracranial aneurysm

Dose
- 1 mg/hour by IV infusion for 2 hours, then 2 mg/hour, provided there is no marked decrease in BP **OR**
- initially up to 0.5 mg/hour by IV infusion (if patient < 70 kg or has unstable BP) **OR**
- 60 mg orally every 4 hours for 7 days (following parenteral administration) **OR**
- 60 mg orally every 4 hours for 10—14 days (oral administration only)

Adverse effects
- hypotension, tachycardia, flushing
- nausea, vomiting
- headache
- rash
- thrombocytopenia
- (IV) infusion site reaction, thrombophlebitis
- (Rare) paralytic ileus, bradycardia, abnormal liver function, sweating, pruritus

Interactions
- (Oral) contraindicated with rifampicin, phenytoin, phenobarbital (phenobarbitone) and carbamazepine
- (IV) not recommended with other calcium-channel blockers or antihypertensive agents
- increased serum levels may occur if given within 4 days of grapefruit juice ingestion
- food delays but does not affect the extent of absorption.
- increased serum levels may occur if given with erythromycin, clarithromycin, ritonavir, fluoxetine and sodium valproate; therefore not recommended together
- (IV) increased risk of nephrotoxicity if given with aminoglycosides, cephalosporins, furosemide or other potentially nephrotoxic agents, and renal function monitoring is recommended
- caution if given with doxorubicin or vincristine
- slightly decreased serum levels may occur if given with nortriptyline
- (IV) may decrease clearance of IV zidovudine
- see also General Interactions of calcium-channel blockers (p. 533)

Nursing considerations/Cautions
- BP should be monitored throughout therapy
- start within 4 days of onset of symptoms and continue for at least 7 days (maximum 14 days)
- decreased dose is recommended if patient weighs < 70 kg or has labile BP
- IV should be continued for at least 5 days post aneurysm clipping
- renal function monitoring is recommended if given IV in those with renal disease
- IV solution is light sensitive, although no protective measures are required if used in artificial or diffuse light
- PVC tubing should not be used because it absorbs nimodipine
- administered via a 'bypass' (3-way stop cock) into a running IV infusion (20 mL/

ANTIHYPERTENSIVE AGENTS

hour initially, increasing to 40 mL/hour with increase in nimodipine) using an infusion pump via a central catheter (CVC). Suitable IV fluids include sodium chloride 0.9%, glucose 5%, Hartmann's solution/lactated Ringer's solution, lactated Ringer's solution with magnesium, Dextran 40, mannitol 10%, human albumin and blood
- administer alone
- all infusion tubing should be changed 24-hourly
- IV solution contains 23.7% alcohol (50 g/daily dose) and therefore should be used with caution in those with alcoholism or impaired alcohol metabolism, impaired liver function or epilepsy, or during pregnancy or breastfeeding
- caution if used in those with known raised intracranial pressure, cerebral oedema, kidney and liver dysfunction or in those with hypotension (systolic BP < 100 mmHg)
- caution if used in those with unstable angina or within 28 days of acute myocardial infarction
- see also General Nursing considerations/Cautions for calcium-channel blockers (p. 533)

Patient education
- patient should be instructed to seek medical advice immediately if any of the following occur:
  - lack of bowel motions, stomach pain or cramping
  - irregular heart rate
- see also General Patient education for calcium-channel blockers (p. 533) and General Patient education for antihypertensive agents (p. 500)

Tablet can be crushed and mixed with water or spoonful of yoghurt or apple puree.

VERAPAMIL
Trade names
Anpec, Cordilox SR, Isoptin, Isoptin SR

Available forms
Tablets: 40 mg, 80 mg, 120 mg, 160 mg;
Tablets (sustained-release): 180 mg, 240 mg;
Ampoules: 5 mg/2 mL

Action
- non-dihydropyridine
- class IV antiarrhythmic agent
- increases AV node refractory period and prolongs conduction time
- dilates coronary arteries and arterioles, inhibits coronary artery spasm
- onset of action 1–5 minutes (IV), 1–2 hours (oral)
- peak effect 1–2 hours (oral)
- duration of action 2 hours (IV), 8–10 hours (oral), 24 hours (controlled-release formulation)
- half-life 2.8–7.4 hours (single dose) increasing to 4.5–12 hours (chronic dosing)
- see also General Actions of calcium-channel blockers (p. 532)

Use
- management of unstable angina pectoris or variant (Prinzmetal's) angina
- prophylaxis and management of arrhythmias (e.g. supraventricular arrhythmias)
- hypertension, hypertensive crises

Dose
- (Hypertension) initially 80 mg orally 2–3 times daily, increasing to 160 mg 2–3 times daily if needed **OR**
- (Hypertension) 120–240 mg orally once daily, increasing dose if needed (SR tablets) **OR**
- (Arrhythmias, hypertensive crisis) 5 mg IV bolus over 2–3 minutes, repeated 5–10 minutes later if necessary, then 5–10 mg/hour by IV infusion (up to 100 mg/day) **OR**
- (Tachyarrhythmias) initially 80 mg orally 2 to 3 times daily, increasing to 160 mg 2–3 times daily if needed (immediate-release tablets) **OR**

- (Angina) initially 80 mg orally 2—3 times daily, increasing to 160 mg 2—3 times daily if needed **OR**
- (Angina) 180—240 mg orally once daily, increasing dose to obtain a response if necessary (sustained-release) (daily maximum 480 mg as 2 divided doses)

Adverse effects
- dyspnoea
- (IV, rare) second- to third-degree AV block, bradycardia, transient asystole
- see also General Adverse effects of calcium-channel blockers (p. 532)

Interactions
- avoid combination with beta adrenoceptor blocking agents (unless under specialist supervision) owing to increased risk of severe bradycardia, heart block and left ventricular failure
- contraindicated IV with beta adrenoceptor blocking agents (unless in ICU setting)
- contraindicated with dabigatran etexilate
- may decrease serum lithium levels if verapamil is introduced to stable lithium therapy; therefore serum levels should be closely monitored
- may increase serum levels of digoxin, carbamazepine, everolimus, sirolimus, tacrolimus, midazolam, doxorubicin, imipramine, theophylline, atorvastatin, simvastatin, ciclosporin, glibenclamide and benzodiazepines increasing risk of adverse effects and/or toxicity
- increased serum levels may result if given with erythromycin, clarithromycin and ritonavir
- added cardiac depressant effects may result if given with class 1c antiarrhythmic agents (e.g. flecainide). Cardiac monitoring is recommended if given together
- disopyramide should be discontinued 48 hours before starting therapy and not restarted within 24 hours of stopping verapamil
- may potentiate effects of neuromuscular blocking agents
- may decrease metabolism of alcohol prolonging its effects
- increased bleeding may occur if given with aspirin
- not recommended with colchicine
- not recommended with quinidine in patients with hypertrophic cardiomyopathy
- may increase serum levels of digoxin which may result in excessive bradycardia or AV block
- excessive cardiac depression may occur if given with inhalation anaesthetics; therefore combination should be given with extreme caution
- phenobarbital (phenobarbitone) and phenytoin may decrease serum verapamil levels
- has an additive effect with other antihypertensives, diuretics, vasodilators or antiarrhythmic medications
- antihypertensive effects may be reduced if given with rifampicin or sulfinpyrazone
- hyperkalaemia and myocardial depression may occur if given with IV dantrolene
- if starting simvastatin or atorvastatin with verapamil, lowest dose should be used in the first instance. If adding verapamil to already existing simvastatin or atorvastatin, statin dose should be reduced
- see also General Interactions of calcium-channel blockers (p. 533)

Nursing considerations/Cautions
- given by slow IV over 2 minutes with continuous BP and ECG monitoring during IV therapy and should be stopped if severe hypotension occurs
- liver enzymes should be monitored regularly throughout therapy
- sustained-release preparations are not considered interchangeable
- have noradrenaline (norepinephrine), isoprenaline, atropine (reversing bradycardia, hypotension), dopamine, digoxin

ANTIHYPERTENSIVE AGENTS

- and calcium gluconate monohydrate 10% solution available during IV administration
- may require digoxin pretreatment in the presence of existing congestive cardiac failure
- ensure that correct formulation of tablets is selected because verapamil is available in sustained-release formulation as well as immediate-release formulation
- caution if given to those with supratentorial tumour as increased intracranial pressure may occur during anaesthetic induction
- caution if used in those with advanced Duchenne's muscular dystrophy or decreased neuromuscular transmission (e.g. myasthenia gravis) owing to decrease in neuromuscular transmission. Can precipitate respiratory muscle failure in patients with progressive muscular dystrophy
- contraindicated in those with atrial flutter or fibrillation with accessory bypass tracts (e.g. Wolff-Parkinson-White syndrome), ventricular tachycardia or decreased liver function
- see also General Nursing considerations/Cautions for calcium-channel blockers (p. 533)

Patient education
- see General Patient education for antianginal agents (p. 58)
- see General Patient education for calcium-channel blockers (p. 533) and General Patient education for antihypertensive agents (p. 500)

Plain tablets can be crushed and mixed with spoonful of yoghurt or apple puree.

(Modified-release tablets) should not be chewed, broken or crushed.

Available in combination with
- (Modified release tablet) verapamil 180 mg + trandolapril 2 mg (Tarka 2/180)
- (Modified release tablet) verapamil 240 mg + trandolapril 4 mg (Tarka 4/240)

CENTRALLY ACTING AGENTS

General Actions of centrally acting agents
- central action by stimulating alpha2 adrenoceptors, causing a reduction in sympathetic tone, resulting in reduced heart rate, peripheral vascular resistance and BP
- decrease both supine (lying down) and standing BP

CLONIDINE
Trade names
Catapres, APO-Clonidine, Clonidine Lupin, MZ Clonidine HCl

Available forms
Tablets: 100 microgram, 150 microgram; Ampoules: 150 microgram/mL

Action
- thought to modify the response of peripheral blood vessels to vasoconstricting and vasodilating stimuli (e.g. noradrenaline (norepinephrine), isoprenaline, angiotensin)
- (Oral) onset of action 0.5–1 hour, peak effect 1-3 hours, duration of action 6–12 hours, half-life 9–26 hours
- see also General Actions of centrally acting agents above

Use
- hypertension
- menopausal flushing
- recurrent vascular headache prophylaxis in adults (frequency > once/mth, not relieved by acute attack therapy)
- acute hypertensive crisis (parenteral)
- (Accepted) ADHD
- (Accepted) managing the symptoms of opioid withdrawal (seek specialist advice)
- (Accepted) adjunct analgesic for acute, chronic and cancer pain (seek specialist advice)
- (Accepted) premedication

Dose
- (Hypertension) initially 75 micrograms orally 2–3 times daily, then increasing gradually by 75-microgram increments to 150–300 micrograms orally 3 times daily if needed (daily maximum 900 micrograms) (150-microgram tablets) **OR**
- (Hypertension) initially 50–100 micrograms orally 2–3 times daily, increasing gradually to daily maximum of 600 micrograms in divided doses (100-microgram tablets) **OR**
- (Hypertensive crisis) 150–300 micrograms IM, may be repeated at 3–6-hour intervals if needed **OR**
- (Hypertensive crisis) 150–300 micrograms diluted in 10 mL sodium chloride 0.9% given slowly IV over 5 minutes, may be repeated at 3–6-hour intervals if needed **OR**
- (Migraine prophylaxis, menopausal flushing) initially 25 micrograms orally each morning and night. If necessary, increasing dose to 50 micrograms twice daily after 2 weeks, and then to 75 micrograms twice daily

Adverse effects
- depression, sleep disturbance, dizziness, sedation, headache, fatigue, anxiety, weakness
- erectile dysfunction
- hypotension
- dry mouth, constipation, nausea, vomiting, anorexia, salivary gland pain
- (Uncommon) reduced lacrimal flow, increased blood glucose levels, bradycardia, nasal dryness, blurred vision, pruritus, rash, urticaria, Raynaud's phenomenon

Interactions
- increased risk of QT prolongation and arrhythmias when IV clonidine is given with high-dose IV haloperidol
- bradycardia may be caused or potentiated if given with cardiac glycosides or beta adrenoceptor blocking agents
- if given with beta adrenoceptor blocking agents and therapy is interrupted, beta adrenoceptor blocking agents should be stopped first, followed by clonidine
- antihypertensive activity may be reduced by TCAs and some antipsychotic agents (with alpha receptor blocking effects)
- not recommended with NSAIDs because they decrease the effects of clonidine
- effects decreased if given with alpha2 adrenoceptor blocking agents (e.g. phentolamine)
- caution if used with other antihypertensive agents
- may potentiate the effects of alcohol, sedatives, hypnotics and other centrally acting agents
- increased risk of bradycardia if given with digoxin or beta adrenoceptor blocking agents

Nursing considerations/Cautions
- IM injection should be given while the patient is supine
- there may be a transient hypertensive response of 5–10 mmHg lasting for about 5 minutes after IV injection (reduced by slower IV administration)
- withdrawal from oral therapy should be gradual over 7 days or more to avoid rebound hypertension, especially if taking high doses
- regular ophthalmological examination is recommended if therapy is prolonged
- score and carefully divide tablet for doses under 100 microgram
- (Migraine) if frequency of attacks decreases significantly, dose should be reduced and gradually stopped
- tablets contain lactose and are not recommended in those with galactose intolerance
- ampoule contains 3.3 mg sodium per ampoule
- should be used for only one indication at a time (e.g. if used for migraine, should

ANTIHYPERTENSIVE AGENTS

not be used as antihypertensive concurrently)
- caution if used in the elderly or those with history of depression, advanced cerebrovascular disease, diabetes mellitus, mild-to-moderate bradyarrhythmias, cerebral or peripheral perfusion disorders, polyneuropathy, history of constipation, recent myocardial infarction or renal insufficiency
- contraindicated in those with sick sinus syndrome, second- or third-degree AV block, severe coronary disease or heart failure

Patient education

- patient wearing contact lenses should be warned about reduced lacrimal flow
- patient should be advised to avoid driving or operating machinery if dizziness or blurred vision are ongoing problems
- those with diabetes mellitus should be instructed to closely monitor blood glucose levels during therapy
- patient should be warned to avoid alcohol during therapy
- see also General Patient education for antihypertensive agents (p. 500)

 Tablet can be dispersed in water or crushed and mixed with spoonful of yoghurt or apple puree (has bitter taste).

 May cause fetal bradycardia and also elevated blood glucose in the newborn; therefore it is used during pregnancy only if the benefits outweigh the risks and other antihypertensives are preferred. Should not be used IV during pregnancy.

 May decrease prolactin secretion and lower milk supply. Clonidine passes into breastmilk. Limited data are available; generally not recommended.

 Caution if used in those with kidney or liver impairment, as half-life is prolonged.

METHYLDOPA

Trade names
Aldomet, Hydopa

Available form
Tablets: 250 mg

Action
- active metabolite thought to stimulate central alpha2 receptors reducing sympathetic outflow to heart, kidneys and peripheral blood vessels
- no direct action on cardiac function, with little effect on kidney function
- may decrease renin activity
- peak effect 4–6 hours (single dose) or 48–72 hours (multiple dosing); duration of action 12–24 hours (single dose) or 24–48 hours (multiple dosing)
- see also General Actions of centrally acting agents (p. 543)

Use
- hypertension

Dose
- (Hypertension) initially 250 mg orally 2–3 times daily for 2 days, then increased/decreased gradually at 2-day intervals as required (daily maximum 3 g)

Adverse effects
- transient drowsiness/sedation, headache, weakness/asthenia, dizziness, lightheadedness, impaired mental acuity
- postural hypotension, oedema and associated weight gain
- bradycardia, carotid sinus hypersensitivity, aggravation of angina, AV block
- depression, mild reversible psychoses, nightmares, anxiety
- nausea, vomiting, dry mouth, sore or 'black' tongue, flatulence, abdominal distension, constipation or diarrhoea, colitis
- fever (usually in first 3 weeks of therapy)
- rash, eczema
- nasal stuffiness
- impotence, decreased libido

- mild arthralgia (with or without joint swelling), myalgia
- abnormal liver function tests, jaundice (with or without fever), hepatitis
- breast enlargement, gynaecomastia, lactation, hyperprolactinaemia, amenorrhoea
- (Prolonged therapy) positive Coombs' test
- (Rare, but serious requiring prompt discontinuation) haemolytic anaemia, leucopenia, thrombocytopenia, bone marrow depression, hepatic necrosis

Interactions

- enhanced hypotension when given with thiazide diuretics and antihypertensive agents
- contraindicated with MAOIs
- bioavailability may be reduced if given with oral iron (or multivitamin preparations containing iron)
- may increase serum lithium levels, increasing the risk of lithium toxicity; therefore serum levels should be closely monitored, especially when starting or stopping therapy or adjusting dose
- antihypertensive effect may be reduced if given with TCAs
- reduced doses of anaesthetic agents may be needed if given together
- may cause fluorescence in urine samples; therefore will interfere with diagnosis of pheochromocytoma

Nursing considerations/Cautions

- urine may darken on exposure to air
- differential blood counts and liver function tests should be monitored for first 6—12 weeks of therapy or if patient has unexplained fever
- if dose increase is required and patient has previously experienced sedation, evening dose should be first increased
- if patient requires blood transfusion and has had positive Coombs' test, retesting using indirect Coombs' test is recommended to prevent possibility of incompatible blood transfusion occurring
- hypertension returns within 48 hours of stopping therapy
- caution if used in those with impaired kidney or liver function or history of depression
- contraindicated in those with active cirrhosis, acute hepatitis, porphyria, pheochromocytoma or paraganglioma, haemolytic anaemia, sulfite sensitivity or methyldopa-induced liver disorder

Patient education

- advise patients that they may feel dizzy on standing when they first start taking this medicine or when the dose is increased. Patients should get up gradually from sitting or lying to reduce risk of falls and fracture
- advise patient that sedation usually lasts 2—3 days when therapy is started or dose is increased
- patient should be warned that fever occasionally occurs in first 3 weeks of therapy
- patient should be instructed to seek medical advice immediately if any of the following occur:
  - any fever (especially in first 12 weeks of therapy)
  - yellowing of eyes or skin, tiredness, loss of appetite, upper abdominal pain, dark urine, pale stools
  - fever, chills, sore throat, mouth ulcers
  - tiredness, pallor, shortness of breath
  - feelings of lowered mood or depression
- instruct patient to separate any iron supplements or vitamins (containing iron) by at least 2 hours from therapy
- see also General Patient education for antihypertensive agents (p. 500)

 Tablet can be dispersed in water or crushed and mixed with spoonful of yoghurt or apple puree.

 Safe to use. It is used to treat hypertension in pregnancy.

ANTIHYPERTENSIVE AGENTS

 Compatible with breastfeeding. Safe in usual dosage

 Caution if used in those with liver dysfunction or previous liver disease.

MOXONIDINE
Trade names
Moxotens, Physiotens, APO-Moxonidine, ARX-Moxonidine, Moxonidine GH, Moxonidine GX, Moxonidine Viatris, Moxonidine-WGR

Available forms
Tablets: 0.2 mg, 0.4 mg

Action
- centrally acting antihypertensive, which differs from others in this class because it has a low affinity for alpha2 adrenoreceptors
- also binds to I_1-imidazoline receptors decreasing sympathetic tone
- decreases systemic vascular resistance reducing arterial BP
- heart rate, cardiac output and stroke volume are unaffected
- half-life 2.2–2.8 hours

Use
- hypertension

Dose
- initially 0.2 mg orally mane, increasing after a 2-week interval to 0.4 mg (single or divided dose, morning and evening). If unsatisfactory response after 2 weeks, dose increased to 0.6 mg (as a divided dose) (single-dose maximum 0.4 mg or daily maximum as divided dose 0.6 mg)

Adverse effects
- asthenia, headache, dizziness, somnolence, sleep disturbance
- anxiety
- vertigo
- dry mouth, diarrhoea, nausea
- (Uncommon) sedation, insomnia, rash, pruritus, urticaria, peripheral oedema
- (Rare) hypotension, postural hypotension, angioedema

Interactions
- hypotensive effect enhanced if given with other antihypertensive agents
- may intensify effects of sedatives, hypnotics and benzodiazepines
- not recommended with TCAs or alcohol

Nursing considerations/Cautions
- if therapy is concurrent with beta adrenoceptor blocking agent and stopping is required, beta adrenoceptor blocking agent should be stopped first, followed by monoxidine several days later to prevent rebound hypertension. BP should be closely monitored during this time
- tablets contain lactose and are therefore not recommended in those with rare hereditary problems of galactose intolerance, Lapp lactase deficiency or glucose–galactose malabsorption
- caution if used in those with history of angioneurotic oedema, severe coronary artery disease, unstable angina, predisposition to AV block (including those with first-degree AV block)
- caution if used in those with moderate kidney impairment (GFR $> 30 < 60$ mL/min, serum creatinine $> 105 < 160$ micromol/L). Dose should not exceed 0.4 mg as daily divided dose or 0.2 mg as single daily dose
- not recommended in those with intermittent claudication, Raynaud's disease/syndrome, Parkinson's disease, epilepsy, depression or glaucoma
- contraindicated in those over 75 years or with heart failure, bradycardia (< 50 beats/min), severe bradyarrhythmias (e.g. sick sinus syndrome), AV block (second or third degree), malignant arrhythmias or severe kidney impairment (GFR < 30 mL/min or serum creatinine > 160 micromol/L)

Patient education
- patient should be instructed to immediately seek medical advice if any unusual swelling of face, eyes, lips,

- inside nose, mouth or throat or shortness of breath or breathing difficulties occur
- see also General Patient education for antihypertensive agents (p. 500)

 Tablet can be dispersed in water or crushed and mixed with spoonful of yoghurt or apple puree.

 Not recommended during pregnancy unless benefits outweigh risks.

 Not recommended during breastfeeding owing to lack of safety data.

 Caution if used in those with moderate kidney impairment. Dose should not exceed 0.4 mg as a daily divided dose or 0.2 mg as a single daily dose. Contraindicated in those with severe kidney impairment.

 Contraindicated in those over 75 years.

DIRECT ACTING VASODILATORS

DIAZOXIDE
Trade name
DBL Diazoxide Solution for Injection BP

Available form
Ampoules: 15 mg/mL

Action
- reduces elevated BP by activation of potassium channels resulting in relaxation of constricted smooth muscle in the peripheral arterioles (vasodilation), which reduces peripheral resistance
- reflex increase in heart rate and cardiac output
- increases blood glucose levels
- onset of action 1 minute, peak effect 2—5 minutes, duration 2—12 hours, long elimination half-life (28 hours)

Use
- hypertensive crises (e.g. acute glomerular nephritis)
- malignant hypertension (emergency management)
- reduce danger of haemorrhage in hypertensive patients undergoing renal biopsy or arteriography
- control of chronic hypertension before starting oral antihypertensive therapy

Dose
- 1—3 mg/kg as an IV bolus over 30 seconds (up to a maximum of 150 mg), may be repeated at 5—15-minute intervals if required **OR**
- 300 mg as an IV bolus over 30 seconds, every 4-24 hrs as needed for up to 5 days

Adverse effects
- transient nausea, vomiting, abdominal cramps
- transient hyperglycaemia
- sodium and water retention (and therefore weight gain, oedema and possibly congestive cardiac failure)
- headache, sensation of warmth, flushing, sweating, lightheadedness, transient weakness, burning/itching, dizziness
- (Local) pain, sensation of warmth along vein
- (Rare) rash, fever, leucopenia, thrombocytopenia, severe hypotension

Interactions
- may potentiate antihypertensive effect of other antihypertensive agents
- diuretics may enhance hyperglycaemic, hyperuricaemic and hypotensive effects of diazoxide
- hyperglycaemic effect may be potentiated if hypokalaemia is present

Nursing considerations/ Cautions
- must be given undiluted IV rapidly over 30 seconds for maximum effect as slow administration may reduce effectiveness

ANTIHYPERTENSIVE AGENTS

- may be repeated at 4–24-hour intervals for up to 5 days if needed, then replaced with oral antihypertensive agent
- avoid extravasation during IV administration as it can cause cellulitis and pain. If extravasation occurs, it is recommended to treat the affected area with cold packs
- not given SC or IM because of high alkalinity
- patient should remain recumbent during and for 30 minutes after IV bolus
- BP is recorded before and at 1-minute intervals after IV bolus for the first 5 minutes, then at 5-minute intervals until BP has stabilised, then hourly
- if patient is ambulant, final BP should be measured while patient is standing
- blood counts are recommended if therapy is prolonged
- serum uric acid should be monitored if patient has a history of hyperuricaemia or gout
- monitor blood glucose levels daily
- diuretic may be necessary if sodium and water retention occur
- has a very long half-life (28 hours); therefore patient should be observed carefully for a longer period if overdosage occurs
- incompatible with hydralazine, lidocaine (lignocaine) and propranolol
- caution if used in those with renal insufficiency, impaired carbohydrate metabolism (including diabetes mellitus), impaired cardiac or cerebral circulation or uraemia (e.g. gout)
- contraindicated in those with hypersensitivity to diazoxide or other thiazide derivatives, or with hypertension caused by mechanical obstruction (e.g. aortic coarctation)

Patient education

- see General Patient education for antihypertensive agents (p. 500)

Safety in pregnancy has not been established and may inhibit uterine contractions if given during labour. Also, enters fetal circulation and may cause fetal bradycardia and hyperglycaemia in the newborn.

Not recommended during breastfeeding owing to lack of safety data.

HYDRALAZINE
Trade names
Alphapress, Apresoline

Available forms
Tablets: 25 mg, 50 mg;
Ampoule: 20 mg

Action
- causes direct relaxation of arteriolar smooth muscle reducing peripheral vascular resistance (little effect on veins)
- reflex increase in heart rate, stroke volume and cardiac output
- causes sodium and fluid retention
- increases renal blood flow and plasma renin activity
- maintains cerebral blood flow
- increased risk of toxicity due to decreased metabolism in some Caucasians and Asians
- onset of action 45 minutes (oral), 10–20 minutes (IV)
- peak effect 1 hour (oral), 15–30 minutes (IV)
- duration of action 3–8 hours, plasma half-life 2-3 hours depending on acetylator phenotype

Use
- moderate-to-severe drug-resistant hypertension (with other antihypertensive agents)
- hypertensive crises (especially in pre-eclampsia and eclampsia) (see Pregnancy, childbirth and breastfeeding, p. 1456)

Dose
- (Hypertension) initially 25 mg orally twice daily, increasing over several

549

weeks, maintenance 50–200 mg in 2 divided doses

Adverse effects
- flushing, tachycardia, palpitations, hypotension, angina, ECG changes
- headache
- arthralgia, myalgia, joint swelling
- stuffy nose
- rash
- peripheral neuritis
- diarrhoea, nausea, vomiting, anorexia
- lupus-like syndrome syndrome (fever, rash, arthralgia, anaemia)
- (Uncommon) proteinuria, anaemia, leucopenia, purpura, agranulocytosis, dizziness, increased lacrimation

Interactions
- caution if given with MAOIs as severe hypotension may occur
- hypotensive effect may be enhanced if given with other antihypertensive agents, vasodilators, diuretics, TCAs, antipsychotic agents or alcohol
- may increase bioavailability of beta-adrenoceptor blocking agents
- enhanced cardiac effects if given with adrenaline (epinephrine)
- hypotensive effect may be antagonised by NSAIDs or oestrogens
- increased hypotension may occur if given just before or after diazoxide

Nursing considerations/Cautions
- daily dose > 100 mg should be avoided to decrease risk of SLE-like syndrome
- (Long-term therapy) urinalysis, full blood examination (FBE) and antinuclear factor (ANF) should be monitored 6-monthly. Microhaematuria and/or proteinuria with positive ANF titres may indicate early SLE-like syndrome
- may cause hypotension during surgery, which should not be corrected with adrenaline (epinephrine) owing to increased heart rate effects
- women are at greater risk of SLE-like syndrome
- not recommended in those with kidney or liver impairment, heart failure or until post-infarction stabilisation has occurred
- caution if used in those with coronary artery disease (beta-adrenoceptor blocking agent should be started at least 3 days before hydralazine) or angina
- caution if used in those with cerebrovascular disease, as ischaemia may occur
- contraindicated in those with SLE or related diseases, severe tachycardia, heart failure with high cardiac output (e.g. thyrotoxicosis), myocardial insufficiency with aortic/mitral valve stenosis, constrictive pericarditis, dissecting aortic aneurysm, cor pulmonale, porphyria, dissecting aortic aneurysm or hypersensitivity to dihydrazine

Patient education
- may cause dizziness, especially at the beginning of treatment; if you experience this, avoid driving or operating machinery
- advise patient to avoid alcohol during therapy
- patient should be instructed to immediately report any:
  - joint pain, fever and skin rash
  - chest pain
- see also General Patient education for antihypertensive agents (p. 500)

 Tablet can be dispersed in water or crushed and mixed with spoonful of yoghurt or apple puree.

 May cause fetal distress and arrhythmias if given during the third trimester and should be used only if benefits are thought to outweigh risks.

 Not recommended during unless benefits are thought to outweigh risks.

 Caution if used in those with liver dysfunction or kidney impairment (CrCl < 30 mL/min). Dose or dosing interval may need to be adjusted to the clinical response to avoid accumulation and adverse effects.

ANTIHYPERTENSIVE AGENTS

MINOXIDIL
Trade names
Loniten, Regaine, Hair A-Gain

Available forms
Tablets: 10 mg;
Topical solution: 20 mg/mL, 50 mg/mL;
Foam: 50 mg/mL

Action
- selectively relaxes arteriolar smooth muscle reducing peripheral vascular resistance, lowering BP (little effect on veins)
- reflex-mediated increase in cardiac output
- increases plasma renin activity
- onset of action 30 minutes, peak effect 2–3 hours, half-life 4–4.5 hours, hypotensive action lasts 24 hours

Use
- as adjunctive therapy with beta adrenoceptor blocking drugs and diuretics in adults with severe refractory hypertension (Loniten)
- alopecia androgenetica (hereditary or common baldness/hairloss) (Hair A-Gain, Regaine) (see Minoxidil in Dermatological agents, p. 1034)

Dose
- (Hypertension) initially 5 mg orally daily, increasing by 5–10 mg at 3-day intervals to 50 mg, then increasing at 25 mg daily increments to 100 mg as a single or divided dose if needed (daily maximum 100 mg)

Adverse effects
- fluid and salt retention, oedema, weight gain
- nausea, vomiting, anorexia
- reversible hypertrichosis, hair colour changes
- pericarditis, tachycardia, pericardial effusion, ECG changes, cardiac tamponade
- (Rare) rash, leucopenia, thrombocytopenia, pleural effusion, breast tenderness

Interactions
- hypotensive effects may be enhanced by other antihypertensive agents
- must be given with a diuretic to avoid fluid retention and a beta adrenoceptor blocking agent to control reflex cardiovascular effects (or methyldopa sesquihydrate or clonidine if beta adrenoceptor blocking agent is contraindicated)

Nursing consideration/Cautions
- (Heart failure) weight, fluid and electrolyte balance should be carefully monitored and diuretic given if fluid retention occurs. Diuretic therapy +/− salt restriction may be recommended if fluid retention occurs
- not recommended for labile or mild hypertension, or for an extended time in those with hypertension improved by surgery or with myocardial infarction until post-infarction stabilisation has occurred
- caution if used in those with unstable or recently diagnosed angina pectoris, pulmonary hypertension with mitral valve regurgitation or those with symptomatic heart failure as deterioration may occur
- caution if used in those with symptomatic heart failure as fluid retention may cause worsening
- contraindicated in those with phaeochromocytoma and pulmonary hypertension caused by mitral valve stenosis

Patient education
- warn patient of unusual growth, thickening and darkening of fine body hair (face, arms and back), which usually occurs within 3–6 weeks of starting therapy and disappears within 1–3 months of stopping. Hair may also show colour change
- patient should be advised that excessive salt and water retention reduce effectiveness; therefore restrict dietary salt and take diuretic if prescribed
- advise patient to immediately report any:

- puffiness or swelling of face, eyes, ankles, hands or feet
- weight gain (especially if > 2 kg)
- increase in heart rate or chest pain
- see also General Patient education for antihypertensive agents (p. 500)

 Tablet can be dispersed in water or crushed and mixed with spoonful of yoghurt or apple puree.

 Not recommended during pregnancy or in women of childbearing potential not using contraception.

Oral minoxidil can cause fetal minoxidil syndrome, which may cause neonatal hypertrichosis (excessive hair growth), congenital heart defects, neurodevelopmental anomalies and kidney, gastrointestinal and limb malformations.

 Not recommended during breastfeeding unless benefits outweigh risks.

SODIUM NITROPRUSSIDE
Trade names
DBL Sodium Nitroprusside Concentrated Injection, Nitroprusside SXP, Sodium Nitroprusside Baxter, Sodium Nitroprusside Medsurge

Available form
Vial: 50 mg/2 mL

Action
- potent short-acting IV agent that relaxes vascular smooth muscle, producing peripheral vasodilation by a direct action on vascular smooth muscle, more active on veins than arteries
- decreases preload and afterload, improving cardiac output
- metabolised to cyanide and cyanmethaemoglobin. Ordinarily, the body deals with cyanide by combining it with thiosulfate to produce thiocyanate, which is excreted in the urine. Cyanide also binds to erythrocytic methaemoglobin and mitochondrial cytochromes. However, when the mitochondrial cytochromes become saturated, there is a switch from aerobic to anaerobic metabolism producing lactic acid
- onset of action/peak effect within minutes, half-life 2 minutes, half-life of thiosulfate 3 days (prolonged if kidney failure exists)
- duration of effect 1–10 minutes after stopping infusion

Use
- hypertensive crises
- elective hypotension to reduce surgical haemorrhage
- short-term management of cardiac failure

Dose
- initially 0.3 microgram/kg/min by IV infusion, then titrated upwards to a maximum of 10 microgram/kg/min if needed

Adverse effects
- (If too rapid reduction in BP) nausea, vomiting/retching, abdominal pain, flushing, sweating, muscle twitching, anxiety, agitation, restlessness, dizziness, headache, palpitations
- excessive postural hypotension, tachycardia, bradycardia, ECG changes
- rash, flushing, skin irritation
- methaemoglobinaemia
- thrombocytopenia
- (Prolonged administration or excessive dose) thiocyanate toxicity (tinnitus, miosis, hyperreflexia, blurred vision, ataxia, headache, nausea, vomiting, shortness of breath, delirium, psychosis, confusion, coma)
- rare but life-threatening cyanide toxicity (hypotension, metabolic acidosis, pink colour (skin, mucous membranes), shallow breathing, decreased reflexes, widely dilated pupils, coma)
- signs of hypothyroidism
- increased intracranial pressure
- (IV site) reddened, venous streaking

Interactions
- hypotensive action enhanced by other antihypertensive agents, inhalation anaesthetics, negative inotropes and most other circulatory depressants

ANTIHYPERTENSIVE AGENTS

- hypertension and pretreatment with antihypertensive agents may sensitise patient to the effects of sodium nitroprusside and therefore risk of cyanide poisoning
- thiocyanate interferes with iodine uptake in thyroid gland

Nursing considerations/Cautions

- protect from light to avoid degradation
- monitor BP closely to avoid life-threatening hypotension. BP should not be allowed to drop rapidly (systolic BP should not be less than 60 mmHg). Venous oxygen level and acid–base balance should be measured frequently. Patient should also be monitored closely for any signs of air hunger, confusion or metabolic (lactic) acidosis, which is indicative of cyanide poisoning. However, acidosis is not a reliable indication of cyanide poisoning because it is a late sign appearing about 1 hour after dangerous cyanide levels have been reached. Patient should also be monitored for retching or vomiting, muscular twitching, sweating and/or agitation as these are signs of a rapid drop in BP
- patient should remain recumbent during infusion to avoid severe postural hypotensive effects
- if severe hypotension occurs, infusion should be stopped and patient placed in a head-down (Trendelenburg) position to maximise venous return
- if BP is not controlled within 10 minutes at maximum infusion rate, therapy should be stopped immediately
- (Elective hypotension for surgery) any pre-existing anaemia and/or hypovolaemia should be corrected before starting therapy
- (Acute congestive heart failure) infusion rate should be titrated to haemodynamic monitoring results and urine output. Oral therapy should be commenced as soon as possible
- BP returns to pretreatment levels within 1–10 minutes of infusion being stopped or slowed
- if patient is receiving maximum rate (10 microgram/kg/min) and has impaired oxygen delivery, methaemoglobin levels should be closely monitored
- dilute concentrated solution in 500 mL glucose 5% (100 microgram/mL) or 1000 mL glucose 5% (50 microgram/mL), depending on the desired concentration
- no other drugs to be added as solution becomes highly coloured (blue, green, dark red), even if small quantities of organic or inorganic substances are mixed with IV solution. If colour occurs, solution should be discarded
- protect from light by wrapping immediately in aluminium foil, black plastic sheeting or some other opaque material. However, it is not necessary to protect drip chamber
- burette, infusion pump or micro-drip regulator should be used to deliver the IV solution
- infusion rate should not exceed 2 microgram/kg/min as this will lead to the accumulation of cyanide ions
- avoid extravasation
- when infusion is stopped, IV tubing should be changed to prevent any extra administration from residual solution in tubing
- simultaneous infusion of sodium thiosulfate pentahydrate (rate 5–10 times rate of sodium nitroprusside infusion) should prevent cyanide poisoning from occurring
- cyanide toxicity may be treated with sodium nitrite (4–6 mg/kg), followed by sodium thiosulfate pentahydrate (150–200 mg/kg). This may be repeated after a 2-hour interval at half the previous dose if needed
- if haemodialysis is used in overdose, it does not remove cyanide, but does remove thiocyanate

- caution if used in the elderly (because of increased sensitivity to hypotension), those with known raised intracranial pressure, hypothyroidism, severe renal or liver dysfunction or hypothermia
- not recommended for compensatory hypertension owing to arteriovenous shunt or coarctation of the aorta
- contraindicated in those with acute congestive heart failure associated with decreased peripheral vascular resistance, arteriovenous shunt or coarctation of the aorta, uncorrected anaemia or hypovolaemia, inadequate cerebral circulation, severe renal disease, congenital optic atrophy or tobacco amblyopia or vitamin B_{12} deficiency disorder

Short-term use for the control of hypertensive crises may be safe provided that the pH and cyanide concentrations in maternal blood are monitored.

Not recommended during breastfeeding unless benefits are thought to outweigh risks. Breastfeeding is not recommended if used > 24 hours.

Renal impairment may reduce excretion of thiocyanate and increase risk of toxicity.

Patients with hepatic dysfunction are at increased risk of cyanide poisoning. Avoid use in severe hepatic impairment.

ANTIMALARIAL AGENTS

Malaria is the major parasitic illness in tropical and subtropical countries. In 2022, there were an estimated 249 million cases globally, resulting in 608,000 deaths across 85 countries, according to the World Health Organization (WHO). The WHO African Region carries the highest burden, with approximately 94% of all malaria cases (233 million) and 95% of malaria deaths (580,000) occurring in this region. Children under five accounted for 80% of all malaria deaths in 2022 (WHO 2024c).

Malaria is spread by *Plasmodium* parasites, transmitted through the bites of infected female *Anopheles* mosquitoes (malaria vectors). Five species are known to cause malaria in humans (*Plasmodium vivax, P. ovule, P. falciparum, P. malariae, P. knowlesi*). *P. vivax* and *P. falciparum* pose the greatest threat, with *P. falciparum* responsible for the most malaria-related deaths worldwide, being most prevalent in Africa (White & Ashley 2018; WHO 2024c).

Initial symptoms of malaria begin 10 to 15 days after the infected mosquito bite and include headache, fatigue, muscle and joint aches, abdominal discomfort and lethargy (similar to symptoms of any simple viral illness), followed by fever, chills, sweating, anorexia, vomiting and worsening malaise. Infections with *P. vivax* or *P. ovule* have cycles of fever spikes, chills and rigors that occur at regular intervals, weeks to months after the first infection. If left untreated or treated ineffectively, the parasites continue to replicate and severe disease may result (especially if due to *P. falciparum*), which may be fatal (White & Ashley 2018; WHO 2024c).

The malarial life cycle

The infected mosquito feeds on a human and, in doing so, injects sporozoites into the bloodstream. The sporozoites enter the liver's hepatocytes where they multiply and develop into exo-erythrocytic (pre-erythrocytic or tissue) schizonts. Schizonts of *P. vivax* and *P. ovule* may lie dormant in the liver and are responsible for relapses (primaquine acts at this point) (White & Ashley 2018).

After 5—16 days, tissue schizonts rupture, releasing merozoites into the bloodstream, where they invade erythrocytes (blood, or erythrocytic, stage) (quinine, mefloquine and proguanil act at this point). Merozoites multiply asexually and mature, causing the erythrocytes to rupture, releasing the matured asexual merozoites (after 48—72 hours), which then invade more erythrocytes and continue the multiplying, maturing and rupturing cycle (this produces the clinical symptoms of slowly rising temperature, shaking chills, rapidly rising temperature and profuse sweating). Within these infected erythrocytes, some merozoites also develop into male and female gametocytes (White & Ashley 2018).

A non-infected mosquito then feeds on the infected human, ingesting male and female gametocytes, which then multiply sexually and develop into sporozoites. Some of these sporozoites migrate to the mosquito's salivary glands and will subsequently infect the next person the mosquito feeds on (the mosquito life cycle is 8—35 days, depending on the species of parasite and temperature) (White & Ashley 2018).

Treatment

Before starting any treatment, it is essential that malaria is confirmed using a diagnostic test (e.g. thick and thin blood smears), rather than relying on symptoms alone. Repeat blood smears every 12—24 hours for 48 hours if the first smears are negative, but malaria is strongly suspected (White & Ashley 2018; WHO 2024c).

Many of the original treatments for malaria were herbal based (such as quinine, extracted from tree bark). Unfortunately, *P. falciparum* developed resistance to chloroquine in the 1950s and since then multiple drug resistance has made prophylaxis and treatment very difficult in many areas of the world. The choice of antimalarial should therefore be based on sensitivity of the infecting parasite, with chloroquine being considered first-line treatment for non-*falciparum* malarias, except in areas (such as Indonesia and Papua New Guinea) where high levels of resistance in *P. vivax* are present (White & Ashley 2018).

The first-line treatment of uncomplicated *P. falciparum* malaria has shifted to artemisinin-based combination therapies (ACTs), e.g. artemether + lumefantrine. ACTs work by combining an artemisinin derivative with another antimalarial drug to reduce parasite load quickly and prevent resistance from developing. These therapies are also suitable for treating other types of malaria, such as *P. vivax*.

Resistance to ACTs has emerged, particularly in Southeast Asia, including Vietnam, Cambodia, Thailand, Laos and Myanmar. This resistance, known as partial artemisinin resistance, reduces the effectiveness of ACTs by slowing the clearance of parasites from the bloodstream. The risk of multi-drug resistance spreading to other regions, particularly sub-Saharan Africa, is a significant concern for global malaria control efforts. The WHO closely monitors these resistance patterns to guide treatment policies and strategies (WHO 2024c)

Prevention

Malaria transmission can be prevented by controlling the vector (mosquito). Successful programs have included the use of insecticide-treated nets for sleeping and spraying indoors with

ANTIMALARIAL AGENTS

insecticides. In 2015, the WHO recommended a large clinical trial be carried out to evaluate a vaccine (RTS, S) against *P. falciparum*, which is currently being piloted in three African countries with promising results including preventing about 4 in 10 cases of malaria in children over a 4-year period (WHO 2023c).

Other agents used for prevention and treatment include doxycycline (see Antibacterial agents, p. 195) and hydroxychloroquine (see Disease-modifying antirheumatic drugs (DMARDS), p. 1045).

General Patient education for people travelling in malarial areas

- prophylactic antimalarial therapy may not always prevent malaria
- travellers should purchase their prophylactic antimalarials from a reputable source before going into a malarious country, as there have been issues with counterfeit and substandard drugs in some countries
- prophylactic antimalarial therapy should be started 2 days to 2 weeks (depending on the drug) before departure and generally continued for 4 weeks after leaving the endemic area (except for atovaquone–proguanil or primaquine, which can be stopped 1 week after leaving the endemic area). Starting the prophylactic antimalarial therapy before departure will allow a therapeutic blood concentration to build up before entering the endemic area, as well as detecting any adverse effects
- avoid being out at dusk or in the early night hours when mosquitoes feed
- wear long sleeves and long pants and avoid dark colours
- avoid using colognes and perfumes because these may attract mosquitoes
- use a recommended insect repellent containing up to 10–35% diethyl-toluamide (commonly known as DEET); however, it is not recommended for young children. Insect repellent containing 7% picaridin can also be used
- use mosquito nets, ensuring that the nets have no holes and are tucked into mattresses
- close windows and doors at night if they do not have screens
- if possible, use pyrethroid mosquito coils at night
- seek medical advice promptly if fever, malaise, headache, backache, muscle ache and/or weakness, vomiting, diarrhoea or cough develop within 1 week of entering a known malarial area.

Malaria and pregnancy

Pregnant women are advised to avoid travelling to malarial areas if possible. Malaria can result in miscarriage and low birthweight, as well as increasing the risk of maternal death (White & Ashley 2019b).

ARTEMETHER AND LUMEFANTRINE

Trade name
Riamet

Available forms
Tablets and Tablets (dispersible): artemether 20 mg/lumefantrine 120 mg

Action
- schizonticide
- both drugs inhibit the conversion of haem (toxic) to haemozoin (non-toxic) and also inhibit nucleic acid synthesis in the parasite
- lumefantrine interferes with polymerisation step

- artemether is a derivative of artemisinin and produces reactive metabolites
- ratio is 1:6 (artemether:lumefantrine)
- artemether has an active metabolite
- antimalarial effect of combination is greater than either substance alone. Clears gametocytes from blood in less than a week and more rapidly than non-artemisinin antimalarial agents
- lumefantrine half-life 2—3 days, artemether half-life 2 hours

Use
- treatment of acute uncomplicated malaria caused by *P. falciparum* in adults, children and infants ≥ 5 kg
- (Dispersible tablets) as above in infants and children between 5 and 35 kg

Dose
- (Adults and children > 12 years and > 35 kg) 4 tablets orally with food at 0 (time of diagnosis), 8, 24, 36, 48 and 60 hours (total of 24 tablets) **OR**
- (Infants, children 3 months—12 years, 5 kg— < 15 kg) initially 1 tablet orally, then 1 tablet after 8 hours, followed by 1 tablet twice daily (morning and evening) for 2 days (total 6 tablets) (dispersible tablets) **OR**
- (Children 3 months—12 years, 15 kg— < 25 kg) initially 2 tablets orally, then 2 tablets after 8 hours, followed by 2 tablets twice daily (morning and evening) for 2 days (total 12 tablets) (dispersible tablets) **OR**
- (Children 3 months—12 years, 25 kg— < 35 kg) initially 3 tablets orally, then 3 tablets after 8 hours, followed by 3 tablets twice daily (morning and evening) for 2 days (total 18 tablets) (dispersible tablets)

Adverse effects
- headache, dizziness, sleep disturbance
- palpitations
- decreased appetite, anorexia, abdominal pain, nausea, vomiting, dyspepsia, diarrhoea
- infection
- myalgia, arthralgia, back pain
- fever, asthenia, fatigue, rigors
- pharyngitis, coughing
- anaemia
- increased liver function tests, splenomegaly
- pruritus, rash, urticaria
- (Rare) QT interval prolongation, hypersensitivity including angioedema

Interactions
- contraindicated with any other agents known to prolong QT interval (such as macrolides, azole antifungals, antipsychotics, some antidepressants, fluoroquinolones and antiarrhythmic agents class IA or III) or cause electrolyte disturbance, especially hypokalaemia or hypomagnesaemia
- contraindicated with other agents metabolised by cytochrome enzyme CYP2D6 (e.g. metoprolol, flecainide, imipramine, amitriptyline, clomipramine)
- contraindicated with rifampicin, carbamazepine, phenytoin and St John's wort
- food (including milk) enhances absorption
- not recommended with other antimalarial agents (as some prolong QT interval)
- caution if used with protease inhibitor antiretroviral agents
- not recommended with grapefruit juice
- may decrease effectiveness of hormonal contraceptives

Nursing considerations/Cautions
- not recommended for malaria prophylaxis or treatment of malaria due to other causes, including complicated malaria (e.g. cerebral malaria)
- a second course may be given for new infection or recurrence
- tablets and dispersible tablets are not bioequivalent
- ECG and blood potassium monitoring are recommended for those with cardiac, renal or hepatic impairment
- caution should be used if given to those with a cardiac history (e.g. bradycardia,

ANTIMALARIAL AGENTS

congestive heart failure, electrolyte disturbances (low potassium or magnesium), cardiac arrhythmias, pre-existing QT interval prolongation) or those taking drugs that are known to prolong the QT interval. ECG and potassium monitoring should occur in such patients before starting and regularly throughout therapy
- caution if used in those with severe liver impairment
- contraindicated in those with severe malaria (WHO definition), with known or family history of prolonged QT interval (or sudden death) or other condition which may prolong QT interval, or those with an electrolyte imbalance (e.g. hypokalaemia, hypomagnesaemia)

Patient education

- the patient should be advised to take tablets whole with food or fluids, as food increases bioavailability, especially that rich in fat such as milk
- instruct the patient that dispersible tablets should be dissolved in water (about 10 mL per tablet), gently stirred and taken immediately. The glass should be rinsed with small amount of water and taken to ensure the total dose is administered
- if the patient vomits within 1 hour of taking tablets, the dose should be readministered
- warn the patient not to drive or operate machinery if dizziness, fatigue or asthenia occurs
- advise the patient to avoid grapefruit juice during therapy
- instruct the patient to seek medical advice immediately if any of the following occur:
  - feeling too unwell to eat or drink
  - unexplained persistent nausea and vomiting
  - irregular or fast heart beat
  - yellowing of skin/eyes, dark urine, tiredness, upper right-sided abdominal pain

- see also General Patient education for people travelling in malarial areas (p. 557)

 Tablets are dispersible in water.

 Limited human data in the first trimester: Should generally be avoided in the first trimester unless other antimalarial drugs are unsuitable or unavailable. Use in second and third trimesters if the benefits outweigh potential risks.

 Small amounts of the drug are excreted into breastmilk, and the effects on the breastfed infant are expected to be minimal. Caution is advised if the infant weighs less than 5 kg.

ATOVAQUONE AND PROGUANIL HYDROCHLORIDE

Trade names
AtovaquoPro Lupin 250/100, Malarone Tablets 250/100, Malarone Junior Tablets 62.5/25

Available forms
Tablets: atovaquone 62.5 mg/proguanil hydrochloride 25 mg, atovaquone 250 mg/proguanil hydrochloride 100 mg

Action
- atovaquone inhibits the mitochondrial electron transport chain in parasites, disrupting the production of adenosine triphosphate and pyrimidine biosynthesis, processes essential for parasite survival and replication
- proguanil is metabolized into cycloguanil, an active metabolite that inhibits plasmodial dihydrofolate reductase, blocking DNA synthesis and cell replication in the parasite
- combined activity is synergistic
- half-life of atovaquone is 2—3 days in adults and 1—2 days in children
- half-life of proguanil and active metabolite is 12—15 hours in both adults and children

- proguanil has active metabolites which have antimalarial actions

Use
- prophylaxis and treatment of *Plasmodium falciparum* malaria

Dose
Prophylaxis
- (Adults, children weighing > 40 kg) 1 tablet (250/100) orally daily starting 1–2 days before entering malaria endemic area and continued for 7 days after leaving area **OR**
- (Children weighing 11–20 kg) 1 tablet (62.5/25) orally daily starting 1–2 days before entering malaria endemic area and continued for 7 days after leaving area **OR**
- (Children weighing 21–30 kg) 2 tablets (62.5/25) orally daily starting 1–2 days before entering malaria endemic area and continued for 7 days after leaving area **OR**
- (Children weighing 31–40 kg) 3 tablets (62.5/25) orally daily starting 1–2 days before entering malaria endemic area and continued for 7 days after leaving area

Treatment
- (Adults, children weighing > 40 kg) 4 tablets (250/100) orally as a single dose for 3 consecutive days **OR**
- (Children weighing 11–20 kg) 1 tablet (250/100) orally as a single dose for 3 consecutive days **OR**
- (Children weighing 21–30 kg) 2 tablets (250/100) orally as a single dose for 3 consecutive days **OR**
- (Children weighing 31–40 kg) 3 tablets (250/100) orally as a single dose for 3 consecutive days

Adverse effects
- diarrhoea, dyspepsia, gastritis, vomiting, abdominal pain, mouth ulcers, anorexia, constipation
- hepatomegaly, elevated liver function tests
- pruritus, hair loss, rash
- fever
- headache, dreams, insomnia
- dizziness, lethargy, asthenia
- backache, myalgia
- visual impairment
- cough
- postural hypotension, palpitations
- anaemia, neutropenia

Interactions
- not recommended with rifampicin, rifabutin, tetracycline or metoclopramide, as they decrease atovaquone plasma levels, reducing antimalarial activity
- if given with metoclopramide or tetracycline, parasitaemia should be closely monitored
- proguanil may potentiate warfarin; therefore the INR should be closely monitored especially when starting or stopping therapy
- serum levels may be decreased if given with efavirenz
- serum levels may be decreased by paracetamol, benzodiazepines, aciclovir, opioids, cephalosporins, antidiarrhoeals or laxatives

Nursing considerations/Cautions
- if a recurrent infection or treatment fails, a different antimalarial agent should be used
- not recommended for treatment of cerebral malaria or other severe manifestations of complicated malaria (e.g. hyperparasitaemia, pulmonary oedema or renal failure)
- not recommended for prophylaxis or treatment of malaria in paediatric patients weighing < 11 kg
- not recommended in those with severe liver impairment
- contraindicated in those with known sensitivity to atovaquone or proguanil, or for prophylaxis in those with severe renal impairment (creatinine clearance < 30 mL/min)

Patient education
- instruct the patient to swallow the tablet whole at same time every day with food or a milky drink

ANTIMALARIAL AGENTS

- warn the patient that the tablet has a bitter taste
- if children have problems swallowing the tablet whole, advise the parent to crush tablet and add to a small amount of milk, which should be taken immediately
- advise the patient that if they vomit within 1 hour of dosing, a repeat dose should be taken. If diarrhoea occurs, normal dosing should occur
- (Prophylaxis) the patient should be advised to start tablets 1 to 2 days before entering a malaria endemic area and continue for 7 days after leaving the area
- see also General Patient education for people travelling in malarial areas (p. 557)

Tablet can be crushed and mixed with a small amount of milk or yoghurt.

Avoid in the first trimester, as limited human data. It may be used in the second and third trimesters if the benefits outweigh the risks. A daily 5 mg folic acid supplement is recommended, particularly because of the proguanil component, which can affect folate metabolism.

Limited human data. Not recommended, especially for infants under 5 kg.

Kidney: contraindicated for prophylaxis if CrCl < 30 mL/min (because of proguanil accumulation). Increased risk of blood dyscrasias; consider alternative antimalarial.

MEFLOQUINE

Trade name
Lariam

Available form
Tablets: 250 mg

Action
- quinoline-methanol antimalarial
- structurally related to quinine
- blood schizonticide that destroys asexual erythrocytic form of *Plasmodium vivax, P. malariae* and most strains of *P. falciparum,* although some resistance has been reported in South-east Asia
- no effect on gametocytes of *P. falciparum*
- half-life about 21 days

Use
- (Treatment) acute attack of *P. falciparum* malaria resistant to conventional antimalarial drugs
- (Orophylaxis) multi-drug-resistant *P. falciparum* in those considered at high risk of malaria

Dose (adults and children more than 45 kg
- (Treatment) initially 750 mg orally, followed by 500 mg 6—8 hours later (total 1250 mg) **OR**
- (Prophylaxis) 250 mg orally as a single weekly dose starting 1 week before exposure and continuing for 2 weeks after leaving the malarial area

Adverse effects
- anorexia, nausea, vomiting, diarrhoea, abdominal pain, mouth ulcers
- tinnitus
- rash, pruritus
- hair loss
- myalgia
- fever, chills
- dizziness, dream disturbances, insomnia, fatigue, headache, vertigo, fuzzy thinking
- visual disturbances
- palpitations, cardiac conduction alterations, bradycardia
- anxiety, depression
- (Uncommon) mood changes, confusion, agitation, hallucinations, paranoia, psychosis, seizures
- (Rare) aplastic anaemia, agranulocytosis, hypersensitivity

Interactions
- may reduce plasma levels of antiepileptics (e.g. valproic acid, carbamazepine, phenobarbital (phenobarbitone), phenytoin), potentially lowering seizure control. Dosage adjustments of antiepileptics may be required

- not recommended with any other agents that are known to prolong the QT interval (e.g. antiarrhythmic agents, beta adrenergic blocking agents, calcium-channel blockers, antihistamines, phenothiazines, tricyclic antidepressants, H_1-receptor blocking agents)
- not recommended with quinine. Concurrent use may lead to ECG abnormalities and increased risk of cardiotoxicity. Use with caution and avoid simultaneous administration
- not recommended with hydroxychloroquine. Increases the risk of convulsions when used with mefloquine. Avoid combining these drugs if possible
- may reduce the effectiveness of the live typhoid vaccine. Complete vaccinations at least 3 days before starting mefloquine
- serum levels may be reduced by rifampicin

Nursing considerations/Cautions

- not recommended for malaria prophylaxis in patients with epilepsy because the risk of seizures is increased
- not recommended in children under 14 years or those adults with cardiac disease
- caution if used in those with impaired liver function, as clearance may be prolonged, increasing the risk of adverse effects
- contraindicated in those with active or history of depression, psychosis, anxiety disorders, schizophrenia or other major psychiatric disorders, epilepsy, severe liver or kidney impairment, or known hypersensitivity to related compounds (e.g. quinine)

Patient education

- advise the patient to immediately seek medical advice if any of the following occur:
  - signs of anxiety, depression, confusion, hallucinations, paranoia or restlessness (these signs may signal more serious psychiatric problems)
  - any visual disturbances or eye problems
  - difficulty sleeping or abnormal/strange dreams
  - seizures (fits)
  - chest pain, irregular heart beat
- the patient should be instructed that malaria prophylaxis with mefloquine should be started at least 1 week before travel commences, as acute psychiatric adverse effects usually occur at the start of therapy
- instruct the patient that the tablet should be swallowed whole with plenty of liquid and taken always on the same day of the week. If the patient vomits within 30 minutes of tablet ingestion, a second full dose should be taken. If vomiting occurs between 30 and 60 minutes, a half dose should be taken
- advise the patient that, because of the long half-life, adverse effects may continue after medication has been withdrawn
- warn the patient against driving a vehicle or operating machinery if dizziness, loss of balance or confusion is a problem
- women of childbearing potential should be counselled to use effective contraceptive throughout therapy and for at least 3 months after taking mefloquine because it may cause fetal abnormalities
- see also General Patient education for people travelling in malarial areas (p. 557)

 Tablet can be crushed and mixed with juice or water or a spoonful of yoghurt, apple puree, jam or honey.

 Use is considered acceptable for malaria treatment because the potential benefits to the mother and fetus outweigh the small risk to the fetus. Use only if the benefit outweighs the risk, especially in the first trimester. Animal studies show teratogenicity at high doses, but human data are limited. Women should use

ANTIMALARIAL AGENTS

contraception during treatment and for 3 months after the last dose.

Limited human studies. Excreted in small amounts into breastmilk. While adverse effects in nursing infants have not been reported, caution is advised.

Hepatic impairment: mefloquine is extensively metabolised in the liver, and its elimination may be prolonged in patients with hepatic impairment, leading to higher plasma levels. Contraindicated in severe hepatic impairment. Regular monitoring of liver function is advised during prolonged use.

PRIMAQUINE
Trade name
Primacin

Available form
Tablets: 7.5 mg

Action
- aminoquinoline
- schizontocide active against exo-erythrocytic forms of *Plasmodium vivax* and *P. ovule* and the primary exo-erythrocytic stage of *P. falciparum*
- prevents transmission of *P. falciparum* by eliminating the reservoir
- more active against the tissue form and gametes than the asexual blood form
- active metabolite longer half-life than parent
- half-life 4.3—7.4 days

Use
- (Radical cure) prevention of relapse of *P. vivax* and *P. ovale* infection
- adjunct treatment for *P. falciparum* infection (gametocytes)

Dose
- (Radical treatment) 15 mg orally daily with food for 14 days, increasing to 30 mg for malaria-resistant strains or where treatment has failed at 15 mg **OR**
- (Radical treatment in those with glucose-6-phosphate dehydrogenase (G6PD) deficiency up to 45 mg once weekly for 8 weeks (with monitoring for haemolysis) **OR**
- (Reduction of *P. falciparum* gametocyte numbers) 45 mg orally with food as a single dose

Adverse effects
- nausea, vomiting, abdominal cramps/pain
- headache, dizziness
- rash, pruritus
- cardiac arrhythmia, QT interval prolongation
- haemolytic anaemia (at high doses or those with G6PD deficiency), methaemoglobinaemia
- (High dose) leucopenia, agranulocytosis, neutropenia

Interactions
- contraindicated with drugs that suppress bone marrow or cause haemolysis
- caution if used with other agents known to prolong QT interval or cause electrolyte imbalance

Nursing considerations/Cautions
- ensure patients are tested for G6PD deficiency before starting primaquine owing to the risk of severe haemolytic anaemia in G6PD-deficient individuals. In cases where G6PD testing is unavailable, careful risk assessment and monitoring are essential
- observe for signs of haemolytic anaemia, such as darkened urine or a sudden drop in haemoglobin or red blood cell count. The drug should be discontinued immediately if these signs occur
- conduct routine blood examinations, including haemoglobin and haematocrit levels, especially for patients at higher risk of haemolysis or other blood disorders, and during prolonged therapy
- ECG monitoring is recommended in those with cardiac disease, a history of arrhythmias, bradycardia, long QT syndrome or uncorrected hypokalaemia or hypomagnesaemia

- administer with food to reduce gastrointestinal upset, as it can cause nausea, vomiting and abdominal discomfort
- tablets contain lactose, so use caution in patients with lactose intolerance
- caution if used in those with a family or personal history of favism because of the increased risk of haemolytic anaemia
- caution if used in those with nicotinamide adenine dinucleotide (NADH) methaemoglobin reductase deficiency, as methaemoglobinaemia may occur
- contraindicated in acutely ill patients with a tendency to granulocytopenia (e.g. rheumatoid arthritis, SLE)
- contraindicated in those with severe G6PD deficiency because haemolytic anaemia may occur. If used in those with moderate G6PD deficiency, close blood monitoring of haemoglobin and haematocrit is recommended
- contraindicated in those with known hypersensitivity to hydroxyquinolines

Patient education

- counsel the patient to take with food to avoid stomach upset
- warn the patient not to drive or operate machinery if dizziness occurs
- advise the patient to seek immediate medical advice if any of the following occur:
  - loss of appetite, back, leg or abdominal pain, reddening or darkening of the urine, pale skin, weakness, fever (haemolytic anaemia)
  - bluish tint to skin, gums, fingernails or around mouth, dizziness, breathing difficulties, weakness (methaemoglobinaemia)
  - rapid or irregular heart beats
- see also General Patient education for people travelling in malarial areas (p. 557)

 Tablet can be crushed and mixed with water or a spoonful of yoghurt or apple puree.

 Contraindicated in pregnant women because of potential harm to the fetus. Even if the mother is G6PD normal, the fetus may not be, increasing the risk of haemolytic anaemia.

 Avoid, as excretion into human milk is unknown. Due to the potential for serious adverse effects, including haemolytic anaemia in nursing infants, a decision should be made to either discontinue breastfeeding or discontinue primaquine therapy, considering the importance of the drug to the mother.

QUININE BISULFATE
Trade name
Quinbisul

QUININE DIHYDROCHLORIDE
Trade name
Quinine Dihydrochloride 6% Sterile Concentrate

QUININE SULFATE
Trade name
Quinate

Available forms
Tablets: 300 mg;
Vial: 600 mg/10 mL

Action
- antimalarial thought to interfere with plasmodial DNA, inhibiting replication
- also leads to accumulation of haem during the erythrocytic stages of infection
- no action on liver stages
- half-life 16 hours (in those with malaria), 11 hours (healthy people)
- half-life prolonged in those with hepatitis or moderate chronic liver disease

Use
- effective against *Plasmodium falciparum* that is resistant to other antimalarial drugs (chloroquine and related 4 aminoquinolines)
- (IV) severe *P. falciparum* malaria

ANTIMALARIAL AGENTS

- (IV) can also be used in the treatment of babesiosis (a malaria-like parasitic disease) (with clindamycin)

Dose
- initially 20 mg/kg by IV infusion over 4 hours (up to 1400 mg) (loading dose), then 10 mg/kg (up to 700 mg) 8—12-hourly after loading dose and repeated 8—12-hourly if needed **OR**
- 600 mg orally 3 times daily after meals for 7—14 days (with pyrimethamine 75 mg and sulfadoxine 1.5 g orally on day 2 of therapy)

Adverse effects
- headache
- fever
- nausea, vomiting, epigastric pain
- (Hypersensitivity reaction) rash, urticaria, pruritus, skin flushing, fever, facial oedema, sweating, dyspnoea, tinnitus, GI distress
- blood dyscrasias, thrombocytopenia, acute haemolysis
- reversible visual disturbances (including photophobia, blurred vision, diplopia, scotomata, disturbed colour vision)
- vertigo, tinnitus, deafness
- apprehension, restlessness, confusion
- syncope
- anuria, uraemia, haemoglobinuria
- hypoglycaemia
- hypoprothrombinaemia
- cardiac rhythm disturbance including ventricular tachycardia, angina
- hepatotoxicity
- cinchonism: initially tinnitus, dizziness, rash and abdominal pain/cramping, followed by (at higher doses) headache, fever, vomiting, apprehension, confusion and convulsions

Interactions
- drug interactions with drugs that are metabolised by CYP3A4, CYP2D6 or those affecting cardiac conduction. Adjust dosages or avoid concomitant use as necessary
- may increase serum digoxin levels, increasing the risk of toxicity; therefore serum levels should be monitored regularly throughout therapy
- risk of toxicity may be increased if given with pyrimethamine
- may enhance effects of anticoagulants; therefore prothrombin time should be monitored regularly especially when starting or stopping quinine
- absorption may be decreased by aluminium-containing antacids
- beverages containing quinine (e.g. tonic water) should be avoided in excess amounts because the risk of adverse effects and toxicity is increased
- may potentiate effects of neuromuscular blocking agents, increasing the risk of respiratory difficulties
- HIV protease inhibitors may have an unpredictable effect on quinine; therefore not recommended together
- may inhibit HMG-CoA reductase inhibitor (statins) metabolism, increasing the risk of toxicity including rhabdomyolysis
- decreased serum levels may result if given with rifampicin; therefore not recommended together
- serum levels may be increased by acetazolamide and sodium bicarbonate (urinary alkalisers), increasing the risk of toxicity
- may potentiate the effects of depolarising and non-depolarising muscle relaxants
- excretion may be increased if given with urinary acidifiers, resulting in decreased serum levels

Nursing considerations/Cautions
- before administering, the patient should be asked about any known sensitivities to quinine or quinidine
- if the patient has atrial fibrillation, digitalisation should be completed before starting quinine
- therapy should be changed from IV to oral as soon as practical
- during IV administration, pulse, BP and blood glucose should be closely monitored

- an IV loading dose is not required if antimalarial agents have been taken in the previous 24 hours
- (IV) diluted in 500 mL glucose 5% or sodium chloride 0.9% and infused slowly over 4 hours
- if IV therapy is required for longer than 48 hours, the maintenance dose should be reduced to 5 mg/kg to avoid accumulation. Serum levels should also be monitored
- not recommended by IM route owing to being highly irritant causing pain, necrosis and abscess formation. However, if an IV route is not available, IM can be used as last resort
- (IV) incompatible with amiodarone, pancuronium, suxamethonium, rocuronium, atracurium, mivacurium, vecuronium, mannitol, ketamine, diuretics especially furosemide (frusemide) and heparin
- discontinue immediately if any haemolytic or hypersensitivity reaction occurs
- solution should be protected from light
- caution if used in those with atrial fibrillation or impaired hepatic or renal function
- contraindicated in those with haemolysis, a history of blackwater fever (dengue fever), diabetes, G6PD deficiency, tinnitus, myasthenia gravis, optic neuritis, hypersensitivity to quinine or quinidine, or previous quinine-induced thrombocytopenia or uraemic syndrome

Patient education

- warn the patient about the bitter taste of tablets
- the patient should be advised to seek medical advice immediately if any of the following occur:
  - flushing, itching, rash, fever, facial swelling, shortness of breath
  - ringing in the ears
  - changes to vision
  - increased heart rate
  - persistent diarrhoea or cramping
  - loss of appetite, back, leg or abdominal pain, reddening or darkening of the urine, pale skin, weakness, fever
- advise the patient that aluminium-containing antacids should be avoided or spaced at least 2 hours apart from quinine
- warn the patient not to drink excess amounts of quinine-containing drinks (e.g. tonic water, bitter lemon)
- see also General Patient education for people travelling in malarial areas (p. 557)

 Tablet can be crushed and mixed with orange juice or a spoonful of yoghurt or apple puree.

 May cause fetal harm, including hearing loss, developmental issues and malformations. It can also induce uterine contractions, increasing the risk of miscarriage. Use should be limited to situations where the benefits clearly outweigh the risks. Its use in treating life-threatening malaria may be justified as the benefits to the mother and fetus outweigh the risks.

 Excreted into breastmilk in small amounts. Infants with G6PD deficiency may be at risk of haemolysis. Weigh the benefits of quinine use for the mother against potential risks to the infant before breastfeeding. If G6PD deficiency cannot be ruled out, avoid breastfeeding.

 Clearance is reduced in patients with renal or hepatic impairment, requiring dosage adjustments and close monitoring of drug levels and potential toxicity.

 Pregnant nurses can handle quinine tablets, but they should take precautions to minimise direct contact. Although

ANTIMALARIAL AGENTS

> quinine poses risks when ingested, handling tablets is generally considered safe if appropriate precautions, such as wearing gloves, are taken to avoid direct skin contact, inhalation of dust or accidental ingestion.
>
> Tablets should not be crushed by pregnant women.

Note
- sulfate and bisulfate salts are used interchangeably

TAFENOQUINE
Trade names
Kodatef, Kozenis

Available forms
Tablets: 100 mg, 150 mg

Action
- aminoquinoline
- exact mechanism of action unknown, but kills developing asexual, developing exoerythrocytic and latent hypnozoites
- long half-life 17 days

Use
- malaria prophylaxis (for up to 6 months) (Kodatef)
- radical cure (prevention of relapse) of *Plasmodium vivax* malaria in patients aged 16 years and over (Kozenis)

Dose
- 200 mg orally once daily for 3 days before travelling to malarial area (loading dose), then 200 mg orally weekly starting 7 days after the last loading dose (maintenance dose) while in malarial area, then 200 mg orally in last week following exit from malarial area 7 days after last maintenance dose (terminal/final dose) (Kodatef) **OR**
- 300 mg orally as single dose on day 1 or 2 of 3-day chloroquine therapy (Kozenis)

Adverse effects
- diarrhoea, nausea, vomiting, gastrointestinal reflux disorder
- headache, migraine, tension headache, dizziness, motion sickness
- back pain
- insomnia, abnormal dreams, nightmares, sleep disorder, depression, depressed mood, anxiety
- vortex keratopathy (corneal deposits)
- increased/abnormal liver enzymes
- (Rare) haemolytic anaemia, methaemoglobinaemia, anaemia
- (Rare) hypersensitivity (can be delayed in onset and/or duration), neurosis, agitation

Interactions
- caution if used with metformin because of an increased risk of lactic acidosis
- caution if used with other agents such as dapsone which may cause haemolysis

Nursing considerations/Cautions
- all patients should be screened for glucose-6-phosphate dehydrogenase (G6PD) deficiency before starting therapy because of the risk of haemolytic anaemia
- contraindicated in those with G6PD deficiency or if G6PD status is unknown
- therapy should be continued only for up to 6 months continuously (Kodatef)
- recommended in those 18 years and over (Kodatef)
- contraindicated in those with current or history of psychosis, delusions or hallucinations
- contraindicated in those with known hypersensitivity to other aminoquinolines

Patient education
- females of reproductive capacity should be counselled to use effective contraception during and for 12 weeks after stopping therapy
- if patient vomits within 60 minutes, the dose can be readministered (but only once) (Kozenis)
- if gastrointestinal disturbances occur, suggest the tablets are taken with food
- the patient should be advised to seek medical attention immediately if any of the following occur:

- pale skin, weakness, dizziness, confusion, dark-coloured urine
- headache, shortness of breath, fatigue, lethargy, confusion, nausea, rapid heart beat
- changes in mood, depression
• see also General Patient education for people travelling in malarial areas (p. 557)

Tablets should be swallowed whole and not chewed or broken apart.

Contraindicated, as no human data. May cause harm to a G6PD-deficient fetus, leading to haemolytic anaemia. Women of childbearing potential should use effective contraception during treatment and for 3 months after the last dose.

Contraindicated, as no human data. Risk of haemolytic anaemia in G6PD-deficient infants. An infant's G6PD status must be confirmed before breastfeeding.

ANTIMIGRAINE AGENTS

Migraine is a common neurological condition affecting about 20.5% of Australians (4.9 million). Women are more than twice as likely to experience migraine than men (probably because of hormonal factors), with females aged 25 to 29 having the highest prevalence of chronic migraine (≥ 15 migraine days/month), and those aged 35 to 39 having the highest rate of episodic migraine. The economic cost of migraine in Australia in 2018 was estimated to be $35.7 billion, made up of health system costs, costs due to lost productivity and other costs (Deloitte Access Economics 2018). However, this does not take into account the impact of migraine on the well-being and quality of life of the person experiencing migraine. Current figures for Australia are not available.

The International Headache Society has the following criteria for migraine, which include: attacks being episodic; the duration of an attack being 4 to 72 hours in length (untreated or unsuccessfully treated); headache being unilateral, throbbing and/or aggravated by movement or routine activity (e.g. walking, climbing stairs); moderate to severe in intensity; causing either nausea/vomiting, or both, photophobia and phonophobia (International Headache Society 2019). Depending on the type of migraine, other symptoms can include sensitivity to smell, confusion, difficulty concentrating, speech disturbance, motor weakness, and stiffness of neck and shoulders (Migraine & Headache Australia 2021). Not all headache disorders respond to the same medication; therefore correct diagnosis is essential in ensuring migraine is promptly treated while other causes of headache are ruled out.

The premonitory phase (predrome) of migraine is defined as non-painful symptoms that precede hours to days before the headache onset and are predictive of impending migraine. These symptoms can include neck stiffness, photophobia, phonophobia, osmophobia, nausea, yawning, sleep disturbance, thirst, food craving, memory impairment, difficulty with concentration, depression and irritability. These premonitory symptoms can also exist during the headache, as well as postdrome, once the headache has resolved (Goadsby 2021). This prodrome stage is followed by aura, with 20% of people experiencing visual symptoms such as flashing or bright zig-zag lights, blind spots or difficulty focusing. There may be a lag between the aura (up to an hour) and headache onset. The headache typically lasts between 4 hours and 3 days and is followed by a post-attack (postdrome) phase which lasts about 24 hours in most people (Migraine & Headache Australia 2021).

Every person diagnosed with migraine should have an action plan for management of an acute attack. The plan should be individualised to include individual differences, such as the presence of nausea or vomiting and time to peak severity. First-line treatment usually involves paracetamol, NSAIDs (e.g. aspirin, diclofenac, naproxen), triptans and antiemetics. It is important that patients understand the importance of optimising treatment by taking medication early. Furthermore, it is also important that the clinician assesses response to treatment by determining factors, such as whether the person was pain free within 2 hours of taking medication, if one dose of medication relieved headache and kept it away for at least 24 hours, and whether taking the medication led to the patient feeling in control of the migraine with minimal to no disruption of daily activities. Not meeting patient expectations on factors such as these leads to non-adherence and dissatisfaction with the management plan (Migraine & Headache Australia 2021).

Prevention of migraine involves a multi-pronged attack, including modification of lifestyle (e.g. regular sleep/wake cycle, regular meals, exercising, reducing stress), identification and avoidance of triggers and risk factors (e.g. excessive caffeine, food additives, certain foods, missed meals, sleep disorders, obesity) and, if needed, the use of preventative medication. Preventative medication may be recommended if acute treatment is needed 3-4 times monthly and should be trialled for 8-12 weeks to determine its effectiveness. The goal of this combined approach is to reduce migraine attack frequency and duration, as well as reducing the severity of symptoms and migraine-related disability. Behavioural therapies, such as relaxation and cognitive behavioural therapy, should also be considered in the overall management plan. It is important to ensure the patient is engaged in any preventative plan (especially pharmacological agents), as the rate of adherence has been shown to be low (Migraine & Headache Australia 2021).

Medication overuse can lead to the development of chronic headaches ('medication overuse headache') in some people, resulting in refractory headaches that are unresponsive to treatment and occur more frequently (daily or almost daily). The definition of 'overuse' is dependent on the medication used. For example, overuse of simple analgesics is considered if taken for 15 or more days per month, whereas antimigraine medications or combination analgesics are considered overused when taken for 10 or more days per month (Goadsby 2021).

ELETRIPTAN HYDROBROMIDE
Trade names
Relpax, Relpax Migraine

Available forms
Tablets: 40 mg, 80 mg

Action
- potent and selective serotonin ($5HT_{1B/1D}$) agonist

ANTIMIGRAINE AGENTS

- $5HT_{1B}$ receptors are thought to mediate intracranial blood vessel constriction
- active metabolite
- half-life about 4 hours

Use
- acute migraine (with or without aura)

Dose
- initially 40–80 mg orally, with a second dose after > 2 hours if migraine recurs (maximum dose 160 mg in 24-hour period)

Adverse effects
- paraesthesia, dizziness, somnolence, headache, asthenia, hypoaesthesia, vertigo
- pharyngitis, throat tightness
- chest tightness/pain/pressure, palpitations, tachycardia
- abdominal discomfort/pain/cramps, dry mouth, dyspepsia, dysphagia, nausea, vomiting
- chills, sensation of warmth/flushing, sweating
- back pain, myalgia, myasthenia, hypertonia
- medication overuse headache (see introduction, above)

Interactions
- contraindicated with or within 48 hours of macrolide antibiotics (erythromycin, clarithromycin), antifungal agents (itraconazole, ketoconazole) or protease inhibitors (ritonavir)
- contraindicated with other $5HT_1$ receptor agonist
- caution if used with selective serotonin reuptake inhibitors (SSRIs), serotonin and noradrenaline (norepinephrine) reuptake inhibitors (SNRIs) or triptans because of the risk of serotonin syndrome
- caution if given with St John's wort

Nursing considerations/Cautions
- a clear diagnosis of migraine should be established and other neurological conditions ruled out before starting therapy in those with no previous history of migraine
- cardiovascular assessment is recommended for those who are at risk of coronary artery disease or myocardial infarction
- caution if used in postmenopausal women, males > 40 years, or those with other risks for coronary artery disease
- not recommended in those under 17 years
- not recommended for hemiplegic, ophthalmoplegic or basilar migraine, or atypical headaches where cerebrovascular vasoconstriction could be harmful
- not recommended for those with heart failure
- contraindicated in those with severe liver impairment, uncontrolled hypertension, coronary artery disease, angina, previous myocardial infarction, ischaemic heart disease, variant (Prinzmetal's) angina, peripheral vascular disease, cerebrovascular accident (CVA) or transient ischaemic attack

Patient education
- warn the patient that the medication should not be used to prevent migraine
- the patient should be advised to take medication early in onset of symptoms during acute migraine attack, although still effective if taken later in an attack
- instruct the patient to swallow tablets whole with water
- advise the patient that, if the first dose is not effective, a second dose is unlikely to relieve migraine during same attack. However, if migraine recurs after initial relief, a second dose can be administered after 2 hours of initial dose (daily maximum 160 mg)
- the patient should be warned against driving or operating machinery if dizziness or drowsiness occurs

Tablet should not be crushed, but can be dispersed in water.

 Safety in pregnancy has not been established; therefore should used during pregnancy only if benefits outweigh risks.

 Excreted in breastmilk; therefore caution if used during breastfeeding. Not recommended within 24 hours of therapy.

 Contraindicated in those with severe liver impairment.

Caution if dose > 40 mg is given to those with renal impairment.

 Doses higher than 40 mg should be used with caution in those over 65 years because of effects on BP.

EPTINEZUMAB
Trade name
Vyepti

Available form
Vial: 100 mg/mL

Action
- humanised immunoglobulin G_1 (IgG_1) that binds to alpha and beta forms of human calcitonin gene-related peptide (CGRP), preventing activation of receptors. Raised CGRP blood levels are associated with migraine
- half-life 27 days

Use
- prevention of migraine

Dose
- 100 mg IV over 30 minutes every 12 weeks, increasing to 300 mg every 12 weeks if needed

Adverse effects
- nasopharyngitis, nasal congestion, rhinorrhea, throat irritation, cough, sneezing, dyspnoea
- fatigue
- hypersensitivity including angioedema, urticaria, flushing, rash, pruritus
- (Infusion site) extravasation
- development of antibodies

Interactions
- do not admix infusion with other drugs

Nursing considerations/Cautions
- therapy should be assessed 3 to 6 months after starting and the dose increased if needed
- the patient should be monitored during and after infusion for any signs of hypersensitivity (e.g. angioedema, urticaria, facial flushing, rash) or anaphylaxis, which may develop within minutes of administration
- the vial should be inspected before use and discarded if there are any visible particles or the solution is cloudy discoloured (colourless to brownish-yellow is normal)
- withdraw 1.0 mL from the vial (100 mg dose) or 1.0 mL from 3 vials (300 mg dose) and inject into a 100 mL bag of sodium chloride 0.9% and gently invert to mix contents (do not shake)
- infuse within 8 hours of dilution
- administer alone
- infuse over 30 minutes using a 0.2—0.22 micron inline or add-on sterile filter
- flush the line with 20 mL sodium chloride 0.9% when infusion is complete
- the vial should be protected from light and stored at 2—8°C. If removed from refrigerator, it should be kept at < 25°C in the original carton and used within 7 days, not returned to the refrigerator

Patient education
- ensure patient understands the importance of receiving infusion every 12 weeks for prevention of migraine
- advise patient that nasopharyngitis commonly occurs after first infusion and decreases with subsequent doses

 Crosses placenta and is not recommended during pregnancy unless benefits to the mother outweigh risks to the fetus.

ANTIMIGRAINE AGENTS

Excreted in breastmilk; therefore breastfeeding is not recommended unless benefits to the mother outweigh risks to the fetus.

ERENUMAB
Trade name
Aimovig

Available form
Prefilled pen (Autoinjector): 70 mg/mL

Actions
- human immunoglobulin G2 (IgG$_2$) (monoclonal antibody) with a high affinity for calcitonin gene-related peptide (CGRP) receptor (CGRP is a neuropeptide that modulates nociceptive signalling and a vasodilator whose levels increase during migraine and return to normal with headache relief)
- half-life 28 days

Use
- prevention of migraine

Dose
- 70 mg SC monthly, increasing to 140 mg if needed

Adverse effects
- constipation (which can become serious with complications), nausea, vomiting
- hypertension, worsening of pre-existing hypertension (especially within 7 days of first dose)
- fatigue
- pruritus
- sinusitis, bronchitis, flu-like symptoms
- (Injection site) pain, redness, pruritus
- antibody development
- (Rare) hypersensitivity

Nursing considerations/Cautions
- initial therapy should be started by a neurologist or migraine specialist
- therapy should be evaluated after 8–12 weeks, then 3–6-monthly
- the patient should be closely monitored for any new hypertension or worsening of pre-existing hypertension (most frequently occurs within 7 days of administration of first dose)
- if the patient is receiving 140 mg, give as two consecutive SC injections
- the first injection should be under medical supervision
- the name and batch number should be recorded in the patient history
- the needle cover contains latex and may cause allergic reaction in those with latex sensitivity
- caution if used in those with a history of constipation or using medications associated with decreased GI motility
- caution if used in those with pre-existing hypertension or at risk for hypertension

Patient education
- instruct the patient that the medication has no effect during an acute attack
- advise the patient to report any constipation, as this may become severe and serious
- the patient should be instructed in the correct administration technique, including:
  - check expiry date and do not use if expired
  - the pen should be at room temperature for 30 minutes before administration
  - the pen should be protected from direct sunlight and not warmed using a heat source (e.g. microwave, hot water)
  - pens should not be returned to fridge once they have reached room temperature
  - SC injections into abdomen (not within 5 cm of the navel), thigh or upper arm
  - injection sites should be rotated and the area not used if skin is broken, reddened, bruised or tender
  - inspect the pen before use and do not use if cloudy, discoloured or contains flakes/particles, or if the

- pen is cracked, broken or has been dropped or white cap is missing
- the site should be cleaned with alcohol wipe and allowed to dry
- remove the white cap from the pen (do not recap) and inject within 5 minutes to prevent solution drying out
- stretch or pinch the skin to make a firm surface, place the pen on skin at 90 degrees and firmly push it down until it stops moving. When ready to inject, press the purple start button and a click should be heard. Keep pushing down on skin (should take about 15 seconds) until window turns yellow, showing the injection is complete
- do not rub the injection site. If there is a small sign of blood, adhesive plaster (e.g. Band-Aid) can be applied
- if 140 mg is required, a second injection will be required using the above steps
- the needle should automatically be covered with a green safety guard when removed from skin
- the pen and white cap should be disposed of safely in a sharps container (not in household waste)
- the pen should not be reused or recycled
- pens should be stored in the original carton in a refrigerator (2—8°C) and protected from sunlight
- if removed from fridge, can be kept at room temperature for up to 14 days but must be discarded after that time if not used
- the pen should not be frozen or shaken

 Safety in pregnancy has not been established; therefore should used during pregnancy only if benefits outweigh risks to the fetus.

FREMANEZUMAB
Trade name
Ajovy

Available form
Prefilled syringe/autoinjector: 225 mg/1.5 mL

Actions
- humanised monoclonal antibody (IgG$_4$) with a high affinity for calcitonin gene-related peptide (CGRP) receptor (CGRP is a neuropeptide that modulates nociceptive signalling and a vasodilator whose levels increase during migraine and return to normal with headache relief)
- derived from recombinant DNA technology using Chinese hamster ovary
- half-life 31 days

Use
- prevention of migraine

Dose
- 225 mg SC once-monthly **OR**
- 675 mg SC 3-monthly

Adverse effects
- (Injection site) pain, induration, erythema, pruritus
- development of neutralising antibodies
- (Uncommon) rash
- (Rare) hypersensitivity

Nursing considerations/Cautions
- initial therapy should be started by a neurologist or migraine specialist
- therapy should be evaluated after 8—12 weeks, then 3—6-monthly
- the patient can be taught to self-administer
- the first self-administered injection should be under medical supervision
- if changing from one dosing regimen to the other, the dose should be given on the next scheduled administration date
- the name and batch number should be recorded in the patient history

ANTIMIGRAINE AGENTS

- contraindicated in those with hypersensitivity to Chinese hamster ovary protein

Patient education

- instruct the patient that the medication has no effect during an acute attack
- advise the patient that injection site reactions usually occur within 1 day of injection and resolve within 5 days
- the patient should be instructed to seek medical advice if any signs of allergy occur, including swelling of lips/tongue/face, trouble breathing, shortness of breath, wheezing, rash, hives or itching
- see Galcanezumab Patient education below for self-administration instructions
- for multiple injections (3-monthly dosing), the same injection site should not be used
- do not administer at the same injection site with any other injectable agents

Crosses the placenta and has a very long half-life, which should be taken into consideration if a women is pregnant or becomes pregnant during therapy. Exposure to the fetus is greatest during the second and third trimesters.

Unknown whether fremanezumab is excreted in breastmilk; therefore consideration should be given to discontinuing breastfeeding or discontinuing therapy.

GALCANEZUMAB

Trade name
Emgality

Available form
Prefilled pen (Autoinjector)/prefilled syringe: 120 mg/mL

Actions
- humanised monoclonal antibody (IgG$_4$) with a high affinity for calcitonin gene-related peptide (CGRP) receptor (CGRP is a neuropeptide that modulates nociceptive signalling and a vasodilator whose levels increase during migraine and return to normal with headache relief)
- derived from recombinant DNA technology using Chinese hamster ovary
- half-life 27 days

Use
- prevention of migraine

Dose
- initially 240 mg SC (loading dose), then 120 mg monthly

Adverse effects
- vertigo
- constipation
- pruritus, rash
- (Injection site) redness, pruritus, bruising, swelling
- (Rare) anaphylaxis, angioedema, urticaria
- antibody development

Nursing considerations/Cautions

- initial therapy should be started by a neurologist or migraine specialist
- therapy should be evaluated after 8—12 weeks, then 3—6-monthly
- for a loading dose of 240 mg, give as two consecutive SC injections
- the first injection should be under medical supervision
- the name and batch number should be recorded in the patient history
- contraindicated in those with hypersensitivity to Chinese hamster ovary protein

Patient education

- instruct the patient that the medication has no effect during an acute attack
- advise the patient that injection site reactions usually occur within 1 day of injection and resolve within 5 days
- the patient should be instructed to seek medical advice if any signs of allergy occur, including swelling of lips/tongue/face, trouble breathing, shortness of breath, wheezing, rash, hives or itching

- the patient should be instructed in the correct administration technique, including:
  - check the expiry date and do not use if expired
  - the pen/syringe should be at room temperature for 30 minutes before administration
  - the pen/syringe should be protected from direct sunlight and not warmed using a heat source (e.g. microwave, hot water)
  - the pen/syringe should not be returned to fridge once it has reached room temperature
  - SC injections into the abdomen (not within 5 cm of navel), thigh or upper arm
  - injection sites should be rotated and an area not used if skin is broken, reddened, bruised or tender
  - do not administer at the same injection site with any other injectable agents
  - inspect the pen/syringe before use and do not use if cloudy, discoloured or contains flakes/particles, or if pen/syringe is damaged in any way
  - the pen/syringe should not be reused or recycled
  - the pen/syringe should be stored in the original carton in refrigerator (2–8°C) and protected from sunlight
  - if removed from fridge, the syringe can be kept at room temperature for up to 7 days, but must be discarded after that time if not used
  - the pen/syringe should not be frozen or shaken
  - dispose of used the pen/syringe safely in a sharps container (not in household waste)

Safety in pregnancy has not been established; therefore should be used only if potential benefits outweigh risks to fetus.

NARATRIPTAN HYDROCHLORIDE

Trade name
Naramig

Available form
Tablets: 2.5 mg

Action
- selective serotonin agonist ($5HT_1$ receptors are found mainly in the cerebral and dural vessels) with little or no effect on other serotonin receptors
- half-life 6 hours

Use
- treatment of acute migraine attack (with or without aura)

Dose
- 2.5 mg orally and, if symptoms recur, a further 2.5 mg may be given after 4 hours (daily maximum 5 mg)

Adverse effects
- palpitations, chest pain/discomfort, chest pressure/heaviness
- warm sensation, feeling of heaviness, numbness
- nausea, vomiting, hyposalivation
- muscle pain, stiffness and tightness
- dizziness, drowsiness, malaise, fatigue, vertigo, headache
- medication overuse headache (see Introduction, p. 570)
- (Rare) severe cardiac events, ischaemic colitis, somnolence, hypersensitivity, peripheral vascular ischaemia, long-term ophthalmological effects

Interactions
- contraindicated with other $5HT_1$ receptor agonists or other triptans
- side-effects may be increased if given with St John's wort; therefore not recommended together
- not recommended with selective serotonin reuptake inhibitors (SSRIs) or serotonin and noradrenaline (norepinephrine) reuptake inhibitors (SNRIs) because of the risk of serotonin syndrome

ANTIMIGRAINE AGENTS

Nursing considerations/Cautions

- a clear diagnosis of migraine should be established and other neurological conditions ruled out before starting therapy in those with no previous history of migraine
- cardiovascular assessment is recommended for those who are at risk of coronary artery disease
- caution if used in postmenopausal women, males > 40 years, or those with other risks for coronary artery disease
- not recommended for hemiplegic, basilar or ophthalmoplegic migraine
- not recommended in those < 12 or > 65 years
- contains sulfonamide; therefore it is contraindicated in those with known hypersensitivity to any sulfonamide
- contraindicated in those with a history of myocardial infarction, ischaemic heart disease, variant (Prinzmetal's) angina, a history of cerebrovascular accident (CVA) or transient ischaemic attacks, peripheral vascular disease, uncontrolled hypertension or severe impaired kidney (creatinine clearance < 15 mL/min) or liver function

Patient education

- ensure that the patient understands therapy is for management of acute migraine, not prevention
- instruct the patient to take early in the onset of headache for best effect
- the patient should be advised that if the dose is not effective, a second dose is unlikely to work during the same attack
- advise the patient to take tablets whole with water
- the patient should be warned not to drive or operate machinery if they experience dizziness, vertigo or drowsiness
- advise the patient to report any pain or purple discolouration of fingers, toes, ears, nose or jaw (peripheral vascular ischaemia)

 Tablet can be dispersed in water, or crushed and mixed with a spoonful of yoghurt or apple puree.

 Safety in pregnancy has not been established; therefore not recommended unless benefits outweigh the risks.

 Breastfeeding should be discontinued for 24 hours after taking naratriptan.

 Dose adjustment required for those with mild-to-moderate renal or liver impairment. Contraindicated in those with severe renal or liver impairment.

PIZOTIFEN MALEATE
Trade name
Sandomigran

Available form
Tablets: 0.5 mg

Action
- serotonin antagonist with anti-bradykinin and antihistamine actions, as well as weak anticholinergic (muscarinic) actions
- action not fully understood, but thought to inhibit reuptake of serotonin by platelets, preventing loss of tone in extracranial blood vessels
- half-life 23 hours

Use
- prophylactically against recurrent typical or atypical migraine, vascular, vasomotor and cluster headaches (Horton's syndrome)

Dose
- initially 0.5 mg orally daily then increasing to 1.5 mg orally daily in single (nightly) or divided doses **OR**
- (Refractory cases) 3–4.5 mg orally daily in 2–3 divided doses

Adverse effects

- sedation, dizziness, somnolence, fatigue
- dry mouth, nausea and less commonly, constipation
- increased appetite, increased weight
- medication overuse headache (see Introduction, p. 570)
- (Rare) seizures, insomnia, anxiety, hypersensitivity reaction, paraesthesia, urticaria, rash, myalgia
- (Withdrawal symptoms) depression, tremor, nausea, anxiety, malaise, dizziness, sleep disorder, decreased weight

Interactions

- CNS effects may be enhanced if given with alcohol, antihistamines (including common cold preparations), sedatives or hypnotics
- not recommended with monoamine oxidase inhibitors (MAOIs) because of prolonged and intensified anticholinergic effects

Nursing considerations/Cautions

- abrupt cessation should be avoided to prevent withdrawal symptoms
- tablets contain lactose; therefore are not recommended in those with severe lactase deficiency, rare hereditary problems of galactose intolerance or glucose–galactose malabsorption
- caution if given to those with narrow-angle glaucoma, prostatic hypertrophy or urinary retention because of anticholinergic effects
- caution in those with epilepsy

Patient education

- instruct the patient that the medication has no effect during an acute attack
- the patient should be advised not to drink alcohol or use common cold preparations
- warn the patient against driving or using machinery if dizziness and sedation are problems
- advise the patient to avoid stopping therapy suddenly

 Tablet can be crushed and mixed with water, or a spoonful of yoghurt or apple puree.

 Not recommended during pregnancy unless benefits outweigh risks.

 Not recommended during breastfeeding unless benefits outweigh risks.

 Caution if used in those with kidney or liver impairment. Dose adjustment may be needed.

RIMEGEPANT

Trade name
Nurtec ODT

Available form
Oral disintegrating tablet 75 mg

Action

- binds to human calcitonin gene-related peptide (CGRP) receptor and antagonises receptor function (CGRP serum levels are raised during migraine and return to normal with pain relief)
- half-life about 11 hours

Use

- acute treatment of migraine (with or without aura) in adults
- prevention of migraine in adults who experience at least 4 migraine episodes per month

Dose

- (Acute migraine) 75 mg orally (daily maximum 75 mg) **OR**
- (Migraine prevention) 75 mg orally every second day (daily maximum 75 mg)

Adverse effects

- nausea (mild to moderate), dyspepsia, epigastric discomfort, abdominal tenderness and pain, abdominal distension
- nasopharyngitis
- drowsiness

- medication overuse headache
- (Rare) hypersensitivity (including dyspnoea and severe rash)

Interactions
- serum levels increased and therefore not recommended with clarithromycin, itraconazole or ritonavir
- serum levels increased and therefore not recommended with diltiazem, erythromycin or fluconazole. Another dose of rimegepant should be avoided within 48 hours if fluconazole is given
- serum levels decreased and therefore not recommended with phenobarbital, rifampicin, St John's wort, bosentan, efavirenz or modafinil
- plasma levels increased and therefore not recommended with ciclosporin or verapamil

Nursing considerations/Cautions
- not recommended in those with end-stage kidney disease (CrCl < 15 mL/min) or on dialysis, or with severe liver impairment

Patient education
- instruct the patient to seek medical advice immediately if they experience any shortness of breath, wheezing or coughing, itching or skin rash
- ensure the patient understands that they should not take any more than one tablet (75 mg) in a 24- hour period (whether this is for prevention or management of acute migraine)
- caution the patient against driving or using machinery, as drowsiness may occur
- advise the patient to use dry hands to carefully remove (not push) the orally disintegrating tablet from foil and then place tablet on or under the tongue to dissolve

Not recommended during pregnancy.

Low secretion into breastmilk; therefore benefits of breastfeeding should be considered versus clinical need for rimegepant by mother.

Not recommended in those with severe liver impairment or end-stage renal disease (CrCl < 15 mL/min).

RIZATRIPTAN BENZOATE
Trade names
APO-Rizatriptan ODT, Maxalt Migraine Relief Wafers, Maxalt Wafers, Rixalt, Rizatriptan AU, Rizatriptan ODT-WGR, Rizatriptan Wafers-10 mg

Available forms
Wafer/Orally Disintegrating Tablet: 5 mg, 10 mg

Action
- selective serotonin ($5HT_{1B/1D}$) agonist that causes selective constriction of extracerebral, intracranial arteries (which have been dilated during migraine attack)
- active metabolite
- onset of action 30 minutes, half-life is 2–3 hours

Use
- acute migraine attack (with or without aura)

Dose
- 10 mg orally; dose can be repeated after 2 hours (maximum dose 30 mg in 24-hour period)

Adverse effects
- chest pain, palpitations, tachycardia
- dry mouth, nausea, vomiting, abdominal pain, diarrhoea, dyspepsia, thirst
- muscle heaviness, muscle pain, neck pain and stiffness, muscle weakness

- dizziness, headache, somnolence, paraesthesia, insomnia, tremor, ataxia, nervousness, vertigo, disorientation, asthenia, fatigue, decreased mental acuity
- flushing, pruritus, sweating
- blurred vision
- pharyngeal discomfort, dyspnoea
- medication overuse headache (see Introduction, p. 570)

Interactions
- contraindicated with or within 2 weeks of monoamine oxidase inhibitors (MAOIs) (selective reversible and non-selective irreversible)
- not recommended with other 5HT$_{1B/1D}$ agonists
- increased risk of serotonin syndrome if given with selective serotonin reuptake inhibitors (SSRIs), serotonin and noradrenaline (norepinephrine) reuptake inhibitors (SNRIs) and triptans and are therefore not recommended together
- increased serum levels may occur if given with propranolol; therefore not recommended together
- caution if used with St John's wort

Nursing considerations/Cautions
- a clear diagnosis of migraine should be established and other neurological conditions ruled out before starting therapy in those with no previous history of migraine
- cardiovascular assessment is recommended for those who are at risk of coronary artery disease
- not recommended in those with basilar or hemiplegic migraine, or atypical headaches
- tablets contain phenylalanine; therefore are not recommended in those with phenylketonuria
- contraindicated in those with uncontrolled hypertension, coronary artery disease, angina, variant (Prinzmetal's) angina, a history of myocardial infarction, ischaemic heart disease, a history of stroke or transient ischaemic attacks or peripheral vascular disease, including ischaemic bowel disease

Patient education
- ensure that the patient understands therapy is for management of acute migraine, not prevention
- the patient should be advised that if the first dose is ineffective in relieving migraine, a second dose is unlikely to be effective
- if migraine recurs within 24 hours, the dose can be repeated as long as there is a 2-hour separation from the last dose and 30 mg daily maximum is not exceeded
- instruct the patient to handle wafer with dry fingers and place on the tongue, allow to dissolve and swallow with saliva

 Wafers can be dissolved on the tongue.

 Recommended during pregnancy only if benefits outweigh risks.

 Excretion in breastmilk is unknown; therefore should be used with caution during breastfeeding.

SUMATRIPTAN
Trade names
APO Health Acute Migraine Relief Sumatriptan, APO-Sumatriptan, Clustran, Imigran, Imigran FDT, Imigran Migraine, Iptam, Iptam Migraine Relief, Phamacor Sumatriptan, Sumagraine, Sumatran, Sumatriptan Generichealth, Sumatriptan Migraine, Sumatriptan Sandoz, Sumatriptan WGR

Available forms
Tablets: 50 mg, 100 mg;
Tablets (fast disintegrating): 50 mg, 100 mg;
Prefilled syringe/Autoinjector: 6 mg/0.5 mL

ANTIMIGRAINE AGENTS

Action
- selective serotonin ($5HT_1$) receptor agonist that selectively constricts cranial blood vessels
- response in 10—15 minutes (SC), 30 minutes (oral)

Use
- acute migraine attack (with or without aura)
- cluster headaches

Dose
- (Migraine, cluster headache) 6 mg SC, followed by a further 6 mg SC at least 1 hour later if symptoms recur (maximum dose 12 mg in 24-hour period) **OR**
- (Migraine) 50—100 mg orally, may be repeated after a 2-hour interval if symptoms recur (maximum dose 300 mg in 24-hour period)

Adverse effects
- (Injection site) transient pain, stinging, burning, erythema, bruising, bleeding, swelling
- transient (and possibly intense) tingling, heaviness, heat/cold, pain or pressure/tightness in any part of the body
- flushing, dizziness, weakness, fatigue, drowsiness, paraesthesia, hypoaesthesia
- dyspnoea
- nausea, vomiting, taste disturbance
- transient increase in BP
- medication overuse headache (see Introduction, p. 570)
- (Rare) severe cardiac events, seizures

Interactions
- contraindicated with or within 2 weeks of stopping monoamine oxidase inhibitors (MAOIs)
- not recommended with or within 24 hours of other $5HT_1$ receptor agonists or St John's wort
- caution and monitoring are recommended if given with selective serotonin reuptake inhibitors (SSRIs) or serotonin and noradrenaline (norepinephrine) reuptake inhibitors (SNRIs) because of the risk of serotonin syndrome

Nursing considerations/Cautions
- a clear diagnosis of migraine should be established and other neurological conditions ruled out before starting therapy in those with no previous history of migraine
- cardiovascular assessment is recommended for those who are at risk of coronary artery disease
- tablets and fast-disintegrating tablets are bioequivalent
- not given IV, only SC
- the first SC dose should be given by medical personnel and then the patient instructed on self-administration
- allergic reaction may occur in those with a hypersensitivity to sulfonamides
- caution if used in those with epilepsy, liver or kidney impairment, or controlled hypertension
- caution if used in those with risk factors for cardiovascular disease (e.g. hypertension, smoking, obesity, diabetes, males > 40 years, menopausal females, hypercholesterolaemia)
- contraindicated in those with hemiplegic, basilar or ophthalmoplegic migraine
- contraindicated in those with a history of myocardial infarction, peripheral vascular disease, ischaemic heart disease, variant (Prinzmetal's) angina, uncontrolled hypertension, cerebrovascular accident (CVA), transient ischaemic attacks or severe liver impairment

Patient education
- ensure that the patient understands therapy is for management of acute migraine, not prevention
- the patient should be adequately educated in the use of the autoinjector, including correct disposal of needles and syringes
- the patient should be advised to use medication when first symptoms occur
- advise the patient that, if the first dose is ineffective in relieving migraine, a second dose is unlikely to be effective.

However, if migraine recurs, a further dose may be taken (24-hour maximum dose and interval (see Dose, above)
- advise the patient that tablets should be swallowed whole with water and they have a bitter taste
- the patient should be warned against driving or using machinery if dizziness and sedation are problems
- instruct the patient not to take multiple forms of sumatriptan during an acute migraine attack
- advise the patient to seek medical advice immediately if any of the following occur:
  - pain in lower stomach, bloody diarrhoea
  - irregular heart rate
  - heaviness, pressure or tightness in any part of the body including throat and heart

Fast-disintegrating tablets can be dispersed in water.

Safety in pregnancy has not been established; therefore should used only if benefits outweigh risks to the fetus.

Secreted in breastmilk; therefore breastfeeding should be avoided within 24 hours of the last dose.

Caution if used in those with impaired liver or renal function. Lower doses are recommended. If appropriate, the first dose should be given under supervision.

Not recommended in those over 65 years.

ZOLMITRIPTAN
Trade names
APO-Zolmitriptan, Zoltrip, Zomig

Available form
Tablets: 2.5 mg

Action
- selective serotonin (5HT$_{1B/1D}$) agonist
- onset of action within 1 hour, half-life 4.7 hours (prolonged in those with liver impairment)
- active metabolite (half-life 5.7 hours)

Use
- acute migraine (with or without aura)

Dose
- initially 2.5 mg orally and, if symptoms persist or recur, a further 2.5 mg may be taken 2 hours after the first dose (maximum dose 10 mg in 24-hour period)

Adverse effects
- nausea, vomiting, dry mouth, abdominal pain, dysphagia, taste disturbance
- dizziness, somnolence, headache, warm/cold sensation, hyperaesthesia, paraesthesia
- asthenia, heaviness/tightness/pain/pressure in throat, neck, limbs or chest
- myalgia, muscle weakness
- palpitations
- (Uncommon) transient increase in BP
- (Very rare) arrhythmias, myocardial infarction, angina, ischaemic colitis
- medication overuse headache (see Introduction, p. xii)

Interactions
- serum levels may increase if given with quinolone antibacterial agents (e.g. ciprofloxacin); therefore dose reduction of zolmitriptan is recommended
- not recommended with or within 24 hours of monoamine oxidase inhibitors (MAOIs) (selective or non-selective)
- caution and monitoring recommended if given with selective serotonin reuptake inhibitors (SSRIs) or serotonin and noradrenaline (norepinephrine) reuptake inhibitors (SNRIs) because of the risk of serotonin syndrome, especially at start of therapy
- contraindicated with or within 12 hours of other 5HT$_{1D}$ receptor agonists
- caution if given with St John's wort

ANTIMIGRAINE AGENTS

Nursing considerations/Cautions

- a clear diagnosis of migraine should be established and other neurological conditions ruled out before starting therapy in those with no previous history of migraine
- cardiovascular assessment is recommended for those who are at risk of coronary artery disease
- if a 2.5 mg dose is ineffective, the dose can be increased to 5 mg for subsequent migraine attacks
- tablets contain phenylalanine and therefore are not recommended in those with phenylketonuria
- not recommended in those with hemiplegic or basilar migraines, or atypical headaches
- not recommended in those aged > 65 years or < 12 years
- contraindicated in those with myocardial infarction, arrhythmias or accessory pathway disorders, ischaemic heart disease, variant (Prinzmetal's) angina, peripheral vascular disease, moderate-to-severe controlled hypertension, uncontrolled mild hypertension, stroke or transient ischaemic attacks, or kidney impairment (creatinine clearance < 15 mL/min)

Patient education

- ensure that the patient understands therapy is for management of acute migraine, not prevention
- instruct the patient to take medication early in onset of headache for best effect
- advise the patient that if first dose is not effective, second dose is unlikely to relieve migraine during same attack
- advise the patient to swallow tablets whole with water
- the patient should be advised against driving and using machinery if dizziness is a problem

 Tablet can be dispersed in water (3–5 minutes), or crushed and mixed with a spoonful of yoghurt or apple puree.

 Safety has not been evaluated; therefore should be given during pregnancy only if benefits outweigh risks to fetus.

 Secreted in breastmilk; therefore should be used with great caution during breastfeeding.

 Maximum dose of 5 mg in 24 hours is recommended in those with severe liver impairment.

 Safety has not been evaluated; therefore not recommended in those over 65 years.

ANTIMYCOBACTERIAL AGENTS

Mycobacteria are a group of slow-growing acid-fast bacilli that are quite different from other Gram-positive or Gram-negative bacteria, with over 150 species identified (Holland 2018). Antimycobacterial agents are a group of antibacterial drugs used in the treatment of tuberculosis (caused by *Mycobacterium tuberculosis*), leprosy (or Hansen's disease, caused by *M. leprae*) and other mycobacterial infections (referred to as non-tuberculous mycobacterial infections), including *M. avium* complex (MAC) and *M. ulcerans* (Buruli ulcer). MAC organisms commonly cause illness in humans, especially those who are immunocompromised and have concurrent lung disease, such as bronchiectasis or chronic obstructive pulmonary disease (COPD). Prolonged multi-drug therapy is recommended for MAC infection (Holland 2018; Reddy & O'Donnell 2018).

In 2022, an estimated 1.30 million people died from tuberculosis (TB), making it the second leading cause of death from a single infectious agent after COVID-19 (WHO 2025). TB remains a preventable and curable disease, yet it continues to impact millions globally. People living with HIV are at a significantly higher risk—between 15 and 21 times more likely—to develop active TB compared with those without HIV. TB most commonly affects the lungs (pulmonary TB), but it can also occur in other parts of the body, such as bones, meninges, lymph glands, the gastrointestinal tract, pericardium, kidneys and urinary tract (extrapulmonary TB). Interestingly, TB affecting the upper airways or pleura is classified as extrapulmonary TB (Raviglione 2018).

People with active pulmonary TB are typically symptomatic, presenting with a persistent cough lasting more than two weeks, chest pain, coughing up sputum or blood, weakness, fever, night sweats, weight loss and anorexia. This form of TB is contagious, spreading through airborne droplets. On the other hand, individuals with latent TB do not display symptoms and are not infectious. It is estimated that approximately one-quarter of the global population has latent TB (WHO 2025). The disease may become activated in the future if the person's immune system becomes weakened, such as through immunosuppressive therapy or other health conditions (Raviglione 2018).

First-line drugs (isoniazid, rifampicin and ethambutol) are used successfully in most patients with TB. Second-line drugs are used when the first-line drugs cannot be used, because of either the adverse effects of, or resistance to, the first-line agents. Second-line drugs include some of the newer macrolide antibacterial agents and also the fluoroquinolones. Before starting any treatment, it is important to take cultures and establish the susceptibility of the organism to the drug(s). Patient education is an important part of treatment to prevent microbial resistance occurring when courses of therapy are not completed, as well as ensuring patients are aware of drug and alcohol interactions and possible adverse effects. Because of the increase in multi-drug-resistant organisms (MDR-TB) worldwide (resistant to both rifampicin and isoniazid), the antimycobacterial agents are not given as monotherapy but rather as part of a multi-drug regimen (generally a 6-month course of four agents) (Reddy & O'Donnell 2018). A test (Xpert MTB/RIF®) is available to detect TB and resistance to rifampicin within 2 hours, with other tests also being developed to test resistance to other first- and second-line TB drugs. Extensively or extreme drug-resistant TB (XDR-TB) now exists in about 58 countries world-wide and occurs when organisms are resistant to second-line drugs in addition to the first-line drugs, with sporadic cases also appearing in Australia (Traver & Cheng 2016; WHO 2025).

With the first case documented in 600 BC, leprosy is a condition that has been recognised since biblical times (WHO 2019b). While global numbers have declined, the disease remains endemic in certain regions, particularly in parts of Asia and Africa (WHO 2019b). While rarely acquired in Australia, Aboriginal and Torres Strait Islanders living in remote areas of Australia (such as in the Northern Territory or Far North Queensland) have the greatest burden of disease, with 20 cases diagnosed between 1989 and 2018 (Hempenstall et al 2019). Droplet transmission, contact with contaminated soil and insect vectors have all been implicated as likely routes of transmission. The disease has a very long incubation period (average 5 years). It generally affects the skin, peripheral nerves and mucous membranes (eyes and upper respiratory tract) to varying degrees, and other organs can be involved (WHO 2019b). Long-term complications include neuropathy, nerve damage (which can lead to paresis, paralysis and muscle atrophy), ulceration, foot drop, destruction of nose cartilage, blindness, impotence and infertility in males, and nerve abscesses (Gelber 2018).

First-line drug treatment for leprosy involves a multi-drug therapy regimen consisting of dapsone, rifampicin and clofazimine. Treatment duration depends on the type of infection: 6 months for cases with fewer skin lesions and 12 months for cases with more extensive infection or nerve involvement. This combination helps to prevent drug resistance, and since its introduction no resistance has developed when used correctly. Thalidomide, a known teratogen, is reserved as a second-line treatment and is used only when other options have been exhausted because of its risks (WHO 2019b).

Leprosy reactional states (Lepra reaction, see Glossary) may occur before diagnosis and treatment have begun or after treatment commences, which may result in patients losing confidence in the treatment regimen as it is perceived to be ineffective (Gelber 2018).

DAPSONE

Trade names
Aczone, Dapsone, Dapsomed

Available forms
Gel: 7.5% (acne vulgaris);
Tablets: 25 mg, 100 mg

Action
* antimycobacterial
* sulfone with actions similar to sulfonamide
* active against a wide range of bacteria which inhibit folic acid synthesis
* bacteriostatic against *Mycobacterium leprae*
* active against *Plasmodium* spp. and *Pneumocystis jirovecii'*
* active metabolite
* half-life of 10–80 hours

Use
* leprosy (as part of a multi-drug regimen)
* dermatitis herpetiformis
* actinomycotic mycetoma

Dose
* (Dermatitis herpetiformis) 50–100 mg orally daily with food (daily maximum 300 mg) **OR**
* (Leprosy) 100 mg (1–2 mg/kg) orally daily with food (with rifampicin) **OR**
* (Actinomycotic mycetoma) 100 mg orally twice daily with food, continued for 2–3 months after symptoms have abated (with streptomycin for the first month and then alternate days)

Adverse effects
* muscle weakness, peripheral neuropathy, reversible sensory impairment
* lepra reaction states (type 1 and type 2 reactions) (see Glossary)
* nausea, vomiting, abdominal pain
* blurred vision, tinnitus, vertigo
* insomnia, headache
* fever
* psychosis
* haemolysis
* phototoxicity
* (Rare) dapsone hypersensitivity syndrome (rash, fever, jaundice, eosinophilia)
* (Rare) agranulocytosis, severe cutaneous reaction, decrease in liver function, jaundice, toxic hepatitis
* (Very rare) aplastic anaemia

Interactions
* great caution if given with other agents that can cause blood dyscrasias or liver impairment, such as folic acid antagonists (e.g. pyrimethamine)
* plasma levels may be increased if given with probenecid, increasing the risk of toxicity
* plasma levels may be decreased if given with rifampicin
* increased risk of methaemoglobinaemia if given with rifampicin because of the increase in active metabolite concentration
* increased serum levels of both dapsone and trimethoprim may occur if given together, increasing the risk of dapsone toxicity

Nursing considerations/Cautions
* any anaemia should be treated before starting therapy
* regular blood count throughout therapy is recommended (weekly for the first month, monthly for 6 months, then twice-yearly, or more regularly if given with other agents that can cause haematological reactions)
* measure liver function before initiating treatment and continue monitoring during treatment to detect hepatotoxicity early.
* patients should be monitored for a 'dapsone reaction' in the first 6 weeks of therapy (persistent rash, fever, jaundice and eosinophilia)
* therapy should be stopped if any blood disorder or dermatological reaction occurs
* caution if given to those with glucose-6-phosphate dehydrogenase (G6PD) deficiency or methaemoglobin reductase deficiency
* caution if used in those with cardiac, hepatic, renal or pulmonary disease

ANTIMYCOBACTERIAL AGENTS

- not recommended in those with porphyria because an acute attack may be induced
- contraindicated in those with hypersensitivity to sulfonamides

Patient education

- the patient should be advised to take tablets whole (not split), with or after food
- instruct the patient to immediately report any of the following:
  - sore throat, fever, pallor, bruises, bleeding under the skin
  - yellowing of eyes or skin, dark urine, pale stools, lethargy, nausea, upper abdominal pain
  - muscle weakness, unusual tiredness
  - severe skin rash
  - tingling, pain, burning sensation, numbness or weakness in the hands and/or feet, bluish fingernails, lips or skin
- warn the patient not to drive or operate machinery if dizziness or blurred vision occurs
- female patients of childbearing potential should be counselled to use adequate contraception to avoid pregnancy during therapy

Tablets can be dispersed in 10–20 mL of water, or crushed and mixed with a spoonful of yoghurt or apple puree.

Contraindicated during pregnancy. Dapsone use during pregnancy, especially near term, carries a risk of neonatal haemolytic anaemia.

Excreted in substantial amounts in breastmilk and may cause haemolytic reaction in infants with G6PD deficiency.

ETHAMBUTOL

Trade names
Ethambutol Lupin, Ethambutol Tablets, Myambutol

Available form
Tablets: 100 mg, 400 mg

Action
- impairs cell metabolism, stops multiplication and causes cell death
- effective against *Mycobacterium* spp.

Use
- first-line drug in treatment of primary and extrapulmonary tuberculosis (TB) (as part of a multi-drug regimen, the exact combination depending on previous treatment and the development of any microbial resistance)

Dose
- (No previous treatment) 15 mg/kg orally daily **OR**
- (Retreatment) initially 25 mg/kg orally daily decreasing to 15 mg/kg after 60 days **OR**
- (Intermittent therapy) initially 15–25 mg/kg orally daily for 2 months (or longer depending on type and extent of disease, and at least one negative sputum sample) then 50 mg/kg orally twice weekly

Adverse effects
- reduced visual acuity, colour vision disturbances (usually reversible) (unilateral or bilateral), visual defects, scotoma
- rash, pruritus, dermatitis
- fever, joint pains
- nausea, vomiting, anorexia, abdominal pain
- malaise, headache, dizziness, confusion, disorientation
- elevated serum uric acid, precipitation of gout
- transient liver function impairment
- anaphylactoid reaction
- (Rare) peripheral neuritis, hallucinations, severe skin reactions

Nursing considerations/Cautions
- should be used only as part of a multi-drug regimen (not monotherapy)
- ophthalmological examinations (including colour discrimination) are recommended before and during therapy (monthly if the dose is greater than 15 mg/kg/day)

- blood counts, kidney and liver function should be monitored regularly throughout therapy
- the maintenance intermittent dose is lower if given with isoniazid
- use with caution in those with gout because it may be exacerbated by elevated uric acid concentrations
- contraindicated in those with optic neuritis (unless benefits of treatment are thought to outweigh risks)

Patient education

- warn the patient It may affect their vision, including causing blurred vision or changes in colour perception. If they notice any changes in eyesight, such as seeing less clearly or difficulty distinguishing colours, they should stop taking ethambutol immediately and contact their health professional. Early detection and stopping the medication can help prevent more serious eye problems
- patients with diabetes should be advised to monitor blood glucose levels closely during therapy
- warn the patient to report immediately and seek medical advice if any of the following occur:
  - visual disturbances such as blurred vision (reversible if the drug is stopped early; however, recovery may take weeks to months after drug is stopped)
  - any weakness, burning sensation, numbness or tingling in hands and/or feet
- advise the patient not to drive or operate machinery if visual problems, dizziness, confusion or disorientation occur

 Tablets can be crushed and mixed with water, apple juice or a spoonful of apple puree, chocolate pudding, peanut butter or jelly if the bitter taste is unpalatable.

 Limited human studies. Risk to the fetus cannot be ruled out.

 Excreted into breastmilk in small amounts, but the risk to a breastfeeding infant is generally considered low.

ISONIAZID
Trade name
Arrotex Isoniazid

Available form
Tablets: 100 mg

Action
- bacteriostatic against mycobacteria only
- resistance may develop in only a few weeks if given alone
- half-life 1–4 hours (this is influenced by whether patient is fast or slow acetylator, which influences the rate of drug metabolism)

Use
- first-line drug in the treatment of pulmonary and extrapulmonary tuberculosis (TB) (as part of a multi-drug regimen)

Dose
- (Treatment) 4–5 mg/kg orally in divided daily doses (300 mg maximum) **OR**
- (TB meningitis) up to 10 mg/kg orally daily for first 1–2 weeks

Adverse effects
- peripheral neuropathy, optic neuritis, convulsions, memory impairment, toxic encephalopathy, toxic psychosis
- nausea, vomiting, epigastric distress, anorexia
- fever, skin eruptions, lymphadenopathy, vasculitis
- fatigue, malaise, weakness
- elevated liver enzymes and bilirubin, jaundice, severe hepatitis
- pyridoxine deficiency, pellagra, metabolic acidosis,
- hyperglycaemia

ANTIMYCOBACTERIAL AGENTS

- gynaecomastia
- pancreatitis
- haemolytic, aplastic or sideroblastic anaemia, agranulocytosis, thrombocytopenia, eosinophilia
- rheumatic syndrome, systemic lupus erythematosus (SLE)-like syndrome

Interactions

- not recommended with hepatotoxic agents
- increased risk of CNS adverse effects if given with disulfiram
- may potentiate anticoagulant activity of warfarin; therefore the prothrombin time should be closely monitored, especially when starting or stopping therapy
- may decrease the excretion of phenytoin, increasing the risk of phenytoin toxicity; therefore blood levels should be monitored throughout therapy
- not recommended with carbamazepine because of the increased risk of isoniazid-induced hepatotoxicity
- may increase serum levels of carbamazepine, increasing the risk of toxicity
- may increase metabolism of paracetamol to hepatotoxic metabolites
- an increased risk of hepatotoxicity if given with rifabutin or rifampicin as part of a multi-drug regimen
- an increased risk of peripheral neuropathies and liver damage if used with alcohol
- may cause false positive on urine glucose determination using Benedict's reagent or Clinitest

Nursing considerations/Cautions

- pyridoxine (vitamin B_6) is often given concurrently to prevent isoniazid-induced peripheral neuropathy or if there is already existing peripheral neuritis
- the risk of peripheral neuritis is greatest in those with poor nutrition, alcohol abuse, uraemia or diabetes or if they are slow acetylators
- liver function should be monitored monthly throughout therapy
- changes in liver enzymes usually occur in the first 4–6 months of therapy
- ophthalmological examination is recommended before starting and regularly throughout therapy
- may be given concurrently with ethambutol or rifampicin to reduce the development of resistance. If used with rifampicin, liver function tests and vitamin D levels should be monitored regularly
- caution if used in those aged 50 or over (increased risk of hepatitis), if drinking alcohol on a daily basis, with diabetes or with kidney impairment
- caution if used in those with liver disorders including hepatitis B and C, alcoholic hepatitis, cirrhosis or who use alcohol regularly
- contraindicated in those with previous adverse reactions during isoniazid therapy, acute liver damage or severe hypersensitivity reactions

Patient education

- advise the patient is best absorbed if taken on an empty stomach – either 1 hour before or 2 hours after a meal.
- warn the patient If they consume tyramine- or histamine-rich foods while taking Isoniazid, they may experience a fast heart beat, dizziness upon standing, flushing, itching, headache or sweating. It is best to avoid foods such as mature cheeses, red wine and dark meat fish (that is not fresh), as they are high in tyramine and histamine
- advise the patient to take isoniazid 1 hour before aluminium-containing antacids
- the patient should be advised to avoid alcohol during therapy
- warn the patient to seek medical advice immediately if any of the following occur:
  - visual disturbances

- numbness or tingling in the hands or feet
- fatigue, weakness, malaise, anorexia, nausea or vomiting
- counsel the patient to avoid driving or operating machinery if visual disturbances or fatigue occur

Can be dispersed in water or crushed and mixed with orange juice or a spoonful of apple puree, chocolate pudding, jelly or peanut butter.

Should be used during pregnancy only if benefits outweigh potential risks. However, preventative therapy should be started soon after childbirth because there is an increased risk of reactivated TB in the new mother. Give with pyridoxine 25 mg daily (the neonate of a mother with TB should also receive isoniazid for 3—6 months).

Secreted in breastmilk, so observe breastfed infants for adverse effects. Give pyridoxine 25 mg daily to mother.

Contraindicated in patients with acute liver disease.

There is an increased risk of hepatotoxicity in patients with hepatic impairment. Use Isoniazid with caution and closely monitor liver function during treatment. Do not start treatment if the alanine aminotransferase (ALT) concentration is greater than 2—3 times the upper limit of normal (ULN).

RIFABUTIN
Trade name
Mycobutin

Available form
Capsules: 150 mg

Action
- ansamycin antibiotic similar to rifampicin, with a wide spectrum of activity
- active against atypical and multi-drug-resistant mycobacteria
- long half-life (45 hours)

Use
- pulmonary tuberculosis (TB) (as part of a multi-drug regimen)
- *Mycobacterium avium* complex (MAC) prophylaxis in patients with advanced HIV (as part of a multi-drug regimen)
- treatment of MAC infections and other atypical mycobacterium infections

Dose
- (MAC prophylaxis) 300 mg orally daily **OR**
- (Non-TB *Mycobacterium* infection) 300—600 mg orally daily for up to 6 months after negative sputum culture **OR**
- (Chronic, multi-drug-resistant pulmonary TB) 300—450 mg orally daily for up to 6 months after negative sputum culture **OR**
- (Newly diagnosed TB) 150—300 mg orally daily for 6 months

Adverse effects
- fever, rash, arthralgia, myalgia
- reversible uveitis (mild to severe), corneal deposits
- nausea, vomiting, jaundice, elevated liver enzymes
- leucopenia, anaemia, neutropenia
- discolouration (red-orange) of urine, skin and body secretions
- breakdown of vitamin K (during pregnancy)
- (Rare) thrombocytopenia, antibiotic-associated pseudomembranous colitis, hypersensitivity

Interactions
- contraindicated with ritonavir
- induces the cytochrome P450 (CYP) enzyme system, especially CYP3A4, which speeds up the metabolism of many drugs. This leads to reduced serum levels and decreased effectiveness of medications such as antiarrhythmics, antiepileptics, antipsychotics, beta blockers, benzodiazepines, calcium-channel blockers, oral hypoglycaemics, methadone, hormonal contraceptives and others. Careful monitoring or dose adjustments are necessary

- increases metabolism and therefore decreases serum levels of atovaquone, benzodiazepines, calcium-channel blockers, clarithromycin, corticosteroids, ciclosporin, dapsone, erythromycin, fluconazole, itraconazole, lidocaine (lignocaine), methadone, midazolam, nevirapine, oestrogens, opioid analgesics, phenytoin, posaconazole, ritonavir, sulfamethoxazole, tacrolimus, theophylline, trimethoprim, warfarin and zidovudine
- significantly reduces the effectiveness of oral contraceptives (combined hormonal contraceptives, including the pill, patch and ring) because it induces liver enzymes that accelerate the breakdown of oestrogen and progesterone. This leads to lower levels of these hormones, reducing contraceptive efficacy.
- increased risk of uveitis if given with clarithromycin, other macrolide antibiotics or fluconazole or related compounds
- plasma levels may be increased by ciprofloxacin, clarithromycin, erythromycin, fluconazole, itraconazole, ritonavir or posaconazole
- caution if given with barbiturates, benzodiazepines, verapamil, beta adrenergic blocking agents, disopyramide, chloramphenicol or antiepileptic agents

Nursing considerations/Cautions

- should be given only as part of a multi-drug regimen
- liver function tests, WBC and platelet counts should be monitored regularly throughout therapy
- if given with indinavir, the dose should be halved and the indinavir dose increased
- if given with clarithromycin, the dose should be decreased to 300 mg daily
- caution if used in those with progressing HIV disease owing to altered gastric pH leading to malabsorption of some drugs
- caution if used in those with severe liver insufficiency or severe kidney impairment (creatinine clearance < 30 mL/min)
- contraindicated in those with known hypersensitivity to other rifamycins

Patient education

- warn the patient their skin may become yellow and urine and body secretions may become red-orange while taking rifabutin. This is usually harmless and should disappear once they stop taking the medication. However, if they notice yellowing of eyes, dark urine or other symptoms of liver problems, they should inform their health professional immediately.
- advise the patient to seek medical advice immediately if any of the following occur:
  - eye pain, red eyes, blurred vision or black floating spots
  - yellowing of eyes or skin, dark urine, pale stools, lethargy, nausea or upper abdominal pain
- rifabutin can reduce the effectiveness of oral contraceptives. It is important to use an additional or alternative form of contraception, such as condoms, while taking this medication to prevent unintended pregnancy.

 Capsules can be opened and the contents mixed with water or a spoonful of apple puree.

 There is no extensive published human data on the safety of rifabutin use during pregnancy. Use can be considered only when rifampicin is unsuitable and the benefits outweigh the risks. It crosses placental barrier. If used during the last few weeks of pregnancy, vitamin K should be given to the mother and infant to reduce the risk of bleeding from hypoprothrombinaemia.

 It may cause loose bowel movements in the baby and discolour breastmilk into a reddish-orange hue. It is important to monitor the baby for any gastrointestinal disturbances or other reactions. Use only when the benefits outweigh the risks.

When CrCl < 10 mL/min, it is recommended to halve the usual dose. This adjustment is necessary to prevent drug accumulation and reduce the risk of toxicity in patients with severely impaired kidney function.

RIFAMPICIN
Trade names
Rifadin, Rimycin

Available forms
Capsules: 150 mg, 300 mg;
Suspension: 100 mg/5 mL;
Vials: 600 mg

Action
- inhibits DNA-dependent RNA polymerase activity
- half-life about 3 hours
- cross-resistance to other rifamycins

Use
- first-line drug in the treatment of tuberculosis (TB) (as part of a multi-drug regimen)
- leprosy (as part of a multi-drug regimen)
- prophylaxis of meningococcal disease and *Haemophilus influenzae* type B

Dose
- (TB) 600 mg orally daily 30 minutes before or 2 hours after food **OR**
- (Leprosy) 450–600 mg orally daily 30 minutes before or 2 hours after food **OR**
- (Meningococcal disease prophylaxis) 600 mg orally daily 30 minutes before or 2 hours after food for 4 days **OR**
- (*H. influenzae* type B prophylaxis) 20 mg/kg orally daily 30 minutes before or 2 hours after food for 4 days (daily maximum 600 mg) **OR**
- 600 mg by IV infusion over 1–3 hours (if unable to take oral preparation)

Adverse effects
- dyspepsia, anorexia, nausea, vomiting, flatulence, diarrhoea, abdominal cramps, sore mouth/tongue
- headache, drowsiness, fatigue, dizziness, decreased concentration, confusion
- visual disturbances, conjunctivitis
- discolouration of sputum, urine, sweat, tears and/or teeth
- muscle weakness, myalgia, myopathy, pain in legs and feet, numbness, ataxia
- rash, fever, flushing, pruritus, urticaria, acne-like lesions
- purpura, eosinophilia, leucopenia, acute haemolytic anaemia
- vitamin K deficiency, hypoprothrombinaemia, vitamin K-dependent coagulopathy
- menstrual disturbances, postpartum haemorrhage, fetal maternal haemorrhage
- lepromatous reaction (when given for leprosy)
- (IV) thrombophlebitis
- (Flu-like syndrome) fever, chills, headache, dizziness, bone pain (occurring during third and sixth month of therapy)
- (Rare) antibiotic-associated pseudomembranous colitis, liver dysfunction, hepatitis, haemolytic anaemia, increased serum uric acid concentrations, thrombocytopenia (reversible if drug stopped early), kidney failure, severe hypersensitivity reactions (including drug reaction with eosinophilia and systemic systems (DRESS)), severe skin reactions, psychosis, cerebral haemorrhage

Interactions
- induces the cytochrome P450 (CYP) enzyme system, especially CYP3A4, which speeds up the metabolism of many drugs. This leads to reduced serum levels and decreased effectiveness of medications such as antiarrhythmics, antiepileptics, antipsychotics, beta blockers, benzodiazepines, calcium-channel blockers, oral hypoglycaemics, methadone, hormonal contraceptives and others. Careful monitoring or dose adjustments are necessary

ANTIMYCOBACTERIAL AGENTS

- significantly reduces the effectiveness of oral contraceptives (combined hormonal contraceptives, including the pill, patch and ring) because it induces liver enzymes that accelerate the breakdown of oestrogen and progesterone. This leads to lower levels of these hormones, reducing contraceptive efficacy
- not recommended with other hepatotoxic agents or hepatitis C antiviral agents
- serum levels may be increased by probenecid and atovaquone
- not recommended with other antibacterial agents causing vitamin K-dependent coagulopathy such as cephalosporins
- increased risk of hepatotoxicity if given with alcohol, isoniazid or halothane
- may decrease serum levels of atovaquone or enalaprilat (active metabolite of enalapril)
- absorption decreased by antacids
- may decrease serum levels of warfarin; therefore increased monitoring of prothrombin is recommended, especially when starting and stopping therapy
- blood glucose control may become disrupted because of decreased serum levels of oral hypoglycaemics (sulfonylureas) when given with rifampicin
- increases metabolism of vitamin D, thyroid hormones and adrenal hormones
- may interfere with some laboratory tests including false positive urine screening for opioids

Nursing considerations/Cautions

- rifampicin is reserved for the treatment of methicillin-resistant *Staphylococcus aureus* (MRSA) and mycobacterial infections, and for the prophylaxis of meningitis and epiglottitis. To prevent the development of resistance, it should not be used indiscriminately
- baseline liver function tests including liver enzymes, bilirubin and creatinine, also full blood count and platelet count, should be measured before starting therapy
- monitor liver function tests regularly if there is pre-existing liver impairment, and immediately if symptoms of hepatic toxicity occur. Rises in aspartate aminotransferase (AST) up to 3—5 times the upper limit of normal (ULN) may be tolerated if the patient is asymptomatic and not jaundiced
- vitamin K supplementation is recommended if vitamin K deficiency or hypoprothrombinaemia occurs
- rifampicin should be stopped and not restarted if thrombocytopenia occurs
- rifampicin with pyrazinamide is not recommended for the treatment of latent TB because of the increased risk of hepatic injury, but is acceptable in combination with other drugs for treating active TB
- IV therapy is indicated for those unable to tolerate oral therapy
- (Leprosy) should be used as part of multi-drug regimen to decrease risk of resistance
- (Leprosy) patient should be assessed for concurrent TB and treated accordingly
- prothrombin time should be monitored daily if the patient is also taking oral anticoagulants, or blood glucose in patients with diabetes taking oral hypoglycaemics
- IV preparation should not be administered IM or SC
- dissolve the vial contents with water for injections, add to 500 mL of glucose 5% or sodium chloride 0.9% and infuse over 1—3 hours
- precipitate may occur if given with IV diltiazem
- (Suspension) contains sodium metabisulfite, which can cause allergic reactions in some people, especially those with asthma or eczema
- use with caution in those with porphyria or pre-existing liver disease
- not recommended for treatment of meningococcal disease
- not recommended as intermittent therapy (less than 2—3 times per week)

- because of increased risk of immunological reactions or anaphylaxis
- contraindicated in those with known hypersensitivity to other rifamycins or with jaundice

Patient education

- advise the patient to inform all health professionals that they are taking rifampicin, because of the long list of drug interactions
- counsel women of childbearing potential taking oral contraceptives to use non-hormonal contraception during therapy to avoid pregnancy
- advise the patient of the importance of continuous therapy (i.e. not stopping therapy) because intermittent therapy may result in hypersensitivity reaction. Rifampicin should not be used less than 2—3 times weekly
- warn the patient that flu-like syndrome commonly occurs between the third and sixth month of therapy
- inform the patient that urine, faeces, sweat, sputum and tears may turn a harmless red-orange colour, and soft contact lenses may become permanently stained
- advise the patient to seek medical advice immediately if any of the following occur:
  - yellowing of eyes or skin, dark urine, pale stools, lethargy, nausea, upper abdominal pain
  - visual disturbances
  - rash, blistering or peeling of skin
  - fever, enlarged glands, rash
  - severe watery diarrhoea, abdominal cramping (even if it occurs several weeks after stopping therapy)
  - white furry, sore mouth or tongue (oral thrush)
  - sore/itchy vagina, discharge (vaginal thrush)
- instruct the patient not to drive or operate machinery if they experience drowsiness, dizziness, visual disturbances or decreased concentration
- warn the patient to avoid alcohol during therapy
- instruct the patient to take oral preparations 30 minutes before or 2 hours after a meal
- advise the patient not to take antacids within 1 hour of taking rifampicin
- patients with diabetes using oral hypoglycaemics (sulfonylureas) should monitor their blood glucose levels closely during therapy

Available as a syrup. Capsules can be opened and mixed with water or a spoonful of apple puree.

Generally considered safe to use during pregnancy and is one of the drugs recommended for treating TB in pregnant women. Crosses the placental barrier. If used during the last few weeks of pregnancy, vitamin K should be given to the mother and infant to reduce the risk of bleeding from hypoprothrombinaemia.

Generally considered safe to use during breastfeeding and can be used when the benefit outweighs the risk. It may cause loose bowel actions in the baby and may discolour breastmilk to a reddish-orange hue. It is important to monitor the baby for any gastrointestinal disturbances or other reactions while using this medication.

Hepatically cleared. Metabolised in the liver and excreted mainly through bile into the faeces. A small portion is excreted in the urine. May worsen hepatic impairment; use cautiously, and a slightly lower dose may be necessary in patients with liver dysfunction.

ANTINEOPLASTIC AGENTS

The characteristics shared by most cancers include the differences between malignant and normal cells (e.g. different cell surface receptors), increased proliferation of the abnormal (or malignant) cells, infiltration of the surrounding tissue and a tendency to metastasise (or spread) to other sites.

In Australia, cancer is one of the five leading causes of death, with different age groups being affected by different cancers. For example, in 2022, while brain cancer was the 4th leading cause of death in all those aged 1 to 14 years, it was the number one cause of death for girls in this age group. For females in the 45 to 64 year age group, four out of five of the leading causes of death were cancer related (breast, lung, colorectal and liver) (AIHW 2024e).

Treatment of cancer involves surgical removal, radiotherapy or chemo-immunotherapy, or a combination of these to remove the malignant cells and prevent more from proliferating, giving a person an overall 71% chance of surviving for 5 years, up from 55% in 2016—20. This number does vary, however, with the type of cancer, stage of diagnosis and/or treatment options (AIHW 2024f).

Very toxic agents, termed antineoplastic agents (also called chemotherapy, cytotoxics or chemotherapeutic agents), are used to inhibit the growth of malignant cells by attacking them at different stages in the cell reproductive cycle. The ideal agent is one that destroys the malignant cells while doing minimal damage to the patient's normal cells. However, because all dividing cells, both malignant and normal, are affected, the use of these agents may be limited because of their effects on rapidly dividing normal cells (e.g. gastrointestinal tract cells, hair follicles, bone marrow cells). Some antineoplastic agents are effective during specific phases of the cell cycle (phase specific), whereas others act throughout the entire cycle (cycle specific) (Knights et al 2023).

Antineoplastic agents can be divided into alkylating agents (e.g. cyclophosphamide), antimetabolites (e.g. methotrexate, mercaptopurine), cytotoxic antibiotics (e.g. doxorubicin), mitotic inhibitors (e.g. vincristine), topoisomerase inhibitors (e.g. etoposide), proteasome inhibitors (e.g. bortezomib), hormonal antineoplastics (e.g. flutamide, tamoxifen, goserilin), immunomodulatory drugs (e.g. checkpoint inhibitors, interferons), non-cytotoxic antineoplastics (e.g. monoclonal antibodies) and other agents such as tyrosine kinase inhibitors and growth factor receptor inhibitors that don't fit into any of the previous classifications (Chu 2024). These agents may be given orally, intravenously, subcutaneously, intrathecally or by regional perfusion, with the maximum tolerated doses being administered. Combinations of high doses of cytotoxic drugs are usually given intermittently (in cycles) to allow normal cells to recover. Because many of the antineoplastic agents are highly emetogenic, antiemetic agents are usually given concurrently to reduce the nausea and vomiting.

General Adverse effects of antineoplastic agents

- headache, migraine, asthenia, malaise, dizziness, depression, insomnia, somnolence, confusion
- loss of appetite, anorexia, nausea, vomiting, dyspepsia, diarrhoea, abdominal pain, flatulence, burping, mucositis, stomatitis, gastrointestinal ulceration and bleeding, weight loss
- anaemia, thrombocytopenia, ecchymosis, leucopenia, neutropenia, febrile neutropenia
- dyspnoea, rhinitis, cough, sinusitis, pneumonia, bronchitis, pharyngitis
- epistaxis
- rash, urticaria, pruritus, alopecia, sweating
- chest or back pain, arthralgia, myalgia, muscle cramps
- abnormal vision, double vision, amblyopia
- tinnitus
- (Flu-like syndrome) fever, chills, rigors
- opportunistic infection (viral, bacterial, fungal)
- palpitations, arrhythmias, tachycardia, heart failure, angina, chest pain
- hypertension, hypotension
- dehydration
- peripheral oedema
- dysuria, haematuria, urinary tract infection
- elevated liver enzymes, hepatitis
- (IV) extravasation, ulceration, soft tissue necrosis

General Interactions of antineoplastic agents

- use with live attenuated vaccines may potentiate replication of vaccine virus, increase the adverse effects of the vaccine virus and/or may decrease the patient's antibody response to the vaccine and can be life threatening
- may decrease antibody response to killed vaccine virus
- it may take 3–12 months for the body to respond normally to vaccine
- close contacts should postpone immunisation with oral polio vaccine (because of viral shedding)
- caution if used with other agents known to cause bone marrow depression or blood dyscrasia, or with radiotherapy
- caution if used with other hepatotoxic, nephrotoxic, neurotoxic or cardiotoxic agents, or those known to produce pulmonary toxicity

General Nursing considerations/ Cautions for antineoplastic agents

- trade name and batch number should be recorded in patient medical history for traceability
- therapy is usually continued until disease progresses, unacceptable toxicity occurs or, for some agents, time or cycle duration (e.g. 24 months, 6 cycles)

ANTINEOPLASTIC AGENTS

- any dehydration or electrolyte imbalance should be corrected before starting therapy
- blood counts (including WBC with differential platelet count) and haemoglobin should be measured before starting and then regularly throughout therapy to monitor bone marrow depression. Liver, kidney and thyroid function should also be closely monitored throughout therapy
- therapy should not be started if bone marrow function is markedly depressed
- if patient has a high tumour burden, blood uric acid, potassium, calcium phosphate and creatinine should be measured 3—4 times in the first week to monitor for tumour lysis syndrome (lysis of a massive number of cells, resulting in the production of large amounts of uric acid from the breakdown of the nucleoproteins and hyperuricaemia)
- cardiac function should be assessed carefully when agents known to be cardiotoxic are to be used. Cardiotoxicity may be delayed and not manifest itself for months after treatment is completed. Depending on the agent, this may include ECG, echocardiogram or measurement of left ventricular ejection fraction (LVEF)
- audiograms are recommended before starting and regularly during therapy with agents known to be ototoxic
- therapy may be interrupted, or the dose reduced or delayed, to manage adverse effects/toxicities
- an adequate interval should be left between cycles of therapy (including radiation therapy) to allow bone marrow to recover
- allopurinol and adequate hydration are used to prevent tumour lysis syndrome
- patient should be closely monitored if severe diarrhoea occurs to prevent dehydration and electrolyte imbalance occurring
- administer alone, ensuring lines are flushed well before and after administration
- prevent extravasation of cytotoxic drugs by ensuring that the IV cannula remains securely in position, thereby avoiding severe pain and tissue damage. If extravasation occurs, elevate limb and apply cold compress for 45 minutes
- observe closely for and report extravasation immediately
- protect the patient from infection by maintaining strict asepsis, standard precautions and a high standard of hygiene
- to reduce risk of infection, the patient may be nursed in a positive-pressure room, as per local protocol
- observe closely for signs of infection, bleeding tendencies, paraesthesia, loss of reflexes, ataxia, mouth ulcers and alopecia
- therapy is usually continued until disease progresses or until unacceptable toxicity occurs
- staff should be aware of any concurrent therapy that may potentiate adverse effects (e.g. therapy with other drugs that are ototoxic, hepatotoxic, nephrotoxic or neurotoxic)
- caution if given within 14—21 days of surgery, as wound healing may be impaired
- when handling any cytotoxic agents, staff should avoid inhaling or having any contact with skin or eyes. If contact occurs, the area should be washed with copious quantities of water

- staff handling cytotoxics should be aware of hospital protocols or guidelines regarding preparation, administration, dealing with spillage, extravasation and disposal of used equipment and patients' body wastes
- pregnant staff should not handle antineoplastic agents
- depending on the patient's immune status, visitors (and staff) may need to be restricted if they display any signs of infections, especially influenza, measles or chicken pox
- staff should be aware of their own immunisation status and ensure that it is up to date to protect immunocompromised patients
- (IV) some antineoplastic agents should be protected from light
- (IV) administer alone via a dedicated line, as many antineoplastic agents have incompatibilities. Lines should be flushed thoroughly after use
- caution if used in those who have had previous exposure to antineoplastic agents or radiotherapy
- caution or contraindicated if used in those with liver, kidney or cardiac impairment
- caution or contraindicated in those with current active infection, herpes zoster or recent chicken pox (including exposure), because severe generalised disease may result
- contraindicated in those with severe pre-existing bone marrow depression. Bone marrow should be allowed to recover before starting treatment

General Patient education for antineoplastic agents

- reassure the patient that nausea and vomiting are transient and that drugs are available to counteract or prevent these adverse effects. Avoiding food for 4–6 hours before therapy may also reduce the severity of nausea and vomiting
- instruct the patient that tablets and capsules should be swallowed whole (not opened, crushed, sucked, broken, chewed or dispersed). If the capsule/tablet is broken or opened, contact with powder should be avoided. If any contact is made with skin or eyes, the area should be thoroughly washed with water. Hands should be washed well after handling tablets or capsules
- advise the patient that if vomiting occurs or a dose is missed the medication should be taken when next scheduled and an additional dose should not be taken
- the patient should be advised that any dental work should be completed before chemotherapy starts or deferred until blood counts return to normal. Good oral hygiene should be encouraged; however, the patient should be advised to take care with a toothbrush, dental floss or toothpicks, as the risk of gingival bleeding is increased
- warn the patient against driving or handling heavy machinery if dizziness, drowsiness, extreme tiredness or lethargy, visual disturbances, headache or pain occurs
- advise the patient that hair will regrow and that a wig may be worn in the mean time. Other options include hats and creative use of scarves. As hair may fall out unevenly (i.e. in clumps), some patients may prefer to shave their head at the start of the alopecia
- instruct the patient to seek medical advice immediately if any of the following occur:

ANTINEOPLASTIC AGENTS

- - fever, chills or other signs of infection
  - persistent bruising or unusual bleeding or black tarry stools
  - cough, hoarseness, side or lower back pain
  - blood in urine, difficulty with urination
  - yellowing of skin/eyes, unusual tiredness, loss of appetite, nausea, upper abdominal pain, dark urine, pale stools
  - unusual tiredness, pallor, shortness of breath on exertion
  - burning sensation in mouth and throat
- advise the patient to avoid contact with those with any infection
- instruct the patient to avoid contact sports or any other activities which may cause bruising or injury during therapy
- the patient should be warned to take care using sharp objects such as nail cutters and razors that may result in bleeding
- the patient should be advised that symptoms of palmar-plantar erythrodysaesthesia syndrome (hand-foot syndrome) can be reduced by keeping hands/feet cool (e.g. wearing loose-fitting socks and shoes, and avoiding sun exposure and hot showers or baths). Other management strategies can include the use of cold compresses or ice packs to wrists and ankles to reduce blood flow to hands and feet, elevating hands and feet, and keeping skin hydrated and protected (e.g. using a good emollient/moisturiser and patting skin dry rather than rubbing with a towel). Activities that cause friction to palms and soles should be temporarily avoided (e.g. jogging, activities that require gripping a tool or device for long periods of time (e.g. chopping vegetables, weeding the garden))
- during therapy and for 1 week after, the patient should be instructed to:
  - flush the toilet twice after use
  - wear gloves and use paper towels and bleach or a large quantity of water to wipe up any body spills
  - wash clothes or bed linen separately if contaminated
  - use a barrier method (e.g. condom) during sexual intercourse
- counsel men about the potential effects of antineoplastic agents on sperm count and the possibility of sperm storage; use of a condom is also recommended during treatment period and in some instances for weeks to months after therapy (manufacturer's instructions should be consulted)
- women should be counselled that antineoplastic agents are not recommended or are contraindicated during pregnancy and it is therefore important to use reliable contraceptive methods (in some cases more than one method is recommended) while undergoing treatment and for a number of months post-therapy (time is dependent on the individual agents)
- counsel women to avoid breastfeeding during treatment, as antineoplastic agents may be secreted into breastmilk, potentially causing severe adverse effects in the infant

In general, antineoplastic capsules should not be opened or tablets crushed, chewed or broken.

Contraindicated or not recommended during pregnancy.

Contraindicated or not recommended during breastfeeding.

ABIRATERONE ACETATE

Trade names
Abiraterone MedTas, Abiraterone Teva, Zyron, Zytiga

Available forms
Tablets: 250 mg, 500 mg

Action
- hormonal antineoplastic (androgen biosynthesis inhibitor)
- active metabolites

Use
- newly diagnosed metastatic hormone-sensitive prostate cancer (with androgen deprivation therapy)
- metastatic advanced prostate cancer (with prednisolone or prednisone) (asymptomatic, mildly symptomatic after failure of androgen deprivation therapy or previously treated with taxanes)

Dose
- 1 g orally daily 1 hour before or 2 hours after food (with 10 mg prednisolone or prednisone for metastatic castration-resistant cancer or 5 mg for hormone-sensitive cancer)

Adverse effects
- peripheral oedema
- cardiac failure, arrhythmias, atrial fibrillation, tachycardia, hypertension
- increased liver enzymes
- hypertriglyceridaemia
- hypokalaemia

Interactions
- not recommended with spironolactone
- not recommended with phenytoin, carbamazepine, rifampicin, rifabutin or phenobarbital (phenobarbitone), as decreased serum levels may occur
- may increase serum levels and hypoglycaemic effects of thiazolinediones and should be used with caution
- combination with prednisolone/prednisone is contraindicated with radium-223 dichloride

Nursing considerations/Cautions
- BP, any fluid retention (e.g. unexplained weight gain or oedema) and serum potassium should be closely monitored during therapy
- liver enzymes should be measured before starting, second-weekly for 12 weeks, then monthly throughout therapy
- if prednisolone or prednisone is withdrawn, the patient should be monitored for any signs of mineralocorticoid excess
- doses of prednisolone or prednisone may need to be increased if the patient undergoes severe stress
- blood glucose levels should be monitored regularly during therapy (because of combination with prednisolone or prednisone)
- caution if used in those affected by increases in BP, hypokalaemia or fluid retention (such as those with recent myocardial infarction or heart failure)
- contraindicated in those with severe liver impairment (Child—Pugh C)
- see also General Nursing considerations/Cautions for antineoplastic agents (p. 596)

Patient education
- if the patient has diabetes, monitoring blood glucose levels should be advised as corticosteroids (prednisolone or prednisone) may cause hyperglycaemia
- see also General Patient education for antineoplastic agents (p. 598)

 Tablets should not be dispersed, crushed or broken.

 Contraindicated in those with severe liver impairment (Child—Pugh Class C)

Available in combination with
- Yonsa Mpred (abiraterone acetate 125 mg with methylprednisolone 4 mg)

ANTINEOPLASTIC AGENTS

ANAGRELIDE

Trade names
Agrylin, Anagrelide APX, Anagrelide Lupin

Available form
Capsules: 0.5 mg

Action
- quinazoline derivative antineoplastic agent that reduces platelet count
- active metabolite
- half-life 3 hours

Use
- essential thrombocytopenia

Dose
- initially 0.5 mg orally twice daily for $\geq$ 7 days, then adjusting dose to lowest effective dose to reduce and maintain required platelet count (daily maximum 10 mg or dose maximum 2.5 mg)

Adverse effects
- abnormal vision, double vision, amblyopia
- (Rare) QT prolongation, pulmonary hypertension
- see also General Adverse effects of antineoplastic agents (p. 596)

Interactions
- caution if given with other agents known to cause QT prolongation or electrolyte imbalance (especially hypokalaemia or hypomagnesaemia)
- caution if used with heparin, as anticoagulant effect may be increased
- may increase effects of milrinone or similar agents
- may inhibit clearance of theophylline, increasing the risk of toxicity
- clearance may be inhibited by fluvoxamine and ciprofloxacin
- caution if used with omeprazole
- enhances the antiplatelet effect of aspirin and should be given only with great caution because of the haemorrhagic risk

Nursing considerations/Cautions
- cardiovascular and cardiopulmonary examinations are recommended before starting therapy
- any electrolyte imbalance (especially hypokalaemia or hypomagnesaemia) should be corrected before starting therapy
- platelet count should be monitored second daily for 7 days, then weekly. Platelet count usually responds to therapy in 7–14 days. Platelet count should be monitored frequently if therapy is interrupted or stopped
- liver function tests, renal function test, electrolytes and full blood count are recommended before starting and regularly during therapy
- plasmapheresis may be more appropriate if immediate platelet reduction is required
- dose should not be increased by more than 0.5 mg weekly
- target platelet count 150–400 $\times$ 10^9/L
- increased risk of renal toxicity if serum creatinine $\geq$ 0.18 mmol/L
- increased risk of thromboembolic events if therapy is suddenly stopped
- caution if used in those with congenital or acquired QT prolongation or electrolyte imbalance
- tablets contain lactose and are therefore not recommended in those with rare hereditary problems of galactose intolerance, Lapp lactase deficiency or glucose-galactose malabsorption
- contraindicated in those with severe liver impairment
- see also General Nursing considerations/Cautions for antineoplastic agents (p. 596)

Patient education
- instruct the patient to seek medical advice immediately if any of the following occur:
  - rapid or irregular heart rate
  - chest pain
  - shortness of breath (initially on exercise, then at rest), chest pressure/pain, pale/blue skin colour, dizziness, fainting, fast pulse or pounding heart beat, swelling of ankles, legs and/or abdominal area

- warn the patient not to drive or operate machinery if visual disturbances occur
- the patient should be advised not to stop therapy abruptly
- see also General Patient education for antineoplastic agents (p. 598)

Capsules may be opened and contents dispersed in water or mixed with spoonful of yoghurt or apple puree.

Caution if used in those with mild-to-moderate liver impairment: the starting dose should be decreased to 0.5 mg daily.

Contraindicated in those with severe liver failure. Those with renal impairment (serum creatinine > 0.18 mmol/L) should be closely monitored during therapy.

ANASTROZOLE

Trade names
Anastrozole Sandoz, Anastrozole-GH, Anastrozole-WGR, Anzole, APO-Anastrozole, Arianna 1, Arimidex

Available form
Tablets: 1 mg

Action
- highly selective non-steroidal aromatase inhibitor that decreases serum estradiol (oestradiol) levels with no effect on formation of adrenal corticosteroids or aldosterone
- half-life 40—50 hours

Use
- early breast cancer (first-line treatment, postmenopausal, oestrogen/progesterone-positive tumour) (adjunctive treatment)
- advanced breast cancer (first-line treatment, postmenopausal, oestrogen/progesterone-positive tumour)
- advanced breast cancer (postmenopausal) (after tamoxifen failure)

Dose
- 1 mg orally daily for up to 5 years

Adverse effects
- hot flushes
- nausea, vomiting, diarrhoea, anorexia
- elevated liver enzymes, hypercholesterolaemia
- headache, asthenia, somnolence
- joint pain/stiffness, bone pain, myalgia
- rash, hair thinning
- vaginal dryness or bleeding
- (Uncommon) urticaria
- (Rare) decreased bone density, osteoporosis, bone fractures

Interactions
- not recommended with tamoxifen, oestrogen-containing products or luteinising hormone-releasing hormone (LHRH) agonists

Nursing considerations/Cautions
- bone density should be measured before starting and regularly throughout therapy, and treatment or prophylaxis therapy started if needed
- 2—3 years of tamoxifen therapy should be completed before switching to anastrozole
- caution if used in those with kidney or liver impairment
- not recommended in premenopausal women or in those with oestrogen/progesterone-negative tumour
- see also General Nursing considerations/Cautions for antineoplastic agents (p. 596)

Patient education
- see General Patient education for antineoplastic agents (p. 598)

Tablet may be dispersed in water or crushed and mixed with a spoonful of yoghurt or apple puree. Mask and gloves should be worn when dispersing or crushing tablet. Pregnant staff must not disperse or crush tablets.

Caution if used in those with severe kidney or severe liver impairment.

Banned in sport.

ANTINEOPLASTIC AGENTS

APALUTAMIDE
Trade name
Erlyand

Available form
Tablets: 60 mg

Action
- hormonal antineoplastic agent that blocks androgen receptors
- active metabolite has one-third the activity of apalutamide

Use
- non-metastatic castration-resistant prostate cancer
- metastatic castration-sensitive prostate cancer

Dose
- 240 mg orally daily (with a gonadotrophin-releasing hormone (GnRH) analogue unless the patient has had bilateral orchiectomy)

Adverse effects
- hot flushes
- depression
- haematuria
- osteopenia, osteoporosis, fractures, increased risk of falls
- hypercholesterolaemia, hyperglycaemia, hypertriglyceridaemia, hyperkalaemia
- hypothyroidism (in those receiving thyroid replacement therapy)
- ischaemic heart disease, heart failure, QT interval prolongation
- (Rare) seizures, serious skin reactions, interstitial lung disease
- see also General Adverse effects of antineoplastic agents (p. 596)

Interactions
- caution if used with agents known to prolong QT interval or cause electrolyte imbalance
- decreased serum level may occur if given with gemfibrozil, itraconazole or rifampicin
- caution if given with warfarin; the INR should be monitored closely if given together
- may decrease serum levels of fexofenadine and rosuvastatin
- may reduce effects of levothyroxine, increasing the risk of hypothyroidism

Nursing considerations/Cautions
- ensure any electrolyte imbalance is corrected before starting therapy
- bone density should be monitored regularly during therapy
- caution if used in those with history of QT prolongation or risk factors for electrolyte imbalance, or a clinically significant cardiac history in the previous six months including severe or unstable angina, myocardial infarction, congestive cardiac failure, thromboembolic event or significant ventricular arrhythmias
- caution if used in those with history of seizures or a history of thyroid dysfunction receiving thyroid replacement therapy
- contraindicated in women

Patient education
- for patients with swallowing difficulties:
  - a 240 mg tablet can be dispersed (without crushing or breaking tablet) in cup with about 10 mL of non-carbonated water. When the tablet has dispersed completely (after about 2 minutes), the suspension should be stirred and added to 30 mL of orange juice, green tea, drinkable yoghurt or apple sauce, stirred again and swallowed immediately. The cup should be rinsed with water and the contents swallowed to ensure the whole dose has been taken
  - a 60 mg tablet can be mixed (not crushed or broken) with 120 mL apple sauce, stirred and mixed well again at 15 minutes and 30 minutes to ensure the tablet has dispersed (no chunks of tablet should remain) and then swallowed immediately. The container should be rinsed with 60 mL water and the contents swallowed, and this repeated again to

ensure the whole dose has been taken
- instruct the patient to seek medical advice immediately if any of the following occur:
  - fits/seizures
  - severe rash with skin blistering or peeling
  - sudden or worsening cough, shortness of breath, difficulty breathing, chest pain
  - chest pain or discomfort, shortness of breath, muscle weakness, numbness or paralysis in any part of the body
- see also General Patient education for antineoplastic agents (p. 598)

 Caution if used in those over 75 years because of an increased risk of serious adverse effects.

ARSENIC TRIOXIDE

Trade names
Arsenic Trioxide-AFT, Arsenic Trioxide Juno, Phenasen

Available form
Vial: 10 mg/10 mL

Action
- antineoplastic agent with unknown action that induces partial differentiation and apoptosis in leukaemic cells
- stored in bone marrow, lung, liver, kidney, heart, hair and nails with hair and nails showing increasing levels of arsenic during therapy
- half-life 92 hours

Use
- induction of remission and consolidation of acute promyelocytic leukaemia (APL) (refractory or relapsed from other therapy) or previously untreated APL (with retinoic acid and/or chemotherapy)

Dose
- (Newly diagnosed APL) 0.15 mg/kg IV over 2 hours on days 9—28 of a 28-day cycle (cycle 1, induction) then, after 3—4 weeks, 0.15 mg/kg on days 1—28 (cycle 2) then, after 3—4 weeks, 0.15 mg/kg for 5 days with 2 days off for 5 weeks (consolidation) (with tretinoin and/or chemotherapy) **OR**
- (Refractory or relapsed APL) 0.15 mg/kg IV over 2 hours until bone marrow remission occurs (induction) then, after 3—4 weeks, 0.15 mg/kg for 25 daily doses for up to 5 weeks (consolidation)

Adverse effects
- cardiac arrhythmia, QT interval prolongation
- APL differentiation syndrome (fever, dyspnoea, weight gain, pulmonary infiltrates, pleural/pericardial effusions (with or without leucocytosis))
- peripheral neuropathy
- see also General Adverse effects of antineoplastic agents (p. 605)

Interactions
- not recommended with agents known to prolong the QT interval (e.g. amiodarone, disopyramide, clarithromycin, sotalol, methadone, ziprasidone) or cause electrolyte disturbances, especially hypokalaemia and hypomagnesaemia (e.g. diuretics, amphotericin B (amphotericin))

Nursing considerations/Cautions
- any electrolyte imbalance should be corrected before starting therapy
- a 12-lead ECG is recommended before starting and then weekly during therapy
- serum electrolytes (especially potassium, calcium and magnesium), creatinine, blood counts and coagulation should be measured before starting and then regularly throughout therapy (more frequent if the patient is unstable)
- (Newly diagnosed APL) 1 mg/kg daily prednisolone/prednisone is recommended for at least 10 days during induction
- female patients of childbearing potential should be tested for pregnancy before starting therapy because of the potential harm to the fetus

ANTINEOPLASTIC AGENTS

- dilute with 100—250 mL sodium chloride 0.9% or glucose 5% for IV infusion
- if the patient shows signs of APL differentiation syndrome, dexamethasone 10 mg IV twice daily should be administered for 3 or more days or until symptoms resolve
- (Refractory/relapsed APL) therapy should be discontinued after 2 months if bone marrow remission does not occur
- caution if used in those with known congenital or acquired prolonged QT syndrome or electrolyte imbalance
- caution if used in those with renal impairment (as arsenic is excreted renally)
- not recommended in those with congestive cardiac failure or in children under 5 years
- contraindicated in those with hypersensitivity to arsenic
- see also General Nursing considerations/Cautions for antineoplastic agents (p. 596)

Patient education

- the patient should be instructed to seek medical advice immediately if any of the following occur:
  - any fever, shortness of breath or weight gain (signs of APL differentiation syndrome)
  - rapid or irregular heart rate or fainting
  - numbness, weakness or tingling in hands or feet
- see also General Patient education for antineoplastic agents (p. 598)

 Caution if used in the elderly because of the increased risk of adverse effects related to renal impairment.

AXICABTAGENE CILOLEUCEL
Trade name
Yescarta

Available form
Suspension bag: $1-2.4 \times 10^6$ anti-CD19 chimeric antigen receptor (CAR) T cells/kg suspension

Action
- CD19 directed genetically modified autologous T-cell immunotherapy prepared from patient's own T cells which have been harvested via leukapheresis and then genetically modified by retroviral transduction to express a CAR

Use
- relapsed or refractory diffuse large B-cell lymphoma
- relapsed or refractory follicular lymphoma (after two or more types of systemic therapy)

Dose
- single IV infusion for a target dose of 2×10^6 anti-CD19 CAR T cells/kg (range 1×10^6 to 2.4×10^6 cells/kg) (maximum 2×10^8 anti-CD19 CAR T cells)

Adverse effects
- cytokine-release syndrome
- neurological toxicity (including encephalopathy, tremor, confusion, aphasia, somnolence)
- bacterial and viral infections, virus reactivation
- hypogammaglobinaemia
- tumour lysis syndrome
- see also General Adverse effects of antineoplastic agents (p. 596)

Interactions
- vaccination with live vaccines is not recommended for at least 6 weeks before lymphodepleting chemotherapy, during therapy and until immune recovery has occurred

Nursing considerations/Cautions
- before collecting cells for therapy, the patient should be screened for hepatitis B and C and human immunodeficiency virus (HIV)
- pregnancy status should be verified before starting therapy in women with childbearing potential
- after infusion, blood counts, uric acid and immunoglobulin levels should be monitored

- severe or life-threatening cytokine-release syndrome should be treated with tocilizumab (see disease-modifying antirheumatic drugs (DMARDs), p. 1073) or tocilizumab and corticosteroids. A minimum of 4 doses of tocilizumab must be readily available in case of cytokine-release syndrome, along with emergency equipment. Treatment and supportive care (e.g. oxygen, fluids, vasopressor and, if life threatening, ventilator support, haemodialysis) must be instituted at first signs of cytokine-release syndrome
- pretreatment involves lymphodepleting chemotherapy (cyclophosphamide 500 mg/m^2 IV and fludarabine 30 mg/m^2 IV on days 5, 4 and 3 before infusion). If the patient has high uric acid levels or high tumour burden, allopurinol (or alternative prophylaxis) should be given before conditioning chemotherapy to reduce the risk of tumour lysis syndrome
- premedication (500–1000 mg paracetamol orally with diphenhydramine 12.5 mg IV or orally (or equivalent)) is recommended 1 hour before infusion
- prophylactic systemic corticosteroids should not be used
- important to coordinate thaw and infusion timing so that infusion is thawed and available for infusion when the patient is ready
- patient identity must be confirmed (matching patient ID with patient identifiers on infusion cassette). When correctly identified, the product bag is removed from the cassette and inspected for any breaks or cracks before thawing. The infusion bag should then be placed in a second sterile bag and then thawed, either in a water bath or by the dry thaw method until there is no visible ice in the infusion bag. The bag should be gently mixed to disperse any cellular clumps. The solution should not be washed, spun down or resuspended before infusion
- a leukodepleting filter should not be used
- given only IV (with a central venous line recommended)
- the line should be primed with sodium chloride 0.9% before and after infusion
- infusion should be via gravity or peristaltic infusion pump
- infusion contains 300 mg sodium
- standard precautions for blood-borne pathogens should be adhered to, and handling and disposal should be as per institution biosafety guidelines
- the patient should be monitored for at least 7 days postinfusion for any signs of cytokine-release syndrome
- the solution must not be irradiated
- contains dimethyl sulfoxide and residual gentamicin, which may cause hypersensitivity reaction in sensitive individuals
- not recommended for primary central nervous system lymphoma
- not recommended in those with active systemic infections or inflammatory disorders

Patient education

- the patient should be instructed to remain within close proximity of the health care facility (< 2 hours) for at least 4 weeks postinfusion
- warn the patient not to drive or operate machinery for at least 8 weeks after infusion owing to the risk of fitting/seizures or other neurological issues
- ensure the patient understands the importance of ongoing monitoring (at least 15 years) for secondary malignancies
- the patient should be advised to immediately seek medical advice if any of the following occur:
  - fever, chills, low blood pressure, which can lead to feeling light-headed or dizzy, or rapid heart rate (signs of cytokine-release syndrome, which can be serious or life threatening)
  - headache, tremor, confusion, difficulty talking, sleepy or drowsiness
  - signs of infection, including fever, chills, swollen glands

- fatigue, confusion, nausea, vomiting, diarrhoea, muscle weakness, cramps or spasms, tingling around mouth or hands/feet, heart beats slower, faster or flutters, fitting (signs of tumour lysis syndrome)
- instruct the patient not to donate blood, organs, tissue or cells for transplantation
- see also General Patient education for antineoplastic agents (p. 598)

AZACITIDINE

Trade names
Azacitidine Accord, Azacitidine Dr Reddy's, Azacitidine Eugia, Azacitidine Juno, Azacitidine MSN, Azacitidine Sandoz, Azacitidine SXP, Azacitidine-Teva, Azadine, Onureg

Available forms
Vial: 100 mg;
Tablets: 300 mg, 400 mg

Action
- pyrimidine analogue antimetabolite that acts on DNA and also has direct cytotoxic action on abnormal haemopoietic cells in bone marrow
- half-life 30 minutes

Use
- acute myeloid leukaemia (AML) (with 20–30% blasts and multilineage dysplasia, stem cell transplant is not recommended)
- AML who achieved complete first remission (CR) or complete remission with incomplete blood count (iCR) recovery after intensive induction therapy or was unable to complete intensive curative therapy
- chronic myelomonocytic leukaemia (CML) (with 10–29% blasts, no myeloproliferative disease)
- intermediate- to high-risk myelodysplastic syndrome (MDS)

Dose
- 75 mg/m^2 SC or IV over 10–40 minutes for 7 days followed by 21-day rest interval (cycle 1), repeated for ≥ 6 cycles (treatment may continue if benefit is noted) **OR**
- (AML with CR or iCR) 300 mg orally daily for 14 days, followed by 14-day rest interval (28-day cycle)

Adverse effects
- (Injection site) pain, redness, rash, inflammation, itching, bruising, induration
- eye/conjunctival haemorrhage
- (Rare) hypersensitivity, interstitial lung disease
- see also General Adverse effects of antineoplastic agents (p. 596)

Nursing considerations/Cautions
- oral and IV therapy are not interchangeable
- patient should be premedicated to prevent nausea and vomiting
- dose reduction is required if severe adverse effects occur
- (Oral) antiemetic is recommended 30 minutes before each dose for first two cycles. If there is no nausea and vomiting, antiemetic prophylaxis can be omitted before subsequent cycles
- (Oral) therapy should be continued until there are no more than 15% blasts in peripheral blood or blood marrow, or until unacceptable toxicity occurs
- (SC) reconstitute with 4 mL water for injections and use within 1 hour (if at room temperature). Can be refrigerated for up to 8 hours, but should be brought to room temperature for at least 30 minutes before SC administration
- (SC) if dose > 4 mL it should be divided and given into separate sites
- (SC) rotate SC injection sites avoiding any areas that are red, tender, hard or bruised. Injections should not be within 2.5 cm of previous injection site
- (IV) reconstitute with 10 mL water for injections, and dilute with sodium chloride 0.9% or lactated Ringer's solution (50–100 mL) and infuse over 10–40 minutes

HAVARD'S NURSING GUIDE TO DRUGS

- (IV) infusion should be completed within 45 minutes of reconstitution
- incompatible with glucose 5% and solutions containing bicarbonate
- (Oral) tablets contain lactose and are therefore not recommended in those with rare hereditary problems of galactose intolerance, total lactase deficiency or glucose—galactose malabsorption
- contraindicated in those with advanced malignant liver tumours or severe kidney impairment (creatinine clearance < 30 mL/min)
- see also General Nursing considerations/Cautions for antineoplastic agents (p. 596)

Patient education

- the patient should be instructed to immediately seek medical advice if the volume of urine decreases or stops altogether
- see also General Patient education for antineoplastic agents (p. 598)

Tablets must not be crushed, broken or chewed.

Contraindicated in those with CrCl < 30 mL/min.

BCG (Non-vaccine)
Trade name
OncoTICE

Available form
Vial: 2–8 × 108 CFU

Action
- immunostimulant that causes inflammatory response resulting in reduction or elimination of non-muscle cancerous lesions in the urinary bladder
- live attenuated *Mycobacterium bovis*

Use
- primary or recurrent bladder cancer (BC) in situ
- adjunct to transurethral resection of high-grade and/or relapsing superficial papillary transitional cell bladder cancer (stage TA or T1)

Dose
- (In situ BC) 50 mL of reconstituted solution instilled into bladder and left in situ for 2 hours if possible, administered weekly for 6 weeks, then monthly for 12 months **OR**
- (Superficial papillary transitional cell bladder cancer) 50 mL of reconstituted solution instilled into bladder and left in situ for 2 hours if possible, administered weekly for 6 weeks, repeated at week 8 and 12, then monthly for 4–12 months

Adverse effects
- dysuria, haematuria, urinary retention, urgency and frequency, bladder cramps/pain, contracted bladder
- cystitis, urinary tract infection, urinary incontinence
- nausea, vomiting, abdominal pain, diarrhoea
- arthralgia, myalgia
- malaise, fatigue
- fever, chills, rigors, flu-like symptoms
- (Rare) systemic disease, hypersensitivity

Interactions
- caution if used with immunosuppressive agents, bone marrow depressants or radiotherapy, as they may interfere with the immune response

Nursing considerations/Cautions

- the patient should be assessed for active tuberculosis (TB) disease before starting therapy using a tuberculin test. If positive, therapy is contraindicated only if there is evidence of active TB infection
- monitor the patient for any signs of BCG infection and toxicity during therapy
- if the patient develops signs of BCG disease, immediate evaluation is recommended, as treatment with antimycobacterial agents may be required
- great care should be taken during reconstitution to avoid contact with or inhalation of the powder. The person

ANTINEOPLASTIC AGENTS

- should wear adequate eye and face protection, gloves, mask and gown during the procedure. Reconstitute the powder with 1 mL of sodium chloride 0.9% and then dilute with 49 mL sodium chloride 0.9% (total volume 50 mL)
- do not shake the solution during reconstitution
- incompatible with hypotonic or hypertonic solution
- if the patient develops a bacterial urinary tract infection (UTI), therapy should be withheld until the UTI has totally resolved to decrease the risk of adverse effects
- not given IV, SC or IM
- therapy should be withheld if the patient is being treated with antibiotics
- caution if used in those with small bladder capacity, as greater irritation may occur
- contraindicated in those with urinary tract infection, febrile illness, gross haematuria, existing active tuberculosis, impaired immune response (including acquired immunodeficiency syndrome (AIDS)), asymptomatic carriers with positive human immunodeficiency virus (HIV) serology, taking corticosteroids or immunosuppressants (including radiotherapy) or within 7–14 days of biopsy or traumatic catheterisation until mucosa has healed
- see also General Nursing considerations/Cautions for antineoplastic agents (p. 596)

Patient education

- the patient should be instructed to:
  - not to drink for 4 hours before instillation
  - empty the bladder, then having the urethral catheter inserted, diluted solution instilled and catheter removed
  - rotate every 15 minutes from left, prone, right and supine for 1 hour while the diluted solution is in the bladder
  - after retaining the solution for another 1 hour (if possible), the patient is asked to void in a seated position
- warn the patient that they may experience a burning sensation with the first void after completion of therapy
- the patient should be instructed to void in a seated position 6 hours after following the procedure, and add an equal volume of household chlorine bleach (e.g. White King) to the toilet. Urine and bleach should be allowed to stand in the toilet for 15 minutes before flushing
- male patients should be advised to either refrain from sexual intercourse or wear a condom for 7 days after treatment

BENDAMUSTINE HYDROCHLORIDE

Trade names
Bendamustine Viatris, Bendamustine Juno, Bendamustine Sandoz, Ribomustin

Available forms
Vial: 25 mg, 100 mg

Action
- alkylating agent (nitrogen mustard analogue) that impairs DNA synthesis and repair
- active against both quiescent and dividing cells
- half-life 28 minutes

Use
- treatment of chronic lymphocytic leukaemia (CLL)
- previously untreated indolent CD20-positive non-Hodgkin lymphoma stage III or IV (with rituximab)
- previously untreated CD20-positive stage III–IV mantle cell lymphoma (with rituximab in those ineligible for stem cell transplantation)
- relapsed/refractory indolent non-Hodgkin lymphoma

Dose
- (CLL monotherapy) 100 mg/m^2 by IV infusion over 30—60 minutes on days 1 and 2, every 4 weeks for up to 6 cycles **OR**
- (Non-Hodgkin lymphoma monotherapy) 120 mg/m^2 by IV infusion over 30—60 minutes on days 1 and 2, every 3 weeks for 6—8 cycles (maximum 8 cycles) **OR**
- (Non-Hodgkin lymphoma, mantle cell lymphoma, combination therapy) 90 mg/m^2 by IV infusion over 30—60 minutes on days 1 and 2 of a 4-week cycle for up to 6 cycles (with rituximab)

Adverse effects
- prolonged lymphocytopenia (for at least 7—9 months after treatment)
- hypokalaemia
- (Infusion reaction) fever, chills, rash, itching
- (Rare) severe skin reaction, anaphylaxis
- see also General Adverse effects of antineoplastic agents (p. 596)

Interactions
- contraindicated with yellow fever vaccination
- an increased risk of myelosuppression if given with other myelosuppressive agents, including ciclosporin and tacrolimus
- caution if used with ciprofloxacin, fluvoxamine or aciclovir

Nursing considerations/Cautions
- the patient should be tested for hepatitis B before starting therapy, as reactivation may occur
- ensure the patient is well hydrated during therapy
- (non-Hodgkin lymphoma, mantle cell lymphoma, combination therapy) therapy should be interrupted if leucocyte and/or platelet counts drop to $< 3 \times 10^9$/L or $< 75 \times 10^9$/L
- serum potassium should be closely monitored during therapy and potassium supplements administered if serum potassium < 3.5 mEq/L; ECG monitoring is also recommended
- reconstitute the powder with 40 mL water for injections (for 100 mg vial) or 10 mL (for 25 mg vial) to given concentration of 2.5 mg/mL and then finally dilute further with sodium chloride 0.9% to a final volume of 500 mL
- contraindicated in those with severe liver impairment (bilirubin > 3 mg/dL), jaundice, severe marrow depression, active infection or within 30 days of major surgery
- see also General Nursing considerations/Cautions for antineoplastic agents (p. 596)

Patient education
- advise the patient to seek medical advice immediately if a severe skin reaction, including peeling and blistering, occurs
- warn the patient that susceptibility to infection will exist for 7—9 months after therapy has stopped
- see also General Patient education for antineoplastic agents (p. 598)

 Not recommended during breastfeeding unless benefits outweigh risks.

 Dose reduction is recommended in those with moderate-to-severe liver impairment. Contraindicated in those with severe liver impairment.

BICALUTAMIDE
Trade names
APO-Bicalutamide, Bicalox, Calutex, Cosamide, Cosudex 50

Available form
Tablets: 50 mg

Action
- non-steroidal hormonal antineoplastic agent (antiandrogen) impairing growth of androgen-dependent tumour cells and regression of prostatic tumours

ANTINEOPLASTIC AGENTS

Use
- locally advanced prostate cancer (with luteinising hormone-releasing hormone (LHRH) agonist therapy)

Dose
- 50 mg orally daily (with LHRH agonist therapy)

Adverse effects
- breast tenderness, gynaecomastia
- decreased libido, erectile dysfunction, impotence
- nocturia, haematuria
- flushing
- (Uncommon) interstitial lung disease
- (Rare) photosensitivity, QT prolongation
- see also General Adverse effects of antineoplastic agents (p. 596)

Interactions
- contraindicated with midazolam
- may increase serum levels of ciclosporin, carbamazepine, calcium-channel blockers, human immunodeficiency virus (HIV) protease inhibitors and 3-hydroxy-3-methylglutaryl coenzyme A (HMG-CoA) reductase inhibitors (statins) and therefore given with caution
- may increase serum levels of warfarin, increasing the risk of bleeding, therefore INR should be closely monitored, especially when starting or stopping therapy
- caution if given with other agents known to prolong the QT interval or cause electrolyte imbalance (especially hypokalaemia and hypomagnesaemia)

Nursing considerations/Cautions
- any electrolyte imbalance should be corrected before starting therapy
- blood glucose levels should be monitored regularly because of the risk of glucose intolerance (when combined with LHRH)
- ECG, electrolyte and liver function monitoring are recommended regularly during therapy
- caution if used in those with moderate-to-severe liver impairment
- caution if used in those with congenital or acquired QT prolongation or electrolyte abnormalities
- not recommended in those with metastatic prostate cancer without LHRH analogues
- contraindicated in females and children
- see also General Nursing considerations/Cautions for antineoplastic agents (p. 596)

Patient education
- advise the patient to seek medical advice immediately if rapid or unusual heart rate occurs
- if the patient has diabetes, recommend close monitoring of blood glucose levels during therapy
- see also General Patient education for antineoplastic agents (p. 598)

Tablet does not disperse easily and is very hard to crush. Crush to a fine powder and mix with yoghurt or apple puree. Gloves and mask should be worn when crushing tablet. Pregnant staff must not crush tablets.

Not recommended during breastfeeding unless benefits outweigh risks.

Available in combination with
- contained in
  - ZolaCos CP with goserelin
  - BiEligard CP with leuprorelin

BLEOMYCIN SULFATE
Trade name
DBL Bleomycin Sulfate for Injection

Available form
Vial: 15,000 IU

Action
- cytotoxic antibiotic that causes breaks in DNA strands, resulting in inhibition of DNA cell synthesis

- most effective during M and G_2 phases of cell division
- bone marrow sparing
- half-life 15—60 minutes (prolonged in those with renal impairment)

Use
- for palliation and treatment adjuvant to surgery and radiation therapy for the following:
  - squamous cell carcinoma of skin, neck, head, oesophagus, penis, larynx and cervix
  - choriocarcinoma and embryonal testicular cancer
  - advanced Hodgkin lymphoma, non-Hodgkin lymphoma
  - mycosis fungoides

Dose
- initially 10,000—20,000 IU/m^2 given 1—2 times weekly IM, IV or SC **OR**
- 15,000 IU IM, IV or SC daily for 7 days, followed by 21 days treatment-free interval, repeated twice (total dose about 300,000 IU)

Adverse effects
- (Pulmonary toxicity) pneumonitis, interstitial fibrosis
- idiosyncratic reaction (similar to anaphylaxis) (hypotension, fever, chills, confusion, wheezing)
- hypoaesthesia, hyperaesthesia, urticaria, swelling, tenderness, pruritus, hyperpigmentation (in areas of pressure or friction including skin folds, nail cuticles, scars and IM injection sites), alopecia
- (IA) dermal lesions in area supplied by artery
- (Injection site) pain, phlebitis
- (Rare) cardiovascular toxicity (including myocardial infarction, haemolytic uraemic syndrome)
- see also General Adverse effects of antineoplastic agents (p. 596); however, it does not cause severe bone marrow toxicity

Interactions
- may decrease serum levels of digoxin and phenytoin
- an increased risk of pulmonary toxicity if given with cisplatin because of cisplatin-induced renal impairment
- caution if given with granulocyte colony stimulating factor (G-CSF) because of potential risk of pulmonary toxicity
- an increased risk of pulmonary toxicity when oxygen is given during surgery (especially long exposure and high concentrations)
- an increased risk of pulmonary toxicity when used before, with or after radiation therapy (especially chest)
- use with other antineoplastic agents as part of combination therapy increases risk of toxicity even at lower bleomycin doses

Nursing considerations/Cautions
- regular physical examination for cough, dyspnoea or basal rales is recommended to detect early signs of lung toxicity. In addition, patient monitoring should also include some of the following:
  - weekly X-rays are recommended, including 4 weeks after stopping therapy
  - lung function tests (including total lung volume, forced vital capacity)
  - baseline and monthly evaluation of carbon monoxide diffusion capacity
  - high-resolution computerised tomography (CT)
- (Lymphoma) a test dose of 1—5 units should be given for the first 2 treatments and the patient should be observed for 4—6 hours. If no reaction (hypotension, fever, chills, wheezing, confusion) occurs, the balance of the dose should then be given
- the patient should be closely observed after the first and second doses for any idiosyncratic reaction (hypotension, fever, chills, wheezing, confusion)
- an increased risk of acute adult respiratory distress syndrome if the patient has surgery/anaesthetic within 6—12 months of therapy. If the patient has

ANTINEOPLASTIC AGENTS

- surgery, the percentage of oxygen should be kept as low as possible, crystalloid fluids restricted and the patient carefully observed for any signs of pulmonary oedema
- more successful if given before irradiation
- note and report fever, dyspnoea and cough, as bleomycin is pulmonary-toxic
- improvement in lymphoma and testicular cancer is usually seen quickly, while squamous cell cancers may take up to 3 weeks to respond to therapy
- if no response is seen after 150,000 IU cumulative dose, therapy should be re-evaluated
- if the response is incomplete, a repeat course may be considered after a treatment-free interval of at least 3–4 weeks and only if there are no signs of lung toxicity
- may be given by IV, IM, SC, IA or intrapleural administration
- IA administration is used when an increased drug concentration at cancer site is required
- reconstitute using 1–5 mL water for injections (for IM or SC) or 5–10 mL (for IV or IA) and give slowly over 10 minutes
- pulmonary toxicity is more likely in those who receive total cumulative doses > 400,000 IU
- incompatible with amino acids, aminophylline, ascorbic acid, dexamethasone, furosemide, hyoscine and riboflavin
- caution if used in those with lung cancer, smokers, those with compromised lung function or if the patient has received previous cytotoxic therapy or radiation therapy (especially chest radiation) because of the increased risk of pulmonary toxicity
- a repeat course is contraindicated if pneumonitis occurs
- contraindicated in those with active lung infection or severely compromised lung function
- see also General Nursing considerations/Cautions for antineoplastic agents (p. 596)

Patient education
- the patient should be advised to seek medical advice immediately if any of the following occur:
  - cough, shortness of breath, difficulty breathing, chest pain related to breathing, wheezing
- see also General Patient education for antineoplastic agents (p. 598)

If patient has creatinine clearance ≤ 40 mL/min, dose reduction by 40–75% is recommended.

Caution if used at adult dose in those over 70 years.

BUSULFAN
Trade names
Busulfan ARX, Busulfex, Myleran

Available forms
Ampoules: 60 mg/10 mL;
Tablets: 2 mg

Action
- non-phase-specific bifunctional alkylating agent
- more selective than nitrogen mustard or folic acid antagonists on myeloid cells

Use
- chronic granulocytic leukaemia (CGL)
- polycythaemia vera, essential thrombocythaemia and myelofibrosis
- conditioning before stem cell transplantation (with other antineoplastic agents) (IV)

Dose
- (CGL) 0.06 mg/kg orally as a single dose (daily maximum 4 mg) (induction), then 0.5–2 mg orally (maintenance) **OR**
- (Polycythaemia vera, essential thrombocythaemia) 4–6 mg orally daily (induction), then 2–3 mg (half induction dose) (maintenance) **OR**

- (Myelofibrosis) initially 2—4 mg orally daily, then dose reduced for maintenance **OR**
- (Conditioning treatment — myeloablative) 3.2 mg/kg IV over 3 hours for 4 days (total dose 12.8 mg/kg) **OR**
- (Conditioning treatment — non-myeloablative) 0.8—6.4 mg/kg IV over 3 hours for 2—4 days

Adverse effects
- lung toxicity
- cardiac toxicity
- liver toxicity, hepatic veno-occlusive disease
- acute graft versus host disease, chronic graft versus host disease
- Fanconi's anaemia
- hyperuricaemia, uric acid nephropathy
- hyperpigmentation (especially in those with dark complexion)
- corneal thinning
- sterility (both sexes)
- (High dose) seizures
- see also General Adverse effects of antineoplastic agents (p. 596)

Interactions
- not recommended with tioguanine (thioguanine) because of the risk of nodular regenerative hyperplasia, portal hypertension and oesophageal varices
- increased risk of toxicity if given with itraconazole or metronidazole
- if given with or within 72 hours of paracetamol, may decrease busulfan clearance
- clearance may be increased if given with phenytoin
- increased risk of pulmonary toxicity if oxygen is given during surgery. The percentage of oxygen should be kept as low as possible
- (High dose) if given with cyclophosphamide, interval of > 24 hours should be allowed to decrease risk of toxicity
- decreased clearance may occur if given with iron chelating agents. They should be stopped before starting therapy with busulfan
- not recommended with other antineoplastic agents or if the patient has had recent radiation therapy
- see also General Interactions of antineoplastic agents (p. 596)

Nursing considerations/Cautions
- (IV) premedication with antiepileptic agents (starting 12 hours before therapy and up to 24 hours after last dose) is recommended with high-dose therapy to decrease the risk of seizures
- (IV) antiemetics are recommended before first high-dose administration and continued throughout therapy
- any hyperuricaemia and/or hyperuricosuria should be corrected before starting therapy
- (CGL) not useful once blast transformation has occurred
- (CGL maintenance therapy) aim to maintain WBC 10,000—15,000/mm^3
- (IV) daily liver function tests are recommended until transplant day 28
- (IV) therapeutic drug monitoring is recommended after the first dose. Blood should not be sampled from the same lumen as busulfan is being administered
- prolonged therapy may lead to pulmonary toxicity
- if surgery and anaesthesia are required, the inspired oxygen concentration should be kept as low as possible
- (IV) if the patient is obese, dose should be based on ideal body weight
- should not be administered via peripheral line. Central venous line is recommended
- not recommended by rapid IV bolus
- must be diluted with sodium chloride 0.9% or glucose 5% for IV infusion to a concentration of 0.5 mg/mL
- IV infusion is given over 2—3 hours
- caution if used in those with epilepsy
- (IV) increased risk of liver toxicity if the patient has received previous radiation therapy ($\geq$ 3 cycles of chemotherapy) or prior stem cell transplant

ANTINEOPLASTIC AGENTS

- increased risk of lung toxicity if used in those with a history of lung or mediastinal radiation
- see also Nursing considerations/Cautions for antineoplastic agents (p. 596)

Patient education

- advise the patient to swallow the tablet whole (without crushing, breaking or chewing)
- warn the patient to avoid paracetamol or paracetamol-containing preparations for at least 72 hours before and after therapy
- the patient should be advised to report any new or worsening unproductive cough (which may be a first sign of lung toxicity)
- the patient (especially if dark complexion) should be warned about skin hyperpigmentation
- see also General Patient education for antineoplastic agents (p. 598)

 Tablet should not be crushed, broken or chewed.

CABAZITAXEL

Trade names
Cabazitaxel Accord, Cabazitaxel Ever Pharma, MSN Cabazitaxel

Available forms
Vial: 60 mg/3 mL, 60 mg/6 mL, 60 mg/1.5 mL

Action
- taxane antimetabolite that inhibits mitotic and cellular functions
- three active metabolites

Use
- hormone refractory metastatic castration-resistant prostate cancer (previously treated with docetaxel) (with prednisolone or prednisone)

Dose
- 20 mg/m^2 IV infusion over 1 hour every 3 weeks (with prednisolone or prednisone 10 mg orally daily)

Adverse effects
- tachycardia, atrial fibrillation
- peripheral neuropathy
- urinary disorder
- pneumonitis, interstitial lung disorder, acute respiratory distress syndrome
- hypersensitivity
- see also General Adverse effects of antineoplastic agents (p. 596)

Interactions
- increased serum levels may result if given with itraconazole, clarithromycin, atazanavir, ritonavir or voriconazole
- decreased serum levels may result if given with phenytoin, carbamazepine, rifampicin, rifabutin, phenobarbital (phenobarbitone) or St John's wort and these are therefore not recommended together
- contraindicated with live or live attenuated vaccines

Nursing considerations/Cautions

- premedication with antihistamine, corticosteroid and H$_2$ antagonist is recommended 30 minutes before infusion. Antiemetic prophylaxis should also be considered at this time
- the patient should be closely observed during first two doses for any signs of hypersensitivity (particularly the first and second infusions)
- ensure the patient is well hydrated during therapy
- dilute the powder using the supplied diluent, taking care to minimise foaming. Allow the solution to stand for 5 minutes before further diluting with sodium chloride 0.9% or glucose 5% to give a concentration of 0.10–0.26 mg/mL
- an inline filter (0.22 microns) is recommended
- caution if used in those who have received pelvic radiation and docetaxel-containing therapy because of the risk of cystisis related to radiation recall phenomenon

- not recommended with PVC bags or bottles or polyurethane tubing, filters or pumps
- contraindicated in those with hypersensitivity to polysorbate 80, previous reaction to cabazitaxel or neutrophil count $\leq$ 1500/mm^3 or severe liver impairment (total bilirubin > 3 upper limit of normal)
- see also General Nursing considerations/Cautions for antineoplastic agents (p. 596)

Patient education

- advise the patient to seek medical advice if any of the following occur:
  - pain, burning, tingling, numbness or weakness of hands or feet
  - rapid or irregular heart rate
  - difficulty breathing, tight chest, cough
  - painful urination, burning sensation, increase in urge or frequency of urination
- see also General Patient education for antineoplastic agents (p. 598)

 Contraindicated in those with severe liver impairment.

CAPECITABINE
Trade names
Capecitabine Sandoz, Capecitabine-DRLA, Xelabine, Xelocitabine

Available forms
Tablets: 150 mg, 500 mg

Action
- fluoropyrimidine antimetabolite that is activated by thymidine phosphorylase in tumours to cytotoxic metabolite fluorouracil (5FU)

Use
- locally advanced or metastatic breast cancer (not responding to taxanes or anthracycline-containing chemotherapy) (with docetaxel)
- advanced or metastatic colorectal cancer
- advanced oesophagogastric cancer (first-line treatment with platinum-based regimen)
- Dukes stage C or high- risk stage B colon cancer (monotherapy or with cisplatin)

Dose
- (Colon, colorectal, breast cancer — monotherapy) initially 1.25 g/m^2 orally twice daily within 30 minutes of meal for 2 weeks, followed by 2-week rest cycle, given as a 3-week cycle **OR**
- (Breast cancer — combination therapy) 1.25 g/m^2 orally twice daily within 30 minutes of meal for 2 weeks (with docetaxel 75 mg/m^2 IV over 1 hour every 3 weeks) followed by a 7-day rest period **OR**
- (Colorectal — combination therapy) 1.0 g/m^2 orally twice daily within 30 minutes of meal for 2 weeks followed by 7-day rest cycle (with oxaliplatin with or without bevacizumab) **OR**
- (Colon cancer adjunct) 1.0 g/m^2 orally twice daily within 30 minutes of meal for 2 weeks followed by 7-day rest cycle (with oxaliplatin IV) **OR**
- (Oesophagogastric cancer) 625 mg/m^2 orally twice daily within 30 minutes of meal continuously for 3-week cycle (with epirubicin and either cisplatin or oxaliplatin) **OR**
- (Gastric cancer) 1.0 g/m^2 orally twice daily within 30 minutes of meal for 2 weeks followed by 7-day rest cycle (with cisplatin IV)

Adverse effects
- myocardial infarction, angina, arrhythmias, cardiac failure, cardiac arrest, ECG changes
- hand—foot syndrome (hand/foot numbness, paraesthesia, tingling, erythema, pain, swelling and, at worst, ulceration, blistering or moist desquamation)
- hyperbilirubinaemia
- see also General Adverse effects of antineoplastic agents (p. 596)

ANTINEOPLASTIC AGENTS

Interactions
- may increase serum levels of phenytoin, increasing the risk of toxicity
- may increase activity of warfarin; therefore INR should be closely monitored, especially when starting or stopping therapy. Changes in coagulation have been seen up to a month after stopping therapy
- increased risk of toxicity if given with folinic acid (calcium folinate)

Nursing considerations/Cautions
- the patient should be well hydrated at the start and during therapy (especially if combined with cisplatin)
- (Colorectal — combination therapy, colon cancer adjunct, gastric cancer) therapy should be started on day 1 evening and finished on day 15 morning of a 21-day cycle
- for metastatic disease, therapy is ongoing
- as adjunct therapy, therapy is for 2 weeks
- caution if used in those with coronary artery disease as there is an increased risk of cardiac toxicity
- contraindicated in those with a known hypersensitivity to fluorouracil or a severe/unexpected reaction to fluoropyrimidine, or those with dihydropyrimidine dehydrogenase (DPD) deficiency or severe kidney impairment (creatinine clearance < 30 mL/min)
- see also General Nursing considerations/Cautions for antineoplastic agents (p. 596)

Patient education
- instruct the patient to swallow tablets whole within 30 minutes of completing meal
- advise the patient to seek medical advice if any of the following occur:
  - painful swelling and redness of hands and/or feet
  - irregular heart rate or chest pain
- see also General Patient education for antineoplastic agents (p. 598)

Tablet should not be crushed, broken or chewed.

Contraindicated in those with severe liver impairment. Dose reduction is recommended for those with mild liver impairment.

Caution if used in those over 65 years as they may be more likely to experience neutropenia or febrile neutropenia.

CARBOPLATIN
Trade names
Carboplatin Accord Solution, DBL Carboplatin Solution for Infusion

Available forms
Solution: 50 mg/5 mL, 150 mg/15 mL, 450 mg/45 mL

Action
- inorganic heavy metal (platinum) that interferes with DNA synthesis
- analogue of cisplatin

Use
- advanced ovarian cancer (epithelial origin)
- small cell lung cancer
- neuroblastoma
- head and neck cancer
- soft tissue sarcoma
- testicular cancer
- paediatric cerebral tumour

Dose
- (Adult) 400 mg/m^2 IV over 15—60 minutes, with at least 4 weeks between infusions

Adverse effects
- peripheral neuropathy, paraesthesia, decreased deep tendon reflexes
- new or worsening hearing loss
- transient sight loss, cortical blindness
- see also General Adverse effects of antineoplastic agents (p. 596)

Interactions
- hepatotoxic, myelotoxic, neurotoxic and ototoxic; therefore should not be given with other drugs with similar adverse effects (e.g. aminoglycosides)
- increased risk of fatigue, myalgia and arthralgia if given with paclitaxel
- pain, asthenia and visual disturbance may occur if given with cyclophosphamide
- increased risk of neurotoxicity and ototoxicity in those previously treated with cisplatin
- not recommended with live or live attenuated vaccines
- may decrease phenytoin serum levels, increasing the risk of seizures

Nursing considerations/Cautions
- incidence and severity of nausea and vomiting can be reduced by premedicating with antiemetic (e.g. metoclopramide, ondansetron), administering as a continual infusion over 24 hours or as divided doses over 5 consecutive days, rather than a single infusion
- a 4-week interval is recommended between treatment cycles
- may be diluted with glucose 5%
- reacts with aluminium (e.g. needles, IV administration sets) to form a black precipitate
- contraindicated in those with known hypersensitivity to platinum-containing compounds or mannitol, severe bleeding tendency, myelodepression or severe renal impairment
- see also General Nursing considerations/Cautions for antineoplastic agents (p. 596)

Patient education
- advise the patient to seek medical advice if any of the following occur:
  - changes in vision
  - new or worsening hearing loss, ringing in ears (tinnitus)
  - pain, burning, tingling, numbness or weakness of hands or feet
- see also General Patient education for antineoplastic agents (p. 598)

Reduced dose recommended for those with renal impairment:
- (creatinine clearance 20–39 mL/min) 250 mg/m^2
- (creatinine clearance < 20 mL/min) 150/m^2

Contraindicated in those with severe renal impairment.

CARMUSTINE
Trade names
BiCNU, Carmustine Lupin, Carmustine Medsurge

Available form
Vial: 100 mg

Action
- alkylating agent (nitrosourea)

Use
- malignant glioma
- multiple myeloma (MM) with prednisolone
- Hodgkin's disease or non-Hodgkin lymphomas (relapsed or failed to respond to primary therapy)

Dose
- 200 mg/m^2 IV every 6 weeks (given as either a single dose or split into 2 doses given on successive days)

Adverse effects
- (IV) pulmonary infiltrates/fibrosis
- brain oedema
- (Rare) pulmonary toxicity
- (IV site) burning, swelling, pain, erythema, skin necrosis
- see also General Adverse effects of antineoplastic agents (p. 596)

Interactions
- not recommended with other agents that affect lung function

Nursing considerations/Cautions
- lung function tests are recommended before starting and regularly throughout therapy

ANTINEOPLASTIC AGENTS

- should be allowed to come to room temperature before reconstitution. Reconstitute using 27 mL water for injections. May be further diluted using sodium chloride (0.9%) or glucose 5%
- given by slow IV infusion over 1–2 hours
- should not be given by rapid infusion
- the dose should not be repeated in less than 6 weeks (until platelets > 100,000/mm^3 and leucocytes > 4000/mm^3)
- caution if used in those with pre-existing lung disease or thoracic irradiation
- see also General Nursing considerations/Cautions for antineoplastic agents (p. 596)

Patient education

- warn the patient that lung problems can occur years after therapy is stopped. The patient should be advised to seek medical advice if new or worsening breathing problems occur
- see also General Patient education for antineoplastic agents (p. 598)

CHLORAMBUCIL

Trade name
Leukeran

Available form
Tablets: 2 mg

Action
- alkylating agent (nitrogen mustard analogue) that interferes with cell replication

Use
- Hodgkin's disease, some forms of non-Hodgkin lymphoma
- chronic lymphocytic leukaemia (CLL)
- Waldenstrom's macroglobulinaemia (lymphoplasmacytic lymphoma)
- advanced ovarian adenocarcinoma
- breast cancer

Dose
- (Hodgkin's disease – monotherapy) 0.2 mg/kg orally 1 hour before or 3 hours after food daily for 4–8 weeks **OR**
- (Non-Hodgkin lymphoma – monotherapy) 0.1–0.2 mg/kg orally 1 hour before or 3 hours after food daily for 4–8 weeks **OR**
- (CLL) 0.15 mg/kg orally 1 hour before or 3 hours after food daily until leucocytes ≤ 10,000/microL, then 0.1 mg/kg orally 1 hour before or 3 hours after food daily from 4 weeks after first course **OR**
- (Waldenstrom's macroglobulinaemia) 6–12 mg orally 1 hour before or 3 hours after food daily until leucopenia occurs, then 2–8 mg daily indefinitely **OR**
- (Advanced ovarian cancer – monotherapy) initially 0.2 mg/kg orally 1 hour before or 3 hours after food daily for 4–6 weeks or 0.3 mg/kg orally 1 hour before or 3 hours after food daily until leucopenia occurs, then 0.2 mg/kg daily for 2–4 weeks with a drug-free interval of 2–6 weeks **OR**
- (Advanced breast cancer – monotherapy) 0.2 mg/kg orally 1 hour before or 3 hours after food daily for 6 weeks

Adverse effects
- seizures
- (Rare) interstitial lung fibrosis
- see also General Adverse effects of antineoplastic agents (p. 596)

Interactions
- caution if given with other agents that increase the risk of seizures
- increased risk of toxicity if given with fludarabine or cladribine
- see also General Interactions of antineoplastic agents (p. 596)

Nursing considerations/Cautions

- (Breast cancer) may be given in combination therapy with prednisolone and either methotrexate or fluorouracil
- caution if used in those with a history of epilepsy or head trauma, prescribed high-dose pulse regimens or children with nephrotic syndrome because of the increased risk of seizure activity
- not recommended in those who have recently undergone radiation therapy or chemotherapy

- contraindicated in those with prior chlorambucil resistance
- see also General Nursing considerations/Cautions for antineoplastic agents (p. 596)

Patient education

- advise the patient to seek medical advice if persistent cough and/or shortness of breath occur
- the patient should be instructed to swallow tablets whole (not crushed, broken or chewed) with a glass of water either 1 hour before or 3 hours after food
- see also General Patient education for antineoplastic agents (p. 598)

Tablet should not be crushed, broken or chewed.

Caution if used in those with renal impairment, as additional myelosuppression may occur. Careful monitoring is recommended.

Dose reduction is recommended in those with severe liver impairment.

CHLORMETHINE

Trade name
Ledaga

Available form
Gel: 160 micrograms/g

Action
- bifunctional alkylating agent that reacts with DNA to form cross-links, causing death of rapidly dividing cells

Use
- topical treatment of mycosis fungoides-type cutaneous T-cell lymphoma

Dose
- apply a thin film to affected area once daily

Adverse effects
- redness, swelling, inflammation, pruritus, blistering, ulceration, skin infection, pain, burning sensation, skin hyperpigmentation
- hypersensitivity reaction
- secondary skin cancers

Nursing considerations/Cautions

- if the patient experiences any skin ulceration, blistering, marked skin redness with swelling, therapy should be stopped and restarted once every 3 days when skin shows improvement. If administration every 3 days is tolerated for at least 1 week, frequency can be increased to every second day for at least 1 week. If tolerated for at least 1 week, administration can resume at one daily application
- contains propylene glycol and butylhydroxytoluene, which can cause contact dermatitis

Patient education

- instruct the patient to immediately seek medical advice if any skin ulceration, blistering, marked skin redness or swelling occurs
- the patient/carer should be instructed in correct use of gel including:
  - gloves must be worn when applying the gel and carefully removed (turning them inside out during removal to avoid contact) and hands washed thoroughly after the gloves have been removed
  - avoid contact with the eyes or mucous membranes (oral mucosa or nasal mucosa). Exposure will cause pain, redness and ulceration and, if eyes are exposed, pain, inflammation, photophobia and blurred vision; if severe, it can result in blindness or irreversible anterior eye injury. If eye or mucous membrane exposure occurs, area should be irrigated with copious amounts of water, sodium chloride 0.9% or balanced salt ophthalmic, irrigating the solution for at least 15 minutes, and medical advice sought immediately

ANTINEOPLASTIC AGENTS

- especially if there is exposure to the eyes
- avoid contact with the face, genitalia, anus and skin folds
- if accidental exposure to non-affected skin occurs, the area should be washed with soap and water for at least 15 minutes
- if clothing is contaminated, it should be removed and washed
- gel should be applied within 30 minutes of removal from the refrigerator and returned immediately after each use (tube placed in original box, which is then placed in a transparent, sealable, plastic bag)
- apply the gel to completely dry skin at least 4 hours before or 30 minutes after showering or bathing
- allow the gel to dry for 5 to 10 minutes
- occlusive dressing should not be applied to the area
- moisturiser or another topical product can be applied to the treated area 2 hours before or 2 hours after the gel has been applied
- fire, flame and smoking must be avoided until the gel has dried. The gel is alcohol based and is flammable
- avoid direct contact of the gel-treated area with other people
- can be stored in refrigerator for up to 60 days, then any unused gel and plastic bag discarded safely
- advise the patient to report any new skin lesions during or after therapy has been stopped

CISPLATIN

Trade names
Cisplatin Accord Concentrate for Infusion, DBL Cisplatin Solution for Infusion

Available forms
Vial: 50 mg/50 mL, 100 mg/100 mL

Action
- inorganic heavy metal (platinum) that inhibits DNA synthesis (also RNA and protein synthesis to a lesser extent)
- properties similar to other alkylating agents
- narrow therapeutic index

Use
- metastatic non-seminomatous germ cell carcinoma
- advanced refractory bladder or ovarian cancer
- refractory squamous cell carcinoma of the head and neck

Dose
- 50–100 mg/m^2 as a single IV infusion over 1–2 hours every 3–4 weeks **OR**
- 15–20 mg/m^2 by IV infusion over 1–2 hours for 5 days every 3–4 weeks

Adverse effects
- nephrotoxicity
- neurotoxicity, including seizures
- peripheral neuropathy and vision loss
- hypertension, arrhythmias, congestive heart failure
- hearing loss, tinnitus
- hypomagnesaemia, secondary hypocalcaemia, hypokalaemia
- (Rare) anaphylaxis
- see also General Adverse effects of antineoplastic agents (p. 596)

Interactions
- not recommended with nephrotoxic medication, especially aminoglycosides and loop diuretics
- contraindicated with live or live attenuated vaccines

Nursing considerations/Cautions

- before starting therapy, renal and liver function, neurological status, full blood count and electrolytes should be measured and repeated regularly during therapy
- any dehydration should be corrected before starting therapy
- the risk of peripheral neuropathy is increased with prolonged therapy
- audiometric hearing tests should be performed before and during therapy
- to decrease nephrotoxicity, pre-treatment hydration with 2 L of glucose 4% in 20%

sodium chloride 0.18% or sodium chloride 0.9% over 2—4 hours and post-treatment hydration 2 L over 6—12 hours. During last 30 minutes of pre-treatment hydration, the patient should also receive 375 mL mannitol 10%
- renal function must return to normal before any further doses are given
- the infusion bag should be protected from light during therapy
- reacts with aluminium (e.g. needles, IV administration sets) to form a black precipitate
- caution if used in those with a history of atopy
- contraindicated in those with known hypersensitivity to platinum-containing compounds or mannitol, cisplatin-induced neuropathy, hearing impairment, renal impairment, bone marrow depression or generalised infections
- see also General Nursing considerations/Cautions for antineoplastic agents (p.596)

Patient education

- the patient should be instructed to seek medical attention if any of the following occur:
  - a decrease in hearing, ringing/buzzing in ears
  - numbness/tingling in feet or hands, burning sensation, weakness
  - fitting
  - blurred vision, altered colour perception
- see also General Patient education for antineoplastic agents (p. 598)

Caution if used in those with pre-existing liver dysfunction.

Caution if used in those with pre-existing renal dysfunction, as elimination half-life may be prolonged.

Contraindicated in those with serum creatinine > 0.2 mmol/L. Repeat courses are not advised until serum creatinine is < 0.14 mmol/L and/or blood urea is < 9 mmol/L.

CLADRIBINE

Trade names
Leustatin, Litak, Mavenclad

Available forms
Vial: 10 mg/5 mL, 10 mg/10 mL; Tablets: 10 mg

Action
- antimetabolite (purine nucleoside analogue)

Use
- hairy cell leukaemia
- Waldenstrom's macroglobulinaemia (lymphoplasmacytic lymphoma) (after failure of alkylating agents)
- B-cell chronic lymphocytic leukaemia (CLL) (after failure of alkylating agents)
- relapsing multiple sclerosis (see Multiple sclerosis, p. 1371) (Mavenclad)

Dose
- (Hairy cell leukaemia) 0.14 mg/kg as SC bolus for 5 days (Litak) **OR**
- (Hairy cell leukaemia) 0.10 mg/kg as IV infusion over 24 hours for 7 days (further courses may be needed) (Litak) **OR**
- (Waldenstrom's macroglobulinaemia) 0.10 mg/kg as SC bolus for 5 days at monthly intervals **OR**
- (B-cell CLL) 0.12 mg/kg as IV infusion over 2 hours on days 1—5 of 28-day cycle (Leustatin)

Adverse effects
- graft versus host disease
- see also General Adverse effects of antineoplastic agents (p. 596)

Interactions
- not recommended with antiviral agents
- an increased risk of infection if given with corticosteroids and therefore not recommended together
- see also General Interactions of antineoplastic agents (p. 596)

Nursing considerations/Cautions
- may be given as SC bolus (with no dilution) or IV

ANTINEOPLASTIC AGENTS

- dilute with 100—500 mL sodium chloride 0.9% and administer by IV infusion over 2—24 hours (depending on use)
- dilution with glucose 5% is not recommended
- low temperatures may cause precipitate, which may redissolve if allowed to warm naturally and shaken vigorously; however, the solution should not be heated or microwaved if frozen — allow to thaw at room temperature
- an increased risk of graft versus host disease if the patient receives a transfusion of a non-irradiated cellular blood product
- if the patient becomes Coombs' positive, there is an increased risk of haemolysis; therefore the patient should be closely monitored
- contraindicated in those under 18 years, or with moderate-to-severe renal impairment (creatine clearance $\leq$ 50 mL/min) or moderate-to-severe liver impairment
- see also General Nursing considerations/Cautions for antineoplastic agents (p. 596)

Patient education

- see General Patient education for antineoplastic agents (p. 598)

 Contraindicated in those with moderate-to-severe renal impairment (CrCl < 50 mL/min) or moderate-to-severe liver impairment (Child-Pugh score > 6).

CLOFARABINE
Trade name
Evoltra

Available form
Vial: 20 mg/20 mL

Action
- purine nucleoside antimetabolite

Use
- acute lymphocytic leukaemia (ALL) in children (relapsed or refractory to at least 2 other regimens)

Dose
- 52 mg/m^2 by IV infusion over 2 hours for 5 consecutive days; cycle repeated after 2—6 weeks

Adverse effects
- haematuria
- tachycardia, pericardial effusion
- hand—foot syndrome (hand/foot numbness, paraesthesia, tingling, erythema, pain, swelling and, at worst, ulceration, blistering or moist desquamation)
- capillary leak syndrome, tumour lysis syndrome
- see also General Adverse effects of antineoplastic agents (p. 596)

Interactions
- not recommended within 5 days of known nephrotoxic agents
- not recommended with hepatotoxic agents
- see also General Interactions of antineoplastic agents (p. 596)

Nursing considerations/Cautions

- IV fluids are recommended with therapy to decrease the risk of tumour lysis syndrome
- prophylactic corticosteroids may decrease the risk of capillary leak syndrome
- a response is usually seen after 1—2 cycles. If no response occurs, use of therapy should be re-evaluated
- inline filter (0.22 micron) is recommended
- dilute with 100—200 mL sodium chloride 0.9% (volume is dependent on surface area of the patient)
- if the child weighs < 20 kg, the infusion time should be increased to > 2 hours to reduce symptoms of anxiety and irritability
- an increased risk of hepatotoxicity in those with a history of haemopoietic stem cell transplant
- not recommended in those > 21 years
- contraindicated in those with severe kidney or liver impairment
- see also General Nursing considerations/Cautions for antineoplastic agents (p. 596)

Patient education

- the patient/parent/carer should be advised to report any:
  - dizziness, lightheadedness, fainting or decreased urine output (which may be suggestive of dehydration)
  - breathing problems
  - rapid heart rate
- see also General Patient education for antineoplastic agents (p. 598)

 Contraindicated in those with severe liver impairment or severe renal insufficiency.

CYCLOPHOSPHAMIDE

Trade names
Cyclonex, Cyclophasphamide-Reach, Endoxan

Available forms
Vial: 500 mg, 1 g, 2 g;
Tablets: 50 mg

Action
- nitrogen mustard analogue
- converted to the active form in the liver that interferes with the growth of susceptible cancers

Use
- (Antineoplastic) treatment of stage III or IV malignant lymphomas, multiple myeloma, leukaemias, advanced mycosis fungoides; less useful in neuroblastoma, retinoblastoma and adenocarcinoma of the ovary, or breast or lung cancer
- (Immunosuppressive) treatment of autoimmune diseases resistant to other treatments; preventing transplantation rejection

Dose
- (Antineoplastic induction) initially 40–50 mg/kg IV in divided doses over 2–5 days (loading dose) **OR**
- (Antineoplastic induction) 1–5 mg/kg orally daily **OR**
- (Antineoplastic maintenance) 1–5 mg/kg orally, 10–15 mg/kg IV every 7–10 days or 3–5 mg/kg IV twice weekly **OR**
- (Immunosuppressive) 1–3 mg/kg orally daily

Adverse effects
- cystitis, haemorrhagic cystitis, haematuria, bladder oedema
- skin hyperpigmentation, nail changes
- (High dose) inappropriate water retention, hyponatraemia, veno-occlusive disease
- see also General Adverse effects of antineoplastic agents (p. 596)

Interactions
- not recommended with grapefruit juice
- an increased risk of bone marrow depression if given with allopurinol or hydrochlorothiazide
- an increased metabolism may occur if given with high-dose phenobarbital (phenobarbitone)
- activation of cyclophosphamide may be inhibited by corticosteroids
- an increased risk of toxicity if given with barbiturates, phenytoin or benzodiazepines
- decreased effects may occur if given with chloramphenicol, imipramine, phenothiazines, potassium iodide or vitamin A
- an increased risk of arrhythmias if given with digoxin
- may potentiate effects of suxamethonium, prolonging apnoea
- an increased risk of hyponatraemia if given with indometacin
- may potentiate effects of insulin or oral hypoglycaemic agents
- an increased risk of cardiotoxicity if given after radiotherapy of chest area or with anthracycline (such as doxorubicin)
- not recommended with alcohol
- an increased risk of veno-occlusive disease if given with busulfan or whole-body irradiation

ANTINEOPLASTIC AGENTS

- may cause false negative on skin tests for candida, mumps and tuberculin, false positive on Papanicolaou test and positive direct antiglobulin (Coombs' test)
- see also General Interactions of antineoplastic agents (p. 596)

Nursing considerations/Cautions

- the risk of cystitis and/or haemorrhagic cystitis is high; therefore high fluid intake (oral or IV) for 24 hours before, during and 24 hours after therapy is recommended. Frequent voiding is recommended
- urine should be tested regularly for red cells (may precede haemorrhagic cystitis)
- in some oncology units, during bone marrow transplantation work-up, continuous bladder washouts are performed during therapy to prevent haemorrhagic cystitis
- mesna (see p. 780) protects the bladder from haemorrhagic cystitis
- caution if used in those with diabetes mellitus
- not recommended in those with porphyria
- contraindicated in those with active infection, depressed bone marrow function, cystitis, acute systemic or urinary infection, urinary outflow obstruction, or drug or radiation-induced haemorrhagic cystitis, or within 8 days of major surgery
- see also General Nursing considerations/Cautions for antineoplastic agents (p. 596)

Patient education

- advise the patient to swallow tablets whole (without breaking crushing or chewing) with a glass of water
- the patient should be advised to void frequently in the 24-hour period after therapy
- instruct the patient to avoid grapefruit and grapefruit juice during therapy
- advise the patient to avoid alcohol during therapy
- warn the patient that darkening of skin or nails may occur during therapy
- if the patient has diabetes, recommend the blood glucose level be closely monitored, as cyclophosphamide can interfere with insulin and hypoglycaemic agents
- the patient should be instructed to seek medical advice immediately if any of the following occur:
  - painful urination, increased frequency of urination
  - blood in urine
  - sudden weight gain, build-up of fluid around abdomen
- see also General Patient education for antineoplastic agents (p. 598)

 Tablets should not be crushed or broken.

 Excreted in the urine; therefore dose adjustment is recommended in those with impaired renal function.

Caution if used in those with impaired liver function, as this is a risk factor for veno-occlusive disease.

 Caution if used in the elderly, especially if prone to infection or if they have diabetes.

CYTARABINE

Trade names
DBL Cytarabine, Pfizer Cytarabine

Available forms
Vial: 100 mg/5 mL, 1 g/10 mL, 2 g/20 mL

Action
- pyrimidine antimetabolite that appears to inhibit DNA synthesis

Use
- induction and maintenance of remission in acute myeloid leukaemia, acute lymphocytic leukaemia, chronic myeloid leukaemia (blast phase)
- non-Hodgkin lymphoma (children)

- meningeal leukaemia (intrathecally)

Dose
- (Monotherapy) 200 mg/m^2 by continuous IV infusion over 24 hours for 5 days, repeated every 2 weeks (induction), then a similar dose but longer intervals between cycles (maintenance) **OR**
- (Meningeal leukaemia) 5–75 mg/m^2 intrathecally daily for 4 days once every 4 weeks or once every 4 days, until CSF is normal, then one additional treatment

Adverse effects
- pancreatitis
- cytarabine (ara-C) syndrome (fever, myalgia, bone pain, rash, malaise, chest pain, conjunctivitis) (within 6–12 hours of administration)
- anaphylaxis
- (Intrathecal) nausea, vomiting, fever and, rarely, paraplegia
- (IV) thrombophlebitis
- see also General Adverse effects of antineoplastic agents (p. 596)

Interactions
- (Intrathecal) an increased risk of severe neurological adverse effects if given with methotrexate
- may decrease effectiveness of methotrexate
- activity may be decreased by methotrexate
- (As part of multi-drug regimen) may decrease serum levels of digoxin; therefore digoxin levels should be closely monitored during therapy
- may antagonise the effects of gentamicin
- may inhibit the antifungal activity of flucytosine
- an increased risk of spinal cord toxicity if given within a few days both intrathecally and IV
- see also General Interactions of antineoplastic agents (p. 596)

Nursing considerations/Cautions
- dilute with sodium chloride 0.9% or glucose 5%
- may also be given SC, IV infusion and, occasionally, intrathecally
- if given SC, injection sites should be rotated
- 100 mg/mL solution is not suitable for intrathecal use
- intrathecal use may result in systemic toxicity so the patient should be closely monitored
- corticosteroids are recommended to treat cytarabine (ara-C) syndrome
- incompatible with heparin, insulin, fluorouracil, penicillins and methylprednisolone
- if precipitate occurs as a result of low temperature, it may be redissolved by warming the solution to 55°C for up to 30 minutes and shaking the solution. The solution should be cooled before administration
- see also General Nursing considerations/Cautions for antineoplastic agents (p. 596)

Patient education
- see General Patient education for antineoplastic agents (p. 598)

Caution if used in those with poor renal function or liver dysfunction, as there is a higher risk of CNS toxicity after high-dose therapy.

Available in combination with
- Vyxeos (cytarabine 100 mg and daunorubicin 44 mg)

DACARBAZINE

Trade name
DBL Dacarbazine for Injection

Available form
Vial: 200 mg

Action
- inhibits DNA synthesis
- has an active metabolite with alkylating properties similar to nitrogen mustard

ANTINEOPLASTIC AGENTS

Use
- metastatic malignant melanoma
- sarcomas

Dose
- 4.5 mg/kg IV over 1 minute daily for 10 days, repeated every 4 weeks if needed **OR**
- 250 mg/m^2 IV over 1 minute daily for 5 days, repeated every 3 weeks if needed

Adverse effects
- (Rare) hepatotoxicity with hepatic vein thrombosis
- (Injection site) severe pain along vein
- see also General Adverse effects of antineoplastic agents (p. 596)

Interactions
- may decrease response to levodopa
- may increase effects of azathioprine, allopurinol and mercaptopurine
- lung toxicity may occur if given before fotemustine
- see also General Interactions of antineoplastic agents (p. 596)

Nursing considerations/Cautions
- prophylactic antiemetic therapy with 5HT3 (e.g. ondansetron) or dexamethasone is recommended
- reconstitute with 19.7 mL water for injections and administer over 1 minute
- see also General Nursing considerations/Cautions for antineoplastic agents (p. 596)

Patient education
- see General Patient education for antineoplastic agents (p. 598)

Metabolised in the liver and excreted 50% unchanged in the urine; therefore dose adjustment is recommended in those with liver or renal impairment.

DACTINOMYCIN (ACTINOMYCIN D)
Trade name
Cosmegen

Available form
Vial: 0.5 mg

Action
- cytotoxic antibiotic

Use
- Wilms' tumour
- rhabdomyosarcoma
- testicular and uterine cancer
- palliative therapy for Ewing's sarcoma and sarcoma botryoides

Dose
- 15 microgram/kg IV daily for 5 days; may be repeated after ≥ 3 weeks if no sign of toxicity **OR**
- 400–600 microgram/m^2 IV daily for 5 days; may be repeated after ≥ 3 weeks if no sign of toxicity **OR**
- (Regional perfusion – lower extremity, pelvis) 50 microgram/kg **OR**
- (Regional perfusion – upper extremity) 35 microgram/kg

Adverse effects
- liver veno-occlusive disease
- (Perfusion technique) oedema, damage to soft tissue of perfused area
- see also General Adverse effects of antineoplastic agents (p. 596)

Interactions
- increased GI disturbance and bone marrow depression may occur if given with radiotherapy
- potentiates the effects of radiation therapy, causing adverse effects at a lower dose of radiation
- radiation therapy potentiates the effects of dactinomycin
- may interfere with assay for antibacterial drug levels
- see also General Interactions of antineoplastic agents (p. 596)

Nursing considerations/Cautions

- lower dose may be required if other chemotherapy or radiation is used at the same time or has been previously used
- may reactivate erythema from previous radiation therapy if given alone
- extremely corrosive; therefore the IV site must be closely monitored to avoid extravasation
- reconstitute using 1.1 mL of preservative-free water for injections. Should not be reconstituted using water for injections containing preservatives (benzyl alcohol or parabens), as precipitate may occur. Can be further diluted with glucose 5% or sodium chloride 0.9% to a concentration not less than 10 microgram/mL
- reconstituted solution is clear gold colour
- not recommended with or within 2 months of irradiation for Wilms' tumour unless benefits outweigh risks because of the high risk of hepatotoxicity
- contraindicated at time of infection with chicken pox or herpes zoster, as generalised disease may occur
- see also General Nursing considerations/Cautions for antineoplastic agents (p. 596)

Patient education

- see General Patient education for antineoplastic agents (p. 598)

DAROLUTAMIDE
Trade name
Nubeqa

Available form
Tablets: 300 mg

Action
- non-steroidal androgen receptor antagonist

Use
- non-metastatic castration-resistant prostate cancer
- metastatic hormone-sensitive prostate cancer (with docetaxel)

Dose
- 600 mg orally twice daily with food (with gonadotrophin-releasing hormone (GnRH) analogue if patient has not had bilateral orchiectomy)

Adverse effects
- fatigue
- pain in extremities
- rash
- decreased neutrophils
- increased aspartate aminotransferase (AST) and bilirubin
- ischaemic heart disease
- seizures

Interactions
- not recommended with rifampicin, carbamazepine, phenobarbital (phenobarbitone) or St John's wort
- increased serum levels may occur if given with itraconazole
- may increase serum levels of rosuvastatin, methotrexate, sulfasalazine, fluvastatin or atorvastatin and are not recommended together

Nursing considerations/Cautions

- (Combination therapy with docetaxel) first 6 cycles of docetaxel should be given within 6 weeks of the start of darolutamide
- tablets contain 176.9 mg lactose and are therefore not recommended in those with rare hereditary conditions of galactose intolerance, Lapp lactase deficiency or glucose—galactose malabsorption
- caution if used in those with recent (within 6 months) cardiac events, including uncontrolled hypertension, stroke, myocardial infarction, severe or unstable angina, coronary or peripheral artery bypass grafts or heart failure

Patient education

- advise the patient to swallow the tablet whole (without chewing, breaking or crushing) with food
- see General Patient education for antineoplastic agents (p. 598)

ANTINEOPLASTIC AGENTS

Tablet should not be crushed or broken.

For those with severe renal impairment, the recommended dose is 300 mg orally twice daily with food.

For those with moderate liver impairment (Child—Pugh B), the recommended dose is 300 mg orally twice daily with food.

DAUNORUBICIN
Trade name
Pfizer Daunorubicin Injection

Available form
Vial: 2 mg/mL

Action
- antineoplastic (anthracycline) antibiotic structurally related to doxorubicin
- antibacterial and immunosuppressive properties
- active metabolite

Use
- acute lymphoblastic (lymphocytic) leukaemia (ALL) and acute myeloblastic leukaemia (AML) (alone or with other antineoplastic agents)
- disseminated neuroblastoma, rhabdomyosarcoma

Dose
- (ALL) 1 mg/kg IV, repeated at 1—4-day intervals if needed **OR**
- (AML) 2 mg/kg IV, repeated at 4—7-day intervals if needed

Adverse effects
- (Acute cardiotoxicity) ECG changes, tachycardia; (delayed cardiotoxicity) cardiac failure, cardiomyopathy
- (IV site) phlebitis, thrombophlebitis, cellulitis, ulceration, necrosis
- see also General Adverse effects of antineoplastic agents (p. 596)

Interactions
- increased skin reaction and mucositis may occur if given with radiation therapy
- increased cardiac toxicity may occur if given with cyclophosphamide
- may worsen cyclophosphamide-induced haemorrhagic cystitis
- any hyperuricaemia should be controlled with allopurinol, not other uricosuric agents because of the risk of uric acid nephropathy
- not recommended with other cardiotoxic agents unless cardiac function can be closely monitored
- increased risk of cardiotoxicity if given with doxorubicin and should not be given if the total cumulative dose of doxorubicin has been given
- not recommended with hepatotoxic agents
- see also General Interactions of antineoplastic agents (p. 596)

Nursing considerations/Cautions
- the total lifetime dose should not exceed 20 mg/kg
- potentially cardiotoxic; therefore ECG and left ventricular ejection fraction should be measured before each course of therapy. Baseline ECHO cardiogram is also recommended. Cardiotoxicity typically appears 1—6 months after starting therapy
- not given IM or SC, or by direct IV injection
- second and subsequent injections are dependent on response
- incompatible with heparin, dexamethasone, aluminium, aztreonam, allopurinol, fludarabine and piperacillin/tazobactam
- should be added to free-flowing IV infusion to reduce the risk of local adverse effects and given over at least 3—5 minutes
- facial flushing and vein streaking will occur if given by rapid IV administration
- an increased risk of cardiotoxicity in those receiving total cumulative dose > 550 mg/m^2 or 400 mg/m^2 if the patient has had chest irradiation (mediastinal or pericardial) or concurrently with cyclophosphamide

- contraindicated in those with hypersensitivity to anthracycline, having previously received full cumulative doses of doxorubicin and/or daunorubicin, cytotoxic radiotherapy, cardiac impairment including myocardial insufficiency, recent myocardial infarction and cardiac arrhythmias, or severe liver (Child—Pugh C) or renal impairment (serum creatinine > 7.9 mg/dL)
- see also General Nursing considerations/Cautions for antineoplastic agents (p. 596)

Patient education

- during administration, advise the patient to immediately report any stinging or burning at the IV site, as this may indicate extravasation
- the patient should be advised that urine may become harmless red colour 2–3 days after administration
- instruct the patient to seek medical advice immediately if any of the following occur:
  - shortness of breath, cough, pink frothy sputum
  - swelling of ankles, legs or abdomen
  - decrease urine output
  - fever, sore throat, any unusual bleeding or bruising
- see also General Patient education for antineoplastic agents (p. 598)

If serum creatinine is > 3.0 mg/dL, the daunorubicin dose should be halved. If serum creatinine is > 7.9 mg/dL, drug is contraindicated.

If patient has mild-to-moderate liver impairment (Child—Pugh A or B):

- bilirubin 1.2 to 3 mg/dL, a dose one-half of starting dose is recommended
- bilirubin > 3 mg/dL, a dose one-quarter of starting dose is recommended.

If patient has severe liver impairment (Child–Pugh C), drug is contraindicated.

Available in combination with
- daunorubicin 44 mg + cytarabine 100 mg (Vyxeos)

DECITABINE + CEDAZURIDINE
Trade name
Inqovi 35/100

Available form
Tablet: decitabine 35 mg/cedazuridine 100 mg

Action
- decitabine is a nucleoside metabolic inhibitor that is phosphorylated and incorporated into DNA leading to hypomethylation, cellular differentiation and/or cell death; however, it has no impact on non-proliferating cells
- cedazuridine inhibits cytidine deaminase (CDA), which is responsible for nucleosides (including decitabine) degradation. CDA is found in large amounts in the liver and gastrointestinal tract limiting nucleoside bioavailability
- combining cedazuridine with decitabine inhibits metabolism of decitabine in the gut and liver by CDA increasing its oral bioavailability
- decitabine half-life 1.2 hours; cedazuridine half-life 6.3 hours

Use
- myelodysplastic syndromes (MDS) intermediate-1, intermediate-2 and high risk (International Prognostic Scoring System groups)
- chronic myelomonocytic leukaemia (CMML)

Dose
- 1 tablet (decitabine 35 mg/cedazuridine 100 mg) orally daily 2 hours before or 2 hours after food, on days 1 to 5 of a 28-day cycle for at least 4 cycles

Adverse effects
- see General Adverse effects for antineoplastic agents (p. 596)

ANTINEOPLASTIC AGENTS

Interactions
- not recommended within 4 hours of agents that modify gastric pH
- should not be administered on the same day as other agents metabolised by cytidine deaminase, such as cytarabine, capecitabine, gemcitabine and azacitidine

Nursing considerations/Cautions
- dose reduction is not recommended in first 2 cycles of therapy
- caution if used in those with severe congestive heart failure or unstable cardiac disease
- see also General Nursing considerations/Cautions for antineoplastic agents (p. 596)

Patient education
- advise the patient to swallow tablet whole (not broken, crushed or chewed) with water on an empty stomach (either 2 hours before or 2 hours after food)
- the patient should be instructed not to take antacids or proton pump inhibitors within 4 hours of therapy
- see also General Patient education for antineoplastic agents (p. 598)

Tablets should not be crushed, broken or dispersed.

Those with moderate renal impairment (CrCl 20–39 mL/min) should be closely monitored because of the increased risk of adverse reactions.

DEGARELIX
Trade name
Firmagon

Available forms
Vial: 80 mg, 120 mg

Action
- hormonal antineoplastic agent (third-generation gonadotrophin-releasing hormone (GnRH) receptor blocker)
- forms depot from SC injections which form a sustained-release formulation

Use
- prostate cancer (androgen deprivation therapy)

Dose
- initially 240 mg SC (given as two 120 mg injections) then, after 4 weeks, 80 mg SC monthly

Adverse effects
- hot flushes, night sweats, chills
- insomnia, headache, dizziness, fatigue
- nausea, constipation
- weight increase
- hypertension
- back pain, arthralgia
- elevated liver enzymes
- (Rare) prolongation of QT interval, decreased bone density, antibody development, hypersensitivity
- (Injection site) pain, redness, swelling, induration, nodule formation

Interactions
- not recommended with agents known to prolong QT interval (e.g. amiodarone, sotalol) or cause electrolyte imbalance (especially hypokalaemia and hypomagnesaemia)

Nursing considerations/Cautions
- observe the patient for at least 60 minutes after administration for any signs of hypersensitivity
- the abdominal area is the preferred SC administration site. The administration site should be rotated, taking care to avoid the waistband or belt region, and not too close to the ribs (i.e. avoiding areas that might be subjected to pressure)
- an SC injection should not be rubbed or massaged after administration, as this may alter release
- reconstitute with water for injections (4.2 mL for 80 mg, 3 mL for 120 mg) and avoid shaking or excessive foaming (may take up to 15 minutes)
- caution if used in those with congenital or acquired QT interval prolongation or electrolyte imbalance
- contraindicated in women and children

- see also General Nursing considerations/Cautions for antineoplastic agents (p. 596)

Patient education
- advise the patient to seek medical advice if any irregular heart rate occurs
- see also General Patient education for antineoplastic agents (p. 598)

DOCETAXEL
Trade names
DBL Docetaxel Concentrated Injection, Docetaxel Accord

Available forms
Vial: 20 mg/2 mL, 80 mg/4 mL, 80 mg/8 mL, 160 mg/8 mL, 160 mg/16 mL

Action
- taxane antimetabolite

Use
- breast cancer (node positive) (adjunctive treatment)
- locally advanced or metastatic breast cancer (where other chemotherapy has failed)
- locally advanced or metastatic non-small cell lung cancer
- metastatic ovarian cancer (when first-line treatment has failed)
- hormone refractory (androgen independent) prostate cancer
- locally advanced squamous cell carcinoma of head and neck

Dose
- (Metastatic breast cancer) 75–100 mg/m^2 IV over 60 minutes every 3 weeks (alone or with capecitabine or trastuzumab) **OR**
- (Breast cancer – adjunctive) 75 mg/m^2 IV over 60 minutes on day 1 of 21-day cycle (in combination with cyclophosphamide) (for 4 cycles) **OR**
- (Non-small cell lung cancer, ovarian cancer) 75–100 mg/m^2 IV over 60 minutes every 3 weeks **OR**
- (Prostate cancer) 75–100 mg/m^2 IV over 60 minutes every 3 weeks (with prednisone or prednisolone 5 mg) **OR**
- (Head and neck cancer) 75–100 mg/m^2 IV over 60 minutes every 3 weeks (with cisplatin, fluorouracil and radiotherapy or chemoradiotherapy)

Adverse effects
- fluid retention
- hypersensitivity
- eye disorders
- (Rare) ototoxicity
- see also General Adverse effects of antineoplastic agents (p. 596)

Interactions
- caution if given with a protease inhibitor such as ritonavir
- bioavailability increased by dexamethasone, clofibrate and phenobarbital (phenobarbitone)
- bioavailability may be decreased by ciclosporin and erythromycin

Nursing considerations/Cautions
- patients should be closely monitored during first and second doses for any signs of hypersensitivity, which can occur at the start, during or just after infusion is stopped
- fluid retention and the risk of hypersensitivity reaction may be reduced by administering dexamethasone (8 mg twice daily orally) for 3 days before starting therapy (or dexamethasone 8 mg orally 12 hours, 3 hours and 1 hour before infusion if treatment is for prostate cancer)
- reconstitute powder using the diluent provided; avoid shaking and allow to stand for 5 minutes before further diluting
- further dilute reconstituted solution or concentrate for infusion with sodium chloride 0.9% or glucose 5%
- if the dose > 200 mg, dilution volume should be greater than 250 mL for a concentration of 0.74 mg/mL or less
- if crystallisation occurs, the solution should be discarded
- contains alcohol, which may need to be considered if the patient is suffering from alcoholism

ANTINEOPLASTIC AGENTS

- caution if used in those with pleural effusion, pericardial effusion and ascites, as fluid retention may worsen these conditions
- contraindicated in those with hypersensitivity to polysorbate 80, severe liver impairment or baseline neutrophil count $< 1.5 \times 10^9$ cells/L
- see also General Nursing considerations/Cautions for antineoplastic agents (p. 596)

Patient education

- advise the patient to seek medical advice immediately if any changes to hearing or vision occur
- see also General Patient education for antineoplastic agents (p. 598)

Contraindicated in those with liver failure.

Reduced dose is recommended in those with elevated transaminases (ALT and/or AST) and increases in alkaline phosphatase levels.

DOXORUBICIN HYDROCHLORIDE
Trade names
Adriamycin, Doxorubicin Accord

DOXORUBICIN HYDROCHLORIDE (LIPOSOMAL)
Trade names
Caelyx, Liposomal Doxorubicin SUN

Available forms
Solution: 10 mg/5 mL, 20 mg/10 mL, 50 mg/25 mL, 200 mg/100 mL

Action
- anthracycline antineoplastic antibiotic
- active metabolites are cytotoxic
- pegylated liposomal formulation increases drug circulation time
- lifetime cumulative dose 550 mg/m^2 body surface area or, if patient is 70 years or over, 450 mg/m^2
- clearance is reduced in those who are obese

Use
- acute leukaemias, soft tissue and bone sarcoma, neuroblastomas, hepatomas, Wilms' tumour, malignant carcinoma of breast, bladder, liver, lung, ovary and thyroid
- Hodgkin's lymphoma, non-Hodgkin lymphoma
- advanced epithelial ovarian cancer (after failed platinum therapy)
- metastatic breast cancer (monotherapy)
- progressive multiple myeloma (MM) (with bortezomib in those who have had or are unsuitable for bone marrow transplant)
- acquired immunodeficiency syndrome (AIDS)-related Kaposi's sarcoma (AIDS KS) (low CD4 counts and extensive mucocutaneous or visceral disease) or where disease has progressed with or intolerant to prior combination chemotherapy
- non-metastatic bladder cancer (intravesicular)

Dose
- (Breast cancer, ovarian cancer) 50 mg/m^2 by IV infusion once every 4 weeks (liposomal formulation) **OR**
- (Multiple myeloma) 30 mg/m^2 by IV infusion on day 4 of bortezomib 3-week cycle (liposomal formulation) **OR**
- (AIDS KS) 20 mg/m^2 by IV infusion over 30 minutes every 2–3 weeks (liposomal formulation) **OR**
- 60–75 mg/m^2 IV over 3–5 minutes at 21-day intervals **OR**
- 30 mg/m^2 IV over 3–5 minutes daily for 3 successive days every 4 weeks **OR**
- 45–100 mg/m^2 via intra-arterial infusion for 1–3 days **OR**
- (Intravesicular) 80 mg/100 mL instilled into bladder monthly

Adverse effects
- cardiotoxicity including cardiac failure

633

- hyperpigmentation (hands, nails, buccal mucosa)
- discoloured urine (red)
- hand–foot syndrome (hand/foot numbness, paraesthesia, tingling, erythema, pain, swelling and, at worst, ulceration, blistering or moist desquamation)
- (Intravesical administration) local transient reactions, including bladder contraction/cramp/pain, chemical cystitis, haematuria, painful micturition, frequency and urgency
- see also General Adverse effects of antineoplastic agents (p. 596)

Interactions

- an increased risk of hepatotoxicity and haemorrhagic cystitis if given with mercaptopurine in those with AIDS KS
- an increased risk of hepatotoxicity if given with high-dose methotrexate
- cyclophosphamide, propranolol or mediastinal radiotherapy given with doxorubicin may increase cardiotoxicity
- may exacerbate cyclophosphamide-induced cystitis
- if given with cytarabine, colitis and necrosis may occur
- calcium-channel blockers may increase risk of cardiotoxicity
- cyclophosphamide, dactinomycin and mitomycin may sensitise the heart to cardiac effects
- an increased risk of cardiotoxicity if given within 7 months of stopping trastuzumab
- may decrease serum levels of phenytoin, phenobarbital (phenobarbitone) and St John's wort
- an increased risk of mucositis if the patient has previously received mucosal irradiation
- an increased risk of hypersensitivity reaction if the patient has recently received clindamycin
- increased serum levels and risk of congestive cardiac failure may occur if paclitaxel is given before doxorubicin
- an increased risk of haematological toxicity, seizures and coma if given with ciclosporin
- the total cumulative dose should be decreased if given with cyclophosphamide, daunorubicin, epirubicin or idarubicin
- see also General Interactions of antineoplastic agents (p. 596)

Nursing considerations/Cautions

- regular ECG monitoring or evaluation of left ventricular ejection fraction is recommended before starting and regularly throughout therapy
- the two formulations of doxorubicin are not interchangeable and have different administration requirements
- (Liposomal formulation) the initial infusion should be given over 90 minutes as follows: 10 mL over 10 minutes, 20 mL over the next 10 minutes, 40 mL over the next 10 minutes and the remainder over 60 minutes. If no reaction is observed, subsequent IV infusions can be given over 1 hour
- (Non-liposomal formulation) IV administration should be given into a freely running infusion over at least 3–5 minutes. Patient facial flushing or local red streaking along vein is indicative that the rate was too fast
- (Non-liposomal formulation) IV push is not recommended because of the risk of extravasation
- the patient is observed for infusion-related reaction, which may occur within minutes of starting the infusion (although it usually occurs with subsequent doses)
- antihistamines, corticosteroids, oxygen and resuscitation equipment should be readily available
- (Liposomal formulation) not recommended IM, SC, IV bolus or undiluted
- (Liposomal formulation) dilute with glucose 5% for IV infusion (250 mL for doses < 90 mg or 500 mL for doses > 90 mg)
- (Liposomal formulation) contains sucrose and is infused in glucose 5%, which may need to be taken into consideration if the patient has diabetes

ANTINEOPLASTIC AGENTS

- (Intravesical) dilute to a concentration of 80 mg in 100 mL and instil via catheter
- incompatible with aminophylline, cefalotin, dexamethasone, diazepam, fluorouracil, furosemide (frusemide), heparin, hydrocortisone and ganciclovir
- the solution will change from red to purple if mixed with aminophylline or fluorouracil
- caution if used in those with impaired cardiac function, prior mediastinal radiation or concurrent cyclophosphamide therapy because of the increased risk of cardiomyopathy
- (AIDS KS) therapy is not recommended in those who have had a splenectomy
- (Non-liposomal formulation) caution if used in obese patients, as clearance may be reduced
- (Intravesicular) contraindicated in those with haematuria, urinary infection, inflamed bladder, invasive bladder tumours or bladder catheterisation because of large intravesical tumour
- contraindicated in those with known hypersensitivity to anthracyclines or anthracenediones, severe arrhythmias, recent myocardial infarction, myocardial insufficiency, persistent myelosuppression or previous severe stomatitis (induced by chemotherapy or radiotherapy), or in those having previously received full cumulative doses of doxorubicin and/or daunorubicin
- (Liposomal formulation) contraindicated for AIDS-related Kaposi's sarcoma that could be effectively treated with alfa interferon or local therapy
- see also General Nursing considerations/Cautions for antineoplastic agents (p. 596)

Patient education

- for patient education related to intravesicular instillation see BCG (non-vaccine) (p. 608)
- advise the patient that hyperpigmentation of hands, nails and buccal mucosa may develop and does not improve when therapy is terminated
- the patient should be warned that urine may be red for 1–2 days after therapy
- instruct the patient to seek medical advice if any of the following occur:
  - shortness of breath
  - swelling of ankles or legs
- see also General Patient education for antineoplastic agents (p. 598)

 For those with liver impairment:
- **(serum bilirubin 20—50 micromol/L) half normal dose is recommended**
- **(serum bilirubin > 50 micromol/L) one quarter of normal dose is recommended.**

 A reduced dose is recommended in the elderly and total cumulative dose should not exceed 450 mg/m^2 of body surface area in those aged 70 and over.

ENZALUTAMIDE
Trade name
Xtandi

Available form
Capsules: 40 mg

Action
- antiandrogen that competitively inhibits androgen binding to androgen receptors
- active metabolites
- half-life 5.8 days

Use
- metastatic hormone-sensitive prostate cancer
- castration-resistant metastatic prostate cancer (previously treated with docetaxel, following androgen deprivation therapy failure (chemotherapy not indicated))
- castration-resistant non-metastatic prostate cancer

Dose
- 160 mg orally once daily

Adverse effects
- bone loss, falls, falls-related injury
- hypertension
- QT interval prolongation
- (Rare) seizures, posterior reversible encephalopathy syndrome (PRES)
- see also General Adverse effects of antineoplastic agents (p. 596)

Interactions
- caution if used with agents that lower seizure threshold
- caution if used with agents known to prolong QT interval or cause electrolyte imbalance (especially hypokalaemia and hypomagnesaemia)
- not recommended with rifampicin and gemfibrozil
- may decrease serum levels and therefore not recommended with warfarin. If used, INR should be closely monitored, especially when starting or stopping therapy
- caution if used with agents with a narrow therapeutic index such as digoxin, colchicine and dabigatran
- may decrease serum levels of omeprazole
- increased risk of liver damage if given with paracetamol
- caution if given with atorvastatin, bisoprolol, cabazitaxel, carbamazepine, ciclosporin, clarithromycin, clonazepam, clopidogrel, dexamethasone, diazepam, digoxin, diltiazem, doxycycline, fentanyl, felodipine, haloperidol, midazolam, nifedipine, phenytoin, prednisolone, primidone, propranolol, ritonavir, simvastatin, tacrolimus, thyroxine, tramadol, valproic acid, verapamil or zolpidem

Nursing considerations/Cautions
- monitor BP regularly during therapy
- caution if used in those with known congenital or acquired QT prolongation or electrolyte imbalance (especially hypokalaemia and hypomagnesaemia)
- not recommended in those with uncontrolled hypertension, recent myocardial infarction (within last 6 months), unstable angina (within last 3 months), class III or IV heart failure or bradycardia
- caution in those with a history of seizures, epilepsy, head injury, stroke, primary brain tumours, brain metastases or alcoholism that may increase risk of seizures. If the patient has a seizure, therapy should be stopped
- contraindicated in women
- see also General Nursing considerations/Cautions for antineoplastic agents (p. 596)

Patient education
- advise the patient to swallow capsules whole (without opening, breaking or chewing)
- the patient should be cautioned about undertaking activities where sudden loss of consciousness/fitting could be dangerous
- instruct the patient to seek medical advice immediately if any of the following occur:
  - confusion, trouble thinking, memory loss, blurred vision, loss of vision, balance or walking problems, decreased strength in arms or legs
  - irregular heart rate
  - fitting/seizures
- see also General Patient education for antineoplastic agents (p. 598)

 Capsules should not be opened or crushed.

EPIRUBICIN HYDROCHLORIDE
Trade names
Epirubicin Accord, Pharmorubicin

Available forms
Solution: 50 mg/25 mL, 200 mg/100 mL

Action
- antineoplastic antibiotic (anthracycline)
- half-life 40 hours
- lifetime cumulative dose 900 mg/m^2

Use
- breast, ovarian, superficial bladder and gastric cancer, small cell lung cancer, soft tissue sarcomas (advanced metastatic), non-Hodgkin lymphoma

ANTINEOPLASTIC AGENTS

- prophylaxis of recurrence after transurethral resection of stage T1 papillary and stage Ta multifocal papillary cancers (grade 2 and 3)

Dose
- 75—90 mg/m^2 IV over 3—20 minutes at 21-day intervals **OR**
- (Breast cancer) up to 135 mg/m^2 (alone) or 120 mg/m^2 (combination therapy) IV over 3—20 minutes every 3—4 weeks **OR**
- (Early breast cancer, node positive, adjunctive therapy) 100—120 mg/m^2 IV over 3—20 minutes every 3—4 weeks **OR**
- (Papillary transitional cell bladder cancer) 50 mg instilled into the bladder every 8 weeks **OR**
- (Prophylaxis after transurethral resection) 50 mg instilled into the bladder weekly for 4 weeks, followed by monthly instillation for 11 months

Adverse effects
- ECG changes, cardiomyopathy, congestive cardiac failure, pericardial effusion
- (IV) thrombophlebitis
- (Intravesical administration) local transient reactions, including bladder contraction/cramp/pain, chemical cystitis, haematuria, painful micturition, frequency and urgency
- see also General Adverse effects of antineoplastic agents (p. 596)

Interactions
- increased risk of cardiotoxicity if given with fluorouracil, cyclophosphamide, calcium-channel blockers, cisplatin, trastuzumab, taxanes or propranolol. A 7-month interval is recommended between stopping trastuzumab and starting epirubicin
- concurrent mediastinal irradiation may potentiate cardiotoxicity
- if paclitaxel is given before epirubicin, serum levels of epirubicin may increase
- see also General Interactions of antineoplastic agents (p. 596)

Nursing considerations/Cautions
- cardiac function should be measured before starting therapy
- cardiac monitoring (ECG, echocardiogram of measurement of left ventricular ejection fraction) is recommended before each cycle of therapy
- maximum lifetime cumulative dose 900 mg/m^2
- not given IM or SC
- IV push is not recommended and the administration should be over 3—20 minutes. Facial flushing and vein streaking will occur if given too rapidly
- incompatible with heparin and alkaline solutions
- solution may gel if refrigerated. Allow the solution to remain at room temperature for at least 2 hours (maximum 4 hours) to come to an infusible consistency
- contraindicated in those who have received full cumulative doses of doxorubicin, daunorubicin, mitozantrone or mitomycin hypersensitivity to other anthracyclines or anthracenediones, severe arrhythmias, myocardial insufficiency, recent myocardial infarction, unstable angina, persistent severe stomatitis or myelosuppression from other drug therapy or radiotherapy, or decreased liver function
- (Intravesical) contraindicated in those with urinary infection, haematuria, inflamed bladder, invasive tumours penetrating the bladder wall or problems associated with catheterisation
- see also General Nursing considerations/Cautions for antineoplastic agents (p. 596)

Patient education
- (Bladder cancer) instruct the patient not to drink fluids for 12 hours before bladder instillation
- the patient should be warned that heart-related adverse effects may occur months after finishing treatment

- advise the patient to seek medical advice if any of the following occur:
  - irregular heart rate, swelling of ankles, shortness of breath
  - (bladder administration) blood in urine, pain on urination, increased frequency or difficulty urinating
- warn the patient that urine may be discoloured red for 1—2 days after treatment
- for intravesical instillation patient education see BCG (non-vaccine) (p. 598)
- see also General Patient education for antineoplastic agents (p. 598)

If serum creatinine > 5 mg/dL, a lower starting dose is recommended.

If serum bilirubin is 20—50 micromol/L, half the normal dose is recommended.

If serum bilirubin > 50 micromol/L, one-quarter the normal dose is recommended.

ERIBULIN MESILATE

Trade name
Halaven

Available form
Vial: 1 mg/2 mL

Action
- halichondrin antineoplastic that inhibits growth phase as well as affecting tumour microenvironment
- half-life 40 hours

Use
- locally advanced or metastatic breast cancer (where disease has progressed despite at least one chemotherapeutic regimen for advanced disease including an anthracycline and a taxane)
- unresectable liposarcoma (after chemotherapy for advanced or metastatic disease)

Dose
- 1.4 mg/m^2 IV over 2—5 minutes on days 1 and 8 of a 21-day cycle

Adverse effects
- peripheral neuropathy
- QT prolongation
- see also General Adverse effects of antineoplastic agents (p. 596)

Interactions
- caution if used with agents known to prolong QT interval and cause electrolyte imbalance (e.g. diuretics) (especially hypokalaemia and hypomagnesaemia)
- caution if used with agents known to have a narrow therapeutic index

Nursing considerations/Cautions
- premedication with antiemetic or corticosteroids is recommended
- may be used undiluted or diluted with 100 mL sodium chloride 0.9%
- should not be diluted with glucose 5%
- contains alcohol (100 mg/dose)
- the dose should be delayed on day 1 or day 8 for up to 7 days if platelets $< 75 \times 10^9$/L or absolute neutrophil count (ANC) $< 1 \times 10^9$/L
- caution if used in those with pre-existing peripheral neuropathy
- not recommended in those with known congenital or acquired QT interval prolongation, or electrolyte imbalance especially hypokalaemia and hypomagnesaemia
- see also General Nursing considerations/Cautions for antineoplastic agents (p. 596)

Patient education
- advise the patient to seek medical advice immediately if any of the following occur:
  - irregular heart rate
  - numbness/tingling in limbs, weakness, tingling or burning sensation
- see also General Patient education for antineoplastic agents (p. 598)

Stage 3 or 4 chronic renal disease: recommended starting dose is 0.7 mg/m^2 IV.

(Mild liver disease, Child—Pugh A) recommended starting dose is 1.1 mg/m^2 IV.

(Moderate liver disease, Child—Pugh B) recommended starting dose is 0.7 mg/m^2 IV.

ANTINEOPLASTIC AGENTS

ETOPOSIDE
Trade names
Etopophos, Etoposide Ebewe, Vepesid

Available forms
Vial: 100 mg, 1 g;
Solution: 100 mg/5 mL;
Capsules: 50 mg, 100 mg

Action
* etoposide phosphate (prodrug) is converted to etoposide (antineoplastic)
* synthetic derivative of podophyllotoxin that inhibits the cell cycle during late S and G_2 phases
* absorption from oral route is variable (50—55% of IV dose)

Use
* small cell lung carcinoma, acute monocytic and myeloblastic leukaemia, Hodgkin's disease, non-Hodgkin lymphoma, testicular tumour

Dose
* 100—200 mg/m^2 orally before food daily, days 1—5 **OR**
* 50—60 mg/m^2 by IV infusion over 30—60 minutes, days 1—5, followed by 14—28 treatment-free days (total dose not exceeding 400 mg/m^2 per course) **OR**
* 50—100 mg/m^2 by IV infusion over 30—60 minutes, days 1—5, every 3—4 weeks (with other antineoplastic agents) **OR**
* 100—150 mg/m^2 by IV infusion over 30—60 minutes, days 1, 3 and 5, every 3—4 weeks (with other antineoplastic agents)

Adverse effects
* injection site reactions
* anaphylaxis (including cardiac arrest)
* see also General Adverse effects of antineoplastic agents (p. 596)

Interactions
* increased serum levels occur if given orally with high-dose ciclosporin
* clearance may be decreased by cisplatin
* may increase INR if given with warfarin; therefore close monitoring is required especially when starting or stopping therapy
* efficacy may be decreased if given with phenytoin or other antiepileptic agents
* may increase risk of anthracycline-induced cardiomyopathy if given with anthracyclines
* seizure control of antiepileptic agents may be decreased if given together
* cross-resistance may exist between etoposide and anthracyclines
* see also General Interactions of antineoplastic agents (p. 596)

Nursing considerations/Cautions
* increased risk of toxicity if the patient has low serum albumin
* not recommended as IV push or bolus, rapid infusion or intracavity injection
* hypotension can be avoided by giving an IV infusion over 30—60 minutes
* reconstitute the powder with 5—10 mL of diluent for a concentration of 10—20 mg/mL
* concentrate for solution must be diluted before administration, usually in 250 mL sodium chloride 0.9% or glucose 5%. The diluted solution should not be greater than 0.4 mg/mL to prevent precipitation occurring
* undiluted concentrate may cause hard plastic to crack and leak
* should not be mixed with alkaline solutions with pH greater than 8
* tablets contain parahydroxybenzoates, which can cause allergic reactions (including delayed reactions)
* caution if used in those with mild-to-moderate liver impairment
* contraindicated in those with severe liver impairment, kidney impairment (creatinine clearance < 15 mL/min), or WBC < 2000 cells/mm^3 or platelet count < 75,000 cells/mm^3 (not due to malignant disease)
* see also General Nursing considerations/Cautions for antineoplastic agents (p. 596)

Patient education

- instruct patient that capsules should be swallowed whole (not chewed or opened) with water either 2 hours before or 1 hour after food
- see also General Patient education for antineoplastic agents (p. 598)

Capsules should not be opened, crushed or broken.

For those with creatinine clearance 15-50 mL/min, 75% of starting dose is recommended.

Contraindicated in those with severe liver dysfunction or CrCl < 15 mL/min.

EXEMESTANE

Trade names
APO Exemestane, Aromasin, Exemestane GH, Exemestane Sandoz, Exemestane-WGR

Available form
Tablets: 25 mg

Action
- hormonal antineoplastic agent (irreversible steroidal, aromatase inactivator)

Use
- early breast cancer (oestrogen receptor positive, postmenopausal) after tamoxifen therapy
- advanced breast cancer (oestrogen receptor positive, postmenopausal after failure of antioestrogen therapy)

Dose
- 25 mg orally once daily with food (for 5 years or tumour relapse in early breast cancer; or in tumour progression in advanced breast cancer)

Adverse effects
- decreased bone density, osteoporosis, fractures
- hot flushes, increased sweating
- fatigue, headache, dizziness, insomnia, depression, asthenia
- anorexia, nausea, vomiting, abdominal pain, diarrhoea, constipation, dyspepsia
- hypertension
- vaginal haemorrhage
- increased weight
- hypercholesterolaemia, increased liver enzymes and bilirubin
- arthralgia, joint and musculoskeletal pain, back and limb pain, osteoarthritis, carpal tunnel syndrome, tendonitis, tenosynovitis
- peripheral oedema
- leukopenia
- rash, alopecia

Interaction
- actions are antagonised if given with oestrogen-containing agents

Nursing considerations/Cautions

- postmenopausal status (such as luteinising hormone (LH), follicle-stimulating hormone (FSH) and estradiol (oestradiol) levels) should be confirmed before starting therapy
- vitamin D levels should be monitored and supplements given if needed
- bone densitometry is recommended before starting and regularly throughout therapy in women who are at risk of osteoporosis. Treatment or prophylaxis for osteoporosis should be started if needed
- caution if used in women with osteoporosis
- not recommended in premenopausal women
- see also General Nursing considerations/Cautions for antineoplastic agents (p. 596)

Patient education

- see General Patient education for antineoplastic agents (p. 598)

Tablet can be dispersed in water (5 minutes or more), or crushed and mixed with a spoonful of yoghurt or apple puree. Mask and gloves should be used to disperse or crush tablets.

Banned in sport.

FLUDARABINE PHOSPHATE

Trade names
Fludara, Fludarabine Ebewe Concentrate, Fludarabine Juno, Fludarabine Phosphate Injection

Available forms
Vial: 50 mg, 50 mg/2 mL;
Tablet: 10 mg

Action
- antineoplastic antibiotic
- purine analogue antagonist that inhibits DNA synthesis
- prodrug of fludarabine

Use
- B-cell chronic lymphocytic leukaemia

Dose
- 25 mg/m^2 by IV injection or IV infusion over 30 minutes for 5 consecutive days every 28-day cycle (until complete or partial remission) **OR**
- 40 mg/m^2 orally daily for 5 consecutive days every 28-day cycle (until complete or partial remission)

Adverse effects
- autoimmune phenomena, haemolytic anaemia
- peripheral neuropathy
- neurotoxicity
- visual disturbances
- (Rare) skin cancers
- see also General Adverse effects of antineoplastic agents (p. 596)

Interactions
- efficacy may be decreased if given with dipyridamole and other adenosine-uptake inhibitors
- may increase intracellular concentrations of cytarabine
- see also General Interactions of antineoplastic agents (p. 596)

Nursing considerations/Cautions
- (IV) reconstitute the powder with 2 mL water for Injections, then further dilute with sodium chloride 0.9% for IV administration (10 mL for IV bolus injection or 100 mL for IV infusion over 30 minutes)
- (Concentrate) dilute in 100–125 mL sodium chloride 0.9% or glucose 5%
- patients receiving fludarabine should receive only irradiated blood transfusions to decrease the risk of transfusion-related graft versus host disease
- may cause reversible worsening or flare-up of pre-existing skin cancer lesions
- contraindicated in those with haemolytic anaemia or creatinine clearance < 30 mL/min
- see also General Nursing considerations/Cautions for antineoplastic agents (p. 596)

Patient education
- advise the patient to swallow tablets whole (without crushing, breaking or chewing)
- instruct the patient to seek medical advice immediately if any of the following occur:
  - numbness, tingling or weakness in arms or legs
  - changes to skin or development of skin lesions
  - confusion, agitation, fitting, changes to vision
- see also General Patient education for antineoplastic agents (p. 598)

 Tablets should not be crushed or broken.

 In those with moderate renal impairment (creatinine clearance 30–70 mL/min), the dose should be reduced in relation to creatinine clearance and close monitoring is recommended.

FLUOROURACIL

Trade names
APOC-5FU Cream, DBL Fluorouracil Solution, Efudix, Fluorouracil Accord, Fluorouracil Ebewe, Fluorouracil Viatris Cream, Tolak 4% Once Daily

Available forms
Vial: 500 mg/10 mL, 1 g/20 mL, 2.5 g/50 mL, 2.5 g/100 mL, 5 g/100 mL;
Cream: 50 mg/g (5%), 40 mg/g (4%)

Action
- uracil analogue that is converted to active metabolite which has antimetabolic properties, interfering with both DNA and RNA synthesis
- half-life 8—22 minutes and dose dependent
- narrow margin of safety; highly toxic

Use
- breast, colon, rectal or stomach cancer (alone or as part of palliative treatment)
- treatment of gastric, pancreas, liver, uterine, cervical, ovarian or bladder cancer
- solar and senile keratosis, Bowen's disease (cream)

Dose
- 15 mg/kg by IV infusion over 4 hours daily until GI side-effects occur, then stop therapy until side-effects recede, then 5—10 mg/kg by IV injection weekly (daily maximum 1 g) **OR**
- 12 mg/kg by IV injection on 3 consecutive days; if no toxic side-effects, then 6 mg/kg on days 5, 7 and 9. If no toxic side-effects, then 5—10 mg/kg by IV injection weekly **OR**
- 5—7 mg/kg by intra-arterial infusion over 24 hours **OR**
- (Cream) apply a thin layer to the lesion 1—2 times daily until the erosive stage (3—4 weeks) **OR**
- (Tolak, cream) apply a thin layer to area of lesions once daily for 4 weeks (as tolerated)

Adverse effects
- severe toxicity (can be life threatening)
- photosensitivity
- neurotoxicity, Wernicke's encephalopathy
- hand—foot syndrome
- (Cream) pain, pruritus, burning, hyperpigmentation, phototoxicity, rash, ulceration, allergy
- see also General Adverse effects of antineoplastic agents (p. 596)

Interactions
- caution if used with leucovorin (folinic acid) because of increased GI toxicity
- decreased bone marrow depression if given with allopurinol; however, increased GI toxicity may occur if given together
- may increase serum levels of phenytoin; therefore serum levels should be closely monitored
- efficacy may be affected if given with methotrexate, metronidazole or folinic acid
- may potentiate necrosis caused by radiation
- myelotoxic effects may be potentiated if given with radiation
- caution if used with warfarin; INR should be closely monitored during therapy, especially when starting or stopping therapy
- may interfere with thiamine (vitamin B_1) metabolism
- may interfere with thyroid function test
- see also General Interactions of antineoplastic agents (p. 596)

Nursing considerations/Cautions
- thiamine levels should be monitored and supplementation recommended if levels are low to prevent onset of Wernicke's encephalopathy
- IV dose should be reduced by one-third to half if the patient has a poor nutritional status, within 30 days of major surgery, WBC < 5000/mm^3 or platelet < 100,000/mm^3
- (IV) dilute with 300—500 mL glucose 5% and infuse over 4 hours
- (IV) incompatible with acidic agents

ANTINEOPLASTIC AGENTS

- (Cream) an occlusive dressing is not recommended for senile or solar keratoses as it may increase penetration and an inflammatory response of adjacent skin
- (Cream) the treatment area should not exceed 23 × 23 cm
- (Cream) not recommended in those who work outdoors for prolonged periods
- (Cream) the number of retreatments is decided by the physician
- caution if used in those who have received high-dose pelvic radiation or therapy with alkylating agents
- not recommended in those who have had a previously documented cardiovascular reaction (e.g. angina, arrhythmia, ST segment change) because of the risk of sudden death
- contraindicated in those with poor nutritional state, are debilitated or with dihydropyrimidine dehydrogenase (DPD) enzyme deficiency
- (Tolak) contraindicated in those with peanut or soya allergy. Also contains hydroxybenzoates, which can cause allergic reactions
- see also General Nursing considerations/Cautions for antineoplastic agents (p. 596)

Patient education

- instruct the patient to seek medical advice immediately if any of the following occur:
  - sore, red or ulcerated mouth or difficulty swallowing within 5–8 days of starting therapy (this can be an early sign of severe toxicity)
  - disorientation, confusion, headache, slurred speech, dizziness, muscle weakness (which may persist after therapy has stopped)
- (Cream) instruct the patient that
  - the cream should not be applied to damaged skin or open wounds
  - the area should be washed, rinsed and dried before applying cream
  - the cream should be applied with gloves or a non-metal applicator
  - avoid application to normal skin, perioral area or nasolabial folds
  - if accidental exposure of the eyes occurs, the eyes should be flushed with copious amounts of water
  - the normal sequence of events is for skin to redden (and appear blotchy), then blister, peel and crack (the reaction peaks at 4 weeks). Redness usually resolves 2–4 weeks after stopping treatment
  - cosmetics and skin preparations should not be applied to same area
  - discard the tube 8 weeks after opening
- warn the patient to avoid or minimise sun exposure during and immediately after therapy
- see also General Patient education for antineoplastic agents (p. 598)

 IV dose should be reduced by one-third to half in those with impaired kidney or liver function.

Available in combination with
fluorouracil 5 mg + salicylic acid 100 mg (Actikerall)

FOTEMUSTINE
Trade name
Muphoran

Available form
Vial: 208 mg

Action
- alkylating agent (nitrogen mustard analogue)

Use
- disseminated malignant melanoma (including cerebral metastases) (alone or as part of combination therapy)

Dose
- initially 100 mg/m^2 by IV infusion over 1 hour or intra-arterial infusion over 4 hours for 3 doses at weekly intervals

(induction), followed by a rest period of 4–5 weeks, then 100 mg/m² every 3 weeks (maintenance)

Adverse effects
- see General Adverse effects of antineoplastic agents (p. 596)

Interactions
- contraindicated with yellow fever vaccine
- caution if given with warfarin; INR should be closely monitored, especially when starting or stopping therapy
- not recommended concurrently with dacarbazine because of the increased risk of pulmonary toxicity and at least a 1-week interval should be allowed between administration of two agents
- not recommended with phenytoin because of the increased risk of seizures, as absorption of phenytoin may be impaired
- see also General Interactions of antineoplastic agents (p. 596)

Nursing considerations/Cautions
- regular ophthalmology examination is recommended before starting and regularly throughout therapy
- should not be given within 4 weeks of other chemotherapy or 6 weeks of nitrosoureas
- if given as part of combination therapy, the induction phase can be omitted
- reconstitute using 4 mL of supplied diluent, then further dilute with glucose 5%
- IV solution should be protected from light during administration
- reconstituted solution contains the equivalent of 2.7 g of 100% alcohol, which may harmful if used in those with alcoholism, liver disease or epilepsy
- contraindicated in those with hypersensitivity to nitrosourea
- see also General Nursing considerations/Cautions for antineoplastic agents (p. 596)

Patient education
- see General Patient education for antineoplastic agents (p. 598)

 Caution if used in those > 60 years, as gastrointestinal toxicity, thrombopenia and leukopenia occur more frequently.

FULVESTRANT
Trade names
Fulvestrant Ever Pharma, Fulvestrant Sandoz, Fulvestrant SXP, Fulvestrant-AFT

Available form
Prefilled syringe: 250 mg/5 mL

Action
- hormonal antineoplastic agent (antioestrogen) which inhibits growth of some oestrogen-sensitive human breast cancer cells

Use
- locally advanced or metastatic hormone receptor (HR)-positive breast cancer (with disease progression after antioestrogen or aromatase therapy) (postmenopausal)
- locally advanced or metastatic hormone receptor (HR)-positive, human epidermal growth factor receptor (HER)-negative breast cancer not previously treated with endocrine therapy (postmenopausal)

Dose
- initially 500 mg slowly IM (as two 250 mg injections in each buttock), then 500 mg after 2 weeks, followed by 500 mg at monthly intervals

Adverse effects
- hot flushes
- headache, asthenia
- anorexia, nausea, vomiting, diarrhoea
- rash
- joint and musculoskeletal pain
- hypersensitivity
- elevated liver enzymes and bilirubin
- injection site reaction
- urinary tract infection
- (Uncommon) liver failure, hepatitis

ANTINEOPLASTIC AGENTS

Interactions
- may interfere with antibody-based oestradiol assay

Nursing considerations/Cautions
- not recommended in men
- caution if used in those with bleeding disorders or thrombocytopenia, or on anticoagulant therapy, because of the risk of bleeding associated with IM administration
- caution if used in those with creatinine clearance < 30 mL/min
- see also General Nursing considerations/Cautions for antineoplastic agents (p. 596)

Caution if used in those with moderate-to-severe liver impairment or CrCl < 30 mL/min.

Banned in sport.

HYDROXYCARBAMIDE (HYDROXYUREA)

Trade names
Hydrea, Hydroxycarbamide Medicianz, Hydroxycarbamide Medsurge

Available form
Capsules: 500 mg

Action
- thought to inhibit DNA synthesis during S phase of the cell cycle
- antimetabolite

Use
- chronic myelocytic leukaemia (CML) (resistant) (pre-treatment phase and palliative care)
- recurrent metastatic or inoperable ovarian cancer

Dose
- (Solid tumours — intermittent therapy) 80 mg/kg orally every third day **OR**
- (Solid tumours — continuous therapy) 20—30 mg/kg orally daily **OR**
- (Head/neck cancer with radiotherapy) 80 mg/kg orally every third day starting at least 7 days before, during and after radiotherapy (depending on any adverse effects) **OR**
- (CML) 20—30 mg/kg orally daily

Adverse effects
- skin ulceration
- exacerbation of post-irradiation erythema
- haemolytic anaemia
- see also General Adverse effects of antineoplastic agents (p. 596)

Interactions
- any uricosuric dose should be adjusted according to increases in the serum uric acid level
- irradiation erythema and mucositis may be worsened by hydroxycarbamide (hydroxyurea)
- may cause falsely elevated results for determination of urea, uric acid and lactic acid
- may cause falsely elevated glucose readings in some continuous glucose monitoring systems
- see also General Interactions of antineoplastic agents (p. 596)

Nursing considerations/Cautions
- (CML) therapy should be reviewed after 6 weeks to assess effectiveness
- hydroxyurea-induced ulcers generally heal when therapy is stopped
- see also General Nursing considerations/Cautions for antineoplastic agents (p. 596)

Patient education
- the patient should be advised to swallow the capsule whole (without opening or crushing)
- instruct the patient to seek medical advice if any skin ulcerations occur
- see also General Patient education for antineoplastic agents (p. 598)

Capsules should not be opened or crushed.

GEMCITABINE

Trade names
DBL Gemcitabine Solution, Gemaccord

Available forms
Vial: 200 mg, 1 g, 200 mg/5.3 mL, 1 g/26.3 mL, 2 g/52.6 mL

Action
- pyrimidine analogue with antimetabolic activity
- cell phase specific (S phase)

Use
- locally advanced or metastatic non-small cell lung cancer (NSCLC)
- locally advanced or metastatic adenocarcinoma of the pancreas
- bladder cancer (monotherapy or with cisplatin)
- recurrent epithelial ovarian carcinoma (relapsed more than 6 months after platinum-based treatment)
- unresectable, locally recurrent or metastatic breast cancer (which has relapsed) (with paclitaxel)
- refractory pancreatic cancer (where fluorouracil was ineffective)

Dose
- (NSCLC, monotherapy) 1 g/m^2 weekly IV over 30 minutes for 3 weeks of a 4-week cycle **OR**
- (NSCLC, combination therapy) 1.25 g/m^2 IV over 30 minutes on days 1 and 8 of a 21-day cycle (with cisplatin) **OR**
- (NSCLC, combination therapy) 1 g/m^2 IV over 30 minutes on days 1, 8 and 15 of a 28-day cycle (with cisplatin) **OR**
- (Pancreatic cancer) 1 g/m^2 weekly IV over 30 minutes for up to 7 weeks, with a 1-week rest interval, then 1 g/m^2 weekly IV for 3 weeks of a 4-week cycle **OR**
- (Bladder cancer — monotherapy) 1.25 g/m^2 IV over 30 minutes on days 1, 8 and 15 of a 28-day cycle **OR**
- (Bladder cancer — combination therapy) 1 g/m^2 IV over 30 minutes on days 1, 8 and 15 of a 28-day cycle (with cisplatin) **OR**
- (Breast cancer — combination therapy) 1.25 g/m^2 IV over 30 minutes on days 1 and 8 of a 21-day cycle (with paclitaxel) **OR**
- (Ovarian cancer — combination therapy) 1 g/m^2 IV over 30 minutes on days 1 and 8 of a 21-day cycle (with carboplatin)

Adverse effects
- (Uncommon) interstitial pneumonitis with pulmonary infiltrates and, rarely, pulmonary oedema and acute respiratory distress syndrome
- see also General Adverse effects of antineoplastic agents (p. 596)

Interactions
- increased risk of interstitial pneumonitis, colitis and oesophagitis if given with or within 7 days of radiotherapy
- see also General Interactions of antineoplastic agents (p. 596)

Nursing considerations/Cautions
- toxicity is increased with prolonged infusion time and with increased dosing frequency
- reconstitute using sodium chloride 0.9% (5 mL for 200 mg vial, 25 mL for 1 g vial), which can be further diluted with sodium chloride 0.9% for infusion
- caution if used in those with liver metastases, a history of hepatitis, or liver cirrhosis or alcoholism, as liver insufficiency may be exacerbated
- see also General Nursing considerations/Cautions for antineoplastic agents (p. 596)

Patient education
- instruct the patient to seek medical advice immediately if any persistent cough, shortness of breath or fever occurs
- see also General Patient education for antineoplastic agents (p. 598)

ANTINEOPLASTIC AGENTS

IDARUBICIN HYDROCHLORIDE
Trade name
Zavedos

Available forms
Solution: 5 mg/5 mL, 10 mg/10 mL

Action
- anthracycline antibiotic analogue of doxorubicin, inhibits nucleic acid synthesis
- half-life 10—35 hours
- active metabolite with long half-life (33—60 hours)

Use
- remission and induction of acute myeloid leukaemia (AML) (untreated, relapsed or refractory patient)

Dose
- 12 mg/m² daily IV over 10—15 minutes for 3 days (with cytarabine IV for 7 days)

Adverse effects
- ECG changes, tachycardia, arrhythmias, congestive cardiac failure, cardiomyopathy
- (Rare) gastrointestinal perforation
- see also General Adverse effects of antineoplastic agents (p. 596)

Interactions
- added myelosuppressive effect if given with or within 14—21 days of radiation therapy
- caution if used with other cardiotoxic agents such as calcium-channel blockers and trastuzumab. If given after trastuzumab, a 7-month interval should be allowed before starting idarubicin
- see also General Interactions of antineoplastic agents (p. 596)

Nursing considerations/Cautions
- cardiac function (including ECG and either echocardiogram or multiple gated acquisition (MUGA)) should be assessed before starting and regularly throughout therapy
- injection given into freely running IV solution over 10—15 minutes
- IV solution is incompatible with heparin or with alkaline drugs
- caution if used in those with pre-existing heart disease or previous irradiation to mediastinal area
- contraindicated in those with recent myocardial infarction, severe arrhythmias, severe myocardial insufficiency or previous treatment with maximum cumulative dose of idarubicin or other anthracyclines or anthracenediones (anthraquinones), hypersensitivity to other anthracyclines or severe liver or renal impairment
- see also General Nursing considerations/Cautions for antineoplastic agents (p. 596)

Patient education
- the patient should be advised that their urine may appear a harmless red colour for 1—2 days after therapy
- instruct the patient to seek medical advice immediately if any of the following occur (even 1—2 months after therapy has stopped):
  - shortness of breath, cough, pink frothy sputum
  - swelling of ankles, legs or abdomen
  - decreased urine output
  - rapid or abnormal heart rate
  - severe abdominal pain
- see also General Patient education for antineoplastic agents (p. 598)

 A 50% dose reduction is recommended if bilirubin levels are 20.4—50.0 micromol/L. Contraindicated in those with severe liver or kidney impairment.

IFOSFAMIDE
Trade name
Holoxan

Available forms
Vial: 500 mg, 1 g, 2 g

Action
- requires activation by microsomal liver enzymes to produce active metabolite, which is an alkylating agent (nitrogen mustard analogue)

Use
- ovarian and cervical tumours

- some response in lung and breast cancers
- sarcomas, lymphomas and germ cell tumours

Dose
- 8—10 g/m² divided into 5 equal doses and administered daily for 5 days given IV, and repeated at 2—4-week intervals **OR**
- 5—6 g/m² IV given over 24 hours (maximum 10 g), repeated at 3—4-week intervals

Adverse effects
- haematuria, haemorrhagic cystitis, tubular dysfunction
- encephalopathy, drowsiness, CNS toxicity
- impaired wound healing
- see also General Adverse effects of antineoplastic agents (p. 596)

Interactions
- an increased risk of bleeding if given with warfarin; therefore INR should be closely monitored when starting or stopping therapy
- hypoglycaemia may be increased if given with sulfonylureas
- increased myelosuppression if given with allopurinol or hydrochlorothiazide
- caution if given with agents acting on the CNS (e.g. antiemetics, opioid analgesics, antihistamines) especially in those with ifosfamide-induced encephalopathy
- efficacy may be decreased by grapefruit and grapefruit juice
- may potentiate muscle relaxant effects of suxamethonium
- effects and toxicity may be increased if given with liothyronine (triiodothyronine), chlorpromazine or disulfiram
- an increased risk of nephrotoxicity, neurotoxicity or myelosuppression if given before or with cisplatin, aminoglycosides, aciclovir or amphotericin B (amphotericin)
- caution if given with bupropion, orphenadrine or cyclophosphamide
- may increase radiodermatitis
- see also General Interactions of antineoplastic agents (p. 596)

Nursing considerations/Cautions
- any electrolyte imbalance, cystitis, outflow disturbance or urinary tract infection should be identified and treated before starting therapy
- renal function, urinary status, urinary sediment and urinary output should be monitored regularly
- urinalysis should be performed before each course, and if haematuria (> 10 RBCs/high- power field) is present the therapy should be postponed until resolved
- haemorrhagic cystitis is a common side-effect; therefore ifosfamide is given with aggressive oral or parenteral hydration
- to prevent bladder toxicity, the uroprotector mesna (see p. 780) should be administered concurrently
- liver function and albumin levels should be closely monitored, as low albumin and liver impairment are risk factors for neurotoxicity; also impaired liver function may lead to increases in metabolite thought to be responsible for nephrotoxicity
- reconstitute with water for injections (13 mL for 500 mg, 25 mL for 1 g and 50 mL for 2 g) to give a concentration of 40 mg/mL, then dilute further for IV infusion
- therapy should not be starting within 2 weeks of surgery
- not recommended within 3 months of nephrectomy or caution if used in unilaterally nephrectomised patients
- caution if used in those who are older or with brain metastases, cerebral symptoms, a history of alcohol abuse, obesity, impaired renal function, pretreated with nephrotoxic before nephrectomy, electrolyte imbalance, postrenal obstruction or are female, due to the increased risk of encephalopathy
- caution if used in those with pre-existing cardiac disorders, those who have had previous irradiation to heart area and/or have been previously treated with anthracyclines

ANTINEOPLASTIC AGENTS

- contraindicated in those with urinary obstruction or bladder inflammation (cystitis)
- see also General Nursing considerations/Cautions for antineoplastic agents (p. 596)

Patient education

- those with diabetes managed with sulfonylurea agents should be warned to monitor blood glucose levels closely during therapy
- the patient should be advised to avoid grapefruit and grapefruit juice during therapy
- instruct the patient to seek medical advice immediately if any of the following occur:
  - blood in urine, bladder pain, difficulty passing urine
  - drowsiness, confusion, hallucinations, fitting (seizure) or loss of consciousness
  - fatigue, chest pain, palpitations, altered heart rate
- see also General Patient education for antineoplastic agents (p. 598)

 Contraindicated in those with severe liver impairment or impaired kidney function and/or obstructions of urine flow.

IRINOTECAN HYDROCHLORIDE TRIHYDRATE (IRINOTECAN HYDROCHLORIDE)
Trade names
Irinotecan Accord, Irinotecan Baxter, Irinotecan Eugia, Meditab Irinotecan

IRINOTECAN (LIPOSOMAL)
Trade name
Onivyde

Available forms
Vial: 40 mg/2 mL, 100 mg/5 mL, 500 mg/25 mL;
Vial (liposomal): 43 mg/10 mL

Action
- topoisomerase1 inhibitor that induces DNA strand break
- active metabolite (SN-38) inhibits topoisomerase1 more potently than irinotecan (parent drug)
- some cholinergic effects
- liposomal formulation prolongs activity at tumour site (Onivyde)

Use
- metastatic carcinoma of the rectum or colon (as first-line treatment or after disease recurrence or progression after initial therapy)
- metastatic pancreatic adenocarcinoma (previously treated with gemcitabine) (with folinic acid and 5FU (fluorouracil))

Dose
- (Rectum or colon cancer — monotherapy) 125 mg/m^2 IV over 90 minutes on days 1, 8, 15 and 22 followed by a 2-week rest interval (6-week cycle). The dose may be increased to 150 mg/m^2 or decreased to 50 mg/m^2 depending on patient tolerance (6-week cycle) **OR**
- (Rectum or colon cancer — monotherapy) 350 mg/m^2 IV over 90 minutes once every 3 weeks, decreasing the dose to 200 mg/m^2 in 50 mg increments if needed (3-week cycle) **OR**
- (Rectum or colon cancer— combination therapy) 125 mg/m^2 IV over 90 minutes on days 1, 8, 15 and 22 followed by a 2-week rest interval (with folinic acid and fluorouracil) (6-week cycle) **OR**
- (Rectum or colon cancer — combination therapy) 180 mg/m^2 IV over 90 minutes on days 1, 15 and 29 followed by a 2-week rest interval (with folinic acid and fluorouracil) (6-week cycle) **OR**
- (Pancreatic adenocarcinoma after gemcitabine) 70 mg/m^2 IV over 90 minutes every 2 weeks (with folinic acid and fluorouracil) (Onivyde) **OR**
- (Pancreatic adenocarcinoma — first-line treatment) 50 mg/m^2 IV over 90 minutes every 2 weeks (with oxaliplatin, folinic acid and fluorouracil) (Onivyde)

649

Adverse effects
- (Cholinergic effects, early, transient) diarrhoea, increased salivation and lacrimation, miosis, sweating, bradycardia, flushing and intestinal hyperperistalsis (causing abdominal cramping)
- colitis, paralytic ileus
- infusion-related reactions
- see also General Adverse effects of antineoplastic agents (p. 596)

Interactions
- not recommended with diuretics (especially during periods of active vomiting or diarrhoea) because of the increased risk of severe dehydration
- not recommended with atazanavir, clarithromycin, gemfibrozil, itraconazole, lopinavir, ritonavir, voriconazole or grapefruit juice, as increased serum levels may occur. Should be stopped for at least 7 days before starting therapy with irinotecan
- may prolong neuromuscular blocking actions of suxamethonium
- may antagonise neuromuscular blockade of non-depolarising blocking agents
- not recommended with St John's wort, phenobarbital (phenobarbitone), phenytoin or carbamazepine, as serum levels may increase. These should be stopped at least 14 days before starting therapy with irinotecan
- an increased risk of myelosuppression and neutropenia if the patient has previously received pelvic/abdominal irradiation
- an increased incidence of akathisia if given with prochlorperazine
- an increased risk of hyperglycaemia and lymphocytopenia if given with dexamethasone
- see also General Interactions of antineoplastic agents (p. 596)

Nursing considerations/Cautions
- liposomal and non-liposomal formulations are not interchangeable
- genotyping for UGT1A1 allele may be useful in identifying patients at increased risk of neutropenia.
- (Pancreatic adenocarcinoma after gemcitabine) for those known to be homozygous for the UGT1A1*28 allele, the recommended starting dose is 50 mg/m^2 for the first cycle and then increasing to 70 mg/m^2 in subsequent cycles if tolerated
- premedication with dexamethasone 10 mg and ondansetron or granisetron is recommended, starting 30 minutes before therapy
- not given as a bolus or undiluted
- IV or SC atropine (0.25—1 g) can be used prophylactically or to relieve cholinergic adverse effects
- (Liposomal formulation) dilute to 500 mL with glucose 5% or sodium chloride 0.9%
- (Non-liposomal formulation) must be diluted with glucose 5% or sodium chloride 0.9% before IV administration to a concentration of 0.12—2.8 mg/mL
- (Onivyde) contains 3.31 mg sodium/mL, which may need to be considered if the patient has sodium restriction
- caution if used in those with asthma, cardiovascular disease, or urinary or GI obstruction because of cholinergic effects
- (Non-liposomal formulation) not recommended in those with fructose intolerance, as the product contains sorbitol
- see also General Nursing considerations/Cautions for antineoplastic agents (p. 596)

Patient education
- advise the patient to have loperamide readily available at the first sign of poorly formed or loose stools
- the patient should be instructed that delayed (or late) diarrhoea (more than 24 hours after treatment) should be treated promptly with loperamide (at the first sign of loose stools) (initially

ANTINEOPLASTIC AGENTS

4 mg, then 2 mg 2-hourly (or 4 mg 4-hourly overnight) until diarrhoea-free for 12 hours) to prevent dehydration and electrolyte imbalance. Loperamide is not recommended for longer than 48 hours because of the increased risk of paralytic ileus. Further, the patient should be instructed to seek medical advice immediately if diarrhoea is not controlled in 24 hours using this regimen
- to help avoid severe diarrhoea, the patient should be encouraged to maintain a low-fat, lactose-free diet and stay well hydrated during therapy
- see also General Patient education for antineoplastic agents (p. 598)

Caution if used in those with kidney impairment and not recommended if patient is on dialysis.

Caution if used in those with liver impairment owing to increased risk of hepatotoxicity.

LETROZOLE
Trade names
ARX Letrozole, Femara, Femolet, Gynotril, Letrozole Actavis, Letrozole GH, Letrozole Sandoz, Letrozole-WGR, Pharmcor Letrozole

Available form
Tablets: 2.5 mg

Action
- non-steroidal aromatase inhibitor that blocks oestrogen-dependent tumour growth

Use
- hormone receptor positive breast cancer (in postmenopausal women)

Dose
- 2.5 mg orally daily (for 5 years or if tumour relapse occurs)

Adverse effects
- see Adverse effects for exemestane (p. 640)

Interactions
- not recommended with tamoxifen, other antioestrogens or oestrogen-containing agents
- increased serum levels may occur if given with itraconazole, voriconazole, ritonavir or clarithromycin
- decreased serum levels may occur if given with phenytoin, rifampicin, carbamazepine, phenobarbital (phenobarbitone) or St John's wort
- may increase serum levels of phenytoin and clopidogrel, increasing the risk of adverse effects

Nursing considerations/Cautions
- see Nursing considerations/Cautions for exemestane (p. 640)

Patient education
- see General Patient education for antineoplastic agents (p. 596)

Banned in sport.

LOMUSTINE
Trade names
CeeNU, Gleostine, Lomustine Capsules

Available form
Capsules: 10 mg, 40 mg

Action
- alkylating agent (nitrosourea)

Use
- palliative treatment of primary, metastatic brain tumours (with surgery and/or radiotherapy and/or chemotherapy)
- Hodgkin's disease (alternative therapy where other therapies were ineffective)

Dose
- 130 mg/m^2 orally 1 hour before or 1 hour after food once every 6 weeks

Adverse effects
- pulmonary fibrosis
- see also General Adverse effects of antineoplastic agents (p. 596)

Interactions
- see General Interactions of antineoplastic agents (p. 596)

Nursing considerations/Cautions
- lung function should be measured before starting and regularly throughout therapy
- pulmonary toxicity symptoms may occur months to years after stopping therapy
- see also General Nursing considerations/Cautions for antineoplastic agents (p. 596)

Patient education
- ensure the patient understands that capsules are taken only once every 6 weeks
- advise the patient that nausea and vomiting are reduced if lomustine is taken on an empty stomach; however, if nausea and vomiting do occur, the patient should ensure that the capsule has not been vomited
- the patient should be advised to swallow capsules whole (without opening or chewing)
- instruct the patient to report any new or worsening cough, shortness of breath or difficulty breathing
- see also General Patient education for antineoplastic agents (p. 598)

 Capsules should not be opened, crushed or chewed.

LURBINECTEDIN
Trade name
Zepzelca

Available form
Vial: 4 mg

Action
- alkylating agent
- binds guanine residues in minor groove of DNA resulting in bending of the helix towards the major groove, which impacts on DNA-binding protein activity leading to eventual cell death
- half-life 51 hours

Use
- metastatic small cell lung cancer (SCLC) that has progressed on or after receiving platinum-containing therapy

Dose
- 3.2 mg/m² by IV infusion over 60 minutes, repeated once every 21 days

Adverse effects
- rhabdomyolysis
- see also General Adverse effects for antineoplastic agents (p. 596)

Interactions
- caution if used with other agents that increase the risk of rhabdomyolysis (e.g. statins)
- serum levels may be increased if given with itraconazole, posaconazole, voriconazole, grapefruit juice, aprepitant, ciprofloxacin, diltiazem, erythromycin, fluconazole, fluvoxamine, imatinib or verapamil, increasing the risk of adverse effects and therefore should not be given together
- serum levels may be decreased if given with carbamazepine, phenytoin, rifampicin, St. John's wort, bosentan, primidone or phenobarbital

Nursing considerations/Cautions
- ensure the absolute neutrophil count is $> 1.5 \times 10^9$/L and platelet count is $> 100 \times 10^9$/L before starting therapy
- pregnancy should be excluded before starting therapy
- the dose can be reduced if adverse reaction warrants; however, therapy should be discontinued if the patient is unable to tolerate 2.0 mg/m² every 21 days
- premedication with corticosteroids (e.g. dexamethasone 8 mg IV or equivalent) and antiemetic (e.g. ondansetron 8 mg IV or equivalent)
- reconstitute using 8 mL water for Injections to give a concentration of

ANTINEOPLASTIC AGENTS

0.5 mg/mL. See manufacturer's information for calculation of required volume. Add this volume to at least 100 mL of sodium chloride 0.9% or glucose 5% and administer over 60 minutes
- not recommended for those with moderate-to-severe liver impairment, severe kidney impairment or end-stage kidney disease
- see also General Nursing considerations/Cautions for antineoplastic agents (p. 596)

Patient education
- instruct the patient to seek medical advice immediately if they experience any muscle pain or stiffness, feeling weak or tired, or urine becomes dark
- see also General Patient education for antineoplastic agents (p. 598)

MELPHALAN
Trade names
Alkeran, Melpha

Available forms
Vial: 50 mg;
Tablets: 2 mg

Action
- alkylating agent (nitrogen mustard derivative)

Use
- palliative treatment of multiple myeloma (MM) and advanced ovarian adenocarcinoma
- advanced breast cancer
- polycythaemia vera

Dose
- (MM) 0.15 mg/kg orally daily in divided doses (with prednisolone 40 mg orally) for 4 days, repeated every 6 weeks **OR**
- (MM) 16 mg/m² by IV infusion over 15—20 minutes every 2 weeks for 4 doses, then every 4 weeks **OR**
- (Advanced ovarian cancer) 0.2 mg/kg orally daily in 3 divided doses for 5 days, repeated every 4—8 weeks **OR**
- (Advanced breast cancer) 0.15 mg/kg or 5 mg/m² orally daily for 4—6 days, repeated every 6 weeks **OR**
- (Polycythaemia vera) 6—10 mg orally daily for 5—7 days, followed by 2—4 mg daily until satisfactory control (remission induction), then 2—6 mg orally once weekly (maintenance)

Adverse effects
- (IV) hypersensitivity
- see also General Adverse effects of antineoplastic agents (p. 596)

Interactions
- increased risk of impaired renal function if given with ciclosporin or cisplatin
- may increase pulmonary toxicity if given with carmustine
- see also General Interactions of antineoplastic agents (p. 596)

Nursing considerations/Cautions
- (MM) IV therapy is indicated when oral therapy is not available or inappropriate
- myelosuppression is greater with IV compared with oral administration
- after reconstitution with 10 mL of supplied diluent, dilute with sodium chloride 0.9% to concentration of ≤ 0.45 mg/mL
- should be completely administered within 60 minutes of reconstitution
- reconstituted solution should not be refrigerated, as a precipitate will form
- (IV) not compatible with solutions containing glucose
- (MM) treatment beyond 12 months does not appear to improve results
- see also General Nursing considerations/Cautions for antineoplastic agents (p. 596)

Patient education
- see General Patient education for antineoplastic agents (p. 598)

Tablets should not be crushed, broken or dispersed.

For those with moderate-to-severe renal impairment, a dose reduction of up to 50% should be considered.

MERCAPTOPURINE MONOHYDRATE

Trade names
Allmercap, Mercaptopurine-Link, Puri-Nethol

Available forms
Tablet: 50 mg;
Oral solution: 20 mg/mL

Action
- purine analogue antimetabolite that interferes with nucleic acid synthesis
- half-life 90 minutes
- active metabolites have a longer life than the parent agent

Use
- acute lymphoblastic and myelogenous leukaemia (remission induction and maintenance), chronic granulocytic leukaemia

Dose
- 2.5 mg/kg orally daily

Adverse effects
- macrophage activation syndrome (high non-abating fever, lymphadenopathy, hepatosplenomegaly, CNS dysfunction, bleeding)
- photosensitivity
- see also General Adverse effects of antineoplastic agents (p. 596)

Interactions
- contraindicated with yellow fever vaccine
- may inhibit the anticoagulant action of warfarin; therefore INR should be closely monitored, especially when starting and stopping therapy
- not recommended with ribavirin, which may decrease the efficacy and increase the toxicity of mercaptopurine
- an increased serum level may occur if given with allopurinol; therefore the dose of mercaptopurine should be decreased to 25%
- the onset of pancytopenia is slowed when taken with unregulated amounts of salicylates, sulfonamides or tranquillisers
- increased serum levels may occur if given with high-dose methotrexate
- caution if given with olsalazine, mesalazine or sulfasalazine (in those with inherited deficiency of thiopurine methyltransferase) because of the risk of increased myelosuppression
- caution if given with infliximab
- dose reduction is required if given with allopurinol
- may interfere with the niacin pathway, resulting in nicotinic acid deficiency/pellagra (especially in those with Crohn's disease)
- see also General Interactions of antineoplastic agents (p. 596)

Nursing considerations/Cautions
- testing for thiopurine methyltransferase (TPMT) enzyme is recommended before starting therapy. Deficiency in TPMT will result in the person being at high risk of severe, life-threatening myelosuppression
- genetic testing for the NUDT15 gene is recommended (especially in children or those of Asian heritage) to reduce the risk of severe leukocytopenia and alopecia
- cross-resistance may exist between mercaptopurine and tioguanine (thioguanine)
- (Oral solution) recommended for paediatric use only
- (Oral solution) contains aspartame and not recommended in those with phenylketouria
- (Oral solution) contains hydroxybenzoates, which may cause allergic reactions (including delayed)
- not recommended in those with Lesch—Nylan syndrome
- not recommended in those with rare hereditary problems of galactose intolerance, complete lactase deficiency or glucose—galactose malabsorption
- see also General Nursing considerations/Cautions for antineoplastic agents (p. 596)

Patient education

- the patient should be advised to standardise when they take tablets (i.e. either before or after food, but not switching between the two)
- the tablet should be swallowed whole, but not with milk or dairy products (either 1 hour before or 2 hours after)
- instruct the patient to limit exposure to sunlight and UV light by wearing long-sleeved clothing, a hat and factor 30+ sunscreen if going outdoors
- if the patient is taking an oral suspension, the following instruction should be given:
  - take suspension 1 hour before or 2 hours after food or dairy products
  - shake the bottle vigorously for at least 30 seconds before using
  - push the bottle adapter firmly into top of bottle
  - two dosing syringes are provided: the orange 5 mL syringe marked 1–5 mL should be used to measure amounts > 1 mL, with each 0.2 mL = 4 mg; the purple 1 mL syringe marked 0.1–1 mL should be used to measure amounts ≤ 1 mL, with each 0.1 mL = 2 mg
  - put the tip of the correct dosing syringe into the bottle adapter, turn the bottle upside down and pull the plunger back to the point on the scale that corresponds with the dose
  - turn the bottle the right way up, withdraw the syringe and gently put the tip into the mouth inside the cheek. Gently squirt suspension into the mouth (not forcefully) and swallow
  - drink a small amount of water to ensure the suspension is not left in the mouth
  - wash the syringe with warm soapy water, rinse well and let it dry completely before reusing
  - wash the hands well after handling the oral suspension and syringe
- discard any unused suspension 8 weeks after opening
- instruct the patient to seek medical advice if they develop any pigmented rash, diarrhoea or any cognitive decline (may be signs of nicotinic acid deficiency)
- see also General Patient education for antineoplastic agents (p. 598)

 Tablets should not be crushed, broken or chewed. Oral liquid is available, however, bioavailability is greater and may require dose adjustment.

 Dose reduction is recommended in those with renal or liver impairment.

METHOTREXATE

Trade names
ARX-Methotrexate, Chexate, DBL Methotrexate Injection, Methoblastin, Methotrexate Accord, Methotrexate Ebewe, Trexject

Available forms
Tablets: 2.5 mg, 10 mg;
Vial: 5 mg/2 mL, 50 mg/2 mL, 500 mg/5 mL, 500 mg/20 mL, 1000 mg/10 mL, 5000 mg/50 mL;
Prefilled syringe: 7.5 mg/0.15 mL, 10 mg/0.2 mL, 15 mg/0.3 mL, 20 mg/0.4 mL, 25 mg/0.5 mL

Action
- inhibits metabolism of folic acid, thereby interfering with DNA and RNA synthesis (cell replication) (especially in rapidly dividing cells such as dermal epithelial, buccal and intestinal cells)

Use
- (With other agents) palliative treatment of acute lymphoblastic leukaemia, Burkitt's lymphoma, advanced lymphosarcoma, advanced mycosis fungoides, prophylaxis and treatment of meningeal leukaemia
- breast cancer, choriocarcinoma, chorioadenoma destruens, hydatidiform mole

- high-dose therapy used for osteogenic sarcoma, acute leukaemias, bronchogenic carcinoma, head and neck epidermoid carcinoma (with calcium folinate)
- unresponsive disabling psoriasis, rheumatoid arthritis (see Disease-modifying antirheumatic drugs (DMARDs), p. 1050)

Dose
- (Trophoblastic neoplasm, hydatidiform mole, chorioadenoma destruens) 15—30 mg IM or orally daily before food for 5 days, may be repeated ≥ 1 week rest interval for 3—5 cycles **OR**
- (Lymphoblastic leukaemia) 3.3 mg/m^2 orally daily (with prednisolone) (remission induction), then 30 mg/m^2 orally twice weekly (maintenance) **OR**
- (Lymphoblastic leukaemia) 30 mg/m^2 IM twice weekly or 2.5 mg/kg IV every 14 days (maintenance) **OR**
- (Lymphoma) 10—25 mg orally daily for 4—8 days, repeated after 7—10 days if needed, repeated for several courses **OR**
- (Mycosis fungoides) 2.5—10 mg orally daily for weeks to months **OR**
- (Mycosis fungoides) 50 mg IM weekly or 25 mg IM twice weekly **OR**
- (Breast cancer) 40 mg/m^2 IV on days 1 and 8 of cyclic chemotherapy (with cyclophosphamide and fluorouracil) **OR**
- (Meningeal leukaemia) 12 mg intrathecally every 2—5 days until CSF cell count returns to normal, then one extra dose

Adverse effects
- interstitial lung disease, pulmonary fibrosis
- (High doses) CNS toxicity, convulsions
- see also General Adverse effects of antineoplastic agents (p. 596)

Interactions
- (Intrathecal) contraindicated with CNS radiotherapy
- contraindicated with acitretin or other retinoids
- contraindicated with alcohol or other hepatotoxic agents (e.g. retinoids, azathioprine, leflunomide, sulfasalazine)
- (Intrathecal) not recommended with nitrous oxide because of an increased risk of toxicity. Caution if used after a recent administration of nitrous oxide
- serum levels (and associated risk of toxicity) may be increased by chloramphenicol, omeprazole, pantoprazole, phenytoin, probenecid, penicillins, salicylates, sulfonamides, sulfonylureas, tetracyclines or aminobenzoic acid; therefore not recommended together
- (High dose) not recommended with NSAIDs owing to an increased risk of myelosuppression and GI toxicity because the half-life of methotrexate is prolonged. Caution should also be used with lower doses of methotrexate
- toxicity may be increased by folate deficiency
- increased risk of myelosuppression and decreased folate levels if given with triamterene
- serum levels may be decreased by colestyramine
- not recommended with vitamin supplements containing folic or folinic acid
- if used with nitrous oxide, may potentiate methotrexate's effects on folate metabolism
- increased risk of bone marrow depression if given with allopurinol, trimethoprim, trimethoprim/sulfamethoxazole or pyrimethamine
- may decrease clearance of theophylline, thereby increasing the risk of toxicity. Theophylline levels should be closely monitored during concurrent therapy
- increased risk of toxicity if given with transfusion of packed red blood cells
- absorption and metabolism may be decreased by tetracycline and nonabsorbable broad-spectrum antibiotics
- may increase plasma levels of mercaptopurine
- increased risk of pancytopenia and interstitial pneumonitis if given with leflunomide
- increased risk of skin cancer if given with psoralen plus ultraviolet A (PUVA) therapy

ANTINEOPLASTIC AGENTS

- may interfere with folic acid detection assay
- see also General Interactions of antineoplastic agents (p. 596)

Nursing considerations/Cautions

- (Choriocarcinoma) effectiveness of therapy is measured by 24-hour urine collection to measure urinary chorionic gonadotrophin hormone levels, which should return to normal after 3 to 4 treatments, followed by complete resolution of measurable lesions at 4–6 weeks. One to two courses is recommended after normalisation of urinary levels (after clinical assessment)
- serum methotrexate levels should be monitored regularly to reduce toxicity, enabling adjustment of dosage, as well as implementation of rescue methods (folinic acid rescue). Patients who are predisposed to elevated and prolonged methotrexate levels include those with pleural effusions, ascites, renal impairment, dehydration, aciduria, GI obstruction and those previously treated with cisplatin
- methotrexate toxicity may not be reversible if folinic acid rescue is not instituted within 42–48 hours of elevated levels
- folinic acid (leucovorin) is given to neutralise the toxic effects of methotrexate (folinic acid rescue). Folinic acid is given orally, IM or IV within 24 hours of methotrexate administration (10 doses 6-hourly) (see Calcium folinate, p. 336)
- if dose > 200 mg, the patient be encouraged to drink plenty of fluids for 2 days after dose, as well as keeping urine alkaline for ≥ 24 hours
- only preservative-free methotrexate should be used for intrathecal administration. Dilute with sodium chloride 0.9% to a concentration of 1 mg/mL
- (Prefilled syringe) used for management of psoriasis and rheumatoid arthritis only
- incompatible with cytarabine, fluorouracil and prednisolone
- (Tablets) contain lactose and are therefore not recommended in those with rare hereditary galactose intolerance, Lapp lactase deficiency or glucose-galactose malabsorption
- caution if used in patients with third-space compartment accumulations (e.g. pleural effusions, ascites), as toxicity may occur owing to methotrexate accumulation. Evacuation of third-space collections before starting therapy is recommended
- contraindicated in those with severe liver or renal impairment, alcoholism or alcoholic liver disease, severe, acute or chronic infections, bone marrow depression or pre-existing blood dyscrasias, or immunodeficiency syndromes
- see also General Nursing considerations/Cautions for antineoplastic agents (p. 596)

Patient education

- instruct the patient to seek medical advice immediately if any dry persistent non-productive cough, shortness of breath, difficulty breathing, chest pain, coughing/spitting up blood occurs
- advise the patient to avoid sun exposure and ensure they wear protective clothing (hat, long-sleeved garment) and sunscreen (SPF 50+)
- see also General Patient education for antineoplastic agents (p. 598)

 Tablets should not be crushed or broken.

 Contraindicated in those with severe kidney disease (CrCl < 30 mL/min), alcoholic liver disease or chronic liver disease.

METHYL AMINOLEVULINATE HYDROCHLORIDE

Trade name
Metvix

Available form
Cream: 160 mg/g

Action
- sensitiser for photodynamic therapy
- after application to skin, photoactive porphyrins accumulate, and after light activation a photochemical reaction destroys target cells

Use
- squamous cell carcinoma (SCC) in situ (Bowen's disease) (where surgery is inappropriate)
- superficial or nodular basal cell carcinoma (BCC) (where surgery is inappropriate)
- facial or scalp actinic keratoses (AK) that are thin or non-hyperkeratotic and non-pigmented (where other therapies are unacceptable)

Dose
- apply cream 1 mm thick to the lesion and 5—10 mm surrounding skin, and cover with occlusive dressing for 3 hours

Adverse effects
- pain, warm sensation, burning, tingling, stinging, erythema, itching, oedema, crusting, ulceration, exudates, blisters, peeling, hypo/hyperpigmentation, bleeding
- allergic contact dermatitis

Nursing considerations/Cautions
- any UV therapy should be discontinued before starting therapy
- (BCC) lesions should be assessed 3 months after treatment for response. If not complete, retreatment is recommended
- (AK) usually requires only one treatment with photodynamic therapy with natural light or red LED light with a suitable lamp
- (BCC, SCC) require two treatments, with a week interval in between, with red LED light with a suitable lamp
- (AK) thick lesions should not be treated
- multiple lesions may be treated at the same time
- protective goggles should be worn by both the patient and the operator during photosensitisation procedure with red light
- (SCC/BCC) should be used only to treat primary lesions
- (SCC/BCC) should be reviewed at 6—12-month intervals to detect any recurrence
- contains hydroxybenzoates (which can cause hypersensitivity) and cetostearyl alcohol and arachis oil, which can cause a local skin reaction (e.g. contact dermatitis)
- caution if used in those with hypertension, as pain associated with procedure may increase BP. BP should be closely monitored
- contraindicated in those with hypersensitivity to peanut oil, porphyria, invasive SCC or morpheaform BCC

Patient education
- the patient should be given the following instructions:
  - avoid getting cream in the eyes
  - sun exposure should be avoided for 2—3 days after treatment
  - any crust or scale should be removed and the lesion roughened (but not to bleeding stage) before application of the cream (with a spatula)
  - (BCC, SCC) after application of the cream, an occlusive dressing should be applied over the lesion/s for 3 hours
  - before exposure to a light source, the cream should be removed and the lesion and surrounding skin cleaned using saline
  - (BCC, SCC) goggles should be worn to protect the eyes during exposure to a red light source
  - if the light source is natural sunlight (for scalp and facial actinic keratosis only), sunscreen (SPF 30+) (but not containing zinc oxide, titanium dioxide or iron oxide) should be applied to all exposed areas 15 minutes before preparation of the lesion(s) (see second instruction) and

ANTINEOPLASTIC AGENTS

application of the cream. No occlusion is needed. Exposure to sunlight should occur within 30 minutes of applying the cream and continue for 2 hours, during which time the person should stay outside and carry out normal activities. After 2 hours, the cream should be washed off and further sun exposure avoided for 2—3 days (see the first instruction)
- warn the patient that a burning sensation generally lasts for only a few hours after therapy
- inform the patient that healthy, untreated skin does not need to be protected during therapy

MIDOSTAURIN
Trade name
Rydapt

Available form
Capsules: 25 mg

Action
- tyrosine kinase inhibitor (including FLT3 and KIT kinase)
- also inhibits mast cell proliferation and survival, and histamine release
- two active metabolites (half-lives 33.4 hours and 495 hours respectively)
- half-life 20.3 hours

Use
- newly diagnosed acute myeloid leukaemia (AML) who are FLT3-mutation positive
- aggressive systemic mastocytosis (ASM)
- systemic mastocytosis with associated haematological neoplasms (SM-AHN)
- mast cell leukaemia (MCL)

Dose
- (AML) 50 mg orally twice daily with food on days 8—21 of induction (with an anthracycline and cytarabine) and consolidation (with cytarabine) cycles, then 50 mg orally twice daily with food (as single agent maintenance therapy) for up to 12 cycles of a 28-day cycle or relapse **OR**
- (Advanced SM) 100 mg orally twice daily with food, continued until clinical response is evident or unacceptable toxicity occurs

Adverse effects
- decrease in left ventricular ejection fraction (LVEF)
- see also General Adverse effects of protein kinase inhibitors (p. 691)

Interactions
- if used with agents that prolong QT interval, regular ECG monitoring is recommended
- contraindicated with rifampicin, carbamazepine, phenytoin, enzalutamide and St John's wort
- see also General Interactions of protein kinase inhibitors (p. 691)

Nursing considerations/Cautions
- prophylactic antiemetics are recommended
- (AML) therapy should be stopped before starting a conditioning regimen for stem cell transplant
- caution if used in those with congestive cardiac failure
- (AML) not recommended as monotherapy for induction or consolidation cycles
- not recommended in children undergoing intensive combined therapy regimens for AML that include an anthracycline, cytarabine and fludarabine
- see also General Nursing considerations/Cautions for protein kinase inhibitors (p. 691)

Patient education
- advise the patient to swallow capsules whole (not opened, crushed or chewed) with food to prevent nausea
- see also General Patient education for protein kinase inhibitors (p. 692)

 Capsules should not be opened, broken or chewed.

MITOZANTRONE
Trade names
Mitozantrone Ebewe, Onkotrone

Available forms
Vial: 20 mg/10 mL, 25 mg/12.5 mL

Action
- non-cell cycle (phase) specific antineoplastic antibiotic (anthracycline)
- half-life 5—18 days

Use
- breast carcinoma (metastatic or locally advanced)
- non-Hodgkin lymphoma
- adult acute non-lymphocytic leukaemia
- blast crisis of chronic myelogenous leukaemia

Dose
- (Breast cancer, non-Hodgkin lymphoma — monotherapy) 14 mg/m^2 IV over 3—5 minutes or by IV infusion over 15—30 minutes once every 3 weeks **OR**
- (Leukaemia (patients with low marrow reserve) — monotherapy) 12 mg/m^2 IV over 3—5 minutes or by IV infusion over 15—30 minutes daily for 5 days, repeated if relapse occurs **OR**
- (Leukaemia — combination therapy) 10—12 mg/m^2 IV over 3—5 minutes or by IV infusion over 15—30 minutes for 3 days with cytosine arabinoside for 7 days. If a second course is required, mitozantrone is given for 2 days with cytosine arabinoside for 5 days **OR**
- (Acute non-lymphocytic leukaemia, chronic myelogenous leukaemia in blast crisis —monotherapy) 12 mg/m^2 IV over 3—5 minutes or by IV infusion over 15—30 minutes for 5 consecutive days (total 60 mg/m^2)

Adverse effects
- congestive cardiac failure, decreased left ventricular ejection fraction (LVEF)
- see also General Adverse effects of antineoplastic agents (p. 596)

Interactions
- (Acute myeloid leukaemia (AML)) clearance may be decreased if given with ciclosporin
- combination with other cytotoxic agents and/or radiation therapy has been associated with t-AML and myelodysplastic syndrome

Nursing considerations/Cautions
- cardiac monitoring is recommended before starting and during therapy
- the dose should be reduced by 2—4 mg/m^2 if given as part of combination therapy
- (Leukaemia) serum uric acid levels should be measured before starting and during therapy, and hypouricaemic therapy instituted to prevent tumour lysis syndrome
- may precipitate if given with heparin
- may cause skin staining. If contact occurs, the area should be washed with copious amounts of water
- dilute to at least 50 mL with glucose 5% or sodium chloride 0.9% and infuse over 15—30 minutes, or can be added to a free-running IV solution
- increased risk of cardiac toxicity if used in those with pre-existing heart disorders, previous treatment with anthracyclines or prior mediastinal radiotherapy
- caution if used in those with severe liver or renal impairment
- contraindicated in those with known hypersensitivity to anthracyclines or sulfite, or who have received substantial anthracycline with abnormal cardiac function (before starting therapy with mitozantrone)
- contraindicated by intrathecal, SC, IM or intra-arterially administration
- see also General Nursing considerations/Cautions for antineoplastic agents (p. 596)

Patient education
- warn the patient that blue/green discolouration of the urine can be expected for 24 hours after treatment and that bluish discolouration of the sclera may also occur
- instruct the patient to seek medical advice immediately if any shortness of

breath, difficulty breathing or swelling of ankles occurs
- see also General Patient education for antineoplastic agents (p. 598)

Contraindicated in those with severe liver impairment and use with caution in those with jaundice.

Caution if used in those with severe kidney insufficiency.

NELARABINE
Trade name
Nelarabine-Reach

Available form
Vial: 250 mg/50 mL

Action
- antimetabolite, purine analogue
- prodrug that is rapidly converted to active form, ara-G, which accumulates in leukaemic blasts inhibiting DNA synthesis leading to cell death
- half-life of nelarabine is 30 minutes and of ara-G is 3 hours

Use
- treatment of relapsing/refractory T-cell acute lymphoblastic leukaemia and T-cell lymphoblastic lymphoma where disease has not responded to and has relapsed after therapy

Dose
- (Adults, adolescents > 16 years) 1,500 mg/m^2 IV over 2 hours on days 1, 3 and 5, then repeated every 21 days **OR**
- (Children, adolescents ≤ 21 years) 650 mg/m^2 IV over 1 hour daily for 5 consecutive days, repeated every 21 days

Adverse effects
- severe somnolence, confusion, coma, convulsions, muscle weakness, ataxia, status epilepticus, peripheral neuropathy, tremor
- hypoglycaemia, hypocalcaemia, hypomagnesaemia, hypokalaemia
- hyperbilirubinaemia, altered liver enzymes
- anorexia
- pleural effusion
- see also General Adverse effects of antineoplastic agents (p. 596)

Interactions
- not recommended with intrathecal therapy or craniospinal irradiation
- immunisation with live vaccine is not recommended
- not recommended with immunosuppressant agents owing to additive effect on immune system

Nursing considerations/Cautions
- blood counts (including platelets) should be monitored regularly
- for patients aged 16 to 21 years, both regimens have been used safely. Decision of which regimen to use should be made by the prescribing physician
- therapy should be discontinued at first signs of neurological events
- IV solution should not be diluted
- transfer the solution to a polyvinyl-chloride (PVC) or an ethyl vinyl acetate (EVA) infusion bag or glass container
- IV hydration is recommended to manage hyperuricaemia in those at risk of tumor lysis syndrome. Allopurinol is recommended for those at risk of hyperuricaemia
- the vial contains 88.51 mg (3.85 mmol) of sodium, which may need to be considered if the patient is on a sodium-restricted diet
- caution if used in those with liver impairment
- if used in those with kidney impairment, careful monitoring for signs of toxicity is recommended

Patient education
- may cause somnolence during and for several days after treatment; therefore the patient should be advised not to drive or operate machinery
- the patient/parent/carer should be instructed to seek medical advice immediately if any of the following occur:

- feeling drowsy or sleepy, headache, dizziness
- abnormal sensation on skin including numbness, prickling or burning, or reduced sensation to touch
- changes to feeling in feet or hands
- muscle weakness or difficulty walking/clumsiness
- feeling disoriented or problems with memory
- blurred vision
- altered or loss of taste
- fitting (seizures)

see also General Patient education for antineoplastic agents (p. 598)

Patients > 65 years are at greater risk of neurological adverse events.

OXALIPLATIN
Trade names
DBL Oxaliplatin Concentrate, Oxaliplatin Accord, Oxaliplatin Baxter, Oxaliplatin Injection, USP

Available forms
Vial (powder): 50 mg, 100 mg;
Vial (concentrate solution): 50 mg/10 mL, 100 mg/20 mL

Action
- platinum-containing analogue of cisplatin that inhibits DNA synthesis (also RNA and protein synthesis to a lesser extent)

Use
- colon cancer (Duke's C) (after resection) (adjuvant therapy with fluorouracil and folinic acid)
- advanced colorectal cancer (with fluorouracil and folinic acid)

Dose
- 85 mg/m^2 IV over 2–6 hours (before fluorouracil) every 2 weeks (for advanced colorectal cancer) or every 2 weeks for 12 cycles (adjuvant for colon cancer) (with fluorouracil and folinic acid)

Adverse effects
- peripheral neuropathy, laryngopharyngeal dysaesthesia, reversible posterior leukoencephalopathy
- intestinal ischaemia
- QT prolongation
- rhabdomyolysis
- allergy/hypersensitivity
- see also General Adverse effects of antineoplastic agents (p. 596)

Interactions
- may increase serum levels of fluorouracil (if given with weekly fluorouracil and 3-weekly oxaliplatin)
- caution if given with statins owing to increased risk of rhabdomyolysis
- not recommended with agents known to prolong QT or cause electrolyte imbalance
- see also General Interactions of antineoplastic agents (p. 596)

Nursing considerations/Cautions
- neurological examination is recommended before each infusion
- any electrolyte imbalance (especially hypokalaemia, hypocalcaemia and hypomagnesaemia) should be corrected before starting therapy
- if patient develops laryngopharyngeal dysaesthesia (e.g. dysphagia, dyspnoea, feeling of suffocation) within 48 hours of infusion, subsequent infusions should be given over 6 hours
- reconstitute powder with 10 mL (for 50 mg vial) or 20 mL (for 100 mg vial) water for injections or glucose 5% and then further dilute with 250–500 mL glucose 5%
- concentrate for infusion should be further diluted with 250–500 mL glucose 5%
- incompatible with chloride-containing solutions. Fluorouracil should not be given via the same infusion line
- do not use with any material containing aluminium

ANTINEOPLASTIC AGENTS

- allergy/hypersensitivity reaction can occur during any cycle of treatment (not just initial infusions)
- re-challenging is contraindicated if the patient experiences an anaphylactic reaction
- caution if used in those with congenital or acquired QT syndrome or predisposition to electrolyte imbalances
- contraindicated in those with a history of peripheral sensory neuropathy with functional impairment, hypersensitivity to platinum-containing preparations or severe renal impairment (creatinine clearance < 30 mL/min)
- see also General Nursing considerations/Cautions for antineoplastic agents (p. 596)

Patient education

- warn the patient to avoid exposure to cold or ingesting cold food or drinks within 48 hours of therapy to decrease the risk of laryngopharyngeal dysaesthesia (e.g. dysphagia, dyspnoea, feeling of suffocation) occurring
- the patient should be instructed to seek medical advice immediately if any of the following occur:
  - weakness, tingling or numbness of arms or feet
  - difficulty swallowing, feeling of suffocation or difficulty breathing
  - headache, memory loss, trouble thinking, loss of vision or other visual disturbances, difficulty walking or muscle weakness
  - rapid or unusual heart rate
  - muscle weakness or pain, fever, dark urine, decreased urination
  - severe abdominal pain
- see also General Patient education for antineoplastic agents (p. 598)

 Contraindicated in those with severe kidney impairment (CrCl < 30 mL/min).

PACLITAXEL
Trade names
Abraxane, Anzatax Injection, Nab-Paclitaxel Juno, Paclitaxel Accord, Paclitaxel Ebewe

Available forms
Vial: 100 mg, 30 mg/5 mL, 100 mg/16.7 mL, 150 mg/25 mL, 300 mg/50 mL

Action
- taxane antimetabolite
- (Abraxane, Nab-Paclitaxel Juno) albumin nanoparticle form of paclitaxel, half-life 13—27 hours
- half-life 3—52.7 hours (dependent on dose and duration of infusion)

Use
- metastatic breast cancer (after anthracycline failure)
- metastatic breast cancer (with trastuzumab) (in those with tumours HER2 overexpression/no previous treatment)
- node-positive breast cancer (adjuvant, sequential to doxorubicin and cyclophosphamide)
- unresectable, locally recurrent or metastatic breast cancer (relapsed after adjunctive chemotherapy including an anthracycline) (with gemcitabine)
- metastatic ovarian cancer (after standard therapy failure)
- ovarian cancer (with platinum agent)
- non-small cell lung cancer (NSCLC) (with carboplatin when surgery and/or radiation are unsuitable)
- metastatic pancreatic adenocarcinoma (with gemcitabine)

Dose
- (Metastatic breast cancer) 260 mg/m^2 IV over 30 minutes every 3 weeks (Abraxane, Nab-Paclitaxel Juno) **OR**
- (Metastatic breast cancer) 175 mg/m^2 IV over 3 hours on day 1, with gemcitabine IV on days 1 and 8 of 21-day cycle **OR**
- (HER2 overexpressive breast cancer) 175 mg/m^2 IV over 3 hours every 3 weeks for 6 cycles (with trastuzumab) **OR**

- (Node-positive breast cancer) 175 mg/m2 IV over 3 hours every 3 weeks for 4 cycles (following doxorubicin cyclophosphamide combined therapy) **OR**
- (Node-positive breast cancer) 175 mg/m^2 IV over 3 hours every 3 weeks for 6 cycles for 4 courses following doxorubicin and cyclophosphamide combination therapy **OR**
- (NSCLC) 100 mg/m^2 IV over 30 minutes on days 1, 8 and 15 of a 21-day cycle (with carboplatin) (Abraxane, Nab-Paclitaxel Juno) **OR**
- (NSCLC, metastatic breast or ovarian cancer) 175 mg/m^2 IV over 3 hours every 3 weeks (up to 9 cycles for metastatic breast or ovarian cancer) **OR**
- (Pancreatic adenocarcinoma) 125 mg/m^2 IV over 30 minutes on days 1, 8 and 15 of a 28-day cycle (with gemcitabine) (Abraxane, Nab-Paclitaxel Juno) **OR**
- (Ovarian cancer) 175 mg/m^2 IV over 3 hours (with cisplatin) every 3 weeks **OR**
- (Ovarian cancer) 135 mg/m^2 IV over 24 hours (with cisplatin) every 3 weeks

Adverse effects
- peripheral neuropathy
- (Metastatic pancreatic cancer) sepsis
- see also General Adverse effects of antineoplastic agents (p. 596)

Interactions
- increased serum levels may occur if given with itraconazole, erythromycin, fluoxetine, imidazole antifungal agents, clopidogrel, gemfibrozil or ritonavir
- decreased serum levels may occur if given with rifampicin, carbamazepine, phenytoin, efavirenz, nevirapine or St John's wort; therefore should be given with caution if used together
- may increase serum levels of doxorubicin and its active metabolite, leading to increased risk of toxicity. Paclitaxel should be given 24 hours after doxorubicin
- if cisplatin is given before paclitaxel, clearance is decreased, leading to increased myelosuppression. Combination also increases the risk of renal failure
- arthralgia and myalgia may be increased if given with filgrastim
- see also General Interactions of antineoplastic agents (p. 596)

Nursing considerations/Cautions
- the albumin form of paclitaxel is not interchangeable with other formulations
- should be given before platinum-containing therapy
- because of the possibility of hypersensitivity, the patient may require pre-medication before each treatment with corticosteroid (e.g. dexamethasone 20 mg orally 12 hours and 6 hours before), antihistamine (e.g. promethazine 25–50 mg IV 30 minutes before paclitaxel) and H$_2$-receptor antagonist (e.g. ranitidine 50 mg IV over 15 minutes 30 minutes before paclitaxel) (not Abraxane)
- patient should be closely observed during the first 30 minutes of infusion for any signs of hypersensitivity (not Abraxane)
- ECG monitoring is recommended if given with doxorubicin or trastuzumab for metastatic breast cancer
- (Metastatic pancreatic cancer) if the patient becomes febrile, broad-spectrum antibiotics are recommended
- (Abraxane, Nab-Paclitaxel Juno) reconstitute the powder by injection of 20 mL sodium chloride 0.9% down the side of the vial (not directly on the powder to prevent foaming), then allow to stand for 5 minutes, and then swirl gently for at least 2 minutes to dissolve the powder. If foaming occurs, allow the vial to stand for at least 15 minutes to allow foam to subside. Reconstituted solution should be milky without visible particles. Dilute further if proteinaceous strands result, administer the infusion via a 15 micron filter
- an inline filter less than 0.15 micron should not be used

ANTINEOPLASTIC AGENTS

- concentrate should be diluted with either glucose 5% or sodium chloride 0.9% to a concentration of 0.3—1.2 mg/mL before administration
- IV administration only
- a micropore filter (0.22 micron or less) is recommended
- (Abraxane, Nab-Paclitaxel Juno) contains 85 mg sodium/vial when reconstituted with sodium chloride 0.9%, which may need to be considered in a sodium-restricted diet
- caution if used in those with pre-existing neuropathy
- not recommended in those with severe liver impairment
- contraindicated in those with hypersensitivity to PEG35 castor oil or with solid tumours and neutrophil count $< 1.5 \times 10^9$/L
- (Abraxane, Nab-Paclitaxel Juno) contraindicated in those with hypersensitivity to albumin
- see also General Nursing considerations/Cautions for antineoplastic agents (p. 596)

Patient education

- instruct the patient to seek medical advice immediately if any of the following occur:
  - numbness or tingling in hands or feet, muscle weakness
  - visual disturbances
- see also General Patient education for antineoplastic agents (p. 598)

(Abraxane, Nab-Paclitaxel Juno) (metastatic breast cancer, NSCLC) for those with moderate-to-severe liver impairment, 20% dose reduction is recommended.

While dose reduction is not required for those > 65 years, close monitoring is recommended because of an increased incidence of serious adverse effects in this age group.

PEGASPARGASE
Trade name
Oncaspar

Available form
Vial: 3750 units

Action
- PEGylated form of L-asparaginase, which converts L-asparagine to aspartic acid and ammonia
- selective destruction of leukaemic cells due to depletion of plasma L-asparagine (leukaemic cells have low levels of asparagine synthetase enzyme to synthesise L-asparagine and are therefore dependent on an extracellular source. Normal cells, however, are less affected by depletion)
- half-life 5.33 days

Use
- acute lymphocytic leukaemia (combination therapy)

Dose
- (Patient > 21 years) 2000 U/m² IM or IV every 2 weeks **OR**
- (Patient ≤ 21 years, body surface area (BSA) > 0.6 m²) 2500 U/m² IM or IV every 2 weeks **OR**
- (Patient BSA < 0.6 m² and infants < 1 year) 82.5 U/kg IM or IV every 2 weeks

Adverse effects
- anaphylaxis, serious hypersensitivity reaction
- pancreatitis, ascites
- hyperglycaemia
- (Children) osteonecrosis (avascular necrosis)
- confusion, somnolence, seizures
- hyperammonaemia
- hyperglycaemia
- hypertriglyceridaemia
- prolonged partial thromboplastin time, increased INR, decrease blood fibrinogen
- liver impairment and, rarely, veno-occlusive disease

- (Uncommon) development of asparaginase antibodies
- see also General Adverse effects of antineoplastic agents (p. 596)

Interactions

- caution if given with other agents that impact coagulation including methotrexate, daunorubicin, corticosteroids, aspirin and NSAIDs
- increased risk of neurotoxicity and anaphylaxis if given concurrently with vincristine. Vincristine should be given before pegaspargase to reduce the risk of toxicity
- may increase the risk of glucocorticoid-induced osteonecrosis in children > 10 years (particularly girls)
- caution if used with warfarin, heparin, dipyridamole, aspirin or NSAIDs, as the impact on coagulation factors is variable
- coagulation parameters are altered if given with prednisolone
- may impair clearance of oral contraceptives and these are therefore not recommended together
- protein- bound drugs such as benzodiazepines, barbiturates, penicillin, warfarin, phenytoin, sodium valproate and NSAIDs may have their toxicity increased
- caution if given with methotrexate or cytarabine, as effects may be variable and dependent on the timing of administration
- see also General Interactions of antineoplastic agents (p. 596)

Nursing considerations/Cautions

- name and batch number should be recorded in the patient's medical history
- baseline coagulation profile, blood counts (with differential) and liver function tests are recommended and repeated regularly during therapy
- premedication with paracetamol, antihistamine (e.g. diphenhydramine) and an H_2 receptor blocker (e.g. famotidine) 30 to 60 minutes before administration is recommended to decrease the risk and severity of infusion-related and hypersensitivity reactions
- for small volumes, IM is the preferred administration route
- reconstitute by adding 5.2 mL water for Injection; swirl gently to dissolve the powder (do not shake)
- for IV, dilute reconstituted solution with 100 mL sodium chloride 0.9% or glucose 5% and administer into a running infusion of either sodium chloride 0.9% or glucose 5% over 1—2 hours
- administer alone
- the patient should be monitored for at least 1 hour after administration. Resuscitation equipment should be readily available in the event of an allergic reaction
- trough asparaginase activity should be measured 2 weeks after administration. If levels are < 0.1 U/mL, consider switching to another asparaginase product, as asparaginase antibodies may have developed
- increased risk of hepatotoxicity in Philadelphia chromosome-positive patients who have combined therapy with protein kinase inhibitor
- children and adolescents (especially girls) should be monitored closely for any signs and symptoms of osteonecrosis
- contraindicated in those with a history of serious reactions to previous asparaginase therapy including thrombosis, pancreatitis or haemorrhagic events, or if the patient has severe liver impairment
- see also General Nursing considerations/Cautions for antineoplastic agents (p. 596)

Patient education

- instruct the patient to seek medical attention immediately if any of the following occur:
  - nausea, vomiting headache, dizziness, rash, lethargy, irritation
  - persistent abdominal pain that radiates through to the back, nausea and

ANTINEOPLASTIC AGENTS

vomiting, bloating, pale-coloured stools, loss of appetite, rapid heartbeat
- joint pain, pain in buttocks, groin, thigh, hip or knee, limited range of movement, limping
- rapid weight gain, fluid retention, tenderness under ribs on right-hand side of the abdomen
- women of childbearing potential should be advised to use a non-oral form of effective contraception during therapy
- see also General Patient education for antineoplastic agents (p. 598)

 Contraindicated in those with severe liver impairment.

PEMETREXED DISODIUM
Trade names
Alimta, DBL Pemetrexed, Pemetrexed Accord, Pemetrexed APOTEX, Pemetrexed Ever Pharma, Pemetrexed Juno, Pemetrexed Sun, Pemetrexed-AFT

Available forms
Vial: 100 mg, 500 mg, 1 g, 100 mg/4 mL, 500 mg/20 mL, 1g/40 mL

Action
- anti-folinic antimetabolite
- active potent metabolites which have a longer half-life than the parent

Use
- malignant pleural mesothelioma (with cisplatin)
- locally advanced or metastatic non-small cell lung cancer (as monotherapy before platinum-based therapy or combination therapy with cisplatin)(not squamous cell)

Dose
- 500 mg/m^2 IV over 10 minutes (day 1 of a 21-day cycle) (with cisplatin)

Adverse effects
- severe rash, radiation recall
- see also General Adverse effects of antineoplastic agents (p. 596)

Interactions
- NSAIDs should not be taken for 5 days before, during or for 2 days after therapy with pemetrexed in those with mild-to-moderate kidney insufficiency, as renal clearance may be decreased
- caution if used with radiation before, during or after therapy because of the risk of radiation pneumonitis
- caution if used with nephrotoxic agents or those that are tubularly secreted, as clearance is decreased, increasing serum levels and the risk of adverse effects
- see also General Interactions of antineoplastic agents (p. 596)

Nursing considerations/Cautions
- the patient should be well hydrated before and during therapy to decrease the risk of severe dehydration when given with cisplatin
- premedication with corticosteroids (e.g. dexamethasone 4 mg orally twice daily, starting the day before, day of and day after therapy) lessens the incidence and severity of rash
- (Powder) reconstitute using sodium chloride 0.9% only (20 mL for 500 mg vial, 4.2 mL for 100 mg vial) and then dilute further with 100 mL sodium chloride 0.9%
- (Concentrate) dilute to 100 mL with sodium chloride 0.9% or glucose 5% and administer as an IV infusion over 10 minutes
- incompatible with calcium-containing diluents (including lactated Ringer's solution)
- caution if used in those with pre-existing cardiovascular risk factors
- not recommended if creatinine clearance < 45 mL/min
- see also General Nursing considerations/Cautions for antineoplastic agents (p. 596)

Patient education
- the patient should be instructed to take prophylactic oral folic acid (350—1000

micrograms) (at least 5 doses in 7 days before, during and 21 days after the last dose) and IM vitamin B_{12} (one dose in week before the first dose, then every 3 cycles) during therapy
- if the patient has mild-to-moderate kidney insufficiency, advise them to avoid taking NSAIDs for 5 days before and up to 2 days after therapy
- see also General Patient education for antineoplastic agents (p. 598)

 Not recommended in those with CrCl < 45 mL/min.

PLITIDEPSIN
Trade name
Aplidin

Available form
Vial: 2 mg

Action
- interacts with eukaryotic elongation factor (eEF1A2), which is overexpressing in some tumour cells, including some multiple myeloma cells
- half-life about 6 days

Use
- relapsed and refractory multiple myeloma (which has received 2–3 previous treatments with or is intolerant to a proteasome inhibitor and immunomodulator) (with dexamethasone)

Dose
- 5 mg/m^2 IV over 3 hours on days 1 and 15 of a 28-day cycle (with dexamethasone 40 mg orally 1 hour before infusion on days 1, 8, 15 and 22 of a 28-day cycle)

Adverse effects
- infusion-related reactions
- muscle weakness, myalgia and, uncommonly, myopathy
- (Uncommon) bradycardia, QT interval prolongation, sinus tachycardia, orthostatic hypotension
- (Injection site) pain, phlebitis, thrombosis
- see also General Adverse effects of antineoplastic agents (p. 596)

Interactions
- caution if used with other agents associated with rhabdomyolysis, such as statins
- not recommended with clarithromycin, itraconazole, voriconazole or grapefruit juice. These should be discontinued for at least 1 week before starting therapy
- caution if used with aprepitant, diltiazem, erythromycin, fluconazole or verapamil
- not recommended with phenytoin, phenobarbital, carbamazepine, rifampicin, rifabutin or St John's wort. These should be discontinued for at least 2 weeks before starting therapy
- caution if given with bosentan or modafinil

Nursing considerations/Cautions
- premedication with ondansetron (8 mg IV) or granisetron (3 mg IV), diphenhydramine (25 mg IV) (or equivalent) and ranitidine (50 mg IV or equivalent) is recommended 30 minutes before infusion. If dexamethasone (40 mg) is stopped owing to adverse effects, it should be included as part of the premedication regimen at 8 mg orally
- emergency equipment and oxygen should be readily available in the event of severe or life-threatening infusion-related reactions
- creatine phosphokinase (CPK) should be measured before each infusion (days 1 and 15) from cycle 1 to cycle 4
- use of an infusion pump and a low-protein filter (0.2 microns) are recommended
- reconstitute using 4 mL diluent (provided) and dilute further with sodium chloride 0.9% or glucose 5% for a total volume of 500 mL (peripheral line) or 250 mL (central venous line)
- caution if used in patients with risk factors for or existing heart disease. Regular ECG monitoring is recommended

ANTINEOPLASTIC AGENTS

- contraindicated in those with hypersensitivity to PEG-35 castor oil or ethanol
- see also General Nursing considerations/Cautions for antineoplastic agents (p. 596)

Patient education

- the patient should be instructed to immediately seek medical advice if muscle weakness or muscle pain, fever or dark urine occurs
- see also General Patient education for antineoplastic agents (p. 598)

Caution if used in those with impaired liver function.

PROCARBAZINE

Trade name
Natulan

Available form
Capsules: 50 mg

Action
- inhibits protein and nucleic acid synthesis
- some immunosuppressant action
- weak monoamine oxidase inhibitor (MAOI) properties

Use
- Hodgkin's disease, other malignant sarcomas including lymphosarcoma and reticulosarcoma

Dose
- initially 50 mg orally daily, then increasing by 50 mg daily to a daily maximum of 250–300 mg after 5–6 days (induction) and this dose maintained for as long as possible, then 50–150 mg daily (maintenance) (to a total of 6 g)

Adverse effects
- severe skin reactions
- see also General Adverse effects of antineoplastic agents (p. 596)

Interactions
- may potentiate barbiturates, psychotropic and sympathomimetic agents due to MAOI (weak) properties
- decreases tolerance to alcohol
- see also General Interactions of antineoplastic agents (p. 596)

Nursing considerations/Cautions

- therapy should be stopped if a severe allergic skin reaction occurs
- contraindicated in those with severe kidney or liver damage
- see also General Nursing considerations/Cautions for antineoplastic agents (p. 596)

Patient education

- advise the patient to swallow capsules whole (without opening, breaking or chewing)
- the patient should be warned about eating certain foodstuffs (see Glossary for 'cheese reaction')
- advise the patient to avoid alcohol during treatment
- see also General Patient education for antineoplastic agents (p. 598)

Capsules should not be opened, broken or chewed.

Contraindicated in those with severe liver or kidney damage. Starting therapy in a hospital setting is recommended in those with liver or kidney impairment.

RADIUM (Ra223) DICHLORIDE

Trade name
Xofigo

Available form
Vial: 6.6 MBq/6 mL

Action
- alpha particle emitting radiopharmaceutical
- mimics calcium and selectively targets areas of bone metastases by forming complexes with bone mineral hydroxyapatite

Use
- treatment of castration-resistant prostate cancer with symptomatic bone

metastases and no known visceral metastatic disease

Dose
- 55 kBq/kg by slow IV over at least 1 minute at 4-week intervals for 6 injections

Adverse effects
- thrombocytopenia, neutropenia, leucopenia, pancytopenia
- diarrhoea, vomiting, nausea
- bone fracture, osteoporosis
- injection site reaction (pain, redness, swelling)

Interactions
- contraindicated with abiraterone acetate and prednisolone/prednisone

Nursing considerations/Cautions
- full blood tests are recommended before starting therapy and before each dose. Baseline blood counts should be absolute neutrophil count (ANC) $\geq 1.0 \times 10^9$/L, platelet count $\geq 100 \times 10^9$/L and haemoglobin ≥ 100 g/L. Blood counts should have recovered to ANC $\geq 1.0 \times 10^9$/L and platelet count $\geq 50 \times 10^9$/L before the next dose is given. If there is no recovery within 6 weeks, therapy should be continued only if benefits outweigh risks
- the dose contributes to the patient's overall long-term cumulative radiation exposure
- patient risk for bone fractures (e.g. osteoporosis, low body weight, medications increasing risk) should be assessed and monitored for least 2 years. Prophylactic denosumab or bisphosphonates should be considered
- should be received, used and administered only by those authorised to handle radiopharmaceuticals
- receipt, storage, use, transfer and disposal are subject to licence and regulation by the Australian Radiation Protection and Nuclear Safety Agency (ARPANSA)
- administration is associated with potential risks to others (including medical staff, care givers and the patient's household contacts). Risks include radiation or contamination from body fluids (e.g. urine, faeces, vomit) and therefore the greatest care should be taken when cleaning up spills
- any unused product or material used in preparation should be treated as radioactive waste and disposed of according to the ARPANSA Code of Practice for disposal of radioactive waste
- should not be diluted or mixed with another solution
- caution if used in those with Crohn's disease or ulcerative colitis
- caution if used in those with pre-existing compromised bone marrow reserve
- any untreated spinal cord compression (imminent or established) or bone fractures should be treated before starting or resuming therapy
- not recommended in women

Patient education
- instruct the patient to
  - flush the toilet twice and then wash the hands after using the bathroom
  - promptly wash the clothes separately if soiled with bodily fluids
  - use gloves if handling bodily fluids and then wash hands
  - practise good personal hygiene for at least 4 weeks after injection

RALTITREXED
Trade name
Tomudex

Available form
Vial: 2 mg

Action
- folic acid analogue antimetabolite
- half-life 37.5 hours

Use
- palliative treatment of advanced colorectal cancer (with distant metastases or unresectable local disease)

Dose
- 3 mg/m^2 IV over 15 minutes, repeated every 3 weeks

Adverse effects
* see General Adverse effects of antineoplastic agents (p. 596)

Interactions
* should not be given with folinic acid or folic acid (or multivitamin preparations containing either substance), as effectiveness will be reduced
* caution if used with nephrotoxic agents that delay clearance
* see also General Interactions of antineoplastic agents (p. 596)

Nursing considerations/Cautions
* reconstitute with 4 mL water for injections, then dilute further with 50—250 mL sodium chloride 0.9% or glucose 5% and gently invert to mix, but prevent foaming
* caution if used in those with mild-to-moderate liver impairment
* not recommended in those with severe liver impairment, clinical jaundice or decompensated liver disease
* contraindicated in those with severe renal impairment (creatinine clearance < 25 mL/min)
* see also General Nursing considerations/Cautions for antineoplastic agents (p. 596)

Patient education
* advise the patient to avoid multivitamin preparations containing folic acid during therapy
* see also General Patient education for antineoplastic agents (p. 598)

(Creatinine clearance 55—65 mL/min) 75% of dose every 4 weeks.

(Creatine clearance 25—54 mL/min) 50% of dose every 4 weeks.

Contraindicated in those with severe kidney impairment (CrCl < 25 mL/min).

ROMIDEPSIN
Trade names
Istodax, Romidepsin-Reach

Available form
Vial: 10 mg

Action
* histone deacetylase inhibitor
* half-life 3.7 hours

Use
* peripheral T cell lymphoma (in patient with ≥ one prior systemic treatments)

Dose
* 14 mg/m^2 IV over 4 hours on days 1, 8 and 15 of 28-day cycle, repeated every 28 days

Adverse effects
* QT interval prolongation, ECG changes
* see also General Adverse effects of antineoplastic agents (p. 596)

Interactions
* caution if used with warfarin as prothrombin time may be prolonged and INR elevated, therefore INR should be closely monitored especially when starting or stopping therapy
* caution if given with agents known to prolong QT interval or cause electrolyte imbalance (especially hypokalaemia, hypocalcaemia or hypomagnesaemia)
* may reduce effectiveness of oestrogen-containing oral contraceptives
* serum levels may be increased by rifampicin and therefore not recommended together

Nursing considerations/Cautions
* ECG is recommended before starting and regularly during therapy
* any electrolyte imbalance should be corrected before therapy is started
* serum potassium and magnesium should be checked before each infusion

671

- reconstitute using 2.2 mL diluent (provided) to given concentration of 5 mg/mL, then dilute further with 500 mL sodium chloride 0.9% and infuse over 4 hours
- caution if used in those with congenital or acquired prolonged QT interval or electrolyte imbalance
- see also General Nursing considerations/Cautions for antineoplastic agents (p. 596)

Patient education

- instruct patient to seek medical advice immediately if irregular or abnormal heartbeat occurs
- female patient should be counselled to use an additional or alternate form of contraception to prevent pregnancy during therapy and for at least 4 weeks after last dose
- see also General Patient education for antineoplastic agents (p. 598)

Dose reduction is recommended in those with moderate to severe liver impairment:
- **for moderate liver impairment, 7 mg/m^2 (50% dose reduction)**
- **for severe liver impairment, 5 mg/m^2 (64% dose reduction)**

TAMOXIFEN
Trade names
Genox, GenRx Tamoxifen, Nolvadex-D, Tamosin, Tamoxifen Sandoz

Available forms
Tablets: 10 mg, 20 mg

Action
- antioestrogen agent which prevents oestrogen binding to oestrogen receptors (although it has also been shown to have some activity on oestrogen-negative tumours, suggesting another mechanism of action)
- active metabolite (which has similar activity to tamoxifen) (half-life 10–14 days)
- half-life 5–7 days

Use
- treatment of breast cancer
- risk reduction of breast cancer in those with moderate-to-high risk

Dose
- (Treatment) initially 20 mg orally daily, increasing to 40 mg if no response **OR**
- (Risk reduction) 20 mg orally daily (for 5 years)

Adverse effects
- hot flushes
- vaginal discharge/bleeding
- endometrial changes (e.g. hyperplasia, polyps, uterine fibroids)
- microvascular flap complications (in delayed breast reconstruction)
- retinopathy, cataract
- thromboembolic events
- paraesthesia, altered taste
- see also General Adverse effects of antineoplastic agents (p. 596)

Interactions
- increased risk of thromboembolic events occurring when given with other cytotoxic agents
- contraindicated with warfarin because of increased anticoagulant effects; therefore INR should be closely monitored, especially when starting or stopping therapy
- decreased efficacy if given with selective serotonin reuptake inhibitors (SSRIs)
- decreased serum levels may occur if given with rifampicin
- not recommended with oral contraceptives or hormone replacement therapy
- no increase in efficacy when given with aromatase inhibitor
- see also General Interactions of antineoplastic agents (p. 596)

Nursing considerations/Cautions

- regular gynaecological examination is recommended
- in premenopausal women, pregnancy should be excluded before starting therapy
- should be stopped during periods of immobility or at least 3 weeks before

ANTINEOPLASTIC AGENTS

- elective surgery because of the increased risk of thromboembolic events
- caution if used in those with hereditary angioedema, as symptoms may be induced or exaggerated
- caution if used in women undergoing delayed microsurgical breast reconstruction, as microvascular flap complications may occur
- not recommended for treatment of McCune Albright syndrome
- (Risk reduction) contraindicated in those with a history of pulmonary embolism or deep vein thrombosis
- see also General Nursing considerations/Cautions for antineoplastic agents (p. 596)

Patient education

- (Risk reduction) ensure the patient is aware that tamoxifen reduces the risk of breast cancer but does not eliminate it altogether and it is important to continue self-examination of breasts and regular mammograms/surveillance
- the patient should be instructed to seek medical advice immediately if any of the following occur:
  - vaginal bleeding or any other gynaecological symptoms such as pelvic pain or pressure
  - visual disturbances
- see also General Patient education for antineoplastic agents (p. 598)

 Tablet can be dispersed in water or crushed and mixed with a spoonful of yoghurt or apple puree. Pregnant staff should not disperse or crush tablets.

 Banned in sport.

TEBENTAFUSP
Trade name
Kimmtrak

Available form
Vial: 0.1 mg/0.5 mL

Action
- bispecific fusion protein made up of T-cell receptor fused to CD3-specific antibody fragment
- T-cell receptor has specificity for gp100 peptide expressed in melanoma cells
- binds to HLA-A*02.01 positive uveal melanoma cells, resulting in lysis of tumour cells

Use
- unresectable or metastatic uveal melanoma (in HLA-A*02.01 positive adults)

Dose
- 20 micrograms (day 1), 30 micrograms (day 8), 68 micrograms (day 15), then 68 micrograms weekly, given by IV infusion over 15–20 minutes

Adverse effects
- cytokine release syndrome
- rash, pruritus, erythema, cutaneous oedema
- see also General adverse effects of antineoplastic agents (p. 596)

Interactions
- caution if used with agents with a narrow therapeutic index such as warfarin and ciclosporin

Nursing considerations/Cautions
- the patient should be adequately hydrated before starting therapy
- preparation of infusion is two-step process involving:
  - step 1: to prevent adsorption of tebentafusp to the infusion bag, a solution of 250 micrograms/mL human albumin in sodium chloride 0.9% is required (consult manufacturer's information for details). The infusion bag should not be shaken but gently inverted multiple times to mix the contents adequately
  - step 2: using a 1 mL graduated syringe, the required volume (20 microgram dose = 0.1 mL; 30 microgram dose = 0.15 mL; 68 microgram dose = 0.34 mL) is

- withdrawn from the vial and added to the 100 mL infusion bag containing sodium chloride 0.9% and albumin 250 micrograms/mL and the bag gently inverted multiple times to mix the contents
- administer via IV infusion over 15–20 minutes using a dedicated line with a low protein-binding 0.2 micron in-line filter
- not to be administered as IV bolus or push
- administer alone
- the first 3 doses should be administered in a health care setting to monitor for cytokine release syndrome (CRS) for at least 16 hours postadministration. Monitoring should include fluid status, oxygenation and vital signs. If the patient experiences CRS, management is dependent on severity of symptoms
- if the patient does not experience hypotension requiring medical intervention, subsequent infusions can be administered in an outpatient or ambulatory setting. The patient should be monitored for at least 30 minutes after each infusion
- therapy should continue until the disease progresses or unacceptable toxicity occurs
- the name of the product and batch number should be clearly recorded in the patient's medical history
- see also General Nursing considerations/Cautions for antineoplastic agents (p. 596)

Patient education

- instruct the patient to seek medical advice immediately if any of the following occur:
  - fever, dizziness, lightheadedness, fatigue, headache, difficulty breathing
  - rash, severe hives, itchy skin, peeling or flaking skin, swelling
- see also General Patient education for antineoplastic agents (p. 598)

TEMOZOLOMIDE

Trade names
APO-Temozolomide, Temizole, Temodal, Temozolomide Juno

Available forms
Capsules: 5 mg, 20 mg, 100 mg, 140 mg, 180 mg, 250 mg

Action
- imidazotetrazine alkylating agent
- rapidly converted to the active compound (monomethyl triazeno imidazole carboxamide)

Use
- newly diagnosed glioblastoma multiforme (with radiotherapy), then as adjunct
- recurrent brain tumours (anaplastic astrocytoma, glioblastoma multiforme) (after standard treatment)
- advanced metastatic malignant melanoma (first-line treatment)

Dose
- (Newly diagnosed glioblastoma multiforme) 75 mg/m^2 orally daily 1 hour before food for 42 days (maximum 49 days) with focal radiotherapy (concomitant phase), then, after a 4-week interval, 150 mg/m^2 orally 1 hour before food for 5 days of a 28-day cycle (cycle 1), then increasing to 200 mg/m^2 for the next 5 cycles depending on toxicity (adjunctive phase) **OR**
- (Recurrent anaplastic astrocytoma or glioblastoma multiforme) 200 mg/m^2 orally 1 hour before food daily (if previously untreated) or 150 mg/m^2 (if previously treated) for 5 days of a 28-day cycle, increasing to 200 mg/m^2 from cycle 2 depending on absolute neutrophil count (ANC) or platelet count (for up to 2 years or disease progression) **OR**
- (Metastatic malignant melanoma) 200 mg/m^2 orally daily 1 hour before food for 5 days of a 28-day cycle (for up to 2 years or disease progression)

Adverse effects
- *Pneumocystis jirovecii* pneumonia (PJP)

ANTINEOPLASTIC AGENTS

- reactivation of hepatitis B
- see also General Adverse effects of antineoplastic agents (p. 596)

Interactions
- clearance may be decreased if given with sodium valproate
- see also General Interactions of antineoplastic agents (p. 596)

Nursing considerations/Cautions
- before starting therapy, the patient should be assessed for hepatitis B status owing to a risk of reactivation
- antiemetic premedication is recommended before administration of temozolomide
- prophylactic antibiotics for PJP are recommended for a 42-day cycle in those receiving radiotherapy concurrently
- contraindicated in those with hypersensitivity to dacarbazine
- see also General Nursing considerations/Cautions for antineoplastic agents (p. 596)

Patient education
- instruct the patient to take 1 hour before food, swallowed whole (not opened, broken or chewed) with water
- see also General Patient education for antineoplastic agents (p. 598)

 Capsules should not be opened, broken or chewed.

THALIDOMIDE
Trade name
Thalomid

Available forms
Capsules: 50 mg, 100 mg

Action
- exact mode of action is unknown
- (Multiple myeloma) inhibits growth and survival of myeloma cells and bone marrow stromal cells, suppresses tumour necrosis factor alpha (TNF-α), inhibits leucocyte migration, shifts the ratio of helper T cells to cytotoxic T cells and blocks growth of blood vessels from tumour
- (Leprosy) appears to block fever and cutaneous symptoms by blocking TNF-α
- does not consistently decrease TNF-α in all disease states
- half-life 5—7 hours

Use
- multiple myeloma (as monotherapy when standard therapies have failed; in combination therapy for untreated multiple myeloma with melphalan and prednisolone in those over 65 years or ineligible for high-dose chemotherapy; or in combination with dexamethasone for induction therapy prior to high-dose chemotherapy with autologous stem cell rescue)
- treatment and maintenance of moderate-to-severe erythema nodosum leprosum (ENL) associated with leprosy

Dose
- (Untreated multiple myeloma) 200 mg orally daily 1 hour after food, for a maximum of 12 cycles of 6 weeks (with prednisolone and melphalan) **OR**
- (Untreated multiple myeloma) 200 mg orally daily 1 hour after food, for 4 cycles of 4 weeks (with dexamethasone) (induction) **OR**
- (Multiple myeloma after failure of standard therapy) initially 200 mg orally daily 1 hour after food, increasing by 100 mg at weekly intervals if necessary (daily maximum 400 mg) **OR**
- (ENL associated with leprosy) initially 100 mg orally daily 1 hour after food, increasing by 100 mg at weekly intervals if symptoms remain uncontrolled (daily maximum 400 mg) (treatment) then the dose reduced if possible to maintain active reaction control (maintenance)

Adverse effects
- teratogenic — severe birth defects
- leucopenia, neutropenia, anaemia, thrombocytopenia
- peripheral neuropathy, paraesthesia, dysaesthesia

- bradycardia, cardiac failure
- orthostatic hypotension, syncope
- depression, confusion, lack of coordination
- drowsiness, dizziness, somnolence, sedation, fatigue, weakness
- fever, asthenia, malaise
- tremor
- nausea, vomiting, dry mouth, constipation
- peripheral oedema
- rash, dry skin, urticaria
- dyspnoea
- delayed wound healing
- (Rare) hypothyroidism, seizures, severe skin reaction, tumour lysis syndrome, reactivation of hepatitis B
- (Multiple myeloma) increased risk of deep vein thrombosis (DVT) and pulmonary embolus (PE)

Interactions

- caution if used with other agents that cause bradycardia such as beta adrenoceptor blocking agents and anticholinesterases
- caution if used with other agents which increase the risk of thromboembolic events (e.g. erythropoietin, oestrogens)
- an increased risk of neutropenia or thrombocytopenia if given with melphalan or prednisolone
- may increase sedative effects of barbiturates, alcohol and chlorpromazine
- may increase effects of morphine derivatives, benzodiazepines, antianxiety agents, hypnotics, sedatives, antidepressants, antihistamines with sedative properties, antipsychotics, baclofen or centrally acting antihypertensive agents
- an increased risk of peripheral neuropathy if used with vincristine
- an increased risk of thromboembolic events (e.g. DVT, PE) and/or thrombosis if used with doxorubicin, melphalan, prednisolone or dexamethasone

Nursing considerations/Cautions

- thalidomide can be prescribed only under a restricted distribution program
- the patient must receive counselling to ensure good understanding of the potential therapy risks and outcomes (as well as alternative therapies), including the contraceptive requirements associated with thalidomide to prevent pregnancy occurring before giving a full, informed and written consent prior to starting therapy. The patient's sexual partner should also receive counselling and information
- females who report having had a hysterectomy or being postmenopausal for more than 2 years should have their status confirmed before starting therapy
- it is suggested that pregnancy testing, prescription issuing and dispensing all occur on the same day. If this is not possible, dispensing of thalidomide should occur within 7 days of a pregnancy test
- it is recommended that women of childbearing potential have a medically supervised pregnancy test either at the time of consultation or 3 days before starting therapy. Pregnancy tests are then recommended weekly during the first month and then monthly (if menstrual cycles are regular) or 2-weekly (if menstrual cycles are irregular) up to 4 weeks after therapy ends. Effective contraception should continue throughout and include the 4 weeks after therapy ends
- therapy should start on day 2 or 3 of the menstrual cycle in those women who have regular cycles and have had a negative pregnancy test and have been using effective contraception for at least 4 weeks
- (ENL) corticosteroids are sometimes added as an adjunct to control moderate-to-severe leprosy-associated neuritis
- (ENL) when symptoms are controlled, therapy may be tapered by 50 mg every 2—4 weeks, with the aim of discontinuing therapy in 3—6 months

ANTINEOPLASTIC AGENTS

- the patient should be monitored for bradycardia and/or syncope and the dose reduced if symptoms occur
- thyroid function tests, WBC count and differential count should be monitored throughout therapy
- therapy should be stopped 7 days before surgery if wound healing may be affected
- if therapy is long term, sensory nerve action potential data should be collected before starting therapy, then 6-monthly. Clinical evaluation for peripheral neuropathy (numbness, tingling, pain) should occur monthly
- if the patient is at increased risk of thromboembolic events (DVT, PE), concurrent therapy with warfarin or low molecular weight heparin is recommended
- if a thromboembolic event occurs, thalidomide should be stopped and anticoagulation therapy started. Thalidomide may be restarted once anticoagulation therapy has stabilised
- (ENL) should not be used in anyone with neuritis unless the benefits are thought to outweigh the risks
- not recommended as those with ENL associated with leprosy with neuritis, as the condition may be aggravated
- caution in those with epilepsy or if other risk factors for seizures exist
- caution if used in those who may experience tumour lysis syndrome
- caution if used in those with hypothyroidism
- caution if used in those with risk factors for myocardial infarction including prior thrombosis, smoking, hypertension and hyperlipidaemia
- caution if used in those with neutropenia. If the count is $< 0.75 \times 10^9$/L neutrophils, therapy should be withheld
- caution if used in those with malignant disease because of an increased risk of thromboembolic events (DVT, PE) (the risk is greatest in the first 5 months of therapy)
- caution if used in combination with corticosteroids in those with previous hepatitis B infection, as reactivation may occur
- contraindicated in those (males and females) who are unable or unwilling to comply with adequate contraception measures throughout therapy
- contraindicated in those under 12 years

Patient education

- the patient should receive adequate information to enable them to give individual, written, fully informed consent for the use of thalidomide showing full understanding of the harm it can cause and the need for contraception during therapy and for 4 weeks after stopping
- advise the patient to swallow tablets whole (not crushed or chewed) with a full glass of water at least an hour after food
- suggest to the patient that the dose could be taken in the evening to overcome drowsiness, sedation and somnolence, which may be problematic during the day
- warn the patient not to drive or operate machinery if drowsiness, dizziness, somnolence, weakness or fatigue occurs
- instruct the patient to avoid alcohol because it may increase drowsiness
- if dizziness or a spinning feeling in the head occurs when getting out of bed (low blood pressure), advise the patient to sit up slowly before standing
- advise the patient to seek medical advice immediately if any of the following occur:
  - any rash or blistering of skin
  - unusual bleeding or bruising, including vomiting blood or experiencing bloody diarrhoea, bloody nose
  - seizures (fitting)
  - slow heart rate, fainting
  - blurred vision, severe headache
  - numbness, tingling, pain or abnormal coordination in hands or feet

- sudden pain in chest or difficulty breathing, shortness of breath
- pain or swelling in the legs, especially lower legs or calves
- fever, severe chills, sore throat, mouth ulcers, tiredness, flu-like symptoms, signs of infection
* instruct all patients not to donate blood during or for 4 weeks after stopping therapy
* counsel male patients not to donate semen during or within 4 weeks of stopping therapy
* male patients should be advised that thalidomide is present in semen and therefore they should not have unprotected sex. Adequate contraceptive methods (latex or polyurethane condoms) must always be used during sexual activity with women of childbearing potential (or who have not been menopausal for at least 1 year); condom use must continue for at least 4 weeks after stopping therapy
* if a male patient is allergic to latex or polyurethane, at least one reliable contraceptive measure (as outlined below) should be utilised by the female partner
* women of childbearing potential (who have not had a hysterectomy or are not postmenopausal for more than 1 year) must use one reliable contraceptive measure (e.g. intrauterine device, hormone contraception, tubal ligation, partner vasectomy) for 1 month before, during and 1 month after stopping therapy. In addition, a second contraceptive measure (e.g. diaphragm, cervical cap, condom) is also recommended during this period of time
* women using oral contraceptives and thalidomide should be advised that there are a number of other medications which reduce the effectiveness of oral contraceptive agents and another form of contraception should be used
* any woman (either taking thalidomide or whose partner is taking thalidomide) who is of childbearing potential and who experiences menstrual irregularities or suspects she is pregnant must seek medical advice immediately
* see also General Patient education (p. 598)

Capsules should not be opened or crushed.

Under no circumstances should thalidomide be used during pregnancy. It is a known human teratogen causing mortality at or just after birth and birth defects that include absence or shortness of limbs, external ear abnormalities, eye abnormalities, facial palsy, congenital heart defects and malformation of alimentary tract, urinary tract and/or genital tract. Birth defects have occurred after taking a single dose of thalidomide.

Contraindicated during breastfeeding.

For patients over 75 years, the recommended starting dose is 100 mg orally daily.

TIOGUANINE (THIOGUANINE)
Trade name
Lanvis

Available form
Tablet: 40 mg

Action
* purine antimetabolite
* derivative of mercaptopurine; however, detoxification is not dependent on xanthine oxidase

Use
* acute myeloblastic leukaemia (AML)
* less commonly, chronic granulocytic leukaemia (during blast crisis or during busulfan-induced thrombocytopenia)

Dose
* 2—2.5 mg/kg daily orally in 1—2 divided doses (to the closest multiple of 20 mg)

Adverse effects
- phototoxicity
- see also General Adverse effects of antineoplastic agents (p. 596)

Interactions
- an increased risk of nodular regenerative hyperplasia, portal hypertension and oesophageal varices if given with busulfan
- caution if given with olsalazine, mesalazine or sulfasalazine
- see also General Interactions of antineoplastic agents (p. 596)

Nursing considerations/Cautions
- testing for thiopurine methyltransferase deficiency is recommended before starting therapy, as low or absent activity may be life threatening. Testing for the NUDT15 gene variant is also recommended to reduce the risk of thiopurine-related severe leucocytopenia and alopecia (especially those of Asian descent who have an increased frequency of the mutation)
- cross-resistance may exist between tioguanine and mercaptopurine
- if remission has not occurred after 2–3 attempts at induction, therapy should be reconsidered
- not effective for solid tumours or chronic lymphocytic leukaemia
- not recommended in those lacking hypoxanthine guanine phosphoribosyltransferase (e.g. in Lesch–Nyhan syndrome), as conversion to the active metabolite will be blocked
- not recommended for maintenance or prolonged therapy because of the risk of hepatotoxicity
- see also General Nursing considerations/Cautions for antineoplastic agents (p. 596)

Patient education
- advise the patient to swallow the tablet whole (without crushing, breaking or chewing)
- the patient should be warned about increased sensitivity to sun and advised to wear protective clothing and sunscreen (SPF 50+) when outdoors
- see also General Patient education for antineoplastic agents (p. 598)

 The tablet should not be crushed, broken or chewed.

 Contraindicated in those with severe kidney or liver impairment.

TISAGENLECLEUCEL
Trade name
Kymriah

Available form
Suspension bag: 1.2×10^6 to 6×10^8 anti-CD19 chimeric antigen receptor (CAR) T cells in 10–50 mL

Action
- CD19-directed genetically modified autologous T-cell immunotherapy prepared from patient's own T cells, which have been harvested via leukapheresis and then genetically modified by retroviral transduction to express a CAR

Use
- relapsed or refractory diffuse large B-cell lymphoma (DLBCL) (after two or more types of systemic therapy)
- B-cell precursor acute lymphoblastic leukaemia (ALL) (refractory, in relapse post-transplant or in second or later relapse) (children and adults < 25 years)

Dose
- (B-cell ALL, weight ≤ 50 kg) $0.2–5.0 \times 10^6$ CAR-positive viable T cells/kg **OR**
- (B-cell ALL, weight > 50 kg) $0.2–2.5 \times 10^8$ CAR-positive viable T cells **OR**
- (DLBCL) $0.6–6.0 \times 10^8$ CAR-positive viable T cells

Adverse effects
- see Adverse effects of Axicabtagene ciloleucel (Yescarta) (p. 691)

Interactions

- not recommended with or within 6 weeks of live virus vaccines
- may cause false positive result on human immunodeficiency virus (HIV) nucleic acid tests. ELISA or Western blot tests for HIV antibodies are recommended instead

Nursing considerations/Cautions

- before collecting cells for therapy, the patient should be screened for hepatitis B and C and HIV
- after infusion, blood counts, uric acid and immunoglobulin levels should be monitored
- therapy should be delayed if the patient has unresolved serious adverse reactions from previous chemotherapy, active uncontrolled infection, active chronic graft versus host disease (GvHD), significant worsening of leukaemia burden or rapid progression of lymphoma after lymphodepleting chemotherapy (see below)
- lymphodepleting chemotherapy is required unless WBC is ≤ 1000 cells/microL within 1 week of infusion. If there are more than 4 weeks between completing lymphodepleting chemotherapy and infusion, and WBC > 1000 cells/microL, the patient should be retreated with chemotherapy
- infusion is recommended 2–14 days after lymphodepleting chemotherapy is completed
- pretreatment involves lymphodepleting chemotherapy:
  - (B-cell ALL) cyclophosphamide 500 mg/m^2 IV daily for 2 days (starting on the same day as fludarabine) and fludarabine 30 mg/m^2 IV daily for 4 days before infusion. If haemorrhagic cystitis occurs with cyclophosphamide, or patient is chemorefractory, then cytarabine 500 mg/mg^2 IV daily for 2 days and etoposide 150 mg/m^2 IV for 3 days (starting on the first day of cytarabine is recommended)
  - (DLBCL) cyclophosphamide 250 mg/m^2 IV daily for 3 days (starting on the same day as fludarabine) and fludarabine 25 mg/m^2 IV daily for 3 days. If haemorrhagic cystitis occurs with cyclophosphamide, or the patient is chemorefractory, then bendamustine 90 mg/m^2 IV for 2 days is recommended
- premedication (paracetamol and diphenhydramine (or other H$_1$ antihistamine)) is recommended 30–60 minutes before infusion. Corticosteroids are not recommended as part of premedication
- severe or life-threatening cytokine-release syndrome should be treated with tocilizumab (see DMARDs, p. 1073) or tocilizumab and corticosteroids. A minimum of 4 doses of tocilizumab must be readily available in case of cytokine-release syndrome, along with emergency equipment. Treatment and supportive care (e.g. oxygen, fluids, vasopressor and, if life threatening, ventilator support, haemodialysis) must be instituted at the first signs of cytokine-release syndrome
- if the patient has high uric acid levels or a high tumour burden, allopurinol (or an alternative) is recommended prophylactically before infusion to reduce the risk of tumour lysis syndrome
- it is important to coordinate thaw and infusion timing so that the infusion is thawed and available for infusion when the patient is ready
- patient identity must be confirmed (matching the patient ID with patient identifiers on the infusion cassette). When correctly identified, the product bag is removed from the cassette and inspected for any breaks or cracks before thawing. The infusion bag should then be placed in a second sterile bag and then thawed, either in a water bath or by the dry thaw method, until there is no visible ice in the infusion bag. The bag

ANTINEOPLASTIC AGENTS

- should be gently mixed to disperse any cellular clumps. If a second bag is used, it should not be thawed until all the contents of the first bag have been infused
- a leukodepleting filter should not be used
- given only IV (with a central venous line recommended)
- the line should be primed with sodium chloride 0.9% before and after infusion
- infused via gravity feed at 10—20 mL/min
- standard precautions for blood-borne pathogens should be adhered to, and handling and disposal should be as per the institution biosafety guidelines
- the patient should be monitored for at least 7 days postinfusion for any signs of cytokine-release syndrome
- contains dextran and dimethyl sulfoxide, which can cause anaphylaxis in sensitive individuals
- not recommended within 4 months of undergoing allogeneic stem cell transplant because of the risk of worsening GvHD
- not recommended in those with HIV because of the risk of loss of HIV viral suppression
- not recommended in those with relapsed CD19-negative leukaemia or primary central nervous system lymphoma

Patient education

- see Patient education for Axicabtagene ciloleucel (Yescarta) (p. 606)

 Banned in sport.

TOPOTECAN HYDROCHLORIDE

Trade names
Hycamtin, Topotecan Accord, Topotecan Injection

Available forms
Vial: 4 mg;
Vial (solution): 4 mg/4 mL

Action
- topoisomerase 1 inhibitor (topoisomerase 1 is involved in replication, transcription and DNA damage repair)

- half-life 2—3 hours

Use
- small cell lung cancer (SCLC) (after failure of first-line treatment)
- metastatic ovarian cancer (after failure of first-line or subsequent treatment)
- recurrent or persistent cervical cancer (with cisplatin) (unsuitable for radiation or surgery)

Dose
- (SCLC, ovarian cancer) 1.5 mg/m^2 IV over 30 minutes for 5 days, repeated every 21 days for at least 4 cycles **OR**
- (Cervical cancer) 0.75 mg/m^2 IV over 30 minutes on days 1, 2 and 3 (with cisplatin on day 1) of a 21-day cycle, for 6 cycles or until disease progression

Adverse effects
- interstitial lung disease
- see also General Adverse effects of antineoplastic agents (p. 596)

Interactions
- see General Interactions of antineoplastic agents (p. 596)

Nursing considerations/Cautions

- reconstitute the powder with 4 mL water for injections and then further dilute with glucose 5% or sodium chloride 0.9% before IV administration
- caution if used in those with interstitial lung disease, pulmonary fibrosis, lung cancer, thoracic irradiation or with use of pneumotoxic agents or colony-stimulating factors, owing to an increased risk of interstitial lung disease
- see also General Nursing considerations/Cautions for antineoplastic agents (p.596)

Patient education

- advise the patient to seek medical advice if any cough, shortness of breath or difficulty breathing occurs
- see also General Patient education for antineoplastic agents (p. 598)

(Monotherapy) (creatinine clearance 0.33—0.66 mL/s) recommended dose is 0.75 mg/m^2

TOREMIFENE
Trade name
Fareston

Available form
Tablet: 60 mg

Action
* triphenylethylene derivative
* antioestrogen agent that binds to oestrogen receptors in a similar way to tamoxifen and clomifene (clomiphene)
* active metabolite with similar antioestrogen properties to the parent drug

Use
* hormone-dependent metastatic breast cancer (postmenopausal)

Dose
* 60 mg orally daily

Adverse effects
* prolongation of QT interval
* (Rare) hypercalcaemia
* see also General Adverse effects of antineoplastic agents (p. 596)

Interactions
* contraindicated with agents that prolong QT interval or cause electrolyte imbalance (especially hypokalaemia and hypomagnesaemia)
* an increased risk of hypercalcaemia if given with thiazide diuretics or other agents that decrease calcium excretion
* decreased serum levels may occur if given with phenobarbital (phenobarbitone), phenytoin or carbamazepine
* not recommended with warfarin. If used together, INR should be closely monitored
* caution if given with antifungal agents, erythromycin or macrolide antibacterial agents, as increased serum levels may occur
* see also General Interactions of antineoplastic agents (p. 596)

Nursing considerations/Cautions
* gynaecological examination is recommended before starting therapy to exclude any endometrial abnormalities, and then repeated annually
* an increased risk of endometrial cancer in those with high BMI (> 30), hypertension, diabetes or a history of hormone replacement therapy
* tablets contain lactose and are therefore not recommended in those with rare hereditary problems of galactose intolerance, Lapp lactose deficiency or glucose—galactose malabsorption
* caution if used in those with severe angina or cardiac insufficiency
* not recommended in those with hypersensitivity to other antioestrogen agents or with severe thromboembolic disease
* contraindicated in those with severe liver failure, pre-existing endometrial hyperplasia or oestrogen receptor-negative tumours
* contraindicated in those with a history of congenital or acquired QT interval prolongation or electrolyte disturbance, clinically relevant bradycardia, heart failure with reduced left ventricular ejection fraction or symptomatic arrhythmias
* see also General Nursing considerations/Cautions for antineoplastic agents (p. 596)

Patient education
* instruct the patient to seek medical advice immediately if any of the following occur:
  * rapid or abnormal heart rate
  * signs of hypercalcaemia including abdominal pain, excessive thirst and urination, muscle pain, weakness, anxiety, depression, confusion, fatigue and loss of concentration
* see also General Patient education for antineoplastic agents (p. 598)

ANTINEOPLASTIC AGENTS

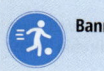
Banned in sport.

TRABECTEDIN
Trade name
Yondelis

Available form
Vial: 1 mg

Action
- binds to minor groove of DNA, causing the helix to bend to the major groove, triggering events affecting transcription factors, DNA-binding proteins and DNA repair pathways, disturbing the cell cycle
- alkylating agent
- half-life 180 hours

Use
- unresectable or metastatic liposarcoma or leiomyosarcoma previously treated with an anthracycline-containing regimen

Dose
- 1.5 mg/ m^2 as IV infusion over 24 hours with 3-week interval between cycles **OR**
- (Japanese patients) 1.2 mg/ m^2 as IV infusion over 24 hours with 3-week interval between cycles

Adverse effects
- (Peripheral line) severe injection site reactions, extravasation, tissue necrosis
- hypersensitivity reaction
- cardiac failure, decreased ejection fraction, right ventricular dysfunction, diastolic dysfunction
- capillary leak syndrome
- (Uncommon) rhabdomyolysis
- see also General Adverse effects for antineoplastic agents (p. 596)

Interactions
- contraindicated with yellow fever vaccine
- not recommended with phenytoin
- increased risk of hepatoxicity if alcohol is used during therapy
- increased serum levels may occur if given with fluconazole, ritonavir, clarithromycin and aprepitant, and therefore not recommended together
- decreased serum levels may occur if given with rifampicin, phenobarbital and St John's wort, and therefore not recommended together
- caution if given with ciclosporin or verapamil as distribution and/or elimination may be altered
- increased risk of rhabdomyolysis with statins
- see also General Interactions for antineoplastic agents (p. 596)

Nursing considerations/Cautions
- patient should receive premedication with corticosteroids (e.g. 20 mg dexamethasone IV) at least 30 minutes before infusion. Antiemetics may also be considered
- monitoring of full blood counts (including differential), liver enzymes and bilirubin, kidney function and creatine phosphokinase (CPK) should occur weekly during first two cycles of treatment, and then at least once between treatments in subsequent cycles
- cardiac assessment, including left ventricular ejection fraction (LVEF) (echocardiogram or multigated acquisition scan (MUGA)) should be conducted before starting and then 2–3 monthly during therapy
- dose should be reduced one level if toxicity occurs, and dose escalation is subsequent cycles is not recommended
- if rhabdomyolysis or capillary leak syndrome occur, therapy should be permanently stopped
- administration through a central line is recommended
- reconstitute using 20 mL water for Injections and then further dilute using either glucose 5% or sodium chloride 0.9% (see manufacturer's

information for calculation for required volume)
- if administration is via a peripheral IV, reconstituted solution should be added to infusion bag ($\geq$ 1000 mL) of either glucose 5% or sodium chloride 0.9%
- if infusion time is > 4 hours, an in-line filter (0.2 micron) should be used
- caution if used in those with existing liver disease
- use with caution if the left ventricular ejection fraction (LVEF) is less than the lower limit of normal, prior cumulative anthracycline dose > 300 mg/m^2, aged > 65 years or with a history of cardiovascular disease due to increased risk of cardiac dysfunction. If used, careful monitoring is recommended
- not recommended in those < 18 years, if bilirubin or liver enzymes (aspartate aminotransferase (AST), alanine aminotransferase (ALT), alkaline phosphatase (ALP)) are elevated at baseline or renal clearance < 30 mL/min or if CPK > 2.5 times upper limit of normal
- see also General Nursing considerations/Cautions for antineoplastic agents (p. 596)

Patient education
- advise the patient to avoid alcohol during therapy
- the patient should be instructed to immediately report any of the following:
  - muscle aches and pain, weakness, stiffness, dark urine
  - fever, rash, nausea, difficulty breathing,
  - unexplained swelling, dizziness, lightheadedness, thirst
  - tiredness, difficulty breathing, swelling of feet or ankles, chest pain, rapid heartbeat
- see also General Patient education for antineoplastic agents (p. 598)

 Not recommended in those with CrCl < 30 mL/min.

Not recommended in those with liver impairment and elevated bilirubin levels.

TRETINOIN
Trade name
Vesanoid

Available form
Capsules: 10 mg

Action
- retinoid, related to vitamin A, which inhibits proliferation of transformed haemopoietic cells, including human myeloid leukaemic cells
- metabolites have longer half lives than the parent drug

Use
- acute promyelocytic leukaemia (induction of remission) (previously untreated or those who have relapsed or are refractory to standard chemotherapy regimens)

Dose
- 45 mg/m^2 orally daily in 2 equal doses, continued for 30–120 days unless disease progression occurs (after remission, consolidation therapy should be started)

Adverse effects
- hyperleukocytosis, retinoic acid syndrome (RAS)
- intracranial hypertension/pseudotumour cerebri
- anxiety, mood alteration, depression
- see also General Adverse effects of antineoplastic agents (p. 596)

Interactions
- contraindicated with vitamin A because of the risk of hypervitaminosis A
- not recommended with other agents that cause intracranial hypertension/pseudotumour cerebri such as tetracyclines
- not recommended with ciclosporin, diltiazem, erythromycin, itraconazole or

verapamil, as increased serum levels may result
- serum levels may be decreased if given with carbamazepine, phenobarbital (phenobarbitone), phenytoin, rifampicin or rifabutin
- caution if used with tranexamic acid because of the increased risk of thrombotic complications

Nursing considerations/Cautions
- a pregnancy test (negative) must be performed 2 weeks before starting and then monthly throughout therapy, as tretinoin is highly teratogenic
- to be eligible for therapy, female patients of childbearing potential must be suffering from life-threatening malignancy, understand the dangers of becoming pregnant (risk of severe fetal malformation) and agree to using effective contraception for 4 weeks before, during and for 4 weeks after stopping therapy
- caution if used in those with a history of depression
- see also General Nursing considerations/Cautions for antineoplastic agents (p. 596)

Patient education
- the patient should be advised to swallow the capsule whole (without opening, crushing or chewing)
- instruct the patient to immediately seek medical advice if any of the following occur:
  - any new or worsening headache
  - fever, difficulty breathing, shortness of breath, sudden weight gain (RAS)
  - anxiety, low mood, depression
  - becoming pregnant
- partners/family members should be aware that depression, anxiety and mood alteration that can occur during therapy and of the importance of encouraging the patient to seek medical advice if this occurs
- ensure a female patient understands the need to use reliable contraception before, during and after therapy, as well as for monthly pregnancy testing, because of tretinoin causing severe fetal malformations if taken during pregnancy
- see also General Patient education for antineoplastic agents (p. 598)

 Capsules should not be opened, crushed or chewed.

Available in combination with
- ReTrieve Cream (tretinoin 0.05%) for management of acne vulgaris
- Acnatac Cream (tretinoin 0.025% + clindamycin 1%) for management of acne vulgaris

TRIFLURIDINE + TIPIRACIL
Trade name
Lonsurf

Available forms
Tablet: trifluridine 15 mg/tipiracil 6.14 mg, trifluridine 15 mg/tipiracil 8.19 mg

Action
- combination of two antineoplastic agents (thymidine-based nucleoside analogue (trifluridine) and thymidine phosphorylase inhibitor (tipiracil) in a ratio of 1 to 0.5.
- trifluridine is rapidly taken up by cancer cells, incorporated into DNA, interfering with function and preventing cell proliferation but is rapidly degraded by thymidine phosphorylase. Therefore the tipiracil is included to stop this step
- combination has antitumour activity against 5-fluorouracil sensitive and resistant colorectal cancer cell lines

Use
- metastatic colorectal cancer (previously treated with, or not considered suitable for fluoropyrimidine-, oxaliplatin- and

irinotecan-based therapy, anti-VEGF agents and anti-EGFR agents)
- metastatic gastric or gastroesophageal junction adenocarcinoma (previously treated with at least 2 previous lines of chemotherapy including a fluoropyrimidine, a platinum, either a taxane or irinotecan, and if appropriate, HER2/neu-targeted therapy)

Dose
- 35 mg/m^2 (based on trifluridine) orally twice daily on days 1 to 5, and 8 to 12 of a 28-day cycle (maximum dose 80 mg)

Adverse effects
- see General Adverse effects of antineoplastic agents (p. 596)

Interactions
- may decrease efficacy of antiviral agents that are human thymidine kinase substrates (e.g. zidovudine)
- increased risk of myelosuppression and haematological toxicity if used in those who received prior radiotherapy

Nursing considerations/Cautions
- a maximum of 3 dose reductions to a minimum of 20 mg/m^2 twice daily are allowed for adverse reactions, However, dose escalations are not permitted once dose has been reduced
- tablets contain lactose and are therefore not recommended in those with rare hereditary problems of galactose intolerance, total lactase deficiency or glucose-galactose malabsorption
- not recommended in those with end-stage renal disease or requiring dialysis, or with moderate-to-severe liver impairment
- not recommended in those under 18 years
- see also General Nursing considerations/Cautions for antineoplastic agents (p. 596)

Patient education
- advise the patient to swallow tablets whole (not to crush, break or chew)
- see also General Patient education for antineoplastic agents (p. 598)

Tablets should not be crushed, broken or dispersed.

Those with moderate renal impairment (creatinine clearance 30–59 mL/min) should be monitored more frequently and the dose adjusted if haematological toxicity occurs.

For those with severe renal impairment (creatinine clearance 15–29 mL/min), a starting dose of 20 mg/m^2 twice daily is recommended, with a dose reduction to 15 mg/m^2 twice daily if needed.

VINBLASTINE SULFATE
Trade name
DBL Vinblastine Injection

Available form
Vial: 10 mg/10 mL

Action
- vinca alkaloid that inhibits cell division and amino acid synthesis
- active metabolite whose activity is greater than the parent
- therapeutic effects are increased when given with other antineoplastic agents
- crosses the blood–brain barrier very poorly

Use
- advanced (stage III and IV) Hodgkin's disease, lymphocytic lymphoma, advanced testicular cancer, mycosis fungoides, Kaposi's sarcoma, histiocytosis X, choriocarcinoma (resistant to other agents), breast cancer (unresponsive to hormone therapy or endocrine surgery)

Dose
- 3.7 mg/m^2 IV once every 7 days (dose 1), then 5.5 mg/m^2 (dose 2), 7.4 mg/m^2 (dose 3), 9.25 mg/m^2 (dose 4), 11.1 mg/m^2 (dose 5) (maximum 18.5 mg/m^2)

Adverse effects
- acute shortness of breath, severe bronchospasm
- see also General Adverse effects of antineoplastic agents (p. 596)

ANTINEOPLASTIC AGENTS

Interactions
- phenytoin serum levels may be decreased, increasing the risk of seizures
- an increased risk of cardiotoxicity if given with bleomycin and cisplatin
- an increased risk of acute pulmonary reaction if given with mitomycin
- bleomycin effectiveness is enhanced when vinblastine is given 4–6 hours before
- erythromycin may increase toxicity
- plasma levels increased if given with cisplatin
- see also General Interactions of antineoplastic agents (p. 596)

Nursing considerations/Cautions
- the patient should be observed for any shortness of breath or bronchospasm, especially if vinblastine is given with mitomycin, and should not be readministered if they occur
- jaw and organ pain (in organ containing tumour) is common
- the next injection should not be given until WBC is at least 4×10^9/L
- not recommended IM, SC or IT (fatal if given intrathecally)
- given as an IV injection or into rapidly flowing IV infusion
- should not be diluted in large volumes (100–250 mL) or given by prolonged infusion
- caution if used in those with cachexia or skin ulceration
- contraindicated in those with vinca alkaloid hypersensitivity
- see also General Nursing considerations/Cautions for antineoplastic agents (p. 596)

Patient education
- see General Patient education for antineoplastic agents (p. 598)

Caution if used in those with a history of liver dysfunction or urate renal stones.

VINCRISTINE SULFATE
Trade names
DBL Vincristine Sulfate, Pfizer (Australia)
Vincristine Sulfate

Available forms
Vial: 1 mg/mL, 2 mg/2 mL, 5 mg/5 mL

Action
- vinca alkaloid that inhibits cell division and also has some immunosuppressant activity
- does not readily cross blood–brain barrier

Use
- acute leukaemias (as part of combination therapy)
- Ewing's sarcoma, Wilms' tumour, Hodgkin's disease, non-Hodgkin lymphoma, neuroblastoma, sarcomas, breast, uterine, cervical and lung (oat cell) tumours, malignant melanoma, rhabdomyosarcoma (with other agents), mycosis fungoides
- idiopathic thrombocytopenic purpura (resistant to other therapies) (not as primary treatment)

Dose
- 0.4–1.4 mg/m² IV over 5–10 minutes weekly

Adverse effects
- acute shortness of breath, severe bronchospasm
- jaw pain
- neurotoxicity
- hyperuricaemia, urate nephropathy
- see also General Adverse effects of antineoplastic agents (p. 596)

Interactions
- serum levels may be increased if given voriconazole
- increases cellular uptake of methotrexate by malignant cells
- clearance may be decreased by nifedipine
- increased risk of myelosuppression if given with allopurinol, prednisolone and

- doxorubicin and these are therefore not recommended together
- may decrease absorption of digoxin, ciprofloxacin or norfloxacin
- may decrease serum levels of phenytoin, increasing the risk of seizures
- severe bronchospasm and acute shortness of breath may occur if given with mitomycin
- therapy should be delayed until any radiation therapy is completed
- earlier onset and/or more severe neurotoxicity if given with itraconazole or fluconazole
- additive neurotoxicity may occur if given with asparaginase or isoniazid
- if given as part of combination therapy with asparaginase, vincristine should be given 12–24 hours before asparaginase to minimise toxicity
- an increased risk of ototoxicity (including permanent hearing impairment) if given with other ototoxic agents such as platinum-containing antineoplastic agents
- thromboembolism and Raynaud's syndrome may occur if given in combination with bleomycin and other agents such as cisplatin and etoposide
- pegfilgrastim and filgrastim should be administered at least 24 hours after receiving vincristine
- see also General Interactions of antineoplastic agents (p. 596)

Nursing considerations/Cautions

- ensure the patient is well hydrated during therapy
- should not be diluted with solutions that raise or lower pH outside the range of 3.5–5.5
- protective clothing should be worn when handling patient urine or faeces for 4–7 days after administration
- may be given IV or into a free-flowing IV infusion line
- caution is used in the elderly, those with neuromuscular disease or previous irradiation owing to the risk of neurotoxicity
- caution if used in those with a history of gout or urate kidney stones
- not recommended for CNS leukaemia, as vincristine has poor blood–brain penetration
- contraindicated via SC, IM or IT route (fatal if given intrathecally)
- contraindicated in those with demyelinating Charcot–Marie–Tooth disease, hypersensitivity to mannitol or other vinca alkaloid, or who have received previous irradiation through ports that include the liver
- see also General Nursing considerations/Cautions for antineoplastic agents (p. 596)

Patient education

- see General Patient education for antineoplastic agents (p. 598)

If direct serum bilirubin > 3 mg/100 mL, dose reduction of 50% is recommended.

Caution if used in the elderly, as they are more prone to neurotoxicity and gastrointestinal side-effects.

VINORELBINE

Trade names
Navelbine, Navelbine Oral, Velabine, Velorelbine Ebewe

Available forms
Vial: 10 mg/mL, 50 mg/5 mL;
Capsules: 20 mg, 30 mg

Action
- vinca alkaloid that inhibits mitosis at metaphase
- active metabolite with activity greater than the parent
- (IV) half-life 38 hours

Use
- advanced breast cancer (after failure of standard treatment) (as monotherapy or part of combination therapy)
- advanced non-small cell lung cancer (NSCLC) (as monotherapy or part of combination therapy)

ANTINEOPLASTIC AGENTS

- completely resected NSCLC stage IB or greater (with cisplatin)

Dose

- (Breast cancer, NSCLC) 60 mg/m² orally with food once weekly for 3 weeks, then increasing to 80 mg/m² (monotherapy) **OR**
- (Breast cancer, NSCLC) 25–30 mg/m² slow IV bolus over 6–10 minutes or IV infusion over 20–30 minutes weekly (monotherapy) **OR**
- (Breast cancer, NSCLC) 25–30 mg/m² slow IV bolus over 6–10 minutes or IV infusion over 20–30 minutes on days 1 and 8, or days 1 and 5 every 3 weeks (combination therapy) **OR**
- (Breast cancer) 60 mg/m² orally with food on days 1 and 8 of a 21-day cycle (cycle 1), then increasing to 80 mg/m² (with capecitabine given orally on days 1–14 of a 21-day cycle) (combination therapy) **OR**
- (Resected NSCLC) 25–30 mg/m² slow IV bolus over 6–10 minutes or IV infusion over 20–30 minutes weekly for 16 weeks (with cisplatin)

Adverse effects

- (IV) acute shortness of breath, severe bronchospasm
- peripheral neuropathy including numbness, paraesthesia
- see also General Adverse effects of antineoplastic agents (p. 596)

Interactions

- contraindicated with yellow fever vaccine and not recommended with other live attenuated vaccines
- severe bronchospasm and acute shortness of breath may occur if given with mitomycin
- an increased risk of neutropenia if given with lapatinib
- may decrease serum levels of phenytoin, increasing the risk of seizure activity
- if given with warfarin, INR should be closely monitored especially when starting or stopping therapy
- not recommended with itraconazole because of an increased risk of neurotoxicity
- not recommended with radiotherapy if the treatment field includes the liver
- caution if used with ciclosporin or tacrolimus because of an increased risk of lymphoproliferation
- see also General Interactions of antineoplastic agents (p. 596)

Nursing considerations/Cautions

- premedication with an antiemetic (e.g. ondansetron) is recommended before oral administration
- dilute before use (50 mL for bolus, 125 mL for infusion) and give by slow IV bolus over 6–10 minutes or a short infusion over 20–30 minutes
- should not be diluted using alkaline solution, as precipitation will occur
- not recommended SC, IM or IT (fatal if given intrathecally)
- (Oral) capsules contain sorbitol and are not recommended in those with rare hereditary problems of fructose intolerance
- contraindicated in those with vinca alkaloid hypersensitivity or requiring long-term oxygen therapy
- (Oral) contraindicated in those who have a significant resection of the stomach or small bowel, with malabsorption syndromes, requiring long-term oxygen therapy or with severe liver impairment
- see also General Nursing considerations/Cautions for antineoplastic agents (p. 596)

Patient education

- instruct the patient that capsules should be swallowed whole with food (not chewed, sucked or opened). The patient should be advised that, if the capsules are accidentally sucked or chewed, the mouth should be rinsed immediately with water or normal saline solution
- the patient should be instructed to seek medical advice immediately if any of the following occur:
  - tingling or numbness of extremities
  - ongoing shortness of breath
- see also General Patient education for antineoplastic agents (p. 598)

Capsules should not be opened, crushed or chewed.

(Breast cancer, NSCLC—monotherapy) for those with moderate liver impairment, dose reduction to 50 mg/m² orally weekly is recommended.

(IV) dose reduction by 33% is recommended in those with severe liver impairment.

VORINOSTAT
Trade name
Zolinza

Available form
Capsule: 100 mg

Action
- histone deacetylase inhibitor (HDAI) 1, 2, 3 and 6

Use
- cutaneous manifestations of cutaneous T-cell lymphoma (progressive, persistent, recurrent disease despite treatment)

Dose
- 400 mg orally daily with food, decreasing the dose to 300 mg daily **OR**
- 300 mg daily for 5 consecutive days if intolerance occurs

Adverse effects
- (Rare) hyperglycaemia, thromboembolism
- see also General Adverse effects of antineoplastic agents (p. 596)

Interactions
- caution if used with warfarin; therefore INR should be closely monitored, especially when starting or stopping therapy
- not recommended with sodium valproate and related agents because of an increased risk of adverse effects

Nursing considerations/Cautions
- ensure the patient is well hydrated and any vomiting or diarrhoea is corrected before starting therapy
- full blood count and electrolytes including electrolytes, glucose and serum creatinine, should be measured every 2 weeks for the first 8 weeks, then monthly during therapy
- caution if used in those with a previous history of thromboembolic events
- contraindicated in those with severe liver impairment

Patient education
- instruct the patient to drink at least 2 L of fluid per day to prevent dehydration
- the patient should be advised to swallow capsules whole (without breaking or chewing) with food
- if the patient has diabetes, blood glucose levels should be monitored closely during therapy
- advise the patient to seek medical advice immediately if any of the following occur:
  - swelling of leg/calf, pain/tenderness in calf/leg, redness, warmth
  - excessive diarrhoea or vomiting
- see also General Patient education for antineoplastic agents (p. 598)

Capsules should not be opened or crushed.

The recommended dose for those with mild liver impairment is 400 mg orally daily with food; for those with moderate liver impairment, the recommended dose is 300 mg orally daily.

PROTEIN KINASE and SMALL MOLECULE INHIBITORS

Introduction
Small molecules such as protein kinase inhibitors exert their effects mainly by entering the cancer cells. They will often inhibit multiple sites having a broader spectrum of activities, desired effects but also adverse effects. They generally have short half-lives requiring at least daily administration (Wellstein & Gioccone 2023).

ANTINEOPLASTIC AGENTS

General Adverse effects of protein kinase inhibitors

- haemorrhage
- infection (bacterial, viral, fungal)
- pneumonitis, interstitial lung disease
- secondary primary malignancies (including skin and non-skin cancers)
- neutropenia, febrile neutropenia, thrombocytopenia, anaemia, leukopenia
- nausea, vomiting, diarrhoea, stomatitis, decreased appetite, abnormal taste, abdominal pain, dry mouth, dyspepsia, constipation
- rash, dry skin, pruritus, palmar–plantar erythrodysaesthesia syndrome (hand–foot syndrome), changes to skin and/or hair colour
- headache, insomnia, dizziness
- hypertension
- dyspnoea, cough, nasopharyngitis
- blurred vision, increase in lacrimation
- fatigue, asthenia, fever
- peripheral oedema
- peripheral neuropathy
- back pain, musculoskeletal pain, arthralgia, muscle spasm, myalgia
- increase in liver enzymes and bilirubin, hepatoxicity
- aneurysm, artery dissection
- hepatitis B reactivation

General Interactions of protein kinase inhibitors

- not recommended with carbamazepine, phenytoin, rifampicin, St John's wort, bosentan, efavirenz, modafinil or rifabutin
- not recommended with azole antifungal agents, clarithromycin, lopinavir, ritonavir, erythromycin, ciprofloxacin, diltiazem, fluconazole, verapamil, aprepitant, imatinib, grapefruit juice or Seville oranges
- caution if used with agents with a narrow therapeutic index such as alfentanil, ciclosporin, everolimus, fentanyl, sirolimus, tacrolimus, digoxin, dabigatran, rosuvastatin and ergot alkaloids
- caution if used with midazolam

General Nursing considerations/Cautions for protein kinase inhibitors

- gene status may need to be confirmed by a validated test before starting targeted therapy
- therapy is generally continued until disease progression or unacceptable toxicity occurs
- full blood counts (with differential), liver, kidney and thyroid function should be monitored before starting and regularly during therapy as needed (e.g. monitoring is usually more frequent at the start of therapy or if levels are not within normal range)
- dermatological assessment is recommended before starting, then 2-monthly during therapy and for 6 months after stopping
- head and neck examination, chest/abdominal CT scan and pelvic (for women) and anal examinations are recommended before starting, during and at the end of therapy
- any hypertension should be controlled before starting therapy and BP monitored regularly
- left ventricular ejection fraction (LVEF) should be monitored regularly in those with cardiac dysfunction
- if the patient is at increased risk of infection, prophylaxis may be considered
- therapy should be stopped if severe dermatological reactions occur
- if the patient has any visual disturbance, urgent ophthalmology review is recommended
- pregnancy status should be verified before starting therapy
- baseline testing for hepatitis B infection is recommended to identify chronic carriers. If the patient has positive hepatitis B serology, consultation with a liver specialist is recommended before starting therapy

- adverse reactions are managed by temporary interruption therapy, dose reduction or stopping therapy altogether. The manufacturer's literature should be consulted for exact details
- pregnant staff should avoid handling tablets or capsules
- caution if used in those at risk for or having risk factors for thromboembolism (especially if the patient has experienced an event in last 6 months)
- caution if used in those with severe liver or kidney impairment. If used, close monitoring is recommended

General Patient education for protein kinase inhibitors

- advise the patient to avoid grapefruit, grapefruit hybrids, star-fruit and Seville oranges (and their juices) during therapy
- warn the patient not to drive or operate machinery if they experience fatigue, dizziness or vertigo during therapy
- the patient should be instructed to consistently take tablets at same time every day (e.g. always at night or always in the morning)
- advise the patient that, if they vomit or misses a dose, an additional dose should not taken
- warn the patient that changes to skin or hair colour may occur and are generally reversible when therapy is stopped
- the patient should be advised to avoid excessive sun exposure and wear protective clothing and sunscreen (SPF 30+) during and for months after stopping therapy
- the patient should be instructed to seek medical advice immediately if any of the following occur:
    - any new or changing skin lesions
    - rash, blistering or peeling skin
    - nausea, loss of appetite, unusual tiredness, upper abdominal pain, yellowing of eyes or skin, itching, pale stools, dark urine
    - fever, chills, or other signs of infection
    - persistent bruising or unusual bleeding, black tarry stools
    - shortness of breath, difficulty breathing, cough, chest pain, fever
    - numbness or tingling in hands or feet, pins and needles sensation, altered sensation, burning sensation
    - blurred vision, changes to vision, visual disturbances
    - fever > 38.5°C
- the patient should be advised that symptoms of palmar–plantar erythrodysaesthesia syndrome (hand–foot syndrome) can be reduced by keeping hands/feet cool (e.g. wearing loose-fitting socks and shoes, and avoiding sun exposure and hot showers or baths). Other management strategies can include the use of cold compresses or ice packs to wrists and ankles to reduce blood flow to hands and feet, elevating hands and feet, and keeping skin hydrated and protected (e.g. using a good emollient/moisturiser and patting skin dry rather than rubbing with a towel). Activities that cause friction to palms and soles should be temporarily avoided (e.g. jogging, activities that require a gripping tool or device for long periods of time (e.g. chopping vegetables, weeding the garden)
- women of childbearing potential should be counselled to use effective contraception during and for some time after stopping therapy (the exact time is dependent on the drug). Some agents may impact on the efficacy of hormonal contraceptives and therefore additional or alternate contraception will be required to prevent pregnancy occurring

There are no adequate or well-controlled studies in pregnant women; therefore protein kinase inhibitors are generally not recommended during pregnancy or in females of reproductive potential not using effective contraception.

It is unknown whether protein kinase inhibitors are excreted into human milk; therefore not recommended during breastfeeding.

ANTINEOPLASTIC AGENTS

ACALABRUTINIB

Trade name
Calquence

Available forms
Capsule: 100 mg;
Tablet: 100 mg

Action
- inhibitor of Bruton's tyrosine kinase (BTK) a signalling molecule that results in activation of B-call proliferation, trafficking, chemotaxis and adhesion and tumour growth)
- active metabolite (half-life 6.9 hours)
- half-life 0.9 hours

Use
- mantle cell lymphoma (MCL) (where at least one prior therapy has been used)
- chronic lymphocytic leukaemia (CLL)

Dose
- (MCL) 100 mg orally twice daily **OR**
- (CLL) 100 mg orally twice daily (monotherapy or in combination with obinutuzumab)

Adverse effects
- atrial fibrillation and flutter
- see also General Adverse effects of protein kinase inhibitors (p. 691)

Interactions
- not recommended with proton pump inhibitors
- H_2-receptor antagonists should be taken 2 hours after acalabrutinib
- if antacids are required, they should be separated by at least 2 hours from acalabrutinib administration
- increased risk of haemorrhage if given with anticoagulants or antiplatelet agents
- see also General Interactions of protein kinase inhibitors (p. 691)

Nursing considerations/Cautions
- (CLL) when given as combination therapy with obinutuzumab, acalabrutinib should be administered first when given on the same day
- therapy should be withheld 3—7 days before and after surgery to decrease risk of bleeding
- ECG is recommended if the patient has any symptoms of atrial fibrillation and flutter
- caution if used in those with pre-existing atrial fibrillation and flutter
- not recommended in those with severe liver impairment (Child—Pugh C or total bilirubin > 3 times upper limit of normal)
- see also General Nursing considerations/Cautions for protein kinase inhibitors (p. 691)

Patient education
- advise the patient that if the dose is missed by more than 3 hours, the next dose should be taken at the scheduled time
- the patient should be instructed to swallow the capsule/tablet whole (without breaking, splitting, chewing or crushing)
- ensure the patient understands that, if an antacid is needed, it should be taken 2 hours apart from medication
- instruct the patient to seek medical advice immediately if any dizziness, fainting, chest pain, rapid or pounding heartbeat (palpitations), or difficulty breathing occurs
- see also General Patient education for protein kinase inhibitors (p. 692)

 Tablets and capsules should not be crushed, broken, split, opened or chewed.

AFATINIB

Trade name
Giotrif

Available form
Tablets: 20 mg, 30 mg, 40 mg, 50 mg

Action
- protein kinase inhibitor blocking epidermal growth factor receptors (EGFR) B1, B2, B3 and B4

693

Use
- treatment of locally advanced or metastatic non-squamous non-small cell carcinoma of the lung (either as first-line treatment or after failed cytotoxic treatment)
- locally advanced or metastatic squamous cell carcinoma (with disease progression or after platinum-based therapy)

Dose
- 40 mg orally daily on an empty stomach. Avoid food for ≥ 3 hours before and ≥ 1 hour after the afatinib dose. Increase to 50 mg daily if well tolerated in the first 3 weeks (daily maximum 50 mg) until disease progresses or it is no longer tolerated

Adverse effects
- renal impairment
- severe diarrhoea
- see also General Adverse effects of protein kinase inhibitors (p. 691)

Interactions
- may increase the availability of rosuvastatin and sulfasalazine
- see also General Interactions of protein kinase inhibitors (p. 691)

Nursing considerations/Cautions
- EGFR mutation should be confirmed by a valid method before starting therapy
- the patient should be well hydrated during therapy
- antidiarrhoeal drugs (e.g. loperamide) should be given at the first sign of diarrhoea. If diarrhoea is severe, IV rehydration with fluid and electrolytes may be required
- tablets contain lactose and are therefore not recommended in those with rare hereditary conditions of galactose intolerance, Lapp lactase deficiency or glucose—galactose malabsorption
- caution if used in females, those of lower body weight or with kidney impairment, as the risk of diarrhoea, skin reactions and stomatitis is increased
- caution if used in those with a history of keratitis, ulcerative keratitis or severe dry eye
- caution if used in those with abnormal left ventricular ejection fraction. Cardiac assessment is recommended before starting therapy if used
- not recommended in those with severe liver or kidney failure or on dialysis
- see also General Nursing considerations/Cautions for protein kinase inhibitors (p. 691)

Patient education
- if the patient is unable to swallow the tablet, instruct them that the tablet can be dropped into 100 mL non-carbonated water only and allowed to dissolve, stirring occasionally over 15 minutes (the tablet should not be crushed or broken). After drinking, the glass should be rinsed with another 100 mL and the remainder drunk. Hands should be washed thoroughly before and after handling the tablet
- instruct the patient to take antidiarrhoeal medication at the first sign of diarrhoea and continue until loose bowel motions have stopped for 12 hours. The patient should be advised to drink plenty of fluids to avoid becoming dehydrated
- advise the patient to seek medical advice immediately if any of the following occur:
  - diarrhoea not controlled after 48 hours of antidiarrhoeal medication or severe diarrhoea (4 or more bowel motions in 24 hours)
  - severe skin reaction such as peeling or blistering of skin
  - blurred vision, eye pain, red eye, tearing, eye inflammation, sensitivity to light
- see also General Patient education for protein kinase inhibitors (p. 692)

 Tablets should not be crushed, split or broken.

ANTINEOPLASTIC AGENTS

ALECTINIB
Trade name
Alecensa

Available forms
Capsule: 150 mg

Action
- tyrosine kinase inhibitor that targets anaplastic lymphoma kinase (ALK) and rearranged during transfection (RET) tyrosine kinase, and therefore inhibits proliferation of cells with ALK fusion proteins
- active metabolite has similar potency and activity to alectinib
- half-life for alectinib 32.5 hours and metabolite 30.7 hours

Use
- anaplastic lymphoma kinase (ALK)-positive advanced or metastatic non-small-cell lung cancer (NSCLC)

Dose
- 600 mg orally twice daily with food

Adverse effects
- gastrointestinal perforation
- bradycardia
- elevated creatine phosphokinase (CPK), myalgia
- haemolytic anaemia
- photosensitivity
- see also General Adverse effects of protein kinase and small molecule inhibitors (p. 691)

Interactions
- caution of used with other agents known to increase risk of GI perforation
- caution if used with digoxin, dabigatran or methotrexate, as increased serum may occur
- see also General interactions of protein kinase and small molecule inhibitors (p. 691)

Nursing considerations/Cautions
- ALK positive NSCLC status must be confirmed by a validated test conducted by an experienced laboratory before starting therapy
- CPK levels should be measured every 2 weeks for the first month and then regularly
- caution if used in those with a history of diverticulitis or gastrointestinal tract metastases because of the increased risk of GI perforation
- see also General nursing considerations/cautions for protein kinase and small molecule inhibitors (p. 691)

Patient education
- advise the patient to swallow capsules whole (not opened, crushed or chewed)
- instruct the patient to seek medical advice immediately if any of the following occur:
  - severe stomach or abdominal pain, fever, chills, vomiting, bloating, rigid abdomen
  - cough, fever, shortness of breath, difficulty breathing
  - slowed heart rate
  - muscle pain, tenderness or weakness
- advise the patient to avoid prolonged sun exposure and to use broad spectrum sunscreen and lip balm (SPF 50+) during therapy and for at least 7 days after therapy is stopped
- see also General Patient education for antineoplastic agents (p. 692)

Capsule can be opened and contents mixed with a spoonful of yoghurt or apple puree. Pregnant staff should not open capsules.

Starting dose for patients with severe liver impairment (Child–Pugh C) should be 450 mg orally twice daily with food. Liver function should be regularly monitored in all patients with liver impairment.

AXITINIB
Trade name
Inlyta

Available forms
Tablets: 1 mg, 3 mg, 5 mg, 7 mg

Action
- tyrosine kinase receptor inhibitor (vascular endothelial growth factor (VEGF) receptor 1, 2, 3)
- receptors are thought to be responsible for tumour growth and metastatic spread

Use
- advanced renal cell carcinoma (where other therapy has failed)

Dose
- initially 5 mg orally twice daily, increasing or decreasing the dose according to patient tolerance

Adverse effects
- hypertension
- impaired wound healing
- (Uncommon) reversible posterior leukoencephalopathy syndrome (RPLS)
- see also General Adverse effects of protein kinase inhibitors (p. 691)

Interactions
- see General Interactions of protein kinase inhibitors (p. 691)

Nursing considerations/Cautions
- the patient should be monitored for any signs of cardiac failure
- urine should be checked for protein before starting and during therapy, and interrupted if moderate-to-severe proteinuria occurs
- any pre-existing hypertension should be controlled before starting therapy
- BP and thyroid function should be measured before starting and regularly during therapy
- increase in dose should occur only if there are no adverse effects and the patient is not being treated with antihypertensive agents
- therapy should be stopped 24 hours before any surgical procedures
- the tablets contain lactose and are therefore not recommended in those with rare hereditary problems of galactose intolerance, Lapp lactase deficiency or glucose—galactose malabsorption
- not recommended in those with untreated brain metastases or recent active GI bleeding
- see also General Nursing considerations/Cautions for protein kinase inhibitors (p. 691)

Patient education
- advise the patient to seek medical advice immediately if any of the following occur:
  - chest pain, coughing, shortness of breath, difficulty breathing
  - leg/calf swelling, pain or tenderness of leg/calf, warmth, redness
  - vomiting blood or coffee ground-like material, black sticky stools, abdominal pain
  - headache, altered mental state, visual disturbances or fitting (seizures)
- see also General Patient education for protein kinase inhibitors (p. 692)

 The tablet should not be crushed, split, broken or chewed.

BINIMETINIB
Trade name
Mektovi

Available form
Tablet: 15 mg

Action
- protein kinase inhibitor that inhibits proliferation and viability or BRAF-mutant melanoma cells
- half-life 8.66 hours

Use
- unresectable or metastatic melanoma with BRAF V600E or V600K mutation (with encorafenib)

Dose
- 45 mg orally twice daily (with encorafenib)

Adverse effects
- retinal pigment epithelial detachment, reduced visual acuity, retinal vein occlusion

ANTINEOPLASTIC AGENTS

- decreased left ventricular ejection fraction (LVEF)
- creatine phosphokinase (CPK) increase and, uncommonly, rhabdomyolysis
- venous thromboembolism
- tumour lysis syndrome
- see also General Adverse effects of protein kinase inhibitors (p. 691)

Interactions
- increased risk of haemorrhage if given with anticoagulants or antiplatelet agents
- see also General Interactions of protein kinase inhibitors (p. 691)

Nursing considerations/Cautions
- BRAF V600 mutant melanoma status should be confirmed by an experienced laboratory before starting therapy
- if dose reduction is required because of adverse reactions, a dose below 30 mg twice daily is not recommended and therapy should be stopped if patient is not able to tolerate this dose
- before starting therapy, LVEF should be measured by echocardiogram or multigated acquisition (MUGA) scan, then repeated 1 month after starting therapy followed by 3-monthly assessments. If the patient becomes symptomatic or LVEF decreases 10% or more from baseline, therapy should be stopped and the patient assessed every 2 weeks until recovery
- creatinine and CPK levels should be monitored monthly for first 6 months of therapy, and then as needed
- the patient should be evaluated each visit for any changes to vision
- if adverse reactions require therapy interruption, both agents should be stopped at the same time unless adverse reactions are primarily related to encorafenib (palmar—plantar erythrodysaesthesia syndrome, uveitis and QTc prolongation)
- caution if used in those with LVEF that is below 50% or below the institutional lower limit of normal
- caution if used in those with a history of or at risk of venous thromboembolism or prior/current cancer associated with RAS mutation
- caution if used in those with risk of retinal vein occlusion including uncontrolled glaucoma, ocular hypertension, uncontrolled diabetes mellitus or a history of hyperviscosity or hypercoagulability syndromes
- not recommended in those with a history of retinal vein occlusion, or with liver impairment (because of combination therapy with encorafenib)
- caution if used in those with high tumour burden, pre-existing kidney insufficiency, oliguria, dehydration, hypotension and acidic urine because of the risk of tumour lysis syndrome
- must not be used if the patient has wild-type BRAF malignant melanoma
- tablets contain lactose and are therefore not recommended in those with rare hereditary problems of galactose intolerance, total lactase deficiency or glucose—galactose malabsorption
- see also General Nursing considerations/Cautions for protein kinase inhibitors (p. 691)

Patient education
- the patient should be instructed to swallow the tablet whole (not chewed, split, broken or crushed)
- advise the patient to maintain good hydration during therapy
- instruct the patient to seek medical advice immediately if any of the following occur:
  - blurred vision, loss of vision, visual changes (e.g. coloured dots or seeing haloes around objects)
  - muscle pain or cramps, stiffness, dark urine
  - cough, difficulty breathing
  - nausea, shortness of breath, muscle cramps, irregular heartbeat, cloudy urine, decreased urine output, tiredness, fitting/seizures
  - feeling dizzy, tired, lightheadedness, short of breath, irregular heartbeat, leg swelling

- see also General Patient education for protein kinase inhibitors (p. 692)

Tablet should not be crushed, broken or dispersed.

Because binimetinib is administered with encorafenib, the combination is not recommended in those with moderate-to-severe liver impairment (Child—Pugh Class B and C).

BORTEZOMIB
Trade names
Bortezom, Bortezomib Accord, Bortezomib Baxter, Bortezomib Eugia, Bortezomib Ever Pharma, Bortezomib Juno, Bortezomib Sandoz, Bortezomib-AFT, Bortezomib-Dr Reddy's, DBL Bortezomib, Velcade

Available forms
Vial: 1 mg, 3 mg, 3.5 mg;
Solution: 2.5 mg/mL, 3.5 mg/1.4 mL

Action
- reverse inhibitor of chymotrypsin-like activity of 26S proteasome preventing signalling cascades within cells resulting in tumour cell death

Use
- multiple myeloma (MM) (progressive disease where at least one therapy was ineffective)
- previously untreated MM (with melphalan and prednisone) (unsuitable for high-dose chemotherapy)
- induction therapy in those with previous untreated MM prior to high-dose chemotherapy and autologous stem cell rescue (< 65 years)
- untreated mantle cell lymphoma (with rituximab, cyclophosphamide, doxorubicin and prednisone)

Dose
- (Previously untreated MM — transplant eligible) 1.3 mg/m^2 SC or IV bolus over 3—5 seconds on days 1, 4, 8 and 11 of a 21-day cycle (with thalidomide and dexamethasone or dexamethasone only) for 3 cycles **OR**
- (Previously untreated MM — transplant ineligible) 1.3 mg/m^2 SC or IV bolus over 3—5 seconds on days 1, 4, 8, 11, 22, 25, 29 and 32 of a 6-week cycle for cycles 1—4, then days 1, 8, 22 and 29 of a 6-week cycle for cycles 5—9 (with melphalan and prednisolone) **OR**
- (Relapsed/refractory MM) 1.3 mg/m^2 SC or IV bolus over 3—5 seconds on days 1, 4, 8 and 11 of a 2-week cycle followed by a 10-day rest period, repeated for 2 additional cycles if response is confirmed **OR**
- (Untreated mantle cell lymphoma) 1.3 mg/m^2 SC or IV bolus over 3—5 seconds on days 1, 4, 8 and 11, followed by a 10-day drug-free interval (for 6 cycles) (with rituximab, cyclophosphamide, doxorubicin and prednisone)

Adverse effects
- peripheral neuropathy
- hypotension
- hyperglycaemia
- new or exacerbation of cardiac failure
- (Uncommon) seizure
- (Rare) acute liver failure, pulmonary disorders, posterior reversible encephalopathy syndrome (PRES), thrombocytopenic purpura
- see also General Adverse effects of protein kinase inhibitors (p. 691)

Interactions
- caution if given with antihypertensive agents, as excessive hypotension may occur
- increased risk of peripheral neuropathy if given with amiodarone, isoniazid, nitrofurantoin, antiviral agents or statins
- not recommended with rifampicin, carbamazepine, phenytoin, phenobarbital (phenobarbitone) or St John's wort
- increased serum levels may occur if given with ritonavir
- caution if used with oral antidiabetic agents. Blood glucose levels should be closely monitored during therapy

ANTINEOPLASTIC AGENTS

Nursing considerations/Cautions

- BP should be monitored during therapy, as hypotension occurs commonly
- the patient should be well hydrated during therapy
- antiviral prophylaxis is recommended to reduce the risk of herpes virus reactivation
- (Relapsed/refractory MM) a minimal 72-hour drug-free interval should be allowed between treatment doses
- (SC) rotate administration sites avoiding areas that are tender, bruised, broken or scarred and not within 2.5 cm of the previous injection site
- (SC) if an injection site reaction occurs, a less concentrated solution (1 mg/mL instead or 2.5 mg/mL) can be used or, alternatively, administer IV
- (IV) reconstitute using 3.5 mL sodium chloride 0.9% (for a 3.5 mg vial) or 1.0 mL sodium chloride 0.9% (for a 1.0 mg vial) for a final concentration of 1 mg/mL for IV bolus administration
- (SC) reconstitute using 1.4 mL sodium chloride 0.9% (for a 3.5 mg vial) for a final concentration of 2.5 mg/mL for SC administration
- do not administer intrathecally
- caution if used in those with diabetes mellitus, as blood glucose levels may become unstable (however, hyperglycaemia may occur in those without diabetes)
- caution if used in those with pre-existing epilepsy, neuropathy, a history of syncope or hypotension, or dehydration
- contraindicated if the patient has a hypersensitivity to mannitol or boron

Patient education

- the patient should be advised to seek medical advice if any of the following occur:
  - new or worsening numbness, pain or burning sensations in hands or feet
  - lightheadedness, dizziness, fainting
  - headache, altered mental state, visual disturbances or fitting (seizures)
  - cough, shortness of breath, breathing difficulties
  - excessive or easy bruising, superficial bleeding (pinpoint-sized reddish-purple spots) into skin resembling a rash (commonly on lower legs)
- if the patient has diabetes, advise them to monitor blood glucose levels closely, as hyperglycaemia occurs with therapy
- see also General Patient education for protein kinase inhibitors (p. 692)

Reduced starting dose is recommended in those with moderate-to-severe liver impairment.

If used in those undergoing dialysis, drug should be administered after completion of dialysis.

BRIGATINIB
Trade name
Alunbrig

Available forms
Tablets: 30 mg, 90 mg, 180 mg

Action
- tyrosine kinase inhibitor (including ALK, ROS1, insulin-like growth factor 1 receptor)
- half-life 25 hours

Use
- anaplastic lymphoma kinase-positive advanced non-small cell lung cancer

Dose
- initially 90 mg orally daily for 7 days, then increasing to 180 mg daily

Adverse effects
- hypertension, bradycardia
- visual disturbances
- elevated creatine phosphokinase and pancreatic enzymes, hyperglycaemia
- peripheral neuropathy
- see also General Adverse effects of protein kinase inhibitors (p. 691)

HAVARD'S NURSING GUIDE TO DRUGS

Interactions
- caution if used with other agents known to cause bradycardia. If given together, the heart rate (HR) should be monitored more regularly
- see also General Interactions of protein kinase inhibitors (p. 691)

Nursing considerations/Cautions
- the patient's ALK-positive status should be confirmed using a validated test before starting therapy
- HR and BP should be monitored throughout therapy
- fasting blood glucose should be measured before starting therapy, then regularly throughout
- if therapy is stopped for 14 days or longer (not related to adverse effects), the dose should be restarted at 90 mg daily for 7 days before increasing to the previously tolerated dose
- an increased risk of pneumonitis and interstitial lung disease in those who have received crizotinib within the last 7 days
- see also General Nursing considerations/Cautions for protein kinase inhibitors (p. 691)

Patient education
- the patient should be advised to swallow the tablet whole (not crushed, split, chewed or broken)
- instruct the patient to seek medical advice immediately if any of the following occur:
  - cough, shortness of breath, tight chest, loss of appetite, weight loss, fatigue, fever, chills
  - slowed heart rate
  - new or worsening visual disturbances
  - unexplained muscle pain, tenderness or weakness
  - numbness/tingling or altered sensation in hands or feet
- if the patient has diabetes, advise close monitoring of blood glucose levels during therapy
- see also General Patient education for protein kinase inhibitors (p. 692)

Tablets should not be crushed, split, chewed or broken.

Severe kidney impairment: dose should be reduced by 50%.

Severe liver impairment: dose should be reduced by 40%.

CABOZANTINIB
Trade name
Cabometyx

Available forms
Tablet: 20 mg, 40 mg, 60 mg

Action
- protein kinase inhibitor that inhibits MET (a hepatocyte growth factor receptor protein) and vascular endothelial growth factor (VEGF) receptors
- half-life 110 hours

Use
- advanced renal cell carcinoma (RCC) as monotherapy in patients who are treatment naive with intermediate or poor risk or following treatment with VEGF-targeted therapy
- advanced RCC in combination therapy with nivolumab (first-line treatment)
- hepatocellular carcinoma (HCC) (previously treated with sorafenib)
- differentiated thyroid carcinoma (DTC) (monotherapy) with locally advanced or metastatic cancer that has progressed during or after treatment with VEGF-targeted therapy and is ineligible for or refractory to radioactive iodine

Dose
- monotherapy
  - (RCC, HCC, DTC) 60 mg orally daily 2 hours before food
  - (DTC, paediatric patients aged 12 years and older)
    - (patient weight < 40 kg) 40 mg orally daily 2 hours before food

ANTINEOPLASTIC AGENTS

- (patient weight $\geq$ 40 kg) 60 mg orally daily 2 hours before food
- RCC, combination therapy with nivolumab
  - 40 mg orally daily 2 hours before food with nivolumab IV either 240 mg every 2 weeks or 480 mg every 4 weeks

Adverse effects

- hepatoxicity, hepatic encephalopathy and, rarely, vanishing bile duct syndrome
- gastrointestinal perforations and fistulas
- aneurysm, artery dissection
- wound complications
- osteonecrosis of the jaw
- palmar–plantar erythrodysaesthesia syndrome (hand–foot syndrome)
- proteinuria
- QT prolongation
- thyroid dysfunction
- posterior reversible encephalopathy syndrome (PRES)
- see also General Adverse effects of protein kinase inhibitors (p. 691)

Interactions

- caution if given with agents known to prolong QT interval or cause electrolyte imbalance
- increased risk of vanishing bile duct syndrome if given with or had prior therapy with checkpoint inhibitors
- caution if used with anticoagulants or antiplatelet agents because of the increased risk of haemorrhage
- caution if used with agents associated with osteonecrosis of the jaw such as bisphosphonates
- may increase serum levels of fexofenadine, dabigatran etexilate, digoxin, colchicine, posaconazole, saxagliptin or sitagliptin, increasing the risk of adverse effects
- increased serum levels may occur if given with ciclosporin, efavirenz or emtricitabine
- caution if given with warfarin; INR should be monitored closely if given together
- decreased absorption may occur if given with cholestyramine
- see also General Interactions of protein kinase inhibitors (p. 691)

Nursing considerations/Cautions

- before staring therapy
  - the patient should be evaluated for hypertension and/or a history of aneurysm before starting therapy. Blood pressure should be well controlled before starting therapy and monitored regularly
  - thyroid and liver function should be evaluated
  - any electrolyte disturbance should be correct, and serum calcium, potassium and magnesium measure regularly
- urine should be tested regularly for protein
- therapy should be stopped 28 days before surgery (including dental surgery or invasive dental procedures) and resumed when wound healing is satisfactory
- caution if used in those with inflammatory bowel disease, tumour infiltration of the GI tract or complications related to previous GI surgery (including delayed or incomplete healing) because of the increased risk of GI perforation and fistulae formation
- caution if used in those who are at risk for or have a history of thromboembolic events including pulmonary embolism and arterial thromboembolism
- caution if used in those with a history of QT prolongation, pre-existing cardiac disease, bradycardia or electrolyte disturbance
- not recommended in those who are at risk for or have severe haemorrhage including tumour invasion of major blood vessels, portal hypertension, thrombocytopenia or liver cirrhosis with oesophageal varices
- not recommended in those with severe kidney or liver impairment, or children with DTC under 12 years
- not recommended in those with rare hereditary problems of galactose

intolerance, Lapp lactase deficiency or glucose-galactose malabsorption
- see also General Nursing considerations/cautions for protein kinase inhibitors (p. 691)

Patient education

- instruct the patient that tablets should be swallowed whole (not crushed) on an empty stomach (not eating anything 2 hours before or 1 hour after taking tablets)
- advise the patient to ensure any dental work is completed before starting therapy. Good oral hygiene is recommended
- the patient should be advised to seek medical attention immediately if any of the following occur:
  - feeling drowsy or confused
  - persistent or recurring diarrhoea, nausea, vomiting, abdominal pain, fever
  - pain in the mouth, jaw and/or teeth, swelling or ulcers inside the mouth, teeth loosening, numbness or heavy feeling in jaw, slow healing after dental surgery or procedure
  - redness, swelling and blistering on the palms or soles of the feet
  - headache, visual disturbances, confusion, altered mental state, fitting/seizures
  - feeling tired, weight gain, dry skin, constipation, feeling cold or weight loss, rapid heartrate and sweating
- see also General Patient education for protein kinase inhibitors (p. 692)

 Tablets should be swallowed whole (not be crushed, broken or chewed) on an empty stomach (not eating anything 2 hours before or 1 hour after taking tablets).

CARFILZOMIB
Trade name
Kyprolis

Available forms
Vial: 10 mg, 30 mg, 60 mg

Action
- tetrapeptide epoxyketone proteasome inhibitor
- selectively and irreversibly binds to active 20S proteasome sites, delaying tumour growth
- half-life $\leq$ 1 hour

Use
- relapsed or refractory multiple myeloma (having received at least one prior therapy as part of combination therapy with dexamethasone, lenalidomide and dexamethasone, or isatuximab and dexamethasone, or daratumumab and dexamethasone

Dose

In combination with lenalidomide and dexamethasone
- (Cycle 1) 20 mg/m^2 IV over 10 minutes (days 1 and 2). If tolerated, dose increased to 27 mg/m^2 on days 8 and 9 (week 2) and repeated on days 15 and 16 (week 3), followed by a 12-day rest period
- (Cycles 2–12) 27 mg/m^2 IV over 10 minutes on days 1, 2, 8, 9, 15 and 16
- (Cycle 13 onward) 27 mg/m^2 IV over 10 minutes on days 1, 2,15 and 16
- lenalidomide 25 mg orally days 1–21
- dexamethasone 40 mg orally or IV on days 1, 8, 15 and 22, administered 30 minutes to 4 hours before carfilzomib

In combination with dexamethasone (weekly dosing)
- (Cycle 1) 20 mg/m^2 IV over 30 minutes (day 1). If tolerated, dose increased to 70 mg/m^2 on day 8 (week 2) and repeated on day 15 (week 3), followed by a 13-day rest period
- (Cycle 2 onward) 70 mg/m^2 IV over 30 minutes on days 1, 8 and 15
- dexamethasone 40 mg orally or IV on days 1, 8, 15 and 22 (cycles 1–9) and days 1, 8 and 15 (cycle 9 onward), administered 30 minutes to 4 hours before carfilzomib

ANTINEOPLASTIC AGENTS

In combination with dexamethasone (twice-weekly dosing)
- (Cycle 1) 20 mg/m^2 IV over 30 minutes (days 1 and 2). If tolerated, dose increased to 56 mg/m^2 on days 8 and 9 (week 2) and repeated on days 15 and 16 (week 3), followed by a 12-day rest period
- (Cycle 2 onward) 56 mg/m^2 IV over 30 minutes on days 1, 2, 8, 9, 15 and 16
- dexamethasone 20 mg IV or orally on days 1, 2, 8, 9, 15, 16, 22 and 23 administered 30 minutes to 4 hours before carfilzomib

In combination with isatuximab and dexamethasone
- (Cycle 1) 20 mg/m^2 IV over 30 minutes (days 1 and 2). If tolerated, dose increased to 56 mg/m^2 on days 8 and 9 (week 2) and repeated on days 15 and 16 (week 3), followed by a 12-day rest period
- (Cycle 2 onward) 56 mg/m^2 IV over 30 minutes on days 1, 2, 8, 9, 15 and 16
- dexamethasone 20 mg IV or orally on days 1, 2, 8, 9, 15, 16, 22 and 23 administered 30 minutes to 4 hours before carfilzomib
- isatuximab 10 mg/kg IV infusion days 1, 8, 15 and 22 (cycle 1), then days 1 and 15 in combination with daratumumab and dexamethasone (weekly dosing)
- (Cycle 1) 20 mg/m^2 IV over 30 minutes (day 1). If tolerated, dose increased to 70 mg/m^2 on day 8 (week 2) and repeated on day 15 (week 3), followed by a 13-day rest period
- (Cycle 2 onward) 70 mg/m^2 IV over 30 minutes on days 1, 8 and 15
- daratumumab 8 mg/kg IV on days 1 and 2 (cycle 1), then 16 mg/kg IV on days 8, 15 and 22 (cycle 1), 16 mg/kg IV on days 1, 8, 15 and 22 (cycle 2), 16 mg/kg IV on days 1 and 15 (cycles 3–6), then 16 mg/kg IV on day 1 (cycle 7 and onward)
- dexamethasone 20 mg orally or IV on days 1, 2, 8, 9, 15, 16, 22 and 23 (cycles 1 and 2), then 20 mg on days 1, 2, 15 and 16, and 40 mg on days 8 and 22 (cycles 3–6); for cycle 7 onwards, 20 mg on days 1 and 2, and 40 mg on days 8, 15 and 22 in combination with daratumumab and dexamethasone (twice-weekly dosing)
- (Cycle 1) 20 mg/m^2 IV over 30 minutes (days 1 and 2). If tolerated, dose increased to 56 mg/m^2 on days 8 and 9 (week 2) and repeated on days 15 and 16 (week 3), followed by a 12-day rest period
- (Cycle 2 onward) 56 mg/m^2 IV over 30 minutes on days 1, 2, 8, 9, 15 and 16
- daratumumab 8 mg/kg IV on days 1 and 2 (cycle 1), then 16 mg/kg IV on days 8, 15 and 22 (cycle 1), 16 mg/kg IV on days 1, 8, 15 and 22 (cycle 2), 16 mg/kg IV on days 1 and 15 (cycles 3–6), then 16 mg/kg IV on day 1 (cycle 7 and onward)
- dexamethasone 20 mg orally or IV on days 1, 2, 8, 9, 15 and 16, and 40 mg on day 22 (all cycles)

Adverse effects
- new or worsening cardiac failure, myocardial infarction, myocardial ischaemia
- hypertension, hypertensive crisis
- acute renal failure
- tumour lysis syndrome
- QT prolongation, ventricular tachycardia
- infusion reactions
- haemorrhage, thrombocytopenia
- venous thrombosis, thrombotic microangiopathy
- (Rare) progressive multifocal leukoencephalopathy (PML), posterior reversible encephalopathy syndrome (PRES)
- see also General Adverse effects of protein kinase inhibitors (p. 691)

Interactions
- increased risk of fatal and serious adverse events if given in combination with melphalan and prednisolone in a newly diagnosed diagnosed multiple myeloma

patient (transplant ineligible) and therefore not recommended together
- not recommended with other agents known to prolong QT interval or cause electrolyte imbalance

Nursing considerations/Cautions

- the dose is calculated on the patient's body surface area (BSA). If BSA > 2.2 m^2, the dose should be based on a BSA of 2.2 m^2. If the patient weight does not change by $>20\%$, no dose adjustment is needed
- antiviral prophylaxis is recommended to reduce the risk of herpes zoster reactivation
- kidney and liver function should be measured before starting and then monthly during therapy
- (Combination with lenalidomide and dexamethasone) thromboprophylaxis is recommended
- adequate hydration is recommended for the cycle (especially if the patient is at risk of tumour lysis syndrome or renal toxicity). Hydration should include both oral and IV fluids — 30 mL/kg/day orally for 48 hours before day 1, cycle 1 and IV 250—500 mL before each dose in cycle 1 and as needed after carfilzomib administration. Oral/IV fluid hydration not required on day when daratumumab is administered
- the fluid balance should be monitored to prevent fluid overload especially in patients at risk of cardiac failure, including those over 75 years or in Asian patients
- serum potassium levels should be measured before starting and then monthly (or more frequently) during therapy, especially if the patient is receiving medication because of the increased risk of hypokalaemia
- blood pressure should be measured and any hypertension controlled before starting therapy. Dose reduction is recommended if hypertension cannot be controlled
- any modifiable risk factors for thromboembolism such as smoking, hypertension and hyperlipidaemia should be managed/minimised and the patient closely monitored during therapy
- the patient should be monitored for any signs or symptoms of infusion reaction during infusion including fever, chills, arthralgia, myalgia, facial flushing or oedema, laryngeal oedema, vomiting, weakness, shortness of breath, hypotension, syncope, bradycardia, chest tightness or angina
- should not be given as IV bolus or push
- reconstitute using water for Injections (5 mL for 10 mg vial; 15 mL for 30 mg vial; 29 mL for 60 mg vial)
- gently swirl or invert for about 1 minute to dissolve the powder but do not shake. If foaming occurs, allow the solution to settle (about 5 minutes) allowing it to become clear
- may be diluted into 50 or 100 mL 5% glucose solution (after withdrawing the calculated amount and discarding)
- do not dilute using sodium chloride 0.9%
- if the patient is a carrier of hepatitis B virus, prophylaxis with antivirals is recommended, with close monitoring during therapy
- not recommended in those with recent myocardial infarction, conduction abnormalities, angina, arrhythmias uncontrolled by medication or heart failure (New York Class III or IV)

Patient education

- advise the patient that infusion-related reactions can occur during administration or up to 24 hours after the infusion has been completed
- instruct the patient to seek medical advice immediately if any of the following occur:
  - shortness of breath, chest pain, arm or leg (particularly calf) swelling or pain, coughing up blood

ANTINEOPLASTIC AGENTS

- headache, fitting/seizures, lethargy, confusion, altered consciousness, visual disturbances, loss of vision
- weakness, clumsiness, difficulty speaking or thinking, visual loss, blurred or double vision
- chest pain, shortness of breath, swelling in ankles and feet, irregular heartbeat, tiredness, dizziness, fainting
- see also General Patient education for protein kinase inhibitors (p. 692)

(Combination therapy with daratumumab and dexamethasone) for patients > 75 years, 20 mg dexamethasone orally or IV weekly after first week.

Increased risk of serious adverse effects especially cardiac failure in those aged 75 years or more.

COBIMETINIB

Trade name
Cotellic

Available form
Tablets: 20 mg

Action
- mitogen extracellular kinase (MEK) protein inhibitor (MEK 1 and MEK 2 kinases are thought to be involved in cell proliferation, cell cycle regulation, cell survival, angiogenesis and cell migration. MEK levels are often high in BRAF mutant tumours)
- half-life 23.1—69.6 hours

Use
- treatment of BRAF V600 mutation positive unresectable or metastatic melanoma (with vemurafenib)

Dose
- 60 mg orally once daily for 21 consecutive days in a 28-day cycle, continued until benefits are no longer obtained or unacceptable toxicity occurs

Adverse effects
- chorioretinopathy, retinal detachment, blurred vision
- decreased left ventricular ejection fraction, hypertension
- photosensitivity, severe rash, skin reactions
- (Rare) rhabdomyolysis
- see also General Adverse effects of protein kinase inhibitors (p. 691)

Interactions
- an increased risk of bleeding if given with antiplatelet agents or anticoagulants
- see also General Interactions of protein kinase inhibitors (p. 691)

Nursing considerations/Cautions
- BRAF V600 mutation should be confirmed before starting therapy
- left ventricular ejection fraction should be measured before starting therapy, after the first month, then 3-monthly until therapy is stopped
- creatine phosphokinase (CPK) levels should be monitored before starting and then regularly during therapy
- if the patient experiences visual disturbances, prompt ophthalmological review is recommended
- caution if used in those with extra risk factors for bleeding such as brain metastases
- see also General Nursing considerations/Cautions for protein kinase inhibitors (p. 691)

Patient education
- advise the patient to swallow the tablet whole (without chewing, breaking, splitting or crushing)
- the patient should be instructed to seek medical advice immediately if any of the following occur:
    - new or worsening visual disturbances, including eye pain and blurred vision
    - sensitivity to sun, including severe sunburn
    - rash or severe skin reactions including blistering

- muscle pain or weakness, difficulty moving arms or legs, nausea, vomiting or abdominal pain
- see also General Patient education for protein kinase inhibitors (p. 692)

The tablet should not be crushed, broken, split or chewed.

CRIZOTINIB
Trade name
Xalkori

Available forms
Capsules: 200 mg, 250 mg

Action
- anaplastic lymphoma kinase (ALK) inhibitor that also inhibits hepatocyte growth factor receptor
- half-life 42 hours

Use
- ALK-positive advanced non-small cell lung cancer
- ROS1-positive advanced non-small cell lung cancer

Dose
- 250 mg orally twice daily

Adverse effects
- bradycardia, QT interval prolongation
- vision loss
- GI perforation
- see also General Adverse effects of protein kinase inhibitors (p. 691)

Interactions
- not recommended with agents that prolong QT interval or cause electrolyte imbalance
- not recommended with other agents that cause bradycardia including beta adrenoceptor blocking agents, digoxin, verapamil, diltiazem and clonidine
- see also General Interactions of protein kinase inhibitors (p. 691)

Nursing considerations/Cautions
- ALK- and ROS1-positive advanced non-small cell lung carcinoma should be confirmed before starting therapy
- monthly BP and pulse rate monitoring is recommended
- caution if used in those with congenital or acquired QT prolongation or electrolyte imbalance. ECG and electrolyte monitoring is recommended if used together
- see also General Nursing considerations/Cautions for protein kinase inhibitors (p. 691)

Patient education
- advise the patient to swallow the capsule whole (without opening, crushing or chewing)
- instruct the patient to seek medical advice immediately if any of the following occur:
    - slow or irregular heart rate
    - cough, shortness of breath, difficulty breathing
    - yellowing of eyes/skin, decreased appetite, weight loss, nausea, upper abdominal pain, dark urine, pale stools
    - dizziness, fainting
    - changes to vision
- see also General Patient education for protein kinase inhibitors (p. 692)

Capsules should not be opened, crushed or chewed.

DABRAFENIB
Trade name
Tafinlar

Available forms
Capsules: 50 mg, 75 mg;
Dispersible tablets: 10 mg

Action
- protein kinase inhibitor that inhibits BRAF enzymes that have been identified in melanoma
- half-life 8 hours

ANTINEOPLASTIC AGENTS

Use
- unresectable stage III or IV (metastatic) melanoma BRAF V600 positive (monotherapy or with trametinib)
- adjunct therapy for melanoma BRAF V600 positive after lymph node resection (with trametinib)
- advanced non-small cell lung cancer (NSCLC) BRAF V600 positive (with trametinib)
- locally advanced or metastatic anaplastic thyroid cancer (ATC) BRAF V600 positive
- low-grade glioma (LGG) in paediatric patients BRAF V600 positive (with trametinib) who require systemic treatment
- high-grade glioma (HGG) in paediatric patients BRAF V600 positive (with trametinib) where disease has progressed following previous treatment and no alternative treatment options are available

Dose
- (Adults) 150 mg orally twice daily 1 hour before or 2 hours after meals (with or without trametinib) OR
- (Children) administered 1 hour before or 2 hours after meals (with trametinib)
  - (26—37 kg) 75 mg orally twice daily
  - (38—50 kg) 100 mg orally twice daily
  - ($\geq$ 51 kg) 150 mg orally twice daily

Adverse effects
- uveitis, iritis
- hyperglycaemia
- renal failure
- (Uncommon) QT interval prolongation, cardiomyopathy
- (Rare) pancreatitis, retinal vein occlusion
- see also General Adverse effects of protein kinase inhibitors (p. 691)

Interactions
- caution if used with agents known to prolong QT interval or cause electrolyte imbalance
- caution if used with 3-hydroxy-3-methylglutaryl coenzyme A (HMG-CoA) reductase inhibitors (statins)
- bioavailability may be decreased if given with proton pump inhibitors, H_2-receptor inhibitors or antacids
- caution if given with warfarin; therefore INR should be closely monitored, especially when starting or stopping therapy
- see also General Interactions of protein kinase inhibitors (p. 691)

Nursing considerations/Cautions
- BRAF V600 mutation should be confirmed before starting therapy
- serum creatinine should be measured regularly during therapy
- (Combination therapy) trametinib is administered as a daily dose with either the morning or the evening dose of dabrafenib
- caution if used in those with glucose-6-phosphate dehydrogenase (G6PD) deficiency, as haemolytic anaemia may occur
- caution if used in those with diabetes, as hyperglycaemia may occur
- caution if used in those with known congenital or acquired QT interval prolongation or electrolyte imbalance (especially hypokalaemia and hypomagnesaemia)
- not recommended in those with BRAF wild-type melanoma
- see also General Nursing considerations/Cautions for protein kinase inhibitors (p. 691)

Patient education
- advise the patient to check their skin regularly for any new or changing skin lesions
- the patient should be instructed to swallow the capsule whole (without opening, crushing or chewing)
- for patients who have swallowing problems, or for children, dispersible tablets can be made into a suspension and swallowed as follows:
  - use 5 mL water for 1—4 tablets or 10 mL water for 5—15 tablets in the dosing cup provided

- it may take 3 minutes or more to dissolve the tablets, resulting in a cloudy white suspension
- the suspension can be taken directly from the dosing cup, from an oral syringe or from a feeding tube
- discard after 30 minutes if prepared and not used
- the patient should be instructed to seek medical advice immediately if any of the following occur:
  - fever $\geq 38.5°$ C
  - any new skin lesions
  - change of vision, photosensitivity, eye pain
  - unexplained abdominal pain
  - excessive thirst, increased frequency or volume of urination
  - irregular heart rate
- caution the patient with diabetes mellitus to monitor blood glucose levels closely, as hyperglycaemia may occur during therapy
- see also General Patient education for protein kinase inhibitors (p. 692)

Capsules should not be crushed, opened or chewed.

Dispersible tablets are available and should be made into a suspension (not crushed, broken or swallowed).

DASATINIB

Trade names
Dasatinib ARX, Dasatinib Dr. Reddy's, Dasatinib Sandoz, Dasatinib SUN, Dasatinib Viatris, Dasatinib-Teva, Sprycel

Available forms
Tablets: 20 mg, 50 mg, 70 mg, 100 mg

Action
- tyrosine, serine/threonine kinase inhibitor which stops replication of tumour cells

Use
- newly diagnosed Philadelphia chromosome positive (Ph+) chronic myeloid leukaemia (CML) (in chronic phase)
- newly diagnosed Ph+ acute lymphoblastic leukaemia (ALL) integrated with chemotherapy
- CML in chronic, accelerated, myeloid or lymphoid blast phase (resistant or intolerant to imatinib)
- Ph+ ALL (resistant or intolerant to other therapies)

Dose
- (CML — chronic phase) 100 mg orally daily **OR**
- (CML — accelerated, myeloid or lymphoid blast phase) 140 mg orally daily **OR**
- (Ph+ ALL — newly diagnosed) 100 mg orally daily **OR**
- (Ph+ ALL — resistant or intolerant) 140 mg orally daily

Adverse effects
- prolongation of QT interval
- fluid retention, pleural or pericardial effusion
- pulmonary arterial hypertension
- severe skin reaction
- see also General Adverse effects of protein kinase inhibitors (p. 691)

Interactions
- not recommended with proton pump inhibitors or histamine H$_2$-receptor antagonists
- not recommended with agents known to prolong QT interval or cause electrolyte imbalance
- absorption is decreased by antacids
- may increase serum levels of simvastatin and ergot alkaloids
- caution if used with antiplatelet or anticoagulant medications
- see also General Interactions of protein kinase inhibitors (p. 691)

Nursing considerations/Cautions
- cardiopulmonary assessment is recommended before starting therapy
- any hypokalaemia or hypomagnesaemia should be corrected before starting therapy (as these may

ANTINEOPLASTIC AGENTS

predispose to prolongation of the QT interval
- chest X-ray is recommended if shortness of breath or cough occurs
- tablets contain lactose and therefore are not recommended in those with galactose intolerance, Lapp lactase insufficiency or glucose—galactose malabsorption
- caution if used in those with congenital or acquired prolongation of the QT interval or electrolyte imbalance (especially hypokalaemia and hypomagnesaemia)
- see also General Nursing considerations/Cautions for protein kinase inhibitors (p. 692)

Patient education

- advise the patient to swallow tablets whole (without crushing, breaking or chewing)
- the patient should be instructed to seek medical advice if any of the following occur:
  - any new or worsening shortness of breath (at rest or on exertion), dry cough or pleuritic chest pains
  - fatigue, shortness of breath
  - irregular heart rate
  - severe skin reaction, especially any peeling or blistering
- instruct the patient to avoid antacids for 2 hours after taking tablets
- see also General Patient education for protein kinase inhibitors (p. 691)

Tablets should not be crushed, broken, chewed or dispersed.

Caution if used in those > 65 years because of an increased risk of pleural effusion, congestive cardiac failure, dyspnoea and gastrointestinal bleeding.

ENCORAFENIB
Trade name
Braftovi

Available forms
Capsules: 50 mg, 75 mg

Action
- ATP-competitive small molecule RAF kinase inhibitor that suppresses the RAF/MEK/ERK pathway in tumour cells expressing mutated forms of BRAF kinase (V600E, V600D, V600K)
- does not inhibit RAF/MEK/ERK signalling in wild-type BRAF cells
- half-life 4—8 hours

Use
- unresectable or metastatic melanoma with a BRAF V600E or V600K mutation (with binimetinib)
- metastatic colorectal cancer with a BRAF V600E mutation (with cetuximab)

Dose
- (Melanoma) 450 mg orally once daily (with binimetinib) **OR**
- (Colorectal cancer) 300 mg orally once daily (with cetuximab)

Adverse effects
- QTc interval prolongation, left ventricular dysfunction
- uveitis, iritis, iridocyclitis
- tumour lysis syndrome
- see also General Adverse effects of protein kinase inhibitors (p. 691)

Interactions
- decreased efficacy of hormonal contraceptives may occur if given together
- may increase serum levels of rosuvastatin, atorvastatin or methotrexate, increasing the risk of adverse effects and toxicity, and should be used with caution
- caution if used with furosemide (frusemide), penicillin, bosentan or posaconazole
- see also General Interactions of protein kinase inhibitors (p. 691)

Nursing considerations/Cautions
- BRAF V600 gene mutation status should be assessed by a validated test before starting therapy
- any electrolyte disturbance should be corrected before starting therapy

709

- ECG and echocardiogram or multigated acquisition (MUGA) are recommended before starting, repeated 1 month later and then at least 3-monthly during therapy to assess for QT interval prolongation and left ventricular function
- (Melanoma) if adverse reactions occur, dose modification for both encorafenib and binimetinib should occur. If encorafenib is stopped permanently, binimetinib should also be discontinued. However, if binimetinib is stopped, encorafenib can be continued at a reduced dose
- (Colorectal cancer) if encorafenib or cetuximab is stopped, the other agent should also be discontinued
- (Melanoma) there is limited information on the use of combined therapy in those who have BRAF V600 mutant melanoma with brain metastases or were previously treated with a BRAF inhibitor for unresectable or metastatic melanoma
- caution if used in those with severe kidney impairment
- not recommended in those with moderate or severe liver impairment
- not recommended in those with wild-type BRAF malignant melanoma or wild-type BRAF colorectal cancer. Giving BRAF inhibitors to those with wild-type BRAF tumours may lead to accelerated tumour growth
- see also General Nursing considerations/Cautions for protein kinase inhibitors (p. 691)

Patient education

- advise the patient to swallow capsules whole without opening, biting or chewing them
- women should be encouraged to use additional or alternative methods of contraception to avoid pregnancy during therapy, as hormonal contraceptives may fail
- the patient should be instructed to seek medical advice if any of the following occur:
  - new or worsening visual disturbances including decreased central vision, blurred vision or loss of vision
  - rapid heart rate, dizzy, fainting, chest pain
- see also General Patient education for protein kinase inhibitors (p. 692)

Capsules should not be opened or crushed.

For those with mild liver impairment (Child—Pugh Class A), 300 mg orally daily is recommended with caution. No dosing recommendations are available for those with moderate-to-severe liver impairment.

ENTRECTINIB

Trade name
Rozlytrek

Available forms
Capsules: 100 mg, 200 mg

Action
- tropomyosin receptor tyrosine kinase inhibitor (TRK) that inhibits TRKA, TRKB and TRKC, as well as ROS1 and ALK, blocking cell proliferation and leading to tumour cell death
- active metabolite (M5), half-life 40 hours
- half-life 20 hours

Use
- advanced non-small cell lung cancer (NSCLC) where tumours are ROS1-positive
- solid tumours that are metastatic and unresectable, previously treated (but disease progressed) and have a neurotrophic tyrosine receptor kinase (NTRK) gene fusion without a known acquired resistance mutation

Dose
- 600 mg orally once daily

Adverse effects
- congestive cardiac failure, QTc interval prolongation
- vision disorders
- skeletal fractures (commonly hip or lower extremity)

ANTINEOPLASTIC AGENTS

- hyperuricaemia
- central nervous system effects (e.g. cognitive impairment, mood disorders, sleep disturbance)
- weight gain
- see also General Adverse effects of protein kinase inhibitors (p. 691)

Interactions
- not recommended with agents known to prolong QT/QTc interval or cause electrolyte disturbance
- see also General Interactions of protein kinase inhibitors (p. 691)

Nursing considerations/Cautions
- gene status must be established before starting therapy — NTRK fusion-positive for solid tumours and ROS1-positive for NSCLC
- QT interval and electrolytes should be assessed before starting and then regularly throughout therapy
- any electrolyte imbalance should be corrected before starting therapy
- if used in those with severe liver impairment, careful monitoring is recommended
- for those with a known history of congestive heart failure, assessment of left ventricular ejection fraction (LVEF) is recommended before starting therapy
- when used in children, the risk of skeletal fractures is higher than in adults and often occurs with minimal or no trauma, whereas in adults they are usually caused by trauma or falls
- caution if used in those with congenital long QT syndrome or are at risk of developing QTc prolongation (e.g. uncontrolled or significant heart disease including recent myocardial infarction, congestive heart failure, unstable angina, electrolyte abnormalities or bradyarrhythmias)
- see also General Nursing considerations/Cautions for protein kinase inhibitors (p. 691)

Patient education
- advise the patient to swallow the capsule whole without biting, chewing or opening
- the patient should be instructed to seek medical advice immediately if any of the following occur:
  - shortness of breath, fatigue, weakness, swelling of feet and ankles, increased heart rate
  - dizziness, insomnia, somnolence, confusion, memory impairment, hallucinations, mental status changes, disturbance in attention
  - bone pain, deformity, change in mobility
  - any new or worsening visual changes including blurred vision, photophobia, double vision and vitreous floaters
  - rapid heart rate, heart pain, dizziness, fainting
- see also General Patient education for protein kinase inhibitors (p. 692)

 Capsules must not be opened or dissolved.

ERLOTINIB HYDROCHLORIDE
Trade names
Erlotinib ARX, Erlotinib Sandoz

Available forms
Tablets: 25 mg, 100 mg, 150 mg

Action
- human growth factor receptor type 1/epidermal growth factor receptor (HER1/EGFR) tyrosine kinase inhibitor

Use
- advanced or metastatic non-small cell lung cancer (NSCLC) (with activating EGFR mutation) (first-line treatment)
- locally advanced or metastatic non-small cell lung cancer (NSCLC) (with activating EGFR mutation) that has not progressed on first-line treatment
- locally advanced, unresectable or metastatic pancreatic cancer (with gemcitabine)

Dose
- (NSCLC) 150 mg orally daily 1 hour before or 2 hours after food, reducing

the dose in 50 mg increments if needed **OR**
- (Pancreatic cancer) 100 mg orally daily 1 hour before or 2 hours after food (with gemcitabine)

Adverse effects
- severe skin reactions
- gastrointestinal perforation
- (Rare) ocular disorders including ulceration, corneal perforation, keratitis, conjunctivitis, abnormal eyelash growth, hypokalaemia, renal failure
- see also General Adverse effects of protein kinase inhibitors (p. 691)

Interactions
- caution if given with warfarin; INR should be closely monitored especially when starting or stopping therapy
- serum levels are decreased in smokers
- increased risk of gastric perforation if given with corticosteroids, NSAIDs and/or taxane-based agents
- solubility decreases as pH increases; therefore not recommended with agents that reduce gastric acid production (e.g. ranitidine or proton pump inhibitors)
- increased risk of myopathy and rhabdomyolysis if used with statins
- see also General Interactions of protein kinase inhibitors (p. 691)

Nursing considerations/Cautions
- EGFR mutation should be confirmed by valid and reliable testing before starting therapy
- tablets contain lactose and therefore not recommended in those with galactose intolerance, Lapp lactase insufficiency or glucose—galactose malabsorption
- caution if used in those with a history of peptic ulceration or diverticular disease because of an increased risk of gastric perforation
- not recommended in those with severe liver impairment
- see also General Nursing considerations/Cautions for protein kinase inhibitors (p. 691)

Patient education
- the patient should be instructed to swallow tablets whole (not crushed, split, chewed or broken) either 1 hour before or 2 hours after food for maximum absorption
- instruct the patient to take erlotinib either 2 hours before or 10 hours after H_2 antagonist (e.g. ranitidine) or proton pump inhibitors (e.g. omeprazole)
- warn the patient not to change smoking habits (i.e. stop smoking) without first consulting their doctor, as this will affect serum levels
- instruct the patient to seek medical advice immediately if any of the following occur:
  - new or worsening cough, shortness of breath and fever
  - severe skin reaction including any peeling or blistering
  - eye pain, abnormally growing eyelashes
  - severe abdominal pain, vomiting blood or coffee ground-like material, black tarry bowel motions, bloody diarrhoea
  - unusual muscle weakness, cramps or contractions, decreased muscle tone
- see also General Patient education for protein kinase inhibitors (p. 692)

Tablets should not be split, crushed, broken or chewed.

Not recommended in those with severe liver impairment.

Caution if used in those with liver impairement because of an increased risk of liver failure.

GEFITINIB
Trade names
Iressa, Cipla Gefitinib

Available form
Tablets: 250 mg

ANTINEOPLASTIC AGENTS

Action
- inhibits epidermal growth factor receptor (EGFR) tyrosine kinase expressed in solid tumours of epithelial origin
- half-life 41 hours

Use
- locally advanced or metastatic non-small cell lung cancers (that express EGFR tyrosine kinase mutation)

Dose
- 250 mg orally daily

Adverse effects
- ulcerative keratitis, keratitis, conjunctivitis, dry eye
- gastrointestinal perforation
- see also General Adverse effects of protein kinase inhibitors (p. 691)

Interactions
- INR should be monitored if given with warfarin, especially when starting or stopping therapy
- efficacy may be reduced if given with agents that increase gastric pH above 5, such as ranitidine
- caution if used with corticosteroids or NSAIDs because of the risk of gastrointestinal perforation
- increased neutropenia may occur if given with vinorelbine
- see also General Interactions of protein kinase inhibitors (p. 691)

Nursing considerations/Cautions
- the EGFR mutation status of the patient should be confirmed using a valid and reliable method before starting therapy
- caution if used in those with history of gastrointestinal ulceration, smoking or bowel metastases, as the risk of gastrointestinal perforation is increased
- see also General Nursing considerations/Cautions for protein kinase inhibitors (p. 691)

Patient education
- instruct the patient that tablets may be dispersed in non-carbonated water if swallowing is difficult. The whole tablet (must not be crushed) should be dropped into water and stirred until dissolved (about 10 minutes) and drunk immediately. The glass should be rinsed and the contents drunk
- advise the patient to seek medical advice if any of the following occur:
  - new or worsening cough, shortness of breath or difficulty breathing
  - eye inflammation, tearing, blurred vision, eye pain, red eye, light sensitivity
  - severe abdominal pain, vomiting blood or coffee ground-like material, black tarry bowel motions, bloody diarrhoea
- see also General Patient education for protein kinase inhibitors (p. 692)

 Tablets should not be crushed, chewed or broken.

 Caution if used in those with mild-to-moderate liver dysfunction.

IBRUTINIB
Trade name
Imbruvica

Available forms
Capsules: 140 mg;
Tablets: 280 mg, 420 mg, 560 mg

Action
- Bruton's tyrosine kinase (BTK) inhibitor that leads to B-cell inhibition
- half-life 4-6 hours

Use
- mantel cell lymphoma (MCL) after ≥ 1 treatment
- previously untreated chronic lymphocytic leukaemia (CLL)/small lymphocytic lymphoma (SLL) (monotherapy or with obinutuzumab or rituximab)
- CLL/SLL (after ≥ 1 treatment) (as monotherapy or with bendamustine and rituximab)

- Waldenstrom's macroglobulinaemia (WM) (after ≥ 1 treatment or as first-line therapy in those unsuitable for chemo-immunotherapy)
- Waldenstrom's macroglobulinaemia (WM) (with rituximab)

Dose
- (MCL) 560 mg orally daily **OR**
- (CLL/SLL, WM) 420 mg orally daily

Adverse effects
- atrial flutter, atrial fibrillation, arrhythmias
- spleen rupture (after interrupting or stopping therapy)
- tumour lysis syndrome
- haemophagocytic lymphohistiocytosis (HLH)
- see also General Adverse effects of protein kinase inhibitors (p. 691)

Interactions
- contraindicated with St John's wort
- not recommended with warfarin or other vitamin K antagonists owing to an increased risk of bleeding
- not recommended with fish oil and vitamin E preparations
- an increased risk of bleeding if given with antiplatelet or anticoagulants agents
- caution if given with digoxin or methotrexate
- see also General Interactions of protein kinase inhibitors (p. 691)

Nursing considerations/Cautions
- when interrupting or stopping therapy, spleen size and disease status should be assessed by clinical examination and ultrasound, as splenic rupture may occur
- the patient should be monitored for any signs of atrial fibrillation or arrhythmias during therapy
- should be withheld 3–7 days pre- and postsurgery
- not recommended in those with atrial fibrillation, acute infections, cardiac risk factors or severe liver impairment
- see also General Nursing considerations/Cautions for protein kinase inhibitors (p. 691)

Patient education
- advise the patient to swallow capsules or tablets with a glass of water (not chewing, crushing, splitting or opening them)
- instruct the patient to seek medical advice immediately if any of the following occur:
  - confusion, trouble thinking, memory loss, blurred vision, loss of vision, balance or walking problems, decreased strength in arms or legs
  - irregular heart rate, shortness of breath
  - left upper abdominal or shoulder tip pain (especially after stopping therapy) (spleen rupture)
  - fever, swollen glands, bruising, rash (signs of HLH)
- see also General Patient education for protein kinase inhibitors (p. 692)

Capsules should not be opened, broken or chewed; tablets should not be crushed, broken or chewed.

For those with mild liver impairment (Child–Pugh Class A), the recommended dose is 280 mg orally daily.

For moderate liver impairment (Child–Pugh Class B), the recommended dose is 140 mg orally daily. Patients should be closely monitored.

IDELALISIB
Trade name
Zydelig

Available forms
Tablets: 100 mg, 150 mg

Action
- phosphatidylinositol 3-kinase (PI3K delta) inhibitor (PI3K delta is hyperactive in B-cell malignancies)
- half-life 8.2 hours

Use
- chronic lymphocytic leukaemia (CLL)/small lymphocytic lymphoma (SLL) (after

ANTINEOPLASTIC AGENTS

relapse where chemoimmunotherapy is not suitable) (with rituximab or ofatumumab)
- refractory follicular lymphoma (in patients who have received two prior therapies, including an alkylating agent and rituximab)

Dose
- 150 mg orally twice daily

Adverse effects
- serious infection
- pneumonitis
- colitis, intestinal perforation
- severe cutaneous reaction
- (Rare) progressive multifocal leukoencephalopathy (PML)
- see also General Adverse effects of protein kinase inhibitors (p. 691)

Interactions
- not recommended with live or live attenuated vaccines
- may increase serum levels of warfarin, midazolam, calcium-channel blockers, some antiarrhythmics, benzodiazepines, 3-hydroxy-3-methylglutaryl coenzyme A (HMG-CoA) reductase inhibitors (statins) or phosphodiesterase 5 (PDE-5) inhibitors, increasing the risk of adverse effects
- see also General Interactions of protein kinase inhibitors (p. 691)

Nursing considerations/Cautions
- the patient should be screened for hepatitis B and hepatitis C before starting therapy
- the patient should be closely monitored for any signs of cytomegalovirus (CMV) infection
- antibiotic prophylaxis against *Pneumocystis jirovecii* is recommended during and for 2–6 months after the last dose
- if the patient presents with colitis, infection causes (e.g. *Clostridium difficile*) should be excluded
- caution if used in those with active hepatitis
- not recommended in those with active infection
- see also General Nursing considerations/Cautions for protein kinase inhibitors (p. 691)

Patient education
- instruct the patient to swallow tablets whole with a glass of water (without chewing, crushing or breaking)
- advise the patient that diarrhoea can occur months after starting therapy
- the patient should be instructed to seek medical advice immediately if any of the following occur:
  - abdominal pain, diarrhoea
  - moderate-to-severe diarrhoea, new or worsening abdominal pain, chills, fever, nausea, vomiting
  - fever, chills, cough, shortness of breath, malaise
  - confusion, trouble thinking, memory loss, blurred vision, loss of vision, balance or walking problems, decreased strength in arms or legs
  - signs of CMV infection including fever, night sweats, sore throat, joint or muscle pain, loss of appetite and/or large mouth ulcers
- see also General Patient education for protein kinase inhibitors (p. 692)

 Tablets should not be crushed, broken or chewed.

 Caution if used in those with liver impairment because of an increased risk of hepatotoxicity.

IMATINIB
Trade names
ARX-Imatinib, Gilmat, Glivec, Imanib, Imatinib GH, Imatinib RBX, Imatinib Sandoz, Imatinib-DRLA, Imatinib Teva

Available forms
Tablets: 100 mg, 400 mg;
Capsules: 100 mg, 400 mg

Action
- inhibits activity of tyrosine kinase (TK), as well as several receptor TKs (KIT), the

receptor for stem cell factor (SCF) coded for by KIT oncogenes, platelet-derived growth factor receptor (PDGFR) and colony-stimulating factor receptor (CSF-1R and others)
* KIT mutation and PDGFR activation have been implicated in a number of conditions including gastrointestinal stromal tumour (GIST), myelodysplastic/myeloproliferative disorder (MDS/MPD), hypereosinophilic syndrome/chronic eosinophilic leukaemia (HES/CEL), dermatofibrosarcoma protuberans (DFSP) and aggressive systemic mastocytosis (ASM)
* active metabolite, half-life 40 hours
* half-life 18 hours

Use
* chronic myeloid leukaemia (CML)
* Philadelphia chromosome positive (Ph+) acute lymphoblastic leukaemia (ALL) (newly diagnosed, relapsed or refractory) (alone or with other agents)
* KIT (CD117)-positive unresectable and/or metastatic malignant GI stromal tumours (GIST) (treatment or as adjuvant therapy post resection to prevent recurrence)
* unresectable, recurrent and/or metastatic DFSP
* MDS/MPD with PDGFR rearrangement (where conventional therapy has failed)
* ASM (where conventional therapy has failed)
* HES and/or CEL

Dose
* (CML — chronic phase) 400 mg orally daily, increasing to 600 mg if no adverse effects occur, and further 400 mg twice daily if no greater than mild toxicity occurs **OR**
* (CML — accelerated phase or blast crisis) 600 mg orally daily, increasing to 400 mg twice daily if no adverse effects occurred **OR**
* (Ph+ ALL) 600 mg orally daily **OR**
* (MDS/MPD) initially 400 mg orally daily, increasing to 600–800 mg if the response is inadequate **OR**
* (ASM) initially 400 mg orally daily, increasing to 600–800 mg if the response is inadequate **OR**
* (Systemic mastocytosis (SM) with eosinophilia) initially 100 mg orally daily, increasing to 400 mg if the response is inadequate and no adverse effects have occurred **OR**
* (HES/CEL) initially 400 mg orally daily, increasing to 600–800 mg if the response is inadequate **OR**
* (GIST) 400 mg orally daily, increasing to 800 mg if disease progression occurs during therapy at 400 mg **OR**
* (GIST — unresectable and/or metastases present) 600 mg orally daily **OR**
* (GIST, adjunctive) 400 mg orally daily (after resection) for up to 3 years **OR**
* (DFSP) 400 mg orally twice daily

Adverse effects
* fluid retention, oedema, pleural effusion, pericardial effusion, pulmonary oedema, ascites
* severe congestive cardiac failure, left ventricular dysfunction
* (HES) cardiogenic shock, left ventricular dysfunction
* hypothyroidism
* phototoxicity
* see also General Adverse effects of protein kinase inhibitors (p. 691)

Interactions
* may increase serum levels of ciclosporin, some benzodiazepines, calcium-channel blockers and 3-hydroxy-3-methylglutaryl coenzyme A (HMG-CoA) reductase inhibitors (statins), increasing the risk of adverse effects
* may inhibit metabolism of paracetamol
* if given with warfarin, INR should be closely monitored especially when starting or stopping therapy
* see also General Interactions of protein kinase inhibitors (p. 691)

Nursing considerations/Cautions
* before starting therapy, the patient should be tested for hepatitis B, as reactivation can occur
* the patient should be weighed and monitored closely for any signs of fluid retention (which can be serious)

ANTINEOPLASTIC AGENTS

- before starting therapy, echocardiogram and serum troponin levels should be measured in those with high eosinophilia levels. If either is abnormal, prophylactic corticosteroids for 1—2 weeks should be considered to prevent hypereosinophilic—cardiac toxicity
- thyroid-stimulating hormone (TSH) levels should be monitored if the patient is taking levothyroxine after thyroidectomy
- doses of 400—600 mg can be given as a single daily dose; a 800 mg dose should be divided and given as 400 mg twice daily
- caution if used in those with pre-existing heart disease
- see also General Nursing considerations/Cautions for protein kinase inhibitors (p. 691)

Patient education

- instruct the patient to take tablets with a large glass of water and food to minimise GI disturbances
- the patient should be advised to avoid paracetamol and paracetamol-containing preparations during therapy
- if tablets cannot be swallowed, advise the patient that they may be dispersed in 50 mL (for a 100 mg tablet) or 200 mL (for a 400 mg tablet) of water or apple juice. Stir well to ensure tablets are dissolved and drink immediately
- instruct the patient to seek medical advice immediately if any of the following occur:
  - rapid weight gain, swelling of ankles, calves or face
  - shortness of breath, difficulty breathing, chest pain, cough
- see also General Patient education for protein kinase inhibitors (p. 692)

Tablets should not be crushed, broken or chewed; capsules should not opened, crushed or chewed.

For those with kidney impairment, the recommended dose is 400 mg orally daily.

For mild-to-moderate liver impairment, the recommended dose is 400 mg orally daily; for those with severe liver impairment, the recommended dose is 300 mg orally daily.

IVOSIDENIB
Trade name
Tibsovo

Available form
Tablet: 250 mg

Action
- small molecule inhibitor of mutant isocitrate dehydrogenase 1 (IDH1) enzymes

Use
- locally advanced or metastatic cholangiocarcinoma with IDH1 R132 mutation after at least one systemic therapy
- acute myeloid leukaemia (AML) that carries the IDH1 R132 mutation (as monotherapy), relapsed and/or refractory AML (monotherapy) or newly diagnosed AML not eligible for intense induction chemotherapy (with azacitidine)

Dose
- 500 mg orally once daily

Adverse effects
- QTc interval prolongation
- (AML) differentiation syndrome
- (Uncommonly) Guillain—Barré syndrome, peripheral neuropathy
- see also General Adverse effects of protein kinase inhibitors (p. 691)

Interactions
- not recommended with agents known to prolong QT interval or cause electrolyte imbalance
- see also General Interactions of protein kinase inhibitors (p. 691)

Nursing considerations/Cautions
- IDH1 mutation must be confirmed by a validated test before starting therapy. If

the patient is negative, they should be retested if they relapse, as IDH1 mutation can emerge during treatment or at relapse
- ECG is recommended before starting therapy to determine the QTc interval time, then monthly
- (AML) differentiation syndrome is associated with rapid proliferation and differentiation of myeloid cells, can be life threatening/fatal and occurs with AML response to treatment (in days or after many months of treatment). Management requires systemic corticosteroids and haemodynamic monitoring. If non-infectious leukocytosis occurs, hydroxycarbamide or leukapheresis is recommended. Corticosteroids should be given for at least 3 days. Tapering of corticosteroids and hydroxycarbamide should occur only when symptoms have resolved, as symptoms can recur if therapy is stopped prematurely
- (AML) therapy should be continued for at least 6 months to determine efficacy
- see also General Nursing considerations/Cautions for protein kinase inhibitors (p. 691)

Patient education
- advise the patient to swallow tablets whole (without crushing, chewing or splitting). Tablets can be taken with or without food; however, if taken with food, a high-fat meal (e.g. bacon, butter, milk, eggs (about 1000 calories and 58 g fat)) should be avoided
- the patient should be instructed to seek medical advice immediately if any of the following occurs:
  - rapid heart rate, chest pain, shortness of breath, fainting
  - fever, dizziness or lightheadedness, shortness of breath, headache, confusion, anxiety, rapid heart rate, rash, rapid weight gain, swelling of arms, legs or face
  - unilateral or bilateral weakness, difficulty breathing, altered sensation, numbness or tingling in hands or feet
- women of childbearing potential should be counselled to use additional or alternative contraception, as the efficacy of hormonal contraception may be affected
- see also General Patient education for protein kinase inhibitors (p. 692)

 Tablets should not be crushed, chewed or split.

LAPATINIB
Trade name
Tykerb

Available form
Tablets: 250 mg

Action
- selective and potent tyrosine kinase inhibitor of both epidermal growth factor (ErbB1) and HER2 (ErbB2) receptors
- half-life 6—14 hours

Use
- hormone-receptor positive metastatic breast cancer in postmenopausal women (tumours overexpressing HER2 where hormonal therapy is indicated) (with aromatase inhibitor)
- advanced or metastatic breast cancer with tumours overexpressing HER2 (where tumours have progressed after treatment with anthracycline, taxane and trastuzumab) (with capecitabine)
- metastatic breast cancer with tumours overexpressing HER2 (where trastuzumab is inappropriate) (first-line treatment with paclitaxel)

Dose
- 1250 mg orally daily at least 1 hour before or after food (with capecitabine) **OR**
- 1500 mg orally daily at least 1 hour before or after food (with paclitaxel or aromatase inhibitor)

Adverse effects
- decreased left ventricular ejection fraction (LVEF), QT interval prolongation

- see also General Adverse effects of protein kinase inhibitors (p. 691)

Interactions
- absorption may be decreased by food and proton pump inhibitors
- caution if given with digoxin, as digoxin toxicity may occur owing to increased serum levels
- increased risk of diarrhoea and neutropenia if given with paclitaxel
- caution if given with agents known to prolong QT interval or cause electrolyte imbalance (especially hypokalaemia and hypomagnesaemia)
- see also General Interactions of protein kinase inhibitors (p. 691)

Nursing considerations/Cautions
- HER2 overexpression and/or HER2 gene amplification should be confirmed by valid and reliable testing before starting therapy
- any electrolyte imbalance (especially hypokalaemia and hypomagnesaemia) should be corrected before starting therapy
- LVEF should be measured by echocardiogram or multi-gated acquisition (MUGA) before starting therapy, then 8—12-weekly
- caution if used in those with known congenital or acquired prolongation of QT interval or electrolyte imbalance (especially hypokalaemia or hypomagnesaemia)
- see also General Nursing considerations/Cautions for protein kinase inhibitors (p. 691)

Patient education
- the patient should be advised to swallow the tablet whole (not crushed, chewed or broken) and avoid food 1 hour before and 1 hour afterwards
- warn the patient that diarrhoea commonly occurs within first 6 days of therapy and lasts 4—5 days. Ensure the patient understands importance of being well hydrated during this time
- instruct the patient to seek medical advice immediately if any of the following occur:
  - change in bowel habits such as increased frequency and consistency
  - new or worsening cough, shortness of breath or difficulty breathing
  - abnormal or rapid heart rate
  - palpitations, shortness of breath, difficulty breathing, swelling of ankle or calf
- see also General Patient education for protein kinase inhibitors (p. 692)

 Tablets should not be crushed, broken or chewed.

 Dose reduction is recommended in those with pre-existing severe liver impairment.

LAROTRECTINIB
Trade name
Vitrakvi

Available forms
Capsule: 25 mg, 100 mg;
Oral solution: 20 mg/mL

Action
- highly selective tyrosine receptor kinase (TRK) inhibitor that targets TRKA, TRKB and TRKC
- half-life about 3 hours

Use
- locally advanced or metastatic solid tumours that have neurotrophic tyrosine receptor kinase (NTRK) gene fusion without acquired resistance mutation, metastatic and unresectable, and have progressed after previous treatment or have no satisfactory alternative therapy

Dose
- (Adults) 100 mg orally twice daily **OR**
- (1 month—18 years) 100 mg/m^2 orally twice daily (maximum dose 100 mg)

Adverse effects
- neurological reactions

- see also General Adverse effects for protein kinase inhibitors (p. 691)

Interactions
- see General interactions for protein kinase inhibitors (p. 691)

Nursing considerations/Cautions
- NTRK gene fusion status must be confirmed by validated test before starting therapy
- capsules and oral solution are bioequivalent
- see also General Nursing considerations/Cautions for protein kinase inhibitors (p. 691)

Patient education
- the patient should be advised to swallow capsule whole without opening, crushing or chewing
- (Oral solution) doses should be rounded to the closest 0.1 mL. For doses less that 1 mL, a 1 mL syringe should be used. For doses over 1 mL, a 5 mL syringe should be used
- the patient should be advised to seek medical advice immediately if any of the following occur:
  - dizziness, walking difficulties, numbness
- see also General Patient education for protein kinase inhibitors (p. 692)

 Capsules should not be opened, chewed or crushed. Oral solution is available.

 Dose reduction by 50% is recommended in those with moderate-to-severe liver impairment.

LENVATINIB
Trade name
Lenvima

Available forms
Capsule: 4 mg, 10 mg

Action
- multiple receptor tyrosine kinase (RTK) inhibitor that inhibits kinase activities of vascular endothelial growth factor (VEGF) receptors (VEGFR1, VEGFR2, VEGFR3), as well as fibroblast growth factor (FGF) receptors, platelet-derived growth factor (PDGF) alpha receptors PDGFR alpha, KIT and RET
- half-life 28 hours

Use
- advanced endometrial carcinoma (EC) (not microsatellite instability high or mismatch repair deficient) where disease has progressed following systemic therapy and not suitable for curative surgery or radiotherapy (with pembrolizumab)
- progressive, locally advanced or metastatic, radioactive iodine refractory differentiated thyroid cancer (DTC)
- advanced renal cell carcinoma (RCC) with pembrolizumab
- advanced RCC where disease has progressed after one VEGF-targeted therapy (with everolimus)
- unresectable hepatocellular carcinoma (HCC) (first-line treatment)

Dose
- (DTC) 24 mg orally daily **OR**
- (RCC, first-line treatment) 20 mg orally daily with pembrolizumab IV over 30 minutes (either 200 mg every 3 weeks or 400 mg every 6 weeks) **OR**
- (RCC, previously treated) 18 mg orally daily with everolimus (5 mg orally daily) **OR**
- (EC) 20 mg orally daily with pembrolizumab IV over 30 minutes (either 200 mg every 3 weeks or 400 mg every 6 weeks) **OR**
- (HCC)
  - (patient weight < 60 kg) 8 mg orally daily **OR**
  - (patient weight ≥ 60 kg) 12 mg orally daily

Adverse effects
- proteinuria, kidney impairment and failure
- hypertension

ANTINEOPLASTIC AGENTS

- aneurysm, artery dissection
- liver failure, hepatic encephalopathy
- arterial thromboembolic events
- wound healing complications
- gastrointestinal perforation, fistula formation, non-gastrointestinal fistula
- QT interval prolongation
- thyroid stimulating hormone suppression
- osteonecrosis of the jaw
- (Uncommon) cardiac failure, decreased left ventricular ejection fraction (LVEF), posterior reversible encephalopathy syndrome (PRES)
- see also General Adverse effects of protein kinase inhibitors (p. 691)

Interactions
- caution if used with other agents that act on renin—angiotensin aldosterone system, as there is an increased risk for acute kidney failure
- an increased risk of GI perforation and fistula (including non-GI) formation if the patient has had previous radiotherapy and surgery
- not recommended with agents that are known to prolong QT interval or cause electrolyte imbalance
- caution if used with bisphosphonates and denosumab because of the increased risk of osteonecrosis of the jaw
- see also General Interactions of protein kinase inhibitors (p. 691)

Nursing considerations/Cautions
- blood pressure should be well controlled before starting therapy. BP monitoring is recommended 1 week after starting, then every 2 weeks for first 2 months, then monthly
- urine should be checked regularly for protein, and therapy may need to be modified if dipstick proteinuria is ≥ 2
- diarrhoea, nausea and vomiting need to be managed early to prevent dehydration and kidney impairment
- if major surgery is planned, therapy may be temporarily interrupted
- caution if used in those with pre-existing kidney impairment and dehydration, and/or hypovolaemia due to diarrhoea, nausea and vomiting
- caution if used in those with hypertension or a history of aneurysm because of the increased risk of aneurysm formation and/or artery dissections
- caution if used in those with worse baseline liver impairment and/or greater liver tumour burden because of the increased risk of liver failure and encephalopathy
- caution if used in those who have had a myocardial infarction, cerebrovascular accident or transient ischaemic attack in the previous 6 months
- see also General Nursing considerations/Cautions for protein kinase inhibitors (p. 691)

Patient education
- advise the patient to swallow capsules whole without crushing, chewing or biting. If there are swallow issues, instruct the patient on dispersal technique including:
    - using only water, apple juice or milk (if the suspension is to be administered via a feeding tube, only water should be used)
    - capsules should be placed in small container (about 20 mL/4 teaspoon capacity) or 20 mL oral syringe
- add 3 mL liquid and wait 10 minutes for capsule shell to disintegrate
- stir or shake for 3 minutes until the capsule is fully disintegrated
- administer the dispersed solution into the mouth or via a feeding tube
- add an extra 2 mL of liquid to the container or oral syringe, swirl/shake and administer. Repeat this step at least twice until no residue is visible
- for feeding tubes $>$ 5 Fr diameter (PVC or PUR tubing) or $>$ 6 Fr diameter (silicone tubing), at least 3 rinses of 2 mL, or at least one 4 mL flush, are required

- the person preparing the suspension should wash their hands thoroughly before and after preparation
- only medication should be in the container at the same time
- if not used immediately, the suspension can be covered and refrigerated for up to 24 hours and then discarded if not used
- warn the patient that diarrhoea commonly occurs early in therapy
- the patient should be advised to seek medical advice immediately if any of the following occur:
  - headache, lethargy, confusion, visual disturbances or seizures/fitting
  - pain in jaw or gums, loose teeth, swelling, jaw numbness, feeling of heaviness in jaw
  - nausea, vomiting, sudden and severe abdominal pain
- in those patients with risk factors for osteonecrosis of the jaw (e.g. poor dental hygiene, chronic periodontal disease, head/neck radiotherapy, as well as treatment with antineoplastic agents and corticosteroids), the patient should be advised to have a dental examination and any necessary treatment before starting therapy, and any invasive dental procedures avoided if possible during therapy
- see also General Patient education for protein kinase inhibitors (p. 692)

Capsules should not be crushed, broken or opened; however, they can be dispersed in water, apple juice or milk. (see patient eduction for instructions). Pregnant staff must not disperse capsules.

Severe kidney impairment (creatinine clearance < 30 mL/min):

- (DTC) 14 mg orally daily
- (RCC, EC) 10 mg orally daily
- not recommended in those with end-stage kidney disease. Severe liver impairment (Child—Pugh C):
- (DTC) 14 mg orally daily
- (RCC, EC) 10 mg orally daily
- (HCC) use not recommended. Close monitoring is recommended.

Increased risk of hepatic encephalopathy in those aged 75 years and older.

LORLATINIB
Trade name
Lorviqua

Available forms
Tablets: 25 mg, 100 mg

Action
- adenosine triphosphate competitive inhibitor of anaplastic lymphoma kinase (ALK) and ROS proto-oncogene 1, receptor (ROS1) tyrosine kinase that addresses mechanisms of resistance after prior treatment with ALK inhibitors
- half-life 23.6 hours

Use
- locally advanced or metastatic ALK-positivenon-small cell lung cancer (NSCLC)

Dose
- 100 mg orally daily

Adverse effects
- hypercholesterolaemia, hypertriglyceridaemia
- hallucinations, changes in cognitive function, mood changes, altered mental status, speech difficulties (central nervous system effects)
- (Uncommon) PR interval prolongation, AV block
- elevated lipase and amylase
- see also General Adverse effects of protein kinase inhibitors (p. 691)

Interactions
- may decrease serum levels of hormonal contraceptives, alfentanil, ciclosporin, ergotamine, fentanyl, midazolam, sirolimus and tacrolimus, and these are therefore not recommended together

ANTINEOPLASTIC AGENTS

- see also General Interactions of protein kinase inhibitors (p. 691)

Nursing considerations/Cautions

- ALK-positive status must be established using a validated test before starting therapy
- serum lipids and cholesterol should be measured before starting, 8 weeks after starting and then regularly during therapy. Lipid-lowering agents may be required
- ECG and measurement of lipase and amylase are recommended before starting therapy and then monthly
- dose reduction may be required if severe adverse effects occur. If the patient is unable to tolerate 50 mg, therapy should be stopped
- not recommended in those with moderate-to-severe liver impairment or severe kidney impairment (creatinine clearance < 30 mL/min)
- see also General Nursing considerations/Cautions for protein kinase inhibitors (p. 691)

Patient education

- advise the patient to swallow tablets whole (without crushing, breaking or chewing)
- the patient should be instructed to seek medical advice immediately if any of the following occur:
    - shortness of breath, difficulty breathing, cough, fever
    - feeling confused, difficulty with speech, mood changes, hallucinations, memory problems
- see also General Patient education for protein kinase inhibitors (p. 692)

Tablets should not be crushed, broken or chewed.

For those with severe kidney impairment, recommended dose is 75 mg orally daily.

NERATINIB
Trade name
Nerlynx

Available form
Tablet: 40 mg

Action
- irreversible inhibitor of three epidermal growth factor receptors (EGFR), including EGFR, HER2 and HER4, thereby inhibiting tumour cell proliferation
- multiple metabolites with varying levels of activity
- half-life 17 hours

Use
- adjunctive treatment of early stage HER2-overexpressed/amplified breast cancer

Dose
- 240 mg orally daily with food for 1 year after completion of trastuzumab therapy **OR**
- dose escalation schedule (to improve tolerance)
    - (days 1–7) 120 mg orally daily with food
    - (days 8–14) 160 mg orally daily with food
    - (day 15 onward) 240 mg orally daily with food

Adverse effects
- diarrhoea, dehydration
- left ventricular ejection fraction (LVEF) dysfunction
- see also General Adverse effects of protein kinase inhibitors (p. 691)

Interactions
- contraindicated with carbamazepine, phenytoin, phenobarbital (phenobarbitone), rifampicin and St John's wort
- contraindicated with diltiazem, erythromycin, fluconazole and verapamil
- not recommended with proton pump inhibitors
- caution if used with sulfasalazine or rosuvastatin

- caution if used with dabigatran, digoxin or fexofenadine. Serum levels should be closely monitored
- see also General Interactions of protein kinase inhibitors (p. 691)

Nursing considerations/Cautions

- liver function tests (including alanine aminotransferase (ALT), aspartate aminotransferase (AST) and total bilirubin) should be measured after 1 week, then monthly for 3 months, and then every 6 weeks or more frequently if needed
- dose escalation schedule is recommended to improve tolerance. If diarrhoea occurs, treatment with antidiarrhoeal, fluids and electrolytes is recommended
- antidiarrhoeal prophylaxis is recommended for first 2 cycles (cycle 56 days) and starting with first dose to achieve 1–2 bowel motions per day
  - days 1–14, loperamide 4 mg orally 3 times daily
  - days 15–56, loperamide 4 mg orally twice daily
  - days 57–365, loperamide 4 mg orally as needed to achieve 1–2 bowel motions per day (daily maximum 16 mg)
  - Additional antidiarrhoeal agents with fluids and electrolytes may be required if diarrhoea continues
- those with kidney impairment are at increased risk of dehydration and complications if diarrhoea occurs
- caution if used in those with significant chronic gastrointestinal disorders with diarrhoea. If used, the patient should be very closely monitored
- caution if used in those with cardiac risk factors. Cardiac monitoring with assessment of LVEF is recommended
- not recommended in those with severe renal impairment or receiving dialysis
- contraindicated in those with severe liver impairment (Child–Pugh C)
- see also General Nursing considerations/Cautions for protein kinase inhibitors (p. 691)

Patient education

- advise the patient to swallow the tablet whole (without crushing, breaking or chewing)
- warn the patient that diarrhoea usually starts in first 1–2 weeks of therapy and is often recurrent
- ensure the patient understands diarrhoea management, including use of an antidiarrhoeal agent (for first 1–2 months titrating the dose to maintain 1–2 bowel motions a day, and then continued prophylactically), diet modification and need for at least 2 L of fluid daily to avoid dehydration
- advise the patient to seek medical advice immediately if diarrhoea does not stop or they feel dizzy or weak (which can be signs of dehydration)
- if antacids are used, advise the patient that there should be a 3-hour interval between antacid and neratinib
- see also General Patient education for protein kinase inhibitors (p. 692)

 Tablets should not be broken, crushed or dispersed.

 Contraindicated in those with severe liver impairment (Child–Pugh Class C).
Caution if used in those with kidney impairment as they are at greater risk of complications related to dehydration due to diarrhoea. Close monitoring is recommended.

 Caution if used in those over 65 years because of the increased risk of dehydration and renal insufficiency.

NILOTINIB
Trade name
Tasigna

Available forms
Capsules: 150 mg, 200 mg

Action
- BCR-ABL tyrosine kinase inhibitor which stops replication of tumour cells

ANTINEOPLASTIC AGENTS

Use
- chronic myeloid leukaemia (CML) (Philadelphia chromosome positive (Ph+)) in chronic or accelerated phase (newly diagnosed, or resistant or intolerant to other therapies)

Dose
- (Newly diagnosed CML (Ph+), chronic phase) 300 mg orally twice daily at least 1 hour before or 2 hours after food **OR**
- (CML, resistant or intolerant to other therapies, chronic or accelerated phase) 400 mg orally twice daily at least 1 hour before or 2 hours after food

Adverse effects
- may prolong the QT interval, ischaemic heart disease, peripheral arterial occlusive disease
- elevated blood glucose and cholesterol
- elevated serum lipase, pancreatitis
- fluid retention
- tumour lysis syndrome
- see also General Adverse effects of protein kinase inhibitors (p. 691)

Interactions
- absorption may be increased by food
- absorption may be decreased by antacids and histamine H_2-receptor antagonists
- not recommended with other agents known to prolong QT interval (e.g. amiodarone, disopyramide, clarithromycin, sotalol, methadone) or cause electrolyte imbalance (especially hypokalaemia and hypomagnesaemia)
- INR should be measured for the first 2 weeks of therapy if given with warfarin
- see also General Interactions of protein kinase inhibitors (p. 691)

Nursing considerations/Cautions
- any hypokalaemia or hypomagnesaemia should be corrected before starting therapy to decrease the risk of QT prolongation
- ECG and blood glucose levels should be taken before starting and regularly throughout therapy
- blood lipids and serum lipases should be measured before starting therapy, 3 and 6 months after starting therapy and then yearly
- hepatitis B status should be evaluated before starting therapy, as reactivation can occur
- therapy may be discontinued after 3 years depending on BCR-ABL transcript levels and the molecular response. If therapy is discontinued, the patient should be closely monitored thereafter
- tablets contain lactose and are therefore not recommended in those with galactose intolerance, lactase insufficiency or glucose—galactose malabsorption
- bioavailability may be reduced in patients with total gastrectomy
- caution if used in those with known congenital or acquired QT prolongation or electrolyte imbalance (especially hypokalaemia and hypomagnesaemia)
- caution if used in those with a history of pancreatitis, pre-existing cardiac history or significant cardiac risk factors
- see also General Nursing considerations for protein kinase inhibitors (p. 691)

Patient education
- if the patient is taking antacids, advise them to take these either 2 hours before or after taking capsules
- instruct the patient to take an H_2-receptor antagonist (e.g. famotidine) 2 hours before or 10 hours after capsules
- if the patient is unable to swallow the capsule whole, suggest that its contents can be sprinkled on a teaspoon of apple sauce and swallowed
- instruct the patient to seek medical advice immediately if any of the following occur:
  - rapid or irregular heart rate
  - pain or discomfort in chest, difficulty breathing, shortness of breath
  - abdominal pain (left upper side), back pain, nausea, vomiting, feeling bloated, loss of appetite, fat in stools
  - sudden unexplained weight gain

- see also General Patient education for protein kinase inhibitors (p. 692)

 Capsule may be opened and added to one teaspoon of apple puree (no other food or yoghurt should be used). Gloves and mask should be worn when opening capsules. Pregnant staff should not open capsules.

NINTEDANIB
Trade name
Ofev

Available forms
Capsules: 100 mg, 150 mg

Action
- tyrosine kinase inhibitor blocking vascular endothelial growth factor receptors, platelet-derived growth factor receptors and fibroblast growth factor receptors kinase activity
- half-life 10—15 hours

Use
- idiopathic pulmonary fibrosis (IPF), or other chronic interstitial lung diseases (ILD)
- locally advanced, metastatic or recurrent non-small cell lung cancer (NSCLC) (after failure of first-line treatment) (with docetaxel)
- slowing rate of pulmonary function decline in those with sclerosis-associated interstitial lung disease (SSc-ILD)

Dose
- (NSCLC) 200 mg orally twice daily with food on days 2 to 21 of a 21-day cycle (with docetaxel given on day 1) **OR**
- (IFP, SSc-ILD) 150 mg orally twice daily with food

Adverse effects
- gastrointestinal (GI) perforation, ischaemic colitis
- hyperbilirubinaemia
- thromboembolic events
- see also General Adverse effects of protein kinase inhibitors (p. 691)

Interactions
- increased risk of GI perforation if given with corticosteroids or NSAIDs
- see also General Interactions of protein kinase inhibitors (p. 691)

Nursing considerations/Cautions
- (NSCLC) nintedanib can be continued alone after starting docetaxel until a clinical response is evident or toxicity occurs
- should not be started within 4 weeks of gastrointestinal surgery
- capsules contain soya lecithin
- caution if used in those who have had previous abdominal surgery, or a history of diverticular or peptic ulcer disease, because of the risk of GI perforation
- caution if used in females, those of low body weight or of Asian race because of the increased risk of elevated liver enzymes
- caution if used in those with active brain metastases because of the increased risk of cerebral haemorrhage
- not recommended in those with an inherited predisposition to bleeding or receiving a full dose of anticoagulant therapy
- not recommended in those who have had recent lung haemorrhage, centrally located tumours with invasion of major blood vessels or necrotic tumours
- not recommended in those with moderate-to-severe liver impairment
- contraindicated in those with hypersensitivity to nintedanib, peanut or soya
- see also General Nursing considerations/Cautions for protein kinase inhibitors (p. 692)

Patient education
- if the patient has problems swallowing, the capsule can be taken with a teaspoon of cold or room temperature soft food such as apple puree or

ANTINEOPLASTIC AGENTS

- chocolate pudding. The capsule must be swallowed whole and not chewed
- caution patient not to use NSAIDs for pain management
- the patient should be instructed to seek medical advice immediately if they experience any moderate-to-severe diarrhoea, new or worsening abdominal pain, chills, fever, nausea or vomiting
- see also General Patient education for protein kinase inhibitors (p. 692)

Capsules should not be opened or chewed.

Not recommended in those with moderate (Child–Pugh Class B) or severe (Child–Pugh Class C) liver impairment.

OLAPARIB
Trade name
Lynparza

Available forms
Tablets: 100 mg, 150 mg

Action
- inhibitor of human poly (ADP ribose) polymerase (PARP) enzymes
- PARP enzymes are needed for efficient single-strand DNA repair
- half-life 15 hours

Use
- epithelial ovarian, fallopian tube or primary peritoneal cancer (monotherapy or combination)
- high-risk HER2-negative early breast cancer previously treated with neoadjuvant or adjuvant chemotherapy (as adjuvant, monotherapy)
- metastatic HER2-negative breast cancer previously treated with chemotherapy
- metastatic pancreatic cancer (as maintenance therapy where disease has not progressed on at least 16 weeks of platinum-based therapy)
- prostate cancer (monotherapy or combination)

Dose
- 300 mg orally twice daily

Adverse effects
- myelodysplastic syndrome, acute myeloid leukaemia
- see also General Adverse effects of protein kinase inhibitors (p. 691)

Interactions
- not recommended with statins
- caution if used with bosentan, efavirenz, modafinil or etravirine, as serum levels may be decreased
- see also General Interactions of protein kinase inhibitors (p. 691)

Nursing considerations/Cautions
- BRCA mutation status should be confirmed by a valid and reliable test before starting therapy
- an increased risk of pneumonitis in those with lung cancer, lung metastasis, underlying lung disease, smoking history, previous radiotherapy or chemotherapy
- not recommended in those with severe kidney disease, end-stage kidney disease or severe liver disease
- see also General Nursing considerations/Cautions for protein kinase inhibitors (p. 691)

Patient education
- advise the patient to swallow tablets whole (not crushed, broken or chewed) with water
- the patient should be instructed to seek medical advice immediately if any of the following occur: pale skin, pin point bleeding under the skin, feeling weak or tired, easy bleeding or bruising, shortness of breath
- see also General Patient education for protein kinase inhibitors (p. 692)

Tablets should not be crushed, broken or chewed.

For those with moderate kidney impairment, the recommended dose is 200 mg orally twice daily.

Not recommended in those with severe renal impairment or end-stage renal disease (CrCl > 30 mL/min).

Not recommended in those with severe liver impairment (Child–Pugh Class C).

PALBOCICLIB

Trade name
Ibrance

Available forms
Tablets: 75 mg, 100 mg, 125 mg

Action
- small molecule inhibitor of cyclin-dependent kinases (CDK) 4 and 6, which are involved in cellular proliferation
- half-life 28.8 hours

Use
- hormone receptor (HR)-positive, human epidermal growth factor receptor (HER2)-negative advanced or metastatic breast cancer in combination with either an aromatase inhibitor as initial endocrine-based therapy, or with fulvestrant in those who have received previous therapy

Dose
- 125 mg orally daily for 21 consecutive days, followed by a 7-day drug-free interval (cycle 28 days) with an aromatase inhibitor or fulvestrant (500 mg IM on days 1, 15 and 29 of cycle, and then monthly)

Adverse effects
- see General Adverse effects of protein kinase inhibitors (p. 691)

Interactions
- see General Interactions of protein kinase inhibitors (p. 691)

Nursing considerations/Cautions
- for pre- or perimenopausal women, a luteinising hormone releasing hormone (LHRH) agonist should also be prescribed
- for men treated with combination therapy with aromatase inhibitor, luteinising hormone releasing hormone (LHRH) agonist is recommended
- see also General Nursing considerations/Cautions for protein kinase inhibitors (p. 691)

Patient education
- see General Patient education for protein kinase inhibitors (p. 692)

Tablet should not be broken, crushed or chewed; however, it may be dispersed in 15 mL boiling water and stirred gently for 2 minutes. Another 15 mL of boiling water and stirred gently for a further 2 minutes. 15 mL of room temperature water should be added and vigorously stirred for 10 seconds. After dose is administered, glass should be rinsed with 15 mL of water to ensure full dose has been taken. Pregnant staff should not disperse tablet.

For those with severe liver impairment, the recommended dose is 75 mg orally daily for 21 consecutive days followed by a 7-day drug-free interval.

PAZOPANIB

Trade name
Votrient

Available forms
Tablets: 200 mg, 400 mg

Action
- multi-target tyrosine kinase inhibitor of vascular endothelial growth factor receptors (VEGFR)
- half-life 30.9 hours

Use
- advanced metastatic renal cell carcinoma (RCC)
- advanced metastatic unresectable soft tissue sarcoma (STS) (with prior chemotherapy)

ANTINEOPLASTIC AGENTS

Dose
- 800 mg orally once daily 1 hour before or 2 hours after food

Adverse effects
- severe and fatal hepatotoxicity
- prolongation of QT interval
- gastrointestinal perforation
- delayed wound healing
- proteinuria, nephrotic syndrome
- posterior reversible encephalopathy syndrome
- see also General Adverse effects of protein kinase inhibitors (p. 691)

Interactions
- not recommended with proton pump inhibitors or other agents that increase gastric pH
- caution if given with simvastatin, as increased serum enzymes (alanine aminotransferase (ALT)) may occur, increasing the risk of hepatotoxicity
- not recommended with agents known to prolong QT interval or cause electrolyte imbalance (especially hypokalaemia or hypomagnesaemia)
- may increase serum levels of dextromethorphan, irinotecan, midazolam, paclitaxel and rosuvastatin, increasing the risk of adverse effects
- see also General Interactions of protein kinase inhibitors (p. 691)

Nursing considerations/Cautions
- liver function tests are recommended before starting therapy, then at weeks 3, 7 and 9, month 3, month 4 and regularly thereafter
- urinalysis should be conducted before starting and regularly throughout therapy to detect any worsening proteinuria that may lead to nephrotic syndrome
- therapy should be stopped 7 days before surgery to decrease the risk of wound-healing complications
- caution if used in those with a history of congenital or acquired QT prolongation or at risk of electrolyte imbalance
- caution if used in those at risk of gastrointestinal perforation or fistula formation
- not recommended in those with severe kidney impairment or severe liver impairment
- see also General Nursing considerations/Cautions for protein kinase inhibitors (p. 691)

Patient education
- instruct the patient to seek medical advice immediately if any of the following occur:
  - irregular or pounding heartbeat, chest pain,
  - headache, fitting (seizures), lethargy, confusion, visual disturbances
  - severe abdominal pain
- see also General Patient education for protein kinase inhibitors (p. 692)

 Tablets should not be crushed, broken or chewed.

 For those with moderate liver impairment, recommended dose is 200 mg orally daily 1 hour before or 2 hours after food. Not recommended in those with severe kidney impairment or severe liver impairment.

PONATINIB
Trade name
Iclusig

Available forms
Tablets: 15 mg, 45 mg

Action
- tyrosine kinase inhibitor that reduces viability of cells with a BCR-ABL mutation
- half-life 22 hours

Use
- chronic, accelerated or blast phase chronic myeloid leukaemia (CML) (resistant to or intolerant of ≥ 2 prior tyrosine kinase inhibitors) or with a T3151 mutation
- Philadelphia chromosome-positive acute lymphoblastic leukaemia (ALL)

(resistant to or intolerant of dasatinib where subsequent imatinib is not appropriate) or with a T3151 mutation

Dose
- (Chronic phase CML) initially 45 mg orally daily, reducing to 15 mg orally daily once a molecular response has been achieved ($\leq 1\%$ BCR-ABL1^{IS}) **OR**
- (Accelerated or blast phase CML, ALL) 45 mg orally daily

Adverse effects
- heart failure
- ocular toxicity
- peripheral neuropathy
- fluid retention (including peripheral oedema, ascites, pleural effusion, pericardial effusion)
- new or worsening hypertension, hypertensive crisis
- thromboembolism, arterial occlusion, retinal arterial occlusion
- peripheral neuropathy
- pancreatitis
- tumour lysis syndrome
- see also General Adverse effects of protein kinase inhibitors (p. 691)

Interactions
- may increase serum levels of digoxin, colchicine, dabigatran, pravastatin, methotrexate, sulfasalazine and rosuvastatin, increasing the risk of adverse effects
- see also General Interactions of protein kinase inhibitors (p. 691)

Nursing considerations/Cautions
- ensure the patient is well hydrated during therapy
- cardiovascular status should be assessed before starting therapy and any identified risk factors managed
- BP should be monitored regularly during therapy
- uric acid levels should be checked before starting therapy and any hyperuricaemia managed
- tablets contain lactose; therefore not recommended in those with lactose intolerance
- caution if used in those with a history of pancreatitis or alcohol abuse
- not recommended in those with history of myocardial infarction, stroke or revascularisation unless benefits outweigh risks
- caution if used in those with severe kidney impairment or end-stage kidney disease
- see also General Nursing considerations/Cautions for protein kinase inhibitors (p. 691)

Patient education
- the patient should be advised to swallow the tablet whole (without crushing, breaking or chewing)
- instruct the patient to seek medical advice immediately if any of the following occur:
  - shortness of breath, chest pain, weakness on one side of body, leg pain or swelling, decreased or blurred vision, speech problems
  - shortness of breath, chest pain, palpitations, fluid retention, dizziness or fainting
  - headache, dizziness, chest pain or shortness of breath
  - nausea, vomiting, abdominal tenderness or discomfort, loss of appetite, yellowing of skin or whites of the eyes
  - leg or calf swelling, weight gain, shortness of breath
  - decreased or blurred vision, changes to vision
- see also General Patient education for protein kinase inhibitors (p. 692)

 Tablets should not be crushed, broken or chewed.

 For those with moderate-to-severe liver impairment, the recommended dose is 30 mg orally daily.

ANTINEOPLASTIC AGENTS

RIBOCICLIB
Trade name
Kisqali

Available form
Tablet: 200 mg

Action
- protein kinase inhibitor that inhibits cyclin-dependent kinases (CDK) 4 and 6
- half-life 29.7—54.7 hours

Use
- hormone receptor (HR)-positive, human epidermal growth factor receptor 2 (HER2)-negative advanced or metastatic breast cancer (in combination with an aromatase inhibitor or fulvestrant as initial endocrine-based therapy or following prior endocrine therapy)

Dose
- 600 mg orally once daily for 21 consecutive days, followed by a 7-day drug free interval (28-day cycle) with either aromatase inhibitor (taken daily for 28 days) or fulvestrant (500 mg on days 1, 15, and 29, and then once monthly)

Adverse effects
- QTc interval prolongation
- severe cutaneous reaction
- blood creatinine increase
- see also General Adverse effects of protein kinase inhibitors (p. 691)

Interactions
- not recommended with tamoxifen because of an increased risk of QT prolongation
- not recommended with agents known to prolong QT interval or cause electrolyte imbalance
- see also General Interactions of protein kinase inhibitors (p. 691)

Nursing considerations/Cautions
- if the woman is pre- or perimenopausal, therapy should be administered with a luteinising hormone-releasing hormone (LHRH) agonist
- before starting therapy, ECG and serum electrolytes (particularly potassium, calcium, phosphate and magnesium), and liver and kidney functions should be measured
- any electrolyte imbalance should be corrected before starting therapy
- caution if used in those with severe kidney impairment
- tablets contain soya lecithin and are not recommended in those with hypersensitivity
- contraindicated in those with congenital long QT syndrome, if the correct QT interval is > 450 milliseconds or are at risk of developing QTc prolongation such as those with significant cardiac disease, recent myocardial infarction, congestive cardiac failure, unstable angina, brady arrhythmias and electrolyte abnormalities
- see also General Nursing considerations/Cautions for protein kinase inhibitors (p. 691)

Patient education
- instruct the patient to swallow tablets whole and not chew, crush or split them

Tablet should not be crushed, chewed or split.

Starting dose of 400 mg orally daily is recommended for those with moderate or severe liver impairment.

RUXOLITINIB
Trade name
Jakavi

Available forms
Tablets: 5 mg, 10 mg, 15 mg, 20 mg

Action
- Janus-associated kinases (JAK1, JAK2) inhibitors (JAK1 dysregulation and JAK2 signalling are associated with polycythaemia and myelofibrosis)
- two major active metabolites contributing about 20% activity

- half-life 3 hours

Use
- disease-related splenomegaly or symptoms of primary myelofibrosis, post-polycythaemia vera myelofibrosis or post-essential thrombocythaemia myelofibrosis
- polycythaemia (in patients resistant or intolerant to hydroxycarbamide (hydroxyurea))
- (Patients 12 years and over) treatment of acute or chronic graft versus host disease with inadequate response to corticosteroids

Dose
- (Myelofibrosis, platelet count 50–100 × 10^9/L) 5 mg orally twice daily **OR**
- (Myelofibrosis, platelet count 100–200 × 10^9/L) 15 mg orally twice daily **OR**
- (Myelofibrosis, platelet count > 200 × 10^9/L) 20 mg orally twice daily **OR**
- (Polycythaemia vera) initially 10 mg orally daily for 4 weeks, increasing at 5 mg increments at $\geq$ 2-week intervals based on response (maximum 25 mg twice daily)
- (Acute graft versus host) 5–10 mg orally twice daily **OR**
- (Chronic graft versus host) 10 mg orally twice daily

Adverse effects
- increased liver enzymes, cholesterol and triglycerides
- herpes zoster (shingles)
- non-melanoma skin cancer
- cardiovascular events
- diverticulitis, GI perforation
- see also General Adverse effects of protein kinase inhibitors (p. 691)

Interactions
- not recommended with fluconazole > 200 mg daily
- see also General Interactions of protein kinase inhibitors (p. 691)

Nursing considerations/Cautions
- liver enzymes, cholesterol and triglycerides should be measured before starting and regularly throughout therapy
- (Polycythaemia vera) therapy should be stopped after 6 months if there has been no reduction in spleen size or improvement in symptoms
- caution if used in those with diverticular disease (especially those receiving corticosteroids, NSAIDs or opioids)
- caution if used in those who are current smokers or with significant cardiac risk factors
- not recommended in those with end-stage kidney disease not receiving dialysis
- see also General Nursing considerations/Cautions for protein kinase inhibitors (p. 691)

Patient education
- advise the patient to swallow the tablets whole (without crushing, breaking or chewing)
- (Myelofibrosis) warn the patient against suddenly stopping therapy, as symptoms of myelofibrosis may return over about 7 days
- the patient should be instructed to seek medical advice immediately if any of the following occur:
  - numbness, itching, tingling or burning pain (which may occur days or weeks before rash appears), flu-like symptoms (usually without fever), rash (usually restricted on one side of body) with blisters (blisters may open, ooze and crust over in 5 days) and a rash that takes 2–4 weeks to heal. Pain may also occur with a rash
  - confusion, trouble thinking, memory loss, blurred vision, loss of vision, balance or walking problems, decreased strength in arms or legs
- see also General Patient education for protein kinase inhibitors (p. 692)

ANTINEOPLASTIC AGENTS

Tablets should not be crushed or broken.

Moderate-to-severe kidney impairment
- **(myelofibrosis) dose should be reduced by 50%**
- **(polycythaemia vera) recommended dose is 5 mg orally twice daily. End-stage kidney disease on dialysis: recommended dose is 10 mg orally after dialysis.**

Liver impairment:
- **(myelofibrosis) dose should be reduced by 50%**
- **(polycythaemia vera) recommended dose is 5 mg orally twice daily.**

SELPERCATINIB
Trade name
Retevmo

Available forms
Capsules: 40 mg, 80 mg

Action
- small molecule inhibitor of rearranged during transfection (RET) receptor tyrosine kinase with activity against human cancer cells derived from multiple tumour types with RET fusion genes and RET mutations
- half-life 22 hours

Use
- locally advanced or metastatic RET fusion-positiveon-small cell lung cancer (NSCLC)

Dose
- (Patient weight < 50 kg) 120 mg orally twice daily
- (Patient weight ≥ 50 kg) 160 mg orally twice daily

Adverse effects
- QT interval prolongation
- hypertension
- hypothyroidism
- impaired wound healing
- tumour lysis syndrome
- see also General Adverse effects of protein kinase inhibitors (p. 691)

Interactions
- caution if given with other agents known to prolong QT interval
- may increase serum levels of cerivastatin, enzalutamide, paclitaxel, repaglinide, sorafenib, rosiglitazone, buprenorphine, selexipag, dasabuvir, montelukast, midazolam, alfentanil, avanafil, darifenacin, darunavir, lovastatin, simvastatin, triazolam or vardenafil, and these are not recommended together
- caution if used with fexofenadine, dabigatran etexilate, colchicine, saxagliptin or digoxin
- see also General Interactions of protein kinase inhibitors (p. 691)

Nursing considerations/Cautions
- any hypokalaemia, hypocalcaemia and hypomagnesaemia should be corrected before starting therapy
- ECG and serum electrolytes should be measured after 1 week of therapy and then monthly for first 6 months, with the frequency of monitoring dependent on risk factors such as the patient developing nausea, vomiting and/or diarrhoea
- thyroid function should be measured before starting and regularly during therapy. Thyroid hormone replacement is recommended if hypothyroidism occurs
- therapy should be stopped for at least 7 days before surgery, and not restarted for at least 2 weeks after major surgery
- caution if used in those with congenital long QT syndrome, acquired long QT syndrome or other conditions that predispose to arrhythmias such as electrolyte imbalance
- see also General Nursing considerations/Cautions for protein kinase inhibitors (p. 691)

Patient education

- the patient should be instructed to:
  - swallow capsule whole (not opening, chewing or crushing capsules) with or without food at the same time every day.
  - if the patient is also taking a proton pump inhibitor (e.g. omeprazole, pantoprazole), they should be instructed to take selpercatinib with a meal
  - if the patient is taking a H$_2$ receptor antagonist (e.g. ranitidine), selpercatinib should be taken either 2 hours before or 10 hours after the H$_2$ receptor antagonist
  - antacids should be taken either 2 hours before or 2 hours after selpercatinib
- see also General Patient education for protein kinase inhibitors (p. 692)

Capsules should not be opened, crushed or chewed.

Patients with severe liver impairment (Child—Pugh class C) should receive 80 mg orally twice daily.

SELUMETINIB
Trade name
Koselugo

Available forms
Capsules: 10 mg, 25 mg

Action
- inhibitor of mitogen-activated protein kinase kinases 1 and 2 (MEK1/2) (MEK inhibition can block proliferation and survival of tumour cells)
- active metabolite
- half-life 6.2 hours

Use
- treatment of neurofibromatosis type 1 with symptomatic, inoperable plexiform neurofibromas (in children aged 2 years and older)

Dose
- 25 mg/m^2 orally twice daily

Adverse effects
- decreased left ventricle ejection fraction (LVEF), sinus tachycardia
- blurred vision, decreased visual acuity
- haematuria, proteinuria
- increased creatine phosphokinase (CPK), myalgia
- see also General Adverse effects of protein kinase inhibitors (p. 691)

Interactions
- may alter effectiveness of hormonal contraceptives
- not recommended with vitamin E supplements, especially in those taking anticoagulant or antiplatelet agents, because of the increased risk of bleeding. INR or prothrombin time should be closely monitored during therapy
- see also General Interactions of protein kinase inhibitors (p. 691)

Nursing considerations/Cautions

- the patient should be assessed for ability to swallow capsule before starting therapy
- LVEF should be measured before starting and at 3-monthly intervals during therapy. If LVEF is reduced, therapy may need to be interrupted, or the dose reduced or discontinued
- ophthalmological evaluation is recommended before starting therapy and if any visual disturbances occur. If retinal pigment epithelial detachment or central serous retinopathy occurs, therapy should be withheld and monitored every 3 weeks until symptoms resolve and resumed at a reduced dose. If retinal vein occlusion occurs, therapy should be stopped permanently
- CPK should be measured before starting and regularly during therapy. If CPK levels increase, the patient should be evaluated for rhabdomyolysis

ANTINEOPLASTIC AGENTS

- a pregnancy test should be performed in women of childbearing potential before starting therapy
- an increased risk of choking in children < 6 years
- not recommended in women of childbearing potential not using contraception
- not recommended in those with severe liver impairment
- not recommended in those who are unable or unwilling to swallow capsule whole
- see also General Nursing considerations/Cautions for protein kinase inhibitors (p. 691)

Patient education

- the patient/parent/carer should be advised that the capsule should be taken on empty stomach with water and should not be chewed, dissolved or opened. Food should not be consumed 2 hours before or 1 hour after administration
- the patient/parent/carer should be instructed to start an antidiarrhoeal agent (e.g. loperamide) at the first signs of unformed loose stool, as well as increasing fluid intake
- warn the patient/parent/carer to avoid vitamin E supplements during therapy. Capsules contain vitamin E (32 mg in 10 mg capsule; 36 mg in 25 mg capsule)
- instruct the patient/parent/carer that:
  - if vomiting occurs, an extra dose should not be given
  - if dose is missed, it should be given only if it is more than 6 hours before the next dose is due
- women of childbearing potential should be counselled to use effective contraception during and for 1 week after stopping therapy. Furthermore, they should be advised that an additional barrier method should be used in addition to a hormonal contraceptive
- male patients with female partners of reproductive age should be counselled to use effective contraception during and for 1 week after stopping therapy
- see also General Patient education for protein kinase inhibitors (p. 692)

Capsule should not be opened, chewed or dissolved.

For moderate liver impairment, the recommended dose is 20 mg/m² orally twice daily.

SORAFENIB TOSILATE (SORAFENIB TOSYLATE)

Trade name
Nexavar

Available form
Tablet: 200 mg

Action
- multi-kinase inhibitor that targets receptors of tyrosine kinase and rapidly accelerated fibrosarcoma (RAF) kinases associated with tumour growth
- active metabolite
- half-life 25–48 hours

Use
- advanced renal cell carcinoma
- advanced hepatocellular carcinoma
- locally advanced or metastatic differentiated thyroid cancer (refractory to radioactive iodine)

Dose
- 400 mg orally twice daily

Adverse effects
- cardiac ischaemia, myocardial infarction, QT prolongation
- (Thyroid cancer) hypocalcaemia, thyroid-stimulating hormone (TSH) suppression
- see also General Adverse effects of protein kinase inhibitors (p. 691)

Interactions
- caution if given with warfarin; INR should be closely monitored especially when starting or stopping therapy
- caution if used with docetaxel or irinotecan

- caution if used with agents known to prolong QT interval or cause electrolyte imbalance (especially hypokalaemia or hypomagnesaemia)
- see also General Interactions of protein kinase inhibitors (p. 691)

Nursing considerations/Cautions

- (Differentiated thyroid cancer) calcium levels and TSH should be monitored during therapy. Thyroxine dose should be adjusted if needed
- caution if used in those with recent myocardial infarction or unstable coronary artery ischaemia
- caution if used in those with known congenital or acquired QT prolongation or electrolyte imbalance
- see also General Nursing considerations/Cautions for protein kinase inhibitors (p. 691)

Patient education

- advise the patient that the tablet should be swallowed whole (not broken, crushed or chewed) on an empty stomach or with a moderate-fat meal
- instruct the patient to seek medical advice if any of the following occur:
    - abnormal or rapid heart rate
    - chest pain that may spread to shoulder or neck
- see also General Patient education for protein kinase inhibitors (p. 692)

 Tablet should not be crushed, broken or chewed.

SOTORASIB
Trade name
Lumakras

Available form
Tablet: 120 mg

Action
- KRAS^{G12C} inhibitor which irreversibly binds to the unique cysteine of KRAS^{G12C}, blocking tumour cell signalling and survival, inhibiting cell growth and promoting selective apoptosis in tumours with the KRAS^{G12C} gene
- half-life 5 hours

Use
- KRAS^{G12C} mutated locally advanced or metastatic non-small cell lung cancer (NSCLC) in those who have received at least one systemic therapy for advanced disease

Dose
- 960 mg orally daily

Adverse effects
- see General Adverse effects of protein kinase inhibitors (p. 691)

Interactions
- not recommended with proton pump inhibitors (e.g. omeprazole) or H$_2$-receptor antagonists (e.g. famotidine)
- may increase serum levels of digoxin, increasing risk of adverse effects
- see also General Interactions of protein kinase inhibitors (p. 691)

Nursing considerations/Cautions

- KRAS^{G12C} mutation should be confirmed by a validated test before starting therapy
- contains lactose and therefore is not recommended in those with rare hereditary problems of galactose intolerance, lactase deficiency or glucose—galactose malabsorption
- see also General Nursing considerations/Cautions for protein kinase inhibitors (p. 691)

Patient education

- advise the patient to swallow tablets whole and not chew, crush or split them. If the patient has problems swallowing, tablets can be dispersed in 120 mL of room temperature water (no other liquids should be used). The resulting mixture will be pale yellow to bright yellow and should be swallowed

ANTINEOPLASTIC AGENTS

immediately or within 2 hours of being dispersed. The glass should be rinsed with another 120 mL of water and swallowed immediately. If the solution is not drunk immediately, it should be stirred before swallowing
- instruct the patient that sotorasib should be taken either 4 hours before or 10 hours after acid-reducing agents such as proton pump inhibitors or H_2-receptor antagonists
- see also General Patient education for protein kinase inhibitors (p. 692)

Tablets should not be crushed, split or chewed; however, tablet can be dispersed in 120 mL of water.

SUNITINIB

Trade names
ARX-Sunitinib, Sunitinib MSN, Sunitinib Sandoz, Sutent

Available forms
Capsules: 12.5 mg, 25 mg, 37.5 mg, 50 mg

Action
- multiple receptor tyrosine kinase inhibitor which stops replication of tumour cells
- active metabolite (half-life 80—110 hours)
- half-life 40—60 hours

Use
- advanced renal cell carcinoma (RCC)
- gastrointestinal stromal tumour (GIST) (after imatinib failure)
- unresectable well-differentiated pancreatic neuroendocrine tumour (NET)

Dose
- (Metastatic RCC, GIST) 50 mg orally daily for 4 consecutive weeks, followed by a 2-week rest interval (6-week cycle) **OR**
- (Pancreatic NET) 37.5 mg orally daily, adjusting in 12.5 mg increments if needed

Adverse effects
- prolongation of QT interval
- osteonecrosis of the jaw
- thromboembolic events, aneurysm, artery dissection
- proteinuria
- hypoglycaemia
- thyroid dysfunction
- (Rare) seizures, necrotising fasciitis
- see also General Adverse effects of protein kinase inhibitors (p. 691)

Interactions
- caution if given with other agents known to prolong QT interval (e.g. amiodarone, clarithromycin, disopyramide, methadone, sotalol) or cause electrolyte imbalance (e.g. diuretics)
- increased risk of osteonecrosis of the jaw if given with or after IV bisphosphonates
- see also General Interactions of protein kinase inhibitors (p. 691)

Nursing considerations/Cautions
- BP should be monitored regularly as hypertension occurs, especially during the early stages of treatment
- urine should be tested for protein regularly during therapy
- any hypomagnesaemia and hypokalaemia should be corrected before starting therapy
- thyroid function should be measured and any imbalance treated before starting therapy
- caution if given in those with known congenital or acquired prolongation of QT interval or at risk of electrolyte imbalance (especially hypokalaemia and hypomagnesaemia)
- not recommended in those who have had a myocardial infarction, severe or unstable angina, coronary artery bypass graft surgery, stroke, pulmonary embolism or transient ischaemic attack in last 12 months
- see also General Nursing considerations/Cautions for protein kinase inhibitors (p. 691)

Patient education
- advise the patient to swallow the capsule whole (not chewed or opened)

- those with diabetes should be warned to monitor blood glucose levels during therapy as hypoglycaemia may occur
- instruct the patient to seek medical advice immediately if any of the following occur:
  - jaw or dental pain, bleeding gums, sores on gums or jaw
  - irregular heart rate
  - cough, shortness of breath, difficulty breathing, swollen calf that is red, warm and tender
- encourage the patient to practise good dental hygiene, including brushing teeth and tongue after meals and before bed, daily flossing to remove plaque and using a mirror to check teeth and gums regularly for any sores or bleeding of the gums
- see also General Patient education for protein kinase inhibitors (p. 692)

 Capsules should not be opened, crushed or chewed.

TALAZOPARIB
Trade name
Talzenna

Available forms
Capsule: 100 microgram, 250 microgram, 350 microgram, 500 microgram

Action
- poly (ADP-ribose) polymerase (PARP)-1, 2 inhibitor

Use
- HER2-negative, locally advanced/metastatic breast cancer with deleterious/suspected deleterious germline BRCA mutation
- combination therapy with enzalutamide for homologous recombination repair (HRR) muted metastatic castration resistant prostate cancer

Dose
- (Breast cancer) 1 mg orally daily **OR**
- (Prostate cancer) 500 micrograms orally daily (with enzalutamide and concurrent luteinising hormone-releasing hormone (LHRH) analogue or prior bilateral orchiectomy)

Adverse effects
- see General Adverse effects of protein kinase inhibitors (p. 691)

Interactions
- see General Interactions of protein kinase inhibitors (p. 691)

Nursing considerations/Cautions
- before starting therapy, BRCA mutation and HRR status should be confirmed using a validated test
- see also General Nursing considerations/Cautions for protein kinase inhibitors (p. 691)

Patient education
- advise the patient to swallow capsules whole (without opening, crushing or chewing)
- see also General Patient education for protein kinase inhibitors (p. 692)

 Capsules should not be opened, crushed or chewed.

TRAMETINIB
Trade name
Mekinist

Available forms
Tablets: 0.5 mg, 2 mg;
Powder for oral solution: 0.05 mg/mL

Action
- protein kinase (MEK) inhibitor
- MEK (mitogen activated extracellular signal regulated kinase) proteins are critical in activating mutated BRAF pathways resulting in tumour growth
- half-life 5.3 days

Use
- BRAF V600-positive unresectable stage III or metastatic stage IV melanoma (with dabrafenib)
- BRAF V600-positive unresectable stage III or metastatic stage IV melanoma (as

ANTINEOPLASTIC AGENTS

- monotherapy, intolerant to or where BRAF inhibitor can't be used)
- adjuvant therapy for BRAF V600-positive melanoma after lymph node resection (with dabrafenib)
- BRAF V600-positive locally advanced or metastatic anaplastic thyroid cancer (with dabrafenib)
- BRAF V600-positive advanced non-small cell lung cancer (with dabrafenib)
- BRAF V600-positivelow-grade glioma (with dabrafenib)(patient aged 12 months or older)
- BRAF V600-positivehigh-grade glioma where disease has progressed and there are no alternate options (with dabrafenib) (patient aged 12 months or older)

Dose
- (Adults) 2 mg orally daily 1 hour before or 2 hours after food (monotherapy or with dabrafenib) **OR**
- (Children) taken 1 hour before or 2 hours after food:
  - (patient weight) 26 to 37 kg) 1 mg orally daily
  - (patient weight 38 to 50 kg) 1.5 mg orally daily
  - (patient weight 51 kg or greater) 2 mg orally daily

Adverse effects
- retinal pigment epithelial detachment, retinal vein occlusion, visual impairment
- left ventricular ejection fraction (LVEF) dysfunction
- see also General Adverse effects of protein kinase inhibitors (p. 691)

Nursing considerations/Cautions
- BRAF V600 mutation should be confirmed using a valid and reliable test
- tablets and powder for oral solution are not bioequivalent nor interchangeable
- LVEF should be evaluated using echocardiogram before starting therapy, 1 month after starting and then 3-monthly
- urgent (within 24 hours) ophthalmological review should be organised if the patient experiences any visual changes
- (Melanoma-adjunctive therapy) treatment should be for 12 months only
- not recommended for BRAF V600 mutation-positive melanoma that has metastasised to brain
- see also General Nursing considerations/Cautions for protein kinase inhibitors (p. 691)

Patient education
- if tablets are being administered, the patient should be advised to swallow them whole (without crushing, breaking or chewing)
- instruct the patient to seek medical advice immediately if any of the following occur:
  - decreased central vision, blurry vision or loss of vision
  - increased heart rate, palpitations, shortness of breath, swelling of ankles, dizziness, lightheadedness
- if the patient is taking dabrafenib as well, the two should be taken at same time (morning or evening)
- if using reconstituted solution, it should be kept refrigerated (not frozen) and discarded 35 days after reconstitution by pharmacist
- see also General Patient education for protein kinase inhibitors (p. 692)

 Tablets should not be crushed, broken or chewed.

VANDETANIB
Trade name
Caprelsa

Available form
Tablet: 100 mg

Action
- tyrosine kinase inhibitor that inhibits vascular endothelial growth factor (VEGF) stimulated endothelial cell migration, proliferation, survival and new blood vessel formation, resulting in an inhibition of tumour growth
- half-life 19 days

Use
- symptomatic or progressive medullary thyroid (in those with unresectable locally advanced or metastatic disease)

Dose
- 300 mg orally daily

Adverse effects
- prolonged QT interval, ventricular arrhythmias (including torsades de pointes), sudden death
- see also General Adverse effects of protein kinase inhibitors (p. 691)

Interactions
- not recommended with other agents known to prolong QT interval or cause electrolyte imbalance
- caution if used with cyclosporin, tacrolimus, docetaxel or bortezomib
- may increase serum levels of dabigatran and digoxin; therefore close monitoring is recommended especially in first 2 months of therapy
- may decrease elimination of metformin, increasing serum levels
- caution if used with warfarin; more frequent monitoring of INR is recommended
- see also General Interactions of protein kinase inhibitors (p. 691)

Nursing considerations/Cautions
- correct any electrolyte imbalance before starting therapy
- before starting, an ECG, potassium, magnesium and calcium levels and thyroid stimulating hormone levels should be obtained and then repeated 1, 3, 6 and 12 weeks after starting therapy, then 3-monthly for at least 12 months
- serum potassium should be maintained at 4 mmol/L or higher, with serum calcium and magnesium maintained within the normal range
- blood pressure should be monitored and, if not able to be controlled with medical management, dose reduction may be necessary
- if patient develops diarrhoea, worsening diarrhoea, dehydration, electrolyte imbalance and/or impaired kidney function, additional ECG, electrolyte and renal function monitoring is recommended to decrease the risk of QTc prolongation
- because vandetanib has a long half-life (19 days), adverse reactions (including prolonged QTc interval) will take time to resolve
- the risk of prolonged QTc interval will continue for some time after therapy is stopped (because of long half-life)
- caution if used in those with history of aneurysm (especially if hypertension is also present) because of the increased risk of aneurysm and artery dissection
- not recommended in those with congenital long QT syndrome, if the corrected QTc interval is > 480 msec, a history of ventricular arrhythmias or torsades de pointes (unless risk factors have been corrected)
- not recommended in those with severe kidney impairment or liver impairment, a recent history of haemoptysis (1/2 teaspoon of red blood), NYHA classification class 2 or greater heart failure
- women of childbearing potential, fertile men (ensure effective contraception including $\geq$ 4 months after last dose)

Patient education
- the patient should be advised that if, they have difficulty swallowing tablets, these can be dispersed in 50 mL of non-carbonated water (tap or still water). No other fluids should be used. The tablet should be dropped into water without crushing and allowed to disperse (about 10 minutes) and then swallowed immediately. The glass should be rinsed with half a glass of water and swallowed
- instruct the patient not to crush the tablet. If the tablet becomes crushed, direct contact should be avoided and, if accidental contact occurs, area should be thoroughly washed

ANTINEOPLASTIC AGENTS

- advise the patient to avoid excessive sun exposure and wear protective clothing and sunscreen (SPF 30+) during and for 4 months after stopping therapy

The tablet should not be crushed; however, it can be dispersed in 50 mL non-carbonated water (no other liquids should be used).

If the patient has creatinine clearance ≥ 30 to < 50 mL/min, the recommended starting dose is 200 mg/day.

VEMURAFENIB
Trade name
Zelboraf

Available form
Tablet: 240 mg

Action
- selective inhibitor of mutated form of BRAF serine–threonine kinase enzyme (mutated BRAF can cause cell proliferation in the absence of growth factors normally required for proliferation)
- very long half-life (about 57 hours)

Use
- metastatic melanoma (unresectable stage IIIc and IV BRAF V600 positive)

Dose
- 960 mg orally twice daily 1 hour before or 2 hours after food

Adverse effects
- phototoxicity
- skin cancers (melanoma, cutaneous squamous cell, non-cutaneous squamous cell)
- uveitis, blurred vision, iritis, photophobia, retinal vein occlusion
- pancreatitis
- QT interval prolongation
- Dupuytren's contracture
- see also General Adverse effects of protein kinase inhibitors (p. 691)

Interactions
- not recommended with agents known to prolong QT interval or cause electrolyte imbalance (such as diuretics)
- not recommended with ipilimumab because of an increased risk of liver injury
- may increase serum levels of caffeine, ciclosporin, clozapine, dextromethorphan, methadone, olanzapine, theophylline and tricyclic antidepressants (TCAs)
- caution if given with warfarin; INR should be closely monitored, especially when starting or stopping therapy
- may potentiate radiation toxicity (given at same time or sequentially)
- efficacy may be reduced if given with amiodarone, ciclosporin, clarithromycin, itraconazole, ritonavir or verapamil
- see also General Interactions of protein kinase inhibitors (p. 691)

Nursing considerations/Cautions
- before starting therapy, BRAF V600 mutation-positive tumour status should be confirmed by an accredited laboratory
- any electrolyte imbalance should be corrected before starting therapy
- skin examination for any lesions should occur before starting, during and for 6 months after completing therapy
- the patient should have ophthalmological examinations before starting and regularly during therapy
- because of the very long half-life, a wash-out period of 8 days may be needed if stopping therapy and starting subsequent treatment
- not recommended in those with congenital or acquired QT prolongation or electrolyte imbalance (especially hypokalaemia and hypomagnesaemia)
- see also General Nursing considerations/Cautions for protein kinase inhibitors (p. 691)

Patient education
- the patient should be instructed to swallow the tablets whole (not chewed, crushed or broken) 1 hour before or 2 hours after meals

- instruct the patient to check skin regularly for any new or changing lesions
- the patient should be instructed to seek medical advice immediately if any of the following occur:
  - any new or changing skin lesions
  - increased sensitivity to sun, severe sunburn or sunburn occurring more easily
  - changes to vision, eye pain, blurred vision, sensitivity to light
  - irregular heart rate
  - unexplained abdominal pain (especially in first 2 weeks of therapy) sometimes with nausea and vomiting
  - thickening or appearance of visible cords, bands or lumps in palm of one or both hands
- see also General Patient education for protein kinase inhibitors (p. 692)

 Tablets should not be crushed, broken or chewed.

VISMODEGIB
Trade name
Erivedge

Available form
Capsule: 150 mg

Action
- small molecule Hedgehog pathway inhibitor that blocks genes responsible for cell proliferation, survival and differentiation
- half-life 4 days

Use
- metastatic or locally advanced basal cell carcinoma (where surgery or other treatment was ineffective or inappropriate)

Dose
- 150 mg orally daily

Adverse effects
- severe skin reactions
- see also General Adverse effects of protein kinase inhibitors (p. 691)

Interactions
- caution if given with statins

Nursing considerations/Cautions
- pregnancy should be excluded using a pregnancy test 7 days before starting therapy. A pregnancy test should be done monthly during therapy
- not recommended in those under 18 years because of a risk of premature fusion of the epiphyses and precocious puberty
- see also General Nursing considerations/Cautions for protein kinase inhibitors (p. 691)

Patient education
- advise the patient to swallow the capsule whole (not chewed or opened)
- the patient should be instructed to seek medical advice immediately if any rash or skin blistering occurs
- all patients should be advised to avoid making blood or blood product donation during therapy and for 24 months after last dose
- male patients should be advised to avoid making semen donation during therapy and for 2 months after last dose
- male patients should be counselled to use condoms with spermicide during sexual intercourse with women during therapy and for 2 months after last dose
- female patients of childbearing potential should be counselled to use two reliable contraceptive methods during therapy and for 24 months after the last dose to avoid pregnancy. The patient should be advised to seek medical advice immediately if pregnancy occurs
- see also General Patient education for protein kinase inhibitors (p. 692)

 Capsules must not be opened, broken or crushed.

ANTINEOPLASTIC AGENTS

Contraindicated during pregnancy and in women of childbearing potential unless two reliable forms of contraception are used during therapy and for 24 months after the last dose.

Breastfeeding is contraindicated during therapy and for 24 months after last dose.

ZANUBRUTINIB

Trade name
Brukinsa

Available form
Capsule: 80 mg

Action
- Bruton's tyrosine kinase (BTK) inhibitor that results in malignant B-cell proliferation inhibition, reducing tumour growth
- half-life 2—4 hours

Use
- Waldenstrom's macroglobulinaemia (WM) (first-line treatment for those unsuitable for chemotherapy, or where one prior therapy has been used)
- mantle cell lymphoma (MCL) where one prior therapy has been used
- marginal zone lymphoma (MZL) where at least one prior anti-CD20 therapy has been used
- chronic lymphocytic leukaemia (CLL) or small lymphocytic lymphoma (SLL) (monotherapy, including those with deletion 17p and/or TP53 mutation)

Dose
- 320 mg orally once daily or 160 mg orally twice daily

Adverse effects
- atrial fibrillation and flutter
- tumour lysis syndrome (particularly those with CLL)
- see also General Adverse effects of protein kinase inhibitors (p. 691)

Interactions
- may decrease serum levels of midazolam
- see also General Interactions of protein kinase inhibitors (p. 691)

Nursing considerations/Cautions
- asymptomatic lymphocytosis is not considered an adverse reaction
- the patient should be assessed for risk of tumour lysis syndrome (e.g. high tumour burden). If deemed at risk, blood uric acid, potassium, calcium phosphate and creatine should be monitored closely in the first week of therapy and the patient given allopurinol and adequate hydration throughout therapy
- see also General Nursing considerations/Cautions for protein kinase inhibitors (p. 691)

Patient education
- instruct the patient to swallow capsules whole with water and not open, break or chew them
- the patient should be instructed to seek medical attention immediately if any of the following occur:
  - nausea, vomiting, diarrhoea, weakness, fatigue, muscle cramps or twitching, numbness or tingling
  - heartbeat that is fast, fluttering or pounding (palpitations), chest pain, weakness, shortness of breath, dizziness
- see also General Patient education for protein kinase inhibitors (p. 692)

Capsules should not be opened, broken or chewed.

If the patient has severe liver impairment, the recommended dose is 80 mg orally twice daily. Patients should be monitored closely for adverse events.

MONOCLONAL ANTIBODIES

Introduction to monoclonal antibodies

A monoclonal antibody is derived from a single B cell, recognises a specific antigen

and can respond to cancer cells in a number of different ways including:
- blocking ligands or cell surface receptors,
- recruiting immune cells and complement to antigen–antibody complexes formed,
- modulating immune cell function, or
- carrying toxins or radionucleotides specifically to cancer cells. Immunoglobulin G1 (IgG_1) is the most commonly used antibody isotype in cancer treatments and is more potent at activating complement pathway or immune cells than IgG_2 or IgG_4 (Wellstein & Atkins 2023).

General Adverse effects for monoclonal antibodies
- immune-related adverse reactions including:
  - pneumonitis or interstitial lung disease
  - colitis, severe diarrhoea, bowel perforation
  - hepatitis
  - endocrinopathies (hypothyroidism, hyperthyroidism, thyroiditis, diabetes mellitus, adrenal insufficiency, hypophysitis/hypopituitarism)
  - nephritis
  - rash (including pemphigoid, Stevens–Johnson Syndrome, toxic epidermal necrolysis, drug rash with eosinophilia and systemic symptoms (DRESS))
  - myocarditis
- increased risk of solid organ transplant rejection
- hyperacute graft-versus-host disease (GVHD), acute GVHD, hepatic veno-occlusive disease
- infusion-related reactions (fever, chills, hypotension, tachycardia, respiratory symptoms, anaphylaxis)
- extravasation-related tissue ulceration and necrosis
- neutropenia, thrombocytopenia, anaemia, leukopenia, febrile neutropenia, pancytopenia, bleeding, haemorrhage
- infection
- hypertension
- peripheral neuropathy
- hyperglycaemia
- tumour lysis syndrome (occurs more commonly in lymphoma, leukaemias and cancers)
- headache, dizziness, insomnia, somnolence
- nausea, vomiting, diarrhoea, abdominal pain, constipation dyspepsia, abnormal taste. stomatitis, dry mouth
- elevated liver enzymes, increased bilirubin, jaundice, abnormal liver function and uncommonly, liver failure
- rash, pruritus, redness, alopecia
- fever, chills, fatigue, asthenia
- peripheral oedema
- dyspnoea, cough
- myalgia, arthralgia, musculoskeletal pain
- hypersensitivity
- (Uncommonly) reactivation of hepatitis B, secondary primary malignancies
- (Rare) progressive multifocal leukoencephalopathy (PML)

General Interactions of monoclonal antibodies
- monoclonal antibodies are not substrates for cytochrome P450 or drug transporters and therefore drug interactions are not expected

General Nursing considerations/ Cautions for monoclonal antibodies
- trade name and batch number should be recorded in the patient's history
- therapy is usually continued until disease progression or unacceptable toxicity occurs. Some agents may have a duration limit such as 12 or 24 months or 6 cycles of therapy
- before starting therapy, blood counts, liver, kidney and thyroid function should be measured and then regularly during therapy. Cardiac function may also be measured and monitored if the drug is

ANTINEOPLASTIC AGENTS

- known to have cardiac effects such as reduced left ventricle ejection fraction (LVEF), or causing or worsening heart failure
- ensure the patient is well hydrated before starting therapy
- premedication is recommended before each infusion to reduce the risk of infusion-related reactions and could include a corticosteroid (e.g. dexamethasone 40 mg orally or IV), antipyretic (e.g. paracetamol 500–1000 mg orally or equivalent), H_2 antagonists (e.g. ranitidine 50 mg IV or equivalent) or oral proton pump inhibitor (e.g. omeprazole) and antihistamine (e.g. diphenhydramine 25–50 mg IV or orally, with IV preferred for at least first 4 infusions). Premedication should be administered 15–60 minutes before infusion
- other causes of immune-related adverse reactions such as infection should be ruled excluded before specific management is started
- the patient should be closely monitored for any immune-related adverse reactions or infusion-related reactions. Depending on the severity of reaction, therapy may be withheld or ceased. Corticosteroids should be given and continued for at least 1 month for immune-related adverse reactions
- dose reduction for management of immune-related adverse reactions is not recommended for some agents
- should not be given as IV push or bolus injection
- monitor IV site for any signs of extravasation. The infusion must be stopped if extravasation occurs and the site monitored for any signs of ulceration or necrosis
- if reconstituting powder, the diluent should be added gently down the side of the vial and then swirled slowly to dissolve contents. The reconstituted vial should be allowed to settle for at least 1 minute until bubbles have gone
- withdraw the calculated volume of diluent from the IV infusion bag (commonly sodium chloride 0.9% or glucose 5%) before adding the volume of medication
- the bag should be gently inverted (not shaken) to ensure thorough mixing
- administer alone, using a 0.20–0.22 micron in-line filter
- for patients at risk of tumour lysis syndrome, prophylactic measures such as the use of antihyperuricaemic agents (e.g. allopurinol, rasburicase), aggressive hydration and correction of any electrolyte imbalances are recommended
- should not be administered if active infection is present
- contraindicated in those with hypersensitivity to Chinese hamster ovary protein, polysorbate 20 or other monoclonal antibodies

General Patient education for monoclonal antibodies

- all patients should be given a 'patient card' that explains what to do in the event of immune-related adverse reaction and encouraged to carry it at all times
- warn the patient that immune-related adverse effects can occur during therapy but also after therapy has been stopped
- advise the patient that, if there are any disturbances to vision or concentration, driving or operating machinery should be avoided
- the patient should be instructed to immediately report any of the following that can occur during or following injection or infusion:
  - nasal stuffiness, cough, throat irritation, runny nose, itchy eyes, wheezing, sneezing, difficulty breathing or feeling short of breath
  - chest pain, coughing
  - eye or skin yellowing, loss of appetite, nausea, vomiting, pain in right upper abdominal area, dark urine
  - increased number of bowel movements, diarrhoea, black stools, stools

- with blood or mucus, severe stomach pain or tenderness, weight loss, loss of appetite
- increased hunger or thirst, needing to urinate more often, weight loss, increased tiredness
- extreme tiredness, rapid heart rate, increased sweating, weight gain or loss, change in mood or behaviour (e.g. irritability forgetfulness), feeling cold
- skin reactions including rash, peeling or blistering
- blurred vision, photophobia, changes to vision
- women of childbearing potential should be counselled to use highly effective contraception during and for 4-6 months after stopping therapy (time is dependent on specific agent)

Human immunoglobulins are known to cross the placental barrier and may be transmitted to the developing fetus, and are therefore not recommended during pregnancy.

Information about excretion into human milk or the effects on the breastfed infant is lacking; therefore monoclonal antibody therapy is not recommended during breastfeeding.

ALEMTUZUMAB

Trade names
Lemtrada, MabCampath

Available forms
Vial: 12 mg/1.2 mL, 30 mg/mL

Action
- IgG$_{1kappa}$ monoclonal antibody specific for cell surface glycoprotein (CD52)

Use
- B-cell chronic lymphocytic leukaemia (where two other therapies were ineffective) (MabCampath)
- treatment of relapsing multiple sclerosis (see Multiple sclerosis, p. 1369) (Lemtrada)

Dose
- initially 3 mg IV on day 1, 10 mg on day 2 and 30 mg on day 3 (if tolerated), then 30 mg IV 3 times weekly on alternate days for a maximum of 12 weeks (daily maximum 30 mg or weekly maximum 90 mg) (MabCampath)

Adverse effects
- hyponatraemia, hypocalcaemia
- conjunctivitis
- vasospasm, flushing
- bronchospasm, haemoptysis
- (IV site) pain, reaction
- (Rare) haemophagocytic lymphohistiocytosis
- see also General Adverse effects of monoclonal antibodies (p. 744)

Interactions
- not recommended within 21 days of other antineoplastic agents
- not recommended with irradiated blood products
- vaccination with live vaccines is not recommended with or within 12 months of finishing therapy

Nursing considerations/Cautions
- BP should be measured during therapy, as transient hypotension occurs commonly
- prophylaxis with an antibacterial agent (e.g. trimethoprim/sulfamethoxazole) and/or antiviral agents (e.g. famciclovir) is recommended during and for 8 weeks after completion of therapy to decrease the likelihood of opportunistic infection
- if adverse reactions occur at 3 mg or 10 mg doses, they should be repeated daily until well tolerated before moving on to the next dose
- if platelet count falls (< 25,000/ microL), therapy should be interrupted and restarted when it recovers
- if therapy is withheld for ≥ 7 days, it should be restarted at a 3 mg dose and gradually escalated
- if retreatment is considered, CD52 gene expression should be checked before starting

ANTINEOPLASTIC AGENTS

- given as an IV infusion over 2 hours
- if an infusion-related reaction occurs, the infusion time can be extended to 8 hours
- contraindicated in those with hypersensitivity to murine proteins or other monoclonal antibodies, with human immunodeficiency virus (HIV) infection or if active secondary malignancies or active infection are present
- see also General Nursing considerations/Cautions for monoclonal antibodies (p. 744)

Patient education
- see General Patient education for monoclonal antibodies (p. 745)

AMIVANTAMAB
Trade name
Rybrevant

Available form
Vial: 350 mg/7 mL

Action
- bispecific monoclonal antibody (IgG₁) directed against epidermal growth factor (EGF) and mesenchymal–epidermal transition (MET) receptors found on the surface of tumour cells
- half-life 11.3 days

Use
- locally advanced or metastatic non-small cell lung cancer (NSCLC) that has an activating epidermal growth factor exon 20 insertion mutation, where the disease has progressed during or after platinum-based chemotherapy

Dose
- (Patient body weight < 80 kg) 1050 mg by IV infusion **OR**
- (Patient body weight ≥ 80 kg) 1400 mg by IV infusion
- dosing schedule:
  - week 1: dose split over two infusions on day 1 and day 2
  - weeks 2–4: full dose on day 1 of each week
  - week 5 onwards: full dose once every 2 weeks starting week 5
- infusion rate is dependent of dose and schedule. Manufacturer's information should be consulted

Adverse effects
- nail-bed infection, nail cuticle fissure, nail disorder, onychoclasis (nail plate separation from nail bed), paronychia
- ocular toxicity
- see also General Adverse effects of monoclonal antibodies (p. 744)

Interactions
- monoclonal antibodies are not substrates for cytochrome P450 or drug transporters and therefore drug interactions are not expected

Nursing considerations/Cautions
- the presence of epidermal-growth factor exon 20 insertion mutation should be established by a validated test before starting therapy
- pre-infusion medications are recommended to decrease the risk of infusion-related reactions and should include antihistamines (e.g. diphenhydramine 25–50 mg IV or oral or equivalent), antipyretic (e.g. 500–1000 mg paracetamol) and glucocorticoid (e.g. dexamethasone 10 mg, methylprednisolone 40 mg or equivalent) administered 15 to 60 minutes before infusion. For week one, days 1 and 2, antihistamine, antipyretic and glucocorticoid should be given but subsequent infusions require only antihistamine and antipyretic
- see also General Nursing considerations/Cautions for monoclonal antibodies (p. 744)

Patient education
- warn the patient that rash commonly occurs in the first 2–4 weeks of therapy
- the patient should be advised to limit sun exposure during and for 2 months after stopping therapy and recommend

protective clothing and sunscreen (SPF 30+) use
- instruct the patient to immediately seek medical advice if any of the following occur:
  - nail infection or nail disorder including nail plate separation from the nail bed
  - dry eyes, blurred vision, itching eyes, visual impairment, eyelashes growing in abnormal positions, redness, eyelid inflammation
- see also General Patient education for monoclonal antibodies (p. 745)

AVELUMAB
Trade name
Bavencio

Available form
Vial: 200 mg/10 mL

Action
- monoclonal antibody (IgG_1) that blocks interaction between PD-L1 (expressed on tumour cells and/or tumour-infiltrating immune cells), restoring antitumour T-cell responses
- half-life 6.1 days

Use
- treatment of metastatic Merkel cell carcinoma

Dose
- 10 mg/kg by IV infusion over 60 minutes every 2 weeks

Adverse effects
- see General Adverse effects of monoclonal antibodies (p. 744)

Interactions
- monoclonal antibodies are not substrates for cytochrome P450 or drug transporters and therefore drug interactions are not expected

Nursing considerations/Cautions
- see General Nursing considerations/ Cautions for monoclonal antibodies (p.744)

Patient education
- see General Patient education for monoclonal antibodies (p. 745)

BEVACIZUMAB
Trade names
Abevmy, Mvasi, Vegzelma

Available forms
Vial: 100 mg/4 mL, 400 mg/16 mL

Action
- monoclonal antibody that selectively binds to vascular endothelial growth factor (VEGF) neutralising it, reducing tumour vascularisation and inhibiting tumour growth
- half-life 18 days (females), 20 days (males)

Use
- metastatic colorectal cancer (combination therapy)
- locally recurrent or metastatic breast cancer (combination therapy)
- advanced and/or metastatic renal cell carcinoma (combination therapy)
- grade IV glioma after relapse or disease progression after standard therapy (combination therapy)
- epithelial ovarian, fallopian tube or primary peritoneal cancer (combination therapy)
- recurrent epithelial ovarian, fallopian tube or primary peritoneal cancer (combination therapy)
- advanced, metastatic or recurrent non-squamousnon-small cell lung (NSCLC) cancer (combination therapy)
- persistent, recurrent or metastatic cervical cancer (combination therapy)

Dose
- (Metastatic colorectal cancer — first-line treatment) 5 mg/kg IV once every 2 weeks or 7.5 mg/kg IV once every 3 weeks **OR**
- (Metastatic colorectal cancer — second-line treatment) 10 mg/kg IV once every 2 weeks or 15 mg/kg IV once every 3 weeks **OR**

ANTINEOPLASTIC AGENTS

- (Breast cancer) 10 mg/kg IV once every 2 weeks or 15 mg/kg IV every 3 weeks **OR**
- (NSCLC) 15 mg/kg IV once every 3 weeks (with carboplatin and paclitaxel) for up to 6 cycles, then as a single agent until disease progresses **OR**
- (Renal cell cancer) 10 mg/kg IV once every 2 weeks (with interferon alfa-2a) **OR**
- (Glioma) 10 mg/kg IV once every 2 weeks or 15 mg/kg IV once every 3 weeks **OR**
- (Epithelial ovarian, fallopian tube or primary peritoneal cancer) 15 mg/kg IV once every 3 weeks (with carboplatin and paclitaxel) for up to 6 cycles, then as a single agent for 15 months or until disease progresses **OR**
- (Recurrent epithelial ovarian, fallopian tube or primary peritoneal cancer) 15 mg/kg IV once every 3 weeks (with carboplatin and gemcitabine) for 6–10 cycles, then as a single agent until disease progresses **OR**
- (Recurrent epithelial ovarian, fallopian tube or primary peritoneal cancer) 15 mg/kg IV once every 3 weeks (with carboplatin and paclitaxel) for 6–8 cycles, then as a single agent until disease progresses **OR**
- (Cervical cancer) 15 mg/kg IV once every 3 weeks (with cisplatin and paclitaxel or paclitaxel and topotecan)

Adverse effects
- impaired wound healing
- thromboembolism
- proteinuria
- peripheral neuropathy
- infusion-related reactions
- (NSCLC) pulmonary haemorrhage, haemoptysis
- (Uncommon) (GI and non-GI) fistulae formation and rarely, GI or gallbladder perforation
- (Rare) hypersensitivity, posterior reversible encephalopathy syndrome (PRES), hand–foot syndrome (hand/foot numbness, paraesthesia, tingling, erythema, pain, swelling and, at worst, ulceration, blistering or moist desquamation), osteonecrosis of the jaw
- (Very rare) hypertensive encephalopathy
- see also General Adverse effects of monoclonal antibodies (p. 744)

Interactions
- caution if given with sunitinib maleate because of an increased risk of microangiopathic haemolytic anaemia
- an increased risk of severe neutropenia if given with liposomal doxorubicin, or platinum- or taxane-based therapy

Nursing considerations/Cautions
- any pre-existing hypertension should be controlled before starting therapy
- dental examination and any dental treatment should be completed before starting therapy
- BP should be monitored during therapy, as hypertension commonly occurs
- the patient should be closely monitored during infusion for any signs of infusion reaction
- therapy is not recommended within 28 days of surgery or until the surgical wound has healed because of an increased risk of wound-healing complications
- urine should be monitored for protein before and during therapy
- not recommended with glucose solutions
- after dilution with sodium chloride 0.9%, give by IV infusion over 90 minutes (first dose) and, if tolerated, the next infusion is given over 60 minutes. If this is tolerated, the next and subsequent infusions are given over 30 minutes
- an increased risk of thromboembolic events if given to those > 65 years with diabetes mellitus or a previous history of thromboembolism
- caution if used in those with bleeding tendencies, congestive cardiac failure or cardiovascular disease

- caution if used in those with a history or symptoms of bowel obstruction, abdominal fistulae or prior pelvic irradiation because of an increased risk of fistulae formation
- contraindicated in those with hypersensitivity to Chinese hamster ovary cell products, other recombinant monoclonal antibodies or untreated CNS metastases
- see also General Nursing considerations/Cautions for monoclonal antibodies (p. 744)

Patient education

- advise the patient to seek medical advice immediately if any of the following occur:
  - headache, altered mental state, visual disturbances or fitting (seizures)
  - cough or spitting blood
  - pain in gums or jaw, swelling or jaw numbness or heavy jaw feeling, loosening of teeth
  - leg/calf swelling, pain or tenderness of leg/calf, warmth, redness
- encourage the patient to practise good dental hygiene, including brushing teeth and tongue after meals and before bed, daily flossing to remove plaque and using a mirror to check teeth and gums regularly for any sores or bleeding of the gums
- see also General patient education for monoclonal antibodies (p. 745)

BLINATUMOMAB

Trade name
Blincyto

Available form
Vial: 38.5 microgram

Action
- bispecific monoclonal antibody that binds to CD19 and CD3
- half-life 2 hours

Use
- treatment of relapsed or refractory B-cell precursor acute lymphocytic leukaemia (ALL)
- treatment of minimal residual disease (MRD) positive B-cell precursor ALL

Dose
- (Relapsed or refractory B-cell precursor ALL, weight > 45 kg) 9 micrograms IV daily for first 7 days, increasing to 28 micrograms IV starting at week 2 through to week 4 (cycle 1), with 28 micrograms IV for subsequent cycles **OR**
- (MRD positive B-cell positive ALL, weight > 45 kg) 28 micrograms IV daily for days 1–28, followed by a 14-day treatment-free interval

Adverse effects
- cytokine-release syndrome (fever, asthenia, headache, hypotension, nausea, increased bilirubin)
- neurological toxicity (encephalopathy, seizures, speech disorders, confusion, disorientation, disturbed consciousness, coordination and balance disorders)
- reactivation of John Cunningham (JC) virus, posterior reversible encephalopathy syndrome (PRES)
- see also General Adverse effects of monoclonal antibodies (p. 744)

Interactions
- vaccination with live vaccine is not recommended for 2 weeks before and during therapy, and after until B-lymphocyte recovery to normal range

Nursing considerations/Cautions
- each cycle is 4 weeks, with a 2-week treatment-free interval between cycles
- hospitalisation is recommended for the first 9 days of the first cycle and the first 2 days of the second cycle (relapsed or refractory ALL) or a minimum first 3 days of the first cycle and first 2 days of the second cycle (MRD positive B-cell positive ALL). Supervision or hospitalisation is also recommended for subsequent treatment cycles
- premedication with dexamethasone IV 20 mg 1 hour before the start of each cycle is recommended

ANTINEOPLASTIC AGENTS

- prophylactically intrathecal chemotherapy is additionally recommended before and during therapy to prevent CNS ALL relapse
- (Relapsed or refractory B-cell precursor ALL) for patient with high tumour burden ($\geq$ 50% leukaemic blasts or > 15,000 microL peripheral blood leukaemic blast cells), prephase treatment with dexamethasone (not exceeding 24 mg daily) is recommended
- see also General Nursing considerations/Cautions for monoclonal antibodies (p. 744)

Patient education

- see General Patient education for monoclonal antibodies (p. 745)

BRENTUXIMAB VEDOTIN
Trade name
Adcetris

Available form
Vial: 50 mg

Action
- CD30-directed antibody-drug conjugate antineoplastic that disrupts microtubules, resulting in the death of CD30-expressing tumour cells

Use
- previously untreated CD30+ peripheral T-cell lymphoma (PTCL) (with cyclophosphamide, doxorubicin and prednisolone)
- treatment of relapsed or refractory CD30+ Hodgkin lymphoma (after autologous stem cell transplant or after $\geq$ 2 therapies when stem cell transplant is not an option)
- cutaneous T-cell CD30+ lymphoma (CTCL) after at least one other systemic treatment

Dose
- 1.8 mg/kg IV over 30 minutes every 3 weeks for 8–16 cycles (about 1 year) (maximum 180 mg)

Adverse effects
- hyperglycaemia
- see also General Adverse effects of monoclonal antibodies (p. 744)

Interactions
- contraindicated with bleomycin because of the increased risk of pulmonary toxicity

Nursing considerations/Cautions
- if the patient's weight > 100 kg, the dose should be calculated according to their ideal weight
- blood glucose levels should be measured before starting and regularly during therapy
- (Previously untreated PTCL) therapy should be started with G-CSF
- reconstitute with 10.5 mL water for injections to give a concentration of 5 mg/mL and then further dilute with 150 mL sodium chloride 0.9%, glucose 5% or lactated Ringer's solution
- caution if used in those with pre-existing GI conditions because of an increased risk of complications, including perforation
- see also General Nursing considerations/Cautions for monoclonal antibodies (p. 744)

Patient education
- caution patient with diabetes mellitus to monitor blood glucose levels closely, as hyperglycaemia may occur during therapy
- see also General Patient education for monoclonal antibodies (p. 745)

CEMIPLIMAB
Trade name
Libtayo

Available form
Vial: 350 mg/7 mL

Action
- monoclonal antibody (IgG4) that binds to programmed cell death-1 (PD-1)

receptors, blocking interaction with ligands PD-L1 and PD-L2 expressed by tumour cells
* half-life 22 days

Use
* monotherapy for metastatic or locally advanced cutaneous squamous cell carcinoma (mCSCC or laCSCC) not suitable for curative surgery or curative radiation
* monotherapy for non-small cell lung cancer (NSCLC) expressing PD-L1 tumour proportion score (TPS) ≥ 50% (determined by validated test) with no EGFR, ALK or ROS1 aberrations, with advanced NSCLC not suitable for surgical resection or definitive chemoradiation, or metastatic NSCLC (first-line treatment)
* combination therapy with platinum-based chemotherapy for NSCLC with no EGFR, ALK or ROS1 aberrations, that is locally advanced not suitable for surgical resection or definitive chemoradiation, or metastatic NSCLC (first-line treatment)
* locally advanced or metastatic basal cell carcinoma (BCC) previously treated with a hedgehog pathway inhibitor or where a hedgehog pathway inhibitor is not appropriate

Dose
* 350 mg by IV infusion over 30 minutes every 3 weeks

Adverse effects
* see General Adverse effects of monoclonal antibodies (p. 744)

Interactions
* caution if used in those with previous exposure to idelalisib and sulfa-containing antibiotics because of an increased risk of Stevens—Johnson syndrome and toxic epidermal necrolysis
* systemic corticosteroids or immunosuppressants (except prednisolone or equivalent ≤ 10 mg/day) should be avoided before starting therapy. However, these can be used after therapy has started to treat immune-related adverse effects

Nursing considerations/Cautions
* PD-L1 expression should be confirmed by a valid test before starting therapy for locally advanced or metastatic NSCLC
* dose reduction for immune-related adverse effects is not recommended; however, dosing may be delayed or discontinued if necessary
* see also General Nursing considerations/Cautions for monoclonal antibodies (p. 744)

Patient education
* see General Patient education for monoclonal antibodies (p. 745)

CETUXIMAB
Trade name
Erbitux

Available form
Vial: 100 mg/20 mL, 500 mg/100 mL

Action
* epidermal growth factor receptor (EGFR) monoclonal antibody whose activity results in decreased neovascularisation of tumours and metastasis
* overexpression of EGFR has been found in a number of human cancers, including rectal and colon
* retinoic acid syndrome (RAS) is a frequently activated family of oncogenes in human cancers
* half-life 70—100 hours

Use
* EGFR-expressing RAS wild-type metastatic colorectal cancer (as monotherapy or as part of combination therapy)
* squamous cell cancer of the neck and head (with radiation (for locally advanced cancer) or platinum-based chemotherapy (for recurrent or metastatic disease))

ANTINEOPLASTIC AGENTS

Dose
- (Weekly dose regimen) initially 400 mg/m^2 by IV infusion over 120 minutes once weekly, then reducing to 250 mg/m^2 by IV infusion over 60 minutes **OR**
- (2-weekly dose regimen) each dose 500 mg/m^2 by IV infusion over 120 minutes, every 2 weeks

Adverse effects
- severe hypomagnesaemia
- keratitis, ulcerative keratitis
- see also General Adverse effects of monoclonal antibodies (p. 744)

Interactions
- not recommended with capecitabine and irinotecan to treat metastatic colorectal cancer
- increased risk of severe diarrhoea if given with capecitabine and oxaliplatin
- increased risk of leucopenia and neutropenia if given with platinum-based therapy
- caution if given with fluoropyrimidines because of an increased risk of cardiac ischaemia (including myocardial infarction and congestive cardiac failure) and hand—foot syndrome
- may increase the risk of local radiation side-effects (e.g. mucositis, radiation dermatitis) if radiation therapy to head and neck is given with cetuximab

Nursing considerations/Cautions
- (Colorectal cancer) RAS mutational status must be evaluated using a validated test method before starting therapy
- cardiovascular assessment before starting therapy is recommended, especially in those > 65 years
- first dose should be given over 2 hours at a rate of 5 mg/mL, then reduced to 60 minutes for the next infusion if no reaction occurred (never greater than 10 mg/min)
- (Squamous cell neck and head cancer) therapy is started 1 week before and continued throughout the course of radiation
- other chemotherapy is not recommended within an hour of completing infusion
- if dilution is required, use sodium chloride 0.9% only
- caution if used in those with a history of keratitis, ulcerative keratitis or severe dry eyes
- not recommended in those with metastatic colorectal cancer with resectable liver metastases
- (Combination therapy with oxaliplatin) contraindicated in those with mutant RAS metastatic colorectal cancer or in those whose status is unknown
- see also General Nursing considerations/Cautions for monoclonal antibodies (p. 744)

Patient education
- see General Patient education for monoclonal antibodies (p. 745)

DARATUMUMAB
Trade names
Darzalex, Darzalex SC

Available forms
Vial: 120 mg/mL;
Vial (concentrate): 100 mg/5 mL, 400 mg/20 mL

Action
- monoclonal antibody (IgG1$_K$) binds to CD38 protein expressed on cell surface of some haematological malignancies
- SC formulation contains recombinant human hyaluronidase
- half-life 20.4 days (multiple myeloma) and 27.5 days (amyloidosis)

Use
- newly diagnosed multiple myeloma:
  - in those eligible for autologous stem cell transplant (ASCT). For use in combination with bortezomib, thalidomide and dexamethasone
  - in those not eligible for ASCT. For use in combination with bortezomib,

melphalan and prednisone; or lenalidomide and dexamethasone
- multiple myeloma:
  - in those who have received at least one prior therapy. For use in combination with bortezomib and dexamethasone, or lenalidomide and dexamethasone
  - in those who have received at least three prior lines of therapy including a proteasome inhibitor (PI) and an immunomodulatory agent, or who are refractory to both a PI and an immunomodulatory agent (as monotherapy)
- light-chain AL amyloidosis with bortezomib, cyclophosphamide and dexamethasone

Dose
- Multiple myeloma, suitable for ASCT, with bortezomib, thalidomide and dexamethasone
  - 1800 mg SC or 16 mg/kg by IV infusion weekly for 8 weeks, then every 2 weeks for weeks (induction). Therapy is then stopped for high-dose chemotherapy and ASCT. Then, 1800 mg SC or 16 mg/kg by IV infusion every 2 weeks for 8 weeks (consolidation) **OR**
- Multiple myeloma, not suitable for ASCT, with bortezomib, melphalan and prednisone
  - 1800 mg SC or 16 mg/kg weekly for 6 weeks, then every 3 weeks for 48 weeks, then every 4 weeks until disease progression **OR**
- Relapsed/refractory multiple myeloma with bortezomib and dexamethasone
  - 1800 mg SC or 16 mg/kg weekly for 9 weeks, then every 3 weeks for 15 weeks, then every 4 weeks until disease progression **OR**
- Multiple myeloma (monotherapy for relapsed/refractory myeloma, or combination therapy with lenalidomide and low-dose dexamethasone)
  - 1800 mg SC or 16 mg/kg weekly for 8 weeks, then every 2 weeks for 8 weeks, then every 4 weeks until disease progression **OR**
- AL amyloidosis
  - 1800 mg SC weekly for 8 weeks, then 2-weekly for 8 weeks, then monthly until disease progression

Adverse effects
- (SC injection-site reaction) redness
- see also General Adverse effects for monoclonal antibodies (p. 744)

Interactions
- may result in positive indirect Coombs' test during and for up to 6 months after therapy has stopped
- may interfere with the determination of complete response and of disease progression on serum protein electrophoresis (SPE) and immunofixation (IFE) assays

Nursing considerations/Cautions
- no dose reduction is recommended but dose may be delayed
- SC formulation should be used only for SC administration
- the first SC dose in daratumumab-naive patients should be administered where resuscitation equipment is readily available
- SC injection is administered over 3–5 minutes into subcutaneous tissue of the abdomen, about 7.5 cm to the right or left of the umbilicus. No other SC administration sites should be used. If pain occurs during administration, the injection can be paused or slowed down to reduce pain. If pain continues, a second administration on the opposite side of the abdomen should be used for the remainder of the injection
- SC injection sites should be rotated and not used if skin is red, bruised, tender, hard or there are scars present
- other SC injections should not be administered into the same SC abdominal site
- if transferring from IV formulation, SC can be used from the next scheduled dose

ANTINEOPLASTIC AGENTS

- the patient should be closely monitored during and after first and second SC injections or IV infusions
- premedication should be given to reduce the risk of infusion-related reactions (IRRs) and administered 1–3 hours before each SC injection and include:
  - corticosteroid — monotherapy: methylprednisolone 100 mg (or equivalent) (first injection), then reducing to 60 mg. For combination therapy, dexamethasone (or equivalent) 20 mg is given before each SC injection (unless part of the combination therapy)
  - antipyretic — oral paracetamol (500–1000 mg)
  - antihistamine — oral or IV diphenhydramine 25–50 mg or equivalent
- postinjection medication is given to reduce the risk of delayed infusion-related reactions and should include:
  - corticosteroid — monotherapy: 20 mg methylprednisolone orally or an equivalent dose of intermediate- or long-acting corticosteroid on each of 2 days after administration. For combination therapy, low-dose oral methylprednisolone ($\leq$ 20 mg) or equivalent on day after administration unless a corticosteroid is part of the combination therapy
- if patient experiences no major infusion-related reactions after three SC injections, the postinjection corticosteroid may no longer be required
- (IV) dilute required volume with sodium chloride 0.9% to 1000 mL (first infusion) or 500 mL (for second and subsequent infusions if no IRR occurred with first infusion)
- (IV) first infusion may be divided into two infusions of 8 mg/kg/day diluted in 500 mL and administered on two consecutive days
- (IV) (weeks 1 and 2) initially 50 mL/hour for the first hour and, if no IRR occurs, increasing in increments of 50 mL/hour (maximum rate 200 mL/hour). (Week 3 and beyond) if no IRR has occurred in previous weeks, infusion can be started at 100 mL/hour, increasing in increments of 50 mL/hour (maximum rate 200 mL/hour). If IRRs have occurred, the previous infusion rate should be used
- if the patient has a history of chronic obstructive pulmonary disease, additional postinjection medication such as short- and long-acting bronchodilators and inhaled corticosteroids may be required
- see also General Nursing considerations/Cautions for monoclonal antibodies (p. 744)

Patient education
- see General Patient education for monoclonal antibodies (p. 745)

DENOSUMAB
Trade names
Corora, Ganvado, Jubbonti, Prolia, Wyost, Xgeva

Available forms
Prefilled syringe: 60 mg/mL;
Vial: 120 mg/1.7 mL

Action
- monoclonal antibody with high affinity and specificity for RANK ligand (essential for formation, function and survival of osteoclast) inhibiting osteoclast formation, thereby decreasing bone resorption and increasing bone mass and strength, as well as decreasing cancer-induced bone destruction
- half-life 14–55 days

Use
- treatment of osteoporosis in postmenopausal women or men with osteopenia receiving androgen-deprivation therapy (see Bone and calcium regulating agents, p. 971) (Corora, Jubbonti, Prolia)
- prevention of skeletal events in those with multiple myeloma or bony metastases from solid tumours, giant cell tumour of bone (recurrent or unresectable) or hypercalcaemia of malignancy (refractory to IV bisphosphonates) (Ganvado, Wyost, Xgeva)

Dose
- (Prevention of skeletal events) 120 mg SC monthly **OR**
- (Giant cell bone tumour, hypercalcaemia of malignancy) 120 mg SC monthly, with extra doses on day 8 and 15 of the first month

Adverse effects
- hypocalcaemia
- (Rare) osteonecrosis of the jaw
- (Rare) atypical femoral fractures, pancreatitis, vertebral fractures (after stopping therapy)
- see also General Adverse effects of monoclonal antibodies (p. 744)

Interactions
- increased risk of osteonecrosis of the jaw if given with corticosteroids
- not recommended with bisphosphonates

Nursing considerations/Cautions
- any hypocalcaemia should be identified and treated before starting therapy, and calcium levels should be closely monitored during therapy, especially during the first weeks of therapy
- supplementation with calcium 500 mg and vitamin D 400 IU orally is generally recommended (unless otherwise contraindicated)
- in those patients with risk factors (e.g. poor dental hygiene, chronic periodontal disease, head/neck radiotherapy as well as treatment with antineoplastic agents and corticosteroids), a dental examination and any necessary treatment should be carried out before starting therapy with bisphosphonate. Invasive dental procedures should be avoided if possible during therapy to prevent osteonecrosis of the jaw occurring
- should not be treated with both formulations concurrently
- should be allowed to come to room temperature for 20—30 minutes before administration
- caution if used in those with growing skeletons or after discontinuation of therapy for giant cell bone tumours, as hypercalcaemia may occur weeks to months after stopping therapy
- caution if used in those with kidney impairment, as the risk of hypocalcaemia increases with the degree of kidney impairment without calcium supplementation. If the patient has severe kidney impairment or is on dialysis, calcium levels should be closely monitored and supplementation with calcium and vitamin D is recommended
- not recommended in those with rare hereditary problems of fructose intolerance
- contraindicated in those with known sensitivity to Chinese hamster ovary proteins, severe untreated hypocalcaemia or unhealed dental or oral surgery lesions

Patient education
- instruct the patient to seek medical advice if any of the following occur:
  - jaw or dental pain
  - persistent or bleeding gums
  - non-healing sores in mouth or jaw
  - new or unusual thigh, hip or groin pain (even if it occurs months after finishing therapy)
- encourage the patient to practise good dental hygiene including brushing teeth and tongue after meals and before bed, daily flossing to remove plaque and using a mirror to check teeth and gums regularly for any sores or bleeding of the gums
- warn the patient not to stop therapy suddenly without seeking medical advice
- see also General Patient education for monoclonal antibodies (p. 745)

 There is an increased risk of developing hypocalcaemia in those with renal impairment. Monitoring calcium levels and supplementation with calcium and vitamin D is recommended.

ANTINEOPLASTIC AGENTS

DINUTUXIMAB BETA
Trade name
Qarziba

Available form
Vial: 20 mg/4.5 mL

Action
- monoclonal antibody (IgG$_1$) that targets carbohydrate moiety of disialoganglioside 2 (GD2) overexpressed on neuroblastoma cells
- neurotoxicity is thought to be related to induction of mechanical allodynia due to reaction with GD2 antigen located on surface of peripheral nerve fibres and myelin
- binds to optic nerve cells
- half-life 190 hours

Use
- treatment of high-risk neuroblastoma patients who have previously received induction chemotherapy and achieved a partial response

Dose
- (Patient weight > 12 kg) total of 100 mg/m^2 per course
- (Patient weight > 5 kg ≤ 12 kg) total of 3.3 mg/kg per course
- continuous infusion over first 10 days of each 35-day course (total 240 hours) at a daily dose of 10 mg/m^2 (patient weight > 12 kg) or 0.33 mg/kg (patient weight > 5 kg ≤ 12 kg) **OR**
- five daily infusions of 20 mg/m^2 (patient weight > 12 kg) or 0.66 mg/kg (patient weight > 5 kg ≤ 12 kg) over 8 hours on first 5 days of each 35-day course

Adverse effects
- neuropathic pain, pain
- hypersensitivity including cytokine release syndrome
- capillary leak syndrome
- impaired visual accommodation, mydriasis, periorbital oedema, eyelid oedema, blurred vision, photophobia
- peripheral neuropathy
- see also General Adverse effects of monoclonal antibodies (p. 744)

Interactions
- corticosteroids are not recommended within 2 weeks before the first course of therapy until 1 week after the final course (except for life-threatening conditions)
- vaccinations should be avoided until 10 weeks after the final course
- not recommended with intravenous immunoglobulin

Nursing considerations/Cautions
- therapy consists of 5 consecutive courses (35 days per course)
- before starting therapy, the patient should have pulse oximetry > 94% on room air, adequate bone marrow function (absolute neutrophil count ≥ 500/microL, platelet count ≥ 20,000/microL, haemoglobin > 8.0 g/dL) adequate liver function (liver enzymes < 5 times upper limit of normal) and adequate kidney function (creatine clearance > 60 mL/min)
- premedication recommended:
  - non-opioid analgesic (e.g. paracetamol or ibuprofen),
  - gabapentin (10 mg/kg/day orally starting 3 days before therapy, increased to 2 × 10 mg/kg/day the next day, then 3 × 10 mg/kg/day the day before the infusion and continued at that dose (maximum dose 300 mg)), and
  - opioid — continuous morphine infusion 0.02–0.05 mg/kg/hour started 2 hours before dinutuximab beta infusion, then 0.03 mg/kg/hour at the same time as dinutuximab beta infusion. For daily infusion schedule, morphine infusion should be continued at decreased rate (0.01 mg/kg/hour) for 4 hours after dinutuximab beta infusion has finished. For continuous infusion schedule, morphine may be weaned over 5 days decreasing dosing rate (e.g. to 0.02 mg/kg/hour, 0.01 mg/kg/hour, 0.005 mg/kg/hour). If continuous morphine infusion is required for more

than 5 days, rate should be gradually reduced by 20% each day after last day of dinutuximab beta infusion
- after weaning off IV morphine, severe neuropathic pain can be managed with oral morphine 0.2–0.4 mg/kg every 4 to 6 hours as needed. For moderate neuropathic pain, tramadol is recommended
- antihistamine (e.g. diphenhydramine IV) is administered about 20 minutes before infusion to decrease risk of hypersensitivity reactions. Antihistamine should be repeated every 4 to 6 hours as needed during infusion
- for continuous infusion, a rate of 2 mL/hour (48 mL/day) via infusion pump is recommended. If 8-hour daily infusion is to be administered, a rate of 13 mL/hour should be used
- the patient should be closely monitored for any signs of allergy or anaphylaxis during infusion, particularly during the first and second treatment courses
- contraindicated in those who have acute grade 3 or 4 or extensive chronic graft-versus-host disease

Patient education

- advise the patient not to drive or use machinery during therapy
- the patient should be warned that pain commonly occurs during the first infusion and decreases over the treatment course
- instruct the patient to immediately report any:
  - fever, itchy hives
  - lightheadedness or dizziness
  - rapid heart rate
  - changes to vision, blurred vision, photophobia
  - weakness, numbness or tingling in extremities
  - diarrhoea, swelling of legs, arms and body
- see also General Patient education for monoclonal antibodies (p. 745)

DOSTARLIMAB
Trade name
Jemperli

Available form
Vial: 500 mg/10 mL

Action
- monoclonal antibody (IgG$_4$) that binds to PD (programmed cell death protein)-1, blocking activity so decreasing tumour growth
- half-life 23.2 days

Use
- treatment of primary advanced or recurrent mismatch repair deficient (dMMR)/ microsatellite instability-high (MSI-H) endometrial cancer (in combination with carboplatin and paclitaxel)
- treatment of primary advanced or recurrent mismatch repair deficient (dMMR) endometrial cancer that has progressed on, or following previous treatment with a platinum-containing regimen (monotherapy)

Dose
- (Endometrial cancer, combination therapy) 500 mg by IV infusion over 30 minutes every 3 weeks for six doses, then 1000 mg every 6 weeks for subsequent cycles **OR**
- (Endometrial cancer, monotherapy) 500 mg by IV infusion over 30 minutes every 3 weeks for four doses, then 1000 mg every 6 weeks for subsequent cycles

Adverse effects
- see General Adverse effects for monoclonal antibodies (p. 744)

Interactions
- monoclonal antibodies are not substrates for cytochrome P450 or drug transporters and therefore drug interactions are not expected

Nursing considerations/Cautions
- (Combination therapy) dostarlimab should be administered before chemotherapy on the same day

ANTINEOPLASTIC AGENTS

- dose reduction for adverse reactions is not recommended, although the dose can be delayed
- see also General Nursing considerations/Cautions for monoclonal antibodies (p. 744)

Patient education
- see General Patient education for monoclonal antibodies (p. 745)

DURVALUMAB
Trade name
Imfinzi

Available forms
Vial: 120 mg/2.4 mL, 500 mg/10 mL

Action
- monoclonal antibody (IgG_{1kappa}) immune checkpoint inhibitor that blocks interaction between PD-L1 and PD-1 and CD80, leading to increased T-cell activation and decreased tumour size (in animal models)

Use
- locally advanced non-small cell lung cancer (NSCLC) (with locally advanced unresectable NSCLC that has not progressed following platinum-based chemoradiation therapy)
- extensive stage small cell lung cancer (SCLC) (with carboplatin or cisplatin)
- locally advanced or metastatic biliary tract cancer (BTC) (with gemcitabine and cisplatin)
- unresectable hepatocellular cancer (HCC) (no prior treatment with PD1/PD-L1 inhibitor) (with tremelimumab)

Dose
- (Locally advanced NSCLC) 10 mg/kg every 2 weeks or 1500 mg every 4 weeks as IV infusion over 60 minutes (monotherapy) **OR**
- (SCLC) 1500 mg every 3 weeks for four cycles as IV infusion over 60 minutes (with chemotherapy), then 1500 mg every 4 weeks as monotherapy **OR**
- (BTC) 1500 mg every 3 weeks for up to eight cycles as IV infusion over 60 minutes (with gemcitabine and cisplatin) then 1500 mg every 4 weeks as monotherapy **OR**
- (HCC) tremelimumab 300 mg as single dose (priming dose) given with durvalumab 1500 mg (day 1, cycle 1) as IV infusion over 60 minutes, then durvalumab 1500 mg given every 4 weeks as monotherapy

Adverse effects
- see General Adverse effects for monoclonal antibodies (p. 744)

Interactions
- monoclonal antibodies are not substrates for cytochrome P450 or drug transporters and therefore drug interactions are not expected

Nursing considerations/Cautions
- (Locally advanced NSCLC) if the patient's weight is less than 30 kg, 10 mg/kg dosage every 2 weeks should be used until the patient's weight increases to > 30 kg
- (ES-SCLC) if the patient's weight is less than 30 kg, they should receive 20 mg/kg every 3 weeks for four cycles (with chemotherapy), then 10 mg/kg every 2 weeks (as monotherapy) until the weight increases to > 30 kg
- (BTC) if the patient's weight is less than 30 kg, they should receive 20 mg/kg every 3 weeks (with chemotherapy), then 20 mg/kg every 4 weeks (as monotherapy) until the weight increases to > 30 kg
- (HCC) if the patient's weight is less than 30 kg, they should receive durvalumab 20 mg/kg and tremelimumab 4 mg/kg until the weight increases to > 30 kg
- no dose reduction or escalation is recommended
- (SCLC, BTC) should be administered before chemotherapy
- (HCC) tremelimumab should be administered first on the same day via different infusion line

- see also General Nursing considerations/Cautions for monoclonal antibodies (p. 744)

Patient education
- see General Patient education for monoclonal antibodies (p. 745)

ELOTUZUMAB
Trade name
Empliciti

Available forms
Vial: 300 mg, 400 mg

Action
- monoclonal antibody (IgG_{1kappa}) that specifically targets signalling lymphocyte activation molecule family member 7 (SLAMF7) protein, which is expressed on multiple myeloma cells, facilitating the interaction with natural killer cells mediating myeloma cell death

Use
- multiple myeloma in those who have received at least one prior therapy (combination therapy with lenalidomide and dexamethasone)

Dose
- 10 mg/kg IV on days 1, 8, 15 and 22 (cycles 1 and 2), then days 1 and 15 (cycle 3 and beyond)
- Infusion rate:
  - (cycle 1, dose 1) 0.5 mL/min for 30 minutes increasing to 1 mL/min for 30 minutes, then 2 mL/min for remainder of infusion
  - (cycle 1, dose 2) 3 mL/min for first 30 minutes, then increasing to 4 mL/min for remainder of infusion
  - (cycle 1, dose 3 and 4, and subsequent cycles) 5 mL/min

Adverse effects
- see General Adverse effects of monoclonal antibodies (p. 744)

Interactions
- may interfere with both serum electrophoresis (SPEP) and immunofixation (IFE) assays impacting on the determination of complete therapy response or relapse

Nursing considerations/Cautions
- reconstitute using water for Injections (13 mL for 300 mg; 17 mL for 400 mg) and allow to stand for 5–10 minutes before dilution with 230 mL of either sodium chloride 0.9% or glucose 5%
- infusion rate should not exceed 5 mL/min
- see also General Nursing considerations/Cautions for monoclonal antibodies (p. 744)

Patient education
- see General Patient education for monoclonal antibodies (p. 744)

 Combination with lenalidomide is contraindicated during pregnancy (see lenalidomide p. 1258).

ENFORTUMAB VEDOTIN
Trade name
Padcev

Available forms
Vial: 20 mg, 30 mg

Action
- monoclonal antibody (IgG_{1kappa}) conjugated to a microtubule-disrupting agent (MMAE) with a protease cleavable linker that binds to Nectin-4-expressing cells where MMAE is released, inducing cell cycle death
- Nectin-4 is expressed on the skin so skin reactions are expected

Use
- locally advanced or metastatic urothelial cancer previously treated with a platinum-containing chemotherapy and a programmed death receptor-1 or programmed death ligand-1 inhibitor

Dose
- 1.25 mg/kg (to a maximum of 125 mg for patients ≥ 100 kg) by IV infusion over

ANTINEOPLASTIC AGENTS

30 minutes on days 1, 8 and 15 of a 28-day cycle

Adverse effects
- skin reactions (mild-to-moderate maculopapular rash, severe reactions include Stevens—Johnson syndrome and toxic epidermal necrolysis)
- hyperglycaemia, diabetic ketoacidosis
- pneumonitis, interstitial lung disease
- peripheral neuropathy
- dry eyes
- skin and soft tissue injury (after extravasation)

Interactions
- caution if given with clarithromycin, diltiazem, erythromycin, itraconazole, ritonavir or verapamil. Although monoclonal antibodies are unlikely to cause drug interaction, MMAE levels may be increased, increasing the risk of adverse effects

Nursing considerations/Cautions
- dose reduction for adverse reactions is recommended
- reconstitute with water for Injections (2.3 mL for 20 mg, 3.3 mL for 30 mg) for 10 mg/mL concentration and then further dilute with glucose 5%, sodium chloride 0.9% or lactated Ringer's solution
- patient must be closely monitored throughout therapy course for skin reactions
- blood glucose levels should be monitored regularly in patients with or at risk of diabetes mellitus or hyperglycaemia
- caution if used in those with pre-existing hyperglycaemia, diabetes mellitus or high BMI ($\geq$ 30 kg/m^2)
- caution if used in those with moderate-to-severe liver impairment
- not recommended in those with end-stage kidney disease
- see also General Nursing considerations/Cautions for monoclonal antibodies (p. 744)

Patient education
- advise the patient to use artificial tears to prevent dry eyes during therapy
- if the patient has diabetes or pre-existing hyperglycaemia, they should be advised to monitor blood glucose levels regularly during therapy
- instruct the patient to seek medical advice immediately if any of the following occur:
  - rash, any skin blistering or peeling
  - numbness, tingling, weakness or pain in hands or feet
  - cough, shortness of breath, difficulty breathing
- if they want to father a child, men should be counselled to have sperm samples frozen and stored before starting therapy, as reproductive function and fertility may be impaired. They should also be advised to use effective contraception during and for up to 6 months after stopping therapy
- see also General Patient education for monoclonal antibodies (p. 745)

GEMTUZUMAB OZOGAMICIN
Trade name
Mylotarg

Available form
Vial: 5 mg

Action
- monoclonal antibody (IgG$_4$) which selectively kills CD33-positive human leukaemic cell line (HL 60) target cells
- half-life 160 hours

Use
- treatment of previously untreated, de novo CD33-positive acute myeloid leukaemia (except acute promyelocytic leukaemia) (combination therapy with anthracycline and cytarabine (AraC))

Dose
- 3 mg/m^2/dose (IV over 2 hours on days 1, 4 and 7 (induction) (maximum dose 5 mg)

Adverse effects
- see General Adverse effects of monoclonal antibodies (p. 744)

Interactions
- see General Interactions of monoclonal antibodies (p. 744)

Nursing considerations/Cautions
- reconstitute and dilute before use
- see also General Nursing considerations/Cautions for monoclonal antibodies (p. 744)

Patient education
- see General Patient education for monoclonal antibodies (p. 745)

GLOFITAMAB
Trade name
Columvi

Available forms
Vial: 2.5 mg, 10 mg

Action
- bispecific monoclonal antibody that binds to CD20 on B-cell surface and CD3 on T-cell surface that results in lysis of CD20-expressing B cells

Use
- relapsed or refractory diffuse large B-cell lymphoma after two or more lines of systemic therapy

Dose
- obinutuzumab 1000 mg by IV infusion at 50 mg/hour, increasing by 50 mg/hour increments (maximum 400 mg/hour) administered 7 days before starting glofitamab (day 1, cycle 1)
- step-up dosing:
  - (cycle 1, day 8) 2.5 mg IV over 4 hours
  - (cycle 1, day 15) 10 mg IV over 4 hours
  - (cycle 2, day 1) 30 mg IV over 4 hours
  - (cycle 3 to 12, day 1) 30 mg over 2 hours

Adverse effects
- cytokine release syndrome (CRS)
- immune effector cell-associated neurotoxicity syndrome (ICANS)
- tumour flare
- see also General Adverse effects of monoclonal antibodies (p. 744)

Interactions
- monoclonal antibodies are not substrates for cytochrome P450 or drug transporters and therefore drug interactions are not expected

Nursing considerations/Cautions
- obinutuzumab is administered as CRS prophylaxis
- step-up dosing schedule should not be skipped
- cycle is 21 days
- see manufacturer's information for dilution table to give final concentration of 0.1 to 0.6 mg/mL
- if the patient experiences CRS during 4-hour infusion (cycle 1, 2), duration can be extended to 8 hours for the next infusion; or if experienced during 2-hour infusion (cycle 3-12), duration can be extended to 4 hours for subsequent infusions
- patients should be closely monitored for signs and symptoms of CRS and ICANS during infusion and for at least 10 hours after the first infusion
- recommended treatment duration is 12 cycles, disease progression or unmanageable toxicity
- if there is a glofitamab-free interval of more than 6 weeks between cycles, pretreatment with obinutuzumab should be repeated, as well as step-up dosing schedule before resuming therapy at 30 mg
- caution if used in those with a history of chronic or recurrent infection
- not recommended for primary CNS lymphoma, active infection or inflammatory disorders
- not recommended in those with moderate-to-severe liver impairment or severe kidney impairment
- see also General Nursing considerations/Cautions for monoclonal antibodies (p. 744)

ANTINEOPLASTIC AGENTS

Patient education
- the patient should be instructed to immediately seek medical attention if any of the following occurs:
  - fever, chills, rapid heart rate, headache, nausea, trouble breathing, lightheadedness or dizziness due to low blood pressure (CRS)
  - headache, dizziness, anxiety, fatigue, difficulty speaking, somnolence, confusion, disorientation, altered consciousness, fitting/seizures (ICANS)
  - localised pain, swelling (tumour flare)
- see also General Patient education for monoclonal antibodies (p. 745)

INOTUZUMAB OZOGAMICIN
Trade name
Besponsa

Available form
Vial: 1 mg

Action
- CD22 antibody-drug conjugate consists of three components: recombinant immunoglobulin (IgG$_{4kappa}$) (inotuzumab), semisynthetic calicheamicin derivative that causes double-stranded DNA breaks and an acid-cleavable linker that joins inotuzumab with the calicheamicin derivative

Use
- relapsed or refractory CD22-positive B-cell precursor acute lymphoblastic leukaemia (ALL)

Dose
- initially 0.8 mg/m^2 (day 1) 0.5 mg/m^2 (day 8) and 0.5 mg/m^2 (day 15) of a 21-day cycle (cycle 1) by IV infusion over 1 hour, then 0.5 mg/m^2 (days 1, 8 and 15) of a 28-day cycle if the patient has achieved complete remission or complete remission with incomplete haematological recovery **OR**
- 0.8 mg/m^2 (day 1) 0.5 mg/m^2 (day 8) and 0.5 mg/m^2 (day 15) of a 28-day cycle if the patient has not achieved complete remission or complete remission with incomplete haematological recovery

Adverse effects
- hepatotoxicity, hepatic venoocclusive disease
- QT prolongation
- increased amylase and lipase
- see also General Adverse effects of monoclonal antibodies (p. 744)

Interactions
- not recommended with other agents known to prolong QT interval

Nursing considerations/Cautions
- liver function tests (e.g. alanine aminotransferase (ALT), aspartate aminotransferase (AST), total bilirubin, alkaline phosphatase) and full blood counts should be monitored before and after each dose or more frequently if abnormal liver tests occur. For patients undergoing stem cell transplantation, liver function should be monitored closely for the first month post-transplant, and regularly thereafter
- before the first dose, if the patient has circulating lymphoblasts, cytoreduction with hydroxyurea, corticosteroids and/or vincristine is recommended to reduce blast count to ≤ 10,000/mm^3
- if complete remission or complete remission with incomplete haematological recovery does not occur within 3 cycles of treatment, therapy should be stopped
- if the patient is not having haematopoietic stem cell transplant (HSCT), 6 cycles of therapy may be given, whereas only 2 cycles are recommended for those who are to have HSCT (however, a third cycle may be given if the patient has not achieved complete remission or complete remission with incomplete haematological recovery)

- therapy interruption is recommended if the patient experiences haematological toxicity or non-haematolgical toxicity (e.g. liver toxicity, veno-occlusive disease, infusion-related reactions)
- the solution is light sensitive and must be protected during reconstitution, dilution and administration using a UV light-blocking cover such as aluminium foil or amber, dark brown or green bags. Infusion line does not need to be protected
- reconstitute using 4 mL water for injections and swirl gently (do not shake), then add to sodium chloride 0.9% for a total volume of 50 mL. Invert gently to mix
- the infusion rate should be 50 mL/hour
- caution if used in those with mild-to-moderate liver disease or a history of liver disease or hepatitis, have experienced mild-to-moderate veno-occlusive liver disease or sinusoidal obstruction syndrome, are older or have undergone stem cell transplantation
- caution if used in those with a history of QT interval prolongation or those with electrolyte disturbances. If used, ECG and electrolyte monitoring is recommended before the start and regularly during treatment
- contraindicated in those with serious ongoing liver disease (e.g. cirrhosis, active hepatitis) or those who have experienced serious or ongoing veno-occlusive liver disease or sinusoidal obstruction syndrome
- see also General Nursing considerations/Cautions for monoclonal antibodies (p. 744)

Patient education

- advise the patient to seek medical advice immediately if any of the following occur:
  - rapid weight gain, upper right abdominal pain, abdominal swelling
  - feeling dizzy or light-headed, abnormal heart rate
  - fever, chills, hot flushes, dizzy or lightheadedness, rash, trouble breathing during or shortly after infusion
- see also General Patient education for monoclonal antibodies (p. 745)

IPILIMUMAB
Trade name
Yervoy

Available forms
Vial: 50 mg/10 mL, 200 mg/40 mL

Action
- recombinant monoclonal antibody that binds cytotoxic T-lymphocyte-associated antigen 4 (CTLA-4) (CTLA-4 is a key regulator of T-cell activity that increases the number of tumour-reactive T-effector cells)
- also increases the antitumour immune response
- half-life about 20 days

Use
- unresectable or metastatic melanoma (previous therapy failed or intolerable) (alone or with nivolumab)
- untreated advanced renal cell (RCC) carcinoma (with nivolumab)
- metastatic or recurrent non-small cell lung cancer (NSCLC) with no EGFR or ALK gene aberrations (with nivolumab and 2 cycles of platinum-double chemotherapy)
- unresectable malignant pleural mesothelioma (MPM) (with nivolumab, first line treatment)
- unresectable advanced, metastatic or recurrent oesophageal squamous cell carcinoma (OSCC) (with nivolumab) in patients with tumour cell PD-L1 expression ≥ 1

Dose
- (Unresectable or metastatic melanoma) 3 mg/kg IV over 90 minutes every 3 weeks for 4 doses or 16 weeks (induction, alone or with nivolumab),

ANTINEOPLASTIC AGENTS

followed by single-agent (nivolumab) therapy (maintenance) **OR**
- (RCC) 1 mg/kg IV over 30 minutes every 3 weeks for 4 doses, then nivolumab alone **OR**
- (NSCLM) 1 mg/kg IV every 6 weeks (with nivolumab every 3 weeks and platinum therapy every 3 weeks) **OR**
- (MPM) 3 mg/kg IV over 30 minutes every 2 weeks, or 360 mg IV over 30 minutes every 3 weeks (with nivolumab every 6 weeks) **OR**
- (OSCC) 1 mg/kg IV every 6 weeks (with nivolumab every 2 or 3 weeks)

Adverse effects
- see General Adverse effects of monoclonal antibodies (p. 744)

Interactions
- immune-related adverse effects occur more commonly when therapy is combined with nivolumab
- not recommended with vemurafenib
- corticosteroids are not recommended before starting ipilimumab therapy; however, they may be used to treat immune-related adverse effects. Corticosteroid therapy should be tapered over at least 1 month
- caution if used with anticoagulants because of an increased risk of GI bleeding

Nursing considerations/Cautions
- (Melanoma) tumour response should be assessed after 4 doses, and if 4 doses are not completed within 16 weeks then therapy should be stopped
- therapy is continued until disease progression, unacceptable toxicity occurs or up to 2 years
- (Combination therapy) if given with nivolumab and/or chemotherapy, nivolumab should be administered first, then ipilimumab at least 30 minutes later, and chemotherapy should be given last (if required)
- not recommended in those with severe active autoimmune disease where further immune activation could be life threatening
- contraindicated in those with hypersensitivity to polysorbate 80
- see also General Nursing considerations/Cautions for monoclonal antibodies (p. 744)

Patient education
- see General Patient education for monoclonal antibodies (p. 745)

ISATUXIMAB
Trade name
Sarclisa

Available form
Vial: 20 mg/mL

Action
- monoclonal antibody (IgG$_1$) that binds to specific CD38 receptors triggering death of CD38-expressing tumour cells
- half-life 28 days

Use
- multiple myeloma where at least two prior therapies (including lenalidomide and a proteasome inhibitor) have been used (combination therapy with pomalidomide and dexamethasone)

Dose
- 10 mg/kg by IV infusion on days 1, 8, 15 and 22 (cycle 1), then days 1 and 15 (cycle 2 and beyond)
- infusion rate:
  - first infusion: 25 mL/hour for the first hour, increasing by 25 mL/hour every 30 minutes if no infusion-related reactions occur in first hour (maximum rate 150 mL/hour)
  - second infusion: 50 mL/hour for 30 minutes and, if no infusion-related reactions occur, the rate can be increased 50 mL/hour for 30 minutes, then by 100 mL/hour every 30 minutes (maximum rate 200 mL/hour)

- subsequent infusions: 200 mL/hour

Adverse effects
- see General Adverse effects of monoclonal antibodies (p. 744)

Interactions
- may result in false positive on indirect Coombs' test
- may be detected on serum protein electrophoresis (SPE) and immunofixation (IFE) assays for monitoring of complete response to therapy

Nursing considerations/Cautions
- blood type and screen test should be performed before starting therapy with phenotyping. If therapy is started, the blood bank should be informed of therapy and interference resolved using dithiothreitol-treated RBC. If emergency transfusion is needed, non-cross-matched ABO/RhD-compatible RBCs can be given
- see also General Nursing considerations/Cautions for monoclonal antibodies (p. 744)

Patient education
- see General Patient education for monoclonal antibodies (p. 745)

NIVOLUMAB
Trade name
Opdivo

Available forms
Vial: 40 mg/4 mL, 100 mg/10 mL, 240 mg/24 mL

Action
- anti-PD-1 monoclonal antibody (human IgG_4)

Use
- unresectable or metastatic melanoma (MM) (monotherapy or with ipilimumab)
- adjunctive treatment of melanoma (stage IIB, IIC, III or IV) after resection (monotherapy)
- locally advanced or metastatic squamous or non-squamousnon-small cell lung cancer (NSCLC)
- unresectable malignant pleural mesothelioma (MPM) (monotherapy)
- intermediate/poor-risk, previously untreated, advanced renal cell carcinoma (RCC) (with ipilimumab)
- advanced clear cell RCC after antiangiogenic therapy (monotherapy)
- advanced RCC (with cabozantinib)
- relapsed or refractory classical Hodgkin lymphoma (cHL) (after stem cell transplant and brentuximab vedotin) (monotherapy)
- recurrent or metastatic squamous cell carcinoma of head and neck (SCCHN) (progressing on or after platinum-based therapy) (monotherapy)
- locally advanced unresectable or metastatic urothelial carcinoma (UC) (after platinum-based therapy) (monotherapy or with gemcitabine and cisplatin)
- hepatocellular carcinoma (HCC) (after sorafenib) (monotherapy)
- oesophageal squamous cell carcinoma (OSCC) (monotherapy, with ipilimumab or fluoropyrimidine and platinum-based combination chemotherapy)
- oesophageal cancer (OC) or gastrooesophageal junction cancer (GOJC) after neoadjuvant chemotherapy (monotherapy)
- HER2-negative advanced or metastatic gastric cancer (GC), gastro-oesophageal junction cancer (GOJC) or oesophageal adenocarcinoma (OAC) (first-line treatment, combined with fluoropyrimidine and platinum-based combination chemotherapy)

Dose
- (MM, NSCLC, RCC, cHL, SCCHN, UC, HCC) (monotherapy) 3 mg/kg IV over 30 minutes every 2 weeks, 240 mg IV over 30 minutes every 2 weeks, or 480 mg IV over 30 minutes every 4 weeks **OR**
- (OSCC, monotherapy or adjuvant therapy for MM, OC) 240 mg IV over 30 minutes every 2 weeks, or 480 mg IV over 30 minutes every 4 weeks **OR**
- (Adjuvant therapy for GOJC and UC) 240 mg IV over 30 minutes every

ANTINEOPLASTIC AGENTS

2 weeks for 16 weeks, then 480 mg IV every 30 minutes every 4 weeks (for up to 12 months without disease progression, disease progression or no longer tolerated) **OR**
- (Combination therapy – metastatic or unresectable melanoma) 1 mg/kg IV over 30 minutes every 3 weeks for 4 doses (on same day as ipilimumab after nivolumab infusion is complete) **OR**
- for combination therapy for other cancers, see manufacturer's information as regimens are complex

Adverse effects
- see General Adverse effects of monoclonal antibodies (p. 744)

Interactions
- increased risk of immune-related adverse effects if given with ipilimumab
- use with corticosteroids is not recommended at start of therapy. If used to treat immune-related adverse effects, corticosteroids can be used and should be tapered slowly when discontinued

Nursing considerations/Cautions
- when given as part of combination therapy, nivolumab should be given first, followed by ipilimumab at least 30 minutes later, followed by platinum-based therapy, if used
- may be used undiluted or dilute with sodium chloride 0.9% or glucose 5% for concentration of 1–10 mg/mL. If patient weight < 40 kg, infusion volume should not be > 4 mL/kg
- contains sodium 2.5 mg/mL
- see also General Nursing considerations/Cautions for monoclonal antibodies (p. 744)

Patient education
- advise the patient to carry a patient alert card at all times
- the patient should be instructed to seek medical advice if any of the following occur:
  - moderate-to-severe diarrhoea, new or worsening abdominal pain, chills, fever, nausea, vomiting
  - any tingling, numbness of hands or feet, burning sensation
  - cough, shortness of breath, difficulty breathing
- see also General Patient education for monoclonal antibodies (p. 745)

Available in combination with
- vailable as Opdualag (nivolumab 240 mg and relatlimab 80 mg)

OBINUTUZUMAB
Trade name
Gazyva

Available form
Vial: 1000 mg/40 mL

Action
- anti-CD20 monoclonal antibody
- half-life 26 days

Use
- previously untreated chronic lymphocytic leukaemia (CLL) (with chlorambucil)
- maintenance of previously untreated follicular lymphoma (FL) (with disease progression, unresponsive or progression after rituximab-containing regimen)
- pretreatment to reduce risk of cytokine release syndrome (CRS) induced by glofitamab

Dose
- (CLL) initially 1000 mg IV over days 1 and 2, then 1000 mg day 8, and 1000 mg day 15 of a 28-day cycle, followed by 1000 mg on day 1 only of subsequent cycles (cycles 2–6) (with chlorambucil) **OR**
- (FL) 1000 mg IV given on days 1, 8 and 15 of a 21- or 28-day cycle (depending on combination therapy) **OR**
- (Prevention of CRS) 1000 mg IV starting at 50 mg/hour, increasing at 50 mg/hour increments to a maximum of 400 mg/

hour, given 7 days before starting glofitamab therapy

Adverse effects
- progressive multifocal leukoencephalopathy (PML)
- worsening of pre-existing cardiac conditions
- see also General Adverse effects of monoclonal antibodies (p. 744)

Interactions
- monoclonal antibodies are not substrates for cytochrome P450 or drug transporters and therefore drug interactions are not expected

Nursing considerations/Cautions
- all patients should be screened for hepatitis B before starting therapy. Therapy should be stopped if reactivation of hepatitis B occurs during therapy
- antihypertensive therapy should be withheld for 12 hours before, during and for 1 hour after therapy to decrease the risk of hypotension occurring
- (Previously untreated FL) can be given as 6 × 28-day cycles (with bendamustine), 6 × 21-day cycles (with CHOP regimen) plus 2 cycles of obinutuzumab alone, or 8 × 21-day cycles (with CVP regimen)
- dilute with sodium chloride 0.9% only
- infusion-related reactions (IRRs) occur most commonly during first 1000 mg dose
- the patient must be closely monitored during infusion period. If a mild-to-moderate reaction occurs, the rate should be slowed and symptoms treated. If the reaction is severe, the infusion should be stopped and symptoms treated. The infusion can be restarted at half the rate that caused the reaction once symptoms have been resolved and then slowly increased. If a second severe reaction occurs, the infusion should be permanently stopped. If life-threatening reactions occur, therapy should be stopped and not restarted
- (CLL, day 1, cycle 1) 1000 mg should be prepared as two infusion bags (100 mg and 900 mg) by diluting 4 mL in a 100 mL infusion bag and 36 mL in a 250 mL infusion bag. Gently invert bags to ensure even distribution **OR**
- (CLL, day 1, cycle 1) administer 100 mg infusion at 25 mg/hour over 4 hours. If there are no modifications or interruptions to infusion due to IRRs, 900 mg infusion can be administered on same day (day 1) starting at a rate of 50 mg/hour for first 30 minutes. If no reaction, the rate can be increased at 50 mg/hour increments every 30 minutes to a maximum of 400 mg/hour **OR**
- (CLL, day 1, cycle 1) if IRRs occur during 100 mg infusion, a 900 mg infusion should be withheld until day 2 and commenced at 50 mg/hour then proceed as outlined in the above point
- (CLL, cycle 1, days 8 and 15; cycles 2—6, day 1) if there is no IRR during the previous infusion and the rate was $\geq$ 100 mg/hour, 1000 mg infusion can be started at 100 mg/hour and increased at increments of 100 mg/hour every 30 minutes to a maximum of 400 mg/hour, monitoring carefully for any IRRs
- (FL, cycle 1, day 1) 1000 mg IV given at 50 mg/hour and increasing in 50 mg/hour increments every 30 minutes to 400 mg/hour (maximum)
- (FL, cycle 1, days 8, 15 and cycles 2—6 or 28 as maintenance) if no IRR occurs and the previous infusion rate $\geq$ 100 mg/hour, infusion can start at 100 mg/hour and increased at 30-minute intervals by 100 mg/hour increments to 400 mg/hour maximum. If the patient experiencesan IRR, infusion should be started at 50 mg/hour and increased at 30-minute intervals at 50 mg/hour increment to 400 mg/hour (maximum)
- (FL) dilute 40 mL in 250 mL of sodium chloride 0.9% and infuse IV

ANTINEOPLASTIC AGENTS

- caution if used in those with pre-existing cardiac or lung conditions because of an increased risk of IRRs
- contraindicated in those with hypersensitivity to murine protein

Patient education
- the patient should be instructed to seek medical advice immediately if any of the following occur:
  - muscle weakness, sensory disturbances, paralysis, aphasia or visual disturbances
  - heart pain, rapid heart rate, swelling of feet or ankles, breathlessness
- also see General Patient education for monoclonal antibodies (p. 745)

PANITUMUMAB
Trade name
Vectibix

Available forms
Vial: 100 mg/5 mL, 400 mg/20 mL

Action
- IgG$_2$ monoclonal antibody with a high affinity for epidermal growth factor receptor (EGFR) inhibiting cell proliferation, interleukin 8 and vascular endothelial growth factor production
- half life 7.5 days

Use
- wild-type RAS metastatic colorectal cancer (mCRC) (monotherapy or combination therapy)

Dose
- 6 mg/kg IV once every 2 weeks (until disease progression or intolerance occurs)

Adverse effects
- phototoxicity, soft tissue toxicity
- severe diarrhoea (when given as combination therapy), dehydration
- ocular toxicity (redness, itching, irritation, dry eyes, increased lacrimation, blepharitis)
- deep vein thrombosis, pulmonary embolism
- see also General Adverse effects of monoclonal antibodies (p. 744)

Interactions
- monoclonal antibodies are not substrates for cytochrome P450 or drug transporters and therefore drug interactions are not expected

Nursing considerations/Cautions
- mutational status of RAS should be determined by valid and reliable testing before starting therapy
- dilute with 100 mL sodium chloride 0.9% to give a concentration of 10 mg/mL
- given as IV infusion over 60 minutes (first infusion) increasing the rate to infuse over 30—60 minutes for the second and subsequent infusions if the first infusion was well tolerated
- if a mild-to-moderate infusion-related reaction occur, the rate can be decreased by 50%
- for doses > 1000 mg, should be diluted with 150 mL and infused over 90 minutes
- not recommended in those with a history of pulmonary fibrosis or interstitial lung disease
- contraindicated with oxaliplatin-based therapy in those in whom RAS gene status is unknown or where mutant RAS mCRC exists
- see also General Nursing considerations/Cautions for monoclonal antibodies (p. 744)

Patient education
- the patient should be advised to limit exposure to the sun during therapy (including wearing protective clothing, sunglasses, hats) and apply sunscreen (SPF 30+) to face, neck, hands, feet, back and chest daily
- instruct the patient to seek medical advice immediately if any of the following occur:

- any new or worsening cough, difficulty breathing or shortness of breath, wheezing
- pain, redness or swelling of calf
- see also General Patient education for monoclonal antibodies (p. 745)

PEMBROLIZUMAB

Trade name
Keytruda

Available form
Vial (concentrate): 100 mg/4 mL

Action
- recombinant monoclonal IgG$_{4kappa}$ antibody that blocks the PD-1 pathway
- half-life 22 days

Use
- unresectable or metastatic malignant melanoma (monotherapy)
- stage IIB, IIC or III melanoma after resection (adjuvant therapy)
- non-small cell lung cancer (NSCLC) (monotherapy or combination therapy)
- urothelial carcinoma (UC) (monotherapy)
- head and neck squamous cell cancer (HNSCC) (monotherapy or combination therapy)
- relapsed or refractory classical Hodgkin lymphoma (cHL) following autologous stem cell transplant (ASCT) or when ASCT or multi-agent chemotherapy is not an option
- primary mediastinal B-cell lymphoma (PMBCL)
- endometrial cancer (EC)
- renal cell carcinoma (RCC)
- colorectal or non-colorectal microsatellite instability-high cancer (MSI-H)
- biliary tract carcinoma (BTC)
- cervical cancer
- breast cancer (triple negative)
- cutaneous squamous cell carcinoma
- gastric or gastro-oesophageal junction cancer
- oesophageal cancer
- tumour mutational burden-high cancer

Dose
- 200 mg IV over 30 minutes every 3 weeks **OR**
- 400 mg IV over 30 minutes every 6 weeks

Adverse effects
- see General Adverse effects of monoclonal antibodies (p. 744)

Interactions
- not recommended with thalidomide analogue and dexamethasone owing to increased mortality if treated for multiple myeloma
- systemic corticosteroids or immunosuppressants should be avoided before starting therapy because they may interfere with activity and efficacy; however, they can be used after starting therapy to treat immune-mediated adverse effects and tapered slowly, or as part of a premedication regimen

Nursing considerations/Cautions
- dose reduction for immune-related adverse reactions is not recommended
- PD-L1 status should be assessed using validated testing before starting therapy
- dilute the required volume with sodium chloride 0.9% or glucose 5% for a final dilution of 1 to 10 mg/mL. Diluted solution may contain translucent to white proteinaceous particles which are of no concern and will be removed by an in-line filter
- caution if used in those with human immunodeficiency virus (HIV), hepatitis B or C, an active infection or a previous history of severe immune-mediated adverse reactions
- contraindicated in those with sensitivity to Chinese hamster ovary protein
- see also General Nursing considerations/Cautions for monoclonal antibodies (p. 744)

Patient education
- see General Patient education for monoclonal antibodies (p. 745)

ANTINEOPLASTIC AGENTS

PERTUZUMAB
Trade name
Perjeta

Available form
Vial: 420 mg/14 mL

Action
* antihuman epidermal growth factor receptor 2 (HER2) monoclonal antibody that inhibits proliferation of tumour cells
* activity improved when used with trastuzumab
* half-life 18 days

Use
* HER2-positive inflammatory or locally advanced or early-stage (either node positive or lesion $\geq$ 2 cm) breast cancer (with trastuzumab)
* HER2-positive metastatic breast cancer (with no prior anti-HER2 or chemotherapy) (with docetaxel, trastuzumab)

Dose
* initially 840 mg IV over 60 minutes, then 420 mg IV over 30—60 minutes every 3 weeks (with trastuzumab and docetaxel) (until disease progression or toxicity occurs (metastatic breast cancer), or 3—6 cycles (early breast cancer before surgery), or maximum 18 cycles, disease progression or toxicity occurs (early breast cancer after surgery))

Adverse effects
* decreased left ventricular ejection fraction
* see also General Adverse effects of monoclonal antibodies (p. 744)

Nursing considerations/Cautions
* positive HER2 gene overexpression should be verified using valid and reliable testing before starting therapy
* left ventricular ejection fraction (LVEF) should be measured before starting and then 3-monthly during therapy
* incompatible with glucose 5%
* during combination therapy, pertuzumab and trastuzumab can be given in any order. If docetaxel is also used, it should be given after pertuzumab and trastuzumab. If anthracycline-based therapy is used, pertuzumab and trastuzumab should be given after the total anthracycline regimen is completed
* caution if used in those previously treated with anthracyclines or radiation to the chest area because of the increased risk of decreased LVEF
* caution if used in those with baseline LVEF $\leq$ 50%, a history of cardiac failure, decreases in LVEF to < 50% during prior trastuzumab adjunct therapy, uncontrolled hypertension, recent myocardial infarction, serious cardiac arrhythmias requiring treatment or doxorubicin total cumulative dose > 360 mg/m^2
* see also General Nursing considerations/Cautions for monoclonal antibodies (p. 744)

Patient education
* advise the patient to seek medical advice if any of the following occur:
  * shortness of breath or tiredness on light physical activity (such as walking)
  * shortness of breath at night, especially when lying flat
  * cough
  * irregular or abnormal heart rate
  * swelling of hands/feet (due to fluid build-up)
* see also General Patient education for antineoplastic agents (p. 745)

POLATUZUMAB VEDOTIN
Trade name
Polivy

Available forms
Vial: 30 mg, 140 mg

Action
* CD79b-targeted antibody—drug conjugate made up of monoclonal antibody (IgG$_1$) and an antimitotic drug that results in killing of malignant B cells
* half-life 4 days

Use
- previously treated diffuse large B-cell lymphoma (in those ineligible for haematopoietic stem cell transplant) (with bendamustine and rituximab)
- previously untreated diffuse large B-cell lymphoma (with rituximab, cyclophosphamide, doxorubicin and prednisolone)

Dose
- (Previously treated patients) 1.8 mg/kg as an IV infusion over 90 minutes every 21 days on day 1 of the cycle with bendamustine and rituximab (given in any order) for 6 cycles **OR**
- (Previously untreated patients) 1.8 mg/kg as an IV infusion over 90 minutes every 21 days with rituximab, cyclophosphamide, doxorubicin and prednisolone for 6 cycles. Prednisolone should be administered first, then rituximab, cyclophosphamide, doxorubicin and polatuzumab can be given in any order. Prednisolone is given on days 1 to 5 of each cycle. Cycles 7 and 8 consist of rituximab as monotherapy

Adverse effects
- peripheral neuropathy
- see also General Adverse effects of monoclonal antibodies (p. 744)

Interactions
- caution if used with rifampicin, phenytoin, carbamazepine, phenobarbital (phenobarbitone) or St John's wort, as serum levels of anti-mitotic drug may be decreased
- caution if used with clarithromycin, cobicistat, itraconazole, ritonavir or voriconazole, as serum levels of the antimitotic drug may be increased

Nursing considerations/Cautions
- if a 90-minute infusion is well tolerated, subsequent infusions can be given over 30 minutes
- reconstitute with water for injections (1.8 mL for 30 mg, 7.2 mL for 140 mg) and then dilute further with either glucose 5% or sodium chloride 0.45% or 0.9% (see manufacturer's information for calculation information)
- not recommended in those with moderate-to-severe liver impairment
- see also General Nursing considerations/Cautions for monoclonal antibodies (p. 744)

Patient education
- instruct the patient to seek medical attention immediately if they experience any pins and needles in extremities, numbness or burning sensation, weakness, changes to sensation in arms or legs/feet, or walking difficulties
- see also General Patient education for monoclonal antibodies (p. 745)

RAMUCIRUMAB
Trade name
Cyramza

Available form
Vial: 100 mg/10 mL

Action
- recombinant IgG$_1$ monoclonal antibody, vascular endothelial growth factor receptor 2 (VEGFR-2) inhibitor
- half-life 14 days

Use
- advanced or metastatic gastric or gastro-oesophageal junction adenocarcinoma (with disease progression after prior platinum and fluoropyrimidine chemotherapy) (combined with paclitaxel, or as monotherapy if paclitaxel is inappropriate)

Dose
- 8 mg/kg IV over 60 minutes every 2 weeks (as monotherapy) **OR**
- 8 mg/kg IV over 60 minutes on days 1 and 15 of a 28-day cycle (before paclitaxel)

Adverse effects
- thromboembolic events (including myocardial infarction, cardiac arrest, cerebral vascular accident)
- gastrointestinal perforation
- hypertension

ANTINEOPLASTIC AGENTS

- impaired wound healing
- proteinuria, nephrotic syndrome
- see also General Adverse effects of monoclonal antibodies (p. 744)

Interactions
- monoclonal antibodies are not substrates for cytochrome P450 or drug transporters and therefore drug interactions are not expected

Nursing considerations/Cautions
- BP should be measured regularly during therapy
- urine should be monitored for protein during therapy. If level ≥ 2/24 hours, urine collection is recommended and therapy should be temporarily stopped and resumed at a lower dose when protein level < 2 g/24 hours
- therapy should be withheld for at least 4 weeks before major surgery
- glucose 5% should not be used as a diluent
- see also General Nursing considerations/Cautions for monoclonal antibodies (p. 744)

Patient education
- advise the patient to seek medical advice immediately if any of the following occur:
  - chest pain, chest heaviness
  - sudden numbness or weakness of arm, leg or face, feeling confused, difficulty speaking or understanding others, difficulty walking, loss of balance or coordination, sudden dizziness
  - severe abdominal pain, nausea, vomiting, fever and chills
- see also General Patient education for monoclonal antibodies (p. 745)

RITUXIMAB
Trade names
Riximyo, Ruxience, Truxima

Available forms
Solution: 100 mg/10 mL, 500 mg/50 mL

Action
- anti-CD20 monoclonal antibody

Use
- previously untreated CD20-positive stage III/IV follicular, B-cell non-Hodgkin lymphoma (NHL)
- relapsed or refractory CD20-positive low-grade or follicular, B-cell NHL
- CD20-positive diffuse large B-cell NHL
- CD20-positive chronic lymphocytic leukaemia (CLL) (with chemotherapy)
- induction of remission of granulomatosis with polyangiitis (GPA) (Wegener's) and microscopic polyangiitis (MPA) (with corticosteroids)
- severe rheumatoid arthritis (with methotrexate) (see Disease-modifying anti-rheumatic drugs (DMARDs), p. 1071)

Dose
- (Relapsed/refractory low-grade follicular NHL) 375 mg/m^2 IV weekly for 4 weeks (monotherapy) on day 1 of each cycle for up to 6 cycles (with cyclophosphamide, hydroxydaunorubicin (doxorubicin), oncovin (vincristine), prednisone (CHOP) chemotherapy) **OR**
- (Relapsed/refractory low-grade follicular NHL — maintenance) 375 mg/m^2 IV once every 12 weeks for up to 2 years **OR**
- (Previously untreated stage III/IV follicular NHL) 375 mg/m^2 IV on day 1 of each chemotherapy cycle (for 8 cycles) **OR**
- (Previously untreated stage III/IV follicular NHL — maintenance) 375 mg/m^2 IV once every 8 weeks for up to 2 years **OR**
- (Diffuse large cell B-cell NHL) 375 mg/m^2 IV on day 1 of each chemotherapy cycle (for up to 8 cycles) (with CHOP chemotherapy) **OR**
- (CLL) 375 mg/m^2 IV on day 1 of first cycle, then 500 mg/m^2 on day 1 of subsequent cycles for 6 cycles (with chemotherapy) **OR**
- (GPA/MPA) 375 mg/m^2 IV weekly for 4 weeks

Adverse effects
- enteroviral meningitis

- see also General Adverse effects of monoclonal antibodies (p. 744)

Interactions
- monoclonal antibodies are not substrates for cytochrome P450 or drug transporters; therefore drug interactions are not expected

Nursing considerations/Cautions
- chemotherapy should always be administered after rituximab
- rapid tumour lysis may occur (with symptoms of hyperkalaemia, hypocalcaemia and hyperuricaemia) within 1–2 hours of the first infusion
- the patient should be monitored during and at least 2 hours after the first infusion for any signs of cytokine-release syndrome (dyspnoea, bronchospasm, hypoxia, chills, fever, rigors, urticaria and angioedema)
- if a severe cytokine syndrome occurs, the infusion should be stopped
- (GPA/MPA) severe vasculitis should be treated with IV methylprednisolone for 1–3 days, followed by prednisolone 1 mg/kg/day orally (up to 80 mg daily), then rapidly tapered when symptoms are controlled
- (GPA/MPA) for the first infusion, the rate should be started at 50 mg/hour and the patient carefully monitored. If no hypersensitivity or infusion-related event occurs, the rate may be increased by 50 mg/hour at 30-minute intervals to a maximum of 400 mg/hour. If a hypersensitivity reaction occurs, the infusion rate should be halved. If no hypersensitivity occurs, subsequent infusions can be started at 100 mg/mL and increased at 100 mg increments at 30-minute intervals to 400 mg/hour maximum
- antibody development has been associated with worsening infusion or allergic reactions after the second infusion
- any concurrent antihypertensive agent may need to be withheld for 12 hours before and during infusion because of an added risk of severe hypotension occurring
- dilute further with sodium chloride 0.9% or glucose 5% to give a concentration of 1–4 mg/mL
- contraindicated in those with murine protein hypersensitivity
- see also General Nursing considerations/Cautions for monoclonal antibodies (p. 744)

Patient education
- warn the patient that reactions (e.g. fever, chills, shivering) may occur after the infusion (especially the first 2 hours of the first infusion) and are transient. They occur less frequently after the first infusion
- instruct the patient to seek medical attention immediately if any headache, stiff neck, fever, altered consciousness, clumsiness or seizures/fitting occurs
- see also General Patient education for monoclonal antibodies (p. 745)

SACITUZUMAB GOVITECAN
Trade name
Trodelvy

Available form
Vial: 180 mg

Action
- Trop-2-directed antibody-drug conjugate which combines monoclonal antibody with small molecule (SN-38) topoisomerase I inhibitor. Conjugate binds to Trop-2-expressing cancer cells where SN-38 is released resulting in DNA damage and cell death
- half-life 23.4 hours (sacituzumab) and 17.6 hours (SN-38)

Use
- unresectable locally advanced or metastatic triple-negative breast cancer (mTNBC) having received at least two prior systemic therapies including one for locally advanced or metastatic disease

ANTINEOPLASTIC AGENTS

- unresectable locally advanced or metastatic hormone receptor (HR)-positive, human epidermal growth factor receptor 2 (HER2)-negative breast cancer having received endocrine-based therapy (including a CDK4/6 inhibitor) and at least two other systemic therapies for locally advanced or metastatic disease

Dose
- 10 mg/kg IV infusion once weekly on days 1 and 8 of a 21-day cycle. First infusion given over 3 hours, subsequent infusions over 1–2 hours if the previous infusion was tolerated

Adverse effects
- severe neutropenia, febrile neutropenia
- severe diarrhoea
- nausea, vomiting
- hypersensitivity
- see also General Adverse effects of monoclonal antibodies (p. 744), but with fewer immune-related adverse reactions

Interactions
- not recommended with UGT1A1 inhibitors (e.g. flunitrazepam, some tyrosine kinase inhibitors) or UGT1A1 inducers (e.g. carbamazepine, phenytoin, phenobarbital, rifampicin, ritonavir)

Nursing considerations/Cautions
- therapy with sacituzumab should not be substituted for or used with other agents containing irinotecan or its active metabolite SN-38
- in addition to premedication to reduce risk of infusion-related reactions, patients should also be given two or three antiemetic drug combinations to prevent chemotherapy-induced nausea and vomiting which could include dexamethasone with either a $5HT_3$ receptor antagonist (e.g. ondansetron) or NK-1 receptor antagonist (e.g. aprepitant)
- if diarrhoea occurs, the cause should be investigated. If not infectious, loperamide should be started immediately (4 mg initially, then 2 mg with each episode of diarrhoea (daily maximum 16 mg)) with fluids and electrolytes as needed
- if the patient experiences an excessive cholinergic response to therapy (e.g. abdominal cramping, diarrhoea, salivation), premedication with atropine is recommended with subsequent infusions
- reconstitute with 20 mL sodium chloride 0.9% only (may require up to 15 minutes to dissolve the powder). Dilute with sodium chloride 0.9% to given final concentration of 1.1 mg/mL to 3.4 mg/mL
- the infusion bag should be protected from light during administration
- if the patient has known reduced uridine diphosphate-glucuronosyl transferase 1A1 (UGT1A1) activity, they should be closely monitored because of the increased risk of acute early onset or unusually severe adverse reactions (particularly neutropenia, febrile neutropenia and anaemia)
- not recommended in those with moderate-to-severe liver impairment
- see also General Nursing considerations/Cautions for monoclonal antibodies (p. 744)

Patient education
- the patient should be instructed to immediately report any of the following:
  - severe diarrhoea including black or bloody stools, diarrhoea that can't be controlled with loperamide within 24 hours, signs of dehydration, nausea and vomiting that prevent adequate fluid intake
  - wheezing, rash, hives, breathing difficulties, fever, chills, face, lips, throat or face swelling
  - fever, chills, shortness of breath, cough, burning or pain on urination
- see also General Patient education for monoclonal antibodies (p. 745)

TECLISTAMAB

Trade name
Tecvayli

Available forms
Vial: 30 mg/3 mL, 153 mg/1.7 mL

Action
* targets CD3 receptors expressed on surface of T cells and B-cell maturation antigen (BCMA) found on the surface of malignant myeloma B-lineage cells, as well as late-stage B cells and plasma cells
* half-life 27 days

Use
* relapsed or refractory multiple myeloma in patients who have had at least three previous therapies (including a proteasome inhibitor, immunomodifier and an anti-CD38 monoclonal antibody)

Dose
* step-up dosing schedule
  * (step-up dose 1, day 1) 0.06 mg/kg SC as single dose
  * (step-up dose 2, day 3) 0.3 mg/kg SC as single dose
  * (first treatment dose, day 5) 1.5 mg/kg SC as single dose
* weekly dosing schedule (1 week after first treatment dose)
  * 1.5 mg/kg SC weekly

Adverse effects
* cytokine release syndrome (CRS)
* immune effector cell-associated neurotoxicity syndrome (ICANS) (mild tremor, confusion, speech hesitancy, deteriorating handwriting, aphasia, agitation, seizures, cerebral oedema)
* hypogammaglobulinaemia
* encephalopathy
* (Injection site) pain, redness, bruising, induration, swelling
* see also General Adverse effects of monoclonal antibodies (p. 744)

Interactions
* vaccination with attenuated live virus vaccines is not recommended for at least 4 weeks before the start, during and for at least 4 weeks after therapy

Nursing considerations/Cautions
* before starting therapy, antiviral prophylaxis for prevention of herpes zoster reactivation should be considered
* therapy should not be started if the patient has an active infection
* SC administration only
* dilution not required
* the solution should come to room temperature for at least 15 minutes before administration, however, it should not be warmed in any way. Gently swirl vial for about 10 seconds (not shaken) and use a transfer needle to remove the required amount
* each injection should not be greater than 2 mL. If a greater dose is required, it should be divided into equal doses in multiple syringes. Transfer needle should be replaced with an appropriate-sized needle for SC administration
* the preferred injection site is the abdomen; however, other subcutaneous sites can be used avoiding scars, tattoos or red, bruised, hard or broken skin. If multiple injections are required, allow at least 2 cm between injection sites
* it is important not to skip step-up doses
* dose delays may be needed to manage toxicity; however, dose reduction is not recommended
* all patients should receive pretreatment medications 1–3 hours before each dose of step-up dosing to reduce the risk of CRS which should include:
  * corticosteroid (oral or IV dexamethasone 16 mg or equivalent)
  * antihistamine (oral or IV diphenhydramine 50 mg or equivalent)
  * antipyretic (oral paracetamol 500–1000 mg)
* pretreatment medications should be repeated if the patient requires repeat doses of step-up dosing schedule due to dose delay or if the patient experiences CRS after a previous dose of teclistamab

ANTINEOPLASTIC AGENTS

- if dose delay occurs and restarting therapy is required, manufacturer's recommendations should be consulted for dosing schedule
- management of CRS is dependent on clinical presentation. If suspected, therapy should be withheld until adverse effects resolves. Management may include antipyretic agents, IV fluids, vasopressors, oxygen, tocilizumab and corticosteroids depending on severity
- immune effector cell-associated neurotoxicity syndrome (ICANS) may occur at the same time or shortly after CRS. Management may include prophylactic antiepileptic agents, corticosteroids and tocilizumab depending on severity

Patient education
- instruct the patient to stay within proximity of the health care facility for at least 48 hours after administration and immediately seek medical advice if any of the following occur:
  - nausea, headache, dizziness, rapid heart rate, difficulty breathing (CRS)
  - headache, feeling confused or less alert, difficulty with speech or writing (ICANS)
- the patient should be advised to keep patient card (information about symptoms of CRS) with them at all times while receiving therapy
- see also General Patient education for monoclonal antibodies (p. 745)

TRASTUZUMAB
Trade names
Herceptin SC, Herzuma, Kanjinti, Ogivri, Trazimera

TRASTUZUMAB EMTANSINE
Trade name
Kadcyla

Available forms
Vial (powder): 60 mg, 100 mg, 150 mg, 160 mg, 420 mg, 440 mg;
Vial (solution): 600 mg/5 mL

Action
- human epidermal growth factor receptor 2 (HER2) recombinant monoclonal antibody
- (Kadcyla) combines HER2 recombinant monoclonal antibody with microtubule inhibitory drug (DM1) and stable thioether linker (both components are active)

Use
- early or locally advanced breast cancer (HER2-positive, after surgery with other chemotherapy and/or radiation therapy)
- metastatic breast cancer (HER2-positive) (monotherapy or with other chemotherapy)
- previously untreated HER2-positive stomach or gastric-oesophageal junction cancer (with cisplatin and fluorouracil or capecitabine)

Dose
- (Early, locally advanced or metastatic breast cancer — 3-week regimen) 8 mg/kg IV over 90 minutes (loading dose), then 6 mg/kg IV over 30 minutes (if loading dose was well tolerated) at 3-weekly intervals **OR**
- (Early or metastatic breast cancer — weekly regimen) 4 mg/kg IV over 90 minutes (loading dose), then 2 mg/kg IV over 30 minutes (if loading dose was well tolerated) at weekly intervals **OR**
- (Advanced gastric cancer) 8 mg/kg IV over 90 minutes (loading dose), then 6 mg/kg over 30 minutes (if loading dose was well tolerated) at 3-weekly intervals **OR**
- (Early, metastatic or locally advanced breast cancer) 600 mg SC over 2–5 minutes every 3 weeks (Herceptin SC) **OR**
- (Early breast cancer) 3.6 mg/kg IV over 90 minutes every 3 weeks, then reducing the IV rate to 30 minutes (if the first infusion was well tolerated) (21-day cycle) for 14 cycles, unacceptable toxicity or disease progression (Kadcyla)

- (Metastatic breast cancer) 3.6 mg/kg IV over 90 minutes every 3 weeks, then reducing the IV rate to 30 minutes (if the first infusion was well tolerated) until disease progression or unacceptable toxicity (Kadcyla)

Adverse effects
- congestive cardiac failure, left ventricular dysfunction
- interstitial lung disease
- (IV) extravasation, tissue necrosis
- see also General Adverse effects of monoclonal antibodies (p. 744)

Interactions
- decreased clearance if given with paclitaxel
- increased risk of cardiac toxicity if anthracyclines or cyclophosphamide have been previously used

Nursing considerations/Cautions
- HER2 testing is required before starting therapy
- cardiac assessment (history, physical assessment, ECHO cardiogram and/or MUGA (multigated acquisition) scan) is recommended before starting, 3-monthly during treatment and 6-monthly for 2 years after stopping therapy
- different formulations of trastuzumab (Herceptin and Kadcyla) are not interchangeable
- the loading dose is given over 90 minutes; if well tolerated, the infusion time can be decreased to 30 minutes
- (Early or locally advanced breast cancer) treatment is for 1 year, disease progression or until unacceptable toxicity occurs
- (Herceptin SC) SC sites should be rotated between right and left thigh and at least 2.5 cm from previous injection sites
- (Herceptin SC) no further dilution is required
- chills and/or fever are common during the first infusion
- (IV) reconstitute using water for injections (3 mL for 60 mg vial, 7.2 mL for 150 mg, 20 mL for 420—440 mg) and swirl gently to dissolve (do not shake), allowing the solution to stand for 15 minutes after reconstitution and then further dilute with 250 mL sodium chloride 0.9%
- (Kadcyla) reconstitute using water for injections (5 mL for 100 mg vial, 8 mL for 160 mg vial) and swirl gently to dissolve (do not shake) and then further dilute with 250 mL sodium chloride 0.45% or sodium chloride 0.9%. If sodium chloride 0.45% is used, no inline filter is required. If sodium chloride 0.9% is used, a 0.22 micron inline filter is required
- incompatible with glucose 5%
- (Ogivri) contains sorbitol and is not recommended in those with hereditary fructose intolerance
- caution if used in those with symptomatic intrinsic lung disease or with extensive tumour involvement of the lungs
- caution if used in those with hypertension, congestive cardiac failure, ventricular dysfunction or coronary artery disease because of the increased risk of cardiac toxicity
- not recommended in those with dyspnoea at rest due to malignancy complications or co-morbidities
- contraindicated in those with left ventricular ejection fraction less than 45%, symptomatic heart failure or hypersensitivity to Chinese hamster ovary cell proteins
- see also General Nursing considerations/Cautions for monoclonal antibodies (p. 744)

Patient education
- advise the patient to seek medical advice if any of the following occur:
  - cough, shortness of breath, difficulty breathing
  - swelling of feet, shortness of breath when lying down or after gentle exercise, such as walking

- pain, ulceration at IV site if extravasation occurs
- see also General Patient education for monoclonal antibodies (p. 745)

TREMELIMUMAB
Trade name
Imjudo

Available forms
Vial: 25 mg/1.25 mL, 300 mg/1.5 mL

Action
- selective monoclonal antibody (IgG$_2$) that blocks CTLA-4 interaction with CD80 and CD86, enhancing antitumour immune activity
- half-life 20.4 days

Use
- unresectable hepatocellular carcinoma (uHCC) previously untreated with a PD-1/PD-L1 inhibitor (with durvalumab)

Dose
- 300 mg IV over 60 minutes (as a single priming dose) with durvalumab (day 1, cycle 1), then durvalumab monotherapy every 4 weeks

Adverse effects
- see General Adverse effects of monoclonal antibodies (p. 744)

Interactions
- monoclonal antibodies are not substrates for cytochrome P450 or drug transporters and therefore drug interactions are not expected

Nursing considerations/Cautions
- if the patient's weight ≤ 30 kg, the tremelimumab dose should be 4 mg/kg
- dose reduction is not recommended
- dilute to a concentration of 0.1–10 mg/mL
- see also General Nursing considerations/Cautions for monoclonal antibodies (p. 744)

Patient education
- see General Patient education for monoclonal antibodies (p. 745)

ANTINEOPLASTIC THERAPY SUPPORT AGENTS

This section contains a heterogenous (diverse) group of agents that are used during or after therapy with antineoplastic agents. Other agents that fulfil a similar supportive role are found in the chapters for Antiemetics (p. 368) and Haemopoietics (p. 1184).

MESNA
Trade name
Uromitexan

Available forms
Tablets: 400 mg, 600 mg;
Ampoules: 400 mg/mL, 1 g/10 mL

Action
- synthetic sulfhydryl detoxifying agent that is rapidly transported to the kidneys where it detoxifies urotoxic compounds; however, does not protect against renal toxicity

Use
- reduce and prevent haemorrhagic cystitis caused by oxazaphosphorine alkylating agents (ifosfamide, cyclophosphamide)

Dose
- (Intermittent alkylating agent therapy) 40% of alkylating agent dose orally 2 hours before alkylating agent therapy and repeated at 2 and 6 hours **OR**
- (Intermittent alkylating agent therapy) initially 20% of alkylating agent dose IV with alkylating agent therapy, followed by oral dose (40% of alkylating agent) given at 2 and 6 hours **OR**
- initially 40% of ifosfamide orally at completion of alkylating agent infusion, repeated at 2 and 6 hours **OR**
- initially 20% of alkylating agent IV over 15–30 minutes with alkylating agent therapy, then same dose repeated IV at 4 and 8 hours (total 3 doses)

Adverse effects
- anorexia, nausea, vomiting, diarrhoea, constipation, bad taste in mouth, flatulence, abdominal pain
- headache, fatigue, dizziness, somnolence
- limb pain, arthralgia, back pain
- flushing, fever, rigors, flu-like symptoms
- pharyngitis, cough
- (Rare) allergic reaction, severe skin reactions
- IV site reaction

Interactions
- may cause false positive to ketones, ascorbic acid (vitamin C) or erythrocytes on urinary dipstick

Nursing considerations/Cautions
- if patient is vomiting or treated with high-dose cyclophosphamide with total body irradiation, oral dose should be replaced with IV dose

ANTINEOPLASTIC THERAPY SUPPORT AGENTS

- urine output should be maintained at 100 mL/hour
- urine should be checked daily (morning) for protein and blood before starting therapy with ifosfamide or cyclophosphamide. If haematuria develops despite therapy, dose of ifosfamide or cyclophosphamide should be decreased or stopped (depending on severity of haematuria)
- repeated with each administration of alkylating agent
- (IV) incompatible with cisplatin, epirubicin, carboplatin and nitrogen mustard
- can be diluted with glucose 5%, sodium chloride 0.9% or lactated Ringer's solution to give concentration 1.5—3 mg/mL and then administered over 15—30 minutes
- if patient has history of urinary tract lesions, previous cystitis related to ifosfamide or cyclophosphamide or irradiation of small pelvis, an increased dose and/or shorter interval may be required as there is a high risk of haemorrhagic cystitis
- caution if given to those with autoimmune diseases because there is an increased risk of anaphylactic reaction. Medical supervision and readily available resuscitation equipment is recommended
- contraindicated in those with hypersensitivity to thiols (e.g. penicillamine, captopril, amifostine)

Patient education

- patient should be advised to avoid driving or operating machinery if dizziness, light headedness or tiredness are ongoing problems

 Tablet can be crushed and mixed with spoonful of yoghurt or apple puree.

 Not recommended in pregnancy owing to no data being available.

 Not recommended when breastfeeding owing to no data being available.

METHOXSALEN
Trade name
Uvadex

Available form
Vial: 200 microgram

Action
- on activation by exposure to UVA light, methoxsalen binds to pyrimidine bases of nucleic acids causing a covalent bond between 2 DNA strands; stops proliferation of lymphocytes
- also suppresses photo-treated T cells
- used with Therakos Cellex photopheresis system, which provides UV light to activate methoxsalen

Use
- extracorporeal (ECP) administration with Therakos Cellex photopheresis system for management of:
  - steroid-refractory or steroid-intolerant chronic graft versus host disease (cGvHD) after allogenic stem cell transplant
  - palliative treatment of skin manifestations of cutaneous T-cell lymphoma (CTCL) that is unresponsive to other treatments

Dose
- dose is calculated according to volume of plasma that is collected in photoactivation bag (displayed on side of photopheresis instrument):
  - treatment volume × 0.017 mL = dose
- (cGvHD) 3 ECP treatments in first week, followed by 2 treatments per week for at least 12 weeks (or as clinically indicated)
OR

- (CTCL) 2 ECP treatments on 2 successive days each month for 6 months, increasing to 2 treatments on 2 successive days every 2 weeks for 12 weeks if skin scores improve after 8 treatments

Adverse effects
- (cGvHD) diarrhoea, nausea, headache, hypertension, sinus/upper respiratory tract infection, fatigue, fever, cough, dyspnoea, anaemia
- (CTCL) nausea, vomiting, hypotension, infection, transient fever, vascular access complication, headache
- (Rare) cataract formation, pulmonary embolism, deep vein thrombosis, allergic reaction

Interactions
- may decrease clearance of caffeine
- decreases activation of paracetamol
- phenytoin may increase metabolism of methoxsalen reducing levels
- caution if given with other medications which may increase sensitivity to light, such as ciprofloxacin, cyclopropamide, doxycycline, haloperidol, isotretinoin, nalidixic acid, and some diuretics

Nursing considerations/Cautions
- should only be administered by medical practitioners trained and experienced in photopheresis
- patient should be informed of risks before starting procedure, especially risk of ocular damage
- photopheresis collection bag should be visually inspected for any signs of haemolysis
- not injected directly into patient
- photopheresis should only be performed where medical emergency equipment is available, as well as volume replacement fluids or volume expanders
- during therapy, patient's eyes should be protected from UVA light by wearing wrap-around UVA-opaque sunglasses
- photopheresis instrument operating manual should be consulted before starting procedure
- (ECP) process involves patient being attached to photopheresis system via a catheter. RBCs are separated from WBCs and plasma with the RBCs and excess plasma returned to patient. The leukocyte-enriched blood and some plasma is collected in the photoactivation bag on the side of the instrument. This instrument shows the volume collected, which is used to calculate the dose required for each session. Methoxsalen is injected into the photoactivation bag followed by the leucocyte-enriched blood circulating through the photoactivation unit, exposing all to UVA light. At the end of the photoactivation, the cells are reinfused into the patient over 15–20 minutes with the whole procedure taking up to 3 hours
- should not be diluted
- should be injected into photopheresis system as soon as drawn up into syringe and discarded if not used with 1 hour
- monitoring of albumin, calcium, haematocrit, haemoglobin, potassium and RBC count is recommended during therapy
- (CTCL) an adequate response is a 25% improvement in skin score that is maintained for at least 4 weeks. Skin scores are calculated based on the severity of lesions in each of 29 body sections, percentage surface area to obtain a regional score, followed by adding all regional scores for an overall lesion score
- (CTCL) number of sessions should not exceed 20 in 6 months
- caution if used in those with liver disease, alcoholism, epilepsy or brain injury/disease due to ethanol content (40.55 mg/mL)
- caution if used in those with liver impairment as prolonged photosensitivity may occur
- not recommended in those who have diseases with sensitivity to light such as porphyria, systemic lupus erythematosus or albinism

ANTINEOPLASTIC THERAPY SUPPORT AGENTS

- contraindicated in those with hypersensitivity to methoxsalen or psoralen compounds or with co-existing melanoma, basal cell or squamous cell carcinoma or aphakia (absence of eye lens)
- photopheresis procedure is contraindicated in those with photosensitive disease, coagulation disorders, previous splenectomy, WBC > 25,000 mm^3, or if unable to tolerate extracorporeal volume loss (e.g. severe anaemia, severe cardiac disease)

Patient education

- advise patient not to drive or operate machinery after photopheresis session
- patient should be instructed to:
  - wear sunglasses for 24 hours after therapy (in addition to during therapy)
  - avoid exposure to sun in 24 after therapy to previous burn injury and premature skin ageing
- men and women of childbearing potential should be counselled to used adequate contraception during and after completion of therapy

Not recommended for pregnancy owing to no safety data being available.

Not recommended when breastfeeding owing to no safety data being available.

Consider use for patients with hepatic impairment.

TELOTRISTAT ETHYL
Trade name
Xermelo

Available form
Tablets: 250 mg

Action
- telotristat ethyl is a prodrug converted to active metabolite telotristat which inhibits serotonin synthesis
- neuroendocrine tumours can cause too much serotonin to be released into the bloodstream, resulting in symptoms such as diarrhoea, abdominal pain, skin flushing, hypotension, rash and weight loss (referred to as carcinoid syndrome)
- by reducing serotonin production, symptoms of carcinoid syndrome are lessened
- terminal half-life is about 11 hours

Use
- carcinoid syndrome diarrhoea (in combination with somastatin analogues (lanreotide or octreotide))

Dose
- 250 mg orally 3 times daily with food

Adverse effects
- constipation, abdominal pain, decreased appetite, flatulence
- elevated liver enzymes
- fatigue, headache
- fever
- peripheral oedema
- depression, depressed mood

Interactions
- if given with octreotide, octreotide should be given at least 30 minutes before telotristat
- loperamide may decrease formation of active telotristat
- may decrease efficacy of amilodipine, atorvastatin, bupropion, carbamazepine, ciclosporin, diltazem, ethinyloestradiol, everolimus, felodipine, midazolam, nifedipine, sertraline, simvastatin, sodium valproate, sunitinib, topiramate, verapamil

Nursing considerations/Cautions

- liver enzymes should be monitored before starting and during therapy, especially if there is any liver impairment present. If liver injury occurs, therapy should be stopped and not restarted until liver enzymes return to normal
- therapy should be reassessed if clinical response is not achieved within 12 weeks
- caution if used in those with mild-to-moderate kidney impairment

- not recommended in those with severe kidney impairment, end-stage renal failure requiring dialysis or severe liver impairment

Patient education

- advise patient not to take double dose if a dose is missed. The subsequent dose should be taken at next scheduled time
- suggest patient take tablet with food, preferably high-fat meal, to improve absorption
- patient should be instructed to drink sufficient water and eat fibre-containing foods to decrease constipation
- warn patient not to drive or operate machinery if fatigue occurs
- patient should be advised to seek medical attention if any of the following occur:
  - nausea, dark urine, yellow skin or eyes, fatigue/tiredness, upper right abdominal pain
  - feelings of sadness or depression
- counsel women of childbearing potential to use effective contraception during therapy to prevent pregnancy occurring

Tablet can be crushed and mixed with water or spoonful of yoghurt or apple puree.

Not recommended during pregnancy due to no safety data being available.

Not recommended when breastfeeding due to no safety data being available.

In those with liver impairment:
- Child—Pugh Class A, dose reduced to 250 mg orally twice daily;
- Child—Pugh Class B, dose reduced to 250 mg orally once daily
- Child—Pugh Class C, use not recommended.

Not recommended in patients with end-stage renal disease requiring dialysis.

GRANULOCYTE COLONY STIMULATING FACTOR (G-CSF)

General Actions of G-CSF
- recombinant human granulocyte colony-stimulating factor (G-CSF), which regulates production and release of neutrophils from bone marrow through action on progenitor (stem) cells

General Uses of G-CSF
- decrease incidence and duration of severe neutropenia (and associated infection) after chemotherapy
- reversal of neutropenia and maintenance of neutrophil counts with antiviral and/or myelosuppressive agents in those with HIV
- severe chronic neutropenia
- mobilisation of peripheral blood progenitor cells (PBPC) for autologous or allogenic bone marrow transplantation
- mobilisation of peripheral blood progenitor cells (PBPC) for allogenic peripheral blood stem cell transplantation in normal volunteers
- after autologous or allogenic bone marrow transplant
- decrease incidence of infection after myelosuppressive therapy in non-myeloid malignancy

General Adverse effects of G-CSF
- splenomegaly
- mild-to-moderate medullary bone pain, back pain, myalgia, arthralgia, pain in extremities
- headache, fatigue, malaise, asthenia, dizziness
- fever
- anorexia, diarrhoea, constipation, stomatitis, abdominal pain
- cough, haemoptysis
- alopecia
- rash, exacerbation of pre-existing skin conditions (e.g. psoriasis)
- leucocytosis, thrombocytopenia, anaemia
- injection site reaction
- reversible elevation of levels of uric acid, lactate dehydrogenase and alkaline phosphatase

- (Uncommon) haematuria, proteinuria
- (Children with chronic severe neutropenia) osteopenia, osteoporosis, decreased bone density
- (Rare) adult respiratory distress syndrome (ARDS), rupture of spleen, hypersensitivity, sickle cell crisis, acute febrile dermatosis (Sweet's syndrome), aortitis, pulmonary haemorrhage, pulmonary infiltrates, glomerulonephritis
- (Very rare) capillary leak syndrome, cutaneous vasculitis

General Interactions of G-CSF
- caution if used with agents known to lower platelet count
- may affect results of bone imaging scans

General Nursing considerations/Cautions for G-CSF
- (Severe chronic neutropenia) diagnosis should be confirmed before starting therapy and other causes of neutropenia eliminated. Before starting therapy, serial blood count (with differential and platelet count) and bone marrow evaluation (morphology and karyotype) should be performed
- trade name should be recorded in patient history
- not recommended with or within 24 hours of chemotherapy
- allow to come to room temperature before use
- avoid vigorous shaking (shaking should be avoided as it will denature protein)
- contraindicated in those with known hypersensitivity to *Escherichia coli*-derived proteins or G-CSF-related products

General Patient education for G-CSF
- warn patient against driving or operating machinery if dizziness is problematic
- patient should be advised to immediately seek medical advice if any of the following occur:
  - pain in shoulder tip or left upper abdominal quadrant
  - unexplained cough, fever, coughing blood or blood-stained sputum, and difficulty breathing (dyspnoea). Chest X-ray is recommended if these symptoms occur
  - fever or painful skin lesions (on arms or legs, sometimes face and neck)
  - blood in urine
- warn patient that mild-to-moderate bone pain commonly occurs at the start of therapy and is controlled with non-opioid analgesics

 Not recommended during pregnancy unless benefits outweigh risks.

 Caution if used during breastfeeding.

FILGRASTIM
Trade names
Nivestim, Zarzio

Available forms
Vial: 120 microgram/0.2 mL, 300 microgram/1 mL, 480 microgram/1.6 mL, 480 microgram/0.8 mL;
Prefilled syringe: 300 microgram/0.5 mL

Action
- effects reversed within 24 hours of stopping therapy and neutrophils return to normal within 4 days
- see also General Actions of G-CSF (p. 784)

Use
- see General Uses of G-CSF (p. 784)

Dose
- (Cancer patients receiving standard chemotherapy; induction/consolidation chemotherapy for acute myeloid leukaemia) 5 microgram/kg/day SC daily
OR
- (Patients with non-myeloid malignancy after chemotherapy) 5 microgram/kg/day SC or as IV infusion over 15–30 minutes for up to 2 weeks until absolute

neutrophil count (ANC) $> 1 \times 10^9$ for 3 consecutive days or 10×10^9/L for 1 day after chemotherapy **OR**
- (Patients with non-myeloid malignancy after high-dose toxic chemotherapy with autologous/allogenic bone marrow or peripheral stem cell transplantation) initially 10 microgram/kg/day by SC/IV infusion over 4—24 hours, then increase, decrease or stop infusion depending on ANC **OR**
- (Patients with myeloid malignancy after high-dose toxic chemotherapy with autologous/allogenic bone marrow or peripheral progenitor cell transplantation) 5 microgram/kg/day following transplant (24 hours after infusion of bone marrow or progenitor cells or cytotoxic therapy) until neutrophil count recovers (up to 28 days) **OR**
- (Autologous progenitor cell collection and therapy) 10 microgram/kg/day daily SC or 24-hour infusion for at least 4 days before first leukapheresis, and continued until last day of leukapheresis. Stem cell collection occurs on day 5 and on consecutive days until sufficient cells have been collected **OR**
- (Autologous stem cell collection and therapy after myelosuppressive chemotherapy) 5 microgram/kg/day SC daily starting 24 hours after chemotherapy until neutrophil count has returned to normal range. Leukapheresis can start when ANC $> 5 \times 10^9$/L and occurs on consecutive days until sufficient cells are collected **OR**
- (Autologous stem cell collection from normal donor) 10 microgram/kg/day SC for 4—5 consecutive days and leukapheresis starting on day 5 and 6 to collect required amount of cells **OR**
- (Congenital severe chronic neutropenia) 12 microgram/kg SC daily or in divided doses **OR**
- (Idiopathic/cyclic severe chronic neutropenia) 5 microgram/kg SC daily or in divided doses **OR**
- (HIV infection) initially 1 microgram/kg/day SC daily, increasing gradually to 5 microgram/kg/day until neutrophil count is achieved and maintained (ANC $\geq 2 \times 10^9$/L), then 300 microgram daily SC 3 times per week, adjusting dose if necessary

Adverse effects
- see General Adverse effects of G-CSF (p. 784)

Interactions
- see General Interactions of G-CSF (p. 785)

Nursing considerations/Cautions
- brands (e.g. Nivestim, Zarzio) should not be substituted without seeking medical advice first
- patient may be taught to self-administer using prefilled syringe
- (Patient with HIV infection) absolute neutrophil count (ANC) is recommended during first 2—3 days, then twice weekly for 2 weeks, then weekly
- (Peripheral blood progenitor cell (PBPC) collection and therapy) neutrophil count should be monitored 4 days after start of therapy, then regular full blood count (including platelet count) is recommended at least 3 times weekly after infusion of PBPCs until haemopoietic recovery. If leucocyte count rises above 100×10^9/L, therapy should be stopped
- (Stem cell collection) prolonged therapy with some chemotherapy agents (e.g. carboplatin, carmustine and melphalan) may decrease stem cell yield
- (Chronic neutropenia) full blood count (with differential) is recommended during initial 4 weeks of therapy and for 2 weeks after any dose adjustment, then monthly for 12 months when patient is clinically stable. If patient has congenital neutropenia, annual bone marrow evaluation is also recommended during therapy
- (Cancer patient receiving myelosuppressive therapy) full blood count (with differential, platelet count and haematocrit) is recommended before chemotherapy and then twice weekly during filgrastim therapy

ANTINEOPLASTIC THERAPY SUPPORT AGENTS

- premature discontinuation of therapy is not recommended
- urinalysis should be conducted regularly during therapy
- for IV or SC infusion, dilute with 25–50 mL glucose 5%. If dilution concentration < 15 microgram/mL, adsorption to plastic may occur. This can be overcome by using albumin (human) to a final concentration of 2 mg/mL
- dilution to < 5 microgram/mL is not recommended
- insertion of CVC line should be avoided
- incompatible with sodium chloride 0.9% as precipitation will occur
- (Patients with non-myeloid malignancy after high-dose toxic chemotherapy with autologous/allogenic bone marrow or peripheral stem cell transplantation) if absolute neutrophil count (ANC) $> 1 \times 10^9$/L for 3 consecutive days, dose should be decreased to 5 microgram/kg/day, then discontinue if ANC remains at that level for 3 consecutive days. If ANC $< 1 \times 10^9$/L, infusion can be resumed at 5 microgram/kg/day. If ANC $< 1 \times 10^9$/L during infusion of 5 microgram/kg/day, dose should be increased to 10 microgram/kg/day
- needle shield contains latex, which may cause reaction in latex-sensitive individuals
- caution if used in those with sickle cell disease or trait (as sickle cell crisis may occur) or if used with chemoradiotherapy
- see also Nursing considerations/Cautions for G-CSF (p. 785)

Patient education

- if patient is going to administer SC, education should include:
  - not administering within 24 hours of chemotherapy, radiotherapy, bone marrow transplant or stem cell transplant
  - injection is under the skin (subcutaneous injection)
  - importance of changing injection sites, including thighs and abdomen, but avoiding navel and waistline
  - not injecting into areas that are red or swollen, into muscle or into the same spot
  - not stopping abruptly or without seeking medical advice
- correct technique, such as:
  - wash and dry hands before start of procedure
  - check name and strength of medication and expiry date (and not using if after expiry date)
  - do not use solution if it is cloudy or coloured, or contains lumps or flakes
  - allow prefilled syringe to come to room temperature before use (about 30 minutes) (not in direct sunlight or using any method, such as hot water or microwave, to warm solution)
  - do not shake solution/syringes. If solution is frothy or bubbly, it should be allowed to sit for a few minutes for froth/bubbles to settle
  - do not mix with any other medications or dilute
  - remove needle cover, taking care not to touch exposed needle
  - check the dose prescribed and find the correct volume mark on syringe barrel, and then carefully push plunger until grey upper edge of plunger reaches correct volume (this will get rid of excess fluid and air)
  - clean area with alcoholic swab and allow to dry
  - pinch skin firmly between thumb and finger
  - push prefilled syringe firmly against pinched skin (at 45–90° angle) and inject
  - withdraw needle, press site gently after injection with cotton wool

- swab to prevent bleeding, but do not rub
- do not recap needle after use
- correct storage
  - store in fridge, but can remain at room temperature for up to 3 days before use
  - do not freeze
- disposal of used equipment
  - do not reuse needles or syringes
  - do not dispose of syringes and needles in the normal household rubbish
  - use puncture-resistant sharps container to dispose of used needles and syringes
  - container should be disposed of as instructed by doctor, pharmacist or nurse
- see also General Patient education for G-CSF (p. 785)

Not recommended unless the benefit outweighs the risk, owing to limited data available.

Not recommended owing to limited data available.

LIPEGFILGRASTIM

Trade names
Lonquex

Available form
Prefilled syringe: 6 mg/mL

Action
- long acting form of filgrastim (p. filgrasti5)
- see also General Actions of G-CSF (p. 784)

Use
- decrease incidence and duration of neutropenia in patients treated with chemotherapy

Dose
- 6 mg SC once per chemotherapy cycle

Adverse effects
- hypokalaemia
- see also General Adverse effects of G-CSF (p. 784)

Interactions
- see General Interactions of G-CSF (p. 784)

Nursing considerations/Cautions
- serum potassium levels should be monitored for hypokalaemia
- contains sorbitol
- see also General Nursing considerations/Cautions for filgrastim and G-CSF (p. 786)

Patient education
- see General Patient education for filgrastim and G-CSF (p. 785)

Not recommended owing to limited data available.

Not recommended owing to limited data available.

PEGFILGRASTIM

Trade names
Pelgraz, Ziextenzo

Available form
Prefilled syringe: 6 mg/0.6 mL

Action
- long-acting form which has been combined with polyethylene glycol (PEG) molecule reducing renal clearance and prolonging persistence compared with filgrastim (p. 785)
- see also General Actions of G-CSF (p. 785)

Use
- cancer patients following chemotherapy to decrease duration of severe neutropenia to reduce incidence of infection

Dose
- 6 mg SC once per cycle given 24 hours after chemotherapy

ANTINEOPLASTIC THERAPY SUPPORT AGENTS

Adverse effects
- see General Adverse effects of G-CSF (p. 784)

Interactions
- see General Interactions of G-CSF (p. 784)

Nursing considerations/Cautions
- can be given 14 days before chemotherapy
- contraindicated in those with hypersensitivity to filgrastim, polyethylene glycol or *E. coli*-derived proteins
- see also General Nursing considerations/Cautions for G-CSF (p. 784)

Patient education
- if patient is going to administer SC, education should include points for filgrastim patient education (p. 787), with the following differences:
    - pull grey needle cap straight out and away from your body
    - pinch skin firmly between thumb and finger
    - insert needle into skin and push plunger slowly until person feels or hears a 'snap' and continue to push all the way down through snap (this is important to ensure full dose)
    - withdraw needle (after releasing plunger, prefilled syringe safety guard will cover injection needle) and press site gently after injection with cotton wool swab to prevent bleeding, but do not rub
    - remove and save label from prefilled syringe
- see also General Patient education for G-CSF (p. 785)

 Not recommended owing to limited data available.

 Not recommended owing to limited data available.

789

ANTI-PARKINSON'S AGENTS

In 1817, James Parkinson described what would become known as Parkinson's disease (PD), and which is now the second most common age-related neurodegenerative disease, behind Alzheimer's disease. PD results from degeneration of the dopaminergic neurones in the substantia nigra, leading to decreased dopamine concentrations in the brain. Other neurones (cholinergic, serotonin, noradrenaline (norepinephrine), olfactory) also degenerate, accounting for the non-dopaminergic symptoms. Symptoms of Parkinsonism become evident when more than 80% of the neurones have degenerated. In most cases, the cause of PD is unknown; however, early-onset PD is thought to run in families. Secondary Parkinsonism has been associated with some drugs (particularly antipsychotic agents, metoclopramide, chlorpromazine, lithium) and also infection, tumour, trauma, stroke or exposure to neurotoxins (e.g. carbon monoxide, manganese) (Douglas & Aminoff 2025).

The four cardinal features of PD are tremor at rest, rigidity/stiffness, bradykinesia (slowing) and gait dysfunction with postural instability. Other motor symptoms include reduced eye blinking, drooling, soft voice, difficulty swallowing, handwriting becoming progressively smaller and cramped, reduced facial expression and freezing (a sudden but temporary inability to move) (Douglas & Aminoff 2025). Non-motor features of PD (thought to be due to the degeneration of non-dopaminergic neurons) include loss of smell, sensory disturbance, mood disorders (e.g. depression (which is very common in PD), anxiety, panic attacks), sleep disturbances (e.g. fragmented, sleep apnoea), orthostatic hypotension, GI (e.g. decreased gastric motility, constipation), genitourinary disturbances, sexual dysfunction and mild cognitive impairment, which may progress to dementia (Lewy body dementia) (Douglas & Aminoff 2025).

Treatment of PD is symptomatic and may involve:
- *pharmacological treatment* — based on restoring the supply of dopamine to the brain
- *management of non-motor and non-dopaminergic features* — this includes management of anxiety, panic attacks, depression, sweating, sensory

issues, freezing and constipation. Other issues can include sleep disturbances, psychosis and dementia
- *non-pharmacological therapy* — involves aids to increase stability and reduce the risk of falling, such as canes and walkers; exercise to maintain and improve function; and access to support groups for both patient and carer. Tai Chi has been shown to improve motor function, functional mobility, balance and depression
- *surgical treatment* — ablative surgery involves destroying small areas of brain tissue responsible for abnormal activity. This has largely been replaced by deep brain stimulation, which uses electrical stimulation to interfere with abnormal activity. This is generally suitable only for those patients with PD who do not have cognitive impairment or psychiatric disorders and have had a good response to levodopa therapy
- A number of other procedures, including gene therapy, are still in the experimental stages (Douglas & Aminoff 2025).

Pharmacological treatment for PD involves a number of different classes of agents, but none actually stops the progression of the disease. The aim of these pharmacological agents is to reduce the symptoms to a manageable level, and include:
- anticholinergics (e.g. benzatropine, benzhexol) are better at alleviating tremor and rigidity than bradykinesia
- catechol-O-methyl transferase (COMT) inhibitors (e.g. entacapone, opicapone) reduce metabolism of levodopa and are therefore adjunctive therapy
- dopaminergic agents
  - levodopa (precursor to dopamine) improves all major features of PD
  - dopamine agonists (e.g. apomorphine, bromocriptine, cabergoline)
  - amantadine (antiviral agent which has dopaminergic activity)
- monoamine oxidase type B enzyme (MAO-B) inhibitors (e.g. selegiline, rasagiline, salfinamide) inhibit the breakdown of dopamine and are useful if there is a declining response to levodopa (Douglas & Aminoff 2025).

ANTICHOLINERGIC ANTI-PARKINSON'S AGENTS

General Actions of anticholinergic anti-Parkinson's agents
- inhibit the action of acetylcholine at the muscarinic receptors of the parasympathetic division of the autonomic nervous system
- reduce production of sweat, saliva, and lacrimal, nasal, bronchial, gastric and intestinal secretions
- reduce GI tone and gastric acid production
- increase heart rate by blocking vagal stimulus
- raise intraocular pressure, cause mydriasis and cycloplegia
- inhibit micturition

General Uses of anticholinergic anti-Parkinson's agents
- all types of Parkinsonism (adjunct)
- prevention or treatment of drug-induced extrapyramidal symptoms

General Adverse effects of anticholinergic anti-Parkinson's agents
- nausea, vomiting, dry mouth, thirst, constipation
- dizziness, headache

- nervousness, euphoria, agitation, delusions, hallucinations, paranoia, impaired memory, confusion, disorientation, drowsiness, sedation
- dry skin, reduced sweating, flushing, heat intolerance, hyperthermia
- rash
- tachycardia or bradycardia, aggravation of pre-existing hypertension
- urinary urgency, difficulty and retention
- mydriasis, photophobia, cycloplegia, blurred vision, raised intraocular pressure, dry eyes
- (Abrupt dose reduction or discontinuation) neuroleptic malignant syndrome, acute exacerbation of Parkinsonism (e.g. anxiety, bradycardia, hypotension, decreased sleep quality)
- (Rare) parotitis, dilation of colon, paralytic ileus, allergic reaction

General Interactions of anticholinergic anti-Parkinson's agents

- may decrease absorption and effects of levodopa
- may increase dopaminergic effects of levodopa
- not recommended with other anticholinergic or antipsychotic agents because of an increased risk of tardive dyskinesia
- may decrease the effects of metoclopramide
- additive anticholinergic effects (including risk of paralytic ileus) may occur if given with other anticholinergic agents, phenothiazines or monoamine oxidase inhibitors (MAOIs)/tricyclic antidepressants (TCAs) with anticholinergic properties
- increased renal tubular absorption, decreased excretion and increased effects may occur if given with carbonic anhydrase inhibitors (e.g. acetazolamide)
- not recommended with alcohol, as serum levels may be decreased
- increased sedation may occur if given with alcohol, hypnotics, sedatives, opioids, barbiturates or cannabinoids
- actions may be antagonised by parasympathomimetic (cholinergic) agents (e.g. acetylcholine)
- caution if used with opioids, as there may be additive effects on GI motility and bladder function

General Nursing Considerations/Cautions for anticholinergic anti-Parkinson's agents

- intraocular pressure should be monitored regularly during therapy
- drug abuse potential is present because of stimulating and euphoric effects
- not recommended in those with tardive dyskinesia (unless patient has concurrent Parkinson's disease) or for prevention of drug-induced Parkinsonism
- caution if given to those with a history of seizures
- caution if used in those with arrhythmias, tachycardia, heart failure, coronary/ischaemic heart disease, mitral valve stenosis or hypertension
- caution if used in those with a history of atherosclerosis or idiosyncrasy to other drugs, as there is an increased risk of nausea, vomiting, confusion, agitation or disturbed behaviour
- caution if given to those with glaucoma, myasthenia gravis, prostatic hypertrophy, urinary retention or obstructive GI disease because of anticholinergic adverse effects
- caution if used during fever, high environmental temperatures, during physical exercise or by those doing manual work in hot environments because of decreased sweating
- contraindicated in those with paralytic ileus, megacolon, narrow-angle glaucoma or tardive dyskinesia

General Patient education for anticholinergic anti-Parkinson's agents

- if dry mouth is a problem, advise the patient to take medication before meals, or if the patient feels nauseous, it may be taken after or with meals

ANTI-PARKINSON'S AGENTS

- advise the patient that thirst and/or dry mouth may be relieved by drinking water, chewing gum or mints or sucking hard sweets
- the patient should be advised to avoid alcohol
- caution the patient to avoid sudden withdrawal of the drug, as it may cause either an exacerbation of the Parkinsonian symptoms or a syndrome similar to neuroleptic malignant syndrome (hyperpyrexia, muscle rigidity, psychological changes, increased serum creatine phosphokinase), which can be life threatening
- the patient should be warned to avoid driving or operating heavy machinery if blurred vision, dizziness or drowsiness occur
- the patient should be advised to report any blurring of vision and to wear dark glasses if there is continuous dilation of pupils
- patients who wear contact lenses should be instructed to use lubricating drops more frequently during therapy, as dry eyes commonly occur
- warn the patient to avoid high environmental temperatures, doing physical exercise or manual work in hot environments because of decreased sweating and risk of overheating and heat stroke
- the patient should be advised to immediately report any fever, heat intolerance or GI problems (especially if also taking phenothiazines, haloperidol or other anticholinergic agents)

Safety in pregnancy has not been established; therefore not recommended.

Excretion in breastmilk is unknown; therefore should be used during breastfeeding with caution.

Caution if given in those with kidney or liver impairment.

Caution if used in those > 60 years because of an increased risk of anticholinergic adverse effects.

BENZATROPINE MESILATE (BENZTROPINE MESYLATE)

Trade names
Benztrop, Benzatropine Injection

Available forms
Tablets: 2 mg;
Ampoules: 2 mg/2 mL

Action/Use
- has both anticholinergic and antihistamine properties
- long duration of action
- main effect is to relieve tremor and rigidity
- onset of action is the same whether given IM or IV
- see also General Actions/Uses of anticholinergic anti-Parkinson's agents (p. 791)

Dose
- (Arteriosclerotic, post-encephalitic or idiopathic Parkinsonism) initially 0.5—1 mg orally, IV or IM, increasing the dose gradually at 0.5 mg increments and 5—6-day intervals (daily maximum 6 mg) **OR**
- (Drug-induced Parkinsonism) 1—4 mg orally or IM 1—2 times daily **OR**
- (Emergency, acute dystonic reaction) 1—2 mg IM or IV stat, repeated if required

Adverse effects
- (Large dose) weakness, inability to move particular muscle groups
- see also General Adverse effects of anticholinergic anti-Parkinson's agents (p. 791)

Interactions
- see General Interactions of anticholinergic anti-Parkinson's agents (p. 792)

Nursing considerations/Cautions/Patient education
- parenteral administration may provide quick results if the patient is psychotic with acute dystonic reactions
- other anti-Parkinson's agents should not be stopped suddenly when starting benzatropine
- therapy is cumulative; therefore should be started with a low dose, increasing at 5—6-day intervals
- some patients may benefit from taking the entire dose at bedtime (i.e. enable them to roll over in bed independently), whereas others prefer divided daily doses
- (Drug-induced Parkinsonism) therapy should be stopped after 1—2 weeks to determine whether continued use is necessary
- caution if used in those with mental disorders, as the condition may become intensified or psychosis may be precipitated
- see also General Nursing considerations/Cautions/Patient education for anticholinergic anti-Parkinson's agents (p. 792)

 Tablet may be dispersed in water, or crushed and mixed with a spoonful of yoghurt or apple puree.

TRIHEXYPHENIDYL (BENZHEXOL) HYDROCHLORIDE
Trade name
Artane

Available form
Tablets: 2 mg, 5 mg

Action/Use
- see General Actions/Uses of anticholinergic anti-Parkinson's agents (p. 791)

Dose
- (Parkinsonism) initially 1 mg orally before or with food, increasing by 2 mg increments at 3—5-day intervals to 6—10 mg daily (in 3 divided doses) according to response. May require 12—15 mg in advanced cases (in 4 divided doses with meals and at bedtime) **OR**
- (Drug-induced Parkinsonism) initially 1 mg orally daily, increasing dose gradually to 5—15 mg orally daily in divided doses until extrapyramidal symptoms are controlled

Adverse effects
- see General Adverse effects of anticholinergic anti-Parkinson's agents (p. 791)

Interactions
- increased risk of euphoria if given with large amounts of caffeine
- effects may be decreased if given with citrus and fruit juices
- additive effects may occur if given with cannabis, barbiturates, opioid analgesics or alcohol (increasing risk of abuse)
- decreased blood levels may occur if given with alcohol
- decreased absorption may occur if given with magnesium hydroxide
- increased risk of dry mouth, blurred vision and urine hesitancy if given with memantine
- see also General Interactions of anticholinergic anti-Parkinson's agents (p. 792)

Nursing considerations/Cautions
- the patient should be advised against ingesting large amounts of caffeine or fruit/citrus juices
- instruct the patient to separate medication by at least 2 hours from magnesium hydroxide (antacid)
- daily doses > 10 mg can be divided into 4 doses (with meals and bedtime)
- (Post-encephalitic Parkinsonism) advise the patient to take medication before meals owing to increased salivation (a small amount of atropine may also be required)

ANTI-PARKINSON'S AGENTS

- abuse potential exists because of stimulant and euphoric effects
- see also General Nursing considerations/Cautions for anticholinergic anti-Parkinson's agents (p. 792)

Patient education

- advise the patient to avoid large amounts of coffee, citrus and fruit juice during therapy
- see also General Patient education for anticholinergic anti-Parkinson's agents (p. 2)

 Tablet can be dispersed in water, or crushed and mixed with a spoonful of yoghurt or apple puree.

CATECHOL-O-METHYL TRANSFERASE (COMT) INHIBITORS

ENTACAPONE

Trade name
Comtan

Available form
Tablets: 200 mg

Action
- inhibits catechol-O-methyltransferase (COMT) in peripheral tissues, reducing metabolism of levodopa by COMT, increasing the amount of levodopa and therefore the amount of dopamine
- short half-life (30 minutes)

Use
- Parkinson's disease (adjunct to levodopa to control motor fluctuations)

Dose
- 200 mg orally (with levodopa—carbidopa or levodopa—benserazide) 4—7 times daily (maximum daily dose 2 g)

Adverse effects
- diarrhoea, nausea, vomiting, dry mouth, abdominal pain, constipation, anorexia
- dizziness, drowsiness, fatigue, headache, vertigo, insomnia, daytime somnolence, nightmares, sudden sleep onset
- falls, pain, back pain, leg cramps
- dyskinesia, dystonia, tremor, aggravated Parkinson's, hyper/hypokinesia
- hallucinations, depression, confusion, paranoia
- discoloured urine
- increased sweating
- postural hypotension, ischaemic heart disease
- (Uncommon) impulse control disorders, including pathological gambling, increased libido, hypersexuality, shopping, eating, repetitive purposeless activity (punding)
- (Rare) rhabdomyolysis, neuroleptic malignant syndrome, elevated liver enzymes, decreased haemoglobin, colitis

Interactions
- contraindicated with non-selective or selective monoamine oxidase inhibitors (MAOIs) (except selegiline at doses less than 10 mg)
- not recommended with tricyclic antidepressants (TCAs), noradrenaline (norepinephrine) reuptake inhibitors, isoprenaline, adrenaline (epinephrine), noradrenaline (norepinephrine), dopamine, dobutamine, methyldopa sesquihydrate, apomorphine or paroxetine
- may form chelates with dietary iron
- may increase levodopa-induced or antihypertensive-induced hypotension
- may require adjustment of other anti-Parkinson's medication to decrease risk of dyskinesia
- may increase bioavailability of levodopa, increasing the risk of dopaminergic adverse effects (especially if combined with benserazide)
- high doses may decrease bioavailability of carbidopa monohydrate
- may increase serum levels of warfarin, increasing the risk of bleeding; therefore INR should be monitored closely,

especially when starting, stopping or altering dose

Nursing considerations/Cautions

- levodopa dose is usually reduced by 10—30% by either decreasing the dose or increasing the dosing interval
- if diarrhoea and anorexia are ongoing, weight should be monitored to prevent excessive loss
- drowsiness is a problem at the start of therapy
- levodopa dose will require adjustment
- tablets contain sucrose and therefore are not recommended in those with fructose intolerance, glucose—galactose malabsorption or sucrase—isomaltase insufficiency
- caution if used in those with ischaemic heart disease
- contraindicated in those with liver impairment, phaeochromocytoma, a previous history of neuroleptic malignant syndrome or rhabdomyolysis (non-traumatic)

Patient education

- instruct the patient to take 2—3 hours apart from meals to prevent binding with dietary iron
- advise the patient to avoid postural hypotension by moving gradually to a sitting or standing position, especially after sleep
- instruct the patient to report any prolonged or persistent diarrhoea
- the patient should be advised not to drive or operate machinery if drowsiness, daytime somnolence, sudden sleep onset or dizziness continues
- family/carers should be asked to observe for:
   - any sudden sleep onset, as patients are often unaware that this occurs and it may be dangerous if the person drives or operates machinery, or
   - persistent/recurring gambling, increase in sexual desires or repetitive behaviours with no purpose
- the patient should be advised to avoid suddenly stopping therapy, as it may cause an exaggeration of the Parkinson's symptoms or may cause overheating, muscle rigidity and psychological changes, which can be potentially life threatening
- the patient should be warned that urine may appear a harmless reddish-brown colour
- see also General Patient education for anticholinergic anti-Parkinson's agents (p. 792)

 Tablet can be dispersed in 20 mL water, or crushed and mixed with a spoonful of yoghurt or apple puree.

 Contraindicated during pregnancy.

 Contraindicated during breastfeeding.

Available in combination with
- levodopa + carbidopa + entacapone (see Levodopa in this chapter p. 805)

OPICAPONE
Trade name
Ongentys

Available form
Capsule: 50 mg

Action
- inhibits catechol-O-methyltransferase (COMT) in peripheral tissues, reducing metabolism of levodopa by COMT, resulting in an increase in levodopa and therefore dopamine

Use
- Parkinson's disease (as an adjunct to levodopa to control motor fluctuations)

Dose
- 50 mg orally at bedtime without food, and at least 1 hour before or after levodopa preparations

ANTI-PARKINSON'S AGENTS

Adverse effects
- dyskinesia, dizziness
- constipation, dry mouth, nausea, vomiting
- decreased weight
- insomnia, abnormal dreams, somnolence
- headache
- hallucination, visual hallucination
- orthostatic hypotension, hypertension
- muscle spasm
- urinary tract infection
- increased liver enzymes
- (Rare) impulse control disorders

Interactions
- contraindicated with non-selective or selective monoamine oxidase inhibitors (MAOIs) (except for rasigiline (up to 1 mg/day) or selegiline (up to 10 mg/day orally or 1.25 mg buccal absorption formulation)
- may interfere with the metabolism of isoprenaline, adrenaline (epinephrine), noradrenaline (norepinephrine), dopamine or dobutamine, potentiating their effects
- caution if used with tricyclic antidepressants (TCAs) and noradrenaline (norepinephrine) reuptake inhibitors (e.g. venlafaxine, desipramine)

Nursing considerations/Cautions
- the levodopa dose may need to be adjusted early in therapy (first days to first weeks) by reducing the dose or extending the dosing interval to prevent dopaminergic adverse effects such as nausea, vomiting, orthostatic hypotension, hallucinations and dyskinesia
- capsules contain lactose and are therefore not recommended in those with rare hereditary problems of galactose intolerance, lactase deficiency or glucose-galactose malabsorption
- not recommended in those with liver impairment or liver cirrhosis
- contraindicated in those with phaeochromocytoma, paraganglioma or other catecholamine-secreting neoplasms, a history of neuroleptic malignant syndrome and/or traumatic rhabdomyolysis

Patient education
- advise the patient to swallow the capsule whole with water, preferably on an empty stomach (2 hours before or after food) and at least an hour before or after levodopa preparation
- warn the patient to move gradually from a sitting to standing position (especially after sleep) to avoid postural hypotension
- the patient should be advised not to drive or operate machinery if dizziness, somnolence or hypotension continues
- if the patient has ongoing loss of appetite, weakness and loss of weight in a short time period, medical advice should be sought and liver function tests recommended
- family/carers should be asked to observe for any persistent/recurring gambling, increase in sexual desires, compulsive spending or buying, binge eating or compulsive eating
- If used in women of childbearing potential, they should be counselled to use adequate contraception (both hormonal and non-hormonal methods are recommended together)

Capsule should be swallowed whole, not chewed, broken or crushed.

Not recommended in pregnancy or in women of childbearing potential not using contraception.

Breastfeeding should be discontinued during therapy.

Not recommended in those with liver impairment or liver cirrhosis.

Caution if used in those > 75 years.

DOPAMINE AGONISTS

General Adverse effects of dopamine agonists
- anorexia, nausea, vomiting, constipation, dyspepsia, indigestion, dry mouth
- dizziness, insomnia, somnolence, sedation, nightmares, drowsiness, lightheadedness, ataxia, abnormal dreams, insomnia, headache, asthenia, fatigue, lethargy
- depression, anxiety, agitation, concentration difficulties, nervousness, elevated mood, hallucinations (visual, auditory), confusion, disorientation
- postural hypotension, peripheral oedema
- rash, pruritus, increased sweating
- dyskinesia, hypokinesia
- (Rare) somnolence, sudden sleep onset
- (Abrupt withdrawal, rare) neuroleptic malignant syndrome, worsening Parkinson's symptoms, drug withdrawal syndrome (apathy, anxiety, depression, fatigue, sweating, pain)
- (Uncommon, high doses) impulse control disorders, including pathological gambling, increased libido, hypersexuality, binge and compulsive eating, repetitive purposeless activity (punding), compulsive spending and buying

General Interactions of dopamine agonists
- not recommended with agents that antagonise dopamine receptors (e.g. metoclopramide, phenothiazines, butyrophenones, thioxanthenes)
- increased risk of adverse effects (e.g. confusion, hallucinations, nightmares, GI disturbances and other atropine-like effects) if given with anticholinergic agents and therefore not recommended together
- caution if given with alcohol and other CNS-depressing agents, as additive CNS effects may occur
- increased risk of dyskinesia, hallucinations and confusion if given with levodopa

General Nursing considerations/ Cautions for dopamine agonists
- before starting therapy, patients should have a cardiovascular assessment (including ECG/echocardiogram), ESR, lung function test, chest X-ray and renal function
- ECG/echocardiogram should be monitored within 3–6 months of starting therapy, then 6–12-monthly
- chest X-ray and ESR are recommended if the patient develops any pulmonary symptoms
- drowsiness is a problem at the start of therapy
- the dose may require adjusting if given with other anti-Parkinson's agents
- observe the patient for suicidal tendencies or depression
- the patient should be carefully monitored for any signs of confusion or hallucinations because this may require cessation of therapy
- avoid abrupt withdrawal of therapy to prevent neuroleptic malignant syndrome, worsening of Parkinson's symptoms, catatonia or delirium
- drug withdrawal syndrome can occur when tapering or discontinuing therapy. If symptoms are persistent or severe, therapy may need to be restarted at the lowest effective dose
- (Drug-induced extrapyramidal symptoms) when symptoms have been controlled, the dose should be gradually decreased and then ceased
- caution if used in those with epilepsy, confusion, psychosis, hallucinations, underlying psychiatric disorders, gastric ulcers or bleeding, cardiovascular disease, congestive heart failure, postural hypotension, narrow-angle glaucoma, prostatic enlargement, kidney or liver impairment, Raynaud's syndrome or recurrent eczema

General Patient education for dopamine agonists
- advise the patient to resume physical activity gradually to avoid injury

ANTI-PARKINSON'S AGENTS

- the patient should be advised to immediately report:
  - any rash
  - swelling of feet or lower limbs
  - feelings of depression or suicidal thoughts
  - changes to vision, blurred vision
- the patient should be advised to avoid suddenly stopping therapy, as worsening of Parkinson's symptoms and/or increase in body temperature, sweating, muscle rigidity or psychological changes may occur, which are potentially life threatening
- patients should be warned to avoid alcohol during therapy
- advise the patient to avoid postural hypotension by moving gradually to a sitting or standing position, especially after sleep
- the patient should be advised not to drive or operate machinery if drowsiness, daytime somnolence, sudden sleep onset or dizziness continues
- family/carers should be asked to observe for any:
  - sudden sleep onset, as patients are often unaware that this occurs and it may be dangerous if the person drives or operates machinery
  - persistent/recurring gambling, increase in sexual desires, pathological gambling, increased libido, binge and compulsive eating, repetitive purposeless activity, compulsive spending or buying
  - change in mood, depression, or expressions of self-harm or suicide

AMANTADINE HYDROCHLORIDE
Trade names
Amantamed, Symmetrel

Available form
Capsules: 100 mg

Action
- thought to stimulate synthesis and release of dopamine (and other catecholamines) in the brain and also delay reuptake
- may alter D_2 receptors
- some anticholinergic activity
- narrow therapeutic index
- (PD) response usually within 24–48 hours and 7 days
- (Influenza) inhibits penetration of the virus (influenza A) into the host cell, preventing viral replication

Use
- Parkinson's disease and other forms of Parkinsonism (not indicated for tardive dyskinesia)
- drug-induced extrapyramidal reactions
- prophylaxis against influenza type A

Dose
- (PD, less than 65 years) initially 100 mg orally daily for 1 week, then increasing to 100 mg orally twice daily **OR**
- (PD, 65 years and over) 100 mg orally daily **OR**
- (Drug-induced extrapyramidal effects) initial treatment should be dosage reduction of the drug causing the effects. If this is not practical, then 100 mg orally 2–3 times daily, discontinuing when symptoms have been controlled **OR**
- (Influenza prophylaxis) 100 mg orally twice daily after food for 10 days

Adverse effects
- palpitations
- mottling of skin (livedo reticularis)
- blurred vision (transient), slurred speech
- (Rare) corneal lesions, seizures
- see also General Adverse effects of dopamine agonists (p. 798)

Interactions
- increased serum levels and toxicity may occur if given with hydrochlorothiazide/triamterene fixed-dose combinations

- see also General Interactions of dopamine agonists (p. 798)

Nursing considerations/Cautions

- adverse effects usually occur within 1—4 days of starting therapy and disappear within 48 hours of stopping
- daily dose should not be exceeded because of the narrow therapeutic index
- effectiveness may diminish after several weeks, but may be regained by temporarily stopping therapy gradually
- abrupt withdrawal is not recommended
- (Influenza) therapy should start immediately after exposure and continue for at least 10 days. Effective for prophylaxis only during administration
- see also General Nursing considerations/Cautions for dopamine agonists (p. 798)

Patient education

- female patients of childbearing potential should be counselled to avoid pregnancy by using effective contraception during and for 5 days after stopping therapy
- see also General Patient education for dopamine agonists (p. 798)

 Capsules are difficult to open and contents are oily and waxy.

 Contraindicated during pregnancy.

 Contraindicated during breastfeeding.

 Those with compromised kidney function or on haemodialysis require dose adjustment by increasing dosing interval according to creatinine clearance (CCl < 15 mL/min: 7-day dose interval; CCl 15—25 mL/min: 3-day dose interval; 26—35 mL/min: 2-day dose interval; 36—75 mL/min: 1-day dose interval; > 75 mL/min: 12-hour dose interval).

APOMORPHINE HYDROCHLORIDE HEMIHYDRATE (APOMORPHINE HYDROCHLORIDE)

Trade names
Apomine, Movapo

Available forms
Ampoules: 20 mg/2 mL, 50 mg/5 mL;
Vial: 100 mg/20 mL;
Prefilled syringes: 50 mg/10 mL;
Multi-dose pen: 30 mg/3 mL

Action

- dopamine agonist acting on pre- and post-synaptic D_2 receptors and antagonising alpha2 adrenergic receptors
- induces vomiting by stimulating chemoreceptor trigger zone (CTZ) in the medulla
- (SC) onset of action within 5 minutes, half-life is approximately 33 minutes

Use

- reduction in severity and number of motor fluctuations in Parkinson's disease refractory to other conventional treatment ('off' phase of the 'on—off' phenomenon, in which the patient fluctuates between mobility and immobility)

Dose

- threshold dose (considered to be the lowest dose that produces an 'unequivocal' motor response compared with baseline)
- after immobility has been provoked and baseline motor assessment has been completed, initially 1.5 mg SC, then observe the patient for 30 minutes for motor response. If there is no/poor response after 40 minutes, give 3 mg SC and observe patient for another 30 minutes. Give a third dose of 5 mg and a fourth dose of 7 mg at 40-minute intervals, if required, observing the patient for 30 minutes as previously (if still no response, patient is thought to be a 'non-responder'; a 10 mg dose can be

ANTI-PARKINSON'S AGENTS

given if the patient had a minimal response at 7 mg)
* (Restarting anti-Parkinsonian treatment) administer threshold dose (as established above) 2.4—3.6 mg SC at first sign of 'off' phase (maximum daily dose 50 mg; maximum single dose 6 mg) and observe for 1 hour **OR**
* initially 1 mg/hour by continuous SC infusion via portable syringe driver pump, increasing as necessary to achieve motor response during waking hours (maximum daily dose 200 mg)

Adverse effects
* (Injection site/continuous SC infusion site) itchy, nodular lesions, local bruising, redness, tenderness, fibrosis and, rarely, necrosis
* nausea, vomiting
* somnolence, drowsiness, sedation
* yawning
* visual hallucinations, confusion
* (Uncommon) increasingly severe 'on' phase dyskinesia, transient postural hypotension, rash
* (Rare) eosinophilia, haemolytic anaemia, impulse control disorders
* (High dose) QT prolongation

Interactions
* Coombs' positive haemolytic anaemia may occur if used in conjunction with levodopa
* not recommended with metoclopramide, as effects of apomorphine may be reduced
* not recommended with ondansetron, dolasetron and granisetron because of risk of toxicity
* increased serum levels may occur if given with entacapone
* not recommended with other agents known to prolong QT interval
* caution if used with clozapine
* may potentiate effects of antihypertensive and cardiac-active medications
* see also General Interactions of dopamine agonists (p. 798)

Nursing considerations/Cautions
* monitoring FBC and hepatic, renal and cardiovascular function during prolonged therapy is recommended
* patient must be hospitalised during pretreatment phase
* domperidone (antiemetic) is started 48—72 hours before treatment (10 mg orally 3 times daily or less if renal insufficiency exists); may be reduced by 10 mg daily at weekly intervals until mild nausea reappears and may be stopped after several weeks
* anti-Parkinsonian medications are stopped to provoke the 'off' phase (immobility) after at least 3 days of hospitalisation
* perform baseline motor assessment (unilateral alternate hand-tapping for 30 seconds, time to walk 12 metres, clinical assessment of tremor and dyskinesia (4-point score) and modified Webster disability scale to assess 12 features of Parkinsonism (maximum disability score 36)). Positive motor response consists of 15% increase in hand-tapping, 25% increase in walking time, 2-point increase in tremor score, or Webster score increase of 3 or more points
* dose for treatment may be further adjusted to response, if needed
* not recommended IV
* when starting therapy, the patient should be closely monitored for adequate therapeutic effects and/or adverse effects
* SC administration sites are usually the thigh and lower abdomen
* prefilled syringe does not require any further dilution. Ampoule is diluted using sodium chloride 0.9% for use in portable syringe-driver pump
* continuous SC infusion via mini pump may be recommended for patients who require 8—10 injections per day, or whose overall control is not satisfactory

- continuous SC infusion is required only during waking hours (unless the patient is experiencing night-time problems)
- infusion sites should be rotated every 12 hours
- liver, kidney, blood and heart function should be regularly monitored during therapy
- an opioid antagonist (e.g. naloxone) may be used to treat overdosage, respiratory or CNS depression, or excessive vomiting
- a prefilled syringe should be discarded 24 hours after opening
- caution if used in those with a predisposition to nausea/vomiting, at increased risk of respiratory depression (including the elderly), or those with endocrine, pulmonary or cardiovascular disease
- contraindicated in those under 18 years
- contraindicated in those with known hypersensitivity to sodium metabisulfite, morphine or related products
- contraindicated in those with dementia or pre-existing neuropsychiatric problems or dementias, at risk of QT interval prolongation, liver/kidney impairment, unstable coronary vascular disease, cerebrovascular disease, respiratory or CNS depression, or in those with Parkinson's disease in which the 'on' response to levodopa is marred by severe dyskinesia, hypotonia or psychotoxicity

Patient education

- the patient/carer should be educated regarding injection technique, importance of site rotation, correct storage information and safe disposal of used needles
- the patient should be warned that injection site reaction (itchy nodules) is common and disappears within 48 hours; however, care should be taken to prevent nodules ulcerating and becoming infected
- warn the patient not to use the solution if it has turned green

- see also General Patient education for dopamine agonists (p. 798)

 Not recommended during pregnancy.

 Not recommended during breastfeeding.

 Contraindicated in those with kidney or liver impairment.

BENSERAZIDE HYDROCHLORIDE

Action
- peripheral inhibitor of dopa decarboxylase, which normally decarboxylates levodopa to dopamine in the tissues, thereby preventing any therapeutic dose from reaching the brain (levodopa but not dopamine can cross the blood—brain barrier). Benserazide prevents this peripheral decarboxylation from occurring, so that the levodopa crosses the blood—brain barrier before conversion to dopamine, allowing substantially lower doses of levodopa to be used (e.g. benserazide and levodopa 200 mg is equal to 1000 mg levodopa alone)
- at therapeutic dose, does not cross the blood—brain barrier

Use
- given with levodopa in the treatment of Parkinson's disease or Parkinsonism

Available in combination with
- levodopa + benserazide (see `levodopa in this chapter p. 805)

BROMOCRIPTINE MESILATE (BROMOCRIPTINE MESYLATE)
Trade name
Parlodel

Available form
Tablets: 2.5 mg

ANTI-PARKINSON'S AGENTS

Action
* ergot derivative with no uterotonic and little vasoconstrictor activity
* stimulates dopaminergic receptors
* inhibits release of prolactin
* elimination half-life 2—8 hours

Use
* mild Parkinson's disease (PD) (as monotherapy or with other anti-Parkinson's agents)
* preventing onset of lactation, hyperprolactinaemia (where surgery and/or radiotherapy are not indicated or have been ineffective) (see Pregnancy, childbirth and breastfeeding, p. 1486)
* acromegaly (adjunctive therapy)

Dose
* (PD) initially 1.25 mg orally 1—2 times daily with food for 7 days, then increasing by 1.25 mg at weekly intervals until a therapeutic response is reached (range 5—40 mg in divided doses 6—8-hourly) **OR**
* (Adjunctive therapy in acromegaly) initially 1.25 mg orally at night, increasing gradually over 7—14 days to 10 mg in 4 divided doses with food (maximum daily dose 40 mg)

Adverse effects
* nausea, vomiting, constipation
* headache, somnolence, dizziness, syncope
* nasal congestion
* (Uncommon) confusion, hypotension, auditory or visual hallucinations
* (Very rare, prolonged therapy) reversible pallor of fingers or toes induced by cold
* (PD, rare) pleural/pericardial effusion/fibrosis, cardiac valvulopathy, retroperitoneal fibrosis, diabetic retinopathy, sudden sleep onset, impulse control disorders, gastric ulceration/bleeding
* (PD, high dose) persistent hallucinations (even after stopping therapy)
* (Acromegaly, high dose) gastric haemorrhage

Interactions
* increased plasma levels may result if given with erythromycin, clarithromycin or octreotide
* not recommended with alcohol
* hypotensive effects may be enhanced if given with antihypertensive agents or other agents known to decrease BP
* increased risk of hypertension and headache if given with sympathomimetic agents
* may alter serum levels of levodopa, increasing the risk of adverse effects
* may have additive effects if given with sumatriptan
* see also General Interactions of dopamine agonists (p. 798)

Nursing considerations/Cautions
* dosage increases are made gradually, starting with the smallest dose, usually over several days, to reduce adverse effects especially hypotension
* decreasing the dose usually stops auditory/visual hallucinations
* (PD) may be given alone or as combination therapy
* (Long-term therapy) women should have regular gynaecological examinations (to monitor for any uterine tumour)
* (PD) regular X-ray monitoring is recommended to detect pulmonary fibrosis
* tablets are not recommended in those with galactose intolerance, severe lactase deficiency or glucose—galactose malabsorption
* caution if used in those with suspected/known peptic ulceration, dementia, Raynaud's phenomenon or impaired liver function
* caution if used in those with diabetes because of the risk of diabetic retinopathy
* caution if used in those with co-existing Parkinson's disease and dementia
* contraindicated in those with hypersensitivity to ergot alkaloids, uncontrolled

hypertension, toxaemia, hypertensive disorders associated with pregnancy (including postpartum), coronary artery disease, severe cardiovascular conditions or serious psychiatric disorders (including history)
* see also General Nursing considerations/Cautions for dopamine agonists (p. 798)

Patient education
* the patient should be advised to immediately report:
  * any shortness of breath, persistent cough or chest pain (pulmonary fibrosis)
  * any loin/flank pain, lower limb swelling or abdominal tenderness (retroperitoneal fibrosis)
  * any vomiting of blood, bloody diarrhoea, red or black bowel motions, or bleeding from the rectum
  * any persistent headache or visual problems
  * any visual or auditory hallucinations
* warn the patient that alcohol may cause nausea, abdominal pain and bloating if used during bromocriptine therapy
* warn patients with acromegaly to immediately report any GI side-effects
* advise the patient to take initial doses at bedtime, to reduce the incidence of hypotension and loss of consciousness
* instruct the patient that gastric irritation can be reduced if taken with or immediately after food
* see also General Patient education for dopamine antagonists (p. 798)

Tablets can be dispersed in water, or crushed and mixed with a spoonful of yoghurt or apple puree.

Use during pregnancy only if benefits outweigh risks.

Not recommended during breastfeeding, as lactation is suppressed/inhibited.

CABERGOLINE
Trade names
Cabaser, Dostamine, Dostinex

Available form
Tablets: 500 microgram, 1 mg, 2 mg

Action
* ergot derivative
* stimulates D_2 dopamine receptors, inhibiting prolactin secretion
* long half-life (63—68 hours)

Use
* Parkinson's disease (PD) (Cabaser)
* inhibiting physiological lactation, hyperprolactinaemia (Dostinex, Dostamine) (see Pregnancy, childbirth and breastfeeding, p. 1488)

Dose
* (PD monotherapy) initially 0.5 mg orally daily, increasing at 1—2-weekly intervals orally to 2—3 mg daily **OR**
* (PD, with levodopa) initially 1 mg orally daily, increasing at 1—2-weekly intervals orally to 2—3 mg daily

Adverse effects
* palpitations, hypertension
* dyspnoea
* (Rare) pleural/pericardial effusion/fibrosis, cardiac valvulopathy, retroperitoneal fibrosis
* see also General Adverse effects of dopamine agonists (p. 798)

Interactions
* not recommended with other ergot alkaloids
* not recommended with macrolide antibacterial agents (e.g. erythromycin)
* hypotensive effects may be enhanced if given with antihypertensive agents or other agents known to decrease BP
* see also General Interactions of dopamine agonists (p. 798)

Nursing considerations/Cautions
* the patient should be screened for any signs of depression or psychiatric history before starting therapy

ANTI-PARKINSON'S AGENTS

- doses of levodopa can be gradually decreased while the dose of cabergoline is increased
- no data exist to show that 1 and 2 mg tablets are bioequivalent at equal doses
- serum creatinine levels should be measured if there is any suspicion of fibrotic disorder
- caution if used in those with severe liver disease
- contraindicated in those with hypersensitivity to any ergot alkaloid
- contraindicated in those with a history of pulmonary, pericardial or retroperitoneal fibrotic disease or anatomical evidence of cardiac valvulopathy
- see also General Nursing considerations/Cautions for dopamine agonists (p. 798)

Patient education

- advise the patient that administration with food may lessen GI disturbances
- the patient should be advised to immediately report:
  - any shortness of breath, persistent cough or chest pain (pulmonary fibrosis)
  - loin/flank pain, lower limb swelling or abdominal tenderness or mass (retroperitoneal fibrosis)
- female patients of childbearing potential should be counselled that pregnancy should be excluded before starting therapy and at least 1 month should elapse between stopping treatment and becoming pregnant
- see also General Patient education for dopamine agonists (p. 798)

 Tablet can be crushed and mixed with water or a spoonful of yoghurt or apple puree.

 Not recommended during pregnancy. If pregnancy occurs, therapy should be stopped to limit fetal exposure.

 Lactation will be suppressed/inhibited and therefore not recommended during breastfeeding.

 Dose reduction required in those with severe liver insufficiency (Child−Pugh score > 10).

CARBIDOPA MONOHYDRATE (CARBIDOPA)

Action
- inhibits peripheral decarboxylation of levodopa, increasing the amount that enters the brain for conversion to dopamine
- does not cross the blood−brain barrier in therapeutic doses

Use
- given with levodopa to treat Parkinsonism

Available in combination with
- levodopa + carbidopa (see Levodopa, below)

LEVODOPA

Available forms
Capsules: levodopa 50 mg/benserazide 12.5 mg, levodopa 100 mg/benserazide 25 mg, levodopa 200 mg/benserazide 50 mg;
Capsules (sustained-release): levodopa 100 mg/benserazide 25 mg;
Tablets: levodopa 100 mg/benserazide 25 mg, levodopa 200 mg/benserazide 50 mg;
Tablets (dispersible): levodopa 50 mg/benserazide 12.5 mg, levodopa 100 mg/benserazide 25 mg;
Tablets: levodopa 100 mg/carbidopa 25 mg, levodopa 250 mg/carbidopa 25 mg;
Tablets (sustained-release): levodopa 50 mg/carbidopa 12.5 mg/entacapone 200 mg, levodopa 200 mg/carbidopa 50 mg;
Tablets (film-coated): levodopa 50 mg/

carbidopa 12.5 mg/entacapone 200 mg, levodopa 75 mg/carbidopa 18.75 mg/entacapone 200 mg, levodopa 100 mg/carbidopa 25 mg/entacapone 200 mg, levodopa 125 mg/carbidopa 31.25 mg/entacapone 200 mg, levodopa 150 mg/carbidopa 37.5 mg/entacapone 200 mg, levodopa 200 mg/carbidopa 50 mg/entacapone 200 mg;
Intestinal cassette gel (plastic): levodopa 20 mg/carbidopa 5 mg/mL

Action
- main therapy for Parkinson's disease since 1960s
- extensively metabolised, mainly to dopamine, but also adrenaline (epinephrine) and noradrenaline (norepinephrine)
- decarboxylation occurs in peripheral tissues, as well as in the CNS, thereby decreasing the amount of levodopa entering the CNS to be converted to dopamine
- peripheral decarboxylation is inhibited by benserazide or carbidopa monohydrate
- controls akinesia and rigidity more effectively than tremor

Use
- all types of Parkinsonism (except drug-induced Parkinsonian symptoms)

Dose
- rarely used alone

Adverse effects
- muscle cramps, hypotonia
- teeth grinding
- delusions
- depression, suicidal ideation
- dyskinesia, hyperkinesia, involuntary movements, freezing episodes
- dark urine, sweat and saliva, rash, hair loss
- (Less frequent) cardiac arrhythmias, palpitations, hypertension and, rarely, chest pain
- (Uncommon) haemolytic and non-haemolytic anaemia, transient leucopenia
- (Late complications) 'wearing-off effect' (deterioration occurs before next dose is due), 'on—off' phenomenon (abrupt but transient fluctuations in severity of symptoms at frequent intervals)
- (Rare) gastrointestinal bleeding and ulceration, melanoma
- (Overdose) muscle twitching, blepharospasm, dystonia, dyskinesia
- (Intestinal gel) dislocation of tube, occlusion, incision site pain and erythema, abdominal pain
- see also General Adverse effects of dopamine agonists (p. 798)

Interactions
- effects enhanced by the peripheral dopa decarboxylase inhibitors, carbidopa monohydrate and benserazide
- not recommended with baclofen, as baclofen toxicity and/or worsening of Parkinsonian symptoms may occur
- contraindicated with or within 14 days of monoamine oxidase inhibitors (MAOIs)
- increased risk of hypertension and dyskinesia if given with tricyclic antidepressants (TCAs)
- not recommended with halothane, as combination may result in arrhythmia
- bioavailability decreased if given with iron-containing products
- effects may be reduced if given with isoniazid, phenothiazines, metoclopramide, benzodiazepine or phenytoin
- caution if given with antihypertensives or other agents known to reduce BP, as symptomatic postural hypotension may occur
- high-protein diet may decrease absorption of levodopa
- increased serum levels may occur if given with penicillamine
- may cause hypotension and/or dyskinesia if given with methyldopa sesquihydrate
- bioavailability may be increased if given with domperidone or catechol-O-methyltransferase (COMT) inhibitors

ANTI-PARKINSON'S AGENTS

- may potentiate effects of adrenaline (epinephrine), noradrenaline (norepinephrine), isoprenaline or dexamphetamine
- (Madopar HBS) absorption decreased if given with antacids
- may cause false positive for urinary ketone bodies and positive Coombs' test; may interfere with uric acid, creatinine and glucose estimation. T-wave increase on ECG
- see also General Interactions of dopamine antagonists (p. 798)

Nursing considerations/Cautions

- GI and cardiovascular adverse effects may be decreased when given with peripheral decarboxylase inhibitor
- conduct monthly FBC and monitor liver, kidney and cardiovascular function during prolonged therapy
- sudden fluctuations of effectiveness of levodopa develop after about 2 years of therapy ('on–off' effect)
- appearance of involuntary movements may be a sign of levodopa toxicity
- levodopa therapy is discontinued at least 2–3 days before surgery and restarted as soon as the patient is able to take oral medications
- dispersible tablets are recommended for those with swallowing difficulties or if rapid onset of action is required
- (Intestinal gel) gel is administered directly into the duodenum, initially via a temporary nasoduodenal/nasojejunal tube to confirm positive clinical response (maximising functional 'on' time and minimising the disabling 'off' periods) before the insertion of a permanent percutaneous endoscopic gastrostomy (PEG) tube (tube placement should be confirmed before administration). Gel is administered continuously using a portable pump (CADD Legacy Duodopa (CE 0473)). Dosage consists of morning bolus dose (100–200 mg over 10–30 minutes), continuous maintenance dose (20–200 mg/hour) and extra boluses (given if patient becomes hypokinetic during the day, usually between 10 and 40 mg). If extra boluses are given more than 5 times per day, the continuous maintenance dose should be recalculated. The morning bolus dose may also require adjusting (maximum levodopa 300 mg (15 mL)). The gel should be administered for a total of 16 hours only, after which the cassette should be discarded, regardless of whether any gel remains in the cassette or not. If the administration continues overnight, the cassette must still be changed after it has been at room temperature for 16 hours. Continuous administration may result in tolerance and reduction of therapeutic effect. If a sudden deterioration in effect (e.g. bradykinesia) is seen, placement of the tube should be checked, as it may become displaced from duodenum into the stomach
- caution if used in those with epilepsy, depression, diabetes, history of psychosis, severe cardiovascular or pulmonary disease, cardiac arrhythmias or myocardial infarction (therapy should be started as an inpatient), asthma, liver, kidney or endocrine disease or history of peptic ulceration
- not recommended for drug-induced extrapyramidal reactions
- (Madopar) contraindicated in those under 30 years
- contraindicated in those with a history of malignant melanoma or suspicious lesion because therapy may activate a malignant melanoma
- contraindicated in those with any hypersensitivity to sympathomimetic amines or with uncompensated cardiovascular, endocrine, kidney, liver or blood disease, narrow-angle glaucoma, active psychosis or psychoneurosis, phaeochromocytoma, hyperthyroidism, Cushing's syndrome, intention tremor or Huntington's chorea

Patient education

- the patient should be advised to take medication 30—60 minutes before food if possible; however, gastric irritation is reduced by taking with or immediately after food, if needed
- instruct the patient to avoid eating a high-protein diet, as this may impair absorption of medication
- (Sustained-release tablets/capsules) advise the patient to swallow whole (not chewed or crushed); however, tablets can be divided without affecting properties. Because the onset of action of sustained-release preparations is long, the patient may also need to take an immediate-release preparation for immediate effects
- instruct the patient that dispersible tablets should be dissolved in 25—50 mL water (solution is milky white) and drunk within 30 minutes, ensuring that solution is well stirred
- advise the patient about the need to continue treatment because it is long-term replacement therapy; maximum improvement may take up to 6 months and is maintained only while therapy continues, so therapy should not be suddenly stopped
- instruct the patient to report any loss of movement (a few minutes to a few hours) that may occur when medication has been taken for a long period of time. This may recur and is called 'on—off' effect. It may require an increase in dose or change of medication
- those with diabetes are advised to monitor blood glucose levels closely during therapy
- warn the patient that a reddish tinge in the urine is harmless; tears and sweat may also appear brown
- the patient/carer should be advised to report any:
  - lowered mood, mental changes or signs of depression or suicidal tendencies
  - appearance of involuntary movements, which may be a sign of levodopa toxicity and should be reported immediately
  - changes in skin lesions (size, shape, colour). Regular skin examination by a dermatologist is recommended
- (Intestinal gel) the patient should be advised to avoid swimming or bathing, as the pump cannot be taken into water. The patient should be warned that disconnecting the pump may result in sudden bradykinesia, which could result in drowning if they are in water
- see also General Patient education for dopamine antagonists (p. 798)

 Plain tablets can be dispersed in water, or crushed and mixed with a spoonful of apple puree.

 Controlled/modified-release tablets/capsules should not be broken or crushed.

 Safety in pregnancy has not been established; therefore benefits to the mother versus risks to the fetus should be considered before use.

 Not recommended during breastfeeding.

 Caution if used in those with kidney or liver impairment. Kidney and liver function tests are recommended during therapy.

Available in combination with

- levodopa 50 mg + benserazide 12.5 mg (Madopar 62.5, Madopar Rapid 62.5)
- levodopa 100 mg + benserazide 25 mg (Madopar 125, Madopar Rapid 125, Madopar HBS)
- levodopa 200 mg + benserazide 50 mg (Madopar)
- levodopa 20 mg/mL + carbidopa monohydrate 5 mg/mL intestinal gel (Duodopa)
- levodopa 100 mg + carbidopa 25 mg (APO-Levodopa/Carbidopa 100/25, Kinson 100/25, SINADOPA 100/25, Sinemet 100/25)

ANTI-PARKINSON'S AGENTS

- levodopa 250 mg + carbidopa 25 mg (APO-Levodopa/Carbidopa 200/25, SINADOPA 200/25, Sinemet 200/25)
- levodopa 200 mg + carbidopa 50 mg (Sinemet CR)
- levodopa 50 mg + carbidopa 12.5 mg + entacapone 200 mg (Carlevent 50/12.5/200, L.C.E. Sandoz 50/12.5/200, Lecteva 50/12.5/200, Stalevo 50/12.5/200)
- levodopa 75 mg + carbidopa 18.75 mg + entacapone 200 mg (Carlevent 75/18.75/200, L.C.E. Sandoz 75/18.75/200, Lecteva 75/18.75/200, Stalevo 75/18.75/200)
- levodopa 100 mg + carbidopa 25 mg + entacapone 200 mg (Carlevent 100/25/200, L.C.E. Sandoz 100/25/200, Lecteva 100/25/200, Stalevo 100/25/200)
- levodopa 125 mg + carbidopa 31.25 mg + entacapone 200 mg (Carlevent 125/31.25/200, L.C.E. Sandoz 125/31.25/200, Lecteva 125/31.25/200, Stalevo 125/31.25/200)
- levodopa 150 mg + carbidopa 37.5 mg + entacapone 200 mg (Carlevent 150/37.5/200, L.C.E. Sandoz 150/37.5/200, Lecteva 150/37.5/200, Stalevo 150/37.5/200)
- levodopa 200 mg + carbidopa 50 mg + entacapone 200 mg (Carlevent 200/50/200, L.C.E. Sandoz 200/50/200, Lecteva 200/50/200, Stalevo 200/50/200)

PRAMIPEXOLE DIHYDROCHLORIDE MONOHYDRATE

Trade names
APO-Pramipexole, Sifrol, Sifrol ER, Simipex, Simipex XR, Simpral

Available forms
Tablets: 125 microgram, 250 microgram, 1 mg;
Tablets (extended-release): 375 microgram, 750 microgram, 1.5 mg, 2.25 mg, 3 mg, 3.75 mg, 4.5 mg

Action
- dopamine agonist that binds selectively to dopamine D_2 and D_3 receptors
- decreases prolactin levels
- half-life 8—12 hours

Use
- Parkinson's disease (alone or with levodopa)
- restless leg syndrome (RLS)

Dose
- (PD) initially 125 micrograms orally 3 times daily, increasing to 250 micrograms orally 3 times daily after 5—7 days, then to 500 micrograms orally 3 times daily after a further 5—7 days, with further increases at weekly intervals if needed (daily maximum 4.5 mg) (immediate-release tablets) **OR**
- (PD) initially 375 micrograms orally daily for 5—7 days, increasing to 750 micrograms orally daily for 5—7 days, then 1.5 mg orally daily for 5—7 days, increasing further if needed at 5—7-day intervals (daily maximum 4.5 mg) (extended-release tablets) **OR**
- (RLS) initially 125 micrograms orally daily 2—3 hours before bedtime, increasing every 4—7 days to 750 micrograms daily if needed (immediate-release tablets)

Adverse effects
- cough, dyspnoea, nasal congestion
- flushing, sweating
- vertigo
- back pain, pain in extremities, arthralgia, muscle cramps, myalgia
- urinary frequency and incontinence
- hallucinations (but more common if given with levodopa)
- axial dystonia (may occur months after starting therapy or dose adjustment)
- retinal degeneration (more than other dopamine agents in patients with PD)
- (Rare) rhabdomyolysis
- (RLS) augmentation (earlier onset of symptoms, increase in severity and

spread of symptoms to other body parts)
- see also General Adverse effects of dopamine agonists (p. 798)

Interactions
- serum levels may be increased by diltiazem, ranitidine, triamterene, verapamil, digoxin or trimethoprim
- see also General Interactions of dopamine agonists (p. 798)

Nursing considerations/Cautions
- if given with levodopa, the dose of levodopa should be reduced by 25% to avoid adverse effects
- if discontinuing therapy, the dose should be gradually reduced at a rate of 750 microgram/day until a 750 microgram daily dose is reached, then reduced by 375 microgram/day
- see also General Nursing considerations/Cautions for dopamine agonists (p. 798)

Patient education
- advise the patient that extended-release tablets should be swallowed whole, and not chewed, crushed or split
- see also General Patient education for dopamine agonists (p. 798)

Plain tablets can be dispersed in water, or crushed and mixed with a spoonful of yoghurt or apple puree.

Extended-release tablets should not be broken or crushed.

Used during pregnancy only if benefits outweigh risks.

May inhibit/suppress lactation; therefore not recommended during breastfeeding.

Dose reduction is required in those with mild kidney impairment (creatinine clearance 20–50 mL/min).

Caution if used in the elderly, as age-related decline in kidney function may result in a prolonged half-life.

ROTIGOTINE
Trade name
Neupro

Available forms
Transdermal patches: 2 mg/24 hour, 4 mg/24 hour, 6 mg/24 hour, 8 mg/24 hour

Action
- non-ergot dopamine agonist that activates D_1, D_2, D_3, D_4 and D_5 (but particularly D_3) receptors in the brain
- decreases prolactin levels

Use
- Parkinson's disease (alone or with levodopa)
- restless leg syndrome (RLS)

Dose
- (Early stage PD) initially 2 mg/24-hour patch applied daily, then increased at weekly intervals of 2 mg/24-hour to an effective dose (maximum 8 mg/24 hours) **OR**
- (Advanced stage PD) initially 4 mg/24-hour patch applied daily, then increased at weekly intervals of 2 mg/24-hour to an effective dose (maximum 16 mg/24 hours). For doses above 8 mg/24 hours, a combination of patches can be used **OR**
- (RLS) initially 1 mg/24 hours, increasing if needed at weekly intervals (maximum 3 mg/24 hours)

Adverse effects
- (Application site) erythema, pruritus, urticaria, rash, irritation, burning, dermatitis, vesicles/papules, exfoliation, swelling, inflammation, discolouration, pain, hypersensitivity
- (RLS) augmentation (earlier onset of symptoms, increase in severity and spread of symptoms to other body parts)

ANTI-PARKINSON'S AGENTS

- increase in systolic and/or diastolic blood pressure, increased heart rate, palpitations, atrial fibrillation
- vertigo
- (PD) weight gain, fluid retention
- (Uncommon) blurred vision, visual impairment, photopsia (flashes of light), elevated liver enzymes
- (Rare) seizures
- see also General Adverse effects of dopamine agonists (p. 798)

Interactions

- see General Interactions of dopamine agonists (p. 798)

Nursing considerations/Cautions

- regular ophthalmology monitoring is recommended
- the patient should be closely monitored for fluid retention and weight gain (especially if pre-existing congestive cardiac failure or kidney insufficiency exists)
- dose reduction is recommended if worsening liver impairment occurs
- (Restless leg syndrome) therapy should be evaluated for effectiveness after 6 months
- contains sodium metabisulfite, which can cause allergic reaction in susceptible people
- contraindicated with cardioversion or magnetic resonance imaging (MRI) owing to the risk of skin burning because of the aluminium backing layer
- see also General Nursing considerations/Cautions for dopamine agonists (p. 798)

Patient education

- patients should be advised to:
  - apply the patch at approximately the same time each day and to leave in place for 24 hours
  - apply the patch to clean, dry, intact skin on upper arms, shoulders, hip, flank (side, between rib and hip), thigh or belly, but not in an area that is rubbed by tight clothing
  - avoid any skin that is red, inflamed, irritated or damaged
  - if applying to a hairy area, skin should be shaved at least 3 days before applying patch
  - rotate application sites daily and do not use the same site within 14 days
  - leave the patch intact when swimming or bathing
  - avoid direct sunlight to any application site rash or irritation until the skin heals
  - avoid external heat (e.g. excessive sunlight, heating pads, sauna, hot bath) to the transdermal patch area
- do not cut transdermal patch into smaller pieces
- if the patch falls off, a new patch should be applied for the rest of the day
- correctly dispose of the used patch (i.e. folded in half without matrix exposed, placed in original sachet and discarded out of the reach of children), as it still contains active substance
- advise the patient not to use any skin products (e.g. creams, oils, powders, lotions) on or near the area where the patch is applied
- instruct the patient to wash the area where patch was applied with water and soap (but not use any alcohol or other dissolving fluids) to remove any residual adhesive
- patients should be advised to report any application site reaction that either spreads beyond the site or persists for more than 2—3 days, or if excessive weight gain/fluid retention occurs
- instruct the patient to seek medical advice if visual changes or disturbances occur
- see also General Patient education for dopamine agonists (p. 798)

 Not recommended during pregnancy.

 Not recommended during breastfeeding. Suppression/inhibition of lactation will occur.

Dose reduction is recommended if worsening kidney or liver impairment occurs in those with pre-existing kidney or liver impairment.

MONOAMINE OXIDASE TYPE B ENZYME (MAO-B) INHIBITORS

General Patient education for MAO-B inhibitors

- warn the patient to avoid driving or operating machinery if dizziness, vertigo, fatigue or hypotension occurs
- advise the patient to avoid postural hypotension by moving gradually to a sitting or standing position, especially after sleep
- advise the patient to resume physical activity gradually to avoid injury
- the patient should be warned not to stop therapy suddenly because it may cause hallucinations and confusion
- the patient should be advised to avoid alcohol during therapy
- the patient should be advised to avoid excessive amounts of foods with a high tyramine content (e.g. aged cheeses, red wine)
- family/carers should be asked to observe for:
  - any signs of depression or altered mood
  - persistent/recurring gambling, increase in sexual desires or repetitive behaviours with no purpose, abnormal buying or selling, or meaningless collecting and sorting of objects

RASAGILINE
Trade names
Alziras, Azilect, Pharmcor Rasagiline, Rasagiline Lupin, Rasagiline Sandoz, Rasagiline-Teva, Rasagiline-WGR

Available form
Tablets: 1 mg

Action
- irreversible monoamine oxidase type B (MAO-B) selective inhibitor thought to cause an increase in extracellular dopamine levels

Use
- idiopathic Parkinson's disease (as monotherapy or as adjunct therapy with levodopa/decarboxylase inhibitor)

Dose
- 1 mg orally daily (with or without levodopa/decarboxylase inhibitor therapy)

Adverse effects
- headache, malaise, dizziness, vertigo, daytime drowsiness, somnolence and (if given with dopamine agonists) sudden sleep onset
- depression, hallucinations
- fever, flu-like symptoms
- neck pain, arthralgia, arthritis, joint or tendon disorder
- angina, peripheral vascular disorder, postural hypotension
- dyspepsia, anorexia, vomiting, tooth disorder
- ecchymosis, leucopenia
- decreased libido, impotence, urinary urgency
- pharyngitis, rhinitis, asthma
- alopecia, contact dermatitis, skin carcinoma (including melanoma), rash
- conjunctivitis, otitis media
- albuminaemia
- (Adjunct therapy) exacerbate dyskinesia, postural hypotension
- (Rare) impulse control disorder, serotonin syndrome (see Glossary), hypertensive crisis, hallucinations

Interactions
- contraindicated with or within 14 days of MAOIs or pethidine
- contraindicated with tramadol, methadone, dextromethorphan, ciprofloxacin or St John's wort
- not recommended with fluoxetine and fluvoxamine. Fluoxetine should be discontinued for 5 weeks before starting therapy with rasagiline. Rasagiline

ANTI-PARKINSON'S AGENTS

should be discontinued for at least 2 weeks before starting therapy with fluoxetine or fluvoxamine
- increased risk of serotonin syndrome (see Glossary) if given with selective serotonin reuptake inhibitors (SSRIs), serotonin and noradrenaline (norepinephrine) reuptake inhibitors (SNRIs) or tricyclic antidepressants (TCAs)
- not recommended with dextromethorphan or sympathomimetic agents (including nasal and cold preparations)
- clearance may be decreased by entacapone
- increased clearance in smokers
- caution if used with alcohol
- may potentiate dopaminergic adverse effects (including exacerbation of pre-existing dyskinesia) if given with levodopa

Nursing considerations/Cautions

- before starting therapy, the patient should be assessed for any skin lesions
- check supine and standing BP regularly for postural hypotension, especially during the first 8 weeks of therapy when it commonly occurs
- if combined with levodopa therapy, a levodopa dose reduction may be considered depending on patient response
- tyramine-containing foods do not need to be restricted during therapy. However, caution is recommended if eating foods containing very high levels of tyramine (e.g. aged cheese)
- the recommended dose should not be exceeded because of the risk of hypertensive crisis
- not recommended in those under 18 years
- contraindicated in those with liver impairment

Patient education

- instruct the patient (or carer) to monitor skin for any new or changes to existing skin lesions, such as a change in colour or size
- if the patient is planning to quit smoking while on therapy, they should be advised to seek medical advice and not stop suddenly
- advise the patient not to take any over-the-counter 'cold and flu' preparations or nasal drops without discussing with the doctor or pharmacist first, as these may interact with therapy
- see also General Patient education for MAO-B inhibitors (p. 812)

Tablet can be dispersed in water, or crushed and mixed with a spoonful of yoghurt or apple puree.

Not recommended during pregnancy unless benefits outweigh risks.

May inhibit lactation. Caution if used during breastfeeding.

Contraindicated in those with liver impairment.

SAFINAMIDE

Trade names
Xadago, ARX-Safinamide

Available form
Tablets: 50 mg, 100 mg

Action
- selectively and reversibly inhibits monoamine oxidase B (MAO-B) enzyme (breaks down dopamine in the brain), thereby increasing brain levels of dopamine
- elimination half-life 20—30 hours, steady state achieved in about 7 days

Use
- Parkinson's disease (as adjunct with levodopa in later stage disease)

Dose
- initially 50 mg orally daily, increasing to 100 mg daily after 14 days if needed

Adverse effects
- nausea, dyspepsia, change in appetite, dry mouth, diarrhoea, abdominal pain/distension
- postural hypotension, peripheral oedema
- gait disturbance, falls
- cataract formation and uncommonly, blurred vision, diplopia, photophobia
- dyskinesia, somnolence, dizziness, headache, vertigo
- fatigue, asthenia
- (Uncommon) hypertriglyceridaemia, hypercholesterolaemia, hyperglycaemia, urinary tract infection, nocturia, dysuria, erectile dysfunction, cough, dyspnoea, palpitations, tachycardia, bradycardia, arrhythmias, sweating
- (Rare) impulse control disorder, serotonin syndrome, suicidal ideation

Interactions
- contraindicated with or within 7 days of monoamine oxidase inhibitors (MAOIs) or pethidine
- not recommended with selective serotonin reuptake inhibitors (SSRIs), serotonin and noradrenaline (norepinephrine) reuptake inhibitors (SNRIs), tricyclic antidepressants (TCAs), tetracyclic antidepressants, opioids or dexamphetamine because of the risk of risk of serotonin syndrome. A washout period of 5 half-lives is recommended when stopping SSRI and starting safinamide
- pre-existing dyskinesia may be exacerbated if given with levodopa and/or dopamine agonists
- caution if used with sympathomimetic agents
- not recommended with dextromethorphan
- may transiently inhibit breast cancer resistance protein (BCRP); therefore a 5-hour interval should be allowed between safinamide and BCRP substrates such as pravastatin, ciprofloxacin, methotrexate, topotecan and diclofenac

Nursing considerations/Cautions
- if discontinuing therapy, a 50 mg daily dose can be stopped without any titration, but 100 mg therapy should be reduced to 50 mg for 7 days before stopping
- tyramine-containing foods do not need to be restricted during therapy
- caution if used in those with moderate liver impairment
- contraindicated in those with severe liver impairment, albinism, retinal degeneration, uveitis, inherited retinopathy or severe progressive diabetic retinopathy

Patient education
- female patients of childbearing potential should be advised to use adequate contraception and avoid pregnancy
- see also General Patient education for MAO-B inhibitors (p. 812)

 Tablets can be crushed and mixed with water or a spoonful of yoghurt or apple puree.

 Not recommended during pregnancy.

 Not recommended during breastfeeding.

 If liver impairment progresses from moderate to severe, therapy should be stopped.

Contraindicated in those with severe liver impairment.

SELEGILINE HYDROCHLORIDE
Trade name
Eldepryl

Available form
Tablets: 5 mg

Action
- selectively and irreversibly inhibits MAO-B enzyme (breaks down dopamine

ANTI-PARKINSON'S AGENTS

in the brain), thereby increasing brain levels of dopamine
- may also inhibit dopamine reuptake
- three active metabolites with half-lives ranging from 2—20 hours

Use
- Parkinson's disease (as monotherapy in early disease, or as adjunct with levodopa in late-stage disease)

Dose
- 5 mg orally twice daily with breakfast and lunch

Adverse effects
- nausea, vomiting, dry mouth
- postural hypotension, syncope
- angina, arrhythmias, bradycardia
- headache, fatigue, dizziness, vertigo, insomnia, sleep disorders
- confusion, hallucinations
- dyskinesia, hypokinesia
- transient increase in liver enzymes (alanine aminotransferase (ALT), aspartate aminotransferase (AST))
- (Rare) impulse control disorder

Interactions
- severe hyper/hypotension may result if given with linezolid or other non-selective monoamine oxidase inhibitors (MAOIs)
- increased tyramine sensitivity may result if given with moclobemide. If given together, a low tyramine diet is recommended (see 'cheese reaction' in Glossary for a list of foods to avoid)
- pethidine is contraindicated with or within 14 days of stopping selegiline
- contraindicated with selective serotonin reuptake inhibitors (SSRIs). Selegiline should be stopped for 2 weeks before starting SSRIs, or SSRIs should be stopped for 5 weeks before starting selegiline
- hypertension may occur if given with dopamine
- increased bioavailability may occur if given with oral contraceptives containing gestodene/ethinylestradiol or levonorgestrel/ethinylestradiol
- increased risk of serotonin syndrome (see Glossary) if given with SSRIs, tricyclic antidepressants (TCAs), clozapine or ecstasy/MDMA (3, 4-methylenedioxymethamphetamine), or other serotonin potentiating agents
- caution if used with tramadol or buprenorphine
- may increase adverse effects of levodopa
- increased risk of CNS toxicity if given with TCAs; therefore these should be stopped 2 weeks before starting selegiline
- not recommended with alcohol
- caution if used with general anaesthetics during surgery owing to increased CNS depression
- caution if used with agents that have a narrow therapeutic index such as digoxin

Nursing considerations/Cautions
- dose of levodopa can be reduced by 10—30% after 2—3 days if levodopa-related adverse effects occur
- check supine and standing BP regularly for postural hypotension
- tyramine-containing foods do not need to be restricted during therapy. However, caution is recommended if eating foods containing very high levels of tyramine (e.g. aged cheese)
- recommended dose should not be exceeded
- caution if used in those with severe kidney or liver dysfunction, labile hypertension, cardiac arrhythmias, severe angina pectoris or psychosis
- not recommended in those with active duodenal or gastric ulcers

Patient education

- see General Patient education for MAO-B inhibitors (p. 812)

Tablets can be dispersed in 10–20 mL water or crushed and mixed with spoonful of yoghurt or apple puree.

Not recommended during pregnancy unless benefits outweigh the risks.

Not recommended during breastfeeding.

Banned in competition.

ANTIPLATELET AGENTS

When a blood vessel is 'damaged', platelets adhere to the site, becoming activated and synthesising factors such as platelet-activating factor, thromboxane A_2, adenosine diphosphate (ADP, which binds to P_2Y_{12} and P_2Y_1 receptors) and thrombin, which cause vasoconstriction and platelet aggregation. Platelet aggregation occurs when the platelet receptors (glycoproteins IIb and IIIa) bind with fibrinogen, linking the platelets together. This process is necessary when haemostasis is required, but can sometimes occur when thrombus formation is not required and the thrombus is, in fact, dangerous and may occlude the vessel, leading to conditions such as myocardial infarction, stroke and peripheral arterial thrombosis (Hogg & Weitz 2018).

Antiplatelet agents inhibit this unwanted thrombus formation by decreasing platelet aggregation. As a group, the antiplatelet agents can be subdivided into aspirin (discussed in Analgesics and non-steroidal anti-inflammatory drugs, p. 15), glycoprotein IIb/IIIa inhibitors and P_2Y_{12} inhibitors. They are used in a range of conditions, including the prevention of thromboembolic events (particularly arterial thrombus, which consists mainly of platelets with little fibrin), ischaemic heart disease and stroke (Hogg & Weitz 2018).

ASPIRIN
Trade names
Aspro Clear Extra Strength, Aspro preparations, Astrix 100, Astrix Tablets, Cardasa, Cardiprin 100, Cartia, Disprin preparations, Solprin, Spren

Available forms
Capsules: 100 mg;
Tablets: 100 mg, 300 mg, 320 mg, 500 mg;
Tablets (enteric coated): 100 mg;
Tablets (effervescent): 300 mg, 500 mg

Action
- aspirin is converted to salicylic acid mainly in the GI tract
- absorption is dependent on formulation (e.g. soluble formulation increases the rate of absorption)
- irreversibly inhibits cyclo-oxygenase (COX) platelet activity (needed for thromboxane synthesis), resulting in prolonged action. It may take 8–12 days (platelet turnover time) after therapy is stopped to fully recover
- half-life of aspirin is about 30 minutes; the half-life of salicylate is dose dependent
- see also General Actions of NSAIDs (p. 11)

Use
- analgesic, anti-inflammatory
- antiplatelet therapy (only on medical advice) for prophylaxis against myocardial infarction, unstable angina, transient ischaemic attacks (TIAs) and stroke (see general points for Analgesics and NSAIDs, p. 10).

Avoid late in pregnancy because of the potential fetal and maternal risks.

Avoid: aspirin is excreted in low levels in breastmilk, which breastfeeding infants eliminate slowly.

Not recommended for children/teenagers because of the Reye's syndrome risk.

P₂Y₁₂ ANTAGONISTS

CLOPIDOGREL
Trade names
Clovix, Iscover, Piax, Plavicor, Plavix, Plidogrel

Available forms
Tablets: 75 mg, 300 mg

Action
- inhibits platelet aggregation by irreversibly binding to hate adenosine diphosphate (ADP) platelet receptors (P₂Y₁₂)
- prodrug which is metabolised to active metabolite in a two-step process
- platelet aggregation occurs within 2 hours
- half-life 6—8 hours (active metabolite 30 minutes)
- platelet function returns to normal within 7 days of stopping therapy

Use
- prevention of vascular ischaemia associated with atherothrombotic events (e.g. myocardial infarction, stroke)
- treatment of unstable angina or non-ST-elevation myocardial infarction (NSTEMI) (with aspirin) to prevent early and long-term atherothrombotic events
- treatment of ST elevation myocardial infarction (STEMI) (with aspirin) to prevent atherothrombotic events

Dose
- (Unstable angina/NSTEMI) 300 mg orally stat (loading dose), then 75 mg orally once daily (with aspirin 75—325 mg daily) **OR**
- (STEMI) 75 mg orally daily (with or without 300 mg loading dose) with aspirin 75—325 mg daily (with or without fibrinolytic agents) commencing as soon as possible after first symptoms

Adverse effects
- dyspepsia, gastritis, diarrhoea
- rash, pruritus
- bleeding
- (Rare) thrombotic thrombocytopenic purpura (TTP), neutropenia, purpura

Interactions
- caution with aspirin or NSAIDs because of the increased risk of GI bleeding
- may interfere with metabolism of phenytoin, tamoxifen, warfarin, fluvastatin and some NSAIDs at high doses
- caution if given with heparin, NSAIDs, antiplatelet agents, warfarin or fibrinolytic agents because of the increased risk of bleeding
- not recommended with omeprazole, esomeprazole, fluvoxamine, fluoxetine, moclobemide, voriconazole, fluconazole, ciprofloxacin, chloramphenicol, carbamazepine or oxcarbazepine

Nursing considerations/Cautions
- should be stopped 5 days before any elective surgery (including coronary artery bypass surgery) if antiplatelet effect is not wanted
- blood counts should be closely monitored if any signs of bleeding occur
- in those who have undergone percutaneous coronary intervention (PCI) with stenting, clopidogrel and aspirin should be continued according to type and reasons for stent

ANTIPLATELET AGENTS

- caution if used in those at increased risk of bleeding due to trauma, surgery or other conditions (e.g. recent transient ischaemic attack or stroke, or at risk of recurrent ischaemic events), or with kidney or liver impairment
- extra caution if the person is at risk of ophthalmic bleeding due to intraocular lesions
- contraindicated in those with any active gastrointestinal or intracranial bleeding or severe liver impairment

Patient education
- warn the patient that any bleeding may take longer to stop compared with before therapy
- the patient should be advised to tell dentists or doctors of their therapy before any invasive procedures (including routine tooth extraction) are undertaken, as bleeding may be prolonged
- advise the patient not to take over-the-counter NSAIDs, as these increase the risk of bleeding
- instruct the patient to immediately report any:
  - unusual or prolonged bleeding or bruising (including abnormal blood noses)
  - red/purple skin blotches
  - vomiting blood, black or bloody bowel motions
- tablets are not scored; therefore the patient should be advised to use a pill cutter to divide the tablet if needed

Tablet can be crushed and mixed with 10 mL of water or given with spoonful of yoghurt or apple sauce. The 300 mg tablet is very hard to crush.

Clopidogrel and its metabolites cross the placenta, so not recommended during pregnancy.

Contraindicated during breastfeeding.

Reduced hepatic function: contraindicated in severe hepatic impairment.

Available in combination with
- clopidogrel 75 mg + aspirin 100 mg tablet (APX-Clopidogrel/Aspirin 75/100, Clopidogrel Winthrop plus Aspirin, Duocover, DuoPlidogrel, Piax Plus Aspirin)

DIPYRIDAMOLE
Trade name
Persantin Ampoules

Available form
Ampoules: 10 mg/2 mL

Action
- antiplatelet agent with coronary vasodilator activity
- P_2Y_{12} receptor inhibitor
- inhibits adenosine uptake by RBC and platelets, increasing levels of circulating adenosine; inhibits cyclic guanosine monophosphate (cGMP)-phosphodiesterase
- half-life 10—12 hours (oral)

Use
- prevention of ischaemic stroke and transient ischaemic attack (with low-dose aspirin or alone)
- alternative to exercise in cardiac imaging

Dose
- (Cardiac perfusion imaging) 0.56 mg/kg infused over 4 minutes (maximum dose 60 mg) **OR**
- (Stress echo) 0.56 mg/kg infused over 4 minutes, followed by 4 minutes of no dose, then 0.28 mg/kg over 2 minutes (if no changes were observed on echo monitoring in real time) (total cumulative dose 0.84 mg/kg over 10 minutes)

Adverse effects
- chest pain, angina, ECG changes, arrhythmias, tachycardia

- hypertension, severe hypotension, labile blood pressure
- headache, dizziness, fatigue
- paraesthesia
- nausea, vomiting, diarrhoea, abdominal pain, dyspepsia
- myalgia
- oedema
- dyspnoea
- hot flushes
- rash, urticaria
- pain
- (Undiluted IV) vein irritation
- (Rare) seizures, non-fatal myocardial infarction, asystole, transient ischaemic attack, AV block, bronchospasm, pulmonary oedema

Interactions
- vasodilating effects decreased by xanthine derivatives (including tea and coffee)
- may counteract anticholinesterase effect of cholinesterase inhibitors (potentially aggravating myasthenia gravis)
- may increase hypotensive effects of antihypertensive agents
- may increase plasma levels and cardiovascular effects of adenosine
- IV dipyridamole is contraindicated in those taking oral dipyridamole

Nursing considerations/Cautions
- ECG and vital signs should be monitored during and 10–15 minutes after administration
- imaging agents should be given within 5 minutes of IV dipyridamole
- should be diluted to 20–50 mL with glucose 5% or sodium chloride 0.45% before being infused
- administer alone
- slow IV aminophylline (50–100 mg over 30–60 seconds) should be administered if bronchospasm or chest pain occurs. Aminophylline is not recommended if variant angina with ST elevation occurs, as it may be worsened by administration of aminophylline. Glyceryl trinitrate (sublingual or intravenous) may also be given if chest pain continues despite administration of aminophylline
- if severe hypotension occurs, the patient should be placed in a supine position with head tilted down (if needed)
- caution if used in those with myasthenia gravis, as dipyridamole may interact with cholinesterase inhibitors
- caution if used in those with left main coronary stenosis, moderate stenotic valvular disease, electrolyte imbalance, severe arterial hypertension (systolic >200 mmHg and/or diastolic > 110 mmHg), tachyarrhythmias, bradyarrhythmias, AV block or cardiomyopathy
- not recommended in those with asthma, hypotension (less than systolic BP 90 mmHg), unexplained syncope or transient ischaemic attacks
- contraindicated in those with unstable angina, uncontrolled cardiac arrhythmias, uncontrolled symptomatic heart failure, acute pulmonary embolus or pulmonary infarction, acute myocardial infarction, acute myocarditis or pericarditis, acute aortic dissection and severe aortic stenosis

Patient education
- advise the patient that side-effects reduce or disappear altogether with continued therapy
- warn the patient against driving or operating machinery if severe headache or dizziness occurs

Should be used during pregnancy only if benefits outweigh risks.

Excreted in human breastmilk. Caution if used during breastfeeding as it appears in breastmilk.

ANTIPLATELET AGENTS

PRASUGREL
Trade name
Prasugrel Lupin

Available form
Tablets: 5 mg, 10 mg

Action
- irreversible P_2Y_{12} receptor inhibitor
- prodrug with active metabolite
- platelet aggregation returned to normal after 7–9 days (single dose) and 5 days (stopping therapy)
- peak concentration within 30 minutes
- half-life of active metabolite is 2–15 hours; however, irreversible binding results in prolonged activity after therapy is stopped

Use
- prevention of atherothrombotic events in patients with unstable angina or non-ST elevation myocardial infarction (NSTEMI) (with aspirin)
- treatment of ST elevation myocardial infarction (STEMI) who will undergo percutaneous coronary intervention (PCI) (with aspirin) to prevent atherothrombotic events

Dose
- initially 60 mg orally (loading dose), followed by 10 mg orally daily (with aspirin 75–325 mg) **OR**
- (Patient weighing < 60 kg) initially 60 mg orally (loading dose), followed by 5 mg orally daily (with aspirin 75–325 mg)

Adverse effects
- bleeding (minor, major)
- hypertension, hypotension, atrial fibrillation, bradycardia, non-cardiac chest pain
- hypercholesterolaemia, hyperlipidaemia
- headache, back pain, pain in extremities
- dyspnoea, cough
- nausea, diarrhoea
- dizziness, fatigue
- leucopenia
- rash
- fever
- peripheral oedema
- (Rare) thrombotic thrombocytopenic purpura (TTP), hypersensitivity, angioedema

Interactions
- caution if used with heparin, oral anticoagulants, NSAIDs or fibrinolytic agents because of increased risk of bleeding

Nursing considerations/Cautions
- for NSTEMI patients, the loading dose should be given at the time of PCI
- therapy should be discontinued for at least 7 days before elective surgery (if antiplatelet effect is not desired)
- caution in those weighing less than 60 kg or who have had recent surgery or trauma, recent/recurrent gastrointestinal bleeding, active peptic ulcer disease, severe liver or kidney impairment
- contains lactose; therefore not recommended in those with galactose intolerance, Lapp lactase deficiency or glucose–galactose malabsorption
- caution if used in those of Asian origin because of an increased risk of bleeding
- not recommended in those over 75 years
- contraindicated in those with active bleeding, a history of stroke or transient ischaemic attack or severe liver failure

Patient education
- advise the patient not to drive or operate machinery if dizziness or fatigue is a problem
- instruct the patient to take tablets whole and not break in half
- advise the patient to report any of the following symptoms immediately:
  - unusual or prolonged bleeding or bruising
  - nosebleeds
  - blue/purple spots under skin or nails
  - vomiting or coughing up blood or dark/black tarry stools

Tablet can be crushed and mixed with water or a spoonful of yoghurt or apple puree.

Should be used during pregnancy only if benefits outweigh risks.

Avoid use, as human data are lacking. Animal studies show that prasugrel metabolites are excreted in rat milk.

Not recommended for patients aged ≥ 75 years because of the increased risk of major bleeding, including life-threatening and fatal bleeding. If the benefits outweigh the risks, a 5 mg maintenance dose may be considered instead of the standard 10 mg dose.

TICAGRELOR

Trade names
ARX-Ticagrelor, Bricalor, Brilinta, Ticalor

Available forms
Tablets: 90 mg;
Orodispersible tablets: 90 mg

Action
- selective and reversible P_2Y_{12} receptor inhibitor
- active metabolite (half-life 6.5—12.8 hours)
- half-life 4.5—12.8 hours

Use
- prevention of atherothrombotic events in those with unstable angina, non-ST elevation myocardial infarction (NSTEMI) or ST elevation myocardial infarction (STEMI) (with aspirin)

Dose
- initially 180 mg orally (loading dose), followed by 90 mg orally twice daily (with aspirin 75—150 mg)

Adverse effects
- epistaxis, bleeding (major, minor)
- dyspnoea, cough
- cardiac failure, atrial fibrillation, bradycardia, chest pain
- hypertension, hypotension
- non-cardiac chest pain, back pain
- increased uric acid, gout, increased creatinine levels
- nausea, vomiting, diarrhoea, constipation, abdominal pain, dyspepsia, gastrointestinal bleeding
- headache, fatigue, dizziness, syncope, vertigo
- fever
- rash
- peripheral oedema
- (Rare) hypersensitivity, angioedema

Interactions
- contraindicated with clarithromycin, ritonavir or atazanavir
- not recommended with clopidogrel or prasugrel
- increased dyspnoea (transient) may occur if given with adenosine
- increased risk of bleeding if given with selective serotonin reuptake inhibitors (SSRIs)
- caution if used with NSAIDs, oral anticoagulants or fibrinolytic agents because of the increased risk of bleeding
- caution if used with agents known to induce bradycardia (e.g. digoxin, beta adrenoceptor blocking agents, verapamil, diltiazem)
- may increase serum levels of ciclosporin and digoxin, increasing the risk of toxicity. Serum levels should be closely monitored if given together
- increased serum levels may occur if given with ciclosporin or digoxin
- decreased serum levels may occur if given with rifampicin, dexamethasone, phenytoin, carbamazepine or phenobarbital (phenobarbitone)
- caution if given with simvastatin (doses > 40 mg daily) because of the increased risk of myopathy and rhabdomyolysis
- caution if used with angiotensin II receptor blocking agents because of the risk of kidney impairment

ANTIPLATELET AGENTS

Nursing considerations/Cautions

- should be discontinued for 5 days before elective surgery
- renal function should be monitored monthly during therapy; uric acid levels should also be monitored regularly
- if switching from clopidogrel, ticagrelor 90 mg should be given 24 hours after the last dose of clopidogrel
- therapy should be continued for at least 12 months
- caution in those with asthma or chronic obstructive pulmonary disorder because of an increased risk of dyspnoea
- caution if used in those without a pacemaker and with sick sinus syndrome, second or third degree A-V block or bradycardia-related syncope because of an increased risk of bradycardia; also use with caution in those with hyperuricaemia or gout, and in those who have coagulation disorders, a history of or recent/active bleeding, recent trauma or surgery, ischaemic stroke, or if the patient weighs less than 60 kg or is aged 75 years or more
- contraindicated in those with active bleeding, a history of intracranial haemorrhage, or moderate-to-severe liver impairment

Patient education

- warn the patient against driving or operating machinery if dizziness or confusion occurs
- the patient should be advised that shortness of breath is a common side-effect of this medication. However, it is still important to seek medical advice if it occurs or worsens
- if unable to swallow tablets, advise the patient to crush the tablet to a fine powder using a mortar and pestle/crushing device and add 100 mL, stir well and pour into a glass. Another 100 mL of water should be added to the mortar and pestle/crushing device, stirred to ensure all fine powder is removed and transferred to a glass and drink 200 mL immediately
- advise the patient to place a dispersible tablet on the tongue, allow to dissolve and swallow with or without water

Available as an orally dispersible tablet (dissolve on the tongue), or the tablet can be crushed and mixed with water.

Not recommended, as limited human data.

Not recommended, as limited human data.

Hepatic impairment: contraindicated in moderate-to-severe hepatic impairment.

GLYCOPROTEIN IIb/IIIa INHIBITORS

TIROFIBAN
Trade names
Aggrastat, Tirofiban Juno Concentrate

Available form
Vial: 12.5 mg/50 mL

Action
- glycoprotein IIb/IIIa receptor inhibitor
- half-life 1.4—1.8 hours, prolonged to 1.9—2.2 hours in those with coronary artery disease

Use
- unstable angina or non-Q wave myocardial infarction in the prevention of cardiac ischaemia (with heparin)

Dose
- 0.4 microgram/kg/min for 30 minutes (with IV bolus of heparin 5000 U), then 0.1 microgram/kg/min (with heparin infusion 1000 U/hour, titrated to aPTT)

Adverse effects
- bleeding (major, minor), thrombocytopenia
- headache
- fever
- nausea
- rash, urticaria

Interactions
- contraindicated with other glycoprotein IIb/IIIa receptor inhibitors
- caution if given with drugs that affect haemostasis such as fibrinolytic agents

Nursing considerations/Cautions
- take the patient history before the procedure to exclude, within the past month, any major surgical procedures or trauma, spinal or epidural anaesthetic, intracranial bleeding, neoplasm or aneurysm, stroke, active internal bleeding, severe uncontrolled hypertension, history or symptoms of aortic dissection or active pericarditis, because these are all contraindications to therapy
- great caution should be taken in patients who have a history of bleeding within the past year
- monitor haemoglobin, haematocrit and platelet count before starting therapy, within 6 hours of loading dose and then daily during therapy
- therapy should be withdrawn if platelet count confirms thrombocytopenia
- activated partial thromboplastin time (aPTT) should be measured before starting and regularly throughout therapy (it should be twice the normal value) and dose adjusted if needed
- patient should be closely monitored after removal of sheath for any signs of bleeding or haematoma formation. Arterial sheath should be removed only when aPTT < 180 seconds or 2–6 hours after stopping heparin therapy
- combination therapy with heparin should be continued for a minimum of 48 hours and may be continued through angiography and for 12–24 hours after if necessary
- monitor urine and faeces for occult blood
- incompatible with IV diazepam
- to dilute, remove 50 mL from 250 mL bag or normal saline 0.9% or glucose 5% and replace with 50 mL of tirofiban to achieve a final concentration of 0.05 mg/mL and administer via infusion pump
- caution if used in those who have had a clinically significant bleed or stroke in the last year, recent epidural procedure, known coagulopathy, platelet disorder or thrombocytopenia, haemorrhagic retinopathy, impaired kidney function (creatinine clearance < 30 mL/min), chronic haemodialysis or platelet count below 150,000 cells/mm^3
- contraindicated in those with or within 30 days of active internal bleeding, within 30 days of severe trauma, major surgery (including epidural or spinal anaesthesia) or haemorrhagic stroke, with thrombocytopenia following previous exposure to tirofiban, bleeding disorders, severe uncontrolled hypertension, a history/symptoms of aortic dissection, acute pericarditis or intracranial haemorrhage, aneurysm, AV malformation or intracranial neoplasm

 Should be used during pregnancy only if benefits outweigh potential risks.

 Avoid use. Excreted in human breastmilk.

 Renal impairment: dose reduction needed in patients with severe renal insufficiency (CrCl < 30 mL/min).

ANTIPROTOZOAL AGENTS

Protozoa are single-celled eukaryotic organisms, some of which are parasitic pathogens that divide within the host, causing various diseases.

Protozoa are generally classified according to their mode of 'locomotion' and include:

- amoebae, which move using pseudopodia (or false feet), and cause, for example, amoebic dysentery
- flagellates, which move by beating their flagellum (whip) in a whip-like movement, and are responsible for giardiasis, trichomonal vaginitis, leishmaniasis and trypanosomiasis
- ciliates, which move by beating cilia (hair-like appendages)
- sporozoans, the adult forms of which do not appear to have any means of movement (e.g. *Plasmodium* spp., see Antimalarial agents, p. 555 (CDC 2016)).

Some human protozoan infections include amoebiasis (second leading cause of death due to parasitic disease), giardiasis, trichomoniasis, toxoplasmosis, leishmaniasis (700,000–1 million new cases and 26,000–65,000 deaths annually), cryptosporidiosis and trypanosomiasis (WHO 2019a).

ATOVAQUONE
Trade names
Atovacue, Wellvone Suspension

Available form
Suspension: 750 mg/5 mL

Action
- selective and potent inhibitor of nucleic acid and ATP synthesis in some parasitic protozoa, particularly *Pneumocystis jirovecii*, *Toxoplasma gondii* and *Plasmodium* spp.
- half-life 2–3 days

Use
- acute treatment of mild-to-moderate *P. jirovecii* pneumonia (PJP) in adults with AIDS who are intolerant of trimethoprim–sulfamethoxazole (co-trimoxazole) therapy

Dose
- 750 mg orally twice daily with food for 21 days **OR**
- 1500 mg orally once daily with food for 21 days (patients with swallowing difficulties or unable to eat 2 meals per day)

Adverse effects
- nausea, vomiting, diarrhoea, abdominal pain, constipation, dyspepsia, oral monilia (thrush)
- rash, pruritus, sweating

- sinusitis
- headache, fever, insomnia, dizziness, asthenia
- anaemia, neutropenia
- increased liver enzymes
- hyponatraemia, hyperglycaemia
- hypersensitivity

Interactions
- plasma levels decreased when given with rifampicin or metoclopramide
- if given with rifabutin, may decrease plasma levels of both drugs
- may decrease metabolism of zidovudine; therefore use with caution
- caution should be used when given with warfarin

Nursing considerations/Cautions
- any patient with lung disease should be carefully evaluated before starting therapy for causes of infection and any other therapies (e.g. antiviral, antibacterial, antifungal, antimycotic) which may have been used in the management of the disease
- not recommended prophylactically, in acute cases of PCP or in those who have failed other treatments for PCP

Patient education
- advise the patient to shake suspension well before use and not to dilute it with any other fluids
- advise the patient to take suspension with food, particularly high-fat meals, because this significantly increases the availability
- warn patient to avoid driving or operating machinery if dizziness occurs
- any diarrhoea should be reported immediately (because this correlates with therapy failure)
- the patient should be advised to report any sore white mouth or tongue (as this may be due to yeast overgrowth and require treatment)

No information on effects of atovaquone administration during human pregnancy. Should not be used during pregnancy unless benefits outweigh potential risks.

Not recommended during breastfeeding.

Available in combination with:
- atovaquone 250 mg + proguanil hydrochloride 100 mg tablet (AtovaquoPro Lupin 250/100, Malarone)
- atovaquone 62.5 mg + proguanil hydrochloride 25 mg tablet (Malarone Junior)

METRONIDAZOLE
Trade names
Baxter Metronidazole Infusion, Flagyl, Flagyl S Suspension, Metrogyl, Metronidazole Intravenous Infusion, Metronidazole Oral Suspension (Reach), Metronide, Rozex Cream and Gel, Zidoval Vaginal Gel

Available forms
IV solution: 500 mg/100 mL;
Tablets: 200 mg, 400 mg;
Suppositories: 500 mg;
Suspension 200 mg/5 mL: ;
Gel: 5 mg/g, 7.5 mg/g;
Cream: 7.5 mg/g;
Vaginal gel: 0.75%

Action
- effective against a wide range of anaerobic organisms (bactericidal, amoebicidal, trichomonacidal) and protozoa
- disrupts DNA and inhibits synthesis of nucleic acids
- metabolite has some antiprotozoal activity
- widely distributed throughout body tissues and reaches therapeutic levels in abscesses, bile, CSF, and synovial and seminal fluid

ANTIPROTOZOAL AGENTS

- inactive against aerobic and facultative anaerobic bacteria
- (IV) half-life 6.3—8.3 hours

Use
- (IV) treatment of severe anaerobic organisms (where oral medication is contraindicated or not possible)
- surgical site prophylaxis where there is potential contamination with anaerobic organisms
- bacterial vaginosis, urogenital trichomoniasis, pelvic abscess/cellulitis, post-delivery sepsis
- amoebiasis (intestinal, extraintestinal)
- anaerobic infections (e.g. septicaemia, osteomyelitis, brain abscess, necrotising pneumonia, giardiasis, acute ulcerative gingivitis, bacteraemia)
- (Topical) rosacea (with associated erythema, papules and pustules)
- postoperative wound infection

Dose
- (Urogenital trichomoniasis, bacterial vaginosis) 2 g as single oral dose **OR**
- (Urogenital trichomoniasis) 200 mg orally 3 times daily for 7 days **OR**
- (Bacterial vaginosis) 400 mg orally 3 times daily for 7 days **OR**
- (Bacterial vaginosis) 2 g orally daily for 3 days **OR**
- (Amoebiasis) 400—800 mg orally 3 times daily for 5—10 days **OR**
- (Giardiasis) 2 g orally daily for 3 days **OR**
- (acute ulcerative gingivitis) 200 mg orally 3 times daily for 3 days **OR**
- (Anaerobic infection) 400 mg orally 3 times daily for 7 days **OR**
- (Surgical prophylaxis) 400 mg orally 1—2 hours before surgery and repeated 8-hourly for 24 hours **OR**
- (Surgical prophylaxis) 500 mg IV just prior to surgery and repeated 8-hourly for 24 hours **OR**
- (Elective colonic surgery) 2 rectal suppositories (1 g) every 8 hours for 48 hours before and after surgery (with bowel preparation) **OR**
- (Anaerobic infection) 2 rectal suppositories (1 g) every 8 hours for 3 days, then 12-hourly if needed **OR**
- (Surgical prophylaxis — appendectomy) 2 rectal suppositories (1 g) at diagnosis, then repeated 8-hourly for 48 hours after surgery **OR**
- 500 mg IV every 8 hours, infused over 30 minutes **OR**
- (Symptomatic bacterial vaginosis) one applicator full (5 g) intravaginally nightly at bedtime for 5 days **OR**
- (Rosacea) apply a thin film of cream or gel to affected area and rub in until absorbed twice daily for 3—9 weeks (gel) or 12—16 weeks (cream)

Adverse effects
- metallic taste, anorexia, nausea, vomiting, dyspepsia, dry mouth, abdominal discomfort/cramping, diarrhoea, constipation, oral mucositis
- rash, pruritus
- hypersensitivity (rash, urticaria, nasal congestion, fever, flushing, dry mouth, angioedema)
- superinfection (including glossitis, stomatitis, furry tongue, vaginitis (*Candida* spp.))
- dysuria, cystitis, pruritus of genital area, pelvic pressure, darkening of urine, dryness of vagina or vulva
- headache, dizziness, insomnia
- vertigo, tinnitus, impaired hearing
- syncope
- seizures, confusion, ataxia, lack of coordination, hallucinations, depression, disorientation, dysarthria
- transient joint pain, weakness
- transient leucopenia
- transient blurry or double vision, changes in vision or acuity or colour vision, optic neuritis
- nasal congestion
- flattened T wave, prolonged QT interval
- (Prolonged administration) peripheral neuropathy, seizures
- (Rare) pancreatitis, abnormal liver function tests, hepatitis, anaphylaxis, aseptic

meningitis, encephalopathy with cerebellar toxicity, pseudomembranous colitis, reversible thrombocytopenia, severe skin reactions
- (IV) thrombophlebitis
- (Vaginal cream) pelvic discomfort
- (Topical) skin irritation, redness, itching, burning, stinging, dryness, aggravated acne/rosacea (transient) eye irritation (if applied too close to eyes)

Interactions
- may result in lithium toxicity in patients on a high dose of lithium
- increased risk of toxicity if used with carmustine or cyclophosphamide
- if taken in combination with alcohol, may produce disulfiram—alcohol reaction (see Glossary)
- may enhance activity of warfarin; therefore prothrombin time should be closely monitored throughout therapy
- may increase serum ciclosporin, busulfan and fluorouracil, increasing risk of toxicity
- plasma levels may be reduced by phenobarbital (phenobarbitone) and phenytoin
- may decrease clearance of phenytoin
- increased risk of psychotic reaction (e.g. acute psychoses, confusion) if given with or within 2 weeks of disulfiram
- transient neutropenia may occur if given with fluorouracil or azathioprine
- increased risk of sodium retention and oedema if given with corticosteroids
- may interfere with laboratory tests (AST, ALT, LDH), triglycerides or glucose determination

Nursing considerations/Cautions
- neurological function (e.g. gait, seizure activity, paraesthesia) and blood counts (e.g. differential leucocyte counts) should be monitored regularly throughout any prolonged therapy (> 10 days) and drug discontinued if leucopenia or neurological symptoms occur
- to reduce the incidence of reinfection, treatment for urogenital trichomoniasis should include sexual partner
- transfer from IV to oral therapy as soon as possible
- oral suspension should not be used to manage acute situations
- suppositories are recommended where oral therapy is contraindicated or not possible
- if retreatment for urogenital trichomoniasis is required, an interval of 4–6 weeks should be allowed and leucocyte count monitored before starting and during therapy
- (Urogenital trichomoniasis) if patient is pregnant and in second or third trimester, 1-day course should not be administered owing to increased risk to fetus
- (Bacterial vaginosis) gonorrohea should be excluded
- IV daily maximum 4 g
- should be administered IV at a rate of 25 mg/min
- administer alone
- incompatible with aluminium
- IV solution contains sodium (310 mg/100 mL) and may result in sodium retention in those predisposed to oedema or taking corticosteroids
- caution if used in those with acute or chronic severe peripheral CNS disease or with impaired liver function
- caution if used in those with Cockayne syndrome because of increased risk of hepatotoxicity. If used, liver function should be assessed before starting, during and after completion of therapy and patient alerted to signs of liver impairment
- contraindicated in those with blood dyscrasias, active organic brain disease or hypersensitivity to imidazoles
- (Topical, vaginal) contraindicated in those with hypersensitivity to hydroxybenzoates

ANTIPROTOZOAL AGENTS

Patient education

- for tablets: instruct patients to take metronidazole with food to reduce stomach upset
- for suspension: metronidazole is best absorbed if taken 1 hour before a meal
- may impair or alter sense of taste
- avoid alcohol during treatment and for at least 24 hours after to prevent a disulfiram-like reaction causing nausea, vomiting, flushing, headaches and palpitations
- warn the patient that the urine may become a harmless dark colour during treatment
- if experiencing dizziness, vertigo, or confusion, avoid driving or operating machinery
- seek immediate medical advice for:
  - weakness in hands/feet, dizziness, numbness, or seizures
  - visual disturbances
  - uncoordinated movements, difficulty speaking, confusion, hallucinations or depression
  - unusual bleeding or bruising
  - frequent infections, fever, chills, sore throat, mouth ulcers or flu-like symptoms
  - sore, white patches in the mouth/tongue (sign of yeast overgrowth)
  - vaginal itching, burning, or white discharge (yeast overgrowth in females)
- (Vaginal cream): ensure the correct insertion technique is understood.
- (Suppository) empty bowel before use and understand the correct insertion technique.
- (Topical) instruct patients in the following:
  - wash hands after application
  - apply cream/gel 20 minutes after cleaning the affected area
  - avoid eye contact
  - do not use drying cosmetics or medicated soaps
  - avoid sunlight or UV radiation; use SPF 30+ and protective clothing
  - moisturiser or cosmetics can be applied after the gel has dried

 Oral suspension is available. Tablets can be dispersed in water or crushed and mixed with spoonful of yoghurt or apple puree.

 Not recommended during first trimester of pregnancy as it enters fetal circulation. If required for trichomoniasis during second or third trimester, therapy should be restricted to those in whom local palliative treatment is ineffective.

 Not recommended during breastfeeding.

 Caution if used in those with liver impairment. If used in patient undergoing dialysis, a further dose is required after completion to maintain therapeutic levels.

PENTAMIDINE

Trade names
DBL Pentamidine Isethionate, Pentamidine-EMC

Available form
Vial: 300 mg

Action
- the exact mechanism of action is unknown although it is thought to interfere with nuclear metabolism
- very low penetration of CNS

Use
- *P. jirovecii* pneumonia (PJP) (first-line treatment in patients with AIDS, second-line treatment in non-AIDS patients)
- most types of trypanosomiasis (second-line treatment)
- visceral and cutaneous forms of leishmaniasis (second-line treatment)
- *Leishmania aethiopica* (first-line treatment)

Dose
- (PCP) 4 mg/kg daily by IV infusion over 60 minutes for 14 days **OR**

- (Visceral leishmaniasis) 3—4 mg/kg by IV infusion over 60 minutes 3 times weekly (alternate days) to a maximum of 10 doses **OR**
- (Cutaneous leishmaniasis) 3—4 mg/kg by IV infusion over 60 minutes 1—2 times weekly until condition resolves **OR**
- (Trypanosomiasis during haemolymphatic stage) 4 mg/kg daily by IV infusion over 60 minutes or on alternate days to a maximum of 7—10 doses

Adverse effects

- severe hypotension, syncope
- cardiac arrhythmias, cardiac arrest, ventricular tachycardia, tachycardia, bradycardia
- dizziness
- nausea, vomiting, taste disturbance
- acute renal failure
- acute pancreatitis, abnormal liver function
- leucopenia, thrombocytopenia, anaemia
- severe hypoglycaemia, sometimes followed by hyperglycaemia, diabetes mellitus
- fever, rash, flushing
- hypocalcaemia, hyperkalaemia, hyponatraemia
- delirium, Jarisch—Herxheimer reaction (malaise, fever, chills, sore throat, myalgia, headache, tachycardia)
- (Local) thrombophlebitis
- (Rare) Stevens—Johnson syndrome (see Glossary)

Interactions

- increased risk of nephrotoxicity if given with other nephrotoxic drugs
- caution if given with hepatotoxic agents

Nursing considerations/Cautions

- the following observations are recommended during therapy:
  - daily serum electrolytes, full blood count (including platelet), serum creatinine and blood urea nitrogen (BUN)
  - fasting blood glucose levels before starting, daily during and at regular intervals after completion of therapy
  - daily urinalysis
  - liver function tests before starting, then weekly (if normal) or every 3—5 days if baseline is elevated or if given with hepatotoxic agents
  - weekly serum calcium levels
  - regular ECG
- the patient should lie down while receiving pentamidine because of hypotensive risk
- monitor BP before and regularly during IV infusion and hourly after completion of infusion until BP is stable
- not recommended by IV push or bolus
- reconstitute with 3—5 mL of water for injections, then dilute further with 50—250 mL of glucose 5% or sodium chloride 0.9%
- administer infusion over at least 60 minutes
- caution if used in those with malnutrition, hyperglycaemia, hypoglycaemia, liver or kidney dysfunction, hypertension, hypotension or blood disorders

Patient education

- warn the patient against driving or operating machinery if dizziness or lightheadedness occurs
- the patient should be advised to avoid alcohol (or reduce consumption) as it will exacerbate dizziness and lightheadedness
- instruct the patient to seek medical advice immediately if any of the following occur:
  - unusual bleeding or bruising
  - flu-like illness, sore throat, fever, chills, mouth ulcers
  - signs of high blood glucose (hyperglycaemia), including increased thirst and urination, tiredness
  - signs of low blood glucose (hypoglycaemia), including trembling/shaking, irritability, lightheadedness
  - peeling of skin
  - dizziness or fainting, slow/fast or irregular heart rate

ANTIPROTOZOAL AGENTS

- fever, chills, headache and muscle pain
- upper abdominal pain
- breathlessness or difficulty breathing
- female patients of childbearing potential should be counselled to use adequate contraception to avoid pregnancy occurring during therapy

Not recommended during pregnancy unless benefits to mother outweigh risks to fetus. Animal studies suggest fetal harm.

Contraindicated during breastfeeding.

Renal impairment: avoid use in patients with severely reduced renal function. If administration is necessary, consider increasing the dosing interval when CrCl is < 10 mL/min to reduce the risk of drug accumulation and toxicity.

PYRIMETHAMINE
Trade name
Daraprim

Available form
Tablets: 25 mg

Action
- antifolate that blocks synthesis of plasmodial nucleic acids by inhibiting dihydrofolate reductase, thereby disrupting protein synthesis and nuclear division
- half-life 90 hours

Use
- toxoplasmosis (usually given with a sulfonamide)

Dose
- adults > 60 kg: 200 mg orally on day 1, then 75 mg once daily
- adults < 60 kg: 200 mg orally on day 1, then 50 mg once daily
- children: 2 mg/kg (max 50 mg) once daily for 3 days, then 1 mg/kg (max 25 mg) once daily
- neonate: 2 mg/kg orally once daily for 2 days, then 1 mg/kg once daily for 2–6 months, followed by 1 mg/kg 3 times a week to complete a 12-month treatment course
- adult: 50 mg orally once a week
- child: 1 mg/kg (max 25 mg) orally once daily
- adult: 25–50 mg orally once daily
- child: 1 mg/kg (max 25 mg) orally once daily

Adverse effects
- nausea, vomiting, diarrhoea, colic
- rash
- headache, dizziness
- anaemia, thrombocytopenia, leucopenia (early in treatment)
- (Less common) dry mouth and/or throat, dermatitis, depression, abnormal skin pigmentation, fever, malaise
- (Rare) convulsions (prolonged therapy or high doses for toxoplasmosis)

Interactions
- increased risk of seizures if given with methotrexate (in children with CNS leukaemia)
- increased risk of bone marrow depression if given with cytostatic agents such as methotrexate, daunorubicin or cytarabine
- may induce hepatotoxicity when given with lorazepam
- may further decrease folate metabolism in those taking folate inhibitors or myelosuppressive agents such as methotrexate, zidovudine, proguanil, trimethoprim or co-trimoxazole
- absorption may be decreased if given with antacids or kaolin
- increased risk of seizures if given with antimalarial agents or methotrexate
- increased risk of megaloblastic anaemia if given in doses > 25 mg/week with trimethoprim/sulfonamide combination

HAVARD'S NURSING GUIDE TO DRUGS

- may increase serum levels if given with agents with low therapeutic index and highly protein bound (e.g. warfarin)

Nursing considerations/Cautions

- folate supplement (folic acid 5 mg or calcium folinate 6 mg daily) is recommended to decrease the risk of bone marrow depression
- monitor blood cell counts weekly during and for 2 weeks after stopping treatment to detect folate deficiency and treat with high-dose calcium folinate if folate deficiency occurs
- treatment for toxoplasmosis should continue for 3–6 weeks. If further treatment is required, a 2-week rest period is required between treatments
- if given with a sulfonamide, the patient should be well hydrated to prevent crystalluria
- tablets contain lactose and are therefore not recommended in those with galactose intolerance, Lapp lactase deficiency or glucose–galactose malabsorption
- caution if used in those with folate deficiency (including megaloblastic anaemia or due to malnutrition) or a history of seizures (loading dose should not be given)

Patient education

- advise the patient to taking antacids within 2 hours of tablets

Tablets can be crushed and mixed with water, yoghurt or apple puree.

Contraindicated during the first trimester of pregnancy. Folate supplementation is recommended if used in the second or third trimester due to vision-threatening eye lesions or rising antibody titres. Toxoplasmosis poses a high risk to the fetus, including malformation and abortion.

Secreted in breastmilk, therefore not recommended during breastfeeding.

Reduced hepatic function: use with caution; increased risk of toxicity. Adjust dose as needed in moderate-to-severe impairment.

Monitor for signs of bone marrow suppression, which may occur more frequently in elderly patients. Hydration is important to prevent crystalluria.

Note

This drug is not marketed in Australia but may be available through the Special Access Scheme.

ANTIPSYCHOTIC AND MOOD-STABILISING AGENTS

Antipsychotic (or neuroleptic) agents are used in the management of schizophrenia, schizoaffective disorders, some forms of bipolar disorder, severe depression and psychotic symptoms of a personality disorder. They do not cure the conditions but can assist in reducing and controlling the psychiatric symptoms such as delusions and hallucinations, as well as disordered thinking, anxiety, confusion, mania and violent or disruptive behaviours.

The antipsychotics are generally classified as typical (first generation) (phenothiazines, butyrophenones and thioxanthenes) or atypical (second generation), which include some of the more recently developed agents, such as clozapine and risperidone. Agents within these groups are not homogeneous and the terminology (first or second generation) tends to be associated with the length of time the agents have been available (e.g. first generation were developed in the 1950s); however, the difference relates to the receptors where they have their main effects. Typical antipsychotic agents inhibit dopamine (D_2) receptors, whereas the atypical antipsychotics also act on serotonin (5-hydroxytryptamine), glutamate, noradrenaline (norepinephrine), histamine and acetylcholine receptors, resulting in not only therapeutic effects but also adverse effects (Radhakrishnan et al 2024).

In general, antipsychotic agents decrease the positive symptoms (e.g. hallucinations, delusions, disorganised speech and behaviour, agitation) of schizophrenia, along with some decrease in hostility and excitement, but have limited impact on negative symptoms (e.g. lack of motivation, self-care, blunted affect, reduced speed output and social withdrawal), cognitive impairment (e.g. impaired memory, planning and social cognition) and mood disturbance (including depression and anxiety), so these aspects require additional management such as support groups, case management, and family support and counselling (Radhakrishnan et al 2024).

Before starting any therapy, a thorough assessment is necessary and medications used only if necessary and then tailored to the patient, starting with the lowest dose and simplest regimen, in combination with non-pharmacological therapies. It is important that the patient understands and agrees to participate in treatment; however, assistance may be required, depending on the level of mental illness experienced by the person.

Antipsychotics generally need to be taken for at least 6 weeks before any clinical improvement is seen; however the full benefit may not become apparent for months. Treatment is often ongoing for many years, and relapses are common when therapy is stopped. Concordance with some of the older antipsychotic agents was poor because of the pronounced side-effects, but this has improved with some of the newer, atypical antipsychotic agents because they have fewer adverse effects. Concordance is complex and can be improved by agreement between patient and doctor on the treatment plan (including discussion of the goals of treatment, advantages and disadvantages of treatment), simplifying the treatment regimen (e.g. once-daily compared with more frequent administration), case management and regular contact with health care professions (such as community mental health nurses), family/friends/significant others involved in therapy (if the patient agrees), provision of clear, written information (and instructions if appropriate), use of reminders (e.g. for appointments, taking medications), monitoring of concordance (e.g. plasma drug levels, counting tablets) or use of long-acting depot preparations which can be administered 2—4-weekly (Radhakrishnan et al 2024).

Recent Royal Commissions in Australia (Aged Care and Disability) have identified the inappropriate use of psychotropic medication to control behaviours of concern, especially in people with cognitive disability or impairment. Standards (such as the Psychotropic Medicines in Cognitive Disability or Impairment Clinical Care Standard) have been been developed to address these issues. For example, management of delirium should be using non-drug methods, unless used short term, and unless there is imminent risk of patient harm to self or others. Furthermore, if possible, informed consent should be sought from the patient and family (Australian Commission on Safety and Quality in Health Care (ACSQHC) 2024; Delirium Clinical Standard 2021).

General Adverse effects of antipsychotics

- neuroleptic malignant syndrome (a rare but potentially fatal reaction to antipsychotic drugs). Symptoms include hyperthermia, muscle rigidity, altered consciousness, tachycardia, labile BP, profuse sweating and arrhythmias. May also include raised creatine phosphokinase, rhabdomyolysis and acute renal failure. Predisposing factors include dehydration, pre-existing organic brain disease and AIDS. Infants and the elderly are particularly susceptible. It is usually managed by discontinuing the antipsychotic drugs and monitoring and treating symptoms
- extrapyramidal reactions or syndrome (may include all or some of the following symptoms and may occur after a single dose, especially in children and young adults):
  - Parkinsonian symptoms: difficulty speaking or swallowing, loss of balance, shuffling gait, rigidity, tremor at rest, mask-like face (occurs commonly in the elderly; usually occurs within 5—30 days of starting therapy; managed with anti-Parkinson's agents, such as benztropine or diphenhydramine)
  - akathisia: motor and mental restlessness (usually occurs within 5—60 days of starting therapy; managed by reducing

ANTIPSYCHOTIC AND MOOD-STABILISING AGENTS

dose, changing drug, or using clonazepam or propranolol)
- acute dystonia: spasm of muscles (tongue, face, neck and back) resulting in facial grimacing, torticollis, oculogyric crisis (commonly occurs in young or patients not previously treated with antipsychotics; usually occurs within 1—5 days of starting medication; usually managed with anti-Parkinson's agents)
- tardive dyskinesia: exaggerated and persistent chewing movements, tongue protrusion, lip smacking, uncontrolled movement of legs/arms (elderly patients are at increased risk; occurs months or years into treatment; may be reversible if recognised early and the drug is stopped)
- anticholinergic effects (may include any of the following: dry mouth, thirst, blurred vision, difficulty with accommodation, urinary retention or urgency retention, constipation, flushing and dryness of skin, decreased sweating, tachycardia, palpitations, arrhythmias, mydriasis, photophobia, cycloplegia and (less commonly) raised intraocular pressure)
- disrupted ability to maintain core temperature, increased sweating
- QT interval prolongation and arrhythmias (the risk is increased in those with bradycardia, hypokalaemia, hypomagnesaemia or a family history of long QT syndrome)
- postural (also referred to as orthostatic) hypotension; may be associated with dizziness, tachycardia and syncope; hypertension sometimes occurs
- raised prolactin levels (and associated symptoms, including galactorrhoea, gynaecomastia, amenorrhoea, menstrual disorders, erectile dysfunction, breast pain, impotence)
- dry mouth, nausea, vomiting, constipation, diarrhoea, dyspepsia, hypersalivation, abdominal pain
- changes in body weight (commonly increased but sometimes decreased)
- headache, dizziness, sedation, drowsiness, somnolence, insomnia, tremor
- restlessness, nervousness, anxiety, fatigue, lethargy, agitation, impaired judgement, thinking and motor skills
- depression, suicide ideation
- decreased seizure control
- hyperglycaemia and, rarely, ketoacidosis or hyperosmolar coma
- altered liver function, increased serum cholesterol and triglycerides
- sleep apnoea
- dysphagia (decreased motility of oesophagus, increasing risk of aspiration), bronchopneumonia
- leucopenia/neutropenia, agranulocytosis
- (Sudden withdrawal effects) vertigo, tachycardia, headache, nausea, vomiting
- (Rare) venous thromboembolism, priapism, intraoperative floppy iris syndrome
- (Very rare) sudden death

General Interactions of antipsychotics

- contraindicated with agents known to prolong the QT interval (such as amiodarone, arsenic trioxide, chlorpromazine, clarithromycin, disopyramide, droperidol, erythromycin, haloperidol, lithium, methadone, pentamidine, sotalol, ziprasidone), those agents which could cause hypokalaemia (e.g. amphotericin B (amphotericin), diuretics, glucocorticoids, stimulant laxatives, tetracosactides) or induce bradycardia (e.g. beta adrenergic blocking agents, calcium-channel blockers, clonidine, digoxin)
- may enhance CNS effects of alcohol, anaesthetics, antidepressants,

antihistamines, barbiturates, benzodiazepines, hypnotics, monoamine oxidase inhibitors (MAOIs), opioid analgesics, sedatives and other CNS active agents
- hypotensive effects of antihypertensive agents (especially those with alpha adrenoceptor blocking properties) may be enhanced if given with antipsychotics
- increased risk of neuroleptic malignant syndrome if antipsychotic agents are given together
- antipsychotic agents are generally not recommended together
- anticholinergic effects of antipsychotics may be enhanced if given with anticholinergic agents
- anticholinergic agents may reduce the effects of antipsychotic agents
- dopamine antagonism reduces effects of cabergoline, bromocriptine and levodopa, and are therefore contraindicated/not recommended together
- caution if given with other agents that lower seizure threshold, as this may increase the risk of seizure activity
- increased risk of sleep apnoea if given with sedatives

General Nursing considerations/ Cautions for antipsychotics

- initial stabilisation should be done under medical supervision, as adverse effects can be unpredictable. Improvement may take days to weeks to achieve and the patient should be closely monitored during this time
- before starting therapy, the patient should be thoroughly medically assessed (including HR, BP, full blood count, electrolyte levels, fasting glucose levels, liver function, full lipid profile, a family history of QT prolongation) to establish any factors which may increase risk of arrhythmias, QT interval prolongation and other adverse effects such as blood dyscrasias
- any hypokalaemia or hypomagnesaemia should be corrected before starting therapy
- liver function, blood counts and serum cholesterol and triglycerides should be monitored regularly throughout therapy
- many antipsychotic agents also have an antiemetic effect; therefore care should be taken, as this may mask symptoms of overdose or obscure diagnosis of other conditions, such as intestinal obstruction or brain tumour
- the patient may experience an increase in temperature during the first 4 weeks of therapy and this must be carefully evaluated and distinguished from neuroleptic malignant syndrome, infection or agranulocytosis
- all psychotic illnesses carry an inherent risk of suicide; therefore patients should be closely observed, especially at the start of therapy. Patients should also have only a small supply of antipsychotic agents to lessen the risk of accidental/ intentional overdose
- the patient should be observed carefully so that a distinction may be made between a return of psychotic behaviour and the onset of extrapyramidal reactions. Rapid mood swings may occur when antipsychotics are used to treat the mania phase of bipolar disorders and should not be used if depression is the major symptom
- therapy should be slowly discontinued over 1–2 weeks before stopping
- caution if used in those with liver impairment, as most antipsychotics are metabolised in the liver, and impairment would lead to increased

- serum levels and therefore increased risk of adverse effects
- caution if used in those with kidney impairment; dose reduction is generally recommended
- caution if used in those with a history of seizures or epilepsy, as seizure threshold may be lowered
- caution if used in those with a risk of aspiration pneumonia or chronic respiratory disorders
- caution if used in those with cardiovascular disease (such as myocardial infarction, heart failure), cerebrovascular disease, predisposition to hypotension (including treatment with antihypertensives) or risk factors for venous or arterial thromboembolic events
- caution if used in those with glaucoma, prostatic hypertrophy, paralytic ileus or urinary retention, as anticholinergic effects may aggravate these conditions
- caution if used in those with diabetes or risk factors for diabetes including obesity. Blood glucose levels should be carefully monitored during therapy
- caution if used in those with hypothyroidism (susceptible to hypothermia), thyrotoxicosis (a higher risk of extrapyramidal adverse effects) or hyperthyroidism (a risk of neurotoxicity)
- caution if used in those with pre-existing low WBC, history of drug-induced leucopenia/neutropenia. FBC should be monitored regularly during first months of therapy and therapy should be stopped if severe neutropenia occurs
- caution if used in those with history or risk factors for sleep apnoea
- caution if used in those with a history of neuroleptic malignant syndrome. If given, the patient should be very closely monitored
- not recommended in elderly patients with dementia-related psychoses (because of the increased risk of stroke and/or death) or organic brain syndrome
- contraindicated in those with prolactin-dependent tumours (including breast cancer and pituitary gland prolactinomas), phaeochromocytoma, liver impairment/failure or active liver disease
- contraindicated in those with severe CNS depression (including drug intoxication), coma, Parkinson's disease, circulatory collapse, congenital/acquired long QT interval, known hypokalaemia or hypomagnesaemia, significant bradycardia or arrhythmias (treated with class IA or III antiarrhythmic agents)

General Patient education for antipsychotics

- the patient/family/carer should be advised that it may take several weeks for there to be improvement in their symptoms and that they should continue to take their medication
- advise the patient that initial drowsiness subsides within weeks of starting therapy
- the patient should be warned against driving a vehicle or operating machinery if drowsy or dizzy, especially in the first few weeks of therapy
- advise the patient to avoid dizziness, lightheadedness and/or fainting (due to postural hypotension) by moving gradually to a sitting or standing position, especially after sleep. Warn the patient that postural hypotension is made worse by prolonged standing, hot baths or showers, hot weather, physical exertion, large meals and drinking alcohol

- instruct the patient to avoid alcohol with therapy because tolerance is reduced
- warn the patient against suddenly stopping therapy because this may cause symptoms such as nausea, vomiting and restlessness. Relapse often occurs
- the patient should be advised to avoid overheating (including strenuous exercise or work and exposure to extreme temperatures) and dehydration, because antipsychotics disrupt the body's ability to control temperature. The patient should also be aware of risks associated with swimming in cold water, and the importance of staying cool in hot weather and ensuring a good oral intake in hot weather
- warn the patient against taking over-the-counter antihistamine preparations because of interactions with antipsychotic medications
- advise the patient to maintain good mouth hygiene, as continued dry mouth may predispose them to tooth decay, gum disease and fungal infection (oral thrush)
- family members/carers should be instructed to monitor the patient closely (especially at the start of therapy or with changes in dose) for any agitation, irritability or change in behaviour, or any signs of depression such as sadness, withdrawal from friends or previously pleasurable activities, or any attempts at self-harm
- the patient should be advised to seek medical advice immediately if any of the following occur:
    - increased thirst, increased urination and weakness
    - sore throat, chills, swollen glands, fever or flu-like symptoms (especially 4—10 weeks after starting therapy)
    - fits/seizures
    - hardness or rigidity of muscles, fever, altered mental state, irregular pulse, sweating
    - unwanted muscle movements of the mouth, tongue, jaw, cheeks, arms or legs
    - worm-like movements of the tongue
    - prolonged and painful penis erection (not returning to the normal flaccid state)
    - sudden fainting for no reason or after exercise/emotional excitement, rapid or erratic heartbeat
- headache, changes in vision
- the patient should be counselled regarding diet, as weight gain is a common adverse effect of most antipsychotic agents
- patients with diabetes should be instructed to monitor blood glucose levels closely during therapy
- advise the patient that any constipation may necessitate increased fluid intake, added dietary roughage or a laxative
- female patients should be counselled to use adequate contraception during therapy to avoid pregnancy

Not recommended during pregnancy unless potential benefits are thought to outweigh risks to fetus. Infants exposed to antipsychotics during the third trimester are at risk of extrapyramidal disturbances and/or withdrawal symptoms after delivery. Newborns should be closely monitored.

Contraindicated/not recommended during breastfeeding.

ANTIPSYCHOTIC AND MOOD-STABILISING AGENTS

AMISULPRIDE

Trade names
Amisulpride Sandoz, Amisulpride WGR, APO-Amisulpride, Solian, Sulprix

Available forms
Tablets: 100 mg, 200 mg, 400 mg;
Suspension: 100 mg/mL

Action
- typical antipsychotic (benzamide) that binds selectively to D_2 and D_3 dopamine receptors (especially presynaptically) with a low affinity for other receptor sites
- has no antiemetic properties
- minimal sedation, hypotensive and anticholinergic effects
- half-life about 12 hours

Use
- acute and chronic schizophrenic disorders (with positive and/or negative symptoms, including those with predominantly negative symptoms)

Dose
- (Acute psychotic episodes) 200—400 mg orally twice daily before meals, increasing if needed (daily maximum 1200 mg) **OR**
- (Predominantly negative symptoms) 50—300 mg orally daily before meals

Adverse effects
- blurred vision
- hypotension and uncommonly, hypertension
- pruritus
- (Uncommon) bradycardia
- see also General Adverse effects of antipsychotics (not anticholinergic effects) (p. 834)

Interactions
- caution if given with other renally excreted agents, such as lithium
- serum level may be increased if given with clozapine
- see also General Interactions of antipsychotics (p. 835)

Nursing considerations/Cautions
- doses of 400 mg or less can be given as a single daily dose
- oral solution contains hydroxybenzoates, which may cause hypersensitivity reactions in sensitive individuals
- contraindicated in children up to puberty
- see also General Nursing considerations/Cautions for antipsychotics (p. 836)

Patient education
- advise the patient that solution should be dispensed using pipette/dosage syringe supplied, which is carefully washed after use
- the patient should be instructed that oral solution can be added to water if desired
- see also General Patient education for antipsychotics (p. 837)

 Oral solution available. Tablet can be crushed and mixed with water or a spoonful of yoghurt or apple puree.

ARIPIPRAZOLE

Trade names
Abilify, Abilify Maintena, Abyraz, APO-Aripiprazole, Aripena, Aripic Aripiprazole, Aripiprazole GH, Aripiprazole Sandoz, Aripiprazole-WGR, Arizole

Available forms
Tablets: 5 mg, 10 mg, 15 mg, 20 mg, 30 mg;
Vial: 300 mg, 400 mg

Action
- atypical antipsychotic
- partial agonist (dopamine D_2 and serotonin $5HT_{1A}$ receptors) and serotonin $5HT_{2A}$ antagonist
- no antiemetic properties, minimal sedation, hypotension and anticholinergic actions
- active metabolite has a half-life of 100 hours
- half-life 75 hours

Use
- acute and maintenance treatment of schizophrenia
- prevention of recurrent mania or mixed episodes associated with bipolar I disorder (monotherapy or combination therapy with lithium or sodium valproate)

Dose
- (Schizophrenia) initially 10—15 mg orally daily, increasing at 2-week intervals if needed (range 10—30 mg daily) **OR**
- (Schizophrenia, prevention of recurrent mania) 400 mg IM monthly **OR**
- (Prevention of recurrent mania) initially 15 mg orally daily (alone or with lithium or sodium valproate), increasing to 30 mg (if needed) for at least 9 weeks

Adverse effects
- rash
- cough, nasal congestion, pharyngolaryngeal pain, nasopharyngitis
- toothache
- peripheral oedema, hypertension
- blurred vision
- arthralgia, muscle stiffness and/or spasm, musculoskeletal pain, myalgia, pain in extremities, back pain
- (Injection site) haematoma, redness, swelling, discomfort/pain, pruritus, induration
- see also General Adverse effects of antipsychotics (p. 834)

Interactions
- increased serum levels may occur if given with amiodarone, ciclosporin, clarithromycin, erythromycin, fluconazole, fluoxetine, itraconazole, paroxetine, ritonavir or grapefruit juice
- decreased serum levels may occur if given with carbamazepine, efavirenz, nevirapine, phenobarbital, phenytoin, primidone, rifabutin, rifampicin or St John's wort
- see also General Interactions of antipsychotics (p. 835)

Nursing considerations/Cautions
- in those who have never taken aripiprazole, oral therapy should be initiated to determine tolerability before starting injectable formulation for maintenance therapy
- (IM) oral therapy (with aripiprazole or another antipsychotic agent) should be continued for 14 consecutive days to maintain therapeutic levels
- (IM) the dose can be decreased to 300 mg if adverse effects occur
- given only IM (not SC or IV) into gluteal or deltoid muscle
- the dose should not be divided
- (Oral) if switching from another antipsychotic agent, this may be done by tapering down over 2 weeks while increasing the dose of aripiprazole, starting on the recommended dose of aripiprazole while tapering down the dose of the other antipsychotic, or starting aripiprazole and stopping another agent
- if switching from another long-acting injectable antipsychotic, it can be replaced at the next scheduled injection with 14 days of oral aripiprazole
- reconstitute using 1.9 mL of water for injections (diluent) for 400 mg or 1.5 mL for a 300 mg dose
- shake well for at least 30 seconds to dissolve powder. Reconstituted solution is opaque and milky in colour
- use a 23-gauge, 1 inch (deltoid) or 22-gauge, 1.5 inch (38 mm) (gluteal) hypodermic needle for a non-obese patient, or a 22-gauge, 1.5 inch (38 mm) (deltoid) or 21-gauge, 2 inch (51 mm) (gluteal) hypodermic needle for an obese patient
- thr solution should be injected slowly and the area not massaged after injection
- injection sites should be rotated
- (IM) if a second or third monthly dose is missed (> 4 weeks but < 5 weeks), the dose should be administered as soon as possible and the monthly regimen resumed; if > 5 weeks has elapsed, the oral dose should be restarted for 14

ANTIPSYCHOTIC AND MOOD-STABILISING AGENTS

- consecutive days with IM injection and then the monthly regimen resumed
- (IM) if a fourth or subsequent monthly dose is missed (> 4 weeks but < 6 weeks), the dose should be administered and the monthly regimen resumed; if > 6 weeks has elapsed, the oral dose should be restarted for 14 consecutive days with IM injection and then the monthly regimen resumed
- tablets contain lactose and are therefore not recommended in those with rare hereditary problems of galactose intolerance, Lapp lactase deficiency or glucose—galactose malabsorption
- not recommended in those under 18 years
- not recommended in those with psychosis related to Alzheimer's disease
- see also General Nursing considerations/Cautions for antipsychotics (p. 836)

Patient education

- the patient should be advised to avoid grapefruit juice
- see also General Patient education for antipsychotics (p. 837)

Tablet can be crushed and mixed with water or spoonful of yoghurt or apple puree. Mask and gloves should be warn to disperse or crush tablet.

ASENAPINE MALEATE

Trade name
Saphris

Available forms
Wafer: 5 mg, 10 mg

Action
- atypical antipsychotic
- dibenzoxepino pyrroles
- binds to dopamine (D_2) and serotonin ($5HT_{2A}$) receptors
- also binds to other serotonin and alpha adrenergic receptors
- no antiemetic properties, minimal sedative, hypotensive and anticholinergic actions
- half-life about 24 hours

Use
- treatment of schizophrenia
- treatment and prevention of acute manic or mixed episodes associated with bipolar I disorder (alone or in combination with lithium or sodium valproate)

Dose
- (Schizophrenia) initially 5 mg orally twice daily, increasing to 10 mg twice daily if needed **OR**
- (Treatment and prevention of manic or mixed episodes in bipolar I disorder: monotherapy) initially 10 mg twice daily, reducing to 5 mg twice daily if needed **OR**
- (Treatment and prevention of manic or mixed episodes in bipolar I disorder: combination therapy) initially 5 mg orally twice daily, increasing to 10 mg twice daily if needed (with lithium or sodium valproate)

Adverse effects
- oral hyperaesthesia/paraesthesia
- see also General Adverse effects of antipsychotics (p. 834)

Interactions
- caution if given with fluvoxamine
- see also General Interactions of antipsychotics (p. 835)

Nursing considerations/Cautions

- not recommended in those under 18 years
- not recommended in those with severe liver impairment
- see also General Nursing considerations/Cautions for antipsychotics (p. 836)

Patient education

- the patient should be given the following instructions regarding administration of wafers:
  - the wafer should not be removed from the blister pack until just before administration
  - hands should be dry
  - the wafer should not be pushed through blister pack

- the tab should be pulled back gently
- the wafer should be placed under the tongue and allowed to dissolve completely without being chewed, crushed or swallowed
- if other medications are administered at the same time, the wafer should be given last
- warn the patient that their mouth may feel numb for up to an hour after using the wafer
- not to eat or drink for 10 minutes after the wafer
- the wafer should be stored in original container, protected from light and moisture and below 30°C
* see also General Patient education for antipsychotics (p. 837)

 The wafer should not be crushed, broken, chewed or swallowed with water.

BREXPIPRAZOLE
Trade name
Rexulti

Available form
Tablet: 1 mg, 2 mg, 3 mg, 4 mg

Action
- atypical antipsychotic
- although its action is not completely understood, thought to modulate serotonin—dopamine activity
- shows affinity for multiple receptors including serotonin, dopamine, noradrenaline (norepinephrine) and histamine
- half-life about 91 hours

Use
- treatment of schizophrenia

Dose
- initially 1 mg orally daily for 4 days, then increasing to 2 mg for 3 days, then 4 mg depending on clinical response and tolerability, maintenance dose 2—4 mg orally daily (daily maximum 4 mg)

Adverse effects
- toothache
- back pain, pain in extremity, muscle spasms, musculoskeletal pain
- tremor
- pruritus
- increased blood creatine phosphokinase, increased triglycerides
- see also General Adverse effects of antipsychotic agents (p. 834)

Interactions
- serum levels may decrease if given with rifampicin, rifabutin, carbamazepine, phenytoin, phenobarbital (phenobarbitone) or St John's wort
- serum levels may increase if given with atazanavir, boceprevir, darunavir, fosamprenavir, itraconazole, ritonavir
- see also General Interactions of antipsychotic agents (p. 835)

Nursing considerations/Cautions
- tablets contain lactose and are not recommended in those with rare hereditary problems of galactose intolerance, Lapp lactase deficiency or glucose—galactose malabsorption
- see also General Nursing considerations/Cautions for antipsychotics (p. 836)

Patient education
- see General Patient education for antipsychotics (p. 837)

 Tablet can be crushed and mixed with water or a spoonful of yoghurt or apple puree.

 Recommended daily dose is 3 mg in those with moderate, severe or end-stage kidney impairment (CrCl < 60 mL/min) or severe liver impairment.

CARBAMAZEPINE
Trade names
Alvoire, Carbamazepine Sandoz, Tegretol

Available forms
Tablets: 100 mg, 200 mg;
Tablets (controlled-release): 200 mg, 400 mg;
Suspension: 100 mg/5 mL

Action
- antipsychotic action thought to be related to its effects on dopamine and noradrenaline
- other actions related to its use in epilepsy and neuralgia (see Carbamazepine in Antiepileptics, p. 392)

Use
- mania, bipolar disorder (as monotherapy or as an adjunct to lithium, other antipsychotic agents or antidepressants)
- epilepsy, neuralgia (see Carbamazepine in Antiepileptics, p. 392)

Dose
- (Mania: monotherapy) 100—200 mg orally twice daily, increasing by 200 mg daily increments to 800—1000 mg/day (week 1) and, if no response in week 2, increasing to 1600 mg daily in divided doses **OR**
- (Maintenance) 100—200 mg twice daily, increasing by 100 mg weekly increments until plasma levels are adequate (4—12 microgram/mL; 17—50 micromol/L)

Adverse effects/Interactions/Nursing considerations/Cautions/Patient education
- suspension or tablets (not sustained release) are recommended for establishing dose for treatment of mania
- see also Adverse effects/Nursing considerations/Cautions/Patient education for antiepileptics (p. 385)

Oral suspension available. Plain tablet can be dispersed in water, or crushed and mixed with a spoonful of yoghurt or apple puree. Mask and gloves should be worn if dispersing or crushing tablets.

Controlled-release tablets should not be crushed, broken or chewed.

Pregnant staff should not crush tablets.

CARIPRAZINE
Trade name
Reagila

Available form
Capsule: 1.5 mg, 3 mg, 4.5 mg, 6 mg

Action
- atypical antipsychotic
- potent dopamine D_3/D_4 receptor partial agonist with preferential binding to D_3 receptors
- partial agonist at serotonin $5HT_{1A}$ receptors
- two major active metabolites
- long half-life (both cariprazine and metabolites)

Use
- treatment of schizophrenia

Dose
- initially 1.5 mg orally daily, increasing by 1.5 mg increments as needed (maximum daily dose 6 mg)

Adverse effects
- see General Adverse effects of Antipsychotics (p. 834)

Interactions
- contraindicated with boceprevir, clarithromycin, cobicistat, itraconazole, posaconazole, ritonavir, telithromycin, voriconazole, diltiazem, erythromycin, fluconazole and verapamil
- contraindicated with carbamazepine, phenobarbital (phenobarbitone), phenytoin, rifampicin, bosentan, efavirenz, etravirine, modafinil and St John's wort
- caution if given with agents that have a narrow therapeutic index such as digoxin and dabigatran
- caution if given with other CNS agents and alcohol

Nursing considerations/Cautions
- because cariprazine and active metabolites have long half-lives, changes in dose may not be reflected in serum levels for some time

- the patient should be monitored closely for adverse effects and treatment response for several weeks after starting therapy and after any dose changes
- if switching from another antipsychotic to cariprazine, gradual discontinuation of the previous treatment is recommended while starting therapy with cariprazine
- if switching from cariprazine to another antipsychotic, the new antipsychotic should be started at its lowest dose while cariprazine is discontinued
- therapy with cariprazine can be stopped immediately; however, it may take 3 to 4 weeks for cariprazine and metabolites to be excreted from the body
- capsules contain Allura red AC (E 129), which may cause allergic reactions in those with hypersensitivity
- not recommended in those with severe kidney or liver impairment
- see also General Nursing considerations/Cautions for antipsychotics (p. 836)

Patient education

- advise the patient to avoid grapefruit and grapefruit juice during therapy
- women of childbearing potential should be advised to avoid pregnancy by using highly effective contraception during therapy and for at least 10 weeks after stopping therapy
- see also General Patient education for antipsychotics (p. 837)

Not recommended during pregnancy and in women of childbearing potential not using effective contraception.

Not recommended during breastfeeding.

CHLORPROMAZINE HYDROCHLORIDE

Trade name
Largactil

Available forms
Tablets: 25 mg, 100 mg;
Syrup: 5 mg/mL;
Ampoules: 50 mg/2 mL

Action
- phenothiazine with typical antipsychotic actions
- alpha adrenergic blocking agent producing hypotension
- dopamine inhibitor
- impairs body temperature regulation
- antiemetic effects; also has sedative and anticholinergic properties, as well as causing hypotension
- stimulates prolactin release

Use
- acute function psychosis (e.g. schizophrenia, mania or psychotic depression)
- schizophrenia (long-term management)
- agitation and/or behavioural disturbance (delirium, dementia) (short term)
- control of nausea and/or vomiting associated with disease, drugs and surgery premedication or terminal illness
- intractable hiccups
- short-term management of agitation, severe depression
- behavioural disturbances (in children with autism or intellectual disability) (with non-pharmacological management program)

Dose
- initially 25 mg orally 3 times daily, increasing gradually if necessary to 25—100 mg orally 3 times daily (maintenance) (daily maximum 600—800 mg) **OR**
- 25—50 mg deep IM 6—8-hourly if needed

Adverse effects
- nasal stuffiness
- rash, urticaria, contact dermatitis, photosensitivity
- decreased cough reflex, respiratory depression
- (Prolonged use) retinopathy
- (IM) postural hypotension, tachycardia
- (IM injection site) pain, irritation, nodule formation
- (Rare) pigmentation of conjunctivae, discolouration of cornea and sclera,

ANTIPSYCHOTIC AND MOOD-STABILISING AGENTS

lens/corneal opacities, severe liver toxicity
- see also General Adverse effects of antipsychotics (p. 834)

Interactions
- plasma level may be increased by propranolol, tricyclic antidepressants (TCAs), selective serotonin reuptake inhibitors (SSRIs), oestrogens, antimalarial agents, ciprofloxacin, fluvoxamine and progestogens
- increased risk of neurotoxicity and extrapyramidal side-effects if given with lithium. Antiemetic effects may mask lithium toxicity if given together
- not recommended with citalopram or escitalopram
- increased CNS effects if given with benzodiazepines, anaesthetics, opioids, barbiturates or lithium
- increased risk of toxicity if given with amitriptyline or other TCAs
- effects may be variable if given with phenytoin; therefore the patient should be closely monitored for any signs of phenytoin toxicity, loss of psychotic control or increase in seizure frequency
- increased risk of QT interval prolongation if given with other antipsychotics, amiodarone, clonidine, diltiazem, disopyramide, IV amphotericin, IV erythromycin, methadone, pentamidine, sotalol, stimulant laxatives, thiazide diuretics, tetracosactides, verapamil or beta adrenergic receptor blocking agents
- use with metoclopramide may increase risk of antipsychotic-induced extrapyramidal effects
- absorption may be decreased when given with food, alcohol, antacids or benztropine, resulting in decreased serum levels
- decreased serum levels may occur if given with phenobarbital (phenobarbitone) or carbamazepine
- may decrease serum levels of phenobarbital (phenobarbitone)
- anticholinergic effects may be increased (e.g. increased risk of heat stroke, severe constipation, paralytic ileus) if given with anticholinergics or atropine
- increased risk of seizures if given with tramadol
- may antagonise anti-Parkinsonian effect of levodopa, bromocriptine and pergolide
- may increase serum levels of sodium valproate and propranolol
- increased hypotension, sedation and respiratory depression may occur if given with pethidine
- may antagonise the effects of antidiabetic agents
- may decrease the effects of amphetamines
- may decrease the effects of anticoagulants; therefore INR should be monitored regularly, especially when starting or stopping therapy
- an increased risk of postural hypotension and extrapyramidal syndrome if given with monoamine oxidase inhibitors (MAOIs) and are therefore not recommended with or within 14 days
- may oppose the action of adrenaline (epinephrine) and clonidine
- adrenaline (epinephrine) should not be used to treat phenothiazine-induced hypotension or in overdose
- an increased risk of transient metabolic encephalopathy if given with desferrioxamine
- may decrease the seizure threshold, requiring adjustment of the antiepileptic dose
- increase the risk of postural hypotension if given with thiazide diuretics
- may cause false positive on a phenylketonuria (PKU) test

Nursing considerations/Cautions
- regular ophthalmological examination and liver function tests are recommended for patients on long-term therapy
- contact dermatitis may be avoided if injectable preparations are handled using plastic or rubber gloves
- give IM injections slowly and deeply to avoid irritating subcutaneous tissues
- rotate IM injection sites

- BP and vital signs should be closely monitored after IM administration
- advise the patient to remain recumbent for at least 1 hour after IM injection to avoid postural hypotension
- syrup is recommended for those with swallowing difficulties or who refuse tablets
- noradrenaline (norepinephrine) should be available for severe hypotension (adrenaline (epinephrine) is contraindicated) and benztropine for severe extrapyramidal side-effects
- (Injection, syrup) contain sodium metabisulfite and sodium sulfite, which may cause allergic-type reactions in susceptible individuals
- (Syrup) contains sucrose and is not recommended in those with fructose intolerance, glucose-galactose malabsorption syndrome or sucrase-isomaltase deficiency
- caution if used in those with chronic respiratory disease or at risk of aspiration pneumonia
- caution if used in children because of the risk of dystonic reactions
- not recommended in children or adolescents with signs suggestive of Reye's syndrome
- not recommended in those with epilepsy, hypoparathyroidism, myasthenia gravis, Parkinson's disease, narrow-angle glaucoma or prostatic hypertrophy
- contraindicated in children under 1 year
- contraindicated in those with hypersensitivity to other phenothiazines (e.g. jaundice, blood dyscrasias), bone marrow depression, severe depression, circulatory collapse, CNS depression (coma or drug intoxication), phaeochromocytoma, liver failure or active liver disease
- see also General Nursing considerations/Cautions for antipsychotics (p. 836)

Patient education

- advise the patient to seek medical advice immediately if any of the following occur:
  - fever or sore throat, gums or mouth, chills or swollen glands, especially between weeks 4 and 10 of therapy (early signs of bone marrow depression)
  - blurred vision or other visual disturbances, including difficulties with night vision or colour vision defects
  - loss of appetite, nausea, vomiting, abdominal pain, fatigue, yellowing of eyes or skin (signs of liver toxicity)
- warn the patient to avoid extreme sun exposure by wearing a hat, long-sleeved clothing and sunscreen (SPF 30+) to avoid exaggerated reaction to sun causing severe sunburn
- instruct the patient that antacids (e.g. aluminium hydroxide or magnesium trisilicate) should be taken either 1 hour before or 2 hours after chlorpromazine
- advise the patient that tablets should not be crushed or broken (syrup is available if tablets are difficult to swallow), as skin contact with crushed tablets may lead to dermatitis
- see also General Patient education for antipsychotics (p. 837)

 Syrup is available. Tablet should not be crushed, broken or chewed.

 If given during the third trimester, an increased risk of neonatal respiratory distress, brady- or tachycardia, agitation, hypo- or hypertonia, tremor, somnolence and/or feeding difficulties.

 Excreted in breast milk; therefore not recommended during breastfeeding unless benefits outweigh risks.

 Contraindicated in those with liver failure or acute liver disease.

 Caution if used in the elderly; starting dose should be half the adult dose.

ANTIPSYCHOTIC AND MOOD-STABILISING AGENTS

CLOZAPINE

Trade names
Clopine, Clozaril, Clozitor, Versacloz

Available forms
Tablets: 25 mg, 50 mg, 100 mg, 200 mg; Oral suspension: 50 mg/mL

Action
- atypical antipsychotic
- tricyclic dibenzodiazepine
- weakly blocks dopamine (D_1 and D_2) receptors
- anticholinergic, antihistamine, antiserotonin with no antiemetic properties
- sedative (inhibits arousal)
- relieves both negative and positive symptoms of schizophrenia
- little or no elevation of prolactin levels
- active metabolite which has weaker action and shorter duration than clozapine
- half-life 14 hours

Use
- treatment-resistant schizophrenia (in those who are unresponsive or intolerant to other antipsychotics)

Dose
- initially 12.5 mg orally 1—2 times daily for day 1, followed by 25 mg orally 1—2 times daily (day 2). If tolerated, then increasing increments of 25—50 mg over 2—3 weeks, up to 300 mg/day. If necessary, further weekly increases of 50—100 mg to a dose of 200—450 mg/day in divided doses, with the larger dose at night (daily maximum 600—900 mg) **OR**
- (Maintenance dose) dose decreased to 150—300 mg orally daily in divided doses

Adverse effects
- fever
- blurred vision
- tachycardia, ECG changes and, less commonly, QT interval prolongation
- (Common) leucopenia, neutropenia, eosinophilia, leucocytosis and, uncommonly, agranulocytosis
- (Rare) myocarditis, cardiomyopathy, myocardial infarction, seizure, sleep apnoea, clozapine-induced gastrointestinal hypomotility
- (Abrupt discontinuation) cholinergic rebound (profuse sweating, headache, nausea, vomiting, diarrhoea)
- see also General Adverse effects of antipsychotics (p. 834)

Interactions
- use with lithium or other CNS active agents may increase the risk of neuroleptic malignant syndrome
- contraindicated with any drugs that may cause bone marrow depression or with long-acting depot antipsychotic agents
- not recommended with carbamazepine owing to added bone marrow depression
- caution if given with other agents with anticholinergic, hypotensive or respiratory depression properties, as additive effects may occur
- plasma levels may be increased when given with azithromycin, azole antifungal agents, caffeine, ciprofloxacin, citalopram, clarithromycin, erythromycin, fluvoxamine, fluoxetine, paroxetine, protease inhibitors, sertraline, venlafaxine or oral contraceptives
- plasma levels may be decreased when given with phenytoin, carbamazepine, rifampicin, St John's wort, nicotine/smoking, pantoprazole or omeprazole, resulting in an exacerbation in symptoms
- increased risk of cardiac and/or respiratory arrest when given with benzodiazepines
- increased risk of seizure and delirium if given with sodium valproate (even in those without epilepsy)
- may antagonise effects of adrenaline (epinephrine) and related products
- see also General Interactions of antipsychotics (p. 834)

Nursing considerations/Cautions
- blood counts (WBC, differential count, absolute neutrophil count (ANC)) should be monitored 10 days before starting, weekly during first 18 weeks and then

monthly and for 1 month after stopping therapy. Additional monitoring is recommended if therapy is interrupted after an initial 18 weeks of therapy
- if the patient has a history of bone marrow disorder, they should be reviewed by a haematologist before starting therapy
- the patient should be screened for constipation before starting therapy and regularly throughout therapy to assess any changes in bowel function (e.g. changes in frequency and nature of bowel movements), as well as any signs of bowel hypo-motility such as nausea, vomiting, abdominal pain/distension, lack of urge to defecate, constipation and inability to defecate. Prompt management is required to prevent more serious gastrointestinal complications such as paralytic ileus, fecal impaction, megacolon and intestinal impaction
- if the patient has been on therapy for more than 18 weeks and treatment is stopped for 4—28 days, blood counts (WBC, ANC) should be monitored weekly for 6 weeks; if the interruption is greater than 28 days, monitoring should be weekly for the next 18 weeks
- doses of up to 200 mg may be given as a single dose at night
- rapid increases in dose should be avoided due to risk of seizures, especially in those with pre-existing epilepsy
- 24-hour washout period should be allowed when changing the patient from conventional antipsychotic therapy to clozapine, after gradual discontinuation over 7 days
- an increased risk of adverse effects if dose > 450 mg/day
- liver function should be regularly monitored in any patient with liver abnormalities
- if therapy is stopped for longer than 2 days, it should be restarted at 12.5 mg 1—2 times daily (day 1) and then titrated upwards more rapidly than the initial titration (within patient tolerance)
- if a family history of cardiac disease exists, cardiac assessment is recommended before starting therapy
- caution if used in those with or at risk of sleep apnoea or stroke
- contraindicated in those with a history of bone marrow disorders (including drug-induced agranulocytosis), alcoholic/toxic psychoses, severe renal/cardiac/liver disease, uncontrolled epilepsy, CNS depression, circulatory collapse, paralytic ileus or if unable to undergo regular blood tests
- see also General Nursing considerations/ Cautions for antipsychotics (p. 836)

Patient education

- advise the patient that fever (above 38°C) occurs commonly during first 4 weeks of therapy; however, the possibility of underlying infection should not discounted
- if the patient is taking an oral suspension, they or a family member/carer should be instructed in correct use, which includes:
  - preparation of the suspension 24 hours before first use to ensure it is adequately dispersed
  - ensuring the suspension is shaken for at least 10 seconds before each use
  - using the oral dispenser/syringe supplied to measure dose accurately
  - the suspension can be taken directly from the dispenser or mixed with water and drunk immediately. No other beverages should be used
  - the dispenser/syringe should be washed with warm soapy water between administrations
  - the suspension should be discarded 90 days after opening (opening date should be written on bottle)
- warn the patient not to suddenly start or stop smoking or drinking coffee/tea/ cola drinks without talking to doctor first, as this will affect blood levels and effectiveness of medication
- the patient should be advised to report immediately any:
  - fever, sore throat, mouth ulcers or other signs of infection or flu-like illness

ANTIPSYCHOTIC AND MOOD-STABILISING AGENTS

- fast or irregular heart rate, shortness of breath, rapid breathing, fatigue, chest pain, fever or flu-like illness (may be signs of cardiomyopathy)
- constipation (early management is important to prevent serious complications)
- see also General Patient education for antipsychotics (p. 837)

Oral suspension is available. Tablet can be crushed (but mask and gloves must be worn) and mixed with water or a spoonful of yoghurt or apple puree.

In patients with cardiovascular, respiratory or hepatic disorders or a history of seizures, the dose should be started at 12.5 mg and increased very slowly, monitoring functions closely.

In the elderly, the dose should be started at 12.5 mg on the first day and subsequent increases limited to 25 mg/day.

DROPERIDOL

Trade names
Droperidol Medsurge, Droperidol Panpharma

Available form
Ampoules: 2.5 mg/mL

Action
- butyrophenone
- antiemetic effect
- onset of action 3—10 minutes (IV, IM), full effect in 30 minutes, duration 2—4 hours
- altered consciousness may last up to 12 hours

Use
- antiemetic, premedication, induction and maintenance of anaesthesia, neuroleptanalgesia
- (Psychiatry) management of severe agitation, aggression or hyperactivity in psychotic disorders or disturbed states, including non-psychotic acute excitation states

Dose

Psychiatry
- 5—25 mg IM 4—6-hourly if needed **OR**
- 25—62.5 mg slow IV infusion over 20 minutes, twice daily **OR**
- (Psychiatric crisis) ≤ 5 mg IM immediately before transferring patient to hospital

Anaesthesia
- (Premedication, diagnostic or minor procedure without anaesthesia) 2.5—10 mg slow IV 30—60 minutes before induction **OR**
- (Adjunct to general anaesthetic) 0.25 mg/kg IM or slow IV with an opioid analgesic and/or general anaesthetic agent to provide a smooth induction **OR**
- (Maintenance) 1.25—2.5 mg slow IV **OR**
- (Adjunct to regional anaesthesia) 2.5—5 mg IM or slow IV when additional sedation is required

Adverse effects
- bronchospasm, laryngospasm, increased depth of respiration
- (Rare) arrhythmia, prolongation of QT interval
- see also General Adverse effects of antipsychotics (p. 834)

Interactions
- contraindicated with drugs known to prolong QT interval or cause significant bradycardia, hypokalaemia or hypomagnesaemia
- may potentiate respiratory depression of opioid analgesics; therefore should be given together with caution using $1/4$ of normal opioid dose
- muscle rigidity may occur if given with opioid analgesic
- adrenaline (epinephrine) may decrease BP when given with droperidol
- may increase effects of barbiturates, general anaesthetics, antipsychotics, benzodiazepines and opioid analgesics
- serum levels may decrease if given with phenytoin, carbamazepine, phenobarbital (phenobarbitone), smoking or alcohol use

Nursing considerations/Cautions

- any electrolyte imbalance should be corrected before starting therapy
- ECG monitoring before the first dose (if possible) is recommended to detect any bradycardia or arrhythmia and up to 7 hours after procedure (if used during surgery). If the patient has acute symptoms, ECG should be performed when symptoms have reduced
- vital signs should be monitored during IV therapy
- slow IV infusion will decrease risk of muscle rigidity (especially respiratory muscles) if given with opioids
- (Anaesthesia) pulmonary arterial pressure may decrease during therapy and this should be considered if these results require clinical interpretation
- may be given in 250 mL of sodium chloride 0.9%, glucose 5% or Ringer's solution and infused over 20 minutes
- (Anaesthesia) caution when repositioning patient because of the risk of orthostatic hypotension
- caution if used in those with ventricular arrhythmias, cardiac disease, a family history of sudden death, kidney/liver failure, respiratory failure, chronic obstructive pulmonary disease (COPD) or electrolyte disturbance (or risk of), including persistent vomiting or diarrhoea
- caution if used in those with a history of epilepsy, epilepsy or risk factors for epilepsy
- not recommended in those with phaeochromocytoma
- contraindicated in those with acute alcohol intoxication (relative contraindication)
- contraindicated in female patients with QT interval > 450 msec or male patients with QT interval > 440 msec, or with acquired or congenital (or a family history of) long QT syndrome
- see also General Nursing considerations/Cautions for antipsychotics (p. 836)

Patient education

- the patient should be warned not to drive or operate machinery for at least 12 hours after administration, as consciousness can remain affected
- see also General Patient education for antipsychotics (p. 837)

FLUPENTIXOL DECANOATE (FLUPENTHIXOL DECANOATE)

Trade name
Fluanxol

Available forms
Ampoule: 20 mg/mL;
Depot Injection: 100 mg/mL

Action
- thioxanthene typical antipsychotic
- non-sedating at low-to-moderate doses
- disinhibiting and mood-elevating properties
- increases prolactin levels
- onset 24—72 hours, symptoms improve for 2—4 weeks
- decanoate allows slow release from oily solution (coconut oil)

Use
- chronic schizophrenia and related chronic psychosis (maintenance therapy)

Dose
- (Patients not previously treated with long-acting depot preparations) 20 mg deep IM (after 5—10 days of test dose of 5—20 mg) **OR**
- (Previously treated patients) 20—40 mg deep IM, then a second dose of 20—40 mg 4—10 days later, then 20—40 mg IM 2—4 weeks later, depending on clinical response and/or side-effects **OR**
- (Concentrated depot preparation) for doses greater than 100 mg IM, fortnightly injections are required; concentrated preparation is recommended to reduce volume required

ANTIPSYCHOTIC AND MOOD-STABILISING AGENTS

Adverse effects
- (IM site) inflammation, abscess
- dysphagia, gingival hypertrophy
- (Uncommon) oculogyric crises
- see also General Adverse effects of antipsychotics (p. 834)

Interactions
- may decrease effects of levodopa and adrenergic agents
- increased risk of extrapyramidal adverse effects if given with metoclopramide
- see also General Interactions of antipsychotics (p. 835)

Nursing considerations/Cautions
- blood counts and liver function tests are recommended during the first months of therapy
- for those not previously treated with a depot long-acting antipsychotic, a test dose of 5–20 mg is recommended. For patients who are elderly, thin, frail or with a family history of extrapyramidal reactions, a 5 mg dose is recommended. For others (long-acting neuroleptic naive), 5–20 mg is recommended
- oral therapy should be continued during the test dose period, but at a reduced dose
- patient should be monitored for 5–10 days after test dose for therapeutic response and/or any adverse effects (especially extrapyramidal reactions)
- not given IV
- given by deep IM injection
- if volume required is greater than 2–3 mL of 20 mg/mL solution, then 100 mg/mL solution should be used
- should not be mixed with any other depot preparations containing sesame oil, as properties may be altered
- not for short-term treatment (less than 3 months)
- fluphenazine decanoate 25 mg = flupentixol decanoate 40 mg and haloperidol decanoate 50 mg = flupentixol decanoate 40 mg
- concentrated solution (100 mg/mL) is recommended in those requiring large volumes (> 2–3 mL) or high doses
- if patient is having surgery, BP should be closely monitored for any hypotensive phenomena
- not recommended in severely agitated psychotic patients, including confused or agitated elderly, as symptoms may be exacerbated
- caution if used in those with liver or kidney damage or insufficiency, severe arteriosclerosis, risk factors for stroke, organic brain syndrome, epilepsy, Parkinsonism, or cerebrovascular or cardiovascular disease
- contraindicated in those with hypersensitivity to thioxanthenes and possible cross-sensitivity to phenothiazines, sensitivity to coconut oil, blood dyscrasias, subcortical brain damage, phaeochromocytoma, circulatory collapse, coma or depressed conscious state due to any cause (e.g. alcohol intoxication, barbiturates, opioids)
- see also General Nursing considerations/ Cautions for antipsychotics (p. 836)

Patient education
- the patient should be advised to immediately report any sore mouth, gums or throat, chills, fever or any flu-like symptoms
- instruct the patient to maintain good dental hygiene throughout therapy, taking care with use of a toothbrush (soft recommended), dental floss or toothpicks, as there is an increased risk of infection, gum bleeding and delayed healing
- see also General Patient education for antipsychotics (p. 837)

HALOPERIDOL
Trade name
Serenace

HALOPERIDOL DECANOATE
Trade names
Haldol Decanoate

Available forms
Tablets: 0.5 mg, 1.5 mg, 5 mg;
Suspension: 2 mg/mL;
Ampoules: 5 mg/mL;
Ampoules (depot): 50 mg/mL

Action
- butyrophenone not related to phenothiazines
- some anticholinergic and sedative actions
- inhibits central action of dopamine (D_2) and noradrenaline (norepinephrine)
- antiemetic
- increase prolactin release
- active metabolite with activity less than haloperidol
- half-life about 24 hours
- decanoate allows slow release from oily solution (sesame oil)

Use
- schizophrenia, psychoses, manic phase of bipolar I disorder
- during alcohol withdrawal (short-term therapy)
- intractable nausea and vomiting related to radiation sickness or cancer (short-term therapy)
- Gilles de la Tourette syndrome
- neuroleptanalgesia

Dose
- (Moderate symptoms) 1—5 mg orally daily as single dose or 2 divided doses **OR**
- (Severe symptoms) 5—15 mg orally daily as single dose or 2 divided doses, increasing up to 20 mg if necessary to achieve control, then reducing to the lowest dose to maintain control **OR**
- (Elderly or debilitated patient) 1—3 mg orally daily as single dose or 2 divided doses **OR**
- (Agitation, aggression with acute psychosis, including alcohol withdrawal) initially 0.5—10 mg IM or IV (slow IV or bolus), followed by further dose half-hourly (slow IV) or hourly (IM) until clinical response is achieved (daily maximum 20 mg) **OR**
- (Maintenance) half of IM/IV dose used to achieve control given as 2 divided doses (morning and evening), with first dose administered 4—8 hours after last controlling dose **OR**
- (Depot IM injection) initially 10—15 times previous oral daily dose, not exceeding 100 mg at 4-week intervals

Adverse effects
- dental caries, periodontal disease, oral thrush
- (Depot injection) local reaction
- (High dose, IV) prolonged QT interval, torsades de pointes
- see also General Adverse effects of antipsychotics (p. 834)

Interactions
- increased risk of hypotension and greater intoxication if given with alcohol
- may inhibit metabolism of tricyclic antidepressants (TCAs), increasing the risk of toxicity and anticholinergic effects
- may result in acute encephalopathic syndrome if given with lithium
- may interfere with anticoagulant action of warfarin
- may enhance CNS effects (e.g. disorientation, memory loss, aggression, confusion) when given in high doses with methyldopa sesquihydrate
- may antagonise the action of adrenaline (epinephrine) and other sympathomimetic agents
- prolonged carbamazepine, phenobarbital (phenobarbitone), phenytoin, St John's wort or rifampicin therapy may decrease plasma levels
- increased serum levels may occur if given with alprazolam, buspirone, chlorpromazine, duloxetine, fluvoxamine, fluoxetine, itraconazole, paroxetine, ritonavir or venlafaxine

ANTIPSYCHOTIC AND MOOD-STABILISING AGENTS

- when given with amphetamines, may decrease stimulant effects of amphetamine and decrease antipsychotic effects of haloperidol
- increased intraocular pressure may occur if given with anticholinergic or anti-Parkinson's agents
- increased risk of hypotension and cardiac arrest if given with propranolol
- anti-Parkinson's agents and haloperidol should not be discontinued simultaneously because of an increased risk of extrapyramidal symptoms
- serum levels may be decreased in those who smoke
- may increase serum levels of dextromethorphan including the risk of adverse effects
- increased risk of Parkinsonism and neuroleptic malignant syndrome if given with olanzapine
- increased risk of seizures if given with tramadol
- may interfere with actions of levodopa
- decreased effect of both haloperidol and cabergoline if given together; therefore not recommended together
- increased serum prolactin levels may occur if given with bromocriptine
- see also General Interactions of antipsychotics (p. 835)

Nursing considerations/Cautions

- children and elderly patients are more sensitive to medication; therefore starting dose should be low and titration gradual
- should be used only short term for acute mania and discontinued as soon as symptoms are relieved
- parenteral medication should be switched to oral as soon as practicable
- dose titration should be rapid and daily dose reduced to the lowest effective dose
- (Depot) before starting therapy with depot long-acting haloperidol, the patient should be stabilised on oral therapy
- (Depot) dose calculated on 10—15 times the previous day's oral dose

- (Depot) short-acting forms may be used to supplement depot preparation during dose adjustment or psychotic symptom exacerbations
- depot injection is given as a deep IM injection using 21-gauge needle
- depot must not be given IV
- 3 mL volume should not be exceeded for IM injection
- ECG is recommended during IV therapy, or if rapid control of an acutely distressed patient is needed or repeated or large doses are given. Parenteral anti-Parkinson medication and resuscitation equipment should be readily available
- serum levels should be monitored if the patient starts or stops smoking
- not recommended in those with bipolar disorder where depression is the predominant feature
- contraindicated in those with known hypersensitivity to sesame products (depot), basal ganglia lesions, CNS depression due to alcohol or depressant drugs, severe depression, previous spastic disease, prolactin-dependent tumours, or patients with pre-existing Parkinsonian symptoms, Parkinson's disease or congenital or acquired long QT syndrome
- see also General Nursing considerations/ Cautions for antipsychotics (p. 836)

Patient education

- the patient should be advised to remain recumbent for at least 1 hour after injection to avoid postural hypotension
- warn the patient not to abruptly start or stop smoking, as this will impact on blood levels and effectiveness of medication
- caution the patient to avoid taking over-the-counter preparations that include dextromethorphan, such as cough mixtures
- instruct the patient to maintain good dental hygiene throughout therapy, taking care with use of toothbrush (soft recommended), dental floss or toothpicks, as there is an increased risk of infection, gum bleeding and delayed healing

- see also General Patient education for antipsychotics (p. 837)

Oral liquid is available. Tablet can be dispersed in water or an acidic drink (not coffee or tea), or crushed and mixed with a spoonful of yoghurt or apple puree. Gloves should be worn to disperse or crush tablets to prevent dermatitis.

(Depot) Lower initial doses with smaller increases at longer intervals are recommended for those with kidney or liver impairment.

(Depot) 12.5—25 mg IM is the recommended dose for transition from oral haloperidol to depot formulation in the elderly patient. The dose can be adjusted by 25 mg at 4-week intervals, to a maximum dose of 150 mg/month.

LITHIUM CARBONATE

Trade names
Lithicarb, Quilonum SR

Available forms
Tablets: 250 mg;
Tablets (slow-release): 450 mg

Action
- lithium ions may compete with sodium ions (which are believed to increase greatly in mania), thereby altering the electrophysiological characteristics of neurones
- thought to inhibit release of dopamine while increasing turnover of noradrenaline (norepinephrine) and serotonin in the brain, decreasing postsynaptic receptor sensitivity resulting in a correction of overactive catecholamines
- proven efficacy in treatment of mania, but little to no effect in those not experiencing mania
- increased tolerance to lithium when patient is in manic phase
- narrow therapeutic index, with therapeutic serum level from 0.8 to 1.6 mmol/L, above which toxic adverse effects may be expected
- half-life 24 hours (adults), 18 hours (adolescents) and up to 36 hours (elderly)
- pregnancy and alkaline urine increase lithium clearance

Use
- prevention and treatment of mania
- prevention and treatment of mania in manic depressive (bipolar) illness (less effective for depressive swing)
- prevention of recurrent unipolar depressive illness
- chronic schizophrenia, schizoaffective illness

Dose

Prophylaxis
- 0.9—1.2 g orally daily in 2 divided doses (SR preparation) (to maintain serum lithium level 0.6—1.0 mmol/L)

Acute episodes
- initially 0.5—1 g orally daily in divided doses (day 1), 1.25—1.75 g orally in divided doses (day 2), 1.5—2 g orally daily in divided doses (day 3). This should achieve serum levels between 0.8 and 1.6 mmol/L (maximum 2 mmol/L). After 7—14 days, the dose should be reduced to maintain therapeutic range (usually 0.5—1 g daily) as a single or divided dose **OR**
- 1.8 g orally daily in 2 divided doses (SR preparation) (to maintain serum lithium level 0.8—1.4 mmol/L)

Adverse effects
- (Initially, disappear with stabilisation of serum level) nausea, diarrhoea, muscle weakness, dazed feeling, vertigo
- (At therapeutic levels)
  - metallic taste, weight gain, constipation, anorexia, transient nausea, diarrhoea, epigastric discomfort/gastritis, increased salivation
  - thirst, polyuria
  - fine hand tremor
  - headache, fatigue, sedation
  - oedema
  - reversible ECG changes, arrhythmias, hypotension, bradycardia

- exacerbation of skin conditions (e.g. acne, psoriasis), rash, alopecia, pruritus
- leucocytosis
- euthyroid goitre, hypercalcaemia, hyperglycaemia, hyperparathyroiditis
- (Toxic/overdose) increased diarrhoea, persistent nausea and vomiting, slurred speech, blurred vision, marked coarse tremor, ataxia, clonic limb movement, muscle twitching, hyperactive deep tendon reflexes, EEG changes, delirium, seizure, stupor, circulatory collapse, coma
- (Rare) nephrogenic diabetes insipidus, hyperthyroidism, hyperparathyroidism

Interactions

- contraindicated with diuretics (loop, thiazide), as excretion of lithium is decreased
- increased risk of toxicity (due to increased serum levels) may result if given with NSAIDs (especially indometacin and piroxicam), metronidazole, methyldopa sesquihydrate, topiramate, angiotensin converting enzyme (ACE) inhibitors, angiotensin II receptor antagonists, calcium-channel blockers, corticosteroids and appetite suppressants
- therapeutic effects of lithium may be reduced by acetazolamide, xanthines (including theophylline and caffeine), urea, sodium-glucose cotransporter 2 inhibitors (SGLT2 inhibitors) (e.g. dapagliflozin, empagliflozin), mannitol and urinary alkalinisers (including sodium bicarbonate) because of increased urinary excretion
- may result in neurotoxicity when given with carbamazepine, methyldopa sesquihydrate, selective serotonin reuptake inhibitors (SSRIs), tricyclic antidepressants (TCAs) or calcium-channel blockers
- may prolong action of neuromuscular blocking agents
- increased risk of delirium, prolonged seizures and/or confusion if given with ECT therapy
- caution if given with SSRIs or other serotonergic agents, as serotonin syndrome may be provoked
- not recommended with other antipsychotic agents owing to potentiation of antipsychotic adverse effects as well as risk of encephalopathic syndrome (weakness, lethargy, fever, tremor, confusion, leucocytosis and extrapyramidal symptoms)
- increased risk of QTc interval prolongation if given with ziprasidone
- increased risk of hypothyroidism and QT prolongation if given with amiodarone
- caution if given with antithyroid drugs or iodides
- excretion may be altered if given with corticosteroids or appetite suppressants

Nursing considerations/Cautions

- therapy should be started in an inpatient setting to closely monitor patient and blood levels
- before starting therapy, the patient should have a thorough assessment, including ECG, serum calcium levels and renal function (e.g. urinalysis, specific gravity, 24-hour urine volume, serum creatinine, creatinine clearance)
- during therapy, regular monitoring of serum calcium levels and thyroid, cardiac and renal functions is recommended
- narrow margin between therapeutic and toxic serum levels necessitates frequent estimations of lithium level, thereby detecting toxicity early and monitoring adherence
- serum levels monitored twice weekly initially, then weekly for 1 month, then monthly for 1 year, and then 4-monthly, with blood samples taken 12 hours after administration of the last dose
- serum levels should also be monitored when starting or stopping other medications, especially those known to increase serum levels
- lithium should be stopped for 24 hours before major surgery. Can be be restarted soon after surgery if electrolytes are normal

- if changing from immediate-release to sustained-release formulation, the same total dose should be given and the patient should be monitored at 1–2-week intervals for therapeutic effects and/or adverse effects and the dose adjusted accordingly
- withdrawal should be gradual over at least 15 days
- overdose/toxicity treatment includes stopping therapy immediately, maintenance of fluid and electrolyte balance and renal function to prevent hypernatraemia, ECG monitoring and control of hypotension and seizures. Activated charcoal does not absorb lithium. Haemodialysis is recommended in cases of severe toxicity; however, rebound increases may occur when haemodialysis is stopped, requiring repeated or prolonged treatment
- caution if given to those with vomiting, diarrhoea, fluid restriction, excessive sweating, dehydration, strenuous exercise, low-salt diet, fever or infection (which might affect electrolyte balance) or during acute mood swings (as lithium requirements may alter)
- caution if used in those who have undergone bariatric surgery. Lithium levels should be closely monitored until weight has stabilised to prevent lithium toxicity
- not recommended in those with Brugada syndrome because of an increased risk of ventricular arrhythmias
- contraindicated in those with cardiovascular or kidney disease, hypothyroidism or conditions associated with hyponatraemia (e.g. Addison's disease, dehydration, low-sodium diet)
- see also General Nursing considerations/Cautions for antipsychotics (p. 836)

Patient education

- the patient should be warned against driving a vehicle or operating machinery if drowsy or dizzy, especially in the first few weeks of therapy
- advise the patient not to take (or suddenly stop taking) over-the-counter NSAIDs without first consulting with their doctor
- the patient should be advised to seek medical attention immediately if any of the following occur:
  - vomiting, diarrhoea, dehydration, fever or infection (as this will increase risk of toxicity occurring)
  - excessive thirst or urination
  - signs or symptoms of toxicity including persistent nausea and vomiting, slurred speech, ataxia (clumsy movements), muscle twitching and seizures (fits)
- the patient, relatives and nurses must memorise or retain a written record of serious adverse effects/toxicity requiring immediate cessation of therapy
- instruct the patient to take with food to minimise nausea, and sustained-release tablets should be taken whole and not broken, crushed, chewed or taken with hot beverages
- ensure the patient has been given information regarding the importance of normal diet with adequate salt intake and a fluid intake of up to 3 L/day, especially if exercising strenuously, leading to increased sweating and therefore sodium loss. Salt intake should not suddenly be restricted
- advise the patient about the need to continue therapy usually for at least 6–9 months before the full benefits are seen
- abrupt changes to caffeine intake can alter lithium serum levels, especially if normal intake is greater than 4 cups of coffee (or caffeine equivalent) per day. The patient should therefore be warned not to eliminate caffeine from diet without first discussing with doctor
- advise the patient against driving or operating machinery if dazed feeling, poor coordination, drowsiness or vertigo occur
- the patient should be advised to avoid alcohol during therapy as drowsiness may be worsened

ANTIPSYCHOTIC AND MOOD-STABILISING AGENTS

- if the patient has pre-existing skin condition such as acne or psoriasis, they should be warned that it may worsen during therapy
- female patients should be counselled regarding avoiding pregnancy during therapy

Plain tablets can be crushed and mixed with water or a spoonful of yoghurt or apple puree.

Slow-release tablets should not be broken, crushed, chewed or taken with hot liquids.

Crosses the placental barrier and enters the fetal circulation, where it may cause thyroid disturbances and/or cardiovascular malformations. Serum lithium levels should be carefully monitored during pregnancy, but it is recommended that therapy be stopped before planning pregnancy.

Not recommended during breastfeeding to avoid infant becoming hypotonic, flaccid and difficult to feed. If the newborn is showing signs of lithium toxicity (e.g. flaccid appearance), fluid therapy should be started.

Caution if used in the elderly, as excretion may be reduced resulting in a longer half-life and increased risk of lithium toxicity.

Pregnant staff should not disperse or crush tablets.

LURASIDONE HYDROCHLORIDE

Trade names
APO-Lurasidone, Latuda, Lavione, Lurasidone Lupin, Lurasidone Sandoz, Lurasidone Sun, Lurisidone-WGR, Pharmcor Lurisidone

Available forms
Tablets: 40 mg, 80 mg

Action
- atypical antipsychotic
- benzisothiazol
- antagonises dopamine (D_2) and serotonin ($5HT_{2A}$) receptors

Use
- management of schizophrenia in adults and adolescents (13—17 years)

Dose
- initially 40 mg orally daily with food, increasing the dose if needed (daily maximum 160 mg (adults) or 80 mg (adolescents))

Adverse effects
- blurred vision
- hypertension, tachycardia
- rash, pruritus
- see also General Adverse effects of antipsychotics (p. 834)

Interactions
- contraindicated with clarithromycin, ritonavir, voriconazole, rifampicin, carbamazepine, phenytoin and St John's wort
- serum levels may be increased by grapefruit or grapefruit juice; therefore not recommended together
- caution if given with diltiazem

Nursing considerations/Cautions
- not recommended in those under 17 years
- not recommended in those with moderate-to-severe kidney or liver impairment
- see also General Nursing considerations/Cautions for antipsychotics (p. 836)

Patient education
- advise the patient not to use with grapefruit or grapefruit juice
- see also General Patient education for antipsychotics (p. 837)

Tablet can be crushed and mixed with water or a spoonful of yoghurt or apple puree.

Initial and daily dose reductions are recommended if used in those with kidney or liver impairment; however, a 20 mg tablet is not available in Australia.

OLANZAPINE
Trade names
APO-Olanzapine, APO-Olanzapine ODT, Noumed Olanzapine, Olanzapine ODT Generichealth, Olanzapine ODT WGR, Olanzapine RBX, Olanzapine Sandoz ODT, Olanzapine Sandoz, Olanzapine-DRLA, Ozin, Pryzex, Pryzex ODT, Zypine, Zypine ODT, Zyprexa, Zyprexa IM, Zyprexa Zydis Wafers

OLANZAPINE PAMOATE MONOHYDRATE
Trade name
Zyprexa Relprevv

Available forms
Tablets: 2.5 mg, 5 mg, 7.5 mg, 10 mg; Wafers (dissolvable/orally disintegrating tablets): 5 mg, 10 mg, 15 mg, 20 mg; Vial: 10 mg;
Vial (prolonged-release): 210 mg, 300 mg, 405 mg

Action
- atypical antipsychotic with mood-stabilising properties
- dopamine antagonist (affinity for D_1, D_2, D_3, D_4, D_5 receptors)
- also shows affinity for cholinergic, serotonergic, histaminic and alpha adrenergic receptors
- increases prolactin level
- half-life is about 33 hours. Half-life is prolonged and clearance is reduced in those > 65 years

Use
- schizophrenia, related psychoses
- schizophrenia maintenance in adults stabilised with oral olanzapine (prolonged-release injectable)
- acute mania associated with bipolar I disorder (alone or with lithium or sodium valproate) (short term)
- prevent recurrence of manic/depressive/mixed episodes associated with bipolar I disorder
- rapid control of agitation and/or disturbed behaviours in patients with schizophrenia or related psychoses where oral therapy is not appropriate
- rapid control in patients with acute mania associated with bipolar I disorder where oral therapy is not appropriate

Dose
- (Schizophrenia) initially 5—10 mg orally daily, increasing to 20 mg if necessary **OR**
- (Acute mania with bipolar disorder: monotherapy) 10—15 mg orally once daily, increasing dose if needed (daily maximum 20 mg) **OR**
- (Acute mania with bipolar disorder with lithium or sodium valproate) 10 mg orally daily, increasing dose if needed (daily maximum 20 mg) **OR**
- (Bipolar disorder prevention) initially 10 mg orally daily (or dose achieved in previous point), increasing dose if needed (range 5—20 mg) **OR**
- (Rapid control of agitation, disturbed behaviours or mania) 5—10 mg IM, followed by 10 mg IM after 2 hours if needed. A further 10 mg IM dose may be given 4 hours after the second injection if needed (maximum daily dose 30 mg)

Schizophrenia maintenance after stabilisation (long-acting formulation)
- (Previous oral dose 10 mg/day) initially 210 mg deep IM every 2 weeks or 405 mg deep IM every 4 weeks for 8 weeks, then 150 mg every 2 weeks or 300 mg every 4 weeks (maintenance) **OR**
- (Previous oral dose 15 mg/day) initially 300 mg deep IM every 2 weeks for 8 weeks, then 210 mg every 2 weeks or 405 mg every 4 weeks (maintenance) **OR**
- (Previous oral dose 20 mg/day) initially 300 mg deep IM every 2 weeks for 8 weeks, then 300 mg every 2 weeks (maintenance)

Adverse effects
- (IM) hypotension, peripheral oedema
- (IM, long-acting formulation) post-injection syndrome (including sedation, confusion, agitation, anxiety, dizziness, cognitive impairment, weakness, ataxia)

ANTIPSYCHOTIC AND MOOD-STABILISING AGENTS

- (Uncommon) secondary amenorrhoea, hypo-oestrogenism, drug reaction eosinophilia and systemic symptoms (DRESS)
- (IM, rare) injection site abscess
- see also General Adverse effects of antipsychotics (p. 834)

Interactions

- increased metabolism may result if taken with carbamazepine or if the patient is a smoker
- increased serum levels may occur if given with fluvoxamine or ciprofloxacin
- increased somnolence when IM olanzapine and IM lorazepam are given together
- see also General Interactions of antipsychotics (p. 835)

Nursing considerations/Cautions

- BP should be regularly monitored throughout therapy, especially if the patient is aged 65 years or over, or if IM dose is 30 mg/24 hours
- if secondary amenorrhoea occurs (lasting more than 6 months), bone loss can be prevented by using prophylactic treatment with bone- and calcium-regulating agents
- wafers are bioequivalent to tablets
- caution when choosing parental formulations: prolonged formulation and immediate formulation are for different uses
- parenteral administration is for short-term use only and oral administration should be recommenced as soon as practicable
- given IM only (not SC or IV)
- before starting maintenance therapy with prolonged formulation, patient tolerability should be determined on oral olanzapine
- (IM, maintenance therapy) the patient must be observed for 2 hours post-injection (including alertness monitored every 30 minutes) for any signs of post-injection syndrome (sedation and/or delirium related to olanzapine overdose). Observation period should be extended if any signs and symptoms occur. The patient should be released only if alert, oriented and free of any signs and symptoms of overdose
- (IM, maintenance therapy) gloves should be worn when reconstituting solution. If the solution makes contact with skin, it should be flushed with water immediately
- wafers contain aspartame; therefore caution if used in those with phenylketonuria
- (Vial 10 mg) should be reconstituted with water for Injections only and administered within 1 hour of reconstitution
- (Vial 10 mg) should not be combined in same syringe as haloperidol, as olanzapine will be degraded
- tablets contain lactose and are not recommended in those with rare hereditary problems of galactose intolerance, Lapp lactase deficiency or glucose—galactose malabsorption
- caution if used in those with diabetes, prostatic hypertrophy, glaucoma, paralytic ileus, kidney/liver impairment, elevated liver enzymes, bone marrow depression, history of or predisposition to seizures, myeloproliferative disorders, cardiovascular disease (with syncope, hypotension and/or bradycardia)
- (IM) contraindicated in those with hypersensitivity to polysorbate 80 or mannitol
- see also General Nursing considerations/Cautions for antipsychotics (p. 836)

Patient education

- the patient should be warned to remain recumbent after injection to avoid postural hypotension
- warn the patient that there is a 2-hour observation period required after

injection with prolonged formulation to monitor for adverse effects
- (IM for maintenance) the patient should be advised not to travel alone post-injection, nor drive or operate heavy machinery
- (IM for maintenance) instruct the patient (carer or family member) to immediately seek medical attention if confusion, irritability, excessive sleepiness, dizziness, disorientation, aggression, anxiety, weakness or difficulty talking or walking occurs
- the patient should be advised to seek medical attention if any rash, dermatitis, fever, chills, headache or enlarged lymph nodes occur
- instruct the patient that the wafer should not be handled directly as it is very fragile and should be placed on the tongue directly from the blister pack and allowed to dissolve, or can be dissolved in liquids (not cola beverages) if preferred
- female patients (premenopausal) should be advised to report any lack of menstruation that occurs for longer than 6 months
- see also General Patient education for antipsychotics (p. 837)

> Available as a wafer or oral disintegrating tablets which can be placed in the mouth and allowed to dissolve or dispersed in water, apple or orange juice, milk or coffee (but not cola). Tablet can be crushed and mixed with water or a spoonful of yoghurt or apple puree. Mask, gloves and glasses should be worn if dispersing or crushing tablets, as contact can cause contact dermatitis.

> Lower starting dose of 150 mg every 4 weeks (long-acting formulation) should be considered in those with kidney or liver impairment.

> Dose should be started at 5 mg orally, or 150 mg IM every 4 weeks (long-acting formulation) in those aged 65 years or more.

PALIPERIDONE

Trade names
Invega, Invega Hafyera, Invega Sustenna, Invega Trinza

Available forms
Tablets (prolonged-release): 3 mg, 6 mg, 9 mg;
Prefilled syringe: 25 mg, 50 mg, 75 mg, 100 mg, 150 mg, 175 mg/0.875 mL, 263 mg/1.315 mL, 350 mg/1.75 mL, 525 mg/2.625 mL, 700 mg/3.5 mL, 1000 mg/5 mL

Action
- benzisoxazole that is an active metabolite of risperidone
- binds to dopamine (D_2) and serotonin ($5HT_{2A}$) receptors
- also binds to other serotonin, histamine and alpha adrenergic receptors, producing moderately high sedation and antihypertensive properties but no antiemetic actions
- half-life 23 hours

Use
- acute and maintenance treatment of schizophrenia
- acute treatment of schizoaffective disorder (alone or in combination with antidepressants and/or lithium or sodium valproate)

Dose
- (Schizophrenia) 6 mg orally daily mane, adjusting dose to 3 or 9 mg after 5 days if needed (maximum daily dose 12 mg) **OR**
- (Schizophrenia) initially 150 mg IM (deltoid) (day 1), then 100 mg IM (deltoid) 7 days later (day 8), followed by 25–150 mg IM (deltoid or ventrogluteal) monthly (maintenance) (monthly formulation) **OR**
- (Schizophrenia) 3.5 times monthly IM dose (above) (first dose given within 7 days of monthly scheduled IM injection), then 3-monthly (dose range 175–525 mg) **OR**
- (Schizophrenia) if monthly IM dose was 100 mg, 700 mg IM (6-monthly formulation) can be given; if monthly IM dose

was 150 mg, 1000 mg IM (6-monthly formulation) should given. Administration with 6-monthly formulation should start when next monthly injection is due (6-monthly formulation) **OR**
- (Schizophrenia) if 3-monthly IM dose was 350 mg, 700 mg IM (6-monthly formulation) can be given; if 3-monthly IM dose was 525 mg, 1000 mg IM (6-monthly formulation) should given. Administration with 6-monthly formulation should start when next monthly injection is due (6-monthly formulation) **OR**
- (Acute exacerbation of schizoaffective disorder) initially 6 mg orally daily mane, increasing at 3 mg daily at 4-day intervals if needed (daily maximum 12 mg)

Adverse effects
- (IM) induration, pain, redness or swelling at injection site
- (IM, very rare) hypersensitivity
- see also General Adverse effects of antipsychotics (p. 834)

Interactions
- not recommended with risperidone (as paliperidone is its active metabolite)
- (Oral) absorption may be delayed if given with metoclopramide
- decreased serum levels may occur if given with carbamazepine
- increased risk of extrapyramidal symptoms if given with psychostimulants such as methylphenidate
- see also General Interactions of antipsychotics (p. 835)

Nursing considerations/Cautions
- tolerability should be established before starting IM paliperidone in those who have never previously used paliperidone (orally) or risperidone (orally or parentally)
- (3-monthly IM formulation) monthly IM formulation should be administered for at least 4 months (with last 2 doses being at the same dose) before switching to 3-monthly formulation
- (3-monthly IM formulation) dose response may not be apparent for several months and this should be taken into consideration if adjusting dose
- (6-monthly IM formulation) recommended for those who have been treated for at least 4 months with monthly IM formulation or at least one 3-month injecting cycle with 3-monthly IM formulation
- (6-monthly IM formulation) doses given 2 weeks before or up to 3 weeks after 6-month dose point are not considered a missed dose. For missed doses, manufacturer's information should be consulted, as the dosing schedule is dependent on previous dose and length of time since last injection
- if switching from monthly to 3-monthly IM dosing, the IM dose should be 3.5 times the monthly dose and administered when the next monthly dose was due, then 3-monthly
- if switching from 3-monthly to monthly IM dosage, the IM dose should be divided by 3.5 and administered 3 months after the last scheduled dose
- if switching from 3-monthly IM formulation to extended-release tablets, administration should start 3 months from the last IM injection, with the oral dose dependent on IM dose (daily dose range 3–12 mg). Manufacturer's information should be consulted
- if switching from 6-monthly to 3-monthly IM dosage, a 700 mg dose decreases to 350 mg dose, and a 1000 mg dose reduces to 525 mg dose, starting 6 months after the last 6-monthly dose, and then given 3-monthly
- if switching from 6-monthly to 1-monthly IM dosage, a 700 mg dose decreases to 100 mg dose, and a 1000 mg dose reduces to 150 mg dose, starting 6 months after the last 6-monthly dose, and then administered monthly
- if switching from 6-monthly IM formulation to extended-release tablets, administration should start 6 months from the last IM injection, with the oral dose dependent on IM dose (daily dose

- range 3—12 mg). Manufacturer's information should be consulted
- if changing from another long-acting injectable antipsychotic agent, therapy can be started at the next scheduled injection and continued monthly
- IM doses should not be divided but given as single IM injection
- given by deep IM only (gluteal or deltoid muscles only)
- injections should be alternated between two deltoid or gluteal muscles
- ensure the syringe is vigorously shaken (for at least 15 seconds) to mix the solution evenly before use within 5 minutes
- (Deltoid administration) a 23-gauge (1 inch) needle is recommended for patients weighing < 90 kg; if the patient weighs > 90 kg, a 22-gauge (1$\frac{1}{2}$ inch) is recommended
- (Gluteal administration) regardless of patient weight, a 22-gauge (1$\frac{1}{2}$ inch) needle is recommended
- (6-monthly formulation) IM administration is to gluteal muscle using a 20-gauge needle that has been provided. No other needle should be used. Future injections should alternate between gluteal muscles
- (6-monthly formulation) if incomplete administration occurs (e.g. needle clogging), the amount remaining in the syringe should not be administered, nor should another dose be given. The patient should be observed closely and oral paliperidone administered if needed until next scheduled 6-montly injection
- (6-monthly formulation) storage of cartons in horizontal position is recommended to improved ability to resuspend highly concentrated solution before use. Manufacturer's instructions should be followed regarding resuspension of solution before administration, as it requires longer and faster shaking than the monthly or 3-monthly formulations
- consult the manufacturer's information if IM doses are missed for the readministration schedule
- increased risk of neuroleptic malignant syndrome if given to those with Parkinson's disease or Lewy body dementia
- caution if used in those with severe liver impairment
- not recommended in those with pre-existing severe gastrointestinal narrowing or motility disorders because of an increased risk of obstruction due to non-conformable tablet coating
- not recommended in those with creatinine clearance < 10 mL/min
- contraindicated in those with hypersensitivity to risperidone
- see also General Nursing considerations/Cautions for antipsychotics (p. 836)

Patient education

- advise the patient to take tablets on an empty stomach or with food, and always take the same way (with or without food, not alternate between the two)
- instruct the patient to take whole (not broken, chewed or crushed) with fluids
- warn the patient that the outer coating of the capsule may appear in stools
- (IM) the patient should be advised to seek medical advice immediately if any fever, abnormally high body temperature, lightheadedness, dizziness or unusual heart rate (fast, slow, irregular) occurs
- see also General Patient education for antipsychotics (p. 837)

Prolonged-release tablets should not be broken, chewed or crushed.

For those with mild-to-moderate kidney impairment, the recommended initial dose is 3 mg orally daily, with increases based on clinical assessment and patient tolerability. For severe kidney impairment, a 3 mg dose should be administered second-daily, with increases to 3 mg orally daily being based on clinical assessment.

For older patients with impaired kidney function, dose adjustments should be based on kidney function.

PERICIAZINE (PERICYAZINE)
Trade name
Neulactil

Available form
Tablets: 2.5 mg, 10 mg

Action
* typical antipsychotic with greater sedating action, and higher antiemetic and anticholinergic properties than other antipsychotic phenothiazines

Use
* severe anxiety and tension
* psychoses (maintenance)

Dose
* (Mild-to-moderate) 15—30 mg orally daily in 2 divided doses, with a larger dose given in the evening **OR**
* (Moderate-to-severe hospitalised patient) 25—75 mg orally daily in 2 divided doses

Adverse effects
* photosensitivity
* see also General Adverse effects of antipsychotics (p. 834)

Interactions
* contraindicated with regional or spinal anaesthetics
* contraindicated with dopaminergic agents (except in patients with Parkinson's disease)
* caution if given with desferrioxamine because of the risk of transient metabolic encephalopathy
* see also General Interactions of antipsychotics (p. 835)

Nursing considerations/Cautions
* caution if used in those with intolerance or hypersensitivity to gluten
* see also General Nursing considerations/ Cautions for antipsychotics (p. 836)

Patient education
* instruct the patient to avoid direct sunlight during therapy, as photosensitivity may occur
* see also General Patient education for antipsychotics (p. 837)

Tablets can be dispersed in water, or crushed and mixed with a spoonful of yoghurt or apple puree. If crushing or dispersing tablets, gloves should be worn, as contact may cause contact dermatitis.

In the elderly, the recommended starting dose should be 10 mg daily in divided doses, increasing if needed to 30 mg daily maximum.

QUETIAPINE
Trade names
APX-Quetiapine, APX-Quetiapine XR, Blooms the Chemist Quetiapine, Delucon, Kaptan, Pharmacor Quetiapine, Quetia, Quetia XR, Quetiapine Sandoz, Quetiapine Sandoz XR, Quetiapine Sandoz Pharma, Quetiapine-DRLA, Quetiapine -WGR, Seroquel, Seroquel XR, Syquet, Tevatiapine XR

Available forms
Tablets: 25 mg, 100 mg, 200 mg, 300 mg; Tablets (modified-release): 50 mg, 150 mg, 200 mg, 300 mg, 400 mg

Action
* atypical antipsychotic agent with high affinity for serotonin ($5HT_2$) and dopamine (D_1 and D_2) receptors
* affinity also for histamine and alpha1 adrenergic receptors
* no antiemetic properties, some sedative and hypotensive properties, low anticholinergic actions
* active metabolite (norquetiapine) which has a half-life of 12 hours
* half-life 7 hours

Use
* schizophrenia
* treatment and maintenance of bipolar I disorder (monotherapy or with lithium or sodium valproate)
* treatment of depressive episodes associated with bipolar disorders

- treatment of acute mania associated with bipolar disorders (monotherapy or with lithium or sodium valproate)
- generalised anxiety disorder
- major depressive disorder (in patients intolerant to or who have had inadequate response to other therapies)

Dose

- (Schizophrenia) initially 50 mg orally (day 1), increasing to 100 mg daily (day 2), 200 mg daily (day 3) and 300 mg daily (day 4) given in 2 divided doses, and then adjusted according to clinical response (usual effective daily dose 300–450 mg) **OR**
- (Schizophrenia) initially 300 mg orally daily (day 1), then 600 mg (day 2) and up to 800 mg (range 400–800 mg daily) (modified-release tablets) **OR**
- (Acute mania in bipolar disorder) initially 100 mg orally (day 1), 200 mg (day 2), 300 mg (day 3), 400 mg (day 4), then increasing by increments not greater than 200 mg daily, up to 800 mg by day 6 if needed, given in 2 divided doses (alone or with lithium or sodium valproate) **OR**
- (Acute mania in bipolar disorder) initially 300 mg orally daily (day 1), then 600 mg (day 2) and up to 800 mg (alone or with lithium or sodium valproate) (modified-release tablets) **OR**
- (Bipolar depression) initially 50 mg orally at bedtime (day 1), then 100 mg (day 2), 200 mg (day 3) and 300 mg (day 4), then increasing at 100 mg daily increments to 600 mg if needed **OR**
- (Bipolar disorder maintenance) 300–800 mg orally daily in 2 divided doses (immediate-release tablets) or single daily dose (modified-release tablets) **OR**
- (Recurrent major depressive disorder) initially 50 mg orally nocte (day 1 and 2), increasing to 150 mg (day 3 and 4), then adjusting dose to clinical response (range 50–300 mg daily) (modified-release tablets) **OR**
- (Generalised anxiety disorder) initially 50 mg orally daily (day 1 and 2), increasing to 150 mg (day 3 and 4), then adjusting dose to clinical response (range 50–150 mg daily) (modified-release tablets)

Adverse effects

- constipation
- sedation
- dry mouth
- transient decrease in thyroid hormone levels
- (Rare) cardiomyopathy, myocarditis, pancreatitis, increased risk of dependence/tolerance
- see also General Adverse effects of antipsychotics (p. 834)

Interactions

- decreased serum levels may occur if given with phenytoin, carbamazepine, phenobarbital (phenobarbitone) or rifampicin
- increased serum levels may occur if given with azole antifungal agents, macrolide antibiotics or protease inhibitors
- not recommended with grapefruit juice, as increased serum levels may occur, increasing the risk of toxicity
- may increase serum levels of lorazepam
- not recommended with medications such as atomoxetine, dexamphetamine and methylphenidate used in the management of attention deficit hyperactivity disorder (ADHD)
- caution if used with other agents that slow intestinal motility because of the risk of constipation and intestinal obstruction
- may cause false positive results for methadone and tricyclic antidepressants (TCAs) in enzyme immunoassays
- see also General Interactions of antipsychotics (p. 835)

Nursing considerations/Cautions

- if switching from immediate-release to modified-release formulation, the dose is equivalent but given as a single daily dose (e.g. 300 mg twice daily immediate-release tablets = 600 mg daily dose of modified-release tablets)

- (Recurrent major depression disorder) if no clinical response after 6 weeks, therapy should be re-evaluated
- (Plain tablets) contain lactose and are not recommended in those with galactose intolerance, Lapp lactase deficiency or glucose—galactose malabsorption
- caution if used in those with a history of constipation or intestinal obstruction
- caution if used in those with a history of alcohol or drug abuse because of the risk of misuse or abuse
- see also General Nursing considerations/Cautions for antipsychotics (p. 836)

Patient education

- instruct the patient that modified-release tablets should be taken whole, not crushed, divided or chewed
- advise the patient that any somnolence usually resolves within the first few weeks of therapy
- the patient should be warned to avoid grapefruit juice during therapy
- the patient should be advised to report any rash or other skin reaction, especially blistering
- see also General Patient education for antipsychotics (p. 837)

 Plain tablets can be crushed and mixed with water or a spoonful of yoghurt or apple puree.

 Modified-release tablets should not be crushed.

 Caution if used in those with liver impairment. Recommended starting dose is 25 mg daily, increasing in 25—50 mg increments as needed and tolerated by the patient

 Caution in the elderly. A slower rate of dose titration and lower daily dose is recommended.

RISPERIDONE
Trade names
APO-Risperidone, Noumed Risperidone, Ozidal, Rispa, Risperdal, Risperdal Consta, Rispernia, Risvan, Rixadone

Available forms
Tablets: 0.5 mg, 1 mg, 2 mg, 3 mg, 4 mg;
Oral suspension: 1 mg/mL;
Vial: 25 mg, 37.5 mg, 50 mg;
Prefilled syringe: 75 mg, 100 mg

Action
- benzisoxazole atypical antipsychotic
- antagonises dopamine (D_2) and serotonin ($5HT_2$) receptors
- also weakly binds to alpha1 and alpha2 adrenergic and H_1 histamine receptors
- no antiemetic properties and moderate hypotensive action
- increases prolactin level
- active metabolite (paliperidone)

Use
- schizophrenia and related psychoses
- management of acute mania associated with bipolar I disorder (short term)
- treatment of behavioural disturbances (with dementia) (up to 12 weeks) (in those not responding to non-pharmacological management strategies)
- treatment of conduct/disruptive behaviour disorders in those with mental retardation or sub-average intellectual functioning (> 5 years)
- behavioural disorders associated with autism
- refractory bipolar I disorder as adjunct treatment with lithium or sodium valproate (4 relapses or more/12 months)
- monotherapy for prevention of recurrence of manic or mixed episodes of bipolar I (following stabilisation on oral risperidone)

Dose
- (Schizophrenia) initially 1 mg orally twice daily (day 1), increased to 2 mg

twice daily (day 2), then increasing gradually if needed (daily dose range 4—6 mg) **OR**
- (Bipolar mania) initially 2 mg orally daily, increasing by 1 mg increments at daily intervals if needed (daily dose range 2—6 mg) **OR**
- (Behavioural disturbance with dementia) initially 0.25 mg orally twice daily, increasing the dose by 0.25 mg increments twice daily every second day if needed **OR**
- (Conduct/disruptive behaviour disorders, body weight $\geq$ 50 kg) initially 0.5 mg orally daily, increasing by 0.5 mg increments every second day if needed (daily maximum 1.5 mg) **OR**
- (Conduct/disruptive behaviour disorders, body weight < 50 kg) initially 0.25 mg orally daily, increasing by 0.25 mg increments every second day if needed (daily maximum 0.75 mg) **OR**
- (Behaviour disorders associated with autism, body weight $\geq$ 20 kg) initially 0.5 mg orally daily (days 1—3), increasing to 1 mg (days 4—14). Clinical response should be assessed at day 14 and, if needed, may be increased at 0.5 mg increments at 2-week intervals (dose range 1—2.5 mg/day but higher dose will be required if body weight is > 45 kg) **OR**
- (Behaviour disorders associated with autism, body weight < 20 kg) initially 0.25 mg orally daily (days 1—3), increasing to 0.5 mg (days 4—14). Clinical response should be assessed at day 14 and, if needed, may be increased at 0.25 mg increments at 2-week intervals (dose range 0.5—1.5 mg/day) **OR**
- (Schizophrenia, refractory bipolar 1 disorder, prevention of manic/mixed episodes in bipolar I disorder) initially 25 mg IM 2-weekly, increasing to 37.5 or 50 mg at intervals of not less than 4 weeks if necessary (maximum dose 50 mg/2-weekly)

Adverse effects
- (Children) salivary hypersecretion, drooling
- rhinorrhoea, cough, nasal stuffiness, rhinitis, nasopharyngitis, dyspnoea, upper respiratory tract infection, sinusitis
- epistaxis
- rash, dry skin
- secondary amenorrhoea
- (IM) pain and, rarely, abscess, cellulitis, ulcer, haematoma or necrosis
- see also General Adverse effects of antipsychotics (p. 834)

Interactions
- carbamazepine and rifampicin may decrease plasma risperidone levels
- plasma levels may be increased if given with phenothiazines, tricyclic antidepressants (TCAs), protease inhibitors, itraconazole, paroxetine, fluoxetine and some beta adrenoceptor blocking agents
- not recommended with psychostimulants (e.g. methylphenidate) owing to an increased risk of extrapyramidal symptoms
- bioavailability may be reduced by topiramate
- increased hypotension may occur if given with antihypertensive agents or TCAs
- caution if given with furosemide (frusemide) (especially in the elderly with dementia) because of the increased risk of mortality
- see also General Interactions of antipsychotics (p. 835)

Nursing considerations/Cautions
- in those not previously treated, oral risperidone is recommended before starting parenteral formulation
- if switching from other antipsychotic agents, gradual discontinuation is recommended before starting risperidone. If the previous antipsychotic agent was administered as depot injection, risperidone should be started at the next scheduled injection
- in stable patients, the oral dose may be administered either daily or twice daily

ANTIPSYCHOTIC AND MOOD-STABILISING AGENTS

- during the first 3 weeks of therapy with slow-release IM preparation, oral therapy should be continued
- (IM) use diluent (in prefilled syringe) and needles provided for administration (drawing up and administration needle — for deltoid a 1-inch hypodermic needle, or for gluteal a 2-inch hypodermic needle is recommended)
- allow components to reach room temperature for 30 minutes before reconstituting
- follow the manufacturer's instructions for use of the safety device
- shake the reconstituted solution well before use to ensure powder is dissolved
- rotate injection sites (alternate gluteals or deltoids, depending on patient preference). Injection site should be inspected before injection and not used if any signs of inflammation exist
- not given IV
- dose increases should not occur more often than monthly
- if secondary amenorrhoea occurs (lasting more than 6 months), bone loss can be prevented by using prophylactic treatment with bone and calcium regulating agents
- when changing from other antipsychotics to risperidone, there should be a gradual discontinuance. If a depot injection has been previously used, risperidone should not be started until the next injection is due
- see also General Nursing considerations/Cautions for antipsychotics (p. 836)

Patient education

- the patient should be warned that it may take up to 3 weeks for a clinical response to increased dose to become apparent
- advise the patient that an oral suspension may be mixed with mineral water, orange juice, milk or coffee but not tea, cola or alcohol
- the patient should be instructed that the oral suspension comes with a calibrated pipette and instructions should be followed regarding its correct use, including rinsing after use before storage
- female patients of menstrual age should be advised to report any lack of menstruation for 6 months or more
- see also General Patient education for antipsychotics (p. 837)

Oral solution is available and can be mixed with mineral water, coffee, low-fat milk or orange juice (not cola-containing drinks, tea or alcoholic beverages).

Tablet can be dispersed in 2.5 mL water and then mixed with a spoonful of yoghurt or apple puree.

For those with kidney or liver impairment, a starting dose of 0.5 mg orally twice daily for 1 week, followed by either 1 mg orally twice daily or 2 mg orally daily for the 2nd week. If a 2 mg daily dose is well tolerated, 25 mg IM every 2 weeks can be administered.

A starting dose of 0.5 mg twice daily is recommended in elderly patients. The dose may then be individually adjusted in 0.5 mg twice-daily increments to 1—2 mg twice daily.

SODIUM VALPROATE
Trade names
APO-Sodium Valproate, Epilim, Epilim IV, Sodium Valproate Juno, Sodium Valproate Sandoz, Sodium Valproate Wockhardt, Valpro EC, Valproate Winthrop

Available forms
Tablets (sustained-release): 200 mg, 500 mg; Tablets (crushable): 100 mg; Suspension: 200 mg/5 mL; Vial: 400 mg

Action
- anticonvulsant, antipsychotic

- thought to raise brain levels of the inhibitory synaptic transmitter gamma aminobutyric acid (GABA), as well as blocking voltage-dependent sodium channels
- half-life 8—12 hours

Use
- mania (where other agents are ineffective or inappropriate)
- epilepsy (see Sodium valproate in Antiepileptics, p. 416)

Dose
- (Mania) initially 600 mg orally daily, increasing by 200 mg/day at 3-day intervals until control is reached (daily maximum 2500 mg) **OR**
- (Mania) up to 10 mg/kg by slow IV injection over 3-5 minutes, followed by 1—2 mg/kg/hour by IV infusion

Adverse effects/Nursing considerations/Cautions/Patient education
- IV administration is recommended for patients normally maintained on sodium valproate where oral therapy is temporarily not possible
- see also General Adverse effects/Nursing considerations/Cautions/Patient education of antiepileptics (p. 385)

Available as a syrup. Immediate-release (plain) tablets can be crushed and mixed with water, or a spoonful of yoghurt or apple puree.

Enteric-coated tablets should not be crushed.

Pregnant staff should not disperse or crush tablets.

ZIPRASIDONE
Trade names
Zeldox, Zeldox IM, Ziprasidone GH, Ziprox

Available forms
Capsules: 20 mg, 40 mg, 60 mg, 80 mg; Vial: 20 mg

Action
- indole derivative unrelated to phenothiazine or butyrophenone antipsychotics
- dopamine (D_2) and serotonin ($5HT_2$) antagonist
- also binds to alpha1 adrenergic and H_1 histamine receptors
- no antiemetic properties, low-to-moderative sedative and hypotensive actions
- half-life 6—10 hours

Use
- schizophrenia and related psychoses
- acute manic or mixed episodes associated with bipolar I disorder (monotherapy, short term)
- (IM) acute management of agitated/disturbed behaviour in schizophrenia and related psychoses where oral therapy is inappropriate (short term)

Dose
- (Schizophrenia, bipolar I disorder) initially 40 mg orally twice daily with food, then increasing at 2-day intervals if needed (daily maximum 160 mg) **OR**
- (Acute management of agitated/disturbed behaviour) 10 mg IM 2-hourly or 20 mg IM 4-hourly (daily maximum 40 mg) (up to 3 days)

Adverse effects
- rash, urticaria and, rarely, severe cutaneous reactions
- 'thick tongue' sensation
- (IM) dizziness, tachycardia, postural hypotension
- see also General Adverse effects of antipsychotics (p. 834)

Interactions
- decreased serum levels may occur if given with carbamazepine, rifampicin or St John's wort
- caution if given with lithium because of an increased risk of arrhythmias
- see also General Interactions of antipsychotics (p. 835)

ANTIPSYCHOTIC AND MOOD-STABILISING AGENTS

Nursing considerations/Cautions
- parenteral therapy should be replaced with oral therapy as soon as possible
- given only IM, not IV
- reconstitute using 1.2 mL water for injections
- not recommended in those under 18 years
- contraindicated in those with recent myocardial infarction (MI) or uncompensated heart failure
- see also General Nursing considerations/Cautions for antipsychotics (p. 836)

Patient education
- advise the patient to seek medical advice if any rash or urticaria develops
- the patient should be advised to swallow capsules whole, without crushing or chewing
- see also General Patient education for antipsychotics (p. 837)

Capsules can be opened and contents added to water and shaken gently for 2 minutes for even dispersion (gloves should be worn).

Pregnant staff should not open capsules.

A reduced dose is recommended in those with mild-to-moderate liver impairment.

ZUCLOPENTHIXOL
Trade name
Clopixol

ZUCLOPENTHIXOL ACETATE
Trade name
Clopixol Acuphase

ZUCLOPENTHIXOL DECANOATE
Trade name
Clopixol Depot

Available forms
Tablets: 10 mg;
Vial: 50 mg/mL, 100 mg/2 mL;
Vial (depot): 200 mg/mL

Action
- thioxanthene
- dopamine receptor (D_1 and D_2) antagonist
- increases serum prolactin levels
- weak anticholinergic properties, no antiemetic action, some sedative properties
- half-life 20 hours
- decanoate allows slow release from oily solution (coconut oil)

Use
- (Tablets) acute and chronic schizophrenia and other psychoses, manic phase of bipolar disorders
- (Acuphase injection) initial treatment of acute psychoses, mania, exacerbation of chronic psychoses
- (Depot) maintenance treatment

Dose
- (Acute schizophrenia, mania, acute agitation, acute psychoses) initially 10—20 mg orally daily, increasing by 10—20 mg every 2—3 days to 75 mg daily if needed **OR**
- (Chronic schizophrenia or psychoses) 20—40 mg orally at bedtime **OR**
- 50—150 mg IM repeated every 2—3 days if necessary (maximum dose 400 mg/course or 4 injections over maximum duration of 2 weeks) **OR**
- (Depot preparation) 200—400 mg IM every 2—4 weeks

Adverse effects
- increased bilirubin
- injection site reaction
- see also General Adverse effects of antipsychotics (p. 834)

Interactions
- may decrease effects of levodopa and adrenergic drugs
- increased risk of extrapyramidal symptoms if given with metoclopramide
- see also General Interactions of antipsychotics (p. 835)

HAVARD'S NURSING GUIDE TO DRUGS

Nursing considerations/Cautions

- dose stabilisation should occur under close medical supervision
- parenteral treatment should not exceed 2 weeks and is then maintained with either oral or depot medication
- sedation occurs up to 2 hours after injection, lasts about 8 hours and then decreases (parenteral)
- if the patient is receiving 100 mg IM, oral treatment is usually started at 40 mg daily as single or divided doses, which can then be increased if necessary
- changing from oral to IM depot formulation, oral daily dose × 8 = depot IM every 2—4 weeks, continuing oral medication at reduced dose for the first week after first depot injection
- if changing from parenteral to depot, the depot injection (200—400 mg) should be given with the last IM parenteral dose
- tablets contain lactose and are therefore not recommended in those with galactose intolerance, Lapp lactase deficiency or glucose—galactose malabsorption
- (Injections) should not be mixed with sesame seed-based formulations

- caution if used in those with severe arteriosclerosis
- contraindicated in those with hypersensitivity to coconut oil (injections) or thioxanthenes, as cross-sensitivity with phenothiazines may exist
- see also General Nursing considerations/Cautions for antipsychotics (p. 836)

Patient education

- the patient should be advised to report any sore throat, chills, fever or flu-like illness
- see also General Patient education for antipsychotics (p. 837)

 Tablet can be crushed and mixed with a spoonful of yoghurt or apple puree, but does not disperse readily in water.

 Half dose is recommended in those with kidney failure or compromised liver function.

 Reduced dose is recommended in elderly patients.

ANTIULCER AGENTS

The cells of the stomach secrete hydrochloric acid and intrinsic factor (from parietal cells), digestive enzymes (pepsinogen, gastric lipase) (from peptic cells), mucus and bicarbonate (from mucus-secreting cells). Hydrochloric acid performs a number of roles, including killing bacteria, denaturing protein and converting inactive pepsinogen to active pepsin, which further degrades protein. Mucus and bicarbonate form a gel-like protective layer, protecting the stomach from acid while also providing lubrication between undigested food and superficial cells. Intrinsic factor (from parietal cells) binds to vitamin B_{12} for absorption in the ileum (Knights et al 2023).

The parietal cells secrete 1–2 litres of hydrochloric acid daily, so it is vital that the mucosal barrier remains intact in order to prevent ulceration from occurring. Factors that impact on the mucosal barrier include blood flow changes, decreased mucus secretion, bacterial infection and damage by alcohol, aspirin, NSAIDs and other agents (Knights et al 2023). This breach in the gastric mucosa allows it to be further attacked, resulting in peptic ulcers (Del Valle 2022).

Peptic ulcers can be divided into duodenal or gastric (depending on their location) and share some common features, including epigastric pain (burning or gnawing) and cause (*Helicobacter pylori* (*H. pylori*) and NSAIDs) (Del Valle 2022):

- *duodenal ulcers* occur most commonly in the first part of the duodenum (within 3 cm of the pylorus) and are often silent, presenting only when complications arise. They are rarely malignant. Epigastric pain usually occurs 90 minutes to 3 hours after eating and is frequently relieved by antacids or food. Pain may wake a person from sleep, occurring in about two-thirds of patients
- *gastric ulcers* tend to occur later in life (peak incidence in the sixth decade), are more common in males and less common than duodenal ulcers. Gastric ulcers may be benign or malignant and should therefore be biopsied. Epigastric discomfort may be caused by food, with nausea, vomiting and weight loss as common symptoms.

Complications of both duodenal and gastric ulcers include bleeding, perforation and gastric outlet obstruction. Furthermore, *H. pylori* infection is associated with an increased risk of gastric cancer (Del Valle 2022; Shakir et al 2023).

Antiulcer agents may be used as either treatment or prophylaxis. Eradication of *H. pylori* and prevention of NSAID-induced disease is the mainstay of ulcer treatment. In Australia, recommended eradication treatment of *H. pylori* involves triple therapy (e.g. proton pump inhibitor, clarithromycin and amoxicillin), usually for 7 days, with alternate regimens available if the patient has a proven penicillin allergy. The outcome of the eradication therapy should be assessed not less than 4 weeks after completion, by either gastroscopy or urea breath test. In an ideal situation, the prior use of macrolides, presence of penicillin allergy and local prevalence of resistance patterns should be considered to guide therapy. Other international guidelines have advocated for quadruple therapy over the standard of clarithromycin-based therapy, given that clarithromycin-resistance rates are generally over the 15% threshold (Shakir et al 2023).

Some antiulcer agents act by either reducing gastric acid secretion or protecting the mucosa from the effects of acid. Reduction of gastric acid secretion occurs by blocking histamine (H_2) receptors (H_2-receptor antagonists) or by acting directly on the parietal cells (proton pump inhibitors). Some prostaglandins inhibit gastrin and gastric acid secretion, as well as protecting the mucosa (cytoprotective agents) (Del Valle 2022). Antacids are generally used to relieve symptoms of dyspepsia and are discussed at the end of this section.

HISTAMINE H_2-RECEPTOR ANTAGONISTS

General Actions of H_2-receptor antagonists
- reduce gastric acid secretion by competitively blocking the action of histamine at histamine H_2-receptor sites of parietal cells, thereby reducing hydrochloric acid
- inhibit both daytime and nocturnal basal (non-stimulated) gastric acid secretion
- inhibit stimulated gastric acid secretion by food, histamine, coffee, insulin and pentagastrin
- cross-sensitivity may exist between members of the histamine H_2-receptor antagonists

General Uses of H_2-receptor antagonists
- treatment and maintenance of gastric and duodenal ulcers (short-term therapy)
- maintenance therapy for chronic benign gastric or duodenal ulcers (up to 12 months)
- persistent gastro-oesophageal reflux disease (commonly known as GORD) (up to 12 months)
- short-term management of heartburn and other GORD symptoms (12 weeks)
- gastrinoma (Zollinger–Ellison syndrome)
- scleroderma oesophagitis (short-term therapy)
- erosive and ulcerative oesophagitis

General Nursing considerations/Cautions for H_2-receptor antagonists
- before starting therapy, any unintentional loss of weight, recurrent vomiting, dysphagia, haematemesis, anaemia, melaena or malignancy should be investigated. It is also recommended that those with ulceration be re-endoscoped 8–12 weeks after starting

ANTIULCER AGENTS

therapy to determine whether the ulcer is healing
- treatment for GORD and associated reflux symptoms should be started only after conservative measures and antacids are unsuccessful
- may increase the risk of developing community-acquired pneumonia in the elderly, those with diabetes or chronic lung disease, or the immunocompromised
- caution when used in those in intensive care units because agents which suppress acid secretion have been associated with nosocomial lung infections
- caution in those with kidney impairment
- contraindicated in those with hypersensitivity to other H_2-receptor antagonists

General Patient education for H_2-receptor antagonists

- the patient should be encouraged to continue treatment for 4—6 weeks, after which a maintenance dose may be prescribed
- antacids may be required for symptomatic relief but should be taken 1 hour apart
- the patient should be advised against driving or operating machinery if drowsiness or dizziness occurs
- the patient should be counselled to:
  - stop (or reduce) smoking
  - limit daily caffeine (coffee, tea, cola, chocolate, cocoa) and alcohol intake
  - if possible, reduce intake of aspirin and other NSAIDs
  - eat small and frequent meals, ensuring meals are eaten slowly

 Not recommended during pregnancy unless the expected benefit outweighs any potential risk.

 Not recommended during breastfeeding unless the expected benefit outweighs any potential risk.

FAMOTIDINE
Trade name
Ausfam

Available form
Tablets: 20 mg, 40 mg

Action
- peak activity 1—3 hours, half-life 2.5—5 hours
- duration of action 10—12 hours
- see also General Actions of H_2-receptor antagonists (p. 872)

Use
- see General Uses of H_2-receptor antagonists (p. 872)

Dose
- (Treatment: duodenal ulcer, benign gastric ulcer) 40 mg orally at night **OR**
- (Maintenance: duodenal ulcer) 20 mg orally at night for up to 12 months **OR**
- (Zollinger—Ellison syndrome) initially 20 mg orally 6-hourly, then dose adjusted and treatment continued, according to clinical need **OR**
- (Treatment and maintenance of GORD) 20 mg orally twice daily

Adverse effects
- headache, dizziness
- constipation, diarrhoea

Nursing considerations/Cautions

- (Duodenal and gastric ulcers) treatment is continued for 4—8 weeks, but duration may be shortened if endoscopy reveals that the ulcer has healed
- see also General Nursing considerations/Cautions for H_2-receptor antagonists (p. 872)

873

Patient education

- see General Patient education for H_2-receptor antagonists (p. 873)

Can be crushed and mixed with water, or given with a spoonful of yoghurt or apple puree.

Not recommended for use in pregnancy and should be prescribed only if clearly needed; weigh the potential benefits from the drug against the possible risks involved.

Breastfeeding women should either stop this drug or stop breastfeeding.

Dosage should be reduced in patients with moderate or severe renal insufficiency.

In elderly patients with decreased renal function, the clearance of the drug may be decreased.

NIZATIDINE

Trade name
Nizac, Tacidine, Tazac

Available form
Capsules: 150 mg, 300 mg

Action
- peak activity 0.5—3 hours, half-life 1—2 hours
- duration of action up to 12 hours
- see also General Actions of H_2-receptor antagonists (p. 872)

Use
- see General Uses of H_2-receptor antagonists (p. 872)

Dose
- (Active duodenal ulcer, benign gastric ulcer, GORD) 150 mg orally twice daily or 300 mg once daily in the evening **OR**
- (Benign gastric ulcer, active duodenal ulcer) 300 mg orally at night or 300 mg once daily in the evening **OR**
- (Maintenance: duodenal ulcer) 150 mg orally at night (for up to 12 months)

Adverse effects
- anaemia, hyperuricaemia
- urticaria, sweating, rash, pruritus
- elevated liver enzymes
- (Rare) reversible confusion, hepatitis, jaundice, impotence, gynaecomastia, fever, eosinophilia, nausea

Interactions
- may increase serum salicylate levels if given with very high doses of aspirin
- may cause false positive test for urobilinogen using Multistix
- nizatidine and other histamine H_2-receptor antagonists can reduce the gastric absorption of drugs whose absorption is dependent on an acidic gastric pH

Nursing considerations/Cautions

- not recommended in those with liver failure
- see also General Nursing considerations/Cautions for H_2-receptor antagonists (p. 872)

Patient education

- advise the patient to immediately seek medical advice if any of the following occur:
  - (men) breast enlargement and impotence
  - yellowing of skin and eyes, loss of appetite, nausea, vomiting, upper abdominal pain, dark urine, pale stools
  - confusion
- see also General Patient education for H_2-receptor antagonists (p. 873)

Capsules can be opened and dispersed in 120 mL water (not apple juice), or contents mixed with yoghurt.

Nizatidine should be used during pregnancy only if the potential benefit justifies the potential risk to the fetus.

In breastfeeding, take into account the importance of the drug to the mother.

ANTIULCER AGENTS

 Not recommended in liver failure.

RANITIDINE HYDROCHLORIDE
Trade names
Chemists' Own Ranitidine, Zantac 150 OTC, Zantac Double Strength, Zantac

Available forms
Tablets: 150 mg, 300 mg

Action
- peak activity 1—3 hours, half-life 1—3 hours
- duration of action up to 4 hours (basal), 13 hours (nocturnal)
- see also General Actions of H_2-receptor antagonists (p. 872)

Use
- see General Uses of H_2-receptor antagonists (p. 872)

Dose
- (Acute treatment: duodenal/gastric ulceration) 300 mg orally at night or 150 mg orally twice daily initially for 4—8 weeks **OR**
- (Maintenance: duodenal/gastric ulceration) 150 mg orally at night **OR**
- (Zollinger—Ellison syndrome) initially 150 mg orally 3 times daily, increasing as necessary to 600—900 mg/day **OR**
- (Oesophagitis: treatment) 300 mg orally at night or 150 mg orally twice daily **OR**
- (Oesophagitis: maintenance) 150 mg orally twice daily (morning and bedtime)

Adverse effects
- headache
- constipation, diarrhoea, nausea, vomiting, abdominal discomfort
- reversible changes in liver function
- rash
- (Rare) reversible confusion, impotence, blurred vision, dizziness, porphyria, hepatitis, jaundice

Interactions
- antacids and high-dose sucralfate (2 g) significantly reduce absorption of ranitidine
- may increase absorption of triazolam, midazolam and glipizide
- may decrease absorption of atazanavir and gefitinib
- prothrombin time should be closely monitored if given with warfarin

Nursing considerations/Cautions
- not recommended in those with porphyria
- see also General Nursing considerations/Cautions for H_2-receptor antagonists (p. 872)

Patient education
- advise the patient to immediately seek medical advice if any of the following occur:
  - (men) breast enlargement (gynaecomastia) and impotence
  - yellowing of skin and eyes, loss of appetite, nausea, vomiting, upper abdominal pain, dark urine, pale stools
  - confusion
  - change in heart rate
- advise the patient that tablets should not be taken with antacids or sucralfate; separate them by at least 2 hours
- see also General Patient education for H_2-receptor antagonists (p. 873)

 The safety of ranitidine in pregnancy has not been established. It should be used during pregnancy only if considered essential, and likewise for nursing mothers.

 Secreted in breastmilk; therefore should be used during breastfeeding only if considered necessary.

 In the elderly, or persons with chronic lung disease, diabetes or the immunocompromised, there may be an increased risk of developing community-acquired pneumonia.

PROTON PUMP INHIBITORS

General Actions of proton pump inhibitors
- reduce gastric acid secretion by inhibiting the enzyme H^+/K^+ATPase (the proton pump) in the parietal cells

- converted to the active form by a high concentration of acid

General Uses of proton pump inhibitors

- treatment of benign gastric and duodenal ulcers
- symptomatic relief of gastro-oesophageal reflux disease (GORD), including treatment and prevention of erosive reflux oesophagitis
- prevention of rebleeding of acute, bleeding gastric or duodenal ulcers after IV treatment
- gastrinoma (Zollinger—Ellison syndrome)
- *Helicobacter pylori* eradication therapy (in combination with antibiotics)
- prophylaxis or treatment of gastric/duodenal ulcers associated with NSAIDs

General Interactions of proton pump inhibitors

- contraindicated with atazanavir, nelfinavir
- may increase absorption of digoxin
- INR/prothrombin time should be monitored if given with warfarin, especially when starting or stopping therapy or changing dose
- may decrease absorption of iron, ampicillin, erlotinib, posaconazole or itraconazole and should therefore be separated from these agents by 2—3 hours to improve absorption
- may increase serum levels of methotrexate (high dose), increasing the risk of adverse effects and toxicity
- caution if used with mycophenolate mofetil in transplant patients
- (Prolonged therapy) caution if used with agents (e.g. diuretics) that cause hypomagnesaemia

General Nursing considerations/Cautions for proton pump inhibitors

- before starting therapy, any unintentional loss of weight, recurrent vomiting, dysphagia, haematemesis, anaemia, melaena or malignancy should be investigated. It is also recommended that those with ulceration be re-endoscoped 8—12 weeks after starting therapy to determine whether the ulcer is healing
- IV therapy is recommended only for short-term therapy where oral administration is not appropriate
- serum magnesium levels should be monitored before starting and then regularly if therapy is expected to be prolonged or if given with agents that can reduce magnesium levels (e.g. diuretics)
- use of proton pump inhibitors increases the risk of fundi gland polyps developing, which increases the chance of GI bleeding or intestinal blockage if large or ulcerated
- an increased risk of GI infection by *Salmonella*, *Campylobacter* and *C. difficile* (in a hospitalised patient); therefore patients should be closely monitored during therapy
- caution if used in those at risk of osteoporosis and bone fracture
- caution if used in those with impaired liver function, as there can be increased availability, decreased plasma clearance and prolonged elimination half-life
- contraindicated in those with hypersensitivity to other proton pump inhibitors

General Patient education for proton pump inhibitors

- the patient should be encouraged to continue treatment for a recommended time (depending on the condition), after which the dose should be stepped down and a maintenance dose may be prescribed
- advise the patient to seek medical advice if symptoms return
- antacids may be required for symptomatic relief, but should be taken 1 hour apart
- the patient should be advised against driving or operating machinery if drowsiness or dizziness occurs
- instruct the patient to immediately seek medical advice if any of the following occur:

ANTIULCER AGENTS

- dizziness, rapid heart rate, confusion, fatigue or tetany (tingling around mouth, hands and feet increasing in intensity, followed by spasm of facial, hand and feet muscles) (signs of hypomagnesaemia)
- lesions appearing on sun-exposed areas of the skin with joint pain
- the patient should be counselled to:
  - stop (or reduce) smoking
  - limit daily caffeine (coffee, tea, cola, chocolate, cocoa) intake
  - if possible, reduce intake of aspirin and other NSAIDs
  - eat small and frequent meals
  - reduce weight
  - assess ongoing use of proton pump inhibitors regularly; if symptoms are well controlled (after at least 4—8 weeks of treatment), consider:stopping treatment (unless the patient has severe oesophagitis or complicated disease, e.g. Barrett's, high risk of GI bleeding)

 Not recommended during pregnancy.

 Not recommended during breastfeeding.

ESOMEPRAZOLE
Trade names
APO-Esomeprazole, Esomeprazole AN, Chemists' Own Heart Burn Relief, Esomeprazole GH, Esomeprazole RBX, Esomeprazole Sun, Esomeprazole Viatris, Esomeprazole-WGR, Guardium Acid Relief, Mepreze, Noumed Esomeprazole, Pharmacy Action 24 Hour Once Daily Heartburn Relief, Zanzole, Esopreze, Nexium, Nexole, Noxicid Caps

Available forms
Vial: 42.5 mg (equivalent 40 mg);
Capsules: 20 mg, 40 mg;
Tablets: 20 mg, 40 mg;
Granules: 10 mg

Action
- half-life about 1 hour
- see also General Actions of proton pump inhibitors (p. 875)

Use
- see General Uses of proton pump inhibitors (p. 876)

Dose
- (GORD with oesophagitis) 40 mg orally or IV daily for 4 weeks; may be repeated for a further 4 weeks for patients who have persistent symptoms or if oesophagitis has not healed **OR**
- (Healed oesophagitis maintenance) 20 mg orally or IV daily **OR**
- (GORD without oesophagitis) 20 mg orally daily for 4 weeks, then 20 mg orally daily when needed **OR**
- (Zollinger—Ellison syndrome) 40 mg orally twice daily, increasing dose if needed **OR**
- (Patients requiring NSAIDs) 20 mg orally daily for up to 4 weeks when starting NSAIDs **OR**
- (Healing of gastric ulceration associated with NSAIDs) 20 mg orally daily for up to 8 weeks **OR**
- (Prevention of gastric/duodenal ulcers associated with NSAIDs) 20 mg orally daily for up to 6 months **OR**
- (Prevention of rebleeding of gastric/duodenal ulcer) 80 mg IV over 30 minutes, followed by 8 mg/hour by IV infusion for 3 days **OR**
- (Prevention of rebleeding of gastric/duodenal ulcer) 40 mg orally daily **OR**
- (*Helicobacter pylori* eradication) 20 mg orally twice daily for 7 days with appropriate antibiotics

Adverse effects
- headache, dizziness
- diarrhoea, flatulence, abdominal pain, nausea, vomiting, constipation, fundic gland polyps

- (Uncommon) dermatitis, pruritus, urticaria, rash, elevated liver enzymes, peripheral oedema
- IV site reaction
- (Prolonged therapy) vitamin B_{12} deficiency
- (Rare) interstitial nephritis, hypomagnesaemia, increased risk of osteoporosis and bone fracture, blood dyscrasias, subacute cutaneous lupus erythematosus

Interactions
- may increase serum levels of phenytoin, citalopram, imipramine, clomipramine, tacrolimus or diazepam
- decreased serum levels may occur if given with St John's wort
- not recommended with clopidogrel
- may interfere with chromogranin A (CgA) estimation for neuroendocrine tumours and should be stopped 5—14 days before measurement
- see also General Interactions of proton pump inhibitors (p. 876)

Nursing considerations/Cautions
- IV therapy is recommended only when oral therapy is inappropriate. Can be continued for up to 10 days, but should be replaced by oral therapy as soon as practicable
- reconstitute with 5 mL sodium chloride 0.9% only and further dilute with 50—100 mL sodium chloride 0.9% for IV infusion administration
- given IV either over 3 minutes or by infusion over 10—30 minutes
- administer alone IV
- see also General Nursing considerations/Cautions for proton pump inhibitors (p. 876)

Patient education
- the patient should be advised to swallow tablets or capsules whole (do not crush or chew); however, if the patient is unable to swallow, tablets and contents of capsules can be dispersed in water only (non-carbonated) and drunk within 30 minutes
- instruct the patient that granules should be used in those with swallowing difficulty or for children. Instructions for using granules should include:
  - disperse granules in non-carbonated water (15 mL for 10 g (1 sachet) or 30 mL for 20 g (2 sachets))
  - contents should be stirred and allowed to thicken
  - stir again and drink within 30 minutes
  - if anything remains, glass should be rinsed and contents swallowed
  - can also be administered via gastric or nasogastric tube after dispersing granules as above. The tube should be flushed well after administration
  - advise the patient that granules should not be chewed or crushed
- see also General Patient education for proton pump inhibitors (p. 876)

 Contents of capsules can be dispersed in water only (non-carbonated) and drunk within 30 minutes.

 Do not crush or chew tablets.

 Esomeprazole should be given to pregnant women only if its use is considered essential.

 No studies in lactating women have been performed; and esomeprazole should not be used during breastfeeding.

Available in combination with
- Esomeprazole 20 mg enteric coated tablets are also available in a combination pack containing: esomeprazole magnesium trihydrate 20 mg, amoxicillin trihydrate 500 mg, clarithromycin 500 mg (Nexium Hp7, Esomeprazole Sandoz Hp7 Combination)

ANTIULCER AGENTS

LANSOPRAZOLE
Trade names
Lanzopran, Zopral, Zopral ODT, Zoton FasTabs, APO-Lansoprazole, APO-Lansoprazole ODT, Lansoprazole ODT GH, Noumed Lansoprazole,

Available forms
Capsules: 15 mg, 30 mg;
Tablets (oral disintegrating): 15 mg, 30 mg

Action/Use
- see General Actions and Uses of proton pump inhibitors (p. 875)

Dose
- (Reflux oesophagitis) 30 mg orally in the morning before food for 4—8 weeks, then 15—30 mg daily (maintenance) **OR**
- (Gastric ulcer) 30 mg orally in the morning before food for 8 weeks **OR**
- (Duodenal ulcer) 30 mg orally in the morning before food for 4 weeks, then 15 mg daily (maintenance) **OR**
- (Acid-related dyspepsia) 15—30 mg orally in the morning before food for 2—4 weeks **OR**
- (*Helicobacter pylori* eradication) 30 mg orally twice daily before food (with appropriate antibiotics; two of the following antibiotics: amoxicillin 1 g twice daily, metronidazole 400 mg twice daily or clarithromycin 250 mg twice daily)

Adverse effects
- headache, dizziness, fatigue, malaise
- depression, confusion, hallucinations
- diarrhoea, abdominal pain, nausea, vomiting, dyspepsia, constipation, flatulence, dry/sore mouth/throat, fundic gland polyps
- rash, urticaria, pruritus
- altered liver enzymes
- (Prolonged therapy) vitamin B_{12} deficiency
- (Rare) interstitial nephritis, hypomagnesaemia, increased risk of osteoporosis and bone fracture, subacute cutaneous lupus erythematosus, blood dyscrasias

Interactions
- caution if given with theophylline, phenytoin or carbamazepine
- absorption decreased by antacids and sucralfate, and should be separated by at least 1 hour
- serum levels may be increased by fluvoxamine
- serum levels may be decreased by St John's wort
- may increase serum levels of tacrolimus
- may decrease serum levels of posaconazole, levothyroxine and liothyronine
- see also General Interactions of proton pump inhibitors (p. 876)

Nursing considerations/Cautions
- not recommended in those with fructose intolerance, glucose—galactose malabsorption or sucrase—isomaltase insufficiency
- contraindicated in those with severe liver impairment
- see also General Nursing considerations/Cautions for proton pump inhibitors (p. 876)

Patient education
- instruct the patient that capsules are enteric coated and should not be chewed or crushed. Capsules may be opened and contents sprinkled on a tablespoon of yoghurt, cottage cheese, apple sauce or strained pears or in fluid (e.g. apple, orange or tomato juice) and swallowed immediately. If fluids are used, the patient should be advised to rinse the glass with a small amount of same fluid and contents swallowed to ensure the full dose is taken
- if the patient has a gastric or nasogastric tube in situ, capsule contents can be sprinkled in 40 mL apple juice (no other fluids) and administered via tube, followed by a flush with apple juice to ensure the full dose is administered
- advise the patient that an orally disintegrating tablet should be placed on the

tongue and gently sucked or swallowed (but not chewed) whole with water
- see also General Patient education for proton pump inhibitors (p. 876)

Capsules are enteric coated and should not be chewed or crushed. Capsules may be opened and the contents sprinkled on a tablespoon of yoghurt, apple sauce or strained pears or in fluid.

Lansoprazole should not be used during pregnancy, unless the benefit clearly outweighs the potential risk to the fetus.

Use in breastfeeding should be avoided.

OMEPRAZOLE

Trade names
Acimax, Losec, Maxor, Maxor Heartburn Relief, Omepral, Ozmep, Pemzo, Probitor, Omeprazole Sandoz, Pharmcor Omeprazole, Omeprazole ADVZ, Omeprazole Caps WGR

Available forms
Vial: 40 mg;
Tablets: 10 mg, 20 mg;
Capsules: 20 mg;
Powder for oral suspension: 2 mg/mL, 4 mg/mL

Action
- onset of action within 60 minutes, peak effect 2 hours, duration of action 3–5 days, half-life 30 minutes
- see also General Actions of proton pump inhibitors (p. 875)

Use
- see General Uses of proton pump inhibitors (p. 876)

Dose
- (Duodenal/gastric ulcer, ulcerative reflux oesophagitis) 40 mg IV over 20–30 minutes once daily **OR**
- (Zollinger–Ellison syndrome) initially 60 mg IV over 20–30 minutes once daily, increasing as needed. Doses greater than 120 mg IV should be given in divided doses **OR**
- (Zollinger–Ellison syndrome) 60 mg orally once daily, adjusting the dose as necessary **OR**
- (Gastro-oesophageal reflux disease (GORD)) 10–20 mg orally daily for a maximum of 4 weeks **OR**
- (Erosive oesophagitis) 20 mg orally daily for 4–8 weeks, then 10–20 mg daily (maintenance therapy) **OR**
- (Erosive oesophagitis refractory to treatment) 40 mg orally daily for 8 weeks **OR**
- (Duodenal/gastric ulcer) 20 mg orally daily for 4–8 weeks, then 10–20 mg daily as maintenance therapy **OR**
- (NSAID-associated ulceration) 20–40 mg orally daily for 4–8 weeks, then 20 mg orally daily as maintenance **OR**
- (*Helicobacter pylori* eradication) 40 mg orally daily, or 20 mg orally twice daily (with appropriate antibiotics)

Adverse effects
- nausea, vomiting, diarrhoea, constipation, flatulence, abdominal pain, fundic gland polyps
- headache, drowsiness, somnolence, insomnia
- (Prolonged therapy) vitamin B_{12} deficiency
- (Rare) interstitial nephritis, hypomagnesaemia, increased risk of osteoporosis and bone fracture, subacute cutaneous lupus erythematosus

Interactions
- may increase serum levels of diazepam, tacrolimus, carbamazepine or phenytoin, increasing the risk of adverse effects including toxicity
- not recommended with St John's wort, as serum levels may be decreased
- not recommended with clopidogrel
- caution if given with digoxin
- not recommended with posaconazole or erlotinib
- serum levels increased by fluvoxamine, voriconazole and clarithromycin

ANTIULCER AGENTS

- contraindicated as combination therapy for *H. pylori* eradication with clarithromycin in those with liver impairment
- may interfere with chromogranin A (CgA) estimation for neuroendocrine tumours and should be stopped 5–14 days before measurement
- see also General Interactions of proton pump inhibitors (p. 876)

Nursing considerations/Cautions
- IV therapy is recommended only in severely ill patients and oral therapy should be resumed as soon as practicable
- if IV therapy is required for > 5 days, the daily dose should be reduced
- (Zollinger–Ellison syndrome) if more than 80 mg orally daily, give in divided doses
- reconstitute powder using 100 mL sodium chloride 0.9% or glucose 5%
- see also General Nursing considerations/Cautions for proton pump inhibitors (p. 876)

Patient education
- advise the patient that tablets and capsules should be swallowed whole with water, not chewed or crushed
- if the patient has difficulty swallowing, tablets can be stirred in non-carbonated water or fruit juice until the pellets are released and then drunk without chewing or crushing the pellets. The glass should be rinsed and drunk to ensure all the pellets have been taken
- see also General Patient education for proton pump inhibitors (p. 876)

If the patient has difficulty swallowing, tablets can be stirred in non-carbonated water or fruit juice until pellets are released and then drunk without chewing or crushing pellets.

Omeprazole use, in pregnancy, in epidemiological studies indicated a higher incidence of cardiac defects compared with controls (more human data required).

It is recommended that omeprazole not be used in nursing mothers.

PANTOPRAZOLE
Trade names
I-Pantoprazole, Ozpan, Panthron, Salpraz, Somac, Somac Injection, Sozol, Topra, Torzole

Available forms
Vial: 40 mg;
Tablets (enteric-coated): 20 mg, 40 mg;
Granules: 40 mg/sachet

Action
- half-life about 1 hour
- see also General Actions of proton pump inhibitors (p. 875)

Use
- see General Uses of proton pump inhibitors (p. 876)

Dose
- (Duodenal ulcer) 40 mg orally or IV daily for 2–4 weeks **OR**
- (Gastric ulcer) 40 mg orally or IV daily for 4–8 weeks **OR**
- (Gastro-oesophageal reflux disease (GORD) – symptomatic relief) 20 mg orally for 4 weeks **OR**
- (GORD – healed reflux oesophagitis maintenance) 20–40 mg orally daily **OR**
- (GORD – treatment of reflux oesophagitis) 20–40 mg orally daily for 4–8 weeks **OR**
- (Lesions refractory to H_2-receptor antagonists) 40 mg orally or IV daily for 4–12 weeks **OR**
- (Prophylaxis of gastroduodenal ulceration in patients taking NSAIDs) 20 mg orally daily **OR**
- (Zollinger–Ellison syndrome) 40 mg orally or IV daily **OR**
- (*Helicobacter pylori* eradication) 40 mg orally twice daily (with appropriate antibiotics)

Adverse effects
- pruritus, rash
- headache, dizziness, fatigue, asthenia
- sweating
- diarrhoea, constipation, flatulence, dry mouth, metallic taste, upper abdominal pain, nausea, vomiting, fundic gland polyps
- (Prolonged therapy) vitamin B_{12} deficiency
- (Rare) interstitial nephritis, hypomagnesaemia, increased risk of osteoporosis and bone fracture, subacute cutaneous lupus erythematosus
- (IV) thrombophlebitis

Interactions
- may increase serum levels of tacrolimus, increasing the risk of toxicity
- may decrease the effects of levothyroxine and liothyronine
- caution if given with fluvoxamine
- see also General Interactions of proton pump inhibitors (p. 876)

Nursing considerations/Cautions
- (Zollinger—Ellison syndrome) the dose should be individually assessed to maintain acid output below 10 mmol/L
- IV therapy should be replaced by oral administration as soon as practicable
- reconstitute the powder using 10 mL sodium chloride 0.9% and then further dilute to 100 mL using sodium chloride 0.9% or glucose 5% or 10%, and then infused over 2—15 minutes
- contraindicated in those with cirrhosis or severe liver disease
- see also General Nursing considerations/Cautions for proton pump inhibitors (p. 876)

Patient education
- the patient should be advised to swallow tablets whole (not chewed or crushed) with a little water before or during breakfast
- (Granules) the patient should be instructed to mix granules with 15—30 mL water, apple or orange juice or apple sauce and drink immediately. The glass should be rinsed and contents swallowed to ensure the entire dose is taken. If the patient has a gastric or nasogastric tube, granules should be emptied into a catheter-tipped syringe connected to the tube, followed by 5 mL of apple or orange (pulp-free) juice or water. The tube should be flushed with water to ensure the full dose has been administered
- see also General Patient education for proton pump inhibitors (p. 876)

 Patients should be advised to swallow tablets whole (not chewed or crushed) with a little water.

 Should be used during pregnancy only if benefits outweigh risks.

 Thought to be excreted in breastmilk; therefore not recommended during breast-feeding unless benefits outweigh risks.

RABEPRAZOLE SODIUM
Trade names
APO-Rabeprazole, Parbezol, Pariet, Razit, Zabep, Noumed Rabeprazole, Rabeprazole Mylan, Rabeprazole Sandoz, Rabeprazole-WGR

Available form
Tablets: 10 mg, 20 mg

Action
- acid suppression starts within 1 hour of administration, maximum effect within 2—4 hours
- see also General Actions of proton pump inhibitors (p. 875)

Use
- see General Uses of proton pump inhibitors (p. 876)

Dose
- (Active gastro-oesophageal reflux disease (GORD)) 20 mg orally daily for 4—8 weeks **OR**

ANTIULCER AGENTS

- (Prevention of GORD relapse) 10—20 mg orally daily **OR**
- (Symptomatic treatment of GORD without oesophagitis) initially 10 mg orally daily, increasing to 20 mg daily for 4 weeks if needed, then decreasing to 10 mg daily when needed **OR**
- (Treatment of gastric/duodenal ulcer) 10—20 mg orally daily for 4—12 weeks **OR**
- (*Helicobacter pylori* eradication) 20 mg orally twice daily (with appropriate antibiotics)

Adverse effects
- nausea, vomiting, diarrhoea, abdominal pain, flatulence, dry mouth, constipation, metallic taste, fundic gland polyps
- headache, dizziness, fatigue, asthenia, insomnia
- cough, rhinitis, pharyngitis, flu-like symptoms
- myalgia, back pain, pain
- chest pain
- rash
- (Prolonged therapy) vitamin B_{12} deficiency
- (Rare) interstitial nephritis, hypomagnesaemia, increased risk of osteoporosis and bone fracture, subacute cutaneous lupus erythematosus

Interactions
- see General Interactions of proton pump inhibitors (p. 876)

Nursing considerations/Cautions/Patient education
- instruct the patient to swallow tablets whole (not crushed or chewed) with water
- see also General Nursing considerations/Cautions/Patient education for proton pump inhibitors (p. 876)

 Tablets must be swallowed whole (not crushed or chewed) with water.

 A decision must be made to discontinue the drug or discontinue breastfeeding.

CYTOPROTECTIVE AGENTS

Cytoprotective agents protect the gastric mucosa and sites of ulceration by various mechanisms; these include increasing mucus and bicarbonate excretion, decreasing acid secretion, and forming acid and pepsin resistance protective coating. They include misoprostol, bismuth sulfate and sucralfate.

MISOPROSTOL
Trade name
Cytotec, GyMiso, Angusta

Available forms
Tablets: 200 microgram; 25 microgram

Action
- synthetic prostaglandin E1 analogue
- acts directly on parietal cells
- reduces gastric acid secretion in the basal state, as well as when stimulated by histamine, food and coffee
- decreases nocturnal acid secretion
- mucosal cytoprotective properties
- active metabolite (half-life 1.5 hours)
- peak effect 30 minutes, half-life 20—40 minutes
- inhibits gastric secretion for 3—6 hours

Use
- treatment of acute gastric and duodenal ulcers
- prophylaxis of stress-induced GI bleeding and lesions (postsurgical intensive care (ICU) patients)
- prophylaxis of gastric ulceration (patients taking NSAIDs at high risk of gastric ulceration)
- pregnancy termination (see Pregnancy, childbirth and breastfeeding, p. 1484) (GyMiso, Angusta)

Dose
- (Duodenal/gastric ulcer treatment) 200 micrograms orally daily after meals and at night (4 times daily) for 4—8 weeks **OR**

- (Prevention of stress-induced bleeding and lesions in ICU) 200 micrograms orally 4-hourly after food for up to 14 days **OR**
- (Prophylaxis of gastric ulceration in patients taking NSAIDs) 100—200 micrograms orally daily with meals and at night (4 times daily), taken with NSAIDs

Adverse effects
- nausea, vomiting, diarrhoea, loose stools, abdominal pain, flatulence, dyspepsia, constipation
- headache
- dizziness
- (Uncommon) uterine cramps, menstrual disorders, dysmenorrhoea, menorrhagia, intermenstrual bleeding, spotting, vaginal haemorrhage (including postmenopausal)
- (Rare) hypotension

Nursing considerations/Cautions
- before starting therapy, any unintentional loss of weight, recurrent vomiting, dysphagia, haematemesis, anaemia, melaena or malignancy should be investigated. It is also recommended that those with ulceration be re-endoscoped 8—12 weeks after starting therapy to determine if the ulcer is healing
- pregnancy must be excluded before commencing therapy
- caution when used in those in ICUs because agents that suppress acid secretion have been associated with nosocomial lung infections
- caution if used in those with asthma (because of the risk of bronchospasm) or those with a predisposition to inflammatory bowel disease, diarrhoea, dehydration, epilepsy or where hypotension may precipitate complications (e.g. cerebrovascular or coronary artery disease)
- not recommended in those under 18 years
- contraindicated in those with known hypersensitivity to prostaglandins

Patient education
- the patient should be warned against driving or operating machinery if dizziness occurs
- advise the patient that diarrhoea is less likely to occur if medication is taken after meals and avoiding magnesium-containing antacids
- women of childbearing potential should receive counselling and written information regarding the importance of adequate contraception before starting therapy

 (Cytotec) can be dispersed in water, or crushed and given with a spoonful of yoghurt or apple puree.

 Contraindicated during pregnancy. May cause uterine contractions, abortion, fetal death and premature birth, as well as incomplete miscarriage.

 Not recommended during breastfeeding, as may cause diarrhoea in newborn.

Note
- contained in MS-2 Step (for pregnancy termination) and GyMiso
- contained in Angusta for induction of labour

SUCRALFATE
Trade name
Carafate

Available form
Tablets: 1 g

Action
- composed of sulfated sucrose and aluminium hydroxide and is non-absorbable
- reacts with acid to produce sticky yellow—white gel which selectively ad-

ANTIULCER AGENTS

heres to the ulcer base, protecting it from potential ulcerogenic properties of acid, pepsin and bile
- complexes with pepsin and bile directly and blocks acid diffusion across the ulcer site
- enhances prostaglandin synthesis, stimulating mucus and bicarbonate production
- protects mucosa for up to 6 hours

Use
- treatment of acute non-malignant gastric and duodenal ulcers
- prevents recurrence of duodenal ulcers

Dose
- (Treatment of gastric/duodenal ulcers) 1 g orally 3 times daily 1 hour before meals and at night for up to 8 weeks **OR**
- (Duodenal ulcer maintenance therapy) 1 g orally twice daily 1 hour before meals for up to 12 months

Adverse effects
- nausea, indigestion, constipation, gastric discomfort, diarrhoea, dry mouth
- obstruction of GI tract (bezoars) (especially patients on parenteral feeding with delayed gastric emptying)
- back pain
- urticaria, rash, pruritus
- headache, dizziness, sleepiness, vertigo
- (Rare) hypophosphataemia

Interactions
- not recommended with citrate preparation because of the risk of increased blood levels of aluminium
- antacids decrease the mucosal binding of sucralfate if taken less than 30 minutes before or after sucralfate
- reduces bioavailability of ciprofloxacin, digoxin, tetracycline, phenytoin, frusemide, proton pump inhibitors and norfloxacin
- may reduce bioavailability of warfarin; therefore INR should be closely monitored, especially when starting or stopping therapy

Nursing considerations/Cautions
- the correct diagnosis is important at the start of therapy to exclude any gastric malignancy
- (Duodenal ulcers) therapy should continue for up to 8 weeks unless healing has been confirmed
- (Gastric ulcers) if no response is seen in 6 weeks, alternative therapy should be considered. However, if the ulcer is large, it may require 8 weeks to achieve healing
- caution if used in those with swallowing difficulties including recent and/or prolonged intubation, dysphagia, a previous history of aspiration, tracheostomy or other conditions which affect gag/cough reflex or oropharyngeal motility
- caution if used in those with phosphate deficiencies
- not recommended in those under 18 years
- not recommended for patients with severely impaired kidney function (contains 190 mg aluminium) or those with actively bleeding peptic ulcers
- contraindicated as long-term therapy in patients receiving dialysis

Patient education
- instruct the patient to take antacids at least 30 minutes before or after sucralfate. Other medications should be taken 2—3 hours before sucralfate
- the patient should be advised not to drive or operate machinery if dizziness, sleepiness or vertigo occurs

 If the person is not at risk of aspiration, tablets can be dispersed in water.

 Not recommended during pregnancy unless benefits outweigh any potential risks.

 Caution if used during breastfeeding.

Sucralfate should be administered carefully in patients with chronic impairment of renal function.

ANTACIDS

Antacids buffer or neutralise hydrochloric acid in the stomach; in the past, acid neutralisation was seen as the main form of peptic ulcer management. Today, however, antacids are now used mainly as symptom relief for dyspepsia, peptic ulcer disease (PUD) and GORD. The major ingredients of antacids include aluminium hydroxide, calcium carbonate, magnesium salts and sodium bicarbonate, either alone or in combination with the magnesium—aluminium combinations, which are the most commonly used (Knights et al 2023). They may be combined with other agents such as alginic acid and simethicone.

ALUMINIUM HYDROXIDE HYDRATE (ALUMINIUM HYDROXIDE)

Trade name
Alu-Tab

Available form
Tablets: 600 mg

Action
- antacid that neutralises gastric hyperacidity
- aluminium hydroxide binds with phosphate ions in the bowel to form insoluble phosphate salts that are excreted by the bowel

Use
- gastric hyperacidity
- relieves symptoms of peptic ulcer (uncomplicated)
- phosphate binding in renal dysfunction

Dose
- 1–2 tablets (600–1200 mg) orally 4 times daily with food

Adverse effects
- constipation, chalky taste
- (Prolonged treatment or high doses) hypophosphataemia (anorexia, malaise, muscle weakness)
- (In chronic renal failure) hyperaluminaemia, dialysis dementia
- intestinal obstruction (in patients who are dehydrated or have reduced bowel motility and develop faecal impaction)

Interactions
- forms a complex with tetracyclines, preventing their absorption
- may reduce absorption of many drugs, but particularly digoxin, indometacin, oral iron, naproxen, penicillin, sulfonamides and vitamins

Nursing considerations/Cautions
- (Chronic therapy) serum calcium, aluminium and phosphate levels should be monitored regularly. For those on maintenance haemodialysis, bimonthly monitoring of serum phosphate levels is recommended
- caution if used in those with renal dysfunction because of the increased risk of hyperalbuminaemia and associated accumulation in bone, lungs and nerve tissue
- contraindicated in those with hypophosphataemia or chronic renal failure (because of the increased risk of aluminium toxicity)

Patient education
- advise the patient to take aluminium-containing antacids 2 hours before or after other medications
- encourage the patient to maintain an adequate fluid intake (within any fluid restriction) during therapy to prevent constipation. If constipation occurs, the patient should be advised to seek medical advice
- the patient should be advised to seek medical advice if symptoms do not improve within a few days

ANTIULCER AGENTS

Caution if used in those with renal dysfunction because of the increased risk of hyperalbuminaemia and associated accumulation in bone, lungs and nerve tissue and toxicity. Avoid use if CrCl < 10 mL/min.

Available in combination with
- aluminium hydroxide, magnesium hydroxide and magnesium trisilicate (Gastrogel liquid)
- aluminium hydroxide 400 mg, magnesium hydroxide 400 mg Simethicone 40 mg, Mylanta 2go Antacid Double Strength Tablets) aluminium hydroxide 200 mg, magnesium hydroxide 200 mg, Simethicone 20 (Mylanta 2go Antacid Original Chewable tablets)

CALCIUM CARBONATE

Action
- antacid that neutralises gastric hyperacidity

Use
- heartburn and indigestion

Adverse effects
- constipation, belching, flatulence, abdominal extension
- (High dose, prolonged use) acid rebound
- (Rare) hypercalcaemia, alkalosis, phosphate depletion, renal calculi, milk—acid syndrome.

Interactions
- may decrease absorption of tetracyclines, fluoroquinolones, salicylates or iron

Nursing considerations/Cautions
- contraindicated in those with severe hypercalcaemia or metabolic acidosis, hyperparathyroidism, kidney impairment (because of increased risk of hypercalcaemia). In hypercalciuria—nephrolithiasis, antacids containing calcium are contraindicated

Patient education
- advise the patient to take calcium-containing antacids 2—3 hours before or after other medications
- the patient should be advised to seek medical advice if symptoms do not improve within a few days

In patients with hypercalcaemia or hypercalciuria—nephrolithiasis, antacids containing calcium are contraindicated. Avoid antacids containing sodium in cirrhosis; they may increase fluid retention.

Available in combination with
- calcium carbonate 550 mg, magnesium hydroxide 110 mg and mannitol 6.7 mg per max daily dose (Mylanta 2go Antacid FastChews Chewable tablets)

MAGNESIUM HYDROXIDE, MAGNESIUM TRISILICATE
Trade names
Magnesium Trisilicate (extemporaneous), Alenic Alka, Foaming Antacid, Gaviscon, Genaton

Available forms
Liquid suspension;
Tablet: 250 mg

Action
- neutralises gastric hyperacidity

Use
- hyperacidity, heartburn; reflux and ulcers

Dose
- 10—20 mL 3 times daily after meals and before bedtime (Gastrogel antacid)

Adverse effects
- diarrhoea, chalky taste, belching
- (Rare) elevated magnesium levels

Interactions
- may form a complex if given with tetracyclines and therefore should be

separated by at least 1–2 hours if given together

Nursing considerations/Cautions

- magnesium trisilicate-containing antacids contain significant amounts of sodium, which should be considered if a sodium-restricted diet is in place
- caution if used in those with existing diarrhoea, as it may be aggravated
- contraindicated in those with kidney impairment because of the increased risk of increased magnesium levels and toxicity

Patient education

- advise the patient to take magnesium-containing antacids 2–3 hours before or after other medications
- the patient should be advised to seek medical advice if symptoms do not improve within a few days

Contraindicated in those with kidney impairment owing to the increased risk of increased magnesium levels and toxicity.

Available in combination with

- aluminium hydroxide, magnesium hydroxide and magnesium trisilicate (Gastrogel liquid)
- aluminium hydroxide 400 mg, magnesium hydroxide 400 mg Simethicone 40 mg, (Mylanta 2go Antacid Double Strength Tablets)
- aluminium hydroxide 200 mg, magnesium hydroxide 200 mg, Simethicone 20 (Mylanta 2go Antacid Original Chewable tablets)
- calcium carbonate 550 mg, magnesium hydroxide 110 mg and mannitol 6.7 mg per max daily dose (Mylanta 2go Antacid FastChews Chewable tablets)
- magnesium trisilicate and Belladonna BPC 1968 (Extemporaneous)

ANTIVENOMS

ANTIVENOMS

General Actions of antivenoms
- snake antivenom is produced by 'milking' venom from the snake and then injecting small quantities repeatedly into horses over 10—12 months. Blood is then removed and the plasma containing antibodies extracted and purified
- monovalent snake antivenom is produced against a single snake (or related) species and a smaller dose is usually required to neutralise the venom. It is, however, important to identify the snake species. It is important to note that Australian snakes are protected species and it is illegal to kill them unless they threaten life
- polyvalent snake antivenom is useful for a broad range of snake species; however, larger doses are required to neutralise the venom
- spider bites are generally less likely to be fatal than snake bites
- spider antivenom is produced in a similar way to snake antivenom, but in different animal species (rabbit, sheep)
- administration of repeated or large dose (> 1 vial) has not been shown to shorten the recovery period

General Uses of antivenoms
- to neutralise specific toxins when envenomation has clearly occurred

General Adverse effects of antivenoms
- anaphylaxis (including hypotension, pallor, angioedema, rash, dyspnoea and cough (because of bronchospasm and laryngeal oedema), urticaria, shock and, less commonly, nausea, vomiting and abdominal pain)
- serum sickness (delayed) occurring 8—13 days later (but can occur 12 hours after second injection of animal protein) (consisting of urticaria, fever, joint pains, enlarged lymph nodes and albuminuria and, less commonly, arthritis, nephritis, neuropathy and vasculitis)
- (Common) fever, chills, headache, hypotension, urticaria, rash
- (Uncommon) arthralgia, myalgia, abdominal pain, nausea, vomiting, diarrhoea, chest pain, cyanosis, angioedema, pain or tenderness at injection sites

General Nursing considerations/Cautions for antivenoms
- antivenom should be used only if there are clear signs of systemic envenomation (usually occur within 2 hours of bite or sting)
- enquire about any previous injections of antivenom (including equine tetanus antitoxin before 1974 in Australia) or any allergies in the patient or family,

- especially asthma, hay fever and infantile eczema, because the risk of anaphylactoid reaction is increased
- suspected snake-bite cases should be observed for at least 6 hours after the bite or removal of the splint and bandage and, in known snake-bite cases, observation should be for 12 hours, preferably in an ICU setting
- the dose for children is the same as the adult dose (as the dose is snake dependent, not weight of victim dependent); however, it should be noted that children can become critically ill faster than adults
- the patient should be carefully monitored for any signs or symptoms of neurotoxicity (flaccid paralysis (within 1–3 hours), ptosis and/or diplopia, dysphagia and, if severe, paralysis of respiratory muscles (3–18 hours)), coagulopathy (regular monitoring of international normalised ratio (INR), activated partial thromboplastin time (aPTT), fibrinogen, platelets), neuromuscular impairment, myolysis (myotoxin destroys muscle cells (rhabdomyolysis) causing pain, weakness, red discolouration of urine and increase in creatine kinase) and nephrotoxicity (resulting from rhabdomyolysis, hypotension and coagulopathy)
- the pressure bandage and splint should not be removed until the antivenom is ready to be administered
- antivenom is diluted in sodium chloride 0.9%, or preferably Hartmann's solution 1 in 10, and given by slow IV infusion without testing for sensitivity to horse serum. Dilution of the antivenom reduces the risk of anaphylactoid reaction
- if the person has a fluid restriction, dilution may be 1 in 5 (with medical advice)
- antivenom is usually not required if envenomation is mild
- IV administration is more likely than SC or IM to cause anaphylaxis
- skin testing is NOT recommended
- IV antihistamine (non-sedating) and 0.25 mL of 1:1000 adrenaline (epinephrine) SC may be used before antivenom administration, but this practice is contentious and is no longer recommended
- have available adrenaline (epinephrine) 1:1000 (drawn up), antihistamines, IV corticosteroid, oxygen, suction and resuscitation equipment whenever antivenom is administered. If anaphylaxis occurs, the antivenom should be stopped immediately and oxygen and IM adrenaline (epinephrine) administered. If there is no response to IM administration, adrenaline (epinephrine) should be readministered IV and repeated at 5-minute intervals if needed
- expired antivenom should not be used
- avoid intravascular injection (when not intended) by withdrawing the syringe plunger
- repeated or larger doses are not generally recommended, as these do not shorten the recovery period
- serial coagulation tests are recommended as indicators of recovery (where venom contains procoagulants or anticoagulants)
- in those with known hypersensitivity (e.g. to horse protein, rabbit or rabbit products, sheep or sheep products), antivenom should be given with caution and patient monitored closely (e.g. airway and vital signs). Antivenom should not be withheld
- because antivenom has been produced from animal plasma, there is always a risk of transmitting infectious agents (possibly unknown) and the patient should be informed of this potential risk before administration
- any deterioration in the patient's condition may indicate the necessity for further administration of antivenom
- envenomation may have significant effects on both mother and fetus and therefore benefits of antivenom should be weighed against risks of envenomation

Patient education for antivenoms

- the patient should be advised to seek medical attention immediately if any signs of delayed serum sickness occur (e.g. rash, fever, joint pain, swollen lymph glands, flu-like illness), as these can be days or weeks after the antivenom was given

Pressure immobilisation first aid technique (Guideline 9.4.8, Australian and New Zealand Committee on Resuscitation, 2025)

- this technique was first developed to manage snake bite as a way to delay the movement of venom from the bite site to the circulation; however, it is suitable for all species of Australian snakes (including sea snakes), funnel-web spiders, blue-ringed octopus and cone shell stings
- this technique is **not** suitable for spider bites (other than funnel-web spider), jelly fish stings, stonefish or other fish stings, scorpion, centipede or beetle bites
- the bitten or stung area should not be washed, cut or excised
- in the event of envenomation, the person should be as immobilised as soon as possible (e.g. not allowed to walk or move limb; if possible, transport such as a stretcher should be brought to the person, rather than the person walking to the stretcher)
- call triple zero (000)
- the bite area should not be washed, as any venom can be used to identify the snake species using a snake venom detection kit
- a wide bandage (e.g. elasticised bandage is preferred over crepe bandage; however, clothing and other material can be torn into wide strips) should be applied to area as soon as possible to reduce venom from spreading through lymphatics. The bandage should be firm, but not tight enough to impair circulation (you should not be able to slide finger between the bandage and skin). Clothing should not be removed, as movement may promote movement of venom into the bloodstream; therefore the limb and patient should be kept as still as possible
- the bandage should be applied upwards from the lower portion of the bitten/stung limb (as this is more comfortable and can be tolerated for longer, even though a small amount of venom may be squeezed upwards). It should be extended as high as possible on the limb (if leg). If an arm or hand is affected, the bandage should start at the fingers and extend upwards, with a splint applied to the elbow. A sling may also be used to immobilise the arm
- if the bite is not on a limb, firm pressure can be applied as long as breathing or chest movement is not restricted. Firm pressure should not be applied to neck or head area
- apply splint to leg (if bitten/stung), and this should then be bound to the limb. A splint can be anything that is firm and at hand (e.g. rolled up newspaper, tree branch, piece of wood)
- if possible, the area of bite should be marked on the bandage so that a venom sample can be accessed for testing without having to remove the compression bandage
- the person should be transported to hospital and the bandage not removed until antivenom is ready for administration (removal may bring on the systemic effects of the venom). The treating doctor should make the decision to remove the bandage
- a snake venom detection kit may be useful in identifying specific venom from snake-bite site, as puncture marks can be difficult to see. The detection kit uses a swab to identify the presence of venom; however, urine can also be used if no venom sample is available (as blood can be unreliable). A snake venom detection kit can detect venom from brown snakes, black snakes, tiger snakes, death adders and taipans

BLACK SNAKE ANTIVENOM

Available form
Vial: 18,000 units

Action
- venom contains neurotoxins, myotoxins, procoagulants and anticoagulants
- local reaction (pain, swelling, redness) is a major feature
- produced from horse plasma
- see also General Actions of antivenoms (p. 889)

Use
- may be used for mulga (King brown) snake, Butler's mulga snake and Papuan black snake
- can also be used for Collett's snake, but tiger snake antivenom is the preferred treatment option

Dose
- 18,000 units diluted 1 in 10 with Hartmann's solution and given IV

Adverse effects/Nursing considerations/Cautions
- not given IM
- see also General Adverse effects/Nursing considerations/Cautions for antivenoms (including pressure immobilisation first aid technique, p. 889)

BOX JELLYFISH ANTIVENOM

Available form
Vial: 20,000 units

Action
- box jellyfish (*Chironex fleckeri*) are found in tropical coastal waters from Gladstone (Queensland) to Broome (Western Australia), but not the Great Barrier Reef from December to March generally, or October to end of May in the Northern Territory
- box jellyfish are transparent and difficult to see in water. They are large (20–30 cm), and weigh up to 6 kg with tentacles $\geq$ 3 metres (containing nematocysts (stinging cells)). Upon contact the nematocysts discharge tubules loaded with venom (which act as mini-harpoons)
- the severity of envenomation is related to the surface area that the tentacles containing nematocysts make contact with and the age of the victim
- in severe cases, death can occur in 20 minutes; however, most cases, while painful, are not life threatening
- the venom contains toxin, which can affect the myocardium and respiratory system as well as causing severe and intense pain
- prepared from sheep plasma

Use
- treat envenomation by box jellyfish

Dose
- 20,000 units diluted 1 in 10 with Hartmann's solution and given IV or 60,000 units IM into 3 separate sites (if IV is not practical)

Adverse effects/Nursing considerations/Cautions
- vinegar (NOT ALCOHOL) should be applied to any tentacles sticking to the skin and first aid measures taken immediately to ensure an adequate airway is maintained. Vinegar will not ease the pain, but will inactivate any stinging cells still present. Any remaining tentacles should be picked off. Cold pack or ice in a dry plastic bag can be applied for pain relief. Fresh water should not be applied to the area, as it may cause further discharge of venom from undischarged nematocysts
- IM administration may be used as emergency treatment pre-hospitalisation
- see also General Adverse effects/Nursing considerations/Cautions for antivenoms (p. 889)

BROWN SNAKE ANTIVENOM

Available form
Vial: 1000 units

ANTIVENOMS

Action
- brown snakes are the most common cause of bites and account for the majority of deaths in Australia
- the venom contains neurotoxins and procoagulants, but local reactions (pain, swelling, redness) rarely occur
- prepared from horse plasma
- see also General Actions of antivenoms (p. 889)

Use
- may be used for all brown snake species (except King brown, which is a black snake), dugite or Western brown (Gwardar) snake bite

Dose
- initial dose is 1000 units slowly IV after dilution of 1:10 with Hartmann's solution

Adverse effects/Nursing considerations/Cautions
- see General Adverse effects/Nursing considerations/Cautions for antivenoms (including pressure immobilisation first aid technique, p. 889)

DEATH ADDER ANTIVENOM

Available form
Vial: 6000 units

Action
- venom contains neurotoxin, with local reactions (pain, redness, swelling) rarely reported
- see also General Actions of antivenoms (p. 889)

Use
- used for death adder species envenomation

Dose
- initial dose is 6000 units by slow IV after dilution 1:10 with Hartmann's solution

Adverse effects/Nursing considerations/Cautions
- see General Adverse effects/Nursing considerations/Cautions for antivenoms (including pressure immobilisation first aid technique, p. 889)

FUNNEL-WEB SPIDER ANTIVENOM

Available form
Vial: 125 units

Action
- funnel-web spiders consist of 30 species in two genera, *Atrax* and *Hadronyche*. The male Sydney funnel-web (*Atrax robustus*) is responsible for most, if not all, of the known funnel-web deaths, which can result within 30 minutes of bite. There have been no recorded deaths since 1980 owing to the availability of the antivenom
- the venom contains neurotoxins
- prepared from rabbit plasma

Use
- treatment of funnel-web spider envenomation

Dose
- 250 units (2 vials) given slowly IV after reconstitution with water for injections

Adverse effects/Nursing considerations/Cautions
- hypersensitivity reactions are not common
- should not be used without clear evidence of systemic envenomation with potential for serious toxic effects
- see also General Adverse effects/Nursing points/Cautions for antivenoms (including pressure immobilisation first aid technique, p. 889)

POLYVALENT SNAKE ANTIVENOM

Available form
Vial: 40,000 units

Action
- contains antivenom against black snakes (18,000 units), tiger (3000 units) and brown snakes (1000 units), taipan (12,000 units) and death adder (6000 units)
- prepared from horse plasma

Use
- for use in Papua New Guinea and Australia (except for Victoria and Tasmania) when the snake has not been definitely identified. In Victoria, a combination of tiger snake and brown snake antivenom is the preferred treatment, whereas in Tasmania the tiger snake antivenom is used in preference to polyvalent antivenom

Dose
- 40,000 units by slow IV after dilution 1:10 with Hartmann's solution

Adverse effects/Nursing considerations/Cautions
- see General Adverse effects/Nursing considerations/Cautions for antivenoms (including pressure immobilisation first aid technique, p. 889)

RED BACK SPIDER ANTIVENOM

Available form
Vial: 500 units

Action/Use
- used for red back spider (*Latrodectus hasselti*) bite
- the venom causes intense pain that can last for days to weeks, redness or red marks and itchiness
- the venom contains alpha latrotoxin causing latrodectism (local pain, local and general sweating, nausea, vomiting, headache, dizziness and malaise, and less commonly, hypertension, hyperthermia, abdominal rigidity and agitation/irritability)
- prepared from horse plasma

Dose
- 500 units IM or 500 units by slow IV after dilution 1:10 with Hartmann's solution (if envenomation is life threatening)

Adverse effects/Nursing considerations/Cautions
- adverse effects are more common if given IV
- ice or cold compress can be applied for up to 20 minutes to decrease the pain of spider bite
- (First aid) pressure immobilisation technique should not be used, as the venom acts slowly
- see also General Adverse effects/Nursing considerations/Cautions for antivenoms (p. 889)

SEA SNAKE ANTIVENOM

Available form
Vial: 1000 units

Action
- sea snakes are commonly found in tropical water $\geq 20°C$
- bite can be painless with no local swelling, although small teeth marks can be obvious
- the venom contains neurotoxins and myotoxins with minor reactions (pain, redness, swelling) reported
- prepared from horse plasma

Use
- used for envenomation due to a variety of sea snakes found in the northern Australian waters

Dose
- 1000 units by slow IV after dilution 1:10 with Hartmann's solution or sodium chloride 0.9%
- (Severe envenomation with myalgia, weakness, trismus, ptosis) 3000—4000 units by slow IV after dilution 1:10 with Hartmann's solution or sodium chloride 0.9%

Adverse effects/Nursing considerations/Cautions
- tiger snake antivenom may also be used if sea snake antivenom is not available
- see also General Adverse effects/Nursing considerations/Cautions for antivenoms (including pressure immobilisation first aid technique) (p. 889)

STONE FISH ANTIVENOM

Available form
Vial: 2000 units

Action
* stonefish are found in tropical Australian waters and prefer calm shallow water where they bury themselves in the sand
* envenomation usually occurs by standing on stone fish buried in sand
* venom contains cardiotoxins, neurotoxins and myotoxins

Use
* envenomation by stone fish (*Synanceia horrida* and *Synanceia verrucosa*) not responding to first aid measures

Dose
* dose given is dependent on the number of puncture wounds and given IM or slowly IV after dilution 1:10 with Hartmann's solution in severe cases
    * (1–2 punctures) 2000 units
    * (3–4 punctures) 4000 units
    * (> 5 punctures) 6000 units

Adverse effects/Nursing considerations/Cautions
* initially, severe pain, redness and swelling occurs at site of puncture, then spreads to limb and local lymph nodes
* first aid includes immersing puncture wounds in hot water (50°C) to relieve pain, as the toxin is heat labile
* tourniquet and/or compression bandage are not recommended
* local anaesthetic injected around puncture site or region may also relieve pain
* see also General Adverse effects/Nursing considerations/Cautions for antivenoms (p. 889)

TAIPAN ANTIVENOM

Available form
Vial: 12,000 units

Action
* taipan venom is thought to be the most potent snake venom worldwide
* the venom contains neurotoxin, myotoxins and procoagulants with minor local reactions (pain, swelling, redness) reported
* prepared from horse plasma

Use
* used for envenomation by coastal taipan (*Oxyuranus scutellatus*) and inland taipan (*Oxyuranus microlepidotus*) (fierce snake)

Dose
* initial dose is 12,000 units slowly IV after dilution 1:10 with Hartmann's solution
* (Severe defibrination) 36,000 units slowly IV after dilution 1:10 with Hartmann's solution

Adverse effects/Nursing considerations/Cautions
* see General Adverse effects/Nursing considerations/Cautions for antivenoms (including pressure immobilisation first aid technique) (p. 889)

TIGER SNAKE ANTIVENOM

Available form
Vial: 3000 units

Action
* venom contains neurotoxin, myotoxin and procoagulants with minor local reactions (pain, swelling, redness) also reported
* prepared from horse plasma

Use
* envenomation due to tiger snakes, as well as copperhead snakes, black snakes, rough-scaled snakes and Collett's snake (red and blue-bellied black snakes)

Dose
* initial dose is 3000 units slowly IV after dilution 1:10 with Hartmann's solution

Adverse effects/Nursing considerations/Cautions
* see General Adverse effects/Nursing considerations/Cautions for antivenoms (including pressure immobilisation first aid technique) (p. 889)

ANTIVIRAL AGENTS

Viruses are true parasites that are unable to replicate independently, requiring a host's metabolic machinery to replicate. Classification of viruses is according to nucleic acid composition (DNA or RNA), whether double or single stranded, and whether a lipoprotein envelope is present or not. Retroviruses are a special class of RNA viruses that have a complex replication mechanism, making them very difficult to treat using standard antiviral agents. Unfortunately, with many viral infections, replication has reached its peak before symptoms are present, making the infection difficult to treat (Knights et al 2023).

Antiviral agents are a broad group of drugs that inhibit viral replication by selectively inhibiting the reproductive pathway of the virus at different stages (e.g. adsorption of the virion into the cell, penetration, uncoating, assembly or release) or they may inhibit transcription or translation steps that are shared with the host cell (Neal 2015). Antiviral drugs can be divided into *antiretrovirals* (those drugs used to treat retroviruses) or *non-retroviral* (drugs used to treat non-HIV viral infections) (Knights et al 2023).

Antiviral (non-retroviral) agents are subdivided into a number of classes:
- DNA polymerase inhibitors (e.g. aciclovir, cidofovir, famciclovir, foscarnet, ganciclovir, valaciclovir, valganciclovir)
- neuraminidase inhibitors (e.g. oseltamivir, zanamivir)
- NS5A inhibitors (e.g. velpatasvir)
- NS5B RNA-dependent RNA protease inhibitors (e.g. sofosbuvir)
- other antiviral agents (e.g. adefovir, amantadine, entecavir, ribavirin) (Knights et al 2023)

Antiretroviral agents are further subdivided depending on their site of action:
- nucleoside reverse transcriptase inhibitors (NRTIs) (prevent viral RNA being converted into viral DNA) (e.g. abacavir, emtricitabine, lamivudine, tenofovir, zidovudine)
- non-nucleoside reverse transcriptase inhibitors (NNRTIs) (block RNA-dependent and DNA-dependent DNA polymerases) (e.g. efavirenz, etravirine, nevirapine, rilpivirine)
- protease inhibitors (PI) (prevent HIV protease from cleaving polypeptide and block maturation of HIV

virus) (e.g. atazanavir, darunavir, lopinavir, ritonavir)
- entry inhibitors (e.g. maraviroc)
- integrase inhibitors (e.g. raltegravir) (Knights et al 2023).

Note
- AIDS: acquired immune deficiency syndrome
- CMV: cytomegalovirus
- HIV: human immunodeficiency virus

ANTIVIRAL (NON-RETROVIRAL) AGENTS

DNA POLYMERASE INHIBITORS

ACICLOVIR
Trade names
Aciclovir Accord, Aciclovir GH, Aciclovir Sandoz, Aciclovir Viatris, Aciclovir-WGR, APO-Aciclovir, ARX-Aciclovir, Blistex Antiviral Cold Sore, Chemists' Own Cold Sore, DBL Aciclovir, Nyal Antiviral Cold Sore, Pharmacy Action Cold Sore, ViruPOS, Xorox, Zovirax Cold Sore

Available forms
Vial: 250 mg, 500 mg;
Tablets: 200 mg, 400 mg, 800 mg;
Tablets dispersible: 200 mg, 400 mg, 800 mg;
Eye ointment: 30 mg/g;
Cream: 50 mg/g

Action
- selectively taken up by herpes virus-infected cell, where it is converted to an active form that inhibits viral replication by interfering with DNA synthesis
- oral form is poorly absorbed, but still reaches therapeutic levels
- (IV) half-life is about 2.5 hours (increasing to 20 hours in those with kidney impairment)
- resistance to therapy may develop

Use
- prophylaxis and treatment of herpes simplex infections (including types 1 and 2, herpes zoster (shingles) (within 72 hours of rash presentation), herpes simplex keratitis, herpes simplex encephalitis)
- advanced HIV disease

Dose
Genital herpes
- (Initial treatment) 200 mg orally 4-hourly (while awake) (total 1 g daily) for 10 days **OR**
- (Chronic suppressive therapy for recurrent genital herpes) 200 mg orally 3 times daily for up to 6 months **OR**
- (Intermittent therapy for recurrent genital herpes) 200 mg orally 4-hourly (while awake) (total 1 g daily) for 5 days, starting at earliest signs of recurrence

Herpes zoster (shingles)
- 800 mg orally 4-hourly (while awake), starting within 72 hours of rash onset and continuing for 7 days **OR**
- (Varicella zoster in immunocompromised patient) 10 mg/kg 8-hourly by slow IV infusion **OR**
- (Severe herpes zoster (shingles) infection) 5 mg/kg 8-hourly by slow IV infusion

Herpes simplex infections
- (Immunocompetent or immunocompromised) 5 mg/kg 8-hourly by slow IV infusion for 5–7 days **OR**
- apply cream in sufficient amount to cover lesion 5 times daily (approximately 4-hour intervals) to mouth lesion for 5–7 days (approximately 4-hour intervals, omitting night-time application), starting at first signs or symptoms (burning, tingling, itching) **OR**
- (Eye infections) 1 cm ointment placed in the lower conjunctival sac 5 times daily (approximately 4-hour intervals) and for

ANTIVIRAL AGENTS

3 days after healing is complete or 14 days (whichever is earlier)

Herpes simplex encephalitis (immunocompetent or immunocompromised)
- 10 mg/kg 8-hourly by slow IV infusion for 10 days

Advanced symptomatic HIV disease
- 800 mg orally 6-hourly (with other antiretrovirals)

Adverse effects
- nausea, vomiting, diarrhoea, abdominal pain, taste alteration, anorexia
- headache, dizziness, lethargy, fatigue, confusion, altered level of consciousness, tremors, somnolence, psychosis, hallucinations, agitation, seizures
- vertigo
- fever
- reversible abnormal liver enzymes and bilirubin
- anaemia, leucopenia, thrombocytopenia
- rash, urticaria, pruritus, photosensitivity, hair loss
- (IV) reversible increased serum urea and creatinine
- (Rare) haematuria, jaundice, hepatitis, coma, encephalopathy, hypotension, dyspnoea, anaphylaxis
- (IV bolus) renal damage
- (Eye ointment) mild stinging, blepharitis and rarely, sensitivity reactions
- (Cold sore cream) (uncommon) mild pain, burning, stinging, skin flaking
- (IV site) inflammation, pain, phlebitis

Interactions
- clearance may be decreased when given with probenecid, increasing risk of crystal precipitation in renal tubules
- serum levels may be increased when given with diuretics (patients aged over 60 years) and mycophenolate mofetil
- caution if used with mycophenolate mofetil, ciclosporin or tacrolimus
- not recommended with nephrotoxic agents
- caution if used with interferon or methotrexate (intrathecally) owing to increased risk of encephalopathy
- may cause increase in theophylline serum levels, increasing the risk of adverse effects

Nursing considerations/Cautions
- (IV) ensure adequate hydration during therapy (especially in elderly patients) to prevent precipitation of crystals in renal tubules
- (IV) urine output should be closely monitored, especially in the first hours after therapy
- IV bolus doses should not be given
- solution should be added to at least 50–100 mL of IV solution and administered over at least 1 hour at a rate of 25 mg/mL using an infusion pump (to avoid renal damage)
- IV site should be closely monitored to avoid extravasation, which may cause inflammation and/or tissue necrosis
- eye(s) or skin should be thoroughly rinsed with water if contact with IV solutions occurs
- doses need to be adjusted for those with renal impairment
- IV solution should not be refrigerated because it causes precipitation and solution should be discarded if this occurs, as crystals will not redissolve at room temperature
- IV solution should not be administered if there are any crystals or it is turbid in appearance
- (Herpes labialis) oral aciclovir is recommended (rather than cream) if the patient is immunocompromised
- caution if used in those with renal disease or impairment, dehydration, neurological abnormalities, significant hypoxia, serious liver or electrolyte abnormalities or in those who have shown neurological changes when using other cytotoxic agents
- contraindicated in those with hypersensitivity to valaciclovir or aciclovir

Patient education

- advise the patient that tablets may be swallowed whole or dispersed in 50 mL water
- those with genital herpes should be advised to avoid sexual intercourse during acute episodes and decrease the risk of transmission by using a condom at other times because viral shedding occurs even when there are no symptoms
- patients with herpes labialis (cold sores) should be instructed to:
  - apply cream at the first signs of cold sore (e.g. area burning, tingling, itching)
  - use gloves when applying cream to prevent spread to other people or other parts of the body
  - avoid kissing to prevent spread to others
  - not use cream on mucous membranes (mouth, eyes, vagina)
  - avoid the cream making contact with their eyes
- patients should be instructed in the correct use of ophthalmic ointment, including:
  - removal of contact lenses during therapy
  - washing hands before and after using ointment
  - applying 1 cm of ointment inside the eyelid of affected eye(s) (without letting the tip of the tube touch the eyelid if possible)
  - closing the eye for 30 seconds
  - noting that vision may be blurred for 5–10 minutes after ointment has been applied and transient stinging may occur
  - allowing vision to clear before driving or operating machinery

 Do not crush; some tablets may be dispersed in at least 50 mL of water for easier swallowing.

 Use only if benefits justify potential risks to the fetus; aciclovir crosses the placenta and safety in pregnant women is not definitively established.

 Use only if benefits outweigh the risks; aciclovir is excreted in breastmilk and may affect the infant.

 Reduced renal function: adjust dosage in patients with reduced renal function; closely monitor for signs of neurological complications because of an increased risk of toxicity.

Available in combination with
- aciclovir 5% w/w + hydrocortisone 1% w/w (Zovirax Duo Cold Sore Cream)

CIDOFOVIR
Trade name
Empovir

Available form
Vial: 375 mg/5 mL

Action
- acyclic nucleoside analogue with activity against cytomegalovirus (CMV)
- selectively inhibits viral DNA polymerase, preventing DNA synthesis and viral replication
- not metabolised and about 70–85% is excreted unchanged in the urine
- probenecid blocks renal clearance and protects kidneys from nephrotoxicity

Use
- CMV retinitis in patients with AIDS (with probenecid)

Dose
- initially 5 mg/kg by IV infusion over 1 hour weekly for 2 weeks (induction), then every 2 weeks (with probenecid) (maintenance)

Adverse effects
- nausea, vomiting, diarrhoea
- headache, asthenia
- fever, chills
- dyspnoea

ANTIVIRAL AGENTS

- proteinuria, increased serum creatinine, renal failure
- neutropenia
- alopecia, rash
- decreased intraocular pressure, uveitis, iritis, decreased visual acuity
- (Rare) acquired Fanconi syndrome (see Glossary)

Interactions

- contraindicated with or within 7 days of other nephrotoxic agents such as aminoglycosides (IV), amphotericin B (amphotericin), foscarnet, pentamidine (IV), NSAIDs and vancomycin
- zidovudine should be temporarily discontinued or the dose decreased on days of cidofovir administration, because probenecid decreases zidovudine clearance
- probenecid interferes with metabolism and excretion of a large number of drugs, leading to increased serum levels and risk of adverse effects or toxicity. Drugs affected include paracetamol, aspirin, aciclovir, angiotensin-converting enzyme (ACE) inhibitors, barbiturates, benzodiazepines, famotidine, furosemide (frusemide), methotrexate, NSAIDs and theophylline

Nursing considerations/Cautions

- serum creatinine, urine protein and WBC count (with neutrophil differential) should be measured 24—48 hours before each administration
- if urine shows ≥ 2+ protein, IV hydration should be administered (see below) and urine retested. If urine continues to show ≥ 2+ protein, therapy should not be continued
- intravenous pre-hydration and oral probenecid are given with each administration; hydration consists of 1 L sodium chloride 0.9% over 1 hour before the cidofovir infusion, and, if tolerated, a second litre over 1—3 hours either with or immediately after cidofovir infusion
- oral probenecid 2 g is given 3 hours before cidofovir infusion, 1 g 2 hours before, then 1 g 8 hours after completion of IV infusion (total 4 g probenecid)
- should be infused into a large vein to allow rapid dilution
- must be diluted in 100 mL of sodium chloride 0.9% and administered using an infusion pump over 1 hour
- regular ophthalmic examinations (especially intraocular pressure monitoring) are recommended during therapy
- contains 57 mg sodium/vial, which may need to be considered if the patient is on a sodium-restricted diet
- contraindicated as direct intraocular injection
- contraindicated in those with renal impairment, creatinine clearance < 55 mL/min, proteinuria (> 100 mg/dL, ≥ 2+), clinically significant hypersensitivity to probenecid or other sulfur-containing products

Patient education

- ensure the patient understands the need for probenecid and hydration before and after therapy to reduce the risk of kidney damage
- the patient should be advised to immediately report any changes to vision
- advise the patient to eat before probenecid to decrease nausea and vomiting
- counsel female patients to use adequate contraception during and for 4 weeks after therapy has stopped to prevent pregnancy occurring
- male patients should be counselled to use barrier method contraception (condom) during and for 12 weeks after stopping therapy

 Contraindicated: should not be used during pregnancy unless absolutely necessary because of potential risks to the fetus.

Excreted in human milk; breastfeeding should be discontinued during treatment.

Contraindicated in those with renal impairment, creatinine clearance (CrCl) < 55 mL/min, proteinuria (>100 mg/dL, 2+).

Monitor renal function closely in elderly patients because of an increased risk of nephrotoxicity.

FAMCICLOVIR
Trade names
APO-Famciclovir, APOhealth Famciclovir Once, Blooms the Chemist Famciclovir Once, Chemists' Own Favic for Cold Sores, Elovax One Dose, Ezovir, Ezovir Cold Sore Relief, Famciclovir-WGR, Famvir, Favic

Available forms
Tablets: 125 mg, 250 mg, 500 mg

Action
* nucleoside analogue that is an orally active prodrug of penciclovir, which targets virus-infected cells inhibiting viral DNA synthesis and therefore viral replication
* orally well absorbed and converted to active metabolite penciclovir in intestinal wall
* half-life 2—3 hours

Use
* treatment of acute herpes zoster (within 72 hours of rash onset)
* treatment and suppression of herpes simplex
* treatment and suppression of recurrent episodes of genital herpes
* treatment of recurrent episodes of herpes labialis (cold sores)

Dose

Immunocompetent patient
* (Herpes zoster) 250 mg orally 3 times daily for 7 days, starting within 48—72 hours of rash onset **OR**
* (Recurrent genital herpes) 125 mg orally twice daily for 5 days, starting during prodromal phase or first onset of lesions **OR**
* (Recurrent genital herpes) 500 mg orally stat, then 250 mg orally 12-hourly for 3 doses **OR**
* (Recurrent genital herpes) 1 g orally twice daily for 1 day **OR**
* (Suppression of recurrent genital herpes) 250 mg orally twice daily **OR**
* (Recurrent herpes labialis (cold sores)) 1.5 g orally stat at first signs of cold sore (tingling, itching, burning) **OR**
* (Recurrent herpes labialis (cold sores)) 750 mg orally twice daily at first signs of cold sore (tingling, itching, burning) for 1 day

Immunocompromised patient
* (Herpes zoster) 500 mg orally 3 times daily for 10 days, starting within 48—72 hours of rash onset **OR**
* (Recurrent genital herpes) 500 mg orally twice daily for 7 days, starting during prodromal phase or first onset of lesions **OR**
* (Suppression of recurrent genital herpes with human immunodeficiency virus (HIV) infection) 500 mg orally twice daily

Adverse effects
* nausea, vomiting, abdominal pain, dry mouth, diarrhoea
* headache, dizziness, anxiety, somnolence, insomnia, fatigue
* nasopharyngitis
* dysmenorrhoea
* back pain
* rash, pruritus
* (Rare) confusion in the elderly

Interactions
* serum level of active metabolite may be increased by probenecid
* caution if given with other agents which are nephrotoxic
* efficacy may be decreased if given with raloxifene

Nursing considerations/Cautions
* (Suppression of recurrent genital herpes) therapy should be reviewed after 12 months
* 125 mg and 250 mg tablets contain lactose and are therefore not recommended in those with galactose

ANTIVIRAL AGENTS

- intolerance, glucose–galactose malabsorption or Lapp lactase deficiency
- caution if used in those with renal impairment
- not recommended for ophthalmic zoster, chicken pox or zoster encephalomyelitis patients

Patient education

- advise the patient against driving or operating machinery if dizziness occurs or is ongoing
- patients with genital herpes should be advised to avoid sexual intercourse during acute episodes and to decrease risk of transmission by using a condom at other times because viral shedding occurs even when the patient is asymptomatic
- (Recurrent genital herpes) advise the patient to start therapy during the prodromal period or as soon as possible after onset of lesions
- (Recurrent herpes labialis (cold sores)) advise the patient to start therapy at the first sign/symptom including tingling, burning or itching at the site

 Tablet can be crushed and mixed with water or a spoonful of yoghurt or apple puree.

 Not recommended during pregnancy unless benefits outweigh risks.

 Avoid, as excretion in human milk is unknown.

 Reduced renal function: dosage adjustment is recommended for patients with impaired renal function. The dosing interval may need to be extended, and dose reduction is suggested based on the degree of renal impairment.

FOSCARNET
Trade name
Foscavir

Available form
Bottle: 6 g/250 mL

Action
- virustatic broad-spectrum antiviral agent that inhibits all human herpes viruses, varicella zoster virus, cytomegalovirus (CMV), Epstein–Barr virus and some retroviruses, including human immunodeficiency virus (HIV)
- viral replication restarts when the drug is discontinued
- chelates bivalent ions such as calcium
- half-life 3.3–6.8 hours

Use
- cytomegalovirus (CMV) retinitis in patients with acquired immunodeficiency syndrome (AIDS)
- aciclovir-resistant herpes simplex virus infection in patients with HIV

Dose
- (CMV retinitis induction and maintenance therapy) 60 mg/kg by slow IV infusion (over 1 hour) 8-hourly for 2–3 weeks (induction), then 90–120 mg/kg IV infusion over 2 hours daily **OR**
- (Herpes simplex virus infections) 40 mg/kg by slow IV infusion (over 1 hour) 8-hourly for 2–3 weeks (or until lesions have healed)

Adverse effects
- anorexia, nausea, vomiting, diarrhoea, dyspepsia, abdominal pain, constipation, GI bleeding, pancreatitis
- paraesthesia, tremor, neuropathy, ataxia, abnormal coordination, hypoaesthesia, involuntary muscle contraction
- aggression, anxiety, confusion, depression, nervousness, agitation
- headache, dizziness, asthenia, fatigue, malaise
- genital ulceration and irritation
- impaired renal function, polyuria, dysuria, decreased creatinine clearance, increased serum creatinine, kidney pain
- abnormal liver function
- hypocalcaemia, hypomagnesaemia, hypokalaemia, hypophosphataemia, hyperphosphataemia, hyponatraemia, hypercalcaemia

- dehydration
- anaemia, leucopenia, thrombocytopenia, granulocytopenia, neutropenia
- chills, fever
- sepsis
- rash, pruritus
- palpitations, tachycardia, hypertension or hypotension, chest pain, ECG abnormalities (including QT interval prolongation)
- seizures (related to impaired electrolyte imbalance)
- (IV site) thrombophlebitis

Interactions
- contraindicated with pentamidine (IV) because it may result in further lowering of calcium levels and both may also cause nephrotoxicity
- caution if given with other drugs known to lower calcium levels
- caution if given with other drugs known to cause QT interval prolongation or electrolyte disturbances
- additive renal toxicity may occur when given with other nephrotoxic drugs (e.g. aminoglycosides, amphotericin B (amphotericin), aciclovir, methotrexate, tacrolimus and ciclosporin)
- renal excretion is impaired when given with drugs that inhibit renal tubular secretion
- not recommended with loop diuretics
- increased risk of renal impairment if given with ritonavir

Nursing considerations/Cautions
- hydration will reduce renal toxicity; therefore 0.5—1 L is recommended before the first infusion to establish diuresis, then 0.5—1 L added to each infusion
- serum electrolytes (especially calcium, magnesium and creatinine) should be monitored before and during therapy
- serum creatinine should be measured every second day during induction and then weekly during maintenance
- the patient should be monitored for any seizure activity
- local irritation and burning sensation may occur if foscarnet contacts eyes or skin, and area should be immediately rinsed with water
- must be given IV only
- if given via peripheral veins, foscarnet should be diluted with glucose 5% or sodium chloride 0.9% to a concentration of 12 mg/mL
- if given via a central vein, a solution of 24 mg/mL does not need further dilution
- administration time should not be less than 1 hour
- if the patient experiences severe nausea or paraesthesia, the infusion rate should be reduced
- an initial induction period of 2—3 weeks is recommended (dependent on clinical response), followed by maintenance therapy as appropriate. Maintenance dose is determined by creatinine clearance
- if the expected response is not achieved, resistance should be considered
- incompatible with a range of drugs (especially those containing calcium); therefore it is recommended that foscarnet be infused alone
- each mL contains 5.5 mg sodium, which may need to be taken into account in those on a sodium-reduced diet
- caution in patients with renal impairment or dehydration
- caution if used in those with pre-existing anaemia, hypomagnesaemia, hypocalcaemia or a history of seizures
- caution if used in those with pre-existing or a history of QT prolongation, electrolyte imbalance (especially hypokalaemia, hyperkalaemia or hypomagnesaemia), bradycardia or cardiac disease
- contraindicated as long-term treatment in those with reasonable prognosis (e.g. bone marrow transplantation)

ANTIVIRAL AGENTS

Patient education
- warn the patient not to drive or operate machinery if any confusion, dizziness, tremor or abnormal coordination occurs
- the patient should be advised to maintain good personal hygiene (washing genital area well after each micturition) to prevent genital irritation and/or ulceration because of the high drug level excreted in the urine
- advise the patient to seek medical advice immediately if any of the following occur:
  - fast, slow or pounding heart rate
  - tingling or numbness of feet or toes
  - fitting (seizures)
  - feeling abnormally tired, pale, lacking in energy, bruising or bleeding easily
- patients (male and female) should be counselled regarding the importance of avoiding pregnancy during therapy. Male patients should be advised to use condoms during therapy and for at least 6 months after stopping

Avoid, as animal studies have shown an increase in skeletal abnormalities at doses lower than human exposure levels, suggesting potential teratogenic effects.

No human data. Passes into the milk of lactating rats at concentrations higher than those in maternal plasma.

Reduced renal function: caution, as dose adjustments are necessary based on creatinine clearance levels. Serum creatinine should be monitored regularly, and adequate hydration maintained to minimise potential renal toxicity.

Elderly patients are more likely to have decreased renal function, and dose selection should be cautious, generally starting at the low end of the dosing range. Regular monitoring of renal function is recommended.

GANCICLOVIR

Trade names
Cymevene, Ganciclovir Lupin

Available form
Vial: 500 mg

Action
- nucleoside analogue that inhibits replication of herpes viruses (e.g. cytomegalovirus (CMV), herpes simplex 1 and 2, Epstein—Barr)
- structurally similar to aciclovir
- plasma half-life is 2.5—3.6 hours
- half-life is prolonged in those with kidney impairment

Use
- palliative and maintenance treatment of CMV retinitis in AIDS or severely immunosuppressed individuals
- treatment of confirmed CMV pneumonitis in bone marrow transplant patients
- prevention of CMV disease in liver, heart and bone marrow transplant patients

Dose
- (CMV retinitis with normal renal function) initially 5 mg/kg 12-hourly by IV infusion over 1 hour for 14—21 days (induction), followed by either 5 mg/kg daily or 6 mg/kg 5 days a week (maintenance) **OR**
- (Prevention of CMV infection in liver transplant patients with normal renal function) initially 5 mg/kg 12-hourly by IV infusion over 1 hour for 7—14 days (induction), followed by either 5 mg/kg for 7 days a week or 6 mg/kg for 5 days a week (for up to 100 days post-transplant) **OR**
- (Prevention of CMV in bone marrow transplant patients with normal renal function) initially 5 mg/kg 12-hourly by IV infusion over 1 hour for 7 days (induction), followed by 5 mg/kg daily for up to 100—120 days after transplant (maintenance) **OR**

- (Prevention of CMV infection in heart transplant patients with normal renal function) 5 mg/kg 12-hourly IV infused over 1 hour for 14 days (induction), followed by 6 mg/kg daily 5 days per week for up to 100 days after transplant (maintenance) **OR**
- (Other transplantation) 5 mg/kg 12-hourly IV infused over 1 hour for 7—14 days (induction), followed by 5 mg/kg for 7 days a week or 6 mg/kg for 5 days a week

Adverse effects
- neutropenia, thrombocytopenia, anaemia, leucopenia, pancytopenia, aplastic anaemia, bone marrow depression
- anorexia, diarrhoea, abdominal pain or distension, dyspepsia, dysphagia, oesophageal candidiasis
- anxiety, headache, confusion
- pruritus
- arthralgia, myalgia
- fever, rigors
- abnormal liver function
- kidney impairment, kidney failure
- infection, sepsis
- lymphadenopathy
- hypertension, hypotension, tachycardia, chest pain
- pleural effusion, cough, dyspnoea, rhinitis
- peripheral neuropathy, hypoaesthesia
- (IV site) phlebitis, pain, inflammation, infection

Interactions
- probenecid may increase plasma half-life, increasing the risk of toxicity
- additive myelosuppression and/or renal impairment may occur when given with some antineoplastic agents (e.g. vinca alkaloids), hydroxycarbamide (hydroxyurea), dapsone, pentamidine, amphotericin B (amphotericin), trimethoprim/sulfonamides, ciclosporin, tacrolimus, mycophenolate mofetil or other nucleoside analogues (e.g. zidovudine)
- zidovudine and ganciclovir should not be given together during ganciclovir induction because severe anaemia and neutropenia may ensue
- not recommended with imipenem—cilastatin owing to risk of seizures

Nursing considerations/Cautions
- CMV retinitis diagnosis should be confirmed by indirect ophthalmoscopy before starting therapy and supported by CMV culture in urine, blood, throat or other sites
- patient should be adequately hydrated before starting IV therapy
- therapy should not be started if neutrophil count is less than 0.5×10^9/L, platelet count is less than 2.5×10^{10}/L or haemoglobin < 80 g/L
- FBC and platelet count should be monitored every second day during first 14 days of therapy, then weekly during maintenance therapy
- serum creatinine or creatinine clearance should be closely monitored if the patient has renal impairment
- if the disease progresses, it can be retreated using induction regimen
- avoid contact with skin or mucous membranes, inhalation or ingestion when handling powder or solution. Wash skin with soap and water or eyes with plain water for at least 15 minutes if contact does occur
- safety glasses and latex gloves should be worn when handling. Preparation, handling and disposal should be according to cytotoxic protocol
- administer alone
- the patient should be monitored for extraocular CMV when treated for CMV retinitis
- regular ophthalmological examination is recommended for both eyes 4—6-weekly during therapy
- reconstitute using water for injections, and then further dilute with glucose 5%, Ringer's lactated solution or sodium chloride 0.9% to 100 mL for infusion (level not greater than 10 mg/mL)

ANTIVIRAL AGENTS

- should be infused in 100 mL of solution over at least 1 hour (not greater than 10 mg/min)
- not administered rapidly or by bolus, as this increases the risk of toxicity
- IM or SC administration will result in severe tissue irritation because of its high pH
- IV site should be closely monitored to avoid phlebitis
- caution if used in those with renal impairment, as dose adjustment will be required (based on creatinine clearance and serum creatinine levels)
- caution if given with valaciclovir or aciclovir because cross-hypersensitivity may exist
- caution if used in those with a history of cytopenia, previous drug-induced cytopenia or exposure to marrow toxic drugs, chemicals or irradiation
- not recommended for congenital or neonatal CMV disease or for treatment of CMV in immunocompetent patients
- not recommended for CMV prophylaxis in donor-negative/receptor-negative transplant patients
- not recommended in the early post-transplant phase of bone marrow transplantation (about 3 weeks post-transplant) until haemopoietic recovery is evident
- contraindicated in those with hypersensitivity to aciclovir, valaciclovir or valganciclovir, or with a neutrophil count $< 0.5 \times 10^9$/L, platelet count $< 2.5 \times 10^{10}$/L or haemoglobin < 80 g/L

Patient education

- the patient should be advised that ganciclovir is not a cure and ophthalmological examinations are recommended every 4–6 weeks during therapy
- warn the patient against driving or operating machinery if any confusion, anxiety or sensory changes occur
- advise the patient to seek medical advice if any of the following occur:
  - numbness or tingling, or decreased sensation in hands or feet
  - worsening eyesight
  - signs of infection, including fever, chills, sore throat, mouth ulcers, swollen glands
  - unusual tiredness or lack of energy, shortness of breath (especially on exertion), pallor
  - unusual bruising or bleeding, purple spots on skin
- patients (male and female) should be counselled regarding the importance of avoiding pregnancy during therapy. Male patients should be advised to use condoms during therapy and for at least 12 weeks after stopping
- male and female patients should be warned that therapy may inhibit fertility during therapy and this may be permanent or temporary

 Contraindicated during pregnancy because of the embryotoxic and teratogenic potential; therefore use adequate contraception during therapy to avoid pregnancy.

 Contraindicated during breastfeeding.

 Reduced renal function: dose adjustments are necessary for patients with impaired renal function, as ganciclovir is primarily excreted by the kidneys.

LETERMOVIR

Trade name
Prevymis

Available forms
Tablets: 240 mg;
Concentrated Injection for infusion: 240 mg/12 mL

Action
- inhibits cytomegalovirus (CMV) DNA-terminase complex required for viral replication

Use
- prophylaxis of CMV infection or disease in adult CMV-seropositive recipients of

allogeneic haematopoietic stem cell transplant

Dose
- 480 mg orally daily, up to 100 days post-transplant (starting no later than 28 days post-transplant) **OR**
- (With ciclosporin) 240 mg orally daily

Adverse effects
- tachycardia, atrial fibrillation
- nausea, vomiting, diarrhoea, abdominal pain
- peripheral oedema
- headache, fatigue
- cough

Interactions
- combination of letermovir and ciclosporin is contraindicated with simvastatin because of an increased risk of myopathy and rhabdomyolysis
- when given with ciclosporin, serum levels of both ciclosporin and letermovir may increase. Ciclosporin levels should be closely monitored during therapy
- may increase serum levels of amiodarone, 3-hydroxy-3-methylglutaryl coenzyme A (HMG-CoA) reductase inhibitors (statins), sirolimus, tacrolimus, repaglinide, rosiglitazone, alfentanil, fentanyl, midazolam or quinidine, increasing the risk of adverse effects
- may decrease serum levels of voriconazole, omeprazole, pantoprazole, phenytoin, warfarin

Nursing considerations/Cautions
- therapy can be started on the day of transplant, or before or after engraftment, but no later than 28 days post-transplant
- if ciclosporin is started after letermovir, the next dose of letermovir should be reduced to 240 mg; if ciclosporin is discontinued, the letermovir dose should be increased to 480 mg, or if ciclosporin is stopped temporarily due to high serum levels, the dose of letermovir does not require changing
- not recommended in those with severe liver impairment or in those with moderate liver impairment with concurrent moderate-to-severe renal impairment

Patient education
- advise the patient that tablets should be swallowed whole, not divided, crushed or broken
- the patient should be advised to seek medical advice if any rapid or fluttering heart rate or swelling of feet and ankles occurs

 Tablets should be swallowed whole and not divided, crushed, or chewed.

 Avoid, as no human data. Embryofetal toxicity was observed in animal studies at maternally toxic exposures. Use only if the potential benefit justifies the potential risk to the fetus.

 Excretion in human milk unknown.

 Not recommended in those with severe liver impairment (Child–Pugh Class C) or in those with moderate liver impairment and concurrent moderate-to-severe kidney impairment.

VALACICLOVIR
Trade names
APX-Valaciclovir, Noumed Valaciclovir, Shilova, Vaclovir, Valaciclovir RBX, Valaciclovir Sandoz, Valaciclovir-WGR, Valtrex, Zelitrex

Available forms
Tablets: 500 mg, 1000 mg

Action
- prodrug that is converted to aciclovir by first-pass intestinal and liver metabolism
- inhibits herpes virus DNA synthesis
- half-life 2.5–3.3 hours
- some resistance has developed

Use
- treatment of herpes zoster (shingles) within 72 hours of onset of rash
- treatment and prevention of genital herpes

ANTIVIRAL AGENTS

- treatment of recurrent herpes labialis (cold sores)
- treatment of ophthalmic zoster
- prevention of cytomegalovirus (CMV) following solid organ transplantation (in those at risk of CMV infection)

Dose
- (Herpes zoster) 1 g orally 3 times daily for 7 days **OR**
- (Herpes labialis (cold sores)) 2 g orally 12 hours apart (total 2 doses) (at first signs of cold sores, including tingling, burning or itching) **OR**
- (Genital herpes) 500 mg orally twice daily for 5–10 days (first presentation) or 5 days (recurrence) **OR**
- (Prevention of genital herpes in immunosuppressed patients) 500 mg orally twice daily **OR**
- (Prevention of genital herpes — fewer than 10 episodes/year) 500 mg orally once daily or in divided doses **OR**
- (Prevention of genital herpes — more than 10 episodes/year) 1 g orally once daily **OR**
- (Reduction of transmission of genital herpes) 500 mg orally daily **OR**
- (Prevention of CMV infection and disease) 2 g orally 4 times daily for 90 days, starting as soon as possible after transplantation

Adverse effects
- (Transplant patients) hallucinations, confusion
- (Prolonged or high dose) thrombotic thrombocytopenic purpura, haemolytic uraemic syndrome
- see also Adverse effects of aciclovir (p. 899)

Interactions
- see Interactions of aciclovir (p. 899)

Nursing considerations/Cautions
- see General Nursing considerations/Cautions for aciclovir (p. 899)

Patient education
- (Herpes labialis (cold sore)) advise the patient to start therapy at the first signs (e.g. tingling, burning, itching) and therapy should not exceed two doses taken 12 hours apart
- the patient/carer/family member should be advised to immediately seek medical advice if the patient displays any confusion or experiences hallucinations
- see also Patient education for aciclovir (p. 900)

 Tablet can be crushed and mixed with a spoonful of jam, yoghurt or apple puree (has a very unpleasant taste).

 Use only if potential benefit justifies potential risk to the fetus.

 Limited data suggest that aciclovir does pass into breastmilk. Caution is advised if valaciclovir is to be administered to a breastfeeding mother.

 Reduced renal function: caution, as adequate hydration should be maintained. Dose reduction may be required based on creatinine clearance.

 Elderly patients are likely to have reduced renal function, and the dose may need adjustment. They should be closely monitored for evidence of neurological side-effects.

VALGANCICLOVIR

Trade names
Valcyte, Valganciclovir Hetero, Valganciclovir Sandoz, Valganciclovir Viatris

Available forms
Tablets: 450 mg;
Oral solution: 50 mg/mL

Action
- prodrug that is converted by intestinal and liver enzymes to ganciclovir
- nucleoside analogue

Use
- treatment of cytomegalovirus (CMV) retinitis in those with acquired immunodeficiency syndrome (AIDS)
- prevention of CMV infection and disease after solid organ transplantation (in those at risk of CMV infection)

Dose
- (Treatment of CMV retinitis in AIDS) 900 mg orally twice daily for 21 days with food (induction), followed by 900 mg orally daily (maintenance) **OR**
- (CMV prevention in solid organ transplantation) 900 mg orally daily with food, starting within 10 days of transplant and continuing up to 200 days after kidney transplantation or 100 days after other solid organ transplantation

Adverse effects
- see Adverse effects of ganciclovir (p. 906)

Interactions
- see Interactions of ganciclovir (p. 906)

Nursing considerations/Cautions
- see Nursing considerations/Cautions for ganciclovir (p. 906)

Patient education
- advise the patient to take tablets with food
- (Oral solution) instruct the patient to use dispenser provided (25 mg graduations) to measure the solution, which should be washed with hot soapy water after use, dried and not used to measure other medications
- patients (male and female) should be counselled regarding the importance of avoiding pregnancy during therapy. Male patients should be advised to use condoms during therapy and for at least 12 weeks after stopping
- male and female patients should be warned that fertility may be inhibited during therapy, and this may be permanent or temporary
- see also Patient education for ganciclovir (p. 907)

Oral solution is available. Tablet should not be crushed, broken or dispersed.

Contraindicated during pregnancy because of the embryotoxic and teratogenic potential; therefore use adequate contraception during therapy to avoid pregnancy.

Contraindicated during breastfeeding.

NEURAMINIDASE INHIBITORS
NS5B RNA-DEPENDENT RNA PROTEASE INHIBITORS

OSELTAMIVIR
Trade names
Oseltamivir Lupin, Talminex, Tamiflu

Available forms
Capsules: 30 mg, 45 mg, 75 mg;
Oral suspension: 6 mg/mL

Action
- neuraminidase inhibitor (prodrug) that is converted to the active form (oseltamivir carboxylate) in the gastrointestinal tract and liver after absorption
- neuraminidase enzyme is required for replication of both influenza A and B strains as it plays a role in viral release from the cells enabling spread to other cells
- active metabolite half-life 6–10 hours (prolonged in those with kidney impairment)

Use
- treatment of influenza A and B (up to 48 hours after onset of first symptoms)
- influenza prophylaxis (although vaccination is the preferred prophylaxis)

Dose
- (Treatment) 75 mg orally twice daily for 5 days, starting within 48 hours of symptom onset **OR**
- (Prophylaxis) 75 mg orally daily for 10 days, starting within 48 hours of exposure

Adverse effects
- nausea, vomiting
- headache
- back pain

ANTIVIRAL AGENTS

Nursing considerations/Cautions
- significantly reduces duration and severity of influenza, as well as reducing risks of secondary infections
- when used prophylactically, protection lasts as long as therapy continues
- effective only against influenza A or B virus
- (Oral suspension) not recommended in those with hereditary fructose intolerance because it contains sorbitol
- caution if used in those with kidney impairment or with underlying respiratory or cardiac conditions and complicated influenza (e.g. pneumonia)
- not recommended in those with end-stage kidney disease (creatinine clearance < 10 mL/min) not undergoing dialysis

Patient education
- advise the patient to avoid contact with skin or eyes. Rinse the area with water if contact occurs
- the patient should be advised to take with food to reduce gastrointestinal adverse effects
- (Oral solution) instruct the patient to shake well before use

 Oral suspension available. Tamiflu capsules can be opened and mixed with a sweetened food (e.g. chocolate syrup) for patients who have difficulty swallowing.

 Limited data suggest no increased risk to the fetus. Use only if potential benefits justify risks to the mother and fetus.

 Limited data indicate low levels of oseltamivir and its active metabolite in breastmilk. Use only if the potential benefit to the mother justifies the possible risk to the nursing infant.

 Reduced renal function: dosage adjustment is recommended in patients with CrCL ≤ 60 mL/min. For treatment, a lower dose is recommended based on severity of renal impairment.

PERAMIVIR
Trade name
Rapivab

Available form
Vial: 200 mg/20 mL

Action
- inhibits influenza virus neuraminidase (enzyme that releases viral particles from infected cells)

Use
- treatment of acute influenza in those who have been symptomatic for up to 2 days

Dose
- 600 mg by IV infusion over 15–30 minutes

Adverse effects
- diarrhoea, constipation
- hypertension
- insomnia
- elevated liver enzymes
- (Rare) allergic reactions, serious skin reactions
- (Rare, children) delirium, abnormal behaviour, hallucinations

Interactions
- live attenuated vaccines are not recommended with 48 hours of peramivir

Nursing considerations/Cautions
- should be given within 2 days of developing influenza symptoms
- dilute vial with sodium chloride 0.9% or 0.45%, glucose 5% or Ringer's lactated solution to a volume of 100 mL
- dose reduction is required in those with creatinine clearance < 50 mL/min
- repeated doses are not recommended as efficacy has not been established
- suitable only for viral illness; bacterial infections may still occur
- not a substitute for vaccination against influenza

Patient education

- suggest that the patient has a yearly influenza vaccination
- advise the patient to seek medical advice immediately if any of the following occur:
  - rash, itching, hives, swelling of face, tongue or lips
  - severe blistering or peeling of skin, mouth sores, fever, fatigue
  - inflamed, red and raised skin and blisters

Limited human data on the effects in pregnancy. Animal studies show potential risks at high doses. Use only if the benefit outweighs the potential risk to the fetus, as influenza infection poses significant risks during pregnancy.

Caution, as excretion in human milk is unknown; however, Rapivab is present in animal milk. Use with caution and consider the benefits of breastfeeding alongside the mother's clinical need for Rapivab.

Reduced renal function: dose adjustments when CrCL < 50 mL/min.

ZANAMIVIR
Trade name
Relenza

Available form
Powder for inhalation: 5 mg/dose

Action
- selective viral neuraminidase inhibitor, preventing release of infective particles and thereby reducing propagation of influenza virus
- neuraminidase enzyme is essential for viral replication as it plays a role in releasing the virus from infected cells, enabling spread
- not metabolised and is excreted unchanged in the urine
- half-life 2.5–5.1 hours (inhalation)

Use
- treatment of influenza (A or B) within 48 hours of symptom onset
- prevention of influenza A or B (where strain is not included in annual influenza vaccine)
- reduces transmission among members of infected person's household

Dose
- (Treatment) 10 mg (2 inhalations) twice daily for 5 days (starting within 48 hours of symptom onset) (daily total 20 mg) **OR**
- (Prevention) 10 mg (2 inhalations) daily for 10 days, which can be increased to 28 days if exposure is > 10 days

Adverse effects
- nausea, vomiting, diarrhoea
- headache
- cough, bronchitis
- (Very rare) bronchospasm, dyspnoea, allergic reaction (facial and oropharyngeal oedema), neuropsychiatric events (e.g. delirium, abnormal behaviour), severe skin reaction

Nursing considerations/Cautions

- maximum benefit if administered within 48 hours of symptom onset
- decreases symptoms and duration of influenza symptoms
- not recommended as routine prevention of influenza
- caution if used in those with asthma or chronic obstructive pulmonary disease (COPD) because of the increased risk of bronchospasm
- contraindicated in those with severe milk protein allergy

Patient education

- the patient should be advised to seek medical advice if any of the following occur:
  - wheezing or shortness of breath
  - abnormal behaviours or mood changes

ANTIVIRAL AGENTS

- if taking with other inhaled medication, instruct the patient that they should be administered before zanamivir
- instruct the patient that medication can be administered only using a Diskhaler device, which is provided, and ensure the patient understands technique for correct use

No human data. Crosses the placenta in animal studies without evidence of harm. Not recommended during pregnancy (especially first trimester).

No data on excretion in human milk. Zanamivir is excreted in animal milk; use with caution in nursing mothers, weighing potential benefits against possible risks to the infant.

NS5B RNA-DEPENDENT RNA PROTEASE INHIBITORS

SOFOSBUVIR
Trade names
Epclusa, Vosevi

Available forms
Tablets: sofosbuvir 400 mg/velpatasvir 100 mg (Epclusa); sofosbuvir 400 mg/velpatasvir 100 mg/voxilaprevir 100 mg (Vosevi)

Action
- (sofosbuvir) NS5B RNA polymerase inhibitor
- (velpatasiv) NSSA protein inhibitor
- (voxilaprevir) NS3/4A protease inhibitor

Use
- chronic hepatitis C (as part of combination antiviral therapy)

Dose
- (Epclusa)(without cirrhosis or with compensated cirrhosis) 1 tablet orally daily for 12 weeks **OR**
- (Epclusa)(decompensated cirrhosis) 1 tablet orally daily with ribavirin (initally 600 mg orally daily) **OR**
- (Vosevi) 1 tablet orally daily with food for 12 weeks

Adverse effects (combination therapy)
- fatigue, headache, insomnia, asthenia, irritability
- nausea, diarrhoea, loss of appetite
- myalgia
- pruritus, rash
- dysglycaemia
- fever, chills, flu-like illness
- anaemia
- (Uncommon) severe depression, suicidal ideation, pancytopenia

Interactions
- (Epclusa) contraindicated with preparations containing velpatasvir and/or sofosbuvir
- (Vosevi) contraindicated with rifampicin and rosuvastatin
- caution if used with HMG-Co reductase inhibitors (statins) as statin levels may increase with associated risk of myopathy. Lowest dose possible should be used if used together
- (Vosevi) may increase concentration of digoxin, ciclosporin and dabigatran increasing the risk of adverse effects. Close monitoring is recommended if used to together
- symptomatic bradycardia may occur if combination therapy (sofosbuvir, peginterferon alfa and ribavirin) is given with amiodarone and these are therefore not recommended together
- not recommended with rifampicin, modafinil, carbamazepine, oxcarbazepine, phenytoin, phenobarbital (phenobarbitone), rifabutin, rifampicin, tipranavir/ritonavir or St John's wort, as they decrease plasma levels of sofosbuvir, velpatasiv and voxilaprevir
- INR should be closely monitored if given with warfarin
- absorption decreased if given with antacids and should be separated by at least 4 hours if used together

Nursing considerations/Cautions

- before starting therapy, the patient should be screened for hepatitis B virus (HBV) co-infection, as reactivation may occur
- if the patient is taking amiodarone (with no other alternative), cardiac monitoring as an inpatient is recommended for the first 48 hours of therapy, then daily as an outpatient or heart rate monitored at home for the first 2 weeks of therapy. If amiodarone is discontinued just before starting therapy, cardiac monitoring as previously described should occur, as amiodarone has a long half-life and a risk of bradycardia would exist
- (Patient with genotype 1, 4, 5 or 6 chronic hepatitis C) given with peginterferon alfa and ribavirin for 12 weeks
- (Patient with genotype 2 chronic hepatitis C) given with ribavirin for 12 weeks
- (Patient with genotype 3 chronic hepatitis C) given with ribavirin for 16 weeks
- (Patient with chronic hepatitis C awaiting liver transplantation) given with ribavirin until liver transplantation occurs
- ribavirin dose is according to weight:
    - < 75 kg: 1000 mg orally in 2 divided doses with food
    - ≥ 75 kg: 1200 mg orally in 2 divided doses with food
- (Combination therapy with ribavirin) therapy should not be started until a negative pregnancy test has been obtained just before starting therapy
- caution if used in those over 65 years
- caution if used in those with pre-existing history of depression or psychiatric illness
- not recommended in those with genotype 1, 4, 5 and 6 HCV infection, HCV/HCB or HCV/human immunodeficiency virus (HIV) co-infection
- not recommended in patients with severe renal failure or decompensated cirrhosis (if combined with peg interferon alfa, contraindicated in those with liver decompensation)
- (Vesovi) not recommended in those with moderate-to-severe liver impairment

Patient education

- warn the patient not to drive or operate machinery if fatigue, asthenia and insomnia occur
- for patients with diabetes, recommend close monitoring of blood glucose levels, as hypoglycaemia may occur
- advise the patient to seek medical advice immediately if any of the following occur:
    - fainting or near fainting, dizziness, lightheadedness, malaise, weakness, excessive tiredness, shortness of breath, chest pains, confusion, memory problems
    - any signs of depression such as sadness, withdrawal from friends or previously pleasurable activities, or any attempts at self-harm
- female patients should be advised to use high-dose oral contraceptive containing at least 30 micrograms of ethinylestradiol combined with norethisterone acetate/norethisterone
- (Combination therapy with ribavirin) counsel female patients regarding the importance of not becoming pregnant during therapy and for 6 months after stopping, including the need for two forms of reliable contraception to be used (one by each partner). Patients should be instructed to conduct monthly pregnancy test during therapy
- (Combination therapy with ribavirin) male patients should be advised regarding the importance of pregnant female partners avoiding any contact with capsules

 Tablet can be crushed and mixed with water, or a spoonful of thickened fluid, yoghurt or apple puree.

 Contraindicated in pregnancy if used in combination with ribavirin because of the risk of birth defects and fetal death.

 Not recommended during breastfeeding.

ANTIVIRAL AGENTS

OTHER ANTIVIRAL DRUGS

ADEFOVIR DIPIVOXIL
Trade name
APO-Adefovir

Available form
Tablets: 10 mg

Action
- nucleoside analogue with an active metabolite (adefovir diphosphate) which inhibits hepatitis B viral DNA reverse transcriptase
- active metabolite (adefovir diphosphate) has half-life of 12–36 hours

Use
- chronic hepatitis B (with evidence of active viral replication and either elevated serum aminotransferases (alanine aminotransferase (ALT), aspartate aminotransferase (AST)) or histologically active disease)

Dose
- 10 mg orally daily

Adverse effects
- abnormal liver function
- kidney failure, abnormal kidney function, nephrotoxicity
- headache, asthenia
- nausea, diarrhoea, flatulence, dyspepsia, abdominal pain
- (Rare) lactic acidosis, severe hepatomegaly with steatosis
- post-treatment exacerbation of hepatitis

Interactions
- increased risk of nephrotoxicity if given with other nephrotoxic agents such as ciclosporin, tacrolimus, vancomycin, aminoglycosides and NSAIDs
- contraindicated with tenofovir disoproxil fumarate, tenofovir alafenamide or formulations containing either of them

Nursing consideratioms/Cautions
- HIV testing is recommended before starting therapy to identify any human immunodeficiency virus (HIV) co-infection because of the risk of viral resistance developing
- monitoring of liver and renal function (including creatinine clearance) is recommended before starting and regularly during therapy
- dosing interval should be adjusted in those with creatinine clearance < 50 mL/min
- caution when discontinuing therapy because severe exacerbation of hepatitis can occur. Liver function should be closely monitored for at least 12 weeks when therapy is stopped
- caution if used in women, the obese or those with prolonged exposure to nucleosides because of the increased risk of lactic acidosis and severe hepatomegaly
- caution if used in those with kidney impairment because of the risk of nephrotoxicity
- caution if used in those > 65 years

Patient education
- warn the patient that exacerbation of hepatitis may occur up to 12 weeks after stopping therapy. If symptoms including upper abdominal pain, tiredness, yellowing of eyes and/or skin, dark urine and pale stools (bowel motions) occur, medical advice should be sought immediately

Tablet can be crushed and mixed with water, or a spoonful of yoghurt or apple puree (has a very bitter taste).

Should be used during pregnancy only if benefits outweigh potential risks.

Excretion in human breastmilk is unknown. Caution is advised, and breastfeeding is not recommended while taking adefovir dipivoxil because of the potential risks to the infant.

Reduced renal function: primarily excreted by the kidneys. Dose adjustment is required for patients with renal impairment, as increased drug exposure can lead to nephrotoxicity. Monitor renal function closely, particularly in patients with baseline renal insufficiency.

 Exercise caution when used in elderly patients, as they may have decreased renal, hepatic or cardiac function and are more likely to be taking other medications. Monitor renal function closely in this population.

ENTECAVIR MONOHYDRATE
Trade names
Entac, Entecavir APO, Entecavir GH, Entecavir RBX, Entecavir Sandoz, Entecavir Viatris, Entecavir-WGR

Available forms
Tablets: 0.5 mg, 1 mg

Action
- deoxyguanosine nucleoside analogue which is selectively active against hepatitis B virus (HBV) polymerase
- little or no activity against other viruses
- phosphorylated to active form that inhibits HBV DNA replication at three stages
- well absorbed on empty stomach but does not undergo extensive metabolism
- half-life 128—149 hours

Use
- chronic hepatitis B (with evidence of active liver inflammation)

Dose
- 0.5 mg orally daily either 2 hours before or 2 hours after a meal **OR**
- (Lamivudine refractory/resistant patient) 1 mg orally daily either 2 hours before or 2 hours after a meal

Adverse effects
- fatigue, headache,
- altered liver enzymes
- (Rare) lactic acidosis, severe hepatomegaly with steatosis

Interactions
- caution if used with agents that reduce kidney function or compete for renal tubular secretion
- caution if given with antiretroviral agents because of the increased risk of lactic acidosis and severe hepatomegaly with steatosis

Nursing considerations/Cautions
- liver function should continue to be monitored for several months after stopping therapy
- tablets contain lactose and are not recommended in those with hereditary problems of galactose intolerance, Lapp lactase deficiency or glucose—galactose malabsorption
- caution if used in those > 65 years
- caution if used in those with renal impairment (creatinine clearance < 50 mL/min)
- caution if used in liver transplant patients receiving immunosuppressants as kidney function may be affected. Kidney function should be closely monitored
- not recommended in those with human immunodeficiency virus (HIV) co-infection, unless being treated with antiretroviral agents

Patient education
- advise the patient to take tablets on an empty stomach, either 2 hours before or after food
- the patient should be warned that acute exacerbation of hepatitis may occur after therapy is stopped
- the patient should be instructed that therapy does not decrease the risk of transmission of hepatitis B virus to others via sexual contact or blood contamination; therefore precautions should be taken (e.g. condoms during sexual contact, not sharing needles)

 Tablet can be dispersed in 10—20 mL of water, or crushed and mixed with a spoonful of yoghurt or apple puree. Mask and gloves should be worn if dispersing or crushing tablets.

 Avoid, as animal studies have shown evidence of fetal harm at high exposures.

ANTIVIRAL AGENTS

 Avoid, as excreted in the milk of rats, but it is unknown if it is excreted in human milk.

 Reduced renal function: dosage adjustment is recommended for patients with a CrCl < 50 mL/min, including those on hemodialysis or continuous ambulatory peritoneal dialysis (CAPD), as entecavir is predominantly excreted by the kidneys. For patients with severe renal impairment, alternative dosing schedules are suggested, but splitting tablets is not recommended for doses lower than 0.5 mg.

RIBAVIRIN
Trade name
Ibavyr

Available form
Capsules: 200 mg

Action
- antiviral agent (nucleoside analogue) that penetrates virus-infected cells and thought to reduce guanosine triphosphate (GTP) storage as well as inhibiting RNA and protein synthesis, thereby inhibiting viral replication and spread to other cells (although the mechanism is not entirely understood)
- no activity against hepatitis C virus (HCV) if used alone
- half-life 9.5 hours after inhalation
- very long half-life (274–298 hours) (multiple dosing) (oral)

Use
- treatment of chronic hepatitis C (in combination therapy with sofosbuvir (see p. 913)

Dose
- (Weight < 75 kg) 500 mg orally twice daily with food (with 400 mg sofosbuvir combination therapy) for 12 weeks (genotype 2), 16 weeks (genotype 3) or until liver transplantation **OR**
- (Weight ≥ 75 kg) 600 mg orally twice daily with food (with 400 mg sofosbuvir combination therapy) for 12 weeks (genotype 2), 16 weeks (genotype 3) or until liver transplantation

Interactions
- because of a very long half-life, interactions with medications may occur up to 2 months after stopping therapy with ribavirin
- not recommended with azathioprine because of an increased risk of myelotoxicity

Nursing considerations/Cautions

Hepatitis C combination therapy
- not given as monotherapy
- (Genotype 3) therapy may be extended to 24 weeks if needed
- complete blood count (with haemoglobin, differential, platelet count, electrolytes, serum creatinine, liver function tests, uric acid, lipid levels), thyroid function and cardiac function are recommended before starting therapy and regularly during combination therapy
- monthly pregnancy testing is required during and for 6 months after stopping therapy for all female patients of childbearing potential or female partners of male patients. Therapy should not be started unless the patient and his/her partner are using two reliable forms of contraception during and for 6 months after therapy has stopped
- caution if used in those with a history of depression
- caution if used in those with pre-existing severe anaemia (e.g. a history of GI bleeding, spherocytosis)
- caution if used in those with pre-existing cardiac disease. If used, ECG monitoring is recommended before starting and regularly during therapy
- not recommended in those with decompensation cirrhosis of the liver, post-liver transplantation or if the patient has co-infection with hepatitis B virus (HBV) or human immunodeficiency virus (HIV)

- contraindicated in men whose partners are pregnant
- contraindicated in those with a history of pre-existing cardiac disease in the previous 6 months, haemoglobinopathies (e.g. thalassaemia, sickle cell anaemia) and renal impairment (creatinine clearance < 50 mL/min)

Patient education

Hepatitis C combination therapy
- warn the patient not to drive or operate machinery if fatigue, headache or depression occurs or is ongoing
- instruct the patient to swallow capsules whole (not opened, broken, crushed or chewed) and take after food
- advise the patient to seek medical advice immediately if any of the following occur:
  - depression, sadness, aggression, mood swings, withdrawal from previously pleasurable activities or friends, thoughts of self-harm or suicide (up to 6 months after therapy has stopped)
  - tiredness, shortness of breath and looking pale
  - unusual bleeding or bruising
- counsel female patients regarding the importance of not becoming pregnant during therapy and for 6 months after stopping, including the need for two forms of reliable contraception to be used (one by each partner). Patients should be instructed to conduct monthly pregnancy tests during therapy
- male patients should be advised regarding the importance of female partners not becoming pregnant during therapy or for 6 months after including the need for two forms of reliable contraception to be used (one by each partner). A male patient's female partner should be instructed to conduct monthly pregnancy tests during therapy

Crushing the tablet may lead to exposure to ribavirin powder, which can be harmful if inhaled or comes into contact with skin or mucous membranes. Tablets should be swallowed whole to ensure appropriate dosing and minimize exposure risks.

Contraindicated in pregnancy because of teratogenicity and a potential for significant embryocidal effects. It is also contraindicated in men whose partners are pregnant. Female patients of childbearing potential and male patients with female partners of childbearing potential must use effective contraception during treatment and for at least 6 months after the last dose.

Excretion in human milk unknown. Due to the potential for adverse effects in the nursing infant, a decision should be made to either discontinue breastfeeding or discontinue ribavirin, considering the importance of the drug to the mother.

Reduced renal function: not recommended when CrCl < 50 mL/min owing to limited pharmacokinetic data and an increased risk of toxicity. Dosage adjustments may be necessary in patients with mild-to-moderate renal impairment.

ANTIRETROVIRAL AGENTS

Retroviruses are RNA viruses that replicate within a host by using an enzyme called reverse transcriptase, which converts their RNA genome into DNA. This DNA is then integrated into the host's cellular DNA, allowing the virus to replicate alongside the host's own genetic material. This intricate replication process makes retroviruses particularly challenging to treat (Knights et al 2023).

General Adverse effects of antiretroviral agents
- headache, dizziness, lethargy, fatigue, asthenia, depression, insomnia, somnolence, dream disturbance, anxiety, concentration level impairment, confusion
- anorexia, nausea, vomiting, diarrhoea, flatulence, abdominal pain, dry mouth, dyspepsia
- fever
- rash

ANTIVIRAL AGENTS

- elevated liver enzymes, elevated cholesterol and triglycerides
- increased risk of opportunistic infections
- (Combination therapy) increased risk of myocardial infarction
- (Rare) (protease inhibitors) spontaneous bleeding in those with haemophilia
- (Rare) lactic acidosis, hepatomegaly
- (Rare) osteonecrosis, lipodystrophy syndrome (redistribution/accumulation of body fat), hyperglycaemia, new onset or exacerbation of pre-existing diabetes mellitus
- (Rare) immune reconstitution syndrome (is an inflammatory reaction to asymptomatic/opportunistic infections (e.g. cytomegalovirus (CMV) retinitis, mycobacterial infections, *Pneumocystis jiroveci* pneumonia (PCP))
- (Nucleoside/nucleotide analogues) mitochondrial dysfunction (in children exposed in utero)

General Interactions of antiretroviral agents

- may increase serum levels and associated risk of myopathy and rhabdomyolysis if given with simvastatin, pravastatin, fluvastatin or atorvastatin
- antacids may decrease absorption
- may decrease serum levels of methadone, increasing the risk of opiate withdrawal syndrome (especially if given with low-dose ritonavir)
- increased risk of hypotension, syncope, visual changes and priapism if given with avanafil, sildenafil or tadalafil
- if given with warfarin, prothrombin time should be closely monitored, especially when starting, stopping or altering dosage

General Nursing considerations/ Cautions for antiretroviral agents

- human immunodeficiency virus (HIV) testing is recommended before starting therapy to identify any HIV disease because of the increased risk of viral resistance to the drug. This should also include cases of needlestick injury involving a known HIV source
- cardiac risk factors (e.g. hypertension, diabetes mellitus, smoking, hyperlipidaemia) should be assessed and treated before starting therapy to decrease risk of myocardial infarction
- liver function should be tested before starting and during therapy
- in patients with concomitant hepatitis B, recurrent hepatitis may occur when therapy is stopped. Monitoring of liver function and markers of hepatitis B virus replication is recommended regularly after therapy is stopped
- the patient should be examined for any signs of lipodystrophy syndrome (e.g. central obesity, buffalo hump, peripheral wasting, breast enlargement, increases in serum cholesterol, triglycerides and blood glucose); therefore serum triglycerides, cholesterol and blood glucose should be monitored throughout therapy
- if one antiretroviral agent (part of combination therapy) is stopped, all the antiretroviral agents should be restarted together
- combination antiretroviral therapy increases the risk of lipodystrophy syndrome
- combination therapy for treatment of HIV infection is common, as resistance occurs quickly to monotherapy. However, it becomes difficult to establish if adverse effects are caused by a single agent, the combination therapy or progression of the disease itself
- cross-resistance between members of a similar group may exist and should be taken into consideration when developing treatment regimens
- (Protease inhibitors) caution if used in those with haemophilia A and B because of the increased risk of bleeding
- (Nucleoside analogues) an increased risk of lactic acidosis and hepatomegaly in women

- caution if used in those who have hepatitis co-infection. Patients should be closely monitored when therapy is stopped for any evidence of exacerbation of hepatitis
- caution if used in those with mild-to-moderate liver impairment (including active hepatitis B or C)
- contraindicated in those with severe liver failure

General Patient education for antiretroviral agents

- therapy with antiretroviral agents does not cure HIV or decrease the risk of transmission of the virus and the patient should therefore be encouraged to continue safe sex practices (e.g. use of condoms) and not share needles
- the patient should be advised to seek medical advice if any of the following occur:
  - fatigue, loss of appetite, skin or eye yellowing, dark urine and upper abdominal tenderness/pain
  - joint aches and/or pain, stiffness or difficulty moving
  - generalised weakness, tiredness, unusual muscle pain, loss of appetite, unexplained weight loss, nausea, vomiting, unusual stomach discomfort, rapid and/or difficulty breathing, shortness of breath, dizziness, lightheadedness
  - signs of infection, such as fever, swollen glands, sore throat
  - very sick with rapid breathing (may be worse in women than men)
  - loss of body fat from arms, legs and face with increased fat on abdomen, breasts and back of neck (buffalo hump)
  - chest pain, which may or may not radiate into neck and/or arm, nausea, sweating, severe anxiety or a sense of impending doom
- the patient should be advised to seek medical advice before taking any prescription or non-prescription drugs (including over-the-counter or herbal preparations), as they may interact with antiretroviral agents
- warn the patient to avoid driving or operating machinery if dizziness, somnolence, fatigue, asthenia or confusion occur
- if the patient has diabetes, advise them to monitor blood glucose levels closely during therapy
- the patient should be warned that some people (especially those who have been HIV-positive for some time) may develop an inflammatory reaction (e.g. fever, pain, redness, swelling) within weeks of starting therapy, which may be a sign of the body's recovery in its ability to fight the infection. The patient should be instructed to discuss any concerns with doctors if this occurs
- some antiretroviral agents decrease the efficacy of oral contraceptives; therefore women of childbearing potential should be advised to use an alternative or additional form of contraception to avoid pregnancy

 To prevent the transmission of HIV to an uninfected child, it is recommended that HIV-positive women refrain from breastfeeding. The use of most antiretroviral agents during breastfeeding is generally discouraged unless the potential benefits are deemed to significantly outweigh the risks.

NUCLEOSIDE REVERSE TRANSCRIPTASE INHIBITORS (NRTIs)

ABACAVIR
Trade name
Ziagen

Available forms
Tablets: 300 mg;
Oral solution: 20 mg/mL

ANTIVIRAL AGENTS

Action
- nucleoside analogue reverse transcriptase inhibitor
- selective against human immunodeficiency virus 1 (HIV-1) and HIV-2
- half-life about 1.5 hours

Use
- HIV infections (with other antiretroviral agents)

Dose
- 300 mg orally twice daily

Adverse effects
- hypersensitivity (may be life threatening)
- myalgia
- dyspnoea, sore throat, cough
- hyperlactataemia
- see also General Adverse effects of antiretroviral agents (p. 918)

Interaction
- caution if given with methadone

Nursing considerations/Cautions
- testing for HLA-B*5701 allele is recommended before starting therapy. Those with a positive allele are at higher risk of hypersensitivity reactions
- if hypersensitivity is suspected, therapy is immediately stopped and should **never** be restarted
- caution if used in women, those who are obese or who have had prolonged exposure to nucleoside analogues, because these factors increase the risk of lactic acidosis and severe hepatomegaly
- (Oral solution) contains sorbitol and is therefore not recommended in those with hereditary fructose intolerance. Sorbitol may also cause diarrhoea and abdominal pain
- see also General Nursing considerations/Cautions for antiretroviral agents (p. 919)

Patient education
- the patient should be advised to immediately stop therapy and seek medical advice if any of the following occur:
- unusual rash, fever, chills, itching, headache, fatigue, muscle pain, nausea, vomiting, diarrhoea, abdominal pain, sore throat, cough or shortness of breath, which may be signs of hypersensitivity (but also adverse effects of the drug) (especially in first 6 weeks of therapy)
- if the patient develops a hypersensitivity reaction (as described above), they should be instructed to **never** take abacavir (or any preparation containing abacavir) again, otherwise a life-threatening reaction can occur within hours
- advise the patient to wear or carry some form of identification, such as a Medic-Alert or Alert card (contained in the medication packet) with details of hypersensitivity
- (Oral solution) instruct the patient to use the supplied dosing syringe to administer the correct dose. The bottle adapter and syringe should be washed after each use
- see also General Patient education for antiretroviral agents (p. 920)

Available as oral solution. Tablet may be crushed and mixed with a spoonful of yoghurt or apple puree. Staff should wear mask and gloves if crushing. Pregnant staff should not crush tablets.

Limited human data. Animal studies showed some evidence of developmental toxicity (such as fetal growth restriction and skeletal malformations) when abacavir was administered at high doses, suggesting potential risks. However, data from the Antiretroviral Pregnancy Registry, with over 2000 reports of abacavir exposure in pregnant women, did not show an increased rate of birth defects compared with the general population.

Abacavir is excreted in breastmilk, which could expose infants to low plasma levels of the drug. The potential for HIV transmission through breastmilk and the risk of adverse reactions in the breastfed infant are significant concerns. It is not recommended for mothers receiving abacavir to breastfeed.

Available in combination with
- abacavir 600 mg + lamivudine 300 mg (Kivexa)
- abacavir 600 mg + lamivudine 300 mg (Abacavir/Lamivudine Viatris)
- abacavir 600 mg + dolutegravir 50 mg + lamivudine 300 mg tablets (Triumeq)

EMTRICITABINE

Action
- synthetic nucleoside analogue
- analogue of cytosine
- effective against HIV-1, HIV-2 and hepatitis B
- half-life about 10 hours

Use
- treatment of human immunodeficiency virus (HIV) (with other antiretroviral agents)

Dose
- 200 mg orally daily

Adverse effects
- rash, skin discolouration (hyperpigmentation of palms and/or soles)
- neutropenia, anaemia
- arthralgia, myalgia
- neuropathy, peripheral neuritis, paraesthesia
- see also General Adverse effects of antiretroviral agents (p. 918)

Interaction
- contraindicated with other preparations containing emtricitabine or lamivudine

Nursing considerations/Cautions
- not available as monotherapy
- increased risk of liver toxicity if given to those with chronic hepatitis B or C treated with combination antiviral therapy
- caution if used in those with kidney impairment, as predominantly excreted via kidney. Adjustment to dosing interval is required depending on creatinine clearance
- see also General Nursing education/Cautions for antiretroviral agents (p. 919)

Patient education
- patient should be advised to seek medical advice immediately if any of the following occur:
  - tingling, numbness or changes to sensation at extremities
  - change in skin colour (palms or soles of feet)

 Avoid, as crosses the placenta in animal studies.

 Excreted in human breastmilk. Avoid breastfeeding because of the potential for HIV transmission and possible adverse effects on the infant, including the risk of viral resistance to emtricitabine.

 Reduced renal function: emtricitabine is primarily eliminated by the kidneys. In patients with CrCl < 50 mL/min, a dosing interval adjustment is required. Emtriva may accumulate in renal impairment, so monitor renal function and adjust dosage as needed.

Available in combination with
- bictegravir + emtricitabine + tenofovir alafenamide tablets (see tenofovir alatenamide p. 924)
- tenofovir disoproxil + emtricitabine tablets (see tenofovir disoproxil p. 925)
- elvitegravir 150 mg + cobicistat 150 mg + emtricitabine 200 mg + tenofovir alafenamide 10 mg (Genvoya)
- emtricitabine 200 mg + rilpivirine 25 mg + tenofovir alafenamide 25 mg (Odefsey)
- darunavir 800 mg + cobicistat 150 mg + emtricitabine 200 mg + tenofovir alafenamide 10 mg (Symtuza)
- tenofovir disoproxil 300 mg + emtricitabine 200 mg + efavirenz 600 mg

ANTIVIRAL AGENTS

(Tenofovir Disoproxil/Emtricitabine/Efavirenz Viatris)

LAMIVUDINE
Trade names
3TC, Lamividine Viatris, Zeffix, Zetlam

Available forms
Tablets: 100 mg, 150 mg, 300 mg;
Oral solution: 10 mg/mL

Action
- active against hepatitis B (HBV), as well as human immunodeficiency virus 1 (HIV-1) and HIV-2
- converted to active metabolite (lamivudine triphosphate), which inhibits HIV reverse transcription by terminating the viral DNA chain
- also inhibits RNA and DNA-dependent DNA polymerase functions
- synergism of antiviral activity when given with zidovudine
- active metabolite half-life 10–15 hours

Use
- treatment of HIV infection (with other antiretroviral agents)
- treatment of chronic hepatitis B

Dose
- (HIV-1 treatment) 150 mg orally twice or 300 mg once daily **OR**
- (HBV) 100 mg daily

Adverse effects
- rash, alopecia
- myalgia, muscle cramps
- hyperlactataemia
- neutropenia, anaemia
- pancreatitis (especially in children)
- neuropathy
- see also General Adverse effects of antiretroviral agents (p. 918)

Interactions
- increased serum levels may occur if given with trimethoprim as part of a trimethoprim/sulfamethoxazole combination
- activity may be decreased by ciprofloxacin, pentamidine or ganciclovir
- not recommended with emtricitabine or formulations that contain emtricitabine
- increased risk of pancreatitis if given with IV pentamidine
- not recommended with other sorbitol-containing medications

Nursing considerations/Cautions
- not recommended as monotherapy
- (Oral solution) contains propylene glycol and hydroxybenzoates, which may cause hypersensitivity reactions in sensitive individuals
- caution if used in those with moderate-to-severe kidney impairment or decompensated liver disease
- caution if used in those with a history of pancreatitis or peripheral neuropathy
- see also General Nursing considerations/Cautions for antiretroviral agents (p. 919)

Patient education
- those with diabetes should be advised that the oral solution contains sucrose (5 mL = 1 g sucrose); therefore blood glucose levels should be closely monitored during therapy if the oral solution is taken
- (HBV) advise the patient that there may be an exacerbation/reactivation of hepatitis if therapy is stopped. Liver function should be monitored for at least 16 weeks after stopping therapy (especially in those with advanced liver disease or transplant recipients)
- advise the patient that the dose for HBV is not appropriate for treatment of HIV
- instruct the patient to immediately seek medical advice if any of the following occur:
  - abdominal pain, nausea and vomiting
  - any weakness, pain, numbness or tingling of feet or hands
- see also General Patient education for antiretroviral agents (p. 920)

Oral solution available. Tablet can be crushed and mixed with water, or a spoonful of yoghurt or apple puree.

 Limited human data; animal studies indicate early embryonic loss. Crosses the placenta. Use only if benefit outweighs risk.

 Excreted in breastmilk and can reach concentrations similar to maternal plasma levels. For women with HIV, breastfeeding is generally not recommended to prevent HIV transmission to the infant.

 Reduced renal function: lamivudine plasma concentrations increase in patients with moderate-to-severe renal impairment because of reduced clearance. Dose adjustments are recommended based on creatinine clearance levels to avoid toxicity. The oral solution is preferred for more precise dosing in patients with significantly impaired renal function.

Available in combination with
- Abacavir 600 mg + Lamivudine 300 mg tablets (Abacavir/Lamivudine Viatris/Kivexa)
- Lamivudine 150 mg + Zidovudine 300 mg tablets (Combivir /Lamivudine/Zidovudine Viatris)
- Dolutegravir 50 mg + Lamivudine 300 mg tablets (Dovato, Triumeq)

TENOFOVIR ALAFENAMIDE
Trade names
Vemlidy

Available in combination with
- Tenofovir alafenamide 10 mg + emtricitabine 200 mg tablets (Descovy 200/10)
- Tenofovir alafenamide 25 mg + emtricitabine 200 mg tablets (Descovy 200/25)
- Tenofovir alafenamide 25 mg + bictegravir 50 mg + emtricitabine 200 mg tablets (Biktarvy)
- Tenofovir alafenamide 10 mg + elvitegravir 150 mg + cobicistat 150 mg + emtricitabine 200 mg tablets (Genvoya)
- Tenofovir alafenamide 25 mg + emtricitabine 200 mg + rilpivirine 25 mg tablets (Odefsey)
- Tenofovir alafenamide 10 mg + darunavir 800 mg + cobicistat 150 mg + emtricitabine 200 mg tablets (Symtuza)

TENOFOVIR DISOPROXIL FUMARATE
Trade names
Viread, Tenofovir ARX, Tenofovir Disoproxil Viatris, Tenofovir GH, Tenofovir Sandoz

Available form
Tablets: 300 mg

Action
- nucleoside reverse transcriptase inhibitor
- prodrug that is converted to tenofovir diphosphate in both resting and activated T cells
- competitively inhibits human immunodeficiency virus (HIV) reverse transcriptase
- bioavailability increases if given with food

Use
- treatment of HIV infection (with other antiretroviral agents)
- treatment of chronic hepatitis B

Dose
- 300 mg orally daily with food

Adverse effects
- decrease in bone density
- nephrotoxicity
- peripheral neuropathy
- (Post discontinuing treatment) reactivation of hepatitis
- see also General Adverse effects of antiretroviral agents (p. 918)

Interactions
- caution if given with other nephrotoxic agents or with agents that increase serum levels (e.g. lopinavir/ritonavir combination)
- contraindicated with other tenofovir disoproxil fumarate-containing agents or tenofovir alafenamide-containing agents or adefovir dipivoxil
- recommended with atazanavir only in combination with ritonavir
- decreased serum levels may occur if given with rifampicin, rifabutin, phenobarbital (phenobarbitone), phenytoin or St John's wort; therefore not recommended together

Nursing considerations/Cautions
- testing for HIV—hepatitis B co-infection is recommended before starting therapy
- discontinuing antihepatitis B therapy in those with advanced liver disease or cirrhosis is not recommended because of the increased risk of liver decompensation
- caution if used as part of a triple nucleoside reverse transcriptase inhibitors (NRTIs) regimen, as viral resistance may occur. Triple regimens therapy should consist of two NRTI agents plus either a non-nucleoside reverse transcriptase inhibitor (NNRTI) or an HIV-1 protease inhibitor
- not recommended in those < 12 years or > 65 years
- see also General Nursing considerations/Cautions for antiretroviral agents (p. 919)

Patient education
- the patient should be advised to take with food
- warn the patient that acute exacerbation/reactivation of hepatitis may occur when therapy is stopped and therefore regular liver function monitoring is recommended
- advise the patient to seek medical advice if any of the following occur:
  - weakness, pain or tingling in hands or feet
  - bone pain
- see also General Patient education for antiretroviral agents (p. 920)

Tablet can be dispersed in 100 mL of water, orange or grape juice, or crushed and mixed with a spoonful of yoghurt or apple puree.

Use during pregnancy only if the potential benefit justifies the risk to the fetus.

Excreted in breastmilk. Use caution, and weigh the benefits of treatment against potential risk to the infant. Consider use only if there are no safer alternatives.

Reduced renal function: adjust dose as clearance is significantly reduced in renal impairment. Monitor renal function closely, especially in patients with a CrCl < 50 mL/min. Avoid use in severe renal impairment unless no alternatives are available, and administer with caution.

Available in combination with
- tenofovir disoproxil 300 mg + emtricitabine 200 mg (Cipla Tenofovir + Emtricitabine/Tenofovir/Emtricitabine 300/200 APX, Tenofovir/Emtricitabine 300/200, ARX, Tenofovir Disoproxil Emtricitabine Viatris, Tenofovir/Emtricitabine Sandoz)
- tenofovir disoproxil 300 mg + emtricitabine 200 mg + efavirenz 600 mg (Tenofovir Disoproxil/Emtricitabine/Efavirenz Viatris)

ZIDOVUDINE
Trade name
Retrovir

Available forms
Capsules: 100 mg, 250 mg;
Syrup: 50 mg/5 mL

Action
- thymidine nucleoside analogue

- converted to zidovudine triphosphate which interferes with RNA-dependent DNA polymerase (reverse transcriptase) inhibiting human immunodeficiency virus (HIV) replication

Use
- treatment of HIV infection (as monotherapy or with other antiretroviral agents)

Dose
- 500—600 mg orally daily in 2—5 divided doses

Adverse effects
- anaemia, neutropenia, leucopenia, pancytopenia
- myalgia, paraesthesia
- dyspnoea
- rash, sweating
- see also General Adverse effects of antiretroviral agents (p. 919)

Interactions
- probenecid may slow renal excretion of zidovudine
- not recommended with ribavirin because of the potential exacerbation of anaemia
- an increased risk of neutropenia if given with paracetamol
- risk of toxicity increases if given with other nephrotoxic or cytotoxic drugs, or those that interfere with white or red blood cell numbers or function, such as pyrimethamine, sulfamethoxazole/trimethoprim, doxorubicin, dapsone, pentamidine (IV), amphotericin B (amphotericin), ganciclovir, flucytosine, vincristine, vinblastine, adriamycin and interferon
- metabolism may be altered by paracetamol, aspirin, indometacin, ketoprofen, naproxen, oxazepam, lorazepam, cimetidine, dapsone, codeine, methadone or morphine
- phenytoin levels should be closely monitored if given together, as serum levels may vary
- absorption may be decreased if given with clarithromycin
- metabolism may be slowed if given with atovaquone
- increased risk of neurotoxicity if given with aciclovir

Nursing considerations/Cautions
- regular blood counts every second week for first 3 months of treatment, then monthly, are recommended
- therapy should be interrupted if the haemoglobin level falls below 7.6 g/dL or the neutrophil count falls below 0.75 $\times$ 10^9/L (or 750/mm^3)
- if the patient develops a rash, evaluation for sensitisation is recommended
- caution if used in those with compromised bone marrow or advanced HIV disease
- contraindicated in those with abnormally low neutrophil counts (below 0.75 $\times$ 10^9/L) or abnormally low haemoglobin level ($<$ 7.5 g/dL)
- see also General Nursing considerations/Cautions for antiretroviral agents (p. 919)

Patient education
- the patient should be advised about the haematological side-effects, which may require treatment by blood transfusion and/or dose modification and the importance of regular blood tests
- warn the patient not to take paracetamol while taking zidovudine
- if given with clarithromycin tablets, instruct the patient to separate by at least 2 hours
- instruct the patient to remain in upright position when taking zidovudine (especially if there are any swallowing difficulties), as oesophageal irritation can occur
- the patient should be advised to seek medical advice if any of the following occur:
  - frequent infection such as fever, chills, sore throat, mouth ulcers or flu-like symptoms

ANTIVIRAL AGENTS

- unusual bleeding or bruising
- shortness of breath on exertion, tiredness, pale appearance (especially in first 2—4 weeks of therapy)
- abnormal rash
- see also General Patient education for antiretroviral agents (p. 920)

Oral solution is available. Capsule can be opened and contents mixed with water, or a spoonful of yoghurt or apple puree. Staff should wear mask and gloves if opening capsule.

Use is recommended only if the expected benefits justify any potential risks to the fetus. Crosses the placenta and may cause mild, transient increases in serum lactate in neonates. Although not teratogenic in animals, it has fetotoxic potential.

Excreted into breastmilk and may expose the infant to the drug. Breastfeeding is not recommended because of the risk of HIV transmission and potential adverse effects on the infant.

Reduced renal function: may accumulate due to reduced glucuronidation in hepatic impairment. Dose adjustments and close monitoring help prevent toxicity.

Available in combination with
- lamivudine 150 mg + zidovudine 300 mg tablet (Combivir/Lamivudine/Zidovudine Viatris)

NON-NUCLEOSIDE REVERSE TRANSCRIPTASE INHIBITORS (NNRTIs)

EFAVIRENZ

Available form
Tablets: tenofovir disoproxil maleate 300 mg, emtricitabine 200 mg, efavirenz 600 mg combination tablet (Tenofovir Disoproxil Emtricitabine Efavirenz Viatris 300/200/600)

Action
- non-nucleoside reverse transcriptase inhibitor of human immunodeficiency virus (HIV)-1 (but not HIV-2)
- blocks RNA-dependent and DNA-dependent DNA polymerases
- viral resistance has occurred when given alone
- onset of action 3—5 hours
- half-life 52—76 hours (single dose) and 40—55 hours (multiple dosing)
- (tenofovir disoproxil) see p. 925 for actions
- (emtricitabine) see p. 922 for actions

Use
- treatment of HIV infections

Dose
- one combination tablet orally 1 hour before or 2 hours after food at night (with other antiretroviral agents)

Adverse effects
- rash
- dizziness, abnormal dreams, impaired concentration
- (Rare) severe depression, suicidal ideation, aggression, paranoia, delusions, psychoses, pancreatitis, severe rash, seizures, QT prolongation
- see also General Adverse effects of antiretroviral agents (p. 918)

Interactions
- contraindicated with midazolam, voriconazole, itraconazole or ergot alkaloids
- contraindicated with St John's wort
- not recommended with sofosbuvir/velpatasvir/voxilaprevir or sofosbuvir/velpatasvir combination
- not recommended with other formulations containing efavirenz
- not recommended with posaconazole, proguanil or atovaquone
- not recommended with alcohol owing to the risk of added CNS effects
- may decrease serum levels of ciclosporin, tacrolimus and sirolimus, reducing efficacy

- caution if given with hepatotoxic agents. If used together, liver function should be closely monitored
- may decrease serum levels of atazanavir, lopinavir/ritonavir, diltiazem, sertraline, bupropion, artemether/lumefantrine, maraviroc, pravastatin, simvastatin, carbamazepine or clarithromycin
- if given with ritonavir, there is an increased risk of adverse effects and liver enzymes should be monitored regularly
- may increase serum levels of ethinylestradiol
- decreased serum levels may result if given with rifampicin, phenytoin, phenobarbital (phenobarbitone), carbamazepine or St John's wort
- bioavailability increased if given with food
- caution if given with warfarin because of variable effects. INR should be carefully monitored, especially when starting and stopping therapy
- may decrease plasma levels of methadone leading to opiate withdrawal symptoms
- not recommended with other agents known to prolong QT interval
- may cause false positive urine cannabinoid test
- see also interactions for tenofovir disoproxil (p. 925) and emtricitabine (p. 922)

Nursing considerations/Cautions

- not available as monotherapy
- cholesterol and triglyceride monitoring is recommended during therapy
- CNS symptoms usually start in first 2 days of therapy and resolve within 1—4 weeks
- increased risk of psychiatric/nervous system symptoms if given to those with a history of mental illness or substance abuse; therefore should be given with caution
- if the patient has (or is suspected of having) hepatitis B or C co-infection or being treated using hepatotoxic agents, liver function monitoring is recommended
- caution if used in those with a history of seizures or moderate-to-severe liver impairment
- contraindicated in those who have previously experienced life-threatening skin reactions
- see also General Nursing considerations/Cautions for antiretroviral agents (p. 919)

Patient education

- the patient and/or significant others/carers should be advised to immediately report any depression, feelings of self-harm, delusion or hallucinations, aggressive behaviour or psychosis
- advise the patient that taking medication at night may alleviate some of the CNS symptoms
- warn the patient that:
  - rash commonly occurs within 1 to 2 days of starting therapy but resolves with continued therapy. If skin blistering, mouth blisters or fever occur, the patient should be advised to seek medical attention immediately
  - symptoms such as dizziness, abnormal dreaming, difficulty sleeping and impaired concentration usually resolve within 2—4 weeks of continued therapy. The patient should be advised not to drive or operate machinery if these occur and/or are ongoing
- patients should be warned to avoid alcohol during therapy
- counsel female patients to use 2 methods of contraception (barrier and oral/hormonal) during and for 12 weeks after stopping therapy to prevent pregnancy
- see also General Patient education for antiretroviral agents (p. 920)

ANTIVIRAL AGENTS

 Combination tablet can be dispersed in at least 20 mL water (takes about 15 minutes) or can be crushed and mixed with spoonful of yoghurt or apple puree.

 Contraindicated during pregnancy.

 Not recommended during breastfeeding.

 Not recommended in those with CrCl < 50 mL/min or with moderate-to-severe liver impairment.

ETRAVIRINE
Trade name
Intelence

Available form
Tablets: 200 mg

Action
- non-nucleoside reverse transcriptase inhibitor of human immunodeficiency virus 1 (HIV-1)
- blocks RNA-dependent and DNA-dependent DNA polymerases
- half-life 30—40 hours

Use
- treatment of HIV-1 infection (in those with evidence of viral replication and resistance to non-nucleoside transcriptase inhibitors and other antiretroviral agents) (as part of combination therapy)

Dose
- 200 mg orally twice daily after food

Adverse effects
- anaemia
- hypercholesterolaemia, hypertriglyceridaemia, hyperlipidaemia, hyperglycaemia
- peripheral neuropathy
- rash
- night sweats
- hypertension
- (Rare) severe skin reactions, hypersensitivity reactions, myocardial infarction
- see also General Adverse effects of antiretroviral agents (p. 918)

Interactions
- not recommended with efavirenz, nevirapine, rilpivirine, unboosted atazanavir, ritonavir, other unboosted protease inhibitors or darunavir/cobicistat
- not recommended with clarithromycin, as increased levels of clarithromycin's active metabolite may occur (which does not have the same efficacy against *Mycobacterium atrium* complex (MAC))
- plasma levels may be decreased by dexamethasone, carbamazepine, phenobarbital (phenobarbitone), phenytoin, rifampicin, maraviroc, dolutegravir or St John's wort, and these are therefore not recommended together
- if given with digoxin, digoxin serum levels should be monitored regularly
- if given with warfarin, INR should be monitored regularly, especially when starting or stopping therapy
- may increase plasma levels of diazepam
- may decrease plasma levels of atorvastatin (but increase plasma levels of active metabolite), simvastatin, rosuvastatin and fluvastatin
- caution if used with ciclosporin, tacrolimus or sirolimus
- may decrease activation of clopidogrel to active metabolite and therefore not recommended together
- caution if boosted etravirine is given with rifabutin
- may decrease serum levels of phosphodiesterase 5 (PDE-5) inhibitors such as sildenafil and tadalafil
- may decrease serum levels of antiarrhythmic agents such as amiodarone, flecainide, disopyramide and lidocaine (systemic)

Nursing considerations/Cautions
- see General Nursing considerations/Cautions for antiretroviral agents (p. 919)

Patient education
- warn the patient that mild-to-moderate rash occurs commonly during the second week of therapy and rarely after week 4

- the patient should be advised to seek medical advice immediately if any of the following occur:
  - severe rash
  - rash with fever, malaise, fatigue, muscle and joint aches, blisters, oral lesions, conjunctivitis
  - chest pain, neck/jaw pain, left arm pain, anxiety, sweating, pallor, nausea, vomiting, indigestion, dizziness
- instruct the patient to swallow tablet whole with water (if possible). If the patient is unable to swallow, advise them that the tablet may be dispersed in water, taking care to stir well and drink immediately. Instruct the patient to rinse the glass well and swallow to ensure a complete dose has been taken
- see also General Patient education for antiretroviral agents (p. 920)

 Tablet can be dispersed in water. Avoid using carbonated or hot beverages.

 Limited human data, but no major embryo-fetal harm was observed in animal studies. Should be used during pregnancy only if the benefits outweigh the risks.

 Excreted in human milk. Due to the potential for HIV transmission and possible adverse effects in breastfed infants, breastfeeding is not recommended.

RILPIVIRINE

Trade name
Edurant

Available form
Tablets: 25 mg

Action
- non-nucleoside reverse transcriptase inhibitor
- blocks RNA-dependent and DNA-dependent DNA polymerases
- effective against human immunodeficiency virus (HIV)-1
- absorption improved if taken with food or high-fat meal
- half-life about 45 hours

Use
- treatment of HIV-1 infection (with other antiretrovirals) in those with viral load ≤ 100,000 copies/mL and treatment naive

Dose
- 25 mg orally daily with food

Adverse effects
- depression
- rash
- (Rare) QT interval prolongation
- see also General Adverse effects of antiretroviral agents (p. 918)

Interactions
- contraindicated with carbamazepine, oxcarbazepine, phenobarbital (phenobarbitone), phenytoin, rifabutin, rifampicin, proton pump inhibitors, dexamethasone (except as a single treatment) or St John's wort
- caution if used with rifabutin, antacids or H_2-receptor antagonists (famotidine, ranitidine, nizatidine), as decreased serum levels may occur
- increased serum levels may occur if given with darunavir/ritonavir, lopinavir/ritonavir, atazanavir/ritonavir, clarithromycin, erythromycin, itraconazole, fluconazole, voriconazole or posaconazole
- not recommended with efavirenz, etravirine or nevirapine
- caution if given with methadone
- caution if given with agents known to prolong QT interval

Nursing considerations/Cautions
- not used as monotherapy
- caution if used in those with moderate liver impairment and not recommended in those with severe liver impairment
- see also General Nursing considerations/Cautions for antiretroviral agents (p. 919)

Patient education
- instruct the patient to take antacids 2 hours before or at least 4 hours after rilpivirine, or for H_2-receptor antagonists

ANTIVIRAL AGENTS

(such as ranitidine) 12 hours before or at least 4 hours after rilpivirine
- advise the patient to take with a meal to help with absorption
- see also General Patient education for antiretroviral agents (p. 920)

Tablet can be dispersed in water, or crushed and mixed with a spoonful of yoghurt or apple puree. Should be administered immediately, as rilpivirine is light sensitive

Use only if the benefits outweigh potential risks. Reduced rilpivirine levels have been observed during pregnancy; monitor viral load closely, and consider alternative antiretroviral therapy if required.

Avoid, as excretion in human milk unknown. Potential for HIV transmission and possible adverse effects in nursing infants.

Available in combination with
- cabotegravir 600 mg/3 mL modified release injection + rilpivirine 900 mg/3 mL modified-release injection (Cabenuva)
- dolutegravir 50 mg + rilpivirine 25 mg tablet (Juluca)
- emtricitabine 200 mg + rilpivirine 25 mg + tenofovir alafenamide 25 mg tablet (Odefsey)

PROTEASE INHIBITORS (PIs)

ATAZANAVIR
Trade name
Reyataz

Available form
Capsules: 200 mg, 300 mg

Action
- human immunodeficiency virus 1 (HIV-1) protease inhibitor
- half-life 6.5—7.9 hours

Use
- treatment of HIV-1 infection (with other antiretroviral agents)

Dose
Therapy-naive patient
- 400 mg orally daily with food **OR**
- 300 mg orally daily (with ritonavir 100 mg daily)

Therapy-experienced patient
- 300 mg orally daily (with ritonavir 100 mg daily)

Adverse effects
- back pain, peripheral neuropathy
- jaundice, scleral icterus, increased bilirubin (asymptomatic)
- prolonged PR interval and, rarely, QT interval prolongation
- rash
- nephrolithiasis, cholelithiasis, haematuria, proteinuria
- see also General Adverse effects of antiretroviral agents (p. 918)

Interactions
- contraindicated with midazolam, rifampicin, alfuzosin, St John's wort, salmeterol, simvastatin, lovastatin, sildenafil (if used for pulmonary arterial hypertension), glecaprevir/pibrentasvir, or ergot alkaloids
- not recommended with efavirenz, nevirapine or voxilaprevir
- atazanavir/ritonavir combination is not recommended with fluticasone or budesonide
- caution if given with other agents which prolong PR interval (e.g. beta adrenoceptor blocking agents, digoxin)
- may increase serum levels of calcium-channel blockers, further prolonging the PR interval. ECG monitoring is recommended if given together
- decreased serum levels may occur if given with histamine H_2-receptor antagonists, proton pump inhibitors,

- phenytoin, phenobarbital (phenobarbitone), carbamazepine, nevirapine, antacids, tenofovir or efavirenz
- increased serum levels may occur if given with ritonavir, other protease inhibitors, itraconazole or voriconazole
- may decrease efficacy of oral contraceptives or hormone replacement therapy by decreasing serum levels of oestradiol
- may increase serum levels of irinotecan, ciclosporin, tacrolimus, sirolimus, clarithromycin, rifabutin, amiodarone, lidocaine (lignocaine), tricyclic antidepressants (TCAs), colchicine, buprenorphine, sildenafil, tadalafil, midazolam (IV) or atorvastatin, increasing the risk of adverse effects and toxicity
- may decrease serum levels of phenytoin, lamotrigine or phenobarbital (phenobarbitone)
- caution if given with warfarin, as serum levels may be increased. INR should be monitored especially when starting or stopping therapy
- caution if given with other agents known to prolong QT interval or cause electrolyte imbalance
- increased risk of bleeding if given with dabigatran, apixaban or rivaroxaban
- see also General Interactions of antiretroviral agents (p. 919)

Nursing considerations/Cautions

- not recommended as monotherapy. Should be given with ritonavir
- should be given 2 hours apart from histamine H_2-receptor antagonists
- dose should be reduced if given with other antiretroviral agents
- tablets contain lactose and therefore not recommended in those with galactose intolerance, glucose—galactose malabsorption or Lapp lactase deficiency
- caution if used in those with pre-existing conduction problems (e.g. AV block), bradycardia, congenital QT syndrome or electrolyte imbalance
- see also General Nursing considerations/Cautions for antiretroviral agents (p. 919)

Patient education

- the patient should be advised that rash commonly occurs in first 3 weeks of therapy and then resolves within 2 weeks of stopping medication
- instruct the patient to seek medical advice immediately if any of the following occur:
  - yellowing of skin or eyes, loss of appetite, unexplained tiredness, upper abdominal pain, dark urine, pale stools
  - pain in right or middle upper stomach, fever, nausea, vomiting, yellowing of eyes/skin
  - pain in kidney area, pain on urination, blood in urine
  - unusual heart rate
  - any numbness, tingling or changed sensation in extremities
- advise the patient to separate by:
  - at least 10 hours if used with an H_2-receptor antagonist such as famotidine
  - if taking antacids, they should be separated by 2 hours before or 1 hour after medication
- see also General Patient education for antiretroviral agents (p. 920)

 Capsules can be opened and the contents mixed with a spoonful of yoghurt or apple puree.

 Use only if the potential benefit justifies the risk. Monitor therapeutic levels because of reduced atazanavir exposure in pregnancy. Avoid combining with drugs that reduce atazanavir levels (e.g. tenofovir, H_2 antagonists); alternative dosing may be needed. Hyperbilirubinaemia may occur and could affect the neonate; consider alternative therapy prepartum.

ANTIVIRAL AGENTS

Avoid, as present in human milk. Due to the potential for HIV transmission and serious adverse reactions in nursing infants, mothers should not breastfeed.

Reduced hepatic function: use cautiously in mild-to-moderate hepatic insufficiency. Contraindicated in severe hepatic impairment. Patients with hepatitis B or C or elevated transaminases at baseline are at higher risk for further liver complications.

Available in combination with
- atazanavir 300 mg + cobicistat 150 mg tablet (Evotaz)

DARUNAVIR
Trade names
Darunavir Juno, Prezista

Available form
Tablets: 600 mg, 800 mg

Action
- human immunodeficiency virus 1 (HIV-1) protease inhibitor
- half-life about 15 hours (when combined with ritonavir)

Use
- treatment of HIV-1 infection (in combination with low-dose ritonavir and other antiretroviral agents)

Dose
- 600 mg orally twice daily with food (with ritonavir 100 mg twice daily) **OR**
- 800 mg orally daily with food (with ritonavir 100 mg daily)

Adverse effects
- drug-induced hepatitis
- rash
- (Rare) severe skin reaction
- see also General Adverse effects of antiretroviral agents (p. 918)

Interactions
- contraindicated with midazolam (oral), alfuzosin, lovastatin, simvastatin, St John's wort, ergot derivatives, rifampicin, flecainide, lidocaine (lignocaine), amiodarone, sildenafil (when used for pulmonary arterial hypertension), lurasidone, dapoxetine, apixaban, ivabradine or colchicine (in those with liver/kidney impairment)
- not recommended with rivaroxaban or dabigatran
- caution if used with other hepatotoxic agents
- caution if given with buprenorphine/naloxone owing to an increase in active metabolite and a risk of opioid toxicity
- caution if given with fentanyl, oxycodone or tramadol, as increased serum levels may occur increasing the risk of respiratory depression
- increased risk of QT prolongation if given with artemether/lumefantrine
- activity is enhanced by ritonavir and is therefore given as combination therapy (low-dose ritonavir)
- may decrease serum levels of etravirine, voriconazole, sertraline or paroxetine
- may decrease serum levels of warfarin; therefore INR should be monitored especially when starting or stopping therapy
- may increase serum levels of bosentan, fluticasone, prednisolone, budesonide, betamethasone, fluconazole, clonazepam, digoxin, calcium-channel blockers, itraconazole, posaconazole, rifabutin, clarithromycin, nevirapine, tenofovir, efavirenz, rilpivirine, carbamazepine, salmeterol, colchicine, atorvastatin, pravastatin, risperidone, quetiapine, carvedilol, metoprolol, sedatives, hypnotics, maraviroc, dasatinib, nilotinib, vinca alkaloids, irinotecan, sildenafil, tadalafil, tricyclic antidepressants (TCAs), domperidone, clotrimazole, ticagrelor, ciclosporin, everolimus, tacrolimus or sirolimus, increasing the risk of adverse effects and toxicity; therefore serum levels should be closely monitored
- may decrease serum levels and efficacy of oral contraceptives and hormone replacement therapy
- serum levels may be decreased if given with oxcarbazepine, modafinil,

HAVARD'S NURSING GUIDE TO DRUGS

dexamethasone, efavirenz, phenobarbital (phenobarbitone) or phenytoin
- serum levels may be increased if given with rifabutin or posaconazole
- not recommended with lopinavir/ritonavir combination

Nursing considerations/Cautions

- not used as monotherapy
- once-a-day dosing is recommended for treatment-naive patients, treatment-experienced patients with no darunavir-resistant mutations and HIV-1 RNA < 100,000 copies/mL, or treatment-experienced but HIV protease-naive patients where HIV-1 genotype is unavailable
- twice-daily dosing is recommended for treatment-experienced patient with at least one darunavir resistance-associated mutation, HIV protease inhibitor treatment-experienced patient where HIV-1 genotype is unavailable or those with plasma HIV-1 RNA ≥ 100,000 copies/mL
- liver function tests should be performed before starting and regularly during therapy
- caution if used in those > 65 years
- caution if used in those with pre-existing liver disease including chronic active hepatitis B or C, and not recommended in those with severe liver impairment
- caution if used in those with sulfonamide allergy
- see also General Nursing considerations/Cautions for antiretroviral agents (p. 919)

Patient education

- the patient should be advised to seek medical advice immediately if any of the following occur
  - any rash (with or without fever), tiredness, muscle/joint ache, blisters or conjunctivitis
  - fatigue, loss of appetite, liver tenderness, nausea, dark urine, yellowing of eyes or skin
- see also General Patient education for antiretroviral agents (p. 920)

 Crush and disperse within 3 minutes in water to form a coarse suspension. If thin fluids cannot be tolerated, mix the crushed tablet with a spoonful of yogurt or apple puree. The 800 mg tablet does not readily disperse and is difficult to crush.

 Caution, as darunavir exposure decreases significantly during the second and third trimesters, especially with once-daily dosing. Lower exposure levels may reduce the drug's effectiveness in managing HIV. Adjustments to dosing frequency or close monitoring of viral load may be necessary to maintain therapeutic levels.

 Caution, as it is unknown whether darunavir is excreted in human breastmilk, but, due to the potential for HIV transmission and adverse effects in nursing infants, breastfeeding is generally not recommended for HIV-positive mothers.

 Reduced hepatic function: use with caution in moderate hepatic impairment; avoid in severe impairment owing to an increased risk of adverse effects and reduced clearance. Regular liver function monitoring is recommended.

Available in combination with

- darunavir 800 mg + cobicistat 150 mg tablet (Prezcobix)
- darunavir 800 mg + cobicistat 150 mg + emtricitabine 200 mg + tenofovir alafenamide 10 mg tablet (Symtuza)

RITONAVIR

Trade name
Norvir

Available form
Tablets: 100 mg

Action

- protease inhibitor of both human immunodeficiency virus 1 (HIV-1) and HIV-2
- HIV protease is needed for viral infectivity and cleaves viral precursor

polypeptide into active viral enzymes and structural proteins. Protease inhibitors prevent polypeptide cleaving and block viral maturation
- 5 metabolites but only one (M2) is active
- half-life 3–5 hours

Use
- treatment of HIV-1 infection (in combination with other antiretroviral agents or as monotherapy if combination therapy is not appropriate)

Dose
- 600 mg orally twice daily with food

Adverse effects
- peripheral neuropathy, paraesthesia, myalgia
- throat irritation, pharyngitis
- altered taste
- rash, and rarely, severe skin reactions
- elevated liver enzymes, cholesterol and triglycerides
- pancreatitis
- prolongation of PR interval
- see also General Adverse effects of antiretroviral agents (p. 918)

Interactions
- contraindicated with diazepam, midazolam, triazolam, flurazepam or zolpidem because of increased sedation and risk of respiratory depression
- contraindicated with ergot alkaloids because of increased risk of ergot toxicity
- contraindicated with amiodarone, bupropion, clozapine, flecainide, pethidine, piroxicam, colchicine, lurasidone, voriconazole, alfuzosin, St John's wort, sildenafil (when used for pulmonary arterial hypertension), simvastatin, lovastatin, salmeterol, fusidic acid, neratinib, apalutamide, venetoclax or rifabutin
- not recommended with glecaprevir/pibrentasvir
- serum levels may be increased by fusidic acid and efavirenz
- may decrease serum levels of bupropion, theophylline, sulfamethoxazole–trimethoprim, warfarin, voriconazole and zidovudine
- may increase serum levels of bosentan, buspirone, clarithromycin, dasatinib, digoxin, efavirenz, fentanyl, fluticasone, maraviroc, nilotinib, quetiapine, vinblastine and vincristine
- increased risk of hepatitis and hepatic decompensation if given with tipranavir (especially in those with hepatitis B or C co-infection)
- increased risk of severe hepatoxicity if given in combination with rifampicin
- increased risk of bleeding if given with rivaroxaban
- not recommended with PDE5 inhibitors (sildenafil, tadalafil)
- doses of clarithromycin > 1 g/day are not recommended with ritonavir
- may produce disulfiram–alcohol-like reaction (see Glossary) if given with disulfiram or metronidazole because the formulation contains alcohol
- may decrease effectiveness of oral contraceptives by decreasing serum levels of estradiol (oestradiol)
- increased risk of Cushing's syndrome and adrenal suppression if given with fluticasone, triamcinolone, budesonide or other glucocorticoids (inhaled, injected or intranasally)
- increased risk of cardiac or neurological adverse events if given with disopyramide
- increased risk of serotonin syndrome if given with fluoxetine
- caution if given with verapamil because of an increased risk of PR interval prolongation
- caution if used with 3-hydroxy-3-methylglutaryl coenzyme A (HMG-CoA) reductase inhibitors (statins) atorvastatin and rosuvastatin

Nursing considerations/Cautions
- caution if used in those with pre-existing prolonged PR interval

- see also General Nursing considerations/Cautions for antiretroviral agents (p. 919)

Patient education

- instruct the patient to take with food
- advise the patient that tablets should be swallowed whole, not chewed, broken or crushed
- the patient should be advised to report any unusual nausea, vomiting and abdominal pain (which may be symptoms of impending pancreatitis)
- counsel female patients to use alternative form of contraception, because oral contraceptives may have reduced effectiveness
- see also General Patient education for antiretroviral agents (p. 920)

Tablets should be swallowed whole. Do not chew, break or crush the tablets, as this may affect the drug's efficacy and tolerability.

Avoid, as limited human data available; animal studies indicate potential developmental toxicity at maternally toxic doses. Use during pregnancy only if the benefits outweigh the risks.

Avoid, as present in human milk. Potential for HIV transmission, development of viral resistance or adverse reactions in the breastfed infant.

Reduced hepatic function: primarily metabolised by the liver. Use with caution in patients with hepatic impairment, as there is an increased risk of hepatic dysfunction, including fatalities, particularly in patients with pre-existing liver disease or co-infection with hepatitis B or C.

Available in combination with

- lopinavir 400 mg/5 mL + ritonavir 100 mg/5 mL oral liquid (Kaletra Oral)
- lopinavir 200 mg + ritonavir 50 mg oral tablet (Kaletra 200/50)
- nirmatrelvir 200/50 mg oral tablet + ritonavir 100 mg tablet (Paxlovid Composite Pack)

ENTRY INHIBITORS

BULEVIRTIDE
Trade name
Hepcludex

Available form
Vial: 2 mg

Action
- blocks entry of hepatitis B virus (HBV) and hepatitis D (HDV)
- half-life 3—7 hours

Use
- treatment of chronic hepatitis HDV in adults with compensated liver disease

Dose
- 2 mg SC daily

Adverse effects
- eosinophilia
- increase in total bile salts
- headache, dizziness, fatigue
- flu-like symptoms
- nausea
- pruritus
- arthralgia
- (Injection site) redness, pruritus, haematoma, swelling, pain, induration
- (Rare) allergic reaction

Interactions
- increased risk of adverse effects if given with pegylated interferons and so should be used with caution

Nursing considerations/Cautions

- reconstitute using 1 mL of water for injections
- SC administration only
- patients may be instructed in self-administration technique
- if the patient discontinues therapy, severe acute exacerbation of HDV and HBV infection may occur. Liver function tests are recommended for several months after stopping therapy. Restarting therapy may be required in some cases

ANTIVIRAL AGENTS

- increase in total bile salts may be greater in those with kidney impairment because bile salts are excreted through the kidneys
- caution if used in those with liver impairment (Child–Pugh B or C), decompensated liver disease or kidney impairment (CrCl less than 60 mL/min), and those over 65 years or under 18 years

Patient education

- warn the patient that hepatitis may be worse when therapy is stopped. Stopping therapy should be discussed with the doctor
- instruct the patient in self-administration including:
  - storing vials in refrigerator before preparation and administration
  - check the expiry date and do not use if the vial is past that date
  - wash hands before reconstituting the solution and administration
  - clean the top of the vial with alcohol wipe and avoid touching with fingers
  - put a longer needle on syringe and reconstitute by adding 1 mL of water for injection to the vial slowly down the side of the vial
  - carefully tap the vial for 10 seconds and then roll it between the hands to dissolve the powder (this can take up to 3 minutes)
  - if bubbles appear in reconstituted solution, gently tap the vial until they disappear. The solution should be clear
  - reconstituted solution should be used immediately
  - change the needle on the syringe to a shorter needle
  - administer by SC injection (at a 45-degree angle) into the upper thigh or lower abdomen avoiding any moles, lesions, scars or tattoos
  - the importance of rotating injection sites
- if a dose is missed, administer as close as possible to the scheduled time. However, if it is almost time for next dose, go back to regular dosing schedule and do not double the dose
- correct disposal of used syringes and vials
- remaining water for injections should be discarded

There are no adequate studies; therefore should be used during pregnancy only if benefits to the mother outweigh potential risks to the fetus.

Secretion into breastmilk is unknown; therefore the benefits of breastfeeding to infant must be weighed against the benefits of therapy to mother.

MARAVIROC

Trade names
Celsentri, Maraviroc Waymade

Available form
Tablets: 150 mg, 300 mg

Action
- chemokine receptor CCR5 antagonist which selectively binds to human cytokine receptor CCR5 blocking interaction between CCR5 and human immunodeficiency virus (HIV) glycoprotein (gp120)
- half-life 13.2 hours

Use
- CCR5 tropic HIV-1 infection (with other retroviral agents)

Dose
- 150 mg, 300 mg or 600 mg orally twice daily (dose depending on co-administered antiretroviral agent)

Adverse effects
- infection (upper respiratory tract, herpes, oesophageal candidiasis, influenza), fever, cough, rhinitis, sinusitis
- rash, pruritus
- myalgia, muscle spasms, arthralgia

- paraesthesia, dysaesthesia
- postural hypotension, syncope, dizziness
- (Uncommon) myocardial infarction, angina
- see also General Adverse effects of antiretroviral agents (p. 918)

Interactions
- caution if used with other agents known to lower blood pressure
- serum levels may be decreased if given with efavirenz, etravirine, rifabutin or rifampicin, and therefore not recommended together
- serum levels may be increased if given with atazanavir, darunavir, ritonavir (or fixed combinations containing ritonavir), lopinavir, clarithromycin or itraconazole increasing the risk of postural hypotension
- not recommended with St John's wort

Nursing considerations/Cautions
- liver function (enzymes and bilirubin) monitoring is recommended before starting and regularly during therapy
- only recommended in those with detectable CCR5 tropic HIV-1; therefore tropism and resistance testing is recommended before starting therapy
- caution in those who are at risk of cardiovascular events, a history of or risk factors for postural hypotension or pre-existing liver disease
- caution if used in those with severe renal insufficiency because of the increased risk of hypotension
- not recommended in those with dual/mixed or CXCR4 tropic HIV-1
- see also General Nursing considerations/Cautions for antiretroviral agents (p. 919)

Patient education
- the patient should be advised to report any signs of frequent infection, such as fever, chills, sore throat, mouth ulcers or flu-like symptoms
- instruct the patient to immediately seek medical advice if chest pain or angina occurs
- warn the patient not to drive or operate machinery if hypotension and dizziness occur
- see also General Patient education for antiretroviral agents (p. 920)

Tablet can be crushed and mixed with water or a spoonful of yoghurt or apple puree.

Use only if the potential benefits outweigh the risks. Safety data for use during pregnancy is limited.

Excretion in human breastmilk is unknown. Consider only if the potential benefit justifies any possible risk.

Reduced renal function: clearance may be reduced. Dose adjustment required. Avoid use in severe renal impairment.

Reduced hepatic function: metabolism may be impaired. Use with caution or avoid in cases of severe hepatic dysfunction.

NIRSEVIMAB
Trade name
Beyfortus

Available form
Prefilled syringe: 50 mg/0.5 mL, 100 mg/mL

Action
- recombinant neutralising human IgG_{1K} monoclonal antibody
- inhibits viral entry process, neutralising the virus and blocking cell-to-cell fusion
- half-life 71 days
- duration of protection is at least 5 months

Use
- prevention of respiratory syncytial virus (RSV) lower respiratory tract disease in neonates/infants born during or entering their first RSV season, or children ≤ 24 months who remain vulner-

ANTIVIRAL AGENTS

able to severe RSV disease through their second RSV season

Dose
- neonates and infants (first RSV season)
  - (weight < 5 kg) 50 mg IM
  - (weight ≥ 5 kg) 100 mg IM
- children up to 24 months at increased risk (second RSV season)
  - 200 mg IM
- children undergoing cardiac surgery with cardiopulmonary bypass
  - (first RSV season, surgery within 90 days of vaccination with nirsevimab) additional dose given based on weights above given when child is stable after surgery
  - (second RSV season, surgery within 90 days of vaccination with nirsevimab) 200 mg IM

Adverse effects
- (Injection site) pain, induration, redness, swelling, oedema
- rash
- fever
- (Rare) hypersensitivity, anaphylaxis

Interactions
- increased risk of bleeding if given with anticoagulants
- palivizumab should not be administered if nirsevimab has been used in the same RSV season
- should not be mixed with other vaccines in the same syringe

Nursing considerations/Cautions
- administered IM into anterolateral aspect of thigh (gluteal muscle is not routinely used owing to the risk of damage to the sciatic nerve)
- if two injections are required (i.e. 200 mg dose), different injection sites should be used
- not indicated for adults
- caution if used in those with thrombocytopenia, bleeding disorders or receiving anticoagulant therapy owing to the risk of bleeding caused by IM injection
- caution if used in those with protein-losing conditions, as clearance is increased possibly reducing protection
- contraindicated in those with a history of hypersensitivity or anaphylactic reactions

Patient education
- advise the parent/carer that rash and fever occur commonly after vaccination and usually within 7–14 days post injection
- instruct the parent/carer to seek medical advice immediately if infant develops any:
  - swelling of lips, face, tongue or throat
  - difficulty breathing or swallowing
  - severe itching, rash or raised bumps (hives)

INTEGRASE INHIBITORS

DOLUTEGRAVIR
Trade name
Tivicay

Available form
Tablets: 10 mg, 25 mg, 50 mg

Action
- human immunodeficiency virus (HIV) integrase inhibitor that blocks the strand transfer step of retroviral DNA integration needed for HIV replication
- half-life about 14 hours

Use
- treatment of HIV-1 infection (with other antiretrovirals) in adults and children (over 12 years) weighing more than 40 kg

Dose
- (No resistance to integrase class) 50 mg orally daily **OR**
- (Resistance to integrase class) 50 mg orally twice daily

Adverse effects
- rash
- (Rare) depression, suicidal ideation
- see also General Adverse effects of antiretroviral agents (p. 918)

Interactions
- plasma levels may be decreased by efavirenz, etravirine, nevirapine, carbamazepine, phenytoin, phenobarbital (phenobarbitone), St John's wort, oxcarbazepine or rifampicin
- plasma levels may be decreased by antacids containing magnesium or aluminium, calcium or iron supplements
- plasma levels may be increased by atazanavir
- may increase serum levels of metformin, increasing the risk of hypoglycaemia

Nursing considerations/Cautions
- liver function tests are recommended especially in those with hepatitis B and/or C co-infection
- caution if used in those with a pre-existing history of depression or other psychiatric illness
- see also General Nursing considerations/Cautions for antiretroviral agents (p. 919)

Patient education
- instruct the patient to immediately seek medical advice if any severe rash or rash with fever, malaise, fatigue, muscle or joint pain, blisters, oral lesions, conjunctivitis or facial swelling occurs
- advise the patient to take aluminium- or magnesium-containing antacids, calcium or iron supplements either 2 hours before or 6 hours after therapy
- if the patient has diabetes treated using metformin, they should be warned to closely monitor blood glucose levels, as there is an increased risk of hypoglycaemia occurring during therapy
- the patient (or carer/family member) should be advised to immediately seek medical advice if any signs of depression, such as sadness, withdrawal from friends or previously pleasurable activities, or any attempts at self-harm, occur
- see also General Patient education for antiretroviral agents (p. 920)

Tablet can be crushed and mixed with water or a spoonful of yoghurt or apple puree.

Avoid: use only if benefits outweigh risks, as a potential risk of neural tube defects when used at conception/early pregnancy. Effective contraception is advised.

Caution, as excreted in breastmilk in small amounts. Use only if benefits outweigh risks.

Available in combination with
- dolutegravir 50 mg + abacavir 600 mg + lamivudine 300 mg tablet (Triumeq)
- dolutegravir 50 mg + lamivudine 300 mg tablet (Dovato)
- dolutegravir 50 mg + rilpivirine 25 mg tablet (Juluca)

RALTEGRAVIR
Trade name
Isentress

Available forms
Tablets: 400 mg, 600 mg

Action
- human immunodeficiency virus (HIV) integrase strand transfer inhibitor (integrase is an HIV encoded enzyme required for viral replication)

Use
- treatment of multi-resistant HIV-1 infection (where current therapy has failed) (with other antiretroviral agents)

Dose
- (Treatment-experienced patients) 400 mg orally twice daily (with other antiretroviral agents) **OR**

ANTIVIRAL AGENTS

- (Treatment-naive patients) 1200 mg orally once daily (with other antiretroviral agents)

Adverse effects
- elevated creatine kinase levels
- (Rare) severe skin reactions
- see also General Adverse effects of antiretroviral agents (p. 918)

Interactions
- serum levels may be decreased by rifampicin, phenytoin, carbamazepine or phenobarbital (phenobarbitone)
- serum levels may be decreased if given with aluminium or magnesium-containing antacids and these are therefore not recommended together
- serum levels may be increased if given with omeprazole
- not recommended with atazanavir

Nursing considerations/Cautions
- 1200 mg dose should be given as 2 × 600 mg NOT 3 × 400 mg
- caution if used in those at risk of myopathy or rhabdomyolysis

Patient education
- (400 or 600 mg tablets) advise the patient that tablets should be swallowed whole, not chewed, crushed or divided
- instruct the patient to separate therapy at least 2 hours from magnesium- or aluminium-containing antacids
- the patient should be advised to immediately seek medical advice if any rash (especially severe or blistering), fever, malaise or fatigue, joint or muscle ache, facial swelling or mouth ulceration/blistering occurs
- see also General Patient education for antiretroviral agents (p. 920)

Do not chew, crush or split the raltegravir 400 mg or 600 mg film-coated tablets.

Limited human data. Use only if benefit outweighs the risk.

Avoid, as excretion in human breastmilk unknown.

BLADDER FUNCTION DISORDER AGENTS

The bladder, a functional internal sphincter and a striated external sphincter, are responsible for the storage and intermittent evacuation of urine. The bladder and internal sphincter are made up of detrusor muscle. The sphincters control continence and, in the male, the internal sphincter is also responsible for preventing the reflux of semen from the urethra during ejaculation. The sphincters relax, allowing the bladder to push the urine into the urethra; this function involves afferent and efferent nerve fibres in the spinal cord. For a person to urinate, there is relaxation of the perineum (voluntary), increased tension in the abdominal wall, contraction of the detrusor muscle and opening of the internal sphincter, followed by relaxation of the external sphincter (Carr 2020).

Causes of bladder function disorder include:

- destruction of the spinal cord below T12, which causes bladder paralysis, resulting in no awareness that the bladder is full
- diseases of the spinal cord, including the nerves that innervate the bladder
- interruption of afferent fibres from the bladder (e.g. diabetes, tabes dorsalis); urinary retention may also occur
- spinal cord lesions above T12 causing neurogenic bladder (e.g. multiple sclerosis, traumatic myelopathy), resulting in accumulation of urine and distension of the bladder
- stretched bladder wall injury, which may occur because of obstruction of the bladder neck (e.g. prostatic hypertrophy) and repeated overdistension of the bladder, resulting in fibroses of the bladder wall increasing bladder capacity; further, contractions are not sufficient to empty the bladder, resulting in residual urine remaining in the bladder (increasing the risk of infection)
- frontal lobe problems resulting in the person ignoring the urge to void because of a confused mental state; and/or
- delay in developing inhibition of micturition, resulting in nocturnal enuresis or urinary incontinence during sleep (Carr 2020).

Agents used in the treatment of bladder function disorders include cholinergic

BLADDER FUNCTION DISORDER AGENTS

agents that stimulate contraction of the bladder and sympathomimetic agents which relax the urinary sphincter, facilitating urination (Carr 2020).

ALFUZOSIN
Trade name
Xatral SR

Available form
Tablets (prolonged-release): 10 mg

Action
- selective alpha1 adrenoreceptor antagonist (alpha1 receptors are found in the trigone of the bladder, urethra and prostate)
- decreases urethral pressure, resulting in decreased resistance to urine flow during micturition
- peak effect 9 hours, half-life 9.1 hours

Use
- treatment of symptoms of benign prostatic hyperplasia

Dose
- 10 mg orally daily immediately after food

Adverse effects
- rhinitis, pharyngitis, upper respiratory tract infection
- headache, dizziness, malaise, asthenia, fatigue
- nausea, abdominal pain, gastralgia, vomiting
- arthralgia
- pruritus
- renal calculi
- (Rare) intraoperative floppy iris syndrome, priapism

Interactions
- contraindicated with other alpha adrenoceptor blocking agents because of an increased risk of postural hypotension
- increased serum levels may occur if given with itraconazole or ritonavir, and are therefore contraindicated together
- caution if used with other antihypertensive agents or agents known to prolong QT interval
- caution if given with nitrates
- not recommended with phenoxybenzamine or labetalol
- increased risk of BP instability if given with general anaesthetics; therefore should be stopped 24 hours pre-surgery
- caution if taken with grapefruit juice, St John's wort or milk thistle

Nursing considerations/Cautions
- blood pressure should be measured before starting and regularly during therapy (especially in those taking concurrent antihypertensive agents)
- patient should be thoroughly assessed for prostate cancer (e.g. digital examination, prostate-specific antigen (PSA) blood test) before starting and regularly during therapy
- should be discontinued 24 hours before surgery
- if cataract surgery is planned, the surgeon should be notified of therapy because of the risk of intraoperative floppy iris syndrome
- caution in those with known hypersensitivity to other alpha adrenoceptor blocking agents
- caution if used in the elderly or those with cardiac disease and/or concurrent treatment with antihypertensive agents
- caution in those with symptomatic orthostatic hypotension or acquired/congenital prolongation of QT interval
- not intended for use in women
- not recommended in those with Parkinson's disease, multiple sclerosis, unstable angina or severe heart disease
- contraindicated in those with history of liver insufficiency or orthostatic hypotension

Patient education
- advise the patient to swallow tablet whole (not crushed, chewed or divided)
- warn the patient against driving or operating machinery if dizziness occurs
- instruct the patient to take care when going from lying or sitting position, as lightheadedness and dizziness may occur. Further, if any dizziness, fatigue, sweating or feeling faint occurs, the

- patient should be advised to lie down until symptoms totally disappear
- advise the patient to avoid grapefruit juice and herbal preparations such as St John's wort during therapy
- the patient should be advised to seek medical advice if any of the following occur:
  - irregular heartbeat or palpitations
  - prolonged painful erection

 Tablet should not be crushed, broken or chewed or dispersed in water.

 Monitor blood pressure in people with renal impairment, as early treatment can cause hypotension.
Contraindicated for people with hepatic insufficiency,

 Caution if used in the elderly, as there is a risk of hypotension and related adverse effect.

BETHANECHOL CHLORIDE

Trade name
Urocarb

Available form
Tablets: 10 mg

Action
- parasympathomimetic agent that is not inactivated by acetylcholinesterase, so has a prolonged action at receptor sites
- produces a rapid but transitory increase in tone and motility of the urinary bladder, stomach and intestine
- effective within 30–90 minutes (oral), duration about 1 hour

Use
- acute postoperative and postpartum urinary retention (non-obstructive)
- neurogenic atony of urinary bladder (with retention)

Dose
- 10–30 mg orally or sublingually 3–4 times daily 1 hour before or 2 hours after food

Adverse effects
- sweating, flushing of skin
- headache, malaise
- abdominal cramps or discomfort, salivation

Interactions
- caution if used with cholinergic agents (e.g. neostigmine), as additive effects may occur
- may counteract actions of sympathomimetic agents (e.g. adrenaline (epinephrine), dobutamine)
- agents with anticholinergic actions (e.g. atropine) may block bethanechol's effects

Nursing considerations/Cautions
- urinary tract infection should be ruled out before starting therapy
- have atropine (0.6 mg) SC available to reverse undesired effects
- contraindicated in those with asthma, hyperthyroidism, hypotension, bradycardia, coronary insufficiency, peptic ulcer, urinary tract infection, epilepsy or Parkinsonism

Patient education
- advise the patient to take on an empty stomach to prevent nausea and vomiting
- female patients of childbearing years should be counselled regarding the need to use adequate contraception to avoid pregnancy during therapy

 Tablet can be placed under the tongue and allowed to dissolve before swallowing, or crushed and mixed with water.

 Not recommended during pregnancy because of a potent excitatory effect on smooth muscle.

BLADDER FUNCTION DISORDER AGENTS

DARIFENACIN HYDROBROMIDE
Trade name
Enablex

Available forms
Tablets (modified-release): 7.5 mg, 15 mg

Action
- selective muscarinic M3 antagonist (M3 receptors appear to control urinary bladder muscle contraction)
- decreases frequency of incontinence, micturition and urgency while increasing functional bladder capacity
- peak effect 6 hours, half-life 12.8—18.7 hours

Use
- treatment of detrusor overactivity (with symptoms of urgency, frequency and/or incontinence)

Dose
- initially 7.5 mg orally daily, increasing to 15 mg daily after 2 weeks if greater symptom relief is required

Adverse effects
- abdominal pain, constipation, dry mouth, dyspepsia, nausea, vomiting, diarrhoea, weight gain
- asthenia, dizziness, headache
- flu-like symptoms
- dry nasal passages, rhinitis, sinusitis, pharyngitis
- arthralgia, back pain
- hypertension
- urinary tract infection, vaginitis
- abnormal vision (including blurred vision), dry eyes
- dry skin
- rash, pruritus
- peripheral oedema

Interactions
- frequency and/or severity of effects increased if given with other anticholinergic agents including anti-Parkinson's agents and tricyclic antidepressants (TCAs)
- caution if given with flecainide or TCAs
- caution if given with agents such as oral bisphosphonates that cause or worsen oesophagitis
- if given with itraconazole, miconazole or ritonavir, the dose should be no greater than 7.5 mg
- caution if given with paroxetine or fluoxetine
- may increase serum levels of digoxin; therefore serum levels should be monitored when starting, stopping or adjusting dose

Nursing considerations/Cautions
- caution if used in those being treated for narrow-angle glaucoma, decreased gastrointestinal motility, gastro-oesophageal reflux, oesophagitis, autonomic neuropathy, hiatus hernia, significant bladder outflow obstruction, risk of urinary retention, severe constipation (< 2 bowel motions/week), gastrointestinal obstructive disorder or pre-existing cardiac disease
- not recommended in those with severe liver impairment
- contraindicated in those with urinary retention, gastric retention or uncontrolled glaucoma

Patient education
- advise the patient that prolonged-release tablets should be swallowed whole, not chewed or crushed
- warn the patient that dry mouth, nose and/or eyes occur commonly but usually disappear with ongoing therapy
- the patient should be advised not to drive or operate machinery if blurred vision, dizziness or drowsiness occurs
- instruct the patient to seek medical advice immediately if any of the following occur:
    - painful red eye with associated loss of vision (may be signs of undiagnosed glaucoma) or
    - diarrhoea (which may be the first sign of intestinal obstruction, especially in those with an ileostomy or colostomy)

Tablets should not be crushed, broken or chewed or dispersed in water.

 Not recommended during pregnancy unless benefits outweigh potential risks.

 Not recommended during breastfeeding unless benefits outweigh potential risks.

 The dose should be no greater than 7.5 mg in those with moderate liver impairment.

DUTASTERIDE
Trade name
APO-Dutasteride, Avodart

Available form
Capsules: 500 microgram

Action
- inhibits conversion of testosterone to 5-alpha dihydrotestosterone (DHT) (which is responsible for development and enlargement of the prostate gland)
- active metabolite
- very long half-life (3—5 weeks), serum levels remain detectable for 4—6 months after stopping therapy

Use
- symptomatic benign prostatic hyperplasia (monotherapy or with alpha adrenoceptor blocking antagonist)

Dose
- 500 micrograms orally daily

Adverse effects
- impotence, decreased libido, ejaculation disorders
- breast enlargement and tenderness
- decrease in prostate-specific antigen (PSA)
- (Rare) increased risk of high-grade prostate cancer, alopecia (mainly body hair), breast cancer and testicular pain/swelling

Interactions
- increased serum levels may occur if given with verapamil and diltiazem

Nursing considerations/Cautions
- patient should be thoroughly assessed for prostate cancer (e.g. digital examination, PSA blood test) before starting and regularly during therapy. It should be noted that dutasteride lowers PSA by almost 50% after 6 months of therapy, even in the presence of prostate cancer. It is recommended that the new PSA baseline is established after 6 months of therapy and then monitored regularly thereafter
- total serum PSA returns to baseline within 6 months of stopping therapy
- may take 6 months of therapy before benefits are apparent
- (Combination therapy with alpha adrenoceptor blocking antagonist) cardiovascular function should be assessed before starting therapy. Dose titration is required to avoid postural hypotension, dizziness and syncope if given with prazosin (but not tamsulosin or alfuzosin)
- caution if used in those with liver disease (because of the very long half-life)
- contraindicated in those with known hypersensitivity to other 5-alpha reductase inhibitors (e.g. finasteride), severe liver impairment, or in women or children

Patient education
- advise the patient to swallow capsules whole without breaking or chewing
- the patient (and female partner/carer) should be advised that women and children should avoid contact with leaking capsules. If contact occurs, the skin should be washed immediately with warm water and soap
- advise the patient to seek medical advice immediately if there are any changes in breast tissue, including lumps or discharge from nipples
- instruct the patient not to donate blood within 6 months of stopping therapy
- the patient should be instructed to wear a condom during sex, as dutasteride has been detected in semen

BLADDER FUNCTION DISORDER AGENTS

- (Combination therapy) warn the patient against driving or operating machinery if dizziness occurs
- (Combination therapy) the patient should be advised to take care getting out of bed or standing from sitting position to avoid dizziness or fainting

Capsules should not be opened, crushed or chewed.

Contraindicated in women. Dutasteride is absorbed through the skin and pregnant women should avoid contact with capsules, as absorption may result in anomalies to a male fetus (i.e. may inhibit the development of male external genitalia).

Available in combination with
- dutasteride 500 microgram + tamsulosin 400 microgram extended-release capsule (Doubluts, Duodarts, Dutatam 500/400)

FINASTERIDE
Trade names
A&M Fintab-1, APO-Finasteride, Finapen, Finasteride GH, Finasteride Viatris, Finasteride-WGR, Finnacar, Finpro, Pharmcor Finasteride, Propecia, Proscar

Available forms
Tablets: 1 mg, 5 mg

Action
- inhibits enzyme (type II 5-alpha reductase) that converts testosterone to dihydrotestosterone (DHT), decreasing amounts circulating and in the prostate gland
- hair follicles also contain type II 5-alpha reductase. Finasteride decreases scalp and serum DHT levels, which may reverse balding
- peak effect 2 hours, half-life 6—8 hours

Use
- benign prostatic hyperplasia (with enlarged prostate)
- male pattern baldness (Propecia)

Dose
- (Benign prostatic hyperplasia) 5 mg orally daily for 6—12 months **OR**
- (Male pattern baldness) 1 mg orally daily (Propecia)

Adverse effects
- impotence, decreased libido, decreased ejaculate, ejaculation disorders, testicular pain
- breast tenderness and enlargement
- rash, pruritus
- depression
- headache
- (Rare) increased risk of high-grade prostate cancer, breast cancer, hypersensitivity reaction

Nursing considerations/Cautions
- the patient should be thoroughly assessed for prostate cancer (e.g. digital examination, prostate-specific antigen (PSA) blood test) before starting and regularly during therapy. It should be noted that dutasteride lowers PSA by almost 50% after 6 months of therapy, even in the presence of prostate cancer. It is recommended that the new PSA baseline is established after 6 months of therapy and then monitored regularly thereafter
- total serum PSA returns to baseline within 6 months of stopping therapy
- therapy should be reviewed after 6—12 months and continued if appropriate. Six months of therapy is required for maximum effects on prostate size and symptom improvement
- symptom improvement is most likely in men with enlarged prostates (> 40 mL on ultrasound examination)
- (Male pattern baldness) effectiveness of treatment (increased hair growth and/or

- decreased further hair loss) may not be apparent for at least 12 weeks
- (Male pattern baldness) efficacy has not been shown in those > 41 years
- tablets contain lactose and are therefore not recommended in those with galactose intolerance, Lapp lactase intolerance or glucose—galactose malabsorption
- caution if used in men with diminished urinary flow and/or large residual volume, as obstruction may occur
- contraindicated in women and children

Patient education

- the patient should be advised that therapy may not decrease symptoms related to prostatic hyperplasia
- advise the patient to seek medical advice immediately if there are any changes in breast tissue including lumps or discharge from nipples
- counsel the patient that tablets should not be handled by pregnant partner because of risk to a male fetus

Tablets can be dispersed in 10—20 mL of water, or crushed and mixed with a spoonful of yoghurt or apple puree.

Pregnant women should not crush or disperse tablets.

The patient should be advised that his sexual partner should avoid exposure to his semen or handling crushed tablets if she is or may become pregnant.

MIRABEGRON

Trade name
Betmiga

Available forms
Tablets (prolonged-release): 25 mg, 50 mg

Action
- beta3 adrenergic agonist that relaxes bladder smooth muscle, increasing mean voided volume per micturition and decreased frequency of non-voiding contractions with no effect on voiding pressure or residual urine
- may enhance urine storage function by stimulating beta3 adrenoceptors in the bladder
- peak activity 3—4 hours, half-life about 50 hours

Use
- symptomatic treatment of urgency, increased micturition frequency and/or urgency incontinence in those with overactive bladder syndrome

Dose
- 25 mg orally daily, increasing to 50 mg if needed

Adverse effects
- hypertension, tachycardia
- nasopharyngitis
- urinary tract infection, urinary retention
- headache, fatigue
- abdominal pain, diarrhoea, constipation, nausea
- upper respiratory tract infection
- arthralgia, back pain
- (Infrequently) blurred vision, dizziness, somnolence, angioedema

Interactions
- may increase serum levels of flecainide and metoprolol
- may increase serum levels of digoxin, increasing the risk of adverse effects; therefore serum levels should be closely monitored
- caution if given with warfarin. INR should be closely monitored, especially when starting or stopping therapy
- caution if given with agents known to prolong QT interval, such as sotalol, amiodarone, haloperidol, erythromycin and clarithromycin

Nursing considerations/Cautions

- BP should be monitored before starting and regularly during therapy (especially if patient is hypertensive)

BLADDER FUNCTION DISORDER AGENTS

- caution if used in those with bladder outlet obstruction or taking antimuscarinic (anticholinergic) agents
- caution if used in those with known prolongation of the QT interval or taking medication that prolongs the QT interval
- caution if used in those with moderate (grade 2) hypertension (systolic BP 160–190 mmHg or diastolic BP 100–109 mmHg)
- not recommended for those with end-stage kidney disease, requiring haemodialysis or with severe liver impairment
- contraindicated in those with severe uncontrolled hypertension (systolic BP ≥ 180 mmHg and/or diastolic BP ≥ 110 mmHg)

Patient education

- advise the patient to swallow tablets whole with liquids but the tablet should not be chewed, crushed or divided
- the patient should be warned not to drive or operate machinery if any dizziness, somnolence or blurred vision occurs
- instruct the patient to seek medical advice immediately if any of the following occur:
  - fast or irregular heartbeat
  - any swelling of face, eyelids, lips, throat or tongue
  - urinary tract infection (burning or pain passing urine, urge to pass urine frequently, cloudy and/or offensive-smelling urine)

Tablets should not be crushed, broken or chewed or dispersed in water.

Not recommended during pregnancy.

Not recommended during breastfeeding.

Recommended dose for patients with severe kidney impairment (eGFR 15–29 mL/min) or moderate liver impairment (Child–Pugh class B) is 25 mg orally daily.
Not recommended in those with end-stage kidney disease or severe liver impairment

OXYBUTYNIN

Trade names
Ditropan, Oxytrol Transdermal System

Available forms
Tablets: 5 mg;
Transdermal patch: 3.9 mg/24 hours

Action
- antispasmodic, anticholinergic
- relaxes smooth muscle in bladder, decreasing urgency and frequency during incontinence and voluntary urination
- greater antispasmodic activity than atropine sulfate monohydrate
- active metabolite has activity similar to oxybutynin on detrusor muscle
- (Tablets) peak activity 1 hour, half-life 2 hours

Use
- treatment of detrusor over activity (frequency, urgency and/or incontinence)

Dose
- 5 mg orally 2–3 times daily (daily maximum 20 mg) **OR**
- 1 transdermal patch twice weekly

Adverse effects
- dry mouth, constipation, nausea, vomiting, diarrhoea
- headache, confusion, drowsiness, dizziness
- urinary urgency, difficulty and retention
- impotence
- flushing and dryness of skin, decreased sweating
- dry eyes, blurred vision
- suppresses lactation

- (Less common) raised intraocular pressure, heat intolerance, hypersensitivity
- (Transdermal patch) pruritus, erythema, rash, vesicles, dry mouth, constipation, dysuria, blurred vision, diarrhoea

Interactions
- additive anticholinergic effects with tricyclic antidepressants (TCAs), phenothiazines, amantadine, digoxin, hyoscine, anti-Parkinson's agents and some antihistamines
- not recommended with alcohol or other sedative agents, as drowsiness may be enhanced
- caution if used with agents that exacerbate oesophagitis (e.g. bisphosphonates)
- may alter absorption of other medications given at the same time because of the effect on GI motility
- metabolism may be inhibited by clarithromycin, isoniazid, erythromycin, verapamil, diltiazem and ritonavir increasing serum levels and risk of adverse effects

Nursing considerations/Cautions
- the patient should be assessed before starting therapy (including cystometry) to determine the cause of bladder dysfunction and to treat any infection (if needed). Cystometry is also recommended regularly to assess effectiveness of therapy
- caution if used in those with significant bladder outflow obstruction, cognitive disorders, Parkinson's disease, prostatic hypertrophy, tachycardia, hypertension, hyperthyroidism, coronary artery disease, congestive cardiac failure, cardiac arrhythmias and hiatus hernia associated with reflux oesophagitis
- caution if used in those with kidney or liver impairment
- caution if used in children, as they may be more sensitive to effects
- not recommended in children with enuresis without definitive evidence of detrusor overactivity
- contraindicated in those with urinary or gastric retention, partial or complete gastrointestinal obstruction, paralytic ileus, intestinal atony, uncontrolled glaucoma or increased intraocular pressure associated with shallow anterior chamber, severe ulcerative colitis, megacolon, toxic megacolon, severe colitis, myasthenia gravis, obstructive uropathy or unstable cardiovascular status in acute haemorrhage

Patient education
- (Transdermal patch) advise the patient about the correct use of transdermal patch, including:
    - use a calendar to record when patch is applied
    - use only one patch at a time
    - apply to clean, dry skin (avoid skin folds or areas that are inflamed, irritated or have rashes)
    - use a different area of skin (stomach area, hips or buttocks) each time and do not reuse the same area within 7 days
    - avoid the waist area, as clothes may rub and cause the patch to roll or be dislodged
    - do not apply to areas that have had oils, lotions or powder applied to them (as these will prevent the patch sticking to skin)
    - do not expose patch to sunlight
    - contact with water (e.g. bathing or showering, swimming, exercising) is acceptable as long as patch is not dislodged during activity
    - if the patch partly rolls up or falls off, it should be pressed back into place. However, if it does not stay on, it should be replaced with a new patch
    - remove the patch slowly to prevent damaging skin
    - wash the area of removed patch with soap and water to remove any adhesive, but do not use alcohol or nail polish remover, as these will irritate skin
    - used patches should be folded together and carefully disposed of

BLADDER FUNCTION DISORDER AGENTS

- the patient should be advised not to drive or operate machinery if blurred vision, dizziness or drowsiness occurs
- warn the patient to take care taking medication during high temperatures or physical exercise, or if febrile, because of increased risk of heat stroke from decreased sweating
- advise the patient to avoid alcohol during therapy
- instruct the patient to immediately report:
  - painful red eye with associated loss of vision (may be signs of undiagnosed glaucoma) or
  - diarrhoea (which may be the first sign of intestinal obstruction, especially in those with an ileostomy or colostomy)

Tablets can be crushed and mixed with water or spoonful of yoghurt or apple puree.

Safety has not been established; therefore not recommended during pregnancy.

May be excreted in breastmilk; therefore not recommended during breastfeeding.

Dose should be started at 2.5 mg in the elderly and slowly increased if needed.

PENTOSAN POLYSULFATE SODIUM

Trade name
Elmiron

Available form
Capsules: 100 mg

Action
- heparin-like derivative similar to glycosaminoglycans
- inhibits formation of activated factor Xa, resulting in anticoagulant activity which is about 1/15 of heparin
- mobilises tissue plasminogen activator, resulting in fibrinolytic activity
- mediates release of lipoprotein lipases
- appears to bind to transitional epithelium in the bladder, coating denuded areas and restoring a normal barrier between bladder epithelium and urine

Use
- treatment of interstitial cystitis

Dose
- 100 mg orally 3 times daily 1 hour before meals or 2 hours after

Adverse effects
- headache, dizziness
- visual disturbances
- peripheral oedema
- nausea, dyspepsia, diarrhoea
- elevated liver function tests
- (Rare) mood swings, suicidal ideation

Interactions
- contraindicated with heparin or oral anticoagulants

Nursing considerations/Cautions
- interstitial cystitis should be confirmed before starting therapy
- complete blood count, prothrombin time (PT), activated partial thromboplastin time (aPTT), liver and renal function tests and serum calcium levels should be monitored regularly during long-term therapy
- if response is not adequate after 6–8 weeks, symptoms recur or new symptoms arise, cystoscopy is recommended
- symptoms may recur when prolonged therapy is discontinued
- caution if used in those with bleeding disorders or at risk of bleeding (e.g. elderly, alcohol-dependent patient)
- not recommended for undiagnosed urogenital bleeding
- contraindicated in those with haemophilia or active or history of bleeding

Patient education
- advise the patient it may take 6–8 weeks before a response is seen

- instruct the patient to take tablets either 1 hour before or 2 hours after meals
- the patient should be warned against driving or operating machinery if dizziness or visual disturbances occur
- instruct the patient to seek medical advice immediately if any of the following occur:
  - worsening of bladder symptoms
  - any ongoing sadness, withdrawal from friends or previously pleasurable activities, or any attempts at self-harm
  - visual disturbances

 Not recommended during pregnancy.

 Not recommended during breastfeeding.

SILODOSIN
Trade name
Urorec

Available forms
Capsules: 4 mg, 8 mg

Action
- selective alpha1A (α_{1A}) adrenoceptor antagonist (mostly located in prostate, bladder base and neck, prostatic capsule and urethra) causing relaxation of smooth muscle in these tissues, decreasing bladder outlet resistance with any impact on detrusor smooth muscle contraction. This results in improvement of lower urinary tract symptoms associated with benign prostatic hyperplasia, including both storage (irritative) and voiding (obstructive) symptoms
- lower affinity for cardiovascular alpha1B (α_{1B}) adrenoceptors
- active metabolite reaches plasma concentrations higher than parent compound and has a longer half-life (18 hours)
- half-life 11 hours

Use
- relief of lower urinary tract symptoms associated with benign prostatic hyperplasia in adult men

Dose
- 8 mg orally daily, swallowed whole with food

Adverse effects
- diarrhoea
- dizziness, headache, insomnia
- urinary tract infection, retrograde ejaculation, erectile dysfunction, loss of libido
- influenza, nasal congestion, nasopharyngitis, sinusitis, rhinitis
- hypertension, orthostatic hypotension, tachycardia
- (Rare) intraoperative floppy iris syndrome

Interactions
- not recommended with other alpha adrenoceptor blocking agents
- not recommended with itraconazole, ritonavir or ciclosporin
- not recommended with strong P-glycoprotein inhibitors such as clarithromycin, erythromycin and verapamil
- caution if used with PDE-5 inhibitors (e.g. sildenafil, tadalafil)
- caution if used with antihypertensive agents

Nursing considerations/Cautions
- the patient should be examined before starting therapy to rule out prostatic cancer which may present with similar symptoms
- if cataract surgery is planned, the surgeon should be notified of therapy because of the risk of intraoperative floppy iris syndrome
- caution if used in those with moderate kidney impairment. A lower starting dose is recommended and caution if the dose is increased to 8 mg
- not recommended in patients with orthostatic hypotension or severe liver impairment

- not recommended in patients who are scheduled for cataract surgery

Patient education

- instruct the patient to take the capsule at the same time every day with food. The capsule should be swallowed whole without chewing, crushing or breaking
- instruct the patient to take care when going from lying or sitting position, as lightheadedness and dizziness may occur. Further, if any dizziness, fatigue, sweating or feeling faint occurs, the patient should be advised to lie down until symptoms totally disappear
- warn the patient not to drive or operate machinery if dizziness occurs
- inform the patient that fertility may be temporarily affected during therapy

Capsules can be opened and contents mixed with apple puree and eaten immediately (however, capsule contents should not be chewed).

SOLIFENACIN SUCCINATE
Trade names
Solicare, Solifenacin Dr Reddy's, Solifenacin Lupin, Solifenacin Sandoz, Solifenacin Viatris, Solifenacin-WGR, Vesicare

Available forms
Tablets: 5 mg, 10 mg

Action
- muscarinic receptor antagonist (muscarinic receptors are important in urinary bladder smooth muscle contraction as well as stimulating salivary secretion)
- peak activity 3—8 hours, half-life 45—68 hours

Use
- treatment of detrusor overactivity (urgency, frequency and/or incontinence)

Dose
- initially 5 mg orally daily, increasing to 10 mg if needed

Adverse effects
- dry mouth, constipation, dyspepsia, abdominal pain, nausea, vomiting
- fatigue, headache, dizziness, insomnia, depression
- blurred vision, dry eyes
- cough, flu-like symptoms
- hypertension
- peripheral oedema
- urinary retention, dysuria, urinary tract infection
- (Rare) QT prolongation, angioedema, anaphylaxis

Interactions
- if given with ritonavir, itraconazole, nelfinavir, ciclosporin or macrolide antibiotics, the dose should not exceed 5 mg daily
- caution if given with verapamil, diltiazem, rifampicin, phenytoin or carbamazepine
- caution if given with agents known to prolong QT interval (or cause electrolyte imbalance, especially hypokalaemia) including erythromycin, sotalol, disopyramide, droperidol, chlorpromazine, haloperidol, amiodarone, amitriptyline and fluconazole
- caution if used with medications that increase the risk of oesophagitis, such as bisphosphonates

Nursing considerations/Cautions

- tablets contain lactose and are therefore not recommended in those with galactose intolerance, Lapp lactase intolerance or glucose—galactose malabsorption
- caution in those who have a history or risk of prolonged QT interval, autonomic

HAVARD'S NURSING GUIDE TO DRUGS

neuropathy, undergoing treatment for narrow-angle glaucoma, risk of decreased gastrointestinal motility, gastrointestinal obstructive disorders, decreased liver or kidney function, clinically significant bladder overflow obstruction or hiatus hernia associated with reflux oesophagitis
* contraindicated in those with urinary or gastric retention, partial or complete gastrointestinal obstruction, paralytic ileus, intestinal atony, uncontrolled glaucoma or increased intraocular pressure associated with shallow anterior chamber, severe ulcerative colitis, megacolon, toxic megacolon, myasthenia gravis, obstructive uropathy, severe liver impairment or on haemodialysis

Patient education

* the patient should be advised to take tablets whole (not crushed or broken) with liquid
* warn the patient to avoid driving or operating heavy machinery if dizziness or blurred vision occurs
* advise the patient to immediately seek medical advice if any of the following occur:
  * worsening of bladder symptoms
  * sudden fainting for no reason or after exercise/emotional excitement, rapid or erratic heartbeat
  * any swelling of lips, tongue or eyes

Tablet can be crushed and mixed with water or a spoonful of yoghurt or apple puree. The crushed tablet has a bitter taste.

Should be used during pregnancy only if potential benefits outweigh risks.

Not recommended during breastfeeding.

TAMSULOSIN HYDROCHLORIDE

Trade names
APO-Tamsulosin SR, Blooms the Chemist Tamsulosin SR, BTC Tamsulosin SR, Flomaxtra, Flosix, Tamsulosin Lupin SR, Tamsulosin Sandoz SR, Tamsulosin-WGR SR

Available form
Tablets (prolonged-/modified-release): 400 microgram

Action
* alpha adrenoceptor blocking agent with no effects on beta adrenoceptors (alpha adrenoceptors are found in the distal urethral sphincter and bladder neck smooth muscle, as well as hyperplastic prostate gland)
* inhibition reduces bladder outflow resistance, improving urinary flow and frequency of micturition, as well as reducing the volume of residual urine in the bladder
* half-life about 15 hours

Use
* benign prostatic hypertrophy

Dose
* 400 micrograms orally daily

Adverse effects
* abnormal ejaculation
* dizziness, insomnia
* blurred vision
* (Uncommonly) postural hypotension, palpitations, headache, rash, pruritus, urticaria
* (Rare) intraoperative floppy iris syndrome (during cataract surgery), priapism, photosensitivity, severe skin reaction

Interactions
* contraindicated with other alpha adrenoceptor blocking agents
* caution if used with paroxetine
* decreased serum levels may occur if given with furosemide (frusemide)
* elimination may be increased by warfarin and diclofenac

BLADDER FUNCTION DISORDER AGENTS

Nursing considerations/Cautions

- prostate cancer and other urological conditions should be ruled out before starting therapy
- if cataract surgery is planned, surgeon should be notified of therapy because of the risk of intraoperative floppy iris syndrome
- caution if used in those with sulfonamide allergy
- not indicated for children or women
- not recommended in those who have experienced angina or myocardial infarction in the previous 6 months
- contraindicated in those with a history of orthostatic hypotension, severe kidney or liver impairment

Patient education

- the patient should be advised to swallow the capsule whole (not broken or chewed)
- warn the patient against driving or operating machinery if dizziness occurs
- instruct the patient to take care when going from a lying or sitting position, as lightheadedness and dizziness may occur. Further, if any dizziness, fatigue, sweating or feeling faint occurs, the patient should be advised to lie down until symptoms totally disappear
- advise the patient to seek medical advice immediately if any of the following occur:
    - prolonged painful erection
    - severe skin reactions, including blistering

 Tablet should not be crushed, broken or chewed or dispersed in water.

Available in combination with

- dutasteride 500 microgram + tamsulosin 400 microgram extended-release capsule (Doubluts, Duodarts, Dutatam 500/400))

TOLTERODINE TARTRATE
Trade name
Detrusitol

Available forms
Tablets: 1 mg, 2 mg

Action
- muscarinic receptor antagonist (anticholinergic) (muscarinic receptors are important in urinary bladder smooth muscle contraction, as well as stimulating salivary secretion)
- active metabolite (same activity as tolterodine)
- half-life 1.9—3.7 hours

Use
- treatment of detrusor overactivity (urgency, frequency and/or incontinence)

Dose
- 1—2 mg orally twice daily

Adverse effects
- dry mouth, abdominal pain, constipation, dyspepsia, vomiting, nausea, diarrhoea, ulcerative stomatitis
- palpitations, hypertension, abnormal ECG
- headache, fatigue, malaise, migraine, somnolence, dizziness
- allergy, acne, pruritus, dry skin
- blurred vision, dry eyes
- abnormal liver enzymes
- asthma, bronchitis, cough, rhinitis, sinusitis
- dysuria, urinary tract infection
- leg pain, pain, arthralgia
- (Rare) prolongation of QT interval

Interactions
- caution if given with agents known to prolong QT interval (or cause hypokalaemia) including erythromycin, sotalol, disopyramide, droperidol, chlorpromazine, haloperidol, amiodarone, amitriptyline and fluconazole

- not recommended with erythromycin, clarithromycin, itraconazole, miconazole, ritonavir
- additive anticholinergic effects with tricyclic antidepressants (TCAs), phenothiazines, amantadine, digoxin, hyoscine, anti-Parkinson's agents and some antihistamines
- may decrease effects of metoclopramide
- serum levels may be increased by fluoxetine

Nursing considerations/Cautions

- if there has been no response after 6 months, consideration to an alternative therapy should be given
- caution in those who have a history or risk of prolonged QT interval, autonomic neuropathy, undergoing treatment for narrow-angle glaucoma, risk of decreased gastrointestinal motility, gastrointestinal obstructive disorders, pyloric stenosis, decreased liver or kidney function, clinically significant bladder overflow obstruction or hiatus hernia associated with reflux oesophagitis
- contraindicated in those with urinary or gastric retention, uncontrolled glaucoma, severe ulcerative colitis, megacolon, toxic megacolon, myasthenia gravis

Patient education

- warn patient to avoid driving or operating heavy machinery if dizziness or blurred vision occur
- advise patient to immediately seek medical advice if any of the following occur:
  - worsening of bladder symptoms
  - sudden fainting for no reason or after exercise/emotional excitement, rapid or erratic heartbeat

 Tablet can be dispersed in water, or crushed and mixed with a spoonful of yoghurt or apple puree.

 Should be used during pregnancy only if potential benefits outweigh risks.

 Not recommended during breastfeeding.

 Dose for those with severe kidney impairment or reduced liver function should be 1 mg twice daily.

BONE AND CALCIUM REGULATING AGENTS

Bone undergoes constant remodelling throughout a person's life and provides the means for mobility (e.g. acts as a lever and site for muscle attachment) and protection (e.g. supporting underlying organs and cavities), as well as acting as a reservoir for many ions necessary for body function (e.g. calcium, phosphorus, magnesium, sodium). Bone is also essential for haematopoiesis where blood cell proliferation and differentiation occur (Bringhurst et al 2023; Knights et al 2023).

Bone remodelling is achieved by two cell types — osteoblasts and osteoclasts. Osteoclasts are responsible for the resorption of old bone, while new bone is deposited by osteoblasts. Bone mass increases and stabilises until about the age of 20—25 years, after which it is lost slowly during the adult years, with this rate increasing in women after menopause. Bone remodelling is a complex interaction of endocrine factors, vitamin D, parathyroid hormone levels, calcitonin and plasma calcium levels (Knights et al 2023).

Paget's disease (osteitis deformans) is a disease of disordered bone remodelling (abnormal osteoclasts increase the rate of bone resorption, followed by a compensatory increase in new bone formation by osteoblasts). This results in bone that is expanded, less compact and more vascular, leading to a decrease in bone strength and increasing the likelihood of bowing, deformity and fractures (Jain & Vokes 2022). It is estimated to affect 3—4% of the middle aged to elderly Australian population (Knights et al 2023). The bones commonly involved include the pelvis, vertebrae, skull, femur and tibia. Pain is generally the most common presenting symptom and results from increased bone vascularity, expanding lytic lesions, fractures, bowing and other deformities (Jain & Vokes 2022). Femur or tibia bowing causes gait abnormalities with associated mechanical stresses, resulting in secondary osteoarthritis of the hip or knee joints. Other serious complications include bone fractures (commonly long bones) and cardiovascular issues (Jain & Vokes 2022).

Osteoporosis is a disease in which the bones lose their density and structural quality, resulting in bones that are weak, fragile and fracture easily. Around 853,600 (3.4%) people in Australia were

estimated to be living with osteoporosis or osteopenia in 2022. The true prevalence, including undiagnosed cases, is likely to be higher than this. In 2022, the prevalence of osteoporosis and osteopenia collectively:
- increased substantially with increasing age, from 0.7% of people aged 35—44, to 17% of people aged 75 and over
- was higher among women compared with men (5.5% and 1.1%, respectively)
- was highest for women aged 75 and over (26%) (AIHW 2024). A number of issues contribute to osteoporosis and fractures, including lifestyle factors (e.g. alcohol abuse, smoking, immobility, inadequate physical activity, falling, previous fractures, genetics, hypogonadal states (e.g. anorexia, bulimia, athletic amenorrhoea), endocrine disorders (e.g. thyrotoxicosis, diabetes mellitus types 1 and 2, gastrointestinal disorders (e.g. malabsorption syndromes), medications (e.g. glucocorticoids, lithium, excessive thyroid hormone, parenteral nutrition, ciclosporin, antiepileptic agents, antidepressants) and a number of other diseases (Lindsay & Samuels 2022). For women, other oestrogen-related risk factors include late menarche (time of first menstrual period), episodic amenorrhoea and early menopause. Age-related bone loss and decreasing sex steroid levels result in osteoporosis in older men compared with women (Knights et al 2023).

Hypercalcaemia can be associated with a number of conditions, including parathyroid conditions, malignancy (e.g. breast, lung and kidney cancer, multiple myeloma, lymphoma, leukaemia), be vitamin D related, or associated with high bone turnover (e.g. hyperthyroidism, immobility), vitamin A intoxication, excessive calcium intake, thiazide or antioestrogen treatment, or with endocrine disease (Khosla 2022). Before starting treatment, it is essential to ensure diagnosis, as a false positive can result from blood collection issues or elevated serum proteins such as albumin. Hypercalcaemia can be asymptomatic or result in fatigue, depression, difficulty concentrating, loss of appetite, nausea, vomiting, constipation, increased urine output, shortened QT interval or, in some, cardiac arrhythmias; it can be life threatening (Khosla 2022).

There are a number of agents used to prevent or treat bone disorders, such as bisphosphonates, parathyroid hormone analogues, calcimimetic agents (increase sensitivity of calcium-sensing receptors), calcitonin, vitamin D analogues, monoclonal antibodies and a selective oestrogen receptor modulator (SERM).

BISPHOSPHONATES

General Actions of bisphosphonates
- incorporated into bone matrix, where they may continue to act for some months, even after therapy has stopped
- inhibit resorption by impairing osteoclast function and decreasing osteoclast numbers
- nitrogen-containing bisphosphonates inhibit bone resorption without inhibiting bone formation (alendronate, ibandronate, pamidronate, risedronate, zoledronic acid)
- low oral availability

General Uses of bisphosphonates
- Paget's disease of the bone
- hypercalcaemia of malignancy (also called tumour-induced hypercalcaemia)
- osteoporosis (prevention and treatment)

BONE AND CALCIUM REGULATING AGENTS

General Adverse effects of bisphosphonates

- abdominal pain/distension, nausea, vomiting, diarrhoea, flatulence, dysphagia, constipation, acid regurgitation, dyspepsia, anorexia, gastritis, taste alteration
- oesophagitis, oesophageal ulcer/erosion
- headache, dizziness, fatigue, malaise, asthenia
- asymptomatic hypocalcaemia, symptomatic hypocalcaemia (tetany, paraesthesia), hypophosphataemia, hypokalaemia, hypomagnesaemia, increased serum creatinine
- bone, joint and muscle pain, muscle cramp
- (Prolonged therapy) atypical stress fractures
- (Rare) conjunctivitis, uveitis, iritis, oesophageal stricture/perforation, renal impairment
- (Rare) osteonecrosis of the jaw (generally occurring in those with cancer (especially those with bony metastases or multiple myeloma), existing periodontal disease, oral trauma, poor oral hygiene or being treated with antineoplastic agents, radiotherapy or corticosteroids. Most cases are associated with dental procedures (e.g. tooth extraction) and symptoms include jaw pain, toothache, altered sensation, recurrent infection (including osteomyelitis), non-healing sores of the mouth/jaw and/or exposed bone)
- osteonecrosis of other bones (including hip, knee, femur, humerus, external auditory canal)

General Interactions of bisphosphonates

- calcium supplements, antacids and other oral medications may decrease absorption of bisphosphonates
- caution if used with NSAIDs because of an increased risk of gastric irritation/ulceration and kidney dysfunction
- should not be given with other bisphosphonates
- caution if given with aminoglycosides, as they may decrease serum calcium
- may interfere with bone scintigraphy examinations

General Nursing considerations/Cautions for bisphosphonates

- osteoporosis should be confirmed (low bone density mass, two or more standard deviations from normal and/or presence of osteoporotic fracture) before starting therapy
- any hypocalcaemia and dehydration should be corrected before starting therapy
- (IV) serum creatinine should be measured before therapy is administered
- calcium and vitamin D supplements are essential in those with Paget's disease or glucocorticoid-induced osteoporosis
- (Tumour-induced hypercalcaemia) rehydration before and after therapy is recommended (especially if patient is older or on concurrent diuretic therapy)
- in those patients with risk factors (e.g. poor dental hygiene, chronic periodontal disease, head/neck radiotherapy, as well as treatment with antineoplastic agents and corticosteroids), a dental examination and any necessary treatment should be carried out before starting therapy with bisphosphonate. Invasive dental procedures should be avoided if possible during therapy
- caution if used in those with history of nephrolithiasis or hypercalciuria, as dietary restriction of calcium may be required during therapy
- not recommended in those with a creatinine clearance of less than 35 mL/min
- caution if used in those with dysphagia, oesophageal diseases/abnormalities, gastritis, duodenitis or gastric ulceration

HAVARD'S NURSING GUIDE TO DRUGS

- contraindicated in those who are unable to sit/stand upright for 30 minutes after taking medication, or have delayed oesophageal emptying (e.g. stricture, achalasia) or hypocalcaemia
- contraindicated in those with hypersensitivity to other bisphosphonates

General Patient education for bisphosphonates

- the patient should be advised to take tablets with plain water (not mineral water, coffee, tea or fruit juices) at least 30 minutes before the first food of the day and to remain upright for at least 30 minutes. Tablets should be swallowed whole and not sucked or chewed
- warn the patient not to take medication at night or lying down because this increases the risk of oesophageal ulceration
- instruct the patient to allow at least 30 minutes before taking any other medications
- advise the patient to avoid milk, calcium-rich foods and antacids for at least 2 hours after taking medication
- the patient should be advised to immediately report any:
  - difficulty or pain with swallowing
  - new or worsening heartburn or chest pain
  - pain in gums or jaw, swelling or jaw numbness or a heavy jaw feeling, loosening of teeth
  - any new or unusual thigh, hip or groin pain
  - visual disturbances (e.g. blurred vision, pain or redness of eyes)
  - ear pain, recurrent or chronic ear infections
- encourage the patient to maintain good dental hygiene during therapy, including brushing teeth after meals and before bed, gentle regular flossing to remove plaque and avoiding the use of alcohol-containing mouthwashes. The patient should also be instructed to keep the mouth moist and regularly check teeth and gums using a mirror and to seek dental advice if there is any tooth or jaw pain or there are loose teeth
- instruct the patient to tell the dentist of therapy before any invasive dental procedures are performed
- the patient taking once-weekly medication should be advised to mark the scheduled day on a calendar as a reminder. If the person forgets to take medication on this day, they should be advised to take it as soon as they remember (in the morning, before food) and then return to the normal scheduled day
- the patient should be advised not to drive or operate machinery if dizziness occurs
- advise the patient to:
  - exercise regularly to build and maintain bone strength
  - eat a balanced diet, including calcium-rich food
  - decrease smoking and/or excessive drinking on a regular basis
- female patients of childbearing potential should be counselled to avoid pregnancy by using adequate contraception during therapy. Patients should also be advised that effects could continue for months after therapy has stopped because bisphosphonates are slowly released from bone

 Tablets should not be chewed or sucked.

 Not recommended/contraindicated during pregnancy.

 Not recommended/contraindicated during breastfeeding.

BONE AND CALCIUM REGULATING AGENTS

ALENDRONIC ACID (ALENDRONATE SODIUM)
Trade names
APO Alendronate, Alendronate Sandoz, Alendronate-WGR, Fonat

Available form
Tablets: 70 mg

Action
- half-life greater than 10 years
- see also General Actions of bisphosphonates (p. 958)

Use
- see General Uses of bisphosphonates (p. 958)

Dose
- (Osteoporosis) 70 mg orally once weekly 30 minutes before food

Adverse effects
- see General Adverse effects of bisphosphonates (p. 959)

Interactions
- use with hormone replacement therapy (HRT) may increase bone mass and reduce bone turnover
- see also General Interactions of bisphosphonates (p. 959)

Nursing considerations/Cautions/Patient education
- see General Nursing considerations/Cautions/Patient education for bisphosphonates (p. 959)

Alendronate has not been studied in pregnant or breastfeeding women, and should therefore not be used.

Available in combination with
- Alendronate 70 mg, Colecalciferol 140 microgram (e.g. Fosamax Plus 70 mg /140 mcg); Alendronate 70 mg, Colecalciferol 70 microgram (e.g. Fosamax Plus 70 mg /70 mcg)

IBANDRONATE
Trade name
Bondronat

Available form
Tablets: 50 mg

Action
- half-life 10–60 hours
- see also General Actions of bisphosphonates (p. 958)

Use
- see General Uses of bisphosphonates (p. 958)

Dose
- (Metastatic bone disease) 50 mg orally daily 30 minutes before food

Adverse effects
- peripheral oedema
- flu-like symptoms
- sore throat, tooth disorder
- increased creatinine
- see also General Adverse effects of bisphosphonates (p. 959)

Interactions
- see General Interactions of bisphosphonates (p. 959)

Nursing considerations/Cautions
- renal function and serum calcium, phosphate and magnesium should be monitored throughout therapy
- (Metastatic bone disease) if patient has renal impairment, dose adjustment is required
- (Tumour-induced hypercalcaemia) dose is dependent on tumour type and severity of hypercalcaemia
- (Tumour-induced hypercalcaemia) repeat treatment may be required if hypercalcaemia recurs if therapy does not sufficiently reduce calcium levels
- see also General Nursing considerations/Cautions for bisphosphonates (p. 959)

Patient education

- see General Patient education for bisphosphonates (p. 960)

Should not be used during pregnancy.

Should not be used during breastfeeding.

If patient has renal impairment, dose adjustment is required (metastatic bone disease).

PAMIDRONATE DISODIUM (DISODIUM PAMIDRONATE)

Trade name
Pamisol

Available form
Solution for injection: 15 mg/5 mL, 30 mg/10 mL, 60 mg/10 mL, 90 mg/10 mL

Action
- biphasic elimination (1.6 hours, 27 hours)
- see also General Actions of bisphosphonates (p. 958)

Use
- see General Uses of bisphosphonates (p. 958)

Dose
- (Paget's disease) 60 mg IV as a single infusion (not exceeding 15—30 mg over 2 hours), but may be repeated when necessary **OR**
- (Lytic bone metastases — breast cancer and multiple myeloma) 90 mg IV infusion (not exceeding 1 mg/min) every 4 weeks, or every 3 weeks if receiving chemotherapy every 3 weeks **OR**
- (Tumour-induced hypercalcaemia) initially 30—90 mg (depending on serum calcium) IV infusion as a single dose or divided doses on consecutive days, over 2—4 hours; may be repeated if hypercalcaemia recurs or serum calcium concentration does not decrease within 2 days

Adverse effects
- rash
- atrial fibrillation, hypertension
- insomnia, somnolence
- anaemia, thrombocytopenia, lymphocytopenia, leucopenia
- hypertension
- (Rare) renal toxicity
- (IV site) redness, swelling, pain, induration, phlebitis
- (Tumour-induced hypercalcaemia) (rare) convulsions
- see also General Adverse effects of bisphosphonates (p. 959)

Interactions
- increased risk of renal dysfunction if given with thalidomide when treating those with multiple myeloma
- caution if used with nephrotoxic agents
- added effect if given with calcitonin to lower serum calcium levels in those with hypercalcaemia
- see also General Interactions of bisphosphonates (p. 959)

Nursing considerations/Cautions
- (Paget's disease) calcium and vitamin D supplements are recommended to prevent hypocalcaemia
- large vein should be used for IV administration to decrease IV site irritation
- not given as IV bolus
- reconstitute using 5—10 mL water for injections and dissolve completely before further diluting using sodium chloride 0.9% or glucose 5%
- for breast cancer, 90 mg is diluted in 250 mL and given over 2 hours; for multiple myeloma 90 mg is diluted in 500 mL and given over 4 hours
- should not be added to IV infusions containing calcium or divalent cations such as Ringer's solution
- serum creatinine should be measured prior to each therapy in those having prolonged therapy, especially if

BONE AND CALCIUM REGULATING AGENTS

- pre-existing (or predisposed to) renal impairment
- serum electrolytes, calcium and phosphate should be monitored regularly after starting therapy
- caution if used in those with liver impairment
- see also General Nursing considerations/Cautions for bisphosphonates (p. 959)

Patient education

- see General Patient education for bisphosphonates (p. 960)

Should not be used during pregnancy.

Should not be used in lactating women.

RISEDRONATE SODIUM
Trade names
Actonel, Actonel EC Once-a-Week, Actonel 150 mg Once-A-Month

Available forms
Tablets: 5 mg, 30 mg, 35 mg, 75mg, 150 mg; Tablets (enteric coated): 35 mg

Action
- biphasic half-life (1.5 hours, 480 hours)
- see also General Actions of bisphosphonates (p. 958)

Use
- see General Uses for bisphosphonates (p. 958)

Dose
- (Osteoporosis) 5 mg orally mane 30–60 minutes before first food/drink **OR**
- (Osteoporosis) 35 mg orally once weekly 30–60 minutes before first food/drink **OR**
- (Osteoporosis) 35 mg orally once weekly (enteric-coated tablets) **OR**
- (Osteoporosis) 150 mg orally monthly 30–60 minutes before first food/drink **OR**
- (Paget's disease) 30 mg orally daily 30–60 minutes before first food/drink for 8 weeks, repeated if treatment fails

Adverse effects
- hypertension
- pharyngitis, rhinitis, flu-like symptoms
- cataract
- infection
- (Uncommon) glossitis, duodenitis
- (Rare) abnormal liver function tests
- see also General Adverse effects of bisphosphonates (p. 959)

Interactions
- see General Interactions of bisphosphonates (p. 959)

Nursing considerations/Cautions/Patient education

- (Actonel EC Once-a-Week) advise the patient that tablet can be swallowed whole with or without food and should not be chewed, cut or crushed
- see also General Nursing considerations/Cautions/Patient education for bisphosphonates (p. 959)

Patients should not chew, cut or crush the tablet because of a potential for oropharyngeal irritation, and because the enteric coating is an important part of the formulation.

Has not been studied in pregnant women and should be used during pregnancy only if the potential benefit justifies the potential risk to mother and fetus.

It is not known whether it is excreted in human milk. Due to the potential for serious adverse reactions in nursing infants from bisphosphonates, a decision should be made whether to discontinue breastfeeding or to discontinue the drug. Take into account the importance of the drug to the mother.

It is not recommended for use in patients with severe renal impairment.

No studies performed to determine safety or efficacy in patients with hepatic impairment.

Available in combination with
- contained in APO-RISEDRONATE/Ca 35/1250 (composite pack) with calcium carbonate

ZOLEDRONIC ACID
Trade names
Aclasta, Deztron, Osteovan, Zometa

Available forms
Solution: 4 mg/5 mL, 4 mg/100 mL, 5 mg/100 mL

Action
- triphasic elimination (0.23 hours, 1.75 hours, 167 hours)
- see also General Actions of bisphosphonates (p. 958)

Use
- see General Uses of bisphosphonates (p. 958)

Dose
- (Bone metastases) 4 mg IV over 15 minutes every 3–4 weeks (4 mg/5 mL solution, 4 mg/100 mL solution) **OR**
- (Hypercalcaemia of malignancy) 4 mg IV over 15 minutes (4 mg/5 mL solution, 4 mg/100 mL solution) **OR**
- (Osteoporosis, Paget's disease, prevention of fractures) 5 mg by IV infusion over 15 minutes once-yearly (5 mg/100 mL solution)

Adverse effects
- post-dose syndrome (also called acute phase reaction) (flu-like symptoms, fever, rigors, flushing, chills, fatigue, bone pain, myalgia, weakness, arthralgia, headache)
- atrial fibrillation, palpitations, hypertension, hypotension
- sweating
- anaemia
- urinary tract infection, urinary retention
- (Uncommon) rash, pruritus, peripheral oedema
- (Injection site) redness, swelling, pain
- see also General Adverse effects of bisphosphonates (p. 959)

Interactions
- caution if used with nephrotoxic agents, aminoglycosides or diuretics
- increased risk of renal dysfunction if given with thalidomide when treating patients with multiple myeloma
- see also General Interactions of bisphosphonates (p. 959)

Nursing considerations/Cautions
- post-dose (acute phase) syndrome symptoms can be reduced by giving paracetamol (not NSAIDs) with IV administration
- (Paget's disease) if retreatment is required, an interval of at least 12 months should be allowed unless clinical symptoms such as bone pain or compression symptoms worsen
- concentrated solution (4 mg/5 mL) should be further diluted using 100 mL sodium chloride 0.9% or glucose 5% and infused over 15 minutes
- 4 mg/100 mL does not require further dilution
- infusion should not be mixed with any other calcium-containing solutions (e.g. Ringer's solution)
- administer alone
- creatinine clearance should be measured before each treatment (especially in those with kidney impairment)
- see also General Nursing considerations/Cautions for bisphosphonates (p. 959)

Patient education
- a patient who experiences post-dose syndrome should be advised that symptoms usually occur within the first 3 days of infusion. Paracetamol (not NSAIDs) can be taken to reduce these adverse effects

BONE AND CALCIUM REGULATING AGENTS

- advise the patient that onset of action is approximately 2—3 months
- see also General Patient education for bisphosphonates (p. 960)

In the absence of adequate available data in human pregnancy, this drug should not be used during pregnancy.

Discontinue in breastfeeding owing to lack of human studies.

OTHER BONE and CALCIUM REGULATING AGENTS

CALCITONIN SALMON (SALCATONIN)
Trade name
Miacalcic

Available form
Ampoules: 50 IU/mL, 100 IU/mL

Action
- synthetic polypeptide hormone structurally identical to salmon calcitonin (called calcitonin salmon (salcatonin)), which is 10—40-fold more potent than human calcitonin in reducing calcium concentrations
- lowers blood calcium concentration by decreasing the rate of bone resorption and increasing urinary calcium, phosphorus and sodium excretion
- thought to also increase osteoclastic activity, thereby promoting bone and collagen formation
- no effect on calcium absorption
- inhibits gastric acid and pancreatic enzyme secretion, stimulates intestinal secretion of water and electrolytes and modifies glucose—insulin relationship
- (Paget's disease) relieves bone pain, lowers skin temperature over affected bones, decreases excessive cardiac output, stabilises hearing and causes regression of bone lesions
- onset of action 15 minutes (IM or SC) or immediately (IV), peak effect 2 hours, duration of action 6—8 hours, half-life 60—90 minutes after s.c. or i.v. administration

Use
- Paget's disease (in those where other treatments are ineffective or unsuitable)
- hypercalcaemia

Dose
- (Paget's disease) 80—100 IU daily or every second day SC or IM, reducing to 50 IU daily when symptoms improve; duration of treatment depends on the therapeutic indication and the patient's response **OR**
- (Hypercalcaemia) 5—10 IU/kg daily by slow IV infusion in 500 mL sodium chloride 0.9% over 6 hours **OR**
- (Hypercalcaemia) 5—10 IU/kg by slow IV injection or infusion in 2—4 divided doses over 24 hours **OR**
- (Hypercalcaemia) 5—10 IU/kg daily IM or SC

Adverse effects
- nausea, vomiting, diarrhoea, abdominal pain, unusual taste
- dizziness, headache, fatigue
- facial flushing, feeling of warmth
- arthralgia
- (Injection site) pain, redness, swelling
- (High dose) development of antibodies
- (Long-term therapy) escape phenomenon
- (Rare) localised or generalised hypersensitivity, visual disturbances, increased risk of malignancy, rash, pruritus

Interactions
- may reduce serum levels of lithium, requiring dose adjustment

Nursing considerations/Cautions
- any dehydration should be corrected before starting therapy

HAVARD'S NURSING GUIDE TO DRUGS

- skin testing using 1:100 diluted solution intradermally is recommended to determine any sensitivity
- treatment duration should be as short as possible in order to reduce the risk of malignancies occurring
- if the patient has kidney impairment, the dose should be reduced
- an IV route is recommended for emergencies or severe cases of hypercalcaemia
- IM is preferable if amount exceeds 2 mL; multiple sites should be used
- nausea and vomiting may be decreased by dividing the daily dose or administering an antiemetic agent at the same time
- escape phenomenon is due to saturation of the receptor sites, not antibody production. Response is restored by stopping therapy for a short period

Patient education
- the patient should be advised not to drive or operate machinery if dizziness, fatigue or visual disturbances occur
- patients should be educated in self-administration: injection technique, rotation of sites, safe handling and disposal of needles, storage requirements

Contraindicated during pregnancy.

Contraindicated during breastfeeding.

A smaller dose may be required in renal impairment.

Use adult dosage with care in the elderly.

CALCITRIOL
Trade names
Calitrol, Rocaltrol, Sical

Available form
Capsules: 0.25 microgram

Action
- active form of vitamin D_3 (colecalciferol) normally formed in the kidneys by a precursor
- regulates bone and calcium homeostasis
- stimulates osteoblastic activity
- active metabolites
- half-life 3—6 hours
- (Uraemia) kidney fails to convert the precursor to the active form

Use
- treatment and prevention of osteoporosis (postmenopausal or corticosteroid-induced)
- hypocalcaemia in patients with uraemic osteodystrophy, hypoparathyroidism, rickets
- vitamin D deficiency

Dose
- (Osteoporosis) initially 0.25 micrograms orally twice daily, increasing to 0.5 micrograms twice daily if needed **OR**
- (Corticosteroid-induced osteoporosis) 0.25—0.75 micrograms orally daily in divided doses (the dose depending on corticosteroid dose) **OR**
- (Uraemic osteodystrophy, hypoparathyroidism, rickets) initially 0.25 micrograms orally daily, increasing by 0.25 micrograms per day at 2—4-week intervals if needed **OR**
- (Uraemic osteodystrophy) 0.25 micrograms orally second daily (if serum calcium is normal or slightly reduced)

Adverse effects
- hypercalcaemia, pruritus, hyperphosphataemia
- drowsiness, weakness, headache
- nausea, diarrhoea, constipation, abdominal pain, decreased appetite

BONE AND CALCIUM REGULATING AGENTS

- rash
- decreased kidney function
- metastatic or ectopic calcification of soft tissue
- (Early signs of vitamin D toxicity (acute)) headache, weakness, somnolence, nausea, vomiting, decreased appetite, abdominal pain, dry mouth, metallic taste, constipation, muscle and bone pain
- (Late signs of vitamin D toxicity (chronic)) muscle weakness, fever, polyuria, polydipsia, dehydration, nocturia, anorexia, weight loss, pancreatitis, photophobia, sensory disturbance, pruritus, decreased libido, increased urea, cholesterol and albumin levels, elevated liver enzymes, hypertension, cardiac arrhythmias, hyperthermia, rhinorrhoea, growth retardation, apathy, conjunctivitis (calcific) and, rarely, overt psychosis

Interactions

- cardiac arrhythmias may occur if given with digoxin
- actions may be counteracted by corticosteroids
- hypermagnesaemia may occur if given with magnesium-containing antacids
- colestyramine or colestipol may decrease absorption
- metabolism may be increased by phenytoin or phenobarbital (phenobarbitone)
- not recommended with vitamin D or derivatives because of the increased risk of hypercalcaemia
- hypercalcaemia may occur if given with thiazide diuretics or calcium supplements
- dose of phosphate-binding agent may require adjusting if given together

Nursing considerations/Cautions

- serum calcium, phosphorus, magnesium and alkaline phosphatase levels and 24-hour urinary calcium and phosphorus levels should be measured twice weekly initially, then 2–4-weekly, then 2–3-monthly for the remainder of therapy
- if the patient becomes immobile, serum calcium levels should be monitored more frequently to avoid hypercalcaemia
- blood samples should be taken without a tourniquet to reduce local calcium effects
- (Hypoparathyroidism) malabsorption may be present requiring an increase in dose
- (Corticosteroid-induced osteoporosis) calcium intake should not be greater than 1 g/day
- caution if changing from ergocalciferol to calcitriol, as it may take months to return to pre-treatment ergocalciferol levels, increasing the risk of overdose occurring
- caution if used in those with kidney failure, as serum phosphate levels may increase
- contraindicated in those with hypercalcaemia or vitamin D toxicity

Patient education

- instruct the patient to immediately seek medical advice if any of the following occur:
    - signs of acute vitamin D toxicity, including headache, weakness, nausea, vomiting, dry mouth, metallic taste and bone/muscle pain
    - signs of hypercalcaemia, including fatigue, depression, confusion, anorexia, nausea, vomiting, constipation, increased urine output and unusual heart rate
- the patient should be advised to maintain adequate daily fluid intake and avoid becoming dehydrated
- the patient should be educated about diet, importance of not exceeding the daily calcium intake (800 mg) by suddenly changing calcium intake and the need to avoid magnesium-containing antacids and vitamin D supplements, including multivitamin preparations, as

these contain both calcium and vitamin D
- warn the patient to avoid driving or operating machinery if drowsiness occurs

 Not recommended during pregnancy unless benefits outweigh risks.

 Not recommended during breastfeeding unless benefits outweigh risks.

 In patients with renal dysfunction, more frequent monitoring is appropriate.

 In elderly patients suffering from ischaemic heart disease, serum calcium levels should be carefully monitored.

CALCIUM CHLORIDE DIHYDRATE (CALCIUM CHLORIDE)
Trade name
Phebra Calcium Chloride Dihydrate 10%

Available form
Vial: 1 g/10 mL

Action
- calcium is an essential element involved in functioning of the heart, nerves and muscle contraction, blood coagulation, absorption of vitamin B_{12}, and storage and release of neurotransmitters and hormones

Use
- hypocalcaemia where a rapid increase in calcium is required (e.g. hypocalcaemic tetany or tetany due to parathyroid deficiency)
- severe hyperkalaemia (as an adjunct to antagonise cardiotoxicity)
- magnesium toxicity
- cardiac resuscitation

Dose
- Each mL of calcium chloride 10% injection contains approximately 0.68 mmol of calcium ions and 1.36 mmol of chloride ions **OR**
- (Hypocalcaemia) an initial dose of 3.5—7 mmol (7—14 mEq) calcium or 0.5—1 g slow IV, at 1—3-day intervals, depending on calcium concentrations **OR**
- (Hyperkalaemia with secondary cardiac toxicity) adults: an initial dose of 1.12—7 mmol (2.25—14 mEq) calcium is recommended, may be repeated after 1—2 minutes if necessary **OR**
- (Magnesium toxicity) 500 mg slow IV, observing patient for signs of recovery before administering any further doses

Adverse effects
- vein irritation
- (Rapid IV) tingling sensation, chalky/calcium taste, hot flushes, sense of oppression (impending doom), decreased BP, bradycardia, cardiac arrhythmias, syncope
- (Rare) hypercalcaemia

Interactions
- contraindicated in patient taking digoxin because of risk of arrhythmias
- may reverse effects of non-depolarising neuromuscular blocking agents
- should not be mixed with carbonates, phosphates, magnesium sulfate, tartrates or tetracyclines
- may reduce effects of calcium-blocking agents
- excretion increased by calcitonin, diuretics and growth hormone
- excretion decreased by parathyroid hormone, thiazide diuretic and vitamin D
- use with calcium- or magnesium-containing agents is not recommended because of the risk of hypercalcaemia or hypermagnesaemia

Nursing considerations/Cautions
- should not be given IM or SC because of the risk of necrosis and tissue sloughing
- administered using a small needle into a large vein at a rate not greater than

BONE AND CALCIUM REGULATING AGENTS

- 0.35–0.7 mmol/min to reduce the risk of adverse effects
- the patient should remain recumbent after administration
- recommended by slow IV administration only, as rapid injection will cause syncope
- IV site should be monitored for any signs of extravasation
- the solution should be warmed to body temperature before administration
- BP should be monitored because vasodilation may occur
- serum and urinary calcium should be closely monitored during therapy
- if patient has hyperkalaemia, constant ECG monitoring is recommended and the dose adjusted if needed
- caution if used in those with cardiac disease
- not recommended in those with renal insufficiency-associated hypocalcaemia
- caution if used in those with respiratory failure, respiratory acidosis or cor pulmonale, or where there is a risk of hypercalcaemia occurring (e.g. dehydration, electrolyte imbalance, kidney impairment)
- contraindicated in those with hypercalcaemia, hypercalciuria or severe renal disease, including renal calculi, in those with sarcoidosis or if the patient is taking digoxin
- (Cardiac resuscitation) contraindicated in those with ventricular fibrillation

Not recommended during pregnancy.

Not recommended during breastfeeding.

High-risk medication — use calcium gluconate for less urgent indications.

CINACALCET
Trade names
Pharmacor Cinacalcet, Cinacalcet Viatris

Available form
Tablets: 30 mg, 60 mg, 90 mg

Action
- reduces parathyroid hormone (PTH) levels by increasing sensitivity of the calcium receptor to extracellular calcium
- reduces serum calcium–phosphorus product and calcium and phosphorus levels
- biphasic half-life (6 hours, 30–40 hours)

Use
- secondary hyperparathyroidism (end-stage kidney disease with dialysis) (adjunctive therapy)
- hypercalcaemia (parathyroid cancer)
- primary hyperparathyroidism (where parathyroidectomy is not possible)

Dose
- (End-stage kidney disease) initially 30 mg orally daily with food, increasing the dose at 2–4 week intervals to a maximum of 180 mg (to achieve a PTH level between 1.5 and 5 times the upper limit of normal) **OR**
- (Parathyroid cancer, primary hyperparathyroidism) initially 30 mg orally twice daily with food, increasing the dose at 2–4-week intervals to 60 mg twice daily, then 90 mg twice daily, then 90 mg orally 3–4 times daily until the calcium level is normal

Adverse effects
- nausea, vomiting, diarrhoea, abdominal pain, dyspepsia, decreased appetite, constipation
- dyspnoea, cough
- headache, dizziness, asthenia, fatigue
- fever
- myalgia, muscle spasm, back pain

- non-cardiac chest pain
- hypertension
- peripheral oedema
- rash
- (Uncommon) hypersensitivity
- (Rare) hypocalcaemia (paraesthesia, myalgia, cramping, tetany, seizures), adynamic bone disease, hypotension, worsening cardiac failure, seizures, gastrointestinal ulceration/bleeding

Interactions
- may increase serum levels of metoprolol, flecainide, vinblastine and tricyclic antidepressants (TCAs), and therefore should be used with caution
- serum levels may be increased by erythromycin or itraconazole
- serum levels may be decreased by rifampicin, phenytoin or St John's wort
- caution if used with other calcium-lowering agents

Nursing considerations/Cautions
- serum calcium levels should be monitored before starting, throughout therapy and during any dose titration. Therapy should not be started if serum calcium is below 8.4 mg/dL (2.1 mmol/mL)
- (Secondary hyperparathyroidism) the serum calcium level should be measured within the first week and intact PTH (iPTH) within 1—4 weeks of starting therapy. When maintenance is achieved, serum calcium should be measured monthly and iPTH levels 1—3-monthly
- (Parathyroid cancer, primary hyperparathyroidism) the serum calcium level should be measured 1 week after starting therapy and the dose adjusted accordingly, then 2—3-monthly when maintenance is achieved
- PTH levels should be measured 12 hours after taking cinacalcet. PTH levels should be maintained above 100 picogram/mL to prevent adynamic bone disease
- if hypocalcaemia occurs (between 7.5 and 8.4 mg/dL), calcium-containing phosphate binder and vitamin D sterol should be started to increase calcium levels. However, if low levels persist, therapy with cinacalcet should be stopped or the dose reduced
- liver function should be monitored regularly if used in those with any liver impairment
- not recommended for those with chronic kidney disease who are not on dialysis
- caution if used in those with epilepsy, as significant decreases in calcium levels may lower seizure threshold
- caution if used in those with hypotension or impaired cardiac function
- caution if used in those with moderate-to-severe liver impairment
- caution if used in those at risk for upper gastrointestinal bleeding (e.g. ulcers, gastritis, severe vomiting)
- contraindicated in those with hypocalcaemia

Patient education
- ensure the patient understands the need to take tablets with or after food to improve availability. The patient should be advised to swallow tablets whole, not chewed or broken
- warn the patient against driving or operating machinery if dizziness occurs
- advise the patient to immediately seek medical advice if any of the following occur:
    - any numbness or tingling around the mouth, muscle pain or cramping
    - seizures (fitting)
    - any signs of worsening heart symptoms
    - rash
    - severe vomiting (especially if blood is present), abdominal or stomach pain

 Tablets should be taken whole and should not be divided.

BONE AND CALCIUM REGULATING AGENTS

Not recommended during pregnancy unless benefits outweigh risks.

Not recommended during breastfeeding unless benefits outweigh risks.

Moderate-to-severe hepatic impairment (Child—Pugh classification) increases cinacalcet drug concentrations by approximately 2 to 4 fold. PTH and serum calcium concentrations should be closely monitored during dose titration of cinacalcet.

DENOSUMAB

Trade names
Prolia, Xgeva

Available forms
Prefilled syringe: 60 mg/mL;
Vial: 120 mg/1.7 mL

Action
* monoclonal antibody (IgG$_2$) with high affinity and specificity for RANK ligand cytokine (essential for formation, function and survival of osteoclast), inhibiting osteoclast formation, thereby decreasing bone resorption and increasing bone mass and strength
* long half-life 28 days

Uses
* treatment of osteoporosis in postmenopausal women
* osteopenia in men after androgen-deprivation therapy for non-metastatic prostate cancer
* increase bone mass in men and women with osteoporosis at risk of fractures (including those due to glucocorticoid therapy)
* prevention of skeletal-related events in patients with multiple myeloma or bone metastases from solid tumours
* treatment of giant cell tumour of the bone (recurrent or unresectable)
* hypercalcaemia of malignancy (not responding to IV bisphosphonates)

Dose
* 60 mg SC 6-monthly (Prolia) **OR**
* 120 mg SC every 4 weeks (Xgeva) **OR**
* (Treatment of giant cell tumour, hypercalcaemia of malignancy) initially 120 mg SC day 8 and day 15 (loading dose), then 120 mg SC every 4 weeks

Adverse effects
* arthralgia, back pain, bone pain, musculoskeletal pain, pain in extremity, osteoarthritis
* nasopharyngitis, bronchitis, cough, dyspnoea
* hypertension, angina
* dizziness, headache, insomnia, fatigue, asthenia
* decreased appetite, nausea, vomiting, diarrhoea, constipation, dyspepsia, decreased weight, abdominal pain
* eczema
* fever
* peripheral oedema
* (SC site) pain
* (After discontinuing therapy) hypercalcaemia, multiple vertebral fractures
* (Rare) osteonecrosis of the jaw (generally occurring in those with cancer (especially bony metastases or multiple myeloma) also being treated with antineoplastic agents and corticosteroids. Most cases are associated with dental procedures (e.g. tooth extraction), periodontal disease, oral trauma, poor oral hygiene or on chemotherapy, radiation therapy or corticosteroids. Symptoms include jaw pain, toothache, altered sensation, recurrent infection (including osteomyelitis), non-healing sores of the mouth/jaw and/or exposed bone)
* (Rare) hypocalcaemia, skin infection (cellulitis), pancreatitis, atypical femoral fractures), hypersensitivity, osteonecrosis of other bones

Interactions
* caution if used with bisphosphonates, glucocorticoids or proton pump

inhibitors because of the increased risk of atypical femoral fractures
- not recommended with other agents containing denosumab

Nursing considerations/Cautions

- any hypocalcaemia should be corrected before starting therapy
- regular serum calcium level monitoring is recommended before starting therapy, within 2 weeks of first administration and then regularly throughout therapy especially if hypocalcaemia is suspected or in those at risk of hypocalcaemia (e.g. severe kidney impairment, history of parathyroid or thyroid surgery, malabsorption syndrome)
- calcium and vitamin D supplements are recommended unless hypercalcaemia is present
- in those patients with risk factors (e.g. poor dental hygiene, chronic periodontal disease, head/neck radiotherapy as well as treatment with antineoplastic agents and corticosteroids), a dental examination and any necessary treatment should be carried out before starting therapy. Invasive dental procedures should be avoided if possible during therapy
- (Xgeva) not recommended in those with rare hereditary problem of fructose intolerance
- not recommended in those under 18 years (unless skeletally mature with giant cell tumour of bone)
- not recommended in those with latex allergy, as the prefilled syringe needle cap contains latex
- caution if used in those with severe kidney impairment (creatinine clearance < 30 mL/min) or on dialysis owing to an increased risk of hypocalcaemia
- caution if used in those with vitamin D deficiency, rheumatoid arthritis or hypophosphatasia because of the increased risk of atypical femoral fractures

- contraindicated in those with severe untreated hypocalcaemia, unhealed lesions from dental/oral surgery or hypersensitivity to Chinese hamster ovary protein

Patient education

- the patient should be advised not to stop therapy without medical advice
- instruct the patient/carer in correct administration technique, including:
  - give as an injection under the skin (subcutaneous) into the upper thigh, belly region (except for 5 cm area around belly button) or upper arm
  - ensure the prefilled syringe is intact when taken from packaging (and hasn't been dropped or damaged in any way), and check the expiry date and solution (should be clear, colourless to slightly yellow)
  - allow it to come to room temperature for 30 minutes before injection to reduce pain (but do not heat by any other means)
  - the prefilled syringe should not be shaken
  - wash hands with soap and water
  - clean the injection site with an alcohol swab and allow it to dry
  - ensure the area to be injected is not tender, bruised, red, hard, scarred or stretch marks are present
  - pull the grey needle cap straight out and away from body, pinch the injection site, insert the needle into skin fold and push the plunger in a slow constant movement until a snap is heard or felt. Continue to push through the snap to inject full dose and then release the thumb and lift syringe from skin
  - the safety guard should automatically cover the needle
  - discard the used syringe into a sharps disposal container
  - a used syringe should not be reused
  - store an unused syringe in fridge but do not freeze. Once the syringe has

BONE AND CALCIUM REGULATING AGENTS

come to room temperature, it should be used within 30 days
- the patient should be advised to use stickers (provided) as a reminder of the next injection date
- advise the patient to seek medical advice immediately if any of the following occur:
  - signs of skin infection (area that is hot, red, swollen, painful/tender)
  - any new or unusual groin, thigh or hip pain
  - pain in gums or jaw, swelling or jaw numbness or a heavy jaw feeling, loosening of teeth or non-healing sores in mouth or jaw
  - numbness or tingling in fingers, toes or around the mouth, muscle twitching, spasm or cramps
  - (after therapy is stopped) excessive thirst, frequent urination, stomach pain, bone pain, muscle weakness, fatigue, confusion, lethargy, anxiety, depression
- warn the patient against driving or operating machinery if dizziness occurs
- the patient should be advised to take calcium (at least 1000 mg) and vitamin D (400 IU) daily
- encourage the patient to maintain good dental hygiene during therapy, including brushing teeth after meals and before bed, gentle regular flossing to remove plaque and avoiding the use of alcohol-containing mouthwashes. The patient should also be instructed to keep the mouth moist, regularly check teeth and gums using a mirror and seek dental advice if any tooth or jaw pain, unhealed sores in mouth/jaw or loose teeth occur
- women of childbearing potential should be counselled to use adequate contraception to avoid pregnancy occurring

 Contraindicated during pregnancy.

 Contraindicated during breastfeeding.

 The safety and efficacy of Prolia has not been studied in patients with hepatic impairment. Caution if used in those with severe kidney impairment.

RALOXIFENE HYDROCHLORIDE

Trade names
Eviista, Fixta 60, Ralovista, Raloxifene GH

Available form
Tablets: 60 mg

Action
- selective (o)estrogen receptor modulator (SERM) that potentiates the effects of oestrogen on bone and lipid metabolism (decreased oestrogen levels lead to increased bone resorption, accelerated bone loss and increased fracture risk)
- antagonises negative effects of oestrogen on uterus and breast tissue, minimising the risk of oestrogen-dependent cancers
- reduces bone absorption and decreases bone turnover caused by oestrogen deficiency
- half-life about 28 hours

Use
- prevention and treatment of osteoporosis (postmenopausal women)
- decreases risk of invasive breast cancer (postmenopausal women at high risk or with osteoporosis)

Dose
- 60 mg orally daily

Adverse effects
- hot flushes, fever, sweating
- headache, depression, insomnia, vertigo

- infection, flu-like symptoms
- conjunctivitis
- rash
- chest pain
- sinusitis, laryngitis, pneumonia, bronchitis, increased cough, pharyngitis
- vaginitis, leucorrhoea, uterine/endometrial disorder, vaginal bleeding
- arthralgia, myalgia, leg cramps, tendon disorder, arthritis
- urinary tract infection, cystitis, urinary tract disorder
- neuralgia
- weight gain, peripheral oedema
- nausea, diarrhoea, vomiting, flatulence, gastric erosion, abdominal pain
- increase serum triglycerides
- deep vein thrombosis, pulmonary embolus, retinal venous thrombosis, stroke, myocardial infarction, acute coronary syndrome

Interactions

- not recommended with colestyramine or colestipol, as absorption will be decreased
- serum levels may be reduced by ampicillin
- may decrease prothrombin time if given with warfarin; therefore should be monitored closely, especially when starting, stopping or changing dose
- lowers serum total and low-density lipoprotein (LDL) cholesterol levels (should be taken into account if given with lipid-lowering agents)
- not recommended with oestrogen or hormone replacement therapy

Nursing considerations/Cautions

- if the patient has a history of oestrogen-induced hypertriglyceridaemia, triglyceride levels should be monitored regularly throughout therapy
- therapy should be stopped if there is prolonged immobilisation. If immobility is due to planned surgery, therapy should be stopped for 3 days before event is planned to occur. Therapy should not be restarted until the patient is fully mobile
- calcium supplementation is recommended if patient's diet is inadequate
- caution if used in women with a history of stroke, atrial fibrillation, transient ischaemic attack or oestrogen-induced hypertriglyceridaemia
- not recommended in those with liver impairment
- contraindicated in males or premenopausal women, or as treatment for invasive breast cancer
- contraindicated in women with or with a history of deep vein thrombosis, pulmonary embolism, retinal vein thrombosis or liver impairment

Patient education

- the patient should be advised to report any unexplained vaginal bleeding immediately
- advise the patient to ensure they have adequate calcium in their diet
- advise the patient to move around regularly during any prolonged travel (especially air travel)
- the patient should be instructed to have a breast examination and mammogram before starting therapy, then regularly during therapy, as raloxifene does not eliminate the risk of breast cancer
- female patients of childbearing potential should be counselled to use adequate contraception to avoid pregnancy during therapy

Tablet can be crushed and mixed with water or spoonful of yoghurt or apple puree.

Mask and gloves must be worn to crush tablets and a closed tablet crusher used. Pregnant staff must not crush tablets.

Contraindicated during pregnancy.

BONE AND CALCIUM REGULATING AGENTS

Contraindicated during breastfeeding.

The use of the drug in patients with hepatic insufficiency is not recommended; further studies need to be done to determine safety and efficacy in this population.

Banned in sport.

ROMOSOZUMAB
Trade name
Evenity

Available form
Prefilled syringe: 105 mg/1.17 mL

Action
- binds to monoclonal antibody sclerostin, a small protein in osteoclasts, inhibiting its activity, increasing bone formation and decreasing bone resorption

Use
- treatment of osteoporosis in postmenopausal women and for increasing bone mass in men with osteoporosis, both at high risk of fracture

Dose
- 210 mg SC once a month for 12 months

Adverse effects
- injection site reactions
- arthralgia
- rash
- (Uncommon) hypocalcaemia, urticaria, cataract formation, cardiovascular events (e.g. myocardial infarction (MI), stroke)
- (Rare) atypical femoral fracture, osteonecrosis of the jaw, angioedema, erythema multiforme

Nursing considerations/Cautions

Administration
- to administer the 210 mg dose, give 2 subcutaneous injections
- patient can be educated in self-administration technique
- to reduce the risk of hypocalcaemia, patients should be adequately supplemented with calcium and vitamin D
- calcium levels should be monitored regularly during therapy
- if the dose is missed, administer as soon as it can be rescheduled. Thereafter, romosozumab can be administered monthly from the date of the last dose.
- full dental assessment and any necessary treatment should be completed before starting romosozumab to minimise the risk of osteonecrosis of the jaw. Risk factors include poor dental hygiene, chronic peridontal disease, radiotherapy to head/neck, or treatment with corticosteroids or antineoplastic agents
- romosozumab's effects on bone resorption do not persist after stopping use
- following treatment with romosozumab, an antiresorptive (e.g. bisphosphonate or denosumab) treatment is recommended
- an improvement in bone mineral density and fracture risk is seen with use for 12 months; however, the early gains in bone formation appear to be lost by 9 months
- efficacy and safety data in men are limited, particularly regarding reduction of fracture risk
- those with severe renal impairment (estimated glomerular filtration rate (eGFR) 15 to 29 mL/min/1.73 m^2) or receiving dialysis are at greater risk of developing hypocalcaemia and should therefore be closely monitored during therapy
- contraindicated in patients with previous myocardial infarction or stroke

Patient education
- see Denosumab (p. 972) for self-administration technique teaching
- ensure the patient understands the importance of maintaining good dental hygiene (e.g. regular tooth brushing and

flossing), including regular dental check-ups, ensuring dentures fit well and telling the dentist about treatment with romosozumab if any procedures such as tooth extraction are planned
- the patient should be advised to take calcium (at least 1000 mg) and vitamin D (400 IU) daily
- advise the patient to seek medical advice immediately if any of the following occur:
  - muscle spasm, twitches or cramps, numbness or tingling in toes, fingers or around the mouth (signs of hypocalcaemia)
  - pressure or pain in chest, shortness of breath, lightheadedness, dizziness, headache, weakness or numbness in face, arm or legs, difficulty talking or walking, loss of balance or changes to vision
  - pain in gums or jaw, swelling or jaw numbness or heavy jaw feeling, loosening of teeth or non-healing sore in mouth or jaw

There are no studies in pregnant women and it is not known whether it can cause fetal harm when administered to a pregnant woman.

It is not known whether the drug is excreted in breastmilk. A decision should be made whether to discontinue nursing or discontinue the drug. Take into account the potential benefit of the drug to the mother or of breastfeeding to the infant.

SODIUM PHOSPHATE

Trade name
Phosphate Phebra

Available form
Tablets (effervescent): 500 mg

Action
- high-dose phosphate supplement
- decreases serum calcium concentration in those with hypercalcaemia, as serum phosphate levels are inversely proportional to serum calcium levels

Use
- hypercalcaemia (associated with hyperparathyroidism, multiple myeloma and metastatic bone disease)
- hypophosphataemia (associated with vitamin D-resistant rickets)

Dose
- (Hypercalcaemia) up to 3 g (6 tablets) orally daily **OR**
- (Vitamin D-resistant rickets) 2—3 g (4—6 tablets) orally daily

Adverse effects
- nausea, vomiting, diarrhoea, abdominal pain
- (Rare) soft tissue calcification, nephrocalcinosis, acute renal failure

Interactions
- absorption may be decreased by antacids or compounds containing calcium, magnesium, iron or aluminium
- increased risk of ectopic soft tissue calcification if given with calcium supplements
- increased risk of hyperphosphataemia due to increased absorption if given with vitamin D supplements

Nursing considerations/Cautions
- dose should be adjusted according to individual requirements
- tablets contain 469 mg sodium (20.4 mmol) and 123 mg potassium (3.1 mmol); therefore caution if used in those with congestive heart failure, hypertension, pre-eclamptic toxaemia, impaired kidney function or electrolyte imbalance

Patient education
- advise the patient that effervescent tablets should be dissolved in half a glass of water and swallowed when fizzing stops. Warn the patient that tablets should not be swallowed whole
- the patient should be warned to avoid calcium and vitamin D supplements (or multivitamin preparations)

BONE AND CALCIUM REGULATING AGENTS

The safety of Phosphate Phebra tablets in human pregnancy has not been formally studied.

The safety of Phosphate Phebra tablets in breastfeeding has not been formally studied.

In patients with impaired renal function, consideration should be given to the sodium and potassium content of Phosphate Phebra tablets before administration.

An excessive dosage has been reported to produce hypocalcaemia in isolated cases, particular care should be taken to ensure appropriate dosage in the elderly.

TERIPARATIDE

Trade names
Forteo, Teriparatide Lupin, Terrosa

Available form
Prefilled pen: 250 microgram/mL

Action
- recombinant human parathyroid hormone (PTH) fragment that activates osteoblasts via specific PTH cell receptors, stimulating formation of new bone
- action is the same as PTH (regulates bone metabolism, renal tubular reabsorption of calcium and phosphate, and absorption of intestinal calcium)
- half-life about 1 hour (SC), 5 minutes (IV)

Use
- osteoporosis (postmenopausal women)
- primary osteoporosis (men at risk of fractures where other agents are unsuitable)
- osteoporosis (associated with glucocorticoid therapy)

Dose
- 20 micrograms daily SC

Adverse effects
- nausea, vomiting, dyspepsia, tooth disorder, constipation, diarrhoea
- leg cramps, arthralgia
- asthenia, dizziness, depression, insomnia, vertigo, headache
- angina, hypertension, syncope, transient hypotension
- increased cough, dyspnoea, pneumonia, pharyngitis, rhinitis
- rash, sweating
- neck pain, muscle spasm
- (Uncommon) hyperuricaemia
- (Rare) antibody development, increased risk of osteosarcoma, exacerbation of hypercalcaemia
- (Injection site) pain, swelling, erythema, pruritus, localised bruising

Interactions
- caution if used with digoxin, as hypercalcaemia may predispose to digoxin toxicity

Nursing considerations/Cautions
- patient should be observed and BP monitored during the first 4 hours of treatment and advised to go slowly from sitting to standing because orthostatic hypotension may occur
- treatment is for 24 months only, after which the patient may commence other therapy for osteoporosis
- if the patient becomes immobile, serum calcium must be closely monitored until fully mobile
- (Males) any primary or secondary hypogonadism should be excluded (and treated) before starting therapy
- calcium and vitamin D supplementation is recommended in those whose diet is inadequate
- should not be used in children or young adults with open epiphyses
- caution if used in those with or with recent urolithiasis because the condition may be exacerbated

- not recommended in those with kidney impairment, hyperparathyroidism, hypercalcaemia or those who have an increased risk of developing osteosarcoma (including those with unexplained alkaline phosphatase levels, open epiphyses or prior skeletal radiation therapy) or who have bone metastases or skeletal malignancies
- contraindicated in those with Paget's disease

Patient education

- the patient needs to be fully informed of length of treatment (24 months only) and the implications of the development of osteosarcoma during animal experiments. The patient should be asked to sign an informed consent form
- advise the patient to go slowly from sitting to standing because dizziness and fainting may occur
- warn the patient that transient low blood pressure may occur during first few treatments, happens within 4 hours of administration and usually resolves spontaneously. However, the patient is advised to lie down during this time
- instruct the patient to maintain adequate amounts of calcium and vitamin D in the diet and add supplements if necessary
- the patient should be instructed that each pen can be used for up to 28 days and then discarded
- educate the patient in self-administration including the correct SC technique, rotation of sites, storage requirements and correct disposal
- the patient should be advised not to drive or operate machinery if dizziness, insomnia or vertigo occurs

Not recommended during pregnancy.
No human studies have been undertaken.

Not recommended during breastfeeding.

Contraindicated in those with severe renal impairment

CARDIAC GLYCOSIDES

Cardiac glycosides increase the force of contraction of the myocardium, producing what is known as a positive inotropic effect. While the term 'digitalis' is used to describe the entire group of cardiac glycosides being obtained from the *Digitalis* (or foxglove) plant, digoxin is the only cardiac glycoside used clinically. In the past, digoxin was considered to be the basis of management for heart failure, but it has been largely replaced by more effective medications, such as angiotensin converting enzyme (ACE) inhibitors, loop and thiazide diuretics, angiotensin II receptor antagonists and beta adrenoceptor blocking agents (beta blockers). Digoxin remains valuable in the management of chronic heart failure in those who have concurrent atrial fibrillation (Knights et al 2023). While milrinone is not a cardiac glycoside, it has a positive inotropic effect by increasing myocardial contraction and therefore has been included in this section.

DIGOXIN
Trade names
Lanoxin, Sigmaxin

Available forms
Tablets: 62.5 micrograms, 250 micrograms;
Elixir (paediatric): 50 micrograms/mL;
IV solution: 500 micrograms/2 mL;
IV solution (paediatric): 50 micrograms/2 mL

Action/Use/Dose/Interactions/Nursing considerations/Cautions/Patient education
- see Digoxin (in Antiarrhythmic agents p. 92)

MILRINONE
Trade names
Milrinone GH, Milrinone-Baxter

Available form
IV solution: 1 mg/mL

Action
- phosphodiesterase 3 (PDE_3) inhibitor which increases cAMP levels, increasing intracellular calcium and the force of contraction (positive inotrope) and improving diastolic function

- not related to digoxin or catecholamines
- vasodilator
- half-life 2.3 hours, duration of action 3—6 hours

Use
- congestive heart failure (short-term (48 hours) management, not responding to other therapy)
- low output states after cardiac surgery (including weaning from bypass pump)

Dose
- 50 microgram/kg by slow IV over 10 minutes (loading dose), then 0.375—0.75 microgram/kg/min by continuous IV infusion (maintenance)

Adverse effects
- ventricular and supraventricular arrhythmias
- hypotension, chest pain
- headache
- infusion site reaction
- (Rare) rash, abnormal liver enzymes
- (Very rare) torsades de pointes (see Glossary)

Nursing considerations/Cautions
- any hypokalaemia or hypotension should be corrected before therapy starts
- use should be restricted to ICU or cardiac units
- heart rate, blood pressure, ECG, renal function, fluid and electrolyte status should be monitored throughout therapy
- infusion rate should be adjusted according to haemodynamic and clinical response
- dose should not exceed 1.13 mg/kg/day
- if severe hypotension occurs, the infusion should be stopped until resolved and restarted at a lower rate if needed
- IV site should be closely monitored to avoid extravasation
- the solution should be further diluted using diluents before use
- incompatible with frusemide (furosemide) or bumetanide because of precipitation in the infusion line
- should not be diluted with sodium bicarbonate
- the infusion should be discarded after 24 hours
- caution if used in those with arrhythmias, including atrial flutter/fibrillation not controlled with digoxin, hypotension, severe renal impairment or previous vigorous treatment with diuretics
- not recommended in those in the acute phase of post-myocardial infarction
- contraindicated in those with severe obstructive aortic or pulmonary valve disease, hypertrophic subaortic stenosis or hypersensitivity to bipyridine

Limited human data. Use only if the benefit outweighs the risk.

Caution, as excretion in human breast-milk is unknown.

Reduced renal function: dosage adjustment required in patients with severe renal impairment. Initiate therapy at a reduced infusion rate according to renal function, monitoring for therapeutic effectiveness and toxicity.

CHOLINERGIC AND ANTICHOLINERGIC AGENTS

The nervous system (NS) is divided into the central nervous system (CNS) and the peripheral nervous system (PNS), which is further divided into the somatic and autonomic nervous systems. The autonomic nervous system (ANS) has two subdivisions — the sympathetic nervous system and the parasympathetic nervous system (Knights et al 2023).

Within the ANS, the sympathetic nervous system primarily manages the body's 'fight or flight' responses (see Sympathomimetic agents, p. 1565). In contrast, the parasympathetic nervous system promotes 'rest and digest' activities, aiding in conserving and restoring energy (Knights et al 2023).

Drugs affecting the parasympathetic nervous system are primarily those that influence acetylcholine (ACh), the main neurotransmitter in the parasympathetic nervous system. These drugs can be classified into parasympathomimetics (cholinergic agonists), which stimulate parasympathetic activity, and parasympatholytics (anticholinergics), which inhibit it. Parasympathomimetics may be used to treat conditions such as dry mouth or glaucoma, while parasympatholytics can treat issues such as overactive bladder or certain gastrointestinal disorders (Knights et al 2023).

Other cholinergic (parasympathomimetic) drugs may be found in the chapters on Eye, ear, nose and throat agents (p. 1128) and Drugs for Alzheimer's disease (p. 50).

CHOLINERGIC (PARASYMPATHOMIMETIC) DRUGS

General Actions of cholinergic agents
- miosis
- decreases heart rate
- bronchoconstriction
- increases gastric and pancreas secretions
- increases in stomach and intestinal motility
- increases skeletal muscle tone
- contracts bladder wall and relaxes trigone and urinary sphincter

General Adverse effects of cholinergic agents
- nausea, vomiting, diarrhoea, abdominal cramps, flatulence, increased peristalsis, increased salivation

- miosis, nystagmus, increased lacrimation
- headache, agitation, fear, slurred speech, drowsiness, dizziness, decreased consciousness
- increased desire to urinate or defecate, involuntary urination or defecation
- muscle cramps and fasciculation, weakness, ataxia
- bradycardia, hypotension, syncope
- rash, urticaria, increased sweating
- dyspnoea, bronchospasm, tight chest, wheezing, increased secretions (bronchial, pharyngeal, oral)
- (Rare) cardiac arrest, coma, convulsions, paralysis, respiratory depression, allergic reaction

NEOSTIGMINE
Trade name
Neostigmine Juno

Available form
Ampoules: 2.5 mg/mL

Action
- reversible cholinesterase inhibitor
- at moderate doses, does not cross the blood–brain barrier
- half-life 47–60 minutes (IV) or 50–91 minutes (IM)
- see also General Actions of cholinergic agents (p. 981)

Use
- reverses effects of non-depolarising neuromuscular blocking agents
- treatment of myasthenia gravis (acute exacerbation)
- prevention and treatment of postoperative intestinal atony and urinary retention

Dose
- (Reversal of non-depolarising muscle relaxants) 0.5–2.5 mg IV (with 0.6–1.2 mg atropine, in separate syringes) slowly IV over 1 minute (maximum dose 5 mg) **OR**
- (Myasthenia gravis) 1–2.5 mg SC or IM daily in several daily doses when greatest strength is required, up to 20 mg daily **OR**
- (Prophylaxis of intestinal atony and urinary retention) 0.25 mg IM or SC before or immediately after operation, repeated 4–6-hourly for 2–3 days **OR**
- (Treatment of urinary retention) 0.5 mg IM or SC and apply heat to lower abdomen. After patient has voided, 0.5 mg IM or SC 3-hourly for at least 5 injections

Adverse effects
- see General Adverse effects of cholinergic agents (p. 981)

Interactions
- may antagonise neuromuscular blockade of aminoglycosides
- prolonged respiratory depression and apnoea may occur if given with suxamethonium
- effects may be decreased if given with corticosteroids
- when concurrent corticosteroids are stopped, increased effect may be seen
- effects may be reversed by atropine
- effects may be decreased if given with quinine, hydroxychloroquine, beta adrenoreceptor antagonists or lithium

Nursing considerations/Cautions
- may be given IV, IM or SC
- 0.5 mg IV = 1–1.5 mg IM or SC
- (Myasthenia gravis) record muscle strength variations because severity can vary and increase risk of over-dosage
- (Myasthenia gravis) duration of action is 2–4 hours
- (Non-depolarising neuromuscular blockage reversal) should not be attempted until spontaneous recovery from paralysis is obvious, and it is recommended that patient is well ventilated with patent airway until normal respiration is achieved

- complete reversal of non-depolarising neuromuscular blocking agents occurs within 5—15 minutes
- have atropine sulfate available to reverse the effects if necessary
- administer alone
- (Bladder dysfunction) if patient has not voided within 1 hour of first dose, catheterisation is recommended
- caution if used in those who have had recent intestinal or bladder surgery, or have asthma, cardiac disease, arrhythmias, bradycardia, recent myocardial infarction or coronary occlusion, hypotension, epilepsy, peptic ulcer, Parkinsonism, vagotonia, kidney impairment, hyperthyroidism or Addison's disease
- contraindicated in those with peritonitis or mechanical obstruction of the intestinal or urinary tract

Use only if the benefits outweigh potential risks; may cause uterine irritability and premature labour near term.

Minimal excretion into breastmilk; adverse effects on the infant are unlikely but should be considered.

Reduced renal function: use with caution; dose adjustment may be necessary, as neostigmine is partly excreted unchanged by the kidneys.

Start at a lower dose, monitoring closely for adverse effects because of increased susceptibility.

Available in combination with
- glycopyrronium 500 microgram/mL + neostigmine 2.5 mg/mL injection (Glyconeo, Novistig)

PYRIDOSTIGMINE
Trade names
Mestinon, Mestinon Timespan

Available forms
Tablets: 10 mg, 60 mg;
Tablets (controlled-release): 180 mg

Action
- cholinesterase inhibitor
- direct effect on skeletal muscle
- onset of action 30—45 minutes, duration 3—6 hours, half-life 1.5—4.25 hours
- see also General Actions of cholinergic agents (p. 981)

Use
- myasthenia gravis

Dose
- 60—180 mg orally 2—4 times daily **OR**
- 180—540 mg orally 1—2 times daily (Timespan tablets)

Adverse effects
- see General Adverse effects of cholinergic agents (p. 981)

Interactions
- may prolong phase I block of depolarising muscle relaxants (e.g. suxamethonium)
- atropine antagonises action of pyridostigmine
- may antagonise neuromuscular blockade of aminoglycosides
- caution if given with aminoglycosides, local and some general anaesthetics, antiarrhythmic agents and other agents known to interfere with neuromuscular transmission in patients with myasthenia gravis
- additive effects may occur if given with dexpanthenol (vitamin B_5)

Nursing considerations/Cautions
- dose and frequency of administration is dependent on severity of disease plus level of physical and/or emotional stress and may vary from day to day
- dose interval should not be less than 6 hours
- lung function (especially vital capacity) should be regularly monitored and the dose adjusted to maintain good respiratory function. Facilities for cardiopulmonary resuscitation, cardiac monitoring, endotracheal intubation and assisted respiration should be

- readily available during dose adjustment
- the patient may become resistant to therapy with prolonged treatment, which may be restored by temporarily discontinuing therapy for several days (under medical supervision)
- lower incidence of adverse effects compared with other anticholinesterases
- if the patient shows little clinical improvement, it may be the result of under- or overdosage. Overdosage may result in cholinergic crisis, whereas underdosage may result in myasthenia crisis
- caution if atropine is used to counteract adverse effects, as it may mask signs of cholinergic or myasthenic crisis
- caution if given to those with epilepsy, asthma, bradycardia, recent coronary occlusion, vagotonia, hyperthyroidism, arrhythmias, peptic ulcers or impaired kidney function
- large doses are not recommended in those with megacolon or decreased GI motility
- contraindicated in those with hypersensitivity to anticholinesterases or bromides, or in those with intestinal or urinary tract obstruction (mechanical)

Patient education

- ensure the patient understands that drug does not restore muscle strength to normal and therefore they are not to increase the dose in order to improve response
- instruct the patient that the dose should be taken when they experience greatest fatigue and have the greatest need (e.g. given 30—45 minutes before meals if the person has problems when eating)
- the patient should be advised that different muscle groups respond differently to therapy, sometimes resulting in weakness of one muscle group and strength in another. Neck muscles and those involved in chewing and swallowing are usually the first to show signs of overdosage, followed by the muscles of the upper extremities and shoulder girdle, with the pelvic girdle, leg muscles and the extraocular muscles being the last to be affected

 Controlled-release tablets should not be crushed. A plain tablet can be crushed and mixed with water, or a spoonful of yoghurt or apple puree.

 Limited data available. The maternal requirement for pyridostigmine in myasthenia gravis may be critical. Cholinergic effects on neonates are rare but possible. Transient muscle weakness may occur in newborn. Use only if potential benefits justify the risks.

 Caution: excretion in human breastmilk unknown. Safety during lactation is not established.

 Reduced renal function: mainly excreted by the kidneys. Lower doses may be necessary, and treatment should be guided by clinical response.

ANTICHOLINERGIC DRUGS

Anticholinergic drugs inhibit the action of acetylcholine at the receptor (muscarinic) sites in the parasympathetic division of the autonomic nervous system. These receptors are found in:

- the CNS, peripheral neurons and gastric parietal cells (neuroparietal or M1 receptors)
- the heart and peripheral neurones (neurocardiac or M2 receptors)
- smooth muscle and glands (smooth muscle—glandular or M3 receptors)
- the eye (ocular or M4 receptors).

Other anticholinergic agents may be found in the chapters on Antiasthma agents, bronchodilators and respiratory agents

CHOLINERGIC AND ANTICHOLINERGIC AGENTS

(p. 97), Eye, ear, nose and throat agents (p. 1128) and Anti-Parkinson's agents (p. 790).

General Actions of anticholinergic agents

- reduce production of sweat, saliva, lacrimal, nasal, bronchial, gastric and intestinal secretions
- reduce stomach and intestinal motility
- reduce gastric acid production
- increase heart rate (by blocking vagal stimulus)
- bronchodilation
- inhibit micturition
- mydriasis, cycloplegia, raises intraocular pressure

General Adverse effects of anticholinergics

- dry mouth, dysphagia, thirst, constipation, nausea, vomiting, taste alteration, bloating
- headache, nervousness, insomnia, confusion, drowsiness, dizziness
- urinary urgency, difficulty and retention
- impotence
- flushing and dryness of skin, decreased sweating
- tachycardia, palpitations, arrhythmias, bradycardia (at high doses)
- mydriasis, photophobia, cycloplegia, blurred vision
- suppresses lactation
- (Less common) raised intraocular pressure, angina, heat intolerance, hypersensitivity, hyperpyrexia
- injection site reaction

General Interactions of anticholinergics

- may delay absorption of other oral agents given at same time
- increased intraocular pressure may occur if given with corticosteroids
- additive anticholinergic effects with disopyramide, tricyclic antidepressants (TCAs), monoamine oxidase inhibitors (MAOIs), phenothiazines, amantadine, antispasmodics, anti-Parkinson's agents, other anticholinergics (e.g. ipratropium) and some antihistamines
- may cause an increase in intraocular pressure if given with corticosteroids
- may antagonise GI effects of metoclopramide
- urinary excretion may be delayed by urinary alkalisers
- increased risk of severe constipation, urinary retention and paralytic ileus if given with opioid analgesics
- may interfere with antipsychotic effectiveness of haloperidol if given to those with schizophrenia
- should not be administered 24 hours before gastric acid secretion test
- mydriasis and cycloplegia caused by anticholinergic may interfere with neuroradiological tests for intracranial neoplasm, subdural haematoma or aneurysm

General Nursing considerations/ Cautions for anticholinergics

- caution if used in the elderly or brain damaged, as there is an increased risk of mental confusion
- caution if used in children or those with Down syndrome, as they have greater sensitivity to effects, whereas those with albinism have reduced sensitivity
- caution if used in those who are febrile, as decreased sweating may lead to hyperpyrexia by inhibiting heat loss
- caution if used in debilitated patients because decreased bronchial secretions may lead to formation of bronchial plug
- caution if used in those with ileostomy or colostomy, as diarrhoea may be sign of incomplete intestinal obstruction
- caution if used in those with diarrhoea, gastric ulcer, GI infection (known or suspected), porphyria, hyperthyroidism, liver, kidney or metabolic impairment, hypertension, cardiac arrhythmias, tachycardia, severe heart disease, ulcerative colitis, paralytic ileus, chronic lung disease, autonomic neuropathy, prostatic hypertrophy, oesophageal reflux or hiatus hernia
- contraindicated in those with hypersensitivity to other anticholinergic

agents, severe ulcerative colitis, toxic megacolon, GI obstructive disease, intestinal atony (in elderly or debilitated patients), closed-angle glaucoma, myasthenia gravis, bladder neck obstruction, tachycardia (because of thyrotoxicosis or cardiac insufficiency), acute haemorrhage (in which cardiovascular status is unstable), prostatic enlargement or fever

General Patient education for anticholinergics

- the patient should be advised not to drive or operate machinery if blurred vision, confusion, dizziness or drowsiness occurs
- warn the patient to take care taking medication during high temperatures or physical exercise or if febrile because of the increased risk of heat stroke from decreased sweating
- caution the patient to keep medications out of reach of infants and young children because they are especially susceptible to toxicity, even from the absorption of eye preparations, so note irritability, dry mouth, tachycardia, mydriasis, fever or rash
- instruct the patient to seek medical advice immediately if any of the following occur:
  - painful red eye with associated loss of vision (may be signs of undiagnosed glaucoma)
  - diarrhoea (which may be the first sign of intestinal obstruction, especially in those with an ileostomy or colostomy)

ATROPINE
Trade names
Atropine Juno Solution, Bridgewest Atropine Injection BP, Atropt 1%, Minims Atropine Eye Drops, Eikance

Available forms
Ampoules: 600 microgram/mL, 1.2 mg/mL; Eye drops: 10 mg/mL (1%)

Action
- more accurately described as antimuscarinic
- well absorbed IM, peak 30 minutes, duration 4–6 hours with longer ocular effects
- salivation inhibited within 30 minutes, peak 1–2 hours, duration 4 hours
- see also General Actions of anticholinergic agents (p. 985)

Use
- premedication before induction of general anaesthesia to reduce salivary and bronchial secretions
- given with anticholinesterase, which reverses the effects of non-depolarising muscle relaxants
- acute myocardial infarction and sinus bradycardia (with associated hypotension and increased ventricular irritability)
- to prevent cholinergic cardiac effects such as bradycardia, hypotension and arrhythmias
- treatment of poisoning by organophosphate insecticides (with anticholinesterase reactivator, e.g. pralidoxime)
- mydriatic and cycloplegic drops (see Eye, ear, nose and throat agents, p. 1128)

Dose
- (Premedication) 0.3–0.6 mg SC or IM, usually with opioid, 30–60 minutes before anaesthesia **OR**
- (Premedication) 0.3–0.6 mg IV immediately before induction of anaesthesia **OR**
- (Reversal of effects of non-depolarising muscle relaxants) 0.6–1.2 mg slowly IV for each 0.5–2.5 mg neostigmine **OR**
- (Cardiopulmonary resuscitation) 0.4–1 mg IV, repeated at 5-minute intervals until the desired heart rate is achieved (total dose maximum 2 mg) **OR**
- (Organophosphate poisoning) initially 1–2 mg IV, then 2 mg IM or IV every 5–60 minutes until symptoms have subsided (and repeated if they

reappear) (total dose of 50 mg in first 24 hours) with a cholinesterase reactivator **OR**
- (Severe organophosphate poisoning) initially 2—6 mg IV, then 2—6 mg IM or IV every 5—60 minutes if necessary (total dose of 50 mg in first 24 hours) with a cholinesterase reactivator

Adverse effects
- see General Adverse effects of anticholinergics (p. 985)

Interactions
- antagonises actions of bethanechol, carbachol, anticholinesterase agents (e.g. neostigmine) and cholinomimetic agents (e.g. pilocarpine)
- may interfere with anti-Alzheimer's agents (e.g. donepezil, rivastigmine)
- see also General Interactions of anticholinergics (p. 985)

Nursing considerations/Cautions
- (Organophosphate poisoning) doses are repeated until signs and symptoms of poisoning disappear and repeated if symptoms reappear
- administer alone
- (Organophosphate poisoning) should be withdrawn slowly when treating severe cases to avoid the recurrence of symptoms such as pulmonary oedema
- incompatible with adrenaline (epinephrine), ampicillin, chloramphenicol, heparin, metaraminol, nitrofurantoin, sodium bicarbonate, sulfadiazine, thiopentone, vitamin B complex with ascorbic acid, and warfarin (may cause precipitation)
- see also General Nursing considerations/Cautions for anticholinergics (p. 985)

Patient education
- see General Patient education for anticholinergics (p. 986)

Use with caution in pregnancy; crosses the placenta and may cause fetal tachycardia.

Not recommended; atropine is excreted in breastmilk and may cause antimuscarinic effects in the infant.

Start at lower doses; elderly patients may experience heightened sensitivity, including confusion and mental disorientation.

Available in combination with
- atropine 19.4 micrograms + hyoscyamine 103.7 micrograms + scopolamine hydrobromide 6.5 micrograms tablet (Donnatab)
- diphenoxylate 2.5 mg + atropine 25 mcg tablet (Lomotil, Lofenoxal)

GLYCOPYRRONIUM (GLYCOPYRROLATE) BROMIDE

Trade names
Glycopyrrolate Accord, Robinul

Available form
Vial: 0.2 mg/mL

Action
- does not cross the blood—brain barrier; therefore there are far fewer CNS-related side-effects than for atropine sulfate monohydrate or hyoscine hydrobromide
- onset of action within 1 minute (IV), action peaks 30—45 minutes (IM), duration of vagal effects 2—3 hours
- see also General Actions of anticholinergic agents (p. 985)

Use
- preoperative or intraoperative use to prevent bradycardia
- preoperative to reduce secretions
- reversal of neuromuscular block

Dose
- (Preoperatively) 0.2–0.4 mg IV or IM before induction of anaesthesia **OR**
- (Intraoperatively) 0.2–0.4 mg IV as a single dose (may be repeated) **OR**
- (Reversal of neuromuscular block) 0.2 mg IV per 1 mg neostigmine or equivalent dose of pyridostigmine

Adverse effects
- see General Adverse effects of anticholinergics (p. 985)

Interactions
- see General Interactions of anticholinergics (p. 985)

Nursing considerations/Cautions
- any tachycardia should be investigated before surgery
- (Neuromuscular blockade) may be administered in the same syringe as anticholinesterase
- stability may be compromised if mixed with dexamethasone, sodium phosphate or a buffered lactated Ringer's solution, as this alters pH
- incompatible with thiopentone, chloramphenicol, diazepam, dimenhydrinate or sodium bicarbonate
- caution if used in those with latex sensitivity (closure system contains dry natural rubber)
- see also General Nursing considerations/Cautions for anticholinergics (p. 985)

Patient education
- see General Patient education for anticholinergics (p. 986)

Safety has not been established; it crosses the placental barrier. Use only if the expected benefit outweighs the potential risk.

Not recommended, as anticholinergic agents may suppress lactation, and it is unknown whether glycopyrronium is excreted in breastmilk.

Reduced renal function: a prolonged effect may occur owing to renal excretion. Dosage adjustment may be required.

Available in combination with
- glycopyrronium 0.5 mg + neostigmine 2.5 mg per mL (Glyconeo, Novistig)

HYOSCINE BUTYLBROMIDE
Trade names
APOHealth Stomach Ease Forte, Buscopan, Busocopan Forte, Gastro-Soothe, Gastro-Soothe Forte, Hyoscine Butylbromide-AFT, Hyoscine Butylbromide SXP, Hyoscine Butylbromide Medsurg, Pharmacy Action Stomach Ease, Releva, Releva Forte, Trust Stomach Ease

HYOSCINE HYDROBROMIDE
Trade names
Kwells, Travacalm HO

Available forms
Ampoule: 20 mg/mL;
Tablets: 150 microgram, 300 microgram, 10 mg, 20 mg

Action
- belladonna alkaloid that has more potent effects than atropine on the iris, ciliary body and some secretory glands, but less potent effects on heart, intestine and bronchial muscle
- produces CNS depression at therapeutic doses, with CNS stimulation at higher doses or in the presence of pain
- does not increase respiratory rate or blood pressure
- (IM) onset of action 30 minutes, duration 4 hours
- known as scopolamine in USA
- see also General Actions of anticholinergics (p. 985)

Use
- premedication (for sedation, amnesia and decreased secretions)
- prevention and treatment of motion sickness

CHOLINERGIC AND ANTICHOLINERGIC AGENTS

- spasm of GI tract, biliary spasm, renal spasm, diagnostic aid in radiology

Dose
- (Premedication) 0.3—0.6 mg SC, IV or IM 30—60 minutes before induction of anaesthesia **OR**
- (Travel sickness) up to 1 mg IM, SC or IV **OR**
- (Travel sickness) 300—600 micrograms orally taken 30—60 minutes before travelling and repeated 4—6-hourly if needed (daily maximum 1.2 mg) (300 microgram tablet) **OR**
- (Antispasmodic) 20 mg orally 4 times daily **OR**
- (Antispasmodic) 20—40 mg IM or slow IV injection (maximum daily dose 100 mg)

Adverse effects
- (Parenteral) anaphylaxis, including shock
- see also General Adverse effects of anticholinergics (p. 985)

Interactions
- may have additive antivagal effects on AV node conduction if given with procainamide
- see also General Interactions of anticholinergics (p. 985)

Nursing considerations/Cautions
- (Buscopan) should not be taken for a prolonged length of time without investigating cause of abdominal pain
- (Buscopan) tablets contain sucrose, which is not recommended in those with rare hereditary fructose intolerance
- (Buscopan Forte) tablets contain lactose, which is not recommended in those with rare hereditary galactose intolerance, Lapp lactase intolerance or glucose—galactose malabsorption
- (Parenteral) may be given IV, IM or SC
- (Parenteral) if given IV, should be diluted with water for injections and administered slowly
- (Parenteral) patient should be closely monitored for any signs of shock or anaphylaxis and emergency equipment readily available
- (Parenteral) incompatible with alkalis
- contraindicated IM in those concurrently taking anticoagulant therapy because of the risk of intramuscular haematoma
- contraindicated in those with porphyria
- see also General Nursing considerations/Cautions for anticholinergics (p. 985)

Patient education
- the patient should be advised to seek medical advice immediately if any of the following occur:
  - abdominal pain or cramps persists or worsens
  - fever, nausea, vomiting, change in bowel movements, blood in stools or fainting
- (Antispasmodic) advise the patient not to take tablets for more than 2—3 days. If symptoms persist, the patient should seek medical advice
- (Motion sickness) tablets may be chewed, sucked or swallowed whole
- see also General Patient education for anticholinergics (p. 986)

 Tablet can be crushed and mixed with water or a spoonful of yoghurt or apple puree.

 If given before onset of labour, it may result in CNS depression in the newborn and may add to risk of newborn haemorrhage due to decreased vitamin K-dependent clotting factors.

 Not recommended during breastfeeding unless benefits outweigh potential risks.

Available in combination with
- Hyoscyamine sulfate dihydrate 103.7 microgram + atropine 19.4 microgram + hyoscine hydrobromide 6.5 microgram tablet (Donnatab)
- Dimenhydrinate 50 mg + hyoscine hydrobromide 0.2 mg + caffeine 20 mg tablet (Travacalm Original)

PROPANTHELINE

Trade name
Pro-Banthine

Available form
Tablets: 15 mg

Action
- does not cross the blood—brain barrier; therefore does not have central effects
- half-life 9 hours
- see also General Actions of anticholinergic agents (p. 985)

Use
- gastric and duodenal ulcers (adjunctive therapy)
- neurogenic bladder, urinary incontinence, hyperhidrosis

Dose
- (Gastric/duodenal ulcer) 15 mg orally 3 times daily 30 minutes before meals and 30 mg at night (maximum daily dose 120 mg) **OR**
- (Other indications) 15—30 mg orally 4 times daily

Adverse effects
- see General Adverse effects of anticholinergics (p. 985)

Interactions
- may increase severity of potassium chloride-induced GI lesions if given with potassium chloride (especially wax matrix preparations)
- absorption may be decreased if given with antacids or absorbent antidiarrhoeals
- may decrease absorption of levodopa
- intestinal motility may be further reduced if given with pyridostigmine
- may increase serum levels of digoxin, increasing the risk of toxicity
- see also General Interactions of anticholinergics (p. 985)

Nursing considerations/Cautions
- see General Nursing considerations/Cautions for anticholinergics (p. 985)

Patient education
- patient should be advised to take 2—3 hours apart from antacids or antidiarrhoeals
- see also General Patient education for anticholinergics (p. 986)

 Tablet can be crushed and mixed with water, or a spoonful of yoghurt or apple puree (tablet has very bitter taste).

 Limited data suggest a possible association with minor malformations. Should be used only if potential benefits outweigh risks.

 Caution: propantheline is incompletely absorbed from the gastrointestinal tract and has poor lipid solubility; minimal secretion in breastmilk. Suppression of lactation may occur. Use only if the potential benefits justify any risk.

 Reduced renal function: dose adjustment may be necessary to avoid accumulation and toxicity.

Reduced hepatic function: caution is advised in patients with hepatic disease owing to reduced drug metabolism, potentially leading to enhanced effects or toxicity. Dose adjustments should be considered.

 Elderly patients may be more susceptible to adverse effects, including urinary retention and risk of glaucoma exacerbation. Monitor closely and advise micturition around the time of dosing to reduce urinary retention.

CORTICOSTEROIDS

The adrenal cortex produces three major groups of steroid hormones, collectively known as corticosteroids (or adrenocorticosteroids):

- Mineralocorticoids (e.g. aldosterone) primarily regulate electrolyte and fluid balance, promoting sodium and water retention while enhancing the excretion of potassium and hydrogen ions. These actions help maintain blood volume and blood pressure.
- Glucocorticoids (e.g. cortisol) influence metabolism by increasing blood glucose levels, breaking down proteins and mobilising fats. They also have significant immunosuppressive and anti-inflammatory effects.
- Androgens (e.g. dehydroepiandrosterone or DHEA) serve as precursors for sex hormones and play a role in regulating reproductive functions and the development of secondary sexual characteristics (Knights et al 2023).

Corticosteroids are synthesised from cholesterol on demand rather than stored for later use. This synthesis and release are regulated by a negative feedback mechanism known as the hypothalamic–pituitary–adrenal (HPA) axis. When the body is stressed, injured or infected, the hypothalamus releases corticotrophin-releasing hormone (CRH, previously known as corticotrophin-releasing factor (CRF)), which stimulates the anterior pituitary gland to secrete adrenocorticotrophic hormone (ACTH). ACTH travels through the bloodstream to the adrenal glands, signalling them to produce and release cortisol. Elevated cortisol levels then exert a negative feedback effect by inhibiting further release of CRH and ACTH, thus 'turning off' the stress response. This regulatory process helps maintain balance but can lead to HPA axis suppression when external corticosteroids are administered over time (Knights et al 2023).

General Actions of corticosteroids

- increase gluconeogenesis and decrease peripheral glucose utilisation, maintaining blood glucose levels and glycogen content in muscle and liver
- increase protein breakdown from muscle and extrahepatic tissue, increasing plasma amino acid levels
- inhibit protein synthesis, delaying wound healing
- promote mobilisation of fatty acid from adipose tissue to plasma;

however, they also increase fat deposition in face, shoulders and abdomen
- decrease calcium absorption from the gut while increasing urinary calcium excretion, inducing increased osteoclastic activity in order to increase blood calcium levels (leading to osteoporosis with prolonged therapy)
- suppress the inflammatory response, including inhibiting inflammatory mediators such as prostaglandins, thromboxanes, prostacyclin and leukotrienes
- cause atrophy of thymus gland, as well as blocking the synthesis and release of cytokines and other immune mediators, and affecting T- and B-lymphocytes, macrocytes and monocytes, resulting in suppression of immune and allergic responses
- inhibit extraneuronal uptake of noradrenaline (norepinephrine) and other catecholamines, potentiating vasoconstriction
- affect mood and behaviour and possibly neuronal/brain excitability, leading to euphoria, depression, insomnia, anxiety and increased motor activity
- (High levels) suppress the HPA axis, decreasing glucocorticoid secretion and long-term adrenal cortex atrophy
- glucocorticoids are well absorbed after oral, topical or local administration

General Uses of corticosteroids
- replacement therapy for primary or secondary adrenocortical insufficiency
- suppress undesirable inflammatory or immune responses in conditions such as:
  - cerebral oedema
  - neonatal respiratory distress syndrome (antenatal prophylaxis)
  - chronic inflammatory conditions of skin, gut, joints, liver
  - allergic conditions (e.g. allergic rhinitis), anaphylaxis, urticaria, drug reaction
  - rheumatic disorders, collagen and dermatological diseases
  - gastrointestinal (e.g. ulcerative colitis, Crohn's disease) and respiratory diseases (e.g. asthma)
  - haematological and neoplastic diseases
  - autoimmune disorders (e.g. systemic lupus erythematosus (SLE), rheumatoid arthritis)
  - prevention of organ or tissue transplantation
  - ophthalmic conditions (e.g. blepharitis and blepharoconjunctivitis (non-infected, allergic conjunctivitis, inflammatory ocular conditions))

General Adverse effects of corticosteroids
- sodium and fluid retention, potassium and calcium depletion, hypokalaemia, negative nitrogen balance
- hypertension, congestive cardiac failure (in susceptible patients), arrhythmias (associated with hypokalaemia)
- muscle wasting, weakness, steroid myopathy, osteoporosis, bone pain, pathological fractures of long bones, vertebral compression fractures, tendon rupture, avascular necrosis
- abdominal distension, indigestion, ulcerative oesophagitis, gastric irritation and ulceration, pancreatitis, diarrhoea, constipation
- headache, dizziness, depression, psychosis, mood swings, personality

changes, euphoria, nervousness, anxiety, insomnia, restlessness, aggravation of pre-existing psychiatric conditions
- delayed wound healing, easy bruising, red/purple striae on thighs/buttocks/shoulders; hirsutism; acne-type eruption on face, chest and back; facial erythema; skin thinning; petechiae; ecchymosis; purpura; increased sweating
- raised intracranial pressure, vertigo, seizures
- menstrual irregularities
- altered number, mobility and motility of sperm
- decreased carbohydrate tolerance, decreased insulin sensitivity, hyperglycaemia, glycosuria, activation of latent diabetes mellitus, hypertriglyceridaemia
- cataract, glaucoma, raised intraocular pressure, increased risk of eye infection, blurred vision
- increased frequency and severity of infection, may mask signs of infection (fever, inflammation)
- development of latent infections, including tuberculosis
- (Cushingoid state) increased appetite, weight gain, obesity, fat redistribution (e.g. moon face, buffalo hump), osteoporosis, hyperglycaemia, negative nitrogen balance, muscle wasting, poor wound healing
- growth restriction in children on prolonged therapy
- increased WBC count
- acute adrenal insufficiency may be precipitated by sudden withdrawal or reduction in dosage or an increase in corticosteroid requirements associated with stress caused by injury, surgery or infection
- (Withdrawal effects) muscle weakness, hypotension, hypoglycaemia, headache, nausea, vomiting, restlessness, muscle and joint pain
- steroid resistance (decreased responsiveness to therapy)
- (IM) pain, sterile abscess formation, hypopigmentation, hyperpigmentation
- (Severe, life threatening) suppression of the HPA axis
- (Rare) anaphylactoid or anaphylactic reaction, pseudotumour cerebri/benign intracranial hypertension, blindness (associated with intradermal administration around face and head)

General Interactions of corticosteroids

- clearance may be increased by rifampicin, phenytoin, carbamazepine, ephedrine, phenobarbital (phenobarbitone) or other barbiturates, decreasing serum levels
- clearance may be decreased by aprepitant, ciclosporin, clarithromycin, diltiazem, erythromycin, isoniazid, itraconazole, ritonavir or grapefruit juice, increasing serum levels and the risk of adverse effects
- response to anticoagulants (heparin and oral) may be altered when given with corticosteroids, therefore prothrombin time should be closely monitored, especially when starting or stopping therapy
- excessive potassium loss and hypokalaemia may occur if used with potassium-depleting diuretics
- may decrease the effects of potassium-sparing agents including diuretics, amphotericin B (amphotericin), xanthines and beta2 agonists
- may enhance potassium depletion caused by amphotericin B (amphotericin), leading to severe hypokalaemia

- may increase the risk of gastric ulceration and bleeding if given with alcohol, aspirin or non-steroidal anti-inflammatory drugs (NSAIDs)
- may decrease plasma levels of salicylates by increasing clearance
- may increase efficacy and risk of toxicity if given with sympathomimetic agents
- CNS adverse effects may be potentiated by CNS active agents such as antianxiety agents and antipsychotics
- hyperglycaemic effect of corticosteroids may counteract hypoglycaemic agents, requiring dose adjustments
- excessive effects may occur if given with oestrogen or oestrogen-containing contraceptives
- increased risk of hypoprothrombinaemia if given with aspirin
- increased risk of arrhythmia or digoxin toxicity associated with hypokalaemia if given with digoxin
- may decrease the effects of somatotrophin
- may antagonise the effects of anticholinesterase (precipitating myasthenic crisis in those with myasthenia gravis)
- increased risk of acute myopathy if high-dose corticosteroids are given with anticholinergics, including neuromuscular blocking agents
- increased serum levels may occur if given with HIV protease inhibitors
- may decrease serum levels of HIV protease inhibitors by increasing metabolism
- may decrease or enhance actions of neuromuscular blocking agents
- may decrease serum levels of isoniazid by increasing metabolism
- may decrease metabolism of ciclosporin, increasing serum levels and the risk of toxicity including convulsions
- metabolism may be decreased by ciclosporin, increasing serum levels of corticosteroid
- not recommended with live attenuated virus vaccination (unless replacement therapy is being used)
- decreased absorption may occur if given with antacids, colestyramine or colestipol and should be separated by 2 hours
- caution if used in those treated with antithyroid agents
- may suppress reaction to skin tests
- may cause false negative reactions using a nitroblue tetrazolium test for systemic bacterial infections
- may decrease I-131 uptake and protein-bound iodine concentration, making it difficult to monitor response to therapy for thyroiditis

General Nursing considerations/Cautions for corticosteroids

- the patient should be monitored for any changes in mood, psychosis or emotional lability
- a salt-restricted diet (< 1 g/day) and potassium supplements may be necessary
- serum electrolytes (especially potassium) should be monitored regularly (especially in those also taking potassium-depleting agents such as thiazide diuretics or with prolonged laxative use)
- check urine for glycosuria; blood glucose monitoring may also be necessary (especially for those with pre-existing diabetes mellitus)
- fluid balance chart (if hospitalised) and daily weight should be monitored to detect fluid retention
- monitor BP and haematological and adrenal functions regularly during therapy

CORTICOSTEROIDS

- IM route is recommended for allergic, dermatological, rheumatic or other conditions such as bursitis that respond to systemic corticosteroids; intralesional injections are recommended for dermatological conditions; intra-/periarticular injections are recommended for treatment of osteoarthritis and rheumatoid arthritis; injection into soft tissue is recommended for bursitis, fibrositis and myositis
- alternate-day oral therapy may be suitable for some patients receiving long-term therapy to minimise adverse effects such as protein catabolism and adrenal suppression and growth suppression in children
- during trauma, surgery or severe illness, the patient will require extra doses of corticosteroids to prevent drug-induced adrenal insufficiency
- select the correct corticosteroid preparation and strength
- rapid IV administration should be avoided as it may cause cardiovascular collapse
- IM preparation given deep into a large muscle mass (e.g. buttock) rather than the deltoid muscle, to avoid subcutaneous atrophy
- a small-bore needle (23 or 25 gauge) should be used for intralesional injections
- care should be taken when injecting into lesions not to produce blanching because this can cause sloughing
- (Osteoarthritis) joint destruction may occur with repeated injections
- may cause tendon rupture if injected directly into a tendon rather than tendon sheath
- suitable intra-articular joints for corticosteroid injections are knee, ankle, wrist, hip, shoulder, elbow and phalangeal joints
- intra-articular corticosteroids are often given with local anaesthetics (e.g. lidocaine (lignocaine), procaine)
- corticosteroids should not be injected into unstable joints, infected or previously infected areas or intravertebral spaces. Joints should be inspected for any signs of intra-articular infection before injection
- infants' and children's growth requires close monitoring during long-term corticosteroid therapy. They should also be closely observed and monitored for any obesity, osteoporosis and/or adrenal suppression
- live attenuated vaccines should not be administered while the patient is undergoing corticosteroid therapy
- long-term follow-up and monitoring is recommended for up to 12 months after discontinuing corticosteroid therapy
- ensure that all relevant medical and nursing personnel are aware that the patient is undergoing corticosteroid therapy, especially if undergoing surgery, as wound healing may be delayed depending on dose, route and duration of therapy (e.g. inhaled corticosteroids have less impact on healing than chronic systemic therapy)
- dose adjustment may be required with disease remission or exacerbation and patient response to emotional or physical stress (e.g. surgery, serious infection, injury)
- (Long-term therapy) transfer from parenteral to oral administration should be considered after weighing risks versus benefits carefully
- not recommended via epidural administration
- soft tissue, intralesional, intra-articular and topical corticosteroids (applied to large areas, when skin is

broken or under occlusive dressings) may produce systemic effects
- caution if used in those with ocular herpes simplex infection because of the increased risk of corneal perforation
- caution if used in postmenopausal women or others at risk of osteoporosis
- caution if used in those with thyroid disease because metabolic clearance of corticosteroid is increased in hypothyroidism and decreased in hyperthyroidism, requiring a dose adjustment of corticosteroid
- caution if used in those with epilepsy, uraemia or diminished cardiac reserve or congestive cardiac failure
- caution if used in those with active or latent tuberculosis (TB), as TB may be reactivated
- caution if used in those with impaired liver function or cirrhosis, the elderly, and those with non-specific ulcerative colitis with a possibility of perforation, abscess or infection
- great caution if used in those with *Strongyloides* (threadworm) infestation, as corticosteroid-induced immunosuppression can lead to hyperinfection and widespread larval migration, resulting in severe enterocolitis and potentially fatal Gram-negative septicaemia
- caution if used in those with renal insufficiency
- not recommended in the management of traumatic brain injury
- corticosteroid therapy is contraindicated (unless a life-threatening situation exists) in those with osteoporosis, marked emotional instability, psychosis/psychoneurosis or peptic ulceration, systemic fungal infections, active or quiescent tuberculosis, acute or chronic infection (including HIV infection or AIDS, measles, chicken pox), ocular herpes simplex, glaucoma (or a family history of), diverticulitis, recent intestinal anastomosis, thromboembolic tendency, diabetes mellitus (or a family history of), myasthenia gravis, pheochromocytoma or hypertension, or in management of hyaline membrane disease after birth
- contraindicated in those with hypersensitivity to other corticosteroid agents
- should be used during pregnancy only after cautious consideration of benefit versus potential risks. Adrenocortical hormones may cause transient postnatal hypoadrenalism in infants and have caused malformations in animal studies
- women should be monitored for adrenal insufficiency during and after labour if treated with corticosteroids during pregnancy

Topical
- topical corticosteroids provide a way of delivering large doses locally without serious systemic effects
- corticosteroid creams and ointments are applied thinly and not rubbed in, preferably after showering or bathing
- lotions are recommended for use on hairy areas such as the scalp
- occlusive dressings are generally not recommended with corticosteroid cream (and especially not if a primary skin infection is present) unless ordered by a doctor, as this increases the risk of absorption and systemic effects. If an occlusive dressing is used, miliaria, folliculitis or pyodermas may occur
- generally not recommended for longer than 7 days

CORTICOSTEROIDS

- should be applied with an applicator, gauze or gloved hand to protect against cutaneous absorption
- should be used alone or in combination with one or more other preparations, such as soothing, cleansing or antibacterial agents or cell growth stimulants, allowing sufficient time between application of individual preparations
- lower strength/potency preparations should be used on the face, with more potent preparations applied to palms, soles and any lichenified areas
- ointments are generally more potent than creams because of their better absorption
- caution if applied to eyelids, as skin is very thin in this area
- caution if applying creams, lotions and ointments to children, as there is an increased risk of systemic absorption and effects because of their higher skin permeability properties and larger surface area to body mass ratio
- not recommended in those with impaired circulation, as skin ulceration may occur
- not recommended on skin that is inflamed, broken or ulcerated (or near chronic ulcerated areas), as systemic absorption may occur
- caution if used in those with psoriasis, as exacerbation of psoriasis or pustular psoriasis may occur during or on withdrawal of therapy
- caution if used in those receiving immunosuppressant therapy or who have impaired T-cell function
- contraindicated in those with hypersensitivity to corticosteroids, perioral dermatitis, skin reaction post-vaccination, viral skin infections (e.g. shingles, chicken pox), acne vulgaris, rosacea, TB or syphilis of the skin or untreated skin infection

Ophthalmic
- corticosteroid eye drops should not be used without a doctor's prescription, as healing is impaired and herpes simplex virus is potentiated, resulting in a dendritic ulcer; cataract may start to form in the lens and intraocular pressure may be increased in some patients
- ocular corticosteroids should not be prescribed for > 2 weeks without supervision from an ophthalmologist, unless facilities for monitoring corneal epithelium and intraocular pressure are readily available
- ocular infections can be masked, enhanced or activated by corticosteroids
- prolonged use may suppress the ocular tissue immune response, leading to the possibility of secondary ocular infection (including fungal)
- take care with any conditions that may cause thinning of the cornea, because perforation may occur
- heavy or prolonged use (> 1 year) of corticosteroids may lead to posterior subcapsular opacities
- may cause increased intraocular pressure in susceptible individuals and pressure should be measured 2–3 weeks after starting corticosteroid therapy, and then as determined by other factors such as the presence of diabetes mellitus
- fungal infections of the cornea may occur with long-term therapy
- pre-existing cataracts and glaucoma may be exacerbated
- caution if used in those with diabetes mellitus, because the therapy may predispose patients to increased intraocular pressure and/or cataract formation

- contraindicated in those with acute superficial herpes simplex keratitis, mycobacterial or viral diseases of the cornea or conjunctiva, TB of the eye, fungal diseases of ocular structures or acute purulent untreated infections, or those with known hypersensitivity to corticosteroid preparations

Withdrawal

- corticosteroid withdrawal should always be gradual to prevent adrenal insufficiency syndrome. The rate of withdrawal is dependent on several factors, including the disease being treated, dose, duration of therapy and the patient's response to therapy (e.g. less likely to occur if dose is lower than 7.5 mg prednisolone (or equivalent) or if therapy is less than 21 days)
- symptoms of adrenal insufficiency precipitated by a sudden withdrawal and/or decrease in dose include headache, malaise, mental changes, restlessness, fever, muscle weakness, muscle and joint pain, dyspnoea, anorexia, nausea, vomiting, hypoglycaemia, hypotension and dehydration (muscle weakness and joint pains may last for 3–6 months after stopping corticosteroids)
- gradual withdrawal allows normal adrenal function to deal with daily needs, but a longer time is required before it can deal with infection, surgery or trauma

General Patient education for corticosteroids

- the patient should be advised to:
    - wear a MedicAlert bracelet or pendant that contains information such as dose and emergency instructions
    - avoid alcohol, NSAIDs (except paracetamol) and aspirin during therapy
    - avoid grapefruit juice
    - reduce sodium intake to less than 1 g/day
    - have an adequate protein intake to counteract any weight loss or muscle wasting
    - have regular medical check-ups during therapy
    - not overuse joint(s) that have been injected
    - not suddenly stop therapy, as adverse effects will occur
    - report infection, inflammation, persistent back ache, chest pain or changes in body shape
    - avoid contact with chicken pox and measles (especially children) and seek medical advice promptly if exposure occurs, as follow-up will be required
    - take antacids or prescribed anti-ulcer agents between meals (but at least 2 hours apart from corticosteroid) to help prevent peptic ulcer development
- warn the patient that corticosteroid therapy may mask signs of infection (fever and inflammation)
- instruct the patient that long-term therapy is ceased gradually over several days, weeks or months to allow return of adequate adrenocortical function, but it may be 1 or 2 years before normal function returns. If the patient becomes stressed (e.g. trauma, illness) during the tapering process, the dose may need to be reintroduced or increased. Patient should also be warned that muscle weakness and joint stiffness may persist for 3–6 months after stopping therapy
- patients on a reduction regimen should be advised to immediately

report any vomiting, weakness or faintness
- the patient needs to be aware that monitoring for up to 12 months after stopping long-term or high-dose corticosteroid therapy is required
- relatives or other household members should also be aware of implications and precautions during corticosteroid therapy, including the need to monitor for any signs of mood changes or depression
- patients with diabetes mellitus should be instructed regarding the need to carefully monitor blood glucose levels during therapy

Topical (cream, ointment, lotion)
- instruct the patient to use topical preparation only as prescribed (amount and frequency) as there is no benefit to more frequent administration or excess amount and it may result in adverse effects
- warn the patient to avoid contact with eyes and wash well with copious amounts of water if contact occurs
- advise the patient that topical corticosteroids should not be used on infected, broken or inflamed areas
- the patient should be instructed to smooth preparation on skin (and not to rub in)
- the patient should be instructed to shake lotion well before application
- instruct the patient to wash hands well after using a topical agent
- advise the patient to allow corticosteroid preparation sufficient time to be absorbed before applying second skin preparation such as a moisturiser

Nasal spray instillation
- if using a nasal spray, instruct the patient in correct use (see Antiasthma agents, bronchodilators and respiratory agents, p. 114)

Eye drop instillation
- instruct the patient in the correct technique for instilling eye drops (see Eye, ear, nose and throat agents, p. 1128)
- advise the patient to seek medical advice immediately if any ocular trauma, infection or surgery occurs, or if they develop conjunctivitis or lid reaction while using the corticosteroid eye preparation

Topical preparations are recommended during pregnancy only in minimal quantities for minimal duration.

Systemic preparations should be avoided during pregnancy unless benefits outweigh risks.

Not recommended in pregnant women with pre-eclampsia, eclampsia or signs of placental damage when used for prophylaxis of hyaline membrane disease in premature infants.

Not recommended during breastfeeding because growth retardation or hypoadrenalism may occur in the infant.

BETAMETHASONE ACETATE, BETAMETHASONE SODIUM PHOSPHATE

Trade name
Celestone Chronodose

Available form
Ampoule: betamethasone acetate 3 mg/mL + betamethasone sodium phosphate 3.9 mg/mL (total betamethasone 5.7 mg/mL)

BETAMETHASONE DIPROPIONATE
Trade names
Diprosone, Diprosone OV, Eleuphrat

BETAMETHASONE VALERATE
Trade names
Antroquoril, Betnovate preparations, Celestone M, Cortival

Available forms
Ampoules: 5.7 mg/mL;
Cream: 0.2 mg/g, 0.5 mg/g, 1 mg/g;
Ointment: 0.2 mg/g, 0.5 mg/g, 1 mg/g;
Lotion: 0.5 mg/mL

Action
- glucocorticoid with much higher potency than hydrocortisone
- combines rapid and depot forms to provide both rapid and steady effect (Celestone Chronodose)
- OV refers to optimised vehicle, which increases penetration and enhances local effects (Diprosone OV)
- see also General Actions of corticosteroids (p. 991)

Use
- see General Uses of corticosteroids (p. 992)

Dose
Parenteral (1 mL = 5.7 mg beclomethasone)
- (Allergic states, collagen diseases) initially 1—2 mL IM, followed by 1 mL weekly **OR**
- (Prevention of respiratory distress syndrome in premature infants) 2 mL IM 24 hours before expected delivery, followed by 2 mL 24 hours later if delivery has not occurred **OR**
- (Bursitis, fibrositis, myositis) initially 1 mL, repeated at 1—2-week intervals injected into bursae, tendon sheath **OR**
- 0.25—2 mL into joint capsules (amount dependent on size of the joint) (intra-articular) **OR**
- (Joint capsule ganglions) 0.5 mL injected directly into ganglion cysts **OR**
- (Intralesional treatment) 0.2 mL/cm^2 intradermally (not exceeding 1 mL/week total)

Topical
- a small amount of cream/ointment applied to affected area 1—3 times daily, may be covered by a dry dressing if necessary **OR**
- (Psoriasis) (pulse dose regimen) up to 3.5 g applied to lesions previously treated for 3 consecutive applications 12 hours apart (e.g. morning, evening, morning) each week (Diprosone OV) **OR**
- (Seborrhoea, scalp psoriasis) part hair with comb and apply lotion directly to scalp twice daily for 4 weeks

Adverse effects
- (Intra-articular) post-injection flare, pain, irritation/discomfort at injection site, sterile abscess formation, hypopigmentation, hyperpigmentation, degeneration of joint with loss of sensation, joint instability (repeated injections), Charcot-type arthropathy (see Glossary)
- (Intradermal/intralesional) local discomfort, sterile abscess formation, hypopigmentation, hyperpigmentation, subcutaneous/cutaneous atrophy
- (Topical) burning, itching, irritation, dryness, erythema
- (Topical) (prolonged/excessive therapy) telangiectasis, skin atrophy, striae
- (Topical) (rare) folliculitis, pustules, hypertrichosis, hypopigmentation, contact or perioral dermatitis, skin maceration, secondary infection, miliaria, acneiform eruptions, visual disturbances
- see also General Adverse effects of corticosteroids (p. 992)

CORTICOSTEROIDS

Interactions
- see General Interactions of corticosteroids (p. 993)

Nursing considerations/Cautions/Withdrawal
- not given IV or SC
- lotion is recommended for areas where hair may impede access to skin conditions
- (Pulse dosing regimen) recommended for patients who have shown at least 80% improvement in lesion/s. If relapse occurs, therapy should return to 1–2 times daily application
- (Celestone M) recommended for maintenance therapy
- (Celestone Chronodose) caution if given IM to those with idiopathic thrombocytopenic purpura
- see also General Nursing considerations/Cautions/Withdrawal for corticosteroids (p. 994)

Patient education
- (Celestone M preparations) instruct the patient that these may be used 2–3 times daily and some conditions (e.g. chronic lichen simplex, hypertrophic lichen planus, atopic dermatitis, chronic eczematous and lichenified hand eruptions, recalcitrant pustular eruptions of palms/soles) are more responsive if occlusive dressing (light gauze covered by transparent film dressing, edges sealed with adhesive tape) is used
- (Osteoarthritis, rheumatoid arthritis) advise the patient that joint pain, soreness and/or stiffness is usually relieved 2–4 hours after injections and relief should last for 1–4 weeks
- see also General Patient education for corticosteroids (p. 995)

 Use with caution. May cross the placenta, potentially causing fetal harm (e.g. cleft palate, growth suppression). Monitor newborns for adrenal suppression.

 Passes into breastmilk and may affect infant growth or adrenal function. Weigh risks and benefits; monitor infants for hypoadrenalism.

 Parental: reduce the dose gradually to avoid adrenal insufficiency. Taper based on clinical response, and monitor during discontinuation.

 Elderly patients may have higher risks of side effects (e.g. osteoporosis, infections). Use the lowest effective dose and monitor carefully.

 Banned in sport for oral, rectal or systemic use. Permitted in sport for intra-articular, local injection and use via anal, respiratory, oromucosal, ocular, nasal, cutaneous/topical and auricular routes.

Available in combination with
- calcipotriol 0.005% + betamethasone dipropionate 0.05% ointment/foam spray (Calcipotriol/Betamethasone Sandoz 50/500, Daivobet 50/500, Enstilar Foam spray, Klarvanta Foam spray)

BUDESONIDE
Trade names
Budamax, Budenofalk, Budenofalk Foam Enema, Cortiment, Entocort, Jorveza, Pulmicort, Rhinocort, Rhinocort Hayfever & Allergy

Available forms
Nebulising solution (respules): 0.5 mg/2 mL, 1 mg/2 mL;
Turbuhaler: 100 microgram/inhalation, 200 microgram/inhalation, 400 microgram/inhalation;
Nasal spray: 32 microgram/dose, 64 microgram/dose;
Capsules: 3 mg;
Orally disintegrating tablets: 1 mg;
Enema: 2 mg;
Tablets (prolonged release): 9 mg

Action
- glucocorticoid related to hydroxyprednisolone, with fewer systemic

effects than beclometasone, although twice as potent

Uses
- (Asthma) symptom preventer and induction of remission in those with mild-to-moderate Crohn's disease (see Antiasthma agents, bronchodilators and respiratory agents, p. 124)

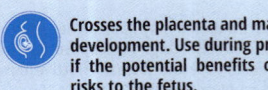

Crosses the placenta and may affect fetal development. Use during pregnancy only if the potential benefits outweigh the risks to the fetus.

Excreted in breastmilk. Exposure to the nursing infant is expected to be low, but use during breastfeeding should be based on the risk-benefit assessment.

If transferring from a higher systemic corticosteroid dose, reduce gradually to avoid symptoms of adrenal suppression or withdrawal. Monitor patients closely.

CLOBETASOL
Trade name
Clobex

Available form
Shampoo: 500 microgram/mL

Action
- see General Actions of corticosteroids (p. 991)

Use
- moderate-to-severe scalp psoriasis

Dose
- apply 7.5 mL to dry scalp, massage well into lesions and leave uncovered for 15 minutes. Rinse hair thoroughly, then wash with normal shampoo and dry as usual

Adverse effects
- skin burning sensation, acne, folliculitis
- (Uncommon) irritation, pruritus, urticaria, skin atrophy, telangiectasis, headache, visual disturbances
- (Prolonged or extensive use, use on broken skin) systemic adverse effects (see General Adverse effects for corticosteroids, p. 992)

Nursing considerations/Cautions/Withdrawal
- for use on scalp only
- recommended for 4 weeks maximum
- if no improvement is seen in 4 weeks, reassessment should be conducted
- not recommended for acne, rosacea or perioral dermatitis
- contraindicated in children < 2 years
- see also General Nursing considerations/Cautions/Withdrawal for corticosteroids (p. 994)

Patient education
- ensure the patient understands instructions for correct use (massage well into lesions on scalp, leave uncovered for 15 minutes and then rinse well, followed by normal washing with shampoo. Hair can be dried normally)
- advise the patient that shampoo should not be applied to other parts of the body
- instruct the patient that, when improvement is seen, frequency of administration can be decreased or changed to other products
- warn the patient to avoid contact with eyes and wash with copious amounts of water if contact occurs
- see also General Patient education for corticosteroids (p. 995)

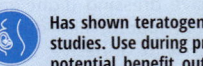

Has shown teratogenic effects in animal studies. Use during pregnancy only if the potential benefit outweighs the risk to the fetus.

Safe to use during breastfeeding, but ensure the breast area is free of corticosteroid before breastfeeding to avoid direct exposure to the infant.

Avoid prolonged use and limit treatment to 4 weeks. Monitor for signs of hypothalamic–pituitary–adrenal (HPA) axis suppression with long-term or excessive application. Gradual discontinuation may be required to avoid adrenal insufficiency.

CLOBETASONE

Trade names
Eumovate, Kloxema

Available form
Cream: 0.5 mg/g (0.05%)

Action
- see General Actions of corticosteroids (p. 991)

Use
- short-term management of mild eczema, dermatitis and other inflammatory skin conditions

Dose
- apply a thin layer to affected area twice daily for up to 7 days

Adverse effects
- (Topical) burning, itching, irritation, dryness, erythema
- (Topical) (prolonged/excessive therapy) telangiectasis, skin atrophy, striae
- (Topical) (rare) folliculitis, pustules, hypertrichosis, hypopigmentation, contact or perioral dermatitis, skin maceration, secondary infection, miliaria, acneiform eruptions, visual disturbances
- (Prolonged or extensive use, use on broken skin) systemic adverse effects (see General Adverse effects of corticosteroids, p. 992)

Interactions
- not recommended with other topical or systemic corticosteroids

Nursing considerations/Cautions/Withdrawal
- not recommended in those with rosacea, acne, pruritus, perioral dermatitis, untreated bacterial, viral or fungal infections or impaired circulation
- see also General Nursing considerations/Cautions/Withdrawal for corticosteroids (p. 994)

Patient education
- advise the patient to seek medical advice if the condition has not improved in 7 days
- instruct the patient that cream should not be applied to face, groin, genitals or between toes
- see also General Patient education for corticosteroids (p. 995)

 Topical corticosteroids can cause fetal harm in animal studies. Use during pregnancy only if the benefits outweigh the risks to the fetus.

 Safe to use; ensure the breast area is free of corticosteroid before breastfeeding to prevent infant ingestion.

 Prolonged use or application over large areas may lead to systemic absorption and Cushing's syndrome. Gradual reduction may be needed to prevent adrenal insufficiency, especially after long-term use.

CORTISONE ACETATE

Trade name
Cortate

Available forms
Tablets: 5 mg, 25 mg

Action
- mineralocorticoid and glucocorticoid activity that is converted to active form (hydrocortisone) in the liver, which has:
    - half-life of about 100 minutes
    - half-life prolonged in those with cirrhosis and shortened in those with thyrotoxicosis
- see also General Actions of corticosteroids (p. 991)

Use
- Addison's disease, allergic disorders, status asthmaticus, angioneurotic oedema, serum sickness, drug sensitisation, giant cell arteritis, periarteritis nodosa, disseminated lupus erythematosus

Dose
- initially 25 mg orally 6-hourly (until remission is achieved), then reduced by 10–20 mg every few days until optimal

maintenance dose is reached (dose is individualised)

Adverse effects/Interactions/Nursing considerations/Cautions/Withdrawal/Patient education

- larger doses may be required in those with acute and severe sensitivity or anaphylaxis
- see also General Adverse effects/Interactions/Nursing considerations/Cautions/Withdrawal/Patient education for corticosteroids (p. 992)

Tablets can be dispersed in water, or crushed and mixed with a spoonful of yoghurt or apple puree.

Can cause fetal harm in animals (e.g. cleft palate, growth retardation). Use during pregnancy only if the benefits to the mother outweigh risks to the fetus.

Excreted in breastmilk; use is not recommended while breastfeeding unless deemed necessary.

Abrupt withdrawal can lead to adrenal insufficiency. Gradual reduction of dosage is necessary to avoid withdrawal effects, particularly after long-term use.

Elderly patients are more susceptible to adverse reactions. Use with caution and adjust dosage if necessary.

Banned in sport.

DESONIDE
Trade name
Desowen

Available form
Lotion: 0.5 mg/g

Action
- see General Actions of corticosteroids (p. 991)

Use
- relief of inflammatory and pruritic signs of dermatoses

Dose
- apply a thin layer to affected area 2—3 times daily for a maximum of 8 weeks

Adverse effects
- (Topical) burning, itching, irritation, dryness, erythema
- (Topical) (prolonged/excessive therapy) telangiectasis, skin atrophy, striae
- (Topical) (rare) folliculitis, pustules, hypertrichosis, hypopigmentation, contact or perioral dermatitis, skin maceration, secondary infection, miliaria, acneiform eruptions, visual disturbances

Nursing considerations/Cautions/Withdrawal/Patient education

- occlusive dressing may be used for psoriasis or recalcitrant conditions management
- advise patient to shake lotion well before use
- see also General Nursing considerations/Cautions/Withdrawal/Patient education for corticosteroids (p. 994)

Topical corticosteroids may be teratogenic in animals. Use during pregnancy only if the potential benefit outweighs the risk to the fetus. Avoid prolonged use and extensive application.

Avoid applying to the breast area to prevent infant ingestion. It is not known if topical corticosteroids are excreted in breastmilk.

Children may absorb larger amounts of desonide through the skin, increasing the risk of systemic effects such as hypothalamic—pituitary—adrenal (HPA) axis suppression and growth retardation. Avoid prolonged use, and limit the amount to the minimum required for effective treatment.

CORTICOSTEROIDS

DEXAMETHASONE
Trade names
Dexmethsone, Maxidex (Eye Drops), Ozurdex

DEXAMETHASONE PHOSPHATE
Trade names
DBL Dexamethasone Sodium Phosphate Injection, Dexamethasone Juno, Dexamethasone Medsurge, Dexamethasone Viatris

Available forms
Tablets: 0.5 mg, 4 mg;
Ampoules: 4 mg/mL, 8 mg/2 mL;
Vial: 8 mg/2 mL;
Eye drops: 0.1%;
Intravitreal implant: 700 microgram

Action
- glucocorticoid that is 25—30 times more potent than hydrocortisone with little mineralocorticoid activity (few sodium and water-retaining properties)
- see also General Actions of corticosteroids (p. 991)

Use
- diabetic macular oedema (DME), oedema due to branch retinal vein occlusion (BRVO), central retinal vein occlusion (CRVO) or non-infectious uveitis of posterior eye segment (intravitreal implant)
- see also General Uses of corticosteroids (p. 992)

Dose
- initially 0.5—10 mg orally daily with food in 3 or 4 divided doses, then reducing 0.5—1 mg daily as maintenance **OR**
- (Cerebral oedema) initially 10 mg IV, then 4 mg IM 6-hourly until symptoms disappear (usually 12 to 24 hours), reducing dose after 2—4 days and stopping over 5—7 days **OR**
- (Acute life-threatening cerebral oedema) initially 50 mg IV, then 8 mg IV 2-hourly for 3 days, 4 mg IV 2-hourly for 1 day, 4 mg IV 4-hourly for the next 3 days, then reducing by 4 mg daily **OR**
- (Cerebral oedema associated with cerebral malignancy) initially 10 mg IV, then 2 mg IM or IV 2—3 times daily (as maintenance) **OR**
- (Severe shock associated with haemorrhage, trauma or surgery) 2—6 mg/kg IV stat, repeated in 2—6 hours if shock persists and usually no longer than 48—72 hours **OR**
- (Severe shock) initially 20 mg IV, followed by 3 mg/kg/day by IV infusion **OR**
- (Intrasynovial, soft tissue injections) 0.4—6 mg into joint or site (depending on size of joint), may be repeated in 3—5 days (bursae) or 2—3-weekly (joints) **OR**
- 700 microgram intravitreal implant, repeated at 5—7-month intervals if needed (DME), or at least 6-month intervals based on visual acuity and/or anatomical parameters (uveitis, retinal vein occlusion (RVO)) **OR**
- 1—2 drops instilled into the conjunctival sac(s) hourly (severe inflammation) or 4—6 times daily (mild inflammation)

Adverse effects
- (Intra-articular) post-injection flare, pain, irritation/discomfort at injection site, sterile abscess formation, hypopigmentation, hyperpigmentation, degeneration of joint with loss of sensation, joint instability (repeated injections), Charcot-type arthropathy (see Glossary)
- (Ophthalmic) transient stinging and burning, irritation, tearing, discharge, itching, eye oedema, eye pain, conjunctival and ocular hyperaemia
- (Ophthalmic, rare) increased intraocular pressure, optic nerve damage, glaucoma, secondary ocular infections, cataract formation, decreased visual acuity, visual disturbances, blurred vision
- (Ophthalmic, long-term therapy) corneal and scleral thinning, corneal perforation
- (Vitreous implant) vitreous floaters/detachment/opacities, anterior chamber

inflammation, ocular hypertension, increased intraocular pressure, cataract, lens opacities, conjunctival oedema, decreased visual acuity
- see also General Adverse effects of corticosteroids (p. 992)

Interactions

- (Ophthalmic) may increase intraocular pressure, decreasing efficiency of antiglaucoma agents
- (Ophthalmic) increased risk of intraocular hypertension if given with anticholinergic agents (in those predisposed to acute-angle closure)
- (Intravitreal implant) increased risk of vitreous haemorrhage if inserted into those taking anticoagulants or antiplatelet agents
- increased serum levels may occur if given with aprepitant. However, prolonged use of dexamethasone may induce aprepitant metabolism, resulting in lowered serum levels
- false negative results for dexamethasone suppression tests may occur if the patient is also treated with indometacin or high doses of benzodiazepines or cyproheptadine
- see also General Interactions of corticosteroids (p. 993)

Nursing considerations/Cautions/Withdrawal

- IM/IV route should be used only for life-threatening situations or acute illness and replaced with oral therapy as soon as possible
- for IV infusion, may be diluted with glucose 5% or sodium chloride 0.9% (as long as sodium restriction is not present)
- (Eye drops) if used for > 10 days, intraocular pressure should be monitored
- (Intravitreal implant) (uveitis, RVO) if vision improves and is maintained, retreatment is not required
- (Intravitreal implant) for DME, retreatment with > 7 implants is not recommended; for RVO, up to 2 implants are recommended; for uveitis, repeat administration is not recommended
- (Intravitreal implant) after insertion, patient monitoring is recommended, including checking optic nerve perfusion, tonometry (within 30 minutes of procedure) and biomicroscopy 2–7 days after injection
- (Intravitreal implant) administration to both eyes concurrently is not recommended
- (Eye drops) not recommended for Sjögren's keratoconjunctivitis
- (Intravitreal implant) caution if used in those who have had cataract surgery or iridectomy because of an increased risk of implant migration into the anterior chamber
- (8 mg/2 mL vial) contraindicated in those with sulfite hypersensitivity
- (Intravitreal implant) contraindicated in those with advanced glaucoma, aphakic eyes with rupture of posterior lens capsule, eyes with anterior intraocular lens, iris or translateral fixated intraocular lens and rupture of posterior lens capsule or active/suspected ocular or periocular infection
- see also General Nursing considerations/Cautions/Withdrawal for corticosteroids (p. 994)

Patient education

- (Intravitreal implant) the patient should be advised to seek medical advice if any of the following occur:
  - pain, redness, lid swelling
  - blurred vision, loss of visual acuity, discharge from the eye, photophobia
  - headache
  - inflammation in and around the eye
- (Intravitreal implant) the patient should be instructed not to drive or operate machinery until visual blurring has cleared after the procedure
- see also General Patient education for corticosteroids (including instillation of eye drops, p. 995)

CORTICOSTEROIDS

Tablets can be crushed and mixed with water or a spoonful of yoghurt or apple puree.

Animal studies have shown that corticosteroids can cause malformations such as cleft palate and skeletal malformations. The potential for adrenal suppression in the newborn should be considered when dexamethasone is administered long term during pregnancy. Only use if the benefit justifies the potential risk to the fetus. Close monitoring is required if used during pregnancy, particularly in cases of pre-eclampsia or fluid retention.

Avoid use, as excreted in breastmilk and could affect the infant, potentially suppressing growth or endogenous corticosteroid production.

Eye drops and intravitreal implants are permitted in sport.

Other preparations are banned in sport via rectal, parenteral or oral use.

Available in combination with:
- framycetin sulfate 0.5% + gramicidin 0.005% + dexamethasone 0.05% (eye/ear drops) (Otodex, Sofradex)

FLUDROCORTISONE
Trade names
Florinef, Fludrocortisone Medsurge

Available form
Tablets: 0.1 mg

Action
- mineralocorticoid with strong glucocorticoid effects similar to hydrocortisone, but with greater effects on electrolyte balance
- duration of action 24–48 hours
- see also General Actions of corticosteroids (p. 991)

Use
- Addison's disease
- salt-losing adrenogenital syndrome

Dose
- (Addison's disease) 0.1 mg orally daily (usually given with cortisone or hydrocortisone) **OR**
- (Salt-losing adrenogenital syndrome) 0.1–0.2 mg orally daily

Adverse effects/Interactions/Nursing considerations/Cautions/Withdrawal
- (Addison's disease) dose can vary from 0.1 mg 3 times weekly to 0.2 mg daily
- (Addison's disease) dose may be reduced by 0.05 mg daily if transient hypertension occurs
- heart failure may be exacerbated if there is fluid and electrolyte imbalance
- not recommended in those with heart disease, hypertension or impaired kidney function
- see also General Adverse effects/Interactions/Nursing considerations/Cautions/Withdrawal for corticosteroids (p. 992)

Patient education
- advise the patient to seek medical advice if any severe or persistent headache, joint pain, dizziness, weakness or swelling of feet or legs occurs
- see also General Patient education for corticosteroids (p. 995)

Tablets can be dispersed in water, or crushed and mixed with a spoonful of yoghurt or apple puree.

May cause fetal harm, including reduced birth weight and adrenal suppression in newborns, especially with long-term use. The risks and benefits should be weighed before use.

Avoid use. May be excreted in breastmilk, potentially affecting the infant's growth and adrenal function. Use with caution in breastfeeding mothers, weighing the benefits to the mother and risks to the infant. Consider alternatives or discontinuing breastfeeding if high doses are required. Monitor the infant for signs of adrenal suppression.

Abrupt withdrawal or rapid dose reduction of fludrocortisone can lead to adrenal insufficiency. When discontinuing or reducing the dose, it should be done gradually to allow adrenal recovery. In situations of stress (e.g. trauma, surgery), additional doses or a return to previous dosing may be necessary. Always monitor for symptoms of adrenal insufficiency during dose adjustments.

The elderly may be more susceptible to adverse effects like hypertension, osteoporosis and fluid retention. Close clinical monitoring is recommended for older adults.

Banned in sport.

FLUOROMETHOLONE
Trade names
Flucon, FML

FLUOROMETHOLONE ACETATE
Trade name
Flarex

Available form
Eye drops: 1 mg/mL (0.1%)

Action
- glucocorticoid that inhibits ocular inflammatory response

Use
- palpebral and bulbar conjunctival inflammation, inflammation of the cornea and anterior segment of the globe

Dose
- 1–2 drops instilled into the conjunctival sac(s) 2–4 times daily. If needed, initial treatment can be 2 drops 1–2-hourly for first 24–48 hours

Adverse effects
- taste disturbance
- transient irritation, tearing, eye pain, ocular hyperaemia, foreign body sensation
- increased intraocular pressure, optic nerve damage, glaucoma
- secondary ocular infections, cataract formation, decreased visual acuity, blurred vision

Interactions
- decreased corneal healing may occur if used with topical NSAIDs
- (Ophthalmic) increased risk of raised intraocular pressure if given with anticholinergics in those at risk of acute-angle closure
- (Ophthalmic) chronic/prolonged use may increase intraocular pressure and decrease efficacy of antiglaucoma agents

Nursing considerations/Cautions/Withdrawal/Patient education

- fluorometholone acetate is more potent than fluorometholone and the two formulations are therefore not interchangeable
- see also General Nursing considerations/Cautions/Withdrawal/Patient education for corticosteroids (p. 994)

Avoid use. Teratogenic and embryocidal effects in animal studies when administered at doses comparable to human use. It should only be used if the potential benefit justifies the potential risk to the fetus.

Use with caution. Unknown whether topical ophthalmic corticosteroids are absorbed systemically in sufficient amounts to be excreted in breastmilk.

Elderly patients may be more susceptible to the adverse effects of corticosteroids, such as increased intraocular pressure and cataract formation, and should be monitored closely during prolonged use.

HYDROCORTISONE
Trade names
Cipla Hydrocortisone, DermAid products, Hydrocortisone Juno, Hydrocortisone Viatris, Hydrocortisone-AFT, Hysone

HYDROCORTISONE ACETATE
Trade names
APOHealth Hydrocortisone 1% Cream, Chemists' Own Skin Irritation Cream, Cortic DS, Pharmacy Action Hydrocortisone Cream, Sigmacort, Siguent Hycor Eye Ointment, Trust Hydrocortic

HYDROCORTISONE SODIUM SUCCINATE
Trade name
Solu-Cortef (100 mg hydrocortisone sodium succinate = 100 mg hydrocortisone)

Available forms
Tablets: 4 mg, 20 mg;
Vial: 100 mg;
Act-O-Vials: 100 mg/2 mL, 250 mg/2 mL, 500 mg/4 mL;
Topical spray: 10 mg/mL;
Topical cream/ointment: 0.5 mg/g (0.5%), 1 mg/g (1%);
Solution: 10 mg/g (1%);
Eye ointment: 1 mg/mL (1%)

Action
- glucocorticoid with some mineralocorticoid properties
- peak concentration achieved in about 1 hour, duration of action 8–12 hours, half-life 1.5–2 hours
- topical products are considered mild potency
- see also General Actions of corticosteroids (p. 991)

Use
- (Topical) facial and flexure dermatitis, psoriasis, nappy dermatitis, minor skin irritation
- see also General Uses of corticosteroids (p. 992)

Dose
- 100–500 mg IV injection or continuous infusion, repeated at 2-, 4- or 6-hourly intervals, depending on severity of the condition and the patient's response **OR**
- (Addison's disease, chronic adrenocortical insufficiency secondary to hypopituitarism) 30 mg orally daily in divided doses with food, increasing to 75–150 mg daily during illness or surgery **OR**
- (Cream, ointment) apply a small amount to the affected area 2–4 times daily **OR**
- (Solution) apply few drops to the affected area 2–3 times daily and massage gently **OR**
- (Topical spray) 1–2 sprays to the affected area 2–3 times daily and massage gently **OR**
- (Eye ointment) apply ointment to the affected eye(s) 2–4 times daily

Adverse effects
- (Topical) slight stinging, burning, itching, irritation, dryness, erythema
- (Topical) (prolonged/excessive therapy) telangiectasis, skin atrophy, striae
- (Topical) (rare) folliculitis, pustules, hypertrichosis, hypopigmentation, contact or perioral dermatitis, skin maceration, secondary infection, miliaria, acneiform eruptions
- (Ophthalmic) transient blurred vision
- (Ophthalmic, uncommon/rare) burning, stinging, redness, tearing, glaucoma, corneal thinning, eye pain, secondary ocular infection, decreased visual acuity
- see also General Adverse effects of corticosteroids (p. 992)

Interactions
- (Ophthalmic) increased risk of raised intraocular pressure if given with anticholinergics in those at risk of acute-angle closure
- (Ophthalmic) chronic/prolonged use may increase intraocular pressure and decrease efficacy of antiglaucoma agents
- see also General Interactions of corticosteroids (p. 993)

Nursing considerations/Cautions/Withdrawal

- (IV) increased risk of hypernatraemia if high-dose therapy is continued beyond 48–72 hours and should be replaced with an agent such as methylprednisolone with little or no salt retention properties
- (Oral) divided doses should be $\frac{2}{3}$ dose in the morning (20 mg) and $\frac{1}{3}$ at about 4 pm (10 mg)
- (IV) reconstitute using water for injections and then dilute with glucose 5% or sodium chloride 0.9% depending on the patient's sodium restriction
- administration rate is dependent on the dose (e.g. 100 mg over 30 seconds, 500 mg or more over 10 minutes)
- ensure the manufacturer's instructions are consulted before using Act-O-Vial system
- frequency of administration can be reduced once condition has improved
- (Solu-Cortef) contraindicated by local, intrathecal or epidural injection
- see also General Nursing considerations/Cautions/Withdrawal for corticosteroids (p. 994)

Patient education

- (Oral) the patient should be advised to take tablets with food or milk to reduce gastric acidity
- (Topical spray) advise the patient to hold spray 10 cm from area to be sprayed
- (Topical) advise the patient to decrease the frequency of administration when inflammation subsides
- instruct the patient in correct eye ointment insertion (see Eye, ear, nose and throat agents, p. 1129), including:
  - allow 10 minutes between ointment and any other topical ophthalmic agent
- see also General Patient education for corticosteroids (p. 995)

Tablets can be dispersed in water, or crushed and mixed with a spoonful of yoghurt or apple puree.

Not recommended during pregnancy unless benefits outweigh risks. Prolonged use may cause fetal abnormalities, including cleft palate and skeletal malformations. Infants born to mothers treated with corticosteroids should be monitored for adrenal insufficiency.

Avoid use, as may be excreted in breastmilk. Potential for serious adverse effects in nursing infants, such as growth suppression and interference with corticosteroid production.

Reduced hepatic function may lead to decreased metabolism and clearance of hydrocortisone, which can enhance its effects. Lower doses may be required, and careful monitoring of the patient's clinical response is recommended.

Gradual reduction of hydrocortisone is essential when discontinuing long-term therapy to prevent adrenal insufficiency. Abrupt withdrawal can lead to a withdrawal syndrome characterised by nausea, vomiting, lethargy, joint pain and hypotension.

May cause more pronounced side-effects, including osteoporosis, hypertension, and glucose intolerance.

Eye ointment and topical preparations are permitted in sport.

Other preparations are banned in sport via rectal, parenteral or oral use.

Available in combination with

- Hydrocortisone 5 mg 0.5% + Cinchocaine 5 mg 0.5% (Proctosedyl rectal suppositories, Proctosedyl rectal ointment)
- Hydrocortisone 1% + Clotrimazole 1% cream (Candacort MiniPak, CandaDerm, Hydrozole, Trimacorte)
- Hydrocortisone 1% + Miconazole nitrate 2% cream (Resolve Plus 1.0)
- Hydrocortisone 0.5% + Miconazole nitrate 2 % cream (Resolve Plus 0.5)
- Hydrocortisone acetate 11.2 mg + clotrimazole 10 mg cream (Canesten Extra

Antifungal Anti-inflammatory Cream, Canesten Plus Antifungal Anti-inflammatory Cream)
- Hydrocortisone 10 mg + ciprofloxacin 2 mg ear drops (Ciproxin HC)
- Hydrocortisone 0.5% + lidocaine (lignocaine) 5% ointment (SOOV IT Ointment)
- Hydorocortisone 1% + aciclovir 5% cream (Zovirax Duo)

METHYLPREDNISOLONE ACEPONATE
Trade names
Advantan, Metvant, Supriad, Tanilone

METHYLPREDNISOLONE ACETATE
Trade names
Depo-Medrol, Depo-Nisolone

METHYLPREDNISOLONE SODIUM SUCCINATE
Trade names
Solu-Medrol

Available forms
Vial: 40 mg/mL, 125 mg, 500 mg, 1 g;
Act-O-Vials: 40 mg/mL, 125 mg/2 mL;
Cream: 1 mg/g;
Ointment: 1 mg/g;
Fatty Ointment: 1 mg/g;
Lotion: 1 mg/g

Action/Use
- potent glucocorticoid
- see also General Actions/Uses of corticosteroids (p. 991)

Dose
- (High dose > 250 mg) 30 mg/kg IV over at least 30 minutes, repeated 4—6-hourly if needed, for up to 48 hours **OR**
- 10—500 mg IV daily (with larger doses being for short-term treatment of acute conditions) **OR**
- (Rheumatoid arthritis, osteoarthritis) 4—80 mg intra-articularly, the dose depending on severity of disease and size of joint, repeated every 1—5 weeks **OR**
- (Bursitis, ganglion, tendinitis, epicondylitis) 4—30 mg into the site, repeated as needed in chronic or recurrent conditions **OR**
- (Adrenogenital syndrome) 40 mg IM every 2 weeks **OR**
- (Rheumatoid arthritis maintenance) 40—120 mg IM weekly **OR**
- (Seborrhoeic dermatitis) 80 mg IM weekly **OR**
- (Multiple sclerosis, acute exacerbation) 160 mg IM daily for 1 week, then 64 mg every second day for 1 month **OR**
- (*Pneumocystis jiroveci* pneumonia (PCP)) 40 mg IV 6-hourly for 5—7 days, then converting to oral tapering regimen (for up to 21 days or the end of antipneumocystis therapy) **OR**
- (Skin lesions) 40—120 mg IM weekly for 1—4 weeks or every 5—10 days (contact dermatitis) **OR**
- (Dermatological conditions) 20—60 mg intradermally into lesions, repeated 1—4 times (interval depends on type of lesions) **OR**
- (Allergic rhinitis) 80—120 mg IM stat (may provide relief in 6 hours, lasting for up to 3 weeks) **OR**
- (Asthma) 80—120 mg IM stat (may provide relief in 6—48 hours, lasting up to 2 weeks) **OR**
- (Cream/ointment) apply thinly to the affected area once daily (twice daily for psoriasis) for up to 12 weeks **OR**
- (Lotion) apply sparingly to the affected area (including scalp) and massage until the lotion disappears for up to 12 weeks

Adverse effects
- (Intra-articular) post-injection flare, pain, irritation/discomfort at injection site, sterile abscess formation, hypopigmentation, hyperpigmentation, degeneration of joint with loss of sensation, joint instability (repeated injections), Charcot-type arthropathy (see Glossary)

HAVARD'S NURSING GUIDE TO DRUGS

- (Intradermal/intralesional) local discomfort, sterile abscess formation, hypopigmentation, hyperpigmentation, subcutaneous/cutaneous atrophy
- (IV, large doses) bradycardia
- (IV, rapid administration) cardiac arrhythmias, circulatory collapse, cardiac arrest
- (Topical) burning, itching, irritation, dryness, erythema, rash
- (Topical) (prolonged/excessive therapy) telangiectasis, skin atrophy, striae
- (Topical) (rare) folliculitis, pustules, secondary infection, miliaria, acneiform eruptions
- see also General Adverse effects of corticosteroids (p. 992)

Interactions

- increased serum levels may occur if given with aprepitant
- increased risk of convulsions if given with ciclosporin
- may alter serum levels of tacrolimus; therefore levels should be monitored especially when stopping methylprednisolone
- see also General Interactions of corticosteroids (p. 993)

Nursing considerations/Cautions/Withdrawal

- the Achilles tendon should not be injected
- (AIDS-related PCP) a diagnosis of PCP should be confirmed because of the potential to mask other untreated lung infection. If the person shows a positive response to skin test for tuberculosis, antimycobacterial therapy should be started with antipneumocystis therapy
- (AIDS-related PCP) adjunctive corticosteroid therapy should be commenced at maximum dose within 72 hours of starting antipneumocystis therapy
- IM injections (250 mg or less) should be injected only into large muscles
- doses of up to 250 mg IV should be given over at least 5 minutes; doses greater than 250 mg should be given over 30 minutes
- high doses (> 250 mg) should be continued for only 48–72 hours until the patient's condition has stabilised
- follow the manufacturer's instructions for reconstitution of powder, as the amount of diluent is dependent on the product's strength and recommended concentration
- reconstituted solution should be diluted with glucose 5% or sodium chloride 0.9% for IV infusion
- administer alone
- ensure the manufacturer's instructions are consulted before using the Act-O-Vial system
- (Topical) if skin shows excessive drying, a change of formulation with a higher fat content (e.g. fatty ointment) is recommended
- (Ointment) suitable for non-weeping, dry, fissured, scaly or hyperkeratinised skin
- (Lotion) suitable for hirsute areas
- see also General Nursing considerations/Cautions/Withdrawal for corticosteroids (p. 994)

Patient education

- (Lotion) the patient should be instructed that lotion should not be used on the axilla, groin or skin folds
- see also General Patient education for corticosteroids (p. 995)

 Should be used during pregnancy only if benefits outweigh risks.

 Excreted in breastmilk and may suppress growth and interfere with endogenous glucocorticoid production in nursing infants. Use in breastfeeding mothers should occur only if the benefits outweigh the potential risks to the infant. If used, the nursing infant should be closely monitored for signs of adrenal suppression or growth disturbances.

 Gradual dose reduction is required, especially following high-dose or long-term therapy.

CORTICOSTEROIDS

Topical preparations are permitted in sport.

Other preparations are banned in sport via rectal, parenteral or oral use.

MOMETASONE FUROATE

Trade names
APOHealth Sensease Nasal Allergy Relief Nasal Spray, Azonaire Hayfever & Allergy Prevention Nasal Spray, Elocon, Glenmark Mometasone Ointment, Nasonex Allergy Nasal Spray, Nasonex Aqueous Nasal Spray, Novasone, Telnasal Allergy Spray, Zatamil

Available forms
Lotion: 1 mg/g;
Cream: 1 mg/g;
Ointment: 1 mg/g;
Hydrogel: 1 mg/mL;
Nasal spray: 50 microgram/dose

Action
* potent topical glucocorticoid
* (Nasal) decreases capillary permeability and mucus production as well as causing vasoconstriction in the nasal mucosa
* see also General Actions of corticosteroids (p. 991)

Use
* psoriasis, dermatitis
* treatment of allergic and perennial rhinitis, prevention of seasonal allergic rhinitis
* prevention and treatment of seasonal or perennial allergic rhinitis
* nasal polyps
* acute rhinosinusitis (without signs/symptoms of severe bacterial infection)

Dose
* (Psoriasis, dermatitis) thin film of cream/ointment/hydrogel applied to the affected area once daily **OR**
* (Psoriasis, dermatitis) apply a few drops of lotion to the affected area, including scalp, massage gently until solution disappears **OR**
* (Allergic rhinitis) initially 2 sprays per nostril (50 micrograms per spray) daily until symptoms are controlled, then reduced to 1 spray per nostril (maximum daily dose 200 micrograms) **OR**
* (Nasal polyps) 2 sprays per nostril (50 micrograms per spray) daily, increasing to twice daily if symptoms are not controlled, then reducing dose (maximum daily dose 400 micrograms) **OR**
* (Acute rhinosinusitis) 2 sprays per nostril (50 micrograms per spray) twice daily for 15 days. If there is no improvement, therapy should be stopped (maximum daily dose 400 micrograms)

Adverse effects
* (Topical) burning, stinging, itching, irritation, dryness, erythema
* (Topical) (prolonged/excessive therapy) telangiectasis, skin atrophy, striae
* (Topical) (rare) folliculitis, pustules, hypertrichosis, hypopigmentation, contact or perioral dermatitis, skin maceration, secondary infection, miliaria, acneiform eruptions
* (Nasal spray) nasal stinging, itching, irritation, epistaxis, sneezing, sore throat, dry mouth, cough, headache, pharyngitis, visual disturbances
* (Nasal spray) (rare) nasal septum perforation, increased intraocular pressure, glaucoma, hypersensitivity, taste/smell disturbances

Nursing considerations/Cautions/Withdrawal

* (Cream) suitable for lesions
* (Ointment) suitable for dry, scaling skin with fissures
* (Lotion) recommended for scalp psoriasis and seborrhoeic dermatitis
* (Nasal spray) not recommended after recent nasal surgery or trauma, as healing may be delayed

- (Nasal spray) contraindicated if severe nasal infection is present, in bleeding disorders or if there is a history of nose bleeding
- (Topical) contraindicated in those with rosacea, perioral dermatitis, viral or fungal skin infection or ulcerative conditions
- see also General Nursing considerations/Cautions/Withdrawal for corticosteroids (p. 994)

Patient education

- (Prevention of seasonal allergic rhinitis) the patient should be advised to start therapy 2—4 weeks before the start of the pollen season
- advise the patient to seek medical advice if any of the following occur:
  - symptoms persist after 7 days of continuous use
  - fever, persistent/severe one-sided face or tooth pain, swelling around eyes
  - worsening of symptoms after an initial improvement
- see also General Patient education for corticosteroids (p. 995)

Use the lowest appropriate dose for the shortest time necessary.

Safe to use; ensure the breast area is free of corticosteroid before breastfeeding.

Use the lowest effective dose owing to a higher risk of skin thinning, osteoporosis and other corticosteroid-related side effects. Monitor for systemic absorption and adjust the dose if necessary.

Permitted in sport.

Available in combination with:
- mometasone furoate + indacterol (Actectura Breezhaler)
- mometasone furoate + indacterol + glycopyrronium (Enerzair Breezhaler)
- mometasone furoate + olopatadine (Ryaltris Nasal Spray)

PREDNISOLONE SODIUM PHOSPHATE
Trade names
Minims Prednisolone Eyedrops

PREDNISOLONE
Trade names
Panafcortelone, Predsolone, Predmix Oral Solution, Predsol Retention Enema and Suppositories, Redipred, Solone

Available forms
Tablets: 1 mg, 5 mg, 25 mg;
Eye drops: 5 mg/mL;
Oral liquid: 5 mg/mL;
Retention enema: 20 mg/100 mL;
Suppositories: 5 mg

Action
- glucocorticoid with greater activity than hydrocortisone but less mineralocorticoid effect (less sodium retention, oedema and electrolyte imbalance)
- peak concentration after 1—2 hours orally, half-life 2—4 hours
- see also General Actions of corticosteroids (p. 991)

Use
- proctitis (haemorrhagic, granular or post-radiation), rectal complications of Crohn's disease
- see also General Uses of corticosteroids (p. 992)

Dose
- initially 20—80 mg orally daily in 2—4 divided doses, as a single dose or on alternate days, reducing gradually to 5—20 mg daily (maintenance) **OR**

CORTICOSTEROIDS

- (Ulcerative colitis, Crohn's disease) contents of 1 disposable enema unit nightly for 2–4 weeks as a retention enema until progressive improvement occurs **OR**
- (Proctitis) suppository inserted twice daily (at bedtime and after morning defecation), with treatment continuing until tissue appears normal **OR**
- 1 drop instilled into the conjunctival sac(s) hourly (for intensive treatment) or 2–4 times daily

Adverse effects
- (Ophthalmic) transient blurred vision or discomfort
- (Ophthalmic, uncommon/rare, prolonged use) glaucoma, secondary ocular infection, visual acuity defect, optic nerve damage, ocular hypertension, ptosis, mydriasis
- (Rectal) mucosal atrophy, itching, burning
- see also General Adverse effects of corticosteroids (p. 992)

Interactions
- topical corticosteroids are not recommended concurrently with oral or IV corticosteroids
- see also General Interactions of corticosteroids (p. 993)

Nursing considerations/Cautions/Withdrawal
- doses > 40 mg are not recommended for prolonged therapy to minimise adverse effects
- alternate-day therapy is recommended for long-term/maintenance treatment providing symptom relief while minimising adrenal suppression and other adverse effects
- (Enema) therapy should not be continued if there is no improvement in condition
- caution if used in those with systemic sclerosis owing to the risk of scleroderma renal crisis with hypertension and decreased urinary output if a daily dose greater than 15 mg is given. BP and renal function should be closely monitored
- (Oral solution) contraindicated in those with hypersensitivity to hydroxybenzoates
- (Rectal) caution if diverticulitis is present or there is any possibility of impending perforation, abscess or other infection
- (Rectal) contraindicated if there is any impaired circulation (as rectal ulceration may occur) or any trauma or infection in the anorectal region
- (Eye drops) contraindicated in those with glaucoma or if any eye infection is present
- see also General Nursing considerations/Cautions/Withdrawal for corticosteroids (p. 994)

Patient education
- advise the patient that 1 mg tablets should not be broken even though they are scored
- (Oral solution) instruct the patient that oral solution should be refrigerated after opening (not frozen) and discarded after 28 days
- (Oral solution) solution can be taken alone or with milk, cordial, soft drink or soft food if needed
- (Rectal) the patient should be advised to stop therapy if irritation, rash or rectal bleeding occurs and seek medical advice
- the patient should be instructed in the correct technique for eye drop instillation (see Eye, ear, nose and throat agents, p. 1129)
- instruct the patient in the correct technique for suppository insertion (see Gastrointestinal agents (miscellaneous) p. 1165)
- ensure the patient understands correct enema instillation technique (see Gastrointestinal agents (miscellaneous) p. 1164)
- see also General Patient education for corticosteroids (p. 995)

Available as oral solution. Tablet can be crushed and mixed with yoghurt or apple puree.

Long-term corticosteroid use during pregnancy can cause low birthweight and potential adrenal suppression in the newborn. Short-term use for preventing respiratory distress syndrome appears safe, but careful risk—benefit analysis is recommended. Use the lowest effective dose of prednisolone for the shortest time necessary.

Excreted in breastmilk, and prolonged use could affect the nursing infant (e.g. suppress growth or adrenal function). Use only after careful consideration of the benefits versus risks, and monitor the infant closely for any adverse effects.

Prednisolone metabolism occurs in the liver. In patients with hepatic impairment, a dosage reduction may be required, and the risk of adverse reactions such as vertebral collapse, hypertension and Cushing's syndrome is increased. Monitor liver function regularly during therapy.

Tapering the dose gradually is recommended to avoid withdrawal symptoms and adrenal insufficiency.

Elderly patients are more susceptible to the side effects of corticosteroids, including osteoporosis, hypertension, and fluid retention. Use the minimum effective dose and monitor closely for adverse effects such as skin thinning, bone loss or susceptibility to infection.

Banned in sport via rectal, parenteral or oral route.

Permitted in sport for intra-articular injection use, local injection and use via anal, respiratory, oral mucosal, ocular, nasal, cutaneous and auricular routes.

Available in combination with
- Prednisolone acetate 1% + phenylephrine hydrochloride 0.12% eye drops (Prednefrin Forte)
- Prednisolone hexanoate 1.9 mg + cinchocaine hydrochloride 5 mg rectal ointment/suppositories (Scheriproct)

PREDNISONE
Trade names
Panafcort, Predsone, Sone

Available forms
Tablets: 1 mg, 5 mg, 25 mg

Action
- synthetic glucocorticoid that is converted in the liver to its active metabolite, prednisolone, within 60 minutes
- duration of action 12—36 hours
- see also General Actions of corticosteroids (p. 991)

Use
- see General Uses of corticosteroids (p. 992)

Dose
- initially 20—80 mg daily in 2—4 divided doses, as a single dose or on alternate days after meals, then 5—20 mg daily (maintenance)

Adverse effects/Interactions/Nursing considerations/Cautions/Withdrawal/Patient education

- advise patient that 1 mg tablets should not be broken even though they are scored
- doses > 40 mg are not recommended for prolonged therapy to minimise adverse effects
- alternate-day therapy is recommended for long-term/maintenance treatment providing symptom relief while minimising adrenal suppression and other adverse effects
- see also General Adverse effects/Interactions/Nursing considerations/Cautions/Withdrawal/Patient education for corticosteroids (p. 992)

Tablets can be dispersed in water (has strong bitter taste), or crushed and mixed with a spoonful of yoghurt or apple puree.

CORTICOSTEROIDS

 Use the lowest effective dose for the shortest time necessary. Long-term corticosteroid use during pregnancy can cause low birthweight and potential adrenal suppression in the newborn. Short-term use for preventing respiratory distress syndrome appears safe, but careful risk–benefit analysis is recommended.

 Excreted in breastmilk, and prolonged use could affect the nursing infant (e.g. suppress growth or adrenal function). Use only after carefully considering the benefits versus risks, and monitor the infant closely for any adverse effects.

 Use with caution in patients with impaired hepatic function, as reduced conversion to active prednisolone may occur, necessitating dose adjustments.

 Use the lowest possible dose and monitor closely because of the increased risk of osteoporosis, fluid retention, hypertension and other adverse effects in elderly patients.

 Banned in sport.

TRIAMCINOLONE ACETONIDE
Trade names
Aristocort, Kenacort-A 10, Kenacort-A 40, Kenalog in Orabase, Tricortone

Available forms
Ampoules: 10 mg/mL, 40 mg/mL;
Cream: 0.2 mg/g;
Ointment: 0.2 mg/g;
Oral paste: 1 mg/g

Action
- moderately potent glucocorticoid with activity similar to prednisolone (4 mg triamcinolone = 5 mg prednisolone)
- see also General Actions of corticosteroids (p. 991)

Use
- see General Uses of corticosteroids (p. 992)

Dose
- initially 60 mg deep IM into buttock, then dose adjusted according to response (range 20—80 mg) (solution strength 40 mg/mL) **OR**
- (Hay fever, pollen asthma unresponsive to other treatment) 40—100 mg IM stat (solution strength 40 mg/mL) **OR**
- 2.5—15 mg depending on size of joint and disease (intra-articular, intrabursal, injection into ganglia or tendon sheath) (solution strength 10 mg/mL) **OR**
- 10—40 mg depending on size of joint and disease (intra-articular, intrabursal, injection into ganglia or tendon sheath) (solution strength 40 mg/mL) **OR**
- (Intradermally) initial dose dependent on specific disease but limited to 1 mg (0.1 mL) per site, repeated weekly or less frequently as needed **OR**
- (Inflamed skin lesions) apply cream or ointment 3—4 times daily to affected area **OR**
- (Mouth ulcers) cover lesion with sufficient paste (about 1 cm) to form a thin film each night, increasing to 2—3 times daily after meals if lesions are severe

Adverse effects
- (Topical) burning, itching, irritation, dryness, erythema
- (Topical) (prolonged/excessive therapy) telangiectasis, skin atrophy, striae
- (Topical) (rare) folliculitis, pustules, hypertrichosis, hypopigmentation, contact or perioral dermatitis, skin maceration, secondary infection, miliaria, acneiform eruptions
- (Intra-articular) post-injection flare, pain, irritation/discomfort at injection site, sterile abscess formation, hypopigmentation, hyperpigmentation, degeneration of joint with loss of sensation, joint instability (repeated injections), Charcot-type arthropathy (see Glossary)
- (Intradermal/intralesional) local discomfort, sterile abscess formation, hypopigmentation, hyperpigmentation, subcutaneous/cutaneous atrophy

- see also General Adverse effects of corticosteroids (p. 992)

Interactions
- see General Interactions of corticosteroids (p. 993)

Nursing considerations/Cautions/Withdrawal
- (Intradermal) if multiple sites are to be injected intradermally, there should be at least 1 cm between sites
- (Ampoules) shake well before use
- (Intra-articular) not recommended for unstable joints
- (Oral paste) contraindicated if bacterial or fungal infection is present in mouth or throat, or in those with viral herpetic oral or intraoral lesions
- (Ampoules) contain benzyl alcohol and are therefore contraindicated in newborn or premature infants
- see also General Nursing considerations/Cautions/Withdrawal for corticosteroids (p. 994)

Patient education
- (Oral paste) advise patient not to rub paste in as it will crumble
- (Cream, ointment) patient should be advised if treating eczematised psoriasis, occlusive non-permeable dressing may be applied over cream or ointment to improve effectiveness
- (Intra-articular) advise patient to seek medical advice if local swelling, restricted joint movement, fever or malaise occurs
- see also General Patient education for corticosteroids (p. 995) and correct instillation of nasal spray (see Anti-asthma agents, bronchodilators and respiratory agents (p. 114))

 Use in pregnancy only if benefits outweigh risks.

 May be excreted in breastmilk. Consider risk versus benefit; long-term use is not recommended during breastfeeding because of the potential for adverse effects in the infant.

 Avoid abrupt cessation after long-term use to prevent adrenal insufficiency. Gradual tapering of dose is recommended to avoid withdrawal symptoms, including fatigue, muscle pain, and hypotension.

 Elderly patients may be more susceptible to adverse effects such as osteoporosis, hypertension and gastrointestinal complications. Use the lowest effective dose and monitor regularly.

 Banned in sport via rectal, parenteral or oral route.

Permitted in sport for intra-articular injection use, local injection and use via anal, respiratory, oral mucosal, ocular, nasal, cutaneous or auricular routes.

Available in combination with
- triamcinolone acetonide 0.09% + neomycin 0.225% + gramicidin 0.0225% + nystatin 90,000 units/mL ear drops (Kenacomb Otic, Otocomb Otic)
- triamcinolone acetonide 0.1% + neomycin 0.25% + gramicidin 0.025% + nystatin 100,000 units/g ointment (Kenacomb)

COUGH SUPPRESSANTS AND EXPECTORANTS

Under normal circumstances, coughing is a protective mechanism that clears the airways of secretions and foreign materials. Combinations of cough suppressants, expectorants, sympathomimetics or analgesics are widely used in various cough and cold preparations that are commonly available as over-the-counter (OTC) preparations. It is important that the patient is aware of the constituents of these preparations because they often have adverse interactions with other medications.

Cough suppressants (antitussives) have a central and/or peripheral action on the cough reflex and are used to suppress irritating unproductive coughs (e.g. dextromethorphan, codeine phosphate and dihydrocodeine).

Although their exact action is unknown, expectorants are thought to increase the volume of secretions in the respiratory tract and therefore facilitate their removal by ciliary action and coughing. Some are thought to have an irritant effect on the gastric mucosa (e.g. ammonium chloride, guaifenesin, ipecacuanha, senega and ammonia).

Decongestants are cough preparations that contain an antihistamine (decreasing capillary permeability) and a sympathomimetic agent (causing vasoconstriction), with the combination resulting in less congested mucous membranes.

AMMONIUM CHLORIDE
Trade name
Nyal Bronchitis Cough Medicine

Available form
Syrup: 110 mg/10 mL

Action
- increases quantity and decreases viscosity of respiratory tract secretions, allowing easier removal by ciliary action and coughing

Use
- expectorant, relief from cough associated with common cold

Dose
- 110 mg (10 mL) orally 4-hourly if needed

Nursing consideration/Caution
- not recommended in children under 6 years

Patient education
- instruct the patient to shake bottle well before use
- the patient should be advised to seek medical advice if symptoms persist after 7 days or if fever and increased bronchial secretions occur

Available in combination with
- ammonium chloride 125 mg/5 mL + diphenlydramine hydrochloride 12.5 mg/5 mL liquid (Benadryl Original Oral Liquid, Codral Dry Cough & Cold with Antihistamine)

BROMHEXINE
Trade names
Bisolvon Chesty Forte Oral Liquid, Bisolvon Chesty Oral Liquid, Bisolvon Chesty Forte Tablets, DuroTuss Chesty Cough Liquid Double Strength, DuroTuss Chesty Cough Liquid Regular, Pharmacy Action Chesty Cough Relief Oral Liquid, Pharmacy Action Chesty Forte Tablets

Available forms
Elixir: 4 mg/5 mL, 8 mg/5 mL;
Tablets: 8 mg

Action
- mucolytic that reduces the viscosity of mucus and promotes flow of thin bronchial secretions, gradually reducing the volume of mucus
- facilitates expectoration, eases cough
- half-life 6.6—31.4 hours (single dose) or 1 hour (multiple dosing)

Use
- breakdown of mucus in those with common cold, influenza or other bronchial conditions causing excessive mucus production

Dose
- (Tablets) initially 8—16 mg orally 3 times daily for 7 days, then 8 mg 3 times daily if needed **OR**
- (Elixir) 8—16 mg (10—20 mL) orally 3 times daily

Adverse effects
- (Occasionally, mild) nausea, vomiting, diarrhoea, indigestion, upper abdominal pain
- headache, dizziness, sweating
- (Rare) hypersensitivity reaction, severe skin reactions

Interaction
- may increase concentration of amoxicillin or erythromycin in bronchial secretions if taken concurrently

Nursing considerations/Cautions
- soluble tablets are not recommended in children under 12 years
- soluble tablets contain fructose and are therefore not recommended in those with fructose intolerance
- (Oral liquid, tablets, sachets) contain lactose and are therefore not recommended in those with Lapp lactase intolerance or glucose—galactose malabsorption
- contains sorbitol, which may cause diarrhoea
- caution if used in those with gastric ulceration or severe kidney/liver disease

Patient education
- the patient should be advised to seek medical attention if any new skin or mucosal lesions occur
- warn the patient to expect an initial increase in the flow of secretions
- instruct the patient to dissolve soluble tablets in either hot or cold water and drink immediately
- the patient should be advised to seek medical advice if symptoms persist after 7 days, or if fever and increased bronchial secretions occur

 Not recommended during the first trimester of pregnancy.

 Not recommended during breastfeeding because there are no available data.

Available in combination with
- contained in Benadryl Chesty Forte (New formulation) Oral liquid, DuroTuss Chesty Cough Liquid Forte, DuroTuss Chesty Cough Liquid Oral, DuroTuss Chesty Cough Liquid plus Nasal Decongestant,

COUGH SUPPRESSANTS AND EXPECTORANTS

DuroTuss Chesty Cough Lozenges, DuroTuss PE Chesty Cough Plus Nasal Decongestant, Robitussin Chesty Cough Forte

DEXTROMETHORPHAN
Trade names
Bisolvon Dry (Oral Liquid), Bisolvon Dry Pastilles, Robitussin Dry Cough Forte

Available forms
Syrup: 10 mg/5 mL, 30 mg/10 mL; Pastilles: 10 mg

Action
- non-opioid antitussive which is centrally acting (medulla)
- metabolised to weak codeine analogue
- no analgesic, sedative or respiratory depressant effects at antitussive dose
- weak serotonergic properties
- onset of action within 60 minutes, duration 3—6 hours
- half-life 1.2—3.9 hours (extended in poor metabolisers)

Use
- relief of dry, irritating, unproductive cough
- (pastilles) also soothe throat

Dose
- 10—20 mg orally 4—6-hourly (10 mg/5 mL) (daily maximum 4 doses, maximum duration 5 days) **OR**
- 30 mg (10 mL) 6—8-hourly (30 mg/10 mL) (maximum duration 5 days) **OR**
- suck 1—3 (10—30 mg) pastilles every 4—6 hours as needed (maximum daily dose 12 pastilles (120 mg))

Adverse effects
- nausea, vomiting, diarrhoea, abdominal pain, constipation
- dizziness, drowsiness, fatigue, confusion, somnolence
- abuse, dependency
- tolerance (with prolonged use)
- (Overdose) confusion, excitation, psychosis, nervousness, restlessness, severe nausea and vomiting, respiratory depression, serotonin syndrome (see Glossary)

Interactions
- contraindicated with or within 14 days of monoamine oxidase inhibitors (MAOIs)
- caution if used with other serotonergic agents, including selective serotonin reuptake inhibitors (SSRIs) and tricyclic antidepressants (TCAs)
- may increase CNS effects if given with alcohol or CNS depressants
- serum levels may increase if given with amiodarone, bupropion, fluoxetine, haloperidol, ritonavir, flecainide or paroxetine, increasing the risk of adverse effects

Nursing considerations/Cautions
- has addictive potential and tolerance may develop with prolonged use
- caution if used in those with tendency towards abuse or dependence (e.g. history of alcohol/drug abuse or psychiatric disorders). Should be used only for a short period of time under medical supervision
- (Bisolvon Dry) contains fructose and is therefore not recommended in those with fructose intolerance
- caution if used in those with liver or kidney impairment or impaired cough reflex (e.g. Parkinson's disease, dementia) or at risk of developing respiratory failure
- not recommended in those with mastocytosis
- not recommended for productive cough with mucus production (e.g. cystic fibrosis, bronchiectasis)
- contraindicated in those with asthma, chronic obstructive pulmonary disease, pneumonia, respiratory failure or depression

Patient education
- advise patient to sip undiluted linctus slowly; it will be more effective if not followed immediately by liquid (e.g. milk or water)

- some oral formulations contain sorbitol, which may cause diarrhoea
- patient should be advised not to drive or operate machinery if drowsiness or dizziness occurs
- warn patient to avoid alcohol while taking this medication
- patient should be advised to seek medical advice if symptoms have not been relieved or fever with increasing bronchial secretions occurs

 Contraindicated during breastfeeding owing to limited information.

Available in combination with
- contained in Benadryl PE Dry Cough and Nasal Congestion Oral Liquid, Codral preparations, Demazin Cold + Flu + Cough Day + Night, Dimetapp preparations, Robitussin Cough & Chest Congestion Syrup

DIHYDROCODEINE
Trade name
Rikodeine Oral Liquid

Available form
Syrup: 19 mg/10 mL

Action
- semi-synthetic opioid with cough suppressant properties

Use
- unproductive or intractable (dry) cough

Dose
- 9.5–19 mg (5–10 mL) orally 4–6-hourly

Adverse effects
- drowsiness, diarrhoea, respiratory depression, sedation

Interactions
- may increase effects of alcohol and CNS depressants therefore not recommended together

Nursing considerations/Cautions
- dose and/or duration of therapy should be limited due to the risk of abuse, misuse and addiction
- risk of addiction is increased in those with personal or family history of substance or alcohol abuse or mental illness, therefore patient should be assessed for any risk factors before starting therapy
- contains sorbitol, which may cause diarrhoea
- caution if used in those with asthma, emphysema, cor pulmonale, chronic obstructive respiratory disease, inflammatory or obstructive bowel disease, biliary tract disorders or pancreatic inflammation
- contraindicated in those with respiratory disease, respiratory depression or hypersensitivity to opioids

Patient education
- the patient should be advised not to drive or operate heavy machinery if drowsiness occurs
- the patient should be advised to seek medical advice if symptoms persist after 7 days or if fever and increased bronchial secretions occur
- warn the patient to avoid alcohol with this medication
- do not use with productive coughs

 Prolonged use late in pregnancy may cause respiratory depression and withdrawal symptoms in newborn.

 Use only if benefit outweighs the risks in breastfeeding because of limited information.

 Dosage should be monitored in people with severe renal disease, as dose accumulation can occur.

Dosage should be reduced in hepatic disease.

GUAIFENESIN

Trade names
Codral Mucus Cough Oral liquid, Robitussin Chesty Cough Oral Liquid, Vicks Cough Syrup for Chest Cough

Available forms
Syrup: 20 mg/mL, 200 mg/15 mL

Action
- increases the volume and reduces the viscosity of bronchial and tracheal secretions
- half-life 60 minutes

Use
- expectorant for productive cough, providing symptomatic relief from congested chest and cough

Dose
- 200—400 mg orally 4-hourly (daily maximum 6 doses)

Adverse effects
- nausea, vomiting, abdominal pain, diarrhoea
- dizziness, headache, drowsiness
- rash
- (Rare) hypersensitivity

Nursing considerations/Cautions
- caution if used in those with porphyria
- not recommended in those with chronic/persistent cough associated with asthma, bronchitis, emphysema, smoker's cough, chronic obstructive pulmonary disease (COPD) or cough associated with excessive secretions
- contraindicated in those under 6 years

Patient education
- the patient should be advised to seek medical advice if symptoms persist after 7 days or if fever and increased bronchial secretions occur

 Not recommended during breastfeeding unless benefits outweigh potential risks owing to limited information.

Available in combination with
- contained in Benadryl Chesty Forte, Benadryl PE Chesty Cough and Nasal Congestion, Codral preparations, DuroTuss Chesty Cough Liquid Forte, DuroTuss Chesty Cough Forte Tablets, Lemsip Multi-Relief, Nyal Chesty Cough Medicine, Robitussin preparations

DERMATOLOGICAL AGENTS

The skin is the largest organ of the body and is subject to a range of disorders, including viral, bacterial and fungal infections, parasitic infestations, cancers, ulcers and allergic reactions, as well as skin-specific conditions, such as disorders of the hair follicles and sebaceous glands, and those of unknown aetiology, such as psoriasis, pityriasis rosea and lichen planus.

Absorption of dermatological agents is influenced by a number of factors, such as age (e.g. skin is thin at the extremes of age), condition and site (e.g. palms and soles of feet have thick layers that are not easily penetrated), metabolism and circulation (i.e. poor circulation impedes healing) and formulation of the agent (e.g. water-soluble drugs are poorly absorbed through the skin; alcohol-containing agents have a drying effect).

Goals of therapy for dermatological agents include:
- treating the cause (e.g. infection)
- relieving symptoms (e.g. redness, pruritus, inflammation), and/or
- restoring and maintaining normal skin function (if possible).

It should be noted that, while dermatological agents are used for their local effects, they may also have systemic effects, especially if applied to large areas, broken skin or under occlusive dressings.

TOPICAL ECTOPARASITICAL AGENTS

Ectoparasites are multicellular organisms that live on or feed off human skin, and include ticks, fleas and mites. Pediculicides are agents which are used to treat lice, while scabicides or acaricides are used to treat mite infestation (Knights et al 2023).

PEDICULOSIS (LICE INFESTATION)

There are three types of lice which cause infestation of the body (body louse), hair (head louse) or pubic area (pubic or crab louse). Lice are small, wingless, bloodsucking organisms that can only crawl (not fly or jump); therefore spread is by close contact. For example, outbreaks of head lice frequently occur in schools, childcare centres and families where children have close contact with each other.

General Patient education for pediculicides
- lice do not distinguish between clean and dirty hair

DERMATOLOGICAL AGENTS

- hair should be checked regularly for head lice (use hair conditioner on dry hair and comb using a fine-toothed comb, looking for lice or eggs (nits))
- children may return to school after treatment for head lice has started
- none of the treatments kill all eggs; therefore treatment must be repeated 7–10 days apart
- all members of the family should be checked for head lice and treated only if head lice/nits are present
- children should be instructed not to share hats, scarves, hair ribbons/bands or combs/brushes
- fine-toothed combs (used for removal of lice/nits) should be washed in hot water and allowed to air dry
- apply lotion/cream/mousse to dry hair and massage into hair to completely cover and wet the hair/scalp
- leave in situ for 10 minutes
- comb out dead lice and nits, starting at the top of the head and lifting a 2 cm section of hair. The comb should be touching the scalp and, using a firm motion, comb away from the scalp towards the end of the hair. Nits/lice should be wiped on tissue before moving to next section of hair
- wash hair with the usual shampoo
- avoid contact with eyes and mucous membranes. If contact occurs, the area should be flushed with water
- gloves should be worn, or wash hands thoroughly after applying lotion
- ensure the patient/parent/carer understands that the lotion should not be swallowed

BENZYL ALCOHOL
Trade name
NeutraLice Advance

Available form
Lotion: 5% w/w

Action
- suffocates lice by blocking respiratory system

Use
- head lice

Dose
- apply a generous amount of lotion to dry hair, rubbing vigorously into hair and scalp, concentrating on areas behind the ears and back of neck. Leave lotion on hair for at least 10 minutes, using the plastic comb provided to remove lice and nits. Wash with water and towel dry

Adverse effects
- skin irritation

Nursing considerations/Cautions
- not recommended in children under 6 months

Patient education
- treatment is required weekly for 3 weeks
- see also General Patient education for pediculicides (p. 1024)

 Considered safe to use when breastfeeding.

SCABIES

Scabies is a highly contagious skin infestation with female mites burrowing under the skin after mating to lay their eggs for 4 to 6 weeks. Mites and eggs are contained in lesions (small, wavy, threadlike, slightly elevated, greyish-white burrows) ranging in length from 1 to 10 mm with a terminal end capped with a small blister. Lesions are commonly found between the toes and fingers, anterior surfaces of wrists and elbows, axillae, lower abdomen, under female breasts and genitalia of both sexes, with face and neck unaffected (Gunning et al 2019).

The main symptom is intense itching, which is usually worse after a hot bath or at night, and scratching may lead to secondary infection. Outbreaks of scabies occur in childcare centres, kindergartens, nursing homes and institutions. Transmission of scabies involves either skin contact with the infected person or infected towels, bedclothes or undergarments (contaminated within past 4—5 days). The incubation period is usually 2—6 weeks (not previously infected) or 1—4 days (re-infection). Diagnosis is via skin scraping (Gunning et al 2019).

General Patient education for scabicides

- ensure the patient understands that the cream/lotion should be applied to skin only and not taken orally
- avoid contact with face, neck and eyes. If contact occurs, the area should be washed thoroughly with water
- solution should be diluted for use in children
- personal garments, towels and bedclothes should be washed in hot water
- blankets should be dry-cleaned or placed in a tumble dryer for 30 minutes on a hot setting
- all members of the household or sexual contacts should be treated at the same time
- a hot bath and gentle scrubbing before application of lotion/cream is recommended to open up burrows; dry thoroughly
- lotion/cream is applied to the whole body from neck to toes, especially in areas known for infestation, but avoiding the face and head. Care should be taken to work cream or lotion into skin folds (especially between fingers and toes, wrists, armpits and genital areas)
- if the area is washed (e.g. hands) during contact time, lotion/cream should be reapplied
- lotion/cream is allowed to dry and remain in situ for 8—24 hours (depending on brand) and then washed off using soap and water
- retreatment is recommended after 5—7 days if mites are still present
- patient is non-infectious within 24 hours of treatment

- itch may persist for up to 4 weeks after treatment (which may be due to reaction to dead mites under the skin rather than treatment failure)

BENZYL BENZOATE

Trade name
McGloin's Benzemul

Available form
Lotion: 250 mg/mL

Action
- ectoparasiticidal

Use
- pediculosis (body lice)
- scabies

Dose
- (Pediculosis) apply lotion thinly to affected area, leave for 24 hours, then remove with soap and water **OR**
- (Scabies) apply lotion thinly to whole body from neck, allow to dry and leave for 24 hours before washing off

Adverse effects
- skin irritation and burning sensation

Nursing considerations/Cautions

- skin testing 10 minutes before general application is recommended to detect any severe skin reaction. If stinging occurs, the solution should be diluted with an equal quantity of water and skin re-tested
- if used in children under 12 years, the lotion should be diluted in equal parts with water, and with 3 parts water if used on children aged 6 months—years.
- (Pediculosis) treatment may be repeated after 7 days if lice are still present. May be repeated multiple times
- (Scabies) re-treatment may be necessary after 5 days if live mites are still present

Patient education

- see General Patient education for scabicides (above)

DERMATOLOGICAL AGENTS

Note
- contained in Anusol with zinc oxide

CROTAMITON
Trade name
Eurax

Available forms
Cream: 10%;
Lotion: 10%

Action
- antipruritic and acaricide with some antiseptic effect, which prevents secondary infection
- duration of effect 6–10 hours

Use
- pruritus (due to insect bites and stings, nettle rash, allergies, prickly heat (miliaria)) or senile, anal and genital pruritus
- itching due to head or pubic lice (lotion)
- scabies

Dose
- (Pruritus) rub gently into affected areas 2–3 times daily **OR**
- (Sscabies infestation) apply thinly and evenly over the whole body (avoiding face and scalp) at bedtime, then repeated daily for 3–5 days depending on response

Adverse effects
- (Uncommon) pruritus
- (Rare) contact dermatitis, rash, eczema, erythema, irritation, angioedema

Nursing considerations/Cautions
- lotion is preferred for use on hairy areas of the body
- contains propylene glycol, which can cause skin irritation, and sorbic acid, cetostearyl alcohol and wool fat, which can cause contact dermatitis in sensitive individuals
- (Children) not recommended for application to whole body

Patient education
- (Pruritus) if itch is not relieved in 5 days, the patient should be advised to seek medical attention
- advise the patient not to reapply more than once daily if washing of the area with soap and water has occurred
- see also General Patient education for scabicides (p. 1026)

 Considered safe to use in pregnancy.

 If breastfeeding, wash the medication from the nipples prior to feeding and reapply after.

PERMETHRIN
Trade name
Lyclear

Available form
Cream: 50 mg/g (5%)

Action
- scabicide that alters conductivity of cells, leading to paralysis

Use
- scabies
- pubic lice

Dose
- (Scabies) (adults, children > 12 years) apply to whole body below neck and wash off 8–12 hours later. Repeat 7 days later
- (Pubic lice) (adults) apply to hair where active lice or eggs are seen, wash after 24 hours, repeat 7 days later

Adverse effects
- burning, stinging, erythema, oedema, eczema, rash, pruritus

Nursing considerations/Cautions
- nursing staff who apply permethrin routinely should wear gloves to avoid hand irritation

- not recommended in the elderly or children under 2 years without medical advice
- contraindicated in those with known hypersensitivity to permethrin, synthetic pyrethroids or pyrethrins

Patient education
- patients should be advised to reapply to hands if handwashing with soap and water has occurred within 8 hours of application
- see also General Patient education for scabicides (p. 1026)

Considered safe to use in pregnancy.

If breastfeeding, wash the medication off nipples prior to breastfeeding and reapply after.

OTHER DERMATOLOGICAL PREPARATIONS

AMINOLEVULINIC ACID
Trade name
Alacare

Available form
Dermal patch: 8 mg

Action
- sensitiser for photodynamic therapy (PDT)
- after application of aminolaevulinic acid hydrochloride, protoporphyrin IX (PPIX) accumulates intracellularly in actinic keratosis lesion. PPIX is a photoactive compound and, when activated in the presence of oxygen, damage is caused to the targeted cells' mitochondria

Use
- treatment of mild-to-moderate actinic keratosis lesion on face and scalp (hairless areas)

Dose
- apply patch to lesion ensuring it is completely covered. Up to 8 lesions can be treated in one session of PDT. Patch(es) left in situ for 4 hours, then removed and lesion(s) exposed to red light

Adverse effects
- (Application site) redness, exfoliation, irritation, pain, pruritus, scab, bleeding, scaling, discharge, discomfort, erosion, hyper/hypopigmentation, swelling, vesicle/pustule formation
- headache

Interactions
- hypericin can increase phototoxic reactions caused by PDT and should therefore be discontinued 2 weeks before therapy. Hypericin-containing products include St John's wort
- phototoxicity may be potentiated if given with etretinate, griseofulvin, iron chelators, methotrexate, phenothiazines, quinolones, St John's wort, sulfonamides, sulfonylureas, tetracyclines, thiazide diuretics or vitamin D analogues
- efficacy may be decreased by tryptophan, glutathione, acetylcysteine, melatonin and methionine
- not recommended with other topical medications

Nursing considerations/Cautions
- any UV therapy should be stopped before starting treatment
- avoid contact with eyes
- should be used only by health professionals experienced in using photodynamic therapies
- if patch does not stick to lesion, it can be fixed with an adhesive strip
- lamp should have filters and mirrors to minimise exposure to heat, blue light and UV radiation
- the light dose is determined by size of light field, distance between lamp and skin surface and illumination time

DERMATOLOGICAL AGENTS

- the patient and operator should wear appropriate protective goggles during illumination period
- untreated skin surrounding lesions does not require protection
- treated lesions should be assessed after 12 weeks
- not recommended for use on very thick, red, scaly, indurated actinic keratosis lesions or in those with moderate brown-to-black skin
- contraindicated in those with porphyria or who have been previously unresponsive to PDT with aminolaevulinic acid preparations, with known photodermatoses or varying pathology (e.g. aminoaciduria, polymorphic light reaction) or diseases/conditions precipitated or aggravated by light exposure (e.g. lupus erythematosus)

Patient education

- advise the patient to avoid sun exposure to the treated lesion site and surrounding area for at least 48 hours post-treatment
- warn the patient about common skin reactions post-treatment. Cooling the area may decrease skin reactions

 No human data; use is not recommended.

 Breastfeeding should be discontinued for 48 hours post-treatment.

BRIMONIDINE
Trade name
Mirvaso

Available form
Gel: 3.3 mg/g

Action
- highly selective alpha2 adrenergic agonist which reduces erythema by direct cutaneous vasoconstriction

Use
- facial erythema of rosacea

Dose
- 5 small pea-sized amounts of cream applied daily to forehead, chin, nose, each cheek

Adverse effects
- erythema, pruritus, flushing, skin-burning sensation, skin warmth, skin irritation, acne, pain
- contact dermatitis, dermatitis, rosacea
- paraesthesia, headache
- blurred vision
- nasal congestion, nasopharyngitis, upper respiratory tract infection
- increased intraocular pressure

Interactions
- contraindicated with monoamine oxidase inhibitors (MAOIs) and tricyclic or tetracyclic antidepressants
- caution if used with CNS depressants (e.g. alcohol, barbiturates, opioids, sedatives or anaesthetics), as additive effects may occur
- caution if used with agents that affect metabolism and uptake of circulating amines (e.g. chlorpromazine, methylphenidate)
- caution if used with antihypertensives and digoxin, as additive cardiac effects may occur
- caution if used with isoprenaline and prazosin, as they may interfere with alpha adrenergic receptor agonists

Nursing considerations/Cautions
- medical diagnosis of rosacea should be made before starting therapy
- before starting therapy, response and tolerance can be determined by applying a small amount of gel daily for at least 7 days
- if therapy is stopped because of adverse effects, it should be recommenced by

using a small amount for at least 1 full day before full face application
- contains methyl parahydroxybenzoate, which may cause allergic reactions, and propylene glycol, which may cause skin irritation
- not recommended for irritated skin or open wounds
- caution if used in those with severe, unstable or uncontrolled cardiovascular disease, depression, cerebral or coronary insufficiency, Raynaud's phenomenon, orthostatic hypotension, thromboangitis obliterans, scleroderma or Sjögren's syndrome
- contraindicated in those under 18 years

Patient education

- instruct the patient not to exceed maximum dose or frequency of application
- the patient should be advised that cooling the treatment area and use of NSAIDs and/or antihistamines may alleviate symptoms of redness and flushing
- advise the patient to wash and dry skin and then smoothly apply cream over all areas of the face, avoiding missing areas
- warn the patient to avoid applying cream to eyes, eyelids, lips, mouth and inner nose membrane. If contact occurs, the area should be washed with copious amount of water
- the patient should be instructed that other creams and lotions (e.g. cosmetics, sunscreen) can be applied after the cream has dried
- advise the patient to avoid excess sunlight or sunlamps, and wear protective clothing and sunscreen with a high protective factor (SPF 30+) when going outdoors

Should be used during pregnancy only if benefits outweigh risks, and use close to delivery should be avoided.

No human data; use is not recommended.

CALCIPOTRIOL WITH BETAMETHASONE 50/500

Trade names
Calcipotriol/Betamethasone Sandoz 50/500, Daivobet 50/500, Enstilar, Klavanta

Available forms
Ointment: calcipotriol 50 microgram/g + betamethasone 500 microgram/g;
Foam spray: calcipotriol 50 microgram and 500 microgram betamethasone

Action
- derived from vitamin D and suppresses proliferation, reversing abnormal keratinocytic changes associated with psoriasis

Use
- chronic stable plaque psoriasis
- psoriasis vulgaris

Adverse effects
- skin and/or scalp irritation, peeling, bullous eruption
- initial exacerbation of psoriasis
- photosensitivity, skin discolouration
- (Uncommon) contact dermatitis, allergic reaction
- (Rare) hypercalcaemia

Interactions
- not recommended with calcium or vitamin D supplements, or other agents which increase availability of calcium

Nursing considerations/Cautions

- serum calcium and renal function should be monitored 3-monthly during therapy. If serum calcium becomes elevated, therapy should be stopped and serum calcium measured weekly until it returns to normal
- dose should not exceed total of 100 g per week
- not recommended for severe extensive psoriasis, generalised pustular psoriasis, guttate psoriasis or erythrodermic exfoliative psoriasis
- not recommended for use on the face; not for use in eyes

DERMATOLOGICAL AGENTS

- contraindicated in those with calcium metabolism disorders

Patient education

- instruct the patient to wash hands immediately after use to avoid transfer to face or other unaffected areas. If contact occurs, the area should be rinsed with water
- the patient should be advised to avoid calcium or vitamin D supplements during therapy
- warn the patient that psoriasis may be exacerbated initially, but this will subside
- the patient should be warned to use the cream/foam spray with caution in skin folds, as this may increase risk of irritation occurring
- advise the patient to avoid excess sunlight or sunlamps and to wear protective clothing and sunscreen with a high protective factor (SPF 30+) when going outdoors
- warn the patient that occlusive dressings should not be used
- advise the patient that the cream/foam spray is not recommended for use on the face
- instruct the patient that refrigeration of the cream is not recommended as it becomes more difficult to spread
- (Foam spray) instruct the patient on the following:
  - shake can well before use
  - holding can at least 3 cm from skin, spray affected area and gently rub in. If unaffected skin is sprayed, wipe foam off immediately
  - if scalp is being treated, hair should be combed to remove any loose scales. Spray foam into palm of hand and then use fingers to apply directly to affected scalp area (minimising application to hair). Hair should not be washed immediately after application. Use a mild non-medicated on dry hair to remove foam (as water dilutes shampoo making the foam difficult to remove). Massage shampoo into scalp, leave for a couple of minutes and then rinse with water
  - no more than 15g should be used in one day (this is the amount fully sprayed in one minute) and not more than 100 g in one week
  - if using cream and foam spray for psoriasis, total amount of calcipotriol should not exceed 15 g in one day or 100 g in one week

 Should be used during pregnancy only if benefits are thought to outweigh risks.

 Caution if used during breastfeeding. Cream/foam spray should not be used on breast.

CRISABOROLE
Trade name
Staquis

Available form
Ointment: 20 mg/g (2% w/w)

Action
- phosphodiesterase-4 (PDE-4) inhibitor that suppresses inflammation and secretion of some cytokines

Use
- mild-to-moderate atopic dermatitis in patients over 2 years old

Dose
- apply a thin layer to affected areas twice daily for up to 28 days

Adverse effects
- application site pain, infection
- eczema, contact dermatitis
- fever
- headache
- cough, nasopharyngitis, upper respiratory tract infection, oropharyngeal pain, sinusitis, asthma, pharyngitis
- vomiting

Nursing considerations/Cautions
- contraindicated in those with hypersensitivity to paraffin, propylene glycol or sodium calcium edetate

Patient education
- instruct the patient (or whoever is applying the ointment) to wash hands after application (unless the hands are being treated)

Recommended during pregnancy only if benefits outweigh risks.

Should not be applied to breasts if the woman is breastfeeding.

DEOXYCHOLIC ACID
Trade name
Belkyra

Available form
Solution for injection: 10 mg/mL

Action
- causes lysis of adipocyte cell membranes, resulting in macrophages being attracted to the area to remove cellular debris and lipids by natural processes

Use
- non-surgical fat removal under chin (submental convexity fullness) for contoured neck profile and jawline

Dose
- 2 mg/cm^2 SC (consisting of up to 50 injections of 0.2 mL spaced 1 cm apart)

Adverse effects
- (Injection site) pain, swelling, haematoma, induration, erythema, pruritus, numbness, bleeding, warmth, bruising, discomfort, discolouration to area, nerve injury
- hypertension
- headache
- nausea
- swallowing difficulties
- (Uncommon) taste alteration, hoarseness
- (Uncommon) alopecia of area (male), urticaria, ulcer formation, hypersensitivity
- (Rare) skin ulceration and necrosis (due to superficial dermal injection)

Nursing considerations/Cautions
- before starting therapy, the patient should be screened for other potential causes for submental (chin) convexity fullness, such as thyromegaly or cervical lymphadenopathy
- should be administered only by a medical practitioner who has good knowledge of submental anatomy, neuromuscular structures and any alterations to anatomy in that particular patient (e.g. due to previous surgery). Needle placement with respect to the mandible is important in reducing potential injury to the marginal mandibular nerve (which could result in paralysis of lip depressor muscle)
- the number of injections and number of treatments is dependent on the patient's fat distribution and treatment goals. Up to 6 single treatments may be given at intervals of at least 4 weeks apart
- patient comfort can be increased by use of topical or injectable local anaesthetic or ice/cold packs
- administer only SC
- the vial should be inverted gently several times before use
- the solution should not be diluted before administration
- pressure may be applied to injection sites to minimise bleeding
- contains 4.23 mg (184 mmol) sodium per mL, which may need to be considered if the patient is on a sodium-restricted diet
- caution if used in those over 65 years, and not recommended in those under 18 years
- caution if there is any inflammation or induration in the area to be injected
- caution if used in patients who have had other procedures to the area, such as surgery, liposuction or other injections, such as Botox

DERMATOLOGICAL AGENTS

- caution if used in those who have excessive skin laxity, prominent platysmal bands or other conditions that may result in suboptimal results
- caution if used in those with bleeding abnormalities or taking antiplatelet or anticoagulant medication because of the risk of excessive bleeding and bruising
- not recommended in patients with previous or current history of dysphagia, as the condition may be exacerbated
- not recommended in patients with mild or extreme submental (chin) fat
- contraindicated if there is infection at the treatment site

Patient education

- the patient should be advised to seek medical attention if any of the following occur:
  - troubling swallowing or taste disturbance
  - uneven smile
  - discolouration or ulceration at the injection site
  - tingling or reduced sensation around the mouth
  - (Male) unusual hair loss around the injection site

Not recommended during pregnancy owing to limited information.

Not recommended while breastfeeding owing to limited information.

IMIQUIMOD
Trade names
Aldara, Aldiq

Available form
Cream: 50 mg/g (5%)

Action
- topical immune response modifier with no direct antiviral activity

Use
- superficial basal cell carcinoma (where surgery is inappropriate)
- solar (actinic) keratosis (face/scalp)
- external genital and perianal warts (condyloma acuminate)

Dose
- (Solar keratosis) apply a thin layer of cream 3 times weekly for 4 weeks. Can be repeated for up to 16 weeks **OR**
- (Superficial basal cell carcinoma) apply a thin layer of cream once a day for 5 consecutive days; continue this for 6 weeks **OR**
- (External genital and perianal warts) apply a thin layer of cream 3 times weekly at bedtime until warts disappear or up to 16 weeks maximum

Adverse effects

(For use in external genital and anal warts)
- (Application site) erythema, oedema, erosion, scabbing, itching, burning or stinging sensation, tenderness, rash, irritation, excoriation/flaking, induration, pain
- headache, flu-like symptoms, myalgia, fatigue
- (Uncommon) infection, hypopigmentation

Interactions
- caution if used with other immunosuppressing agents

Nursing considerations/Cautions

- repeat courses are not recommended if the patient is immunocompromised
- efficacy may be reduced in those with HIV (although the reason for this is unclear)
- not recommended on broken skin; therefore the area should be allowed to heal before starting therapy
- not recommended for urethral, intravaginal, cervical, rectal or intra-anal warts

Patient education

- advise the patient that it usually takes 8–10 weeks for warts to disappear, but may clear sooner
- the patient should be advised to seek medical attention if warts recur

- instruct the patient that sexual (genital, anal, oral) contact should be avoided while the cream is on the skin
- if the skin reaction is severe, advise the patient to wash the area with mild soap and water and stop therapy for several days until irritation has settled, and then restart (there is no need to make up missed doses)
- the cream may weaken condoms and vaginal diaphragms; therefore alternative forms of contraception are recommended during therapy
- advise the patient to select 3 days for therapy (e.g. Monday, Wednesday and Friday or Tuesday, Thursday and Saturday), as this will improve adherence with the therapy regimen
- instruct the patient to avoid application of excessive cream, as this will only increase the risk of irritation
- if severe irritation occurs, advise the patient that the area can be covered with a non-occlusive dressing (such as cotton gauze or cotton underwear), but an occlusive dressing should not be used
- female patients should be advised to avoid applying cream near the vaginal opening, as skin reactions on the mucosal membrane may occur resulting in pain and/or swelling, which may further result in difficulty passing urine
- uncircumcised male patients with wart(s) under the foreskin should be instructed to retract the foreskin and clean the area daily to prevent foreskin tightness and stricture, which may occur with cream use. Patients should be advised to immediately report any local skin reactions (induration, swelling, erosion, ulceration) or difficulty retracting the foreskin
- instruct the patient as follows:
  - cream is available in single-use sachets or pump
  - after removing the protective cap, the pump should be primed until cream appears in the nozzle
  - 4 pump actuations = 250 mg sachet (and is sufficient to cover an area of 20 cm^2)
  - hands should be washed thoroughly before and after cream application
  - wash the application area with mild soap, rinse and dry
  - apply cream and rub in until not visible
  - leave the cream on wart(s) for 6—10 hours (overnight) and then wash off with mild soap and water
  - the patient should not bathe or shower while cream is on the skin
  - replace the protective cap on pump
  - the pump should be discarded 4 weeks after opening

No human data; use is not recommended, seek medical advice before use.

No human data; use is not recommended, seek medical advice before use.

MINOXIDIL
Trade names
Hair A-Gain, Men's Regaine Extra Strength, Women's Regaine

Available forms
Liquid: 20 mg/mL (2%), 50 mg/mL (5%); Foam: 50 mg/mL (5%)

Action
- (Topical) stimulates hair growth, although the exact mechanism of action is unknown

Use
- alopecia androgenetica (hereditary/common baldness) (in healthy males and females)

Dose
- (Solution) 1 mL (2% solution for females, 5% solution for males) applied and massaged gently into scalp twice daily (maximum daily dose 2 mL) **OR**
- (Foam — male) up to $^1/_2$ capful (depending on size of hair loss) applied and massaged gently into scalp twice daily **OR**

DERMATOLOGICAL AGENTS

- (Foam — female) up to $\frac{1}{2}$ capful (depending on size of hair loss) applied and massaged gently into scalp once daily

Adverse effects
- (Topical) dermatitis, rash, acne, redness, scaling, burning, itching, dry skin/scalp, transient hair shedding
- headache, peripheral oedema, dyspnoea, pruritus, rash
- (Rare) (women) hypertrichosis (including facial hair growth)
- (Rare) allergic reactions

Interactions
- not recommended with topical retinoids, topical corticosteroids or other skin preparations
- caution if given with other vasodilators
- not recommended with other topical scalp preparations

Nursing considerations/Cautions
- the scalp should be examined before starting therapy for any signs of infection or inflammation and, if they exist, therapy should not be started until conditions have resolved
- therapy should be discontinued after 6 months if no regrowth has occurred
- not recommended for any areas of the body other than the scalp
- not recommended in those with heart disease
- contraindicated in those with hypersensitivity to other formulations of minoxidil or propylene glycol or ethanol
- contraindicated in those with non-familial baldness, unexplained hair loss, scalp inflammation or if any pain, infection or irritation of scalp exists
- contraindicated in those over 65 years or under 18 years

Patient education
- ensure the patient understands that foam/lotion should be applied to the scalp only (no other parts of the body)
- warn the patient that there may be some transient hair loss at the start of therapy (first 2—6 weeks)
- the patient should be advised to immediately report any fluid retention or unexplained weight gain, swollen feet or hands, chest pain, rapid heartbeat, faintness or dizziness
- warn the patient not to drive or operate machinery if dizziness occurs
- instruct the patient that hair and scalp should be dry before applying the lotion/foam
- advise the patient not to use the hair dryer to speed up the drying process, because heat may decrease effectiveness
- instruct the patient to wash hands thoroughly after applying lotion/foam
- (Lotion) the patient should be instructed to use the dropper applicator and apply to the centre of the affected area first (not exceeding 2 mL daily dose) regardless of size of bald spot, massaged gently into the scalp and then left for at least 2 hours (up to 4 hours)
- (Foam) instruct patient to hold the can upside down and press the nozzle down to dispense up to $\frac{1}{2}$ capful into the palm, massage gently into scalp and then leave for at least 2 hours (up to 4 hours)
- (Foam) warn the patient that hands should be cold when using foam, otherwise it will melt on contact with warm hands. Rinse hands under cold water and ensure they are dry before using foam
- warn the patient that hair regrowth usually takes at least 4 months of twice-daily application for males (once per day for females) to become noticeable and, when therapy is discontinued, hair growth will stop and pretreatment appearance will be restored in 3—4 months
- the patient should be advised to allow 1 hour before applying protective headgear (e.g. bicycle or motorbike helmet)

- warn the patient to avoid contact with eyes, mucous membranes or abraded skin. If contact occurs, the area should be washed with copious quantities of cold water

Insufficient human data available; use is not recommended.

Insufficient human data available; use is not recommended.

Note
- minoxidil is also available as Loniten (tablets) for use as adjunctive therapy for hypertension unresponsive to multiple therapies

PIMECROLIMUS
Trade name
Elidel

Available form
Cream: 10 mg/g (1%)

Action
- anti-inflammatory, ascomycin macrolactam derivative calcineurin inhibitor

Use
- atopic dermatitis (eczema) (short-term management of signs and symptoms, or intermediate long-term management of emerging or resolving lesions where corticosteroids are not yet warranted, no longer needed or not recommended) in those over 3 months of age

Dose
- apply a thin layer to the affected area and rub in completely twice daily for up to 6 weeks

Adverse effects
- transient skin burning/warmth sensation
- irritation, pruritus, erythema, folliculitis
- lymphadenopathy
- (Rare) skin cancer, lymphoma, hypersensitivity, allergic reactions

Nursing considerations/Cautions
- any bacterial or fungal infection should be treated during therapy. If infection continues, pimecrolimus should be ceased until infection is controlled
- not recommended if an acute viral skin infection (e.g. cold sore) is present, on skin post-vaccination
- not recommended with phototherapy
- not recommended for skin areas where skin cancer has been removed, affected by premalignant changes (e.g. actinic keratoses), or in those with Netherton syndrome or generalised erythroderma (severely inflamed, damaged skin), or if immunocompromised
- contraindicated in those with hypersensitivity to macrolactams

Patient education
- instruct the patient that the cream should be completely rubbed in
- the patient should be warned that a feeling of warmth and/or burning sensation is common on application and is transient
- advise the patient/carer to avoid excess sunlight or sunlamps, and to wear protective clothing and sunscreen with a high protective factor (SPF 30+) when going outdoors
- the patient should be instructed to apply cream only to areas that are eczematous
- instruct the patient to avoid using excessive amounts of cream. In an adult, a fingertip of cream is sufficient to cover an area equivalent to two hands
- the patient/carer should be instructed to wash hands after application
- warn the patient to avoid contact with eyes, nose or mouth, areas of viral infection (such as cold sores), areas post-vaccination or breasts (if breastfeeding)
- advise the patient that treatment should be restarted at the first sign of recurrence (e.g. itching, scratching, persistent redness, thickening of skin)

DERMATOLOGICAL AGENTS

- if using a moisturiser, the patient should be instructed to use it after pimecrolimus cream. If having a shower or bath, use moisturiser first, then apply pimecrolimus cream
- ensure the patient/carer understands that occlusive dressings over cream are not recommended
- advise the patient to seek medical advice if any of the following occur:
  - condition worsens
  - condition shows no improvement after 6 weeks
  - any skin infection occurs

Insufficient human data available; use is not recommended.

Insufficient human data available; use is not recommended. If used, should not be applied to breast area.

PODOPHYLLOTOXIN
Trade name
Condyline Paint

Available form
Paint: 5 mg/mL

Action
- antimitotic agent that causes necrosis of wart tissue

Use
- anogenital warts (condylomata acuminate) in males and females

Dose
- sufficient paint using the provided applicator to cover wart is applied twice daily for 3 consecutive days, with 4 drug-free days, repeated initially for 4 weeks; if the wart is not removed, seek medical advice

Adverse effects
- tenderness, pain, itching, smarting, burning, erythema, superficial epithelial ulceration, skin discolouration
- (Males) inflammation of glans and foreskin (balanoposthitis)

Nursing considerations/Cautions
- medical supervision is recommended for lesions in females or if > 4 cm² in males
- increased risk of systemic adverse effects with prolonged use, involvement of an extensive area of skin, if the skin is friable or bleeding, or if applied to recently biopsied skin. This risk is also increased if applied to mucous membrane or healthy skin
- treatment can be repeated for a total of 5 weeks if needed
- contraindicated in those with open surgical wounds, inflamed or bleeding lesions, or in children

Patient education
- instruct the patient to wash their hands before and after applying the paint
- the patient should be advised to wash the area thoroughly with soap and water and dry before application of paint; allow the paint to dry after applications
- warn the patient to avoid contact with eyes and mucous membranes; rinse with water immediately if contact occurs
- instruct the patient to apply using applicator supplied
- the patient should be advised that local irritation may increase on day 2 or 3 of therapy as the wart starts to respond (i.e. becomes necrotic), but it will decrease with ongoing treatment
- warn the patient to apply paint to the wart only and avoid healthy surrounding tissue, because prolonged exposure may harm healthy skin or increase the risk of systemic absorption
- instruct the patient to discard the paint solution 6 weeks after opening

Contraindicated during pregnancy.

Contraindicated while breastfeeding.

DISEASE-MODIFYING ANTIRHEUMATIC DRUGS (DMARDS)

Arthritis refers to a variety of joint diseases, including common forms such as osteoarthritis (OA), rheumatoid arthritis (RA), juvenile idiopathic arthritis and spondyloarthropathies (e.g. ankylosing spondylitis). As of 2022, an estimated 3.7 million Australians (or 15% of the population) are living with some form of arthritis. RA affects approximately 514,000 people, or 2% of the population (AIHW 2024f).

RA is a chronic autoimmune disease primarily characterised by inflammation and thickening of the synovial membrane (synovitis), which leads to tissue destruction, cartilage erosion and potential tendon rupture. While RA is known for affecting the small joints of the hands and feet, it can also impact the entire body, including organs such as the heart, lungs, nerves and eyes. Common symptoms include joint pain, swelling, stiffness and loss of function. The disease often follows an unpredictable and rapidly progressing course, even with treatment (AIHW 2024f).

Early diagnosis and treatment with disease-modifying antirheumatic drugs (DMARDs) are critical for slowing disease progression and achieving remission. Studies show that early DMARD use improves long-term functional outcomes and quality of life compared with older treatment approaches, which primarily relied on non-steroidal anti-inflammatory drugs (NSAIDs) for initial management.

DMARDs represent a diverse category of drugs that help manage autoimmune diseases by modifying the underlying disease process, rather than merely relieving symptoms. While their mechanisms are not fully understood, they are primarily used for treating RA but are also employed in managing other autoimmune conditions such as Crohn's disease, psoriatic arthritis and systemic lupus erythematosus.

DMARDs are generally categorised into:
- *Conventional DMARDs*: examples include methotrexate, gold and sulfasalazine. These are often the first line of treatment in RA.
- *Immunosuppressants*: this group includes drugs such as ciclosporin, azathioprine and leflunomide, which modulate the immune response to prevent further joint damage.
- *Cytokine modulators*: these drugs, such as abatacept, anakinra and rituximab, specifically target cytokines,

DISEASE-MODIFYING ANTIRHEUMATIC DRUGS (DMARDS)

which are molecules that promote inflammation.

- *TNF-α antagonists*: these include adalimumab and infliximab, which specifically inhibit tumour necrosis factor alpha (TNF-α), a substance that plays a major role in inflammatory processes in RA (Knights et al 2023). The onset of action for DMARDs is often slow, requiring weeks or months before significant clinical improvement is observed. They are commonly used alone or in combination with other DMARDs, NSAIDs or corticosteroids to manage inflammation and control disease progression (Knights et al 2023).

Adjunctive treatment for RA should encompass a multidisciplinary approach that includes physiotherapy, occupational therapy and a structured exercise regimen tailored to maintain joint flexibility, muscle strength and overall mobility. These therapies can significantly improve daily functioning and help manage pain and stiffness.

Patient education is also important, ensuring that individuals with RA are empowered with knowledge about their condition and treatment options. Access to support services, such as those offered by organisations like Arthritis Australia, provides emotional support and resources to help manage the chronic nature of RA. Support services often include counselling, peer support groups and information on managing the disease in everyday life, improving both physical and mental health outcomes for patients (Arthritis Australia 2024).

CONVENTIONAL DMARDs

AURANOFIN

Trade name
Ridaura

Available forms
Tablets: 3 mg;
Capsules: 3 mg

Action
- synthetic gold complex that decreases inflammation, levels of rheumatoid factor and elevated immunoglobulin levels
- may slow progression of joint erosion
- anti-inflammatory action
- clinical improvement seen in 3—4 months after initiation of therapy (although some people may take longer)
- half-life increased from about 17 days to 26 days after 6 months of therapy

Use
- rheumatoid arthritis (unresponsive or intolerant to non-steroidal anti-inflammatory drugs (NSAIDs)

Dose
- initially 6 mg orally daily with food, increasing to 9 mg in 3 divided doses if needed after 4—6 months

Adverse effects
- diarrhoea or loose stools, constipation, flatulence
- anorexia, nausea, vomiting, abdominal pain/cramps, dyspepsia, distorted taste, stomatitis, glossitis
- conjunctivitis
- rash, pruritus, phototoxicity
- hair loss
- leucopenia, granulocytopenia, anaemia, thrombocytopenia
- haematuria, proteinuria, increased blood urea and serum creatinine, nephrotoxicity
- increased liver enzymes
- (Rare) ulcerative enterocolitis

Interactions

- contraindicated with other agents causing blood dyscrasias or bone marrow depression
- contraindicated with leflunomide
- contraindicated with clozapine, antimalarial agents, penicillamine or immunosuppressants
- caution if used with warfarin or clonidine
- may increase effects of radiotherapy
- caution if given with angiotensin converting enzyme (ACE) inhibitors owing to a risk of vasomotor reaction (see Glossary)
- increased risk of nephrotoxicity and/or haemotoxicity if given with alcohol, aminoglycosides, amphotericin B, penicillins, phenytoin, sulfonamides, NSAIDs or aciclovir
- may increase serum levels of phenytoin, increasing the risk of adverse effects, including skin reactions; therefore phenytoin levels should be closely monitored
- delayed hypersensitivity may occur if given with aspirin or penicillins
- absorption may be decreased if given with prokinetic agents (e.g. loperamide) or laxatives
- caution if given with theophylline

Nursing considerations/Cautions

- diabetes, heart failure or hypertension should be controlled or corrected before starting therapy
- renal and liver function tests, blood count (with differential white cell count), haemoglobin and complete urinalysis (with urinary protein levels) should be performed before starting therapy
- monthly blood counts (with differential white cell count), platelet count and urinary protein levels are recommended
- ophthalmological examination is recommended periodically throughout therapy
- annual chest X-ray is recommended
- GI symptoms are dose related and those with low bodyweight are at greatest risk
- auranofin-induced diarrhoea can be controlled by decreasing the dose
- daily dose > 9 mg is not recommended
- overlap or washout period not required if transferring from injectable gold preparations
- tablets contain lactose and are therefore not recommended in those with galactose intolerance, Lapp lactase deficiency or glucose—galactose malabsorption
- caution if used in those with inflammatory bowel disease, a history of bone marrow depression or atopy, or liver/kidney dysfunction
- not recommended in those with porphyria, systemic sclerosis or Sjögren's syndrome
- not recommended in those who have undergone recent radiotherapy
- contraindicated in those with previous toxicity or sensitivity to gold or heavy metals, severe liver/kidney disease, severe chronic dermatitis, bone marrow depression, bone marrow aplasia, haematological disorders or gold-induced pulmonary fibrosis, necrotising enterocolitis or systemic lupus erythematosus (SLE)

Patient education

- the patient should be warned that diarrhoea is a common adverse effect, especially in those of low bodyweight
- advise the patient to avoid alcohol during therapy
- instruct the patient to avoid exposure to strong direct sunlight and, if outdoors, they should wear protective clothing and SPF 30+ sunscreen
- the patient should be advised to seek medical advice immediately if any of the following occur:
  - diarrhoea with rectal bleeding or rectal bleeding alone
  - any metallic taste, sore throat or tongue, mouth ulceration, easy bruising, bleeding gums, blood nose, heavy menstrual bleeding, bleeding

DISEASE-MODIFYING ANTIRHEUMATIC DRUGS (DMARDS)

under the skin resembling purple rash (sign of impending toxicity)
- itching (pruritus), rash (early sign of intolerance)
- counsel women of childbearing age to use adequate contraception during and for at least 6 months after stopping therapy because gold is slowly excreted from the body, which may have negative effects on a developing fetus

Tablet can be dispersed in water, or crushed and mixed with a spoonful of yoghurt or apple puree.

Limited human data. Evidence of fetal damage has been seen in animal studies; significance in humans is uncertain. Women of childbearing potential should use effective contraception during treatment.

Not recommended during breastfeeding. Gold is slowly excreted from the body after stopping therapy; this should be taken into account if a woman wants to breastfeed.

Contraindicated in progressive renal disease.

Contraindicated in moderate or severe hepatic impairment. Liver function tests should be monitored regularly in all patients.

Elderly patients may be more susceptible to adverse effects. Close monitoring of renal and hepatic function is recommended. Start at the lower end of the dosing range and adjust as needed.

CICLOSPORIN (CYCLOSPORIN)
Trade names
APO-Ciclosporin, Cequa, Ciclosporin-WGR, Ikervis, Neoral, Sandimmun IV

Available forms
Capsules: 10 mg, 25 mg, 50 mg, 100 mg; Oral solution: 100 mg/mL; Ampoules: 50 mg/mL; Eye drops: 0.1%

Action
- potent immunosuppressive agent (calcineurin inhibitor)
- thought to act by blocking both lymphocytes and antigen-triggered lymphokine release by activated T cells
- half-life 6.3 hours, increasing to 20.4 hours in those with severe liver disease

Use
- prevent or delay organ rejection after transplantation
- prevention of graft versus host disease in organ transplantation
- induction and/or maintenance of remission in nephrotic syndrome (when other therapies have been ineffective or inappropriate and renal function is still intact)
- severe, active rheumatoid arthritis (when other therapies have been ineffective or inappropriate)
- severe psoriasis (when other therapies have been ineffective or inappropriate)
- severe atopic dermatitis (when other therapies have been ineffective or inappropriate)

Dose
- (Rheumatoid arthritis) 3 mg/kg daily orally in 2 divided doses for first 6 weeks of therapy (which may be continued to 12 weeks for full effectiveness). If there is no clinical response in 4—8 weeks, the dose may be increased by 0.5—1.0 mg/kg/day at 1—2-month intervals to 5 mg/kg/day maximum. If the patient has been stable for at least 3 months, the dose may be decreased by 0.5 mg/kg/day at 1—2-month intervals to achieve the lowest effective dose **OR**
- (Psoriasis) 2.5 mg/kg orally daily in 2 divided doses, increasing to 5 mg/kg if there is no clinical response in 4 weeks (daily maximum 5 mg/kg) **OR**
- (Nephrotic syndrome) 2.5—5 mg/kg/day, decreasing to lowest effective dose (maintenance) **OR**
- (Atopic dermatitis) initially 2.5—5 mg/kg orally daily in 2 divided doses, reducing

1041

dose gradually when satisfactory response has been achieved **OR**
- (Organ transplantation) initially 10–15 mg/kg orally 4–12 hours pre-transplant, continued for 1–2 weeks postoperatively, then gradually reduced to 2–6 mg/kg/day as single or 2 divided doses (maintenance) **OR**
- (Organ transplantation) 3–5 mg/kg/day by IV infusion over 2–6 hours, started 4–12 hours pre-transplant, then starting oral dosing as soon as possible post-transplant

Adverse effects
- hypertension
- fluid retention and oedema, weight increase
- hyperkalaemia, hyperuricaemia, hypomagnesaemia, hyperlipidaemia
- fever, flushing
- tremor, fatigue, burning sensation in hands and feet (initially)
- muscle cramps, myalgia
- headache/migraine, paraesthesia, convulsions
- hirsutism, rash, acne
- dysmenorrhoea/amenorrhoea (reversible)
- gingival hypertrophy
- anorexia, nausea, vomiting, diarrhoea, abdominal pain, peptic ulceration
- anaemia, leucopenia
- increased susceptibility to or aggravation of infection (local or general)
- impaired renal function, hepatic dysfunction, acute pancreatitis
- increased risk of malignancy
- (IV) anaphylactoid reactions

Interactions
- increased risk of nephrotoxicity when low-dose ciclosporin is given with NSAIDs, requiring regular monitoring of kidney function
- may increase serum levels of sirolimus, everolimus and anthracyclines (e.g. doxorubicin), increasing the risk of toxicity
- may lead to increase in blood pressure if given with recombinant human erythropoietin
- increased risk of nephrotoxicity if given with tacrolimus
- increase in BP may result if given with recombinant human erythropoietin
- caution if given with lercanidipine, as serum level of both agents may be increased
- increased risk of hyperkalaemia if given with potassium-containing or potassium-sparing medications, including potassium-sparing diuretics, angiotensin converting enzyme (ACE) inhibitors and angiotensin II receptor antagonists
- not recommended with UVB irradiation or psoralen plus ultraviolet A (PUVA) photochemotherapy because of increased risk of skin cancer development
- reversible renal impairment may occur if given with fenofibrate or other fibric acid derivatives
- not recommended with other known nephrotoxic drugs such as aminoglycosides, amphotericin B (amphotericin), ciprofloxacin, colchicine, histamine H_2 antagonists, melphalan, methotrexate, NSAIDs, trimethoprim and vancomycin. If used together, serum creatinine and renal function should be closely monitored
- serum levels may be increased if given with allopurinol, amiodarone, azole antifungal agents, cholic acid, colchicine, danazol, diltiazem, doxycycline, grapefruit juice, imatinib, macrolide antibiotics, metoclopramide, methylprednisolone (high dose), oral contraceptives, protease inhibitors, verapamil or voriconazole, increasing the risk of toxicity
- not recommended with atorvastatin or simvastatin because of an increased risk of muscle toxicity (muscle pain, weakness, myositis, rhabdomyolysis) due to decreased clearance. Caution if used

DISEASE-MODIFYING ANTIRHEUMATIC DRUGS (DMARDS)

- with pravastatin, fluvastatin or rosuvastatin
- may increase serum levels of repaglinide, increasing the risk of hypoglycaemia occurring
- serum levels may be decreased if given with barbiturates, bosentan, carbamazepine, ciprofloxacin, isoniazid, octreotide, orlistat, oxcarbazepine, phenytoin, rifampicin, St John's wort or sulfamethoxazole/trimethoprim (IV)
- not recommended with thiazide or loop diuretics because of the increased risk of hyperuricaemia and gout. Serum uric acid levels should be monitored if any signs of gout occur
- not recommended with live or live attenuated vaccines
- caution if used with alcohol
- an increased risk of gingival hyperplasia if given with nifedipine or amlodipine
- may decrease clearance (and therefore increase blood levels) of ambrisentan, bosentan, colchicine, dabigatran, digoxin, etoposide, prednisolone or statins, and increasing the risk of toxicity

Nursing considerations/Cautions

- capsules and oral solution are bioequivalent; however, changing between brands should be done carefully. Ciclosporin serum level, serum creatinine level and blood pressure should be measured at 2, 4 and 8 weeks (or within 4–7 days if used for transplant) after changeover. If blood pressure or creatinine levels are greater than the pre-changeover levels, decreasing the dose is recommended
- any infections should be identified and treated before starting therapy
- adverse effects are more common when ciclosporin is used for transplant patients than when used for other conditions because the dose is higher
- routine serum ciclosporin levels should be monitored in transplant patients, but not required in non-transplant patients unless indicated by risk of adverse reactions or potential drug interaction
- blood taken to measure routine serum levels should be taken immediately before the next dose is due and the collection time recorded
- blood pressure should be monitored regularly throughout therapy and hypertension treated with appropriate antihypertensive medication if it occurs. However, diuretic therapy should be avoided. If hypertension cannot be controlled, ciclosporin therapy should be stopped
- blood lipids should be measured before starting therapy and after 4 weeks of therapy. If lipids increase, the dose should be decreased and a fat-reduced diet commenced
- creatinine levels should be measured twice before and every 2 weeks during the first 3 months of therapy, then monthly. Doses should then be adjusted accordingly. Therapy should stop if reducing the dose does not reduce creatinine levels within 1 month. Creatinine levels should be measured more frequently when the dose of ciclosporin is increased or if the patient is taking NSAIDs concurrently
- serum bilirubin and urea should be measured before starting and regularly throughout therapy
- serum potassium levels should be monitored regularly, as should serum uric acid levels in high-risk patients (e.g. gout) and serum magnesium (as hypomagnesaemia increases risk of neurotoxicity)
- (Nephrotic syndrome) the dose is dependent on renal function. If improvement is not seen in 12 weeks, therapy should be stopped
- (Nephrotic syndrome) renal biopsy is recommended if therapy continues for 12 months
- (Psoriasis) any unusual lesions should be biopsied before starting therapy to decrease risk of cancer occurring

- (Psoriasis) if there is no improvement within 6 weeks of therapy at 5 mg/kg/day, therapy should be stopped
- (Atopic dermatitis) active herpes infection and skin infections should be treated before starting therapy
- (Atopic dermatitis) lymphadenopathy should be monitored during therapy. If lymphadenopathy is present after skin improves with therapy, a biopsy is recommended to rule out lymphoma
- (Atopic dermatitis) course can be continued for up to 12 months if tolerated
- (Atopic dermatitis) not recommended with PUVA photochemotherapy
- (Rheumatoid arthritis) patients appear to be at greater risk of nephrotoxicity
- (Rheumatoid arthritis) discontinue therapy if there is no improvement in 6 months where maximum tolerable dose has been achieved for 3 months
- (Organ transplant) if given as part of triple or quadruple drug therapy with other immunosuppressants (including corticosteroids), a decreased dose may be used (e.g. renal transplant patients may require a dose less than 5 mg/kg/day if given with corticosteroid)
- IV should be used only if the patient is unable to tolerate oral formulation
- (IV) a glass container should be used if available
- care should be taken during IV administration because the solution is highly irritant and can cause tissue damage if extravasation occurs
- IV concentrate should be diluted using sodium chloride 0.9% or glucose 5% to 1:20—1:100 concentration and infused over 2—6 hours
- any unused diluted solution should be discarded after 48 hours
- (Oral solution) 0.1 mL solution = 10 mg ciclosporin
- solution and capsules contain up to 12—13% v/v alcohol, while IV concentrate contains 34% v/v, which may need to be considered in patients with epilepsy, alcohol abuse problems or if pregnant or breastfeeding
- (Oral) caution if used in those with malabsorption problems, as reaching a therapeutic level may be difficult
- not recommended in those with severe heart, lung or peripheral vessel complications
- (Non-transplant use) contraindicated in those with uncontrolled hypertension or infection, primary or secondary immunodeficiency, impaired baseline renal function with serum creatinine greater than 200 micromol/L (nephrotic syndrome use), any renal impairment (other uses), or any existing malignant or premalignant conditions
- (IV) contraindicated in those with hypersensitivity to polyoxyethylated castor oil

Patient education

- advise the patient to avoid heavy alcohol use while taking ciclosporin, especially red wine
- instruct the patient to take doses 12 hours apart at the same time each day
- caution the patient to swallow capsules whole, with or without food
- advise the patient that the oral solution comes with two syringes (1 mL and 4 mL). The 1 mL syringe should be used for doses less than or equal to 1 mL, while the 4 mL syringe is used for doses between 1 mL and 4 mL
- instruct the patient to dilute oral solution of ciclosporin with apple or orange juice (not grapefruit) or a soft drink and stir well before drinking immediately. The glass should be rinsed with more juice or soft drink to ensure the whole dose is taken
- warn the patient to avoid grapefruit juice during therapy
- instruct the patient that the dose-dispensing syringe should not come into contact with juice or soft drink when diluting the solution and should

- be wiped clean, not rinsed with water or other fluids
- the patient should be advised to avoid foods high in potassium (e.g. sweet potatoes, potatoes, bananas, milk, spinach) and potassium-containing or potassium-sparing medications to avoid an increase in potassium levels
- counsel the patient to avoid excessive unprotected sun exposure because of an increased risk of skin cancer and to wear a hat, use SPF 30+ sunscreen and wear protective clothing if sun exposure cannot be avoided
- educate the patient regarding care of teeth and gums during therapy
- instruct the patient to discard the oral solution 2 months after opening
- advise the patient that the oral solution should be stored in a cool dark place (20−25°C), but not refrigerated. Oily components of ciclosporin may solidify below 20°C and a jelly-like substance may also result. This is reversible at warmer temperatures and does not affect the safety or efficacy

An oral solution is available. Capsules should not be opened or crushed. They are designed to be swallowed whole to ensure proper release and absorption.

May cause immunosuppression in the infant. The experience with using ciclosporin in pregnancy is still limited. Use only if the potential benefit justifies the potential risk to the fetus.

Passes into breastmilk. Mothers receiving treatment with ciclosporin should not breastfeed their infants.

Reduced renal function: may impair renal function. Serum creatinine should be monitored regularly, and dosage should be adjusted to avoid toxicity.

Reduced hepatic function: monitor liver function regularly, as ciclosporin may cause increases in serum bilirubin and liver enzymes. If liver dysfunction is detected, dose adjustments may be required.

Use with caution, starting at the low end of the dosing range, considering the greater frequency of decreased hepatic, renal or cardiac function, and concomitant diseases or other drug therapy in the elderly.

HYDROXYCHLOROQUINE

Trade names
APO-Hydroxychloroquine, Hydroxychloroquine GH, Hequinel, Plaquenil, Rusquen

Available form
Tablets: 200 mg

Action
- aminoquinoline antimalarial that has unknown therapeutic actions in rheumatoid arthritis and systemic and discoid lupus erythematosus
- active against erythrocytic forms of *Plasmodium vivax* and *Plasmodium malariae* and most strains of *Plasmodium falciparum* (not gametocytes of *P. falciparum*)
- does not prevent relapses because it is not active against exo-erythrocytic phases
- stops acute attacks and lengthens the time between treatment and relapses (*P. vivax*, *P. malariae*). With *P. falciparum*, complete cure may be possible if the organism is not resistant to hydroxychloroquine
- not effective against chloroquine-resistant strains of *P. falciparum*
- onset of action: may take 2−6 months before benefits are apparent

Use
- rheumatoid arthritis
- systemic and discoid lupus erythematosus (mild)
- treatment and suppression of malaria

Dose
- (Lupus erythematosus) initially 400−800 mg orally daily for several weeks, reducing to a maintenance dose of 200−400 mg daily **OR**
- (Rheumatoid arthritis) initially 400−600 mg orally daily with food,

increasing the dose slowly after 5–10 days until an optimal dose is achieved without adverse effects for 4–12 weeks, reducing to a maintenance dose of 200–400 mg daily when clinical improvement is established (daily maximum 6 mg/kg) **OR**
- (Acute malaria treatment) initially 800 mg orally, then 400 mg 6–8 hours later, followed by 400 mg daily for 2 consecutive days or 800 mg as a single oral dose (total dose 2 g) **OR**
- (Malaria suppression/prophylaxis) 400 mg orally as a single weekly dose starting 2 weeks before exposure and continuing for 8 weeks after leaving a malarial area (if unable to start 2 weeks before exposure, 2 doses of 400 mg are taken 6 hours apart)

Adverse effects
- nausea, abdominal pain, diarrhoea, vomiting, anorexia
- blurred vision
- rash, pruritus, skin dryness, increased skin pigmentation
- alopecia
- headache
- hypoglycaemia
- (Uncommon) vertigo, tinnitus, corneal or retinal changes, photophobia, halos, dizziness, nerve deafness, bleaching of hair
- (Rare) bone marrow depression, muscle weakness, decreased/absent deep tendon reflexes, exacerbate or precipitate porphyria, cardiomyopathy, seizures
- (Very rare) suicidal behaviours, extrapyramidal disorder

Interactions
- incompatible with monoamine oxidase inhibitors (MAOIs)
- use with digoxin may increase plasma digoxin levels, leading to toxicity; therefore digoxin levels should be closely monitored during therapy
- may enhance hypoglycaemic action of insulin or oral hypoglycaemic agents
- may lower convulsive threshold, increasing the risk of seizures. This is enhanced if given with other antimalarial agents
- may impair antiepileptic effect, so should be used with caution
- caution if given with antiarrhythmic agents because of the risk of inducing ventricular arrhythmias
- may increase serum levels of ciclosporin

Nursing considerations/Cautions
- because the effect of hydroxychloroquine accumulates, maximum clinical effects may take several months to be achieved; however, side-effects may appear much earlier
- ophthalmological examination (colour vision, fundoscopy, visual fields) should be done before starting therapy and continued every 6 months during treatment or more often in those at high risk (e.g. dose > 6 mg/kg, elderly, kidney/liver impairment, visual problems in previous 8 years, low body weight). Visual disturbances/retinal changes can continue to occur after therapy has stopped
- patients on long-term therapy should have regular full blood counts, blood glucose levels and testing of knee and ankle reflexes to monitor muscle strength. If any weakness occurs, medication should be stopped
- if rash appears, the drug should be withdrawn and recommenced at a lower dose
- (Rheumatoid arthritis) any corticosteroid and/or salicylate dose may be decreased once hydroxychloroquine has been used for several weeks. Gradual reduction in corticosteroid dosage is recommended
- (Rheumatoid arthritis) therapy should be stopped if there is no clinical improvement (e.g. improved mobility, decreased joint swelling) in 6 months
- patients should be monitored for any signs of cardiomyopathy

DISEASE-MODIFYING ANTIRHEUMATIC DRUGS (DMARDS)

- caution if used in those with diabetes, kidney or liver impairment, quinine sensitivity or glucose-6-phosphate dehydrogenase (G6PD) deficiency
- not recommended in those with porphyria or psoriasis, as symptoms may become exacerbated, or in those with severe GI, neurological or blood disorders
- contraindicated in those with pre-existing maculopathy, hypersensitivity to 4-aminoquinolone compounds or as long-term therapy in children under 6 years

Patient education

- the patient should be advised to seek medical advice if any of the following occur:
  - visual disturbances (e.g. blurred vision, changes to night vision, light flashes or streaks)
  - rash, itchiness, dry skin or changes to pigmentation
- advise the patient that visual disturbance may occur or progress after therapy has ceased
- warn the patient about the dangers of driving or operating machinery if blurred vision occurs
- the patient should be advised to wear sunglasses in strong sunlight
- inform the patient that clinical effect may take months to be noticeable; however, adverse effects may occur sooner
- if the patient has diabetes, they should be instructed to monitor blood glucose levels closely, as hydroxychloroquine may cause hypoglycaemia. The dose of antidiabetic medications may need to be adjusted accordingly
- (Malaria prophylaxis) the patient should be advised to take the dose on same day of each week to increase likelihood of adherence to the regimen

 Tablet can be crushed (has a bitter taste) and mixed with water or a spoonful of yoghurt or apple puree.

 Avoid use: not recommended during pregnancy unless benefits outweigh the risks. May cause CNS damage, ototoxicity, retinal haemorrhage and abnormal retinal pigmentation in newborn. (Note: this is the recommendation for use as an antimalarial.)

 Excreted in breastmilk. Use with caution. Use only when benefits outweigh the risks.

 Use in renal impairment: dose reduction may be necessary.

Use in hepatic impairment: metabolised by the liver. Dose reduction may be necessary.

 Elderly patients may have an increased risk of ocular toxicity. Use with caution. More frequent ophthalmological monitoring may be necessary.

LEFLUNOMIDE
Trade names
APO-Leflunomide, Arava, Ataris, Leflunomide Generichealth, Leflunomide Sandoz, Leflunomide-WGR, Lunava

Available forms
Tablets: 10 mg, 20 mg

Action
- immunomodulating and immunosuppressant actions
- weak anti-inflammatory properties
- converted to active metabolite by first-pass metabolism in the gut wall and liver
- active metabolite has a long half-life of approximately 1—4 weeks
- clinical improvement may occur in 4 weeks, and usually occurs in 4—6 months

Use
- active rheumatoid arthritis
- active psoriatic arthritis

Dose
- initially 100 mg orally daily for 3 days (loading dose), then 10—20 mg daily (maintenance)

Adverse effects
- rash, hair loss (reversible), pruritus, dry skin, hair and skin discolouration
- allergic reaction
- diarrhoea, abdominal pain, dyspepsia, nausea, anorexia, vomiting, mouth ulceration, stomatitis, weight loss, dry mouth, altered taste
- sleep disorder
- anxiety
- reversible elevation of liver enzymes (alanine aminotransferase (ALT), aspartate aminotransferase (AST))
- urinary tract infection
- flu-like symptoms
- hypertension, chest pain, angina, tachycardia
- respiratory infection, bronchitis, cough, pharyngitis, sinusitis, rhinitis, pneumonia
- dizziness, headache, migraine
- paraesthesia, asthenia
- blurred vision
- hypokalaemia
- arthralgia, leg cramps, synovitis, tenosynovitis, back pain, neck pain, tendon rupture
- (Rare) haematological disorder, hepatitis, jaundice, severe infection
- (Very rare) severe skin reaction, interstitial lung disease, peripheral neuropathy

Interactions
- colestyramine and activated charcoal rapidly decrease plasma levels
- may increase plasma levels of rifampicin and phenytoin
- excessive alcohol intake should be avoided
- vaccination with live or live attenuated vaccines should be avoided during and for at least 6 months after finishing therapy
- not recommended with other agents that are hepatotoxic or haemotoxic/myelotoxic (e.g. methotrexate). If used together, increased monitoring of adverse effects is recommended
- caution if given with NSAIDs (including cyclo-oxygenase-2 (COX-2) inhibitors) because of increased risk of hepatotoxicity
- increased risk of peripheral neuropathy if used with other neurotoxic agents
- if given with warfarin, INR should be closely monitored
- may alter efficacy of combined oral contraceptives (ethinylestradiol, levonorgestrel)
- may increase serum levels of repaglinide, pioglitazone, paclitaxel or rosiglitazone
- may decrease efficacy of theophylline or duloxetine
- caution if used with benzylpenicillin, cefaclor, ciprofloxacin, indometacin (indomethacin), furosemide (frusemide), ketoprofen or zidovudine
- may increase serum levels of rifampicin, doxorubicin, methotrexate, sulfasalazine, daunorubicin, topotecan or 3-hydroxy-3-methylglutaryl coenzyme A (HMG-CoA) reductase inhibitors (e.g. rosuvastatin, simvastatin), increasing risk of toxicity or adverse effects

Nursing considerations/Cautions
- before starting, every 4 weeks for 6 months and then 6—8-weekly during therapy, the patient should have a full blood count (including differential white cell count), platelet count and liver function tests
- the patient should be carefully evaluated for any active or latent tuberculosis and closely monitored for any reactivation
- BP should be monitored before starting and throughout therapy
- treatment should be immediately ceased if ulcerative stomatitis is evident
- because of the long half-life (1—4 weeks) of the active metabolite, recovery from any adverse effects may take some time after ceasing therapy

DISEASE-MODIFYING ANTIRHEUMATIC DRUGS (DMARDS)

- the risk of adverse effects when given with methotrexate may be lessened by avoiding giving the loading dose
- (Washout procedure) leflunomide is stopped, then colestyramine 8 g orally 3 times daily or 50 g orally activated charcoal 4 times daily for 11 days total. Colestyramine and activated charcoal may both interfere with oral contraceptives, and therefore barrier forms of contraception should also be used. Plasma levels should be measured twice, 2 weeks apart after washout
- caution if used in those over 60 years or with diabetes mellitus because of the increased risk of peripheral neuropathy
- caution if used in those with kidney impairment
- contraindicated in those with severe immunodeficiency states, impaired bone marrow function, blood dyscrasias, significant anaemia, severe uncontrolled infection, liver impairment, severe hypoproteinaemia or those who have (or had) severe skin reactions (e.g. Stevens–Johnson syndrome, toxic epidermal necrolysis or erythema multiforme)

Patient education

- the patient should be advised to swallow the tablet whole with water, at the same time every day
- warn the patient to avoid excessive alcohol intake
- instruct the patient to seek medical advice immediately if any of the following occur:
    - sore throat, rash, excessive tiredness or flu-like symptoms
    - persistent cough, coughing up blood, fatigue or weight loss
    - fever, cough, breathing difficulties
    - pins & needles, numbness or weakness in arms or legs
    - recurring or persistent painful mouth ulcers
    - skin reaction
- caution the patient against driving or operating machinery if dizziness or blurred vision occurs
- the patient should be warned that clinical improvement may take 4 weeks; however, it may take longer
- before starting treatment, pregnancy must be excluded
- if a female patient is undergoing washout procedure prior to conception (see above), advise her to use a barrier method of contraception in addition to oral contraceptive, as failure may occur because of the colestyramine or activated charcoal
- counsel women of childbearing potential to use reliable contraception during therapy and the importance of telling their doctor if menstruation is delayed
- men and women are advised that levels of active metabolite should be below 0.02 mg/L on two separate tests taken 14 days apart before considering pregnancy after a washout procedure (see Nursing considerations above)

 Tablet should not be crushed or broken. Can be dispersed in 10–20 mL water (2–7 minutes dispersion time). The person handling the tablet should wear disposable gloves.

 Contraindicated during pregnancy, as teratogenic and may cause serious birth defects. Very high risk of causing permanent damage to the fetus. Women of childbearing potential must use effective contraception during treatment and until the drug is completely eliminated from the body. If pregnancy occurs, initiate a drug washout procedure using cholestyramine or activated charcoal to reduce plasma levels.

 Contraindicated during breastfeeding. Leflunomide and its metabolites pass into breastmilk.

Use in renal impairment: Monitor renal function closely. Dose adjustment may be necessary.

METHOTREXATE

Trade names
ARX-Methotrexate, Chexate, DBL Methotrexate, Methoblastin, Methotrexate Accord, Methotrexate Ebewe, Trexject

Available forms
Tablets: 2.5 mg, 10 mg;
Vial: 5 mg/2 mL, 50 mg/2 mL, 500 mg/5 mL, 500 mg/20 mL, 1000 mg/10 mL, 5000 mg/50 mL;
Prefilled syringe: 7.5 mg/0.15 mL, 7.5 mg/0.3 mL, 10 mg/0.2 mL, 10 mg/0.4 mL, 15 mg/0.3 mL, 15 mg/0.6 mL, 20 mg/0.4 mL, 20 mg/0.8 mL, 25 mg/0.5 mL, 25 mg/mL

Action
- antimetabolite antineoplastic agent
- inhibits metabolism of folic acid, thereby interfering with cell replication (especially in rapidly dividing cells such as dermal epithelial cells, and buccal, urinary bladder and intestinal cells)
- (Rheumatoid arthritis) decreases swelling, pain and stiffness in rheumatoid arthritis, but does not induce remission or affect bone erosion
- (Psoriasis) the rate of epithelial cell production in skin is increased; therefore methotrexate's action is due to its interference with this process
- may accumulate in third-space compartments (e.g. pleural effusions, ascites), resulting in prolonged half-life and toxicity
- onset of action may take 3—6 weeks, peak activity 1—4 hours (oral), 0.25—1 hour (IM) and 0.25—1.5 hours (SC)

Use
- antineoplastic chemotherapy (see Antineoplastic agents, p. 595)
- severe psoriasis that is unresponsive to other treatments
- severe rheumatoid arthritis that is unresponsive to other treatments

Dose

Rheumatoid arthritis
- 7.5 mg orally once weekly. May be increased by 15 mg/week after 6 weeks if there is no response (weekly maximum 20 mg). Once a response is established, the dose should be decreased to the lowest that produces a clinical effect **OR**
- 2.5 mg orally for 3 doses at 12-hourly intervals weekly. May be increased by 15 mg/week after 6 weeks if there is no response (weekly maximum 20 mg). Once a response is established, the dose should be decreased to the lowest that produces a clinical effect **OR**
- initially 7.5 mg SC weekly, increasing by 2.5 mg weekly (maximum 20—25 mg/weekly), then reduce to the lowest effective dose as maintenance

Psoriasis
- (Patient weight ≥ 70 kg) 10—25 mg IM or IV once weekly, gradually increasing to achieve an optimal response, but not exceeding 50 mg/week. Once a response is established, the dose should be decreased to the lowest that produces a clinical effect **OR**
- initially 7.5 mg SC weekly, then increasing gradually to 20—25 mg/weekly, then reducing to the lowest effective dose as maintenance **OR**
- 10—25 mg orally once weekly, increasing gradually until an adequate response is achieved (weekly maximum 50 mg) **OR**
- 2.5 mg orally for 3 doses at 12-hourly intervals weekly, gradually increasing to achieve an optimal response, but not exceeding 30 mg/week. Once a response is established, the dose should be decreased to the lowest that produces a clinical effect **OR**
- 2.5 mg orally for 4 doses at 8-hourly intervals weekly, gradually increasing to achieve an optimal response, but not exceeding 30 mg/week. Once a response is established, the dose should

be decreased to the lowest that produces a clinical effect **OR**
- 2.5 mg orally daily for 5 days, followed by 2-day rest period, gradually increasing to achieve an optimal response, but not exceeding 6.25 mg/day. Once a response is established, the dose should be decreased to the lowest that produces a clinical effect

Adverse effects
- nausea, abdominal pain, diarrhoea, anorexia, vomiting, haematemesis, melaena, GI ulceration
- ulcerative stomatitis, mucositis (gingivitis, pharyngitis, glossitis)
- decreased serum albumin, altered liver function
- rash, pruritus, urticaria, acne, dermatitis, photosensitivity, hyperpigmentation/depigmentation
- nail changes
- hair loss (reversible)
- cystitis, haematuria, dysuria, proteinuria, urogenital dysfunction, renal failure
- dry non-productive cough, dyspnoea, pneumonia, interstitial pneumonitis, pulmonary fibrosis
- menstrual dysfunction, infertility, transient oligospermia, azotaemia
- abortion, fetal defects, fetal death
- osteoporosis, arthralgia, myalgia
- bone marrow depression, neutropenia, leucopenia, pancytopenia
- hypotension, pericarditis, pericardial effusion, thromboembolic events
- malaise, fatigue, chills and fever, headache, dizziness, drowsiness, paraesthesia
- tinnitus
- blurred vision, eye discomfort
- decreased resistance to infection
- increased risk of secondary tumour formation, increased risk of infection
- (High and prolonged therapy) hepatotoxicity, haemorrhagic enteritis, liver fibrosis and cirrhosis
- (Psoriasis) burning, erythema (1—2 days after treatment), skin ulceration and, rarely, anaphylactoid reactions
- (Rare) tumour lysis syndrome (if a rapidly growing tumour is present), severe skin reactions

Interactions
- (Intrathecal) contraindicated with CNS radiotherapy
- contraindicated with acitretin or other retinoids
- contraindicated with alcohol or other hepatotoxic agents (e.g. retinoids, azathioprine, leflunomide, sulfasalazine)
- contraindicated with live or live attenuated vaccines
- not recommended with other disease-modifying antirheumatic drugs (DMARDs)
- serum levels (and associated risk of toxicity) may be increased by salicylates, sulfonamides, sulfonylureas, phenytoin, penicillins, ciprofloxacin, tetracyclines, chloramphenicol, probenecid, proton pump inhibitors (e.g. omeprazole, pantoprazole) or aminobenzoic acid; therefore not recommended together
- (High dose) not recommended with NSAIDs owing to an increased risk of myelosuppression and GI toxicity because the half-life of methotrexate is prolonged. Caution should also be used with lower doses of methotrexate
- toxicity may be increased by folate deficiency
- serum levels may be decreased by colestyramine
- the risk of toxicity is increased if given with other antineoplastic agents
- (Antineoplastic agent) not recommended with vitamin supplements containing folic or folinic acid
- (Rheumatoid arthritis) folic acid or folinic acid may decrease adverse effects but also decrease the efficacy of methotrexate and should not be administered on the same day
- if used with nitrous oxide, may potentiate methotrexate's effects on folate metabolism

HAVARD'S NURSING GUIDE TO DRUGS

- increased risk of bone marrow depression if given with allopurinol, trimethoprim, trimethoprim/sulfamethoxazole or pyrimethamine
- (Use in psoriasis) an increased risk of skin ulceration if given with amiodarone
- may decrease the clearance of theophylline, thereby increasing the risk of toxicity. Theophylline levels should be closely monitored during concurrent therapy
- may impair absorption of phenytoin, increasing the risk of seizures
- may be antagonised by asparaginase
- (IV infusion) an increased risk of toxicity if given with transfusion of packed red blood cells
- absorption and metabolism may be decreased by chloramphenicol, tetracycline or non-absorbable broad-spectrum antibiotics
- may increase plasma levels of mercaptopurine
- an increased risk of pancytopenia and hepatotoxicity if given with leflunomide
- an increased risk of soft tissue necrosis and osteonecrosis if given with radiotherapy
- half-life may be increased if given with probenecid or phenylbutazone
- an increased risk of skin cancer if given with psoralen plus ultraviolet A (PUVA) therapy
- may interfere with folic acid detection assay

Nursing considerations/Cautions

- pregnancy should be excluded before starting therapy
- adverse effects are generally dose related
- SC administration is for psoriasis and rheumatoid arthritis therapy only
- if switching from oral to parenteral administration, a dose reduction may be required because of variable methotrexate bioavailability after oral administration. No dose adjustment is required if switching from IM to SC route or vice versa
- (SC, rheumatoid arthritis) therapeutic response occurs after 4–8 weeks
- (SC, psoriasis) therapeutic response occurs after 2–6 weeks
- (SC) first self-administration should be under medical supervision
- (IM or IV, psoriasis) a single 5–10 mg IV or IM dose may be given as a test dose before starting therapy to identify any patient idiosyncrasies. Complete blood counts with platelets should be evaluated 7–10 days later
- full blood count (with differential and platelet count), haematocrit, renal function test, liver function test (including serum albumin and prothrombin time), urinalysis (urine should be alkaline), hepatitis B or C infection testing and chest X-ray should all be completed before, during (4–8-weekly) and after therapy. Liver biopsy may be recommended if the patient has history of excessive alcohol use, chronic hepatitis B or C infection or a persistently abnormal liver function test. Testing should be more frequent if changing dosage or if dehydration occurs, increasing the risk of elevated levels
- the patient should be closely monitored for any lung symptoms. Lung function tests are recommended if methotrexate-induced lung disease is suspected
- (Psoriasis) liver biopsy is recommended before and during therapy (2–4-monthly), after a cumulative dose of 1.5 g and then after each additional 1–1.5 g
- liver biopsy and/or bone marrow aspiration is recommended for those receiving high-dose or long-term therapy
- (Rheumatoid arthritis) hepatotoxicity is related to the age of first dose and duration of therapy
- urine should be kept alkaline during therapy
- pregnant staff should be cautioned not to handle methotrexate
- tablets contain lactose and are therefore not recommended in those with

galactose intolerance, Lapp lactase deficiency or glucose—galactose malabsorption
- (IV) incompatible with cytarabine, fluorouracil and prednisolone
- caution if used in those with inactive chronic infections (e.g. TB, herpes zoster, hepatitis B or C), as these may be reactivated
- caution if used in those who are debilitated or at extremes of age (young, elderly)
- contraindicated in those with poor nutrition, bone marrow depression, blood dyscrasias, severe liver or kidney impairment, alcoholic or alcoholic liver disease, immunodeficiency syndromes, blood dyscrasias, peptic ulcer disease, ulcerative colitis or severe acute or chronic infection

Patient education

- it is important to ensure the patient has a good understanding of the dosing regimen, as accidental daily dosing (instead of weekly) may be fatal
- caution the patient not to crush or chew tablets, and to swallow tablets with a full glass of water
- hands should be washed immediately after handling tablets
- advise the patient to avoid alcohol during therapy
- (SC, psoriasis, rheumatoid arthritis) the patient can be taught to self-administer:
  - See p. 1059 in General education for TNF-α antagonists for self-administration education. The following should also be included:
    - if the patient's weight > 100 kg, the administration site should be upper thigh only
    - if the patient has psoriasis, advice should include avoiding injections into psoriatic lesion
    - if a carer is administering the injection, disposable gloves should be worn and hands washed before and after administration
  - if any spills occur, the area should be cleaned with paper towels, which are disposed of in a 'sharps container' and area
  - if any solution makes contact with eyes or skin, it should be washed with copious amounts of water and medical attention sought
- (Psoriasis) warn the patient that burning and redness is common in the psoriatic area for 1—2 days post-therapy
- (Rheumatoid arthritis) the patient should be advised that improvement may be seen in 3—6 weeks after starting therapy, and improvement seen for a further 12 weeks or more
- (Rheumatoid arthritis) warn the patient that symptoms may worsen within 3—6 weeks of stopping therapy
- advise the patient to maintain good hydration throughout therapy and seek medical advice if any vomiting, diarrhoea or stomatitis (sore inflamed gums, inside of lips, cheeks or tongue) occurs that might lead to dehydration
- instruct the patient to immediately seek medical advice if any of the following occur:
  - dry persistent non-productive cough, fever, chest pain, shortness of breath (lung disorder)
  - fever, sore throat, chills (signs of infection)
  - vomiting, diarrhoea, inflamed gums or mouth ulcers
  - headache, shortness of breath, dizziness, looking pale (signs of anaemia)
  - blood in urine or bowel motions, black tarry bowel motions, black vomit, pinpoint red spots on skin (bleeding disorders or internal bleeding)
  - pain or difficulty urinating, lower back or side pain (possible kidney disorder)
- the patient should be advised to avoid people with infections if possible

- instruct the patient to avoid excessive sun exposure or sunlamps, as photosensitivity reaction may occur, or to wear a hat and long-sleeved shirt/garment and SPF 30+ sunscreen to protect the skin if sun exposure cannot be avoided
- caution the patient not to drive or operate machinery if dizziness, drowsiness, blurred vision or fatigue occurs
- advise pregnant women that they should not handle tablets
- before treatment begins, all patients (male and female) should be counselled regarding potential benefits and risks of therapy, including effects on reproduction, and the importance of using effective contraception throughout therapy and for a minimum of 3 months after therapy has stopped. Female patients should be instructed to seek medical advice immediately if menstruation does not occur and pregnancy is suspected

Tablet should not be broken or crushed. Tablet can be dispersed in 10–20 mL of water.

Contraindicated during pregnancy. Has been proven to cause fetal death and/or congenital abnormalities, as well as severe and/or toxic adverse effects. Women of childbearing potential must use effective contraception during treatment and for at least six months after cessation.

Use in males: men should use reliable contraception during treatment and for at least three months after stopping methotrexate.

Contraindicated during breastfeeding as passes into breastmilk.

Use in renal impairment: contraindicated in severe renal impairment, CrCl < 10 mL/min. In mild to moderate renal impairment, dosage adjustments may be necessary. Monitor renal function closely.

Contraindicated in chronic hepatic disease.

Disposable gloves should be worn by staff dispersing tablet. Pregnant staff should not disperse tablet.

PENICILLAMINE
Trade name
D Penamine

Available forms
Tablets: 125 mg, 250 mg

Action
- degradation product of penicillin
- forms a stable complex (chelate) with heavy metals such as copper, lead, gold and mercury
- reduces urinary levels of cystine by combining with cystine to form a more soluble, readily excretable complex, so reducing formation of cystine calculi
- effect in rheumatoid arthritis is due to unknown action
- half-life about 90 hours

Use
- severe active rheumatoid arthritis (rarely used)
- Wilson's disease (deficiency of copper-binding protein)
- treatment of heavy metal poisoning
- treatment of cystinuria (where high fluid regimens are not adequate or as an adjunct to them)

Dose
- (Rheumatoid arthritis) up to 250 mg orally daily in divided doses 1 hour before or 2 hours after food for 1 month, then increasing by the same amount monthly to a maximum of 1500 mg daily. The dose is then lowered to achieve the lowest effective dose (maintenance dose) **OR**
- (Wilson's disease) 1500–2000 mg orally daily 1 hour before or 2 hours after meals **OR**

DISEASE-MODIFYING ANTIRHEUMATIC DRUGS (DMARDS)

- (Heavy metal poisoning) 250–1000 mg orally in divided doses 1 hour before or 2 hours after meals **OR**
- (Cystinuria) 750–1000 mg orally in divided doses 1 hour before or 2 hours after meals (maximum daily dose 2 g) **OR**
- (Cystinuria) 500 mg orally before retiring, followed by free fluids during the day

Adverse effects
- erythematous or maculopapular rash, fever, joint pains, urticaria, lymphadenopathy
- impaired taste (reversible), anorexia, nausea, vomiting, diarrhoea, cheilosis, glossitis
- drug fever (in second or third week of therapy)
- tinnitus
- hair loss
- hepatic dysfunction, pancreatitis
- proteinuria, nephrotic syndrome
- iron-deficiency anaemia (prolonged use), agranulocytosis, thrombocytosis, eosinophilia, leukocytosis, leucopenia, thrombocytopenia
- impaired wound healing, increased skin friability (at pressure points), purpuric skin lesions
- increased excretion of other heavy metals
- (Rarely) pyridoxine deficiency, reversible optic neuritis, breast enlargement (male and female), glomerulonephritis (Goodpasture's syndrome) (see Glossary)

Interactions
- enhances urinary excretion of copper, lead, zinc, gold, mercury and other heavy metals
- may potentiate isoniazid
- contraindicated in those taking antimalarial agents or receiving gold therapy for arthritis

Nursing considerations/Cautions
- neurological examination is recommended before starting therapy
- blood count (including WBC count, differential cell count and direct platelet count) should be measured weekly for the first 4 weeks, then every second week for 5 months, then monthly. Urinalysis should occur at the same time. Skin and mucous membranes should also be assessed for any allergic reaction. Therapy should be stopped if there is fever or reaction in urine, blood or skin appears, or if the blood count declines over three successive tests
- if albumin > 2 g/day, therapy should be stopped
- liver function should be monitored 6-monthly for 18 months
- annual ophthalmological examination is recommended
- (Rheumatoid arthritis) if no response occurs in 6 months at full maintenance dose, therapy should be discontinued
- should be discontinued at least 6 weeks before any surgery, as penicillamine may interfere with collagen cross-links and therefore interrupt the healing process
- (Cystinuria) annual chest X-ray is recommended
- may require daily prophylactic pyridoxine (25 mg) if central and/or peripheral nervous system symptoms occur
- (Wilson's disease, lead poisoning) if the patient is vomiting or unable to swallow, parenteral EDTA is recommended
- (Wilson's disease) some clinical deterioration may occur at the start of therapy before improvement
- iron supplementation may be required if iron deficiency occurs
- caution if used in penicillin-hypersensitive patients because cross-allergy may occur

Patient education
- instruct the patient to check temperature, skin and urine each day before taking medication and any fever, chills, bruising, bleeding, rash, sore throat, proteinuria or haematuria should be

reported immediately to the doctor because it indicates the need to stop the drug
- (Rheumatoid arthritis) warn the patient that it may take 6—8 weeks for a response to be seen
- warn the patient that drug fever (with or without skin reactions) commonly occurs in the first 2—3 weeks of therapy
- advise the patient against abrupt withdrawal of therapy
- instruct the patient to take medication on an empty stomach (1 hour before or 2 hours after food, and at least 1 hour apart from other medication, milk or snacks)
- the patient should be advised to immediately seek medical advice if any of the following occur:
  - visual disturbances
  - becoming pale and tired, short of breath
  - developing muscle weakness, double vision or drooping eyelids
- female patients should be counselled regarding the need to avoid becoming pregnant while taking medication

Tablet can be crushed and mixed with water or a spoonful of apple puree (NOT yoghurt).

Avoid use. It has been associated with fetal malformations, such as cutis laxa, because of its effects on collagen and its chelating properties.

Avoid use. Limited human data. No data on its concentration in breastmilk are available.

Reduced renal function: use cautiously. It may lead to further renal toxicity, including nephrotic syndrome and proteinuria. Regular monitoring of renal function (e.g. proteinuria and albuminuria) is recommended. Discontinue treatment if proteinuria exceeds 2 g per day or haematuria develops.

Elderly patients may be at increased risk of adverse effects, particularly haematological or renal toxicity, owing to decreased physiological reserve.

Use the lowest effective dose and monitor renal function, blood counts and liver function regularly. Gradual dose escalation may reduce the incidence of side effects.

Pregnant staff should not crush or disperse tablet.

SULFASALAZINE
Trade names
Pyralin EN, Salazopyrin, Salazopyrin EN-Tabs

Available forms
Tablets: 500 mg;
Tablets (enteric-coated): 500 mg

Action
- broken down in the colon by bacteria to 5-aminosalicylic acid and sulfapyridine, producing an anti-inflammatory effect by its action on prostaglandin synthesis, leukotrienes and arachidonic acid metabolites
- onset of action may take 6—12 weeks

Use
- ulcerative colitis and Crohn's disease (see Gastrointestinal agents (miscellaneous), p. 1166)
- rheumatoid arthritis (unresponsive to other drug therapy)

Dose
- (Rheumatoid arthritis) initially 500 mg orally at night for 1 week, 500 mg twice daily for 1 week, 500 mg in the morning and 1 g at night for 1 week, then 1 g twice daily for 1 week (to daily maximum of 3 g) **OR**
- (Ulcerative colitis, Crohn's disease) initially 1—2 g orally 4 times daily after meals, then 500 mg 4 times daily

Adverse effects/Interactions/Nursing considerations/Cautions/Patient education
- see sulfasalazine in Gastrointestinal agents (miscellaneous) p. 1166)

DISEASE-MODIFYING ANTIRHEUMATIC DRUGS (DMARDS)

Do not crush enteric-coated tablets.

Safe: while sulfasalazine is classified as safe for use during pregnancy, it inhibits the absorption and metabolism of folic acid, potentially leading to folic acid deficiency and serious blood disorders such as macrocytosis and pancytopenia. There have been reports of neural tube defects in babies born to mothers exposed to sulfasalazine during pregnancy, although a causal link has not been definitively established. To reduce the risk, supplementation with folic acid during pregnancy is recommended, and sulfasalazine should be used only if clearly needed, with close monitoring.

Passes into breastmilk in negligible amounts; however, its metabolite, sulfapyridine, reaches concentrations of about 40% of maternal serum levels in breastmilk. Although the risk of kernicterus in breastfed infants is low, caution is advised, particularly in breastfeeding premature infants or those deficient in glucose-6-phosphate dehydrogenase. Monitor for possible adverse effects such as bloody stools or diarrhoea in the infant, and weigh the benefits to the mother against potential risks to the infant.

Reduced renal function: contraindicated, as an increased risk of crystalluria, haematuria and nephrotoxicity. Regular monitoring of renal function (including urinalysis) is required during treatment, especially in the first three months. Ensure adequate fluid intake to reduce the risk of crystal formation in the urinary tract.

Reduced hepatic function: contraindicated, as may worsen liver function and lead to hepatotoxicity, including hepatitis and liver failure. Liver function tests must be performed before initiating treatment and regularly during therapy. Discontinue sulfasalazine if any signs of hepatotoxicity or worsening hepatic function occur.

Elderly patients may be more susceptible to adverse reactions, especially haematological and hepatic toxicity. Start with the lowest effective dose and monitor closely for toxicity, including blood counts, liver function and renal function. Adjust doses based on tolerance and overall health status.

TUMOUR NECROSIS FACTOR ALPHA (TNF-α) ANTAGONISTS

General Actions of TNF-α antagonists
- tumour necrosis factor alpha (TNF-α) antagonists are recombinant monoclonal antibodies (IgG_1) designed to neutralise the activity of TNF, a pro-inflammatory cytokine involved in various autoimmune and inflammatory diseases.
- TNF plays a significant role in joint inflammation and erosion, particularly in rheumatoid arthritis (RA), psoriatic arthritis, ankylosing spondylitis and psoriasis. In these conditions, elevated TNF levels are found in the synovial fluid (for RA) and in the affected tissues (e.g. psoriatic plaques).
- by blocking the interaction of TNF with its receptors, TNF-α antagonists reduce the inflammatory response and help slow the progression of tissue destruction. These agents are often combined with other treatments, such as methotrexate or corticosteroids, to enhance their efficacy in controlling disease activity.

General Adverse effects of TNF-α antagonists
- (Infusion site reaction) erythema, pain, itching, swelling
- headache, fatigue, fever, dizziness, vertigo, asthenia
- flushing

HAVARD'S NURSING GUIDE TO DRUGS

- nausea, vomiting, abdominal pain, diarrhoea, dyspepsia
- upper and lower respiratory tract infections, pneumonia, dyspnoea, sinusitis, pharyngitis, nasopharyngitis, cough
- viral infection
- other infections (urinary tract, soft tissue, joints, reproductive tract, ear, oral, fungal)
- chest pain, hypertension
- rash, pruritus, urticaria, dry skin, increased sweating
- autoantibody development
- (Long-term) development of malignancy and blood dyscrasias
- (Rare) reactivation of tuberculosis, demyelinating diseases, peripheral neuropathy, transverse myelitis, seizure disorders, new or worsening psoriasis, aplastic anaemia, pancytopenia, worsening heart failure, lupus-like syndrome, hypersensitivity

General Interactions of TNF-α antagonists

- contraindicated with anakinra, abatacept, other cytokine modulators and other TNF-α antagonists because of an increased risk of infection
- not recommended with live or live attenuated vaccines

General Nursing considerations/Cautions for TNF-α antagonists

- before starting therapy, all patients should be:
  - screened for any signs of infection. This should include screening for hepatitis B and C, and tuberculosis (TB) (clinical history, chest X-ray, skin tuberculin test), as these can become reactivated. If latent TB is diagnosed, it should be treated with appropriate antimycobacterial agents before starting therapy. If active TB is found, therapy should not be started
  - asked about any travel to areas at high risk of TB or endemic mycoses (e.g. histoplasmosis)
  - examined for skin cancer
  - checked to ensure their immunisations are up to date before starting therapy
- any infection should be identified, treated and controlled before starting therapy
- before starting therapy, full blood count, creatinine and liver function tests are recommended and should be repeated if signs of infection or blood dyscrasias occur
- trade name and batch number should be recorded in the patient history
- infusion-related reactions occur more frequently in those who develop autoantibodies
- do not mix with other agents in the syringe
- the patient may be taught to self-administer medication SC. They should be educated about rotation of sites, injection technique, storage requirements and safe disposal of used needles
- rotate injection sites (thigh or abdomen) avoiding skin that is reddened, bruised, tender or hard or within 3 cm of previous injection sites
- if undergoing surgery, the patient should be closely monitored for any signs of infection
- needle covers of prefilled syringes contain latex and should not be handled by or administered to anyone with a latex sensitivity
- therapy should be stopped if new, serious infection develops
- if switching from one biological agent to another, the patient should be carefully monitored for any signs of infection
- development of autoantibodies may worsen or induce lupus-like syndrome
- cardiac status should be closely monitored in those with mild congestive cardiac failure and stopped if there is any worsening
- caution if used in those who live or travel to areas where mycoses are endemic. Fungal infection should be suspected if the person develops a serious systemic infection

DISEASE-MODIFYING ANTIRHEUMATIC DRUGS (DMARDS)

- caution if used in those aged 65 years or more, as they are at increased risk of infection and malignancy
- caution if used in those who have recently been diagnosed with CNS or peripheral demyelinating disease, on concurrent immunosuppressive therapy (as there is an increased risk of infection) or with mild heart failure (as it may be worsened)
- caution if used in those with chronic or recurring infection or conditions that may predispose them to infection, including asthma or poorly controlled diabetes
- caution if used in heavy smokers or those with chronic obstructive pulmonary disease (COPD), as there is an increased risk of lung, neck and head cancer
- contraindicated in those with serious or untreated infections (including active tuberculosis), sepsis, moderate-to-severe heart failure, lupus-like syndrome and history of blood dyscrasias

General Patient education for TNF-α antagonists

- patients should be counselled to immediately seek medical advice if they develop any:
  - persistent cough, coughing up blood, loss of weight or low-grade fever (signs of TB)
  - persistent fever, bruising, bleeding, pallor
  - numbness or tingling in arms or legs
  - changes to skin lesions (new ones appearing or existing ones changing in size or appearance)
- advise the patient to have regular skin examinations (self-examination and by qualified health professional)
- warn the patient that needle covers of prefilled syringes and pens contain latex
- the patient may be taught to self-administer medication SC. Information should include:
  - if not confident about the techniques, do not attempt to self-inject
  - do not inject through clothing
  - wash hands before self-injecting
  - collect the prefilled syringe/auto-injector and alcohol pad
  - check the expiry date before using and do not use if after month/year shown
  - the solution should be checked to ensure that the colour has not changed and that there are no particles present. If cloudy, discoloured or if flakes are present, the syringe should not be used
  - allow the syringe to come to room temperature before administration (15–30 minutes) (this will reduce pain). It should not be warmed in any other way, such as in a water bath or microwave
  - choose an injection site (thigh or stomach) 3 cm away from the previous injection site or navel (do not choose an area that is red, tender, hard, bruised, scarred or has broken skin)
  - it is important to rotate or change injection sites so that the area does not become too painful. Areas should be rotated between thigh and stomach
  - clean the injection site using alcohol wipe, wiping the area in a circular motion
  - don't touch this area again before injecting
  - gently invert, but do not shake, the syringe before administration. If the solution looks frothy, it should be allowed to rest until it clears before using
  - remove the cap from the needle (being careful not to touch the needle or let it touch any surface)
  - grasp the cleaned skin area with one hand, gently but firmly
  - with the other hand, hold the syringe at 45–90-degree angle with the grooved side up
  - using a quick, short motion, push the needle completely into skin

- release the skin and push the plunger to completely inject solution (may take 2–5 seconds)
- when the syringe is empty, remove needle from skin
- using thumb and a piece of gauze or cottonwool ball (not the alcohol swab), apply pressure (but do not rub) over the injection site for 10 seconds
- can apply a plaster (e.g. Band-Aid) if required
- the syringe should not be recapped; dispose of according to instructions (e.g. the patient may have been supplied with a sharps container for safe disposal)
- protect prefilled syringes from light before use and store them at 2–8°C, but not frozen
- if travelling, ensure syringes are kept at the correct temperature
- if injection site reactions occur, applying a cold pack to site will relieve any pain, swelling or itching

ADALIMUMAB

Trade names
Abrilada, Adalicip, Amgevita, Hadlima, Humira, Hyrimoz, Yuflyma

Available forms
Prefilled syringe: 20 mg/0.2 mL, 20 mg/0.4 mL, 40 mg/0.4 mL, 40 mg/0.8 mL, 80 mg/0.8 mL;
Prefilled pen: 40 mg/0.4 mL, 40 mg/0.8 mL, 80 mg/0.8 mL

Action
- long half-life 10–20 days
- see also General Actions of TNF-α antagonists (p. 1057)

Use
- moderate-to-severe rheumatoid arthritis (alone or with methotrexate)
- moderate-to-severe psoriatic arthritis (unresponsive to other disease-modifying antirheumatic drugs (DMARDs))
- active ankylosing spondylitis
- moderate-to-severe polyarticular juvenile idiopathic arthritis (over 2 years of age) (unresponsive to other DMARDs) (alone or with methotrexate)
- moderate-to-severe plaque psoriasis
- moderate-to-severe Crohn's disease (inadequate response to conventional therapies or intolerant/unresponsive to infliximab)
- moderate-to-severe ulcerative colitis (inadequate response to conventional therapies)
- moderate-to-severe non-infectious intermediate posterior uveitis (inadequate response to corticosteroids)
- moderate-to-severe hidradenitis suppurativa (HS) (acne inversa) (inadequate response to conventional therapies)

Dose
- (Rheumatoid arthritis) 40 mg SC fortnightly (or weekly if not given concurrently with methotrexate) **OR**
- (Psoriatic arthritis, ankylosing spondylitis) 40 mg SC fortnightly **OR**
- (Psoriasis) initially 80 mg SC, then 1 week later 40 mg SC, repeated fortnightly **OR**
- (Polyarticular juvenile idiopathic arthritis) 20 mg SC fortnightly (weight 10 kg to < 30 kg) or 40 mg SC fortnightly (weight 30 kg or more) **OR**
- (Crohn's disease, ulcerative colitis, HS) initially 160 mg SC as 4 injections (day 0), or 80 mg SC as 2 injections (day 0) and repeated on day 1, followed by 80 mg as 2 injections on day 14 (induction), then 40 mg SC on day 28 and continuing fortnightly (maintenance) **OR**
- (Uveitis) initially 80 mg SC, then 40 mg SC fortnightly starting 1 week after initial dose

Adverse effects
- visual impairment, conjunctivitis, eye swelling
- impaired healing
- nail disorder
- cough, asthma

DISEASE-MODIFYING ANTIRHEUMATIC DRUGS (DMARDS)

- migraine
- musculoskeletal pain, muscle spasm
- paraesthesia
- tachycardia, oedema
- depression, anxiety, insomnia
- elevated liver enzymes
- gastrointestinal haemorrhage, gastro-esophageal reflux disease (GORD)
- haematuria, renal impairment
- leucopenia, thrombocytopenia, anaemia, neutropenia
- hyperlipidaemia, hypokalaemia, hypocalcaemia, hypophosphataemia, hyperglycaemia, increased uric acid, abnormal serum sodium
- prolonged activated partial thromboplastin time (aPTT)
- see also General Adverse effects of TNF-α antagonists (p. 1057)

Interactions
- see General Interactions of TNF-α antagonists (p. 1058)

Nursing considerations/Cautions
- (Uveitis) because of the association between uveitis and central demyelinating disorders, neurological assessment is recommended before starting therapy
- (Ulcerative colitis) if the patient has a previous history or is at risk of dysplasia or colon cancer (e.g. long-standing ulcerative colitis or primary sclerosing cholangitis), screening for dysplasia (e.g. colonoscopy, biopsy) is recommended before starting and regularly during therapy
- (Psoriasis) not recommended with phototherapy or other systemic agents
- (Uveitis) can be given with corticosteroids and/or non-biological immunotherapy. Corticosteroid dose may be tapered 2 weeks after starting therapy
- (HS) antibiotic therapy may be continued if necessary
- (HS) therapy should be stopped after 12 weeks if there is no clinical response
- (Crohn's) aminosalicylates, corticosteroids and/or azathioprine or mercaptopurine can be continued during therapy
- (Ankylosing spondylitis, psoriatic arthritis) glucocorticoids, salicylates, NSAIDs or DMARDs can be continued during therapy
- see also General Nursing considerations/Cautions for TNF-α antagonists (p. 1058)

Patient education
- patients can be instructed to self-administer using a prefilled syringe or pen. (For patient education for a prefilled syringe see p. 1059.) For a prefilled pen, the instructions are as follows:
  - leave at room temperature for 15–30 minutes before administration, but do not use any other method to warm (e.g. microwave, water bath)
  - check expiry date and do not use if it has passed
  - hold the pen with the grey cap pointing up (viewing solution through the window)
  - ensure solution is clear, colourless and contains no particles
  - do not remove the grey or plum-coloured caps until ready to inject
  - follow the instructions on p. 1059 for choosing and rotating sites, cleaning skin and handwashing
  - remove the grey cap and discard, exposing the white needle sleeve
  - remove the plum cap and discard, revealing the activation button
  - it is important not to put the pen down as this might activate and release the solution
  - with the free hand, pinch clean skin at the injection site and hold firmly
  - place the white end of pen at 90 degrees (right angle) to the skin, pressing down slightly and observing the window
  - when ready to inject, press the plum-coloured button. A click will be heard as the needle is released and a small prick felt. Keep pressing, holding the pen steady for about 10 seconds to complete injection. A yellow

HAVARD'S NURSING GUIDE TO DRUGS

- indicator will move into the window during the injection and will stop moving when the injection is complete
- lift the pen away from injection site and discard into a sharps-disposal container
- if there is a drop of blood at the injection site, press the site with gauze or a cotton wool ball but do not rub the injection site
- store pen at 2–8°C but do not freeze. Pen can be stored at room temperature (< 25°C) for up to 14 days (write down the date of removal from fridge) and protected from the light. If not used in this time, the pen should be discarded and not refrigerated again. This is important if the patient is travelling
- women of childbearing age should be counselled to use adequate contraception during and for 5 months after stopping therapy
- if the newborn has been exposed to adalimumab during pregnancy, live vaccines should not be administered for at least 5 months after the last administration
- see also General Patient education for TNF-α antagonists (p. 1059)

Crosses the placenta and may affect the immune system of a newborn exposed in utero, increasing the risk of infection.

Women of childbearing potential should use effective contraception during treatment and for at least 5 months after the last dose.

Thought to be safe during breastfeeding, as excretion into breastmilk is very low. The benefits of breastfeeding should be weighed against the mother's clinical need for adalimumab.

Elderly patients may be more prone to infections and adverse effects because of immunosuppression and comorbidities. No dose adjustments are needed, but careful monitoring for infections and adverse effects is recommended, especially in frail patients.

CERTOLIZUMAB
Trade name
Cimzia PEGOL

Available forms
Prefilled syringe: 200 mg/mL;
Prefilled pen: 200 mg/mL

Action
- immunomodifier
- recombinant humanised antibody fragment (Fab)
- expressed in *Escherichia coli* and conjugated (pegylated) to polyethylene glycol (PEG), increasing half-life
- high affinity for human tumour necrosis factor alpha (TNF-α), which is a pro-inflammatory cytokine that plays a central role in the inflammatory process
- long half-life (14 days)

Use
- moderate-to-severe rheumatoid arthritis (RA) (alone or with methotrexate)
- active ankylosing spondylitis (unresponsive or intolerant to at least one nonsteroidal anti-inflammatory drug (NSAID))
- active psoriatic arthritis (unresponsive to other disease-modifying antirheumatic drugs (DMARDs))
- moderate-to-severe plaque psoriasis

Dose
- (All uses) initially 400 mg (2 injections of 200 mg) SC at weeks 0, 2 and 4, then either 200 mg SC second-weekly or 400 mg SC monthly (maintenance) (alone or with methotrexate)

Adverse effects
- prolonged activated partial thromboplastin time (aPTT)
- anaemia, eosinophilia
- conjunctivitis
- gastritis
- abnormal liver function
- back ache, muscle spasm, pain in extremities
- oropharyngeal pain
- see also General Adverse effects of TNF-α antagonists (p. 1057)

DISEASE-MODIFYING ANTIRHEUMATIC DRUGS (DMARDS)

Interactions
- may interfere with some coagulation assays, resulting in falsely elevated aPTT
- see also General Interactions of TNF-α antagonists (p. 1058)

Nursing considerations/Cautions
- (RA) if there is no response within 12 weeks, use should be re-evaluated
- (Psoriasis) if there is no response within 16 weeks, use should be re-evaluated
- see also General Nursing considerations/Cautions for TNF-α antagonists (p. 1058)

Patient education
- patients can be instructed to self-administer using a prefilled syringe or pen. For patient education for a prefilled syringe see p. 1059. For a prefilled pen, instructions are similar to those for adalimumab (p. 1061) with the following differences:
  - hold the pen firmly by the black handle and remove clear cap
  - the injection should occur within 5 minutes of cap removal
  - holding the pen firmly by the black handle, press down firmly on skin at 90 degrees. A click will be heard starting the injection and a second click is heard (this may take up to 15 seconds). The window on the side of the pen should then be orange, indicating the injection is complete.
- counsel female patients about the importance of using adequate contraception to avoid pregnancy during and for at least 5 months after stopping therapy
- see also General Patient education for TNF-α antagonists (p. 1059)

Use with caution during pregnancy. Minimal transfer to the fetus; however, potential effects on the newborn's immune system should be considered. Women of childbearing potential should use effective contraception during treatment and for at least 5 months after the last dose.

Safe to use. Minimal transfer into breastmilk.

ETANERCEPT
Trade names
Brenzys, Enbrel, Erelzi, Nepexto

Available forms
Vial: 25 mg
Prefilled syringe: 50 mg/mL;
Autoinjector: 50 mg/mL

Action
- reaches maximum concentration in 24–96 hours after SC administration
- long half-life (about 80 hours)
- see also General Actions of TNF-α antagonists (p. 1057)

Use
- rheumatoid arthritis (unresponsive to other disease-modifying antirheumatic drugs (DMARDs)) (alone or with methotrexate)
- active polyarticular course juvenile chronic arthritis (unresponsive to other DMARDs)
- psoriatic arthritis (unresponsive to other DMARDs)
- active ankylosing spondylitis
- moderate-to-severe chronic plaque psoriasis
- non-radiographic axial spondyloarthritis (inadequate response to non-steroidal anti-inflammatory drugs (NSAIDs))

Dose
- (Rheumatoid arthritis, polyarticular juvenile chronic arthritis, psoriatic arthritis, ankylosing spondylitis, axial spondyloarthritis) 50 mg SC weekly or 25 mg SC twice weekly 3–4 days apart
OR

- (Plaque psoriasis) 50 mg SC weekly or 25 mg SC twice weekly 3—4 days apart. The dose may be increased to 50 mg SC twice weekly for up to 12 weeks if necessary, then reduced

Adverse effects
- (Rare) uveitis, inflammatory bowel disease, autoimmune hepatitis
- (Very rare) fatal pancytopenia, aplastic anaemia
- see also General Adverse effects of TNF-α antagonists (p. 1057)

Interactions
- do not administer live vaccines concurrently with etanercept
- caution if given with sulfasalazine, as a decrease in WBC may occur
- not recommended with cyclophosphamide
- see also General Interactions of TNF-α antagonists (p. 1058)

Nursing considerations/Cautions
- (Vial) reconstitute powder by gently injecting water for injections into the vial using the vial adapter attached to the syringe and swirl gently, avoiding vigorous agitation or shaking
- (Vial) a clear and colourless solution should result within 10 minutes of reconstitution
- (Vial) the solution should not be filtered, nor used if discoloured, cloudy or containing particulate matter
- (Vial) use within 6 hours of reconstitution
- subcutaneous injection; rotate injection sites
- caution if used in those with diabetes, as there is an increased risk of hypoglycaemia, necessitating a decreased dose in hypoglycaemic medication
- caution in those with moderate-to-severe alcoholic hepatitis
- live vaccines in the newborn infant. Generally not recommended for infants exposed in utero until 16 weeks after the mother's last dose.
- see also General Nursing considerations/Cautions for TNF-α antagonists (p. 1058)

Patient education
- inform the patient that injection site reaction reduces after initial 4 weeks
- if the patient has diabetes, they should be instructed to monitor blood glucose levels closely, as etanercept may cause hypoglycaemia. The dose of hypoglycaemic medications may need to be adjusted accordingly
- advise the patient to seek medical advice immediately if they are exposed to chickenpox or shingles during therapy
- the prefilled syringe/autoinjector can be stored at up to 25°C for 4 weeks; however, it should be discarded if not used in that time or if exposed to high temperature
- see also General Patient education for TNF-α antagonists (p. 1059)

Avoid use. Safety during pregnancy has not been established. Crosses the placenta and has been detected in infant serum. There may be an increased risk of infections in the newborn. Women of childbearing potential should use effective contraception during treatment and for 3 weeks after the last dose.

Excreted in human milk in low levels. Weigh the benefits of breastfeeding against the potential risks to the infant.

GOLIMUMAB
Trade name
Simponi

Available forms
Prefilled syringe/injector pen: 50 mg/0.5 mL, 100 mg/mL

DISEASE-MODIFYING ANTIRHEUMATIC DRUGS (DMARDS)

Action
- half-life 9—15 days
- see also General Actions of TNF-α antagonists (p. 1057)

Use
- moderate-to-severe active rheumatoid arthritis (with methotrexate)
- active, progressive psoriatic arthritis (alone or with methotrexate)
- active ankylosing spondylitis
- moderate-to-severe ulcerative colitis (unresponsive to other treatments)
- non-radiographic axial spondyloarthritis (inadequate response to non-steroidal anti-inflammatory drugs (NSAIDs))

Dose
- (Rheumatoid arthritis, psoriatic arthritis, ankylosing spondylitis, axial spondyloarthritis) 50 mg SC monthly **OR**
- (Ulcerative colitis) initially 200 mg SC, 100 mg SC after 2 weeks, then 100 mg SC monthly

Adverse effects
- constipation
- elevated liver enzymes
- bone fractures
- see also General Adverse effects of TNF-α antagonists (p. 1057)

Interactions
- see General Interactions of TNF-α antagonists (p. 1058)

Nursing considerations/Cautions
- the long half-life should be taken into consideration if the patient is undergoing surgery
- (Post-surgery) the patient should be closely monitored during and after therapy for any signs of infection
- (Ulcerative colitis) because of the increased risk of bowel cancer and dysplasia, colonoscopy and biopsy are recommended before starting therapy and at regular intervals in those with long-standing ulcerative colitis, primary sclerosing cholangitis or a previous history of colon dysplasia or cancer
- (Ulcerative colitis) the corticosteroid dose may be tapered during maintenance therapy according to clinical practice guidelines
- patients with active rheumatoid arthritis (especially if treated previously with immunosuppressant agents) are at increased risk of leukaemia and lymphoma, and should be carefully monitored during and after therapy
- see also General Nursing considerations/Cautions for TNF-α antagonists (p. 1058)

Patient education
- if multiple injections are required, different sites should be used
- women of childbearing potential should be counselled to use reliable contraception during therapy and for 6 months post-therapy, and also the importance of telling their doctor if menstruation is delayed
- see also General Patient education for TNF-α antagonists (p. 1059)

Not recommended during pregnancy. Women of childbearing potential should use effective contraception during treatment and for 6 months after the last dose. Live vaccines should not be administered to infants within 6 months of stopping therapy.

Not recommended during breastfeeding and should not be commenced within 6 months of stopping therapy.

INFLIXIMAB
Trade names
Inflectra, Remicade, Remsima, Renflexis

Available form
Vial: 100 mg

Action
- half-life 8—9.5 days

- see also General Actions of TNF-α antagonists (p. 1057)

Use
- moderate-to-severe Crohn's disease (in patients over 6 years) to induce and maintain remission (unresponsive to conventional treatment)
- moderately severe-to-severe active ulcerative colitis (unresponsive to conventional treatment)
- treatment of refractory fistulising Crohn's disease
- rheumatoid arthritis (with methotrexate)
- ankylosing spondylitis
- psoriatic arthritis (unresponsive to other disease-modifying antirheumatic drugs (DMARDs)) (alone or with methotrexate)
- severe plaque psoriasis (unresponsive to other conventional treatment)

Dose
- (Rheumatoid arthritis) initially 3 mg/kg IV over 2 hours, then 3 mg/kg IV given at 2 and 6 weeks after the first infusion, then 3 mg/kg IV 8-weekly (with methotrexate). The dose may be increased by 1.5 mg/kg incrementally to a maximum of 7.5 mg/kg for optimal response **OR**
- (Ankylosing spondylitis) initially 5 mg/kg IV over 2 hours, then 5 mg/kg IV given at 2 and 6 weeks after the first infusion, followed by 5 mg/kg IV 6-weekly **OR**
- (Psoriatic arthritis, plaque psoriasis) 5 mg/kg IV over 2 hours, then 5 mg/kg at 2 and 6 weeks after the initial dose, then 8-weekly (maintenance) **OR**
- (Moderate-to-severe Crohn's disease, refractory fistulating Crohn's disease, ulcerative colitis) initially 5 mg/kg by IV infusion over 2 hours, then 2 and 6 weeks after initial infusion (induction), followed by 5 mg/kg by IV infusion 8-weekly (maintenance)

Adverse effects
- see General Adverse effects of TNF-α antagonists (p. 1057)

Interactions
- see General Interactions of TNF-α antagonists (p. 1058)

Nursing considerations/Cautions
- for doses > 6 mg/kg, infusion should be > 2 hours
- gently add 10 mL water for injections down the inside of the vial, swirl gently and avoid shaking to dissolve; foaming may occur
- allow the solution to stand for 5 minutes before administering
- the solution may be clear and colourless to light yellow
- it should be diluted to 250 mL with sodium chloride 0.9%, gently mixed and then given as an IV infusion (rate not greater than 2 mL/min) over at least 2 hours
- a filter (micron size 1.2 or less) should be added to the infusion set
- administer alone
- the patient should be carefully observed for at least 2 hours post-infusion (especially after the first and second dose), because infusion reactions are most likely to occur during this time
- if an infusion reaction occurs, the infusion should be slowed or stopped until symptoms subside, then started at a lower rate
- paracetamol, antihistamines, corticosteroids, adrenaline (epinephrine) and artificial airway should be readily available for infusion reaction
- premedication with paracetamol, hydrocortisone and/or antihistamine may prevent mild and transient effects of infusion reaction
- in adult patients who have tolerated three 2-hour infusions and are receiving maintenance therapy, consideration may be given to decreasing the infusion time (no less than 1 hour). If an infusion reaction occurs, subsequent infusions should be at a slower rate

DISEASE-MODIFYING ANTIRHEUMATIC DRUGS (DMARDS)

- readministration after a 16-week drug-free interval is not recommended because of an increased risk of hypersensitivity reaction
- (Refractory fistulating Crohn's disease, ulcerative colitis) if there is no response after initial 3 doses, therapy should be stopped
- (Crohn's disease — maintenance) the dose can be increased to 10 mg/kg if response is inadequate
- (Rheumatoid arthritis) clinical response is usually seen within 12 weeks. The dose may be increased if response is inadequate or lost
- contraindicated in those with hypersensitivity to other murine proteins
- see also General Nursing considerations/Cautions for TNF-α antagonists (p. 1058)

Patient education

- women of childbearing age should be counselled to use adequate contraception during and for 6 months after stopping therapy
- see also General Patient education for TNF-α antagonists (p. 1059)

Not recommended during pregnancy. Women of childbearing potential should use effective contraception during treatment and for 6 months after the last dose.

Caution advised: present at low levels in human milk. Limited data suggest low risk, but potential effects on the infant are not fully known. Administration of live vaccines to a breastfed infant is not recommended unless infant infliximab serum levels are undetectable.

CYTOKINE MODULATORS

General Adverse effects of cytokine modulators

- headache, dizziness, fatigue, asthenia, paraesthesia, insomnia
- nausea, abdominal pain, diarrhoea, dyspepsia, mouth ulceration, stomatitis
- infection (lower respiratory, urinary tract, upper respiratory), rhinitis, herpes simplex, herpes zoster
- limb pain, back pain, myalgia, arthralgia
- hypertension, chest pain
- development of antibodies
- (Uncommon) hypersensitivity, anaphylaxis, reactivation of hepatitis B, non-melanoma skin cancers, malignancies
- (Rare) chronic inflammatory, demyelinating polyneuropathy, multiple sclerosis

General Interactions of cytokine modulators

- not recommended with tumour necrosis factor (TNF) inhibitors, rituximab or anakinra
- not recommended with or within 3 months of live or live attenuated vaccine

General Nursing considerations/ Cautions for cytokine modulators

- the patient should be screened for any signs of infection before starting therapy. This should include screening for hepatitis B and tuberculosis (clinical history, chest X-ray, skin tuberculin test). If latent tuberculosis is diagnosed, it should be treated with appropriate antimycobacterial agents before starting therapy
- patients with previous tuberculosis should be closely monitored for any reactivation
- regular skin examinations are recommended
- if changing from a tumour necrosis factor (TNF) blocking agent, the patient should be closely monitored for any sign of infection
- vaccinations should be up to date before starting therapy
- needle covers of prefilled syringes contain latex and should not be handled by or administered to anyone with a latex sensitivity

- caution if used in those ≥ 65 years, as they are at greater risk of infections and malignancy
- caution if used in those with moderate-to-severe kidney impairment
- caution if used in those with a previous history or at increased risk of skin cancers
- caution if used in those with chronic obstructive pulmonary disease (COPD), as respiratory symptoms (cough, dyspnoea, rhonchi) may be exacerbated
- not recommended in those with active (including chronic or localised) infection and caution if used in those with chronic or recurrent infection, those who have been exposed to TB, a history of serious or opportunistic infection, or have lived or travelled in areas of endemic TB or endemic mycoses

General Patient education for cytokine modulators

- the patient should be counselled to immediately seek medical advice if they develop:
- (signs of TB) persistent cough, coughing up blood, unexplained weight loss, loss of energy or low-grade fever
- any new skin spots, including spots that have changed, become larger, bleed or don't heal
- (abdominal symptoms) stomach ache or pain that does not go away, change in bowel habits
- (infections symptoms) fever, sweating or chills, muscle aches
- (anaemia-related symptoms) tiredness, headache, shortness of breath when exercising, looking pale
- if the patient has pre-existing COPD, they should be advised to immediately report to the doctor any worsening symptoms, trouble breathing, cough or development of pneumonia
- advise the patient to have regular screening for any skin cancers, avoid sunburn and wear sunscreen (SPF 30+), long-sleeved clothing and a hat when outdoors
- warn the patient not to drive or operate machinery if dizziness, fatigue or insomnia occurs
- women of childbearing age should be advised to use adequate contraception during therapy

ABATACEPT

Trade name
Orencia

Available forms
Vial: 250 mg;
Prefilled syringe: 125 mg/mL;
Autoinjector: 125 mg/mL

Action
- modulates key co-stimulatory signal required for full activation of T-lymphocytes which are found in the synovium of those with rheumatoid arthritis
- (Rheumatoid arthritis) half-life about 14 days (IV, SC)

Use
- moderate-to-severe rheumatoid arthritis (with methotrexate) (intolerant or unresponsive to other disease-modifying antirheumatic drugs (DMARDs) or never previously treated with methotrexate)
- moderate-to-severe active polyarticular juvenile idiopathic arthritis (unresponsive to other DMARDs) (alone or with methotrexate)
- active psoriatic arthritis (inadequate response to DMARDs) (alone or with non-biological DMARDs)

Dose
- (Rheumatoid arthritis, psoriatic arthritis) (patient weight < 60 kg) 500 mg, (60—100 kg) 750 mg or (> 100 kg) 1 g IV over 30 minutes given 2 and 4 weeks after initial infusion, then monthly **OR**

DISEASE-MODIFYING ANTIRHEUMATIC DRUGS (DMARDS)

- (Rheumatoid arthritis) initially 500 mg, 750 mg or 1 g IV (loading dose) (according to body weight, as above) then 125 mg SC within 24 hours of loading dose, then weekly **OR**
- (Rheumatoid arthritis, psoriatic arthritis) 125 mg SC weekly **OR**
- (Polyarticular juvenile idiopathic arthritis) (patient weight < 75 kg) 10 mg/kg IV over 30 minutes given 2 and 4 weeks after initial infusion, then monthly (if patient weight is > 75 kg, regimen for rheumatoid arthritis is followed (maximum 1 g))

Adverse effects
- (IV infusion-related reaction — within 1 hour) dizziness, hypotension, nausea, headache, flushing
- (IV peri-infusion reaction — up to 24 hours of infusion) dizziness, nausea, vomiting, flushing, rash
- (SC) local injection site reaction including redness, pruritus, haematoma
- cough
- rash, alopecia
- elevated liver enzymes
- increased BP
- (Uncommon) leucopenia, thrombocytopenia
- see also General Adverse effects of cytokine modulators (p. 1067)

Interactions
- may cause a falsely elevated blood glucose reading on the day of IV infusion (not SC injection) (if test strips contain glucose dehydrogenase pyrroloquinoline quinone, as this reacts with maltose in the solution)
- see also General Interactions of cytokine modulators (p. 1067)

Nursing considerations/Cautions
- if switching from IV to SC therapy, first SC dose should be given when monthly IV dose is due
- patients should be monitored during and after infusion for any signs of infusion-related events
- patient may be taught to self-administer medication SC. They should be educated about rotation of sites, injection technique, storage requirements and safe disposal of used needles. First self-administration should be done under supervision
- rotate injection sites (thigh or abdomen) avoiding skin that is reddened, bruised, tender or hard or within 3 cm of previous injection sites
- (Polyarticular juvenile idiopathic arthritis) vaccinations should be up to date before starting therapy
- IV dosage dependent on body weight
- (IV) reconstitute by gently injecting 10 mL water for injections into vial, swirl gently, avoiding vigorous agitation or shaking to prevent foaming. After reconstitution, vial should be vented with a needle to dispel any foam formed. Reconstituted solution should be clear and colourless to pale yellow. This should be added to a 100 mL bag of 0.9% sodium chloride, first removing the equivalent amount of sodium chloride (e.g. if 4 vials have been reconstituted totalling 40 mL, then 40 mL of sodium chloride should be removed before adding the reconstituted solution). Bag should be gently inverted, not shaken
- (IV) administer alone
- (IV) contains 8.6 mg sodium per vial, which may need to be considered for those on a sodium-controlled diet
- see also General Nursing considerations/Cautions for cytokine modulators (p. 1067)

Patient education
- warn the patient that hair loss may occur
- for SC self-administration instructions, see General Patient education for TNF-α antagonists (p. 1068)

HAVARD'S NURSING GUIDE TO DRUGS

- if the newborn has been exposed to abatacept during pregnancy, live vaccines should not be administered for at least 5 months after last administration
- see also General Patient education for cytokine modulators (p. 1068)

Not recommended during pregnancy. Evidence of adverse effects on the fetus observed in animal studies.

Not recommended during breastfeeding and for at least 14 weeks after the last dose.

Elderly patients may have a higher incidence of infections. Use with caution and monitor closely for adverse effects.

ANAKINRA (RBE)
Trade name
Kineret

Available form
Prefilled syringe: 100 mg/0.67 mL

Action
- recombinant, non-glycosylated human interleukin-1 receptor antagonist (interleukin-1 is thought to play a part in both inflammatory and immunological responses, including the degradation of cartilage and stimulation of bone resorption)
- half-life 4—6 hours

Use
- active rheumatoid arthritis (with methotrexate) (unresponsive to other disease-modifying antirheumatic drugs (DMARDs))

Dose
- 100 mg daily SC (same time every day)

Adverse effects
- mild injection site reaction (erythema, ecchymosis, inflammation, pain)
- elevated total cholesterol levels
- depression
- rash, pruritus
- (Uncommon) transient elevation of liver enzymes
- (Rare) neutropenia, thrombocytopenia, bone fractures
- see also General Adverse effects of cytokine modulators (p. 1067)

Interactions
- caution if given with agents that have narrow therapeutic index (e.g. warfarin). Serum levels should be closely monitored, especially when starting or stopping therapy
- see also General Interactions of cytokine modulators (p. 1067)

Nursing considerations/Cautions
- baseline blood counts (WBC, platelets, absolute neutrophil count) should be measured before starting, monthly for 6 months and then every 4 months throughout therapy
- patient may be taught to self-administer medication SC. They should be educated about rotation of sites, injection technique, storage requirements and safe disposal of used needles. The first self-administration should be done under supervision
- not recommended in those with severe renal impairment
- contraindicated in those with known hypersensitivity to *Escherichia coli*-derived products or if the patient is neutropenic (ANC $< 1.5 \times 10^9$/L)
- see also General Nursing considerations/Cautions for cytokine modulators (p. 1067)

Patient education
- for SC self-administration instructions, see General Patient education for TNF-α antagonists (p. 1068)
- if the patient is experiencing discomfort at the administration site, advice can include rotation of sites, cooling the site

DISEASE-MODIFYING ANTIRHEUMATIC DRUGS (DMARDS)

after administration with cold cloth, ensuring the solution is at room temperature before administration and, if prescribed, the use of topical corticosteroids or antihistamines
- see also General Patient education for cytokine modulators (p. 1068)

Should be used during pregnancy only if the benefits outweigh the potential risks.

Caution advised. Should be used only when if the benefits outweigh the potential risks.

Reduced renal function: dose adjustment required when CrCl < 30 mL/min; use with caution when CrCl 30–50 mL/min.

Severe hepatic impairment: use with caution; monitor liver function tests regularly.

RITUXIMAB
Trade names
Riximyo, Ruxience, Truxima

Available forms
Vial: 100 mg/10 mL, 500 mg/50 mL

Action
- murine/human anti-CD20 monoclonal antibody that depletes B lymphocytes
- action in rheumatoid arthritis may be due to suppression of inflammation by reducing B-lymphocyte-induced T-cell activation and cytokine production

Use
- relapsed or refractory CD20 positive diffuse large B-cell non-Hodgkin lymphoma, chronic lymphocytic leukaemia, severe granulomatosis with polyangiitis (Wegener's), microscopic polyangiitis
- severe rheumatoid arthritis (unresponsive or intolerant to tumour necrosis factor alpha (TNF-α) antagonists) (with methotrexate)

Dose
- (Rheumatoid arthritis) 1 g by IV infusion, then 1 g by IV infusion 2 weeks later (with methotrexate) (see General Nursing considerations/Cautions section regarding rate of administration)

Adverse effects
- acute infusion reactions (hypo/hypertension, nausea, rash, pruritus, urticaria, chills, fever, rhinitis, throat irritation, flushing)
- hypercholesterolaemia
- transient hypophosphataemia, hyperuricaemia
- transient neutropenia
- (Rare) progressive multifocal leukoencephalopathy (PML), severe bronchospasm, hypoxia, dyspnoea, acute respiratory failure
- see also General Adverse effects of cytokine modulators (p. 1067)

Interactions
- see General Interactions of cytokine modulators (p. 1067)

Nursing considerations/Cautions
- premedication with paracetamol/salicylate/NSAID, antihistamine and glucocorticoid (e.g. methylprednisolone 100 mg IV) is recommended 30–60 minutes before the infusion to reduce the severity and frequency of an infusion-related reaction
- the patient should be monitored during and at least 2 hours after the first infusion for any signs of cytokine release syndrome (dyspnoea, bronchospasm, hypoxia, chills, fever, rigors, urticaria and angioedema).
- if severe cytokine release syndrome occurs, the infusion should be stopped
- ensure emergency treatment for anaphylaxis (adrenaline (epinephrine), antihistamine, corticosteroid) is readily available

- for the first infusion, the rate should be started at 50 mg/hour and the patient carefully monitored. If no hypersensitivity or infusion-related event occurs, the rate may be increased by 50 mg/hour at 30-minute intervals to a maximum of 400 mg/hour. If hypersensitivity reaction occurs, the infusion rate should be halved. If no hypersensitivity occurs, subsequent infusions can be started at 100 mg/mL and increased at 100 mg increments at 30-minute intervals to 400 mg/hour maximum
- if no serious infusion reaction has occurred, a more rapid infusion may be given for second and subsequent infusions using 4 mg/mL in 250 mL volume. The rate can be started at 250 mg/hour for first 30 minutes, then 600 mg/hour for next 90 minutes. The infusion will be completed in 2 hours using this rate
- (RA) response is usually seen in about 16 weeks
- (RA) further courses may be given. Repeat courses should not be given at intervals less than 16 weeks
- antibody development has been associated with worsening infusion or allergic reactions after the second infusion
- any concurrent antihypertensive agent may need to be withheld for 12 hours before and during the infusion because of added risk of severe hypotension occurring
- reconstitute with 4 mL water for injections, then dilute further with 50—250 mL sodium chloride 0.9% or glucose 5% and gently invert to mix, but prevent foaming
- administer alone
- not given as SC, IV push or bolus
- the patient should be carefully monitored for any signs or symptoms that might suggest progressive multifocal leukoencephalopathy (PML) (e.g. cognitive, neurological or psychiatric symptoms). If signs occur, therapy should be stopped and further evaluation including MRI, CSF testing and repeat neurological assessments completed
- contains sodium chloride (100 mg vial = 52.6 mg sodium; 500 mg vial = 263.2 mg sodium), which may need to be considered if the patient is on a sodium-reduced intake
- patients with cardiovascular disease (including arrhythmias) or previous serious reaction to other biological therapy or rituximab, should not be given rapid (2-hour) IV infusion and should be closely monitored during infusion
- not recommended in patients who are severely immunocompromised (CD4 or CD8 are very low)
- contraindicated in those with murine protein hypersensitivity
- see also General Nursing considerations/Cautions for cytokine modulators (p. 1067)

Patient education

- warn the patient that reactions (e.g. fever, chills, shivering) may occur after the infusion (especially within the first 2 hours of the first infusion) and are transient. They occur less frequently after the first infusion
- the patient/carer/family members should be advised to seek medical advice immediately if any confusion, disorientation, memory loss, changes in moving, talking and/or walking, decreased strength, increased weakness or blurred or loss of vision occurs
- women of childbearing potential should be counselled to use adequate contraception during and for 12 months after stopping therapy
- see also General Patient education for cytokine modulators (p. 1068)

Not recommended during pregnancy unless benefits outweigh risks. Crosses the placenta, especially during the second and third trimesters.

Adequate contraception should be used during and for 12 months after stopping therapy.

Excreted in human milk. Potential for serious adverse reactions in nursing infant, including B-cell depletion.

DISEASE-MODIFYING ANTIRHEUMATIC DRUGS (DMARDS)

> Discontinue breastfeeding during rituximab treatment and for several months after the last dose.

 Reduced renal function: associated with renal toxicity, including acute renal failure, especially in patients with pre-existing renal conditions. Regular monitoring of renal function is recommended during treatment.

TOCILIZUMAB
Trade name
Actemra

Available forms
Vial: 80 mg/4 mL, 200 mg/10 mL, 400 mg/20 mL;
Prefilled syringe: 162 mg/0.9 mL;
Prefilled pen: 162 mg/0.9 mL

Action
- recombinant humanised monoclonal antibody of IgG_1 that binds to interleukin-6 receptors, which are thought to be involved in the pathogenesis of inflammatory disease including rheumatoid arthritis and juvenile idiopathic arthritis
- produced by recombinant DNA technology using mammalian Chinese hamster ovary cell culture
- (IV) long half-life (11–13 days) and even longer in younger patients with juvenile arthritis (up to 23 days)

Use
- moderate-to-severe rheumatoid arthritis (RA) (either alone or in combination with methotrexate or other non-biological disease-modifying antirheumatic drugs (DMARDs))
- active systemic juvenile idiopathic arthritis (sJIA) (> 2 years) (alone or with methotrexate)
- moderate-to-severe polyarticular juvenile idiopathic arthritis (pJIA) (> 2 years) (alone or with methotrexate)
- giant cell arteritis (GCA)
- cytokine release syndrome (CRS)

Dose
- (RA) 8 mg/kg by IV infusion over 1 hour every 4 weeks (maximum 800 mg) (alone or with methotrexate and/or other non-biological DMARD) **OR**
- (RA) 162 mg SC weekly (alone or with methotrexate and/or non-biological DMARD) **OR**
- (sJIA < 30 kg) 12 mg/kg by IV infusion over 1 hour every 2 weeks (alone or with methotrexate) **OR**
- (sJIA ≥ 30 kg) 8 mg/kg by IV infusion over 1 hour every 2 weeks (alone or with methotrexate) **OR**
- (pJIA < 30 kg) 10 mg/kg by IV infusion over 1 hour monthly (alone or with methotrexate) **OR**
- (pJIA ≥ 30 kg) 8 mg/kg by IV infusion over 1 hour monthly (alone or with methotrexate) **OR**
- (pJIA < 30 kg) 162 mg SC every 3 weeks (alone or with methotrexate) **OR**
- (pJIA ≥ 30 kg) 162 mg SC every 2 weeks (alone or with methotrexate) **OR**
- (GCA) 162 mg SC weekly or every 2 weeks (with tapering corticosteroids or alone after corticosteroids have been discontinued) **OR**
- (CRS) 8 mg/kg (if patient weight ≥ 30 kg) or 12 mg/kg (if patient weight < 30 kg) by IV infusion over 1 hour (alone or with corticosteroids) (800 mg maximum per infusion)

Adverse effects
- IV infusion reaction (hypo/hypertension, nausea, headache, dizziness, rash, urticaria)
- SC site reaction (erythema, pruritus, pain, haematoma)
- cough, dyspnoea
- weight increase
- rash, pruritus, urticaria
- leucopenia, neutropenia
- hypercholesterolaemia, hypertriglyceridaemia
- hypofibrinogenaemia
- (sJIA) (rare) macrophage activation syndrome
- (CRS) elevated liver enzymes, cytopenias

HAVARD'S NURSING GUIDE TO DRUGS

- (Rare) GI perforation, hepatotoxicity
- see also General Adverse effects of cytokine modulators (p. 1067)

Interactions

- may decrease serum levels of simvastatin
- caution if given with atorvastatin, calcium-channel blockers, theophylline, warfarin, phenytoin, ciclosporin or benzodiazepines, especially when starting or stopping therapy, as serum levels may be altered
- caution if used with other hepatotoxic agents
- see also General Interactions of cytokine modulators (p. 1067)

Nursing considerations/Cautions

- ensure the correct formulation is selected for administration, as IV and SC formulations are not interchangeable
- if absolute neutrophil count (ANC) < 0.5 × 10^9/L, therapy should not be started
- IV dose is adjusted according to liver enzymes, ANC and platelet count
- the patient should be monitored during and for 30 minutes after infusion for any signs of infusion reaction, which can occur up to 24 hours after completion
- serum lipids (low-density lipoprotein (LDL), high-density lipoprotein (HDL), total cholesterol) should be measured 4—8 weeks after starting therapy, then regularly or (pJIA) 12-weekly
- ensure emergency treatment (adrenaline (epinephrine), antihistamine, corticosteroid) and resuscitation equipment are readily available
- (RA) an increased risk of cardiovascular disorders; therefore should be thoroughly assessed for any risk factors (e.g. hypertension, hyperlipidaemia) before starting therapy. Serum lipids should be monitored 4—8-weekly during the first 6 months of therapy
- (RA, GCA) liver enzymes (ALT, AST), neutrophil and platelet count should be measured 4—8-weekly during the first 6 months of therapy, then 12-weekly or (sJIA, pJIA) at time of second infusion, then 4—8-weekly (pJIA) or (sJIA) 2—4-weekly
- it is recommended that all patients (and especially those with sJIA) are up to date with vaccinations; these should be completed before starting therapy
- (GCA) if the condition relapses, corticosteroid therapy may be restarted or the dose increased according to clinical need
- (CRS) if there is no improvement after the first dose, up to 3 further doses may be given at intervals not less than 8-hourly
- (RA, sJIA, pJIA ≥ 30 kg) dilute to a total volume of 100 mL with sodium chloride 0.9% and administer over 1 hour or (sJIA, pJIA < 30 kg) to a total volume of 50 mL. An equivalent amount of sodium chloride should be removed from the infusion bag first before adding tocilizumab
- instruct the patient on SC administration technique. The first SC injection should be under medical supervision
- contains 26.55 mg (1.17 mmol) of sodium per maximum dose of 1200 mg, which may need to be taken into consideration if the patient is on a sodium-restricted diet
- caution if used in those with history of diverticulitis or intestinal ulceration because of the risk of GI perforation
- caution if used in those with liver impairment or active liver disease
- caution if used in those with low neutrophil (ANC < 2 × 10^9/L) or platelet count (< 100 × 10^9/L)
- contraindicated in those with hypersensitivity to other recombinant human or humanised antibodies or Chinese hamster ovary cell products, or if active severe infection is present
- see also General Nursing considerations/Cautions for cytokine modulators (p. 1067)

Patient education

- warn the patient/carer that infusion-related reaction (headache, rash, hives,

diarrhoea, arthralgia, stomach pains) may occur up to 24 hours after infusion
- for SC self-administration instructions for a prefilled syringe, see General Patient education for TNF-α antagonists (p. 1059), with the following difference:
  - allow the syringe to stand at room temperature for 25—30 minutes and injection should be completed within 5 minutes
- for SC self-administration instruction for a prefilled pen, instructions are similar to those for adalimumab (see Patient education for adalimumab, p. 1061) (read those instructions first) with the following differences:
  - allow the pen to come to room temperature for at least 45 minutes (not in direct sunlight, nor using any other means such as microwave or a water bath)
  - hold the pen with green cap pointing down and view the solution through the window on the side (should be clear and colourless to pale yellow)
  - remove the green cap and discard
  - pinch skin to make a fold, hold the needle guard against skin at 90 degrees
  - unlock the green activation button by pressing the pen firmly against skin until the needle shield is pushed in
  - press the green activation button until a click is heard. Continue pressing it until a purple indicator in the window has stopped moving (a second click may be heard) — the injection may take up to 10 seconds. When the purple indicator has stopped, remove the pen from skin (at 90 degrees). The needle shield should move into place and cover the needle
  - do not rub the injection site. If there is any blood, press gauze or a cotton ball on the site to stop the bleeding. A small dressing such as a Band-Aid can be used if needed
  - the injection should be completed within 3 minutes of removing the green cap
- see also General Patient education for cytokine modulators (p. 1068)

Limited human data. Animal studies have shown adverse effects, so it should be used only if the potential benefits justify the potential risks.

Not recommended during breastfeeding owing to limited human data.

Reduced hepatic function: use with caution. May elevate liver enzymes. Regular monitoring of liver function is recommended, and dose adjustments may be needed for patients with liver enzyme elevations.

TOFACITINIB
Trade name
Xeljanz

Available forms
Tablets: 5 mg, 10 mg;
Oral Solution: 1 mg/mL

Action
- Janus kinase (JAK1—3) inhibitor (these cytokines are thought to have a role in immune function modulation)
- peak activity in 0.5—1 hour, rapid half-life about 3 hours

Use
- treatment of moderate-to-severe active rheumatoid arthritis (RA) (with or without non-biological disease-modifying anti-rheumatic drugs (DMARDs)) in patients who have intolerance or inadequate response to methotrexate
- active psoriatic arthritis (PA) (with conventional DMARDs) in patients who have had inadequate response to DMARDs
- moderate-to-severe ulcerative colitis (UC) in patients where response has been lost or who are intolerant to other therapies

Dose
- (RA, PA) 5 mg orally twice daily **OR**
- (UC) initially 10 mg orally twice daily for 8 weeks (induction), then 5 mg orally twice daily (maintenance)

Adverse effects
- anaemia, neutropenia, lymphocytosis
- hypercholesterolaemia, hyperlipidaemia
- altered liver enzymes
- increased heart rate
- fever
- cough
- peripheral oedema
- acne
- (Uncommon) prolongation of the PR interval
- (Rare) interstitial lung disease, gastrointestinal perforation
- see also General Adverse effects of cytokine modulators (p. 1067)

Interactions
- not recommended with other agents that decrease heart rate or prolong the PR interval such as antiarrhythmics, beta adrenoceptor blocking agents, alpha2 agonists, cholinesterase inhibitors, some calcium-channel blockers, some HIV protease inhibitors and digoxin
- serum levels may be increased by fluconazole
- serum levels may be decreased by rifampicin
- contraindicated with ciclosporin
- not recommended with tacrolimus
- see also General Interactions of cytokine modulators (p. 1067)

Nursing considerations/Cautions
- before starting, a full blood count (including differential white cell count), platelet count and liver function tests are recommended, then monitoring:
  - lymphocytes, neutrophils and haemoglobin after 4–8 weeks, then 3-monthly
  - lipids after 4–8 weeks
  - liver function routinely
- therapy should not be started if ALC $< 0.75 \times 10^9$/L, ANC $< 1 \times 10^9$/L or Hb < 90 g/L
- (UC) if adequate clinical response is not achieved by week 8, an induction dose (10 mg twice daily) can be used for an extra 8 weeks (16 weeks total). If there is no clinical response after this time, therapy should be stopped. If clinical benefit is not maintained on 5 mg twice-daily maintenance dose, this can be increased to 10 mg twice daily
- caution if used in those with low heart rate (< 60 beats/min), a history of arrhythmias or syncope, sick sinus syndrome, SA or AV block, ischaemic heart disease or congestive cardiac failure
- caution if used in those with or at risk of interstitial lung disease, especially Asian patients, who are at greater risk of interstitial lung disease, herpes zoster, elevated liver enzymes, opportunistic infections and decreased white blood counts
- caution if used in those at risk of gastrointestinal perforation (e.g. history of diverticulitis)
- caution if used in those with kidney impairment. Dose adjustment is required if GFR ≤ 50 mL/min
- contraindicated in those with severe liver impairment
- see also General Nursing considerations/Cautions for cytokine modulators (p. 1067)

Patient education
- if the patient is Asian, warn of the increased risk of infection and lung problems
- advise the patient to seek medical advice if any of the following occur:
  - change in heart rate
  - stomach pain/ache that does not go away, change in bowel habits
  - dry persistent cough, shortness of breath, fatigue
- women of childbearing potential should be counselled to use adequate contraception during therapy

DISEASE-MODIFYING ANTIRHEUMATIC DRUGS (DMARDS)

- see also General Patient education for cytokine modulators (p. 1068)

 Tablet should not be crushed or broken.

 Not recommended during pregnancy or in women wanting to become pregnant. Effective contraception should be used during and after stopping therapy.

 Not recommended, during breastfeeding.

 Not recommended in those over 65 years and should be used only if no other alternative treatment is available.

UPADACITINIB

Trade name
Rinvoq

Available forms
Tablets: 15 mg, 30 mg, 45 mg

Action
- Janus kinase (JAK1–3) inhibitor (these cytokines are thought to have a role in immune function modulation)
- half-life 9–14 hours

Use
- treatment of moderate-to-severe rheumatoid arthritis (RA) in patients who are intolerant to or have had inadequate response to one or more disease-modifying antirheumatic drugs (DMARDs)
- treatment of moderate-to-severe active ulcerative colitis (UC) or Crohn's disease (CD) with inadequate/lost response or intolerance to conventional/biological therapy

Dose
- (RA) 15 mg orally daily (as monotherapy or with methotrexate or other conventional DMARDs)
- (Crohn's disease) induction 45 mg daily for 12 weeks then reassess
- (UC) induction 45 mg daily for 8 weeks then reassess

Adverse effects
- serious infections (e.g. pneumonia, cellulitis, bacterial meningitis), reactivation of tuberculosis and herpes zoster, oral/oesophageal candidiasis, cryptococcosis, pneumocytosis, bronchitis, nasopharyngitis, sinusitis, urinary tract infection
- neutropenia, lymphopaemia, anaemia
- elevated lipids (total cholesterol, low-density lipoprotein (LDL) cholesterol, high-density lipoprotein (HDL) cholesterol
- increased liver enzymes, elevated creatine phosphokinase (CPK)
- headache, dizziness
- hypertension
- cough
- fever
- diarrhoea, nausea, vomiting
- (Rare) thrombosis (deep vein thrombosis, pulmonary embolism, arterial thrombosis), non-melanoma skin cancer, increased risk of malignancy

Interactions
- contraindicated with biological DMARDs
- not recommended with other JAK inhibitors or potent immunosuppressants (e.g. azathioprine, ciclosporin, tacrolimus) because of the added immunosuppression
- caution if used with itraconazole, posaconazole, voriconazole or clarithromycin
- therapeutic effect may be decreased if given with rifampicin or phenytoin

Nursing considerations/Cautions
- the patient should be screened for any signs of infection before starting therapy. This should include screening for hepatitis

B and tuberculosis (clinical history, chest X-ray, skin tuberculin test). If latent tuberculosis is diagnosed, it should be treated with appropriate antimycobacterial agents before starting therapy
- before starting therapy neutrophil, lymphocyte and haemoglobin levels should be monitored and not started if the absolute lymphocyte count (ALC) < 500 cells/mm^3, absolute neutrophil count (ANC) < 1000 cells/mm^3 or haemoglobin < 8 g/dL. Therapy should be interrupted if neutrophil, lymphocyte and haemoglobin levels fall below these levels and restarted once they return to normal
- lipids and liver enzymes should be monitored before starting and regularly throughout therapy
- patients with previous tuberculosis should be closely monitored for any reactivation
- therapy should be interrupted if the patient develops a serious or opportunistic infection and restarted once the infection has been treated and controlled
- regular skin examinations are recommended
- vaccinations should be up to date before starting therapy
- caution if used in those with severe kidney impairment
- not recommended in those with severe liver impairment
- not recommended in those with active (including chronic or localised) infection and caution if used in those with chronic or recurrent infection, those who have been exposed to tuberculosis (TB), have history of serious or opportunistic infection, or have lived or travelled in areas of endemic TB or endemic mycoses

Patient education

- the patient should be counselled to immediately seek medical advice if they develop:
  - persistent cough, coughing up blood, unexplained weight loss, loss of energy or low-grade fever (signs of TB)
  - any new skin spots, including spots that have changed, become larger, bleed or don't heal
  - symptoms of infection such as fever, sweating or chills, muscle aches
  - tiredness, headache, shortness of breath when exercising, looking pale
  - swelling, pain, redness, warmth in the calf area
  - shortness of breath, rapid breathing, sudden sharp chest pain made worse on coughing or deep breathing, rapid heart rate, coughing up pink frothy sputum, sweating
  - cold pulseless limb, muscle pain or spasm in affected area, numbness or tingling in area
- advise the patient to have regular screening for any skin cancers, avoid sunburn and wear sunscreen (SPF 30+), long-sleeved clothing and a hat when outdoors
- warn the patient not to drive or operate machinery if dizziness occurs
- women of childbearing age should be advised to use adequate contraception during therapy

 Modified-release tablets should not be crushed, broken, divided, or chewed. Swallow tablets whole with or without food.

 Contraindicated during pregnancy. Women of reproductive potential should use effective contraception during treatment and for at least 4 weeks after the final dose.

 Not recommended during breastfeeding owing to lack of human data.

 Reduced hepatic function: not recommended for patients with severe hepatic impairment. No dose adjustment is needed for mild or moderate hepatic impairment, but monitoring is advised.

DIURETICS

Diuretics increase the rate of urine formation by reducing the reabsorption of sodium, chloride and water by the renal tubules, either by interfering with active transport mechanisms or by altering tubular permeability. Uses for diuretics include treatment of hypertension, oedema (e.g. acute and chronic congestive cardiac failure), chronic renal failure, nephrotic syndrome and cirrhosis (Knights et al 2023).

Classes of diuretics include:

- *aldosterone receptor antagonists* (e.g. eplerenone, finerenone, spironolactone) block the action of aldosterone at its receptor sites in the distal convoluted tubule and collecting ducts of the kidney, reducing sodium reabsorption and potassium excretion at the end of the distal tubule and the collecting duct
- *loop diuretics* (e.g. bumetanide, furosemide (frusemide)) limit the amount of sodium reabsorbed in the peritubular capillaries surrounding the loop of Henle, with reabsorption of calcium and magnesium also blocked
- *thiazide diuretics* (e.g. chlortalidone, hydrochlorothiazide, indapamide) interfere with sodium chloride reabsorption in the distal tubules, leading to increased excretion of sodium, chloride and water

General Nursing considerations/Cautions for diuretics

- excessive doses or diuresis may result in electrolyte imbalances, requiring close observation
- regularly monitor the patient's fluid intake, output and weight to assess fluid balance and diuretic effectiveness
- look for signs of dehydration, especially during hot weather or in vulnerable patients
- note any increase or reduction in oedema, indicating the effectiveness of the diuretic therapy
- check both supine and standing BP regularly to detect postural hypotension, a common side effect of diuretics
- look for symptoms of electrolyte imbalance such as anorexia, nausea, vomiting, dry mouth, thirst, excessive diuresis, oliguria, weakness, lethargy, restlessness, muscle pain or cramps, fatigue, hypotension, tachycardia and arrhythmias
- observe for signs of low sodium levels, such as lethargy, weakness, anorexia, nausea and cognitive slowing

- observe for symptoms of low potassium, including drowsiness, muscle weakness or cramps, paraesthesia, cardiac arrhythmias or ECG changes. This is especially critical in patients taking digoxin, as hypokalaemia can lead to digoxin toxicity
- if signs of hypovolaemia or dehydration are observed, diuretic should be stopped and fluid, electrolyte and/or acid—base imbalance corrected
- diuretics can impair glucose tolerance, so patients with diabetes mellitus should be closely monitored for any changes in blood sugar control

General Patient education for diuretics

- expect to urinate more frequently
- take the diuretic early in the day to avoid nocturia (waking up at night to urinate). If prescribed twice daily, take the second dose around midday, but never after 6 pm to avoid sleep disruption
- take the diuretic with or right after meals to minimise nausea or gastrointestinal side effects
- ensure you drink enough fluids, especially after exercise or exposure to hot environments, to avoid dehydration. However, if your health professional has advised any fluid restrictions, be sure to follow them carefully
- to avoid dizziness or faintness when standing up, move slowly from lying down or sitting, especially after sleeping. Postural hypotension can be worsened by prolonged standing, hot baths or showers, hot weather, physical exertion, large meals and alcohol. If faintness occurs, sit or lie down immediately
- if you experience dizziness, drowsiness, lethargy, faintness or confusion, avoid driving or handling heavy machinery until you feel better
- non-potassium-sparing diuretics, such as thiazides (e.g. hydrochlorothiazide) and loop diuretics (e.g. furosemide), can lead to hypokalaemia (low potassium levels) by promoting the excretion of potassium in the urine. Over time, this potassium loss can become significant, especially in cases of long-term or high-dose use. If you are on long-term, high-dose, non-potassium-sparing diuretics, incorporate potassium-rich foods into your diet, such as apricots, avocados, bananas, rockmelon, dates, grapefruit, oranges, potatoes, prunes, raisins, spinach, strawberries, and fruit juices like orange, grapefruit, prune and pineapple juice
- contact your healthcare provider immediately if you experience:
  - weak and rapid pulse, clammy skin, rapid breathing, dry mouth or nose, reduced urination
  - nausea, vomiting, headache, confusion, fatigue, restlessness, irritability, muscle weakness or cramps, seizures or coma
  - weakness, muscle cramps, heart palpitations
  - numbness or tingling in hands, feet or lips, muscle cramps or spasms, seizures, facial twitching, muscle weakness, lightheadedness or slow heart rate
- always refer to your healthcare professional's instructions and ask if you have any concerns or questions about your medication

DIURETICS

 Diuretics are banned in sport. Diuretics can cause rapid loss of water weight, which can give athletes in weight-class sports (e.g. boxing, wrestling or martial arts) an advantage by helping them quickly meet weight requirements; Diuretics can mask the presence of other prohibited substances in urine samples by diluting the urine.

CARBONIC ANHYDRASE INHIBITORS

ACETAZOLAMIDE
Trade names
Acetazolamide Powder for Injection (USP), Diamox, Glaumox Powder for Injection

Available forms
Tablets: 250 mg;
Vial: 500 mg

Action
- sulfonamide derivative that inhibits carbonic anhydrase
- reduces intraocular pressure by inhibiting the secretion of aqueous humour
- thought to slow abnormal, paroxysmal excessive discharges from CNS neurons
- increases bicarbonate excretion in the renal tubules, leading to increased sodium, potassium and water excretion, resulting in alkaline diuresis

Use
- adjunctive treatment in chronic simple (open-angle) glaucoma, secondary glaucoma and preoperatively in acute closed-angle glaucoma (see Antiglaucoma agents, p. 462)
- some types of epilepsy (see Antiepileptics, p. 388)
- cardiac- and drug-induced oedema (adjunct)

Dose
- (Cardiac failure induced oedema) initially 250—375 mg (5 mg/kg) orally or IV each morning. If response is not sustained, then therapy should be continued on alternate days or for 2 days, followed by a rest day if there is not a continued weight loss **OR**
- (Drug-induced oedema) 250—375 mg orally or IV for 1—2 days, alternating with a rest day

Adverse effects
- paraesthesia with tingling feeling in extremities and face
- fatigue, headache, dizziness, flushing, drowsiness, malaise
- anorexia, nausea, vomiting, diarrhoea
- polyuria, polydipsia, thirst
- fever
- depression, excitement, confusion, ataxia
- abnormal liver function
- crystalluria, renal colic, renal calculi
- transient myopia
- (Uncommon) convulsions
- (Rare) allergic skin reactions, photosensitivity, tinnitus, hearing disturbances
- (Rare, but occasionally fatal) blood dyscrasias, anaphylaxis, anaphylactoid reaction
- (Prolonged therapy) electrolyte imbalance (hypokalaemia, metabolic acidosis, hyponatraemia, osteomalacia, hypoglycaemia, hyperglycaemia)
- (Injection site) pain

Interactions
- may potentiate effects of oral anticoagulants and folic acid antagonists
- increased risk of osteomalacia if given with chronic phenytoin therapy
- risk of cardiac glycoside toxicity may be increased by acetazolamide-induced hypokalaemia
- use with salicylates may result in severe metabolic acidosis
- may decrease serum levels of lithium or primidone
- increased risk of renal calculi if given with sodium bicarbonate
- may prevent urinary antiseptic effect of methenamine hippurate
- not recommended with other carbonic anhydrase inhibitors

- may increase effects and duration of amphetamines by decreasing excretion
- may increase or decrease blood glucose levels; therefore treatment with hypoglycaemic agents may be affected
- may increase serum levels of ciclosporin or phenytoin, increasing risk of adverse effects and toxicity
- caution if used with antihypertensive agents
- increased risk of anorexia, tachypnoea, lethargy and coma if given with high-dose aspirin
- may interfere with HPLC assay method for theophylline
- may give false negative or decreased result for urinary protein, serum non-protein and serum uric acid

Nursing considerations/Cautions

- FBC, platelet count and serum electrolytes should be monitored before starting and regularly throughout therapy
- effectiveness as a diuretic diminishes with continuous use
- hypokalaemic acidosis corrected by administering bicarbonate and/or potassium
- increasing dose does not increase diuresis (or may decrease diuresis), and may increase risk of dizziness, drowsiness and/or paraesthesia
- therapy should be stopped if any skin reactions occur
- IV route is recommended only when oral route cannot be used
- reconstitute vial using 5 mL water for injections
- caution if used in those with diabetes mellitus or impaired glucose tolerance
- caution if used in those with a predisposition to electrolyte and acid–base imbalance, such as those with renal impairment
- contraindicated in those with pre-existing depression of serum sodium and/or potassium levels, glomerular filtration rate < 10 mL/min, kidney/liver dysfunction, suprarenal gland failure or hyperchloraemic acidosis; long-term administration contraindicated in those with chronic, non-congestive angle-closure glaucoma
- contraindicated in those with hypersensitivity to sulfonamide or related products
- see also General Nursing considerations/Cautions for diuretics (p. 1079)

Patient education

- advise patient against taking high doses of aspirin during therapy
- those with diabetes should be advised to closely monitor blood glucose levels during therapy
- see also General Patient education for diuretics (p. 1080)

 Tablet can be crushed and mixed with water or spoonful of yoghurt or apple puree.

 Not recommended during pregnancy (especially during first trimester) owing to inadequate human data.

 Not recommended during breastfeeding, as it is secreted in low levels in breastmilk, posing a potential risk to breastfed infant.

 Banned in sport.

LOOP DIURETICS

General Actions of loop diuretics

- also known as high-ceiling diuretics
- potent diuretics that inhibit sodium, potassium and chloride reabsorption in the proximal and distal renal convoluted tubules, but mainly in the ascending limb of the loop of Henle, resulting in increased water excretion

DIURETICS

- some direct vascular effect, which may be due to reduced response to angiotensin II and noradrenaline (norepinephrine) (both vasoconstrictors)
- rapid onset of action

General Uses of loop diuretics
- oedema associated with heart failure, cirrhosis, nephrotic syndrome and renal impairment
- acute pulmonary oedema (where other diuretics have been ineffective)

General Adverse effects of loop diuretics
- electrolyte imbalance (hyperglycaemia, hypokalaemia, hypomagnesaemia, hyponatraemia, metabolic acidosis, increased creatinine and blood urea nitrogen (BUN))
- hypovolaemia, dehydration (thirst, dizziness, headache, dry mouth, visual disturbances)
- urinary retention
- deafness, tinnitus, vertigo, sense of fullness in the ears
- anorexia, nausea, vomiting, dysphagia, abdominal pain/discomfort, diarrhoea
- malaise, fatigue, confusion, apprehension, headache
- hypotension, dizziness, syncope
- muscle cramps, weakness, musculoskeletal pain, arthralgia
- blurred vision
- hyperuricaemia, precipitation of gout
- rash, pruritus, urticaria
- fever, chills
- (Rare) blood dyscrasias

General Interactions of loop diuretics
- not recommended with lithium because lithium serum levels and toxicity are increased
- effects of antihypertensive agents may be enhanced
- loop diuretic-induced hypokalaemia may increase risk of toxicity and arrhythmias of digoxin
- increased risk of ototoxicity and nephrotoxicity if given with aminoglycosides
- effects may be inhibited by probenecid
- caution if used with angiotensin receptor antagonists or ACE inhibitors because of increased risk of first-dose hypotension (severe)
- effects reduced by NSAIDs and may predispose patient to kidney failure, especially in the presence of pre-existing hypovolaemia
- increased risk of nephrotoxicity if given with cisplatin
- increased risk of hypokalaemia if given with potassium-lowering agents (e.g. thiazide diuretics)
- profound diuresis and electrolyte imbalance may occur if given with thiazide diuretics
- may reduce glucose tolerance in patients with diabetes mellitus, necessitating dose adjustment of insulin and/or oral hypoglycaemics

General Nursing considerations/ Cautions for loop diuretics
- ensure electrolyte imbalances are corrected before starting therapy, as loop diuretics can worsen these conditions
- regularly monitor serum electrolytes (especially potassium) and blood urea nitrogen (BUN); consider potassium supplements or encourage potassium-rich foods, particularly in patients undergoing long-term therapy
- encourage dietary salt (if permitted) to prevent hyponatraemia and hypochloraemia
- discontinue therapy in patients with renal disease if oliguria develops or if there is a significant increase in BUN or serum creatinine levels
- if excessive diuresis or electrolyte loss occurs, stop the therapy to prevent further complications
- advise patients with diabetes to monitor blood glucose levels more frequently, as diuretics may impair glucose control
- use caution with excessive dosing or frequent administration, especially in

- elderly patients, as they are more prone to dehydration and electrolyte disturbances
- exercise caution in patients with advanced liver cirrhosis, as sudden electrolyte imbalances can precipitate hepatic encephalopathy and coma
- monitor patients with severe myocardial disease who are treated with digoxin for signs of arrhythmias, as hypokalaemia can increase the risk
- be cautious with patients with renal impairment or severely decompensated liver cirrhosis with ascites, as these conditions can worsen with loop diuretic therapy
- be mindful of the risk of urinary retention in patients with prostatic hypertrophy and impaired micturition
- use caution in patients with gout, predisposition to hypotension, hepatorenal syndrome, hypoproteinaemia, diabetes mellitus or systemic lupus erythematosus, as these conditions may be precipitated or exacerbated by loop diuretics
- contraindicated in patients with hypersensitivity to sulfonamides or loop diuretics, as cross-sensitivity may occur
- contraindicated in patients with anuria, complete renal shutdown, hepatic coma or pre-coma, or conditions causing severe electrolyte depletion until the imbalance is corrected
- see also General Nursing considerations/Cautions for diuretics (p. 1079)

General Patient education for loop diuretics

- seek advice from your health professional if hearing loss or ringing in ears (tinnitus) occurs
- instruct patient with diabetes to closely monitor blood glucose levels, as impaired glucose tolerance may occur
- see also General Patient education for diuretics (p. 1080)

 Used during pregnancy only if potential benefits outweigh risks and then at the lowest possible dose to achieve desired results. Loop diuretics enter fetal circulation and/or may cause fetal electrolyte disturbances and neonatal thrombocytopenia.

 Banned in sport.

BUMETANIDE
Trade name
Burinex

Available form
Tablets: 1 mg

Action
- effect on distal tubule is small
- decreases uric acid excretion, thereby increasing uric acid level
- onset of action 30 minutes (oral), peak effect in 1–2 hours, duration approximately 4–6 hours, half-life 60–90 minutes
- diuretic effect: 1 mg bumetanide = 40 mg furosemide (oral)
- diuretic effect is dose related and increasing dose produces diuresis
- see also General Actions of loop diuretics (p. 1082)

Use
- see General Uses of loop diuretics (p. 1083)

Dose
- 1 mg orally daily (morning or early evening) (daily maximum 10 mg) **OR**
- 1 mg orally 4–5-hourly to achieve diuresis in refractory patients (daily maximum 10 mg) **OR**
- 1 mg orally daily (morning or evening) on alternate days (daily maximum 10 mg) **OR**
- 1 mg orally daily for 3–4 days, followed by 1–2 drug-free days (daily maximum 10 mg)

Adverse effects
- dyspnoea, cough
- peripheral oedema

DIURETICS

- (High-dose, prolonged therapy) increased creatinine, hyperuricaemia, azotaemia
- see also General Adverse effects of loop diuretics (p. 1083)

Interactions

- increased risk of electrolyte imbalance and cardiotoxicity if given with class III antiarrhythmic agents (e.g. amiodarone)
- increased sensitivity to neuromuscular blocking agents may occur if hypokalaemia results
- caution if used with proton pump inhibitors owing to increased risk of hypomagnesaemia
- see also General Interactions of loop diuretics (p. 1083)

Nursing considerations/Cautions

- tablets contain lactose and are not recommended in those with hereditary problems of galactose intolerance, Lapp lactase deficiency or glucose—galactose malabsorption
- contraindicated in those with hypersensitivity to furosemide, as cross-sensitivity may exist
- see also General Nursing considerations/Cautions for diuretics (p. 1079) and General Nursing considerations/Cautions for loop diuretics (p. 1083)

Patient education

- see General Patient education for diuretics (p. 1080) and General Patient education for loop diuretics (p. 1084)

Tablet can be crushed and mixed with water or spoonful of yoghurt or apple puree.

Avoid use during pregnancy; it may cause fetal electrolyte disturbances and possible neonatal thrombocytopenia.

Limited data on use during breastfeeding. Caution is recommended as it may reduce milk supply, though it's unlikely to suppress lactation significantly. Use at the lowest effective dose and monitor both milk supply and infant health.

Higher doses are often needed in renal impairment, but kidney function may worsen. Monitor electrolytes and creatinine closely.

FUROSEMIDE (FRUSEMIDE)
Trade names
APO-Frusemide, Frusemix, Frusemix-M, Furosemide-Baxter, Furosemide-WGR, Lasix, Lasix High Dose, Noumed Furosemide, Uremide, Urex Forte

Available forms
Ampoules: 20 mg/2 mL, 40 mg/4 mL, 250 mg/25 mL;
Tablets: 20 mg, 40 mg, 500 mg;
Oral solution: 10 mg/mL

Action
- also known as a high-ceiling diuretic
- sulfonamide
- diuresis onset within 1 hour (oral), peak 1—2 hours, duration 6—8 hours
- diuresis onset within 10—15 minutes (IM), 5 minutes (IV), peak 30 minutes, duration 2 hours (IM, IV)
- biphasic half-life is about 100 minutes (prolonged in those with kidney or liver impairment or in newborns)
- oral bioavailability is about 50% of IV (e.g. 20 mg IV = 40 mg oral)
- oral bioavailability may be reduced in those with severe heart failure or renal impairment
- see also General Actions of loop diuretics (p. 1082)

Use
- treatment of severe hypercalcaemia (with adequate rehydration)
- oliguria or oedema in patients with severely impaired renal function (high-dose formulations)
- see also General Uses of loop diuretics (p. 1083)

Dose
- (Oedema) initially 20—80 mg orally daily, increasing by 20—40 mg at 6—8-hourly

intervals until required diuresis is seen (maximum daily dose 400 mg) **OR**
- (Hypertension) initially 40 mg orally twice daily, then add antihypertensive agent if response is unsatisfactory **OR**
- (Oedema) 20–40 mg IM or IV slowly; may be repeated in 2 hours if necessary **OR**
- (Acute pulmonary oedema) initially 40 mg IV slowly, increasing to 80 mg if there is no response within 1 hour **OR**
- (Cerebral oedema) 20–40 mg IV 3 times daily **OR**
- (Oedema in patients with severely impaired renal function) 250 mg diluted with 250 mL sodium chloride 0.9%, glucose 5% or lactated Ringer's solution and infused over 60 minutes at a rate not greater than 4 mg/min. A second infusion of 500 mg diluted as above may be given 1 hour after completion of first infusion if diuresis of 40–50 mL/hour has not occurred (maximum daily dose 1000 mg) (high-dose IV formulation) **OR**
- (Oedema in patients with severely impaired renal function) (after no response to conventional therapy) initially 250 mg orally daily, increasing by 250 mg every 4–6 hours until required diuresis of at least 2.5 L/day occurs (maximum daily dose 1000 mg) (high-dose oral formulation)

Adverse effects
- increased serum cholesterol and triglyceride levels
- decreased serum calcium and, rarely, tetany
- (Uncommon) impaired glucose tolerance
- transient increase in blood urea, creatinine and uric acid, gout
- (Rapid administration) ototoxicity
- (Rare) exacerbation/activation of SLE, vasculitis, acute pancreatitis, cholestasis, jaundice
- (Very rare, IV) anaphylaxis
- see also General Adverse effects of loop diuretics (p. 1083)

Interactions
- increased risk of hypotension and/or decreased renal function may occur if given with ACE inhibitors. Furosemide (frusemide) should be stopped or dose decreased for 3 days before starting therapy with ACE inhibitors or angiotensin II receptor antagonists
- (IV) not recommended within 24 hours of chloral hydrate, as sweating, flushing, nausea, tachycardia and increased BP may occur
- (IV) may increase serum levels of theophylline
- not recommended with cisplatin (increased risk of ototoxicity)
- increased risk of nephrotoxicity if given with cisplatin (unless furosemide (frusemide) is given in low doses and fluid balance is positive)
- increased risk of ototoxicity and nephrotoxicity if given with some cephalosporins (especially in high doses)
- (Oral) absorption may be decreased by sucralfate
- increases risk of salicylate toxicity if given with high-dose salicylate therapy
- may result in excessive loss of potassium if given with corticosteroids or amphotericin B (amphotericin)
- effect may be antagonised by indometacin, aspirin and other NSAIDs, as well as increased risk of renal failure if hypovolaemia also exists
- may potentiate or antagonise neuromuscular blocking agents, depending on dosage of both agents
- response may be decreased if given with antiepileptic agents
- effects may be reduced if given with phenytoin, methotrexate or probenecid
- may decrease elimination of phenytoin, methotrexate and probenecid, resulting in elevated serum levels
- caution if used with risperidone, as toxicity may result (especially in the elderly)
- furosemide (frusemide)-induced hypokalaemia or hypomagnesaemia may

DIURETICS

- increase toxicity to agents that prolong the QT interval
- corticosteroids, laxatives (prolonged use) and liquorice (large amounts) predispose the patient to hypokalaemia, and excessive potassium loss may occur if given with furosemide (frusemide)
- increased risk of gouty arthritis if given with ciclosporin
- may reduce effects of adrenaline (epinephrine) and noradrenaline (norepinephrine)
- (High dose) caution if given with levothyroxine. If given together, thyroid hormone levels should be monitored regularly
- may increase deterioration of renal function if given to those with radio-contrast nephropathy
- see also General Interactions of loop diuretics (p. 1083)

Nursing considerations/Cautions

- any fluid, electrolyte or acid—base imbalance should be corrected before starting therapy with parenteral furosemide (frusemide)
- IM route is generally not recommended unless both oral and parenteral routes are not available
- (250 mg/25 mL) should not be given as IV bolus
- (High-dose formulations, IV or oral) test dose of 40—80 mg IV over 2—5 minutes may be given to test diuretic response before administration
- not mixed with other drugs for injection or infusion
- should not be added to tubing of already running IV infusion
- may precipitate if added to solutions of pH less than 5.5
- add only to sodium chloride 0.9%, glucose 5% or compound sodium lactate for infusion and use within 24 hours (high-dose formulation)
- for hypervolaemic patients, high-dose formulation may be administered undiluted or in a small volume (50 mL) using a volumetric pump to ensure 4 mg/min limit is not exceeded (to prevent ototoxicity)
- parenteral therapy should be replaced with oral (high-dose) therapy as soon as practicable
- maximum injection and infusion rate 4 mg/min (or 2.5 mg/min if renally impaired) to avoid hearing impairment/ototoxicity
- monitor vital signs and fluid balance (input and output) if given parenterally
- oral salt restriction is not recommended
- if starting therapy with ACE inhibitor, furosemide (frusemide) should be stopped or dose decreased for 3 days prior
- recommended to discontinue furosemide (frusemide) 7 days before elective surgery
- (IV) if stored at low temperatures, crystals may form in solution. These can be dissolved by warming solution to 40°C
- (Oral solution) available in two formulations, so manufacturer's instructions should be followed regarding correct storage conditions
- (Oral solution) contains sorbitol, which may cause diarrhoea
- (Oral solution — not requiring refrigeration) contains alcohol (0.5 g/5 mL), which may be harmful in those with alcoholism, children or those with epilepsy or liver disease
- (High-dose formulations) recommended for use in those with greatly reduced glomerular filtration rate ($<$ 20 mL/min but $>$ 5 mL/min)
- (High-dose formulation) contraindicated in those with impaired renal function, severe dehydration or electrolyte imbalance, or hypotension
- (High-dose formulation) contraindicated in those with normal renal function because of increased risk of severe fluid and electrolyte loss, or hepatitis, cirrhosis, existing or impending hepatic coma or nephrotoxic agent induced renal failure

- see also General Nursing considerations/Cautions for loop diuretics (p. 1083) and General Nursing considerations/Cautions for diuretics (p. 1079)

Patient education

- advise patient to take tablets or oral solution on empty stomach
- patient should be advised to separate furosemide by at least 2 hours from sucralfate
- see also General Patient education for loop diuretics (p. 1084) and General Patient education for diuretics (p. 1080)

Available as oral solution. Tablet can be dispersed in water or crushed and mixed with water or spoonful of yoghurt or apple puree.

Avoid use unless absolutely necessary. It may cause electrolyte disturbances in the fetus, possible neonatal thrombocytopenia and reduced placental blood flow, potentially affecting fetal growth. If used, close monitoring of fluid balance, electrolytes and fetal development is essential.

Little data available; use with caution. It is unlikely to significantly suppress lactation, but higher doses may reduce milk production owing to its diuretic effects.

Higher doses may be needed in renal impairment, but it can worsen kidney function; monitor electrolytes and creatinine. Increased risk of nephrotoxicity when combined with nephrotoxic drugs, especially in renal impairment. Contraindicated in anuria.

CHLORTALIDONE

Trade name
Hygroton

Available form
Tablets: 25 mg

Action
- see General Actions of thiazide diuretics (p. 1091)

- thiazide-related; thiazide-like diuretic.
- onset of diuresis 2–3 hours, peak effect in 4–24 hours, duration 48–72 hours, half-life 24–55 hours

Use
- see General Uses of thiazide diuretics (p. 1091)

Dose
- (Oedema) up to 50 mg orally daily or on alternative days **OR**
- (Chronic stable congestive heart failure) initially 25–50 mg orally daily or 100 mg every second day, then either 12.5–50 mg daily or 25–50 mg every second day (maintenance) **OR**
- (Hypertension) initially 12.5–25 mg orally daily; if ineffective after 3–4 weeks, may be combined with anti-hypertensive agent

Adverse effects
- see General Adverse effects of thiazide diuretics (p. 1091)

Interactions
- see General Interactions of thiazide diuretics (p. 1092)

Nursing considerations/Cautions

- not recommended as first-line treatment in those with diabetes mellitus or hypercholesterolaemia
- see also General Nursing considerations/Cautions for thiazide diuretics (p. 1092) and diuretics (p. 1079)

Patient education

- see General Patient education for thiazide diuretics (p. 1093) and diuretics (p. 1080)

Tablets can be dispersed in water, or crushed and mixed with a spoonful of yoghurt or apple puree.

Avoid use, as limited human data. Diuretics can cause placental hypoperfusion and may affect fetal electrolyte

DIURETICS

balance, causing thrombocytopenia, bone marrow depression and jaundice.

Avoid use, as excreted in human breast-milk.

Reduced renal function: contraindicated and ineffective when CrCl is < 30 mL/min; thiazides may precipitate azotaemia.

Reduced hepatic function: use cautiously in patients with hepatic impairment, as minor fluid and electrolyte imbalances may precipitate hepatic coma, especially in those with liver cirrhosis.

Elderly patients may experience slower elimination; closely monitor serum electrolytes and adjust the dosage as needed.

HYDROCHLOROTHIAZIDE
Trade name
Dithiazide

Available form
Tablets: 25 mg

Action
- low-ceiling diuretic, thiazide
- onset of action within 2 hours, peak action in 4 hours, duration 6—12 hours, half-life 2.5 hours
- see also General Actions of thiazide diuretics (p. 1091)

Use
- premenstrual tension (PMT) with oedema
- see also General Uses of thiazide diuretics (p. 1091)

Dose
- (Oedema) 25—100 mg once or twice daily. Intermittent therapy (e.g. alternate days or 3—5 days per week) may help avoid excessive response and electrolyte imbalance. Maximum recommended daily dose is 200 mg **OR**
- (Hypertension) 12.5—50 mg orally daily, as a single or divided dose. Adjust dosage based on blood pressure response. Maximum recommended daily dose is 100 mg **OR**
- (Premenstrual tension with oedema) 25—50 mg orally once or twice daily from the first morning of symptoms until the onset of menses

Adverse effects
- acute transient myopia, acute secondary angle-closure glaucoma, increased risk of non-melanoma skin cancers
- see also General Adverse effects of thiazide diuretics (p. 1091)

Interactions
- see General Interactions of thiazide diuretics (p. 2)

Nursing considerations/Cautions
- caution if used in those with penicillin allergy owing to increased risk of acute secondary angle-closure glaucoma
- caution if used in patients with a history of non-melanoma skin cancers
- see also General Nursing considerations/Cautions for thiazide diuretics (p. 1092) and General Nursing considerations/Cautions for diuretics (p. 1079)

Patient education
- advise patient to seek medical advice immediately if any eye pain, blurred vision or changes to vision occur (especially at the start of therapy)
- instruct patient to check skin regularly for any new or changing skin lesions and to seek medical advice immediately if any occur. Patient should also be advised to avoid exposure to sunlight or UV light and ensure protection with sunscreen (SPF 30+), hat and long-sleeved garments
- if used for PMT, counsel patient to start therapy when symptoms start, up to the start of period
- see also General Patient education for thiazide diuretics (p. 1093) and General Patient education for diuretics (p. 1080)

Available in combination with

- hydrochlorothiazide + candesartan (see candesartan in Antihypertensive agents p. 515)
- hydrochlorothiazide + enalapril (see enalapril in Antihypertensive agents p. 508)
- hydrochlorothiazide 12.5 mg + fosinopril 20 mg (Fosetic)
- hydrochlorothiazide + irbesartan (see irbesartan in Antihypertensive agents p. 515)
- hydrochlorothiazide + olmesartan medoximil (see olmesartan medoximil in Antihypertensive agents p. 517)
- hydrochlorothiazide + telmisartan (see telmisartan in Antihypertensive agents p. 518)
- hydrochlorothiazide + valsartan (see valsartan in Antihypertensive agents p. 519)
- hydrochlorothiazide + valsartan + amlodipine (see valsartan in Antihypertensive agents p. 519)

Used only if benefits outweigh risks, and at the lowest effective dose. Thiazides can cross into fetal circulation, potentially causing electrolyte imbalances and neonatal thrombocytopenia. They may also reduce uteroplacental perfusion owing to decreased maternal blood volume.

Not recommended during breastfeeding.

Renal: less effective as diuretics when CrCl < 30 mL/min, but may still lower BP via vasodilation at low doses. Contraindicated in anuria.

Hepatic: contraindicated in hepatic precoma/coma.

Banned in sport.

INDAPAMIDE HEMIHYDRATE

Trade names
DapaTabs, Insig, APO-Indapamide SR, Natrilix SR, Odaplix SR, Tenaxil SR

Available forms
Tablets: 2.5 mg;
Tablets (sustained-release): 1.5 mg

Action
- thiazide-related; thiazide-like diuretic
- onset of action 30 min–2 hours, peak effect 1–3 hours, biphasic half-life 14 and 25 hours
- antihypertensive effect may be due to decreased vascular reactivity to pressor amines
- see also General Actions of thiazide diuretics (p. 1091)

Use
- see General Uses of thiazide diuretics (p. 1091)

Dose
- (Hypertension) 1.5 mg orally each morning (SR formulation) **OR**
- (Hypertension) 2.5 mg orally each morning

Adverse effects
- (Rare) severe skin reaction
- see also General Adverse effects of thiazide diuretics (p. 1091)

Interactions
- increased risk of antihypertensive effects if given with baclofen
- not recommended with disopyramide, amiodarone, sotalol, some antipsychotic agents, erythromycin (IV), pentamidine and moxifloxacin owing to risk of QT prolongation and cardiac arrhythmias
- if given with iodinated contrast media, patient should be well hydrated to prevent acute renal failure
- see also General Interactions of thiazide diuretics (p. 1092)

Nursing considerations/Cautions

- optimum hypotensive effect is seen in approximately 4—6 weeks
- hypotensive effect may continue for up to 1—2 weeks after stopping therapy
- tablets contain lactose and are therefore not recommended in those with rare hereditary problems of galactose intolerance, Lapp lactase deficiency or glucose—galactose malabsorption
- see also General Nursing considerations/Cautions for thiazide diuretics (p. 1092) and General Nursing considerations/Cautions for diuretics (p. 1079)

Patient education

- instruct patient to seek medical advice immediately if any of the following occur:
  - rapid or irregular heartbeat
  - skin rash with purple spots and some blistering, mainly on legs, arms, neck and around ears
- see also General Patient education for thiazide diuretics (p. 1093) and General Patient education for diuretics (p. 1080)

Available in combination with

- indapamide + perindopril (see perindopril erbumine/arginine in Antihypertensive agents p. 510)

 Sustained-release tablets should not be chewed or broken. They must be swallowed whole so it released slowly over time.

THIAZIDE AND THIAZIDE-RELATED DIURETICS

General Actions of thiazide and thiazide-related diuretics

- chemically related to sulfonamides
- increase excretion of sodium and chloride ions and water, principally in the proximal segment (diluting) of the distal tubule
- increase excretion of potassium, magnesium and bicarbonate ions
- reduce calcium excretion
- ineffective if creatinine clearance is less than 30 mL/min
- will not lower blood pressure in normotensive patients
- some vasodilator activity

General Uses of thiazide and thiazide-related diuretics

- oedema, including cirrhosis with ascites
- hypertension (as primary therapy in those with creatinine clearance > 30 mL/min or combined with antihypertensive agents)
- mild-to-moderate stable, chronic heart failure (creatinine clearance > 30 mL/min)

General Adverse effects of thiazide and thiazide-related diuretics

- electrolyte disturbances (hyperglycaemia, hypochloraemia, hypokalaemia, hyponatraemia, hypomagnesaemia, impaired glucose tolerance, hyperuricaemia, alkalosis)
- hypovolaemia, dehydration
- dizziness, vertigo, headache, asthenia, fatigue
- blurred vision
- reversible tinnitus and hearing loss (rarely permanent)
- weakness, muscle cramps
- polyuria
- hypotension
- rash, urticaria, photosensitivity
- male impotence
- increased serum total cholesterol, low-density lipoprotein (LDL) cholesterol and triglyceride levels, decreased high-density lipoprotein (HDL) cholesterol
- anorexia, mild GI disturbances, dry mouth
- (Rare) blood dyscrasias
- (Rare) hypersensitivity reactions, attack of gout, hypercalcaemia, glycosuria, activation or exacerbation of systemic lupus erythematosus

General Interactions of thiazide and thiazide-related diuretics

- thiazide diuretic-induced hypokalaemia or hypomagnesaemia may increase sensitivity of heart to digoxin, increasing risk of cardiac arrhythmias
- not recommended with lithium because it may increase serum levels and toxicity of lithium
- orthostatic hypotension may be enhanced when given with alcohol, barbiturates, opioid analgesics, sedatives or imipramine-related antidepressants
- may impair glucose tolerance and hypoglycaemic control in those with diabetes; therefore adjustment to insulin and/or oral hypoglycaemic agent may be required
- decreased antihypertensive effect may occur if given with corticosteroids
- increased risk of renal impairment if given with angiotensin converting enzyme (ACE) inhibitors and NSAIDs (including cyclooxygenase-2 (COX-2) inhibitors and high-dose aspirin)
- may potentiate the hypotensive effect of antihypertensive agents (especially ACE inhibitors)
- absorption may be reduced by colestyramine
- increased effects may occur if given with anticholinergic agents (owing to decreased GI motility and gastric emptying rate)
- increased hyperglycaemic effect if given with diazoxide
- increased risk of adverse effects if given with amantadine
- decreased diuretic and antihypertensive effects may occur if given with indometacin and some other NSAIDs
- increased risk of hypersensitivity reaction if given with allopurinol
- increase in hypokalaemia may occur if given with corticosteroids, adrenocorticotrophic hormone (ACTH), beta2 agonists or amphotericin B (amphotericin)
- caution if used with potassium-sparing diuretics owing to alterations to serum potassium levels
- may increase serum calcium level if given with vitamin D or calcium salts
- increased risk of hyperuricaemia and gout-like complications if given with ciclosporin
- caution if given with tacrolimus or ciclosporin owing to risk of increased plasma creatinine
- not recommended with metformin if plasma creatinine is > 15 mg/L (men) or 12 mg/L (women) owing to risk of lactic acidosis
- may interfere with parathyroid function tests; therefore should be discontinued before test

General Nursing considerations/Cautions for thiazide and thiazide-related diuretics

- any induced electrolyte imbalance should be corrected before therapy starts
- serum electrolytes and blood urea nitrogen (BUN) should be monitored regularly (especially potassium) and potassium supplements added if needed (or patient encouraged to eat potassium-rich food) (especially if patient is on long-term therapy)
- should be stopped for 2–3 days before starting antihypertensive therapy with ACE inhibitors or angiotensin II inhibitors
- discontinue before parathyroid function tests
- sulfonamide derivatives may activate or exacerbate systemic lupus erythematosus (SLE) in susceptible patients; therefore should be given with caution
- caution if used in the elderly, as they are more susceptible to electrolyte imbalance and orthostatic hypotension
- caution if used in those with diabetes mellitus or if receiving treatment (diet/combination) for hypercholesterolaemia with renal or liver impairment

- contraindicated in those with anuria, severe oliguria, severe kidney or liver failure (including hepatic pre-coma and coma, cirrhosis), untreated Addison's disease, refractory hypokalaemia, hyponatraemia or hypercalcaemia, history of gout or uric acid calculi, pregnancy-related hypertension, creatinine clearance less than 30 mL/min and conditions involving potassium loss or heart failure with significant oedema
- contraindicated in those with thiazide or sulfonamide sensitivity
- see also General Nursing considerations/Cautions for diuretics (p. 1079)

General Patient education for thiazide and thiazide-related diuretics

- regular blood tests may be needed to monitor electrolytes and kidney function
- increased urination is common, especially in the first few weeks
- avoid vitamin D and calcium supplements unless directed by your doctor
- avoid NSAIDs like ibuprofen, as they can reduce the diuretic's effectiveness and harm kidney function
- refrain from alcohol use during treatment
- protect your skin from the sun with clothing, hats and SPF 30+ sunscreen. Avoid tanning beds and seek help from your health professional if severe sunburn occurs
- see also General Patient education for diuretics (p. 1080)

Use only if benefits outweigh risks, and at the lowest effective dose. Thiazides can cross into the fetal circulation, potentially causing electrolyte imbalances and neonatal thrombocytopenia. They may also reduce uteroplacental perfusion owing to decreased maternal blood volume.

Not recommended during breastfeeding.

Banned in sport.

DIURETICS

ALDOSTERONE RECEPTOR ANTAGONISTS

AMILORIDE WITH HYDROCHLOROTHIAZIDE

Trade name
Only available in combination with hydrochlorothiazide (Moduretic)

Available form
Tablets: 5 mg/50 mg

Action
- potassium-sparing diuretic (antikaliuretic diuretic agent) that increases excretion of sodium in the distal convoluted tubule but conserves potassium
- does not antagonise aldosterone; therefore does not require aldosterone to be present to be effective
- mild diuretic and antihypertensive effect when used alone
- onset of action about 2 hours, peak action 6–10 hours, duration 24 hours, half-life 17–26 hours
- see also Hydrochlorothiazide (p. 1089)

Use
- oedema due to heart failure, hepatic cirrhosis or nephrotic syndrome
- hypertension

Dose
- (Oedema) initially 5–10 mg amiloride/50–100 mg hydrochlorothiazide daily; may be increased up to a maximum of 20 mg amiloride/200 mg hydrochlorothiazide daily; after diuresis, gradually reduce to the lowest effective dose
- (Hypertension) 5 mg amiloride/50 mg hydrochlorothiazide once daily

Adverse effects
- nervous system: dizziness, weakness, headache, fatigue, paraesthesia
- gastrointestinal: anorexia, nausea, vomiting, abdominal pain, flatulence, dry mouth, thirst, diarrhoea
- dermatological: mild rash, pruritus, alopecia

- reproductive system: impotence, decreased libido
- urinary system: polyuria, dysuria, bladder spasm, increased micturition
- cardiovascular: hypotension, palpitations, arrhythmias
- respiratory: cough, dyspnoea
- musculoskeletal: joint pain, back pain, pain in extremities
- hepatic (rare): jaundice

Interactions
- not recommended use with other potassium-sparing diuretics (such as spironolactone) or potassium supplements, as this increases the risk of high potassium levels (hyperkalemia)
- higher risk of hyperkalaemia if used with medicines like ciclosporin, tacrolimus, angiotensin II receptor blockers or ACE inhibitors
- increased risk of hyperkalaemia and kidney failure when taken with NSAIDs
- avoid using with lithium owing to the potential for lithium toxicity caused by increased lithium levels in the blood

Nursing considerations/Cautions
- renal function and electrolyte levels should be checked before starting and regularly throughout therapy (especially if patient is taking NSAID concurrently)
- observe for features of hyponatraemia and hyperkalaemia
- discontinue for 3 days prior to patients with diabetes having a glucose tolerance test
- caution if used in those with known or suspected diabetes mellitus (especially if uncontrolled) because of increased risk of hyperkalaemia
- caution if potassium serum levels > 3.5 mmol/L
- caution if used in those with respiratory or metabolic acidosis or liver cirrhosis
- contraindicated in those with hyperkalaemia (> 5.5 mmol/L), anuria, acute renal failure, severe progressive renal failure or diabetic nephropathy
- see also General Nursing considerations/Cautions for diuretics (p. 1079)

Patient education
- take this medicine once daily in the morning. If prescribed twice daily, take the first dose in the morning and the second before 6 pm
- you may feel dizzy when standing. Rise slowly from sitting or lying down, and sit or lie down if dizziness occurs
- avoid foods high in potassium (such as apricots, avocados, bananas, rockmelon, dates, grapefruit, oranges, potatoes, prunes, raisins, spinach, strawberries and watermelon, and orange, grapefruit, prune and pineapple juice)
- avoid potassium supplements
- seek medical attention immediately if you experience muscle weakness, tiredness, nausea, slow heart rate, weak pulse, numbness, or tingling in your hands or feet, as these may be signs of high potassium levels (hyperkalaemia)
- see also General Patient education for diuretics (p. 1080)

 Tablet can be dispersed in water or crushed and mixed with spoonful of yoghurt or apple puree.

 Not recommended during pregnancy unless the expected benefit outweighs any potential risk. Maternal use may result in electrolyte disturbance in the fetus.

 Limited data available. Avoid use.

 Banned in sport.

Available in combination with
- amiloride 5 mg + hydrochlorothiazide 50 mg tablet (Moduretic)

DIURETICS

EPLERENONE

Trade names
APO-Eplerenone, Espler, Inspra, Inpler

Available forms
Tablets: 25 mg, 50 mg

Action
- selective mineralocorticoid receptor antagonist that competitively inhibits aldosterone
- peak concentration within 1.5 hours, half-life 3—5 hours

Use
- to decrease risk of cardiovascular death in patients with heart failure/left ventricle impairment (within 3—14 days of myocardial infarction) (adjunct)
- to decrease risk of mortality and morbidity in those with chronic heart failure and left ventricular systolic dysfunction (adjunct)

Dose
- initially 25 mg orally daily, increasing to 50 mg within 4 weeks of starting therapy according to serum potassium levels

Adverse effects
- hypotension, syncope
- myocardial infarction, angina, non-cardiac chest pain
- dehydration
- dizziness
- nausea, vomiting, diarrhoea, constipation, flatulence
- hyperkalaemia, increased blood urea
- abnormal kidney function, increased creatinine
- muscle spasm, musculoskeletal pain
- cough
- pruritus
- infection

Interactions
- contraindicated with other potassium sparing diuretics owing to the risk of hyperkalemia
- contraindicated with CYP3A4 inhibitors (e.g. fluconazole, itraconazole, erythromycin, clarithromycin, verapamil and ritonavir), which can increase eplerenone levels leading to hyperkalemia and other adverse effects
- not recommended with ciclosporin or tacrolimus owing to risk of hyperkalaemia and renal impairment
- increased risk of hyperkalaemia if given with trimethoprim
- increased risk of hypotension if given with prazosin, alfuzosin, TCAs or baclofen
- not recommended with lithium
- caution if given with NSAIDs owing to risk of reduced antihypertensive effect, hyperkalaemia and renal impairment
- caution if given with ACE inhibitors or angiotensin II receptor antagonists owing to risk of hyperkalaemia
- St John's wort, rifampicin, carbamazepine, phenytoin and phenobarbital may decrease eplerenone serum levels (CYP3A4 inducers), and concurrent use is not recommended

Nursing considerations/Cautions
- serum potassium should be measured before starting therapy, after first week and first month, then regularly and the dose adjusted accordingly
- if serum potassium level is $\geq$ 6 mmol/L, therapy should be stopped and restarted at 25 mg second-daily when serum potassium level has fallen to below 5.5 mmol/L
- chronic heart failure should be reassessed after 12 months to determine effectiveness of therapy
- caution if used in those with diabetes mellitus (with cardiac failure post myocardial infarction)
- contraindicated in those with hyperkalaemia (> 5.5 mmol/L when starting therapy), moderate-to-severe kidney impairment (glomerular filtration rate < 30 mL/minute) or severe liver impairment

Patient education
- advise patient to avoid foods high in potassium (such as apricots, avocados,

bananas, rockmelon, dates, grapefruit, oranges, potatoes, prunes, raisins, spinach, strawberries and watermelon, and orange, grapefruit, prune and pineapple juice) and potassium supplements
- patient should be advised to seek medical advice immediately if they experience any muscle weakness, tiredness, nausea, slow heart rate or weak pulse, numbness or tingling in the hands or feet (signs of hyperkalaemia)
- see also General Patient education for diuretics (p. 1080)

Tablets can be crushed and mixed with water or a spoonful of yoghurt or apple puree.

Not recommended during pregnancy unless benefits outweigh risks.

Not recommended during breastfeeding unless benefits outweigh risks.

Renal: the manufacturer contraindicates the use of eplerenone if eGFR < 30 mL/min/1.73 m^2 owing to an increased risk of hyperkalemia. Dose reduction is recommended if eGFR is 30–50 mL/min/1.73 m^2.

Hepatic: eplerenone is contraindicated in severe hepatic impairment.

Banned in sport.

SPIRONOLACTONE
Trade names
Aldactone, Spiractin, Spironolactone Viatris

Available forms
Tablets: 25 mg, 100 mg

Action
- competitive inhibitor of aldosterone in the distal convoluted tubule that increases sodium and water excretion but decreases potassium excretion
- effect is directly related to plasma concentration of circulating aldosterone
- does not interfere with renal tubule transport of sodium and chloride
- does not inhibit carbonic anhydrase
- has both diuretic and antihypertensive effects
- moderate antiandrogen effects
- active metabolite (canrenone) (half-life 18–20 hours)
- onset of action 24–48 hours, peak response in 48–72 hours, effects last 3 days after discontinuation, half-life 1.5 hours

Use
- oedema associated with congestive heart failure and hepatic cirrhosis and ascites
- diagnosis and treatment of primary hyperaldosteronism
- adjunctive therapy in malignant hypertension (excessive aldosterone secretion, hypokalaemia and metabolic acidosis)
- female hirsutism
- essential hypertension
- prevention and treatment of diuretic-induced hypokalaemia (when other measures are ineffective or inappropriate)
- nephrotic syndrome

Dose
- (Essential hypertension) 50–100 mg orally daily as a single or divided dose **OR**
- (Oedema — congestive heart failure) initially 100 mg orally daily as a single or divided dose, increasing to 200 mg if needed, then reducing to 25–200 mg daily (maintenance) **OR**
- (Cirrhosis — sodium:potassium ratio > 1) 100 mg orally daily **OR**
- (Cirrhosis — sodium:potassium ratio < 1) 200–400 mg orally daily **OR**
- (Hypokalaemia) up to 100 mg orally daily **OR**
- (Female hirsutism) 50–200 mg orally daily in divided doses for 12 months as either continuous therapy or 3 weeks of

DIURETICS

therapy followed by 1 drug-free week **OR**
- (Malignant hypertension) initially 100 mg orally daily, increasing at 2-weekly intervals to 400 mg daily (with other antihypertensive agents) **OR**
- (Nephrotic syndrome) 100—200 mg orally daily **OR**
- (Primary hyperaldosteronism diagnosis — long test) 400 mg orally daily for 3—4 weeks **OR**
- (Primary hyperaldosteronism diagnosis — short test) 400 mg orally daily for 4 days

Adverse effects
- headache, drowsiness, confusion, ataxia, lethargy, drug fever, malaise, dizziness
- rash, urticaria, pruritus
- nausea, vomiting, gastritis, gastric bleeding, gastric ulceration, abdominal cramp, diarrhoea, constipation
- alopecia, hypertrichosis
- electrolyte disturbance: hyponatraemia (tachycardia, hypotension, oliguria), hyperchloraemia, hyperkalaemia (paraesthesia, muscle weakness, fatigue, flaccid paralysis, bradycardia, serum potassium > 5.5 mmol/L, ECG changes)
- (Prolonged or high-dose therapy) (females) menstrual disturbances, postmenopausal bleeding, breast pain, changes to libido, benign breast neoplasm
- (Prolonged or high-dose therapy) (males) gynaecomastia, impotence, decreased libido
- abnormal liver function
- (Female hirsutism, cyclical dosing) menstrual irregularities (in women with previously regular cycles)
- (Rare) agranulocytosis, thrombocytopenia, severe skin reactions

Interactions
- contraindicated with eplerenone
- increased risk of hyperkalaemia if given with indometacin or ACE inhibitors
- diuretic effect may be weakened by NSAIDs, in particular aspirin, indometacin or mefenamic acid
- may increase half-life of digoxin increasing serum levels and risk of toxicity
- not recommended with other potassium sparing diuretics or potassium supplements, angiotensin II inhibitors, aldosterone blockers, potassium-rich diet, NSAIDs, heparin, low molecular weight heparins or ACE inhibitors owing to risk of hyperkalaemia
- may potentiate action of other diuretics and antihypertensive agents; therefore doses should be reduced
- caution if used with noradrenaline (norepinephrine) as vascular response is reduced
- hyperkalaemic metabolic acidosis may occur if given with colestyramine or ammonium chloride
- may interfere with assay for digoxin plasma levels

Nursing considerations/Cautions
- (Primary hyperaldosteronism diagnosis) correction of hypokalaemia and hypertension is evidence for diagnosis of hyperaldosteronism (long test)
- (Primary hyperaldosteronism diagnosis) if serum potassium increases during therapy and then decreases when stopped, this is suggestive evidence for hyperaldosteronism (short test)
- monitor fluid intake, output and body weight and note increase or decrease in oedema
- check BP at start, then regularly during therapy
- maximum effect for essential hypertension may not be seen for up to 2 weeks
- serum electrolytes should be monitored regularly and therapy stopped if serum potassium > 5 mEq/L or serum creatinine > 4 mg/dL
- (Heart failure) potassium and creatinine levels should be measured 1 week after starting therapy, then monthly for 3 months, then 4 times for 1 year and 6-monthly when increasing dose
- observe for features of hyponatraemia and hyperkalaemia

- (Hirsutism) cyclical dosing of 3 weeks with 1 week drug free may decrease menstrual irregularities in women with previously regular cycle
- (Hirsutism) clinical improvement may be seen in 3–6 months, but should be continued for at least 12 months initially
- (Essential hypertension only) dose of diuretic or antihypertensive agent should be decreased by 50% when aldosterone is added and then doses adjusted according to response
- caution if used in those with kidney or liver impairment
- caution if used in the elderly as they are at greater risk of electrolyte imbalance and hypotension
- not recommended in those with severe heart failure
- contraindicated in those with anuria, acute renal failure, significant renal impairment, Addison's disease or pre-existing hyperkalaemia (> 5 mmol/L)

Patient education

- instruct patient to take with food or immediately after to increase absorption
- advise patient to avoid foods high in potassium (such as apricots, avocados, bananas, rockmelon, dates, grapefruit, oranges, potatoes, prunes, raisins, spinach, strawberries and watermelon, and orange, grapefruit, prune and pineapple juice) and potassium supplements
- patient should be advised to seek medical attention immediately if any of the following occur:
  - muscle weakness, tiredness, nausea, slow heart rate or weak pulse, numbness or tingling in hands or feet (signs of hyperkalaemia)
  - (male) breast enlargement or inability to get or maintain erection
  - (female) menstrual changes
  - changes in sex drive
  - breast pain, breast lump
  - excessive hair growth
  - hair loss or thinning
  - yellowing of skin or eyes
- (Female hirsutism, cyclical dosing) warn female patients that menstrual cycle may become irregular during therapy
- female patients of childbearing potential should be counselled to use adequate contraceptive measures throughout therapy and advise doctor immediately if pregnancy occurs
- also see General Patient education for diuretics (p. 1080)

Mask and gloves must be worn if crushing tablets, which should then be mixed with water or spoonful of yoghurt or apple puree.

Contraindicated during pregnancy. Has antiandrogenic effects, which can potentially cause demasculinisation of a male fetus. Spironolactone blocks androgen receptors and inhibits the synthesis of male hormones, which can interfere with the development of male genitalia during pregnancy.

Generally considered safe but use with caution. Low levels in breastmilk, minimal risk to the infant.

Banned in sport.

OSMOTIC DIURETICS

GLUCOSE
Trade name
Glucose 50%

Available form
Vial: 25 g/50 mL (50%)

Action
- monosaccharide
- strongly hypertonic solution that promotes diuresis by increasing osmotic pressure of glomerular filtrate
- metabolised to carbon dioxide and water releasing energy

DIURETICS

- cerebrospinal fluid (CSF) pressure reduced for 2–4 hours after injection

Use
- reduce CSF pressure and/or oedema caused by acute alcohol intoxication or delirium tremens
- severe hypoglycaemia (from insulin excess)

Dose
- (Acute hypoglycaemia) 12.5–25 g (25–50 mL) by slow IV injection at 3 mL/minute, then evaluate response

Adverse effects
- fever
- venous thrombosis, phlebitis, extravasation, thrombophlebitis
- generalised flush, local pain, vein irritation (if given too rapidly)
- precipitate vitamin B deficiency, oedema, hypokalaemia, hypophosphataemia, hypomagnesaemia
- exacerbation of diabetes mellitus
- (Overdosage) hyperglycaemia, glycosuria
- (Rare) anaphylaxis

Nursing considerations/Cautions
- patient should be closely monitored for:
  - signs of dehydration, including observation of skin (decreased skin turgor) and tongue (dry), and haematocrit measurement
  - signs of fluid overload or electrolyte imbalance including hyperglycaemia
- prolonged administration may affect insulin production
- (Acute hypoglycaemia) after desired response has been achieved, patient should be commenced on oral feeding to prevent relapse
- hypertonic solution is for IV use only
- injection should be given slowly to avoid thrombosis
- should be given using small-bore needle to avoid venous trauma
- tourniquet should be removed as soon as venipuncture is completed
- warming patient's arm and the IV solution may decrease risk of thrombosis
- flushing may occur owing to rapid administration and should subside in about 10 minutes
- should not be administered with blood or blood products because agglutination may occur
- caution if used in those with carbohydrate intolerance, thiamine deficiency (e.g. chronic alcohol abuse), diabetes mellitus, severe malnutrition, thiamine deficiency, hypokalaemia, hypophosphataemia, hypomagnesaemia, haemodilution, sepsis or trauma
- contraindicated in those with diabetic coma (while blood glucose is excessively high), anuria, at risk of or after ischaemic stroke, intracranial or intraspinal haemorrhage, delirium tremens with dehydration, or hypersensitivity to corn or corn products
- contraindicated in those with glucose–galactose malabsorption syndrome

 Safety has not been established. Use only when the potential benefits outweigh the risks to the fetus.

 Not used during breastfeeding unless expected benefit outweighs any potential risk.

 Banned in some sports and not others.

MANNITOL
Trade name
Osmitrol Intravenous Infusion

Available forms
Solution: 10% w/v, 20% w/v

Action
- pharmacologically inert
- hyperosmotic agent
- produces osmotic diuresis by inhibiting tubular reabsorption of water and enhancing sodium and chloride

excretion by increasing osmolarity of glomerular filtrate
- alters plasma osmotic pressure, lowering intraocular and cerebrospinal fluid pressures

Use
- promoting diuresis (prevention and/or treatment of acute renal failure before it becomes irreversible)
- reducing intracranial pressure (ICP) and oedema
- reducing raised intraocular pressure (where other treatments are ineffective)
- promoting urinary excretion of toxic substances by forced diuresis

Dose
- 50—100 g/24 hours by IV infusion to maintain urine output of at least 30—50 mL/hour **OR**
- (Reduce intraocular pressure) 1.5—2 g/kg body weight infused over 30 minutes using 20% solution (may be given 1—1.5 hours preoperatively) **OR**
- (ICP reduction) 0.25 g/kg body weight by IV infusion 6—8-hourly **OR**
- (Prevention of acute renal failure — oliguria) 50—100 g as a 10% or 20% solution by IV infusion (during surgery) **OR**
- (Oliguria treatment) 100 g as 20% solution by IV infusion **OR**
- (Adjunct treatment to intoxication) 10—20% solution, depending on fluid requirements and urinary output

Adverse effects
- fluid and electrolyte imbalance, hyponatraemia, hypernatraemia, acidosis
- dehydration (oedema, cramps, thirst, dry mouth), hypovolaemia, haemoconcentration
- hypotension, hypertension, tachycardia, chest pain, arrhythmia, pulmonary oedema, congestive cardiac failure
- excessive diuresis, urinary retention, acute renal failure, osmotic nephrosis
- nausea, vomiting
- headache, dizziness, raised intracranial pressure
- chills, fever
- blurred vision
- urticaria
- hypersensitivity reaction (rhinitis, angioedema, allergic reaction, anaphylaxis)
- CNS toxicity (confusion, lethargy, coma)
- (injection site) pain, necrosis, inflammation, rash, thrombophlebitis

Interactions
- increased risk of renal failure if given with nephrotoxic agents
- effects may be potentiated by diuretics
- may increase excretion of lithium and methotrexate
- increased risk of nephrotoxicity if given with ciclosporin
- caution if given with aminoglycosides owing to risk of ototoxicity
- may enhance effects of neuromuscular blocking agents
- may decrease effects of oral anticoagulants
- increased risk of digoxin toxicity if mannitol-induced hypokalaemia occurs
- may cause false positive for blood ethylene glycol concentrations

Nursing considerations/Cautions
- cardiovascular evaluation is recommended before starting therapy
- rapid infusion of hypertonic solutions is not recommended
- administration should be via large peripheral veins or central line to decrease venous irritation
- IV site should be closely monitored to avoid extravasation
- infusion rate should be regulated to maintain a urine output of 30—50 mL/hour or as directed
- monitor vital signs during infusion, noting changes in heart and respiratory rate and BP
- monitor fluid intake and output carefully, noting signs of circulatory overload, excessive diuresis or urinary retention
- monitor serum electrolytes (especially sodium and potassium), acid—base

DIURETICS

- balance, renal function and osmolarity levels closely during mannitol administration
- patient should be monitored for any signs of hypersensitivity reaction and infusion stopped immediately if any signs occur
- test dose should be given before therapy if the patient has marked oliguria or inadequate renal function (may require 1 or 2 test doses of 0.2 g/kg over 3–5 minutes to produce urine flow of 30–50 mL/hour). No more than 2 test doses should be given
- no more than 50 g of mannitol should be administered at any one time
- (ICP reduction) rebound increase in ICP may occur 12 hours after mannitol administration
- should not be administered with blood or blood products because agglutination may occur
- incompatible with cefepime, cilastatin and imipenem
- should not be administered with solutions containing potassium or sodium chloride
- any crystals formed at low temperature can be redissolved by warming solution to approximately 70°C, then allowing it to cool to room temperature before administration via an IV administration set containing a filter. Solution should not be microwaved
- caution if used in the elderly, children, women and those with psychogenic polydipsia owing to increased risk of developing hyponatraemia (which may lead to acute symptomatic hyponatraemic encephalopathy)
- not recommended in children < 12 years
- not recommended in acute traumatic brain injury or acute shock
- not recommended for those in shock and/or kidney dysfunction until fluid and electrolyte balance has been restored
- contraindicated in those with established anuria (due to severe kidney disease), pre-existing plasma hyperosmolarity, blood–brain barrier disturbance, severe heart failure, severe pulmonary congestion or frank pulmonary oedema, active intracranial bleeding (except during craniotomy), severe dehydration or if there was no response to test dose(s) or hypersensitivity to mannitol
- contraindicated in those with progressive renal damage/dysfunction, progressive heart failure or pulmonary congestion after mannitol therapy has been started

Not used during pregnancy unless expected benefit outweighs any potential risk.

Mannitol is primarily renally cleared. Renal impairment increases the risk of renal failure; dose reduction is recommended. Contraindicated in renal failure.

Banned in sport.

Also available as

- mannitol 40 mg powder for inhalation (for cystic fibrosis) (Bronchitol Powder for Inhalation)
- mannitol powder for inhalation in hard capsules composite pack; Each capsule contains 0 mg, 5 mg, 10 mg, 20 mg or 40 mg of mannitol. The delivered dose from each of the 5, 10, 20 and 40 mg capsules is approximately 3, 8, 16, and 31 mg, respectively (test for asthma) (Aridol Diagnostic Kit)

DRUG DEPENDENCE

Any drug (prescribed, over-the-counter (OTC) or recreational) has the capacity to be abused or misused. *Drug abuse* is defined as 'self-administration of a drug in chronically excessive quantities in a manner that deviates from approved medical or social patterns in a given culture resulting in physical or psychological harm', while *drug misuse* is considered to be 'inappropriate or indiscriminate use of drugs' (Knights et al 2023). Factors leading to drug abuse and dependence include sociocultural (e.g. drug availability, peer-group pressure), personality (e.g. rebelliousness, tolerance of deviance, school performance, genetic predisposition to dependence, antisocial tendencies, depression) and pharmacological factors (e.g. drug's CNS effects provide relief from problems and/or achieve pleasure) (Knights et al 2023).

Physical dependence occurs when the body progressively adapts to a drug, producing tolerance whereby the same dose produces a smaller effect. Many drugs given at therapeutic doses can result in physical dependence and also withdrawal symptoms if the drug is suddenly stopped. Physical dependence, tolerance and withdrawal symptoms are natural biological phenomena and not suggestive of addiction, which is compulsive drug taking (Knights et al 2023). The distinction between addiction and dependence is an important one for health professionals to understand as it is the underlying reason for many patients with pain being undermedicated, especially with opioid analgesics.

ACAMPROSATE
Trade names
Acamprosate Viatris, Acamprosate-WGR, APO-Acamprosate, Campral

Available form
Tablets (enteric coated): 333 mg

Action
- structurally similar to neuromediators gamma amino butyric acid (GABA) and taurine
- decreases voluntary intake of alcohol without affecting food and fluid intake
- appears to reduce elevation of brain concentration of glutamate during withdrawal from ethanol, although mechanism of action is not completely understood
- half-life 13–28 hours

DRUG DEPENDENCE

Use
- maintenance of abstinence in alcohol-dependent patients (combined with counselling)

Dose
- (weight ≥ 60 kg) 666 mg (2 tablets) orally 3 times daily **OR**
- (weight < 60 kg) 666 mg (2 tablets) orally each morning, 333 mg (1 tablet) orally at midday and at night

Adverse effects
- nausea, vomiting, abdominal pain, diarrhoea
- pruritus, rash
- decreased libido, frigidity, impotence

Interaction
- bioavailability decreased by food

Nursing considerations/Cautions
- tablets should be swallowed whole
- treatment should be started after alcohol withdrawal period, maintained even if relapse occurs and continued for up to 1 year
- should be used in combination with counselling
- patients should be monitored for any signs of depression or suicidal ideation
- tablets contain 33.3 mg of calcium; therefore caution should be observed in those who may need to limit calcium intake
- not recommended in those over 65 years
- contraindicated in those with severe kidney or liver failure

Patient education
- advise patient to swallow tablets whole, not crush or break them
- patient (or partner/family member) should be advised to report any thoughts/talk about self-harm, harm to others, suicide or death or recent attempts at self-harm or change in mood including signs of depression

 Tablet should not be crushed, chewed or broken.

 No human data; use is not recommended.

 No human data, use is not recommended.

 Renal impairment slows acamprosate elimination, increasing concentrations. Contraindicated if serum creatinine > 120 micromol/L. Contraindicated in severe hepatic impairment (Child—Pugh class C) owing to limited data, though not metabolised by the liver.

BUPRENORPHINE
Trade names
B-Patch, Bupredermal, Buvidal Monthly, Buvidal Weekly, Norspan Transdermal Patch, Sublocade, Subutex, Temgesic

Available forms
Sublingual tablets: 200 microgram, 400 microgram, 2 mg, 8 mg;
Transdermal patches: 5 mg, 10 mg, 15 mg, 20 mg, 25 mg, 30 mg, 40 mg;
Ampoules: 300 microgram/mL;
Modified-release solution (prefilled syringe): 8 mg/0.16 mL, 16 mg/0.32 mL, 24 mg/0.48 mL, 32 mg/0.64 mL, 64 mg/0.18 mL, 96 mg/0.27 mL, 100 mg/0.5 mL, 128 mg/0.36 mL, 160 mg/0.45 mL, 300 mg/1.5 mL

Action
- synthetic opioid that has both opioid agonist and antagonist properties
- more potent than morphine and longer acting (6—8 hours IM, IV or sublingual, 7 days of transdermal patches)
- active metabolite (norbuprenorphine)
- half-life about 35 hours (sublingual)

Use
- moderate-to-severe pain (short-term management), opioid dependence (detoxification or maintenance) (see Opioid analgesics, p. 1435)

Available in combination with
buprenorphine + naloxone combination (see buprenorphine in Opioids p. 1435)

BUPROPION
Trade name
Zyban SR

Available form
Tablets (sustained-release): 150 mg

Action
- selectively inhibits noradrenaline (norepinephrine) and dopamine reuptake
- originally developed as an antidepressant
- an unknown mechanism increases the ability to refrain from smoking
- has equivalent efficacy to nicotine replacement therapy but not as efficacious as varenicline; therefore considered second-line management
- use with nicotine replacement therapy does not improve efficacy
- half-life is about 20 hours
- three active metabolites (half-life range 20—37 hours)

Use
- nicotine dependence (short-term adjunct with counselling)

Dose
- initially 150 mg orally daily (for 3 days), then 150 mg orally twice daily for 7—9 weeks (daily maximum 300 mg)

Adverse effects
- headache, dizziness, insomnia, abnormal dreams, agitation, anxiety, asthenia, impaired concentration, tremor, nervousness
- anorexia, nausea, vomiting, dry mouth, constipation, altered taste sensation, abdominal pain, mouth ulcers
- urticaria, rash, pruritus, sweating, flushing
- neck pain, myalgia, arthralgia
- rhinitis, pharyngitis, sinusitis, epistaxis
- visual disturbances, increased intraocular pressure, glaucoma, mydriasis
- fever
- (Uncommon) hypertension, tachycardia, tinnitus
- (Rare) seizures, depression, psychosis, mania, suicidal ideation

Interactions
- contraindicated with or within 14 days of monoamine oxidase inhibitors (MAOIs)
- increased risk of hypertension if used with nicotine replacement therapy
- may decrease efficacy of tamoxifen
- caution if given with ifosfamide, cyclophosphamide, ticlopidine, clopidogrel or orphenadrine
- may reduce tolerance to alcohol and increase risk of neuropsychiatric adverse effects
- caution if given with St John's wort
- decreased serum levels may occur if given with phenytoin, phenobarbital (phenobarbitone), carbamazepine, efavirenz or ritonavir
- may increase serum levels of sodium valproate, increasing the risk of adverse effects
- lowers seizure threshold; therefore not recommended in those taking antidepressants, antipsychotic agents, antihistamines (sedating), corticosteroids (systemic), theophylline, tramadol, antimalarials, sedatives, stimulants, anorectic agents or those with high alcohol intake
- caution if used with tricyclic antidepressants (TCAs), selective serotonin reuptake inhibitors (SSRIs), antipsychotic agents, some beta adrenoceptor blocking agents or antiarrhythmic agents
- smoking cessation itself may alter pharmacokinetics of some medications taken concurrently
- may decrease serum levels of digoxin
- increased risk of neuropsychiatric adverse effects if given with amantadine or levodopa; therefore should be given together with caution
- may result in false positive results in some rapid urine drug screening tests

DRUG DEPENDENCE

Nursing considerations/Cautions

- before starting therapy, the patient should be assessed for any factors that might lower seizure threshold, such as medications known to lower threshold, head trauma, diabetes, use of stimulants or anorectic agents, or excessive use of alcohol or sedatives
- the patient should start therapy while they are still smoking to allow sufficient time for therapy to have its therapeutic effect. If they are still smoking after 7 weeks, it is unlikely that therapy will be of benefit
- may be combined with nicotine replacement program (although this does increase the risk of hypertension occurring) and, if used together, blood pressure should be monitored weekly
- should be part of a multifaceted program that includes counselling
- caution if used in those with psychiatric disorders (e.g. bipolar disorder) because neuropsychiatric symptoms may be precipitated or exacerbated
- caution if used in those with renal impairment, raised intracranial pressure, at risk of glaucoma, a history of head trauma, epilepsy, diabetes, high alcohol or sedative intake, recent myocardial infarction or unstable heart disease
- caution if used in those with liver impairment (especially liver cirrhosis). The dose should not be greater than 150 mg every second day
- contraindicated in those with a history of seizures, CNS tumour, abrupt withdrawal from alcohol or benzodiazepines, or current or a history of eating disorder

Patient education

- the patient should be warned not to drive or operate heavy machinery if dizziness, visual disturbance or impaired concentration occurs
- instruct the patient that insomnia can be reduced by not taking the second dose close to bedtime (but at least 8 hours after last dose)
- advise the patient to take tablets whole, not broken or crushed
- the patient should be advised not to exceed the recommended dose
- counsel the patient to avoid alcohol during therapy, as this may increase the risk of having a seizure
- advise the patient to report any insomnia, dry mouth or seizures (as these signs may indicate high drug or metabolite levels)
- the patient (or partner/family member) should be advised to report any thoughts/talk about self-harm, harm to others, suicide or death, or recent attempts at self-harm or change in mood including signs of depression
- counsel the patient to identify other strategies to help quit including other activities (e.g. eating healthy snacks, exercise, drinking water slowly, chewing sugar-free gum) that take their mind off smoking, as well as identifying other situations (such as socialising with other friends that smoke, drinking alcohol, reducing coffee intake) where smoking is a 'normal' activity for that person

 Tablets should not be crushed, broken or chewed.

 Insufficient human data available; therefore use is not recommended during pregnancy.

 Not recommended for use while breast-feeding unless benefits outweigh potential risks.

 Patients with renal impairment may need a lower dose because bupropion is excreted through the kidneys.

> Patients with hepatic impairment should be monitored for adverse effects and dose reduction should be considered in those with liver cirrhosis.

Available in combination with
- bupropion 90 mg + naltrexone 8 mg tablets (Contrave 8/90)

DISULFIRAM
Trade name
Antabuse

Available form
Tablets (effervescent): 200 mg

Action
- interferes with alcohol metabolism by inhibition of aldehyde dehydrogenase, causing an accumulation of acetaldehyde, resulting in the 'aldehyde' or 'disulfiram—alcohol' reaction (intense flushing starting at face, throbbing headache, nausea, vomiting, sweating, palpitation, difficulty breathing)
- prodrug
- inert in small doses
- half-life about 10 hours
- effect may persist for 7—14 days

Use
- deterrent to alcohol consumption in the management of chronic alcoholism (as part of a multidiscipline, holistic management strategy)

Dose
- initially 100 mg orally daily on waking (at night if sedation is a problem) for 1—2 weeks, increasing dose to a maximum of 300 mg daily if needed. For maintenance it is recommended to decrease to 200 mg daily for 6 weeks to 6 months as necessary

Adverse effects
- drowsiness, lassitude
- peripheral neuropathy, polyneuritis (numbness, tingling, pain or weakness in feet/hands)
- optic neuritis (eye pain, tenderness, visual changes)
- (During first 1—2 weeks) metallic or garlic aftertaste, fatigue, headache, acne rash, stomach upset, seizures
- (Rare) mood and psychotic changes, altered liver function tests, jaundice, hepatitis

Interactions
- contraindicated with metronidazole
- contraindicated with alcohol and alcohol-containing preparations (e.g. cough syrup, vinegar)
- use with phenytoin may result in increased levels of phenytoin and associated risk of toxicity
- use with isoniazid may result in ataxia and changes in mood
- effects of diazepam may be prolonged
- may prolong prothrombin time, requiring dose adjustments of oral anticoagulants (e.g. warfarin)
- may increase toxicity of morphine, pethidine, amphetamines and barbiturates

Nursing considerations/Cautions
- should be part of a multifaceted program that includes counselling
- therapy commences only after abstinence from alcohol for 24 hours
- intensity of reaction is proportional to the amount of alcohol ingested
- duration of reaction is dependent on ethanol concentration in the blood, but the disulfiram reaction can occur within 5—10 minutes of alcohol ingestion and last for 2—4 hours or longer (in severe cases, until there is no alcohol in blood)
- disulfiram reaction is treated using IV ascorbic acid (1 g) and chlorpromazine (5—100 mg IM). Patient should be closely monitored and any hypotension, hypoxia, fluid or electrolyte imbalance treated using supportive measures, including elevation of foot of bed by 20—25 cm

DRUG DEPENDENCE

- if therapy is prolonged, liver function monitoring and FBC are recommended regularly
- caution if used in those with diabetes, epilepsy, hypothyroidism, impaired liver or kidney function, heart disease, asthma or allergic contact dermatitis
- contraindicated in those with severe myocardial disease, ischaemic heart disease, uncompensated heart failure, previous CVA, severe personality disorder, suicide risk, psychosis/psychotic state, or serious organic brain damage

Patient education

- patient and relatives or responsible household member must be counselled and understand the basis of treatment and be educated about the disulfiram—alcohol reaction (e.g. intense flushing, sensation of heat, sweating, palpitations, tachycardia, pounding headache, hyperventilation, dyspnoea) and its consequences before starting therapy
- patient should be strongly cautioned against taking alcohol or alcohol-containing preparations, including some cough syrups, sauces, vinegar and food prepared in wine. Alcohol-based backrubs and aftershave lotions should also be avoided
- warn patient to avoid alcohol during therapy and for at least a week after stopping as disulfiram—alcohol reaction can occur for up to 3 weeks post-therapy
- advise patient that effervescent tablets should be dissolved in water
- patient should be advised not to drive or operate machinery if drowsiness, visual changes or numbness/tingling in feet occur
- warn patient that during first 1—2 weeks of therapy a number of side-effects (e.g. metallic or garlic aftertaste, fatigue, headache, acne, rash, stomach upset, seizures, impotence) may occur, but these subside after this time
- instruct patient to seek medical advice immediately if any of the following occur:

- weakness, tiredness, loss of appetite, nausea, vomiting, dark urine, abdominal pain or yellowing of skin or eyes
- numbness, tingling, pain or weakness in hands or feet
- eye pain or tenderness or changes in vision
- mood changes or abnormal thoughts

 Tablet can be dissolved in water or crushed and mixed with spoonful of yoghurt or apple puree.

 Contraindicated during pregnancy.

 No human data, use is not recommended.

 Contraindicated if patient has advanced renal disease. Contraindicated if patient has advanced liver disease, as hepatic toxicity has been reported.

METHADONE

Trade names
Aspen Methadone Syrup, Biodone Forte, Methadone-AFT, Physeptone

Available forms
Oral liquid: 5 mg/mL;
Tablets: 10 mg;
Vials: 10 mg/mL

Action
- synthetic opioid with properties similar to morphine but less hypnotic
- duration of action 4—24 hours (oral, IM or IV)
- long half-life of 15 hours in non-tolerant (opioid-naive) people, increasing to 22 hours with chronic use (with variation of 15—60 hours being reported)

Use
- severe pain (especially visceral), substitution therapy in the treatment of opioid dependence (Biodone Forte) (see Opioid analgesics, p. 1444)

NALTREXONE

Trade names
ARX-Naltrexone, Naltrexone GH

Available form
Tablets: 50 mg

Action
- opioid antagonist related to naloxone which blocks physical dependence to opioids
- produces some pupillary constriction by unknown mechanism
- does not cause disulfiram-like reaction when used as part of an alcohol dependence program
- elimination half-life 4 hours
- active metabolite (half-life about 13 hours)

Use
- part of alcohol dependence program
- adjunctive treatment in maintenance of abstinence from opioids

Dose
- (Alcohol dependence) 50 mg orally daily for up to 12 weeks **OR**
- (Opioid dependence) initially 25 mg orally daily, increasing to 50 mg daily if no signs of withdrawal occur

Adverse effects
- nausea, vomiting, decreased appetite, diarrhoea, constipation, increased thirst, abdominal pain/cramps
- headache, dizziness, nervousness, fatigue, anxiety, lethargy, irritability, low mood
- insomnia, somnolence
- joint and muscle pain
- rash
- chills
- (Large doses) hepatotoxicity
- (Rare) depression, suicidal ideation

Interactions
- not recommended with other hepatotoxic agents
- not recommended with neuroleptic agents, barbiturates, benzodiazepines, antianxiety agents, hypnotics, sedatives, centrally acting antihypertensives, sedating antidepressants, sedating antihistamines, baclofen and thalidomide
- may counteract effects of any opioid-containing preparations (including cough/cold preparations, antidiarrhoeals or combination analgesics)
- may increase rate and extent of absorption of acamprosate

Nursing considerations/Cautions
- naloxone (Narcan) challenge test should not be performed if patient's urine is positive for opioids or there are any clinical signs of opioid withdrawal
- if there is any concern that the patient is still using opioids or has used in the last 7–10 days, urine should first be tested for the presence of opioids. Naloxone (Narcan) challenge test should then be performed: 0.2 mg naloxone (Narcan) IV and observe patient for signs of withdrawal for 30 seconds, then further 0.6 mg IV and observe for 20 minutes. Alternatively, 0.8 mg SC and observe for 20 minutes for signs of withdrawal. Signs and symptoms of withdrawal include nausea, vomiting, abdominal cramps, yawning, sweating, weeping eyes, stuffy nose, rhinorrhoea, opioid craving, dysphoria, disrupted sleep, sweating, fidgeting, pupil dilation, inability to concentrate or focus, piloerection (goose bumps), anxiety, feeling of skin crawling, fasciculations, change in BP, pulse or temperature, muscle aches or cramps. If test is positive, therapy should not begin. Retest 24 hours later and if test is still positive then therapy should not begin. If negative, therapy may begin
- risk of hepatotoxicity is increased if dose > 50 mg daily, especially if therapy is prolonged
- treatment should be ceased if there are any signs of hepatitis
- patient should be closely monitored throughout therapy because risk of suicide is increased in those with a substance abuse problem

DRUG DEPENDENCE

- if patient requires opioid analgesic in an emergency situation, a larger than usual dose may be needed to obtain the required analgesic effect, greatly increasing the risk of deeper and more prolonged respiratory depression. Respiratory status should be closely monitored during this time
- motivation and social supports as part of a treatment plan are required for successful withdrawal and ongoing abstinence
- tablets contain lactose and are therefore not recommended in those with rare hereditary galactose intolerance, Lapp lactase or glucose malabsorption
- caution if used in those with liver or kidney impairment
- contraindicated in those who are currently receiving or have a dependence on opioids, experiencing opioid withdrawal, have failed the naloxone (Narcan) challenge test, have a positive urine test for opioids or have acute hepatitis or hepatic failure

Patient education
- caution patient against driving or operating machinery if dizziness or drowsiness occur
- patient should be advised to seek medical advice immediately if loss of appetite, lethargy or tiredness, abdominal pain, dark urine, pale bowel motions or yellowing of eyes or skin occurs
- counsel patient regarding the risk of opioid sensitivity and therefore increased risk of overdose and death if they stop therapy and resume heroin (opioid) habit at previous level

Insufficient human data available; use is not recommended.

Due to limited data available, caution is advised for use when breastfeeding.

Caution advised for use in patients with renal impairment as drug is primarily excreted in urine. Contradicted in patients in liver failure or with acute hepatitis. When given in high doses, hepatocellular injury has been reported.

Available in combination with
- Naltrexone 8 mg + bupropion 90 mg tablets (Contrave 8/90)

NICOTINE
Trade names
Amcal Nicotine preparations, Herron Nicaway Lozenges, Nicabate preparations, Nicorette preparations, Nicotinell preparations, Pharmacy Care Nicotine preparations, QuitX preparations

Available forms
Transdermal patches: 7 mg/day, 14 mg/day, 21 mg/day, 10 mg/16 hours, 15 mg/16 hours, 25 mg/16 hours;
Lozenges: 1.5 mg, 2 mg, 4 mg;
Chewing gum: 2 mg, 4 mg;
Inhalator: 15 mg;
Oral spray: 1 mg/spray

Action
- the main alkaloid found in tobacco which is rapidly absorbed through skin and respiratory tract
- acts on nicotinic receptors in the peripheral and central nervous systems
- cardiovascular effects include vasoconstriction, tachycardia and increased BP
- stimulates the cerebral cortex, resulting in alertness and increased cognitive performance, and produces 'stimulating' and 'reward/pleasure' effects in different parts of the brain. In low doses, produces stimulant effects. At high doses, reward effects are produced
- all formulations are equally efficacious
- evidence suggests combination nicotine replacement therapy is more effective than monotherapy

Use
- treatment of nicotine dependence, as an aid to the cessation of smoking

1109

Dose

- (Transdermal patch (e.g. Nicabate, QuitX) initially a patch of 21 mg/day applied daily for 4—6 weeks, then 14 mg/day for 2—4 weeks and finally 7 mg/day for the last 2—4 weeks **OR**
- (Transdermal patch (e.g. Nicabate, QuitX), < 10 cigarettes/day, weighing less than 45 kg or having cardiovascular disease) initially a patch of 14 mg/day applied daily for 4—6 weeks, decreasing gradually to 7 mg/day for the last 2—8 weeks **OR**
- (Transdermal patch (e.g. Nicorette), > 15 cigarettes per day) initially a patch 22.5 cm^2 (25 mg/16 hours) applied in the morning and removed each night for 8 weeks, then reducing to 13.5 cm^2 (15 mg/16 hours) for 2 weeks and finally 20 cm^2 (10 mg/16 hours) for 2 weeks **OR**
- (Transdermal patch (e.g. Nicorette), < 15 cigarettes per day) initially 13.5 cm^2 (15 mg/16 hours) applied in the morning and removed each night for 8 weeks, then reducing to 20 cm^2 (10 mg/16 hours) for 4 weeks **OR**
- (Chewing gum) one piece of gum when the person feels the urge to smoke, normally 8—12 pieces of 2 mg strength gum or 8—10 pieces of 4 mg strength gum per day for 12 weeks, then reducing amount over the next 4 weeks (daily maximum 40 mg) **OR**
- (Inhalator) 3—6 cartridges daily taking puffs that mimic normal cigarette smoking for 12 weeks, then reducing the dose over 6—8 weeks (daily maximum 6 cartridges) **OR**
- (Lozenge) 1 lozenge orally 1—2-hourly for 6 weeks, then 1 lozenge orally 2—4-hourly for 3 weeks, then 1 lozenge 4—8-hourly for 3 weeks, then 1 lozenge when strongly tempted to smoke for the next 12 weeks (daily maximum 15—20 lozenges depending on cigarette habit) **OR**
- (Oral spray) 1—2 sprays when the person feels the urge to smoke (up to 64 sprays per 24 hours) for 6 weeks, then decreasing the number of sprays over the next 3 weeks (to about half the previous number), then further reducing the number of sprays to no more than 4 per day for 3 weeks

Adverse effects

- headache, dizziness, nervousness, tremor, sleep disturbances including insomnia and abnormal dreams
- nausea, vomiting, dyspepsia, flatulence, abdominal pain, diarrhoea, dry mouth, constipation
- palpitations
- increased sweating
- cough, dyspnoea, pharyngitis
- arthralgia, myalgia
- nicotine withdrawal syndrome (craving, irritability, anxiety, impaired concentration, dizziness, nausea, vomiting, abdominal pain, sweating, flushing, confusion)
- (Chewing gum) hiccups, jaw muscle ache, sore mouth/throat, diarrhoea
- (Transdermal patch) erythema, urticaria, itching, rash, swelling, pain, burning, tingling, numbness, heavy sensation at application site or surrounding limb and, uncommonly, hypersensitivity
- (Inhaler) mouth/throat irritation, cough, nasal congestion, hiccups
- (Lozenge) hiccups, mouth/throat irritation and ulceration, burning sensation, dry mouth, bloating, belching, dysphagia, heartburn, indigestion
- (Oral spray) mouth/throat irritation, hiccups, cough, mouth ulcers, gum bleeding, nasopharyngitis

Interactions

- cessation of smoking may alter response to concurrently used medications, with or without nicotine substitutes
- smoking increases metabolism (and decreases blood levels) of caffeine, theophylline, insulin, fluvoxamine, olanzapine, clomipramine, clozapine, paracetamol, oestrogens, prazosin, labetalol, lidocaine (lignocaine), warfarin and imipramine, and therefore ceasing smoking will lead to increased blood levels. Other agents

DRUG DEPENDENCE

that require close monitoring include antiepileptics, furosemide (frusemide), propranolol, H$_2$-antagonists, isoprenaline, phenylephrine and nifedipine
- may enhance effects of adenosine

Nursing considerations/Cautions

- if the person relapses on monotherapy, combination (e.g. a transdermal patch plus gum/lozenge/oral spray/inhaler) may be used. However, only 2 mg strength (not 4 mg strength) lozenge/gum should be used as combination therapy
- (Transdermal patches) are available in a variety of strengths, so ensure the correct strength is selected (e.g. a patch labelled 21 mg/day means that a total of 21 mg of nicotine is absorbed over 24 hours). Dimensional measures (cm^2) refer to the drug releasing area, not the patch size
- (Oral spray) therapy should be stopped when the patient is using only 2–4 sprays per day. Regular use for longer than 6 months is not recommended
- (Chewing gum) contains sorbitol, which is not recommended in those with hereditary fructose intolerance and may have laxative effect in others
- (Chewing gum) caution if used by those with dentures (as chewing may be difficult) or if oral inflammation is present
- (iInhalator) offers an alternative to patches and gum that addresses behavioural dependence ('hand-to-mouth' action) as well as physical dependence
- (Inhaler/inhalator) caution if used in those with asthma or chronic throat conditions
- (Lozenge) contains 15 mg sodium per lozenge, which may need to be considered in those on a low-sodium diet
- (Lozenge) contains aspartame and is therefore contraindicated in those with phenylketonuria
- (Lozenge) caution if used in those with any oral inflammation
- (Transdermal patches) caution if used in those with a history of dermatitis
- caution if used in those with diabetes when nicotine replacement therapy is started, as carbohydrate metabolism may be affected and therefore impact on blood glucose levels. Vasoconstriction may also reduce insulin absorption
- combination therapy (using more than one nicotine preparation at the same time) is not recommended in those with known cardiovascular disease
- (Oral spray) caution if used in those with active gastric/duodenal ulcers or oesophagitis, as symptoms may become exacerbated
- caution if used in those with moderate-to-severe liver or kidney impairment, uncontrolled hypertension, vasospasm, heart failure, stable angina, cerebrovascular disease or occlusive peripheral arterial disease
- caution if used in those with hyperthyroidism or pheochromocytoma
- caution if used in those with susceptibility to angioedema and/or urticaria
- (Nicabate P) contraindicated in those who smoke < 10 cigarettes/day or weigh < 45 kg
- (Transdermal patches) contraindicated in those with chronic dermatological conditions such as urticaria and psoriasis
- (All nicotine products) contraindicated in those who are non-tobacco users, within 3 months of myocardial infarction, in those who have unstable angina, variant (Prinzmetal) angina, severe cardiac arrhythmias or acute phase of stroke

Patient education

- advise the patient of counselling facilities that may assist, such as Quitline (Australia: 13 78 48; New Zealand: 0800 778778)

- instruct the patient to keep nicotine-containing products out of reach of children and ensure used products are safely disposed of, because poisoning in children can be fatal
- a patient with diabetes should be advised to monitor blood glucose levels during therapy, as well as after quitting smoking altogether
- warn the patient that if they continue to smoke while using nicotine-containing products (or using multiple products concurrently), the risk of adverse effects (especially cardiovascular) is greatly increased
- the patient should be cautioned against abrupt withdrawal from nicotine products to avoid withdrawal syndrome (dysphoria, depression, insomnia, irritability, anger, frustration, anxiety, impaired concentration, impatience, restlessness, decreased heart rate, increased appetite and weight gain)
- nicotine is dangerous in small children and can be fatal. Patients should be warned to keep nicotine replacement therapy products out of reach of children

Transdermal patches
- advise the patient to:
    - rotate sites daily (using upper thigh, upper body and upper outer arm)
    - apply to clean, non-hairy skin
    - avoid areas that are red, irritated or broken skin or creases
    - the same application site should not be reused within 7 days to avoid adverse skin reaction
    - bathing, swimming and showering are permissible as long as the patch is correctly applied
    - wash hands thoroughly after application or removal of the patch
    - avoid contact with eyes or sensitive skin
    - remove the transdermal patch if undergoing MRI procedure
    - discard used patches safely (folded in half with sticky side innermost)
- Nicorette patches should be applied in the morning and removed at night (16-hour use), whereas QuitX and Nicabate are left on the skin for 24 hours. However, if the person is experiencing sleep disturbance, the patch may be removed at bedtime
- withdrawal from patches should be gradual, beginning at about 12 weeks and being completed by approximately week 16. Withdrawal consists of reducing patch strength over a number of weeks (e.g. for a person starting on a 30 cm^2 patch, reduce to a 20 cm^2 patch for 2 weeks, followed by a 10 cm^2 patch for 2 weeks before final withdrawal). Soft gum or lozenges may be used with the patches during this withdrawal period
- the patient should be advised that if they continue to smoke or chew nicotine-containing gum while using transdermal patches, they are at risk of greater adverse effects because of the added amount of nicotine
- instruct the patient to stop using patches and seek medical advice if they experience persistent (4 days) or severe local skin reactions at application site or generalised skin reactions, including rash, hives or urticaria

Chewing gum
- gum is available in different strengths, so ensure that the correct strength is selected, with 4 mg gum recommended for those who smoke > 20 cigarettes/day
- the patient should be instructed in the correct use of the gum before starting therapy, including:
    - use only 1 piece of chewing gum at a time and no more than 20 pieces/day (2 mg) or 10 pieces/day (4 mg)
    - use 1 piece of chewing gum per hour only
    - chew the gum slowly until a strong taste or slight tingling is felt
    - when this occurs, the gum should be placed under the tongue or between the cheek and gums until the taste or tingling has disappeared

DRUG DEPENDENCE

- chewing may then be slowly resumed and the procedure repeated until the effects are no longer felt (about 30 minutes)
- avoid rapid chewing as this may result in hiccups, nausea or irritation to the mouth/throat
- any nicotine swallowed is destroyed by the liver
- if indigestion or heartburn occurs with 4 mg gum, changing to 2 mg gum, chewing slowly and increasing frequency of use (if needed) may reduce symptoms
- instruct the patient to avoid acidic drinks (e.g. coffee, soft drinks) for 15 minutes before using the gum, because the acid interferes with nicotine absorption
- the patient should be warned that overdose may occur if multiple pieces of gum are chewed together or in rapid succession
- after 3 months, the patient should be advised to reduce the number of pieces chewed daily gradually to 1—2 pieces/day and then stop completely
- if therapy extends beyond 9 months, the patient should be advised to seek medical advice, as alternative strategies may be required for successful quitting to occur
- warn the patient that, because of mannitol and sorbitol content in the gum, excessive use may result in diarrhoea
- advise the patient that gum (2 mg) may be used with transdermal patches

Inhaler/Inhalator
- instruct the patient on correct use including:
  - a sealed cartridge is put into the mouthpiece, which is then reassembled and seals both ends of the broken cartridge. Nicotine is vaporised and absorbed as air is inhaled through the cartridge
  - technique depends on the person's preference and smoking habit (e.g. can be used intensely or using a slower technique)
- each cartridge equals 7 cigarettes (about 80 puffs)
- if craving is not relieved, the number of puffs, size of puffs or how often used should be increased (however, not greater than 6 cartridges over 24 hours)
- an opened cartridge should be used for only 24 hours and then discarded
- the patient should be instructed not to eat or drink during inhaler therapy
- instruct the patient to avoid acidic drinks (e.g. coffee, soft drinks) for 15 minutes before using the inhaler, because the acid interferes with nicotine absorption

Lozenge
- those who have their first cigarette of the day more than 30 minutes after waking should be advised to use 2 mg strength lozenge; however, if the person has their first cigarette of the day less than 30 minutes after waking, a 4 mg strength lozenge should be used
- advise the patient that lozenges should not be chewed or swallowed whole. The lozenge should be placed in the mouth and allowed to dissolve over 20—30 minutes, moving lozenge from one side of the mouth to the other
- the patient should be advised to use only one lozenge at a time
- the patient should be instructed to refrain from eating or drinking until the lozenge is totally dissolved
- instruct the patient to avoid acidic drinks (e.g. coffee, soft drinks) for 15 minutes before using lozenge, because the acid interferes with nicotine absorption
- after 12 weeks of therapy, the patient should be counselled to take 1 lozenge if smoking urge is strong

Oral spray
- ensure the patient understands how to use oral spray, including:
  - prime the device before first use, or if unused for 2 days, by pointing the nozzle away from their self or anyone else and pressing several times until a fine spray occurs

- pointing spray nozzle towards the open mouth (as close as possible) and pressing to release one spray (avoiding the lips)
- avoid inhaling while spraying to prevent spray in the throat
- not swallowing for a few seconds after spraying
- if a second spray is required, repeat the above steps
- avoid contact with eyes. If this occurs, the eye should be rinsed thoroughly with water
- ensure the device is safely closed after each use
- advise the patient not to use more than 2 sprays per episode and no more than 64 sprays in 24 hours (4 sprays per hour over 16 hours)
- may be combined with transdermal patches (no more than 2 sprays per hour, or 32 sprays per day)
- instruct the patient to avoid acidic drinks (e.g. coffee, soft drinks) for 15 minutes before using oral spray, because the acid interferes with nicotine absorption

Nicotine is harmful to the fetus, but the risk from nicotine replacement therapy appears to be lower than that from smoking. Nicotine affects fetal breathing and has a dose-dependent impact on placental circulation. Lozenges and gum are preferred, as the daily dose is lower than for patches.

Nicotine is found in breastmilk. Patches are not recommended during breastfeeding. Gum or lozenges should be used just after breastfeeding to allow the maximum time between therapy and breastfeeding.

VARENICLINE

Trade names
Pharmacor Varenicline, Varenapix
Varenicline Lupin, Varenicline Sandoz,
Varenicline Viatris

Available form
Tablets: 0.5 mg, 1 mg

Action
- has both agonist (alleviating craving and withdrawal symptoms) and antagonist (blocking reward and reinforcing effects of smoking) activity
- highly selective, binding to alpha4 beta2 receptor, thereby blocking nicotine from binding to the same site
- as efficacious as combination nicotine replacement therapy (NRT) but greater efficacy than monotherapy NRT
- considered first-line treatment
- half-life 10–58 hours

Use
- aid to smoking cessation

Dose
- 0.5 mg orally daily (for 3 days), then 0.5 mg orally twice daily (for 4 days), then 1 mg orally twice daily (for remainder of therapy)

Adverse effects
- nausea, vomiting, dyspepsia, dry mouth, diarrhoea, constipation, flatulence, abdominal pain/distension, altered taste, increased or decreased appetite, weight gain
- headache, fatigue, dizziness, somnolence, insomnia, abnormal dreams, nightmares, agitation, irritability, disturbed attention
- nasopharyngitis, sinusitis, cough, dyspnoea
- rash, pruritus
- back pain, arthralgia, myalgia
- (Uncommon) altered mood, abnormal thinking, restlessness, decreased libido
- (Uncommon) hypertension, chest pain
- (Rare) seizures, angioedema, severe skin reactions, sleepwalking

Interactions
- smoking impacts on pharmacokinetics of many agents and this should be considered when ceasing smoking, as dose adjustments may be necessary
- increased risk of adverse effects if taken with NRT

DRUG DEPENDENCE

- caution if used with alcohol, as it may increase the risk of neuropsychiatric adverse effects as well as increasing alcohol's effects

Nursing considerations/Cautions

- before starting therapy, the patient should set a target date to stop smoking and therapy started 1—2 weeks before the target date. Alternatively, the patient can start therapy and stop smoking between days 8 and 35
- therapy should go for 12 weeks: for those who successfully stop smoking in this time, 1 mg twice daily is recommended for a further 12 weeks to reinforce abstinence; for those not successful in 12 weeks (or who relapse), factors contributing to failure should be identified and dealt with before recommencing therapy
- stopping smoking may be associated with exacerbation of underlying psychiatric diseases and these should be identified before starting therapy
- caution if used in those with a history of seizures or cardiovascular disease

Patient education

- instruct the patient to take tablets whole (not divided or chewed) with a glass of water; if feeling nauseous take with food.
- the patient should be advised not to drive or operate machinery if fatigue, dizziness and sleep problems are ongoing problems
- warn the patient that, when therapy is stopped, increased irritability, an urge to smoke, depression and/or insomnia commonly occur
- counsel the patient to identify other strategies to help quit including other activities (e.g. eating healthy snacks, exercise, drinking water slowly, chewing sugar-free gum) that take their mind off smoking, as well as identifying other situations (such as socialising with other friends who smoke, drinking alcohol, reducing coffee intake) where smoking is a 'normal' activity for that person
- the patient (or partner/family member) should be advised to report any thoughts/talk about self-harm, harm to others, suicide or death or recent attempts at self-harm, or a change in mood including signs of depression, agitation and/or anxiety
- advise the patient to seek medical advice immediately if any of the following occur:
  - rash or sudden severe itching
  - severe painful red blisters, chills, fever, feeling unwell
  - swelling of face, lips, eyes, throat
  - fitting (seizures)
  - sleepwalking
  - any new or worsening heart symptoms including chest pain
- warn the patient that the intoxicating effects of alcohol may be increased, as well as increasing the risk of neuropsychiatric adverse effects such as altered mood or abnormal thinking

Tablet can be dispersed in water or crushed and mixed with a spoonful of yoghurt or apple puree.

No human data; use is not recommended in pregnancy.

No human data; use is not recommended while breastfeeding.

Reduce the dose in patients with severe renal impairment if creatine clearance (CrCl) < 30 mL/min because of increased exposure to drug.

ERECTILE DYSFUNCTION AGENTS

Sensory or mental stimulation begins penile erection, as impulses from the brain and local nerves cause relaxation of the corpora cavernosa muscles, allowing blood to flow in. This causes an increase in pressure, resulting in expansion of the penis. The erection is maintained because the tunica albuginea traps the blood. When the penile muscles contract, the inflow of blood is stopped and the outflow channels open, thereby reversing the erection. Therefore normal erection is dependent on intact autonomic and somatic nerves, arterial blood flow and neurotransmitter (nitric oxide) to ensure it is initiated, sustained and then reversed (Sorensen et al 2025).

Erectile dysfunction is defined as the consistent inability to attain or maintain a sufficiently rigid penile erection for sexual intercourse (Sorensen et al 2025). It is a common condition that, if left untreated, can impact negatively on a person's quality of life. While not life threatening in itself, erectile dysfunction can be an early sign of more serious vascular problems. Erectile dysfunction is thought to occur for one or more of three reasons:

- failure to initiate (psychogenic, endocrinological or neurogenic)
- failure to fill (arteriogenic), and/or
- failure to store adequate blood volume within lacunar network (veno-occlusive dysfunction).

Commonly, conditions implicated in the development of erectile dysfunction include penile problems (e.g. injury to the penis); problems with the muscles, fibrous tissues, veins or arteries (arteriogenic) (reduced arterial blood flow from progressive vascular disease is the most common cause) in or near the corpora cavernosa; diabetes mellitus; obesity; heart disease; hypertension; general systemic inflammatory diseases (e.g. rheumatoid arthritis); chronic alcoholism; neurological diseases (e.g. multiple sclerosis) and spinal cord injury. Surgery or radiation therapy (e.g. prostate or bladder surgery for cancer), commonly prescribed medications (e.g. antihypertensive agents, diuretics, selective serotonin reuptake inhibitors (SSRIs), tricyclic antidepressants (TCAs), lithium and phenothiazines) and recreational agents (e.g. alcohol, cocaine, marijuana) can also produce erectile dysfunction as an adverse effect. Furthermore, smoking, hormonal abnormalities and psychological (psychogenic) factors (e.g. stress, anxiety, guilt, depression, anger) are also implicated (Sorensen et al 2025).

It is important that underlying causes are investigated and treated (if possible) before starting therapy with erectile dysfunction agents. This includes taking a history to identify comorbidities (e.g. diabetes, cardiac or peripheral vascular disease), lifestyle (e.g. alcohol intake, smoking), medication review and physical examination (e.g. cardiovascular and neurological examinations, genitalia examination to identify any abnormalities). Blood tests may also be conducted for lipid profile, glucose and testosterone levels.

Treatment should be patient focused. Lifestyle modification and decreasing cardiac risk factors are critical and should include smoking cessation, reduction of alcohol intake, diet, exercise and management of other medical issues such as diabetes, hypertension and dyslipidaemia. Management strategies can include hormonal replacement, vasoactive therapy (e.g. using phosphodiesterase type 5 (PDE-5) agents, injectable medications), vacuum erection devices, penile prosthetic surgery (e.g. implant) and sexual health therapy or psychological counselling (Sorensen et al 2025).

INTRACAVERNOSAL ADMINISTRATION

General Adverse effects of intracavernosal administration

- pain (including burning sensation or tension) in penis during erection, penile fibrosis, prolonged erection (lasting 4–6 hours), priapism (erection lasting > 6 hours)
- (Injection site) bleeding, haematoma, oedema, inflammation, itching, swelling

General Interactions of intracavernosal administration

- increased risk of bleeding if given with anticoagulants
- not recommended with other erectile dysfunction agents

General Nursing considerations/Cautions for intracavernosal administration

- medical causes of erectile dysfunction should be examined before use of erectile dysfunction agents and penile fibrosis should be excluded
- first injection should be administered by medical personnel and the patient educated in self-administration techniques
- the dose should be sufficient for erection, lasting no longer than 1 hour for satisfactory sexual intercourse
- contraindicated in women or children
- contraindicated in men who are predisposed to priapism (e.g. leukaemia, sickle cell anaemia), have a deformed penis (e.g. angulation, cavernosal fibrosis, Peyronie's disease), penile fibrosis or a penile implant, or if sexual activity is not advisable or contraindicated

General Patient education for intracavernosal administration

- the patient should be advised to visit a specialist regularly to establish efficacy and dose, as well as for examination for penile fibrosis
- instruct and assess the patient (or partner) in:
  - correct self-injection technique
  - reconstitution of powder or dialling of dose
  - not injecting more than once daily or 3 times per week
  - cleaning area with alcohol swab before injection

- rotating injection sites, not using midline or underside of penis for injection, and taking care to avoid veins
- not using bent needles or attempting to straighten bent needles, because this increases the risk of needle breakage during administration. If needle breakage occurs, the patient should attend the emergency department immediately
- performing an injection while upright, standing or slightly reclining
- massaging after injection to help the solution distribute through the penis
- applying pressure to the injection site for 5 minutes or until bleeding stops
- using equipment once only
- safe disposal of injection equipment
* in titrating dose, the patient should be advised to halve the dose if erection lasts for more than 1 hour
* small amounts of blood may be present at the injection site and the patient should be advised about the possibility of blood-borne diseases and their spread
* counsel patient regarding the need to use barrier methods (e.g. condom) to protect against sexually transmitted or blood-borne diseases
* instruct the patient to seek medical attention immediately if:
  - an erection lasts for longer than 4 hours. The patient should be advised to empty their bladder, try walking around, take a shower and avoid sexual contact before seeking medical attention
  - any new or increased penile pain, penile bending or nodule formation in shaft occurs

ALPROSTADIL (prostaglandin E1)
Trade names
Caverject Impulse, Neupedix, Prostin VR

Available forms
Disposable syringe device (powder and diluent): 10 microgram, 20 microgram; Ampoules: 500 microgram/mL (for treatment of ductus arteriosus)

Action
- vasodilator, prevents platelet aggregation
- relaxes trabecular smooth muscle and dilates cavernosal arteries, inducing erection in men with erectile dysfunction, with erection starting 5—20 minutes after administration and duration being dose dependent

Use
- erectile dysfunction in adult men (treatment and diagnosis) (see p. 1116)
- to maintain patency of the ductus arteriosus in neonates with congenital heart failure until surgery is possible

Dose
- (Erectile dysfunction treatment) initially 2.5—5.0 micrograms intracavernosally, increasing by 2.5—5.0 microgram increments until a satisfactory response is achieved (usually 10—20 micrograms) (no more than once daily or 3 times per week) **OR**
- (Erectile dysfunction diagnosis) initially 2.5 micrograms intracavernosally, increasing by 2.5 microgram increments

Adverse effects/Interactions
- see General Adverse effects/Interactions of intracavernosal administration (p. 1117)

Nursing considerations/Cautions
- starting dose is dependent on cause of erectile dysfunction. If the cause is unknown or due to neurogenic/psychogenic causes, the starting dose is 2.5 micrograms, increasing in 2.5 microgram increments. If cause is arteriogenic (or other cause), the starting dose is 5 micrograms with increments of 5 micrograms
- contains benzyl alcohol
- see also General Nursing considerations/Cautions for intracavernosal administration (p. 1117)

ERECTILE DYSFUNCTION AGENTS

Patient education
- instruct the patient that reconstituted solution can be refrigerated for up to 24 hours if not used
- the patient (and partner) should be advised not to inhale particles or expose skin to alprostadil
- see also General Patient education for intracavernosal administration (p. 1117)

 Semen may contain small amounts of alprostadil, which stimulates uterine smooth muscle. Use of condoms is therefore recommended if the partner is pregnant.

Note
- Prostin VR and Neupedix are not used for erectile dysfunction

PAPAVERINE HYDROCHLORIDE
Trade name
(DBL Papaverine Hydrochloride Injection)

Available forms
Ampoule: 120 mg/10 mL

Action
- relaxes arteriolar smooth muscle, leading to penile erection
- spasmolytic effect is pronounced in coronary, cerebral, pulmonary and peripheral vessels
- relaxes smooth muscles of bronchial, GI, biliary and urinary tracts
- direct inotropic effect, increasing myocardial oxygen consumption, decreasing myocardial excitability, prolonging refractory period and depressing myocardial conductivity
- erection within 10 minutes of injection, duration > 1 hour, short half-life 1–2 hours

Use
- erectile dysfunction treatment

Dose
- initially 15 mg intracavernosally, increasing or decreasing the dose to achieve required result (up to 60 mg) **OR**
- (Erectile dysfunction caused by spinal cord injury) initially 5 mg intracavernosally, then titrating the dose to required response

Adverse effects
- liver function abnormalities
- headache, flushing, heat sensation in pelvis, dizziness
- retinal irritation (seeing sparks or flashes)
- tachycardia, hypotension
- syncope, vasovagal reaction
- allergic reaction, urticaria
- tolerance (with long-term use)
- impaired ejaculation, loss of penile sensation, thrombophlebitis
- (High dose) cardiac arrhythmias, apnoea
- see also General Adverse effects of intracavernosal administration (p. 1117)

Interactions
- may be potentiated by CNS depressants
- may result in synergistic action if given with morphine
- may interfere with levodopa; therefore not recommended for use together
- not recommended with alprostadil because of the risk of dizziness and syncope
- see also General Interactions of intracavernosal administration (p. 1117)

Nursing considerations/Cautions
- if the patient does not respond to a 60 mg dose, other therapies should be considered
- if erection lasts longer than 4 hours, the dose should be reduced
- if tolerance occurs with long-term use, an increase in dose may be required
- baseline and 6-monthly liver function tests are recommended in those males who have liver disease or a history of alcohol abuse
- patients with psychogenic erectile dysfunction are more likely to respond to lower doses, while higher doses may be required in those with vasculogenic erectile dysfunction

- incompatible with lactated Ringer's solution, as precipitate will form
- caution in those males who have liver impairment, cardiac conduction disorders or unstable cardiovascular disease
- contraindicated in men with complete AV block
- see also General Nursing considerations/Cautions for intracavernosal administration (p. 1117)

Patient education

- advise the patient to take care rising from a lying or sitting position or when climbing stairs because of the risk of postural hypotension
- the patient should be instructed to seek medical advice immediately if any of the following occur:
  - rapid or unusual heart rate, fainting
  - yellowing of eyes or skin, dark urine, upper abdominal pain, lethargy, nausea, loss of appetite, light bowel motions
- see also General Patient education for intracavernosal administration (p. 1117)

 ECG is recommended in the elderly before starting therapy to rule out any cardiac conduction disorders.

PHOSPHODIESTERASE TYPE 5 (PDE5) INHIBITORS

General Actions of PDE5 inhibitors

- sexual stimulation leads to an increase in nitrous oxide levels that leads to an increase in cyclic guanosine monophosphate (cGMP), which relaxes smooth muscle
- inhibits specific phosphodiesterase type 5 (main phosphodiesterase in human corpora cavernosa) (commonly known as a PDE5 inhibitor) that breaks down cGMP, resulting in relaxation of smooth muscle and flow of blood into penile tissue, producing an erection
- effective in a broad range of reasons for erectile dysfunction, including psychogenic, diabetic, vasculogenic, post-radical prostatectomy (nerve-sparing procedures) and spinal cord injury
- may also inhibit phosphodiesterase type 6, involved in phototransduction cascade in the retina

General Adverse effects of PDE5 inhibitors

- headache, flushing, dizziness
- dyspepsia, diarrhoea
- nasal and sinus congestion, rhinitis
- urinary tract infection
- abnormal vision (including increased sensitivity to light, blurred vision, colour tinge in vision)
- rash
- (Uncommon) angina, tachycardia, palpitations, transient hypotension, dyspnoea, hearing impairment, tinnitus
- (Rare) myocardial ischaemia, arrhythmias, non-arteritic anterior ischaemic optic neuropathy (NAION), prolonged erection, priapism, allergic reaction

General Interactions of PDE5 inhibitors

- contraindicated with nitrates (via any route), including glyceryl trinitrate, isosorbide salts, sodium nitroprusside, amyl nitrite and nicorandil
- serum levels may be increased if given with clarithromycin, erythromycin, itraconazole, ritonavir or voriconazole; therefore contraindicated together
- increased risk of hypotension if given with riociguat; therefore contraindicated together
- serum levels may be decreased if given with rifampicin, phenobarbital (phenobarbitone), phenytoin, bosentan or carbamazepine
- caution if given with alpha adrenoceptor blocking agents (e.g. prazosin), as hypotension may occur. The patient should be haemodynamically stable for introduction of PDE5 inhibitor therapy, which should be started at the lowest dose

ERECTILE DYSFUNCTION AGENTS

- not recommended with alcohol
- serum levels may be increased by grapefruit juice

General Nursing considerations/Cautions for PDE5 inhibitors

- the patient should have a thorough medical and physical examination (especially cardiovascular assessment) before starting therapy. Reasons for erectile dysfunction should be investigated before starting therapy
- if the patient has not engaged in sexual intercourse for some time, cardiovascular assessment is recommended before starting therapy
- erectile dysfunction agents are not indicated for use in women
- caution if used in men with severe kidney impairment, cardiovascular disease with left ventricular outflow obstruction (e.g. aortic stenosis), coronary revascularisation, predisposition to priapism (e.g. sickle cell anaemia, leukaemia, multiple myeloma), deformity of the penis, diabetic retinopathy, bleeding disorders, active peptic ulceration, conditions that are sensitive to hypotension or multiple system atrophy (with impaired blood pressure control)
- contraindicated in those men for whom sexual activity is not recommended owing to heart failure, unstable angina or uncontrolled arrhythmias, recent stroke (within 6 months) or myocardial infarction (90 days), hypertension (BP > 170/110), hypotension (BP < 90/50), severe liver impairment (Child-Pugh C), known hereditary degenerative retinal disorders (e.g. retinitis pigmentosa), or if they have had vision loss due to NAION or hypersensitivity to PDE5 inhibitors

General Patient education for PDE5 inhibitors

- warn the patient not to exceed daily dose and use only once per day
- the patient should be advised not to combine therapies for erectile dysfunction
- instruct the patient to take medication about 1 hour before intending to have sex
- advise the patient against driving or operating machinery if dizziness or visual disturbances occur
- warn the patient that substantial consumption of alcohol with therapy may result in dizziness, fainting and hypotension
- instruct the patient to avoid grapefruit juice for 24 hours before use
- the patient should be advised to stop therapy and immediately seek medical advice if any of the following occur:
  - loss of vision to one or both eyes occurs (NAION)
  - changes to vision (blurring, sensitivity to light, blue tinge)
  - decrease or loss of hearing, or ringing/buzzing in the ears
  - persistent headache
  - unusual heart rate or chest pain
  - prolonged erection lasting longer than 4 hours (as damage to penile tissue may occur)
- ensure the patient understands that alcohol may impair the ability to obtain an erection

AVANAFIL

Trade name
Spedra

Available forms
Tablets: 50 mg, 100 mg, 200 mg

Action
- active metabolites
- half-life 6—17 hours
- see also General Actions of PDE5 inhibitors (p. 1120)

Use
- erectile dysfunction in adult males

Dose
- 100 mg orally once daily 15—30 minutes before sexual activity (maximum daily dose 200 mg)

Adverse effects
- back ache, muscle tightness
- nasopharyngitis, sinusitis, bronchitis, influenza
- hypertension
- see also General Adverse effects and Interactions of PDE5 inhibitors (p. 1120)

Interactions
- caution if used with vasodilators or antihypertensive agents because of the risk of symptomatic hypotension (e.g. dizziness, lightheadedness, syncope or near syncope)
- not recommended with bosentan or grapefruit juice
- increased serum levels may occur if given with erythromycin, amprenavir, aprepitant, diltiazem, fluconazole, fosamprenavir or verapamil. If used together, avanafil dose should be restricted to 100 mg every 48 hours
- see also General Interactions of PDE5 inhibitors (p. 1120)

Nursing considerations/Cautions
- the dose can be decreased to 50 mg or increased to 200 mg once daily if needed
- contraindicated in those with severe liver impairment (Child—Pugh C), severe kidney impairment (creatinine clearance < 30 mL/min), chronic kidney disease stage 4 or end-stage kidney failure
- see also General Nursing considerations/Cautions for PDE5 inhibitors (p. 1121)

Patient education
- advise the patient to avoid grapefruit juice for at least 24 hours before taking avanafil
- warn the patient that onset of activity may be delayed if taken with food
- see also General Patient education for PDE5 inhibitors (p. 1121)

 Tablets can be crushed and mixed with water or spoonful of yoghurt or apple puree.

SILDENAFIL
Trade names
(APX-Sildenafil, Noumed, Revatio, Silcap, Sildatio PHT, Sildenafil, Sildenafil Generichealth, Sildenafil Lupin, Sildenafil PHT ARX, Sildenafil Sandoz, Sildenafil Sandoz PHT, Vasafil, Vedafil, Viagra, Wafesil)

Available forms
Tablets: 20 mg, 25 mg, 50 mg, 100 mg;
Wafers: 25 mg, 50 mg;
Vial: 10 mg/12.5 mL

Action
- phosphodiesterase type 5 (PDE5) is also found in pulmonary vascular smooth muscle; therefore in those with pulmonary hypertension it can lead to selective vasodilation of pulmonary vascular bed and some vasodilation of systemic circulation
- active metabolite (half-life 4 hours)
- half-life 3—5 hours
- see also General Actions of PDE5 inhibitors (p. 1120)

Use
- erectile dysfunction in adult males (Noumed, Silaran, Silcap, Sildatio, Vasafil, Vedafil, Viagra, Wafesil)
- pulmonary arterial hypertension (PAH) (WHO functional classes II and III) to improve exercise capacity or secondary to connective/collagen tissue disease (Revatio, Sidatio PHT, Sildenafil PHT ARX, Sildenafil Sandoz PHT)

Dose
- (Erectile dysfunction) 25—100 mg orally once daily 1 hour before sexual activity (maximum daily dose 100 mg) **OR**
- (Erectile dysfunction) initially 50 mg sublingually once daily 1 hour before sexual activity (maximum daily dose 100 mg) (wafers) **OR**

ERECTILE DYSFUNCTION AGENTS

- (PAH) 20 mg orally 3 times daily **OR**
- (PAH) 10 mg by IV bolus 3 times daily

Adverse effects
- (PAH) myalgia, cough, fever, epistaxis, vertigo
- fluid retention, weight increase, paraesthesia
- (IV) flushing, flatulence
- see also General Adverse effects of PDE5 inhibitors (p. 1120)

Interactions
- (PAH) serum levels may be decreased by bosentan
- (PAH) may increase serum levels of bosentan
- (PAH) not recommended with other PDE5 inhibitors
- (PAH) increased risk of epistaxis if given with a vitamin K antagonist such as warfarin
- (PAH) contraindicated with ritonavir
- (PAH) caution if used with other agents used for management of pulmonary arterial hypertension
- see also General Interactions of PDE5 inhibitors (p. 1120)

Nursing considerations/Cautions
- (PAH) therapy should be initiated and monitored only by a physician experienced in management of PAH
- (PAH) IV administration is recommended in those who are temporarily unable to take oral therapy but are haemodynamically stable
- (PAH) blood pressure should be carefully monitored during IV administration
- (PAH) therapy should be stopped gradually and the patient carefully monitored during this period
- (PAH) caution if used in those with bleeding disorders, active peptic ulceration or over 65 years
- (PAH) not recommended if the patient is clinically or haemodynamically unstable, under 18 years or with pulmonary veno-occlusive disease
- (PAH) not recommended in those with severe pulmonary hypertension (functional class IV) or with PAH with previous episode of non-arteritic anterior ischaemic optic neuropathy (NAION)
- (PAH) contraindicated in those with severe liver impairment (Child—Pugh class C)
- see also General Nursing considerations/Cautions for PDE5 inhibitors (p. 1121)

Patient education
- the patient should be warned that absorption will be decreased if taken with a high-fat meal and therefore will take longer to work
- advise the patient not to take with grapefruit juice
- (Wafers) instruct the patient on the following:
    - take 30—60 minutes before sexual activity
    - do not remove wafer from foil until just before administration
    - do not push wafer through foil packet. Peel backing off carefully and tap wafer out gently
    - handle wafer with dry hands
    - rinse mouth with water before administration to ensure mouth is moist
    - do not chew, suck, swallow, eat or drink until wafer has totally dissolved
    - (one-wafer dose) place wafer under tongue and allow to dissolve (this may take 2—3 minutes)
    - (two-wafer dose) place wafers under tongue on opposite sides and allow to dissolve
- see also General Patient education for PDE5 inhibitors (p. 1121)

Available as a sublingual wafer which will dissolve in the mouth. Tablet can be dispersed in water and mixed with strong-flavoured drink to disguise taste, or crushed and mixed with a spoonful of yoghurt, apple puree, honey or jam.

(PAH) caution if used during pregnancy, as no adequate or controlled studies have been conducted in pregnant women.

(PAH) excreted in small amounts in breastmilk; therefore not recommended during breastfeeding.

(Erectile dysfunction) in those with kidney or liver impairment, starting dose of 25 mg should be considered, increasing to 50–100 mg depending on tolerance and efficacy.

(Erectile dysfunction) a starting dose of 25 mg should be considered, increasing to 50–100 mg depending on tolerance and efficacy.

TADALAFIL
Trade names
(Adcirca, APO-Tadalafil, Cialis, Cidala, Cilatil, Cipla Tadalafil, Tadacip, Tadalaccord, Tadalafil GH, Tadalafil Sandoz, Tadalca, Tadalis)

Available forms
Tablets: 5 mg, 10 mg, 20 mg

Action
- phosphodiesterase type 5 (PDE5) is also found in pulmonary vascular smooth muscle, therefore in those with pulmonary hypertension it can lead to selective vasodilation of the pulmonary vascular bed and some vasodilation of systemic circulation
- half-life 17.5 hours (prolonged to 22 hours in those over 65 years)
- see also General Actions of PDE5 inhibitors (p. 1120)

Use
- erectile dysfunction in adult males
- moderate-to-severe lower urinary tract symptoms associated with benign prostatic hyperplasia
- pulmonary arterial hypertension (PAH) (WHO functional classes II and III) to improve exercise capacity, idiopathic PAH, or PAH secondary to connective/collagen tissue disease (Adcirca)

Dose
- (Erectile dysfunction, on-demand dosing) 10–20 mg orally 30–60 minutes prior to sexual activity once daily only (daily maximum 20 mg) **OR**
- (Erectile dysfunction) 2.5–5 mg orally once daily **OR**
- (Benign prostatic hyperplasia) 5 mg orally daily **OR**
- (PAH) 40 mg orally daily

Adverse effects
- myalgia, back pain, pain in extremities
- epistaxis
- (Over 75 years) diarrhoea, dizziness
- (PAH) abnormal or excessive menstrual bleeding
- see also General Adverse effects of PDE5 inhibitors (p. 1120)

Interactions
- (PAH) not recommended with other PDE5 inhibitors
- absorption may be decreased if given with an aluminium- or magnesium-containing antacid
- see also General Interactions of PDE5 inhibitors (p. 1120)

Nursing considerations/Cautions
- (PAH) therapy should be initiated and monitored by a physician experienced in management of PAH
- (Benign prostatic hyperplasia) prostate cancer and other causes for lower urinary tract symptoms should be excluded before starting therapy
- tablets contain lactose; therefore not recommended in those with rare hereditary problems of galactose intolerance, Lapp lactase deficiency or glucose–galactose malabsorption
- (PAH) caution if used in those who could be affected by vasodilation such as those with severe left ventricular outflow obstruction, fluid depletion, autonomic hypotension or resting hypotension
- (PAH) not recommended in those with pulmonary veno-occlusive disease, severe liver cirrhosis or severe renal impairment

ERECTILE DYSFUNCTION AGENTS

- (PAH) not recommended in those with severe kidney or liver impairment (Child–Pugh Class C)
- (PAH) not recommended in those under 18 years
- caution if used in those with creatinine clearance ≤ 50 mL/min
- see also General Nursing considerations/Cautions for PDE5 inhibitors (p. 1121)

Patient education

- (Daily dosing) advise the patient to take the dose at the same time every day
- patients 75 years and older should be cautioned to take care driving or using machines, as dizziness may occur
- see also General Patient education for PDE5 inhibitors (p. 1121)

Tablet can be crushed and mixed with water or a spoonful of yoghurt or apple puree.

(PAH) Should be used during pregnancy only if benefits are thought to outweigh risks.

Excreted in breastmilk; therefore caution if used during breastfeeding.

(PAH) Starting dose of 20 mg daily is recommended in those with mild-to-moderate kidney impairment or liver impairment (Child–Pugh Class A and B).

If prescribed for males 75 years and older, assessment of other illnesses, any renal impairment and other medications should be conducted to determine benefit versus risk of hypotensive events.

OTHER AGENTS

DAPOXETINE
Trade name
Priligy

Available form
Tablets: 30 mg

Action
- selective serotonin reuptake inhibitor (SSRI)
- ejaculation is mediated by the sympathetic nervous system and action is thought to be due to inhibition of serotonin uptake and potentiation at pre- and postsynaptic receptors
- equipotent active metabolite
- half-life 19 hours (with similar half-life for active metabolite)

Use
- treatment of premature ejaculation in men (18–64 years) who have intravaginal ejaculatory latency time < 2 minutes; persistent or recurrent ejaculation with minimal sexual stimulation before, on or shortly after penetration and before the patient wishes; marked personal distress; interpersonal difficulty as a consequence of premature ejaculation and poor control over ejaculation

Dose
- 30 mg orally 1–3 hours before sexual activity (daily maximum 30 mg)

Adverse effects
- syncope (with or without prodromal symptoms)
- orthostatic/postural hypotension
- headache, dizziness, somnolence, insomnia, disturbed dreams, irritability, anxiety, fatigue, restlessness, disturbed attention, tremor
- paraesthesia
- back pain
- blurred vision
- tinnitus
- flushing, sweating
- nausea, diarrhoea, dry mouth, vomiting, constipation, abdominal pain, flatulence, dyspepsia
- nasopharyngitis, influenza, sinusitis, yawning
- cough
- erectile dysfunction, decreased libido
- (Uncommon) depression, loss of libido, tachycardia, visual disturbances, eye pain, mydriasis, bleeding

Interactions

- contraindicated with or within 14 days of stopping monoamine oxidase inhibitors (MAOIs) because of increased risk of serotonin syndrome. MAOIs should not be administered within 7 days of stopping dapoxetine
- contraindicated with or within 14 days of stopping SSRIs, serotonin and noradrenaline (norepinephrine) reuptake inhibitors (SNRIs), tricyclic antidepressants (TCAs) or serotonergic agents such as linezolid, sumatriptan, tramadol, tryptophan, fentanyl, lithium and St John's wort. These agents should not be administered within 7 days of stopping dapoxetine
- contraindicated with azole antifungal agents (e.g. itraconazole) and HIV retroviral agents (e.g. ritonavir, atazanavir)
- not recommended with phosphodiesterase type 5 (PDE5) inhibitors because of the increased risk of postural hypotension
- increased serum levels may occur if given with erythromycin, clarithromycin, aprepitant, verapamil, diltiazem or fluconazole, increasing the risk of adverse effects
- use with alcohol should be avoided
- not recommended within 24 hours of consuming grapefruit juice
- caution if given with agents that lower seizure threshold
- caution if given with other centrally acting agents
- caution if used with other vasodilating agents such as alpha adrenergic receptor antagonists and nitrates because of the increased risk of postural hypotension
- caution if used with agents known to affect platelet function (e.g. atypical antipsychotics, phenothiazines, TCAs, aspirin, antiplatelet agents, NSAIDs, anticoagulants)

Nursing considerations/Cautions

- the patient should be evaluated for any depressive or psychiatric disorder before starting therapy
- before starting therapy, an orthostatic test should be performed to assess the patient for orthostatic hypotension
- risk versus benefit of therapy should be evaluated after 12 weeks or 6 doses (whichever comes first)
- syncope (with or without prodromal symptoms) can occur at any time, but commonly occurs within 3 hours of taking dapoxetine, after the first dose or after procedures such as blood taking
- not recommended in those under 18 years
- not recommended in those with history of mania/hypomania, bipolar disorder, depressive disorder, schizophrenia or unstable epilepsy
- caution if used in those with a history of bleeding disorders, with epilepsy or history of seizures, mild liver impairment, raised intraocular pressure or narrow-angle glaucoma, or mild-to-moderate kidney impairment
- caution if used in men with other forms of sexual dysfunction, as the condition might worsen
- not recommended in those with underlying structural cardiovascular disease (e.g. carotid stenosis, coronary artery disease, valvular heart disease), a history of orthostatic reaction, or severe kidney impairment
- contraindicated in those with significant cardiac disease (e.g. heart failure, second- or third-degree AV block, sick sinus syndrome) not treated with pacemaker, significant ischaemic heart disease or valvular disease, or moderate-to-severe liver impairment

Patient education

- advise the patient to take the tablet whole with at least 1 full glass of water to avoid a bitter taste
- warn the patient not to exceed 1 tablet per day, as this increases risk of side-effects such as fainting
- counsel the patient against using recreational drugs (e.g. ecstasy, LSD,

ERECTILE DYSFUNCTION AGENTS

- ketamine, narcotics, benzodiazepines) with dapoxetine because of combined side-effects
- the patient should be advised not to drink alcohol because of an increased risk of fainting and accidental injury
- advise the patient to avoid grapefruit juice within 24 hours of dapoxetine
- warn the patient to take care not to stand up quickly after prolonged lying or sitting, as lightheadedness, dizziness and fainting may occur
- warn the patient about syncope (loss of consciousness), which may occur with or without warning signs (including nausea, dizziness, lightheadedness, sweating). If symptoms occur, the patient should lie down (so head is lower than body) or put their head between the knees until symptoms have passed
- instruct the patient to avoid driving, operating machinery or other situations where injury could occur if syncope or other side-effects (e.g. dizziness, blurred vision, somnolence, disturbance in attention) occur

Tablet can be dispersed in 5—20 mL water, or crushed and mixed with a spoonful of yoghurt or apple puree.

LIDOCAINE (LIGNOCAINE)
Trade name
(Stud 100 Desensitising Spray For Men)

Available form
Metered dose spray: 9.6%

Action
- local anaesthetic

Use
- local surface penile desensitiser to delay ejaculation

Dose
- 3—8 sprays applied to head and shaft of penis 5—15 minutes before intercourse (maximum daily dose 24 sprays)

Adverse effects
- rash, irritation

Nursing considerations/Cautions

- caution if used in those with liver or kidney disorders
- contraindicated if the partner is pregnant, if either partner is allergic to local anaesthetics or if skin is broken or inflamed

Patient education

- instruct the patient that the number of sprays and timing before intercourse will depend on individual needs
- warn the patient not to apply spray to any broken or inflamed skin
- the patient should be advised to wash spray off after intercourse
- warn the patient that therapy should be stopped if either partner develops rash or irritation
- instruct the patient that therapy should be used for only 12 weeks without medical supervision
- instruct the patient to avoid spray contact with eyes or nostrils. If contact occurs, the area should be thoroughly washed with water

Contraindicated if the partner is pregnant.

EYE, EAR, NOSE AND THROAT AGENTS

THE EYE

Many eye conditions require treatment with drugs, which are most commonly applied topically. Conditions such as glaucoma are particularly dependent on antiglaucoma agents that help manage intraocular pressure, which, if left untreated, can lead to optic nerve damage and peripheral vision loss (see Antiglaucoma agents, p. 460). For macular degeneration, drugs aim to slow progression; infections are commonly treated with antibiotic or antiviral eye drops, and inflammation often requires anti-inflammatory agents. Diagnostic agents, such as fluorescein and Bengal rose, highlight damaged tissue. In contrast, mydriatic and cycloplegic agents facilitate an examination by dilating the pupil and temporarily paralysing the eye's focusing ability; ocular decongestants provide symptomatic relief from redness and tearing, often associated with irritation or allergic reactions (Knights et al 2023).

It should also be noted that there are a number of systemic medications that have ocular adverse effects, such as blurred or impaired vision, dry eyes, nystagmus, raised intraocular pressure, diplopia, optic neuritis and cataract formation. Conversely, ocular agents can have systemic effects after nasolacrimal absorption and include bradycardia, hypo/hypertension, palpitations, nausea, sweating and tremors (Knights et al 2023).

General Nursing considerations/ Cautions for eye preparations

Instillation of eye drops
- patient should be sitting or lying comfortably
- select correct drug preparation including strength, and check which eye is to be treated
- check expiry date before use
- wash hands before instilling
- ensure contact lenses are removed, if worn
- shake drops before use
- evert lower lid and ask patient to look up
- instil correct number of drops into the lower conjunctival sac, midway between the inner and outer canthus, avoiding contact between the container and the skin or lashes
- ask patient to close the eye gently and not squeeze the lids or rub eyes
- systemic absorption may be reduced by compressing the lacrimal sac (tear duct) for 2 minutes after instilling the drops
- when separate solutions of a miotic and adrenaline (epinephrine) are to be instilled, adrenaline (epinephrine) is instilled 2—10 minutes after the miotic
- allow 5—10 minutes between preparations if instilling one or more antiglaucoma agents.

EYE, EAR, NOSE AND THROAT AGENTS

Insertion of eye ointment
- crust or exudate should be cleaned from lid margins, first using cooled boiled water or sterile saline solution, if available
- patient should be sitting or lying comfortably
- advise patient that the ointment may cause blurred vision
- select correct drug preparation and check which eye is to be treated
- wash hands before insertion
- ensure contact lenses are removed, if worn
- the first centimetre of ointment from the tube should be discarded onto a sterile swab to prevent contamination of the eye
- evert lower lid and ask the patient to look up
- starting at the inner canthus, squeeze the tube and insert the ointment along the lower fornix, ending at the outer canthus, avoiding contact of the container with the skin or lashes
- ask patient to close the eye gently to spread ointment over the eye

General Patient education for eye preparations
- advise patient that eye drops should not be instilled if soft or gas-permeable contact lenses are in situ. Lenses should be removed before instillation and reinserted after at least a 15-minute interval
- patient should be instructed to thoroughly wash their hands before handling contact lenses and ensure that the correct solution is used with the particular lens type (i.e. either hard lens, soft lens or gas permeable)
- warn patient that many eye preparations contain benzalkonium chloride (preservative), which can cause irritation and also discolours soft contact lenses
- advise patient to report if the eye drops cause burning or visual disturbances
- the presence of pus and other exudates can decrease the effectiveness of anti-infective agents, therefore advise patient to cleanse the eye with saline or cooled boiled water
- patient should be escorted to and from an ophthalmological examination in which cycloplegic mydriatic drops are used for retinoscopy, because accommodation is paralysed for several hours. They should be advised not to drive or operate machinery during this time
- instruct patient to write the expiry date on eye preparations and discard accordingly (usually 28 days)
- advise patients that eye preparations are for one patient only
- patients should be warned not to stop treatment suddenly
- patients should be instructed to seek medical advice if eye infection does not show some improvement within 24–48 hours of starting eye drops or completely clear after 7 days
- instruct patient in correct technique for instilling eye drops, including:
  - do not allow tip of dispensing container to touch the eye as it may cause injury and/or contaminate the eye drops
  - if the container is new, remove the protective seal, otherwise it is important to check the expiry date
  - wash hands thoroughly with soap and water
  - remove lid/cap and hold container upside down in one hand between thumb and forefinger or index finger
  - using other hand, gently pull down on lower eyelid to form a pouch/pocket and tilt head back, looking up
  - place tip of container close to lower eyelid (taking care not to make contact between tip and eye). Squeezing bottle gently, release one drop into pouch/pocket formed between eye and eyelid, taking care not to allow tip to touch eye
  - gently close eye, but do not blink or rub eye

- while eye is closed, place index finger against inside corner of eye and press against nose for about 2 minutes (this stops medicine from draining through tear duct into nose and throat)
- blot any excess solution from around the eye with a tissue
- replace lid/cap tightly
- wash hands again to remove any residue
• instruct patient in correct eye ointment application, including:
  - check expiry date
  - wash hands thoroughly before applying eye ointment
  - tilt head back gently and gently pull lower eyelid down
  - squeeze 1.5 cm of eye ointment inside lower eyelid (however, do not allow tip of tube to touch eye, eyelid or lashes)
  - release eyelid slowly and close eyes gently for 1–2 minutes or blink a few times to help spread the ointment over the eye
  - blot any excessive ointment from around the eye with a tissue
  - wash hands thoroughly after finishing applying eye ointment

CYCLOPLEGIC AND MYDRIATIC DROPS

General Actions of cycloplegic and mydriatic drops
- acetylcholine typically induces miosis (pupil constriction) and supports accommodation (near vision focusing). However, antimuscarinic (anticholinergic) drugs inhibit acetylcholine's effects, leading to mydriasis (pupil dilation) and blocking the ciliary muscle function. This results in a loss of accommodation, known as cycloplegia, which prevents the eye from focusing on near objects.

General Adverse effects of cycloplegic and mydriatic drops
- dilation of the pupil (resulting in photophobia and loss of accommodation)
- blurred vision, irritation, redness, follicular conjunctivitis, vascular congestion, oedema, contact dermatitis, transient stinging, photophobia
- increased intraocular pressure
- (Uncommon) CNS disturbance (ataxia, incoherent speech, hallucinations, hyperactivity, disorientation, seizures) (children are particularly susceptible)
- (Rare, systemic absorption) dry mouth, thirst, flushing, dry skin, blurred vision, rapid and irregular pulse, fever, lack of coordination, atrial fibrillation, drowsiness, confusion, decreased bladder tone, increased risk of urinary retention (especially in older men), decreased GI motility, which may lead to constipation

General Interactions of cycloplegic and mydriatic drops
- increased risk of convulsions and extrapyramidal symptoms if systemic absorption occurs and if given with phenothiazines, antiemetics or barbiturates
- if systemic absorption occurs, may potentiate actions of other anticholinergic agents
- may interfere with antiglaucoma actions of carbachol or pilocarpine

General Nursing considerations/Cautions for cycloplegic and mydriatic drops
- intraocular pressure and estimation of anterior chamber depth should be measured before starting therapy
- atropine is never put into an eye without a doctor's prescription, because its effects cannot be reversed quickly and it will cause an increase in intraocular pressure in susceptible patients
- systemic absorption of atropine or atropine-like drugs can result in toxicity,

EYE, EAR, NOSE AND THROAT AGENTS

- including increased pulse and respiratory rate, hypotension, restlessness, confusion, delirium and coma
- atropine-like agents can increase intraocular pressure in patients predisposed to glaucoma
- caution if used in the elderly as they are more sensitive to effects and also more prone to adverse effects
- caution if used in those who have had severe reactions to systemic atropine in the past
- caution if atropine or atropine-like agents are used in high ambient temperatures because of the risk of hyperpyrexia (especially in children)
- caution if used in those with Down syndrome or predisposed to narrow-angle (angle-closure) glaucoma or with anatomically narrow angles
- contraindicated in those with or suspected of narrow-angle (angle-closure) glaucoma
- see also General Nursing considerations/Cautions for eye preparations (p. 1130)

General Patient education for cycloplegic and mydriatic drops

- warn patient not to drive while pupils are dilated
- patient should be warned that eyes may be sensitive to light and that sunglasses should be worn outside
- see also General Patient education for eye preparations (p. 1128), which includes instructions on eye drop instillation

ATROPINE SULFATE
Trade names
Atropt, Eikance, Minims Atropine Eye Drops

Available form
Eye drops: 10 mg/mL (1%)

Action
- belladonna alkaloid that blocks acetylcholine
- dilates pupil (mydriasis), paralyses accommodation (cycloplegia)
- maximum mydriatic effects in 30—40 minutes, duration 7—12 days
- maximum cycloplegic effects in 3—6 hours, duration 7—14 days
- see also General Actions of cycloplegic and mydriatic drops (p. 1130)
- for other actions of atropine sulfate monohydrate, see General Actions of anticholinergic agents (p. 985)

Use
- diagnostic procedures requiring mydriasis and cycloplegia

Dose
- 1 drop into eye(s) as required

Interactions
- if systemic absorption occurs, may decrease gastric motility increasing risk of adverse effects and/or toxicity if given with potassium supplements, potassium citrate or antimyasthenics (e.g. neostigmine, pyridostigmine)
- see also General Interactions of cycloplegic and mydriatic drops (p. 1130)

Adverse effects/Nursing considerations/Cautions/Patient education
- infants and young children are especially susceptible to atropine toxicity, even from the absorption of eye preparations, so note irritability, dry mouth, tachycardia, mydriasis, fever and rash
- onset and duration of action is prolonged in patients with heavily pigmented eyes
- not recommended in infants under 3 months
- not recommended in those with keratoconus or synechiae between iris and lens
- see also General Adverse effects/Nursing considerations/Cautions/Patient education for cycloplegic and mydriatic drops (p. 1130)

 While atropine sulfate may be systemically absorbed after ocular administration, no significant effects on the fetus have been reported. Use only if the potential benefits outweigh the risks, especially in early pregnancy.

Small amounts of systemically absorbed atropine sulfate may pass into breastmilk, potentially causing rapid pulse, fever or dry skin in infants. Minimise use and avoid breastfeeding immediately after administration.

Elderly patients may be more sensitive to the anticholinergic effects of atropine, increasing the likelihood of systemic side effects such as confusion, drowsiness and dry mouth. Monitor closely, particularly if the patient is using other anticholinergic medications.

CYCLOPENTOLATE HYDROCHLORIDE

Trade names
Cyclogyl, Minims Cyclopentolate Eye Drops

Available forms
Eye drops: 5 mg/mL (0.5%), 10 mg/mL (1%)

Action
- anticholinergic with rapid action but shorter duration than atropine sulfate monohydrate (p. 986)
- maximum mydriatic effect 30—60 minutes, duration 24 hours
- maximum cycloplegic effect 25—75 minutes, duration 6—24 hours

Use
- diagnostic procedures requiring mydriasis and cycloplegia
- treatment of uveitis

Dose
- (Refraction, examination of back of eye) 1 drop (0.5% but 1% in heavily pigmented eyes) to affected eye(s), followed 5 minutes later by 1 drop **OR**
- (Anterior/posterior uveitis, breakdown of posterior synechiae (adhesion)) 1—2 drops (0.5%) to affected eye(s) 6—8 hourly

Adverse effects
- (Children) psychotic reactions and behavioural disturbances (more common than with other anticholinergic agents)
- (Rare) seizures, acute psychosis
- see also General Adverse effects of cycloplegic and mydriatic drops (p. 1130)

Interactions
- see General Interactions of cycloplegic and mydriatic drops (p. 1130)

Nursing considerations/Cautions
- infants should be observed for at least 30 minutes after instillation for any behavioural or psychotic reactions
- caution if used in children with epilepsy
- (1% solution) not recommended in young children
- see also General Nursing considerations/Cautions for cycloplegic and mydriatic drops (p. 1130)

Patient education
- patient should be advised that full recovery will take approximately 24 hours
- see also General Patient education for cycloplegic and mydriatic drops (p. 1131)

Use only if the potential benefits outweigh risks, particularly in early pregnancy.

Due to the potential for anticholinergic effects in infants, including rapid pulse, fever and gastrointestinal symptoms, use only if clearly necessary.

Elderly patients may be more sensitive to the anticholinergic effects of atropine, increasing the likelihood of systemic side effects such as confusion, drowsiness and dry mouth. Monitor closely, particularly if the patient is using other anticholinergic medications.

PHENYLEPHRINE

Trade name
Minims Phenylephrine Eye Drops

Available forms
Eye drops: 25 mg/mL (2.5%), 100 mg/mL (10%)

EYE, EAR, NOSE AND THROAT AGENTS

Action
- sympathomimetic agent that causes mydriasis by direct stimulation of alpha adrenoceptors (alpha1 and alpha2)
- no cycloplegic action or effect on intraocular pressure
- mydriasis occurs in 10–90 minutes, recovery 5–7 hours

Use
- mydriasis for diagnostic or therapeutic purposes

Dose
- (Diagnostic) (2.5%, 10%) 1 drop to each eye, repeated once only after 1 hour

Adverse effects
- (Rare) significant increase in BP, aneurysm, arrhythmias
- see also General Adverse effects of cycloplegic and mydriatic drops (p. 1180)

Interactions
- may reverse action of antihypertensive agents
- absorption is increased if ocular hyperaemia is present
- increased risk of arrhythmias if given with or within several days of stopping TCAs
- increased risk of arrhythmias if given with digoxin
- not recommended with or within 3 weeks of MAOIs

Nursing considerations/Cautions
- local anaesthetic eye drops may be used before phenylephrine to reduce stinging
- caution if used in those with hyperthyroidism, asthma, arteriosclerosis, hypertension, cardiovascular problems, aneurysms, tachycardia or long-standing insulin-dependent diabetes mellitus
- caution if used in those with closed-angle glaucoma (unless treated with iridectomy) or narrow-angle glaucoma sensitive to mydriatic-provoked glaucoma
- not recommended if corneal epithelium is damaged because of risk of increased absorption
- contraindicated in those with hypersensitivity to sodium metabisulfite
- (10% solution) contraindicated in children and elderly
- see also General Nursing considerations/Cautions for cycloplegic and mydriatic drops (p. 1180)

Patient education
- patients should be warned that they may experience transient floaters for 30–45 minutes after administrations
- see also General Patient education for cycloplegic and mydriatic drops (p. 1180)

 Use only if the potential benefits outweigh the risks, particularly in the early stages of pregnancy.

 Given the potential for systemic absorption and possible effects on the infant, use only if the potential benefits outweigh the risks.

 The use of phenylephrine 10% is contraindicated in elderly patients because of an increased risk of systemic toxicity. For those requiring phenylephrine, the 2.5% concentration should be used. Monitor closely for cardiovascular effects, including hypertension and arrhythmias, as elderly patients are more susceptible to these adverse effects.

Available in combination with
- phenylephrine hydrochloride 0.12% + prednisolone acetate 1% eye drops (Prednefrin Forte)

TROPICAMIDE
Trade names
Minims Tropicamide, Mydriacyl

Available forms
Eye drops: 5 mg/mL (0.5%), 10 mg/mL (1%)

Action
- anticholinergic with action and adverse effects similar to those of atropine sulfate monohydrate but with more rapid onset and shorter duration
- mydriasis occurs in 20—40 minutes, duration 6 hours
- maximum cycloplegia occurs within 30—40 minutes, recovery in 2—6 hours

Use
- diagnostic purposes

Dose
- (Examination of fundus) 1—2 drops 0.5% solution 15—20 minutes before examination of the fundus **OR**
- (Refraction examination) 1—2 drops 1% solution, repeated after 5 minutes; may be repeated after 20—30 minutes if necessary

Interactions
- effects may be enhanced if given with other agents with anticholinergic effects
- may interfere with hypotensive effects of carbachol, pilocarpine or ophthalmic cholinesterase inhibitors

Adverse effects
- (Children) CNS disturbances
- see also General Adverse effects of cycloplegic and mydriatic drops (p. 1130)

Nursing considerations/Cautions
- those with heavily pigmented irises may require more doses or higher-strength solution
- contains benzalkonium chloride, which may cause eye irritation
- caution if eye is inflamed as increased absorption may occur
- (1% solution) not recommended in infants
- see also General Nursing considerations/Cautions for cycloplegic and mydriatic drops (p. 1180)

Patient education
- see General Patient education for cycloplegic and mydriatic drops (p. 1181)

 Use only if the potential benefits justify the risks.

 Due to the potential for systemic absorption, use only if the potential benefits justify the risks.

Compress the tear duct for 1 minute following application to reduce systemic absorption.

 Elderly patients may be more sensitive to the anticholinergic effects of tropicamide, increasing the likelihood of systemic side effects such as confusion, drowsiness and dry mouth. Monitor closely, particularly if the patient is using other anticholinergic medications.

MIOTICS AND OCULAR DECONGESTANTS

ACETYLCHOLINE CHLORIDE
Trade name
Miochol-E

Available form
Vial: 20 mg/2 mL

Action
- parasympathomimetic
- very short-acting chemical transmitter that acts directly on cholinergic synapses and neuroeffector junctions
- activates neuromuscular junctions of parasympathetic fibres in the iris sphincter, resulting in very rapid miosis
- rapidly inactivated by acetylcholinesterase to choline and acetic acid

Use
- rapid miosis during ocular surgery (e.g. placement of intraocular lens after cataract surgery), penetrating keratoplasty, iridectomy

EYE, EAR, NOSE AND THROAT AGENTS

Dose
- 0.5–2 mL by gentle intraocular irrigation (instilled into anterior chamber with or after sutures are secured)

Adverse effects
- (Uncommon) corneal clouding or oedema (infrequent)
- (Systemic, rare) bradycardia, hypotension, flushing, sweating, breathing difficulties

Nursing considerations/Cautions/Patient education
- reconstitute using diluent provided
- if used after cataract surgery, should only be used after placement of intraocular lens
- solution is prepared immediately before use and the remainder discarded after use as it becomes rapidly unstable
- see also General Nursing considerations/Cautions for eye preparations (p. 1128) and General Patient education for eye preparations (p. 1129)

The effects on fetal development are unknown, so use during pregnancy only if the potential benefit justifies the possible risk to the fetus.

Given the possibility of systemic absorption, use only if essential.

Elderly patients may be more susceptible to adverse effects from acetylcholine chloride because of age-related systemic vulnerabilities. Use the lowest effective dose and monitor for signs of systemic effects, such as bradycardia or hypotension.

CARBACHOL
Trade name
Miostat

Available form
Vial: 150 microgram/1.5 mL (0.01%)

Action
- parasympathomimetic agent that stimulates the parasympathetic nervous system, but is not inactivated by acetylcholinesterase
- causes contraction of ciliary muscle, resulting in accommodation for near vision
- miosis occurs in 2–5 minutes
- decreases intraocular pressure

Use
- miosis during surgery

Dose
- (Miosis during surgery) 50 micrograms (0.5 mL of 0.01% solution) gently instilled into anterior chamber before or after securing sutures

Adverse effects
- blurred vision, redness, eye pain
- (Uncommon) headache, increased intraocular pressure
- (Rare) retinal detachment, corneal clouding, persistent bullous keratopathy and postoperative iritis (after cataract extraction)

Nursing considerations/Cautions
- patient should be carefully monitored as therapy may increase surgically induced intraocular inflammation
- vial stopper contains latex, which may cause allergic reaction in sensitive individuals
- caution if used in those with acute heart failure, asthma, active peptic ulceration, hyperthyroidism, GI spasm, urinary tract obstruction or Parkinson's disease

Patient education
- patient should be advised to wait until vision has cleared before driving or operating machinery

Due to limited human data, use only if the potential benefits outweigh the potential risks to the fetus.

Given the potential for systemic absorption, use only if the potential benefits outweigh the potential risks.

 Elderly patients may be more susceptible to side effects of carbachol, particularly if they have underlying cardiac or respiratory conditions. Use the lowest effective dose, and monitor for any signs of systemic cholinergic effects, including flushing, sweating or epigastric distress.

LODOXAMIDE
Trade name
Lomide Eye Drops 0.1%

Available form
Eye drops: 1 mg/mL (0.1%)

Action
* mast cell stabiliser that inhibits IgE-mediated (immediate) hypersensitivity reaction
* inhibits increase in cutaneous vascular permeability, but has no vasoconstricting, antihistamine or anti-inflammatory activity

Use
* seasonal allergic conjunctivitis (prophylaxis and treatment)
* vernal keratoconjunctivitis

Dose
* 1 drop in each eye 4 times daily at regular intervals

Adverse effects
* transient burning/stinging/discomfort, ocular pruritus, blurred vision, lid margin crusting, dry eye, tearing, hyperaemia
* (uncommon) warm sensation, headache, nausea, dizziness, dry nose, sneezing, rash

Nursing considerations/Cautions
* (Vernal keratoconjunctivitis) contact lenses should not be worn
* eye drops contain benzalkonium chloride, which can cause eye irritation and also discolours soft contact lenses
* not recommended in children under 4 years

Patient education
* (Prophylaxis of seasonal allergic conjunctivitis) advise patient to begin therapy about a week before start of allergy season and continue for duration of season
* emphasise the need to use drops as directed to be effective. Improvement in symptoms may be seen in a few days, but some patients may require longer (4 weeks)
* warn patient that some transient stinging or burning may occur when drops are first instilled; however, if this continues, advise patient to seek medical advice
* if patient normally wears soft contact lenses, instruct patient to remove before instilling eye drops and not to reinsert for at least 15 minutes
* advise patient to wait at least 10 minutes after instilling medication before instilling any other eye drops
* see also General Patient education for eye preparations (p. 1129)

 Use only if the potential benefits justify the potential risk to the fetus

 Given the possibility of systemic absorption, a risk to the breastfed infant cannot be excluded. Use only if the potential benefits justify the potential risks.

NAPHAZOLINE
Trade names
Albalon, Murine Clear Eyes, Naphcon Forte, Optrex Eye Drops, Systane Red Eyes

Available forms
Eye drops: 0.12 mg/mL (0.012%), 0.1 mg/mL (0.01%), 1 mg/mL (0.1%)

Action
* sympathomimetic agent

EYE, EAR, NOSE AND THROAT AGENTS

Use
- minor irritation (redness and dryness)

Dose
- 1–2 drops to affected eye(s) 3–4-hourly (Albalon, Systane Red Eyes) or up to 4 times daily (Murine, Naphcon Forte, Optrex Eye Drops)

Adverse effects
- raised intraocular pressure with pupil dilation
- transient stinging, blurred vision, hyperaemia, eye irritation, oedema, eye pain
- (Systemic, rare) drowsiness, hypersensitivity

Interactions
- contraindicated with MAOIs
- caution if used with methyldopa sesquihydrate or TCAs

Nursing considerations/Cautions
- caution if used in men with prostatic enlargement
- caution if used in those with hypertension, hyperthyroidism, diabetes mellitus or cardiac disease
- caution if used on inflamed eyes, as hyperaemia increases systemic absorption
- contraindicated in those with narrow-angle glaucoma or anatomically narrow angle
- see also General Nursing considerations/Cautions for eye preparations (p. 1128)

Patient education
- instruct patient that eye drops should not be used for more than 2 weeks
- if condition does not improve in 48 hours or symptoms recur, patient should be advised to seek medical advice
- see also General Patient education for eye preparations (p. 1129)

Use only if the potential benefit justifies the possible risk.

Use only if the potential benefit justifies the possible risk.

Available in combination with
- naphazoline 0.025% + pheniramine 0.3% (Naphcon-A, Visine Allergy)
- naphazoline 0.05% + antazoline 0.5% (Albalon-A)

TETRYZOLINE
Trade names
Murine Sore Eyes, Visine Advanced, Visine Clear

Available form
Eye drops: 0.5 mg/mL (0.05%)

Action
- sympathomimetic with marked alpha adrenergic activity
- conjunctival decongestant

Use
- minor eye irritation

Dose
- 1–2 drops to affected eye(s) up to 4 times daily

Adverse effects
- eye pain, blurred vision, hyperaemia

Nursing considerations/Cautions
- contraindicated in those with narrow-angle glaucoma, anatomically narrow angle, or if serious eye infection is present
- contraindicated in children under 6 years
- see also General Nursing considerations/Cautions for eye preparations (p. 1128)

Patient education
- advise patient to seek medical advice if symptoms persist for more than 72 hours
- see also General Patient education for eye preparations (p. 1129)

Use during pregnancy only if the potential benefits justify potential risks to the fetus.

 Due to the risk of systemic absorption, exercise caution and consider using only if essential.

 Elderly patients may be more susceptible to the vasoconstrictive and drying effects of tetryzoline, which can exacerbate conditions such as dry eye or cardiovascular issues. Use the lowest effective dose and monitor for any signs of systemic effects, such as increased blood pressure.

AGENTS USED FOR MACULAR DEGENERATION

General Adverse effects of macular degeneration treatment agents

- (Very common) conjunctival or retinal haemorrhage, eye pain, vitreous floaters, vitreous detachment, intraocular inflammation, eye irritation, foreign body sensation, increased lacrimation, blepharitis, ocular hyperaemia, dry eye, ocular pruritus, subretinal fibrosis, vitritis
- (Common) retinal degeneration or detachment, retinal tear, decreased visual acuity, vitreous haemorrhage, blurred vision, eyelid pain or oedema, conjunctival hyperaemia, corneal abrasion, eye discharge, photophobia, iritis, uveitis, iridocyclitis, subcapsular cataract, conjunctivitis
- transient increased intraocular pressure
- (Rare) arterial thromboembolic events, endophthalmitis, retinal detachment, hypersensitivity

General Nursing considerations/ Cautions for macular degeneration treatment agents

- should be administered only by a qualified ophthalmologist who is experienced in intravitreal injection
- intraocular pressure and optic nerve head perfusion should be measured immediately after intravitreal injection
- bilateral treatment at the same time may increase risk of systemic exposure and is generally not recommended
- dose interval should not be less than 1 month
- treatment should be withheld if intraocular surgery is planned or performed within the previous or next 28 days
- treatment should be withheld if rhegmatogenous retinal detachment or stage 3 or 4 macular holes occur
- if a retinal break occurs, dose should be withheld and not restarted until break has been repaired
- treatment should be withheld (and not resumed until next scheduled interval) if there is a decrease in visual acuity (decrease of $\geq$ 30 letters compared with last assessment), a subretinal haemorrhage involving fovea centre occurs or if haemorrhage is $\geq$ 50% of total lesion area
- caution if used in those with poorly controlled glaucoma
- caution if used in those with a history of stroke or transient ischaemic attack (TIA) owing to increased risk of thromboembolic events
- caution if used in those with risk factors for retinal pigment epithelial tears
- contraindicated in those with ocular or periocular infection, or active severe intraocular inflammation

General Patient education for macular degeneration treatment agents

- do not to drive or operate machinery until visual function has recovered post-injection and any associated eye examinations
- advise the patient to seek advice from their health professional if any of the following occur immediately:
  - severe eye pain, redness, significant blurring of vision or increased sensitivity to light

EYE, EAR, NOSE AND THROAT AGENTS

- a sudden decrease in vision or noticeable swelling of the eyelid in the treated eye
- sensation of 'floaters' (seeing specks or strings in your vision) or other visual disturbances, such as dark spots or blurring
- increased tear production or excessive tearing from the treated eye
- weakness, numbness or tingling in your limbs or face, or difficulty with swallowing or speaking (signs of a stroke)
- chest pain and pain that spreads to shoulders and neck (signs of heart attack)

AFLIBERCEPT

Trade name
Eylea

Available forms
Vial: 4 mg/0.1 mL 8 mg/0.07 mL
Prefilled syringe: 2 mg/0.5 mL

Action
- anti-vascular endothelial growth factor (VEGF), placental growth factor monoclonal antibody fragment
- antineovascularisation action

Use
- neovascular (wet) age-related macular degeneration (AMD)
- visual impairment due to diabetic macular oedema (DME)
- visual impairment secondary to central retinal vein occlusion (CRVO), branch retinal vein occlusion (BRVO) or myopic choroidal neovascularisation (myopic CNV)

Dose
- (Wet AMD) 2 mg by intravitreal injection monthly for 3 consecutive months, followed by 1 injection every 2 months, then treatment interval adjusted based on visual and/or anatomical outcomes **OR**
- (DME) 2 mg by intravitreal injection monthly for 5 consecutive months, followed by 1 injection every 2 months for 12 months, then treatment interval adjusted based on visual and/or anatomical outcomes **OR**
- (BRVO, CRVO) 2 mg by intravitreal injection monthly for 3 consecutive months, then treatment interval adjusted based on visual and/or anatomical outcomes **OR**
- (Myopic CNV) 2 mg by intravitreal injection, dose repeated if disease persists

Adverse effects
- (Injection site) irritation, pain, haemorrhage
- see also General Adverse effects for macular degeneration treatment agents (p. 1138)

Nursing considerations/Cautions
- (Wet AMD) dosing interval can be extended from every 2 to every 3 months once visual acuity is optimised and there is no active disease present
- not recommended in those with clinical signs of irreversible ischaemic visual function loss
- see also General Nursing considerations/Cautions for macular degeneration treatment agents (p. 1138)

Patient education
- see General Patient education for macular degeneration agents (p. 1138)

Not recommended. Aflibercept may pose risks to fetal development. Animal studies have shown reproductive toxicity, including fetal malformations, at systemic doses. For aflibercept 2 mg, effective contraception should be used during treatment and for at least 3 months after the last injection. For aflibercept 8 mg, contraception should continue for at least 4 months.

Not recommended. The potential for adverse effects on a breastfed child cannot be excluded.

BROLUCIZUMAB

Trade name
Beovu

Available form
Prefilled syringe: 6 mg/0.05 mL

Action
- anti-vascular endothelial growth factor (VEGF) that suppresses endothelial cell proliferation, reducing neovascularisation and decreasing vascular permeability
- monoclonal antibody fragment

Use
- treatment of neovascular (wet) age-related macular degeneration

Dose
- 6 mg by intravitreal injection every 4 weeks for 3 doses, then according to disease activity (for active disease, every 8 weeks; for no disease activity, every 12 weeks)

Adverse effects
- hypersensitivity reaction
- see also General Adverse effects for macular degeneration treatment agents (p. 1138)

Interactions
- not recommended with other VEGF agents (ocular or systemic)

Nursing considerations/Cautions
- patient should be assessed 16 weeks after starting therapy
- see also General Nursing considerations/Cautions for macular degeneration treatment agents (p. 1138)

Patient education
- women of childbearing potential should be counselled to use effective contraception during and for at least 4 weeks after stopping therapy
- see also General Patient education for macular degeneration treatment agents (p. 1138)

Not recommended. Brolucizumab has potential risks for fetal development owing to VEGF inhibition effects, which may impact embryofetal development and reproductive health. Women of childbearing potential are advised to use effective contraception during treatment and for at least 1 month after the last injection.

Not recommended during therapy or for at least 4 weeks after stopping therapy.

RANIBIZUMAB

Trade name
Lucentis

Available forms
Vial: 2.3 mg/0.23 mL;
Prefilled syringe: 1.65 mg/0.165 mL

Action
- recombinant monoclonal antibody fragment that targets vascular endothelial growth factor A

Use
- neovascular (wet) age-related macular degeneration (AMD)
- visual impairment due to diabetic macular oedema (DME)
- treatment of proliferative diabetic retinopathy (PDR)
- visual impairment secondary to retinal vein occlusion (RVO)
- visual impairment due to choroidal neovascularisation (CNV) secondary to pathological myopia
- visual impairment due to macular oedema secondary to retinal vein occlusion (RVO)

Dose
- initially 0.5 mg by intravitreal injection monthly until visual acuity has optimised or there are no signs of active disease. For AMD, DME, PDR and RVO, 3 or more monthly injections are usually required

EYE, EAR, NOSE AND THROAT AGENTS

Adverse effects
- nasopharyngitis, cough, flu-like syndrome
- anaemia
- nausea
- rash, urticaria, pruritus, erythema
- arthralgia
- headache, anxiety, stroke
- urinary tract infection
- (Injection site) haemorrhage, pain
- see also General Adverse effects of macular degeneration treatment agents (p. 1138)

Nursing considerations/Cautions
- (Vial) 5-micrometre filter (supplied) should be used when drawing up solution
- (Prefilled syringe) attach 30-gauge $^1/_2$ inch needle for intravitreal injection
- administer alone
- intraocular pressure should be monitored pre- and post-injection (60 minutes)
- patient should be reviewed 1 week post-injection to allow early treatment of infection if it occurs
- treatment may be fixed (monthly) or variable (patient is seen regularly and treated when disease is active)
- (CNV) patient may require only 1–2 injections per year; however, some patients require more
- (Macular oedema due to RVO) if no improvement to visual acuity is seen after 3–4 injections, therapy may be stopped
- if given with laser photocoagulation therapy, a 30-minute interval should be allowed between the two therapies with injection administered first
- caution if used in those with type 1 diabetes mellitus, especially those with HbA1c > 12% or uncontrolled hypertension
- not recommended in patients with RVO with clinical signs of irreversible ischaemic visual function loss

- increased risk of stroke or myocardial infarction (arterial thromboembolic events) in patients with prior events.
- see also General Nursing considerations/Cautions for macular degeneration treatment agents (p. 1138)

Patient education
- counsel female patient of childbearing potential to use adequate contraception during and for 12 months after stopping therapy
- see also General Patient education for macular degeneration treatment agents (p. 1138)

Not recommended. Effective contraception recommended during and for 3 months post-treatment.

Avoid breastfeeding during and for at least 1 month post-treatment owing to unknown effects on infant VEGF levels.

OTHER OPHTHALMIC AGENTS

LIFITEGRAST
Trade name
Xiidra

Available form
Eye drops: 50 mg/mL (5%)

Action
- targets interaction between lymphocyte function-associated antigen-1 (LFA-1) (protein found on leukocytes that mediates immune and inflammatory responses) and intercellular adhesion molecule-1 (ICAM-1). ICAM-1 is normally found in low levels in leucocytes but is thought to increase when inflammatory cytokines are present, including dry eye conditions

Use
- moderate-to-severe dry eye disease where artificial tear use has not been sufficient

Dose
- 1 drop to affected eye(s) twice daily

Adverse effects
- eye irritation, eye pain, eye pruritus, increased lacrimation, blurred vision
- altered taste
- headache
- (Rare) allergic reactions

Nursing considerations/Cautions
- comprehensive examination is recommended before starting therapy to determine reason for symptoms that may be reversible and treatable
- see also General Nursing considerations/Cautions for eye preparations (p. 1128)

Patient education
- see General Patient education for eye preparations (p. 1129)

 May be used during pregnancy if needed.

 Caution if used during breastfeeding.

OCRIPLASMIN
Trade name
Jetrea RTU

Available form
Vial: 375 microgram/0.3 mL

Action
- ocular proteolytic enzyme developed by recombinant DNA technology
- acts against vitreous body and vitreoretinal interface proteins (e.g. laminin, fibronectin, collagen) dissolving protein matrix responsible for abnormal vitreomacular adhesion. Tight protein binding leads to vitreomacular traction, visual impairment and/or macular holes
- half-life several hours

Use
- treatment of vitreomacular traction, including when associated with macular hole diameter ≤ 400 micrometres

Dose
- 0.125 mg (0.1 mL) injected into mid-vitreous of affected eye

Adverse effects
- blurred vision, vitreous floaters, eye pain, photopsia (perceived flashes of light), conjunctival haemorrhage, decreased visual acuity, visual impairment, macular oedema, photophobia, ocular discomfort, iritis, vitreous detachment, dry eye, eye pruritus/irritation, foreign body sensation, increased lacrimation
- intraocular inflammation/infection, intraocular haemorrhage, increased intraocular pressure
- dyschromatopsia (yellowish vision)
- (Uncommon) long-term loss of visual acuity
- lens subluxation, phacodonesis (lens tremulous)
- new or enlarged macular holes

Interactions
- remains in the eye for several days after intravitreal injection; therefore administration of other agents to treated eye is not recommended, as activity of both agents may be affected

Nursing considerations/Cautions
- before treatment, a complete clinical picture (patient history, clinical examination and investigations including optical coherence tomography) should be obtained
- patient monitoring after injection (between 2 and 7 days) is recommended to detect any inflammation, infection or increase in intraocular pressure
- patient should be monitored for any loss of visual acuity, especially in first week after treatment
- for intravitreal use only

EYE, EAR, NOSE AND THROAT AGENTS

- both eyes should not be treated concurrently or within 7 days of initial injection
- repeat administration to same eye is not recommended
- allow to thaw at room temperature before use (about 2 minutes), then dilute with 0.2 mL sodium chloride 0.9%, gently swirl and use within 15 minutes of reconstitution
- caution if used in those with non-proliferative diabetic retinopathy, history of uveitis or significant eye trauma
- not recommended in those with large diameter macular holes (> 400 micrometres), high myopia (> 8 dioptre spherical correction or axial length > 28 mm), aphakia, history of rhegmatogenous retinal detachment, lens zonule instability, recent ocular surgery or intraocular injection (including laser therapy), proliferative diabetic retinopathy, ischaemic retinopathies, retinal vein occlusion, exudative age-related macular degeneration or vitreous haemorrhage
- not recommended in those with panretinal disease associated with electroretinography (ERG) findings (e.g. retinitis pigmentosa, chorioderaemia)
- contraindicated in those with active or suspected ocular or periocular infection

Patient education

- patient should be advised of risk of transient loss of visual acuity during first week after treatment
- instruct patient not to drive or operate machinery if any visual disturbances occur (and these are most likely in first 7 days after treatment)

Use only if benefits outweigh potential risks.

Consider only if benefits outweigh potential risks.

THE EAR

Ear conditions include infections (bacterial and fungal), ear wax accumulation, pain, inflammation, allergic reactions, hearing loss and balance problems. Treatments often involve drugs such as anti-inflammatories (including analgesics, topical anaesthetics and corticosteroids), antibacterial and antifungal agents, as well as analgesics and decongestants (Knights et al 2023). While specific agents like corticosteroids, antibacterial, antifungal agents and NSAIDs are covered in other sections, it is essential to note that some drugs — such as aminoglycosides, salicylates and loop diuretics — can induce ear-related side effects such as tinnitus or ototoxicity (Knights et al 2023).

General Nursing considerations/ Cautions for ear preparations

- some systemic absorption may occur
- contraindicated if there is inflammation or perforation of the tympanic membrane

Instillation of ear drops

- patient should sit or lie comfortably
- select the correct preparation and strength, and check which ear is to be treated
- cleanse ear canal before instilling ear drops
- ensure that drops are at room temperature before instillation, as cold solution may provoke dizziness
- with the affected ear uppermost, pull the auricle upwards and backwards to straighten the external auditory canal (for children, pull the auricle downwards)
- instill required number of drops into the canal without touching the ear with the dropper, and return dropper to bottle without washing
- press the tragus over the meatus
- position is maintained for 2—3 minutes so that the drops reach the ear drum
- saturated wick may be used for the first 24—48 hours

General Patient education for ear preparations

- warn patient not to drive or operate machinery if dizziness or lightheadness occurs
- advise patient to stop use if any pain or inflammation is experienced
- patient should be advised to seek medical advice if pain or irritation occurs, or condition continues
- instruct patient in correct instillation technique for ear drops, including:
  - check expiry date
  - if the ear drops are new, break safety cap and open
  - wash hands thoroughly with soap and water
  - hold bottle upside down in one hand (between thumb and middle finger)
  - tilt head to one side with affected ear facing up (it may be easier in a sitting or lying position)
  - place dropper tip close to (but not touching) ear and gently tap or press base of container to release drops
  - continue holding head in the same position for 1 minute to allow drops to reach deeper into the ear
  - repeat for other ear if needed
  - replace cap on bottle and close tightly
  - wash hands to remove any residue
- warn patient that feeling of drops flowing deeper into ear may be unpleasant
- advise patient that a bad taste in the mouth may occur after using ear drops
- patient should be advised to note opening date and discard after that date (e.g. 28 days)

WAX SOFTENERS (Cerumenolytics)

Wax softeners, also known as cerumenolytics, are agents used to soften or break down ear wax (cerumen), making it easier to remove. They are often recommended when ear wax buildup causes discomfort, in those with hearing difficulties, or with the sensation of blockage in the ear.

CARBAMIDE PEROXIDE
Trade name
Ear Clear for Ear Wax Removal

Available form
Ear drops: 65 mg/mL

Action
- breaks down into hydrogen peroxide and urea upon contact with human ear wax. Hydrogen peroxide releases oxygen, which creates tiny bubbles that help to break down and loosen the wax, making it easier to remove

Use
- wax removal

Dose
- tilt head to one side and instil 5–10 drops in affected ear(s) twice daily for up to 4 days

Nursing considerations/Cautions/Patient education

- not recommended for children under 12 years
- not recommended for swimmer's ear, inflamed tissue or itching in the ear canal
- not recommended if there is any dizziness, ear perforation or ear pain, or within 6 weeks of ear surgery
- see also General Nursing considerations/Cautions for ear preparations (p. 1143), including instillation advice, and General Patient education for ear preparations (p. 1144)

DOCUSATE SODIUM
Trade name
Waxsol

Available form
Ear drops: 0.5%

EYE, EAR, NOSE AND THROAT AGENTS

Action
- penetrates ceruminous mass, reducing solid mass to semi-solid, allowing it to be removed normally by physiological process or syringing process

Use
- softening or loosening of ear wax to help in removal

Dose
- fill affected ear(s) for 2 nights preceding syringe procedure

Nursing considerations/Cautions/ Patient education

- do not use if the patient has a perforated eardrum, ear pain, swelling, or an inflamed ear.
- see also General Nursing considerations/Cautions for ear preparations (p. 1143), including instillation advice, and General Patient education for ear preparations (p. 1144)

Safe.

Safe.

THE NOSE

Olfaction (sense of smell) receptors are found on the top of the nasal cavity, and synapse to the olfactory bulb, forming the olfactory tract passing through the temporal lobe of the cortex and to the limbic system and hypothalamus. Decreased lack of smell (hyposmia) resulting from colds, rhinitis and nasal passage obstruction is common and may result in food becoming tasteless (because it can't be smelt) (Knights et al 2023). A number of drugs can decrease or impair smell, including calcium-channel blockers (nifedipine, diltiazem), some diuretics (e.g. acetazolamide, spironolactone), some antimicrobial agents (e.g. ciprofloxacin, metronidazole), corticosteroids (e.g. prednisolone) and antiepileptics (e.g. carbamazepine, phenytoin) (Knights et al 2023).

Drugs administered into the nasal passages aim to treat infections, sinusitis and rhinitis, and alleviate nasal congestion. They may treat underlying issues and/or provide symptom relief in the nasal cavity.

General Nursing considerations/ Cautions for nasal preparations

Instillation of nasal drops
- ask patient to blow nose
- have the patient recumbent, but with a pillow under the shoulders so that the neck is hyperextended (if possible) to prevent entry of drops into the throat
- select correct preparation and strength
- ask patient to breathe through the mouth
- instill the prescribed volume of drops into each nostril, turning the head to the same side as the nostril being dealt with
- maintain the position for several seconds to enable wide coverage of the nasal mucosa
- excessive use of topical sympathomimetic nasal decongestants can lead to drug-induced rhinitis and rebound nasal congestion

General Patient education for nasal preparations

- if using a nasal spray, instruct the patient to:
  - ensure nasal spray is primed for use if new, dust cover has been left off or device has been unused for some time (priming instructions vary from nasal spray to nasal spray, but essentially involve vigorously shaking container (with cap on) for 10 seconds and then priming by releasing 6–7 sprays until spray is uniform)
  - blow nose
  - insert spray adapter/nozzle into nostril while closing other nostril
  - tilt head slightly forwards keeping nasal spray container upright

- avoid tilting head back as this will result in bitter smell/taste
- depress pump while breathing gently and slowly through the nostril
- repeat procedure in same nostril if second spray per nostril is required
- remove adapter/nozzle from nostril and repeat in other nostril
- after prescribed amount has been delivered, remove adapter/nozzle from nostril and wipe with tissue
- wash spray adapter/nozzle regularly with warm water
- reprime with 2 sprays after cleaning
- if nozzle/adapter becomes blocked, pins or other sharp devices should not be used to unblock device as it may become damaged and not deliver the required amount of nasal spray
- nasal spray should be vigorously shaken for at least 10 seconds before each use
- replace dust cap after each use

SYMPATHOMIMETIC NASAL DECONGESTANTS

General Actions of sympathomimetic nasal decongestants
- sympathomimetic agent that stimulates alpha adrenergic receptors, causing vasoconstriction of the small arterioles of the nasal passage
- vasoconstriction reduces blood flow to the area, leading to decreased swelling and congestion in the nasal passages, relieving nasal congestion associated with colds, allergies and sinusitis.

General Uses of sympathomimetic nasal decongestants
- temporary relief of nasal congestion (colds, influenza, allergy, sinusitis)

General Adverse effects of sympathomimetic nasal decongestants
- burning/stinging in nose or throat
- sneezing
- nose/mouth/throat dryness or irritation
- increase in nasal discharge, epistaxis
- nausea, taste disturbance
- headache, insomnia, tiredness, dizziness, lightheadedness
- nervousness, tremors
- hypertension, palpitations, reflex bradycardia
- rebound congestion
- (Rare) allergy

General Interactions of sympathomimetic nasal decongestants
- not recommended with or within 2 weeks of MAOIs or TCAs
- not recommended with other cold or cough medications

General Nursing considerations/Cautions for sympathomimetic nasal decongestants
- caution if used in those with heart disease (including angina), diabetes mellitus, hypertension, prostatic enlargement, congenital porphyria or thyroid disease
- not recommended in children under 6 and used in those 6—11 years only with medical advice
- contraindicated in those with hypersensitivity to other nasal decongestants or with narrow-angle glaucoma
- contraindicated in those with recent transsphenoidal hypophysectomy, transnasal or transoral surgical procedures where the dura mater has been exposed
- see also General Nursing considerations/Cautions for nasal preparations (p. 1145)

General Patient education for sympathomimetic nasal decongestants
- instruct patient that nasal decongestant should not be used for more than 3—5 days because rebound nasal congestion may occur
- advise patient to avoid contact with eyes
- patient should be advised not to share preparations to prevent spreading infection

EYE, EAR, NOSE AND THROAT AGENTS

- advise patient not to exceed recommended dose
- see also General Patient education for nasal preparations (p. 1145), including instillation advice

Not recommended during pregnancy.

Not recommended during breastfeeding.

Use only if the potential benefit outweighs the risk to the fetus.

Use cautiously and only if benefits to the mother justify potential risks to the infant.

Use with caution in elderly patients because of increased susceptibility to adverse effects such as hypertension and dizziness.

OXYMETAZOLINE
Trade names
APOHealth Decongestant Nasal Spray, Chemists' Own Decongestant, Dimetapp 12 Hour Nasal Spray, Drixine Decongestant Nasal Spray, Drixine No Drip Formula, Logicin Rapid Relief Nasal Spray, Pharmacy Action Nasal Decongestant Spray, Trust Decongestant, Vicks Sinex Nasal Spray

Available forms
Metered-dose nasal spray: 500 microgram/mL;
Squeeze spray: 500 microgram/mL

Action
- action in 5—10 minutes, duration 5—6 hours, gradual decline over next 6 hours
- see also General Actions and Uses of sympathomimetic nasal decongestants (p. 1146)

Dose
- 1—3 sprays in each nostril twice daily 10—12-hourly (not exceeding twice in 24 hours) (Dimetapp) **OR**
- 1—2 sprays to each nostril 2—3 times daily (Logicin, Vicks Sinex) **OR**
- 2—3 sprays in each nostril twice daily (Drixine)

Uses/Adverse effects/Interactions/Nursing considerations/Cautions/Patient education
- see General Nursing considerations/Cautions for sympathomimetic nasal decongestants (p. 1146) and General Patient education for sympathomimetic nasal decongestants (p. 1146)

TRAMAZOLINE
Trade names
Spray Tish, Spray Tish Menthol

Available form
Metered-dose nasal spray: 82 microgram/dose

Action
- action within 5 minutes, duration up to 8 hours
- see also General Actions and Uses of sympathomimetic nasal decongestants (p. 1146)

Dose
- 1—2 sprays in each nostril up to 4 times daily

Uses/Adverse effects/Interactions/Nursing considerations/Cautions
- contraindicated in those with rhinitis sicca (dry disease of nasal mucosa forming crusts and scabs) or with hypersensitivity to benzalkonium chloride (preservative)
- see also General Nursing considerations for sympathomimetic nasal decongestants (p. 1146)

Patient education
- do not use for more than 5 days, as it may worsen symptoms (rebound congestion)
- instruct patient that pump should be reprimed if not used for 2 weeks
- see also General Patient education for sympathomimetic nasal decongestants (p. 1146)

Should not be used in the first trimester. In the second and third trimesters, use only if the potential benefits outweigh the risks.

Use with caution as excretion in human breastmilk unknown.

XYLOMETAZOLINE

Trade names
Flo Rapid Relief, Otrivin Menthol Spray, Otrivin Nasal Drops Adult, Otrivin Nasal Drops Junior, Otrivin Nasal Spray Adult, Otrivin Nasal Spray Junior, Sudafed Xylo Nasal Decongestant

Available forms
Metered-dose nasal spray (adult): 1 mg/mL;
Nasal drops (adult): 1 mg/mL;
Metered-dose nasal spray (junior): 0.5 mg/mL;
Nasal drops (junior): 0.5 mg/mL

Action
- action within few minutes, duration up to 10—12 hours
- see also General Actions and Uses of sympathomimetic nasal decongestants (p. 1146)

Dose
- (Nasal spray, adult) 1 spray to each nostril 2—3 times daily **OR**
- (Nasal drops, adult) 2—3 drops to each nostril 2—3 times daily (8—10-hourly)

Uses/Adverse effects/Interactions/Nursing considerations/Cautions/Patient education
- should not be used for more than 3 days
- (Flo Rapid Relief) can be used for up to 12 weeks after opening
- see also General Nursing considerations for sympathomimetic nasal decongestants (p. 1146) and General Patient education for sympathomimetic nasal decongestants (p. 1146)

Available in combination with
- xylometazoline hydrochloride 0.05% + ipratropium bromide 0.06% (Otrivin Plus Nasal Spray)

THE OROPHARYNX

The mouth contains the four main taste receptors (sour, sweet, bitter and salty), where the information is received and relayed via the taste pathways through the pons and medulla to the thalamus and on to the cerebral cortex, where taste is perceived (Knights et al 2023).

Some drugs can alter, decrease or impair the sense of taste including ACE inhibitors (e.g. captopril, enalapril), antineoplastic agents (e.g. fluorouracil, methotrexate, bleomycin, doxorubicin), nicotine, some antidepressants, antiepileptics and anti-Parkinson's agents, NSAIDs and antimicrobial agents (Knights et al 2023).

Agents are introduced into the mouth and throat to treat mouth ulcers, infections and inflammation.

General Nursing considerations/Cautions for mouth and throat preparations
- ensure that analgesic or anaesthetic agents are given to patients with painful mouth ulcers a few minutes before eating
- do not give anything to drink if the patient has had the pharynx anaesthetised until at least 1 hour after application to prevent aspiration of fluid
- mouth washes are beneficial before as well as after meals

General Patient education for mouth and throat preparations
- patient should be advised not to eat or drink within 15 minutes of applying mouth gel
- instruct patient that lozenges should not be chewed, but allowed to dissolve slowly
- advise patient to remove dentures when necessary to allow access to ulcers
- instruct patient that rinsing/gargling solution should not be swallowed, but spat out after gargling, and that rinsing/gargling solution is generally used undiluted, but if stinging/burning occurs it may be diluted with water

EYE, EAR, NOSE AND THROAT AGENTS

ANTI-INFECTIVE AGENTS

CETYLPYRIDINIUM CHLORIDE
Trade name
Cepacol

Available form
Solution: 500 microgram/mL

Action
- antibacterial

Use
- sore, irritated, inflamed or infected throat or mouth
- after dental treatments

Dose
- gargle or rinse 10–15 mL for 10–15 seconds and expel every 2–3 hours **OR**
- (Dental treatments/plaque reduction) rinse for 10–15 seconds after brushing teeth and meals

Nursing considerations/Cautions/Patient education

- the patient should be advised not to swallow the solution
- instruct the patient to seek medical advice if symptoms persist, recur or worsen, or if other symptoms (fever, headache, vomiting, nausea) develop
- see also General Nursing considerations/Cautions/Patient education for mouth and throat preparations (p. 1146)

CHLORHEXIDINE GLUCONATE
Trade names
Pharmacy Select Chlorhexidine Mouthwash, Rivacol Chlorhexidine 0.2% Mouthwash, Savacol Mouth & Throat Rinse

Available form
Solution: 2 mg/mL (0.2%)

Action
- antiseptic

Use
- mouth ulcer, minor throat infection
- plaque reduction and prevention of gingivitis

Dose
- (mouth ulcer, throat infection) rinse or gargle 10 mL for 1–2 minutes 3 times daily after meals **OR**
- (dental hygiene) rinse or gargle 10 mL for 1–2 minutes daily

Adverse effects
- teeth staining, taste alteration

Nursing considerations/Cautions/Patient education

- patient should be advised not to swallow solution after rinsing or gargling
- instruct patient to seek medical advice if symptoms persist, recur or worsen or if other symptoms (fever, headache, vomiting, nausea) develop
- (children under 10 years) dilute solution (5 mL in 5 mL warm water)
- see also General Nursing considerations/Cautions for mouth and throat preparations (p. 1148) and General Patient education for mouth and throat preparations (p. 1148)

 Safe.

Available in combination with
- chlorhexidine gluconate 18 mg/15 mL + benzydamine hydrochloride 22.5 mg/15 mL (Difflam-C Sore Throat Gargle & Mouth Solution + Antiseptic)

 Not recommended during pregnancy.

POVIDONE—IODINE
Trade names
Betadine Sore Throat Gargle, Betadine Sore Throat Gargle — Ready To Use, Difflam Sore Throat Gargle with Iodine Concentrate

Available forms
Solution (diluted): 10 mg/mL;
Solution (undiluted): 75 mg/mL (7.5%)

Action
- topical microbicidal antiseptic

Use
- sore throat

Dose
- (Undiluted preparations) dilute according to directions (1 mL solution to 20 mL water) and gargle for up to 30 seconds 3—4-hourly daily **OR**
- (Diluted preparation) 15 mL gargled for 30 seconds 3—4-hourly

Adverse effects
- allergy

Interactions
- not recommended with hydrogen peroxide mouthwash

Nursing considerations/Cautions/Patient education
- do not swallow —gargle only
- contraindicated in those with hypersensitivity to iodine, thyroid disease or within 4 weeks of thyroid cancer treatment
- if the condition does not improve in 2 days, the patient should be advised to seek medical advice
- see also General Nursing considerations for mouth and throat preparations (p. 1146) and General Patient education for mouth and throat preparations (p. 1146)

 Not recommended during pregnancy.

 Not recommended during breastfeeding.

FIBRINOLYTIC AGENTS

Thrombosis is the formation of a clot that may occlude either the arterial circulation (and may lead to myocardial infarction or peripheral ischaemia) or the venous circulation (and may lead to pulmonary embolism or deep vein thrombosis). Blood stasis is often a cause of venous thrombi because it allows platelets and fibrin to build up, which also makes these thrombi amenable to treatment with fibrinolytic agents. Because arterial thrombi consist mainly of platelets, fibrinolytic agents are not as effective (Hogg & Weitz 2018).

Fibrinolytic agents (also known as thrombolytic agents) activate plasminogen to form the proteolytic enzyme plasmin, which breaks down fibrin and therefore dissolves the clot wherever it can be reached by the plasmin. Fibrinolytic agents have a greater impact on haemostasis compared with anticoagulants, resulting in bleeding that is more severe and difficult to control (in part, because the clots may be located in areas that are not amenable to compression) (Knights et al 2023). Some agents, such as alteplase, are fibrin specific and have little or no effect on circulating unbound plasminogen, whereas the fibrin non-specific agents affect circulating unbound plasminogen as well as fibrin-bound plasminogen. Potency is generally expressed in units that are not comparable between agents in this class.

General Adverse effects of fibrinolytic agents

- minor or major bleeding (intracranial, internal or superficial)
- (IV site) haemorrhage
- arrhythmias (associated with reperfusion), tachycardia or bradycardia
- hypotension
- (Rare) anaphylactoid reaction (rash, urticaria, bronchospasm, laryngeal oedema, periorbital oedema, angioedema), cholesterol embolus, seizures

General Interactions of fibrinolytic agents

- increased risk of bleeding if given before, during or within 24 hours of anticoagulants (INR > 1.3), antiplatelet agents or other fibrinolytic agents, and these agents are therefore not recommended/contraindicated together

General Nursing considerations/Cautions for fibrinolytic agents

- treatment should be started as soon as possible after onset of symptoms

- should be used only in a hospital setting by experienced doctors with facilities that allow monitoring and have readily available resuscitation equipment
- any recent puncture sites should be carefully observed for bleeding
- IM injections, arterial punctures, venipuncture and undue patient handling should be avoided during therapy; however, if arterial puncture is necessary, choose a site that can be manually compressed and apply pressure for 30 minutes; a pressure dressing should be applied and the site frequently observed
- the patient should be closely monitored for:
  - any signs of cholesterol embolism, including 'purple toe' syndrome, gangrenous digits, livedo reticularis (see Glossary), hypertension, myocardial infarction, bowel infarction and rhabdomyolysis
  - any signs of bradycardia or ventricular irritability, as this can become life threatening. Antiarrhythmic agents should be readily available
  - any signs of angioedema (during infusion and for 24 hours after)
- the patient should be advised to report any visual disturbances that might be indicative of ophthalmic bleeding
- should not be mixed with any other drugs
- diluent should be added gently to the vial to reconstitute it and the solution should not be shaken or vial inverted. If reconstituted solution is further diluted, the infusion bag should not be agitated, but should be gently inverted to ensure even mixing of solution
- do not administer if any discolouration or particulate matter is present
- discard any unused solution
- should be administered via a dedicated line/lumen and infusions given via infusion pump
- infusion should be stopped if significant bleeding occurs
- fibrinolytic agents are generally not recommended within 10 days of surgery or trauma unless exceptional circumstances exist (e.g. pulmonary embolus) where risk versus benefit must be carefully weighed
- (Acute myocardial infarction) generally not recommended in those with only ST depression on ECG, except in those with true posterior infarct (tall R waves with marked ST depression in leads V1 to V3)
- caution if used in those with left heart thrombus (e.g. mitral stenosis, atrial fibrillation) as there is an increased risk of thromboembolism
- consider analysis of benefits versus risks in patients with the following conditions, who have increased risk of adverse effects: within 6 months of transient ischaemic attacks or ischaemic stroke, over 75 years of age, over 70 years of age with hypertension, mitral stenosis with atrial fibrillation, diabetic haemorrhagic retinopathy, recent head or cranial trauma, pregnancy, septic thrombophlebitis, occluded arteriovenous cannula at seriously infected site, recent minor traumas within 10 days (e.g. biopsy, IM injections), systolic BP > 160 mmHg, indwelling urethral catheter in situ, open tuberculosis or low body weight (< 60 kg)
- contraindicated in those with bleeding disorders (or within last

6 months), coagulation problems, intracranial bleed, neoplasm (likely to bleed), intracranial or spinal surgery, recent head trauma, aneurysm, severe uncontrolled hypertension (systolic BP > 180 mmHg, diastolic > 110 mmHg), within 10 days of obstetric delivery (or abortion), prolonged or traumatic cardiopulmonary resuscitation (> 2 minutes) within 10 days, organ biopsy or puncture of the subclavian or jugular vein, within 12 weeks of major surgery, significant trauma or ulcerative GI disease, oesophageal varices, acute pancreatitis, arterial aneurysm, arterial/venous malformation, subacute bacterial endocarditis, pericarditis, severe liver or kidney disease/dysfunction (especially if associated with coagulation problems), a recent history of stroke (< 6 months), diabetic haemorrhagic retinopathy or other haemorrhagic ophthalmic conditions

ALTEPLASE
Trade name
Actilyse

Available forms
Vial: 10 mg, 50 mg

Action
- recombinant tissue plasminogen activator (r-tPA) which acts on fibrin in thrombus with little or no effect on circulating unbound plasminogen
- minimal systemic effects
- duration of fibrinolytic effect 4 hours
- (Acute myocardial infarction) reperfuses occluded vessels in approximately 90 minutes in most patients

Use
- acute myocardial infarction (within 12 hours of onset of symptoms)
- pulmonary embolism
- acute ischaemic stroke within 4.5 hours of onset of symptoms (and exclusion of intracranial bleed)

Dose
- (Pulmonary embolus) 100 mg IV given as a 10 mg IV bolus over 1–2 minutes, then remaining 90 mg over 2 hours (not exceeding 1.5 mg/kg if weight is < 65 kg) **OR**
- (Myocardial infarction) 10 mg IV bolus over 1–2 minutes, 50 mg by IV infusion over 60 minutes, then 40 mg over the next 2 hours (not exceeding 1.5 mg/kg if weight is ≤ 65 kg) **OR**
- (Myocardial infarction, weight > 65 kg) 100 mg IV given as a 15 mg IV bolus over 1–2 minutes, 50 mg by IV infusion over 30 minutes, then 35 mg over the next 60 minutes **OR**
- (Myocardial infarction, weight < 65 kg) 100 mg IV given as a 15 mg IV bolus over 1–2 minutes, then 0.75 mg/kg by IV infusion over 30 minutes, then 0.5 mg/kg over the next 60 minutes **OR**
- (Acute ischaemic stroke) 0.9 mg/kg (maximum 90 mg) by IV infusion over 60 minutes, with 10% of total dose as initial IV bolus

Adverse effects
- nausea, vomiting
- fever
- see also General Adverse effects of fibrinolytic agents (p. 1151)

Interactions
- increased risk of anaphylactoid reaction if given with angiotensin converting enzyme (ACE) inhibitors
- (Acute ischaemic stroke) increased risk of bleeding if the patient has been pretreated with aspirin
- see also General Interactions of fibrinolytic agents (p. 1151)

Nursing considerations/Cautions
- (Pulmonary embolus) diagnosis should be confirmed before starting therapy. Any underlying deep vein thrombosis should also be treated, taking into

- consideration that lysis of any deep vein thrombi may cause re-embolisation; therefore the patient should be closely monitored
- (Acute ischaemic stroke) intracranial haemorrhage should be excluded (e.g. CT scan) before starting therapy
- (Acute ischaemic stroke) BP monitoring is recommended during therapy and 24 hours postinfusion
- trade name and batch number should be recorded in patient medical notes
- reconstitute using water for injections (without preservatives). Dissolve the powder by swirling the vial gently to prevent excessive foaming. Allow to stand for several minutes to allow any foaming to settle and clear, then dilute with sodium chloride 0.9% only
- when reconstituting 50 mg vial, use the transfer cannula (provided) to inject water for injections into the vial
- solutions containing preservatives or carbohydrates (e.g. glucose) should be avoided for reconstitution or dilution, as this increases turbidity of the fluid
- administer alone
- (Acute myocardial infarction, pulmonary embolism) usually given with IV heparin to reduce risk of reocclusion. An IV bolus of 5000 units is given before the start of fibrinolytic therapy or within the first hour, followed by infusion of 1000 units/hour for 24–48 hours, adjusted according to activated partial thromboplastin time (aPTT) (1.5–2.5 of normal limits, 50–70 seconds)
- aspirin 160 mg should be started immediately and continued (160–325 mg daily) for the first few months after myocardial infarction
- heparin and alteplase infusions should be stopped immediately if uncontrolled bleeding occurs
- readministration should be undertaken with great caution because there is a possibility of antibody formation and hypersensitivity reaction
- stopper contains latex, which may cause hypersensitivity reaction in sensitive individuals
- increased risk of intracranial bleeding if total dose $>$ 100 mg (myocardial infarction, pulmonary embolus) or $>$ 90 mg (acute ischaemic stroke)
- (Acute ischaemic stroke) caution if used in those who have received previous aspirin therapy, have uncontrolled diabetes, who have had a prior stroke, late presentation, have small asymptomatic cerebral aneurysms or are over 80 years
- (Acute ischaemic stroke) contraindicated if $>$ 4.5 hours have elapsed since onset of symptoms or if onset time is unknown, in those showing minor neurological deficit showing improvement or in those with severe stroke, if seizure occurred with stroke, within 48 hours of heparin therapy or elevated aPTT, combination of prior stroke and diabetes, within 12 weeks of previous stroke or head trauma, if platelet count is $<$ 100,000/mm^3, systolic BP $>$ 185 mmHg or diastolic BP $>$ 110 mmHg, blood glucose $<$ 50 mg/dL (2.8 mmol/L) or $>$ 400 mg/dL (22.2 mmol/L), or if the patient is aged less than 18 or greater than 80 years or with an intracranial bleed (including symptomatic subarachnoid bleed with normal CT)
- (Myocardial infarction, pulmonary embolus) contraindicated in those with haemorrhagic stroke, stroke of unknown origin or within 6 months of ischaemic stroke or transient ischaemic attack
- contraindicated in those with hypersensitivity to gentamicin (traces may remain from the manufacturing process)
- see also General Nursing considerations/Cautions for fibrinolytic agents (p. 1151)

Should be used in pregnancy only when the benefits outweigh the risks. Animal studies have shown placental haemorrhage resulting in prematurity and fetal loss.

Avoid use, as no human data are available.

FIBRINOLYTIC AGENTS

 Patients > 80 years have an increased risk of intracranial hemorrhage and a reduced net benefit from alteplase treatment. Treatment decisions in the elderly should carefully weigh the risks and benefits, particularly considering advanced age and stroke severity.

TENECTEPLASE
Trade name
Metalyse

Available forms
Vial: 40 mg (8000 IU), 50 mg (10,000 IU)

Action
- genetically engineered tissue plasminogen activator (tPA), similar to alteplase, although structural differences make it fibrin specific
- biphasic elimination with initial half-life about 18.5—29.5 minutes and terminal half-life 42—206 minutes
- improves blood flow within 90 minutes of injection
- no antibody formation has been observed

Use
- thrombolysis for acute myocardial infarction within 12 hours of onset of symptoms

Dose
- 30—50 mg (6000—10,000 IU) as a single IV bolus (dose is weight dependent)

Adverse effects
- nausea, vomiting
- fever
- see also General Adverse effects of fibrinolytic agents (p. 1151)

Interactions
- see General Interactions of fibrinolytic agents (p. 1151)

Nursing considerations/Cautions
- reconstitute using water for injections (provided in prefilled syringe), swirling gently to dissolve the powder, avoiding excessive foaming
- given as a single bolus injection over 10 seconds
- should be injected only into IV lines containing sodium chloride 0.9%
- incompatible with glucose solutions
- administer alone
- heparin is usually started with a 4000—5000 IU bolus, then continued at 800—1000 IU/hour IV infusion for at least 48—72 hours to maintain activated partial thromboplastin time (aPTT) at 50—75 seconds
- aspirin (150—325 mg) is usually started as soon as possible after onset of symptoms and continued daily until discharge
- caution if used in those ≥ 75 years
- contraindicated in those with gentamicin or polysorbate 20 hypersensitivity
- see also General Nursing considerations/Cautions for fibrinolytic agents (p. 1151)

 Should be used in pregnancy only when the benefits outweigh the risks. Thrombolytic agents may cause placental haemorrhage and subsequent fetal loss or prematurity.

 Caution, as limited human data.

 Use with caution in elderly patients (≥75 years) because of a higher risk of intracranial hemorrhage and other bleeding complications. The benefits and risks should be carefully evaluated.

GASTROINTESTINAL AGENTS (MISCELLANEOUS)

Numerous agents exert their effects on the GI tract, including agents from the following drug classes covered in other sections of this book:
- antidiarrhoeal agents
- antiemetics
- antiulcer agents (including antacids)
- laxatives
- topical rectal medication

Gastrointestinal agents that do not fall into these categories are included in this section. They include agents used in inflammatory bowel disorders and those for enzyme replacement

MEBEVERINE HYDROCHLORIDE
Trade names
Colese, Colofac, APO-Mebeverine

Available form
Tablets: 135 mg

Action
- antispasmodic
- non-specifically relaxes vascular, cardiac and other smooth muscle

Use
- management of irritable bowel syndrome (IBS) symptoms

Dose
- 135 mg orally 3 times daily before or with food until desired effect is achieved, then gradually decrease the dose

Adverse effects
- dizziness, headache, insomnia, general malaise
- indigestion, heartburn, anorexia, constipation
- decreased pulse rate
- (Rare) hypersensitivity, angioedema

Nursing considerations/Cautions
- liver function tests are recommended if the patient develops gastrointestinal symptoms or jaundice
- contains lactose (Colese: 100 mg/tablet; Colofac: 80 mg/tablet) and should not be given to patients with lactose intolerance
- not recommended in those with galactose intolerance, Lapp lactase deficiency or glucose—galactose malabsorption
- caution if used in those with cardiac arrhythmias, AV heart block, angina or ischaemic heart disease, or advanced liver or kidney dysfunction

Patient education
- warn the patient that it may take several weeks before desired effects are achieved
- the patient should be advised not to drive or operate machinery if dizziness occurs

GASTROINTESTINAL AGENTS (MISCELLANEOUS)

Not to be used during pregnancy unless the expected benefit outweighs any potential risk.

Not to be used during breastfeeding unless the expected benefit outweighs any potential risk.

TEDUGLUTIDE
Trade name
Revestive

Available form
Vial: 5 mg

Action
- analogue of GLP-2 (peptide secreted by L-cells of distal intestine) (GLP-2 increases intestinal and portal blood flow, decreases intestinal motility and inhibits gastric acid secretion)
- binds to GLP-2 receptors, releasing mediators such as insulin-like growth factors (IGF-1), nitric oxide and keratinocyte growth factor (KGF)
- preserves mucosal integrity by promoting repair and normal intestine growth, increasing villus height and crypt depth
- half-life is 1.1 hours (in patients with short bowel syndrome)

Use
- treatment of patients (adult and paediatric patients 2 years of age and above) with short bowel syndrome (who are dependent on parental support)

Dose
- 0.05 mg/kg SC daily

Adverse effects
- abdominal pain and distension, nausea, vomiting, flatulence, diarrhoea, loss of appetite
- colonic polyps, pancreatitis, small intestinal stenosis, intestinal obstruction
- cholecystitis
- fatigue, headache, insomnia
- fever
- arthralgia
- nasopharyngitis, flu-like illness
- cough, dyspnoea
- peripheral oedema, congestive cardiac failure
- (Injection site) haematoma, erythema
- (Uncommon) increase in blood amylase and lipase, pancreatic duct stenosis, pancreas infection, fluid overload, antibody development

Interactions
- caution if used with benzodiazepines, opioid analgesics, digoxin or antihypertensive agents

Nursing considerations/Cautions
- not for IM or IV administration
- reconstitute using 0.5 mL water for injections, giving a concentration of 10 mg/mL
- when reconstituting, the vial should not be shaken but can be rolled between the palms and turned gently upside down once, and used within 3 hours of reconstitution
- reconstituted solution should not be shaken or frozen or used if cloudy or containing particles
- the patient should be stable for 4 or more weeks on parental nutrition before starting therapy
- therapy should be started under medical supervision
- bilirubin and alkaline phosphatase should be measured before starting and regularly during therapy
- colonoscopy of the whole colon with removal of any polyps is recommended before starting therapy (up to 6 months), and then within 1–2 years after starting therapy, and then every 5 years (or more often for patients at high risk of colorectal polyps). If polyps are found, removed and found to be colorectal cancer, therapy should be stopped
- the patient should be closely monitored for any signs of small bowel and hepatobiliary malignancy
- the patient should be monitored for any fluid overload, especially at the start of therapy. Parenteral nutrition needs should be assessed and re-evaluated

- during the first months of therapy to minimise the risk of fluid overload
- therapy should be continued in those patients who have been weaned off parenteral nutrition
- when therapy is stopped, fluid and electrolyte levels should be carefully monitored, as discontinuation may result in fluid and electrolyte imbalance and potential dehydration
- should be administered only SC, rotating sites (thigh, upper arm or abdomen)
- in patients with active non-gastrointestinal malignancy or at risk of malignancy, the decision to start therapy should be based on risk versus benefit
- caution if used in those with a history of cardiovascular disease (e.g. cardiac insufficiency, hypertension)
- contraindicated in those with active gastrointestinal (gastrointestinal tract, hepatobiliary, pancreatic) malignancy or with a history of gastrointestinal malignancy within lthe ast 5 years

Patient education

- the patient should be instructed to seek medical advice immediately if any of the following occur:
  - sudden weight gain, swollen ankles, difficulty breathing (fluid overload)
  - upper abdominal pain which spreads to right shoulder or back, abdominal tenderness, nausea, vomiting, fever (cholecystitis)
  - upper abdominal pain radiating to the back, abdominal pain that is worse after eating, abdominal tenderness, nausea, vomiting, rapid pulse (pancreatitis)
  - intermittent crampy abdominal pain, loss of appetite, vomiting, abdominal swelling, inability to pass gas or have bowel movements (intestinal obstruction)

 Should be used during pregnancy only if benefits outweigh risks.

 Should be used during breastfeeding only if benefits outweigh risks.

URSODEOXYCHOLIC ACID

Trade names
Ursodox GH, Ursofalk, Ursosan, APO-Ursodeoxycholic Acid

Available forms
Capsules: 250 mg;
Tablets: 500 mg;
Suspension: 50 mg/mL

Action
- alters bile salt composition, decreasing the concentration of more toxic bile salts and increasing bile acid output and bile flow
- half-life 3.5—5.8 days

Use
- chronic cholestatic liver disease (including associated with primary sclerosing cholangitis (PSC), primary biliary cholangitis (PBC) and cystic fibrosis (CF)-related cholestasis)

Dose
- (PSC) 10—16 mg/kg/day orally in 2—3 divided doses, increasing to 20 mg/kg/day if needed **OR**
- (CF-related cholestasis) up to 20 mg/kg/day orally in 2—3 divided doses **OR**
- (PBC, non-CF chronic cholestasis) 12—16 mg/kg/day orally in 2—3 divided doses until liver function improves, then decreasing to a single nightly dose

Adverse effects
- diarrhoea, nausea, vomiting, right upper abdominal pain
- increased pruritus
- sleep disturbance
- increased cholestasis
- (Rare) allergic reaction, calcification of gallstones, hepatitis, cirrhosis, urticaria

Interactions
- absorption may be inhibited by colestyramine, colestipol, charcoal and antacids containing aluminium hydroxide or aluminium oxide

GASTROINTESTINAL AGENTS (MISCELLANEOUS)

- may increase absorption of ciclosporin; therefore ciclosporin serum levels should be closely monitored
- may decrease the absorption of ciprofloxacin

Nursing considerations/Cautions

- liver enzymes (aspartate aminotransferase (AST), alanine aminotransferase (ALT) and glutamyl transferase) should be measured monthly for the first 3 months, then 3-monthly
- if the patient weighs less than 34 kg or is unable to swallow, suspension is recommended
- (PBC) if pruritus increases initially, the dose should be decreased to 250 mg daily, then slowly increased at weekly intervals
- 5 mL suspension contains 11.39 mg sodium, which may need to be considered if the patient is on a sodium-restricted diet
- not recommended in those with acute gallbladder or bile duct inflammation, or obstruction of the common bile duct or cystic duct

Patient education

- advise the patient to swallow capsules and tablets whole
- the patient should be advised to separate by 2 hours from colestyramine, colestipol, charcoal and some antacids
- instruct the patient to shake the suspension well before use and discard 4 months after opening
- warn the patient to seek medical advice immediately if right-sided upper abdominal pains occurs or if itching (pruritus) gets worse

Tablet can be crushed or capsule opened and dispersed in water or mixed with spoonful of yoghurt or apple puree.

Suspension is available for those with swallowing difficulties.

Not recommended in the first month of pregnancy.

Not recommended during breastfeeding.

AGENTS USED IN INFLAMMATORY BOWEL DISEASE

Australia has one of the highest incidence rates of inflammatory bowel disease (IBD) in the developed countries. With 179,420 Australians living with IBD in 2025, the incidence of IBD is increasing globally, and the growth in Australia is outpacing similar nations (Crohns and Colitis Australia 2025). IBD is made up of Crohn's disease and ulcerative colitis. *Crohn's disease* may affect the entire intestine and causes inflammation of both the mucosal and the submucosal layers, while *ulcerative colitis* affects the colon and rectum and, in severe cases, abscesses may erode the colon wall, leading to perforation (Wright et al 2018). Early diagnosis and management is vital in inducing and maintaining remission rather than just symptom control, as subclinical inflammation may lead to intestinal damage (Wright et al 2018).

Aminosalicylic acid-based agents (e.g. sulfasalazine, mesalazine) are used to induce remission and prevent relapse in mild-to-moderate ulcerative colitis; however, these are less efficacious in Crohn's disease. For moderate-to-severe disease, corticosteroids such as prednisolone are used for remission of active disease (see Corticosteroids, p. 1014). Immunomodifying agents (such as azathioprine) are recommended for maintenance of remission in moderate-to-severe Crohn's disease or ulcerative colitis not responding to other treatment. More recently, anti-tumour necrosis-α factor (e.g. adalimumab, infliximab) (see DMARDs, p. 1060) and monoclonal antibodies (e.g. vedolizumab, ustekinumab) have been used for induction and maintenance of remission.

BALSALAZIDE SODIUM

Trade name
Colazide

Available form
Capsules: 750 mg

Action
- aminosalicylate
- prodrug, active metabolite is mesalazine, which is an intestinal anti-inflammatory agent action on colonic mucosa
- onset of action 1–2 hours

Use
- treatment of mild-to-moderate ulcerative colitis, and maintenance of remission in those intolerant to sulfasalazine

Dose
- initially 2.25 g (3 capsules) 3 times daily until remission or 12 weeks, then 1.5 g (2 capsules) twice daily (maintenance)

Adverse effects
- abdominal pain, diarrhoea, nausea, vomiting, dyspepsia, anorexia, constipation, dry mouth
- headache, fatigue, dizziness
- arthralgia, back pain, myalgia
- flu-like illness, dyspnoea
- rectal bleeding
- aggravated ulcerative colitis
- pruritus
- (Rare) blood dyscrasias

Interactions
- caution if used with digoxin; therefore plasma levels should be closely monitored during therapy, especially when starting or stopping therapy
- caution if used with agents with a narrow therapeutic range if secreted in the renal tubules
- caution if given with warfarin
- may impair the absorption of folic acid
- may increase the risk of myelosuppression if given with mercaptopurine or azathioprine
- caution if given with oral antibacterial agents

Nursing considerations/Cautions
- blood counts, blood urea nitrogen (BUN), creatinine and urine analysis is recommended during therapy
- rectal or oral corticosteroids can be used at the same time if needed
- caution if used in those with asthma, a history of kidney disease or mild kidney impairment, or mild-to-moderate liver impairment
- not recommended in those under 18 years
- contraindicated in those with hypersensitivity to mesalazine or salicylates, severe liver impairment, moderate-to-severe kidney impairment, or those with bleeding tendency or active peptic ulceration

Patient education
- advise the patient to seek medical advice if any unexplained bruising, bleeding, sore throat, fever or tiredness occurs

The prolonged-release tablet that can be dispersed in water, or open the capsule and disperse the contents in 10–20 mL of water. Can be mixed with apple puree or yoghurt.

Not recommended during the first stages of pregnancy unless the expected benefit outweighs any potential risk, and contraindicated in the last weeks of pregnancy.

Renal toxicity has been observed. Balsalazide is therefore contraindicated in patients with moderate-to-severe renal impairment and caution should be exercised when administering balsalazide to patients with mild renal impairment or a history of renal disease.

Balsalazide should be used with caution in patients with mild-to-moderate hepatic impairment.

GASTROINTESTINAL AGENTS (MISCELLANEOUS)

ETRASIMOD
Trade name
Velsipity

Available form
Tablet: 2 mg

Action
* sphingosine 1-phosphate (S1P) receptor modulator
* high affinity for S1P receptors 1, 4 and 5
* partially and reversibly block lymphocytic capacity to leave lymphoid organs, resulting in a decreased number of lymphocytes in peripheral blood, lowering the number of activated lymphocytes in tissue including intestines

Use
* treatment of moderate-to-severe ulcerative colitis (UC) who have had inadequate response, loss of response or intolerance to conventional, biological or Janus kinase (JAK) inhibitor therapies

Dose
* 2 mg orally daily

Adverse effects
* lymphopenia, neutropenia, anaemia
* fever
* urinary tract infection
* hypercholesterolaemia
* headache, dizziness
* bradycardia
* blurred vision, decreased visual acuity, visual impairment
* hypertension
* increased liver enzymes
* (Uncommon) macular oedema, AV block
* (Rare) progressive multifocal leukoencephalopathy (PML), malignancies, respiratory difficulty

Interactions
* not recommended with rifampicin
* not recommended with fluconazole, clarithromycin, itraconazole or ritonavir
* not recommended with phototherapy with UV-B radiation or PUVA (psoralen ultraviolet A) photochemotherapy
* caution if used in with beta adrenergic blocking agents, calcium-channel blockers, agents that prolong QT interval, Class Ia and Class III antiarrhythmic agents owing to additive effects
* beta adrenergic blocking agents and antiarrhythmic agents can be started after etrasimod therapy has been in place for at least 7 consecutive days
* if live attenuated vaccine is required, it should be administered at least 4 weeks before starting therapy
* caution if used with antineoplastic agents or immunosuppressants (including corticosteroids) because of added effects on immune system

Nursing considerations/Cautions
* therapy should not be started until any active infection has been treated
* ECG, blood pressure monitoring and liver function tests and bilirubin level testing are recommended before starting therapy (or within last 6 months)
* complete blood count (with lymphocyte count) should be monitored before starting and regularly through therapy. Treatment should be interrupted if absolute lymphocyte count $< 0.2 \times 10^9$/L and restarting considered when counts $> 0.5 \times 10^9$/L
* ophthalmic assessment (e.g. evaluation of fundus and macula) is recommended before starting therapy in those with a history of uveitis, retinal disease or diabetes mellitus. All patients should have an ophthalmic examination if they experience any change in vision
* pregnancy must be excluded before starting therapy
* immunisations should be updated before starting therapy. If the patient dose not have a health care professional-confirmed history of varicella (chickenpox) or without documentation of full course of vaccination against varicella zoster (VZV) virus, they should be tested for VZV antibodies; a full course of VZV vaccination is recommended if the patient is antibody negative

- if switching from an immunosuppressive medication, consideration should be given to an appropriate washout period to prevent additive immune effects
- lymphocyte count usually returns to normal within 1 to 2 weeks of stopping therapy and this should be considered if the patient is started on an immunosuppressive medication because of the potential additive immune effects
- cardiology advice is recommended before starting therapy in patients who have significant QT prolongation, arrhythmias requiring treatment with Class Ia or Class III antiarrhythmic agents, ischaemic heart disease, heart failure, a history of cardiac arrest, cerebrovascular disease, uncontrolled hypertension, a resting heart rate less than 50 beats/min, a history of symptomatic bradycardia, recurrent cardiogenic syncope, severe untreated sleep apnoea, or a history of Mobitz type I second-degree AV block (without pacemaker)
- in patients with pre-existing cardiac conditions, monitoring for signs and symptoms of symptomatic bradycardia (hourly pulse rate and blood pressure) is recommended for 4 hours after the first dose. An ECG should also be conducted at the start and end of the four-hour period. If the patient has heart rate < 45 beats/min or the ECG shows signs of new-onset second-degree or higher AV block, additional monitoring is recommended
- caution if used in those with severe respiratory disease such as pulmonary fibrosis, asthma and chronic obstructive pulmonary disease
- not recommended in those with severe liver impairment
- contraindicated in those who have a recent (previous 6 months) history of myocardial infarction, unstable angina pectoris, stroke, transient ischaemic attack, decompensated heart failure (requiring hospitalisation or NYHA Class III/IV heart failure), history or presence of Mobitz type II second-degree or third-degree AV block, sick sinus syndrome of SA block (without pacemaker), or with active malignancies

Patient education

- the patient should be instructed to seek medical advice immediately if any of the following occur:
  - fever, chills, sweating, cough, body aches and pains, sore throat
  - nausea, vomiting, abdominal pain, fatigue, loss of appetite, dark urine, yellowing of skin and/or whites of the eyes, pale bowel motions
  - progressive weakness on one side of body, clumsiness, visual disturbances, confusion, personality changes (signs of PML)
  - changes to vision
  - any new or changes to skin lesions
- warn the patient that lymphocyte levels may remain low for up to 2 weeks after therapy is stopped, meaning they need to be vigilant to monitor for any infection
- the patient should be advised to have a regular skin examination to identify any new or changing lesions
- advise the patient to avoid excessive sun exposure and wear SPF 30+ sunscreen, a hat and long sleeves
- women of childbearing potential should be counselled to use effective contraception during and for 10 days after stopping therapy

 Contraindicated during pregnancy owing to reports of fetal and embryonic harm at clinical doses. Women of childbearing potential must use effective contraception during treatment and for 10 days after discontinuation. Pregnancy must be excluded prior to initiating therapy.

 Contraindicated during breastfeeding owing to lack of human studies.

GASTROINTESTINAL AGENTS (MISCELLANEOUS)

 Caution if used in those over 65 years because of decreased liver, kidney and/or cardiac function. Regular monitoring is recommended.

MESALAZINE
Trade names
Asacol, Mesalz, Mesasal, Mezavant, Pentasa preparation, Salofalk preparations

Available forms
Tablets: 250 mg, 500 mg, 800 mg, 1.6 g;
Tablets (modified release): 500 mg, 1 g, 1.2 g;
Granules (modified release): 500 mg/sachet, 1 g/sachet, 1.5 g/sachet, 2 g/sachet, 3 g/sachet, 4 g/sache;
Suppositories: 1 g;
Enema: 2 g/60 mL, 4 g/60 mL;
Enema (foam): 1 g

Action
- active component of sulfasalazine (5-aminosalicylic acid)
- anti-inflammatory action by inhibiting prostaglandin synthesis, chemotactic leukotriene synthesis and leucocytic motility

Use
- acute inflammatory large bowel disease
- maintenance of remission of ulcerative colitis and Crohn's disease in patients intolerant to sulfasalazine
- ulcerative proctitis, ulcerative proctosigmoiditis

Dose
- (Ulcerative colitis) 1.5—3 g orally daily in 1—3 divided doses 30—60 minutes before food (treatment), then 250 mg orally 3 times daily (maintenance of remission) **OR**
- (Crohn's disease) 2.4—4.8 g orally once daily (induction of remission), then 2.4 g daily (maintenance) (prolonged-release tablets) **OR**
- (Crohn's disease — maintenance) 250 mg orally 3 times daily **OR**
- (Ulcerative colitis) 2.4—4.8 g orally daily in single or divided doses (induction of remission), then 1.6—2.4 g orally daily (maintenance of remission) (modified-release tablets) **OR**
- (Ulcerative colitis) up to 4 g once daily or in divided doses (induction of remission), then 1.5—2 g daily in divided doses (maintenance) (Pentasa — prolonged-release tablets, granules) **OR**
- (Crohn's disease) up to 4 g daily in divided doses (treatment), then 4 g daily (maintenance) (Pentasa — prolonged-release tablets, granules) **OR**
- (Ulcerative colitis) 2—4 g enema/foam enema nightly per rectum (acute treatment and maintenance) **OR**
- (Ulcerative proctosigmoiditis, left-sided ulcerative colitis) 1 g enema nightly per rectum (Pentasa) **OR**
- (Ulcerative proctitis) 1 g rectally at bedtime (suppository)

Adverse effects
- nausea, vomiting, diarrhoea, abdominal pain, flatulence, dyspepsia, exacerbation of ulcerative colitis
- headache, neuropathy, fatigue, asthenia
- fever
- hypertension
- rash, alopecia, pruritus, urticaria
- arthralgia, myalgia, back pain
- decreased sperm count, impaired sperm motility
- haematuria, ketonuria
- chest pain
- (Transient) changes in liver function tests
- (Rare) interstitial nephritis, reversible pancreatitis, colitis, blood dyscrasias, myocarditis, pericarditis, hypersensitivity, kidney failure, photosensitivity

Interactions
- not recommended with anticoagulants, as effects may be potentiated; therefore prothrombin time should be closely monitored
- may potentiate effects of sulfonylureas, increasing the risk of hypoglycaemia; therefore blood glucose levels should be closely monitored

- may delay excretion of methotrexate, increasing the risk of toxicity
- may antagonise probenecid and sulfinpyrazone
- may decrease the effects of rifampicin, furosemide (frusemide) and spironolactone
- not recommended with lactulose or similar drugs that lower gastric or stool pH and prevent the release of mesalazine
- increased risk of nephrotoxicity if given with nephrotoxic agents including NSAIDs and azathioprine
- increased risk of myelosuppression if given with azathioprine, thioguanine or mercaptopurine
- increased risk of gastric adverse effects if given with glucocorticoids

Nursing considerations/Cautions

- kidney (including urinalysis) and liver function and differential blood counts should be monitored before starting, monthly for 3 months, then 3-monthly
- if the patient weighs less than 40 kg, a half-dose should be given
- (Acute ulcerative colitis) remission usually occurs in about 8 weeks
- (Foam enema) contains sodium metasulfite and therefore should be used with caution in those with allergies or asthma
- (Salofalk granules) contain aspartame and therefore not recommended in those with phenylketonuria
- (Pentasa enema) contains sodium metabisulfite and therefore should be used with caution in those with allergies or asthma
- (Asacol) not recommended in those with galactose intolerance, Lapp lactase deficiency or glucose—galactose malabsorption
- caution if used in patients with pre-existing skin conditions (e.g. eczema, dermatitis) owing to an increased risk of photosensitivity reaction
- caution if given to patients with renal impairment or renal failure (with proteinuria and elevated blood urea nitrogen (BUN)), hypersensitivity to sulfasalazine or liver impairment, or predisposed to myocarditis or pericarditis
- caution in those with organic/functional obstruction of upper GI tract, as this may delay onset of action of tablets or granules
- contraindicated in those with hypersensitivity to salicylates or sulfasalazine, severe kidney impairment, active peptic ulcer or bleeding tendency
- of limited benefit in Crohn's disease

Patient education

- warn the patient that empty tablet shells may appear in faeces. If an intact tablet is present, medical advice should be sought
- instruct the patient to place granules on the tongue, not crushed or chewed, and then wash them down with water or juice. They may also be dispersed in 50 mL of cold water
- (Enema) warn the patient that enema may cause staining to clothing and fabrics
- (Enema) ensure the patient understands correct instillation technique, including:
  - bowel should be emptied before instillation
  - wash hands with soap and water
  - cut along dotted line of enema pack, taking care not to damage bottle
  - shake bottle for 30 seconds
  - remove applicator cap
  - lie on left side with left leg outstretched and right leg bent
  - guide applicator into rectum and squeeze bottle gently until empty
  - remove and remain lying down for at least 30 minutes
  - wash hands and try not to open bowels until next morning if possible
- (Foam enema) ensure the patient understands the following:
  - 2 g = 2 applications
  - empty the bowel before application

GASTROINTESTINAL AGENTS (MISCELLANEOUS)

- use foam enema at room temperature (20–25°C)
- wash hands thoroughly with soap and water
- shake for 15 seconds after fitting the applicator to the canister
- remove safety tab under the pump dome, twist dome until the semicircular gap is underneath in line with the nozzle
- insert applicator into the rectum (while standing with one foot on floor and other on chair/stool)
- push the pump dome and hold for 5 seconds and then release to administer one application (1 g) and wait 15 seconds
- after second administration, the applicator should be left in the rectum for 30 seconds before withdrawal
- remove applicator from the canister and dispose of appropriately
- wash hands
- instruct the patient to store the canister away from direct sunlight, flames or sparks. The canister should not be frozen or refrigerated or punctured when empty
- (Suppository) instruct the adult patient in the correct technique for suppository insertion, including:
  - the need to empty the bowel if possible before suppository insertion
  - wash hands with soap and water
  - if the suppository feels soft, place it (unwrapped) in the fridge or hold it under cold water to firm it up
  - put on disposable glove, if wanted
  - remove wrapper from the suppository and moisten slightly by dipping in cool water
  - lie on one side with knees raised to chest
  - push the suppository (blunt end first) gently into the rectum, taking care not to break suppository
  - remain lying down for a few minutes to allow the suppository to dissolve
  - wash hands thoroughly after insertion
- advise the patient to seek medical advice if any of the following occur:
  - unusual bleeding or bruising, fever, chills, sore throat, mouth ulcers
  - severe stomach ache and/or cramps, fever, rash, severe headache
  - skin rash, hives, itching
  - yellowing of eyes or skin, itching, upper abdominal pain, lethargy, loss of appetite, nausea, dark urine, pale stools
- male patients should be counselled regarding the possibility of transient reduction in sperm and sperm mobility during therapy
- female patients should be counselled to use contraception and avoid pregnancy occurring during therapy

 Granules are recommended for those with swallowing difficulties.

 Not recommended during the first stages of pregnancy unless the expected benefit outweighs any potential risk. Contraindicated in the last weeks of pregnancy.

 Not recommended during breastfeeding.

 Check renal and liver function at baseline; repeat every 3 months in the first year, then every 6 months.

OLSALAZINE SODIUM

Trade name
Dipentum

Available forms
Capsules: 250 mg;
Tablets: 500 mg

Action
- consists of 2 molecules of 5-aminosalicylic acid
- cleaved by bacteria in the colon to the clinically active form
- poorly absorbed by the GI tract

Use
- ulcerative colitis (in those intolerant to sulfasalazine)

Dose
- (Treatment of acute ulcerative colitis) initially 250 mg orally daily after meals (day 1), then increasing by 250 mg per day to 2 g orally daily in divided doses after meals (capsules) **OR**
- (Treatment of acute ulcerative colitis) initially 500 mg orally daily after meals (day 1), then increasing by 500 mg per day to 2 g orally daily in divided doses (tablets) **OR**
- (Maintenance of remission) 500 mg orally twice daily after meals
- if no response is achieved with 2 g and the medicine is well tolerated, the total dose may be increased to 3 g/day

Adverse effects
- nausea, diarrhoea, abdominal pain, upset stomach, dry mouth
- headache, dizziness, insomnia, mood swings, irritability
- blurred vision, dry eyes, watery eyes
- fever, chills
- rash, urticaria, photosensitivity, alopecia
- dysuria, haematuria, proteinuria, impotence, menorrhagia
- arthralgia, myalgia, joint pain
- (Rare) blood dyscrasias, hepatitis, pancreatitis, peripheral neuropathy, angioedema, rectal bleeding/discomfort, interstitial lung disease, nephritis

Interactions
- not recommended with salicylates or low molecular weight heparins because of the increased risk of bleeding
- prothrombin time should be closely monitored if given with warfarin; however, they are not recommended together
- increased risk of myelosuppression if given with mercaptopurine or tioguanine
- increased risk of Reye's syndrome if given within 6 weeks of varicella vaccine

Nursing considerations/Cautions
- bioequivalence of capsules and tablets has not been established
- a single dose should not be greater than 1 g
- the daily dose can be increased to 3 g if needed
- kidney function (serum creatinine) should be measured before starting therapy, 3-monthly for the first year, 6-monthly for the next 4 years, then yearly for life
- caution if used in those with known allergies, asthma or impaired kidney or liver function
- contraindicated in those with hypersensitivity to salicylates, bleeding tendency/blood dyscrasias, peptic ulcer or erosive gastritis

Patient education
- warn the patient that diarrhoea occurs commonly during therapy
- advise the patient that tablets should not be divided
- the patient should be advised not to drive or operate machinery if dizziness occurs
- instruct the patient to seek medical advice if any of the following occur:
  - diarrhoea (as watery diarrhoea requires dose reduction)
  - fever, chills, sore throat, mouth ulcers, unusual bleeding or bruising

 Not to be used during pregnancy unless the expected benefits outweigh any potential risks.

 Not to be used during breastfeeding unless the expected benefits outweigh any potential risks.

SULFASALAZINE
Trade names
Pyralin EN, Salazopyrin, Salazopyrin EN-Tabs

Available forms
Tablets: 500 mg;
Tablets (enteric-coated): 500 mg

Action
- broken down in the colon by bacteria to 5-aminosalicylic acid and sulfapyridine,

GASTROINTESTINAL AGENTS (MISCELLANEOUS)

producing an anti-inflammatory effect by its action on prostaglandin synthesis, leukotrienes and arachidonic acid metabolites
- onset of action may take 6—12 weeks

Use
- ulcerative colitis
- treatment of active Crohn's disease with colonic involvement
- rheumatoid arthritis (unresponsive to non-steroidal anti-inflammatory drugs (NSAIDs))

Dose
- (Ulcerative colitis, Crohn's disease) initially 1—2 g orally 4 times daily after meals, then 2 g daily in four divided doses. as maintenance **OR**
- (Rheumatoid arthritis) initially 500 mg daily; increase the daily dose by 500 mg each week to a maximum of 3 g daily in divided doses. Maintenance: 2—3 g daily in 2 or 3 doses.

Adverse effects
- anorexia, nausea, vomiting, diarrhoea
- fever, headache, pallor
- erythema, pruritus, rash
- reversible oligospermia, proteinuria, haematuria, crystalluria
- (Rare) hypersensitivity reaction (including drug rash with eosinophilia and systemic symptoms (DRESS)), agranulocytosis, aplastic anaemia, microcytosis, pancytopenia, folate deficiency

Interactions
- may potentiate oral anticoagulants, methotrexate and sulfonylureas, increasing the risk of adverse effects
- reduces absorption and metabolism of folic acid, resulting in folic acid deficiency, macrocytosis and pancytopenia
- reduces the absorption of digoxin; therefore serum levels should be monitored
- increased blood levels may occur in patients taking oral anticoagulants, indometacin, sulfinpyrazone, urinary acidifiers or salicylates
- decreased absorption may occur if given with antacids or ferrous sulfate heptahydrate
- increased risk of bone marrow depression and leucopenia if given with azathioprine or mercaptopurine
- activity may be decreased if given with para-aminobenzoicacid-type local anaesthetics
- increased GI disturbances (especially nausea) may occur if given with methotrexate

Nursing considerations/Cautions
- therapy should be discontinued if serious infection develops
- enteric-coated tablets are available if GI intolerance is experienced
- monitor blood counts (including differential white cell count), liver function tests and renal function analysis (including urinalysis) before starting therapy, second-weekly for 3 months and then every 3 months
- adverse effects are mainly dose dependent
- encourage adequate fluid intake to reduce risk of crystalluria and stone formation
- serious skin reactions are most likely to occur in the first 4 weeks of therapy
- caution if given to those with glucose-6-phosphate dehydrogenase (G6PD) deficiency (as the risk of haemolytic anaemia is increased) or severe allergy, bronchial asthma, atopic disease or recurring or chronic infection
- not recommended in those with blood dyscrasias or impaired liver or kidney function
- contraindicated in those with any allergy/hypersensitivity to sulfonamide or salicylate derivatives, intestinal/urinary obstruction, porphyria or blood dyscrasias

Patient education
- instruct patients that enteric-coated tablets should not be crushed or broken but rather swallowed whole with plenty of water

- advise the patient to allow a 2-hour interval if taking antacids
- (Inflammatory bowel disease) the patient should be advised that no more than 8 hours should elapse between overnight doses
- warn the patient that urine may become orange-yellow colour if alkaline
- instruct the patient to immediately report any:
  - sore throat, fever, pallor
  - swollen glands
  - skin rash
  - pinpoint bleeding on the skin (purpura)
  - yellow-orange discolouration of skin, urine and other body fluids
- instruct the patient to drink plenty of water during therapy
- counsel male patients about reversible male infertility (effects reversed within 8—12 weeks of stopping therapy), and female patients regarding potential harm to a developing fetus

Enteric coated tablets should not be crushed or broken.

Plain tablet can be crushed and mixed with water or spoonful of yoghurt or apple puree. Mask and gloves should be warn if crushing tablet.

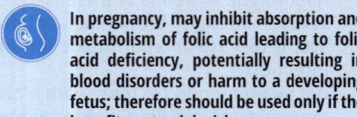

In pregnancy, may inhibit absorption and metabolism of folic acid leading to folic acid deficiency, potentially resulting in blood disorders or harm to a developing fetus; therefore should be used only if the benefits outweigh risks.

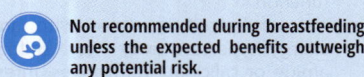

Not recommended during breastfeeding unless the expected benefits outweigh any potential risk.

Monitor blood counts (including differential white cell count), liver function tests and renal function analysis (including urinalysis) before starting therapy, second-weekly for 3 months and then every 3 months.

VEDOLIZUMAB (rch)
Trade name
Entyvio

Available forms
Vial: 300 mg
Prefilled pen: 108 mg/0.68 mL

Action
- humanised IgG_1 monoclonal antibody that binds to alpha4 beta7 (α4 β7) integrin (integrin α4β7 is expressed on leucocytes including T-lymphocytes that migrate into GI tract, causing inflammation)
- selectively inhibits α4β7 integrin, preventing inflammation

Use
- moderate-to-severe ulcerative colitis or Crohn's disease in those with inadequate response or intolerant to conventional therapy or tumour necrosis factor alpha (TNF-α) antagonist

Dose
- 300 mg by IV infusion over 30 minutes, repeated after 2 and 6 weeks, then every 8 weeks and **OR**
- 108 mg SC every two week

Adverse effects
- infusion-related reaction (including flushing, hypertension, increased heart rate, rash, urticaria, bronchospasm, dyspnoea)
- nausea
- nasopharyngitis, upper respiratory tract infection, cough, bronchitis, influenza
- arthralgia, back pain, pain in extremities
- rash, pruritus
- fever
- fatigue, headache, dizziness
- oropharyngeal pain
- (Rare) progressive multifocal leukoencephalopathy, increased liver enzymes, hypersensitivity reaction, development of anti-vedolizumab antibodies, malignancy

Interactions
- not recommended with live or attenuated live vaccines or within 3 months of stopping vedolizumab

GASTROINTESTINAL AGENTS (MISCELLANEOUS)

- caution if used with or within 12 weeks of natalizumab
- not recommended concurrently with biological immunosuppressants

Nursing considerations/Cautions

- not given via IV bolus or push
- reconstitute using 4.8 mL of water for injections, vial swirled gently for at least 15 seconds to dissolve the powder. Reconstituted solution should be allowed to sit for 20 minutes to allow any foam to settle. The vial can be swirled further if needed. If not fully dissolved, wait another 10 minutes. Invert the reconstituted solution 3 times before withdrawing 5 mL and adding to 250 mL sodium chloride 0.9%, and then gently mixing the infusion bag before administration
- administer alone
- the trade name and batch number should be recorded in the patient's medical records
- caution if used in those with controlled severe infection or history of severe infection
- not recommended in those under 18 years
- contraindicated in those with active severe infections (including active TB), sepsis and serious abscesses
- all patients should be carefully screened for history or symptoms of tuberculosis (TB), including detailed medical history and possible previous exposure to TB. Chest X-ray and tuberculin skin test (Mantoux) may also be performed (however, there is a risk of false negative skin test occurring in patients who are severely ill or immunocompromised)
- any patient with latent TB should be treated with antimycobacterials before starting therapy
- any other active infections should be treated before starting therapy
- the patient should be up to date with current immunisation guidelines before starting therapy
- the patient should be reviewed for signs of clinical response within 12–14 weeks of starting therapy. If no response is seen within 14 weeks, therapy should not be continued
- the patient should be closely monitored during and after infusion for any signs of infusion reaction, which can occur up to several hours post-infusion. If an infusion reaction occurs, the infusion should be slowed or stopped until symptoms subside, then started at a lower rate. Infusion reactions have occurred after 2 hours and more than 2 days after infusion
- paracetamol, antihistamines, corticosteroids, adrenaline (epinephrine) and artificial airway should be readily available for infusion reaction
- premedication with paracetamol, hydrocortisone and/or antihistamine may prevent mild and transient effects of an infusion reaction
- the patient should be carefully monitored for any signs of symptoms that might suggest progressive multifocal leukoencephalopathy (e.g. cognitive, neurological or psychiatric symptoms). If signs (progressive one-sided weakness, clumsiness, visual disturbances, changes to thinking, memory or orientation, confusion, personality changes) occur, therapy should be stopped and further evaluation including MRI, CSF testing and repeat neurological assessments completed
- patient may be started on SC therapy as maintenance following at least 2 IV infusions, with the first SC injection given in place of the next IV infusion and then continued every two weeks
- prefilled syringe should be removed from fridge 30 minutes before administration and allowed to come to room temperature

Patient education

- instruct the patient to carry a Patient Alert Card at all times
- the patient should be advised to seek medical advice immediately if any of the following occur:
  - recurrent or persistent infection
  - persistent fever, pallor, unexplained bleeding or bruising (blood dyscrasia)

- persistent cough, weight loss and low-grade fever (possible TB)
- progressive one-sided arm or leg weakness, clumsiness or loss of balance, blurred or double vision, disorientation, confusion, personality changes, difficulty speaking, persistent numbness, decreased or loss of sensation
- women of childbearing age should be counselled to use adequate contraception during and for 18 weeks after stopping therapy to avoid pregnancy

 Not recommended during pregnancy unless benefits are thought to outweigh risks.

 Not recommended during breastfeeding unless benefits are thought to outweigh risks.

ENZYME REPLACEMENT

Pancreatic enzyme replacement is used when the pancreas is unable to produce sufficient amounts of the enzymes necessary for the digestion of fats, carbohydrates and proteins. Conditions requiring enzyme replacement therapy include cystic fibrosis, chronic pancreatitis or after pancreatectomy (MacNaughton & Sharkey 2023). The goal of pancreatic enzyme replacement therapy for those with cystic fibrosis is to improve nutritional status and growth while controlling maldigestion symptoms (such as steatorrhoea). Currently marketed pancreatic enzyme replacement preparations differ in their composition, enzymatic activities, formulation, stability and bioavailability.

PANCRELIPASE
Trade names
Creon Capsules, Creon Micro, Panzytrat 25000

Available forms
Capsules: contain lipase, protease and amylase;
Enteric-coated granules

Action
- mimics the enzymes that assist in the digestion of fats to fatty acids and glycerol, proteins to amino acids and carbohydrates to dextrins and sugars

Use
- malabsorption caused by pancreatic insufficiency, including cystic fibrosis and chronic pancreatitis, and after some types of abdominal surgery (e.g. post-pancreatectomy, gastric bypass surgery)

Dose
- usually 1 capsule orally with meals and 1 capsule with snacks (6 capsules daily) **OR**
- (Cystic fibrosis. Children < 4 years): initially 1000 lipase U/kg/meal
- (Cystic fibrosis ≥ 4 years) 500 lipase units/kg of body weight with meal (titrating the dose to the disease severity, control of steatorrhoea and maintenance of good nutritional status) **OR**
- (Patients with pancreatic insufficiency due to other causes) 25,000–40,000 BP units of lipase (5–8 scoops of granules) with meals and half-dose with snacks, adjusting the dose if necessary (max: 10,000 lipase U/kg/day or 4000 lipase U/g fat intake)

Adverse effects
- skin reaction (rash, pruritus, urticaria)
- diarrhoea, constipation, abdominal pain or distension, nausea, flatulence
- (High dose) fibrosing colonopathy

Interactions
- not recommended with antacids

Nursing considerations/Cautions
- patients with a history of gastrointestinal complications should be closely assessed for risk of fibrosing colonopathy
- 1 measuring scoop = 100 g of granules = 5000 units of lipase
- the dose should be adjusted according to food and disease severity; however,

GASTROINTESTINAL AGENTS (MISCELLANEOUS)

- a rapid increase in dose is not recommended owing to risk of constipation
- the dose should not exceed 10,000 lipase units/kg/day or 4000 lipase units/g fat intake
- of porcine origin, and therefore should not be given to patients who have cultural or religious objections, such as those of the Muslim or Jewish faith
- contraindicated in those with hypersensitivity to porcine protein, in early stages of acute pancreatitis or in acute attack of chronic pancreatitis

Patient education

- advise the patient that capsules should not be crushed or chewed, although if swallowing is problematic capsules may be opened and contents sprinkled on food and eaten immediately
- instruct the patient that the capsule content should not be sprinkled on food with a pH greater than 5.5 (e.g. milk, icecream) because the protective coating may dissolve
- if antacids are necessary, the patient should be advised to allow at least 1 hour between antacids and pancrelipase
- instruct the patient to use the measuring scoop provided for administration of granules (1 measuring scoop = 100 g of granules = 5000 units of lipase)
- advise the patient that granules may be sprinkled on small amount of acidic soft food (pH < 5.5) such as apple sauce or mashed banana and eaten immediately (not stored) without chewing or crushing granules, followed by water or juice to ensure the entire dose has been swallowed
- the patient should be instructed to ensure they drink sufficiently to prevent dehydration and constipation from occurring
- advise the patient (especially if they have cystic fibrosis) to immediately seek medical advice if severe or prolonged abdominal pain occurs

 Capsules can be opened and granules sprinkled on food and eaten immediately without chewing or crushing granules.

 Not to be used during the first trimester of pregnancy.

 Not to be used during breastfeeding unless the expected benefit outweighs any potential risks.

GENERAL ANAESTHETICS

General anaesthetic agents cause a loss of sensation associated with a reversible loss of consciousness and absence of pain (Knights et al 2023). There is no one anaesthetic agent that can produce muscle relaxation, abolition of reflexes, unconsciousness and analgesia, so several agents are used together during a procedure. Combinations of intravenous and inhaled drugs (balanced anaesthesia techniques) minimises their adverse effects. The choice of anaesthetic is determined by the type of intervention that the patient needs (Eilers & Yost 2024).

The anaesthetic procedure is made up of the following:
- *premedication* — given to reduce anxiety, apprehension and pain, to decrease secretions and sometimes to produce sedation and amnesia. Premedication agents also assist with induction of anaesthesia and are usually given 30—60 minutes (IM or SC) or IV just before induction. Agents given as premedications include opioid analgesics (e.g. morphine, fentanyl), benzodiazepines (e.g. midazolam, flunitrazepam), phenothiazines (e.g. prochlorperazine, promethazine), H_2-receptor antagonists (e.g. ranitidine) and anticholinergics (e.g. atropine, glycopyrronium (glycopyrrolate) bromide, hyoscine)
- *induction* — render the patient unconscious and unreactive to stimuli, usually by means of a short-acting barbiturate or benzodiazepine given IV, often with a short-acting muscle relaxant to allow intubation
- *maintenance* — unconsciousness is maintained, usually with an inhalation anaesthetic, and supplemented with IV analgesics and muscle relaxants
- *reversal* — anticholinesterases (e.g. neostigmine) are used to reverse the effects of the non-polarising muscle relaxants
- *recovery* — recovery period lasts until the patient is fully conscious, has stable cardiovascular status, is able to maintain airway unaided and is comfortable

There are two groups of general anaesthetics:
- *inhalation anaesthetics* (including gases (e.g. nitrous oxide) and volatile liquids (e.g. desflurane)
  - mixed with oxygen, allowing administration by inhalation where they rapidly reach a concentration in the blood and brain

GENERAL ANAESTHETICS

- to depress the CNS, causing anaesthesia
- lung function is critical for effectiveness
- abolish both superficial and deep reflexes
- good anaesthetic agents, but not very useful as analgesics, requiring combination with other agents such as opioid analgesics
- rapid recovery when administration is stopped
- allergic reactions uncommon (Knights et al 2023)
- *intravenous anaesthetics* (e.g. thiopental and propofol)
  - can be used for induction and maintenance of general anaesthesia, conscious sedation, induce amnesia and as an adjunct to inhalation anaesthetics
  - induce unconsciousness and suppress reflexes rapidly, allowing external control of airway
  - reduce the amount of inhalation agent required
  - allow prompt recovery
  - minimal analgesic properties (except ketamine) or muscle relaxation actions
  - have amnesic properties (especially midazolam)
  - commonly cause hypersensitivity reactions
  - may cause hypotension, laryngospasm and respiratory failure after overdosage or prolonged administration (Knights et al 2023)

Dose

- doses have not been stated for each drug because anaesthetic agents are generally given by anaesthetists and are calculated for individual patients using body weight or mass and can also be based on the procedure required, patient's physical condition and patient's response

General Adverse effects of general anaesthetics

- cardiovascular and respiratory depression
- (During induction) coughing, breath holding, apnoea, laryngospasm, bronchospasm, increased salivary secretions, hiccups
- involuntary muscle movements, shivering
- (Halogenated anaesthetic) dose-dependent hypotension
- decreased reflexes
- postoperative nausea and vomiting, headache, convulsions
- kidney and liver toxicity
- (Halogenated anaesthetic) intraoperative hyperkalaemia and/or hyperglycaemia
- increased intracranial pressure (in those with space-occupying lesions)
- (Rare) hypersensitivity, malignant hyperthermia/hyperpyrexia (see Glossary)
- (Rare) hepatitis, jaundice

General Interactions of general anaesthetics

- additive CNS depressant effects if given with opioid analgesic, resulting in lower general anaesthetic dose being required
- alcohol, antihistamines, antianxiety agents, opioid analgesics, sedatives and hypnotics intensify cardiovascular, respiratory and CNS depressant effects
- cardiovascular suppression may be enhanced if given with calcium-channel blockers, beta-adrenergic blocking agents or angiotensin converting enzyme (ACE) inhibitors

General Nursing Considerations/Cautions for general anaesthetics

- some long-term therapy (e.g. aspirin, oral anticoagulants) may require a change of dose or cessation before surgery
- dose adjustments may be necessary for patients with chronic conditions, such as diabetes and hypertension
- (halogenated anaesthetic) repeated administration within a short period of time is not recommended and, if undertaken, great caution is needed
- potassium levels should be closely monitored in those with latent or overt neuromuscular disorders to avoid development of cardiac arrhythmias
- hyperventilation before or during anaesthesia prevents an increase in intracranial pressure
- repeat administration within short period of time should be undertaken with great caution
- if the patient is a heavy or regular alcohol user, close monitoring is recommended. as alcohol withdrawal syndrome may occur. Anaesthetic requirements may also be increased
- caution if used in those with mitochondrial disorders
- caution if used in those with myasthenia gravis, as these people are very sensitive to agents that depress respiration
- caution if used in those with latent or overt neuromuscular disorders, as cardiac arrhythmias may occur
- caution if used in those with space-occupying brain lesions or those at risk of raised intracranial pressure, as intracranial pressure or CSF may be increased
- caution if used in those with hypovolaemia or hypotension, who are haemodynamically unstable, with kidney/liver impairment, cardiac or respiratory diseases/impairment (where bronchoconstriction may occur), hypertension or in those who are debilitated
- contraindicated in those with history/risk of malignant hyperthermia/hyperpyrexia
- contraindicated in those who developed jaundice, liver dysfunction, unexplained fever, or leucocytosis after exposure to halogenated anaesthetics
- contraindicated as the sole agent for general anaesthesia induction

General Patient education for general anaesthetics

- the patient should be advised to avoid alcohol in the immediate postoperative period
- instruct the patient to have an adult to escort them home
- warn the patient that their intellectual functioning may decrease or be clouded for 2—3 days after a general anaesthetic; therefore it is recommended that they do not drive, operate machinery, make important decisions or sign legal documents during this time
- alert the patient that they may experience mood changes for up to 6 days after an anaesthetic

 All general anaesthetics cross the placenta and may potentially depress the CNS and respiratory system of the newborn. Caution should be taken if the fetus is known to be compromised and the anaesthetic agent selected carefully, if used at all. Many general anaesthetics are uterine relaxants and decrease placental blood flow.

GENERAL ANAESTHETICS

 Breastfeeding is not recommended for 12 hours after an anaesthetic agent and any milk produced during this time should be discarded.

DESFLURANE
Trade names
Piramal Desflurane, Suprane

Available form
Liquid for inhalation: 240 mL, 250 mL

Action
- non-flammable volatile liquid agent given by inhalation (halogenated anaesthetic)
- similar to isoflurane
- fast washout from the body allowing rapid recovery
- excreted mainly via lungs

Use
- maintenance of surgical anaesthesia

Adverse effects
- pharyngitis
- (Rare) QT prolongation
- see also General Adverse effects of general anaesthetics (p. 1173)

Interactions
- may potentiate actions of non-depolarising muscle relaxants
- recovery from neuromuscular blockade is longer for desflurane than isoflurane
- anaesthesia is more pronounced when given with nitrous oxide
- interacts with dry carbon dioxide absorbents to form carbon monoxide and carboxyhaemoglobin in some patients
- see also General Interactions of general anaesthetics (p. 1173)

Nursing considerations/Cautions
- caution if used in those with coronary artery disease or where increase in heart rate or blood pressure is undesirable, in order to avoid myocardial ischaemia
- caution if used in those with history of QT prolongation
- not recommended in pregnancy termination
- not recommended for mask induction because of respiratory adverse effects
- contraindicated in those with hypersensitivity to halogenated anaesthetics or as inhalational induction agent in children
- see also General Nursing considerations/Cautions for general anaesthetics (p. 1174)

Patient education
- see General Patient education for general anaesthetics (p. 1174)

 Should be used during pregnancy only if the potential benefit justifies the potential risk to the fetus.

 Not indicated for use in nursing mothers because it is not known whether it is excreted in human milk.

ISOFLURANE
Trade name
Aerrane

Available forms
Liquid for inhalation: 1 mL/mL

Action
- non-flammable volatile liquid agent given by inhalation (halogenated anaesthetic)
- slightly irritating to mucous membranes
- ether smell
- rapid induction and recovery
- excreted via lungs
- analgesic and muscle relaxant properties, as well as profound respiratory depressant
- peripheral vasodilation
- stimulates secretions weakly

Use
- induction and maintenance of surgical anaesthesia (usually with nitrous oxide and oxygen)

1175

Dose
- (Anaesthesia) a starting concentration of 0.5% administered by inhalation is recommended. Concentrations of 1.3–3.0% usually bring about surgical anaesthesia within 7–10 minutes

Adverse effects
- shivering, sweating, chills
- delirium, asthenia, fatigue
- (During induction) agitation, retching
- hypotension, cardiac arrhythmias
- myalgia
- increased WBC count
- increased liver enzymes and bilirubin, liver dysfunction, hepatitis
- rash
- (Uncommon) nightmares, mood changes
- (Rare) QT prolongation
- see also General Adverse effects of general anaesthetics (p. 1173)

Interactions
- contraindicated with or within 15 days of monoamine oxidase inhibitors (MAOIs)
- not recommended with isoprenaline, adrenaline (epinephrine) or noradrenaline (norepinephrine) because of the risk of ventricular arrhythmia. Adrenaline (epinephrine) used for haemostatic action (SC, gingival) should also be limited
- increased respiratory depression may occur if given with opioid analgesic (including as premedication) or other respiratory depressants
- caution if used with beta adrenergic receptor blockers owing to increased hypotension and negative inotropic effects
- decreases requirements for neuromuscular blocking agents
- caution if used with calcium-channel blockers, as marked hypotension may occur
- may potentiate actions of non-depolarising muscle relaxants
- anaesthesia is more pronounced when given with nitrous oxide
- increased risk of hepatotoxicity if given with isoniazid. Should be stopped 7 days before and restarted 15 days after administration of isoflurane
- increased risk of hypersensitivity if given with dexamphetamine and related agents, appetite suppressants or ephedrine and related products. Should be stopped several days before isoflurane administration
- interacts with dry carbon dioxide absorbents to form carbon monoxide
- increased risk of severe hypotension and delayed emergence if used in those treated long term with St John's wort
- see also General Interactions of general anaesthetics (p. 1173)

Nursing considerations/Cautions
- caution if used in those with a history of QT prolongation
- caution if used in those with coronary artery disease (especially those with subendocardial ischaemia)
- contraindicated in those undergoing obstetric procedures
- see also General Nursing considerations/Cautions for general anaesthetics (p. 1174)

Patient education
- see General Patient education for general anaesthetics (p. 1174)

 Insufficient information is available to recommend use in pregnancy or obstetrics.

 Potential risks and benefits for each specific patient should be carefully considered before isoflurane is administered to nursing women.

 Acute renal failure and oliguria have been reported; may be secondary to hypotension.

GENERAL ANAESTHETICS

 Cases of mild, moderate and severe postoperative hepatic dysfunction or hepatitis with or without jaundice, including fatal hepatic necrosis and hepatic failure, have been reported with isoflurane.

KETAMINE HYDROCHLORIDE
Trade names
Ketalar, Ketamine Solution for Injection

Available forms
Vial: 200 mg/2 mL, 250 mg/5 mL, 10 mg/mL

Action
- non-barbiturate short-acting general anaesthetic agent (dissociative anaesthetic that causes amnesia and dissociation from surroundings/event)
- non-competitive antagonist at N-methyl-D-aspartate (NMDA) receptors, increasing extracellular glutamate in prefrontal cortex
- pharyngeal and laryngeal reflexes remain intact
- marked analgesic properties, but transient minimal respiratory depression
- active metabolite
- induction of anaesthesia in 30 seconds (IV) usually and lasts 5–10 minutes
- induction of anaesthesia in 3–4 minutes (IM) and lasts 12–25 minutes

Use
- induction of anaesthesia
- diagnostic or short painful surgical operations not requiring skeletal muscle relaxation
- to supplement low-potency agents such as nitrous oxide
- chronic and postoperative pain

Adverse effects
- involuntary muscle movement (may resemble seizures)
- hypotension, hypertension, bradycardia, tachycardia, cardiac arrhythmias
- emergence reactions (pleasant or unpleasant, including vivid dreams, nightmares, hallucinations, irrational behaviour, confusion, delirium)
- postoperative nausea, vomiting, anorexia, hypersalivation, laryngospasm
- (Rapid IV, high dose) respiratory depression, apnoea
- diplopia, nystagmus, slightly increased intraocular pressure
- abuse/dependence potential
- (Misuse) severe urinary tract symptoms
- (Rare) anaphylaxis
- (Injection site) pain, erythema, rash

Interactions
- prolonged recovery time may occur if given with barbiturates and/or opioid analgesics
- increased half-life may occur if given with halogenated anaesthetics or benzodiazepines, resulting in prolonged recovery
- increased risk of bradycardia, hypotension and/or decreased cardiac output if given with high-dose halogenated anaesthetics (especially if given rapidly or in high doses)
- may antagonise hypnotic effect of thiopental
- increased risk of hypertension and tachycardia may result if given with thyroxine
- increased risk of hypotension if given with antihypertensive agents. Cardiac function should be monitored if given together
- seizure threshold may be decreased if given with theophylline
- increased risk of CNS and respiratory depression may occur if given with alcohol, phenothiazines, muscle relaxants or some antihistamines
- decreased dose may be required if given with antianxiety agents, sedatives or hypnotics
- may potentiate neuromuscular blocking effect and respiratory depression if given with atracurium

Nursing considerations/Cautions
- given IV or IM
- emergence reaction usually lasts for a few hours, but in some patients has lasted up to 24 hours postoperatively

- great care should be taken not to disturb or overstimulate the patient during recovery to avoid emergence reaction
- risk of emergence reaction is decreased if given IM
- severe emergence reaction can be treated with low dose of short-acting or ultra-short-acting barbiturate
- cardiac monitoring is recommended in those with hypertension or cardiac decompensation
- should not be mixed in the same syringe as barbiturates as precipitation will occur
- respiratory depression may occur if given by rapid IV injection; therefore should be given over at least 1 minute
- caution if used in those with alcohol abuse problems or who are intoxicated or have known raised intracranial pressure, glaucoma, schizophrenia, acute psychosis, porphyria, epilepsy, hyperthyroidism or receiving thyroid hormone replacement, lung or upper respiratory tract infection, hydrocephalus, head injury or intracranial mass
- caution if used in those with hypovolaemia, dehydration or who have cardiac disease, moderate hypertension or arrhythmias
- not recommended as sole agent for surgery or diagnostic procedures of pharynx, larynx or bronchial tree, as pharyngeal and laryngeal reflexes are active
- contraindicated in those with severe/poorly controlled hypertension, severe cardiovascular disease, heart failure, recent myocardial infarction, history of stroke, kidney or liver impairment, cerebral trauma or haemorrhage or intracerebral mass
- see also General Nursing considerations/Cautions for general anaesthetics (p. 1174)

Patient education

- see General Patient education for general anaesthetics (p. 1174)

METHOXYFLURANE
Trade name
Penthrox

Available form
Liquid for inhalation 3 mL

Action
- non-flammable volatile anaesthetic with mildly pungent odour
- powerful inhalation analgesic. Onset of analgesia occurs after a few breaths; intermittent use provides analgesia for 20–30 minutes
- slower metabolism and longer half-life than other halogenated anaesthetics
- renal toxicity limits use as anaesthetic

Use
- self-administration to haemodynamically stable, conscious patients (under supervision of trained staff) in trauma situations
- in monitored, conscious patients requiring analgesia for short surgical procedures (e.g. dressing changes)

Adverse effects
- cough, oropharyngeal pain
- dry mouth, nausea, vomiting
- retrograde amnesia, drowsiness, dizziness, euphoria, somnolence, anxiety, depression
- sensory neuropathy
- feeling drunk, increased risk of falls and accident
- fever, headache or migraine
- back pain
- sweating
- elevated liver enzymes
- hypotension, hypertension
- rash
- (Rare) hepatic damage, nephrotoxicity, malignant hyperthermia/hyperpyrexia

Interactions
- use with tetracyclines may result in fatal renal toxicity
- may enhance renal toxicity of gentamicin, colistin or amphotericin B (amphotericin)

GENERAL ANAESTHETICS

- increased metabolism may occur if given with barbiturates, alcohol, isoniazid, phenobarbital or rifampicin
- caution if given with adrenaline (epinephrine) or noradrenaline (norepinephrine)
- increased risk of hypotension if given with beta adrenergic blocking agents
- caution if used with CNS depressants, as added depression may occur

Nursing considerations/Cautions

Penthrox inhaler
- patients using an inhaler should be supervised by trained personnel at all times
- an activated carbon (AC) chamber should be inserted on top of the inhaler
- loosen the lid of the methoxyflurane bottle (bottom of inhaler can be used for this) and pour contents into the inhaler, which is tipped at 45°, while rotating
- place wrist loop over the patient's wrist
- instruct the patient to inhale through the mouthpiece with the first few breaths being gentle, then breathing normally (exhaled breath goes through AC chamber, which absorbs exhaled methoxyflurane)
- if stronger analgesia is required, the patient can cover the dilutor hole with a finger during inhalation

General
- health workers regularly exposed to methoxyflurane should be aware of occupational health and safety guidelines for inhalational agents
- cumulative doses should be less than 6 mL/day or 15 mL/week to avoid nephrotoxicity; therefore not recommended on consecutive days
- caution if used in those with decreased renal blood flow, urine output or glomerular filtration rate
- caution if used in those with diabetes (especially in those who are obese, poorly controlled, have polyuria or kidney impairment) because of the increased risk of nephropathy
- not recommended for use in toxaemia of pregnancy because of the possibility of existing kidney impairment
- not recommended as an anaesthetic agent because of the risk of nephrotoxicity
- not recommended in those with methoxyflurane or halothane-induced liver damage
- contraindicated in those with renal failure/impairment, sensitivity to fluorinated anaesthetics, respiratory depression, cardiovascular instability, head injury, loss of consciousness or a history/family history of adverse reactions following anaesthetics including malignant hyperthermia/hyperpyrexia
- see also General Nursing considerations/Cautions for general anaesthetics (p. 1174)

Patient education
- the patient should be instructed in use of the inhaler before starting (take gentle breaths initially, then normal inhalation and exhalation) and the expected effects (relief of pain/discomfort within 6–10 breaths; however, pain may not be totally eliminated)
- instruct the patient to use the inhaler intermittently rather than continuously
- advise the patient of a fruity smell of the agent
- the patient should be warned to take care as a pedestrian and not to drive or operate machinery until the doctor advises that normal activities can be resumed

Caution should be exercised when used by pregnant women. There are limited studies in humans. However some anaesthetic/analgesic/sedation drugs have been reported to have adverse effects in early life and late pregnancy.

Caution should be exercised when methoxyflurane is administered to a nursing mother.

Methoxyflurane impairs renal function in a dose-related manner owing to the effect of the released fluoride on the distal tubule.

Advisable not to administer methoxyflurane to patients who have shown signs of liver damage, especially after previous methoxyflurane or halothane anaesthesia.

Caution should be exercised in the elderly because of a possible reduction in blood pressure or heart rate.

NITROUS OXIDE

Actions
- colourless gas given by inhalation
- although non-flammable, supports combustion
- strong analgesic properties (thought to be mediated through opioid receptors); however, it has weak anaesthetic and muscle relaxant properties
- inhaled and absorbed by lungs and has low solubility in blood and tissue
- excreted unchanged through the lungs
- often combined with other (volatile) anaesthetics to enhance effects
- rapid onset of action and recovery time

Use
- used with other agents in induction and maintenance of surgical anaesthesia
- used with oxygen in dentistry
- used with oxygen in obstetrics by self-administration

Adverse effects
- hypoxia (unless adequate oxygen administered)
- mild cardiac depression
- nausea, vomiting
- delerium
- prolonged (> 6 hours) administration leads to bone marrow depression, neurological effects

Nursing considerations/caution
- supplied in blue metal gas cylinder
- increased risk of hypoxia if inadequate oxygen is given
- supplementary oxygen is usually given for 3—5 minutes to clear nitrous oxide from lungs at end of anaesthesia

PROPOFOL
Trade names
Diprivan, Fresofol 1% Injection, Fresofol 1% MCT/LCT, Propofol-Lipuro 1% and 2%, Provive 1%

Available forms
Prefilled syringe: 500 mg/50 mL;
Ampoule: 10 mg/mL;
Bottle: 20 mg/mL;
Vial: 10 mg/mL

Action
- non-barbiturate hypnotic
- short-acting IV agent with onset of action approximately 30 seconds
- no analgesic effects
- effects thought to be mediated through gamma aminobutyric acid (GABA) receptors
- onset of action within 30 seconds, duration 3—5 minutes, recovery usually within 5—10 minutes
- rapid elimination phase with a half-life of 30—60 minutes, followed by a slower final phase — elimination half-life 3—8 hours.

Use
- induction and maintenance of general anaesthesia in adults
- sedation of mechanically ventilated adult patients in intensive care setting
- monitored conscious sedation for surgical/diagnostic procedures

Adverse effects
- involuntary muscle movement, shivering, twitching, tremors, hiccups
- cough
- hypotension, bradycardia (sometimes profound), hypertension
- postoperative nausea, vomiting
- respiratory depression, transient apnoea
- increased intracranial pressure
- headache, euphoria
- flushing, rash

GENERAL ANAESTHETICS

- raised serum triglycerides
- (Injection site) pain, burning, stinging, tingling, phlebitis
- (Rare) (prolonged therapy > 48 hours, high dose > 5 mg/hour) (intensive care) propofol infusion syndrome (cardiac failure, arrhythmias, metabolic acidosis, rhabdomyolysis, kidney failure), urine discolouration, hyperkalaemia, potential for abuse

Interactions
- increased sedation and respiratory depression may occur if given with other CNS depressants, including fentanyl
- decreased dose may be required if given after premedication with opioid analgesics and/or benzodiazepines, barbiturates, chloral hydrate or droperidol
- decreased dose may be used when adjunct to regional anaesthesia
- lower dose may be required when used as an adjunct to regional anaesthetic techniques

Nursing considerations/Cautions
- do not use if emulsion is separated or discoloured
- shake well before use
- emulsion is formulated for IV injection or infusion
- not recommended as rapid bolus injection
- calorific value is similar to Intralipid 10% (1.0 mL = 1.1 kcal)
- urine may become discoloured with prolonged use
- incompatible with atracurium and mivacurium
- prefilled syringe should be administered using syringe driver
- compatible with glucose 5% if dilution is required
- administer alone
- caution if used in those with epilepsy as there is an increased risk of seizures during recovery period
- caution if used in those with hyperlipidaemia or a disorder of fat metabolism
- not recommended for obstetric anaesthesia
- contraindicated in those with known hypersensitivity to egg lecithin, peanut, glycerol, soya oil or sodium hydroxide, sodium oleate or sodium edetate
- contraindicated in children under 16 years in intensive care or for monitored conscious sedation for surgery or diagnostic procedures
- see also General Nursing considerations/Cautions for general anaesthetics (p. 1174)

Patient education
- warn the patient that urine may become discoloured if administration has been prolonged
- see also General Patient education for general anaesthetics (p. 1174)

 General anaesthetics cross the placenta and carry the potential to produce CNS and respiratory depression especially in the compromised fetus. Possible teratogenic effects; therefore propofol should not be used in pregnancy.

 Do not use in breastfeeding. Safety to the child has not been established if used during breastfeeding.

 Caution should be applied in patients with cardiac, respiratory, renal or hepatic impairment, or in hypovolaemic or debilitated patients.

SEVOFLURANE
Trade names
Sevorane, Piramal Sevoflurane, Sevoflurane

Available form
Liquid for inhalation: 100 mL, 250 mL

Action
- inhalation anaesthetic
- volatile, non-flammable liquid
- faster induction and emergence than isoflurane, but slightly slower than desflurane
- excreted mainly via lungs

- pleasant smell
- half-life 15—23 hours

Use
- induction and maintenance of general anaesthesia

Adverse effects
- fever, hypothermia
- hypotension, bradycardia, tachycardia
- agitation, headache, somnolence, dizziness
- (Rare) cardiac arrhythmias, QT prolongation
- see also General Adverse effects of general anaesthetics (p. 1173)

Interactions
- may potentiate the actions of non-depolarising muscle relaxants
- anaesthesia is more pronounced when given with nitrous oxide
- increased risk of respiratory depression if given with opioid analgesics or other respiratory depressing agents
- caution if used with isoprenaline, adrenaline (epinephrine) or noradrenaline (norepinephrine) because of the risk of ventricular arrhythmias
- not recommended with or within 14 days of monoamine oxidase inhibitors (MAOIs)
- caution if given with calcium-channel blockers because of the risk of additive negative inotropic effects and marked hypotension
- a decreased dose may be required if given with benzodiazepines or opioid analgesics
- increased metabolism may occur if given with alcohol or isoniazid
- increased risk of hypotension and chills if given with alfentanil

Nursing considerations/Cautions
- caution if used in those with cardiac arrhythmias or a history of QT prolongation
- contraindicated in those with hypersensitivity to other halogenated anaesthetics or with rebreathing apparatus containing Baralyme
- see also General Nursing considerations/Cautions for general anaesthetics (p. 1174)

Patient education
- see General Patient education for general anaesthetics (p. 1174)

 Sevoflurane should be used during pregnancy only if clearly needed.

 Caution should be exercised when sevoflurane is administered to a breastfeeding woman.

 Caution is recommended when using sevoflurane in patients with renal insufficiency.

Caution and use of clinical judgement when sevoflurane is used in patients with underlying hepatic conditions or under treatment with drugs known to cause hepatic dysfunction.

 Malignant hypothermia may occur when used in susceptible individuals.

THIOPENTAL SODIUM
Trade name
Omegapharm Thiopental Sodium

Available forms
Ampoules: 470 mg;
Powder for injection

Action
- very short-acting IV barbiturate with poor analgesic and muscle-relaxing properties
- depresses the myocardium and respiration
- decreases intracranial pressure, laryngeal reflexes and lower oesophageal sphincter tone
- accumulates in fatty tissue if repeated doses are given
- recovery usually occurs within 10—30 minutes
- half-life 3—8 hours (single dose)

Use
- induction of anaesthesia before other anaesthetic agents

GENERAL ANAESTHETICS

- anaesthesia of short duration
- control convulsions (short term)
- supplement to regional anaesthesia or nitrous oxide

Adverse effects
- hiccups, sneezing
- prolonged somnolence
- tachycardia, cardiac arrhythmias
- (Rare) anaphylactic reaction
- see also General Adverse effects of general anaesthetics (p. 1173)

Interactions
- increased risk of hypotension if given with diazoxide, diuretics, antihypertensives, ketamine (high dose, rapid IV administration) or phenothiazines
- may be antagonised by aminophylline
- alcohol and CNS depressants may increase depressant and hypotensive effects
- increased risk of respiratory depression and hypotension when given with ketamine
- action may be prolonged by probenecid
- increased CNS depressant effect may occur if given with IV magnesium sulfate heptahydrate
- increased effects if given with benzodiazepines
- decreased analgesic effect if given with opioid analgesics
- may decrease uptake of sodium iodide by thyroid

Nursing considerations/Cautions
- small test dose (25—75 mg) is usually given to test tolerance and sensitivity with patient observed for 1 minute post-administration
- extravasation and intra-arterial injection should be avoided
- may form a precipitate with acidic solutions (e.g. suxamethonium)
- caution if used in those who are debilitated or with severe cardiovascular disease, hypotension, shock, excessive premedication, Addison's disease, liver or kidney dysfunction, myxoedema, myasthenia gravis, severe anaemia, severe uraemia, increased intracranial pressure, asthma, endocrine insufficiency, muscular dystrophies or myotonias
- contraindicated in those with hypersensitivity to barbiturates, status asthmaticus, inadequate airway maintenance perioperatively, porphyria, constrictive pericarditis, respiratory depression/impairment, mouth, jaw and/or neck inflammation
- contraindicated if suitable veins are not available
- see also General Nursing considerations/Cautions for general anaesthetics (p. 1174)

Patient education
- the patient should be advised that they may experience the taste sensation of garlic after thiopentone is given and before onset of anaesthesia
- see also General Patient education for general anaesthetics (p. 1174)

 Hypnotic effect is prolonged in renal and hepatic dysfunction.

 For older patients, recovery of cognitive and psychomotor functions is generally slower than in younger patients.

HAEMOPOIETIC AGENTS

Erythropoiesis is the process of producing new red blood cells, and it occurs in the bone marrow in adults (and the liver and spleen in the fetus). A haematopoietic stem cell must undergo several steps to become a mature erythrocyte, and it requires adequate nutrients, including iron, vitamin B_{12} and folate. These steps are controlled by the hormone erythropoietin (also known as EPO or epoetin), which is produced in the kidneys (Hendrick 2017).

Haemopoietic agents are termed erythropoietin-stimulating agents (ESA) and are similar to human erythropoietin but are produced by recombinant DNA technology. They are used to increase the production of erythrocytes, primarily in anaemia due to causes such as chronic renal failure and during chemotherapy with agents that cause bone marrow depression. Unfortunately, ESA are also used illegally in some sports to improve aerobic performance and have led to the deaths of athletes (Knights et al 2023). EPO and ESA are banned in all sports, both in and out of competition (WADA 2025a).

General Actions of haemopoietic agents

- glycoproteins produced by recombinant technology
- ESA that stimulates production and differentiation of erythroid stem cells and stimulates proliferation and maturation of red blood cells, causing increased haemoglobin formation
- haemoglobin levels may take 2–10 weeks to rise
- endogenous erythropoietin production is impaired in chronic renal failure, resulting in anaemia

General Adverse effects of haemopoietic agents

- flu-like symptoms, fever, chills
- headache, dizziness, asthenia, fatigue
- insomnia, depression, anxiety
- hypertension (including increase in BP in normotensive patient, or aggravation of existing hypertension), hypotension
- non-cardiac chest pain
- peripheral oedema, fluid overload
- dyspnoea, cough, bronchitis, upper respiratory tract infection
- arthralgia, myalgia, limb or back pain
- mild rash, urticaria, pruritus, alopecia
- anorexia, nausea, diarrhoea, vomiting, abdominal pain, constipation
- (Dialysis patients) haemodialysis graft occlusion/shunt thrombosis
- increased liver enzymes, decreased serum ferritin and transferrin
- (Injection site) pain

HAEMOPOIETIC AGENTS

- pure red cell aplasia, anaemia, neutralising antibody development
- (Rare) myocardial ischaemia/infarction, cerebrovascular haemorrhage/infarction, transient ischaemic attacks, deep vein thrombosis, pulmonary emboli, retinal thrombosis, hypertensive encephalopathy, seizures, hyperkalaemia, tumour growth
- (Rare) anaphylactoid reactions, angioedema, severe skin reactions

General Nursing considerations/Cautions for haemopoietic agents

- ESAs are not equivalent and should not be substituted without authorisation from treating doctor
- any hypertension should be controlled before starting therapy
- potentially correctable anaemia should be investigated and treated before considering use of ESA
- folic acid and vitamin B_{12} deficiencies should be excluded before starting therapy, as effectiveness may be reduced
- monitor haemoglobin, serum iron, ferritin and total iron-binding capacity before starting, then monthly for first 3 months, then 3-monthly
- blood pressure, platelet count and serum potassium and phosphate levels should be monitored throughout regular therapy. Any elevated potassium levels should be treated
- if blood pressure cannot be controlled during therapy (with standard measures), therapy should be withheld until haemoglobin level falls, to decrease the risk of hypertensive encephalopathy and seizures
- the lowest dose possible should be used and haemoglobin level should not be allowed to rise above 120 g/L and increase the rate not more than 10 g/L over 2 weeks to reduce the risk of cardiovascular/thrombotic events
- (Chronic renal failure) 200−300 mg oral iron daily is recommended if serum ferritin < 100 nanogram/mL or serum transferrin < 20%
- (Non-myeloid malignancies) 200−300 mg oral iron daily is recommended if transferrin saturation < 20%
- (Autologous predonation) 200 mg oral iron daily is recommended for several weeks before donation
- for dialysis patients, IV is the preferred route
- first SC injection should be done by health professional/under supervision and then the patient may be taught to self-administer
- for non-dialysis patients, the SC route is recommended to avoid peripheral vein puncture
- rotate SC sites
- volumes greater than 1 mL should be given in different SC sites
- IV route should be used only by health professionals
- administer alone
- do not dilute
- guidelines for autologous predonation cover principles for blood donation, including that haemoglobin should be ≥ 110 g/L and volume of blood withdrawn should not be greater than 12% of person's estimated blood volume
- any vigorous shaking should be avoided, as it will denature the protein
- pure red cell aplasia is associated with neutralising antibodies (to native erythropoietin) and results in loss of response; therefore any loss of response should be investigated and therapy ceased if neutralising antibodies are found
- (Non-myeloid malignancies) recommended to treat anaemia in cancer patients only when anaemia

is due to chemotherapy. ESA have been associated with increased mortality and should be used only if blood transfusion is considered inappropriate
- (Chronic renal failure) caution in those who are hyporesponsive, as there is an increased risk of cardiovascular events and mortality
- (Chronic renal failure, dialysis) caution if used in those with hypotension or if arteriovenous fistulae shows any signs of complications, as there is an increased risk of shunt thrombosis
- caution if used in those with pre-existing hypertension, ischaemic vascular disease, refractory anaemia, epilepsy or history or seizures, CNS infections, brain tumours/metastases, chronic liver failure, thrombocytosis, porphyria or gout
- not recommended in those with active malignant disease not receiving chemotherapy or radiation therapy
- contraindicated in those with known sensitivity to mammalian cell-derived products (e.g. Chinese hamster ovary protein used in DNA recombinant technology)
- contraindicated in those with uncontrolled hypertension or severe cardiovascular disease, or who have developed pure red cell aplasia after treatment with erythropoietin, or those scheduled for elective surgery who have severe coronary, peripheral, arterial, carotid or cerebrovascular disease, recent (within 4 weeks) myocardial infarction or cerebrovascular accident, or if scheduled for surgery and cannot receive antithrombotic therapy

General Patient education for haemopoietic agents

- advise the patient to seek medical advice immediately if any of the following occur:
    - rapid pulse, difficulty breathing, feeling faint, sweating
    - swelling of face, lips, mouth, tongue or throat
    - shortness of breath
    - rash or hives
- the patient should be advised of the importance of maintaining dietary restrictions and continuing to take antihypertensive medication throughout therapy
- warn the patient not to drive or operate machinery if dizziness or changes to blood pressure occur
- the patient should be instructed to immediately seek medical advice if stabbing, severe migraine/headache occurs
- the patient should be advised that ESA are not necessarily equivalent and should not be switched or the dose changed without consulting the doctor
- if the patient is going to self-administer SC, education should include:
    - injection is under the skin (SC)
    - importance of rotating injection sites, including thighs and abdomen, but avoiding navel and waistline
    - do not inject into areas that are red or swollen, into muscle or into the same spot as previous injection
    - correct technique, such as:
        - wash and dry hands before start of procedure

HAEMOPOIETIC AGENTS

- check name and strength of medication and expiry date (and do not use if after expiry date)
- allow prefilled syringe/pen to come to room temperature before use (about 30 minutes) (not in direct sunlight or using any method such as hot water or microwave to warm solution)
- do not shake solution/syringes
- do not mix with any other medications or dilute
- clean area with alcoholic swab and allow to dry
- pinch skin firmly between thumb and finger
- push prefilled syringe/pen firmly against pinched skin and inject
- press site gently after injection with cotton wool swab to prevent bleeding, but do not rub
- correct storage
  - store in fridge, but can remain at room temperature for up to 3 days before use
- disposal of used equipment
  - do not recap needles
  - do not reuse needles, pens or syringes
  - syringes, pens and needles should not be disposed of in normal household rubbish
  - use puncture-resistant sharps container to dispose of used needles and syringes
  - container should be disposed of as instructed by doctor, pharmacist or nurse
- (Chronic renal failure) female patients of childbearing potential should be counselled that menses may restart with therapy and therefore adequate contraception may be needed to prevent unwanted pregnancy occurring

 Banned in sport at all times (in and out of competition). Misuse by healthy people may lead to an excessive increase in packed cell volume, increasing the risk of cardiovascular and thrombotic events.

DARBEPOETIN ALFA
Trade name
Aranesp

Available forms
Prefilled syringe: 10 microgram/0.4 mL, 20 microgram/0.5 mL, 30 microgram/0.3 mL, 40 microgram/0.4 mL, 50 microgram/0.5 mL, 60 microgram/0.3 mL, 80 microgram/0.4 mL, 100 microgram/0.5 mL, 150 microgram/0.3 mL;
Prefilled pen: 20 microgram/0.5 mL, 40 microgram/0.4 mL, 60 microgram/0.3 mL, 80 microgram/0.4 mL, 100 microgram/0.5 mL, 150 microgram/0.3 mL

Action
- terminal half-life is 3 times longer than erythropoietin
- half-life 12—40 hours (IV) or 35—39 hours (SC, chronic renal failure) or 124—144 hours (SC, non-myeloid malignancy)
- see also General Actions of haemopoietic agents (p. 1184)

Use
- anaemia associated with chronic renal failure
- prevention and treatment of anaemia in those with non-myeloid malignancies receiving chemotherapy where blood transfusion is not appropriate

Dose
- (Chronic renal failure: on dialysis) initially 0.45 microgram/kg SC or IV weekly, increasing dose by 25% at monthly intervals if response is inadequate (i.e. if haemoglobin increase < 10 g/L in 4 weeks) and iron stores are adequate. For maintenance, dose should be given weekly or every 2 weeks to maintain target haemoglobin **OR**

- (Chronic renal failure: no dialysis) initially either 0.45 microgram/kg SC weekly, 0.75 microgram/kg SC every 2 weeks or 1.5 microgram/kg SC monthly, increasing dose by 25% at monthly intervals if response is inadequate (i.e. if haemoglobin increase < 10 g/L in 4 weeks) and iron stores are adequate. For maintenance, dose should be given weekly, every 2 weeks or monthly to maintain target haemoglobin **OR**
- (Non-myeloid malignancies) 500 micrograms (or 6.75 microgram/kg) every 3 weeks SC or 2.25 microgram/kg SC weekly, increasing to 4.5 microgram/kg weekly if haemoglobin response is less than 10 g/L after 1 month, continuing for 4 weeks after the end of chemotherapy or until haemoglobin concentration normalises. If no/poor response after 9 weeks, further treatment is unlikely to be beneficial

Adverse effects
- see General Adverse effects of haemopoietic agents (p. 1184)

Nursing considerations/Cautions
- the needle cover of the prefilled syringe contains latex and is not recommended in those with known latex allergy
- (Chronic renal failure) if changing from 2–3 times weekly recombinant human erythropoietin (r-HuEpo), once-weekly darbepoetin is recommended. If changing from once-weekly r-HuEPO, 2-weekly darbepoetin is recommended. The dose of darbepoetin should be based on r-HuEPO dose and administered via the same route
- (Chronic renal failure) haemoglobin should be measured every 1–2 weeks
- (Chronic renal failure) if no response or the response is not maintained, other causes of anaemia should be investigated
- (Chronic renal failure) dose changes during maintenance period should not occur more often than every 1–2 weeks
- (Chronic renal failure) as haemoglobin (Hb) approaches 120 g/L, the dose should be decreased by 25%. If Hb continues to increase, therapy should be stopped until the Hb level has decreased and then restarted at 25% lower than previous dose
- (Non-myeloid malignancy) therapy should not be started until Hb < 100–110 g/L
- (Non-myeloid malignancy) as Hb approaches 120 g/L, the dose should be decreased by 25–50%. If Hb > 120 g/L, therapy should be stopped until Hb decreases to 110 g/L and then restarted at 25–50% lower than previous dose
- (Non-myeloid malignancy) therapy should be continued for 4 weeks post-chemotherapy or until Hb approaches 120 g/L
- if changing the oute of administration, the same dose should be used and Hb monitored, with subsequent dose adjustment if needed
- see also General Nursing considerations/Cautions for haemopoietic agents (p. 1185)

Patient education
- if the patient is going to self-administer, ensure that each prefilled syringe type is demonstrated so the patient is confident in administration technique
- see also General Patient education for haemopoietic agents (p. 1186)

No human data. Use during pregnancy only if the benefit justifies potential risk.

Caution, as limited human data. Use only if the benefit justifies potential risk.

EPOETIN ALFA
Trade name
Eprex

Available forms
Prefilled syringe: 1000 IU/0.5 mL, 2000 IU/0.5 mL, 3000 IU/0.3 mL, 4000 IU/0.4 mL, 5000 IU/0.5 mL, 6000 IU/0.6 mL, 8000 IU/0.8 mL, 10,000 IU/mL, 20,000 IU/0.5 mL, 30,000 IU/0.75 mL, 40,000 IU/mL

HAEMOPOIETIC AGENTS

Action
- also known as EPO
- half-life 4—6 hours (increasing to 6—9 hours in those with renal failure)
- see also General Actions of haemopoietic agents (p. 1184)

Use
- anaemia associated with chronic renal failure
- prevention and treatment of anaemia in those with non-myeloid malignancies receiving chemotherapy where blood transfusion is not appropriate
- elective surgery (expecting moderate blood loss (900—1800 mL)) in those with mild-to-moderate anaemia (haemoglobin (Hb) 100—130 g/L)
- augment autologous blood collection

Dose
- (Chronic renal failure, anaemia: correction phase) initially 50 IU/kg IV over 1—2 minutes 3 times weekly, increasing to 75 IU/kg if Hb has not increased by 10 g/L after 1 month, increasing by 25 IU/kg 3 times weekly at monthly intervals to achieve an Hb concentration of not greater than 120 g/L (maximum dose 3 × 200 IU/kg/week) **OR**
- (Chronic renal failure, anaemia: maintenance phase) maintenance phase is individually tailored, usually 75—300 IU/kg IV or SC weekly to maintain target Hb (maximum dose is less than the maintenance maximum dose) **OR**
- (Elective surgery) 600 IU/kg SC weekly for 3 weeks before surgery and on day of surgery **OR**
- (Elective surgery where lead time is less than 3 weeks) 300 IU/kg SC daily for 10 consecutive days before surgery, on the day of surgery and for 4 days after surgery, stopping when Hb reaches 150 g/L regardless of the number of doses given **OR**
- (Autologous pre-donation program) 300—600 IU/kg IV twice weekly for 3 weeks (with 200 mg oral iron) **OR**
- (Non-myeloid malignancies) initially 150 IU/kg SC 3 times weekly for 1 month, then adjusting the dose according to Hb and reticulocyte count

Adverse effects
- see General Adverse effects of haemopoietic agents (p. 1184)

Interactions
- may increase heparin required during dialysis to prevent clotting in the dialyser
- serum level of ciclosporin should be closely monitored and dose adjusted if necessary if given together
- caution if used with agents that decrease erythropoiesis, as effectiveness will be reduced

Nursing considerations/Cautions
- (Elective surgery) antithrombic therapy is recommended
- (Chronic renal failure) administer after completion of haemodialysis
- (Chronic renal failure) IV route is recommended for patients who undergo dialysis; SC is suggested for non-dialysis patients
- if converting from the SC to the IV route, the same dose should be given and the Hb monitored, and dose adjusted if needed
- (Chronic renal failure) if Hb approaches 120 g/L, the dose should be decreased by 25%. If Hb continues to increase, therapy should be stopped until Hb level has decreased and then restarted at 25% lower than the previous dose. If Hb increases by > 10 g/L in any 2-week period, the dose should be decreased, or the dosing interval increased or both
- slow injection may prevent flu-like symptoms
- (Elective surgery) therapy should not be started if Hb > 130 g/L because of an increased risk of postoperative thrombotic vascular events
- (Non-myeloid malignancies) therapy should not be started unless Hb < 100—110 g/L
- caution if used in patients with chronic liver failure
- see also General Nursing considerations/Cautions for haemopoietic agents (p. 1185)

Patient education
- see General Patient education for haemopoietic agents (p. 1186)

Use during pregnancy should be considered only if the potential benefit justifies any possible risk.

Caution, as excretion in human breastmilk is unknown. Consider only if the potential benefit justifies any possible risk.

Caution in those with chronic liver failure.

EPOETIN BETA
Trade name
NeoRecormon

Available forms
Prefilled syringe: 2000 IU/0.3 mL, 3000 IU/0.3 mL, 4000 IU/0.3 mL, 5000 IU/0.3 mL, 6000 IU/0.3 mL, 10,000 IU/0.6 mL

Action
- half-life is 4–12 hours (IV) or 13–28 hours (SC)
- see also General Actions of haemopoietic agents (p. 1184)

Use
- anaemia associated with chronic renal failure
- prevention and treatment of anaemia in those with non-myeloid malignancies receiving chemotherapy where blood transfusion is not appropriate
- increase yield of autologous blood (pre-donation) to avoid use of homologous blood
- prevention of anaemia in premature infants (less than 34 weeks gestation and weight 750–1500 g)

Dose
- (Chronic renal failure: correction) 60 IU/kg/week SC either as single weekly dose or 7 divided doses given daily, increasing at monthly intervals by 60 IU/kg/week if haemoglobin (Hb) increase is not adequate (< 1.5 g/L/week) **OR**
- (Chronic renal failure: correction) 120 IU/kg/week IV over 2 minutes in 3 divided doses, increasing to 240 IU/kg/week after 1 month if Hb increase is not adequate (< 1.5 g/L/week). If the response still remains inadequate, further increases by 60 IU/kg/week at monthly intervals may be needed **OR**
- (Chronic renal failure: maintenance) dose is initially halved and then adjusted to maintain Hb between 100 and 120 g/L, given as either a single weekly dose or up to 7 divided doses (weekly maximum 720 IU/kg) **OR**
- (Autologous pre-donation program) 400–1600 IU/kg/week IV over 2 minutes or 300–1200 IU/kg/week SC given in 2 divided doses for a maximum of 4 weeks **OR**
- (Anaemia in non-myeloid malignancy) 450 IU/kg/week SC as a single weekly dose or in 3–7 divided doses. If response is inadequate after 4 weeks, the dose should be increased to 900 IU/kg/week **OR**
- (Prevention of anaemia in premature infants) 750 IU/kg/week SC in 3 divided doses (starting by day 3 of life) for 6 weeks

Adverse effects
- overhydration
- menstrual disorders
- leucopenia, thrombocytopenia
- lower respiratory tract infection, infection
- see also General Adverse effects of haemopoietic agents (p. 1184)

Nursing considerations/Cautions
- (Non-myeloid malignancy) therapy should be continued for up to 4 weeks after the end of chemotherapy. If Hb falls by more than 10 g/L during next cycle of chemotherapy in spite of therapy with epoetin beta, further treatment is not warranted
- (Prevention of anaemia in premature infants) less effective if a premature infant has had blood transfusion

HAEMOPOIETIC AGENTS

- (Prevention of anaemia in premature infants) oral iron (2 mg/day) should be started as soon as possible (by day 14 at the latest). If serum ferritin < 100 nanogram/mL or there are other signs of iron deficiency, oral iron dose should be increased to 5—10 mg/day
- increase in heparin may be required in dialysis patients to prevent occlusion of dialysis system/shunt thrombosis
- dose adjustments should be no more frequent than monthly and dependent on Hb (maintaining Hb < 120 g/L)
- (Non-myeloid malignancy) not recommended if Hb > 110 g/L
- caution if used in those with refractory anaemia (with blasts in transformation), thrombocytosis or chronic liver failure
- contains phenylalanine; therefore not recommended in those with severe phenylketonuria
- contraindicated in those with angina pectoris or a history of thromboembolic disease (autologous blood collection), or who have suffered myocardial infarction or stroke in the preceding 4 weeks
- see also General Nursing considerations/Cautions for haemopoietic agents (p. 1185)

Patient education

- see General Patient education for haemopoietic agents (p. 1186)

No human data. Animal studies show fetal weight reductions are likely linked to maternal polycythaemia but no direct embryotoxic, fetotoxic or teratogenic effects. Use during pregnancy only if the benefit justifies potential risk.

Caution, as limited human data.

EPOETIN LAMBDA
Trade name
Novicrit

Available forms
Prefilled syringe: 1000 IU/0.5 mL, 2000 IU/mL, 3000 IU/0.3 mL, 4000 IU/0.4 mL, 5000 IU/0.5 mL, 6000 IU/0.6 mL, 8000 IU/0.8 mL, 10,000 IU/mL

Action
- similar to epoetin alfa
- half-life 2.5—6.7 hours (IV) or 24 hours (SC)
- see also General Actions of haemopoietic agents (p. 1184)

Use
- anaemia associated with chronic renal failure
- prevention and treatment of anaemia in those with non-myeloid malignancies receiving chemotherapy where blood transfusion is not appropriate
- patients with anaemia (Hb > 100 ≤ 130 g/L) scheduled for elective surgery where moderate blood loss (900—1800 mL) is expected to reduce exposure to allogeneic blood transfusion
- augment autologous blood collection in patients scheduled for major elective surgery

Dose
- (Elective surgery scheduled) 600 IU/kg SC over 1—2 minutes weekly for 3 weeks before surgery and on day of surgery (total 4 doses) (with 200 mg oral elemental iron daily) **OR**
- (Elective surgery, shortened lead-in time) 300 IU/kg SC over 1—2 minutes daily for 10 consecutive days before surgery, day of surgery and 4 days post-surgery (total 15 doses) **OR**
- (Autologous pre-donation program) 300—600 IU/kg IV over 1—2 minutes twice weekly for 3 weeks (with 200 mg oral elemental iron daily) **OR**

- (Chronic renal failure) initially 50 IU/kg IV over 1—2 minutes 3 times weekly. If haemoglobin (Hb) does not increase by 10 g/L after 4 weeks, dose may be increased to 75 IU/kg IV over 1—2 minutes 3 times weekly to achieve Hb not greater than 120 g/L (correction) (maximum weekly dose 3 × 200 IU/kg), then 75—300 IU/kg weekly IV over 1—2 minutes (maintenance) to maintain Hb in target range **OR**
- (Non-myeloid malignancies) initially 150 IU/kg SC over 1—2 minutes 3 times weekly. If Hb has increased by 10 g/L or reticulocyte count $\geq$ 40,000 cells/microlitre above baseline after 4 weeks, dose continues at 150 IU/kg. If Hb increases < 10 g/L and reticulocyte count < 40,000 cells/microlitre above baseline, dose is increased to 300 IU/kg. After a further 4 weeks at 300 IU/kg, if there is no improvement in Hb or reticulocyte count, therapy should be discontinued, as response is unlikely

Adverse effects
- seizures
- see also General Adverse effects of haemopoietic agents (p. 1184)

Interactions
- effects may be decreased if given with agents that decrease erythropoiesis
- may increase serum levels of ciclosporin; therefore blood levels should be closely monitored during therapy

Nursing considerations/Cautions
- blood pressure and prodromal neurological symptoms of seizures should be closely monitored during therapy (especially in first 3 months)
- if the patient is on dialysis, administration should be after completion
- if the patient experiences flu-like symptoms, administration can be slowed to 5 minutes
- (Non-myeloid malignancy) therapy should not start until Hb < 100—110 g/L
- (Elective surgery) therapy should be stopped if Hb is 150 g/L regardless of the number of doses given
- see also General Nursing considerations/Cautions for haemopoietic agents (p. 1185)

Patient education
- the patient should be advised against driving or operating machinery during the first 3 months of therapy because of the increased risk of seizures
- see also General Patient education for haemopoietic agents (p. 1186)

Use only if clearly needed, weighing potential risks. Animal studies show no teratogenic effects, but higher doses may affect fertility and fetal development. Not recommended for pregnant surgical patients in autologous blood pre-donation programs.

Caution, as excretion in human breastmilk is unknown. Use only if clearly needed. In lactating surgical patients in autologous blood pre-donation programs, use is not recommended.

METHOXY POLYETHYLENE GLYCOL EPOETIN BETA

Trade name
Mircera

Available forms
Prefilled syringes (with colour-coded plunger): 30 microgram/0.3 mL (aqua), 50 microgram/0.3 mL (yellow), 75 microgram/0.3 mL (red), 100 microgram/0.3 mL (turquoise), 120 microgram/0.3 mL (lime), 200 microgram/0.3 mL (purple), 360 microgram/0.6 mL (salmon)

Action
- chemically synthesised erythropoiesis-stimulating agent (ESA) with longer half-life (15—20 times) than erythropoietin
- longer half-life allows monthly administration

- increase in haemoglobin is usually seen 7–15 days after administration
- see also General Actions of haemopoietic agents (p. 1184)

Use
- anaemia associated with chronic kidney disease

Dose
- (Chronic kidney disease, not currently receiving ESA, not on dialysis) initially 1.2 microgram/kg SC monthly **OR**
- (Chronic kidney disease, not currently receiving ESA, no dialysis) initially 0.6 microgram/kg IV or SC every second week **OR**
- (Chronic kidney disease, not currently receiving ESA, dialysis) initially 0.6 microgram/kg IV or SC every second week **OR**
- (Chronic kidney disease, receiving ESA) initial dose is dependent on previous weekly dose:
  - darbepoetin alfa < 40 microgram/week or epoetin < 8000 IU/week, starting dose 120 microgram/month
  - darbepoetin alfa 40–80 microgram/week or epoetin 8000–16,000 IU/week, starting dose 200 microgram/month
  - darbepoetin alfa > 80 microgram/week or epoetin > 16,000 IU/week, starting dose 360 microgram/month

Adverse effects
- see General Adverse effects of haemopoietic agents (p. 1184)

Nursing considerations/Cautions
- if changing the route of administration, haemoglobin (Hb) should be closely monitored to ensure it remains in target range
- Hb should be monitored 2-weekly until stable and then regularly to maintain target (100–120 g/L). If Hb increase is < 10 g/L over 4 weeks, the dose should be increased by 25–50%. Further increases of 25–50% may be required at monthly intervals to achieve target Hb
- if Hb approaches 120 g/L, the dose should be decreased by 25%. If Hb continues to increase, therapy should be stopped until the Hb level has decreased, and then restarted at 25% lower than previous dose. If Hb increases by > 10 g/L in any 2-week period, the dose should be decreased or the dosing interval increased, or both
- dose adjustments should be no more frequent than monthly
- when converting from epoetin or darbepoetin alfa, administration can be monthly or every 2 weeks
- see also General Nursing considerations/Cautions for haemopoietic agents (p. 1185)

Patient education
- see General Patient education for haemopoietic agents (p. 1186)

Not recommended during pregnancy unless potential benefits to mother outweigh risks to fetus. Animal studies suggest developmental issues in rats and rabbits.

Not recommended during breastfeeding, as excretion in breastmilk is unknown. Animal studies suggest adverse effects.

HAEMOSTATICS

Haemostasis is the process of stopping bleeding from a damaged blood vessel and occurs in three steps: (1) constriction of the blood vessel, (2) platelet plug formation and (3) clot (mainly fibrin) formation. Once vessel repair has started, the fibrin clot is broken down by the action of plasmin on the fibrin (fibrinolysis). For clot formation to occur, a series of steps (the clotting cascade) involving an intrinsic or extrinsic pathway (which converge to a common pathway) must occur (Arruda & High 2018). Deficiency in coagulation factors results in inadequate clot formation and continued bleeding.

Examples of coagulation factor deficiencies include:
- haemophilia A (also called 'classic' haemophilia), a genetically transmitted deficiency of factor VIII affecting males (although transmitted by females), which occurs in mild, moderate or severe forms (Arruda & High 2018)
- haemophilia B (also called 'Christmas disease'), a deficiency of factor IX, occurring less commonly than haemophilia A and also occurring in mild, moderate or severe forms (Arruda & High 2018)
- von Willebrand disease (VWD), the most common inherited bleeding disorder and a deficiency of von Willebrand's factor, which circulates in the blood attached to factor VIII, binding platelets to minor ruptures in blood vessels. There are three types of VWD, with type 2 having four subtypes (Konkie 2018).

Bleeding associated with coagulation factor deficiencies is sometimes spontaneous, as a result of mild trauma or associated with surgical or dental procedures. Bleeding into joints (haemarthrosis) can become chronic, leading to joint damage (e.g. synovial thickening and synovitis) and deformity (Arruda & High 2018). Management using haemostatic agents may be prophylactic (to prevent spontaneous bleeding or bleeding associated with a surgical or dental procedure) or it may be to treat the bleeding when it occurs.

Some haemostatic agents act by inhibiting the breakdown of the fibrin clot, whereas others replace the missing coagulation factors, with the aim of both types of agents being to reduce blood loss.

ELTROMBOPAG OLAMINE

Trade name
Revolade

Available forms
Tablets: 25 mg, 50 mg

Action
- thrombopoietin (TPO) receptor agonist, resulting in proliferation of megakaryocytes from bone marrow stem cells
- pharmacokinetics influenced by race and gender, with those from East Asia having increased plasma levels when compared with Caucasians. Plasma levels in females > males
- half-life 21–32 hours, prolonged in those with idiopathic thrombocytopenic purpura (ITP)

Use
- treatment of ITP (in those patients who are intolerant or had ineffective response to corticosteroids and immunoglobulins)
- chronic hepatitis C-associated thrombocytopenia that prevents initiation of interferon-based therapy
- severe aplastic anaemia (SAA) (with standard immunosuppressive therapy)
- refractory SAA (where response to immunosuppressive therapy was ineffective)

Dose
- (Chronic ITP) initially 50 mg orally daily, then adjusting dose in 25 mg daily increments at intervals of at least 2 weeks to maintain platelet count $\geq 50 \times 10^9$/L for at least 4 weeks (daily maximum 75 mg) **OR**
- (Hepatitis C-associated thrombocytopenia) initially 25 mg orally daily, adjusting dose in 25 mg intervals at 2-week intervals to achieve target platelet count to start interferon therapy (daily maximum 100 mg) **OR**
- (SAA) 150 mg orally daily for 6 months, with dose adjustment according to platelet count (with immunosuppressive therapy) **OR**
- (Refractory SAA) 50 mg orally daily with dose adjustment of 50 mg increments every 2 weeks according to platelet count (daily maximum 150 mg)

Adverse effects
- diarrhoea, nausea, vomiting
- pharyngolaryngeal pain, pharyngitis
- myalgia, back pain, musculoskeletal chest pain, musculoskeletal pain, muscle spasms, bone pain
- alopecia, rash, phototoxicity
- elevated liver enzymes, elevated bilirubin
- paraesthesia
- menorrhagia
- thromboembolic/thrombotic events, bone marrow reticulin formation, bone marrow fibrosis, cytogenic abnormalities
- dry eye, cataract formation

Interactions
- serum levels may be decreased by lopinavir/ritonavir combination or with dietary calcium (e.g. dairy products)
- may increase serum levels of rosuvastatin, increasing the risk of toxicity
- chelates polyvalent cations, including aluminium, calcium, iron, magnesium, selenium and zinc

Nursing considerations/Cautions
- (ITP, East Asian patients) dose should be started at 25 mg daily
- (East Asian patients) dose should be started at 75 mg daily (SAA) or 25 mg (refractory SAA)
- platelet count usually increases within 1–2 weeks of starting therapy
- any loss in response should be investigated
- (ITP, refractory SAA, hepatitis-associated thrombocytopenia) liver function should be measured before starting therapy, then 2-weekly during dose adjustment and then monthly once maintenance has been established. If abnormal liver enzymes occur, testing

should be carried out within 3–5 days and therapy discontinued if levels are elevated ($\geq$ 3 times upper limit of normal (ULN) or baseline), progressive or persist for $\geq$ 4 weeks, or if clinical symptoms or an increase in direct bilirubin also exist
- (SAA) liver function should be measured before starting and regularly throughout therapy. If liver enzymes (alanine aminotransferase (ALT)) are $> 6 \times$ ULN, therapy should be discontinued and restarted at the same dose when ALT $< 5 \times$ ULN. If ALT again increases to $> 6 \times$ ULN with reason (e.g. sepsis, azole therapy), therapy should be again stopped and ALT measured every 3–4 days, and restarted at a reduced dose (25 mg less than previous dose) when ALT $< 5 \times$ ULN. If ALT remains $> 6 \times$ ULN, therapy should be stopped. If ALT $< 5 \times$ ULN, therapy should be restarted at reduced dose. If ALT again increases to $> 6 \times$ ULN, dose should be reduced by 25 mg daily until ALT $< 5 \times$ ULN
- peripheral blood smears and full blood count (with white blood cell count differential) should be assessed before starting and weekly during therapy until platelet count is stable for at least 4 weeks, and then monitored monthly
- blood smears should be checked for any red blood cell abnormalities or cytopenia and therapy should be stopped if abnormalities are found
- platelet count returns to baseline within 14 days of discontinuing therapy, increasing risk of bleeding. Platelet count should be monitored for 4 weeks after stopping therapy
- (ITP) if platelet count does not increase to expected level with 4 weeks of therapy at maximum dose, stopping therapy is recommended
- (Hepatitis C-associated thrombocytopenia) if there is no response after 12 weeks, therapy should be stopped
- (Refractory SAA) therapy should be stopped if no response is evident in 16 weeks, if new cytogenic abnormality appears, if there is an excessive platelet response or if liver abnormalities occur
- (Refractory SAA) if platelet count $> 50 \times 10^9$/L, Hb > 100g/L and absolute neutrophil count (ANC) $> 1 \times 10^9$/L for more than 8 weeks, the dose should be reduced by 50%. If counts remain stable after 8 weeks at reduced dose, therapy can be stopped and blood counts monitored regularly
- (ITP, liver impairment) dose adjustment intervals should be 3 weeks
- baseline ocular examinations should be performed before starting therapy, then regularly throughout monitoring for signs and symptoms of cataracts
- (Hepatitis C-associated thrombocytopenia) therapy should be started in patients with chronic hepatitis C only where thrombocytopenia prevents interferon therapy from being initiated or limits the ability to maintain optimal interferon therapy
- (Hepatitis C-associated thrombocytopenia) platelet count should be monitored weekly before starting and during interferon therapy until platelet count is stable, then monthly (and should include full blood count, platelet count and peripheral blood smears)
- (Hepatitis C-associated thrombocytopenia) therapy should be stopped when interferon therapy is ceased
- caution if used in those with liver or kidney impairment, advanced age or at risk of thromboembolism (e.g. prolonged periods of immobilisation, malignancies, surgery, trauma, obesity, smoking, factor V Leiden, antithrombin III (AT III) deficiency or antiphospholipid syndrome)

Patient education

- advise the patient that dairy products, antacids and mineral supplements should be taken at least 4 hours apart from medication. Tablets can be taken with food with little or no calcium

HAEMOSTATICS

- instruct the patient to avoid unnecessary UV exposure, including direct sunlight or artificial sources (such as tanning beds). Sunscreen, a hat and protective clothing are recommended to avoid sunburn
- the patient should be advised to seek medical advice immediately if any of the following occur:
  - yellowing of eyes or skin, dark urine, tiredness, loss of appetite, right upper stomach pain
  - swelling or pain/tenderness in legs

Tablet may be crushed and mixed with water or spoonful of apple puree. Tablet does not disperse readily

Not recommended during pregnancy unless benefits are thought to outweigh risks.

Not recommended during breastfeeding unless benefits outweigh risks.

FIBRINOGEN
Trade name
RiaSTAP

Available form
Vial: 1 g

Action
- coagulation factor I derived from human plasma
- converted to haemostatic clot in the presence of thrombin, activated coagulation factor XIII and calcium ions

Use
- acute bleeding episodes in patients with congenital fibrinogen deficiency (e.g. afibrinogenaemia, hypofibrinogenaemia)

Dose
- (Fibrinogen level not known) initially 70 mg/kg IV, dose then adjusted according to target level (e.g. 1 g/L for minor event such as epistaxis, intramuscular bleeding or menorrhagia or 1.5 g/L for major event such as head trauma or intracranial haemorrhage). Target levels should be maintained for at least 3 days after minor bleeding or for 7 days after major bleeding **OR**
- calculated according to following equation: Dose of fibrinogen (mg/kg body weight) = [Target level (g/L) − measured level (g/L)] / 0.017 (g/L per mg/kg body weight)

Adverse effects
- fever
- thromboembolic events
- (Uncommon) allergic/anaphylactic reactions

Nursing considerations/Cautions
- fibrinogen level should be measured before starting therapy and during dose adjustment
- dose is dependent on severity of disorder, location and extent of bleeding, and clinical condition of patient
- normal fibrinogen level 2.0–4.5 g/L, with bleeding occurring at levels of 1.0 g/L and below
- the patient should be closely monitored during infusion for any signs of allergy or thrombosis
- product is made from human plasma, which may contain infectious agents such as viruses. Current manufacturing processes are effective against HIV, hepatitis B, hepatitis C and hepatitis A
- contains 164 mg (7.1 mmol) sodium per vial, which may need to be considered in those with sodium-restricted diet
- vial and water for injections should be at room temperature before reconstitution. Reconstitute by adding 50 mL water for injections to the vial and swirling gently (avoid shaking vial) until the solution is clear and colourless
- administer alone
- the rate should not exceed 5 mL/min
- the name and batch number of product should be recorded in patient notes
- caution if used in those with coronary heart disease, myocardial infarction,

- liver impairment, peri- or postoperative patients, or those at risk of thromboembolic events or disseminated intravascular coagulation
- caution if used in those with congenital dysfibrinogenaemia because of increased risk of thrombosis

No human data. Used during pregnancy only if the benefits are thought to outweigh risks.

No human data. Used during breastfeeding only if the benefits are thought to outweigh risks.

Available in combination with
- fibrinogen 5.5 mg + thrombin 2 IU/cm sponge (TachoSil)
- fibrinogen + aprotonin + Factor VIII + calcium chloride dihydrate syringe (Artiss, Tisseel VH S/D)

ROMIPLOSTIM
Trade name
Nplate

Available forms
Vial: 375 microgram (extractable dose 250 microgram/0.5 mL), 625 microgram (extractable dose 500 microgram/mL)

Action
- thrombopoietin (TPO) mimetic class agent
- increases platelet production by binding to and activating thrombopoietin receptor, similar to the action of endogenous thrombopoietin

Use
- thrombocytopenia (in those with chronic idiopathic thrombocytopenia (ITP), who have been splenectomised with inadequate response or have not been splenectomised with inadequate response, or where immunoglobulins and corticosteroids are inappropriate)

Dose
- initially 1 microgram/kg SC weekly, then adjusting dose at weekly intervals and increments of 1 microgram/kg (to maintain platelet count $\geq 50 \times 10^9$/L but $\leq 200 \times 10^9$/L) (maximum weekly dose 10 microgram/kg)

Adverse effects
- anaemia, thrombocytopenia, idiopathic thrombocytopenic purpura
- haematoma, petichiae, ecchymosis
- nosebleed
- hypertension
- diarrhoea, nausea, vomiting, abdominal pain, bleeding gums or mouth, constipation
- headache, dizziness, paraesthesia, fatigue, asthenia, anxiety, insomnia, confusion
- peripheral oedema
- fever
- rash, pruritus
- arthralgia, myalgia, back/leg pain, muscle spasm, musculoskeletal pain, chest pain, pain
- toothache
- hypokalaemia
- upper respiratory tract infection, cough, dyspnoea, nasopharyngitis, sinusitis, bronchitis, nasal congestion, rhinorrhoea
- urinary tract infection
- development of neutralising antibodies (inhibitors)
- (Rare) increase in bone marrow reticulum, thrombotic/thromboembolic events, progression of existing myelodysplastic syndromes, hypersensitivity

Nursing considerations/Cautions
- before starting and during therapy, peripheral blood smears and blood count should be monitored for any red blood cell abnormalities or cytopenia. Therapy should be stopped if abnormalities are found. Blood counts should be monitored for at least 4 weeks after stopping therapy
- platelet count should be measured weekly until the count is stable at $\geq 50 \times 10^9$/L for at least 4 weeks without any dose adjustment

HAEMOSTATICS

- if the maximum weekly dose of 10 microgram/kg is reached for 4 weeks without platelet improvement, therapy should be stopped
- if, after initial response, there is a failure to maintain or there is a loss of the platelet response, causative factors may be the development of neutralising antibodies or increased bone marrow reticulin
- thrombocytopenia may recur when therapy is stopped
- the patient may be taught to self-administer once the platelet count has been stable for 4 weeks. After 4 weeks of self-administration, the patient's technique for reconstitution and administration should be checked
- should be administered using a syringe with 0.01 graduations
- reconstitute using sterile water for injections (0.72 mL for 375 mg vial and 1.2 mL for 625 mg vial), swirl gently and invert the vial until solution is clear and colourless; however, do not shake the vial
- caution if used in those with severe liver or kidney impairment, or with known or acquired factors for thromboembolism including factor V Leiden, antiphospholipid syndrome, advanced age, prolonged immobilisation, malignancy, surgery, trauma, smoking and obesity
- contraindicated in those with hypersensitivity to *Escherichia coli* (*E. coli*) products

Patient education

- warn the patient against driving or operating machinery if dizziness, numbness or fatigue occurs
- if the patient is going to self-administer SC, education should include:
  - injection is under the skin (SC)
  - importance of rotating injection sites, including thighs and abdomen, but avoiding navel and waistline
  - not injecting into areas that are red or swollen, into muscle or into the same spot as the previous injection
- correct technique, such as:
  - wash and dry hands before start of procedure
  - checking name and strength of medication and expiry date (and not using if after expiry date)
  - reconstituting powder using water for injections as demonstrated by the nurse or physician
  - swirling the vial gently to dissolve powder (but not shaking) until the solution is clear and colourless
  - cleaning the area with alcoholic swab and allowing to dry
  - pinching the skin firmly between thumb and finger
  - pushing the syringe against the pinched skin and injecting solution
  - pressing the site gently after injection with a cotton wool swab to prevent bleeding, but do not rub
- correct storage
  - the powder should be stored in a fridge but not frozen
  - after reconstituting the powder, the solution can be kept in fridge for up to 24 hours if not given immediately
  - any unused solution should be discarded
- disposal of used equipment
  - not recapping needles
  - using a puncture-resistant sharps container to dispose of used syringes
  - the container should be disposed of as instructed by a doctor, pharmacist or nurse

Avoid: animal studies showed some risks, including stillbirths and reduced pup survival at high doses. Romiplostim may cross the placenta. Use only if the benefit outweighs the risk to the fetus.

Avoid, as limited human data.

TRANEXAMIC ACID

Trade names
Cyklokapron, Tranexamic Acid Solution for Injection, Zamic

Available forms
Tablets: 500 mg;
Ampoule: 500 mg/5 mL, 1 g/10 mL

Action
- competitive inhibitor of plasminogen activation
- inhibits fibrinolysis by reducing the conversion of plasminogen to plasmin (high doses)
- half-life about 2 hours

Use
- hereditary angioneurotic oedema
- hyphaema (short term)
- in patients with established coagulopathies having minor procedures
- menorrhagia
- (IV) reduce blood loss peri- and post-surgery (cardiac surgery, total knee arthroplasty, total hip arthroplasty)

Dose
- (Traumatic hyphaema) 1—1.5 g orally 8-hourly for 6—7 days **OR**
- (Known coagulopathy: cervical conisation) 1—1.5 g orally 8—12-hourly for 12 days postoperatively **OR**
- (Known coagulopathy: prostatectomy) 1 g orally 6 hours preoperatively, followed by 1 g 3—4 times daily until macroscopic haematuria disappears **OR**
- (Known coagulopathy: dental procedures) 25 mg/kg orally 2 hours before the procedure (with factor VIII and IX), followed by 25 mg/kg 3—4 times daily for 6—8 days **OR**
- (Hereditary angioneurotic oedema) 1—1.5 g orally 2—3 times daily (continuously or until symptoms subside) **OR**
- (Menorrhagia) 1 g orally 4 times daily, increasing to 1.5 g 4 times daily if necessary for a total of 4 days, starting with onset of visible bleeding **OR**
- (Cardiac surgery, after anaesthetic induction, before skin incision) 15 mg/kg IV bolus (loading dose), then 4.5 mg/kg/hour IV infusion for duration of surgery (0.6 mg/kg of infusion dose may be given as part of priming volume of heart—lung machine) **OR**
- (Total knee arthroplasty) 15 mg/kg IV bolus (before release of tourniquet), then 15 mg/kg IV bolus 8-hourly for 2 doses (last bolus given 16 hours after initial dose) **OR**
- (Total hip arthroplasty) 15 mg/kg IV bolus (before skin incision), then 15 mg/kg IV bolus 8-hourly for 2 doses (last bolus given 16 hours after initial dose)

Adverse effects
- nausea, vomiting, diarrhoea
- dermatitis
- (Rapid IV) dizziness, hypotension
- (IV) cardiogenic shock, renal failure, respiratory failure, stroke, myocardial infarction, arrhythmias
- (Rarely) colour vision impairment, altered vision, giddiness, thromboembolic events, seizures, death

Interactions
- not recommended with factor IX complex concentrates or anti-inhibitor coagulant concentrates because of the increased risk of thrombosis

Nursing considerations/Cautions
- IV bolus should not exceed 50 mg/min to avoid dizziness and/or hypotension
- should be discontinued if the patient develops a colour vision or other vision defect, as these may be indicative of retinotoxicity
- (Menorrhagia) the patient should be reassessed after 3 months of therapy
- (Prostatectomy) treatment > 14 days is not recommended
- if treatment is to be prolonged (> 7 days), a baseline ophthalmological examination (visual acuity, colour vision, eyeground and visual fields) is recommended before starting and regularly throughout therapy
- (IV) should not be mixed with blood or penicillin

HAEMOSTATICS

- use with caution if blood exists in body cavities (pleural space, joint spaces, urinary tract), because undissolvable clots may occur, or in those with disseminated intravascular coagulation (DIC) or impaired kidney function
- should be used in those at high risk of thrombosis only if benefits outweigh risks and under close medical supervision
- (Menorrhagia) not recommended in females with irregular menstrual bleeding due to an unknown cause
- not recommended for haematuria caused by renal parenchymal disease
- contraindicated in those with a history/risk of thrombosis (unless treated with anticoagulants), active thromboembolic disease, subarachnoid haemorrhage or acquired disturbance of colour vision

Patient education

- the patient should be advised to immediately seek medical advice if any of the following occur:
  - visual disturbances, including colour vision
  - dizziness, lightheadedness, rapid heart rate, weakness, sweating, cold, clammy skin, restlessness

Tablet can be dispersed in water (2–5 minutes), or can be crushed and mixed with a spoonful of yoghurt or apple puree.

Should be used during pregnancy only if the benefits outweigh potential risk.

Caution if used during breastfeeding.

Renal impairment: clearance reduced, increasing the risk of accumulation. Dose adjustment is recommended based on renal function. In severe impairment (eGFR < 30 mL/min), avoid use if possible. Monitor renal function and adjust dosing accordingly.

COAGULATION FACTORS

Coagulation factors treat coagulation factor deficiencies and may be produced by recombinant technology or extracted from human plasma. Recombinant technology consists of taking the human coagulation factor and expressing it in non-human cells (e.g. hamster kidney cells). The coagulation factors produced are expressed as international units (IU), but each coagulation factor has its own discrete units, which are therefore not interchangeable.

FACTOR VII

Activated factor VII (factor VIIa) is essential in the coagulation cascade as it activates factor X to factor Xa. This activation initiates the conversion of prothrombin to thrombin, which then converts fibrinogen to fibrin, forming a clot. For factor VIIa to be effective, it must bind with tissue factor (TF), a protein exposed on cells at the site of blood vessel injury, to localise and start the clotting process at the site of injury.

EPTACOG ALFA
Trade name
NovoSeven RT

Available forms
Vial: 1 mg (50,000 IU), 2 mg (100,000 IU), 5 mg (250,000 IU), 8 mg (400,000 IU)

Action
- recombinant coagulation factor VIIa

Use
- treatment and prophylaxis of bleeding in patients with inhibitors to coagulation factors VIII or IX

- treatment and prophylaxis of bleeding in patients with congenital deficiency of factor VII
- Glanzmann's thrombasthenia (with GPIIb-IIIa and/or HLA antibodies, refractory to platelet transfusion)

Dose

Inhibitors to clotting factors VIII or IX

- (Bleeding control) 35–120 microgram/kg by IV bolus over 2–5 minutes 2–3-hourly until bleeding is controlled, then 3–12-hourly if treatment is still needed **OR**
- (Mild-to-moderate bleeding episodes) 90 microgram/kg by IV bolus over 2–5 minutes at 3-hourly intervals for 2–3 doses **OR**
- (Mild-to-moderate bleeding episodes) 270 microgram/kg by IV bolus over 2–5 minutes stat **OR**
- (Surgical prophylaxis) 35–120 microgram/kg by IV bolus over 2–5 minutes 2–3-hourly for 1–2 days, then 2–6-hourly if treatment is still needed **OR**
- (Prophylaxis to decrease frequency of bleeding episodes) 90 microgram/kg daily by IV bolus over 2–5 minutes for up to 12 weeks

Congenital factor VII deficiency

- 15–30 microgram/kg 4–6-hourly until haemostasis is achieved

Glanzmann's thrombasthenia

- 80–120 microgram/kg for at least 3 doses 2.5 hours apart

Adverse effects

- fever, headache
- nausea
- pruritus, urticaria, rash
- (Rare) (injection site) reaction, pain
- (Rare) anaphylaxis, neutralising antibody production (inhibitors), thromboembolic events, disseminated intravascular coagulation (DIC)

Interactions

- not recommended with prothrombin complex concentrate or recombinant coagulation factor XIII
- may shorten prothrombin time if given at 15–30 microgram/kg 4–6-hourly

Nursing considerations/Cautions

- prothrombin time and factor VII coagulant activity should be measured before starting and regularly throughout therapy. If expected level is not reached or uncontrolled bleeding continues, this may be due to development of neutralising antibodies and should be investigated
- patient should be closely monitored for any sign of thrombosis or unwanted activation of the coagulation system (e.g. inducing DIC)
- if bleeding is severe, administration of coagulation factor VIII or IX inhibitors is recommended
- reconstitute using provided solvent/diluent (1.1 mL for 1 mg vial, 2.1 mL for 2 mg and 5.2 mL for 5 mg), swirling gently to dissolve until the solution is clear
- administer alone
- not recommended in those with fructose intolerance, glucose malabsorption or sucrase–isomaltase insufficiency
- caution if used in those with advanced atherosclerotic disease, crush injury, septicaemia, DIC, coronary heart disease, liver disease or after major surgery because of the increased risk of a thromboembolic event
- caution if used in those with platelet and/or blood product sensitivity
- contraindicated in those with a known hypersensitivity to mouse, hamster or bovine proteins or factor VIIa complexes

 Animal studies show no harm, but human data is lacking. Use only if benefits outweigh risks.

 Excretion in breastmilk unknown. Use with caution, considering benefits and risks.

 Reduced renal function: use with caution. Adjust dose if necessary; monitor renal function closely.

HAEMOSTATICS

> Reduced hepatic function: caution advised. Adjust dose and monitor liver function.

 Increased risk of thromboembolic events. Monitor closely; consider dose adjustments.

FACTOR VIII

Factor VIIIa acts as a cofactor for factor IXa, accelerating the conversion of factor X to factor Xa. Factor Xa then catalyses the transformation of prothrombin to thrombin, which subsequently converts fibrinogen to fibrin, leading to clot formation.

EFMOROCTOCOG ALFA
Trade name
Eloctate

MOROCTOCOG ALFA
Trade name
Xyntha

OCTOCOG ALFA
Trade name
Advate

RURIOCTOCOG ALFA PEGOL
Trade name
Adynovate

Available forms
Vial: 250 IU, 500 IU, 750 IU, 1000 IU, 1500 IU, 2000 IU, 3000 IU, 4000 IU

Action
* recombinant coagulation factor VIII
* (Rurioctocog alfa pegol) octocog alfa has been conjugated with percutaneous endoscopic gastrostomy (PEG) reagent to extend plasma half-life
* (Efmoroctocog alfa) recombinant fusion protein of factor VIII bonded to IgG$_1$ prolonging half-life

Use
* treatment and prophylaxis of bleeding in patients with haemophilia A

Dose
* dose is calculated to determine amount required for a given response or the response expected from a given amount. The formula used is:
* (Mild muscle or oral bleeding, early haemarthrosis) 10—20 IU/kg IV repeated 12—24-hourly for 1—3 days until bleeding and pain resolves **OR**
* (Mild-to-moderate bleeding) 20—30 IU/kg IV repeated 24—48-hourly until bleeding and pain resolves (Eloctate) **OR**
* (Moderate muscle bleeding, bleeding into oral cavity, known trauma, definite haemarthrosis) 15—30 IU/kg IV, repeated 12—24-hourly for 3 or more days, until bleeding resolves **OR**
* (Major/significant bleed, fractures, head trauma) initially 30—50 IU/kg IV, repeated 8—24-hourly until bleeding resolves **OR**
* (Major bleed) 40—50 IU/kg IV every 12—24 hours until bleeding resolves (Eloctate) **OR**
* (Perioperative, minor surgery) 30—50 IU IV bolus within 1 hour of surgery, with additional dosing 12—24-hourly if needed **OR**
* (Perioperative, minor surgery including tooth extraction) 25—40 IU/kg IV, repeated every 24 hours if needed (Eloctate) **OR**
* (Perioperative, major surgery) preoperatively 40—60 IU IV bolus (verifying 100% activity has been achieved before surgery), then 40—60 IU 8—24-hourly (depending on desired level of factor VIII and state of healing) **OR**
* (Long-term prophylaxis) 10—50 IU/kg IV 3 to 5 times weekly **OR**
* (Long-term prophylaxis) 65 IU/kg IV weekly (Eloctate)

Adverse effects
* (Injection site) inflammation, pain
* headache, chills, flushing, sweating, fever

1203

- dizziness, tremor
- nausea, vomiting, altered taste, abdominal pain
- rash, urticaria, pruritus
- dyspnoea
- palpitations
- fatigue, malaise
- development of neutralising antibodies (inhibitors)
- (Uncommon/rare) allergy, hypersensitivity

Nursing considerations/Cautions

- 1 IU is equal to the concentration of factor VIII in 1 mL of fresh human plasma (pooled) (WHO standard)
- dose, frequency and duration of therapy is dependent on the patient's weight, site and extent of bleeding, severity of disorder, titre of inhibitors and desired concentration of factor VIII. For example, the minimum plasma factor VIII activity required will be different for minor surgical procedures than for major surgical procedures or life-threatening haemorrhage
- the risk of developing neutralising antibodies is highest in the first 20 days of exposure (but can occur after 100 days) and therefore the patient should be closely monitored (clinical observation and laboratory values), which may result in bleeding not being controlled
- blood levels for factor VIII should be measured 3–6 hours after the start of IV infusion and then daily using one-stage clotting assay
- if switching between factor VIII products, therapeutic response should be closely monitored
- if bolus administration results in an increase in pulse rate, the rate should be decreased or temporarily stopped
- (Advate) can be given as bolus injection at a rate not greater than 10 mL/min or by continuous infusion for 500 IU, 1000 IU or 1500 IU doses (by syringe driver at a rate of 0.4 mL/hour or greater)
- (Advate) initial reconstitution should be with 5 mL of diluent until no hypersensitivity is established. If no hypersensitivity occurs, diluent volume can be reduced to 2 mL
- reconstitution should occur at room temperature and according to the manufacturer's specific instructions (different products are not interchangeable in terms of use or reconstitution instructions)
- add the diluent provided (amount according to manufacturer's instructions) to the powder and swirl gently to dissolve
- the solution should be used within 3 hours of reconstitution
- (Adynovate) contains 10 mg sodium per vial, which may need to be taken into consideration in those who have a low-sodium diet
- not recommended in those with von Willebrand disease
- contraindicated in those with a known hypersensitivity to mouse, hamster or bovine proteins

Patient education

- the patient should be advised to immediately report any skin reaction (such as hives), chest pain/tightness, wheezing, flushing, feeling faint or difficulty breathing
- ensure the patient/carer understands and is able to demonstrate correct administration technique, including reconstitution of the powder, use of the connection device (provided), attaching the infusion needle, administration rate, safe disposal of used needles and cleaning requirements if any blood is spilled
- if the patient is planning travel, ensure they understand the importance of having adequate supply for length of trip

HAEMOSTATICS

No adequate studies in pregnant women. Use only if necessary, considering potential risks.

Excretion in human breastmilk is unknown. Use with caution and only if the potential benefit outweighs any risk.

FACTOR VIII
Trade name
Biostate

Available forms
Vial: (contains 1:2.4 ratio of factor VIII to von Willebrand factor): 250/600 IU, 500/1200 IU, 1000/2400 IU

Action
- human purified coagulation factor VIII plus von Willebrand factor complex (promotes platelet aggregation and adhesion on damaged endothelium and carrier protein for precoagulant protein factor VIII)

Use
- treatment and prophylaxis in those with factor VIII deficiency caused by haemophilia A
- treatment of bleeding associated with von Willebrand disease (where desmopressin is ineffective or contraindicated)

Dose
Haemophilia A
- (Minor haemorrhage) 10—15 IU/kg IV 12—24-hourly for 1—2 days **OR**
- (Moderate-to-severe haemorrhage) 15—40 IU/kg IV 8—24-hourly for 1—4 days **OR**
- (Life-threatening haemorrhage) initially 50—60 IU/kg IV, then 20—25 IU/kg 8—12 hourly (days 2—10) **OR**
- (Minor surgery) 20—30 IU/kg IV stat (loading dose preoperatively), followed by 20—25 IU/kg twice daily (days 1—3), then 20—30 IU daily **OR**
- (Major surgery) 40—50 IU/kg IV stat (loading dose preoperatively), followed by 20—25 IU/kg 8—12-hourly (days 1—3), 15—20 IU/kg 8—12-hourly (days 4—6), then 10—20 IU/kg twice daily **OR**
- (Dentistry) 35—40 IU/kg IV stat (loading dose preoperatively), followed by 25—30 IU/kg twice daily for 1—3 days (maintenance) **OR**
- (Prophylaxis) 25—40 IU/kg IV 3 times weekly

von Willebrand disease
- (Spontaneous bleeding) initially 10—20/25—50 IU/kg IV, then 10—20 IU/kg IV 12—24-hourly until bleeding stops (usually 2—4 days) **OR**
- (Minor surgery) 25/60 IU/kg IV daily until healing is complete (usually 2—4 days) **OR**
- (Major surgery) initially 25—35/60—80 IU/kg IV, then 15—25/30—60 IU/kg IV 12—24-hourly, usually 5—10 days until healing is complete **OR**
- (Prophylaxis) 10—15/25—40 IU/kg IV 1—3 times per week

Adverse effects
- hypersensitivity (tachycardia, chest pain/discomfort, back pain)
- altered taste
- fever, headache
- abnormal liver enzymes
- development of neutralising antibodies (inhibitors)
- (Rare) allergy, anaphylactic reaction, thromboembolic events, thrombophlebitis

Nursing considerations/Cautions
- for surgical indications, the loading dose is given day before the procedure
- the risk of developing neutralising antibodies is greatest in the first 20 days (although in some it will develop after 100 days of exposure) or in those who are switching from one factor VIII product to another who have previ-

ously had > 100 exposure days with a previous development of neutralising antibodies. If bleeding is not controlled or target levels not reached, investigation for neutralising antibodies is recommended
- immunisation with hepatitis A and hepatitis B vaccines is recommended for those with no antibodies to these viruses before administration of factor VIII
- product is made from human plasma, which may contain infectious agents such as viruses. Current manufacturing processes are effective against HIV, hepatitis B, hepatitis C and hepatitis A
- the vial should be allowed to reach room temperature before reconstitution. The appropriate amount of water for injections should be drawn into the syringe and attached to the preparation device. A plastic cannula of the preparation device is then inserted into the stopper using a push and twist action, and water is drawn into the vial by vacuum. Contents are gently swirled to dissolve without excessive frothing (2–5 minutes to produce clear solution)
- the name and batch number should be recorded for each treatment
- reconstituted solution should not be refrigerated
- if clots or gel form, it should not be used (return to Australian Red Cross Lifeblood)
- administer over at least 5 minutes (or as tolerated). The infusion rate should not exceed 6 mL/min
- administer alone
- do not mix with whole bleed
- any spills should be cleaned with sodium hypochlorite 1% for 15 minutes
- the patient and/or family member can be instructed in preparation and administration
- caution if used in those with allergy to factor VIII and/or von Willebrand factor concentrates or human albumin
- contraindicated in those with a history of anaphylaxis or severe systemic response to factor VIII or von Willebrand factor preparations

Patient education

- the patient should be advised to immediately report any skin reaction (such as hives), chest pain/tightness, wheezing, flushing, feeling faint or difficulty breathing
- ensure the patient/carer understands and is able to demonstrate the correct administration technique, including reconstitution of powder, use of connection device (provided), attaching the infusion needle, administration rate, safe disposal of used needles and cleaning requirements if any blood is spilled
- if the patient is planning travel, ensure they understand the importance of having an adequate supply for the length of trip

Avoid, as increases risk of bleeding during delivery. There is no available experience for use in pregnant women with von Willebrand disease or haemophilia A.

Limited human data.

FACTOR VIII INHIBITOR BYPASSING FRACTION
Trade name
Feiba-NF

Available forms
Vial: 500 IU, 1000 IU, 2500 IU

Action
- blood coagulation factor complex
- contains factors II, IX and X (mainly non-activated), factor VII (activated) and 1–6 units of factor VIII coagulation antigen
- those with haemophilia A and B can acquire inhibitors to factor VIII or IX during factor VIII or IX replacement therapy. This prevents the formation of

HAEMOSTATICS

- the complex that catalyses Xa production
- generates Xa and thrombin without needing factor VIIIa–IXa complex, bypassing inhibitory action of factor VIII or IX inhibitors

Use
- routine prophylaxis, control of spontaneous bleeding or in surgery in those with haemophilia A or B with neutralising antibodies (inhibitors)

Dose
- (Joint, muscle and soft tissue haemorrhage — minor-to-moderate bleed) 50–75 IU/kg IV 12-hourly until bleeding resolves (pain decreases, reduction in swelling or joint mobilisation) (daily maximum 200 IU/kg) **OR**
- (Joint, muscle and soft tissue haemorrhage — major bleed) 100 IU/kg IV 12-hourly until bleeding resolves (pain decreases, reduction in swelling or joint mobilisation) (daily maximum 200 IU/kg) **OR**
- (Mucous membrane haemorrhage) 50 IU/kg IV 6-hourly, increasing to 100 IU/kg if bleeding does not stop (daily maximum 200 IU/kg) **OR**
- (Other severe haemorrhage) 100 IU/kg IV 12-hourly, reducing to 6-hourly if needed (daily maximum 200 IU/kg) **OR**
- (Surgery) 50–100 IU/kg IV up to 6-hourly (daily maximum 200 IU/kg) **OR**
- (Routine prophylaxis) 70–100 IU/kg IV 3–4 times weekly, adjusting dose on clinical response (daily maximum 200 IU/kg)

Adverse effects
- hypersensitivity reaction
- dizziness, headache
- hypotension
- rash
- hepatitis B surface antibody positive
- (Rare) thrombotic and thromboembolic events, allergic and anaphylactoid reactions

Interactions
- not recommended with antifibrinolytic agents because of the risk of a thrombotic event. If required, they should be administered 12 hours apart
- may decrease active immunity from live attenuated vaccine if given together
- may interfere with Coomb's test (antiglobulin test)

Nursing considerations/Cautions
- increased risk of thromboembolic events if high doses are given; therefore dose should not exceed 100 IU/kg (as a single dose) or 200 IU/kg (daily maximum)
- dose is independent of the patient's inhibitor titres
- the patient should be monitored carefully for any signs including changes in BP, pulse rate, respiratory distress, chest pain and cough. If these occur, the infusion should be stopped and diagnostic tests conducted to determine whether disseminated intravascular coagulation (DIC) is present (decreased fibrinogen, decreased platelet count and/or presence of fibrin-fibrinogen degradation product, significantly prolonged thrombin time, prothrombin time or partial thromboplastin time)
- the infusion rate should not exceed 2 IU/kg/min
- the vial should be allowed to reach room temperature before reconstitution. An appropriate amount of water for injections should be drawn into the syringe and attached to the preparation device. A plastic cannula of the preparation device is then inserted into the stopper using a push and twist action and water drawn into the vial using a vacuum. The contents are gently swirled to dissolve without excessive frothing
- the solution should not be refrigerated and should be used within 3 hours of reconstitution

HAVARD'S NURSING GUIDE TO DRUGS

- the product is made from human plasma, which may contain infectious agents such as viruses. Current manufacturing processes are effective against HIV, hepatitis B, hepatitis C and hepatitis A
- appropriate vaccination (hepatitis A and B) should be considered if the patient is receiving regular or repeated therapy
- contains sodium (80—200 mg/vial), which may need to be taken into consideration in those who have a low-sodium diet
- caution if used in those with liver impairment
- caution if used in those with DIC, advanced arterial disease, crush injury, septicaemia, arterial or venous thrombosis, or if receiving concurrent therapy with recombinant factor VIIa
- contraindicated in those with normal coagulation, DIC, fibrinolysis, coronary heart disease, acute thrombosis and/or embolism
- contraindicated during cardiac surgery involving cardiopulmonary bypass and procedures involving extracorporeal membrane oxygenation (ECMO) because of a high risk of thrombotic adverse events

Patient education
- the patient should be advised to immediately report any skin reaction (such as hives), chest pain/tightness, wheezing, flushing, feeling faint or difficulty breathing

Should be used during pregnancy only if benefits outweigh risks. Pregnancy and the postpartum period confer an increased risk of thromboembolic events, and some pregnancy complications are associated with DIC.

Caution, as it is unknown whether FEIBA NF components are excreted in human milk. Use only if the potential benefit justifies any possible risk, especially considering the postpartum period's increased thromboembolic risk.

Use with caution in elderly patients, especially those with additional risk factors for thromboembolic events.

EMICIZUMAB
Trade name
Hemlibra

Available forms
Vial: 30 mg/mL, 60 mg/0.4 mL, 105 mg/0.7 mL, 150 mg/mL

Action
- humanised monoclonal antibody immunoglobulin G4 (IgG$_4$) whose structure bridges activated factor IX and factor X to restore function of missing activated factor VIII
- does not induce or enhance development of neutralising antibodies (inhibitors)
- produced by recombinant DNA technology in Chinese hamster ovary cells
- long half-life resulting in effects on coagulation assays persisting for up to 6 months after therapy has been stopped

Use
- prophylaxis to prevent bleeding in those with haemophilia A

Dose
- 3 mg/kg SC once weekly for 4 weeks, then either 1.5 mg/kg SC weekly, 3 mg/kg SC every 2 weeks or 6 mg/kg SC monthly

Adverse effects
- (Injection site) redness, pain, pruritus
- fever
- headache
- diarrhoea
- arthralgia, myalgia
- (Uncommon) thrombotic microangiopathy, thrombosis, skin necrosis, thrombophlebitis

Interactions
- increases the risk of microangiopathy and thrombotic events if given with

HAEMOSTATICS

activated prothrombin complex concentrate (cumulative dose > 100 IU/kg/24 hours) for 24 hours or more. If given together, the patient should be monitored closely for any signs of thrombotic microangiopathy or thromboembolism
- caution if given with activated factor VII or factor VIII, as lower doses may be required
- may interfere with intrinsic pathway clotting-based tests

Nursing considerations/Cautions

- store at 2–8°C. Can be kept at room temperature (below 30°C) for up to 7 days.
- protect from light and do not shake.
- any bypassing agents (e.g. Feiba-NF) should be discontinued 24 hours before starting therapy. If required during prophylaxis with emicizumab, the doctor should discuss dose with the patient, as this may be lower than used without emicizumab prophylaxis. However, it should be avoided unless there are no other treatment options or alternatives available. The initial dose should not exceed 50 IU/kg and the total dose not greater than 100 IU/kg in first 24 hours
- factor VIII prophylaxis therapy can be continued for first 7 days of therapy
- trade name and batch number of product should be recorded in the patient's medical notes
- SC injection sites should be rotated, avoiding any areas that are hard, tender, red, bruised or scarred, or there are moles present
- injection of other SC agents should be at different anatomical sites
- the patient may be taught to self-administer
- if the patient develops thrombotic microangiopathy, supportive care with or without plasmapheresis and haemodialysis is recommended. Improvement in the patient;s condition should be seen within a week
- contraindicated in those with known hypersensitivity to hamster-derived proteins

Patient education

- self-administration instruction should include rotation of injection sites, preparation of skin and solution, injection technique, correct storage and disposal advice
- ensure the patient understands the importance of following the doctor's instruction regarding use of a bypassing agent (e.g. Feiba NF), as serious adverse effects may occur if instructions are not followed
- the patient should be advised to immediately seek medical advice if any of the following occur:
  - confusion, weakness, arm or leg swelling, yellowing of skin and eyes, abdominal or back pain, nausea, vomiting, or urinating less (may be signs of thrombotic microangiopathy)
  - swelling, warmth, redness or pain (may be signs of blood clot in veins near skin surface)
  - headache, face numbness, eye pain or swelling, vision impairment (may be signs of blood clot in eye blood vessel)
  - blackening of skin

Limited data; use only if benefits justify the potential risks.

Excretion in human milk is unknown. Consider the benefit of breastfeeding against the clinical need for emicizumab.

FACTOR IX

Factor IX is synthesised by the liver and is involved in the intrinsic pathway for blood coagulation. Factor XIa activates factor IX, which then activates factor X (in the presence of factor VIIIa). This leads to the conversion of prothrombin to thrombin and the formation of a fibrin clot.

FACTOR IX
Trade name
MonoFIX-VF

Available forms
Vial: 500 IU, 1000 IU

Action
- human purified coagulation factor IX
- contains heparin sodium
- half-life is about 24 hours

Use
- treatment and prophylaxis of bleeding in patients with haemophilia B (Christmas disease)

Dose
- (Minor haemorrhage) 20–30 IU/kg IV daily for 1–2 days **OR**
- (Moderate-to-severe haemorrhage) 30–50 IU/kg IV 1–2 times daily for 1–5 days **OR**
- (Minor surgery, including dental extraction) 40–60 IU/kg IV stat (loading dose), then 15–40 IU/kg 1–2 times daily for 7–10 days **OR**
- (Major surgery) 70–100 IU/kg IV stat (loading dose), then 20–90 IU/kg 1–2 times daily for 10–12 days **OR**
- (Prophylaxis) 25–40 IU/kg IV twice weekly

Adverse effects
- injection site reaction
- nausea, altered taste
- dizziness
- clammy skin
- thrombocytopenia (because of the heparin component)
- development of neutralising antibodies (inhibitors)
- (Rare) allergy, anaphylactic reaction, fever, thrombosis, disseminated intravascular coagulation (DIC)

Nursing considerations/Cautions
- any coagulation test results should be carefully interpreted in view of the heparin content
- made from human plasma; therefore it carries a potential risk of transmission of infectious agents (despite the manufacturing process which removes and inactivates a number of known viruses, including HIV, hepatitis B and C viruses)
- hepatitis A and hepatitis B vaccination is recommended for patients who have no antibody titre to hepatitis A or B
- plasma factor IX levels should be monitored in those with severe haemorrhage or undergoing surgery
- if expected activity is not achieved or bleeding is not controlled, blood assay for factor IX neutralising antibodies (inhibitors) should be performed
- vial contains 50–140 IU heparin per reconstituted 500 IU vial or 100–280 IU per reconstituted 1000 IU vial
- vial should be allowed to reach room temperature before reconstitution. Appropriate amount of water for injections should be drawn into syringe and attached to preparation device. A plastic cannula of the preparation device is then inserted into the stopper using a push and twist action and water drawn into the vial using vacuum. Contents are gently swirled to dissolve without excessive frothing (2–5 minutes to produce clear solution)
- should not be refrigerated once reconstituted
- if clots or gel form or a vacuum is not present in the vial, it should not be used (return to Australian Red Cross Lifeblood)
- administer alone at a rate not greater than 3 mL/min
- spillage should be cleaned using sodium hypochlorite 1% for 15 minutes
- not indicated for treatment of factor II, VII or X deficiency or in those with

HAEMOSTATICS

- haemophilia A with factor VIII neutralising antibodies (inhibitors)
- caution if used in those with previous severe reaction to factor IX concentrates or in those with fibrinolysis, myocardial infarction, DIC or liver disease

Use only if the potential benefit justifies the risk. Contains heparin; therefore it may increase the risk of fetal loss or premature birth due to maternal haemorrhage.

Excretion in breastmilk unknown; use only if benefit justifies risk to the infant.

Available in combination with
- Prothrombin, Factor IX, Factor X (Prothrombinex-VF)

NONACOG ALFA
Trade name
BeneFIX

Available forms
Vial: 250 IU, 500 IU, 1000 IU, 2000 IU, 3000 IU

Action
- recombinant coagulation factor IX

Use
- treatment and prophylaxis of bleeding in patients with haemophilia B (Christmas disease)

Dose
- (Patients aged ≥ 15 years) dose calculated using the following formula: number of factor IX IU required (IU) = weight (kg) × desired factor IX increase (% or IU/dL) × 1.1 dL/kg

Adverse effects
- reaction at IV site
- (Uncommon) headache, dizziness, tremor
- (Uncommon) nausea, altered taste
- (Uncommon) cough, dyspnoea
- (Rare) allergy, anaphylaxis, thrombosis, fever, burning sensation in jaw/skull, chest tightness, GI upset
- development of neutralising antibodies (inhibitors)

Nursing considerations/Cautions
- initial 10–20 doses should be given under medical supervision because of the risk of allergic reaction
- patient changing from plasma-derived factor IX products to nonacog (alfa) should be instructed that recovery may be slower and higher doses may be required
- length of therapy is dependent on reason for administration:
    - (minor bleeding) given 12–24-hourly for 1 to 2 days
    - (moderate bleeding) given 12–24-hourly for 2–7 days (until bleeding stops, healing occurs)
    - (major bleeding) given 12–24-hourly for 7–10 days
- (Prophylaxis) may be given as a regular schedule (2–3 times weekly)
- reconstitute by injecting diluent provided (in prefilled syringe) into vial, swirling gently until dissolved and then drawing clear solution back into syringe using vial adapter. Administer using provided infusion kit
- during administration, blood should not be allowed to enter syringe containing reconstituted solution. If this occurs, syringe, tubing and solution should be discarded
- should be administered at a rate of 1–2 mL/min IV
- administer alone
- reconstituted solution should be used as soon as possible to decrease time spent in plastic syringe as solution absorbs PVC from syringe surface
- caution if used in those with liver disease, post-surgically or with signs/risk of fibrinolysis, DIC or thromboembolic events
- contraindicated in those with known allergy to hamster protein

No human studies. Use only if benefits outweigh the risks.

 Unknown if excreted in breastmilk; use with caution.

NONACOG GAMMA
Trade name
Rixubis

Available forms
Vial: 250 IU, 500 IU, 1000 IU, 2000 IU, 3000 IU

Action
- recombinant coagulation factor IX
- specific activity is $\geq$ 200 IU factor IX/mg

Use
- treatment and prophylaxis of bleeding in patients with haemophilia B (Christmas disease)

Dose
- ($\geq$ 12 years of age) calculated using the following formula: number of factor IX IU required (IU) = weight (kg) × desired factor IX increase (% or IU/dL) × 1.1 dL/kg
- (< 12 years of age) calculated using the following formula: number of factor IX IU required (IU) = weight (kg) × desired factor IX increase (% or IU/dL) × 1.4 dL/kg
- (Routine prophylaxis in those with moderate-to-severe haemophilia B, $\geq$ 12 years and previously treated) 40–60 IU by IV bolus infusion twice weekly **OR**
- (Routine prophylaxis in those with moderate-to-severe haemophilia B, < 12 years and previously treated) 40–80 IU by IV bolus infusion twice weekly

Adverse effects
- altered taste
- pain in extremity
- rash, urticaria
- (Rare) hypersensitivity, allergy, anaphylaxis, thromboembolism, disseminated intravascular coagulation (DIC)
- development of neutralising antibodies (inhibitors), nephrotic syndrome

Nursing considerations/Cautions
- factor IX activity levels should be monitored using a one-stage clotting assay to confirm adequate factor IX levels have been achieved and maintained
- risk of hypersensitivity is highest in those previously untreated and with high-risk gene mutations
- length of therapy is dependent on reason for administration:
  - (minor bleeding) given daily until bleeding resolves
  - (moderate bleeding) given daily for 3–4 days or until bleeding stops and healing occurs
  - (life-threatening bleeding) given 8–12-hourly until threat has resolved
  - (minor surgery, including tooth extraction) repeated daily after bolus, continued until healing occurs
  - (major surgery) repeated 8–24-hourly after bolus until adequate healing occurs, then for at least another 7 days (to maintain factor IX activity of 30–60% IU/dL)
- neutralising antibodies (inhibitors) may develop and should be suspected if plasma factor IX activity levels are not achieved or bleeding is not controlled with the expected dose. If this occurs, factor IX inhibitor concentration levels should be measured
- those with high levels (titres) of factor IX inhibitors are at increased risk of severe hypersensitivity or anaphylaxis if re-exposed to factor IX
- only plastic syringes should be used
- allow the vial and diluent (water for injections) to come to room temperature before reconstitution
- reconstitute by using diluent provided (water for injections) and following manufacturer's instructions
- should be administered by IV bolus at a rate that is comfortable for the patient (up to 10 mL/min)

HAEMOSTATICS

- should not be given by continuous IV infusion
- administer alone
- the solution should be used within 3 hours of reconstitution
- the patient/carer may be taught administration technique
- caution if used in those with liver disease, postsurgically or with signs/risk of fibrinolysis, DIC or thromboembolic events
- contraindicated in those with known allergy to hamster protein

Patient education

- advise the patient to immediately seek medical advice if any rash/hives, itching, throat tightness, chest pain/tightness, difficulty breathing, lightheadedness, dizziness, nausea or fainting occurs (especially if early in therapy)
- ensure the patient/carer understands and is able to demonstrate the correct administration technique including reconstitution of the powder, use of the connection device (provided), attaching the infusion needle, administration rate, safe disposal of used needles and cleaning requirements if any blood is spilled
- if the patient is planning travel, ensure they understand the importance of having adequate supply for length of trip

 Limited data: used during pregnancy only if benefits outweigh risks.

 Used in breastfeeding only if benefits outweigh risks.

EFTRENONACOG ALFA
Trade name
Alprolix

Available forms
Vial: 250 IU, 500 IU, 1000 IU, 2000 IU, 3000 IU

Action
- long-acting fusion protein made up of factor IX and IgG$_1$, resulting in a longer plasma half-life

Use
- prophylaxis and treatment of bleeding in patients with haemophilia B

Dose
- (Minor-to-moderate bleed) 30—60 IU/kg IV, repeated every 48 hours until bleeding has resolved **OR**
- (Surgical prophylaxis — minor surgery including uncomplicated dental extraction) 50—80 IU/kg IV, repeated after 24—48 hours if needed **OR**
- (Major bleed; surgical prophylaxis — major surgery) initially 100 IU/kg IV, then 80 IU/kg after 6—10 hours, then daily for 3 days, may be extended to every 48 hours after day 3 if needed **OR**
- (Prophylaxis) 50 IU/kg IV weekly or 100 IU/kg IV every 10 days

Adverse effects
- headache, dizziness
- oral paraesthesia
- obstructive uropathy
- (Uncommon) haematuria, renal colic
- (Uncommon) decreased appetite, breath odour, altered taste
- development of neutralising antibodies (inhibitors), nephrotic syndrome
- (Rare) allergic reaction, anaphylaxis, thromboembolic events

Nursing considerations/Cautions

- factor IX activity levels should be monitored using a one-stage clotting assay to confirm adequate factor IX levels have been achieved and maintained
- neutralising antibodies (inhibitors) may develop and should be suspected if plasma factor IX activity levels are not achieved or bleeding is not controlled with the expected dose. If this occurs, factor IX inhibitor levels should be measured
- the patient may be taught to self-administer

- allow the vial and diluent (water for injections) to come to room temperature before reconstitution
- reconstitute by using the diluent provided (water for injections) and following the manufacturer's instructions
- swirl vial gently to dissolve but do not shake

Patient education

- advise the patient to immediately seek medical advice if any rash/hives, itching, throat tightness, chest pain/tightness, difficulty breathing, lightheadedness, dizziness, nausea or fainting occurs (especially if early in therapy)
- ensure the patient/carer understands and is able to demonstrate the correct administration technique, including reconstitution of the powder, use of the connection device (provided), attaching the infusion needle, administration rate, safe disposal of used needles and cleaning requirements if any blood is spilled
- if the patient is planning travel, ensure they understand the importance of having an adequate supply for length of trip

Use only if the benefit outweighs the risk; effects on the fetus are unknown.

Caution, as unknown whether excreted in milk; use only if necessary.

FACTOR XIII

Factor XIII is the last enzyme in the blood coagulation cascade. When vessel wall damage occurs, factor XIII is activated by thrombin at the site and is responsible for haemostasis maintenance through cross-linking of fibrin and other proteins at the fibrin clot. In the plasma, it circulates as two A-subunits and two B-subunits, which are held together by non-covalent bonds.

CATRIDECACOG
Trade name
NovoThirteen

Available form
Vial: 2500 IU

Action
- recombinant coagulation factor XIII A-subunit produced in yeast cells

Use
- prophylaxis of bleeding in patients with congenital factor XIII A-subunit deficiency

Dose
- 35 IU/kg IV monthly, with any dose adjustment based on factor XIII activity level

Adverse effects
- nausea, diarrhoea, gastroenteritis
- fever
- headache
- rash
- nasopharyngitis, sinusitis, upper respiratory tract infection, nasal congestion, oropharyngeal pain
- cough
- confusion
- arthralgia, back pain, musculoskeletal pain, myalgia, extremity pain, limb pain
- leucopenia, aggravated neutropenia
- injection site pain
- neutralising antibody development (inhibitors)
- allergic reaction, anaphylaxis

Interaction
- not recommended with factor VII-containing products

Nursing considerations/Cautions

- not recommended for bleeding prophylaxis in those with congenital factor

HAEMOSTATICS

- XIII B-subunit deficiency; therefore it is important that the subunit deficiency is identified before starting therapy
- monitoring factor XIII activity using standard factor XIII assay technique is recommended
- neutralising antibodies (inhibitors) may develop and should be suspected if plasma factor XIII activity levels are not achieved or bleeding is not controlled with expected dose. If this occurs, factor XIII inhibitor levels should be measured
- reconstitute using the provided vial adapter and diluent (water for injections) using the manufacturer's instructions
- swirl the solution gently to dissolve but do not shake, as this causes foaming
- the solution should be clear, colourless and used within 3 hours of reconstitution
- if dilution of the reconstituted solution is needed (e.g. for children under 24 kg), 6 mL of sodium chloride 0.9% is recommended
- caution if used in those with a predisposition to thrombosis, as fibrin stabilisation effect may lead to increased risk of vessel occlusion
- caution if used in those with severe liver impairment. Factor XIII activity levels should be closely monitored if used
- may contain traces of yeast; therefore not recommended in those with known yeast hypersensitivity
- not recommended in those with known neutralising antibodies to factor XIII without close monitoring

Patient education

- advise the patient to immediately seek medical advice if any rash/hives, itching, throat tightness, chest pain/tightness, difficulty breathing, lightheadedness, dizziness, nausea or fainting occurs (especially if early in therapy)

No human data; use only if needed for replacement therapy, as the risk is unknown.

Excretion in human milk unknown. Weigh the benefits of breastfeeding and therapy continuation.

HYPOTHALAMIC AND PITUITARY HORMONES

The hypothalamus and pituitary gland are located inferior to the midbrain and work in unison to regulate the synthesis and release of hormones throughout the body. The pituitary gland (also called the hypophysis) is linked to the hypothalamus via a stalk (the infundibulum) (Tortora & Derrickson 2021).

The hypothalamus secretes a range of hormones and releasing factors, including thyrotrophin-releasing hormone (TRH), gonadotrophin-releasing hormone (GnRH), somatostatin (also called growth hormone release-inhibiting hormone (GHRIH)), growth hormone-releasing hormone (GHRH), corticotrophin-releasing hormone (CRH), substance P and prolactin release-inhibiting factor (PRIH). The secretion of hormones and releasing factors is controlled or regulated by a series of complex feedback mechanisms. In turn, all of these hormones and releasing factors regulate the synthesis and secretion of hormones from the anterior pituitary (Tortora & Derrickson 2021).

The pituitary gland itself is divided into two distinct lobes — the anterior pituitary (adenohypophysis) and the posterior pituitary (neurohypophysis). The anterior pituitary secretes a number of hormones that have their effects on various target organs throughout the body, producing other hormones, which are part of the feedback loop to the hypothalamus and/or pituitary, regulating further synthesis and release. Hormones secreted from the anterior pituitary include:

- human growth hormone (GH) (somatotrophin) (stimulates growth and regulates metabolism), secretion stimulated by GHRH
- thyroid-stimulating hormone (TSH, or thyrotrophin) (stimulates secretion of hormones from the thyroid gland), secretion stimulated by TRH
- adrenocorticotrophic hormone (ACTH) (stimulates secretion of glucocorticoids, mineralocorticoids and, to a lesser extent, sex hormones from the adrenal cortex), secretion stimulated by CRH
- gonadotrophins, such as follicle-stimulating hormone (FSH) (stimulates maturation of ovarian follicles and oestrogen production in females and sperm production in males) and luteinising hormone (LH) (stimulates ovulation and oestrogen

HYPOTHALAMIC AND PITUITARY HORMONES

production in females and testosterone production in males), secretion stimulated by GnRH
- prolactin (promotes lactation), secretion stimulated by prolactin-releasing hormone (PRH)
- melanocyte-stimulating hormone (stimulates production of the melatonin that darkens the skin), secretion stimulated by CRH (Tortora & Derrickson 2021).

The posterior pituitary is responsible for only two hormones and their release is mediated by the sympathetic and parasympathetic nervous systems:
- oxytocin (stimulates uterine smooth muscle contraction, as well as stimulating milk ejection from mammary glands. Role in non-pregnant female is unknown) and
- antidiuretic hormone (ADH, or vasopressin) (regulates reabsorption of water in the renal tubules, decreasing urine production) (Tortora & Derrickson 2021).

A number of hypothalamic and pituitary hormone-related agents are discussed in the Pregnancy, childbirth and breastfeeding section (p. 1456).

GONADOTROPHIN-RELEASING HORMONE

GOSERELIN
Trade names
Zoladex 3.6 mg Implant, Zoladex 10.8 mg Implant

Available forms
Subcutaneous implant: 3.6 mg, 10.8 mg

Action
- gonadotrophin-releasing hormone (GnRH) agonist, which causes the release of luteinising hormone (LH) from the pituitary gland (also called luteinising hormone-releasing hormone (LHRH))
- (Chronic administration) inhibits gonadotrophin (LH) production, resulting in gonadal suppression and regression of sex organs
- (Males) testosterone concentration decreases to within castrate range, resulting in prostate tumour regression and symptom improvement
- (Females) serum estradiol (oestradiol) levels decrease to postmenopausal levels
- implant releases consistent doses over at least 28 days

Use
- advanced prostate cancer (palliative management of stages C or D (metastatic or locally advanced), suitable for hormonal manipulation or as adjunctive treatment with radiotherapy)
- advanced breast cancer in premenopausal women
- early breast cancer (as adjunct therapy in premenopausal or perimenopausal women)
- assisted reproduction (in preparation for controlled ovarian superstimulation)
- endometrial thinning (prior to endometrial ablation)
- endometriosis (visually proven) (to reduce size and number of lesions, as well as relieving pain)
- uterine fibroids (to reduce size and symptoms, including pain)

Dose
- (Prostate cancer) 3.6 mg SC implant into anterior abdominal wall every 28 days **OR**
- (Prostate cancer) 10.8 mg SC implant into anterior abdominal wall 3-monthly **OR**
- (Early breast cancer, alternative to combination chemotherapy) 3.6 mg SC implant into anterior abdominal wall every 28 days for 2 years **OR**
- (Early breast cancer, as adjunct post-combination chemotherapy) 3.6 mg SC

implant into anterior abdominal wall every 28 days for 5 years **OR**
- (Advanced breast cancer) 3.6 mg SC implant into anterior abdominal wall every 28 days **OR**
- (Endometrial thinning) 3.6 mg SC implant into anterior abdominal wall followed by surgery 28 days later, or course of 2 implants 28 days apart with surgery within 14—28 days of second implant **OR**
- (Benign gynaecological disorders) 3.6 mg SC implant into anterior abdominal wall every 28 days for 6 months **OR**
- (Uterine fibroids) 3.6 mg SC implant into anterior abdominal wall every 28 days for 3—6 months

Adverse effects
- (Injection site) pain, haematoma, bleeding and, rarely, vascular injury
- decrease in bone density
- (Males) flushing, sweating, gynaecomastia, breast tenderness, decreased libido, erectile dysfunction, decreased glucose tolerance, change in BP, cardiac failure, myocardial infarction, paraesthesia, spinal cord compression, rash, bone pain, arthralgia, weight increase
- (Males — after radiotherapy) incontinence, urinary frequency
- (Females) headache, flushing, sweating, decreased libido, mood changes, depression, breast enlargement, vaginal dryness, change in BP, arthralgia, paraesthesia, alopecia, rash, acne, weight increase
- (Temporary) increase in bone pain (in patients with bony metastases), increase in signs and symptoms of breast cancer (in patients with breast cancer)
- (Rare) hypersensitivity reactions, ovarian hyperstimulation syndrome (OHSS) (if given with gonadotrophins), QT prolongation
- (Endometrial thinning) increased risk of cervical tearing during procedures

Interactions
- increased risk of QT prolongation if given with agents known to prolong QT interval (e.g. Class IA and Class III anti-arrhythmic agents (e.g. amiodarone, sotalol)) or cause electrolyte imbalance (especially hypokalaemia and hypomagnesaemia) (e.g. diuretics)
- increased risk of bleeding when implant is inserted if patient is taking anticoagulants

Nursing considerations/Cautions
- any electrolyte imbalance should be corrected before starting therapy
- any osteoporosis risk should be assessed before starting therapy and bone density measured if any significant risk factor exists. Risk factors include family history, slight build, heavy smoker, low dietary calcium intake, chronic immobility, chronic anovulatory menstrual disturbances and taking glucocorticoids
- blood glucose levels and/or glycosylated haemoglobin (HbA1c) should be monitored regularly during therapy (especially in those with existing diabetes mellitus)
- (Benign gynaecological conditions) therapy should not exceed 6 months, nor should it be repeated
- implant should be visible in applicator window
- plunger should not be withdrawn when needle is in position
- plunger should be fully depressed to ensure implant enters SC site
- SC sites should be rotated
- injections should not be omitted or delayed, because serum testosterone concentration will rise
- 10.8 mg implant is not for use in females
- (Endometriosis) patient should be assessed after 6 months for any risk of osteoporosis and a 2-year interval should be allowed between repeat courses

HYPOTHALAMIC AND PITUITARY HORMONES

- caution if used in those with cancer who are at risk of spinal cord compression or ureteric obstruction. These patients should be closely monitored for the first 4 weeks of therapy
- caution if used in those with polycystic ovarian syndrome because of the increased risk of OHSS
- caution if used in those with congenital long QT syndrome, congestive heart failure, frequent electrolyte imbalance or taking agents that prolong QT interval, as androgen deprivation may also prolong QT interval
- contraindicated in those with known hypersensitivity to LH agonist analogues

Patient education

- male patients with pre-existing diabetes mellitus should be warned that there may be a loss of glycaemic control and blood glucose levels should be monitored frequently, especially at the start of therapy
- patients with advanced cancer and/or bony metastases should be warned that they may experience an increase in bone pain or other symptoms for up to 2 weeks at the start of therapy
- the patient should be instructed to immediately seek medical advice if any of the following occur:
  - bone pain
  - numbness, tingling or weakness of legs or arms

Contraindicated for use during pregnancy.

Contraindicated for use when breastfeeding.

Banned in sport but may be permitted in sport for females only; caution advised.

Available in combination with
- contained in ZolaCos CP with bicalutamide

LEUPRORELIN (LEUPROLIDE)
Trade names
Eligard, Lucrin Depot

Available forms
Dual-chamber syringe: 7.5 mg, 22.5 mg, 30 mg, 45 mg

Action
- analogue of gonadotrophin-releasing hormone (GnRH) that inhibits growth of some hormone-dependent tumours
- (Central precocious puberty (CPP)) suppresses pituitary gonadotrophins and peripheral sex steroids, and stops progression of secondary sex characteristics

Use
- advanced prostatic cancer (stages C or D, palliative treatment)
- CPP in children

Dose
- (Advanced prostatic cancer) 7.5 mg IM monthly (depot) **OR**
- (Advanced prostatic cancer) 22.5 mg IM 3-monthly (depot) **OR**
- (Advanced prostatic cancer) 30 mg IM 4-monthly (depot) **OR**
- (Advanced prostatic cancer) 45 mg IM 6-monthly (depot) **OR**
- (CPP) 30 mg IM 3-monthly (depot)

Adverse effects
- hot flushes, sweating, clamminess, night sweats
- dizziness, headache, asthenia, fatigue, malaise, vertigo, insomnia, depression
- (Children) emotional lability, tearfulness
- paraesthesia, neuromuscular disorders
- decreased testicular size, testicular pain, gynaecomastia/breast tenderness, decreased libido, erectile dysfunction
- urinary frequency, urgency and retention, nocturia, haematuria, incontinence
- rash, pruritus, alopecia, acne
- general pain, arthralgia, bone pain, myalgia, joint disorders
- peripheral oedema, oedema
- nausea, vomiting, GI disorders, gastroenteritis/colitis, weight gain
- hyperglycaemia

HAVARD'S NURSING GUIDE TO DRUGS

- decreased bone density
- flare phenomenon (increased bone pain, ureteric obstruction and spinal cord compression)
- (Rare) spinal cord compression, ureteric obstruction, myocardial infarction, stroke, convulsions
- (Very rare) pituitary apoplexy (rare condition in those with pituitary adenoma caused by infarction of the pituitary gland, which can occur within hours or weeks of the first dose; symptoms include sudden headache, vomiting, visual disturbances, altered mental state and, sometimes, cardiovascular collapse)
- (Injection site) pain, burning, stinging, redness, mild bruising

Interactions
- increased risk of QT prolongation if given with agents known to prolong QT interval (e.g. Class IA and Class III antiarrhythmic agents (e.g. amiodarone, sotalol))

Nursing considerations/Cautions
- flare phenomenon/reaction can be reduced by use of non-steroidal antiandrogen agent
- blood glucose levels and glycosylated haemoglobin (HbA1c) should be monitored regularly during therapy
- serum testosterone and prostate-specific antigen levels should be measured regularly during therapy
- (CPP) must be diagnosed and therapy supervised by paediatric endocrinologist
- rotate injection sites
- depot preparations have different release properties and are not interchangeable, nor should part doses be used
- manufacturer's instructions should be followed for preparation and administration of depot preparations
- (Eligard) product should be allowed to come to room temperature before reconstitution (to reduce pain) and then used within 30 minutes
- caution if used in men with urinary tract obstruction or metastatic vertebral lesions, epilepsy, history of seizures, CNS disorders or tumours
- caution if used in those with or at risk of QT prolongation, electrolyte abnormalities or congestive cardiac failure

Patient education
- the patient should receive adequate education in correct use of equipment, correct SC injection technique, importance of rotating sites, storage information and safe disposal of used equipment before self-administration can begin
- patients with pre-existing diabetes mellitus should be warned that there may be a loss of glycaemic control and blood glucose levels should be monitored frequently, especially at start of therapy
- warn the patient that symptoms (especially bone pain) may initially worsen in first 1 to 2 weeks of therapy (especially if bony metastases are present)
- advise the patient to seek medical advice immediately if any of the following occur:
    - any sudden headache, visual disturbance, vomiting or altered mental state
    - weakness, tingling or numbness of arms or legs
    - blood in the urine or difficulty passing urine
    - chest pain or irregular heart rate
- warn the patient against driving or operating machinery if dizziness, vertigo, fatigue or paraesthesia occur

 Contraindicated during pregnancy.

 Contraindicated when breastfeeding.

 Banned in sport; females may be exempt but caution advised.

1220

HYPOTHALAMIC AND PITUITARY HORMONES

GROWTH HORMONE RELEASE-INHIBITING FACTOR

General Adverse effects of growth hormone release-inhibiting factor
- (Injection site, transient) redness, swelling, stinging, pain, burning, irritation, rash
- anorexia, nausea, vomiting, abdominal pain, bloating, flatulence, dyspepsia, loose stools, diarrhoea, constipation, discolouration of stools, steatorrhoea, decreased weight
- impaired glucose tolerance, hyperglycaemia, hypoglycaemia
- thyroid dysfunction, hypothyroidism
- headache, dizziness, weakness, fatigue, asthenia
- pruritus, rash, transient alopecia
- bradycardia
- reduced gallbladder motility, cholelithiasis, elevated liver enzymes, decreased pancreatic enzymes

General Interactions of growth hormone release-inhibiting factor
- may decrease or delay absorption of ciclosporin
- dose of insulin/oral hypoglycaemic agents may need adjustment when therapy is commenced
- increased risk of bradycardia if given with beta adrenoceptor blocking agents or other agents that decrease heart rate
- caution if given with agents that have a low therapeutic index

General Patient education for growth hormone release-inhibiting factor
- the patient should receive adequate education in correct use of equipment, correct SC injection technique, the importance of rotating sites, storage information and safe disposal of used equipment before self-administration can begin
- the patient with diabetes mellitus should be advised to closely monitor blood glucose levels during therapy as there is an increased risk of hypo- or hyperglycaemia
- warn the patient to avoid driving or operating machinery if dizziness or weakness occurs
- instruct the patient to seek medical advice immediately if any of the following occur:
  - feeling more thirsty or tired than usual, dry mouth
  - feeling hungry, shaky or sweating more than usual, confusion
  - severe or sudden abdominal pain, high fever, yellowing of skin or eyes, loss of appetite, itchy skin
  - slow heart rate
  - any sudden headache, visual disturbance, vomiting or altered mental state

LANREOTIDE
Trade names
Mytolac, Somatuline Autogel

Available forms
Prefilled syringe (prolonged-release solution): 60 mg/0.5 mL, 90 mg/0.5 mL, 120 mg/0.5 mL

Action
- somatostatin analogue with a long duration of action
- inhibits secretion of growth hormone (GH), serotonin and gastroenteropancreatic (GEP) peptides (gastrin, insulin, glucagon, secretin, motilin, pancreatic polypeptide and vasoactive intestinal peptide)
- inhibits secretion of insulin and glucagon

Use
- acromegaly (after surgery and/or radiotherapy where GH and insulin-like growth factor 1 (IGF-1) levels remain high or unresponsive to dopamine agonist treatment)
- carcinoid tumour

- management of symptoms of GEP neuroendocrine tumours (unresectable, locally advanced or metastatic disease)

Dose
Acromegaly
- (Not previously treated) initially 60 mg SC every 28 days, then dose increased or decreased according to GH/IGF-1 levels

Carcinoid tumour
- 60—120 mg SC every 28 days, with dose adjusted according to response

GEP neuroendocrine tumours
- 120 mg SC every 28 days

Adverse effects
- myalgia, musculoskeletal pain
- see also General Adverse effects of growth hormone release-inhibiting factor (p. 1221)

Interactions
- see General Interactions of growth hormone release-inhibiting factor (p. 1221)

Nursing considerations/Cautions
- gallbladder ultrasound is recommended when starting therapy and then 6-monthly
- thyroid function tests are recommended if there are any signs of decreasing thyroid function during therapy
- (Carcinoid tumour) obstructive intestinal tumour should be excluded before starting therapy
- should be given deep SC into upper outer quadrant of buttocks or, if self-administered, the upper outer thigh
- blood glucose levels should be monitored when starting therapy or adjusting dose (especially in those with pre-existing diabetes)
- kidney and liver function monitoring is recommended in those with renal/hepatic dysfunction
- heart rate monitoring is recommended in those with underlying cardiac disease
- caution if used in those with bradycardia

Patient education
- see General Patient education for growth hormone release-inhibiting factor (p. 1221)

 Not recommended when pregnant because limited studies in humans are available.

 Contraindicated when breastfeeding.

OCTREOTIDE
Trade names
Octreotide Acetate Omega, Octreotide GH, Octreotide Sun, Sandostatin, Sandostatin LAR

Available forms
Vial/Prefilled syringes (modified-release solution): 10 mg, 20 mg, 30 mg;
Vial: 0.05 mg/mL, 0.1 mg/mL, 0.5 mg/mL

Action
- synthetic analogue of somatostatin (growth hormone (GH) inhibitor) with prolonged duration of action
- inhibits secretion of GH, serotonin and gastroenteropancreatic (GEP) peptides (gastrin, insulin, glucagon, secretin, motilin, pancreatic polypeptide and vasoactive intestinal peptide)

Use
- treatment of acromegaly (inadequately controlled by surgery, radiotherapy or dopamine agonists, unfit or unwilling to undergo surgery, or until radiotherapy becomes fully effective)
- management of symptoms of GEP endocrine tumours (e.g. carcinoid tumours and vasoactive intestinal peptide-secreting tumours)
- reduction of complications post-pancreatic surgery
- treatment of advanced neuroendocrine tumours of midgut

HYPOTHALAMIC AND PITUITARY HORMONES

Dose
Acromegaly
- initially 0.05—0.1 mg SC 8—12-hourly, then dose adjusted monthly depending on clinical symptoms, tolerance and GH and/or insulin-like growth factors (IGF) (maximum daily dose 1.5 mg) **OR**
- (Patients controlled with octreotide SC) 20 mg IM monthly for 3 months, starting the day after octreotide SC, then reducing to 10 mg monthly (if symptoms are controlled) or increasing to 30 mg monthly (if symptoms are only partially controlled) (modified-release preparation)

GEP endocrine tumour
- initially 0.05 mg SC 1—2 times daily, increasing gradually to 0.2 mg 3 times daily (depending on tolerance and clinical response) **OR**
- (Patients controlled with octreotide SC) 20 mg IM monthly for 3 months with previous SC dose for first 2 weeks of therapy with modified-release preparation, then reduced to 10 mg monthly (if symptoms controlled) or increased to 30 mg monthly (if symptoms only partially controlled) (modified-release preparation) **OR**
- (Patients not previously treated with octreotide) 0.1 mg SC 3 times daily for 2 weeks, then assess suitability for modified-release preparation

Complications after pancreatic surgery
- 0.1 mg SC 3 times daily for 7 consecutive days starting 1 hour before surgery

Advanced neuroendocrine tumour of midgut
- 30 mg IM monthly (modified-release preparation)

Adverse effects
- dyspnoea
- (Prolonged use) biliary sludge, hyperbilirubinaemia, decreased vitamin B_{12} levels, thrombocytopenia
- (Rare) hypersensitivity, acute pancreatitis, liver/biliary dysfunction, QT prolongation, arrhythmias, ECG changes, increase in size of pre-existing GH-secreting pituitary tumour
- see also General Adverse effects of growth hormone release-inhibiting factor (p. 1221)

Interactions
- may increase bioavailability of bromocriptine
- caution if given with agents that prolong QT interval (e.g. disopyramide, amiodarone, sotalol, some antipsychotic agents, some antibacterial agents (e.g. IV erythromycin, pentamidine, clarithromycin), antifungal agents or some antihistamines) or agents that cause hypokalaemia or hypomagnesaemia (e.g. diuretics)
- see also General Interactions of growth hormone release-inhibiting factors (p. 1221)

Nursing considerations/Cautions
- gallbladder ultrasound is recommended before starting therapy and at 6—12-month intervals and any symptomatic gallstones treated
- (Acromegaly) those not previously treated with octreotide should be commenced on SC preparation to assess response, then switched to IM preparation
- (Acromegaly) monthly assessment of GH and/or IGF-1 levels, clinical symptoms and biochemical markers should occur. If no change after 3 months, therapy should be stopped
- (GEP endocrine tumours) SC doses may be required in addition to IM modified preparation for first 8 weeks of therapy until therapeutic levels are reached and symptoms are controlled
- (Sandostatin LAR) allow the provided diluent and vial to come to room temperature, then the diluent should be injected slowly down the side of the vial (but not directly onto the powder), allow

2–5 minutes undisturbed (or longer if needed) for powder to become wet, then swirl very gently to form an even, milky suspension. Withdraw the required amount without inverting the vial. Change the needle before IM administration
- rotate injection sites
- IM injection into deltoid muscle is not recommended because of pain and discomfort
- (Long-term therapy) thyroid function, blood glucose levels and vitamin B_{12} levels should be monitored regularly in those with a history of or at risk of vitamin B_{12} deficiency
- patient should be monitored regularly for any signs or symptoms of the GH-secreting tumour increasing in size (e.g. visual field defects)
- caution if used in those with cardiovascular disease, history of gallstones or vitamin B_{12} deficiency, or those with concurrent bleeding gastro-oesophageal varices
- caution if used in those with liver cirrhosis, as half-life may be increased

Patient education

- if the patient is experiencing gastrointestinal adverse effects, suggest injecting between meals and at bedtime to reduce them
- female patients treated for acromegaly should be advised that fertility may be restored during therapy and contraception should be used to avoid pregnancy if not wanted
- see also General Patient education for growth hormone release-inhibiting factor (p. 1221)

Not recommended when pregnant because of limited studies in humans available.

Contraindicated when breastfeeding.

This drug may fall into a category that is banned in sports; caution advised.

PASIREOTIDE
Trade names
Signifor, Signifor LAR

Available forms
Ampoule (for SC injection): 300 microgram/mL, 600 microgram/mL, 900 microgram/mL; Vial (for IM injection): 20 mg, 40 mg, 60 mg

Action
- somatostatin analogue
- has a high binding affinity for four of the five human somatostatin receptor subtypes, which are expressed in many tissues, especially neuroendocrine tumours (secreting hormones such as adrenocorticotrophic hormone (ACTH) in Cushing's syndrome)

Use
- treatment of adults with Cushing's syndrome where surgery has failed or is unsuitable
- treatment of adults with acromegaly where surgery is not an option or has not been curative or inadequately controlled with other somatostatin analogues

Dose
- (Cushing's syndrome) initially 600 micrograms or 900 micrograms SC twice daily, then dose titrated to 300–900 micrograms SC twice daily **OR**
- (Acromegaly) initially 40 mg IM every 4 weeks, increasing to 60 mg if growth hormone (GH) and/or insulin-like growth factor 1 (IGF-1) levels are not controlled after 12 weeks, or decreased by 20 mg increments if adverse reactions or over-response to treatment (IGF-1 < lower normal limit) occur (modified-release preparation)

Adverse effects
- myalgia, arthralgia, back pain, muscle spasm
- fever
- nasopharyngitis, bronchitis, influenza, upper respiratory tract infection, cough, oropharyngeal pain
- hypokalaemia
- prolonged QT interval

HYPOTHALAMIC AND PITUITARY HORMONES

- hypocortisolism
- see also General Adverse effects of growth hormone release-inhibiting factors (p. 1221)

Interactions

- may increase availability of bromocriptine
- increased serum levels may occur if given with ciclosporin, verapamil and clarithromycin
- caution if given with agents that prolong QT interval (e.g. disopyramide, amiodarone, sotalol, some antipsychotic agents, some antibacterial agents (e.g. IV erythromycin, pentamidine, clarithromycin), antifungal agents or some antihistamines) or agents that cause hypokalaemia or hypomagnesaemia (e.g. diuretics)
- see also General Interactions of growth hormone release-inhibiting factors (p. 1221)

Nursing considerations/Cautions

- any hypokalaemia or hypomagnesaemia should be corrected before starting therapy
- baseline ECG is recommended before starting and then after 21 days of therapy
- blood glucose levels (BGL) (HbA1c and/or fasting plasma glucose levels) should be measured before starting therapy, then weekly for 8–12 weeks, then regularly afterwards
- cortisol levels should be closely monitored during therapy, especially in the first 8 weeks, as temporary glucocorticoid therapy or interruption of pasireotide therapy may be required if hypocortisolism occurs
- electrolyte levels (especially potassium and magnesium) and pituitary function (e.g. thyroid-stimulating hormone (TSH), free thyroxine (T4), GH, IGF-1) should be measured before starting and then regularly during therapy
- liver function should be monitored before starting, then after first 2–3 weeks, monthly for 3 months and then regularly during therapy. If transaminases are elevated (after second test to confirm results), more frequent monitoring is recommended until pretreatment levels are reached. If jaundice or other signs of liver impairment develop, therapy should be stopped
- heart rate should be monitored (especially at the start of therapy and if patient is taking other agents that cause bradycardia)
- (Cushing's syndrome) response to therapy (decrease in urinary free cortisol and/or improvement in signs and symptoms) should be determined after 8 weeks
- if the patient has uncontrolled diabetes mellitus, intense antidiabetic therapy is recommended before starting pasireotide therapy. Additional BGL monitoring is also suggested
- if hyperglycaemia develops during therapy, antidiabetic therapy should be started or adjusted to control BGL. If hyperglycaemia persists, pasireotide dose should be reduced or therapy stopped
- (Cushing's syndrome) dose should be started at 300 micrograms twice daily for those with moderate liver impairment to a maximum of 600 micrograms twice daily
- (Cushing's syndrome) a starting dose of 600 mg twice daily should be considered for those with diabetes mellitus
- (Cushing's syndrome) patient can be instructed to self-inject
- (Acromegaly) IM injection sites should be alternated between left and right gluteal muscles
- (Acromegaly) injection kit (powder, prefilled syringe containing diluent, vial adapter and injection needle) should be allowed to come to room temperature for at least 30 minutes before administration
- (Acromegaly) manufacturer's instructions should be followed to reconstitute the solution, including shaking the vial

in a horizontal position for at least 30 seconds after addition of diluent
* (Acromegaly) to avoid sedimentation occurring, the syringe may be shaken gently to maintain a uniform suspension
* caution if the patient has poor glycaemic control (HbA1c > 8%), as there is an increased risk of severe hyperglycaemia and ketoacidosis
* caution and monitoring is recommended if the patient has cardiac disease and/or risk factors for bradycardia (e.g. a history of clinically significant bradycardia or acute myocardial infarction, high-grade heart block, congestive cardiac failure, unstable angina, ventricular tachycardia/fibrillation)
* caution if used in those at risk of QT prolongation including congenital long QT syndrome, or uncontrolled or significant cardiac disease
* not recommended for treatment of paediatric Cushing's syndrome or in those under 18 years
* contraindicated in those with severe liver impairment

Patient education
* advise the patient to seek medical advice immediately if any of the following occur:
  * weakness, fatigue, loss of appetite, nausea, vomiting, hypotension (light-headedness, dizziness or fainting), hyponatraemia (nausea, vomiting, headache, confusion, loss of energy and fatigue, irritability, restlessness, muscle weakness/cramps/spasms or fitting), hypoglycaemia (cool pale skin, fatigue, drowsiness, unusual tiredness, sweating, shaking, anxiety, crying, vomiting, headache, excessive hunger, visual changes, palpitations, confusion)
* see also General Patient education for growth hormone release-inhibiting factor (p. 1221)

 Should be used during pregnancy only if benefits outweigh risks.

 Not recommended when breastfeeding owing to limited human data available.

PEGVISOMANT
Trade name
Somavert

Available forms
Vial: 10 mg, 15 mg, 20 mg

Action
* growth hormone (GH) analogue that has been structurally altered to produce GH receptor antagonist, which binds to GH receptor sites blocking endogenous GH from binding, resulting in decreased levels of insulin-like growth factor 1 (IGF-1)
* protein is bonded to propylene glycol

Use
* acromegaly (in patient with inadequate response to surgery, radiation or medical therapy or where these therapies are inappropriate)

Dose
* initially 80 mg SC (loading dose), then 10 mg SC daily, with dose adjustments of 5 mg daily according to serum IGF-1 (daily maximum 30 mg)

Adverse effects
* injection site reaction
* chest pain, peripheral oedema
* pain, back pain
* dizziness, paraesthesia
* hypertension
* diarrhoea, nausea
* influenza, sinusitis, respiratory infections
* abnormal liver function
* rash, erythema, pruritus, urticaria
* (Rare) increase in size of pre-existing GH-secreting pituitary tumour

Interactions
* caution if used with opioids as higher doses of pegvisomant may be required

in order to achieve appropriate IGF-1 suppression
- dose of insulin or oral hypoglycaemic agent may require adjustment especially at the start of therapy

Nursing considerations/Cautions

- before starting therapy, patient should have liver function tests and not start if any signs of liver disease are present. Liver function tests are recommended at least every 6 months after IGF-1 levels have become normal
- serum IGF-1 level should be measured before starting therapy, then every 4–6 weeks
- because pegvisomant is structurally similar to GH and may cross-react in commercially available assays, serum GH levels should not be used to monitor treatment. Dose adjustments should only be based on serum IGF-1 levels
- reconstitute using 1 mL water for injections (provided)
- SC injection sites should be rotated daily to prevent lipohypertrophy
- caution if used in the elderly or those with diabetes mellitus

Patient education

- see General Patient education for growth hormone release-inhibiting factor (p. 1221)

Caution if used during breastfeeding, as limited data are available.

GROWTH HORMONE

SOMATROGON
Trade name
Ngenla

Available forms
Prefilled pen: 24 mg/1.2 mL, 60 mg/1.2 mL

Action
- long-acting recombinant human growth hormone (HGH) designed to mimic the effects of natural growth hormone (GH) in the body
- promotes skeletal and cell (increasing number and size of muscle cells) growth
- stimulates protein, carbohydrate, mineral and lipid metabolism

Use
- to improve growth in children who have low levels of GH

Dose
- Child: 0.66 mg/kg weekly given via subcutaneous injection

Adverse effects
- (Injection site) pain, redness, swelling, headaches and febrile illness
- (Common) hyperglycaemia, rash
- (Uncommon) adrenal insufficiency, generalised rash

Interactions
- this is a new drug so unreported interactions may occur

Nursing considerations/Cautions

- safety of somatrogon has not been established in patients under 3 years of age
- monitor growth rate closely in the first year of treatment, regular monitoring of insulin-like growth factor-1 (IGF-1) concentrations is recommended during treatment
- must be given only via subcutaneous injection (abdomen, thighs, buttocks or upper arms), rotating the site weekly
- contraindicated in patients with active tumours and/or malignancy
- contraindicated for growth promotion if epiphyses are closed
- watch for limping, as this may indicate development of a slipped capital epiphysis

Patient education

- the patient should receive adequate education in correct use of equipment, correct injection technique, importance of rotating sites, storage information

- and safe disposal of used equipment before self-administration can begin
- the patient should not shake the pen, as shaking can damage the medicine
- the patient should take the medication at the same time each week, and not take double doses to make up for a missed dose
- if travelling, the patient should keep medication in an insulated container with ice brick

 Not recommended when breastfeeding, as insufficient human data are available.

SOMATROPIN (SOMATOTROPHIN/ SOMATOTROPIN)
Trade names
Genotropin, Genotropin GoQuick, Genotropin MiniQuick, Norditropin FlexPro, Omnitrope, Saizen, SciTropin A

Available forms
Prefilled pen: 5 mg/1.5 mL, 6 mg/1.03 mL, 10 mg/1.5 mL, 12 mg/1.5 mL, 15 mg/1.5 mL, 20 mg/2.5 mL;
Cartridge solution: 5 mg/1.5 mL, 10 mg/1.5 mL;
Cartridge (with syringe of diluting solution): 6 mg, 12 mg, 20 mg;
Two-compartment cartridge (with preservative): 5 mg, 12 mg;
Two-compartment cartridge (without preservative): 0.4 mg, 0.6 mg, 0.8 mg, 1 mg, 1.2 mg, 1.4 mg, 1.6 mg, 1.8 mg, 2 mg;
Vial: 3 mg, 4 mg, 8 mg, 10 mg

Action
- human growth hormone (GH) is normally secreted at night during sleep, promoting growth through action of insulin-like growth factors (IGF)
- synthetic human GH produced by recombinant DNA technology with therapeutic equivalence to human GH
- normalises insulin-like growth factor 1 (IGF-1)
- promotes skeletal and cell (increasing number and size of muscle cells) growth
- stimulates protein, carbohydrate, mineral and lipid metabolism
- increases retention of sodium, potassium and phosphorus
- gender differences, with adult females requiring higher doses than males for GH deficiency
- choose the appropriate patient, dose and management; only to be undertaken by those specialised in this field
- special approval is required for the prescribing of this medication
- 1 mg = 3 IU

Use
- decreased or failed secretion of pituitary GH, resulting in short stature
- growth disturbance associated with gonadal dysgenesis (Turner's syndrome)
- adults with severe deficiency of GH
- paediatric patients with Prader–Willi syndrome (to treat short stature and improve body composition)
- growth disturbance in children with chronic renal insufficiency (height or growth velocity ≤ 25th percentile)

Dose
- (Children, GH deficiency) initially 0.175–0.255 mg/kg/week SC divided into either 7 daily doses, 6 doses or 3 doses given on alternate days, then gradually titrated to desired response (maximum weekly dose 0.26 mg/kg) **OR**
- (Adults, GH deficiency) initially 0.04 mg/kg/week SC divided into 7 daily doses, then increased gradually to maximum dose 0.08 mg/kg/week **OR**
- (Turner's syndrome) 0.3–0.35 mg/kg/week SC divided into 6–7 daily doses, preferably in the evening (with concurrent sex steroid therapy) **OR**
- (Turner's syndrome) 0.045–0.05 mg/kg/day SC, increasing dose in following year if response is not satisfactory **OR**
- (Prader–Willi syndrome) 0.035–0.05 mg/kg SC daily **OR**

HYPOTHALAMIC AND PITUITARY HORMONES

- (Chronic renal insufficiency) 0.045–0.05 mg/kg SC daily (up to the time of renal transplant)

Adverse effects
- (Injection site) pain, redness, swelling
- (Adults, common) paraesthesia/abnormal sensation, muscle stiffness, peripheral oedema, facial oedema, arthralgia, myalgia, localised muscle pain, hyperglycaemia (mild), dyspnoea, sleep apnoea, hypertension, carpal tunnel syndrome, insomnia, gynaecomastia
- (Adults, uncommon) headache, muscle weakness, glycosuria
- (Children) scoliosis, slipped epiphysis of hip, mild transient urticaria at the injection site, mild and transient oedema
- (Children, uncommon) muscle stiffness, arthralgia, myalgia, peripheral oedema
- (Turner's syndrome) otitis media, ear disorders, hypothyroidism, peripheral oedema
- antibody formation
- rash, pruritus, urticaria
- (Rare) lipoatrophy (SC), antibody formation
- (Rare) myositis, benign intracranial hypertension, diabetes mellitus
- (Very rare, children) leukaemia, pancreatitis, gynaecomastia

Interactions
- large doses of glucocorticoids may inhibit growth promotion effects
- dose adjustment of insulin or oral hypoglycaemic agents may be necessary
- caution if used with thyroid hormones, as GH preparations may alter triiodothyronine (T3) and thyroxine (T4) concentrations
- larger dose may be required in adult women on oral oestrogen therapy
- may decrease plasma levels of ciclosporin, some antiepileptic agents and sex steroids

Nursing considerations/Cautions
- before starting therapy, pituitary function (including provocation tests) should be investigated thoroughly
- fasting insulin and IGF-1 levels should be measured before starting therapy and then twice yearly
- urine testing and/or blood glucose levels should be monitored regularly in all patients (as insulin resistance can occur with GH therapy). If the patient is at risk of developing diabetes, oral glucose tolerance testing is also recommended
- regular growth monitoring and measuring of biochemical markers are recommended throughout therapy
- any other pituitary hormone deficiencies or pituitary tumours should be treated before starting therapy (especially in adults)
- any antitumour therapy should be completed before starting therapy with somatotropin
- thyroid function test is recommended after start of therapy, along with any dose adjustment (especially in those receiving treatment with thyroid hormones), as hypothyroidism can develop with therapy
- if GH deficiency is due to malignant disease treatment, the patient should be closely monitored for any malignancy relapse
- (Childhood GH deficiency) GH level should be retested before starting treatment as an adult
- may also be given IM, although SC is the preferred route
- (Prader–Willi syndrome) diagnosis should be confirmed by genetic testing before starting therapy
- (Prader–Willi syndrome) evaluation of any upper respiratory obstruction and sleep apnoea should occur before starting therapy. Therapy should be interrupted if any signs of airway obstruction, including onset or worsening of snoring
- (Prader–Willi syndrome) any respiratory infection should be diagnosed as soon as symptoms appear and treated aggressively

- (Prader—Willi syndrome) a calorie-controlled diet is also recommended with GH therapy
- (Turner's syndrome) girls should have regular ear examinations, including hearing tests, as they have an increased risk of ear or hearing disorders
- (Chronic renal insufficiency) conservative treatment for renal insufficiency should be established and maintained before starting therapy
- (Chronic renal insufficiency) growth retardation should be established for at least 1 year before starting therapy
- (Chronic renal insufficiency) treatment should be stopped if renal transplantation is to occur
- reconstitution should be with provided diluents and according to manufacturer's instructions
- some solutions are stable for 14—28 days after reconstitution if refrigerated at 2—8°C. However, some need to be used within 24 hours of reconstitution. It is important to read and follow the manufacturer's instructions with regard to storage requirements
- do not shake the vial vigorously, as protein will be denatured
- (Genotropin) bioequivalence between formulations has not been demonstrated
- (Humatrope) not indicated for use in those with Prader—Willi syndrome
- caution if used in those who have had renal allograft (who have experienced two or more episodes of rejection), as there is an increased risk of kidney rejection
- caution if used in those with diabetes mellitus due to decreased insulin sensitivity and glucose intolerance. Any existing antidiabetic therapy may require adjustment
- (Humatrope, Genotropin) contraindicated in those with known sensitivity to metacresol or glycerol
- contraindicated in those with evidence of active tumours, children with closed epiphyses, acute respiratory failure, active proliferative or severe non-proliferative diabetic retinopathy, acute critical illness (following trauma, burns or surgery), or those with Prader—Willi syndrome (with severe obesity or severe respiratory impairment, including sleep apnoea)

Patient education

- the patient should receive adequate education in correct use of the equipment (differs from brand to brand), correct injection technique, the importance of rotating sites, storage information and safe disposal of used equipment before self-administration can begin
- the parent/carer should be advised to observe children for any limping (which may indicate slipped epiphyses of the hip)
- instruct the patient to seek medical advice if any of the following occur:
  - any muscle pain or severe pain at the injection site (disproportional to injection) (as this may require changing to a metacresol-free preparation)
  - any nausea/vomiting, severe or recurrent headaches or visual problems (signs of intracranial hypertension)
  - weakness or numbness of legs or arms
- female patients taking oral oestrogen therapy should be advised not to stop oestrogen therapy suddenly without seeking medical advice

 Used during pregnancy only if clearly needed, as limited data are available.

 Used when breastfeeding only if benefit outweighs the risks, as limited data are available.

 Banned in sport.

SOMATOSTATIN ANALOGUES

ANTIDIURETIC HORMONE (ADH)

ARGIPRESSIN
Trade names
Pitressin, Argipressin Medsurge

Available form
Ampoule: 20 U (pressor units)/mL

Action
- direct antidiuretic action on the distal renal tubule by increasing permeability to water reabsorption
- causes contraction of smooth muscle of the GI tract and vascular bed (especially capillaries, small arterioles and venules)

Use
- symptomatic control of diabetes insipidus
- prevention and control of abdominal distension
- dispelling gas shadows in abdominal X-rays

Dose
- (Abdominal distension) initially 0.25 mL (5 units) IM or SC, increasing to 0.5 mL (10 units) if needed, given 3—4-hourly **OR**
- (Abdominal radiography) 0.5 mL (10 units) IM or SC given twice, once at 2 hours, then 30 minutes before films are exposed **OR**
- (Diabetes insipidus) 0.25—0.5 mL (5—10 units) IM or SC 2—3 times daily

Adverse effects
- pallor
- nausea, vomiting, abdominal cramping, flatulence
- tremor, sweating, pounding in head, vertigo
- urticaria, bronchial constriction
- arrhythmias, angina, peripheral vasoconstriction
- (Rare) water intoxication, anaphylaxis (shortly after injection), gangrene

Interactions
- antidiuretic effect may be potentiated by carbamazepine, urea, fludrocortisone or tricyclic antidepressants (TCAs)
- antidiuretic effect may be reduced by noradrenaline (norepinephrine), lithium, heparin or alcohol
- caution if given with H_2 antagonists, as bradycardia and heart block may occur

Nursing considerations/Cautions
- the patient should be closely monitored for any signs of anaphylaxis after administration
- should not be given by IV administration
- SC or IM doses should not exceed 0.75 mL
- (Radiology) enema before first dose may be recommended by radiologist
- caution if given to those with epilepsy, migraine, asthma, toxaemia associated with pregnancy, nephritis (with arterial hypertension), goitre (with cardiac complications), coronary thrombosis, angina or arteriosclerosis
- not recommended in those with vascular disease, especially coronary artery disease, as angina or myocardial infarction may be precipitated (depending on dose)
- contraindicated in those with chronic nephritis (with nitrogen retention)

Patient education
- the patient should be advised to immediately report any drowsiness, listlessness or headache (signs of water intoxication)
- warn the patient to avoid driving or operating machinery if vertigo, pounding in head or tremor occurs

 Not recommended during pregnancy because of limited data available.

 Not recommended during breastfeeding unless benefits outweigh risks because of limited data available.

Banned in sport.

DESMOPRESSIN
Trade names
Minirin Melt, Minirin Tablets, Nocdurna

DESMOPRESSIN ACETATE
Trade names
Minirin Injection, Minirin Nasal Spray, Octostim Injection

Available forms
Metered-dose nasal spray: 10 microgram/dose;
Tablets: 200 microgram;
Ampoules: 4 microgram/mL, 15 microgram/mL;
Sublingual wafers: 25 microgram, 50 microgram, 60 microgram, 120 microgram, 240 microgram

Action
- synthetic analogue of vasopressin, but with greater antidiuretic activity, more prolonged action and less pressor activity
- acts on renal collecting tubules, increasing permeability to water reabsorption
- high doses increase factor VIII coagulant activity and von Willebrand factor activity, and also release of plasminogen activator
- reduces skin bleeding time by unknown mechanisms
- slight oxytocic effect
- vasodilatory effect reducing BP

Use
- diabetes insipidus
- nocturia due to nocturnal polyuria (in adults who wake ≥ 2 times per night, unresponsive to lifestyle measures)
- diagnostically to determine renal concentrating capacity
- before dental or minor surgery in mild and moderate haemophilia A and von Willebrand disease to increase factor VIII levels
- bleeding in patients with platelet dysfunction (e.g. congenital or drug-induced dysfunction)
- primary nocturnal enuresis (in those aged 6 or more who are refractory to enuresis alarm)

Dose
- (Diabetes insipidus) 10—40 micrograms intranasally daily or in 2 divided doses **OR**
- (Diabetes insipidus) 1—4 micrograms IM or IV daily or in 2 divided doses (Minirin) **OR**
- (Diabetes insipidus) initially 100 micrograms orally 3 times daily, increasing dose according to response, then 100—200 micrograms 3 times daily (maintenance) **OR**
- (Diabetes insipidus) initially 60 micrograms sublingually 3 times daily, then 60—120 micrograms 3 times daily (maintenance) **OR**
- (Diagnostic) 40 micrograms intranasally as a single dose **OR**
- (Diagnostic) 4 micrograms IM as a single dose (Minirin) **OR**
- (Nocturnal enuresis) initially 20 micrograms intranasally at night, then adjusting dose as needed to 10—40 micrograms (maintenance) **OR**
- (Nocturnal enuresis) initially 120 micrograms sublingually at night, increasing to 240 micrograms if needed **OR**
- (Nocturnal enuresis) initially 200 micrograms orally at bedtime, increasing to 400 micrograms if needed **OR**
- (Adult nocturia) 25 micrograms (women) or 50 micrograms (men) sublingually daily 1 hour before bed (Nocdurna) **OR**
- (Mild-to-moderate bleeding — haemophilia A or von Willebrand disease) 0.4 microgram/kg IV, diluted to 10—100 mL with sodium chloride 0.9% and infused

HYPOTHALAMIC AND PITUITARY HORMONES

over 15—20 minutes 30 minutes before procedure (with tranexamic acid). This may be repeated 12-hourly if cover is needed and response is adequate **OR**
- (Non-surgical bleeding in patients with platelet dysfunction) 0.3 microgram/kg IV, diluted to 50 mL with sodium chloride 0.9% and infused over 30 minutes (RBC transfusion may also be given to improve haemostasis in uraemic patients). This may be repeated 12-hourly if cover is needed and response is adequate **OR**
- (Before general surgery (except cardiac surgery) in patients with platelet dysfunction) 0.3 microgram/kg IV, diluted to 50 mL with sodium chloride 0.9% and infused over 30 minutes, given 30 minutes before surgery **OR**
- (Before cardiac surgery in patients with platelet dysfunction) 0.3 microgram/kg IV, diluted to 50 mL with sodium chloride 0.9% and infused over 30 minutes when cardiopulmonary bypass is complete and protamine has been given

Adverse effects
- (Diabetes insipidus) headache, cold, increased weight, dizziness, sore throat, depression
- (Nocturnal enuresis) headache, respiratory disorders, coughing, sore throat, nasal congestion, asthma, vomiting, abdominal pain and cramping, nausea, diarrhoea, fever, flu-like symptoms, allergy, earache, ear infection
- (Nasal preparations) headache, nausea, abdominal pain, nasal congestion, rhinitis, flushing, nosebleed, upper respiratory infection, insomnia, nightmares, aggression, nervousness, labile mood
- (Rare) water intoxication, hyponatraemia, oedema

Interactions
- additive antidiuretic effects may result if given with tricyclic antidepressants (TCAs), selective serotonin reuptake inhibitors (SSRIs), chlorpromazine, carbamazepine or sulfonylurea antidiabetic agents, increasing the risk of water retention and hyponatraemia
- NSAIDs may induce water retention and hyponatraemia; therefore increased effect may be expected if given together
- increased plasma levels may occur if given with loperamide
- magnitude (not duration) of response may be increased if given with indometacin

Nursing considerations/Cautions
- fluid balance should be restored before starting therapy and therapy not started if the patient is dehydrated or overhydrated
- (Haemophilia) fluid restriction is required and the patient should be weighed daily. If weight increases gradually or there is a decrease in serum sodium (< 130 mmol/L) or plasma osmolality (< 270 mOsm/kg), further fluid restriction will be required and therapy interrupted
- bladder dysfunction and outlet obstruction should be investigated and ruled out as the cause of primary nocturnal enuresis before starting therapy
- if the patient becomes acutely unwell during therapy (e.g. systemic infection, fever, gastroenteritis) leading to electrolyte and/or fluid imbalance, therapy should be stopped
- (Diabetes insipidus) dose is determined by adequate sleep and adequate, but not excessive, water turnover
- (Diagnostic purpose) fluid should be restricted to 500 mL for 1 hour before and 8 hours after administration
- (Diabetes insipidus) serum and urinary sodium and osmolality should be closely monitored during therapy
- (Diabetes insipidus) if the patient develops headache, nausea/vomiting, weight gain (and convulsions in severe cases), therapy should be stopped, the dose adjusted and fluids restricted

- (signs and symptoms of water intoxication and hyponatraemia)
- (Diabetes insipidus) usually given as 2 divided doses, but a single dose may be administered if the patient tolerates it and diabetes insipidus is controlled adequately
- (Platelet dysfunction) skin bleeding time should be monitored before surgery and during therapy. Prolonged bleeding may indicate a risk of increased blood loss
- (Nocturnal enuresis) serum electrolytes should be monitored if therapy continues for more than 7 days
- (Nocturnal enuresis, nasal preparations) therapy should be interrupted if the patient has nasal infection and/or rhinorrhoea, as therapy may be ineffective or unreliable
- (Nocturnal enuresis) therapy should be continued for 4–12 weeks and then stopped for 1 week to establish the effectiveness of treatment
- baseline blood tests (VIII:C or VIIIR:Ag assays) should be carried out before and repeated 20 minutes after infusion for haemophilia A or von Willebrand disease
- IV/IM dose is 1/10th of intranasal dose
- 15 microgram/mL solution is recommended for IV use only
- caution should be taken to prevent hyponatraemia from occurring, especially in those at high risk (e.g. those with cystic fibrosis or cardiac failure, at risk of intracranial pressure, elderly patients or those taking medications that may affect fluid balance or induce syndrome of inappropriate secretion of antidiuretic hormone)
- caution is used in those with other causes of urinary frequency (e.g. multiple sclerosis, urge incontinence) or in those with diabetes mellitus or kidney impairment (creatinine clearance < 50 mL/min)
- not recommended in patients who are dehydrated or overhydrated
- (Minirin tablets) contain lactose and are therefore not recommended in those with Lapp lactase deficiency, rare hereditary problems of galactose intolerance or glucose–galactose malabsorption
- contraindicated to treat bleeding in patients with type IIB von Willebrand disease
- contraindicated in those with psychogenic/habitual polydipsia (resulting in urine output > 40 mL/kg/24 hours), hyponatraemia, moderate/severe kidney insufficiency (creatinine clearance < 50 mL/min), syndrome of inappropriate secretion of antidiuretic hormone (SIADH) or cardiac insufficiency or other conditions requiring diuretic therapy

Patient education

- advise the patient to immediately report any sudden or severe headache, lethargy, malaise, dizziness, confusion, blackouts, fitting, nausea/vomiting or sudden weight gain (signs of water retention)
- (Nasal spray) patients with nasal infections or rhinorrhoea (runny nose) should be instructed to stop therapy until the condition resolves, as intranasal absorption will be ineffective/unreliable
- instruct the patient in intranasal pump spray use, including:
    - priming pump by pressing at least 4 times before first use (or until even spray is achieved)
    - priming pump by pressing several times if not used in past 2 days to achieve even spray
    - intranasal pump spray delivers 10 micrograms per dose. If a smaller dose is needed, a rhinyle delivery system should be used. Doses greater than 10 micrograms should be administered into each nostril (i.e. 20 microgram dose = 10 micrograms per nostril)
- (Nocturnal enuresis) advise the patient/parent/carer that fluid intake should be

HYPOTHALAMIC AND PITUITARY HORMONES

limited 1 hour before and at least 8 hours after administration to prevent water retention/hyponatraemia from occurring
- (Oral wafers) the patient should be advised to place the wafer under the tongue and allow it to dissolve

Available as dissolvable wafers. Tablets can be dispersed in 10–20 mL water or crushed and mixed with spoonful of yoghurt or apple puree.

Should be used during pregnancy only if benefits outweigh risks; seek advice from specialist.

Should be used during breastfeeding only if benefits outweigh risks, because of limited data available.

Tablets, wafers or nasal sprays are contraindicated with patients with renal impairment (CrCl < 50 mL/min).

Consider dosages, as elderly patients have an increased risk of hyponatraemia.

TERLIPRESSIN
Trade names
Glypressin Solution, Terlipressin Ever Pharma Solution for Injection

Available forms
Ampoule: 0.85 mg/8.5 mL;
Vial: 0.85 mg/5 mL, 1.7 mg/10 mL

Action
- synthetic vasopressin analogue
- prodrug that is converted to active lysine vasopressin
- dose-dependent reduction of portal venous pressure and marked vasoconstriction
- increases mean arterial pressure, with reflexic decrease in heart rate
- minimal effects on fibrinolytic system in those with cirrhosis

Use
- treatment of bleeding oesophageal varices
- treatment of hepatorenal syndrome type 1 (reduced renal perfusion and glomerular filtration with preserved tubular function) in patients considered for renal transplant

Dose
- (Bleeding oesophageal varices) initially 1.7 mg by slow IV 4-hourly until bleeding is controlled, then adjusting dose to 0.85 mg IV 4-hourly if patient weight < 50 kg or adverse effects occur **OR**
- (Treatment of hepatorenal syndrome type 1) 0.85 mg by slow IV injection 6-hourly, increasing dose to 1.7 mg after 3 days if serum creatinine has not decreased from baseline levels by at least 30% for 7–14 days (with albumin 20%)

Adverse effects
- headache, anxiety
- facial pallor
- bradycardia, hypotension, peripheral vasoconstriction, peripheral ischaemia, hypertension, arrhythmias, chest pain
- fluid overload, pulmonary oedema
- fever
- pain in extremities
- abdominal pain, diarrhoea, vomiting, flatulence
- wheezing, bronchospasm, dyspnoea, respiratory failure, pneumonia
- (Rrare) prolonged QT interval, torsade de pointes, cardiac failure
- (IV site) necrosis

Interactions
- caution if used with agents that can prolong QT interval (e.g. Class IA or III antiarrhythmic agents, erythromycin, some antihistamines and tricyclic antidepressants (TCAs)) or cause hypokalaemia or hypomagnesaemia (e.g. diuretics), as cardiac arrhythmias may be induced
- may increase hypotensive effect of non-selective beta adrenoceptive blocking agents
- caution if used with other agents known to cause bradycardia (e.g. propofol), as

HAVARD'S NURSING GUIDE TO DRUGS

heart rate and cardiac output may be lowered

Nursing considerations/Cautions

- fluid balance and electrolytes (especially serum creatinine) should be monitored daily during therapy
- IV site should be closely monitored to prevent necrosis
- (Bleeding oesophageal varices) therapy should not continue for more than 48 hours
- therapy should be continued until hepatorenal syndrome has been resolved for at least 2 days, patient undergoes dialysis or liver transplant, or if serum creatinine remains at or above baseline for 7 days
- dose should not be increased in those with significant ongoing adverse effects (such as pulmonary oedema) or pre-existing cardiovascular disease
- incompatible with glucose solutions
- administer by slow IV bolus, ensuring line is flushed with sodium chloride 0.9% before and after terlipressin
- caution if used in those with kidney insufficiency
- caution if used in those with uncontrolled hypertension, cardiac arrhythmias, coronary artery disease, previous myocardial infarction or cerebral/peripheral vascular disease
- caution if used in those with a history of QT interval prolongation or electrolyte abnormalities (hypokalaemia, hypomagnesaemia)
- caution if used in those who are morbidly obese or have peripheral venous hypertension, as they are at increased risk of infusion site necrosis
- caution if used in those with severe asthma or chronic obstructive pulmonary disease (COPD), as smooth muscle constriction may occur
- not recommended in those with unstable angina or recent acute myocardial infarction

 Contraindicated during pregnancy.

 Considered safe to use when breastfeeding.

 Banned ingredient in all sports.

IMMUNOMODIFIERS

As the name suggests, immunomodifiers are drugs that modify the immune system in some way. They are used in a range of conditions, the prime ones being the prevention and treatment of organ rejection after transplantation, and the treatment of autoimmune diseases such as rheumatoid arthritis, psoriasis and multiple sclerosis.

The success of allograft transplantation can, in part, be directly attributed to the use of immunomodifiers such as ciclosporin and, more recently, the interferons and monoclonal antibodies, which have decreased the risk of graft rejection.

Unfortunately, suppression of the immune system carries with it the increased risk of bacterial, viral and fungal infection, and may also increase the risk of developing neoplasms.

General Adverse effects of immunomodifiers

- increased risk of developing malignancies (especially skin)
- increased risk of infections (viral, bacterial and/or fungal)
- reactivation of chronic infection (e.g. tuberculosis (TB), hepatitis)
- hypersensitivity reaction (e.g. headache, dizziness, malaise, fever, rigors, myalgia, arthralgia, nausea, vomiting, diarrhoea)

General Interactions of immunomodifiers

- use of live attenuated vaccines should be avoided and be given only 6 months after stopping immunosuppressive therapy. Close contacts should not be vaccinated with live poliomyelitis vaccine. If the patient is exposed to chicken pox or measles, immunoglobulin should be given immediately
- lower doses are usually required if given with corticosteroids or other immunomodifiers
- decreases efficacy of other vaccinations (especially if given with corticosteroids)

General Nursing considerations/Cautions for immunomodifiers

- all patients should be carefully screened for history or symptoms of TB or hepatitis, including detailed medical history and possible previous exposure to TB
- chest X-ray and tuberculin skin test (Mantoux) may also be performed (however, there is a risk of a false negative skin test occurring in

patients who are severely ill or immunocompromised)
- any patient with latent TB should be treated with antimycobacterials before starting therapy with immunomodifier(s)
- patient's immunity to varicella zoster virus (chicken pox, herpes zoster (shingles)) should be assessed (including serological testing) before starting therapy because the response to the virus may be severe if exposed and unprotected
- any other active infections should be treated before starting therapy with immunomodifier
- caution if used in those with a history of hepatitis B infection or positive for hepatitis B surface antigen for > 6 months because of the risk of reactivation

General Patient education for immunomodifiers

- instruct the patient to seek medical advice if any of the following occur:
  - recurrent or persistent infection
  - persistent fever, pallor, unexplained bleeding or bruising, shortness of breath on exertion (blood dyscrasia)
  - persistent cough, weight loss and low-grade fever (possible TB)
  - contact with anyone suffering from chicken pox or shingles
- warn the patient to limit exposure to direct sunlight and UV light, wear protective clothing (including hat and sunglasses) and use sunscreen with a high protective factor (SPF 30+) to decrease the risk of skin cancers
- advise the patient to immediately report any new or changes to existing moles, cysts, polyps or unusual lumps

ANTITHYMOCYTE GLOBULIN (EQUINE)
Trade name
Atgam

ANTITHYMOCYTE GLOBULIN (RABBIT)
Trade name
Thymoglobuline

Available forms
Ampoules: 250 mg/5 mL;
Vial: 25 mg

Action
- purified, concentrated gamma globulin (IgG) derived from horse or rabbit plasma
- lymphocyte selective immunosuppressant that reduces circulating thymus-dependent T-lymphocytes, as well as those in the spleen and lymph nodes

Use
- renal transplant (to delay onset of allograft rejection)
- treatment of steroid-resistant moderate-to-severe renal transplant rejection
- treatment of refractory or relapsing aplastic anaemia

Dose
- (Delaying rejection of renal transplant) 15 mg/kg daily by IV infusion for 14 days, then every second day for 14 days, starting within 24 hours of transplant (total 21 doses) (Atgam) **OR**
- (Treatment of rejection of renal transplant) 10—15 mg/kg daily by IV infusion for 14 days, starting when rejection has been diagnosed. Additional doses on alternate days can be given (total 21 doses) (Atgam) **OR**
- (Prevention of renal transplant graft rejection) 1—1.5 mg/kg IV daily for 3—9 days after transplantation (cumulative dose 3—13.5 mg/kg) **OR**

IMMUNOMODIFIERS

- (Treatment of steroid-resistant moderate-to-severe renal transplant graft rejection) 1.5 mg/kg IV daily for 7—14 days post-transplant (cumulative dose 10.5—21 mg/kg) **OR**
- (Refractory or relapsing aplastic anaemia) 2.5—3.75 mg/kg IV daily for 5 consecutive days (cumulative dose 12.5—18.75 mg/kg)

Adverse effects
- fever, chills, shivering, night sweats
- leucopenia, thrombocytopenia
- rash, pruritus, urticaria, weal, flare
- arthralgia, chest/back/flank pain
- peripheral oedema
- hyperkalaemia
- nausea, vomiting, diarrhoea, stomatitis, dysphagia
- dyspnoea
- headache, malaise, dizziness, asthenia
- hypotension, hypertension, tachycardia
- abnormal renal function tests
- pain at infusion site, clotted arteriovenous fistula, peripheral thrombophlebitis
- (Uncommon) anaphylactoid reaction, anaphylaxis, serum sickness, antibody development
- (Rare) cytokine-release syndrome, lymphoma, lymphoproliferative disorders
- see also General Adverse effects of immunomodifiers (p. 1237)

Interactions
- see General Interactions of immunomodifiers (p. 1237)

Nursing considerations/Cautions
- usually given with azathioprine and corticosteroids
- white blood cell and platelet counts should be monitored during and after therapy
- premedication with corticosteroids, antipyretic and/or antihistamine 1 hour before infusion is recommended to decrease likelihood and/or severity of infusion-related reaction
- name and batch number of product should be recorded in the patient's medical history
- (Atgam) skin testing is recommended using undiluted solution pricked into skin initially. If there is no reaction (weal) after 10 minutes, 0.02 mL of diluted solution (1:1000 with sodium chloride 0.9%) given intradermally and area read after 10 minutes. A sodium chloride control should also be injected. A positive reaction is a weal 3 mm or larger (compared with sodium chloride control) and this indicates an increased risk of allergic reaction. However, allergic reactions can occur with a negative skin test, and it does not predict delayed serum sickness reaction
- the patient should be observed throughout infusion
- adrenaline (epinephrine), antihistamines, corticosteroids and resuscitation equipment must be readily available in the event of an allergic reaction
- administer alone
- (Atgam) should be diluted before use. A suitable IV solution container should be inverted and antithymocyte globulin solution injected directly into solution (not allowing it to make contact with air) and the container gently inverted to mix solution. The solution (diluted or undiluted) should not be shaken as it will become denatured
- (Atgam) suitable IV solutions include sodium chloride 0.9%, glucose 5% with sodium chloride 0.45% and glucose 5% with sodium chloride 0.225%
- (Atgam) not recommended for dilution using glucose-only solutions (as precipitation may occur) or highly acidic solution (become unstable)
- (Thymoglobuline) if the patient is obese, the dose should be calculated on ideal weight, not actual weight
- (Thymoglobuline) the vial should be allowed to come to room temperature for 30 minutes before reconstituting
- (Thymoglobuline) reconstitute powder with 5 mL water for injections, injecting diluent gently down side of vial and gently tilting or rolling to dissolve the powder. Vial should not be inverted,

shaken or swirled, as the protein will be denatured
- (Thymoglobuline) dilute reconstituted solution with 50—500 mL (50 mL/vial) of either sodium chloride 0.9% or glucose 5% and gently invert the infusion bag to ensure even distribution
- (Thymoglobuline) precipitation will occur if added to glucose 5% containing heparin and hydrocortisone
- may be administered via high-flow central vein, existing vascular shunt or arterial—venous fistula using inline filter (0.2—1 micron)
- (Thymoglobuline) first dose should be administered over 6 hours, and subsequent doses over 4 hours
- (Atgam) infusion should be over at least 4 hours
- (Atgam) solution may be clear, colourless to light brown in colour and may develop flaky deposit when stored
- repeat courses should be given with great caution because of an increased risk of hypersensitivity reaction
- contraindicated in those with hypersensitivity to equine gamma globulin (immunoglobulin) (Atgam) or rabbit protein hypersensitivity (Thymoglobuline), or if the person has acute or chronic infection

Patient education

- the patient should be advised that the possibility of transmitting infectious diseases (e.g. human immunodeficiency virus (HIV), viral hepatitis), while remote, does exist
- warn the patient not to drive or operate machinery if dizziness, malaise or hypotension occurs
- see also General Patient education for immunomodifiers (p. 1238)

Not recommended; only limited data are available.

Use during when breastfeeding only if benefits outweigh risks; only limited data are available.

APREMILAST
Trade name
Otezla

Available forms
Tablets: 10 mg, 20 mg, 30 mg

Action
- phosphodiesterase 4 inhibitor (phosphodiesterase 4 is thought to be involved in the inflammatory process), resulting in a decrease in pro-inflammatory cytokines (e.g. interleukin-23) and increase in anti-inflammatory cytokines (e.g. interleukin-10)
- elimination half-life 9 hours

Use
- active psoriatic arthritis
- moderate-to-severe plaque psoriasis in those who are candidates for phototherapy or systemic therapy

Dose
- initially 10 mg orally daily (day 1), then 10 mg twice daily (day 2), 10 mg (morning) and 20 mg (night) (day 3), 20 mg orally twice daily (day 4), 20 mg (morning) and 30 mg (night) (day 5), then 30 mg twice daily

Adverse effects
- decreased appetite, diarrhoea, nausea, vomiting, weight loss, frequent bowel motions, abdominal pain, gastroesophageal reflux disease (GORD), dyspepsia, gastroenteritis
- headache, migraine, tension headache, fatigue, insomnia
- depression, lowered mood
- upper respiratory tract infection, bronchitis, nasopharyngitis, sinusitis
- cough

IMMUNOMODIFIERS

- back pain, arthralgia
- hypertension
- urinary tract infection
- hypersensitivity

Interactions
- serum levels decreased by phenytoin, rifampicin, carbamazepine, phenobarbital (phenobarbitone) and St John's wort

Nursing considerations/Cautions
- renal function should be assessed before starting therapy
- weight should be monitored during therapy and if there is clinically significant weight loss, interruption to therapy should be considered
- caution if used in those with a history of depression and/or suicidal ideation
- caution if used in those with severe kidney impairment; dose should be reduced to 30 mg daily
- caution if used in those aged > 65 years or those at risk of volume depletion or hypotension, as they should be closely monitored for diarrhoea, nausea and vomiting
- tablets contain lactose and are therefore not recommended in those with rare hereditary problems of galactose intolerance, Lapp lactase deficiency or glucose–galactose malabsorption

Patient education
- advise the patient to swallow tablets whole, not chewed, broken or divided
- warn the patient (and carer/family member) to immediately seek medical advice if there is any change in mood, sadness or thoughts of self-harm

Tablets should not be crushed or broken.

Contraindicated during pregnancy, as no safety data are available.

Contraindicated when breastfeeding, as no safety data are available.

In renal impairment patients, consider starting on a reduced dose if CrCl < 30 mL/min.

AVACOPAN
Trade name
Tavneos

Available form
Capsule: 10 mg

Action
- selective antagonist of human complement 5a receptor (C5aR1 or CD88) that completely inhibits interaction between C5aR1 and anaphylatoxin C5a, reducing pro-inflammatory effects (neutrophil activation, migration and adherence to small blood vessel inflammation, vascular endothelial cell retraction and permeability)
- does not decrease formation of membrane attack complex (C5b-9) or terminal complement complex (TCC) needed for fighting infections with encapsulated bacteria such as *Neisseria* species
- half-life 21 days

Use
- treatment of antineutrophil cytoplasmic autoantibody (ANCA)-associated vasculitis (granulomatosis with polyangiitis and microscopic polyangiitis) in combination with a rituximab- or cyclophosphamide-based regimen

Dose
- 30 mg orally twice daily with food in combination with rituximab or cyclophosphamide-based regimens

Adverse effects
- headache
- nausea, vomiting, diarrhoea, gastroenteritis, upper abdominal pain
- upper respiratory tract infection, nasopharyngitis, pneumonia, lower respiratory tract infection, influenza, bronchitis, sinusitis, rhinitis, otitis media
- herpes zoster, oral herpes

- urinary tract infection
- elevated liver enzymes and total bilirubin
- decreased white cell count, neutropenia
- (Uncommon) angioedema
- (Rare) vanishing bile duct syndrome, increased risk of malignancies

Interactions

- not recommended with grapefruit or grapefruit juice
- serum levels may be decreased if given with carbamazepine, enzalutamide, mitotane, phenobarbital (phenobarbitone), phenytoin, rifampicin or St John's wort, and these are therefore not recommended together
- caution if used with clarithromycin, itraconazole, ketoconazole, lopinavir/ritonavir, posaconazole, ritonavir or voriconazole, as serum levels may be increased, increasing the risk of adverse effects
- caution if used with bosentan, efavirenz or modafinil
- caution if used with agents that have a narrow therapeutic index such as ciclosporin, fentanyl, sirolimus, tacrolimus and alfentanil
- caution if used with dabigatran etexilate owing to PEG-40 hydrogenated castor oil content in the capsule
- an increased risk of cardiac disorders if given in combination with cyclophosphamide or azathioprine

Nursing considerations/Cautions

- the patient should be assessed for any serious infections such as tuberculosis, hepatitis B, hepatitis C and HIV
- liver function (enzymes alanine aminotransferase (ALT), aspartate aminotransferase (AST) and bilirubin) and white blood cells should be measured before and during therapy. If ALT or AST is > 3 times above upper limit of normal (ULN), therapy should be reassessed. Therapy should be stopped temporarily if ALT or AST is > 5 ULN. WBC $< 2 \times 10^9$/L, neutrophils $< 1 \times 10^9$/L or lymphocytes $< 0.2 \times 10^9$/L, or the patient develops an active serious infection that requires hospitalisation. Therapy can be restarted when values return to normal; however, liver enzymes and bilirubin should be closely monitored
- therapy should not be started if WBC $< 3.5 \times 10^9$/L, neutrophils $< 1.5 \times 10^9$/L or lymphocytes $< 0.5 \times 10^9$/L
- those with granulomatosis with polyangiitis or microscopic polyangiitis should be given *Pneumocystis jirovecii* pneumonia prophylaxis during therapy
- combination therapy may include rituximab IV for 4 weekly doses, or IV/oral cyclophosphamide for 13–24 weeks followed by oral azathioprine or mycophenolate mofetil, and glucocorticoids as needed
- caution if used in those with a history of tuberculosis, hepatitis B, hepatitis C or HIV infection
- caution if used in those with an eGFR below 15 mL/min/1.73 m^2, requiring dialysis, or undergoing plasma exchange
- not recommended in those under 17 years
- not recommended in those with severe liver impairment (Child–Pugh C)

Patient education

- advise the patient to swallow the capsule whole with water and food (capsules should not be opened, chewed or crushed)
- the patient should be instructed to avoid grapefruit and grapefruit juice during therapy
- instruct the patient to seek medical advice immediately if any of the following occur:
  - unexpected bleeding or bruising
  - nausea, fatigue, upper abdominal pain, loss of appetite, itching, dark urine, yellowing of skin or whites of the eyes, light-coloured bowel motions
  - infection
  - swelling of face, lips, tongue or throat tightness, or difficulty breathing

IMMUNOMODIFIERS

- women of childbearing potential should be counselled to use effective contraception during and for 1 week after stopping therapy

Capsules should not be crushed, chewed or opened.

Avoid use in pregnancy because of the risk of potential fetal harm (based on animal studies).

Avoid use, as excretion in human milk is unknown; therefore potential risk to the infant cannot be excluded. Discontinue breastfeeding or medicine based on the benefit–risk assessment.

Not recommended in those with severe liver impairment (Child–Pugh Class C).

AZATHIOPRINE

Trade names
Azapin, APO-Azathioprine, Azathioprine Sandoz, Azathioprine-WGR, Imazan, Imuran, Noumed Azathioprine, Thioprine

Available forms
Tablets: 25 mg, 50 mg;
Vial: 50 mg

Action
- imidazole, with immune response suppression
- derivative of mercaptopurine (see Antineoplastic agents, p. 654)
- therapeutic effects may become apparent only after weeks to months of therapy when used for other conditions
- half-life about 5 hours

Use
- organ transplantation (with corticosteroids and/or other immunosuppressive agents)
- chronic autoimmune diseases (e.g. severe rheumatoid arthritis, systemic lupus erythematosus (SLE)) (with or without corticosteroids and/or other immunosuppressive agents)

Dose
- (Transplantation) initially 5 mg/kg IV or orally 1 hour before or 3 hours after food daily, then reducing to 1–4 mg/kg IV or orally daily as maintenance **OR**
- (Other conditions) initially 1 mg/kg IV or orally 1 hour before or 3 hours after food daily, then increasing by 0.5 mg/kg/day over several weeks (maximum daily dose 2.5 mg/kg), then dose reduced as appropriate

Adverse effects
- skin rash
- anaemia, leucopenia, thrombocytopenia
- nausea, vomiting, sores on mouth and lips, diarrhoea, GI discomfort, altered taste or smell
- pancreatitis
- (Renal transplantation with corticosteroids) reversible alopecia
- (Uncommon) decreased liver function, hepatotoxicity, formication (sensation of ants on skin), meningitis
- (Rare) reversible pneumonitis, progressive multifocal leucoencephalopathy (PML) (if given with other immunosuppressants), exacerbation of myasthenia gravis, macrophage activation syndrome
- see also General Adverse effects of immunomodifiers (p. 1237)

Interactions
- dose reduction (to one-quarter) may be required if given with allopurinol or related substances
- may increase neuromuscular blockade of suxamethonium
- may decrease neuromuscular blockade of non-depolarising neuromuscular blocking agents such as pancuronium or vecuronium
- may inhibit anticoagulant activity of warfarin, requiring increase in dosage; therefore the INR should be closely monitored, especially when starting or stopping therapy or with any dose adjustment
- caution if given with angiotensin converting enzyme (ACE) inhibitors and

captopril owing to increased susceptibility to leucopenia
- myelosuppressive effects may be enhanced if given with indometacin, penicillamine or other bone marrow depressing agents and therefore not recommended together
- caution if given with olsalazine, mesalazine or sulfasalazine
- metabolism may be impaired by furosemide (frusemide) or febuxostat
- clearance may be altered by phenytoin, phenobarbital (phenobarbitone), rifampicin or erythromycin
- not recommended with ribavirin
- dose adjustment may be required if given with high-dose methotrexate
- caution if given with infliximab
- see also General Interactions of immunomodifiers (p. 1237)

Nursing considerations/Cautions

- testing for thiopurine methyltransferase deficiency is recommended before starting therapy
- IV should be used only when oral route is impractical or unavailable. Oral therapy should replace IV as soon as possible
- any dental work should be completed before the start of therapy or postponed until therapy is completed and/or blood counts have returned to normal
- blood counts (including platelet count) should be monitored weekly for the first 8 weeks (or more frequently if the dose is high or renal/liver disorder is present), then monthly
- should be handled as per cytotoxic protocol
- reconstitute powder using 5–15 mL water for injections and then dilute with 20–200 mL sodium chloride 0.9%, sodium chloride 0.45% or sodium chloride (0.18%) and glucose (4%) solution
- reconstituted solution may be given over at least 1 minute, followed by at least 50 mL of suitable dilution fluid (see the previous point) if the patient is unable to tolerate large volumes of fluid
- administer alone
- avoid extravasation
- withdrawal should be gradual and under supervision
- caution if used in those with myasthenia gravis, as the condition may become exacerbated
- caution if used in those with thiopurine methyltransferase deficiency, as they are sensitive to myelosuppressive effects
- not recommended in those with hypersplenism or Lesch—Nyhan syndrome (hypoxanthine-guanine-phosphoribosyl transferase deficiency) or with liver dysfunction (regular blood counts and liver function tests are recommended)
- contraindicated in those with known hypersensitivity to mercaptopurine or with rheumatoid arthritis treated previously with alkylating agents (e.g. cyclophosphamide, melphalan) (because of an increased risk of neoplasm development)
- see also General Nursing considerations/Cautions for immunomodifiers (p. 1238)

Patient education

- the patient should be advised to report immediately any infection, unexpected bruising or bleeding, black tarry stools or blood in urine or stools
- (Renal transplantation with corticosteroids) warn the patient that alopecia (hair loss) occurs commonly but in most cases is reversible even with continuation of therapy
- advise the patient that tablets should be swallowed whole, not crushed or chewed
- counsel the patient to use adequate contraception during therapy to avoid pregnancy occurring
- see also General Patient education for immunomodifiers (p. 1238)

 Tablets are cytotoxic and should not be crushed or broken.

IMMUNOMODIFIERS

 Use only if benefit outweighs the risk in pregnancy.

 Considered safe in breastfeeding but if high doses are taken consider avoiding breastfeeding for 4 hours after.

 Patients with renal impairment (CrCl < 30 mL/min) should be started on a reduced dose.

Consider a lower dose in hepatic patients and increase monitoring.

BARICITINIB
Trade name
Olumiant

Available forms
Tablets: 2 mg, 4 mg

Action
- selective and reversible inhibitor of Janus kinases (JAK1 and JAK2) (Janus kinases are enzymes that relay signals from cell surface receptors to a number of cytokines and growth factors involved in haematopoiesis, inflammation and immune function)

Use
- treatment of moderate-to-severe rheumatoid arthritis in those who are intolerant to or have had an inadequate response to one or more disease-modifying antirheumatic drugs (DMARDs) (as monotherapy or with cDMARDs)
- treatment of moderate-to-severe atopic dermatitis (AD) in adults who are candidates for systemic therapy
- treatment of alopecia areata (AA) in adults where other treatments have failed

Dose
- 2—4 mg orally daily

Adverse effects
- thrombocytosis
- nausea, vomiting, upper abdominal pain, increased weight
- fatigue, headache, depression
- oropharyngeal pain
- upper respiratory tract infection, urinary tract infection, pharyngitis, vulvovaginal candidiasis, influenza
- elevated creatine phosphokinase (CPK), hypercholesterolaemia
- deep venous thrombosis, pulmonary embolism
- see also General Adverse effects of immunomodifiers (p. 1237)

Interactions
- not recommended with other JAK inhibitors or biological DMARDs
- see also General Interactions of immunomodifiers (p. 1237)

Nursing considerations/Cautions
- before starting therapy, lipids, absolute neutrophil count (ANC), absolute lymphocyte count (ALC), haemoglobin and liver function should be measured, and then regularly during treatment. Treatment should be interrupted if ANC, ALC, haemoglobin or liver transaminases become abnormal. Any hyperlipidaemia should be treated if it develops
- caution if used in those with risk factors for deep vein thrombosis or pulmonary embolism (e.g. older age, obesity, history of either, undergoing surgery, immobilisation)
- caution if used in those with moderate renal impairment; 2 mg dose is recommended
- caution if used in the elderly and those with diabetes because of the increased risk of infection
- not recommended in patients with severe and end-stage renal impairment
- see also General Nursing considerations/Cautions for immunomodifiers (p. 1238)

Patient education
- advise the patient to seek medical advice immediately if any of the following occur:
  - any shortness of breath or sudden chest pain, cough, lightheadedness, dizziness, rapid heart rate

1245

- sudden painful or tender leg swelling, increased limb warmth, skin discolouration
- female patients of childbearing potential should be counselled to avoid pregnancy by using effective contraception during and for at least 1 week after stopping therapy

Tablets should not be crushed or broken.

Should be used in pregnancy only if benefits outweigh risks to fetus. Female of childbearing potential should be counselled to use effective contraception during therapy and for at least 1 week after stopping

Not recommended when breastfeeding, as no safety data are available.

In renal impairment patients, if eGFR <60 mL/min/1.73 m^2 reduce the dose. Not recommended for use if eGFR < 30 mL/min/1.73 m^2, as this medication is renally excreted.

Not recommended for use with the elderly (65 and over) owing to the increased risk of infections, malignancy and higher cardiovascular events.

BASILIXIMAB

Trade name
Simulect

Available form
Vial: 20 mg

Action
- recombinant IgG$_{1kappa}$ that binds to the CD25 antigen on activated T-lymphocyte surface preventing interleukin 2 binding and production of T cells
- does not cause cytokine release or myelosuppression
- half-life 4—10.4 days

Use
- prophylaxis of acute organ rejection (renal transplantation)

Dose
- 20 mg as IV bolus or infusion over 20—30 minutes 2 hours before transplantation, then 20 mg IV 4 days after transplantation

Adverse effects
- pain
- fever
- headache, insomnia
- peripheral oedema, general oedema
- nausea, vomiting, diarrhoea, constipation, abdominal pain
- anaemia
- hyperkalaemia
- hypertension
- antibody development
- see also General Adverse effects of immunomodifiers (p. 1237)

Interactions
- see General Interactions of immunomodifiers (p. 1237)

Nursing considerations/Cautions
- the first dose should be given only when it is certain that transplantation will occur (with immunosuppressive therapy)
- the second dose should not be given if there is severe hypersensitivity or if the patient experiences postoperative complication(s)
- reconstitute using 5.0 mL water for injections and then dilute with at least 50 mL sodium chloride 0.9% or glucose 5% for IV infusion
- not recommended for other organ transplantation except kidney
- contraindicated in those with hypersensitivity to murine antibody preparations
- see also General Nursing considerations/Cautions for immunomodifiers (p. 1238)

Patient education
- ensure female patients receive adequate counselling regarding the importance of using adequate contraception during and for 16 weeks after stopping therapy to avoid pregnancy occurring. They should also be advised

IMMUNOMODIFIERS

- to seek immediate medical advice if they think they may be pregnant
- see also General Patient education for immunomodifiers (p. 1238)

Not recommended in pregnancy because no safety data are available.

Not recommended when breastfeeding because no safety data are available.

BELIMUMAB
Trade name
Benlysta

Available forms
Vial: 120 mg, 400 mg

Action
- human B-lymphocyte stimulator neutralising antibody
- B-lymphocyte stimulator is a member of the tumour necrosis factor (TNF) family that inhibits B-cell apoptosis and stimulates differentiation of B cells into immunoglobulin-producing plasma cells and is overexpressed in those with systemic lupus erythematosus (SLE)
- belimumab is a human $IgG_{1\gamma}$ monoclonal antibody that inhibits survival of B cells, reducing differentiation

Use
- add-on therapy in those with active autoantibody-positive SLE with a high degree of disease activity (ANA titre $\geq$ 1:80 or anti-dsDNA titre $\geq$ 30 IU/mL) despite standard treatment

Dose
- 10 mg/kg by IV infusion over 60 minutes on days 0, 14 and 28, then monthly

Adverse effects
- infusion-related reaction (fatigue, fever, dizziness, headache, shortness of breath, hypertension)
- fever
- headache, migraine, fatigue, insomnia
- nausea, diarrhoea
- arthralgia
- nasopharyngitis, bronchitis, pharyngitis
- leucopenia
- depression and less commonly, suicidal ideation and behaviour
- hypersensitivity, anaphylaxis, angioedema
- (Rare) progressive multifocal leukoencephalopathy (PML)
- see also General Adverse effects of immunomodifiers (p. 1237)

Interactions
- see General Interactions of immunomodifiers (p. 1237)

Nursing considerations/Cautions
- premedication with oral antihistamines with or without antipyretic may be given
- the patient should be closely monitored during and after administration for any signs of hypersensitivity
- the risk of hypersensitivity is highest during first 2 days of therapy, decreasing with duration. However, delayed sensitivity has occurred
- if the patient presents with signs of neurological deterioration, referral to a neurologist is recommended, as it may be a sign of PML
- therapy should be re-evaluated if there has been no improvement in 6 months
- allow vial to come to room temperature for 10–15 minutes before administration
- reconstitute 120 mg vial with 1.5 mL of water for injections and 400 mg vial with 4.8 mL to give a concentration of 80 mg/mL
- water for injections should be added to the side of the vial to avoid frothing. Gently swirl (not shake) for 60 seconds every 5 minutes to dissolve the powder. This usually takes 10–15 minutes, but may take up to 30 minutes
- reconstituted solution should be further diluted to 250 mL with sodium chloride 0.9% (withdraw and discard a volume equal to the amount to be added). Gently invert the infusion bag to ensure the solution is adequately mixed
- not compatible with glucose 5%
- not given as IV push or bolus

- administer alone
- caution if used in a patient with chronic infection, and therapy should not be started if the patient is currently receiving therapy for chronic infection
- caution if used in those with a history of malignancy or depression
- caution if used in those with a history of multiple drug allergies or significant hypersensitivity, as there is an increased risk of hypersensitivity or infusion-related reaction
- see also General Nursing considerations/Cautions for immunomodifiers (p. 1238)

Patient education

- advise the patient to seek medical advice immediately if any of the following occur:
  - rash, nausea, fatigue, muscle pain, headache, facial swelling (which may occur up to 5 days after administration)
  - changes in mood, sadness or signs/talk of self-harm
- women of childbearing potential should be counselled to use adequate contraception during and for at least 4 months after stopping therapy
- see also General Patient education for immunomodifiers (p. 1238)

 Not recommended during pregnancy because limited data are available.

 Not recommended when breastfeeding because limited data are available.

DUPILUMAB

Trade name
Dupixent

Available forms
Prefilled syringe: 200 mg, 300 mg

Action
- recombinant IgG$_4$ monoclonal antibody that inhibits interleukin-4 and interleukin-13 (which are known to be cytokines involved in atopic disease)

Use
- treatment of moderate-to-severe atopic dermatitis in those who are candidates for chronic systemic therapy
- as add-on maintenance therapy in those with moderate-to-severe asthma with type 2 inflammation (elevated eosinophils of FeNO (fractional exhaled nitrous oxide))

Dose
- (Atopic dermatitis) initially 600 mg SC, followed by 300 mg every second week **OR**
- (Asthma) initially 400 mg SC, followed by 200 mg every second week **OR**
- (Oral corticosteroid-dependent asthma or with co-morbid moderate-to-severe atopic dermatitis) initially 600 mg SC, followed by 300 mg every second week

Adverse effects
- conjunctivitis (allergic, bacterial), keratitis, eye pruritus, blepharitis, dry eye
- herpes simplex
- oropharyngeal pain
- (Asthma) eosinophilic conditions (e.g. eosinophilic pneumonia, vasculitis)
- injection site reactions (redness, oedema, pruritus)
- (Rare) hypersensitivity

Interactions
- see General Interactions of immunomodifiers (p. 1237)

Nursing considerations/Cautions

- any helminth infestation should be treated before starting therapy
- 600 mg or 400 mg doses should be given as two injections consecutively into different injection sites
- trade name and batch number should be recorded in the patient's medical history or dispensing record
- the patient can be taught to self-administer. The first dose should be given under medical supervision
- (Atopic dermatitis) not recommended for episodic use

IMMUNOMODIFIERS

- see also General Nursing considerations/ Cautions for immunomodifiers (p. 1238)

Patient education

- (Asthma) ensure the patient understands that dupilumab is not for management of acute asthma, acute asthma exacerbations, acute bronchospasm or status asthmaticus
- (Asthma) warn the patient not to stop corticosteroid therapy when starting therapy with dupilumab
- see patient education for icatibant (p. 1256) for self-administration instructions for self-administration instructions
- advise the patient that if a dose is forgotten it can be administered within 7 days from the missed dose and then the previous dosing schedule resumed. If the missed dose is not given within 7 days, advise the patient to wait until next dose is due
- the patient should be instructed to seek medical advice if any of the following occur:
  - new or worsening eye symptoms
  - (asthma) rash, worsening lung symptoms, flu-like symptoms, pins and needles or numbness to arms or legs

Should be used during pregnancy only if benefits outweigh risks because no safety data are available.

Should be used when breastfeeding only if benefits outweigh risks because no safety data are available.

ECULIZUMAB

Trade name
Soliris

Available form
Vial: 300 mg/30 mL

Action

- monoclonal antibody hybrid (IgG$_2$-IgG$_{4kappa}$) specifically binds to complement protein C5 inhibiting its cleavage to C5a and C5b, preventing generation of terminal complement complex C5b-9
- genetic mutation in those with paroxysmal nocturnal haemoglobinuria leads to abnormal blood cells that are deficient in terminal complement inhibitors, causing these blood cells to be sensitive to terminal complement-mediated destruction with ensuing anaemia, fatigue, difficulty in function, pain, dark urine, kidney disease, shortness of breath and blood clots. In atypical haemolytic uraemic syndrome, complement activity regulation impairment leads to uncontrolled terminal complement activation, resulting in platelet activation, endothelial cell damage and thrombotic microangiopathy
- mean elimination half life 11.3 ± 3.4 days

Use

- haemolysis reduction in paroxysmal nocturnal haemoglobinuria (PNH)
- treatment of atypical haemolytic uraemic syndrome (aHUS)
- neuromyelitis optica spectrum disorder (NMOSD) in those with are anti-aquaporin-4 antibody positive (adjunct therapy)

Dose

- (PNH) initially 600 mg IV over 25–45 minutes weekly for 4 weeks, followed by 900 mg IV (week 5), then 900 mg IV every 12–16 days (depending on monitoring results) **OR**
- (aHUS, NMOSD) initially 900 mg IV over 25–45 minutes weekly for 4 weeks, followed by 1200 mg (week 5), then 1200 mg IV every 12–16 days (depending on monitoring results)

Adverse effects

- headache, insomnia, dizziness
- fatigue
- fever
- nausea, vomiting, abdominal pain, diarrhoea, altered taste, decreased appetite,
- oropharyngeal pain

- herpes infection, respiratory tract infection, cough, pneumonia, bronchitis, nasopharyngitis, flu-like illness
- urinary tract infection
- hypertension
- dry skin, rash, pruritus, alopecia
- arthralgia, myalgia, pain in extremities
- leucopenia, lymphopenia, anaemia
- infusion-related reaction
- (Uncommon) meningococcal infection

Interaction
- not recommended with etrasimod owing to added immunosuppression

Nursing considerations/Cautions
- all patients must be vaccinated against meningococcal disease at least 2 weeks before starting therapy. If vaccination has occurred less than 2 weeks before starting therapy, prophylactic antibiotics are recommended until 2 weeks after vaccination
- if patient is < 18 years, additional vaccination against *Haemophilus influenzae* and *Streptococcus pneumoniae* is also required
- patients should be closely monitored postvaccination for signs of their underlying disease (e.g. haemolysis), as vaccination may activate complement (and the complement-mediated diseases)
- if patient misses multiple doses, re-induction should be considered
- extra doses may be required if patient is undergoing plasmapheresis, plasma exchange or plasma infusion
- (NMOSD) given as an adjunct to other immunosuppressive therapy
- all patients should be monitored for at least one hour postinfusion
- requires further dilution to concentration of 5 mg/mL (for 600 mg, add 60 mL diluent; 900 mg, add 90 mL diluent; 1200 mg, add 120 mL diluent). Diluents include sodium chloride 0.9%, sodium chloride 0.45%, glucose 5% or Lactated Ringer's solution
- infusion bag should be gently inverted before administration using gravity feed, syringe pump or infusion pump and delivered over 25-45 minutes
- if infusion is slowed (e.g. adverse reaction occurs), infusion must be completed with 2 hours
- should not be given as IV bolus or push
- administer alone
- (PNH) the patient should be monitored for signs and symptoms of intravascular haemolysis, including serum lactate dehydrogenase (LDH) levels, which may result in dose adjustment (e.g. dosing schedule reduced from 14 days to 12)
- (aHUS) the patient should be monitored for thrombotic microangioplasty by measuring platelet count, serum lactate dehydrogenase (LDH) and serum creatinine, which may result in dose adjustment (e.g. dosing schedule reduced from 14 days to 12)
- (PNH) if therapy is stopped, the patient should be monitored for at least 8 weeks to detect any haemolysis. If serious haemolysis occurs, treatment may include blood transfusion, exchange transfusion, anticoagulation, corticosteroids or restarting therapy
- (aHUS) if therapy is stopped, the patient should be monitored to detect any severe thrombotic microangiopathy complications. If they occur, treatment may include restarting therapy, anticoagulation, respiratory support (with ventilation if needed) or renal support with dialysis
- (NMOSD) if therapy is stopped, the patient should be monitored for relapse
- contains 5 mmol sodium/30 mL which may need to be considered if the patient is on a sodium-restricted diet
- caution if used in those with active systemic infection
- contraindicated in those with hypersensitivity to murine products, unresolved *Neisseria meningitidis* infection or not currently vaccinated against *N. meningitidis* (unless receiving appropriate prophylactic antibiotics until 2 weeks after vaccination)

Patient education

- ensure that the patient understands that therapy is life long
- the patient should be provided with 'Patient safety information' card and advised to carry it at all times, and shown to any health professionals who may be involved in their care
- warn patients not to drive or operate machinery if they experience any dizziness or vertigo
- patients should be instructed to seek medical advice immediately if any of the following occur (as they may be signs of meningococcal disease):
  - fever > 39°C
  - headache with nausea or vomiting
  - headache with fever and/or stiff neck/back
  - rash
  - confusion
  - severe muscle aches with flu-like symptoms
  - sensitivity to light
- patients should also be instructed to seek medical advice if any of the following occur:
  - tiredness, headache, shortness of breath on exercising, dizziness, looking pale
  - confusion or change in alertness
  - chest pain or angina
  - dark urine
  - blood clots
  - decreased urination, fitting/seizures (for aHUS)
- female patients of childbearing capacity should be counselled to use adequate contraception during and for up to 5 months after stopping therapy to avoid pregnancy occurring

 There are risks to mother and fetus of both treated and untreated PNH and aHUS; therefore should be used during pregnancy only after careful risk evaluation of benefits versus risks.

 There is insufficient information available regarding the effect of eculizumab on the breastfed infant.

EVEROLIMUS
Trade names
Afinitor, Certican, Everocan

Available forms
Tablets: 0.25 mg, 0.5 mg, 0.75 mg, 1 mg, 5 mg, 10 mg;
Dispersible tablets: 2 mg, 3 mg, 5 mg

Action
- protein kinase mTOR inhibitor
- inhibits proliferation of activated T cells by binding to T-cell growth factor receptor sites, thereby blocking the G_1 stage of the cell cycle
- narrow therapeutic index

Use
- prevention of organ rejection in those at risk after receiving allogeneic renal or heart transplant (with ciclosporin and corticosteroids) or liver transplant (with tacrolimus with corticosteroids) (Certican, Everocan)
- treatment of advanced HER2-negative hormone receptor-positive breast cancer in postmenopausal women (after letrozole or anastrozole failure), advanced renal cancer (after sorafenib or sunitinib failure), well or moderately differentiated progressive unresectable or metastatic neuroendocrine tumours (of pancreatic origin), tuberous sclerosis complex (TSC) associated with subependymal giant cell astrocytoma (SEGA) (requiring therapeutic intervention but not suitable for curative surgery), TSC with renal angiomyolipoma (not requiring immediate surgery, TSC with refractory seizures (as adjunct) (Afinitor))

Dose
- (Renal or heart transplant) initially 0.75 mg orally twice daily starting as soon as possible after transplantation (Certican, Everocan) **OR**

- (Liver transplant) 1 mg orally twice daily starting 4 weeks post-transplant (Certican, Everocan) **OR**
- (Breast cancer, renal cancer, neuroendocrine tumours, TSC with renal angiomyolipoma) 10 mg orally daily (Afinitor) **OR**
- (TSC with SEGA) 4.5 mg/m^2 orally daily (rounded to nearest strength of tablet) (Afinitor) **OR**
- (TSC with refractory seizures, aged ≥ 6 years) 5 mg/m^2 orally daily (rounded to nearest strength of tablet) (Afinitor Dispersible)

Adverse effects

- leucopenia, neutropenia, thrombocytopenia, anaemia, pancytopenia, thrombotic microangiopathies
- epistaxis
- hypertension
- decreased appetite, nausea, vomiting, abdominal pain, diarrhoea, stomatitis, constipation, oropharyngeal pain, mouth ulcers, oral mucositis, decreased weight, altered taste, dry mouth, dyspepsia, dysphagia, gastritis, flatulence
- hypokalaemia
- dehydration
- fever
- headache, insomnia, anxiety, fatigue, asthenia, irritability, aggression
- abnormal liver enzymes
- peripheral oedema, lymphoedema
- pain, myalgia, arthralgia
- hypercholesterolaemia, hyperlipidaemia, hypertriglyceridaemia
- cough, dyspnoea, pleural effusion, pneumonitis
- nasopharyngitis
- hypophosphataemia
- acne, rash, pruritus, dry skin, nail disorder
- impaired wound healing, lymphocele
- proteinuria, renal failure
- decreased testosterone, erectile dysfunction
- menstruation irregularities, amenorrhoea, menorrhagia, ovarian cyst, vaginal bleeding
- hyperglycaemia, new onset diabetes mellitus
- angioedema
- renal graft thrombosis
- (Rare) interstitial lung disease/non-infectious pneumonitis
- see also General Adverse effects of immunomodifiers (p. 1237)

Interactions

- not recommended with itraconazole, voriconazole, clarithromycin, ritonavir, rifampicin or rifabutin
- may increase renal toxicity of ciclosporin
- serum levels may be increased by ciclosporin, fluconazole, itraconazole, posaconazole, erythromycin, clarithromycin, verapamil, diltiazem, metoclopramide, bromocriptine, danazol or aprepitant
- not recommended with grapefruit, grapefruit juice, star fruit or Seville oranges
- serum levels may be decreased by St John's wort, carbamazepine, phenobarbital (phenobarbitone), rifampicin, phenytoin, rifabutin, dexamethasone, prednisolone, prednisone, efavirenz or nevirapine
- caution if used with other agents which affect renal function
- increased risk of angioedema if given with angiotensin converting enzyme (ACE) inhibitors
- may increase bioavailability of midazolam
- increased risk of thrombotic microangiopathy, thrombotic thrombocytopenic purpura and/or haemolytic uraemic syndrome if given with calcineurin inhibitors (e.g. ciclosporin, tacrolimus)
- increased risk of acute rejection if not given with either ciclosporin or tacrolimus
- increased risk of serious infection if everolimus/corticosteroid/ciclosporin combination is given with antithymocyte globulin (rabbit) in heart transplant patients

IMMUNOMODIFIERS

- see also General Interactions of immunomodifiers (p. 1237)

Nursing considerations/Cautions

- renal function (including urine protein, serum creatinine, blood urea nitrogen (BUN)), serum lipids, full blood count and blood glucose levels should be monitored regularly during therapy
- therapeutic serum levels should be monitored regularly during therapy (especially in those with liver impairment)
- (TSC with SEGA, TSC with seizures) therapeutic levels should be measured 1–2 weeks after starting therapy or altering dose
- if the patient is treated for pneumonia with antibiotics and does not show improvement, interstitial lung disease/non-infectious pneumonitis should be considered
- increased risk of hypertension, pneumonitis and/or hyperglycaemia if used in Asian patients
- Afinitor and Afinitor Dispersible tablets are not interchangeable, nor should they be mixed together to achieve the dosage
- (Afinitor) if switching between formulations, the dose should be estimated to the closest mg and serum levels measured 2 weeks later
- (TSC with SEGA) SEGA volume should be measured 12 weeks after starting therapy and the dose adjusted accordingly
- (TSC with SEGA, TSC with refractory seizures) once dosage has stabilised, trough concentration should be measured every 3–6 months if patients have changing surface area (e.g. growth) or 6–12-monthly if the surface area is stable
- (Afinitor) dose interruption, reduction or stopping is recommended if the patient develops adverse effects (e.g. non-infectious pneumonitis, stomatitis, thrombocytopenia)
- caution if used in those with severe refractory hyperlipidaemia, or impaired kidney or liver function
- caution if used in perisurgical period, as delayed wound healing may occur
- tablets contain lactose and are not recommended in those with galactose intolerance, Lapp lactase deficiency or glucose–galactose malabsorption
- (Afinitor) not recommended in children with cancer, TSC with renal angiomyolipoma, TSC with SEGA (if under 1 year) or TSC with refractory seizures (if under 2 years)
- (Afinitor) not recommended in those under 18 years with liver impairment and TSC with SEGA or TSC with refractory seizures
- (Afinitor) not recommended in those with severe liver impairment. Dose reduction is recommended with mild-to-moderate liver impairment
- contraindicated in those with hypersensitivity to sirolimus
- see also General Nursing considerations/Cautions for immunomodifiers (p. 1238)

Patient education

- instruct the patient to take tablets whole, not chewed or broken, and to consistently take either with or without food (but not switch between the two) and at the same time
- (Dispersible tablets) advise the patient that dispersible tablets should not be swallowed whole, chewed or crushed
- (Dispersible tablets) the patient should be given the following instructions regarding dispersion of tablets:
  - (using syringe) place the dose (up to 10 mg) in a 10 mL syringe and add 5 mL water and 4 mL air. If the dose is greater than 10 mg, a second syringe should be used. Allow the syringe to stand (tip up) in a container for 3 minutes until the tablet has dispersed into suspension. The syringe should then be inverted five times to mix the suspension and then drunk. A further 5 mL water and 4 mL of air should be added to the

syringe, swirled to suspend any remaining particles and drunk
- (using glass) place the tablet (up to 10 mg) in 25 mL water and allow to disperse for 3 minutes, stir gently with a spoon and drink. A further 25 mL water should be added to the glass, stirred with the same spoon to resuspend any remaining particles and drunk
- if mouth ulcers or oral mucositis occur, the patient should be advised not to use alcohol, hydrogen peroxide, iodine or thyme-containing mouthwashes as they may make the condition worse. Antifungal preparations should be used only if fungal infection exists
- the patient should be instructed to avoid grapefruit, grapefruit juice, star fruit or Seville oranges during therapy
- advise the patient to seek medical advice if any persistent or worsening cough, wheezing, difficulty breathing or shortness of breath occurs
- counsel the patient regarding the importance of avoiding pregnancy during therapy, including the need to use adequate contraception before starting, during and for 8 weeks after therapy is stopped
- see also General Patient education for immunomodifiers (p. 1238)

 Tablets should not be crushed or broken. Mask and gloves should be worn when dispersing tablets.

 Not recommended during pregnancy unless benefits outweigh risks.

 Not recommended during breastfeeding or for 2 weeks after last dose.

GUSELKUMAB
Trade name
Tremfya

Available form
Prefilled syringe/pen: 100 mg/mL

Action
- human IgG$_1$ monoclonal antibody that selectively binds to interleukin-23 (known to be elevated in the skin of those with plaque psoriasis)

Use
- treatment of moderate-to-severe plaque psoriasis in those who are candidates for systemic therapy or phototherapy

Dose
- 100 mg SC at weeks 0, 4 and then every 8 weeks afterwards

Adverse effects
- diarrhoea, gastroenteritis
- upper respiratory tract infection, herpes simplex infections, tinea
- arthralgia
- headache, migraine
- injection site reactions
- (Uncommon) hypersensitivity, rash, urticaria

Interactions
- see General Interactions of immunomodifiers (p. 1237)

Nursing considerations/Cautions
- the trade name and batch number should be recorded in the patient's medical history
- the patient may be taught to self-administer. The first injection should be under medical supervision
- see also General Nursing considerations/Cautions for immunomodifiers (p. 1238)

Patient education
- see Patient education for icatibant (p. 1256) for self-administration instructions
- see General Patient education for immunomodifiers (p. 1238)

 Not recommended in pregnancy because no safety data are available.

IMMUNOMODIFIERS

 Not recommended in when breastfeeding because no safety data are available.

C1 ESTERASE INHIBITOR
Trade names
Berinert, Cinryze

Available forms
Vial: 500 IU, 2000 IU, 3000 IU

Action
- belongs to serine protease inhibitor group (that includes antithrombin III) and inhibits activated serine proteinases (C1r and C1s), kallikrein and coagulation factors XIIa and XIa
- inhibits complement system, contact system, fibrinolytic system and coagulation cascade
- produced from human plasma
- long elimination half-life (> 60 hours)

Use
- treatment of acute attacks in those with hereditary angioedema
- preprocedure prevention in those with C1 esterase deficiency
- prevention of angioedema in those experiencing frequent attacks who are intolerant to or inadequately protected by oral therapy

Dose
- (Acute attack treatment) 20 IU/kg as slow IV injection at 4 mL/min (Berinert IV) **OR**
- (Treatment of acute attack) 1000 IU IV at 1 mL/min at first sign of attack, with a second dose given if no response after 60 minutes (Cinryze) **OR**
- (Routine prophylaxis) 1000 IU IV at 1 mL/min every 3–4 days, adjusting interval according to response (Cinryze) **OR**
- (Routine prophylaxis) 60 IU/kg SC twice weekly (every 3–4 days) (Berinert SC) **OR**
- (Preprocedure prevention) 1000 IU IV at 1 mL/min within 24 hours of medical, dental or surgical procedure (Cinryze)

Adverse effects
- nausea, vomiting, altered taste, abdominal pain
- headache, dizziness
- rash, erythema, pruritus
- nasopharyngitis
- flushing
- muscle spasms, pain
- peripheral oedema
- fever
- hypersensitivity
- (Injection site) redness, pain, bruising, irritation, haematoma and, uncommonly, burning sensation, thrombosis, phlebitis
- (Uncommon) thrombotic events
- (Rare) allergic reaction, anaphylaxis

Nursing considerations/Cautions
- if the patient has a known allergy tendency (e.g. asthma), antihistamines and corticosteroids should be given prophylactically
- (Cinryze, acute attack) second dose is more likely to be required if the patient has severe attack, laryngeal attack or if treatment has been delayed
- contains 486 mg of sodium/100 mL (Berinert) or 11.5 mg (Cinryze), which may need to be considered as part of salt-restricted diet
- patient can be taught to self-administer with first injection under medical supervision
- because it is derived from human plasma, there is a theoretical risk, although remote, of transmission of infectious material such as viruses
- reconstituted using diluent provided (water for injections) and manufacturer's instructions
- (IV) administer alone
- do not shake solution, as this will denature protein
- name and batch number of product should be recorded in patient history
- caution if used in those at risk of thrombotic events (including presence of indwelling catheter)
- not recommended for treatment of capillary leak syndrome (Berinert IV)

Patient education
- caution the patient against driving or operating machinery if dizziness persists

- instruct the patient in the correct self-administration technique, including reconstitution of solution, administration and correct disposal of used needles. It is important to ensure the patient understands the importance of seeking medical attention immediately if any laryngeal swelling or airway obstruction occurs
- counsel the patient regarding the medication being a human plasma derivative and the theoretical risk of transmission of infectious material

Recommended during pregnancy only if the benefit outweighs the risk owing to limited data.

Recommended when breastfeeding only if the benefit outweighs the risk owing to limited data.

ICATIBANT
Trade names
Cipla Icatibant, Firazyr, Fyzant, Icatibant Lupin

Available form
Prefilled syringe: 30 mg/3 mL

Action
- selective antagonist at bradykinin type 2 receptors
- hereditary angioedema attacks are accompanied by bradykinin release, which is responsible for many of the clinical symptoms (subcutaneous and/or submucosal oedema of upper respiratory tract, skin and GI tract)

Use
- symptomatic treatment of hereditary angioedema attack (in adults with C1 esterase inhibitor deficiency)

Dose
- 30 mg SC slowly. If symptoms recur or are not relieved, a further 30 mg SC can be given after 6 hours, and repeated again if necessary (daily maximum 90 mg at 6-hour intervals)

Adverse effects
- (Injection site) irritation, erythema, swelling, burning sensation, itching, pain
- prolonged prothrombin time, increase in blood creatine phosphokinase (CPK) and transaminases, and uncommonly abnormal liver function tests, hyperglycaemia, hyperuricaemia
- dizziness, headache and uncommonly fatigue, asthenia
- fever
- rash, pruritus, erythema and uncommonly urticaria
- nausea and uncommonly, vomiting, weight increase
- (Uncommon) hot flush
- (Uncommon) cough, asthma, nasal congestion, pharyngitis
- (Uncommon) herpes zoster
- (Uncommon) muscle spasm

Interactions
- may antagonise actions of angiotensin converting enzyme (ACE) inhibitors (which are not recommended for those with hereditary angioedema because of the risk of inducing an attack)

Nursing considerations/Cautions
- the patient may be taught to self-administer. The first injection should be under medical supervision
- caution if used in those with acute ischaemic heart disease, unstable angina pectoris or within weeks of having a stroke

Patient education
- the patient should be advised to seek medical attention immediately if an attack involves the face, lips, throat or voice box area or the patient has difficulty breathing (regardless of response to self-injection)
- advise the patient to seek medical advice if there is no resolution in an attack within 2 hours of self-injection

IMMUNOMODIFIERS

- instruct the patient in the correct SC self-administration technique, including:
  - the patient has demonstrated SC administration and is comfortable with the technique
  - remove the syringe from the fridge 30–45 minutes before injection and allow the solution to come to room temperature but do not warm in any way
  - check the prefilled syringe for any signs of particles or cloudiness (and do not use if these are present)
  - check the expiry date and do not use if the date has passed
  - do not shake the syringe
  - rotate injections sites (abdomen (at least 5 cm from navel), thighs (front, avoiding area 5 cm above knees and below groin) and upper arms (fleshy area at back)
  - do not inject into skin that is red and inflamed, has stretch marks, is scarred, tender or bruised or has psoriasis
  - wash hands with soap and water
  - clean the injection site with alcohol and allow to dry for at least 10 seconds (and do not touch the site again)
  - remove the needle cover and hold the syringe in the dominant hand (similar to holding a pencil)
  - pinch skin between thumb and index finger (about 5 cm fold) and insert the needle at 45–90-degree angle
  - release skin and push the plunger down to inject the entire content of the syringe
  - release the plunger and remove syringe
  - if there is blood present, press with cotton ball or gauze but do not rub the injection site
  - safely dispose of the syringe (e.g. sharps container, puncture-proof hard plastic or glass container with lid) and store container out of reach of children. When full, see advice from the pharmacist or doctor regarding disposal
  - prefilled syringes should be used only once
  - store unused syringes in the fridge but do not freeze
  - if a vial of powder and diluent (water for injections) requires mixing, this must be done carefully and according to directions, taking care not to shake the solution in order to mix it
  - nothing else should be mixed in the same syringe
- instruct the patient to inject slowly
- warn the patient against driving or operating machinery if dizziness, asthenia or fatigue occurs

 Not recommended in pregnancy, as no safety data available.

 Breastfeeding is not recommended within 12 hours of therapy.

IXEKIZUMAB
Trade name
Taltz

Available form
Autoinjector/prefilled syringe: 80 mg/mL

Action
- IgG$_4$ monoclonal antibody with high affinity for proinflammatory cytokine IL-17A (IL-17A plays a major role in excess keratinocyte proliferation and activation in psoriasis)
- half-life 13 days (plaque psoriasis); clearance increases as body weight increases

Use
- moderate-to-severe plaque psoriasis
- active psoriatic arthritis (in patients who have not responded to or are intolerant to other disease-modifying antirheumatic drugs (DMARDs))

Dose
- (Plaque psoriasis) initially 160 mg SC (week 0), then 80 mg SC every 2 weeks

1257

for 12 weeks (weeks 2, 4, 6, 8, 10, 12), then 80 mg SC monthly **OR**
- (Psoriatic arthritis) initially 160 mg SC, then 80 mg SC monthly

Adverse effects
- upper respiratory tract infection, nasopharyngitis, rhinitis, influenza
- nausea
- oropharyngeal pain
- tinea
- conjunctivitis
- oral candidiasis
- transient neutropenia
- (Injection site) pain, redness
- (Rare) anaphylaxis, angioedema, urticaria, development of antibodies

Interaction
- not recommended with live vaccines

Nursing considerations/Cautions
- if the patient has psoriatic arthritis and moderate-to-severe plaque psoriasis, the dosage for plaque psoriasis should be used
- the patient should be assessed for TB before starting therapy. Anti-TB therapy should be considered for patients with latent or active TB if adequate treatment cannot be confirmed. Patients must be closely monitored for any signs of TB
- the patient can be taught to self-administer
- caution if used in those with Crohn's disease or ulcerative colitis, as exacerbation of the condition may occur
- caution if used in those with clinically important chronic or active infection

Patient education
- advise the patient to seek medical advice if any of the following occur:
  - fever, flu-like symptoms, night sweats, cough that lasts for weeks, shortness of breath, fatigue, unintentional weight loss, coughing up blood
- instruct the patient in correct SC self-administration technique (see Patient education for icatibant, p. 1256). Warn the patient not to shake the autoinjector/prefilled syringe
- warn the patient not to use the solution if it has been frozen
- the autoinjector/prefilled syringe should be stored at 2−8°C and protected from light. If not refrigerated and unused for 5 days, the autoinjector/prefilled syringe should be discarded

Not recommended in pregnancy, as limited safety data are available.

Not recommended when breastfeeding, as no safety data are available.

LENALIDOMIDE
Trade names
Cipla Lenalidomide, Lenalidomide Dr Reddy's, Lenalidomide Sandoz, Lenalidomide Viatris, Lenalidomide-Teva, Revlimid, Lenalide

Available forms
Capsules: 5 mg, 10 mg, 15 mg, 25 mg

Action
- immunomodulator with antiangiogenic, antineoplastic and pro-erythropoietic properties
- inhibits growth of some haemopoietic tumour cells (including multiple myeloma plasma tumour cells), increases T-cell and natural killer cell-mediated immunity, increases number of natural killer T cells, inhibits monocyte production of pro-inflammatory cytokines and inhibits formation of micro vessels
- structurally related to thalidomide and carries the same risk of teratogenic effects

Use
- treatment of multiple myeloma (MM) (with dexamethasone) in patients where disease has progressed despite one treatment
- treatment of newly diagnosed multiple myeloma (with dexamethasone and bortezomib) in patients ineligible for

IMMUNOMODIFIERS

- autologous stem cell transplantation or as induction before stem cell transplantation in those who are eligible
- treatment of relapsed or refractory mantle cell lymphoma
- treatment of transfusion-dependent anaemia due to low or intermediate-1 risk myelodysplastic syndromes (MDS) (associated with deletion 5q cytogenetic abnormality, with or without other cytogenetic abnormalities)

Dose

- (Previously treated MM) initially 25 mg orally daily (1 hour before or 2 hours after food) on days 1—21 of a 28-day cycle (with dexamethasone 40 mg orally daily on days 1—4, 9—12 and 17—20 for 4 cycles, then decreasing dexamethasone to 40 mg orally daily on days 1—4 only of a 28-day cycle) (with dose adjustment dependent on platelet and absolute neutrophil count (ANC)) and continued until disease progression or unacceptable toxicity occurs **OR**
- (Newly diagnosed MM, not eligible for stem cell transplant) initially 25 mg orally daily on days 1—14 of a 21-day cycle (with dexamethasone 20 mg orally daily on days 2, 4, 5, 8, 9, 11 and 12 of a 21-day cycle and bortezomib IV or SC 1.3 mg/m^2 on days 1, 4, 8 and 11 of a 21-day cycle), then 25 mg orally daily on days 1—21 of a 28-day cycle (with dexamethasone 40 mg orally daily on days 1, 8, 15 and 22 of a 28-day cycle) **OR**
- (Newly diagnosed MM, not eligible for stem cell transplant, ≤ 75 years, no renal impairment) initially 25 mg orally daily on days 1—21 of a 28-day cycle (with dexamethasone 40 mg orally daily on days 1, 8, 15 and 22 of a 28-day cycle) **OR**
- (Newly diagnosed MM, eligible for stem cell transplant) 25 mg orally daily on days 1—14 of a 21-day cycle (with dexamethasone 20 mg orally daily on days 2, 4, 5, 8, 9, 11 and 12 of a 21-day cycle and bortezomib IV or SC 1.3 mg/m^2 on days 1, 4, 8 and 11 of a 21-day cycle) **OR**
- (Newly diagnosed MM, eligible for stem cell transplant) 25 mg orally daily on days 1—21 of a 28-day cycle (with dexamethasone 20 mg orally daily on days 1—4 and 9—12 of a 28-day cycle and bortezomib IV or SC 1.3 mg/m^2 on days 1, 4, 8 and 11 of a 28-day cycle) **OR**
- (Newly diagnosed MM, post stem cell transplant) 10 mg orally daily for days 1—28 of a 28-day cycle for repeated cycles. If tolerated, the dose may be increased to 15 mg orally daily after 12 weeks **OR**
- (MDS) initially 10 mg orally daily on days 1—21 of a 28-day cycle (with dose adjustment dependent on platelet and ANC) **OR**
- (Relapsed or refractory mantle cell lymphoma) 25 mg orally daily on days 1—21 of a 28-day cycle, continued until disease progression or unacceptable toxicity occurs

Adverse effects

- neutropenia, thrombocytopenia, anaemia, leucopenia, febrile neutropenia, pancytopenia
- atrial fibrillation, tachycardia, hypotension, hypertension, chest pain, cardiac failure, myocardial infarction
- peripheral oedema
- dyspnoea, cough, oropharyngeal pain, dysphonia
- anorexia, nausea, vomiting, diarrhoea, abdominal pain, constipation, dyspepsia, altered taste, dry mouth, weight decrease, toothache
- headache, fatigue, asthenia, insomnia, depression, dizziness, tremor
- vertigo
- syncope
- fever
- muscle weakness, muscle spasm, myalgia, arthralgia, bone pain, musculoskeletal pain, back pain, pain in extremities
- hyperglycaemia, hypocalcaemia, hypokalaemia, hypomagnesaemia, iron overload

- transient altered liver enzymes, hyperbilirubinaemia, liver damage
- hypothyroidism and, less commonly, hyperthyroidism
- thromboembolism (deep vein thrombosis (DVT), pulmonary embolus (PE))
- kidney failure
- rash, pruritus, dry skin, increased sweating
- peripheral neuropathy, paraesthesia, neuralgia
- (Rare) angioedema, severe dermatological reactions, tumour lysis syndrome, tumour flare reaction, progressive multifocal leukoencephalopathy (with dexamethasone)
- see also General Adverse effects of immunomodifiers (p. 1237)

Interactions
- caution if given with other agents that increase the risk of thrombosis
- (MM) increased the risk of thromboembolism when given with dexamethasone
- caution if used with agents that impair liver function
- not recommended with combined oral contraceptives or hormone replacement therapy because of the increased risk of thromboembolism
- caution if given with other myelosuppressive agents
- caution if given with warfarin; therefore INR should be closely monitored especially when starting or stopping therapy
- may increase serum levels of digoxin increasing the risk of toxicity; therefore serum levels should be monitored during therapy

Nursing considerations/Cautions
- only doctors and pharmacists who are registered with the restricted distribution program can prescribe and dispense lenalidomide to patients who meet all the requirements and are registered with this program. Patients must be fully aware of the consequences if pregnancy occurs and be willing to abide by the conditions (e.g. pregnancy testing, contraception) before, during and after completion of treatment
- to be eligible for therapy, a female patient (or female partner of male patient) is considered to no longer be of childbearing potential if she:
  - is over 50 years and has been naturally amenorrhoeic for 1 year (however, amenorrhoea postchemotherapy does not rule out childbearing potential)
  - has premature ovarian failure (confirmed by specialist gynaecologist)
  - has had a hysterectomy or bilateral salpingo-oophorectomy
  - has uterine agenesis, Turner syndrome or XY genotype
- it is recommended that women of childbearing potential should have a pregnancy test before starting therapy, weekly during the first month and then monthly (if menstrual cycles are regular) or 2-weekly (if menstrual cycles are irregular)
- (MM, MDS) complete blood count (including white blood cell count with differential, platelet count, haemoglobin and haematocrit) should be performed before starting therapy, then weekly for 8 weeks, and then monthly
- (Newly diagnosed MM, transplant ineligible) complete blood count (including white blood cell count with differential, platelet count, haemoglobin and haematocrit) should be performed before starting therapy, then weekly for the first 2 cycles of treatment, then day 1 and 15 of cycle 3 and monthly thereafter
- (Newly diagnosed MM, with dexamethasone and bortezomib) complete blood count (including white blood cell count with differential, platelet count, haemoglobin and haematocrit) should be performed before starting therapy, then weekly for the first cycle of treatment, then before the start of each subsequent cycle, and then monthly afterwards

IMMUNOMODIFIERS

- (Mantle cell lymphoma) complete blood count (including white blood cell count with differential, platelet count, haemoglobin and haematocrit) should be performed before starting therapy, then weekly for the first cycle of treatment, every 2 weeks (for cycles 2—4), then before the start of each subsequent cycle
- ANC and platelet count should be measured before starting therapy
- (MM) if ANC $< 1.0 \times 10^9$/L and/or platelet count $< 75 \times 10^9$/L (or $< 30 \times 10^9$/L depending on bone marrow infiltration by plasma cells), therapy should not be started
- (Newly diagnosed MM) if ANC $< 1.5 \times 10^9$/L and/or platelet count $< 50 \times 10^9$/L, therapy should not be started
- (MDS) if ANC $< 0.5 \times 10^9$/L and/or platelet count $< 50 \times 10^9$/L, therapy should not be started
- thyroid and renal function monitoring is recommended before starting and regularly during therapy
- (MM, eligible for stem cell transplant) up to 8 cycles of 21 days or 6 cycles of 28-day treatment are recommended. Autologous stem cell transplant should occur within 4 cycles
- tablets contain lactose and are not recommended in those with galactose intolerance, lactase deficiency or glucose—galactose malabsorption
- caution if used in those with hypertension, congestive cardiac failure, electrolyte imbalance or infection, as they are at increased risk of atrial fibrillation
- caution if used in those with hypertension, hyperlipidaemia or if a smoker, because of the increased risk of myocardial infarction
- caution if used in those with high tumour burden (e.g. previously treated mantle cell lymphoma) because of the increased risk of tumour lysis syndrome or tumour flare syndrome
- caution if used in those with liver or renal impairment (dose reduction is recommended in those with renal impairment)
- caution if used in those who have undergone solid organ transplantation because of the increased risk of organ rejection
- an increased risk of venous and arterial thromboembolism (when given with dexamethasone); therefore caution if used in those with a history of thrombosis or with risk factors such as smoking, hypertension or hyperlipidaemia
- not recommended in those who have experienced thalidomide-induced rash
- not recommended for management of chronic lymphocytic leukaemia owing to increased mortality
- contraindicated if ANC $< 1.0 \times 10^9$/L or platelet count $< 75 \times 10^9$/L (or $< 30 \times 10^9$/L depending on bone marrow infiltration by plasma cells) (MM), ANC $< 1.0 \times 10^9$/L or platelet count $< 50 \times 10^9$/L (newly diagnosed MM) or if ANC $< 0.5 \times 10^9$/L (MDS)
- contraindicated in women of child-bearing potential unless all conditions have been met

Patient education

- the patient should be advised to take capsules at the same time every day and swallow whole (not opened, chewed or divided) with water 1 hour before or 2 hours after food
- the patient should be advised that if dose is missed by more than 12 hours it should not be taken. The next dose should be taken at the normal time the next day
- the patient must receive counselling to ensure good understanding of the potential therapy risks and outcomes (i.e. risks to an unborn child), and contraceptive requirements associated with lenalidomide before giving a full and written consent prior to starting therapy. The patient's sexual partner should also receive counselling and information

- important patient advice should include:
  - do not drive or operate machinery if fatigue, dizziness, blurred vision and/or somnolence occurs
  - seek medical advice if any of the following occur:
    - any shortness of breath, chest pain or arm/leg swelling (symptoms of DVT and PE)
    - febrile illness (neutropenia)
    - bleeding and nosebleeds
    - rash, especially if accompanied with fever and/or swollen glands
    - any numbness, tingling or pain in hands or feet
  - do not donate blood during therapy or within 1 week of stopping therapy
  - a male patient must not donate semen during or within 1 week of stopping therapy
  - male patients should be advised that lenalidomide is present in semen and therefore adequate contraceptive methods (latex or polyurethane condoms) must be used during sexual activity with women of childbearing potential (or who have not been menopausal for at least 2 years); condom use must continue for at least 4 weeks after stopping therapy
  - explain the importance of having a medically supervised pregnancy test at the time of consultation (or within 3 days prior to visit) to exclude pregnancy before the start of therapy, with a medically supervised pregnancy test repeated every 4 weeks, including when therapy is stopped
  - women of childbearing potential (who have not had a hysterectomy, salpingo-oophorectomy or are not > 50 years and postmenopausal for more than 1 year) must use one reliable contraceptive measure (e.g. intrauterine device, hormone implant or depot contraception, tubal ligation, partner vasectomy (with two negative semen analyses), oral progesterone-only contraceptive pill) for 1 month before, during and 1 month after stopping therapy
  - copper-releasing intrauterine devices (IUD) are not recommended because of the risk of infection (at the time of insertion) and menstrual blood loss, which can compromise female patients with neutropenia or thrombocytopenia
  - a combined oral contraceptive pill is not recommended because of the increased risk of venous thrombotic event
  - any woman (either taking lenalidomide or whose partner is taking lenalidomide) who is of childbearing potential and who experiences menstrual irregularities or suspects she is pregnant must seek medical advice immediately

 Teratogen — capsules must not be opened or crushed.

 Under NO circumstances should lenalidomide be used during pregnancy because of its relationship to thalidomide. Thalidomide is a known human teratogen causing mortality at or just after birth and birth defects, which include absence or shortness of limbs, external ear abnormalities, eye abnormalities, facial palsy, congenital heart defects and malformation of the alimentary tract, urinary tract and/or genital tract.

 Not recommended when breastfeeding, as no safety data are available.

 In renal impairment: patient's dose must be reduced

MYCOPHENOLATE MOFETIL
Trade names
APO-Mycophenolate, ARX-Mycophenolate, CellCept, Cellplant, Ceptolate, Mycophenolate Accord, Mycophenolate GH, Mycophenolate Sandoz, Noumed Mycophenolate, Pharmcor Mycophenolate

MYCOPHENOLATE SODIUM
Trade names
Myfortic, Mycotex

Available forms
Capsules: 250 mg;
Tablets: 500 mg;
Tablets (enteric coated): 180 mg, 360 mg;
Oral solution: 1 g/5 mL;
Vial: 500 mg

Action
- immunosuppressant
- selectively inhibits inosine monophosphate dehydrogenase thereby inhibiting proliferation of T and B cells, decreasing monocyte and lymphocyte recruitment to chronic inflammatory sites
- narrow therapeutic index
- metabolised to the active form (mycophenolic acid)

Use
- prevention of solid allogeneic organ rejection
- lupus nephritis (WHO class III, IV or V) (induction and maintenance)

Dose
- (Renal transplant) 1 g orally or IV over 2 hours twice daily **OR**
- (Cardiac transplant) 1.5 g orally or IV over 2 hours twice daily **OR**
- (Liver transplant) initially 1 g IV over 2 hours twice daily, then 1.5 g orally twice daily **OR**
- (Other transplant) 1–1.5 g orally or IV over 2 hours twice daily **OR**
- (Renal transplant) 720 mg orally twice daily, starting within 48 hours of transplantation (enteric-coated capsules) **OR**
- (Lupus nephritis) 720 mg orally twice daily (with corticosteroids) (induction), then dose reduction once the clinical response has been achieved (Myfortic)

Adverse effects
- anorexia, diarrhoea, loose stools, constipation, dyspepsia, nausea, vomiting, oral thrush, gastritis, flatulence, GI thrush, abdominal pain/tenderness/distension, oesophagitis and, uncommonly, GI ulceration and haemorrhage and, rarely, perforation
- headache, dizziness, fatigue, anxiety, asthenia, insomnia, tremor
- arthralgia, myalgia
- hypertension, hypotension
- cough, dyspnoea, dyspnoea on exertion
- hyperlipidaemia, abnormal liver function tests, hepatitis
- elevated blood creatinine
- peripheral oedema
- hypocalcaemia, hypokalaemia, hyperuricaemia, hyperkalaemia, hypomagnesaemia
- fever
- leucopenia, thrombocytopenia, anaemia, neutropenia
- (IV site) phlebitis, thrombosis
- (Rare) progressive multifocal leukoencephalopathy, pure red cell aplasia
- see also General Adverse effects of immunomodifiers (p. 1237)

Interactions
- not recommended with azathioprine because of the increased risk of bone marrow depression
- caution if given with aciclovir or valaciclovir, as combination may lead to increased serum levels of both agents
- absorption may be decreased if given with aluminium/magnesium hydroxide, phosphate binders or colestyramine
- caution if used with proton pump inhibitors
- dose reduction may be required if given with ganciclovir in those with renal impairment
- not recommended with live attenuated virus vaccines
- caution if given with tacrolimus or sirolimus
- availability may be reduced if given with iron or iron supplements
- serum levels may be decreased by rifampicin and telmisartan

- may decrease the efficacy of combined oral contraceptives
- caution if given with ciprofloxacin or amoxicillin with clavulanic acid and metronidazole, as serum levels may decrease

Nursing considerations/Cautions

- therapy should be started within 24 hours of transplantation
- therapy should be changed from IV to oral as soon as possible
- blood counts should be measured weekly for the first month, twice monthly for 2 months, then monthly for the first year. Therapy should be interrupted and/or the dose decreased if the absolute neutrophil count (ANC) $< 1.5 \times 10^9$/L
- pregnancy should be excluded before starting therapy in female patients using 2 urine or serum pregnancy tests. The second test should be performed 8–10 days after the first test and just before the start of therapy. Pregnancy tests should be repeated if there is any gap in contraception
- therapeutic serum levels should be monitored regularly during therapy
- (IV) reconstitute using glucose 5% only and dilute according to the manufacturer's instructions to a concentration of 6 g/mL and administer by IV infusion over 2 hours
- (IV) not recommended by rapid or bolus IV
- (IV) administer alone
- (IV) incompatible with sodium chloride 0.9% and Ringer's or lactated Ringer's solution
- (IV) reconstituting should be gentle, avoiding foaming
- if oral solution is given via nasogastric tube, the tube should have a diameter of not less than 1.7 mm
- preparations are not equivalent nor interchangeable (2 g mycophenolate mofetil = 1.44 g mycophenolate sodium)
- (Oral suspension) caution if used in those with phenylketonuria, as the suspension contains aspartame
- caution if used in those with chronic renal impairment (dose should not be greater than 1 g twice daily in those with severe renal impairment), GI disease or Lesch–Nyhan syndrome (hypoxanthine–guanine–phospho-ribosyl transferase deficiency)
- caution if used in those over 65 years because of an increased risk of adverse effects
- contraindicated in those with hypersensitivity to mycophenolate, mycophenolic acid or polysorbate 80 (if given IV)
- see also General Nursing considerations/Cautions for immunomodifiers (p. 1238)

Patient education

- instruct the patient to take iron supplements 3 hours after mycophenolate preparations
- the patient should be advised to take antacids 2 hours apart from mycophenolate preparations
- advise the patient to swallow enteric-coated capsules whole, without chewing or breaking them
- ensure the patient understands the importance of consistently taking medication in relation to food (i.e. always before food or always after, not mixing the two) to ensure consistent absorption
- advise the patient and carer to seek medical advice if any confusion, apathy, one-sided paralysis, difficulty walking or cognitive impairment occurs
- all patients should be advised not to donate blood during or for 6 weeks after stopping therapy
- (Male patient) instruct the patient not to donate semen during or for 90 days after stopping therapy
- warn the patient not to drive or operate machinery if dizziness, fatigue or anxiety occurs
- (Male patient) counsel the patient regarding the need to wear a condom during and for 13 weeks after stopping therapy (regardless of whether he has had a vasectomy or not), as there is a risk of transmission in seminal fluid. The

IMMUNOMODIFIERS

- female partner of a male patient should also be counselled regarding the need to use highly effective contraception during and for 13 weeks after their partner has ceased therapy
- ensure female patients of childbearing potential understand the importance of using two forms of highly effective contraception before, during and 6 weeks after therapy to avoid pregnancy and to seek medical advice immediately if pregnancy occurs. Patients should be warned that combined oral contraceptives may not be effective during therapy
- see also General Patient education for immunomodifiers (p. 1238)

Oral solution is available. Capsule should not be opened or tablets broken or crushed.

Under NO circumstances should this be used during pregnancy because it is a known human teratogen and fetal loss and/or congenital abnormalities may occur.

Contraindicated during breastfeeding because of inconsistent available data. Another drug is recommended.

In renal impairment patients: if CrCl < 25 mL/min consider adjusting the dose, additional plasma concentration monitoring is required.

PALIVIZUMAB

Trade name
Synagis

Available form
Vial: 100 mg/mL

Action
- IgG$_1$ monoclonal antibody that has inhibitory activity against respiratory syncytial virus (RSV)

Use
- prevention of serious respiratory tract disease caused by RSV in high-risk children (e.g. bronchopulmonary dysplasia, prematurity (< 35 weeks gestation), significant congenital heart disease)

Dose
- 15 mg/kg IM monthly, starting at the beginning of the RSV season

Adverse effects
- upper respiratory infection, rhinitis, cough, wheeze, bronchiolitis, pneumonia, dyspnoea, pharyngitis, flu-like symptoms, apnoea, croup
- otitis media
- fever
- rash, eczema, fungal dermatitis
- diarrhoea, vomiting, oral thrush, gastroenteritis, constipation, flatulence, feeding abnormalities
- conjunctivitis
- pain
- viral, bacterial and fungal infections
- nervousness, somnolence
- coagulation disorder, haemorrhage, thrombocytopenia, anaemia
- hypokalaemia
- elevated liver enzymes
- failure to thrive
- hypotonia
- (Rare) anaphylaxis, allergic reaction
- injection site reaction

Interactions
- may interfere with immune-based RSV diagnostic test and viral culture assays

Nursing considerations/Cautions
- the first dose should be given before the start of the RSV season
- use may be delayed if the child has severe acute infection or acute febrile illness, unless the RSV risk is high
- if a child develops RSV, monthly injections are still recommended to prevent reinfection
- adrenaline (epinephrine) (1:1000), corticosteroid, antihistamines, oxygen and resuscitation equipment should be readily available in the event of anaphylaxis
- a volume greater than 1 mL should be given as divided IM doses

- the gluteal muscle is not routinely used for IM injection in children
- the solution should not be diluted for IM administration
- not recommended for use in adults
- caution if given IM to those with thrombocytopenia or coagulation disorder
- contraindicated in those with known hypersensitivity to other recombinant monoclonal antibodies

PIRFENIDONE

Trade names
ARX-Pirfenidone, Esbriet, Pirfenidet, Pirfenidone Dr. Reddy's, Pirfenidone Sandoz

Available forms
Tablets: 267 mg, 801 mg

Action
- antifibrotic, anti-inflammatory immunomodifier

Use
- treatment of idiopathic pulmonary fibrosis

Dose
- 267 mg orally 3 times daily with food (days 1—7), then 534 mg 3 times daily (days 8—14), then 801 mg 3 times daily (day 15 onwards)

Adverse effects
- nausea, vomiting, diarrhoea, anorexia, dyspepsia, abdominal pain, gastro-esophageal reflux disease (GORD)
- weight loss
- upper respiratory tract infection, sinusitis
- photosensitivity, rash
- angioedema, anaphylaxis
- dizziness, fatigue, headache, insomnia
- arthralgia

Interactions
- contraindicated with fluvoxamine
- not recommended with other agents known to cause photosensitivity
- decreased serum levels in smokers
- caution if given with ciprofloxacin, as increased serum levels may occur
- decreased serum levels may occur if given with omeprazole or rifampicin

Nursing considerations/Cautions
- liver function (alanine aminotransferase (ALT), aspartate aminotransferase (AST) and bilirubin) should be measured before starting therapy, then monthly for 6 months and 3-monthly for the remainder of the treatment
- patient weight should be monitored during therapy and dietary advice recommended if weight loss of clinical significance occurs
- if therapy is interrupted for 14 or more consecutive days, it should be restarted by undergoing the initial 2 weeks of titration up to the recommended daily dose. If therapy is interrupted for less than 14 days, the dose can be resumed at the previous recommended dose without titration
- caution if used in those with mild, moderate or severe kidney impairment or mild-to-moderate liver impairment
- contraindicated in those with a history of pirfenidone-induced angioedema, severe liver impairment, end-stage liver disease, severe kidney impairment (creatinine clearance < 30 mL/min) or end-stage kidney disease requiring dialysis

Patient education
- instruct the patient not to drive or operate machinery if dizziness or fatigue occurs
- remind the patient to take capsules or tablets with food to reduce gastrointestinal adverse effects
- the patient should be advised to avoid or minimise exposure to direct sunlight and sunlamps during therapy. If sun exposure cannot be avoided, instruct the patient to wear protective clothing and sunscreen (SPF 30+)

IMMUNOMODIFIERS

- encourage the patient to stop smoking before and during therapy, and discuss any changes to smoking habit with the doctor
- advise the patient to seek medical advice immediately if any of the following occur:
  - swelling of face, lips and/or tongue
  - rash or photosensitivity (exaggerated sunburn)
  - dizziness
  - weight loss
  - fatigue, loss of appetite, right upper quadrant abdominal pain, dark urine, yellowing of skin and/or whites of the eyes

 Tablet can be crushed and mixed with water, or a spoonful of yoghurt or apple puree.

 Not recommended during pregnancy; no human safety data available.

 Not recommended when breastfeeding because no safety data are available.

 In renal impairment patients this medication is contraindicated if CrCl < 30 mL/min or the patient is receiving dialysis.

Contraindicated in patients with severe hepatic impairment and end-stage liver disease as this medication is eliminated via hepatic metabolism.

PLERIXAFOR
Trade names
Mozobil, Plerixafor ARX, Plerixafor Eugia, Plerixafor-AFT

Available form
Vial: 24 mg/1.2 mL

Action
- CXCR4 chemokine receptor antagonist
- stem cells secrete CXCR4 and migrate to bone marrow through a chemo-attractant effect of stromal cell-derived factor-1β (SDF-1β) produced by bone marrow stromal cells. CXCR4 is thought to assist in binding the stem cells in the marrow
- by using a CXCR4 receptor antagonist, leukocytosis is induced and mature and stem cells appear in the circulation

Use
- mobilise stem cells to peripheral blood for collection and subsequent autologous transplantation in those with lymphoma and multiple myeloma (with granulocyte-colony stimulating factor (G-CSF))

Dose
- therapy is initiated after G-CSF (10 microgram/kg) has been given daily for 4 days, then plerixafor 0.24 mg/kg SC 6–11 hours before apheresis for 2–4 consecutive days (but up to 7 days)

Adverse effects
- (Postinjection reaction) urticaria, periorbital swelling, dyspnoea, hypoxia
- nausea, vomiting, diarrhoea, abdominal pain, flatulence
- headache, dizziness, insomnia, abnormal dreams, fatigue
- arthralgia
- (Uncommon) vasovagal reaction (orthostatic hypotension and/or syncope)
- (Injection site) pain, redness
- (Rare) myocardial infarction, splenic enlargement

Nursing considerations/Cautions
- WBC and platelet count should be monitored during therapy and apheresis
- patient should be closely monitored for 60 minutes for any postinjection reactions or hypotension and/or syncope
- injection-related reaction can be treated using antihistamines, corticosteroids, hydration and oxygen
- the abdomen is the preferred SC injection site
- caution if used in those with moderate-to-severe kidney impairment (dose should be reduced to 0.16 mg/kg)
- caution if used in those with neutrophil count > 50×10^9 cells/L
- not recommended in those with leukaemia

- not recommended for haemopoietic stem cell mobilisation and harvest in those with leukaemia

Patient education
- advise the patient to immediately report any left upper abdominal pain and/or shoulder pain (may be a sign of a spleen problem)
- warn the patient that a vasovagal reaction may occur up to 1 hour after injection
- the patient should be advised not to drive or operate machinery if dizziness, fatigue or vasovagal reaction occurs
- female patients of childbearing capacity should be counselled to use adequate contraception during therapy to prevent pregnancy from occurring

Not recommended during pregnancy, as this is teratogenic in animals and no human safety data are available.

Not recommended when breastfeeding as no human safety data are available.

POMALIDOMIDE
Trade names
Pomalidomide Sandoz, Pomalyst, Pomolide

Available forms
Capsules: 1 mg, 2 mg, 3 mg, 4 mg

Action
- thalidomide analogue with direct anti-myeloma tumouricidal activity, has immunomodulatory activities and inhibits stromal cells support for multiple myeloma tumour cell growth
- inhibits proliferation and induces apoptosis of haematopoietic tumour cells
- inhibits proliferation of lenalidomide-resistant multiple myeloma cell lines and synergises with dexamethasone in both lenalidomide-sensitive and lenalidomide-resistant cell lines to induce apoptosis
- enhances T-cell and natural killer cell-mediated immunity, inhibiting production of pro-inflammatory cytokines by monocytes
- half-life about 9.5 hours

Use
- relapsed refractory multiple myeloma (with dexamethasone) in patients who have received two or more prior treatments (including both lenalidomide and bortezomib) with disease progression
- relapsed or refractory multiple myeloma (with dexamethasone and bortezomib) patients who have received one prior treatment regimen (including lenalidomide)

Dose
- 4 mg orally daily on days 1−21 (of 28-day cycle) with dexamethasone 40 mg orally on days 1, 8, 15 and 22 (of 28-day cycle) **OR**
- 4 mg orally daily on days 1−14 (of 21-day cycle) with dexamethasone 20 mg on days 1, 2, 4, 5, 8, 9, 11 and 12, and bortezomib 1.3 mg/m^2 IV or SC on days 1, 4, 8 and 11 (for cycles 1 to 8), then dexamethasone 20 mg orally daily on days 1, 2, 8 and 9, and bortezomib 1.3 mg/mg^2 IV or SC on days 1 and 8 (for cycle 9 and onwards)

Adverse effects
- dizziness, fatigue, tremor, insomnia, depression
- peripheral neuropathy, paraesthesia
- syncope
- constipation, diarrhoea, nausea, vomiting, decreased weight, altered taste, abdominal pain, stomatitis, dry mouth, abdominal distension
- fever
- peripheral oedema
- anaemia, neutropenia, febrile neutropenia, thrombocytopenia, leucopenia
- pneumonia, upper and lower respiratory tract infection, bronchitis, nasopharyngitis
- dyspnoea, cough, pulmonary embolism
- rash
- atrial fibrillation, hypotension, hypertension
- cataract
- non-cardiac chest pain

IMMUNOMODIFIERS

- bone pain, back pain, muscle spasm, muscular weakness
- hyperkalaemia, hypokalaemia, hyperglycaemia, hypermagnesaemia, hypophosphataemia, hypocalcaemia
- elevated liver enzymes and bilirubin
- urinary retention, renal failure
- deep vein thrombosis
- (Rare) angioedema, severe dermatological reactions, malignancies, tumour lysis syndrome, interstitial lung disease, pneumonitis

Interactions
- caution if used with warfarin. INR should be monitored during therapy, especially when starting, stopping or altering dose
- effectiveness reduced by smoking

Nursing considerations/Cautions
- only doctors and pharmacists who are registered with the restricted distribution (i-access) program can prescribe and dispense pomalidomide to patients who meet all requirements and are registered with this program
- unless other contraindicated, anticoagulation therapy (e.g. aspirin, warfarin, heparin, clopidogrel) is recommended to decrease the risk of thromboembolic events
- blood counts should be monitored weekly for the first 8 weeks, then monthly during therapy
- liver function should be monitored regularly during therapy
- therapy should be started only when the platelet count $\geq 50 \times 10^9$/L and neutrophil count $\geq 1.0 \times 10^9$/L. Dose modification or interruption to therapy is required for haematological issues such as a fall in platelets or a fall in absolute neutrophil count (ANC)
- to be eligible for therapy, a female patient (or female partner of male patient) is considered to no longer be of childbearing potential if she:
  - is over 50 years and has been naturally amenorrhoeic for ≥ 1 year (however, amenorrhoea post-chemotherapy does not rule out childbearing potential)
  - has premature ovarian failure (confirmed by specialist gynaecologist)
  - has had a hysterectomy or bilateral salpingo-oophorectomy
  - has uterine agenesis, Turner syndrome or XY genotype
- it is recommended that women of childbearing potential should have a pregnancy test before starting therapy, weekly during the first month and then monthly (if menstrual cycles are regular) or 2-weekly (if menstrual cycles are irregular)
- if the patient > 75 years, the dexamethasone dose should be decreased
- if pregnancy occurs in a female treated with pomalidomide or she has a male partner taking pomalidomide, therapy should be stopped and the woman referred to a physician specialising/experienced in teratology for evaluation and advice
- caution if used in those with peripheral neuropathy
- caution if used in those with renal impairment or high tumour burden because of an increased risk of tumour lysis syndrome
- contraindicated in females of childbearing potential and male patients unless all of the conditions of the i-access program have been met
- contraindicated in those who have had previous allergic reactions to thalidomide or lenalidomide

Patient education
- instruct the patient to take capsules at the same time every day and swallow whole (not chewed, broken, opened or divided). If powder from capsules makes contact with skin, the skin should be immediately washed with soap and water. If the powder makes contact with mucous membranes, the area should be flushed well with water
- the patient should be advised that if a dose is missed by more than 12 hours it

- should not be taken. The next dose should be taken at the normal time on the next day
- advise the patient to stop smoking before starting therapy. However, any changes to smoking habit during therapy should be discussed with the doctor, as smoking alters the effectiveness of pomalidomide
- the patient must receive counselling to ensure good understanding of the potential therapy risks and outcomes (i.e. risks to unborn child), and contraceptive requirements associated with pomalidomide before giving a full and written consent prior to starting therapy. The patient's sexual partner should also receive counselling and information
- important patient advice should include:
  - do not drive or operate machinery if fatigue, dizziness, blurred vision and/or somnolence occurs
  - seek medical advice immediately if any of the following occur:
    - any shortness of breath, sudden chest pain, cough or arm/leg swelling/tenderness, discolouration or warmth of limb (symptoms of deep vein thrombosis (DVT) and pulmonary embolism (PE))
    - febrile illness (neutropenia)
    - unusual bruising or bleeding, nosebleeds
    - numbness, tingling or pain in hands or feet
    - fever, chills, muscle/joint pain, headache, cough, shortness of breath, fatigue, loss of appetite
- do not donate blood during therapy or within 1 week of stopping therapy (all patients with multiple myelomas are permanently excluded from donating blood in Australia)
- male patients must not donate semen during or within 1 week of stopping therapy
- male patients should be advised that pomalidomide is present in semen and therefore adequate contraceptive methods (latex or polyurethane condoms) must be used during sexual activity with women of childbearing potential (or who have not been menopausal for at least 2 years); condom use must continue for at least 4 weeks after stopping therapy
- emphasise the importance of having a medically supervised pregnancy test at the time of consultation (or within 3 days prior to visit) to exclude pregnancy before the start of therapy, with a medically supervised pregnancy test repeated every 4 weeks, including when therapy is stopped
- women of childbearing potential (who have not had a hysterectomy, salpingo-oophorectomy or are not $\geq$ 50 years and postmenopausal for more than 1 year) must use one reliable contraceptive measure (e.g. intrauterine device, contraceptive hormonal implant, tubal ligation, partner vasectomy (with 2 negative semen analyses), progesterone-only pills, medroxyprogesterone acetate depot) for 1 month before, during and 1 month after stopping therapy
- copper-releasing intrauterine devices (IUD) are not recommended because of the risk of infection (at time of insertion) and menstrual blood loss, which can compromise female patients with neutropenia or thrombocytopenia
- combined oral contraceptive pills are not recommended because of the increased risk of venous thromboembolism
- any woman (either taking pomalidomide or whose partner is taking pomalidomide) who is of childbearing potential and who experiences menstrual irregularities or suspects she is pregnant must seek medical advice immediately

IMMUNOMODIFIERS

- emphasise the importance of not sharing this medication with anyone and returning any unused capsules to the pharmacist at the end of therapy

Teratogen — capsules must not be opened or crushed.

Contraindicated during pregnancy. Women of childbearing potential should be counselled regarding the use of effective contraception during therapy and for 4 weeks after last dose to avoid pregnancy occurring.

Contraindicated during breastfeeding.

RISANKIZUMAB

Trade name
Skyrizi

Available forms
Prefilled syringe: 75 mg/0.83 mL, 150 mg/mL

Action
- humanised immunoglobulin G_1 (IgG_1) monoclonal antibody that selectively binds to interleukin-23 (subunit p19) (known to be involved in inflammation and immune response)

Use
- treatment of moderate-to-severe plaque psoriasis in those who are candidates for systemic therapy or phototherapy

Dose
- 150 mg SC at week 0, week 4 and every 12 weeks afterwards

Adverse effects
- upper respiratory tract infection, tinea infection, folliculitis
- headache, fatigue
- injection site reaction
- (Rare) hypersensitivity

Interactions
- see General Interactions of immunomodifiers (p. 1237)

Nursing considerations/Cautions
- the patient may be taught to self-administer. The first injection should be under medical supervision
- see also General Nursing considerations/Cautions for immunomodifiers (p. 1238)

Patient education
- advise patients that some vaccines are not suitable to be used when on this medication and speak to their doctor
- see also Patient education for icatibant (p. 1256) for self-administration instructions
- see also General Patient education for immunomodifiers (p. 1238)

Should be used during pregnancy only if benefits outweigh risks.

Excretion in breastmilk is unknown; therefore should be used during breastfeeding only if benefits outweigh risks.

SECUKINUMAB

Trade name
Cosentyx

Available forms
Prefilled pen: 150 mg/mL;
Prefilled syringe: 75 mg/0.5 mL

Action
- monoclonal antibody IgG_{1kappa} that inhibits interleukin 17A, which is a pro-inflammatory cytokine that is involved in normal inflammatory and immune responses
- half-life 17—41 days (in those with plaque psoriasis)

Use
- treatment of moderate-to-severe plaque psoriasis in those who are candidates for systemic or phototherapy
- psoriatic arthritis (where previous response to a disease-modifying anti-rheumatic drug (DMARD) was inadequate)

- ankylosing spondylitis

Dose
- (Plaque psoriasis) initially 300 mg SC at weeks 0, 1, 2, 3 and 4, followed by 300 mg monthly (as maintenance) **OR**
- (Psoriatic arthritis, ankylosing spondylitis) initially 150 mg SC at weeks 0, 1, 2, 3 and 4, followed by 150 mg monthly (as maintenance)

Adverse effects
- nasopharyngitis, rhinitis, pharyngitis, upper respiratory tract infections, rhinorrhoea
- oral herpes
- diarrhoea
- urticaria
- elevated liver enzymes, cholesterol and triglycerides
- (Uncommon) conjunctivitis, neutropenia, sinusitis, otitis externa
- (Rare) antibody development
- see also General Adverse effects of immunomodifiers (p. 1237)

Interactions
- see General Interactions of immunomodifiers (p. 1237)

Nursing considerations/Cautions
- 300 mg dose is given as 2 SC injections of 150 mg
- prefilled pen cap contains a latex derivative, which may cause a reaction in latex-sensitive individuals
- the patient may be taught to self-administer. The first administration should be under medical supervision
- caution if used in those with active Crohn's disease, as it may be exacerbated by therapy
- caution if used in those with chronic infection or a history of recurrent infection
- contraindicated in those with active infection such as tuberculosis. The infection should be treated before starting therapy
- see also General Nursing considerations/Cautions for immunomodifiers (p. 1238)

Patient education
- instruct the patient in SC self-administration technique (see Patient education for icatibant, p. 1256) including avoiding injecting into areas not affected by psoriasis
- see also General Patient education for immunomodifiers (p. 1238)

 Should be used during pregnancy only if benefits outweigh risks owing to limited data. If used during pregnancy, infants should not be vaccinated with live vaccines for at least 16 weeks after mother's last dose.

 Caution if used during breastfeeding, as no human safety data are available.

Note
- 75 mg/0.5 mL prefilled syringe is available for use in children

SIROLIMUS
Trade name
Rapamune

Available forms
Oral solution: 1 mg/mL;
Tablets: 0.5 mg, 1 mg, 2 mg

Action
- selective immunosuppressant agent that inhibits T-cell activation
- blocks calcium-dependent and calcium-independent intracellular signals that cause T-cell activation, suppressing immune-mediated reactions (e.g. allograft rejection)
- long half-life (46—78 hours)

Use
- prevention of organ rejection in those at mild-to-moderate risk after receiving a renal transplant (with ciclosporin and corticosteroids)

Dose
- initially 6 mg orally (as soon as possible after transplantation) (loading dose), followed by 2 mg orally daily (with

ciclosporin and corticosteroids). After 2–4 months, ciclosporin is gradually withdrawn over 4–8 weeks; sirolimus dose should be adjusted to maintain blood concentration of 12–20 nanogram/mL (daily maximum 40 mg)

Adverse effects
- peripheral oedema, oedema and rarely, lymphoedema
- delayed wound healing, wound dehiscence, lymphocele
- fever
- tachycardia, thromboembolism (deep vein thrombosis (DVT), pulmonary embolism (PE)), hypertension, pericardial effusion
- nausea, abdominal pain, diarrhoea, stomatitis, constipation, ascites, pancreatitis
- anaemia, thrombocytopenia, leucopenia, neutropenia, haemolytic uraemic syndrome, and uncommonly, thrombotic thrombocytopenic purpura
- abnormal liver function tests, elevated liver enzymes and creatinine
- hypertriglycidaemia, hyperlipidaemia, hypophosphataemia, hypokalaemia, hyperglycaemia
- arthralgia, bone necrosis
- epistaxis
- pleural effusion, pneumonia, pneumonitis
- acne, rash
- pyelonephritis, proteinuria
- headache
- pain
- amenorrhoea, menorrhagia, ovarian cyst
- (Rare) interstitial lung disease, pneumonitis, angioedema
- see also General Adverse effects of immunomodifiers (p. 1237)

Interactions
- not recommended with grapefruit juice
- long-term therapy with ciclosporin is not recommended
- increased risk of angioedema if given with angiotensin converting enzyme (ACE) inhibitors
- serum levels may increase if given with voriconazole, fluconazole, itraconazole, clarithromycin, erythromycin, ciclosporin, metoclopramide, bromocriptine, danazol, diltiazem, verapamil or protease inhibitors (e.g. ritonavir); therefore not recommended together
- serum levels may be decreased if given with rifampicin, rifabutin, phenytoin, phenobarbital (phenobarbitone), carbamazepine or St John's wort; therefore not recommended together
- caution if given with other agents that impair kidney function
- increased risk of rhabdomyolysis if given with 3-hydroxy-3-methylglutaryl coenzyme A (HMG-CoA) reductase inhibitors (statins) or ciclosporin
- see also General Interactions of immunomodifiers (p. 1237)

Nursing considerations/Cautions
- renal function, serum cholesterol and triglyceride levels should be monitored throughout therapy (especially during concurrent ciclosporin therapy)
- urine should be monitored for traces of protein
- combined therapy with ciclosporin should not exceed 3 months post-transplantation
- when measuring blood levels, same dose should be maintained for 3 days (with loading dose) or 7–14 days (without loading dose) to achieve a steady state before adjusting dosage
- blood levels should be measured 7–14 days after switching between different tablet strengths (e.g. 2 mg to 5 mg tablets)
- 2 mg of oral solution = 2 × 1 mg tablets and are therefore interchangeable
- a new loading dose may be required if a large dose increase is necessary; calculated according to the following formula: loading dose = 3 × (new maintenance dose − current maintenance dose)
- if the calculated dose is greater than 40 mg daily maximum dose, the dose should be split into two loading doses given over 2 days. Trough level should be measured 3–4 days after new loading dose

- antimicrobial prophylaxis should be given for 12 months to prevent *Pneumocystis jirovecii* pneumonia (PJP) and for 3 months to prevent cytomegalovirus (CMV) infection
- increased risk of delayed wound healing if used in those with BMI > 30 kg/m^2
- caution if used in those with severe liver impairment, as clearance will be decreased and a lower maintenance dose required
- not recommended for liver or lung transplantation
- see also General Nursing considerations/Cautions for immunomodifiers (p. 1238)

Patient education

- advise the patient to take tablets or oral solution consistently either with or after food, but not switch between the two
- instruct the patient to swallow tablets whole, not broken or chewed
- the patient should be advised to withdraw the dose from the bottle using a syringe, then add to a glass or plastic cup and mix thoroughly with at least 60 mL of water or orange juice (no other liquids should be used) and drink immediately. The glass should be refilled with at least 120 mL of water or orange juice, stirred thoroughly again and drunk
- instruct the patient to discard any oral solution 4 weeks after opening
- the patient should be advised that it is common for the solution to appear white to off-white when mixed with water or orange juice
- the patient should be warned to avoid grapefruit juice during therapy
- instruct the patient to take 4 hours after ciclosporin and at the same time every day consistently with or without food
- warn the patient that refrigerating the solution may result in a harmless haze, which disappears when the solution is allowed to stand at room temperature
- if the solution comes into contact with skin or mucous membranes (e.g. eyes), skin should be washed with soap and water or the eyes rinsed with water
- advise the patient to seek medical advice immediately if any of the following occur:
    - any shortness of breath, sudden chest pain, cough or arm/leg swelling/tenderness, discolouration or warmth of limb (symptoms of DVT and PE)
    - febrile illness (neutropenia)
    - unusual bruising or bleeding, nosebleeds
    - fever, chills, muscle/joint pain, headache, cough, shortness of breath, fatigue, loss of appetite
- counsel female patients of childbearing potential regarding the importance of using reliable contraception during and for 12 weeks after stopping therapy to avoid pregnancy and seeking medical advice if pregnancy occurs
- see also General Patient education for immunomodifiers (p. 1238)

 An oral solution is available. Tablet should not be divided, broken or crushed.

 May cause immunosuppression in infant; therefore should be used during pregnancy only if benefits outweigh risks. Reliable contraception should be used during therapy and for 12 weeks after last dose.

 Not recommended for use when breastfeeding owing to lack of safety data.

 Consider dosage of patients with a kidney transplant, as more adverse events are recorded when GFR is < 40 mL/min.

In patients with renal impairment consider reducing dose.

SPESOLIMAB
Trade name
Spevigo

Available form
Vial: 450 mg/7.5 mL

IMMUNOMODIFIERS

Action
- monoclonal immunoglobulin G$_1$ (IgG$_1$) antibody with a high affinity for IL36R that prevents the activation of pro-inflammatory and pro-fibrotic pathways (strong link between IL36R signalling and skin inflammation)
- reduces levels of C-reactive protein, interleukin (IL)-6, T-helper cell mediated cytokines, keratinocyte-medicated inflammation, neutrophilic mediators and pro-inflammatory cytokines

Use
- generalised pustular psoriasis

Dose
- 900 mg by IV infusion over 90 minutes. If flare symptoms persist, a second 900 mg dose can be given one week after the initial dose

Adverse effects
- urinary tract infection
- upper respiratory tract infection
- pruritus
- (Injection site) redness, swelling, pain, induration, warmth
- fatigue
- (Rare) hypersensitivity, drug reaction with eosinophilia and systemic symptoms (DRESS), peripheral neuropathy

Interactions
- live vaccines should not be given for at least 16 weeks after therapy is completed
- therapy should not be started within 4 weeks of live vaccine administration

Nursing considerations/Cautions
- any infection should be treated before starting therapy
- patient should be assessed for tuberculosis (TB) before starting therapy. If the patient has latent TB or a history of TB without adequate confirmation of treatment, anti-TB therapy should be considered before starting spesolimab
- if the patient develops mild-to-moderate infusion-related reaction, the infusion should be stopped and treatment with systemic antihistamines and/or corticosteroids considered. The infusion can be restarted at a slower rate on resolution of symptoms
- to prepare IV infusion, remove 15 mL from a 100 mL container of sodium chloride 0.9% and then add 15 mL (two vials) of spesolimab and mix gently (do not shake)
- administer alone, using a sterile, non-pyrogenic, low protein binding in-line filter (0.2 microns)
- flush the IV line before and after administration of spesolimab with sodium chloride 0.9%
- if the infusion is slowed or stopped, total time should not exceed 180 minutes
- record the trade name and batch number in the patient's medical history

Patient education
- the patient should be instructed to seek medical attention immediately if any of the following occur:
  - cough (with or without phlegm), chest pain, fever, chills, night sweats, weight loss
  - numbness or tingling in arms or legs, muscle weakness
  - serious infection with fever, chills, weakness, rapid heart rate

Human IgG is known to cross the placental barrier; therefore not recommended in pregnancy unless benefits clearly outweigh potential risks to the fetus.

Unknown if excreted in breastmilk; therefore a decision needs to be made to discontinue or continue breastfeeding.

TACROLIMUS
Trade names
Advagraf XL, Pacrolim, Prograf, Tacrograf

Available forms
Capsules: 0.5 mg, 1 mg, 5 mg;
Capsules (extended release): 0.5 mg, 1 mg, 3 mg, 5 mg;

Ampoule: 5 mg/mL;
Ointment: 0.1%

Action
- macrolide lactone that inhibits lymphocyte formation thought to be responsible for graft rejection
- suppresses T-cell activation, T-helper cell dependent B-cell proliferation and lymphokine formation
- half-life about 43 hours

Use
- adjunct to lung, heart, liver or kidney allograft transplantation
- moderate-to-severe atopic dermatitis (not adequately controlled or intolerant to conventional therapy) or to prolong flare-free intervals

Dose
- (Liver transplantation) 0.10–0.20 mg/kg orally daily 1 hour before food in 2 divided doses (Prograf, Pacrolim, Tacrograf) or single dose (Advagraf XL), starting 6 hours after liver transplantation **OR**
- (Liver transplantation) 0.01–0.05 mg/kg by IV infusion over 24 hours (if oral administration is not possible) **OR**
- (Kidney transplantation) 0.15–0.30 mg/kg orally daily 1 hour before food in 2 divided doses (Prograf, Pacrolim, Tacrograf) or single dose (Advagraf XL), starting within 24 hours of kidney transplantation **OR**
- (Kidney transplantation) 0.04–0.06 mg/kg by IV infusion over 24 hours (if oral administration is not possible) **OR**
- (Lung transplantation) 0.10–0.30 mg/kg orally daily 1 hour before food in 2 divided doses (Prograf, Pacrolim, Tacrograf) or single dose (Advagraf XL), starting 24 hours after lung transplantation **OR**
- (Lung transplantation) 0.01–0.05 mg/kg by IV infusion over 24 hours (if oral administration is not possible) **OR**
- (Heart transplantation) 0.075 mg/kg orally daily 1 hour before food in 2 divided doses (Prograf, Pacrolim, Tacrograf) or single dose (Advagraf XL), starting 24 hours after lung transplantation **OR**
- (Heart transplantation) 0.01–0.02 mg/kg by IV infusion over 24 hours (if oral administration is not possible) **OR**
- (Moderate-to-severe atopic dermatitis) apply thin layer to affected area twice daily until lesion clears (for flare-up), then once daily two days per week (e.g. Monday, Thursday) once lesions have cleared or mildly affected. May increase to twice daily if flare recurs

Adverse effects
- tremor, headache, abnormal dreams, insomnia, depression, anxiety, confusion, dizziness, disorientation, seizures, asthenia, mood disorder, depression, hallucination
- paraesthesia, peripheral neuropathy
- anorexia, diarrhoea, nausea, vomiting, dyspepsia, flatulence, abdominal pain/distension, constipation, stomatitis, bloating, gastrointestinal ulceration and perforation
- fever
- hypertension, tachycardia, fluid overload, ventricular/septal hypertrophy (cardiomyopathy), heart failure, arrhythmias, QT interval prolongation
- thromboembolic and ischaemic events, peripheral vascular disease
- renal dysfunction, renal failure, oliguria, bladder/urethral symptoms
- abnormal liver function tests, cholestasis, jaundice, hepatitis, ascites
- hyperkalaemia, hypomagnesaemia, hyperphosphataemia, hyperuricaemia, hypokalaemia, hypocalcaemia, hyponatraemia, hyperglycaemia, diabetes mellitus, post-transplant diabetes mellitus
- hypercholesterolaemia, hyperlipidaemia, hypertriglyceridaemia
- anaemia, leucopenia, thrombocytopenia, leukocytosis, pure red cell aplasia
- pruritus, rash, acne, sweating, alopecia
- blurred vision, photophobia, eye disorder
- tinnitus
- arthralgia, myalgia, muscle cramps, limb and back pain

IMMUNOMODIFIERS

- dyspnoea, pleural effusion, cough, nasal congestion, pharyngitis
- neurotoxicity (e.g. tremor, headache, insomnia, seizures, motor function changes, mental status changes), posterior reversible encephalopathy syndrome (PRES) (e.g. headache, visual disturbances, altered mental state)
- primary graft dysfunction
- anaphylaxis, allergic reaction
- (Ointment) burning, pruritis, warmth, pain, irritation, oedema
- see also General Adverse effects of immunomodifiers (p. 1237)

Interactions

- contraindicated with ciclosporin, because of additive nephrotoxicity and increase in ciclosporin half-life. An interval of 24 hours should be allowed between stopping one therapy and starting the other and ciclosporin blood levels should be closely monitored
- contraindicated with potassium-sparing diuretics
- oral tacrolimus is not recommended with topical tacrolimus use
- caution if used with other nephrotoxic agents such as aminoglycosides, amphotericin B (amphotericin), cotrimoxazole, vancomycin, NSAIDs, aciclovir, ganciclovir or ibuprofen
- increased risk of hyperkalaemia if potassium supplements or potassium-sparing diuretics are given
- caution if given with other agents known to prolong QT interval
- serum levels may increase if given with grapefruit juice
- caution if given with mycophenolate products. Mycophenolate serum levels should be monitored during therapy
- increased serum level may occur if given with amiodarone, amphotericin B (amphotericin), bromocriptine, clarithromycin, clotrimazole, cortisone, danazol, dapsone, diltiazem, erythromycin, ethinylestradiol, fluconazole, gestodene, itraconazole, lidocaine (lignocaine), methylprednisolone (high dose) midazolam, nelfinavir, nifedipine, omeprazole, prednisolone (high dose), ritonavir, tamoxifen, telaprevir, verapamil or voriconazole
- may increase serum levels of phenytoin, increasing the risk of toxicity
- decreased serum level may occur if given with dexamethasone, rifampicin, sodium bicarbonate, aluminium hydroxide, magnesium oxide, phenobarbital (phenobarbitone), carbamazepine, phenytoin, isoniazid or St John's wort
- absorption may be increased by metoclopramide. Serum levels of tacrolimus should be closely monitored
- see also General Interactions of immunomodifiers (p. 1237)

Nursing considerations/Cautions

- oral administration should start as soon as possible. The first oral dose should be given 8—12 hours after stopping IV infusion
- for the first few months after transplantation, BP, ECG, visual status, blood glucose, creatinine, urea and electrolyte concentrations (especially potassium), urinary output, haematology, coagulation, liver and renal function tests should be monitored frequently
- if switching from ciclosporin, therapy should be started 12—24 hours after stopping ciclosporin. If ciclosporin serum levels are high, therapy should not be started and ciclosporin levels closely monitored
- the patient should not be switched between different formulations of tacrolimus once effective dosage has been established
- trough serum levels should be measured 12 hours after immediate-release preparations or 24 hours after extended-release capsules
- care should be taken when selecting dose/formulations of tacrolimus, as medication errors have resulted in the past
- refrigerating IV solution may result in a harmless haze, which disappears when

- the solution is allowed to stand at room temperature
- if IV solution comes into contact with skin or mucous membranes (e.g. eyes), the skin should be washed with soap and water or the eyes rinsed with water
- not recommended as an IV bolus
- IV concentrate should be diluted using glucose 5% or sodium chloride 0.9%
- IV solution is incompatible with PVC plastic
- caution if used in those with neurological or CNS disorders (because they can be exacerbated), diabetes mellitus, pre-existing heart disease, liver or kidney impairment, renal/liver dysfunction, fluid overload or hypertension
- caution if given to those who have previously received polyoxyethylene hydrogenated castor oil or have an allergic predisposition, because they have an increased risk of anaphylaxis
- caution if used in those with congenital or acquired QT prolongation
- contraindicated in those with known hypersensitivity to other macrolides or polyoxyethylene hydrogenated castor oil (found in Prograf Concentrated Injection)
- see also General Nursing considerations/Cautions for immunomodifiers (p. 1238)

Patient education

- instruct the patient to take tablets on an empty stomach either 1 hour before or 2 hours after food
- advise the patient to avoid grapefruit juice during therapy
- the patient should be advised to avoid a high-potassium diet during therapy
- warn the patient against driving or operating machinery if visual disturbances, dizziness or hallucinations occur
- the patient should be advised to seek medical advice immediately if any of the following occur:
  - numbness or tingling in hands or feet (signs of peripheral neuropathy)
  - tremor
  - headache, insomnia, changes in motor function, sensory function, mental status or fitting (signs of neurotoxicity)
  - headache, altered mental state, visual disturbances or fitting (signs of PRES)
  - yellowing of eyes/skin, tiredness, loss of appetite, nausea, vomiting, dark urine, upper abdominal pain (jaundice, hepatitis)
  - palpitation, abnormal heart rate
  - severe abdominal pain, nausea, vomiting, fever, chills (GI perforation signs)
- see also General Patient education for immunomodifiers (p. 1238)

Immediate-release capsules only — capsules can be opened and contents dispersed in water.

Tacrolimus is excreted in breastmilk and therefore breastfeeding is not recommended during therapy.

TILDRAKIZUMAB

Trade name
Ilumya

Available form
Prefilled syringe: 100 mg/mL

Action
- IgG$_{1/kappa}$ monoclonal antibody that binds specifically to interleukin 23 (subunit p19) (which is involved in inflammatory and immune responses)

Use
- moderate-to-severe plaque psoriasis (in those eligible for systemic therapy)

Dose
- 100 mg SC at week 0, 4 and every 12 weeks afterwards

Adverse effects
- headache, fatigue
- nausea, diarrhoea
- nasopharyngitis, sinusitis
- arthralgia, back pain, pain in extremity

IMMUNOMODIFIERS

- (Injection site) pain
- see also General Adverse effects of immunomodifiers (p. 1237)

Interactions
- see General Interactions of immunomodifiers (p. 1237)

Nursing considerations/Cautions
- patient may be taught to self-administer. First injection should be under medical supervision
- caution if used in those with chronic infection or history of recurrent infection
- see also General Nursing considerations/Cautions for immunomodifiers (p. 1238)

Patient education
- female patient of childbearing potential should be counselled to use effective contraception during and for at least 17 weeks post therapy
- see also Patient education for icatibant (p. 1256) for self-administration instructions
- see also General Patient education for immunomodifiers (p. 1238)

Not recommended during pregnancy unless benefits outweigh risks; limited available data.

Not recommended when breastfeeding; no available data.

USTEKINUMAB
Trade names
Steqeyma, Stelara

Available forms
Prefilled syringe: 45 mg/0.5 mL (SC); Vial: 130 mg/26 mL (IV)

Action
- IgG$_{1kappa}$ monoclonal antibody that binds to interleukin (IL) 12 and 23, interrupting signalling and cytokines involved in psoriasis

Use
- treatment of moderate-to-severe plaque psoriasis in those who are candidates for phototherapy or systemic therapy and over 18 years
- active psoriatic arthritis (with methotrexate) (in those with inadequate response to non-biological disease-modifying antirheumatic drugs (DMARDs))
- moderate-to-severe active Crohn's disease or ulcerative colitis (in those with inadequate or lost response)

Dose
- (Plaque psoriasis, psoriatic arthritis) 45 mg SC at weeks 0 and 4 and then 3-monthly **OR**
- (Plaque psoriasis, psoriatic arthritis, patient weight > 100 kg) 90 mg SC at weeks 0 and 4 and then 3-monthly **OR**
- (Crohn's disease, ulcerative colitis) initially 260 mg (weight ≤ 55 kg), 390 mg IV (weight > 55 kg but ≤ 85 kg) or 520 mg (weight > 85 kg) by IV infusion over 1 hour, then 90 mg SC after 8 weeks, then 90 mg SC every 12 weeks

Adverse effects
- upper respiratory tract infection, nasopharyngitis, sinusitis
- dizziness, headache, fatigue and, less commonly, depression
- pruritus
- oropharyngeal pain
- nausea, vomiting, diarrhoea
- back pain, myalgia, arthralgia
- (Injection site) redness, pain
- antibody development
- (Rare) reversible posterior leukoencephalopathy syndrome
- see also General Adverse effects of immunomodifiers (p. 1237)

Interactions
- caution if given with medications with a narrow therapeutic index. Serum levels should be closely monitored if used together
- see also General Interactions of immunomodifiers (p. 1237)

1279

Nursing considerations/Cautions

- (Plaque psoriasis) if the response is inadequate, therapy may be increased to every 8 weeks
- (Psoriatic arthritis) if no response after 28 weeks, therapy should be re-evaluated
- (Crohn's disease) if therapy is interrupted, it may be resumed with SC administration every 8 weeks
- (Crohn's disease, ulcerative colitis) if response is inadequate during the maintenance period, the frequency can be reduced to every 8 weeks
- the patient may be instructed to self-inject SC. The first self-administration should be under medical supervision
- (IV) calculate the number of vials required (and therefore volume). Withdraw and discard the volume to be added from a 250 mL sodium chloride 0.9% infusion bag (e.g. if 3 vials are required (390 mg), 78 mL should be discarded). Add the required volume, gently invert the infusion bag (do not shake) and infuse over 1 hour
- caution if used in those receiving or have undergone allergy treatment especially for anaphylaxis
- caution if used in those > 60 years, with prolonged use of immunosuppressants or a history of PUVA therapy because of the increased risk of non-melanoma skin cancer
- not recommended in those with a past history of malignancy
- contraindicated if active clinically important infection is present (e.g. tuberculosis)
- see also General Nursing considerations/Cautions for immunomodifiers (p. 1238)

Patient education

- warn the patient against driving or operating machinery if dizziness occurs
- advise the patient to seek medical advice if any headache, seizures, confusion or visual disturbances occur
- counsel female patients of childbearing potential of the importance of using effective contraception during and for 15 weeks after stopping therapy
- see also instructions for SC self-administration (see Patient education for icatibant, p. 1256)
- see also General Patient education for immunomodifiers (p. 1238)

Not recommended for use in pregnancy because of the limited safety data available. If used during pregnancy, a 6-month waiting period after birth is recommended before the infant is vaccinated using live vaccines.

Not recommended when breastfeeding because of the limited safety data available.

INTERFERONS

General Actions of interferons

- naturally occurring, small protein molecules produced and secreted by cells in response to viral infections or to various synthetic and biological inducers
- bind to specific cell surface receptors that are linked to inner cell networks that control enzyme activity, cell proliferation and immune activity enhancement (e.g. inhibit viral replication in virus-infected cells; enhance activity of macrophages and lymphocytes)
- produced by recombinant DNA technology

General Adverse effects of interferons

- flu-like symptoms (including fever, malaise, chills, sweating, fatigue, myalgia, arthralgia, loss of appetite, headache)
- drowsiness, somnolence, insomnia, dizziness, depression, anxiety, confusion, impaired concentration, nervousness
- vertigo
- nausea, vomiting, anorexia, diarrhoea, abdominal pain, weight loss, taste alteration, dry mouth
- anaemia, leucopenia, thrombocytopenia

IMMUNOMODIFIERS

- elevated liver enzymes, hypertriglyceridaemia
- reversible alopecia, pruritus, dry skin
- arthralgia, myalgia
- visual disturbances, retinopathy, retinal haemorrhage, cotton wool spots, retinal artery or vein thrombosis, optic neuropathy
- palpitations, transient hypotension or hypertension, chest pain, arrhythmias, oedema, cyanosis
- (Alfa interferons, uncommon) cough, dyspnoea, pneumonia, pneumonitis, pulmonary infiltrates
- (Alfa interferons) graft rejection
- (Uncommon) altered liver function tests, elevated liver enzymes
- thyroid dysfunction
- (Rare) hypersensitivity reaction (including bronchospasm, urticaria, anaphylaxis, angioedema), suicidal ideation, hyperglycaemia, diabetes mellitus, jaundice, hepatitis, seizures, development of anti-interferon antibodies, injection site reaction, exacerbation of psoriasis
- see also General Adverse effects of immunomodifiers (p. 1237)

General Nursing considerations/Cautions for interferons

- the patient should be well hydrated before and during therapy (especially during the initial stages of treatment) to prevent fluid depletion and hypotension
- monitor blood cell counts (with WBC differential, platelet count), electrolytes, serum creatinine, serum protein, serum lipids, thyroid and liver function before therapy, then at monthly or appropriate intervals during treatment. Ophthalmological examination is also recommended. Furthermore, ECG is recommended in those with pre-existing cardiac disease or advanced cancer
- (Hepatitis B or C) liver biopsy should be performed before starting treatment to exclude other causes of hepatitis and determine extent of disease
- paracetamol 0.5–1 g can be taken orally 30 minutes before the administration of interferon to alleviate symptoms of fever and headache, then up to 1 g 4 times daily
- chest X-ray is recommended if the patient develops a cough, dyspnoea or other respiratory symptoms
- any persistent fever should be investigated thoroughly
- all patients should be monitored for any signs of depression or suicidal ideation
- at the discretion of the doctor, the patient may be educated to self-administer medication. The first self-administered injection should be done under medical supervision
- ensure the administered product name and batch number is documented in the patient's medical history
- when reconstituting the solution, care should be taken to avoid foaming or shaking the solution when dissolving
- administer alone
- patients with chronic hepatitis not caused by hepatitis B or C should not be treated with interferon therapy
- (Alfa interferons) caution if used in those with liver or other organ transplant because of an increased risk of graft rejections
- caution if used in those with diabetes mellitus, because antidiabetic therapy may need adjusting to control blood glucose levels, as well as an increased risk of retinopathy and ketoacidosis occurring
- caution if used in those with psoriasis, as the disease may be exacerbated
- caution if used in those with severe bone marrow suppression because of an increased risk of infection and/or bleeding
- caution if used in those with pre-existing cardiac disease; lung disease; severe kidney, liver or myeloid dysfunction; thyroid disease; history of seizures; compromised CNS function or neuropsychiatric disorders, including depression
- contraindicated in those with hypersensitivity to interferons (natural or

recombinant), autoimmune disease, autoimmune hepatitis, chronic hepatitis with advanced decompensated liver disease or cirrhosis, or chronic hepatitis recently treated with immunosuppressive therapy
- contraindicated in neonates and children under 3 years because of the benzyl alcohol content
- see also General Nursing considerations/Cautions for immunomodifiers (p. 1238)

General Patient education for interferons

- advise the patient not to change brands without the doctor's supervision
- warn the patient about alopecia, which sometimes continues for weeks after stopping therapy
- patients should be advised not to drive or operate machinery if adverse effects such as dizziness, confusion, somnolence, visual disturbance or fatigue occur
- instruct the patient/family member/carer in correct administration (see Patient education for icatibant, p. 1256)
- the patient should be advised to seek medical advice immediately if any of the following occur:
  - loss or decrease in vision
  - increase in thirst and urination
  - persistent fever
  - fever, cough and difficulty breathing
  - depression, sadness, loss of appetite, withdrawal from friends or previously pleasurable activities, ideas of or attempts at self-harm or thoughts of suicide

INTERFERON GAMMA 1B
Trade name
Imukin

Available form
Vial: 2 million IU (100 microgram)/0.5 mL

Action
- see General Actions of interferons (p. 1280)

Use
- chronic granulomatous disease (as adjunct therapy) to decrease the frequency of serious infections

Dose
- (Patient surface area ≤ 0.5 m^2) 30,000 IU (1.5 microgram)/kg SC 3 times weekly **OR**
- (Patient surface area > 0.5 m^2) 1 million IU (50 microgram)/m^2 SC 3 times weekly

Adverse effects
- see General Adverse effects of interferons (p. 1280)

Interactions
- caution if given with other hepatotoxic, myelosuppressive and/or nephrotoxic agents
- not recommended with vaccines or other heterologous serum protein preparations owing to unexpected effects on the immune system

Nursing considerations/Cautions
- the patient or carer can be taught the correct administration technique. The first injection should be under medical supervision
- the vial stopper contains rubber, which causes an allergic reaction in those with latex allergy
- caution if used in those with compromised CNS function, as there is an increased risk of gait disturbance, dizziness or decreased mental function (especially if high doses are administered)
- see also General Nursing considerations/Cautions for interferons (p. 1281)

Patient education
- instruct the patient in the correct SC administration technique (see Patient education for icatibant, p. 1282)

- advise the patient/carer to seek medical advice if any dizziness, gait disturbance or change in mental function occurs
- see also General Patient education for interferons (p. 1282)

Should be used during pregnancy only if benefits outweigh risks. Limited safety data available.

Not recommended when breastfeeding because no safety data are available.

PEGINTERFERON ALFA 2A

Trade name
Pegasys

Available forms
Prefilled syringe: 135 microgram/0.5 mL, 180 microgram/0.5 mL

Action
- combination (termed pegylated) of recombinant interferon alfa 2a and monomethoxy polyethylene glycol (PEG reagent), prolonging the half-life
- see also General Actions of interferons (p. 1280)

Use
- chronic hepatitis B (with evidence of viral replication, liver inflammation and compensated liver disease)
- chronic hepatitis C (in those not receiving previous interferon therapy or who have failed interferon alfa therapy (alone or with ribavirin) and with compensated liver disease)

Dose
- (Chronic hepatitis B) 180 micrograms SC weekly for 48 weeks **OR**
- (Chronic hepatitis C — treatment naive) 180 micrograms SC weekly for 24—48 weeks (depending on viral genotype) (with ribavirin 0.8—1.2 g orally daily depending on patient weight) **OR**
- (Chronic hepatitis C — non-responder or relapsed) 180 micrograms SC weekly for 48—72 weeks (depending on viral genotype) (with ribavirin 1—1.2 g orally daily depending on patient weight) **OR**
- (Human immunodeficiency virus (HIV) —hepatitis C co-infection) 180 micrograms SC weekly for 48 weeks (alone or with ribavirin 800 mg orally daily)

Adverse effects
- (Hepatitis C, combined with ribavirin, children 5—17 years) inhibited growth, decreased weight
- see also General Adverse effects of interferons (p. 1280)

Interactions
- not recommended with Chinese herbal medicine Xiao-Chai-Hu (also known as sho-saiko-to) because it may increase the risk of pulmonary symptoms
- may decrease metabolism of theophylline leading to increased serum levels and risk of toxicity
- may increase serum levels of methadone
- increased risk of severe anaemia and neutropenia if given with zidovudine
- increased risk of myelotoxicity if given with azathioprine

Nursing considerations/Cautions
- (Hepatitis C, combined with ribavirin, children 5—17 years) growth and weight of children should be monitored regularly during therapy
- dose may be decreased if moderate-to-severe adverse effects occur
- therapy may be discontinued if there has been no response after 12 weeks
- (HIV-hepatitis C co-infection) patient should be closely monitored during therapy for any signs of liver decompensation (e.g. ascites, variceal bleeding, encephalopathy) and therapy should be stopped if this occurs
- (Hepatitis B) disease exacerbation (transient increase in serum ALT) occurs commonly during therapy which may require dose reduction or interruption to therapy

- contraindicated in those with hypersensitivity to E. coli-derived products, polyethylene glycol or HIV—hepatitis C co-infection with cirrhosis (unless due to medication-related indirect hyperbilirubinaemia), autoimmune hepatitis, decompensated cirrhosis, thalassaemia or sickle cell anaemia
- see also General Nursing considerations/Cautions for interferons (p. 1281)

Patient education

- instruct patient in correct SC administration technique (see Patient education for icatibant, p. 1256)
- see also General Patient education for interferons (p. 1282)

(Used alone) Should be used during pregnancy only if benefits outweigh risks. Women should be counselled to use effective contraception during therapy. (With ribivirin) Contraindicated during pregnancy.

Use with caution because limited data are available.

For those with severe kidney impairment, dose should be reduced to 135 micrograms weekly, as recommended, and patient should be closely monitored.

LAXATIVES

Constipation is difficult to define define because normal bowel habits vary considerably from person to person. However, can be described as a common, heterogeneous disorder characterised by multiple symptoms and pathophysiological mechanisms. It involves infrequent bowel movements, difficulty passing stools and a sensation of incomplete evacuation (Camilleri & Murray 2026). Chronic constipation results from factors such as inadequate dietary fibre or fluid intake, or from disordered colonic transit or anorectal function resulting from advanced age, medications (e.g. calcium-channel blockers, some antidepressants), colonic obstruction (e.g. diverticular disease, tumour), anal fissure, painful haemorrhoids, pelvic floor dysfunction, neurological disease (e.g. multiple sclerosis, Parkinson's disease), psychiatric disorders (e.g. depression) and endocrine-related diseases (e.g. hypothyroidism, hypercalcaemia) and lifestyle factors such as low-fibre diet, inadequate fluid intake and lack of physical activity (Camilleri & Murray 2026).

Laxatives, also known as aperients, purgatives, cathartics or evacuants, promote defaecation. Given orally, by suppository or evacuant enema, laxatives are also used to reduce straining, to reduce pain in anorectal disorders and before surgery, and in radiological or endoscopic procedures (Sharkey & Wallace 2018).

Most laxatives act by increasing the retention of fluid in the colon and/or altering motility. Bulk-forming laxatives are hydrophilic, causing an increase in faecal mass and resulting in stimulation of peristalsis. *Stimulant* (irritant) *laxatives* stimulate accumulation of water and electrolytes, which increases intestinal motility. *Osmotic* (non-absorbable inorganic salts or sugars) *laxatives* are poorly absorbed, concentrated solutions that increase intracolonic osmotic pressure, causing decreased absorption of fluid in the bowel and resulting in a fairly rapid, semifluid evacuation. *Emollient laxatives* (faecal softeners) soften faeces by decreasing surface tension and increasing penetration of intestinal fluids into the faecal mass, while *prokinetic agents* act primarily on motility (Sharkey & Wallace 2018).

General Uses of laxatives
- prophylactically to prevent straining during defecation (e.g. haemorrhoids, anal fissures)
- short-term management of constipation

- bowel evacuation before investigational procedures (proctoscopy, sigmoidoscopy, colonoscopy, radiology) or surgery

General Adverse effects of laxatives

- (Common) nausea, abdominal bloating/discomfort, flatulence
- (Less common) vomiting, abdominal cramps, rectal irritation, proctitis
- (Prolonged use or overdose) diarrhoea, excessive loss of water and electrolytes, especially potassium
- (Rare) intestinal impaction

General Nursing considerations/Cautions for laxatives

- sufficient lubrication will be produced by warming the suppository in the hand before removing it from the foil wrapper
- the entire suppository does not need to dissolve to be effective
- suppositories are effective within 20–60 minutes of insertion
- a microenema is usually effective within 5–15 minutes
- (Enemas/suppositories) are not recommended in those with anal fissures, ulcerative proctitis with mucosal damage or ulcerated haemorrhoids
- (All laxatives) are contraindicated in those with intestinal obstruction, faecal impaction, bowel perforation (frank or suspected), gastric retention, paralytic ileus, undiagnosed abdominal pain and/or nausea/vomiting (including suspected appendicitis), acute surgical abdomen, undiagnosed rectal bleeding, toxic megacolon, toxic colitis or colonic atony

General Patient education for laxatives

- warn the patient not to drive or operate machinery if any dizziness or fatigue occurs
- advise the patient that laxatives should be used only as a short-term management measure
- the patient should be advised to seek medical advice before taking laxatives if bowel habits have changed suddenly over 2 weeks. Medical advice should also be sought if constipation continues for 7 days or more despite treatment, or if rectal bleeding occurs
- warn the patient to avoid the 'laxative habit' and encourage normal bowel function by increasing fibre and fluid intake, and regular exercise
- the patient should be warned not to take the laxative in powdered form, because oesophageal obstruction may occur
- instruct the patient that it may take 24–48 hours for normal bowel habits to return
- the patient should be instructed in the correct technique for insertion of an enema, including:
  - lying on the left side with knees drawn up
  - lubricating the tip of the enema and gently inserting into the rectum, discontinuing the procedure if there is any resistance
  - maintaining the position until the urge to evacuate the bowel is strong
  - not retaining the enema for a prolonged length of time
- instructions for insertion of a suppository include:
  - washing the hands thoroughly before insertion
  - removing the foil wrapper
  - lying on the left side with knees drawn up towards chest
  - gently inserting the suppository (pointed end first) into the rectum

LAXATIVES

BULK-FORMING LAXATIVES

General Actions of bulk-forming laxatives

- increase the volume, bulk and moisture of faeces by absorbing water, distending the bowel, so stimulating peristalsis
- generally consist of natural plant gums that are not broken down by normal digestive processes
- do not interfere with absorption of food, but do require adequate fluids for maximal effect
- effective in 12—24 hours, although the full effect may take 2—3 days
- also improve stool consistency for those with diarrhoea or colonoscopy/ileostomy patients

ISPAGHULA
Trade name
Fybogel

Available form
Powder: 3.5 g/sachet

Dose
- 1 sachet (3.5 g) orally twice daily morning and evening after meals

Use/Adverse effects
- see General Uses/Adverse effects of laxatives (p. 1285)

Interactions
- advise the patient to take oral medication 2 hours before or after oral laxative therapy

Nursing considerations/Cautions

- contains aspartame; therefore caution should be used if given to those with phenylketonuria
- caution if used in those with dysphagia
- see also General Nursing considerations/Cautions for laxatives (p. 1286)

Patient education

- instruct the patient that sachet should be stirred into 250 mL glass of water or fruit juice and drunk immediately
- suggest to patient to increase water consumption
- advise the patient it may take several days to come into effect
- see also General Patient education for laxatives (p. 1286)

Powder can be stirred into a 250 mL glass of water or fruit juice, or mixed with half cup of yoghurt or apple puree.

Considered safe to use in pregnancy.

Considered safe to use when breastfeeding.

PSYLLIUM
Trade name
Metamucil

Available forms
Powder: 3.4 g/7 g, 3.4 g/5.9 g, 3.4 g/11 g

Use
- constipation
- lower cholesterol

Dose
- (Constipation) 2 level medicinal teaspoons (5 mL spoon) 1—3 times daily in 250 mL of cool water, followed by an additional glass of water **OR**
- (Cholesterol) 2 level medicinal teaspoons (5 mL spoon) orally 3 times daily

Adverse effects
- see General Adverse effects of laxatives (p. 1286)

Interactions
- advise the patient to take oral medication 2 hours before or after oral laxative therapy

Nursing considerations/Cautions

- contains aspartame; therefore not recommended in those with phenylketonuria (Metamucil Smooth Texture)
- caution if used in those with dysphagia

- see also General Nursing considerations/Cautions for laxatives (p. 1286)

Patient education
- advise the patient to drink generous amounts of water to prevent laxative swelling and blocking throat or oesophagus
- see also General Patient education for laxatives (p. 1286)

Available in combination with
- contained in GIT 1, Herb-a-lax, Lax-Active

OSMOTIC LAXATIVES

General Actions of osmotic laxatives
- not absorbed, but action is via osmotic effect which causes an increase in fluid volume in the lumen, which accelerates transfer to gut contents, thereby increasing defecation

COLON ELECTROLYTE LAVAGE

Trade names
ColonLYTELY, Glycoprep, Macrovic Powder, Molaxole, Movicol preparations, Moviprep, Plenvu

Available forms
Powder: 68.58 g/sachet, 70 g/sachet, 123 g/2 sachets (A & B)

Action
- polyethylene glycol—electrolyte solution that cleanses bowel by inducing diarrhoea, while causing little change in water and electrolyte balance
- polyethylene glycol (macrogel) acts as an osmotic agent
- electrolyte combinations vary between preparations
- action usually within 1—4 hours of administration
- see also General Actions of osmotic laxatives (above)

Use
- short-term management of constipation (under supervision)
- bowel preparation before investigational procedures (proctoscopy, sigmoidoscopy, colonoscopy, radiology) or surgery

Dose
- (Evening before morning investigation or surgery or morning before afternoon investigation) dissolve sachet in water (according to instructions), then 250 mL orally every 10 minutes until 3—4 L have been consumed or rectal effluent is clear **OR**
- (Constipation) 2 L over 2 hours (may be dissolved in cordial or fruit juice) **OR**
- (Constipation) initially 1 sachet daily dissolved in 125 mL water, increasing to 2—3 sachets if needed **OR**
- (Constipation — ready-to-use solution) 1 sachet daily, increasing to 2—3 sachets, if needed **OR**
- (Nasogastric) 20—30 mL per hour **OR**
- (Before barium enema) 2 L orally (with 10 mg bisacodyl) the night before the procedure **OR**
- (Faecal impaction) 8 sachets over 6 hours for up to 3 days (if the patient has cardiac impairment, the dose should be reduced to 2 sachets per hour) (daily maximum 8 sachets) (Movicol)

Adverse effects
- rhinorrhoea, skin reactions
- see also General Adverse effects of laxatives (p. 1286)

Interactions
- any oral medications taken within 1 hour may not be absorbed
- may reduce the effect of benzylpenicillin
- caution if used with calcium-channel blockers, diuretics or other agents that may affect electrolyte levels
- may interfere with oral contraceptive

Nursing considerations/Cautions
- any dehydration should be corrected before starting therapy
- the patient is to fast for 3—4 hours before administration
- (Endoscopy/colonoscopy) no solid food should be taken on the day prior to the procedure. Only clear, sugar-free liquids are allowed
- reconstitute powder using 250 mL water for 15.546 sachet, 1 L water for 68—70 g

LAXATIVES

- sachet or 3 L for 200—210 g sachet (other clear fluids may be allowed by the doctor)
- (Moviprep) to reconstitute, mix sachet A and sachet B together with 1 L water and then drink over 1—2 hours; repeat with a second litre
- (Nasogastric) rate should be decreased if the patient experiences nausea and/or bloating
- (Nasogastric) observe the patient closely if there is an impaired gag reflex or if unconscious
- (ColonLYTELY) no additional flavouring should be added unless instructed by the doctor
- contains aspartame; therefore not recommended in those with phenylketonuria
- first bowel action occurs about 1 hour after starting solution
- preparation is considered to be complete when the patient is passing clear fluid from the bowel
- caution if used in a patient with severe ulcerative colitis, diabetes, impaired kidney function (creatinine clearance < 30 mL/min), pre-existing electrolyte imbalance or dehydration, congestive cardiac failure, thyroid disease, impaired gag reflex, at risk of arrhythmias, unconscious or semiconscious, or prone to aspiration/regurgitation, or in the elderly
- contraindicated in those with stoma or weight < 20 kg
- see also General Nursing considerations/Cautions for laxatives (p. 1286)

Patient education

- advise the patient that the mixture may be more palatable if refrigerated and can be kept for up to 72 hours
- the patient should be advised to slow their drinking rate if nausea and bloating become severe
- if patients are ordered to take clear fluids only as part of bowel preparation, these may include water, tea or coffee (without milk or non-dairy creamer), soft drinks (non-carbonated) or cordials (but no red or purple colouring as these may interfere with investigations), strained fruit juice (no pulp), strained soup or clear broth
- advise the patient to seek medical advice immediately if any swelling, shortness of breath or fatigue occurs
- for constipation, instruct the patient that Movicol powder requires dilution in 125 mL water, but Movicol Ready-to-Take solution can be taken directly from sachet without dilution
- the patient should be advised to take fluids orally before and after bowel preparation to prevent dehydration
- female patients should be counselled regarding possible oral contraceptive failure during therapy and should be advised to use an alternative form of contraception during this time to avoid unwanted pregnancy occurring

 Used during pregnancy only if benefits outweigh the risks.

LACTULOSE

Trade names
Actilax, Chemists' Own Constipation Relief, Dulose

Available form
Syrup: 3.34 g/5 mL

Action

- administered orally as 50% w/w syrup, which is poorly absorbed from the gastrointestinal tract
- metabolised in the colon by bacteria to acetic and lactic acids
- reduces colon pH to 5.0, causing ammonia to be trapped as ammonium, so that less ammonia is absorbed into the blood and is instead excreted in the faeces (this is thought to be mechanism of action in portal systemic encephalopathy (PSE))
- change in osmotic pressure and colon acidification increase the water content

of stools, promoting peristalsis and evacuation
- also thought to promote growth of healthy promoting bacteria (probiotic action) while potentially suppressing pathogenic bacteria (e.g. *Escherichia coli, Clostridium*)

Use
- chronic constipation
- treatment and prevention of PSE (including hepatic pre-coma and coma)

Dose

Chronic constipation
- initially 15—30 mL orally daily after breakfast for 3 days (increasing to 45 mL daily if necessary), then 10—25 mL daily.

PSE
- initially 30—45 mL orally 3—4 times daily, adjusting dose every 1—2 days to produce 2—3 soft stools daily **OR**
- 30—45 mL orally hourly for 24—48 hours for more rapid response, then 30—45 mL 3—4 times daily **OR**
- (Acute) 50 mL orally 1—2-hourly until 2 soft stools are produced, then decreasing to 30—45 mL orally 3—4 times daily **OR**
- 300 mL diluted with 700 mL water/sodium chloride 0.9% and given as retention enema, repeated 4—6-hourly until the patient is able to take orally

Interactions
- avoid other laxatives during lactulose therapy because loose stools resulting from their use may be mistaken for adequate lactulose dosage
- caution if given with neomycin (conflicting information about interaction)

Adverse effects
- see General Adverse effects of laxatives (p. 1286)

Nursing considerations/Cautions
- (PSE) overall management should include dietary protein restriction, correction of any fluid and/or electrolyte imbalance, bowel cleansing and sterilisation, provision of nutritional/caloric needs and treatment of underlying liver disease
- use cautiously in those with diabetes, especially if therapy is prolonged
- caution if used in those with lactose intolerance
- caution if used in those undergoing electrocautery procedures during colonoscopy or proctoscopy. Bowel should be thoroughly cleansed with non-fermentable solution before procedure
- not recommended in those with rare hereditary problems of galactose intolerance, Lapp lactase deficiency or glucose—galactose malabsorption
- contraindicated in those with galactosaemia
- see also General Nursing considerations/Cautions for laxatives (p. 1286)

Patient education
- advise the patient that solution may be taken undiluted or diluted with water, milk or fruit juice
- the patient should be advised that it may take 24—48 hours before a result is seen
- instruct the patient to seek medical advice if painful abdominal symptoms occur
- see also General Patient education for laxatives (p. 1286)

SODIUM PHOSPHATE

Trade names
Fleet Ready-to-Use-Enema, Phospho-Soda

Available forms
Oral solution: 23.1 g/45 mL; Enema: 26 g/133 mL

Action
- see General Actions of osmotic laxatives (p. 1288)

Use
- constipation (under supervision)
- bowel preparation for colon X-ray or colonoscopy

LAXATIVES

postoperatively, or relief of faecal/barium impaction

Dose
* contents of 1 disposable enema unit (133 mL) **OR**
* 15 mL mixed with 250 mL of clear fluids and drunk, repeated twice more in next 20 minutes (first dose), followed by at least 3 glasses (250 mL) of clear fluids. Second dose is repeated as per first dose 10–12 hours later (timing is dependent on whether procedure is morning or afternoon)

Adverse effects
* (Rare) nephrocalcinosis associated with renal insufficiency or renal failure, seizures, QT prolongation
* see also General Adverse effects of laxatives (p. 1286)

Interactions
* caution if given with diuretics, NSAIDs, calcium-channel blockers, angiotensin converting enzyme (ACE) inhibitors, angiotensin receptor blockers, lithium or other agents that may affect electrolyte balance and increase risk of QT prolongation
* not recommended with colon electrolyte lavage solutions containing polyethylene glycol (macrogol)

Nursing considerations/Cautions
* any electrolyte imbalance should be corrected before starting therapy, especially in those with pre-existing electrolyte abnormalities
* calcium and phosphate levels should be closely monitored
* the patient should be monitored for any signs of dehydration, as life-threatening dehydration and/or electrolyte imbalance can occur
* the enema should be warmed to body temperature
* repeat administration of bowel preparation is not recommended within 7 days
* (Enema) contains 4.4 g sodium
* (Oral solution) caution if used in those on salt restriction, as oral solution contains 4.82 mEq sodium and 12.45 mEq/mL phosphate
* caution if used in those with pre-existing dehydration (including taking diuretics), at risk of hyponatraemia (e.g. syndrome of inappropriate antidiuretic hormone secretion (SIADH), inadequate treatment of hypothyroidism, electrolyte imbalance), diabetes, heart disease or renal impairment
* caution if used in those at risk of hyponatraemia, as risk of seizures is increased
* caution if used within 3 months of cardiac surgery or acute myocardial infarction
* caution if used in those with inflammatory bowel disease, as an acute exacerbation of the condition may occur
* (Phospho-soda) not recommended in children under 18 years
* not recommended in patients with a colostomy, because of the increased risk of hypocalcaemia, hyperphosphataemia, hypernatraemia or acidosis
* contraindicated in those with imperforate anus, faecal impaction, kidney impairment, fluid/electrolyte disturbance (or at risk of), congestive cardiac failure, ascites, unstable angina, gastric retention, paralytic ileus, bowel obstruction, severe chronic constipation, bowel perforation, acute colitis, active inflammatory disease, congenital or toxic megacolon or hypomotility syndrome
* contraindicated in those with hypersensitivity to sodium phosphate salt
* see also General Nursing considerations/Cautions for laxatives (p. 1285)

Patient education
* advise the patient to drink only clear fluids for 12 hours before first dose
* the patient should be instructed to avoid laxative use (with any type of laxative) for 7 days after procedure
* instruct the patient to seek medical advice if there is no return of liquid after

1291

- enema administration or no bowel motion within 6 hours of taking oral solution
- if patients are ordered to take clear fluids only as part of bowel preparation, these may include water, tea or coffee (without milk or non-dairy creamer), soft drinks (carbonated or non-carbonated) or cordial (but no red or purple colouring, as these may interfere with investigations), strained fruit juice (no pulp), strained soup or clear broth
- if the patient has diabetes, frequent monitoring of blood glucose levels is recommended. Adjustment to insulin and/or oral hypoglycaemic agents may be required
- (Phospho-soda) ensure the patient understands that the solution must be diluted before use
- see also General Patient education for laxatives (p. 1286)

 Used during pregnancy only if benefits clearly outweigh risks.

 Considered safe to use when breastfeeding.

 Contradicted in patients with renal failure because of increased further risk of renal damage.

SORBITOL

Trade name
Sorbisol

Available form
Syrup: 70% sorbitol solution (14 g/20 mL)

Action
- osmotic laxative, similar to lactulose
- see also General Actions of osmotic laxatives (p. 1288)

Use
- relief of constipation

Dose
- initially 20 mL daily, increasing to 20 mL 3 times daily if needed either 1 hour before or 3 hours after food; dose may then be reduced

Adverse effects
- see General Adverse effects of laxatives (p. 1286)

Interactions
- effectiveness may be reduced by antacids and opioid analgesics
- if used with stimulant laxatives, diarrhoea may occur

Nursing considerations/Cautions
- (Chronic use) electrolytes should be monitored regularly with prolonged use
- caution if used in those with insulin-dependent diabetes. If the patient has adequate insulin reserves and is stabilised on insulin there should be an impact on blood glucose levels. However, an increase in blood glucose levels may occur if the patient has insulin-depleted reserves
- contraindicated in those with fructose intolerance
- see also General Nursing considerations/Cautions for laxatives (p. 1286)

Patient education
- advise the patient to avoid refrigeration of syrup, as crystals may form. Warm to room temperature and shake the bottle if this occurs
- warn the patient that eating fructose-containing foods (e.g. apples, pears) at the same time may cause diarrhoea
- see also General Patient education for laxatives (p. 1286)

Available in combination with
- contained in Microlax enema and Micolette micro-enema
- contained in Carbosorb XS with charcoal

STIMULANT LAXATIVES

General Actions of stimulant laxatives
- promote accumulation of water and electrolytes in lumen and stimulate sensory nerve endings in mucosa, resulting in increased peristalsis of colon

LAXATIVES

- primary effect is on small and large intestines, hence the tendency to cause cramping
- often used as preparation for bowel procedures and surgery

BISACODYL
Trade names
Bisalax, Dulcolax, Lax-Tab, Petrus Bisacodyl Suppositories

Available forms
Suppositories: 10 mg;
Tablets: 5 mg;
Micro-enema: 2 mg/mL

Action
- tablet onset of action in 6—8 hours (empty stomach), increasing to 10—12 hours (with food). Suppository onset of action is 20—60 minutes and onset of action for enema is 5—10 minutes
- see also General Actions of osmotic laxatives (p. 1288)

Use
- constipation

Dose
- 10 mg orally at night, or 30 minutes before breakfast (for effect 6—8 hours later) **OR**
- 1 enema rectally after breakfast (on days where defecation is desired) **OR**
- 10 mg (1 suppository) rectally

Adverse effects
- see General Adverse effects of laxatives (p. 1286)

Interactions
- not recommended within 1 hour of antacids or milk

Nursing considerations/Cautions
- sufficient lubrication will be produced by warming the suppository in the hand before removing it from the foil wrapper
- suppositories are effective within 20—60 minutes of insertion; an enema is usually effective within 5—15 minutes; tablets are effective within 6—8 hours
- enema should be warmed to body temperature
- (Dulcolax) tablets contain lactose and are therefore not recommended in those with hereditary conditions of galactose intolerance, Lapp lactase deficiency or glucose—galactose malabsorption
- (Tablets) not recommended in children under 6 years
- see also General Nursing considerations/Cautions for laxatives (p. 1286)

Patient education
- instruct the patient that tablets should be swallowed whole, not chewed or broken, as it is enteric coated
- the patient should have no antacids or milk within 60 minutes of taking tablets

Tablet must be swallowed whole.

Considered safe to use for occasional doses when pregnant.

Considered safe to use when breast-feeding.

Available in combination with
- contained in Go Kit and Glycoprep-C combination pack as complete bowel preparation before abdominal radiographic examination

GLYCEROL
Trade names
Colxyl Glycerol Suppositories for Adults, Petrus Glycerol Suppositories BP

Available forms
Suppository: 2.8 g (adult), 1.4 g (child), 700 mg (infant)

Dose
- insert 1 suppository high into rectum against the rectal wall and allow it to remain for 15—30 minutes

Nursing considerations/Cautions/Patient education

- entire suppository does not have to dissolve to be effective
- also has an osmotic effect
- see also General Nursing considerations/Cautions/Patient education for laxatives (p. 1286)

SENNOSIDES A AND B (formerly known as Senna)
Trade names
Bekunis Senna Tablets, Laxettes with Senna, Laxettes with Sennosides, Senna-Gen, Senokot

Available forms
Tablets: 7.5 mg, 12 mg, 20 mg; Chocolate squares: 12 mg

Dose
- (Senokot) 2—4 tablets orally at night **OR**
- (Laxettes with Senna) initially 1—2 tablets daily with water at bedtime, increasing to 3 tablets if needed **OR**
- (Laxettes with Sennosides) 1—3 squares orally daily at bedtime **OR**
- (Bekunis Senna Tablets) 1—2 tablets daily before bedtime

Nursing considerations/Cautions/Patient education

- acts within 8—12 hours
- advise patient that tablets should be swallowed whole
- increase water consumption
- see also General Nursing considerations/Cautions/Patient education for laxatives (p. 1286)

Available in combination with
- docusate sodium 50 mg + sennoside B 8 mg tablet (APOHealth Laxative with Softener, Chemists' Own Laxative and Senna, Coloxyl with Senna, Co-Senna, Herron Sennesoft, Pharmacy Action Colox-Senna, Trust ColoxEase)

FAECAL SOFTENERS

General Actions of faecal softeners
- soften faeces by decreasing surface tension
- onset of action 1—3 days

General Uses of faecal softener
- constipation

DOCUSATE
Trade names
Coloxyl Tablets

Available forms
Tablets: 50 mg, 120 mg

Dose
- 240 mg orally daily after evening meal (120 mg tablets) **OR**
- 100—150 mg orally twice daily (50 mg tablets)

Nursing considerations/Cautions/Patient education

- see General Nursing considerations/Cautions/Patient education for laxatives (p. 1285)

 Considered safe to use in pregnancy.

 Considered safe to use when breastfeeding.

Available in combination with
- see docusate sodium + sennosides (under Sennosides A & B)

Note
- can also be used to soften ear wax (Waxsol).

PARAFFIN, LIQUID
Trade names
Agarol, Little Parachoc

Available forms
Suspension: 2.5 mL/5 mL, 4.83 mL/15 mL

LAXATIVES

Dose
- 15–40 mL orally at bedtime, increasing or decreasing dose by 5 mL to produce soft stool without oily leakage

Nursing considerations/Cautions/Patient education
- see General Nursing considerations/Cautions/Patient education for laxatives (p. 1286)

POLOXAMER (formerly known as poloxalkol)
Trade name
Coloxyl Infant Drops

Available form
Drops: 10%

Action
- increases penetration of fluid into faeces, softening stools

Use
- faecal softener for children and infants

Paediatric dose
- (< 6 months) 10 drops (0.3 mL) orally 3 times daily **OR**
- (6–18 months) 15 drops (0.5 mL) orally 3 times daily **OR**
- (18 months–3 years) 25 drops (0.8 mL) orally 3 times daily

Adverse effects
- see General Adverse effects of laxatives (p. 1286)

Interactions
- not recommended with other laxatives

Nursing considerations/Cautions
- effective within 2–3 days
- chronic use should be avoided, as this may increase potassium loss from the intestine, leading to electrolyte imbalance
- contraindicated if appendicitis or intestinal obstruction is suspected, or if undiagnosed rectal bleeding or abdominal pain is present
- see also General Nursing considerations/Cautions for laxatives (p. 1286)

Patient education
- advise the parent/carer to give the dose orally 3 times daily in a feeding bottle or in fruit juice
- instruct the parent/carer to use the syringe (provided) to measure dose accurately and then rinse with warm water after use

SODIUM PICOSULFATE
Trade name
Dulcolax SP Drops

Available form
Drops: 7.5 mg/mL

Action
- hydrolysed by bacteria in the colon to form the active ingredient, which stimulates the colon and increases motility, decreasing transit time and softening stool

Use
- constipation

Dose
- initially 10 drops (5 mg) orally at night, increasing to 20 drops (10 mg) if needed

Adverse effects
- dizziness, syncope
- (Rare) skin reactions
- see also General Adverse effects of laxatives (p. 1286)

Interactions
- increased risk of electrolyte imbalance if given with diuretics or corticosteroids
- decreased action may occur if given with broad-spectrum antibiotics
- if electrolyte imbalance occurs, it may result in increased sensitivity to digoxin
- efficacy decreased if given with bulk-forming laxatives

- may increase bowel transit time, which will impact on orally administered medications
- caution if used with NSAIDs, tricyclic antidepressants (TCAs), selective serotonin reuptake inhibitors (SSRIs), carbamazepine and antipsychotic agents, as these may increase water retention and/or electrolyte imbalance

Nursing considerations/Cautions

- (Dulcolax SP Drops) contraindicated in those with fructose intolerance
- see also General Nursing considerations/Cautions for laxatives (p. 1286)

Patient education

- advise the patient to ensure that other medications are taken 2 hours before or at least 6 hours after sodium picosulfate
- (Drops) the patient should be advised not to shake bottle and to use the dropper provided for correct dosage. Water can be added

Available in combination with

- contained in Picosalax, Picoprep, Picolax and Prep Kit C

OTHER AGENTS

METHYLNALTREXONE

Trade name
Relistor

Available form
Vial: 12 mg/0.6 mL

Action

- opioid antagonist with selectivity for mu opioid receptors (> kappa receptors) and no significant interaction with delta receptors
- peripherally acting as is not able to cross blood–brain barrier; therefore has no effect on opioid-mediated analgesic effect
- terminal half-life about 8 hours

Use

- opioid-induced constipation in those with advanced illness where response to laxative therapy has been inadequate

Dose

- (Weight 38 to < 62 kg) 8 mg SC every second day **OR**
- (Weight 62–114 kg) 12 mg SC every second day **OR**
- (< 38 kg or > 114 kg) 0.15 mg/kg SC every second day

Adverse effects

- abdominal pain, flatulence, nausea, diarrhoea
- dizziness
- sweating
- (Rare) gastrointestinal perforation (stomach, duodenum, colon)

Interactions

- caution if given with NSAIDs, corticosteroids or bevacizumab, as there may be an increased risk of gastrointestinal perforation

Nursing considerations/Cautions

- no known risk of abuse and/or dependence
- dosing interval can be increased if needed
- only given SC
- administer alone
- rotate administration; sites and areas that are scarred, tender, inflamed or bruised should not be used
- caution if used in those with advanced illness/disease (e.g. cancer, peptic ulcer, pseudo obstruction) which may impact on integrity of GI wall, as there may be increased risk of bowel perforation
- caution if used in those with GI tract lesions, active diverticular disease, faecal impaction, colostomy or peritoneal catheter
- not recommended in those with severe liver impairment or end-stage kidney disease requiring dialysis
- not recommended in those with postoperative ileus or those who have undergone gastrointestinal resection

- contraindicated in those with known or suspected mechanical GI obstruction or acute surgical abdomen

Patient education
- instruct the patient to seek medical advice if severe, persistent diarrhoea or severe or persistent abdominal pain occurs
- advise the patient that action usually occurs within 30 minutes; therefore they should remain near toilet facilities
- warn the patient to avoid driving or operating machinery if dizziness occurs

Not recommended during pregnancy unless clearly needed because of limited data available.

Not recommended when breastfeeding because limited data are available.

For those with CrCl < 30 mL/min, dose should be reduced by one-half. Not recommended for those with end-stage renal impairment on dialysis.

PRUCALOPRIDE
Trade names
Resotrans, Rospride

Available forms
Tablets: 1 mg, 2 mg

Action
- 5HT$_4$ agonist
- decreases small bowel transit time, increasing gastric emptying with no impact on colon transit time

Use
- chronic functional constipation that has not been relieved after therapy with laxatives from two or more different classes at highest tolerated dose for ≥ 6 months

Dose
- 2 mg orally daily **OR**
- (Adults > 65 years) initially 1 mg orally daily, increasing to 2 mg if needed **OR**
- (Adults with kidney or liver impairment) 1 mg orally daily

Adverse effects
- headache, dizziness, fatigue
- decreased appetite, nausea, diarrhoea, abdominal pain, abdominal distension, vomiting, dyspepsia, rectal bleeding, flatulence, unusual bowel sounds
- polyuria
- (Uncommon) palpitations, rectal bleeding, tremor, migraine
- (Rare) suicidal ideation

Interactions
- if diarrhoea results after use, failure of oral contraceptives may occur
- decreased effectiveness if given with atropine-like agents
- caution if used with agents that prolong QT interval

Nursing considerations/Cautions
- thorough assessment should be conducted before starting therapy to exclude any secondary causes of constipation
- if therapy is not effective after 4 weeks, the patient should be reassessed
- the patient should be reassessed after 12 weeks of therapy
- tablets contain lactose and are not recommended in those with galactose intolerance, Lapp lactase deficiency or glucose—galactose malabsorption
- caution if used in those with arrhythmias, ischaemic cardiovascular disease, severe liver or kidney impairment
- not recommended in those with constipation due to secondary causes such as endocrine, neurological or metabolic disorders or related to opioid use
- contraindicated in those with renal impairment requiring dialysis, intestinal perforation or obstruction, paralytic ileus, acute inflammatory intestinal conditions (e.g. Crohn's disease), ulcerative colitis, toxic megacolon or recent bowel surgery

Patient education

- warn the patient to avoid driving or operating machinery if dizziness or fatigue occurs
- advise the patient to seek medical advice if any tremor, rectal bleeding or pounding heart sensation occurs
- the patient should be warned that abdominal pain, nausea and/or diarrhoea commonly occur at the start of therapy, but these symptoms abate with continued therapy
- family members or carers should be advised to monitor the patient closely and seek medical advice immediately if any lowered mood, talk of self-harm or self-harm behaviours occur
- females of childbearing years should be counselled to use adequate contraception to avoid pregnancy during therapy

 Tablet can be dispersed in water or crushed and mixed with a spoonful of yoghurt or apple puree.

 Not recommended during pregnancy because of limited data available.

 Not recommended when breastfeeding because of limited data available.

 Contraindicated in patients undergoing renal dialysis; reduced dose required if CrCl < 30 mL/min.

LIPID REGULATING AGENTS

Atherosclerosis describes the process by which plaque is deposited in moderate- to large-sized arteries, resulting in narrowing of the lumen over a period of years to decades. Plaque is comprised of cholesterol, lipid, collagen and modified monocytes. Atherosclerosis may predispose a person to coronary artery disease (e.g. myocardial infarction, angina pectoris), cerebrovascular disease (e.g. stroke, transient cerebral ischaemia), peripheral vascular disease (e.g. intermittent claudication, gangrene) and/or renal artery insufficiency, depending on the location and severity of the plaque deposition (Knights et al 2023).

Cholesterol is essential in the production of steroid hormones (adrenocorticosteroids) and is produced from carbohydrates, proteins and lipids from the diet. Chylomicrons transport cholesterol and fatty acids from the GI tract to the liver. Oversupply of cholesterol from the diet in the form of saturated fat and/or a hereditary factor causing the overproduction of cholesterol leads to high serum levels of cholesterol known as hypercholesterolaemia (Knights et al 2023).

Lipids (e.g. triglycerides, cholesterol) are transported from the liver in the blood, in complexes called lipoproteins. The liver synthesises approximately two-thirds of the total plasma lipoproteins. Low-density lipoproteins (LDLs) are responsible for transporting cholesterol to the arteries, where it is deposited, whereas high-density lipoproteins (HDLs) transport cholesterol from peripheral cells to the liver, where it is processed into bile salts. The liver contains LDL receptors which remove LDLs from the plasma — the main mechanism for controlling LDL levels. The number of LDL receptors can be modulated. High levels of HDL are considered to be beneficial (preventing accumulation of cholesterol in artery walls), whereas high levels of LDLs are harmful and predispose a person to the development of atherosclerosis (Knights et al 2023).

Large amounts of triglycerides (and small amounts of cholesterol) are transported via very-low-density lipoproteins (VLDL). Lipoprotein lipase (an enzyme found in the endothelium of adipose and muscle tissue capillaries) releases the triglycerides from the VLDL, resulting in a short-lived intermediate-density lipoprotein (IDL), which is then either returned to the liver or converted to LDL (Knights et al 2023).

Apolipoproteins are proteins found on the surface of the lipoproteins and appear to confer properties on the lipoprotein. These apolipoproteins are classified using a letter and Roman numeral (e.g. A-I, A-II). Apolipoprotein A-I appears to confer the beneficial effects of HDL, whereas apolipoprotein C-II deficiency in VLDL results in impaired triglyceride metabolism and hypertriglyceridaemia (Knights et al 2023).

Dyslipidaemias (hyperlipidaemias) are disorders in which there are elevated levels of triglycerides (hypertriglyceridaemia), cholesterol (hypercholesterolaemia) or both (mixed lipidaemia). Primary hyperlipidaemia is subdivided into six subgroups (I, IIa, IIb, III, IV and V), with the different types carrying differing risks of atherosclerosis and being amenable to treatment by different classes of lipid regulating agents. For example, IIa (familial hypercholesterolaemia) has elevated LDL and cholesterol levels and may be managed using a statin, bile acid binding resin or a combination of both. Secondary causes of dyslipidaemia include disease (e.g. diabetes mellitus, obesity, hypothyroidism, nephrotic syndrome), excess alcohol consumption and some medications (e.g. thiazide diuretics, corticosteroids) (Knights et al 2023).

Management should include appropriate dietary modification (low in cholesterol, and saturated and total fats), correction of any underlying disease (diabetes mellitus, hypothyroidism, alcoholism), avoidance of precipitating factors (smoking, obesity, hypertension) and lifestyle changes (e.g. increasing physical activity) before instituting drug therapy.

Lipid regulating agents can be divided into several classes:

- hydroxymethylglutaryl co-enzyme A (HMG-CoA) reductase inhibitors (statins) (atorvastatin, fluvastatin, rosuvastatin, pravastatin, simvastatin), which are used to treat hypercholesterolaemia or mixed hyperlipidaemia
- fibrates (fenofibrate, gemfibrozil), which are used to treat hypertriglyceridaemia or mixed hyperlipidaemia
- bile acid binding agents (e.g. colestyramine), which are used to treat hypercholesterolaemia or combined hyperlipidaemia
- PCSK9 inhibitors (e.g. alirocumab, evolocumab)
- other agents (e.g. nicotinic acid, ezetimibe, omega-3 fatty acids)

HMG-CoA REDUCTASE INHIBITORS (STATINS)

General Actions of statins
- HMG-CoA reductase is the rate-limiting enzyme that converts 3-hydroxy-3-methylglutarylco-enzyme A to mevalonate (precursor of sterols, including cholesterol). Statins reversibly inhibit HMG-CoA reductase, reducing cholesterol synthesis and increasing the number of liver LDL receptors, thereby reducing LDL concentration
- also thought to have an effect on endothelial function, modify inflammatory response, decrease platelet aggregation, modify thrombus formation, stabilise atherosclerotic plaque, decrease smooth muscle cell migration and proliferation, increase fibrolytic action and decrease C-reactive protein
- effect on LDL cholesterol is dependent on specific statin and dose
- reach peak concentration within 5 hours

General Uses of statins
- hypercholesterolaemia (types IIa, IIb) (adjunct to diet)
- mixed hyperlipidaemia

LIPID REGULATING AGENTS

- prevention of cardiovascular disease in those with two or more risk factors

General Adverse effects of statins

- GI symptoms: constipation, flatulence, dyspepsia, abdominal pain, nausea, diarrhoea
- headache, dizziness, asthenia, fatigue
- (muscle symptoms) myopathy (muscle aching or weakness with increase in CPK), myalgia (common) rhabdomyolysis (rare), hypersensitivity, interstitial lung disease (long-term therapy), haemorrhagic stroke, immune-mediated necrotising myopathy (very rare)
- insomnia, nightmares
- rash, pruritus
- hyperglycaemia
- elevated liver enzymes and creatine kinase (CK) levels
- (high dose) increase risk of type 2 diabetes

General Interactions of statins

- contraindicated with sodium fusidate because of increased risk of rhabdomyolysis. Statin should be stopped for at least 7 days longer than sodium fusidate therapy
- increased serum levels may occur if used with ciclosporin, erythromycin, clarithromycin, antifungal (azole) agents or diltiazem, increasing risk of myalgia and/or rhabdomyolysis
- caution if used with fibrates or nicotinic acid
- caution if used with spironolactone as it may decrease levels or activity of naturally occurring steroid hormones
- if given within 4 hours of colestyramine, decreased serum levels may result

General Nursing considerations/Cautions for statins

- contraindications: avoid in people with active liver disease, unexplained elevated ALT/AST or a history of myopathy from lipid lowering agents
- address and treat secondary hypercholesterolemia causes (e.g. poorly controlled diabetes, hypothyroidism, liver disease) before starting therapy; encourage weight loss and diet changes
- lipid levels should be monitored regularly, initially at 4 weeks, and the dose should be adjusted as needed
- liver function tests should be performed before starting therapy, at 6 and 12 weeks, then twice yearly
- if conditions predisposing to rhabdomyolysis occur (e.g. trauma, severe infection, major surgery, uncontrolled epilepsy), withhold statin
- check CK before starting in patients with renal impairment, hypothyroidism, history of muscle disorders, alcohol abuse or age > 70 owing to myopathy risk; avoid testing after strenuous exercise
- use with caution: in history of liver disease, impaired liver function or substantial alcohol consumption; in patients > 65 years, females or with uncontrolled hypothyroidism (increased myopathy risk); in those with renal impairment, monitor renal function and CK levels regularly; in patients at risk of diabetes, closely monitor blood glucose levels during therapy
- ophthalmological testing is recommended after 5 years of therapy
- statins with short half-life (fluvastatin, pravastatin, simvastatin) should be taken in the evening to maximise efficiency as cholesterol synthesis in the liver is at its maximum between midnight and 2 am

General Patient education for statins

- advise patient to seek medical advice immediately if any of the following occur:
  - muscle pain, cramps, tenderness or weakness (not related to exercise), malaise, dark (resembling the color of cola) urine or fever
  - non-productive cough, difficulty breathing, fatigue, weight loss or fever

- itching, yellowing of skin or eyes, loss of appetite, tiredness, dark urine
- advise patient to take medication at least 1 hour before or 4 hours after colestyramine
- patient should be warned against drinking large amounts of alcohol because of increased risk of liver damage
- women of childbearing potential should be counselled to use adequate contraception during therapy

 Use statins cautiously in renal impairment owing to the risk of myopathy and rhabdomyolysis. Adjust dosages as needed and monitor renal function and CK levels regularly.

ATORVASTATIN

Trade names
APO-Atorvastatin, Atomed, Atorvachol, Atorvastatin SZ, Atorvastatin-WGR, Blooms the Chemist Atorvastatin, BTC Atorvastatin, Lipitor, Lorstat, Noumed Atorvastatin, Pharmacor Atorvastatin, Torvastat, Trovas

Available form
Tablets: 10 mg, 20 mg, 40 mg, 80 mg

Action
- second-generation synthetic statin
- active metabolites
- elimination half-life 15—30 hours
- see also General Actions of statins (p. 1300)

Use
- hypercholesterolaemia
- hypertensive patients with additional risk factors for heart disease
- see General Uses of statins (p. 1300)

Dose
- initially 10 mg orally daily, titrating dose at 4-week intervals (range 10—80 mg)

Adverse effects
- nasopharyngitis
- muscle spasm, joint swelling
- (rare) haemorrhagic stroke
- see also General Adverse effects of statins (p. 1301)

Interactions
- serum level may be increased by HIV protease inhibitors, clarithromycin, itraconazole, diltiazem, boceprevir and grapefruit juice (especially excessive amounts > 1.2 L/day)
- caution if given with colchicine owing to increased risk of myopathy
- may affect efficacy of oral contraceptives containing norethisterone and ethinylestradiol
- serum levels may be decreased by antacids (magnesium or aluminium hydroxide)
- caution if given with phenytoin, rifampicin or efavirenz as effect may be variable
- if given 1 hour after rifampicin, decreased serum levels may occur. However, if given simultaneously, no effect on serum levels
- not recommended with St John's wort
- caution if given with digoxin. If given together, serum digoxin levels should be closely monitored
- see also General Interactions of statins (p. 1301)

Nursing considerations/Cautions
- patient should be assessed for history of stroke or transischaemic attacks (TIAs) within last 6 months before starting therapy because of increased risk of haemorrhagic stroke
- see also General Nursing considerations/Cautions for statins (p. 1301)

Patient education
- seek medical advice promptly if you have dark urine or muscle pain
- patient should be advised to avoid grapefruit during therapy
- instruct patient to take 2 hours apart from antacids
- see also General Patient education for statins (p. 1301)

LIPID REGULATING AGENTS

Tablet can be dispersed in water (5–6 minutes) or crushed and mixed with spoonful of yoghurt or apple puree.

Avoid using statins during pregnancy (and in women planning to conceive); specialists may consider statins for women at very high risk of heart attack or stroke. Although statins have a theoretical risk of harming the fetus, inadvertent use early in pregnancy is unlikely to be harmful.

Avoid breastfeeding. Atorvastatin may be excreted into breastmilk, which could lead to exposure of the nursing infant. There is limited research on the effects of atorvastatin on breastfed infants.

Available in combination with:
- atorvastatin 10 mg + amlodipine 5 mg tablet (Caduet 5/10, Cadivast 5/10)
- atorvastatin 10 mg + amlodipine 10 mg tablet (Caduet 10/10, Cadivast 10/10)
- atorvastatin 20 mg + amlodipine 5 mg tablet (Caduet 5/20, Cadivast 5/20)
- atorvastatin 20 mg + amlodipine 10 mg tablet (Caduet 10/20, Cadivast 10/20)
- atorvastatin 40 mg + amlodipine 5 mg tablet (Caduet 5/40, Cadivast 5/40)
- atorvastatin 40 mg + amlodipine 10 mg tablet (Caduet 10/40, Cadivast 10/40)
- atorvastatin 80 mg + amlodipine 5 mg tablet (Caduet 5/80, Cadivast 5/80)
- atorvastatin 80 mg + amlodipine 10 mg tablet (Caduet 10/80, Cadivast 10/80)
- atorvastatin 10 mg + ezetimibe 10 mg tablet (Atozet 10/10, Ezetast 10/10, Ezetimide/Atorvastatin GH 10/10)
- atorvastatin 20 mg + ezetimibe 10 mg table (Atozet 20/10, Ezetast 20/10, Ezetimide/Atorvastatin GH 20/10)
- atorvastatin 40 mg + ezetimibe 10 mg tablet (Atozet 40/10, Ezetast 40/10, Ezetimibe/Atorvastatin GH 40/10)
- atorvastatin 80 mg + ezetimibe 10 mg tablet (Atozet 80/10, Ezetast 80/10, Ezetimibe/Atorvastatin GH 80/10)

FLUVASTATIN
Trade name
Lescol XL

Available form
Tablets (prolonged-release): 80 mg

Action/Use
- elimination half-life 0.5–2.3 hours
- see also General Actions/Uses of statins (p. 1300,1301)

Dose
- (Lipid lowering) 80 mg orally nocte **OR**
- (Post-coronary transcatheter therapy) 80 mg orally nocte

Adverse effects
- see General Adverse effects of statins (p. 1300)

Interactions
- bioavailability may be increased if given with ranitidine or omeprazole
- bioavailability may be decreased if given with rifampicin
- if given with warfarin, INR should be monitored, especially when starting, stopping or altering dose
- may increase plasma levels of phenytoin, increasing the risk of toxicity
- increased plasma levels may occur if given with phenytoin
- increased risk of myalgia and/or rhabdomyolysis if given with colchicine
- see also General Interactions of statins (p. 1301)

Nursing considerations/Cautions
- see General Nursing considerations/Cautions for statins (p. 1301)

Patient education
- patients should be advised that prolonged-release tablets should be swallowed whole, not broken, crushed or chewed
- seek medical advice if you notice dark urine or experience muscle pain, tenderness or weakness.

- see also General Patient education for statins (p. 1301)

 Prolonged-release tablets should be swallowed whole, so do not break, crush or chew.

 Avoid using statins during pregnancy (and in women planning to conceive); specialists may consider statins for women at very high risk of heart attack or stroke. Although statins have a theoretical risk of harming the fetus, inadvertent use early in pregnancy is unlikely to be harmful.

 Avoid breastfeeding while taking fluvastatin, as it may be excreted into breastmilk and potentially expose the nursing infant to the drug. There is limited research on the effects of fluvastatin on breastfed infants.

PRAVASTATIN

Trade names
Cholstat, Lipostat, Pravachol, APX-Pravastatin, Auro-Pravastatin, Pravastatin Sandoz, Pravastatin-WGR

Available form
Tablets: 10 mg, 20 mg, 40 mg, 80 mg

Action
- half-life 1.3—2.8 hours
- see also General Actions of statins (p. 1300)

Use
- hypercholesterolaemia
- previous myocardial infarction with normal cholesterol levels, unstable angina
- (Adolescents) heterozygous familial hypercholesterolaemia
- see also General Uses of statins (p. 1300)

Dose
- (Lipid lowering) initially 10—20 mg orally nocte, increasing at 4-week intervals to 80 mg daily if necessary **OR**
- (Coronary heart disease, prevention of myocardial infarction) 40 mg orally nocte **OR**
- (Heterozygous familial hypercholesterolaemia, 8—13 years) 20 mg orally nocte **OR**
- (Heterozygous familial hypercholesterolaemia, 14—18 years) 40 mg orally nocte

Adverse effects
- dyspnoea
- visual disturbances, including blurred vision
- see also General Adverse effects of statins (p. 1301)

Interactions
- see General Interactions of statins (p. 1301)

Nursing considerations/Cautions
- not recommended for hypertriglyceridaemia
- not recommended for homozygous familial hypercholesterolaemia
- see also General Nursing considerations/Cautions for statins (p. 1301)

Patient education
- slightly more effective when taken in the evening;, take in the evening
- warn patient against driving or operating machinery if blurred vision occurs
- see also General Patient education for statins (p. 1301)

 Tablet can be crushed and mixed with water (but does not disperse readily) or spoonful of yoghurt or apple puree.

 Do not crush or disperse the tablet if you are pregnant.

 Avoid using statins during pregnancy (and in women planning to conceive); specialists may consider statins for women at very high risk of heart attack or stroke. Although statins have a theoretical risk of harming the fetus, inadvertent use early in pregnancy is unlikely to be harmful.

 Avoid breastfeeding while taking pravastatin, as it may be excreted into breastmilk, potentially exposing the nursing infant to the drug. There is limited research on the effects of pravastatin on breastfed infants.

LIPID REGULATING AGENTS

ROSUVASTATIN
Trade names
APO-Rosuvastatin, APX-Rosuvastatin, Blooms Rosuvastatin, BTC Rosuvastatin, Cavstat, Crestor, Crosuva, Noumed Rosuvastatin, Rostor, Pharmcor Rosuvastatin, Rosuvastatin Intas, Rosuvastatin Lupin, Rosuvastatin RBX, Rosuvastatin Sandoz, Rosuvastatin-WGR

Available form
Tablets: 5 mg, 10 mg, 20 mg, 40 mg

Action
- hypercholesterolaemia
- high risk of coronary heart disease, with or without hypercholesterolaemia
- metabolite has some activity
- elimination half-life 14—26 hours
- see also General Actions of statins (p. 1300)

Use
- see General Uses of statins (p. 1300)

Dose
- (Lipid lowering) initially 5—10 mg orally daily, increasing at 4-week intervals if needed (daily maximum 20 mg) **OR**
- (Lipid lowering, Asian patients) initially 5 mg orally daily, increasing at 4-week intervals if needed (daily maximum 20 mg) **OR**
- (Prevention of cardiovascular disease) 20 mg orally daily

Adverse effects
- see General Adverse effects of statins (p. 1301)

Interactions
- may decrease serum levels if given with antacids
- caution if used with HIV protease inhibitors
- (Asian patients) contraindicated with fibrates
- see also General Interactions of statins (p. 1301)

Nursing considerations/Cautions
- 40 mg tablets are contraindicated in those with predisposition to myopathy or rhabdomyolysis
- tablets contain lactose and are therefore not recommended in those with rare hereditary problems of galactose intolerance, Lapp lactase deficiency or glucose—galactose malabsorption
- see also General Nursing considerations/Cautions for statins (p. 1301)

Patient education
- seek immediate medical advice if you have dark urine or muscle pain
- instruct patients to take rosuvastatin 2 hours apart from antacids
- see also General Patient education for statins (p. 1301)

 Tablet can be dispersed in water or crushed and mixed with spoonful of yoghurt or apple puree.

 Avoid using statins during pregnancy (and in women planning to conceive); specialists may consider statins for women at very high risk of heart attack or stroke. Although statins have a theoretical risk of harming the fetus, inadvertent use early in pregnancy is unlikely to be harmful.

 Avoid breastfeeding. May be excreted into breastmilk, which could lead to exposure of the nursing infant. There is limited research on the effects on breastfed infants.

Available in combination with:
- rosuvastatin 5 mg tablet + ezetimibe 10 mg tablet (Ezalo Composite Pack 10 mg + 5 mg, Ezecrest Composite Pack 10 mg + 5 mg, Ezetimide-Rosuvastatin Sandoz Composite Pack 10 mg + 5 mg, Pharmcor Ezetimide-Rosuvastatin Composite Pack 10 mg + 5 mg, Rosuzet Composite Pack 10 mg + 5 mg)
- rosuvastatin 10 mg tablet + ezetimibe 10 mg tablet (Ezalo Composite Pack 10 mg + 10 mg, Ezecrest Composite Pack 10 mg + 10 mg, Ezetimide-Rosuvastatin Sandoz Composite Pack 10 mg + 10 mg, Pharmcor Ezetimide-Rosuvastatin Composite Pack 10 mg + 10 mg, Rosuzet Composite Pack 10 mg + 10 mg)

- rosuvastatin 20 mg tablet + ezetimibe 10 mg tablet (Ezalo Composite Pack 10 mg + 20 mg, Ezecrest Composite Pack 10 mg + 20 mg, Ezetimide-Rosuvastatin Sandoz Composite Pack 10 mg + 20 mg, Pharmcor Ezetimide-Rosuvastatin Composite Pack 10 mg + 20 mg, Rosuzet Composite Pack 10 mg + 20 mg)
- rosuvastatin 40 mg tablet + ezetimibe 10 mg tablet (Ezalo Composite Pack 10 mg + 40 mg, Ezecrest Composite Pack 10 mg + 40 mg, Ezetimide-Rosuvastatin Sandoz Composite Pack 10 mg + 40 mg, Pharmcor Ezetimide-Rosuvastatin Composite Pack 10 mg + 40 mg, Rosuzet Composite Pack 10 mg + 40 mg)

SIMVASTATIN

Trade names
APO-Simvastatin, Lipex, Noumed Simvastatin, Simvar, Zimstat, Zocor

Available form
Tablets: 5 mg, 10 mg, 20 mg, 40 mg, 80 mg

Action
- prodrug requires activation in the liver
- active metabolites
- decreases cholesterol levels by 30–50%
- half-life 2–3 hours
- see also General Actions of statins (p. 1300)

Use
- heterozygous familial hypercholesterolaemia (adolescents, 10–17 years)
- see also General Uses of statins (p. 1300)

Dose
- (Lipid lowering) initially 10–20 mg orally nocte, increasing at 4-week intervals if needed (daily maximum 80 mg) **OR**
- (Heterozygous familial hypercholesterolaemia, adolescents, 10–17 years) initially 10 mg orally nocte, increasing to maximum of 40 mg if needed **OR**
- (Coronary heart disease) 40–80 mg orally nocte

Adverse effects
- transient hypotension
- (Uncommon) peripheral neuropathy, paraesthesia
- see also General Adverse effects of statins (p. 1301)

Interactions
- contraindicated with gemfibrozil, ciclosporin, danazol, clarithromycin, erythromycin, HIV protease inhibitors and azole antifungals
- caution if used with warfarin; INR should be closely monitored, especially when starting or stopping therapy
- grapefruit juice should be avoided as it can increase blood levels of simvastatin, potentially leading to a higher risk of adverse effects
- caution if given with digoxin. If given together serum digoxin levels should be closely monitored
- increased risk of rhabdomyolysis if given with amiodarone, verapamil, diltiazem, amlodipine or nicotinic acid (niacin) ($\geq$ 1g/day)
- caution if given with colchicine in those with renal insufficiency
- (Asian patients) not recommended with niacin ($\geq$ 1 g/day)
- see also General Interactions of statins (p. 1301)

Nursing considerations/Cautions
- risk of myopathy increases with dose; 80 mg dose should only be used in patients with high risk of cardiovascular complications who have not achieved treatment goals and where benefits outweigh risks
- see also General Nursing considerations/Cautions for statins (p. 1301)

Patient education
- seek medical advice if you have dark urine or muscle pain
- avoid grapefruit juice during therapy

LIPID REGULATING AGENTS

- report any numbness or tingling in hands or feet
- see also General Patient education for statins (p. 1301)

Tablet can be crushed and mixed with water or spoonful of yoghurt or apple puree.

Avoid using statins during pregnancy (and in women planning to conceive); specialists may consider statins for women at very high risk of heart attack or stroke. Although statins have a theoretical risk of harming the fetus, inadvertent use early in pregnancy is unlikely to be harmful.

Avoid breastfeeding. Simvastatin may be excreted into breastmilk, which could expose the nursing infant to the drug. There is limited research on the effects of simvastatin on breastfed infants.

Available in combination with:
- simvastatin 10 mg + ezetimibe 10 mg tablet (APO-Ezetimibe/Simvastatin 10/10, Ezisim 10/10, Ezetimibe/Simvastatin Sandoz, 10/10, Ezetimibe/Simvastatin-WGR 10/10, Ezetorin 10/10, EzSimva GH 10 mg/10 mg, Pharmcor Ezetimibe Simvastatin 10/10, Vytorin 10/10, Zimybe 10/10)
- simvastatin 20 mg + ezetimibe 10 mg tablet (APO-Ezetimibe/Simvastatin 10/10, Ezisim 10/20, Ezetimibe/Simvastatin Sandoz, 10/20, Ezetimibe/Simvastatin-WGR 10/20, Ezetorin 10/10, EzSimva GH 10 mg/20 mg, Pharmcor Ezetimibe Simvastatin 10/20, Vytorin 10/20, Zimybe 10/20)
- simvastatin 40 mg + ezetimibe 10 mg tablet (APO-Ezetimibe/Simvastatin 10/10, Ezisim 10/40, Ezetimibe/Simvastatin Sandoz, 10/40, Ezetimibe/Simvastatin-WGR 10/40, Ezetorin 10/10, EzSimva GH 10 mg/40 mg, Pharmcor Ezetimibe Simvastatin 10/40, Vytorin 10/40, Zimybe 10/40)
- simvastatin 80 mg + ezetimibe 10 mg tablet (APO-Ezetimibe/Simvastatin 10/10, Ezisim 10/80, Ezetimibe/Simvastatin Sandoz, 10/80, Ezetimibe/Simvastatin-WGR 10/80, Ezetorin 10/10, EzSimva GH 10 mg/80 mg, Pharmcor Ezetimibe Simvastatin 10/80, Vytorin 10/80, Zimybe 10/80)

BILE ACID BINDING AGENTS

General Actions of bile acid binding agents
- cholesterol is the major precursor of bile salts. Bile acid binding agents bind cholesterol containing bile acids in the intestine, preventing them from being reabsorbed. This increases hepatic LDL receptor activity, promoting hepatic uptake and subsequent breakdown of plasma LDL cholesterol for conversion to replacement bile acids, thus lowering the plasma cholesterol concentration

General Uses of bile acid binding agents
- hypercholesterolaemia (adjunctive therapy)
- mixed hyperlipidaemia
- diarrhoea (ileal resection or disease)
- relief of pruritus (itch) associated with biliary obstruction and primary biliary cirrhosis

General Adverse effects of bile acid binding agents
- constipation, faecal impaction, haemorrhoids or aggravation of pre-existing haemorrhoids
- (Less common) nausea, vomiting, anorexia, abdominal pain and distension, heartburn, indigestion, flatulence, diarrhoea, steatorrhoea
- (Less common) headache, migraine, sinus headache, dizziness, fatigue
- (Less common) reduced absorption of fat-soluble vitamins, increased risk of bleeding (hypoprothrombinaemia, vitamin K), night blindness (vitamin A) and osteoporosis (vitamin D)

- (Less common) rash, irritation of skin, tongue and perianal area
- (Prolonged use) hyperchloraemic acidosis

General Interactions of bile acid binding agents
- may reduce or delay absorption of thyroid hormones, warfarin, digoxin, phenobarbital (phenobarbitone), tetracycline, propranolol, benzylpenicillin, gemfibrozil, furosemide (frusemide), mycophenolate mofetil, mycophenolate sodium, inorganic iron and oral phosphate supplements

Nursing considerations/Cautions
- any secondary causes of hypercholesterolaemia (e.g. poorly controlled diabetes mellitus, hypothyroidism, obstructive liver disease, alcoholism, nephrotic syndrome, dysproteinaemia, drug therapy) should be identified and treated before starting therapy, as well as weight reduction and diet modification
- baseline cholesterol and triglyceride levels should be established, then monitored during therapy
- GI function should be evaluated before starting therapy to identify any risks for severe constipation and/or faecal impaction
- if therapy is prolonged, supplementary fat-soluble vitamins A and D may be required and, if there is a bleeding tendency, vitamin K
- therapy should be discontinued if cholesterol level does not fall or triglyceride levels increase
- caution in those with pre-existing constipation (reduced dose required) or if > 60 years
- contraindicated in those with complete biliary obstruction

General Patient education for bile acid binding agents
- advise patient that powder/granules must not be taken in dry form
- patient should be instructed to place prescribed amount of sachet contents on the surface of 100–150 mL (for 4 g sachet) or 200–300 mL (for 8 g sachet) of water, milk, carbonated beverage (taking care with excess foaming/frothing), tomato or fruit juice, thin soups, cereals, apple sauce or puree, pears, peaches, fruit cocktail or crushed pineapple in a large glass. Stir vigorously or shake in Questran Lite shaker (for colestyramine only) until the mixture is evenly suspended. Rinse glass after use and drink contents to ensure total dose is taken
- advise patient that for better absorption take other oral drugs either 1 hour before or 4–6 hours after
- addition of cereal bran and good fluid intake is recommended to minimise constipation
- patient should be advised to seek medical advice if constipation occurs

COLESTYRAMINE
Trade name
Questran Lite

Available form
Powder: 4 g

Action
- insoluble in water
- not absorbed by GI tract and not affected by digestive enzymes
- decreases cholesterol levels by about 20–40%
- see also General Actions of bile acid binding agents (p. 1307)

Use
- see General Uses of bile acid binding agents (p. 1307)

Dose
- (Lipid lowering) initially 4 g (1 sachet) orally daily, increasing over next 2–4 weeks to the required dose **OR**
- (Other uses) 12–16 g orally daily

Adverse effects
- (Uncommon) osteoporosis
- see also General Adverse effects of bile acid binding agents (p. 1307)

LIPID REGULATING AGENTS

Interactions
- caution if given with aldosterone antagonists (e.g. spironolactone) because of increased risk of hyperchloraemic acidosis
- may interfere with oestrogen metabolism
- see also General Interactions of bile acid binding agents (p. 1308)

Nursing considerations/Cautions
- (Diarrhoea use) response should be seen within 3 days
- large doses (24 g per day) may interfere with fat absorption and result in steatorrhoea
- those with phenylketonuria should be advised that colestyramine contains phenylalanine (16.8 mg/4 g colestyramine)
- see also General Nursing considerations/Cautions for bile acid binding agents (p. 1308)

Patient education
- advise patient to avoid holding in mouth for prolonged length of time to avoid tooth decay or discolouration
- see also General Patient education for bile acid binding agents (p. 1308)

Avoid use. Cholestyramine binds to various substances, including fat-soluble vitamins, which may reduce their absorption in the mother. The potential impact of this reduction on fetal development remains unclear.

Colestyramine is not absorbed from the mother's gastrointestinal tract. However, it may reduce the absorption of fat-soluble vitamins, which could potentially affect breastmilk quality.

FIBRATES

General Actions of fibrates
- activate peroxisome proliferator-activated receptors (PPARs) to modulate lipoprotein synthesis and breakdown
- stimulate lipoprotein lipase, reducing the amount of triglyceride in VLDL and chylomicrons
- stimulate liver to increase LDL uptake and therefore LDL clearance
- reduce plasma triglycerides
- moderately increase HDL
- variable effect on LDL concentrations

General Uses of fibrates
- types II, III, IV and V dyslipidaemia
- mixed hyperlipidaemia
- dyslipidaemia associated with type 2 diabetes
- hypercholesterolaemia (second line)

General Adverse effects of fibrates
- GI disturbances: nausea, vomiting, diarrhoea, constipation, dyspepsia, abdominal pain, flatulence
- rash
- elevated liver enzymes and CPK
- gallstone formation
- (Uncommon) photosensitivity reaction
- (Uncommon) myopathy, myalgia, myositis
- (Rare) rhabdomyolysis, hepatitis, pancreatitis, hypersensitivity
- (Rare) anaemia, leucopenia, thrombocytopenia

General Interactions of fibrates
- contraindicated with other fibrates
- not recommended with statins because of increased risk of myopathy and rhabdomyolysis
- may enhance effects of oral anticoagulants; therefore INR should be carefully monitored, especially when starting, stopping or altering doses
- caution if used with ciclosporin
- increased risk of myotoxicity if given with colchicine

General Nursing considerations/Cautions for fibrates
- contraindicated in those with photoallergy/phototoxic reaction to other fibrates or ketoprofen

- contraindicated in those with liver/ renal dysfunction, primary biliary cirrhosis, liver function abnormalities, existing gallbladder disease or chronic/acute pancreatitis (except due to hypertriglyceridaemia)
- any secondary causes of hypercholesterolaemia (e.g. poorly controlled diabetes mellitus, hypothyroidism, obstructive liver disease, alcoholism, nephrotic syndrome, dysproteinaemia, drug therapy) should be identified and treated before starting therapy, as well as weight reduction and diet modification
- ineffective in patients with raised cholesterol but normal triglyceride levels
- baseline liver function tests (including liver enzymes, serum lipids, lipoproteins and ratios) should be performed before starting, 3-monthly for first 12 months and then regularly throughout treatment
- if HDL-C levels become severely depressed, therapy should be stopped and restarted when the levels return to baseline
- full blood count should be measured before starting and regularly during first 12 months of therapy
- if not effective in 12 weeks at maximum dose, a different or adjunct therapy should be considered
- caution if used in those with hepatobiliary disease
- increased risk of myopathy and/or rhabdomyolysis if given to those over 70 years, history of hereditary muscular disorders, kidney impairment, hypoalbuminaemia, hypothyroidism or high alcohol intake

General Patient education for fibrates

- seek immediate medical attention if you experience yellowing of the skin or eyes, tiredness, loss of appetite, abdominal pain or dark urine; muscle pain, cramps, tenderness or weakness; malaise or fever; sudden intense pain in the upper right abdomen, severe pain below the breastbone, pain between the shoulder blades or right shoulder tip; vomiting
- avoid consuming large quantities of alcohol while taking this medication
- do not drive or operate machinery if you experience dizziness or vertigo
- avoid direct UV exposure; wear protective clothing, a hat, sunscreen (SPF 30+), and sunglasses when outdoors

 Use of fibrates during pregnancy should be avoided owing to limited human data, except on specialist advice in cases of severe hypertriglyceridaemia with a risk of pancreatitis.

 There are no data on fibrates and breastfeeding; avoid breastfeeding.

 Fibrates are contraindicated in patients with severe renal impairment, hepatic impairment, primary biliary cirrhosis, or if gallstones or gallbladder disease are present.

FENOFIBRATE

Trade names
APO Fenofibrate, ARX-Fenofibrate, BTC Fenofibrate, Fenofibrate RBX, Fenofibrate-WGR, Fenocol, Fenofibrate Cipla, Fenofibrate Sandoz, Fenofibrate Viatris, Lipidil

Available form
Tablets: 48 mg, 145 mg

Action
- active metabolite (fenofibric acid) which has half-life of about 20 hours
- significantly reduces triglyceride levels by 20—50%
- some uricosuric effect, decreasing uric acid levels by about 25%
- see also General Actions of fibrates (p. 1309)

Use
- decreases progression of diabetic retinopathy in those with type 2 diabetes and existing diabetic retinopathy

LIPID REGULATING AGENTS

- see also General Uses of fibrates (p. 1309)

Dose
- (Dyslipidaemia, diabetic neuropathy) 145 mg orally daily with food

Adverse effects
- increase in serum creatinine
- (Uncommon) headaches
- (Rare) urticaria, rash, pulmonary embolism, deep vein thrombosis
- see also General Adverse effects of fibrates (p. 1309)

Interactions
- reversible renal impairment may occur if given with ciclosporin. Renal function should be monitored carefully
- caution if used with pioglitazone
- caution if used with agents that have a narrow therapeutic index
- see also General Interactions of fibrates (p. 1309)

Nursing considerations/Cautions
- contraindicated in children, patients with photoallergy to ketoprofen and those allergic to peanuts, arachis oil, or soya lecithin.
- use 48 mg capsules only for reduced doses in kidney impairment.
- 3 x 48 mg tablets are bioequivalent to one 145 mg tablet.
- monitor creatinine clearance (CrCl) during the first 12 weeks and regularly after that, especially in elderly patients or those with diabetes.
- not recommended for those with lecithin hypersensitivity or hereditary issues like fructose/galactose intolerance, Lapp lactase deficiency, or glucose–galactose malabsorption.
- see also General Nursing consderations/Cautions for fibrates (p. 1309)

Patient education
- avoid sun exposure; wear protective clothing and use sunscreen.
- seek medical advice if you notice dark (brown) urine or experience muscle pain, tenderness, or weakness.

- see also General Patient education for fibrates (p. 1310)

Tablet does not disperse readily in water and is hard to crush. Tablets can be crushed and mixed with apple sauce or yogurt.

Limited human data; avoid use unless for severe hypertriglyceridaemia with a risk of pancreatitis. Contact a pregnancy drug information centre for guidance.

No data available; fenofibrate should not be administrated to breastfeeding women.

Reduced renal function: use with caution in renal impairment (CrCl < 60 mL/min). Start with 48 mg once daily for CrCl 30–60 mL/min; may increase to 96 mg once daily, if needed, after checking renal function and lipids.

GEMFIBROZIL

Trade names
Ausgem, Lipigem

Available form
Tablets: 600 mg

Action
- decreases triglycerides
- slight decrease in total cholesterol, increase in HDL
- onset of action 2–5 days, peak effect 4 weeks
- half-life about 1.5 hours
- see also General Actions of fibrates (p. 1309)

Use
- see General Uses of fibrates (p. 1309)

Dose
- 600 mg orally twice daily 30 minutes before the morning and evening meal

Adverse effects
- acute appendicitis, altered taste
- atrial fibrillation
- fatigue, vertigo, headache, dizziness
- eczema
- (Rare) subcapsular bilateral cataracts, urticaria, pruritus

- see also General Adverse effects of fibrates (p. 1309)

Interactions
- caution if given with hypoglycaemic agents as hypoglycaemia may occur
- see also General Interactions of fibrates (p. 1309)

Nursing considerations/Cautions
- contraindicated in those with type I hyperlipoproteinaemia
- see also General Nursing considerations/Cautions for fibrates (p. 1309)

Patient education
- swallow tablets whole before meals. If not tolerated, they can be taken with food.
- do not drive or operate machinery if you experience dizziness or vertigo.
- patients with diabetes should closely monitor BGLs during therapy, as hypoglycaemia may occur
- women of childbearing potential should use effective contraception during therapy to avoid pregnancy
- see also General Patient education for fibrates (p. 1310)

Contraindicated during pregnancy. Use only on specialist advice for severe hypertriglyceridemia with risk of pancreatitis. Contact a pregnancy drug information center for guidance.

No data available; gemfibrozil should not be administered to breastfeeding women.

ICOSAPENT ETHYL

Trade name
Vazkepa

Available form
Capsule: 998 mg

Action
- stable ester of omega-3 fatty acid eicosapentaenoic acid (EPA)
- antiplatelet, anti-inflammatory and antioxidant effects
- reduces macrophage accumulation, improves endothelial function, increases fibrous cap thickness/stability
- alters development, progression and stabilisation of atherosclerotic plaque
- improves lipoprotein profile by suppressing cholesterol, fatty acid and triglyceride synthesising enzymes

Use
- reduces risk of cardiovascular events in adult statin-treated patients at high cardiovascular risk with elevated triglycerides (>1.7 mmol/L), established cardiovascular disease or diabetes, and at least one other cardiovascular risk factor

Dose
- 1,996 g (2 tablets) orally twice daily with or after meal

Adverse effects
- constipation, altered taste, belching
- back pain, arthralgia
- peripheral oedema
- atrial fibrillation or flutter
- bleeding (including epistaxis, haematuria, gastrointestinal bleeding, contusion)
- gout
- rash
- (Uncommon) hypersensitivity

Interactions
- increased risk of bleeding if given with antiplatelet agents, anticoagulants or aspirin

Nursing considerations/Cautions
- if patient has liver impairment, liver enzymes (ALT and AST) should be measured before starting therapy and regularly during treatment
- capsules contain sorbitol and maltitol and are not recommended in those with hereditary problems of fructose intolerance
- capsules contain soya lecithin and are not recommended in those with allergy to soya or peanuts
- caution if used those with a history of atrial fibrillation or atrial flutter

LIPID REGULATING AGENTS

- caution if used in those with hypersensitivity to fish or shellfish, as icosapent ethyl has been extracted from fish oil

Patient education

- advise the patient to swallow capsules whole with or after meal
- the patient should be instructed to seek medical advice if any of the following occur:
  - bruising easily or unable to stop bleeding, bloody nose, blood in urine
  - irregular heart beat or palpitations, dizziness, fainting, chest discomfort, shortness of breath

 Capsules should not be broken, crushed, chewed or dissolved.

 Avoid use unless clearly needed, as there are limited human data. Animal studies show no fetal harm at clinically relevant doses; therefore use only if potential benefits to the mother outweigh risks to the fetus.

 Excretion in human milk is unknown; however, the active metabolite (EPA) is found in milk and therefore a potential risk to the infant cannot be excluded. Discontinue breastfeeding or drug based on benefit–risk assessment.

INCLISIRAN
Trade name
Leqvio

Available form
Prefilled syringe: 284 mg/1.5 mL

Action
- cholesterol lowering double-stranded small interfering ribonucleic acid (RNA) conjugated to increase uptake into hepatocytes, leading to low-density lipoprotein cholesterol (LDL-C) receptor recycling, increasing LDL-C uptake and resulting in lower LDL-C levels in the blood
- half-life 9 hours

Use
- adjunct to diet and exercise to lower LDL-C in adults with heterozygous familial hypercholesterolaemia or atherosclerotic cardiovascular disease, or at high risk of cardiovascular event, with statin or statin and other lipid lowering agent in those who unable to reach LDL-C goal on maximum statin dose
- patient who are statin intolerant (monotherapy or in combination with other lipid lowering agents)

Dose
- 284 mg SC, repeated after 3 months, then 6-monthly

Adverse effects
- (Injection site) pain, redness, rash
- back pain, arthralgia, lower extremity pain
- diarrhoea
- bronchitis, nasopharyngitis
- urinary tract infection
- cough, dyspnoea
- headache, dizziness
- angina
- anti-drug antibody development

Nursing considerations/Cautions
- SC administration only (abdomen, thighs or upper arm), rotating sites and not injecting into areas that have active inflammation, infection, sunburn, rash, lesion or scarring
- if dose if missed by less than 3 months, administration should continue according to schedule. If dose is missed by more than 3 months, schedule should be restarted with initial dosing
- if switching from a proprotein convertase subtilisin/kexin type 9 (PCSK9) inhibitor (e.g. alirocumab, evolocumab) to inclisiran, administer a last dose of PCSK9 inhibitor and then, when the next dose is due, replace with inclisiran

 Animal studies have not shown fetal harm, but data in pregnant women are limited. Use only if the potential benefit justifies the potential risk.

Human data are lacking; therefore a risk to the breastfeeding infant cannot be excluded.

Caution if used in severe kidney impairment. Not recommended in those with end-stage kidney disease or severe liver impairment (Child-Pugh class C)

PROPROTEIN CONVERTASE SUBTILISIN/KEXIN TYPE 9 (PCSK9) INHIBITORS

General Actions of PCSK9 inhibitors
- monoclonal antibody (IgG$_2$) that has high affinity for proprotein convertase subtilisin/kexin type 9 (PCSK9)
- inhibits circulation PCSK9 from binding to low-density lipoprotein receptor (LDLR) on liver cell surface preventing PCSK9-mediated LDLR degradation, increasing liver levels of LDLR, resulting in an associated decrease in serum low-density lipoprotein cholesterol (LDL-C)
- maximum inhibition occurs 4–8 hours after administration, peak concentration 3–4 days

General Adverse effects of PCSK9 inhibitors
- (Injection site) redness, pain, bruising
- nasopharyngitis, influenza, upper respiratory tract infection, cough, sinusitis, bronchitis, flu-like illness
- back pain, arthralgia, myalgia, muscle spasms, pain in extremity
- headache, fatigue, dizziness, insomnia
- nausea, diarrhoea, constipation, gastroenteritis, upper abdominal pain
- hypertension, angina
- rash, urticaria, pruritus
- diabetes mellitus, gout
- antibody development
- (Rare) hypersensitivity (e.g. angioedema, urticaria, vasculitis)

General Interactions of PCSK9 inhibitors
- clearance may be increased by statins

General Nursing considerations/Cautions for PCSK9 inhibitors
- patient may be instructed to self-administer
- caution if used in those with severe liver impairment or severe/very severe kidney impairment
- contraindicated in those with hypersensitivity to hamster ovary protein or polysorbate

General Patient education for PCSK9 inhibitors
- advise patient to seek medical advice immediately if there are any skin reactions, including swelling, itching or hives
- instructions for SC administration should include the following:
  - SC injections are given under the skin
  - injection sites include upper arm, thigh and abdomen, and sites should be rotated
  - injections should not be given into skin that is tender, red, sunburnt, bruised, hard, broken or inflamed
  - prefilled pen/syringe should be allowed to come to room temperature for at least 30–40 minutes before administration; however, it should not be warmed in other ways
  - prefilled pen/syringe should not be shaken
  - no other injections should be given into the same site
  - if prefilled pen/syringe is removed from refrigerator, it should be used within 30 days

LIPID REGULATING AGENTS

- store in refrigerator but do not freeze
- used pen/syringe should be disposed of into puncture-resistant container

Avoid use. No human data.

No human data available, but it is unlikely to be absorbed by the nursing infant.

ALIROCUMAB
Trade name
Praluent

Available form
Prefilled syringe: 75 mg/mL, 150 mg/mL

Action
- see also General Actions for PCSK9 inhibitors (p. 1314)
- half-life 17—20 days (or 12 days if given with a statin)

Use
- primary hypercholesterolaemia (as adjunct to diet and exercise in adults with heterozygous familial or non-familial hypercholesterolaemia at moderate to very high cardiovascular risk)
- as monotherapy or in combination with statin or other lipid-lowering agents in patients with primary hypercholesterolaemia unable to reach LDL-C goals with maximum dose of statin, if intolerant to statin or statin is contraindicated
- reduce risk of cardiovascular events (e.g. myocardial infarction, stroke, unstable angina requiring hospitalisation) in those with established cardiovascular disease in combination with statin or other lipid-lowering agent

Dose
- initially 75 mg SC every 2 weeks, increasing to 150 mg SC every 2 weeks if further LDL-C reduction is required **OR**
- 300 mg SC monthly

Adverse effects
- oropharyngeal pain
- peripheral oedema
- musculoskeletal pain
- palpitations
- epistaxis
- haematuria
- increase in liver enzymes
- see also General Adverse effects of PCSK9 inhibitors (p. 1314)

Interactions
- see General Interactions of PCSK9 inhibitors (p. 1314)

Nursing considerations/Cautions
- patient can be taught to self-administer (see General Patient education for PCSK9 inhibitors p. 1314)
- see LDL-C levels should be measured before starting therapy, after 4—8 weeks and during dose titration
- see also General Nursing points/Cautions for PCSK9 inhibitors (p. 1314)

Patient education
- if dose is missed, advise patient to administer within 7 days of missed dose and then resume previous administration schedule
- if dosing schedule is every 2 weeks and dose is missed and not administered within 7 days, advise patient that administration should be delayed until next scheduled injection. If dosing schedule is monthly and dose is not administered within 7 days, advise patient to administer dose and then start a new schedule based on this date
- for 300 mg dose, instruct patient to administer two 150 mg injections into 2 different injection sites

Not recommended during pregnancy unless benefits outweigh risks to fetus.

Not recommended during breastfeeding.

EVOLOCUMAB

Trade name
Repatha

Available form
Prefilled pen: 140 mg/mL,

Action
- half-life 11–17 days
- see also General Actions for PCSK9 inhibitors (p. 1314)

Use
- primary hypercholesterolaemia (heterozygous familial or non-familial hypercholesterolaemia (HeFH) (adjunct to diet, exercise and/or statin and other lipid lowering therapies)
- homozygous familial hypercholesterolaemia (with other lipid lowering therapies)
- prevention of cardiovascular events in those with established cardiovascular disease with statin or other lipid lowering agents

Dose
- (Primary hypercholesterolaemia or prevention of cardiovascular disease) 140 mg SC every 2 weeks or 420 mg SC once monthly **OR**
- (Homozygous familial hypercholesterolemia) initially 420 mg SC monthly, increasing dose to 420 mg SC every 2 weeks if no response after 12 weeks

Adverse effects
- nausea, gastroenteritis
- see also General Adverse effects of PCSK9 inhibitors (p. 1314)

Interactions
- see General Interactions of PCSK9 inhibitors (p. 1314)

Nursing considerations/Cautions
- patient can be taught to self-administer (see General Patient education for PCSK9 inhibitors p. 1314)
- (Homozygous familial hypercholesterolaemia) if patient is having apheresis, dose can be started at 420 mg SC every 2 weeks to correspond with apheresis schedule
- see also General Nursing considerations/Cautions for PCSK9 inhibitors (p. 1314)

Patient education
- if 420 mg dose is required, dose should be given as 3 SC injections, which should be consecutively within 30 minutes
- see also also General Patient education for PCSK9 inhibitors (p. 1314)

 Avoid use. No human data.

 No human data available, but it is unlikely to be absorbed by the nursing child.

OTHER LIPID LOWERING AGENTS

EICOSAPENTAENOIC ACID ETHYL ESTER (EPA)/DOCOSAHEXAENOIC ACID ETHYL ESTER (DHA)

Trade name
Omacor

Available form
Capsules: 1 g

Action
- omega-3 fatty acids
- docosahexaenoic acid is an omega-3 fatty acid and a natural component of fish oil found in oily fish such as mackerel, salmon and tuna
- omega-3 fatty acids are thought to reduce formation of VLDL and accelerate metabolism of VLDL to LDL, thereby reducing triglyceride levels, but may also potentially increase LDL levels
- also thought to upregulate metabolism of fatty acids in the liver

LIPID REGULATING AGENTS

Use
- hypertriglyceridaemia (type IV and V as monotherapy; type IIb (with statin))

Dose
- (Hypertriglyceridaemia) 4 g orally daily with glass of water

Adverse effects
- GI disturbances: abdominal pain, dyspepsia, gastroesophageal reflux disease (GORD), belching, nausea, vomiting, abdominal distension, flatulence, diarrhoea, constipation, taste disturbance
- headache
- mildly elevated ALT
- (Uncommon) headache, dizziness, hypotension, angina, rash

Interactions
- increased bleeding time may occur if given with aspirin or warfarin; therefore INR should be monitored carefully, especially when starting or stopping therapy

Nursing considerations/Cautions

- lipids should be closely monitored during therapy, especially LDL in those with type IV or V dyslipidaemia
- caution if used in those with sensitivity or allergy to fish
- caution if used in those with liver impairment. Liver function should be monitored during therapy especially if daily dose > 4 g
- not recommended for exogenous hypertriglyceridaemia (type 1 hyperchylomicronaemia)
- contraindicated in those with hypersensitivity to soya, including soya milk, soya beans or peanuts

Patient education

- advise patient to swallow capsules whole with water; however, they can take the capsules with food if GI disturbances occur

Capsules should not be opened or crushed.

Avoid use. No human data.

Avoid use. No human data.

EZETIMIBE
Trade names
APO-Ezetimibe, ARX-Ezetimibe, BTC Ezetimibe, Ezemichol, Ezetimibe GH, Ezetimibe Sandoz, Ezetimibe-WGR, Ezetrol, Pharmacor Ezetimibe, Zient

Available form
Tablets: 10 mg

Action
- cholesterol absorption inhibitor
- inhibits absorption of cholesterol in the small intestine, decreasing the amount of intestinal cholesterol reaching the liver, resulting in reduced liver cholesterol stores and increasing clearance in the blood
- does not increase bile acid excretion (as with bile acid binding agents)
- does not inhibit liver cholesterol synthesis (as with statins)
- conjugated to active compound in liver
- does not inhibit absorption of fat-soluble vitamins or nutrients
- reduce LDL by about 18% with little impact on triglyceride or HDL levels
- half-life of both parent and conjugated compound is about 22 hours

Use
- (Adult) primary hypercholesterolaemia (alone or with statin)
- (Adult) homozygous familial hypercholesterolaemia (with statin)
- (Adolescent, 10—17 years) heterozygous familial hypercholesterolaemia (with simvastatin) (adjunctive therapy)

1317

HAVARD'S NURSING GUIDE TO DRUGS

- (Adolescent, 10—17 years) homozygous familial hypercholesterolaemia (with simvastatin) (adjunctive therapy)
- prevention of cardiovascular disease in patients with coronary heart disease and history of acute coronary syndrome (with statin)

Dose
- 10 mg orally daily (with or without statin)

Adverse effects
- elevated liver enzymes
- headache, fatigue
- abdominal pain, diarrhoea, flatulence and uncommonly, dyspepsia, gastrointestinal reflex disease, decreased appetite
- (Uncommon) cough, muscle spasm, neck pain
- (With statin) myalgia
- (With fenofibrate) abdominal pain

Interactions
- not recommended with fibrates (other than fenofibrate)
- caution if used with ciclosporin; therefore ciclosporin levels should be closely monitored during therapy
- decreased plasma level may occur if given within 4 hours of colestyramine
- contraindicated with fenofibrate in those with gallbladder disease
- increased risk of myopathy and/or rhabdomyolysis if given with statin
- if given with warfarin, INR should be closely monitored especially when starting and stopping therapy

Nursing considerations/Cautions
- any secondary causes of hypercholesterolaemia (e.g. poorly controlled diabetes mellitus, hypothyroidism, obstructive liver disease, alcoholism, nephrotic syndrome, dysproteinaemia, drug therapy) should be identified and treated before starting therapy, as well as weight reduction and diet modification
- liver function tests should be performed at start and regularly throughout therapy if given with a statin
- not recommended in those with impaired liver function
- not recommended in children under 10 years or in premenarchal girls or prepubertal boys
- contraindicated with fenofibrate in those with gallbladder disease
- contraindicated with statin in those with active liver disease or unexplained raised serum transaminases

Patient education
- report any muscle pain, cramps, tenderness or weakness (not caused by exercise), malaise or fever
- if the patient is taking a bile acid sequestrant like cholestyramine, they should take ezetimibe either 2 hours before or 4 hours after

 Tablet can be crushed and mixed with water or spoonful of yoghurt or apple puree.

 Avoid use, no clinical data.

 Avoid use. Ezetimibe appears in very low amounts in breastmilk and emerging data shows it is likely safe for breastfeeding. However, avoid using ezetimibe combined with a statin (e.g. atorvastatin, rosuvastatin) while breastfeeding.

Available in combination with:
- ezetimibe + atorvastatin tablets (see atorvastatin in this chapter p. 1303)
- ezetimibe + simvastatin tablets (see simvastatin in this chapter p. 1307)
- ezetimibe + rosuvastatin composite pack (see rosuvastatin in this chapter p. 1305)

NICOTINIC ACID
Trade name
Nicotinic Acid

Available form
Tablets: 250 mg

LIPID REGULATING AGENTS

Action
- also known as niacin
- inhibits synthesis of lipoproteins (very-low-density lipoprotein (VLDL)) in the liver, thereby decreasing low-density lipoprotein (LDL) and cholesterol. The cholesterol level decreases by 10—20%, while triglycerides decrease by 40—80%
- promotes lipoprotein lipase activity
- decreases mobilisation of free fatty acids from adipose tissue, increasing sterol in the faeces
- a vasodilator at therapeutic levels (not nutritional dose)
- an essential dietary element (water-soluble B complex vitamin (vitamin B_3, niacin); see Vitamins, minerals and electrolytes, p. 1638)
- elimination half-life 45 minutes

Use
- hypercholesterolaemia and hypertriglyceridaemia
- hyperlipoproteinaemia types II, IIB, III, IV and V (adjunctive therapy)
- pellagra (severe deficiency of niacin — vitamin B_3)

Dose
- (Lipid lowering/hypertriglyceridaemia) initially 250 mg orally 3 times daily after meals, increasing by 250 mg every fourth day to a daily maximum of 3—4.5 g **OR**
- (Pellagra) 250 mg orally twice daily after meals

Adverse effects
- vasodilation, flushing, headache, pounding head, heat sensation
- atrial fibrillation, cardiac arrhythmias (if coronary heart disease), hypotension
- dry skin, urticaria, rash, pruritus, hyperpigmentation (brown), hyperkeratosis
- nausea, vomiting, diarrhoea, flatulence, heartburn
- activation of peptic ulcer
- jaundice, impaired liver function, ascites, hepatomegaly
- decrease in glucose tolerance, hyperglycaemia
- hyperuricaemia
- hypothyroidism
- toxic amblyopia
- nervousness

Interactions
- vasodilation and hypotensive effects may be enhanced by antihypertensive drugs, including adrenergic blocking agents
- may require increased insulin or oral hypoglycaemic requirement in patients with diabetes
- caution if used with alcohol, as delirium and/or lactic acidosis may occur
- may have increased and prolonged effect if given with aspirin, increasing the risk of toxicity
- flushing and warm sensation may be reduced by aspirin or clonidine
- increased risk of myopathy, rhabdomyolysis and acute renal failure if given with statins
- increased flushing and dizziness may occur if used with transdermal nicotine
- may cause false positive result for blood bilirubin or urinary glucose (Benedict's agent) or falsely elevated urinary catecholamines

Nursing considerations/Cautions
- plasma cholesterol and triglyceride levels should be monitored regularly and dose adjusted accordingly
- liver function monitoring is recommended at 4—6-week intervals during the first 3 months of therapy or after any increase in dose, then 3-monthly for 1 year and annually thereafter
- glucose tolerance should be monitored regularly and the diet adjusted and/or oral hypoglycaemic dose also adjusted if needed
- serum uric acid levels should be monitored regularly during long-term therapy
- caution if used in those with history of peptic ulceration or gastrointestinal irritation

- contraindicated in patients with recent myocardial infarction and should be stopped immediately if the patient has a myocardial infarction during therapy
- contraindicated in those with liver dysfunction, peptic ulcers, diabetes mellitus, gout or hyperuricaemia, or in large doses in those with heart or gallbladder disease, glaucoma, arterial bleeding or a sudden fall in peripheral vascular resistance

Patient education

- take with or soon after food to reduce stomach upset.
- flushing and stomach upset usually subside in 2–6 weeks but can return if multiple doses are missed
- patient should be warned that vasodilation occurs approximately 20 minutes after administration and may persist for 20–60 minutes
- advise patient to seek medical advice immediately if there is fever, malaise, yellowing of skin and eyes, dark urine or abdominal pain
- counsel patient about use of alcohol, hot drinks and aspirin during therapy. Alcohol and hot drinks increase flushing and itching
- if patient is concurrently using nicotine replacement therapy (e.g. nicotine patches), they should be advised of the increased risk of flushing and/or dizziness, especially when driving or operating machinery
- patients with diabetes should be warned to monitor blood glucose levels closely, as insulin and/or oral hypoglycaemic dose may be altered
- women of childbearing potential should be counselled to use adequate contraception during therapy to avoid pregnancy

Tablet can be dispersed in water, or crushed and mixed with yoghurt or apple puree.

Contraindicated during pregnancy.

Contraindicated during breastfeeding

Reduced renal function: CrCl 10–30 mL/min: start with half the usual dose. CrCl <10 mL/min: Start with one-quarter of the usual dose. Reduce dose when CrCl is below 30 mL/min, as adverse reactions are more common in severe renal impairment.

LOCAL ANAESTHETICS

Local anaesthetics are a group of chemically related agents that produce a reversible loss of sensation (without a loss of consciousness), as well as producing a local analgesic action without loss of control. They are administered either topically (e.g. lotions, creams, lozenges, sprays) or parenterally, but not orally (Knights et al 2023).

General Actions of local anaesthetics
- amide type or ester type
- block or diminish nerve conduction reversibly by inhibiting depolarisation and ion (sodium) exchange (membrane stabiliser)
- do not produce loss of consciousness
- ester-like local anaesthetics are rapidly metabolised by plasma enzyme to p-aminobenzoic acid (PABA) metabolites, which may cause allergic reaction in some people
- amide-like local anaesthetics are not metabolised to PABA metabolites and are less likely to cause allergic reactions
- onset and duration of action is dependent on the agent's lipid solubility, volume and concentration, local blood flow and speed of injection, as well as the patient's liver, kidney and cardiovascular function. Short-acting local anaesthetics (e.g. benzocaine, cocaine) have a duration of 30–60 minutes, intermediate-acting local anaesthetics (e.g. prilocaine, lidocaine (lignocaine)) have a duration of 30 minutes to 4 hours, while long-acting local anaesthetics (e.g. bupivacaine, tetracaine (amethocaine)) have a duration of action 3–10 hours
- most local anaesthetics produce vasodilation, therefore the addition of vasoconstrictors (usually adrenaline (epinephrine) or felypressin) decreases blood flow in the area and prolongs the anaesthesia by reducing absorption
- half-life is generally short (1–2 hours)

Surface or topical anaesthesia
- blocks sensory nerve endings in the skin, mucous membranes and the eye

Infiltration anaesthesia
- solution is injected into and around site causing nerve endings (but not motor nerves) to become anaesthetised

Intravenous regional anaesthesia (Bier's block)
- specialised technique for anaesthesia of the upper limbs

Nerve block anaesthesia
- sensory nerve pathways are blocked by injecting into or around nerve trunks or ganglia supplying the affected area
- single nerves or nerve trunks emerging from spinal cord (paravertebral) may be blocked
- epidural and spinal blocks are specialised central nerve blocks. Analgesia can be enhanced if co-administered with an opioid
- dermatome assessment is used to monitor levels and extent of analgesia

Spinal anaesthesia
- regional anaesthesia blocking transmission in spinal nerves in contact with the anaesthetic agent
- agent is injected intrathecally after lumbar puncture procedure
- the somatic level of anaesthesia depends on the specific gravity of the anaesthetic solution and the position of the patient

General Uses of local anaesthetics
- procedures where patient's cooperation and consciousness are needed or wanted
- minor procedures where general anaesthetic is not warranted or hazardous
- sympathetic blockade
- postoperative analgesia

General Doses for local anaesthetics
- dose is dependent on site, vascularity of area, number of neuronal segments to be blocked, individual tolerance and technique, as well as other factors, including age, weight, and kidney and liver function

General Adverse effects of local anaesthetics
- hypotension, bradycardia
- headache, dizziness, drowsiness, nervousness
- tremor, twitching, shaking
- blurred or double vision
- tinnitus
- nausea, vomiting
- increased temperature, chills/rigors
- slurred speech, numbness of tongue
- (Uncommon) muscle rigidity and/or muscle twitching
- (Injection site) inflammation, haematoma, nerve injury, abscess formation, necrosis
- (Spinal or epidural anaesthesia) hypotension, headache, backache, paraesthesia, neuropathy, infection, autonomic dysfunction
- (Epidural or intrathecal blockade) hypotension, bradycardia
- (Epidural or spinal anaesthesia) epidural/spinal haematoma
- (Uncommon) convulsions, unconsciousness, severe hypotension, cardiovascular collapse, bradycardia and possible cardiac arrest
- (Rare, spinal anaesthetic) high or total blockade (resulting in respiratory or cardiovascular depression/arrest)
- (Rare, intrathecal) paraesthesia, anaesthesia, motor weakness, paralysis, loss of bladder control
- (Rare) allergic dermatitis, anaphylaxis (more common with ester-type local anaesthetics), bronchospasm

General Interactions of local anaesthetics
- amide-type local anaesthetics should be used with caution with antiarrhythmic agents, because the cardiac effect may be potentiated
- caution if used with other amide local anaesthetics or chemically related agents as adverse effects are additive
- not recommended with agents that prolong QT interval or cause dysrhythmias
- (Epidural/spinal) increased hypotension can occur if given with antihypertensive agents

LOCAL ANAESTHETICS

- (Spinal/epidural anaesthesia) increased risk of epidural/spinal haematoma if given to patients on anticoagulant therapy with low-molecular-weight heparins/heparinoids or if taking other agents that affect haemostasis (e.g. NSAIDs, antiplatelet agents, other anticoagulant agents)

General Nursing considerations/ Cautions for local anaesthetics

- before receiving local anaesthetic agent, patient should have any hypoxia, hypotension, fluid or acid—base imbalance corrected to decrease risk of toxic reactions
- monitor heart rate, respiratory rate, oxygen saturation, level of consciousness and BP of patients during and for at least 4 hours after spinal anaesthesia
- (Spinal/epidural anaesthesia) patients should be closely monitored for any neurological impairment
- test doses are sometimes given if large dose or epidural anaesthesia is to be administered
- nurse patient in a recumbent position
- have equipment (including oxygen) available for assisted ventilation and mucus extraction in the event of emergency resuscitation. Diazepam and/or thiopentone should be readily available for convulsions and/or vasopressors for bradycardia and hypotension
- local anaesthetics react with some metals and may cause local irritation if injected after being in contact with them; therefore the local anaesthetics should not have prolonged contact with metal bowls, cannulae or syringes with metal parts
- adrenaline (epinephrine) must not be used when producing a nerve block in an appendage such as the digits, ears, nose or penis, because these are supplied by end arteries and therefore subject to gangrene
- spinal cord may be damaged if spinal anaesthetic contains adrenaline (epinephrine)
- caution if used in the head and neck area as systemic adverse effects may occur and respiratory and cardiovascular function should be closely monitored
- all local anaesthetics should be used with caution in those with known drug allergy or sensitivity
- not recommended in those with porphyria unless no safer alternative is available
- caution if epidural anaesthetics are used in those with impaired cardiovascular function
- caution if local anaesthetics are used in those with predisposition to malignant hyperthermia or pre-existing neurological condition
- caution if used in those with renal or liver impairment, epilepsy, partial or complete heart block or conduction disorders, severe bradycardia, shock, hyperthyroidism or digoxin intoxication
- (Spinal/epidural) contraindicated in those with CNS or spinal disease, including meningitis, spinal fluid block, syphilis, poliomyelitis, TB or metastatic lesions of the spinal cord, uncorrected hypotension or cranial/spinal haemorrhage
- contraindicated in those with myasthenia gravis, Stokes—Adams syndrome or Wolff-Parkinson-White syndrome, impaired cardiac conduction, severe shock, known deficiency in plasma cholinesterase activity, serious disease or infection of CNS, or uncorrected hypotension

- contraindicated for extensive surgery requiring large doses that could be toxic
- contraindicated for IV regional anaesthesia (Bier's block) or obstetric paracervical block (due to increased risk of fetal bradycardia and acidosis)
- contraindicated if there is infection or inflammation at the site of the proposed injection or if the patient has septicaemia

General Patient education for local anaesthetics

- patient should be advised to avoid driving or operating machinery until any possible impaired coordination, dizziness, drowsiness or other adverse effects have resolved
- warn patient about temporary loss of sensation and muscle function after infiltration and nerve block injection and should not drive after procedure

Should be used during pregnancy (not obstetric use) only if benefits outweigh risks as local anaesthetics cross the placenta rapidly.

ARTICAINE HYDROCHLORIDE
Trade names
Articadent Dental with Adrenaline – injection (Articaine, Adrenaline (Epinephrine)), Septanest – injection (Articaine, Adrenaline (Epinephrine))

Action
- amide type, similar to prilocaine and lidocaine (lignocaine)
- onset of action 1–6 minutes, duration about 68 minutes, half-life about 1.8 hours
- adrenaline (epinephrine) added as vasoconstrictor to reduce bleeding and prolong tissue concentration
- see also General Actions of local anaesthetics (p. 1321)

Use
- local or regional anaesthesia, for simple and complex dental procedures

Adverse effects
- neuropathy: neuralgia, hypoaesthesia/numbness (oral and perioral), hyperesthesia, dysaesthesia
- gingivitis
- tachypnoea, followed by bradypnoea and apnoea
- decreased heart rate and blood pressure
- facial oedema
- see also General Adverse effects of local anaesthetics (p. 1322)

Interactions
- contraindicated with or within 2 weeks of monoamine oxidase inhibitors (MAOIs), with tricyclic antidepressants (TCAs) or phenothiazines because of the risk of prolonged hypotension or hypertension
- caution if used with sympathomimetic, agents or with agents whose therapeutic actions may be antagonised by adrenaline (epinephrine)
- interactions with adrenaline (epinephrine) include adrenergic blocking agents, antiarrhythmics, thyroid hormones, ergot-type oxytocic drugs, sympathomimetic vasopressors, phenothiazines and other neuroleptics
- toxicity of local anaesthetics is additive
- see also General Interactions of sympathomimetic agents (p. 1322)

Nursing considerations/Cautions

- contains sodium metasulfite; therefore contraindicated in those with hypersensitivity to sulfites
- contraindicated IV
- contraindicated in children under 4 years
- not recommended (because of adrenaline (epinephrine)) in those with diabetes or untreated thyrotoxicosis and use with caution in those with

LOCAL ANAESTHETICS

- hypertension, cardiac disease, cardiac conduction abnormalities or epilepsy
- contraindicated in those with hypersensitivity to amide-type local anaesthetics
- see also General Nursing considerations/Cautions for local anaesthetics (p. 1323)

Patient education

- see General Patient education for local anaesthetics (p. 1324)

In renal impairment the lowest dose leading to efficient anaesthesia should be used.

In those over 70 years of age the lowest dose leading to efficient anaesthesia should be used.

BUPIVACAINE HYDROCHLORIDE MONOHYDRATE (BUPIVACAINE HYDROCHLORIDE)

Trade names
Bupivacaine Spinal Heavy BNM, Marcain, Marcain Epidural, Marcain Spinal 0.5%, Marcain Spinal 0.5% Heavy, Pfizer (Australia) Bupivacaine Hydrochloride Injection BP

Available forms
Vial: 50 mg/20 mL, 100 mg;
Ampoules: 20 mg/4 mL;
Infusion bag: 125 mg/100 mL

Action

- long-acting amide with duration up to 12 hours (peripheral nerve block) and 2–5 hours (single epidural injection)
- four-fold potency and toxicity of lidocaine (lignocaine)
- onset of action 10–15 minutes (topical and/or infiltration), 15–30 minutes (nerve block)
- duration of action 3–4 hours (infiltration), 2–6 hours (minor nerve block), 7–14 hours (major nerve block), 3–4 hours (epidural)
- half-life 2–5.5 hours
- accumulation may occur with repeated doses

Use

- surgical anaesthesia (epidural block, infiltration, caudal and regional nerve block)
- analgesia (epidural)

Adverse effects/Interactions/Patient education

- see General Adverse effects/Interactions/Patient education for local anaesthetics (p. 1322)

Nursing considerations/Cautions

- contraindicated IV
- contraindicated in those with pernicious anaemia combined with subacute degeneration of the spinal cord
- contraindicated in those with hypersensitivity to amide-type local anaesthetics
- see also General Nursing considerations/Cautions for local anaesthetics (p. 1323)

Available in combination with

- may be combined with adrenaline (epinephrine) (Bupivadren, Bupivacaine with Adrenaline, Marcain with Adrenaline (epinephrine))

LEVOBUPIVACAINE HYDROCHLORIDE

Trade name
Chirocaine

Available forms
Ampoule: 25 mg/10 mL, 50 mg/10 mL, 75 mg/10 mL;
Infusion bags: 250 mg/200 mL

Action

- amide, which is equipotent to bupivacaine
- onset of action 10–15 minutes (infiltration), 15–30 minutes (nerve block)

- duration of action 3—4 hours (infiltration), 2—6 hours (minor nerve block), 7—14 hours (major nerve block), 3—4 hours (epidural)
- half-life 2—3 hours

Use
- surgical anaesthesia (epidural, intrathecal, peripheral nerve block, local infiltration, peribulbar block in ophthalmic surgery)
- pain management (epidural)

Adverse effects
- hypotension
- nausea and vomiting
- anaemia
- pruritus
- fetal distress, delayed delivery
- see also General Adverse effects of local anaesthetics (p. 1322)

Interactions
- increased serum levels and risk of toxicity may occur if given with rifampicin, phenytoin, phenobarbital (phenobarbitone), clarithromycin, erythromycin, ritonavir, omeprazole, azole antifungal agents or verapamil
- see also General Interactions of local anaesthetics (p. 1322)

Nursing considerations/Cautions
- (Epidural) test dose (3—5 mL) is recommended, followed by patient monitoring (HR, BP, verbal contact) 5 minutes after dose. If accidental IV administration has occurred, HR will increase immediately, or, if given intrathecally, the patient will show signs of spinal block
- not given as rapid IV bolus
- not recommended if fast onset of action is required
- (Epidural analgesia) not recommended for > 24 hours after test dose
- (7.5 mg/mL solution) contraindicated for obstetric use because of the increased risk of cardiotoxicity
- contraindicated in those with hypersensitivity to amide-type local anaesthetics

- see also General Nursing considerations/Cautions for local anaesthetics (p. 1323)

Patient education
- see General Patient education for local anaesthetics (p. 1324)

 Some local anaesthetic drugs are excreted in human milk.

 Should be used with caution in patients with severe hepatic disease.

LIDOCAINE (LIGNOCAINE)
Trade names
Lignocaine 2% Gel, Lidocaine-Baxter Solution for Injection, LMX4, Mucosoothe, Nervoderm, Seda Lotion, Stud 100 Desensitising Spray for Men, Versatis, Xogel Dental gel, Xylocard, Xylocaine preparations, Ziagel Dental gel

Available forms
Ampoules: 10 mg/mL, 20 mg/mL, 50 mg/5 mL;
Aerosol pump: 10 mg/actuation;
Dental gel: 50 mg/g;
Gel (sterile or preserved): 20 mg/g (2%);
Oral solution: 5 mg/mL (2.5%), 20 mg/mL (2%);
Topical ointment: 50 mg/g;
Transdermal patch: 50 mg/g (5%);
Cream: 40 mg/g (4%)

Action
- amide-type local anaesthetic with Class I antiarrhythmic action
- onset of action 1—5 minutes (infiltration or topical), 5—15 minutes (nerve block, other administration methods)
- duration of action (dependent on concentration and increases when used with a vasoconstrictor) 0.5—1 hour (topical), 1—2.5 hours (infiltration), 1—2 hours (minor nerve block), 3—4 hours (major nerve block), 1—3 hours (epidural)
- half-life 90—120 minutes (doubled in those with liver dysfunction)

LOCAL ANAESTHETICS

- active metabolites
- (Transdermal patch) hydrogel protects hypersensitive area with lidocaine (lignocaine) diffusing into skin, providing analgesia

Use
- local and regional anaesthesia by infiltration, regional anaesthesia, nerve block, epidural and caudal anaesthesia
- surface anaesthesia of mucous membranes (e.g. endoscopy, cystoscopy, urethral catheterisation, ear, nose and throat procedures)
- ventricular arrhythmias (see Antiarrhythmic agents, p. 79)
- erectile dysfunction (see Erectile dysfunction agents, p. 1116)
- relief of pain or discomfort of mucous membranes of mouth, pharynx and upper gastrointestinal tract (e.g. post-tonsillectomy, mouth ulcers, dental scaling procedures, fitting new dentures)
- (Transdermal patch) relief of neuropathic pain (postherpetic neuralgia)
- cutaneous anaesthesia (before venipuncture or IV catheter insertion) or temporary pain relief (e.g. associated with minor burns, non-blistered sunburn, insect bites, sore nipples)

Dose
- (Transdermal patch) apply patch to affected area once daily, leaving in situ for 12 hours (maximum of 3 patches) **OR**
- (Oral solution) 15 mL of undiluted solution either swished (mouth) or gargled (pharynx) for 30 seconds every 3 hours if needed (daily maximum 120 mL) (2% oral solution) **OR**
- (Cutaneous) 1—2.5 g cream applied to skin for 30 minutes before procedure **OR**
- (Cutaneous) apply thin layer to unbroken skin 3—4 times daily as needed **OR**
- (Dental ointment) apply thin layer to oral mucosa and wait 3—5 minutes before procedure **OR**
- (Topical — lotion) apply to affected area (mouth ulcer, sore gum) 2-hourly

Adverse effects
- (Transdermal patch) burning, redness, pain and pruritus at application site, headache, nausea, rash, nasopharyngitis
- (Cream) redness, itching, irritation, rash
- (Aerosol spray) sore throat, hoarseness, loss of voice
- (Dental ointment) numb tongue
- see also General Adverse effects of local anaesthetics (p. 1322)

Interactions
- metabolism of IV lidocaine (lignocaine) may be decreased by propranolol and metoprolol, increasing the risk of toxicity
- increased cardiac depressant effects may occur if given with phenytoin
- metabolism of lidocaine (lignocaine) may be increased by antiepileptic agents
- may prolong duration of suxamethonium
- caution if given with antiarrhythmic agents because of added cardiac effects
- decreased clearance and therefore increased serum levels if given IV when using amiodarone or cimetidine
- half-life may be prolonged if given in acute severe alcohol intoxication
- decreases minimum effective concentration of inhalation anaesthetics such as nitrous oxide
- caution if given with other amide local anaesthetics
- if given IM, may cause a rise in creatine kinase (CK) for 48 hours, which may interfere with myocardial infarction diagnosis
- may cause elevated creatinine levels when enzymatic estimation is used
- see also General Interactions of local anaesthetics (p. 1322)

Nursing considerations/Cautions
- excessive doses and/or short interval between doses can result in elevated serum levels and increase the risk of adverse effects

- avoid contact with eyes. Area should be washed well with copious amount of water if contact occurs
- (Cream) 1 g cream = 5 cm squeezed from a 5 g tube or 3.5 cm from a 30 g tube
- (Cream) cream may be covered with occlusive dressing if needed and left undisturbed for 30 minutes. Cream can then be removed using gauze and area prepared as per usual protocol for venipuncture or IV cannulation
- (Transdermal patch) no more than 3 patches should be used at one time and there should be a 12-hour drug-free interval between applications
- (Gel/oral solution) caution if applied topically to traumatised mucosa or if infection is present at the application site
- (Aerosol pump) prime pump spray before use
- prolonged use or application to a large body area is not advised
- (Oral solution) not recommended in infants and children for teething pain
- not recommended in those with porphyria
- (Mucosoothe oral gel) contraindicated in those with hypersensitivity to hydroxybenzoate
- see also General Nursing considerations/Cautions for local anaesthetics (p. 1323)

Patient education

- the patient should be warned not to exceed recommended dose or shorten intervals between doses
- see also General Patient education for local anaesthetics (p. 1324)

Oral solution/spray

- instruct the patient to shake the bottle well before use
- advise the patient to swish (if mouth is painful) or gargle (if pharynx is painful) 15 mL solution undiluted for 30 seconds. If the pharynx is involved, the solution may be swallowed after gargling
- the patient should be instructed not to eat or drink within 60 minutes of oral solutions because of the increased risk of biting and damaging numbed mucous membranes or burning if hot food or liquid is ingested

Cream

- instruct the patient that cream should not be applied to wounds, mucous membranes, irritated or broken skin or areas of atopic dermatitis

Ointment

- if used for sore nipples, the patient should be instructed to wash the area well before breastfeeding
- (Dental ointment) advise the patient not to exceed daily maximum (8.5—10 g) or single dose (2.5 g = 7.5 cm length of ointment)
- (Dental ointment) if inserting new dentures, the patient should be instructed to apply ointment to the denture surface that will make contact with gum and not to eat or drink for at least 1 hour afterwards

Transdermal patch

- ensure the patient understands that transdermal patches should be applied for 12 hours only when pain is greatest (e.g. if pain is worse at night, patch should be applied for night coverage)
- instruct the patient in the following:
  - separate protective liner and apply to hairless skin (trim hair with scissors if needed but do not shave area)
  - if skin folds, scars, inflamed or irritated areas should not be used. Herpetic lesions should be completely healed if the patch is applied in that area
  - do not apply to mucous membranes
  - avoid contact with eyes
  - the patch can be cut into smaller pieces (before removing the liner) to better fit painful area; however, no more than 3 patches in total can be used at one time

LOCAL ANAESTHETICS

- press the patch to the skin for about 10 seconds to ensure the patch adheres well
- wash hands thoroughly before and after applying the patch
- if possible, avoid bathing or showering with the patch in place and allow skin to cool down before applying the patch if bathing or showering first
- avoid the area with the patch making contact with external heat sources such as electric blanket or heating pads
- used patches should be disposed of appropriately as they still contain lidocaine (lignocaine)
- used and unused patches should be kept out of the reach of children at all times
- store patches in a cool place to avoid extremes of temperature and humidity but do not refrigerate or freeze

Available in combination with
- lidocaine HCl monohydrate 5 mg/spray (5%, 50 mg/mL), phenylephrine HCl 500 microgram/spray (0.5%, 5 mg/mL) (Co-Phenylcaine Forte)
- lidocaine (lignocaine) HCl 0.66%, aminacrine HCl 0.05% (Medijel)
- lidocaine (lignocaine), chlorhexidine acetate 0.1% (Hemocane Ointment)
- lidocaine 25 mg and prilocaine 25 mg (EMLA cream 5%)
- lidocaine (lignocaine) hydrochloride 20 mg/mL (2%), Adrenaline (epinephrine) 12.5 microgram/mL (Lignospan Special)
- lidocaine hydrochloride monohydrate 4% w/v and fluorescein sodium 0.25% w/v. (Minims Lidocaine and Fluorescein eye drops)
- also available in other preparations such as Difflam PlusAnaesthetics Sore Throat Lozenges and Spray, Juvederm preparations, Numit, Oraqix (periodontal gel), Paxyl sunburn relief spray, SM-33, SM-33 Adult formula, SOOV-IT, Strepsils Plus Anaesthetic lozenges, Virasolve

MEPIVACAINE HYDROCHLORIDE
Trade names
Scandonest 3%, ATO-Mepivacaine

Available form
Cartridge: 66 mg/2.2 mL

Action
- amide-type local anaesthetic with anaesthetic properties greater than procaine
- onset is more rapid than procaine and slightly more rapid than lidocaine (lignocaine)
- onset of action 5—10 minutes (infiltration), 5—15 minutes (nerve blockade)
- duration of action 1—2.5 hours (infiltration), 1—2 hours (minor nerve block)
- equipotent to lidocaine (lignocaine) but less toxic

Use
- infiltration or nerve block (dental procedures)

Adverse effects
- see General Adverse effects of local anaesthetics (p. 1322)

Interactions
- contraindicated with or within 2 weeks of monoamine oxidase inhibitors (MAOIs) or with tricyclic antidepressants (TCAs)
- lower dose required if given with sedatives or antianxiety agents
- increased risk of toxicity if given with beta adrenoreceptor blocking agents
- increased risk of seizures, bradycardia and long sinoatrial arrest if given with amiodarone
- additive cardiac depression may occur if given with phenytoin
- see also General Interactions of local anaesthetics (p. 1322)

Nursing considerations/Cautions

- contraindicated IV if given
- contraindicated in those with hypersensitivity to amide-type local anaesthetics
- contraindicated if there is a possibility that a general anaesthetic may be required to complete the procedure
- see also General Nursing considerations/Cautions for local anaesthetics (p. 1323)

Patient education

- see General Patient education for local anaesthetics (p. 1324)

Safe use during pregnancy has not been established; however, it has been used extensively for dental procedures during pregnancy, with no proven increase in frequency of malformations or of harmful effects to mother or fetus.

ATO-Mepivacaine 3% should be used with caution in patients with renal or hepatic disease.

Elderly patients should be given reduced doses commensurate with their age and physical condition.

Available in combination with
- contained in Scandonest 2% Special (with adrenaline (epinephrine))

PRILOCAINE HYDROCHLORIDE
Trade names
Citanest, Prilotekal

Available forms
Ampoules: 5 mg/mL (0.5%), 20 mg/mL (2%)

Action
- amide local anaesthetic with similar onset and potency as lidocaine (lignocaine), but less vasodilator activity and CNS toxicity
- active metabolite, which may be responsible for methaemoglobinaemia if prilocaine is given in large doses
- onset of action 5—10 minutes (infiltration), 5—15 minutes (nerve blockade)
- duration of action 1—2.5 hours (infiltration), 1—2 hours (minor nerve block), 3—4 hours (major nerve block), 1—3 hours (epidural)
- half-life about 2 hours

Use
- local or regional anaesthesia (infiltration, intravenous regional anaesthesia, nerve block, major plexus block, epidural and subarachnoid block)

Adverse effects
- (High dose) methaemoglobinaemia, cyanosis
- see also General Adverse effects of local anaesthetics (p. 1322)

Interactions
- risk of methaemoglobin formation may be increased if given with sulfonamides, antimalarial agents or some nitric compounds
- see also General Interactions of local anaesthetics (p. 1322)

Nursing considerations/Cautions

- skin testing for suspected hypersensitivity is of limited value
- the patient should be observed closely for any cyanosis of lips and/or nails (sign of methaemoglobinaemia; see Action)
- (Epidural) test dose (3—5 mL) is recommended (preferably with 15 micrograms adrenaline (epinephrine)), followed by patient monitoring (HR, BP, verbal contact) 5 minutes after dose. If accidental IV administration has occurred, HR will increase immediately or, if given intrathecally, patient will show signs of spinal block
- increased risk of methaemoglobinaemia if given in high doses to those with hypoxia (e.g. that due to severe anaemia, cardiac insufficiency)

LOCAL ANAESTHETICS

- caution if using pulse oximetry, as methaemoglobinaemia (even at low levels) may interfere with readings
- may precipitate in alkaline solutions
- not recommended as obstetric paracervical or pudendal block because of the risk of methaemoglobinaemia in neonate
- not recommended in infants < 6 months because of the increased risk of methaemoglobinaemia
- contraindicated in those with congenital or idiopathic methaemoglobinaemia or with hypoxaemia
- contraindicated in those with hypersensitivity to amide-type local anaesthetics
- see also General Nursing considerations/Cautions for local anaesthetics (p. 1323)

Data lacking in pregnancy — the drug should not be used in pregnant women, or those likely to become pregnant, unless the expected benefit outweighs any potential risk.

In impaired renal function, toxicity due to accumulation may develop with prolonged or repeated administration.

In impaired hepatic function, caution should be exercised with repeated doses.

A reduction in dosage may be necessary for elderly patients, especially those with compromised hepatic and/or cardiovascular function.

Available in combination with
- contained in 3% Citanest Dental with Octapressin (with felypressin)
- Lidocaine (lignocaine) 25 mg, prilocaine 25 mg (EMLA Patch)
- Lidocaine (lignocaine) 25 mg and prilocaine 25 mg (EMLA cream 5%.)
- Lidocaine (lignocaine) 25 mg/g, prilocaine 25 mg/g (Oraqix Periodontal gel)
- other preparations include Numit 5% and Oraqiz with lidocaine (lignocaine)

ROPIVACAINE HYDROCHLORIDE
Trade names
Naropin, Ropibam, Ropivacaine Kabi,, Ropivacaine ReadyfusOR, Ropivacaine Actavis, Ropivacaine-AFT

Available forms
Ampoules: 2 mg/mL, 5 mg/mL, 7.5 mg/mL, 10 mg/mL

Action
- amide with both anaesthetic and analgesic properties
- vasoconstriction at lower concentrations and vasodilation at higher concentrations
- duration and intensity is not improved by adrenaline (epinephrine)
- similar analgesic potency to bupivacaine, but less potent for motor block
- onset of action 10—15 minutes (infiltration), 15—30 minutes (nerve block)
- duration of action 3—4 hours (infiltration), 2—6 hours (minor nerve block), 7—14 hours (major nerve block), 3—4 hours (epidural)
- two-phase half-life (14 minutes, 4 hours) due to biphasic absorption

Use
- epidural block, minor nerve block and infiltration, major nerve block, intrathecal anaesthesia
- postoperative pain management

Adverse effects
- urinary retention, oliguria
- back pain, pain, chest pain
- dyspnoea
- (Rare) cardiac arrest/arrhythmia, spinal/epidural haematoma
- see also General Adverse effects of local anaesthetics (p. 1322)

Interactions
- clearance may be decreased if given with fluvoxamine and ciprofloxacin leading to increased serum level, duration and risk of toxicity; therefore not recommended together
- ECG monitoring is recommended if given with Class III antiarrhythmic agents such as amiodarone
- see also General Interactions of local anaesthetics (p. 1322)

Nursing considerations/Cautions
- (Epidural) test dose (3—5 mL) is recommended (preferably with 15 microgram/mL adrenaline (epinephrine)) followed by patient monitoring (HR, BP, verbal contact) 5 minutes after dose. If accidental IV administration has occurred, HR will increase immediately, or if given intrathecally, patient will show signs of spinal block
- skin testing is thought to be of limited value
- administered slowly (25—50 mg/minute)
- if given by two or more routes, total dose should be calculated to avoid toxicity
- precipitation may occur if added to alkaline solution
- increased risk of spinal/epidural haematoma if procedure is traumatic or repeated, or if an indwelling epidural catheter is used
- not recommended as a paracervical block during pregnancy
- caution if used in those with acute porphyria (if given at all) or severe liver impairment
- contraindicated IV
- contraindicated in those with hypersensitivity to amide-type local anaesthetics
- see also General Nursing considerations/Cautions for local anaesthetics (p. 1323)

Patient education
- see General Patient education for local anaesthetics (p. 1324)

 Should be used during pregnancy only if the potential benefit justifies the potential risk to the fetus.

 Elderly, young or debilitated patients, including those with partial or complete heart conduction block, advanced liver disease or severe renal dysfunction, should be given reduced doses commensurate with their age and physical condition.

LOCAL ANAESTHETIC EYE DROPS

General Actions of local anaesthetic eye drops
- reversibly blocks propagation and conduction of nerve impulses, stabilising membrane and preventing generation of action potential

General Adverse effects of local anaesthetic eye drops
- transient stinging or burning sensation, tearing, blurred vision
- conjunctival redness
- corneal damage (prolonged administration)
- allergic conjunctivitis
- (Uncommon) severe keratitis
- (Rare) hypersensitivity, allergic reactions

General Interactions of local anaesthetic eye drops
- ester-type local anaesthetics may be blocked by anticholinesterases, prolonging activity
- ester-type local anaesthetics may enhance neuromuscular blockade of suxamethonium chloride

General Nursing considerations/Cautions for local anaesthetic eye drops
- local anaesthetics should never be put into an eye without a doctor's prescription, because healing is impaired and secondary bacterial infection is possible
- should be administered only by a clinician

LOCAL ANAESTHETICS

- systemic absorption can be reduced by compressing the lacrimal sac at the medial canthus for 60 seconds during and after instillation
- if more than one ophthalmic agent is to be used, a 5-minute interval should be allowed between instillations, with eye ointment applied last
- prolonged use will slow wound healing, prevent reflex ocular protection and mask progression of keratopathy
- any remaining solution should be discarded (single patient use only) to prevent transmission of infection
- for topical ophthalmic application only and should not be injected
- caution if used in the elderly or children
- not recommended after corneal staining
- repeated instillation is contraindicated because of the risk of corneal damage
- caution if used in those with known allergies, epilepsy, cardiac disease, hyperthyroidism, myasthenia gravis or respiratory disease
- contraindicated in those with known allergy or hypersensitivity to ester-type local anaesthetics or in premature babies
- topical anaesthetics mask the protective mechanism of pain
- use for short procedures only (< 20 minutes)
- increase corneal permeability and intraocular bioavailability of other topical drugs

General Patient education for local anaesthetic eye drops

- warn the patient that burning/stinging may occur for up to 30 seconds after instillation
- instruct the patient that the eye should be protected from dust and bacterial contamination while anaesthetised (e.g. eye may be covered with a patch until the blink reflex returns)
- warn the patient not to drive or operate machinery until normal sensation returns to the eye(s)
- the patient should be advised not to touch or rub eye(s) until the anaesthetic effect has worn off

OXYBUPROCAINE HYDROCHLORIDE

Trade name
Minims Oxybuprocaine

Available form
Eye drops: 4 mg/mL (0.4%)

Action
- ester-type local anaesthetic
- onset of action 1 minute, peak response 1–15 minutes, duration 20–30 minutes, full sensation returns in 40 or more minutes
- see also General Actions of local anaesthetic eye drops (p. 1332)

Use
- anaesthesia for short ophthalmological procedures

Dose
- (Tonometry) 1 drop to affected eye(s) 1 minute before procedure **OR**
- (Fitting contact lens) 1 drop, followed 90 seconds later by 1 drop **OR**
- (Removal of foreign body, minor surgery) 3–6 drops to affected eye(s) **OR**
- (Pterygium surgery) 1 drop per minute to affected eye(s) for 10 minutes **OR**
- (Deeper anaesthesia) 1 drop at intervals of greater than 90 seconds

Adverse effects
- (Rare) nausea, vomiting, dysphagia
- see also General Adverse effects of local anaesthetic eye drops (p. 1332)

Interactions
- see General Interactions of local anaesthetic eye drops (p. 1332)

Nursing considerations/Cautions
- contraindicated if eye infection is present

- see also General Nursing considerations/Cautions for local anaesthetic eye drops (p. 1332)

Patient education
- see General Patient education for local anaesthetic eye drops (p. 1333)

To be used during pregnancy only if benefits outweigh risks.

To be used during breastfeeding only if benefits outweigh risks.

PROXYMETACAINE HYDROCHLORIDE
Trade name
Alcaine Eye Drops 0.5%

Available form
Eye drops: 5 mg/mL (0.5%)

Action
- ester-type local anaesthetic
- onset of action within 30 seconds, duration of action 15 minutes or more
- see also General Actions of local anaesthetic eye drops (p. 1332)

Use
- short ophthalmic procedures requiring short anaesthesia (e.g. minor surgery, tonometry, removal of foreign body, conjunctival scraping for diagnostic procedures)

Dose
- (Tonometry) 1–2 drops just before evaluation **OR**
- (Minor surgical procedure (e.g. foreign body or suture removal)) 1–2 drops every 5–10 minutes for 1–3 doses **OR**
- (Prolonged anaesthesia (e.g. cataract extraction)) 1–2 drops every 5–10 minutes for 3–5 doses

Adverse effects
- see General Adverse effects of local anaesthetic eye drops (p. 1332)

Interactions
- see General Interactions of local anaesthetic eye drops (p. 1332)

Nursing considerations/Cautions
- avoid contact with skin, as contact dermatitis may occur
- contains preservative benzalkonium chloride, which may cause eye irritation as well as discolouring and depositing on soft contact lenses
- see also General Nursing considerations/Cautions for local anaesthetic eye drops (p. 1332)

Patient education
- advise the patient to avoid wearing contact lenses until local anaesthesia has worn off
- see also General Patient education for local anaesthetic eye drops (p. 1333)

To be used during pregnancy only if clearly needed.

TETRACAINE (AMETHOCAINE) HYDROCHLORIDE
Trade name
Minims Amethocaine Eye Drops

Available forms
Eye drops: 5 mg/mL (0.5%), 10 mg/mL (1%)

Action
- ester-type local anaesthetic
- onset of action 10–20 seconds, duration 10–20 minutes, but 1% solution can have a duration up to 1 hour
- see also General Actions of local anaesthetic eye drops (p. 1332)

LOCAL ANAESTHETICS

Dose
- 1 drop to affected eye(s), may be repeated as necessary

Adverse effects
- see General Adverse effects of local anaesthetic eye drops (p. 1332)

Interactions
- contraindicated with sulfonamides
- see also General Interactions of local anaesthetic eye drops (p. 1332)

Nursing considerations/Cautions
- see General Nursing considerations/Cautions for local anaesthetic eye drops (p. 1332)

Patient education
- see General Patient education for local anaesthetic eye drops (p. 1333)

Safety for use in pregnancy has not been established; therefore should be used only when considered essential.

It is not known whether tetracaine and/or its metabolites are excreted in breastmilk; therefore should be used only when considered essential.

Should be used with caution in the elderly, as this group is more susceptible to the effects of local anaesthetics.

1335

METABOLIC DISORDERS AGENTS

Inborn errors of metabolism (IEMs) are disorders in which a single gene defect causes a significant block in the metabolic pathway, generally with an accumulation of macromolecules in tissues and cells, with associated morbidity and mortality. In the past, these were considered rare, but with better detection (such as genetic sequencing) these disorders are increasing in incidence. In Australia, the combined incidence of IEMs is estimated to be between 1 in 1500 and 1 in 4000 live births. This range reflects the variability in detection rates and the inclusion of different disorders in newborn screening programs (Goel et al 2010).

Many causes, including disorders of amino acid, purine and carbohydrate metabolism and lysosomal storage diseases, can cause these inborn errors of metabolism disorders. For example, about 50 different lysosomal storage diseases have been identified, including Tay—Sachs disease, Fabry disease, Gaucher disease and Niemann—Pick disease (Hopkins & Grabowski 2019).

Treatments include enzyme replacement therapy, dietary restrictions of precursor, enzyme inhibition of precursor or removal of accumulated substrate using either pharmacological agents or dialysis (Thomas et al 2020).

AGALSIDASE ALPHA
Trade name
Replagal

Available form
Vial: 3.5 mg/3.5 mL

Action
- alpha galactosidase A enzyme that hydrolyses glycosphingolipids (e.g. globotriaosylceramide (GL-3, also called Gb3)) to ceramide and galactose
- in Fabry disease, there is a deficiency in alpha-galactosidase which leads to an accumulation of glycosphingolipids (especially GL-3 (Gb3)) in tissues and fluids, ultimately resulting in narrowing and thrombosis of arteries and arterioles, peripheral neuritis, renal failure, myocardial and cerebral infarction
- enzyme replacement produced by recombinant DNA technology

Use
- long-term enzyme replacement therapy in those with alpha galactosidase A deficiency (Fabry disease)

Dose
- 0.2 mg/kg by IV infusion over 40 minutes every 2 weeks

METABOLIC DISORDERS AGENTS

Adverse effects
- infusion-related reaction (commonly, rigors/chills, headache, nausea, fever, flushing, fatigue and uncommonly (more serious) fever, rigors, tachycardia, urticaria, nausea, vomiting, angioedema, throat tightness, stridor, swollen tongue)
- peripheral oedema, tachycardia, palpitation, hypertension
- flushing, acne, erythema, pruritus, rash
- cough, throat tightness, hoarseness, dyspnoea, rhinorrhoea, pharyngitis, nasopharyngitis, flu-like symptoms
- headache, dizziness, tremor, fatigue, malaise, asthenia
- paraesthesia, hypoaesthesia
- increased lacrimation
- tinnitus, aggravation of pre-existing tinnitus
- neuropathic pain
- myalgia, back and limb pain, arthralgia, joint swelling
- taste alteration, nausea, vomiting, diarrhoea, abdominal pain/discomfort
- antibody development
- (Rare) hypersensitivity, anaphylaxis

Interactions
- not recommended with amiodarone or gentamicin

Nursing considerations/Cautions
- infusion-related reactions usually occur in first 2—4 months of therapy
- the infusion can be interrupted for 5—10 minutes until infusion-related reaction subsides and then restarted
- if infused-related reaction occurs, pretreatment with antihistamine and/or corticosteroid 1—24 hours before next infusion is recommended
- administer alone
- standard 0.2 micron filter is recommended
- dilute with 100 mL sodium chloride 0.9% before IV administration
- do not shake solution, as protein will be denatured
- not recommended in children under 6.5 years

Patient education
- warn the patient/carer that infusion-related reactions commonly occur within first 2—4 months of therapy
- advise the patient to avoid driving or operating machinery if dizziness occurs

Limited human data. Animal studies have not shown harm to the fetus. Use only if clearly needed during pregnancy.

Caution, as excretion in human milk unknown. Due to potential risks, caution is advised.

AGALSIDASE BETA (RCH)
Trade name
Fabrazyme

Available forms
Vial: 5 mg, 35 mg

Action
- alpha galactosidase A enzyme that hydrolyses glycosphingolipids (e.g. globotriaosylceramide (GL-3) also called Gb3) to ceramide and galactose
- in Fabry disease, there is a deficiency in alpha galactosidase which leads to an accumulation of glycosphingolipids (especially GL-3 (Gb3)) in tissues and fluids, ultimately resulting in narrowing and thrombosis of arteries and arterioles, peripheral neuritis, renal failure, and myocardial and cerebral infarction
- enzyme replacement produced by recombinant DNA technology

Use
- long-term enzyme replacement therapy in those with alpha galactosidase deficiency (Fabry disease)

Dose
- 1 mg/kg by IV infusion every 2 weeks

Adverse effects
- infusion-related reaction (pallor, tachycardia, chest discomfort/pain, chills, fever, feeling hot or cold, headache, dizziness, somnolence, pruritus, urticaria)
- injection site reaction

- nausea, vomiting, abdominal pain
- palpitations, tachycardia, peripheral oedema, hypertension
- flushing
- oral or facial oedema
- asthenia, malaise, paraesthesia, lethargy, fatigue
- dyspnoea, nasal stuffiness, throat tightness, cough, wheezing
- rash, erythema, pruritus, urticaria
- pain in extremities, myalgia, back pain or spasm, arthralgia, muscle tightness, musculoskeletal stiffness
- increased lacrimation
- development of anti-drug antibodies

Interactions
- not recommended with amiodarone or gentamicin

Nursing considerations/Cautions

- resuscitation equipment should be readily available in the event of infusion-related reaction or anaphylaxis
- initial infusion rate should be no greater than 15 mg/hour to decrease the risk of infusion-related reactions. If the rate is tolerated and no reactions occur, it may be gradually increased over subsequent infusions
- pretreatment with antipyretics (e.g. paracetamol, ibuprofen) and/or antihistamines (e.g. diphenhydramine) is recommended 60 minutes before infusion in those who have experienced a single mild-to-moderate infusion-related reaction. The infusion rate should be 10 mg/hour
- if the patient has experienced previous infusion-related reaction (a single severe event or recurrent moderate-to-severe events), corticosteroids are recommended 13 hours, 7 hours and 1 hour before infusion (in addition to pretreatment as described in the previous point)
- slowing the IV rate or temporarily stopping the infusion will improve infusion-related reactions
- reconstitute the vial(s) using water for injections for a final concentration of 5 mg/mL (see manufacturer's recommendations), then further dilute using sodium chloride 0.9% and administer by IV infusion
- administer alone
- an inline low protein binding 0.2 micron filter can be used
- IgG antibody testing is recommended before starting therapy, 3-monthly for 18 months, then 6-monthly
- caution if given to a patient who has experienced infusion-related reaction or in those with liver impairment
- not recommended in children under 8 years

Patient education

- warn the patient to avoid driving or operating machinery if dizziness or somnolence occurs

 Caution if used during pregnancy.

 Not recommended during breastfeeding.

ALGLUCOSIDASE ALFA (RHU)
Trade name
Myozyme

Available form
Vial: 50 mg

Action
- lysosomal enzyme replacement for Pompe disease
- Pompe disease is a glycogen storage disease (type II) caused by deficiency of lysosomal acid alpha glucosidase, which breaks down lysosomal glycogen resulting in an accumulation of glycogen in various tissues, including cardiac and skeletal muscle

METABOLIC DISORDERS AGENTS

Use
- long-term treatment of patients with Pompe disease (acid alpha glucosidase deficiency)

Dose
- 20 mg/kg by IV infusion every 2 weeks

Adverse effects
- infusion-related reaction (hypo/hypertension cyanosis, tachycardia, bradycardia, pallor, flushing, peripheral coldness, tachypnoea, wheezing, throat tightness, hypoxia, dyspnoea, cough, respiratory tract irritation, decreased oxygen saturation, angioedema, urticaria, rash, erythema, periorbital oedema, pruritus, sweating)
- fever
- rhinorrhoea, respiratory distress/failure, rhinitis, cough, tachypnoea
- tachycardia, bradycardia
- pneumonia, otitis media, upper respiratory tract infection, ear infection, pharyngitis, gastroenteritis, oral candidiasis, bronchiolitis, nasopharyngitis
- rash, urticaria
- diarrhoea, vomiting, constipation, upper abdominal pain, gastro-oesophageal reflux disease
- anaemia
- antibody development
- (Rare) hypersensitivity, anaphylaxis, severe cutaneous reaction, nephrotic syndrome

Nursing considerations/Cautions
- resuscitation equipment should be readily available in the event of infusion-related reaction or anaphylaxis
- antibody levels (IgG) should be measured 3-monthly during therapy
- initial infusion rate should not exceed 1 mg/kg/hour, which may then be increased by 2 mg/kg/hour every 30 minutes if the patient tolerates it and no infusion-related reactions occur. A maximum rate of 7 mg/kg/hour should not be exceeded
- the infusion rate should be slowed or stopped if infusion reactions occur
- if the patient has experienced an infusion-related reaction, decreasing the rate and/or pretreatment with antihistamines and/or corticosteroids is recommended for next infusion
- do not shake the reconstituted or diluted solution, as protein will be denatured
- vial(s) should be allowed to reach room temperature for 30 minutes before reconstitution. Reconstitute using 10.3 mL water for injections, slowly injecting it down the inside wall of the vial to prevent foaming, giving a concentration of 5 mg/mL. Reconstituted solution may contain thin white strands or translucent fibres, which are removed by the inline filter without losing any strength or affecting the purity of the solution
- reconstituted solution should be protected from light
- airspace should be removed from the infusion bag to minimise particle formation, as the solution is sensitive to air—liquid interface, then dilute the reconstituted solution in sodium chloride 0.9% to give a final concentration of 0.5–4 mg/mL taking care to avoid foaming in the infusion bag. Invert gently to mix thoroughly
- a standard inline 0.2 micron filter is recommended
- administer alone
- the infusion solution should be protected from light during administration
- there is an increased risk of hypersensitivity reactions in those with infantile or late-onset Pompe disease; therefore it should be given with great caution

Patient education

- warn the patient/carer that recurrent reaction including flu-like symptoms or combination of chills, fever, muscle or bone pain and fatigue may occur after the infusion has finished and last for a few days in some patients
- advise the patient/carer to immediately seek medical advice if any skin reactions occur

Limited data from post-marketing reports indicate no association with miscarriage or adverse fetal outcomes. Untreated Pompe disease may worsen in pregnancy.

Caution, as excreted in breastmilk. Consider interrupting breastfeeding during infusion and for 24 hours afterward to minimise infant exposure.

ALPHA-1-PROTEINASE INHIBITOR

Trade name
Prolastin C Solution for Infusion

Available form
Vial (solution): 1 g/20 mL

Action

- increases serum alpha1 proteinase inhibitor levels in those with congenital alpha1 antitrypsin deficiency and with clinically significant emphysema (FEV$_1$ < 80%)
- congenital alpha1 antitrypsin deficiency is a hereditary disorder characterised by low serum and lung levels of alpha1-P1 proteinase inhibitor. Those with levels < 11 micrometres are at increased risk of developing emphysema, with levels of 9–23 micrometres considered to be at moderate risk
- smoking increases the risk of developing emphysema in those with the deficiency

Use
- congenital alpha1 antitrypsin deficiency

Dose
- 60 mg/kg IV weekly at a rate of 0.08 mL/kg/min

Adverse effects
- rash, pruritus, urticaria
- diarrhoea, nausea
- fatigue, headache, dizziness
- fever, chills, flu-like illness
- nasopharyngitis, exacerbation of chronic obstructive pulmonary disease (COPD), dyspnoea
- arthralgia
- urinary tract infection
- tachycardia
- hypersensitivity reaction

Nursing considerations/Cautions

- treatment should be started and monitored by respiratory doctor in conjunction with other appropriate therapies
- for therapy to commence, patient must be diagnosed with alpha1 antitrypsin deficiency based on genotype, clinical symptoms of emphysema and alpha1 antitrypsin level < 11 micrometres
- for IV administration alone
- should be administered alone, within 3 hours of preparation
- recommended dose of 60 mg/kg should take about 15 minutes to administer
- (Solution) the vial should be allowed to come to room temperature and carefully inspected. It should contain few protein particles and be clear to slightly opalescent, colourless or pale yellow/green/brown and not discoloured or cloudy
- may contain trace amounts of IgA, which will increase risk of hypersensitivity reaction in those with selective or severe IgA deficiency
- derived from pooled human plasma collected from donors and carries the

METABOLIC DISORDERS AGENTS

- risk of transmissible infectious agents. Risk versus benefit should be discussed with patient before prescription or administration of solution
- contraindicated in those with IgA deficiency and antibodies against IgA, or those with history of anaphylaxis or other systemic reactions to alpha1 proteinase inhibitor

Patient education
- the patient should be counselled to avoid smoking with this condition to decrease the risk of developing emphysema

 Should be given during pregnancy only if benefits outweigh risks.

 Caution if used during breastfeeding.

ASFOTASE ALFA
Trade name
Strensiq

Available forms
Vial: 18 mg/0.45 mL, 28 mg/0.7 mL, 40 mg/mL, 80 mg/0.8 mL

Action
- recombinant human tissue non-specific alkaline phosphatase (ALP)
- produced by recombinant DNA technology using mammalian Chinese hamster ovary cell culture
- promotes skeletal mineralisation in patients with hypophosphatasia
- hypophosphatasia is a rare, serious and potentially fatal genetic disorder caused by loss of function mutation in the gene encoding tissue non-specific alkaline phosphatase (TNSALP). Deficiency in TNSALP enzymatic activity leads to increased concentrations of TNSALP substrates, including inorganic pyrophosphate (PPi). Elevated extracellular PPi levels block hydroxyapatite crystal growth inhibiting bone mineralisation and causing accumulation of unmineralised bone matrix (rickets and bone deformations in children) and osteomalacia (bone softening) when growth plates have closed, along with muscle weakness
- half-life 1.06—3.62 days

Use
- enzyme replacement in paediatric-onset hypophosphatasia

Dose
- 2 mg/kg 3 times per week or 1 mg/kg 6 times per week SC

Adverse effects
- craniosynostosis, increased intracranial pressure
- ectopic calcifications (conjunctival and corneal calcification, nephrocalcinosis)
- weight gain
- headache
- tooth loss, dental caries
- vomiting, diarrhoea, constipation, gastro-oesophageal reflux disease
- respiratory tract infection, nasopharyngitis, pneumonia, otitis media, rhinitis, influenza
- cough, oropharyngeal pain
- conjunctivitis
- anaemia
- pain in extremity, arthralgia, back pain
- injection site reaction (redness, rash, pruritus, pain, papule, nodule, atrophy, cellulitis)
- localised lipodystrophy including lipoatrophy and lipohypertrophy
- development of antidrug antibodies
- hypersensitivity

Interaction
- may interfere with routine measurement of serum alkaline phosphatase

Nursing considerations/Cautions

- regular monitoring for increased intracranial pressure (including fundoscopy for signs of papilloedema) is recommended for patients < 5 years
- before starting therapy, ophthalmology examination and renal ultrasound are recommended, then regularly throughout treatment
- serum parathyroid hormone and calcium levels should be monitored regularly, and calcium and vitamin D supplements given if needed
- dietary advice is recommended to avoid disproportionate weight gain
- not given IM or IV
- maximum 1 mL per SC injection site
- SC sites should be rotated and monitored regularly for any signs of potential reactions
- response should be regularly reviewed especially when progressing to adolescence or adulthood
- the patient can be taught to self-administer after supervision
- caution if readministered to a patient who has previously experienced hypersensitivity reaction. If administered, it should be under medical supervision with emergency equipment readily available
- contraindicated in those with hypersensitivity to Chinese hamster ovary protein

Patient education

- the patient should be advised to seek medical attention immediately if any hypersensitivity reaction occurs, including difficulty breathing, choking sensation, swelling around eyes and dizziness, which can occur within minutes of administration
- ensure the patient has been instructed in SC administration, including:
  - the injection technique
  - the importance of rotating injection sites including abdomen, thigh, buttock and upper arm
  - correct disposal of sharps, including not reusing needles
  - correct storage (refrigerated but removed an hour before administration)
- female patients of childbearing potential should be counselled to use reliable contraception during therapy and if pregnancy occurs, doctor should be informed immediately

 Not recommended during pregnancy or in women of childbearing potential not using contraception.

 Caution, as excretion in human breastmilk is unknown.

BETAINE
Trade name
Cystadane

Available form
Dissolvable powder: 1 g/g

Action
- antihomocysteine agent (elevated homocysteine blood levels may cause cardiovascular thrombosis, osteoporosis, skeletal abnormalities and optic lens dislocation)
- reduces homocysteine levels by 20–30% of pretreatment levels
- betaine occurs naturally in the body and some foods, such as seafood, spinach, beets and cereals

Use
- adjunct in management of homocystinuria
- decrease raised homocysteine levels in patients with cystathionine beta synthase (CBS) deficiency type of homocystinuria
- increase methionine and S-adenosylmethionine levels in patients with methylenetetrahydrofolate reductase (MTHFR) deficiency and cobalamin co-factor metabolism type of homocysteine

METABOLIC DISORDERS AGENTS

Dose
- initially 3 g orally twice daily, increasing gradually until plasma homocysteine is undetectable (maximum 20 g daily)

Adverse effects
- nausea, diarrhoea, gastrointestinal distress
- (CBS deficiency) cerebral oedema

Nursing considerations/Cautions
- plasma homocysteine levels should be monitored throughout therapy
- response is usually seen within a week of starting therapy
- can be given with folate, vitamin B_6 and vitamin B_{12}
- (CBS deficiency) plasma methionine levels should be monitored during therapy and kept below 1000 micromol/L. Dietary modification and reduced betaine dose may be required

Patient education
- instruct the patient to use provided scoop (1 g) to measure the required amount and dissolve in 120—180 mL water, then drink immediately

Should be used during pregnancy only if clearly necessary, and the benefits outweigh the potential risks.

Avoid, as excretion in human breastmilk is unknown, though its metabolic precursor, choline, is present in high levels in human milk.

CARGLUMIC ACID
Trade name
Carbaglu

Available form
Tablets (for oral solution): 200 mg

Action
- *N*-acetylglutamate (NAG) analogue
- NAG is a naturally occurring activator of carbamoyl phosphate synthetase 1 (CPS1) (first enzyme in urea cycle); therefore, if deficiency occurs, the urea cycle is not triggered resulting in elevated levels of ammonia
- half-life up to 28 hours

Use
- treatment of hyperammonaemia due to NAG synthase primary deficiency or organic acidaemias (e.g. due to isovaleric acidaemia, methylmalonic acidaemia or propionic acidaemia)

Dose
- (Acute hyperammonaemia) initially 100—250 mg/kg orally or via nasogastric tube daily in 2—4 divided doses (rounded to closest 100 mg), titrating to plasma ammonia levels and clinical symptoms

Adverse effects
- anaemia
- ear infection, infection, influenza, pneumonia, nasopharyngitis, tonsillitis
- abdominal pain, diarrhoea, vomiting, taste perversion, decreased weight, anorexia
- asthenia, headache, somnolence
- rash
- fever, sweating
- cardiac murmur, decreased oxygen saturation
- hyperglycaemia

Nursing considerations/Cautions
- therapy can be started as early as the first day of life, as acute symptomatic hyperammonaemia can be life threatening
- regular neurological and cardiac status assessment, laboratory tests (kidney, liver and blood) and clinical response to treatment should be monitored regularly during therapy to maintain plasma levels of ammonia and amino acids within normal levels

- individual responsiveness should be tested before starting long-term therapy (e.g. in a comatose child, 100—250 mg/kg daily is given and ammonia plasma levels measured before each administration. Should normalise within a few hours of starting therapy)
- protein restriction during acute phase and protein supplementation during maintenance phase may be required and, if needed, dietetic advice is recommended
- if administration is via a nasogastric tube, a 200 mg tablet should be dissolved in 5—10 mL water and then administered via the nasogastric tube, followed by water to flush the tube

Patient education

- advise the patient/parent/carer that tablets should not be swallowed whole or crushed. Each 200 mg tablet should be dissolved in 5—10 mL water and given before meals or feed. If undissolved particles remain, the container should be rinsed with 5—10 mL water and swallowed immediately (tablets do not completely dissolve)
- warn the patient/parent/carer that suspension has a slightly acidic taste

Tablets should not be crushed or swallowed whole. Tablets should be dispersed in water immediately before use. Ensure complete delivery by rinsing the mixing the container with additional water to take any remaining particles.

Carglumic acid should be used during pregnancy only if clearly needed, and the benefits outweigh the potential risks.

Contraindicated during breastfeeding.

CERLIPONASE ALFA
Trade name
Brineura

Available form
Vial: 150 mg/5 mL

Action
- recombinant form of human tripeptidyl peptidase 1 (TPP1)
- inactive proenzyme (zymogen) form of a protease that is activated in the lysosome
- inadequate levels of TPPI cause CLN2 disease resulting in neurodegeneration, loss of neurological function (e.g. decline of motor and language functions) and death during childhood

Use
- treatment of neuronal ceroid lipofuscinosis type 2 (CLN2) disease (also known as TPP1 deficiency)

Dose
- (2 years and older) 300 mg by intracerebroventricular infusion every second week at a rate of 2.5 mL/hour

Adverse effects
- device-related infection (including meningitis)
- hypersensitivity, anaphylactic reactions
- fever
- low CSF protein
- ECG abnormalities, bradycardia
- vomiting, constipation, diarrhoea, dysphagia, abdominal pain, tongue or oral mucosa blistering
- upper respiratory tract infection, nasopharyngitis, rhinitis, viral infection, pharyngitis, tonsillitis, cough
- seizures
- tremor, headache, insomnia, irritability
- rash, urticaria
- development of anti-drug antibodies

Nursing considerations/Cautions

- not to be administered via any route other than intracerebroventricular infusion.

METABOLIC DISORDERS AGENTS

- Strict aseptic technique is required to prevent infection, and the product should not be shaken or mixed with any other drug products
- the first dose should be given at least 5 to 7 days after intracerebroventricular access device (surgically implanted reservoir and catheter) implantation
- medical support and equipment should be readily available in the event of anaphylaxis occurring
- pretreatment with antihistamines +/− an antipyretic 30—60 minutes before the infusion is recommended
- if the patient is unable to tolerate the infusion, the dose may be reduced by 50% and/or the infusion rate decreased
- if the infusion is stopped because of hypersensitivity reaction, it should be restarted at 50% of the initial infusion rate at which the reaction occurred
- the child should be closely monitored for any increase in intracranial pressure (headache, nausea, vomiting, decreased mental state) during infusion, and the infusion stopped or rate slowed if these occur
- vital signs should be monitored before start of infusion, during infusion and postinfusion. Longer monitoring is recommended in children under 3 years
- ECG is recommended during infusion if the child has any history of conduction disorders of the heart (including bradycardia and structural heart disease). If the child has no cardiac history, a 12-lead ECG is recommended every 6 months
- strict aseptic techniques must be adhered to during administration to prevent device-related infection occurring
- cerliponase alfa and flushing solution should be thawed at room temperature for about 60 minutes before administration (it should not be thawed or warmed in any other way)
- the vials should not be shaken
- when thawed, cerliponase alfa should be clear to slightly opalescent and colourless to pale yellow (thin translucent fibres or opaque fibres may be present but these are removed by the inline filter). Flushing solution should be clear and colourless
- cerliponase alfa and flushing solution should not be refrozen if not used
- a programmable syringe pump and 0.2 micron inline filter must be used for administration
- after infusion of cerliponase alfa, a calculated amount of flushing solution must be used to ensure the full dose has been administered and maintain patency of the device
- to administer:
  - one unused sterile syringe should be labelled 'Brineura' and, using aseptic technique, the required volume should be removed from the vial
  - the solution should not be diluted or mixed with any other agents
  - the amount of flushing solution should be determined to ensure the complete dose is administered (flush volume should be calculated by adding priming volume of all infusion components including access device)
  - one unused sterile syringe should be labelled 'flushing solution' and the calculated dose removed from the vial using aseptic technique
  - the infusion line should be primed with cerliponase alfa solution
  - the scalp should be closely inspected for signs of potential infection or access device leakage or failure (e.g. swelling, scalp erythema, extravasation of fluid, scalp bulging around or above access device site) (and not administered if any occur)
  - the scalp should be prepared according to workplace policy and the port needle inserted into the access device

- the empty sterile syringe (no larger than 3 mL) should be attached to the port needle and 0.5 to 1 mL of CSF should be withdrawn to check patency of the access device. The CSF sample should be sent for infection monitoring
- the infusion set should be connected to the port needle and secured
- the syringe with 'Brineura' should be placed in the syringe drive pump and the program set to deliver an infusion rate of 2.5 mL/hour and the infusion commenced
- when complete, the syringe containing flushing solution should be placed in the syringe drive pump and set at the same rate
- when the infusion is complete, the port needle should be removed and gentle pressure and dressing applied to the infusion site
- contains 17.42 mg sodium per vial (including flushing solution), which may need to be considered if the patient requires a sodium-controlled diet
- contraindicated in CLN2 patients with ventriculo-peritoneal shunts, if there is any sign of infection or evidence of access device leakage or failure, or if patient has sensitivity to Chinese hamster ovary cells

Patient education
- parents should be instructed to seek medical advice immediately if the child develops fever, nausea, vomiting, headache, neck stiffness, becomes sensitive to light and/or has changes in mental status (e.g. becomes sleepy, confused or irritable)

Should be administered to a pregnant woman only if clearly needed, and if the potential benefits outweigh the risks.

Due to the potential for adverse effects in a breastfed infant, breastfeeding should be discontinued during treatment.

ELIGLUSTAT
Trade name
Cerdelga

Available form
Capsules: 84 mg

Action
- Gaucher disease is a lysosomal storage disease in which there is a deficiency of acid β-glucosidase resulting in accumulation of glucosylceramide (GL-1), especially in the liver, spleen and bone marrow
- potent and specific inhibitor of GL-1 synthase in order to reduce the rate of synthesis to match the impaired rate of catabolism, preventing accumulation and the associated clinical manifestations

Use
- long-term management of patients with Gaucher disease (type 1)

Dose
- (CYP2D6 intermediate (IM) and extensive metabolisers (EM)) 84 mg orally twice daily **OR**
- (CYP2D6 poor metabolisers (PM)) 84 mg orally once daily

Adverse effects
- headache, dizziness
- palpitations
- dyspepsia, upper abdominal pain, diarrhoea, nausea, constipation, gastro-oesophageal reflux, abdominal distension, gastritis
- arthralgia
- fatigue

Interactions
- contraindicated in CYP2D6 immediate or extensive metabolisers who are taking paroxetine, fluoxetine, bupropion, duloxetine, moclobemide, tipranavir/ritonavir, cinacalcet with itraconazole, posaconazole, voriconazole, clarithromycin, cobicistat, indinavir, lopinavir, tipranavir/ritonavir, grapefruit juice, fluconazole, ciprofloxacin, erythromycin, ciclosporin, diltiazem, verapamil,

METABOLIC DISORDERS AGENTS

- imatinib, atazanavir/ritonavir, darunavir, darunavir/ritonavir or aprepitant (dose dependent)
- contraindicated in CYP2D6 poor metabolisers who are taking itraconazole, posaconazole, voriconazole, clarithromycin, cobicistat, lopinavir, tipranavir/ritonavir or grapefruit juice
- not recommended with grapefruit or grapefruit juice
- not recommended with class IA or class III (e.g. amiodarone, sotalol) antiarrhythmic agents
- decreased serum levels may occur if given with rifampicin, carbamazepine, phenobarbital (phenobarbitone), phenytoin, rifabutin or St John's wort and not recommended in CYP2D6 immediate, extensive or poor metabolisers
- may increase serum levels of digoxin, colchicine, dabigatran, phenytoin, pravastatin, metoprolol, amitriptyline, imipramine, clomipramine, dextromethorphan, atomoxetine, flecainide or phenothiazines

Nursing considerations/Cautions

- before starting therapy, patients should be genotyped to determine metabolic status for CYP2D6
- in patients switching from enzyme replacement therapy to eliglustat, disease progression should be monitored at 6-monthly intervals. If there is a suboptimal response, reinstitution of enzyme replacement therapy or an alternative treatment should be considered
- contains lactose, therefore are not recommended in those with rare hereditary problems of galactose intolerance, Lapp lactase deficiency or glucose–galactose malabsorption
- not recommended in those with congestive cardiac failure, recent acute myocardial infarction, bradycardia, heart block, ventricular arrhythmias or structural heart disease associated with arrhythmias, long QT syndrome
- not recommended in those who are CYP2D6 ultra-rapid metabolisers or whose status is indeterminate
- not recommended in those with moderate-to-severe kidney impairment or end-stage renal disease
- contraindicated in those with liver impairment who are intermediate or poor CYP2D6 metabolisers

Patient education

- instruct the patient to avoid grapefruit and grapefruit juice during therapy
- advise the patient to swallow capsules whole with glass of water
- warn the patient not to drive or operate machinery if dizziness is an ongoing problem

Capsules should not be crushed, dispersed in water or opened.

Eliglustat should be used during pregnancy only if the potential benefit justifies the risk.

Excretion in human milk is unknown. Breastfeeding should be discontinued during treatment, or eliglustat should be avoided, depending on the importance of the drug to the mother.

Reduced renal function: not recommended for CYP2D6 EMs with end-stage renal disease, or for IMs and PMs with any renal impairment. No adjustment needed for CYP2D6 EMs with mild-to-moderate impairment.

Reduced hepatic function: contraindicated in CYP2D6 EMs with moderate-to-severe impairment and in IMs/PMs with any impairment. Dose adjustments may be needed for CYP2D6 EMs with mild impairment if used with certain inhibitors.

ELOSULFASE ALFA (RCH)
Trade name
Vimizim

Available form
Vial: 1 mg/mL

Action
* purified human enzyme produced by recombinant DNA technology in Chinese hamster ovary
* mucopolysaccharidosis type IVA is characterised by absence or reduction in N-acetylgalactosamine-6-sulfatase activity, leading to accumulation of glycosaminoglycans (GAGs) resulting in cellular, tissue and organ dysfunction

Use
* treatment of mucopolysaccharidosis type IVA (MPS IVA — Morquio A syndrome)

Dose
* 2 mg/kg IV over 4 hours once per week

Adverse effects
* infusion reactions
* headache
* nausea, vomiting, diarrhoea, abdominal pain
* fever, chills
* otitis media, ear infection
* chest discomfort
* oropharyngeal pain, dyspnoea, throat irritation
* headache, dizziness, paraesthesia, somnolence, agitation
* neck pain, myalgia
* urticaria, flushing
* corneal opacity
* development of neutralising antibodies
* (Infusion site) pain
* (Rare) spinal/cervical cord compression, anaphylaxis, hypersensitivity

Nursing considerations/Cautions
* the patient should be assessed for any acute febrile or respiratory illness before infusion because of an increased risk of severe hypersensitivity reaction. Therapy should be postponed if illness is present
* evaluation of airway patency is recommended before starting therapy, as sleep apnoea is common in MPS IVA patients. If the patient is using supplemental oxygen or continuous positive airway pressure (CPAP) to manage sleep apnoea, these should be immediately available in the event of an emergency
* infusion-related reactions occur more frequently in first 12 weeks of therapy and the incidence decreases with time
* pretreatment with antihistamine with or without antipyretic is recommended before infusion to decrease the risk of infusion-related reaction
* the patient should be monitored for any signs of hypersensitivity or anaphylaxis. Hypersensitivity reaction occurs within 30 minutes of starting or up to 6 days after completing infusion, while anaphylaxis commonly occurs within 30 minutes of starting and up to 3 hours after completion
* if an infusion-related reaction occurs, the infusion should be slowed or stopped and/or additional antihistamines, antipyretics and/or corticosteroids administered
* calculate the total amount required and round up to the whole next vial
* the vials should be removed from refrigerator but not warmed artificially or shaken
* withdraw and discard a volume of sodium chloride 0.9% from infusion bag (equal to volume to be added). Add the required volume of elosulfase alfa slowly to the infusion bag, taking care not to agitate it. The infusion bag should be gently rotated (not shaken) to evenly distribute the solution

METABOLIC DISORDERS AGENTS

- dilute with sodium chloride 0.9% to a final volume of 100 mL (if weight < 25 kg) or 250 mL (if weight ≥ 25 kg)
- if the final volume is 100 mL, the initial infusion rate should be 3 mL/hour, increasing to 6 mL/hour after 15 minutes, then increasing further by 6 mL/hour at 15-minute intervals until a maximum rate of 36 mL/hour is reached if tolerated by the patient
- if the final volume is 250 mL, the initial infusion rate should be 6 mL/hour, increasing to 12 mL/hour after 15 minutes, then increasing further by 12 mL/hour at 15-minute intervals until a maximum rate of 72 mL/hour is reached if tolerated by the patient
- should be administered using a low protein binding infusion set with low protein binding 0.2 micron inline filter
- administer alone
- each vial contains 8 mg sodium (plus sodium in infusion solution), which may need to be taken into account if the patient is on sodium-controlled diet
- contains sorbitol and is not recommended in those with rare hereditary problems of fructose intolerance
- not recommended in those under 5 or over 65 years
- contraindicated in those with hypersensitivity to Chinese hamster ovary protein

Patient education
- the patient should be advised not to drive or operate machinery if dizziness occurs
- advise the patient to immediately seek medical advice if any of the following occur:
  - back pain, numbness or paralysis, urinary or faecal incontinence
  - cough, redness, throat tightness, hives, flushing, rash, difficulty breathing, lightheadedness or fainting, chest discomfort with nausea, abdominal pain, retching or vomiting

Not recommended during pregnancy unless benefits outweigh risks. No human data.

Avoid, as excretion in human milk is unknown.

GALSULFASE
Trade name
Naglazyme

Available form
Vial: 5 mg/5 mL

Action
- mucopolysaccharidosis VI is characterised by a lack of N-acetylgalactosamine4-sulfatase, resulting in an accumulation of glycosaminoglycan (GAG) substrate (dermatan sulfate) throughout the body, leading to widespread cellular, tissue and organ dysfunction
- provides an exogenous enzyme to be taken up into lysosomes and increasing catabolism of GAG
- half-life about 9 hours (first week) increasing to 26 hours by week 24 of therapy

Use
- long-term enzyme replacement therapy in patients with mucopolysaccharidosis VI (also called Maroteaux—Lamy syndrome or N-acetylgalactosamine 4-sulfatase deficiency)

Dose
- 1 mg/kg body weight IV once weekly over 4 hours

Adverse effects
- apnoea, respiratory distress, dyspnoea, laryngeal oedema, pharyngitis, nasal congestions
- conjunctivitis
- chest pain

- fever, chills, rigors
- malaise
- abdominal pain
- rash
- anaphylaxis, allergic reactions
- immune-mediated reaction (e.g. membranous glomerulonephritis)
- infusion-related reaction (serious or severe)
- onset or worsening of cervical cord compression
- development of antidrug antibodies

Nursing considerations/Cautions

- medical staff and resuscitation equipment should be readily available
- airway patency should be assessed before starting therapy
- pretreatment with antihistamines +/− antipyretics is recommended before infusion to decrease the risk of infusion-related reactions. Patients who use supplemental oxygen or continuous positive airway pressure (CPAP) should have them readily available during infusion in the event of infusion reaction or extreme sleepiness/drowsiness related to antihistamine
- if infusion-related reactions occur, the infusion rate should be stopped or slowed and additional administration of antihistamine, antipyretic and possibly corticosteroid is recommended
- the infusion rate should be set to run the infusion over at least 4 hours using an infusion pump. Initially the rate should be set at 6 mL/hour for the first hour and then, if well tolerated, the rate can be increased to 80 mL/hour for the last 3 hours. If an infusion reaction occurs, the rate can be extended
- when calculating the number of vials required according to patient weight, the amount should be rounded to the next whole vial
- vials should be allowed to come to room temperature before administration (but should not be heated)
- dilute with sodium chloride to a final volume of 250 mL by withdrawing and discarding a volume of sodium chloride equal to the volume of the vials to be added. The infusion bag should be gently rotated to mix but not shaken or agitated
- vials should not be shaken, as this will denature protein
- a 0.2 micron inline filter should be used
- contains 18.5 mg sodium per vial (and is given in sodium chloride 9 mg/mL), which may need to be taken into consideration if a patient is on a sodium-restricted diet
- caution if used in patients who have experienced anaphylaxis or allergic reactions previously to galsulfase. During re-challenge, trained personnel and emergency equipment must be readily available
- caution if used in patients susceptible to fluid volume overload (e.g. weighing less than 20 kg, compromised cardiac and/or respiratory system, acute underlying respiratory illness) because of the risk of acute cardio-respiratory failure

Patient education

- the patient/carer should be advised that anaphylaxis and allergic reactions can occur during and up to 24 hours after infusion
- advise the patient/carer to seek medical attention immediately if any back pain, limb paralysis, urinary or faecal incontinence occurs

 Use only if benefits outweigh potential risks.

 Use with caution and consider benefits of treatment to the mother versus potential risk to the infant.

METABOLIC DISORDERS AGENTS

IDURSULFASE
Trade name
Elaprase

Available form
Vial: 6 mg/3 mL

Action
- iduronate-2-sulfatase replacement therapy for Hunter syndrome
- Hunter syndrome is caused by insufficient levels of iduronate-2-sulfatase (lysosomal enzyme). Iduronate-2-sulfatase breaks down glycosaminoglycan dermatan sulfate and heparin sulfate; therefore insufficient enzyme levels result in glycosaminoglycan build-up in lysosomes at cell, tissue and organ level and, subsequently, organ dysfunction and tissue destruction

Use
- long-term treatment of Hunter syndrome (mucopolysaccharidosis II)

Dose
- 0.5 mg/kg by IV infusion weekly

Adverse effects
- (IV site) reaction, swelling
- infusion-related reactions (rash, urticaria, pruritus, fever, headache, nausea, vomiting, wheezing, hypertension and flushing)
- headache
- fever
- cyanosis, arrhythmias, tachycardia, hypotension, hypertension, chest pain
- wheezing, dyspnoea, tachypnoea, bronchospasm, hypoxia
- nausea, abdominal pain, dyspepsia, swollen tongue
- erythema, rash, pruritus, urticaria
- facial oedema, peripheral oedema
- antibody development
- (Rare) hypersensitivity, late emergent (biphasic) anaphylactoid/anaphylactic reactions

Nursing considerations/Cautions
- the patient should be assessed for any signs of acute febrile respiratory illness before infusion and therapy delayed if signs exist
- some patients may experience a late emergent or biphasic anaphylactic reaction where the person has a second reaction about 24 hours after the first; therefore prolonged observation is recommended
- resuscitation equipment should be readily available in the event of infusion-related reaction or anaphylaxis
- if infusion-related reactions occur, the infusion rate should be slowed or stopped, or administration of antihistamines, antipyretic, low-dose corticosteroid or beta agonist nebulisation
- should be diluted in 100 mL of sodium chloride 0.9%
- an inline low protein binding filter (0.2 micron) can be used
- the diluted solution should be administered within 3 hours. Initial infusion rate should be 8 mL/hour for the first 15 minutes, then increasing by 8 mL/hour at 15-minute intervals if tolerated by the patient. Infusion rate should not exceed 100 mL/hour
- if a 3-hour infusion is well tolerated, the infusion time can be gradually decreased for subsequent infusions. The minimum time for infusion should not be less than 1 hour. Infusion time can be increased if the patient experiences infusion-related reactions; however, this should not be greater than 8 hours
- an infusion time of less than 3 hours is not recommended in children under 5 years
- infusion in the home environment by a health professional may be considered if the patient is tolerating infusions well, has received at least 6 months of treatment and has been infusion-related reaction free for that period of time, as well as having stable airway disease. The health professional must be adequately trained in cardiopulmonary resuscitative measures, have ready access to emergency services

- and be trained to recognise and manage serious infusion-related reactions, hypersensitivity reactions and medical emergencies
- caution if used in those with acute respiratory disease or compromised respiratory function, as respiratory compromise may occur as a result of infusion reaction
- caution if used in those who are at risk of fluid overload, acute respiratory disease or compromised cardiac/respiratory function. Fluid restriction and prolonged observation is recommended if used in these patients
- caution if used in children with a severe form of Hunter syndrome because of an increased risk of developing neutralising antibodies and infusion-related reactions, as well as showing a reduced response to therapy
- not recommended in those over 65 years

Patient education

- warn the patient/carer that second infusion-related reactions may occur within 24 hours of the first and it is important to seek medical advice immediately

Limited human data. Use only if benefits to the mother outweigh potential risks to the fetus.

Not recommended, as excretion in human milk is unknown. Consider risks and benefits before use in lactating women.

IMIGLUCERASE (RCH)
Trade name
Cerezyme

Available form
Vial: 400 U

Action
- a recombinant macrophage (variant of human beta glucocerebrosidase) that catalyses hydrolysis of glucocerebroside (derived from haemopoietic cell turnover) to glucose and ceramide
- a deficiency of glucocerebrosidase results in an accumulation of glucocerebroside in tissue macrophages, which become swollen (Gaucher cells)
- Gaucher cells are commonly found in the liver, spleen and bone marrow, as well as the lung, kidney and intestine
- consequences include anaemia, thrombocytopenia, hepatosplenomegaly and debilitating skeletal complications such as osteonecrosis, osteopenia with secondary pathological fractures, remodelling failure, osteosclerosis and bone crisis

Use
- long-term enzyme replacement for those with non-neuronopathic (type 1) or chronic neuronopathic (type 3) Gaucher disease (with anaemia, thrombocytopenia, bone disease, hepatomegaly or splenomegaly)

Dose
- 2.5 U/kg 3 times weekly — 60 U/kg every 2 weeks by IV infusion over 1–2 hours

Adverse effects
- (IV site) discomfort, pruritus, burning, swelling, sterile abscess
- infusion-related reactions (pruritus, flushing, urticaria, angioedema, chest discomfort, dyspnoea, coughing, cyanosis, hypotension)
- nausea, abdominal pain, vomiting, diarrhoea
- rash
- chills, fever
- backache
- tachycardia
- fatigue, headache, dizziness
- transient peripheral oedema
- development of immunoglobulin G (IgG) antibodies

METABOLIC DISORDERS AGENTS

- (Rare) anaphylactoid reactions, hypersensitivity, pulmonary hypertension

Nursing considerations/Cautions

- dose and frequency of administration are dependent on the severity of disease
- regular monitoring for the development of IgG antibodies is recommended during first 12 months of therapy. Development of antibodies increases the risk of hypersensitivity reactions
- if the patient has experienced infusion-related reaction, decreasing the rate and/or pretreatment with antihistamines and/or corticosteroids is recommended for the next infusion
- if the patient develops respiratory symptoms, evaluation for pulmonary hypertension is recommended
- reconstitute with water for injections, mixing gently and avoiding frothing, then dilute further with sodium chloride 0.9% (100–200 mL), rotating the infusion bag gently to ensure even distribution before administration
- an inline low protein binding filter (0.2 micron) can be used
- diluted solution should be administered within 3 hours
- not recommended in the management of type 2 or type 3 Gaucher disease or acute bone crises associated with Gaucher disease
- caution if given to those with IgG antibodies or previous hypersensitivity reactions to imiglucerase
- not recommended in those with hypersensitivity to Chinese hamster ovary cells

Patient education

- warn the patient to avoid driving or operating machinery if dizziness occurs

While post-marketing data from over 150 pregnancies suggest it may be used to manage Gaucher disease during pregnancy, a risk–benefit assessment is required for each case. Pregnancy may worsen Gaucher symptoms, so careful monitoring is essential.

Excretion in human milk unknown. Likely to be digested in the infant's gastrointestinal tract, but caution is recommended.

LARONIDASE (RCH)
Trade name
Aldurazyme

Available form
Vial: 500 U/5 mL

Action
- lysosomal enzyme alpha L-iduronidase required for glycosaminoglycan catabolism deficiency results in mucopolysaccharide (lysosomal) storage disorder. Deficiency in this enzyme results in accumulation of glycosaminoglycan and associated cell, tissue and organ dysfunction
- enzyme replacement produced by recombinant DNA technology

Use
- long-term enzyme replacement therapy for those with mucopolysaccharidosis (alpha-L-iduronidase deficiency) for treatment of non-neurological manifestations

Dose
- 100 U/kg weekly by IV infusion

Adverse effects
- infusion-related reaction (commonly fever, headache, flushing and rash and, less commonly, cough, bronchospasm, dyspnoea, urticaria, angioedema, pruritus)
- injection site reaction and pain, abscess formation
- upper respiratory tract infection
- corneal opacities
- thrombocytopenia
- bilirubinaemia
- hyperreflexia, paraesthesia

1353

- rash
- hypotension, oedema, chest pain
- cough, oxygen desaturation/hypoxia, dyspnoea, tachypnoea, cyanosis, angioedema, facial/laryngeal oedema
- erythema
- feeling cold
- development of immunoglobulin G (IgG) antibodies
- anaphylaxis, allergic reaction

Interaction
- not recommended with procaine

Nursing considerations/Cautions/ Patient education

- patient should be assessed before administration, as acute illness may increase the risk of infusion-related reactions
- resuscitation equipment should be readily available in the event of infusion-related reaction or anaphylaxis
- pretreatment with antipyretics (e.g. paracetamol, ibuprofen) and/or antihistamines (e.g. diphenhydramine) is recommended 60 minutes before infusion to decrease infusion-related reactions
- slowing the IV rate or temporarily stopping infusion will lessen infusion-related reactions
- the volume of infusion is dependent on weight ($\leq$ 20 kg total of 100 mL > 20 kg total of 250 mL)
- initial infusion rate is 2 U/kg/hour, the rate doubling every 15 minutes for the first hour (if tolerated), to a maximum of 43 U/kg/hour and the maximum rate maintained for the remainder of infusion (2–3 hours)
- do not shake the solution, as protein will be denatured
- allow the vial(s) to come to room temperature while calculating the amount required. Withdraw and discard this amount of sodium chloride 0.9% from the infusion bag. Gently withdraw the required amount from the vial(s) and slowly add to the sodium chloride infusion bag, taking care not to agitate the solution. Gently rotate the infusion bag to ensure distribution and administer IV
- the infusion set should contain an inline low protein 0.2 micron filter
- administer alone
- not recommended in children under 5 years or those over 65 years
- caution if used in those with compromised lung function or acute respiratory disorders, as infusion-related reactions may compromise respiration and require extra monitoring and/or support

Not recommended during pregnancy unless the benefits outweigh risks.

Exercise caution if administering to nursing women because of the potential for adverse effects in the infant.

MERCAPTAMINE (CYSTEAMINE) BITARTRATE

Trade name
Cystagon

Available forms
Capsules: 50 mg, 150 mg

Action
- cystinosis causes abnormal transport of cystine out of lysosomes, which may result in accumulation of cystine in organs, especially the kidneys. The cystine crystals damage the kidneys, retina, muscles and CNS, resulting in photophobia, failure to grow, rickets and kidney failure
- cysteamine converts cystine into cysteine and cysteine–cysteamine compound, which can be removed
- half-life 1.5 hours

Use
- management of nephropathic cystinosis

Dose
- (Patients > 12 years and > 50 kg) initially 0.2–0.3 g/m^2 orally daily in 4 divided doses, increasing over 4–6 weeks to 2 g

METABOLIC DISORDERS AGENTS

daily in 4 divided doses (maintenance) **OR**

(Patients < 12 years) initially 0.2–0.3 g/m^2 orally daily in 4 divided doses, increasing over 4–6 weeks to 1.3 g/m^2 daily in 4 divided doses (maintenance)

Adverse effects
- fever
- lethargy
- diarrhoea, nausea, vomiting, anorexia, bad breath, constipation, dyspepsia, abdominal pain, GI bleeding/ulceration
- rash, urticaria
- hair colour changes
- (Uncommon) abnormal liver function, reversible leucopenia, anaemia, kidney failure, seizures, dehydration, somnolence, depression, lethargy, encephalopathy, headache, confusion, dizziness, nervousness
- (Rare) benign intracranial hypertension (pseudotumour cerebri), papilloedema, serious skin reactions

Nursing considerations/Cautions
- leucocyte cysteine levels should be monitored 5–6 hours after administration and levels should be kept at less than 1 nanomol of half cystine/mg protein. Levels should be repeated 3-monthly
- therapy should be stopped if a rash develops and restarted at a lower dose after the rash has cleared and slowly titrated to therapeutic dose if possible
- blood counts and liver function tests should be monitored regularly throughout therapy
- eyes should be examined regularly during therapy
- contraindicated in those with hypersensitivity to mercaptamine (cysteamine) or penicillamine

Patient/carer education
- the patient/carer should be warned that GI symptoms are common at the start of therapy
- if the patient is an adult, they should be advised not to drive or use machinery if drowsiness or decreased alertness occurs
- if the patient is a child, they should be advised to be careful when partaking in activities such as bike riding and climbing trees if dizziness or decreased alertness occur
- if the patient is child under 6 years, the parent/carer should be instructed to sprinkle the contents of capsules over food to decrease the risk of aspiration by trying to swallow a capsule whole
- advise patients/carers to seek medical advice if any of the following occur:
  - nausea, vomiting, loss of appetite, stomach pain or vomiting blood
  - rash
  - skin lesions (resembling stretch marks), leg pain, bone fractures or deformities or joint problems
  - fitting, depression, excessive sleepiness
  - headache, ringing or whooshing in ears (tinnitus), dizziness, nausea, double or blurry vision, loss of vision, pain behind eye or on eye movement

 Capsules can be opened and the contents mixed with water or a spoonful of smooth food such as yoghurt.

 No human data, but animal studies suggest teratogenic and fetotoxic effects. Use during pregnancy only if the potential benefit justifies the risk to the fetus.

 Caution is advised when administered during breastfeeding because of the potential risks.

MIGALASTAT
Trade name
Galafold

Available form
Capsules: 123 mg

Action
- Fabry disease is a progressive X-linked lysosomal storage disorder that causes a deficiency of lysosomal enzyme alpha galactosidase A (α-Gal A) that is needed for glycosphingolipid substrate metabolism. Deficiency in the enzyme results in accumulation of substrate in organs and tissues leading to morbidity and mortality
- selectively and reversibly binds with some mutant forms of α-Gal A stabilising these in the endoplasmic reticulum leading to restoration of α-Gal A
- elimination half-life 3—5 hours

Use
- long-term treatment of Fabry disease in adults and adolescents over 16 years who have amenable mutations of α-Gal A

Dose
- 123 mg orally every second day at same time of day at least 2 hours apart from food.

Adverse effects
- palpitations
- vertigo
- nausea, diarrhoea, abdominal pain, constipation, dry mouth, urge to defecate, dyspepsia, weight increase
- fatigue, headache, dizziness
- muscle spasm, myalgia, torticollis, extremity pain
- paraesthesia, hypoaesthesia
- depression
- proteinuria
- dyspnoea, epistaxis
- rash, pruritus

Interactions
- not recommended at the same time as enzyme replacement therapy

Nursing considerations/Cautions
- kidney function, ECG and biochemical markers should be monitored at least 6-monthly
- not recommended for patients with non-amenable mutations
- not recommended in patients with severe kidney insufficiency
- not recommended in women of childbearing potential who are not using contraception

Patient education
- advise the patient that capsules should be taken at least 2 hours after food and food and caffeine should not be consumed within 2 hours of taking medication
- instruct the patient that capsules should not be taken on 2 consecutive days
- the patient should be advised not to drive or operate machinery if dizziness is an ongoing problem
- women of childbearing potential should be advised to use adequate contraception during therapy

Capsules should not be opened or crushed.

Not recommended during pregnancy.

Should be used during breastfeeding only if benefits outweigh risks.

Reduced renal function: dose adjustment may be required. Monitor renal function closely; avoid in severe renal impairment unless necessary, as clearance may be reduced, potentially increasing toxicity risk.

Reduced hepatic function: metabolism may be affected, necessitating dose adjustment. Avoid in severe hepatic impairment if possible; monitor liver function and signs of toxicity closely.

Consider a lower starting dose because of the potential for increased sensitivity and slower metabolism. Monitor closely for side-effects and adjust dose accordingly.

MIGLUSTAT

Trade name
Zavesca

Available form
Capsules: 100 mg

Action
- glucosylceramide synthase inhibitor
- beta glucocerebrosidase catalyses hydrolysis of glucocerebroside (derived from haemopoietic cell turnover) to glucose and ceramide
- deficiency of glucocerebrosidase results in an accumulation of glucocerebroside in tissue macrophages, which become swollen (Gaucher cells) and are commonly found in the liver, spleen and bone marrow, as well as the lung, kidney and intestine
- consequences of Gaucher disease include anaemia, thrombocytopenia, hepatosplenomegaly and debilitating skeletal complications such as osteonecrosis, osteopenia with secondary pathological fractures, remodelling failure, osteosclerosis and bone crisis
- neurological characteristics of Niemann–Pick type C disease are thought to be due to accumulation of glycosphingolipids in neurones and glial cells
- half-life 6–7 hours

Use
- mild-to-moderate type 1 Gaucher disease (where enzyme replacement is not an option)
- treatment of progressive neuropathy in Niemann–Pick type C disease

Dose
- (Type 1 Gaucher disease) 100 mg orally 3 times daily **OR**
- (Niemann–Pick type C disease) 200 mg orally 3 times daily

Adverse effects
- thrombocytopenia
- weight loss, anorexia, diarrhoea, flatulence, abdominal pain, nausea, constipation, vomiting, dyspepsia, abdominal distension/discomfort
- muscle spasm
- tremor, insomnia, decreased libido, peripheral neuropathy, headache, dizziness, paraesthesia, hypoaesthesia, ataxia, fatigue, asthenia
- abnormal nerve conduction tests
- decreased fertility, increased number of abnormal sperm

Nursing considerations/Cautions
- regular monitoring of vitamin B_{12} is recommended during therapy, as deficiency occurs commonly in those with Gaucher disease
- neurological examination should be conducted before starting therapy, then at 6-monthly intervals
- regular blood counts are recommended
- dose reduction may be required because of diarrhoea
- enzyme replacement therapy is standard management of type 1 Gaucher disease
- any pre-existing tremor should be assessed before starting therapy
- (Niemann–Pick type C disease) 6-monthly patient assessment is recommended to evaluate neurological manifestations and benefits of treatment
- (Niemann–Pick type C disease) weight and growth should be monitored in children
- not recommended in those with severe kidney impairment (creatinine clearance (CrCl) < 30 mL/min)
- not recommended in those with severe type 1 Gaucher disease (Hb < 90 g/L, platelet < 50×10^9/L, active bone disease)

Patient education
- warn the patient to avoid driving or operating machinery if dizziness or tremor occurs
- the patient/carer should be warned that tremor commonly occurs in first month of therapy and usually resolves within

4—12 weeks (although dose reduction is sometimes required)
- the patient/carer should be advised to decrease lactose or sucrose-containing foods or take tablets on empty stomach to reduce GI side-effects, especially diarrhoea
- advise the patient/carer to report any:
  - numbness or tingling in hands or feet
  - tremor
- counsel male patients to use reliable contraception during and for 12 weeks after stopping therapy because of an increased incidence of abnormal sperm production and decreased fertility
- female patients should be advised to use effective contraception to avoid pregnancy occurring during therapy

Capsules should not be crushed, as this may affect drug absorption and efficacy.

Contraindicated, as animal studies have shown adverse effects. Effective contraception is recommended for both men and women during treatment and for 3 months following discontinuation in men.

Due to potential risks, it is recommended to avoid use during breastfeeding.

Reduced renal function: primarily excreted via the kidneys. Dose adjustment is recommended for patients with mild-to-moderate renal impairment (CrCl 30—70 mL/min). Use is not recommended in severe renal impairment (CrCl < 30 mL/min) owing to limited clinical data.

If capsules are opened, mask and safety glasses should be worn and pregnant staff must not handle.

NITISINONE
Trade names
Nityr, Orfadin

Available forms
Capsules: 2 mg, 5 mg, 10 mg, 20 mg;
Oral suspension: 4 mg/mL;
Tablets: 2 mg, 5 mg, 10 mg

Action
- competitive 4-hydroxyphenylpyruvate dioxygenase inhibitor which prevents accumulation of toxic intermediates (succinylacetone, succinylacetoacetate) from tyrosine metabolism (which further inhibit porphyrin synthesis pathway and accumulation of 5-aminolevulinate)

Use
- treatment of hereditary tyrosinaemia type 1 (with dietary restriction of tyrosine and phenylalanine)

Dose
- (Patients weighing > 20 kg) initially 1 mg/kg/day divided orally after food in 2 divided doses, decreasing to once daily if urine succinylacetone is undetectable after 4 weeks of therapy. Dose may need to be increased to 1.5 mg/kg/day in 2 divided doses if urine succinylacetone is detectable after 4 weeks of therapy (maximum 2 mg/kg/day)

Adverse effects
- thrombocytopenia, leucopenia, granulocytosis
- conjunctivitis, corneal ulcers and opacity, keratitis, photophobia, eye pain
- increased liver enzymes, hepatomegaly, liver failure
- (Uncommon) rash, pruritus, dermatitis

Interactions
- may increase serum levels of warfarin and phenytoin, increasing the risk of adverse effects. If given together, serum levels should be closely monitored

METABOLIC DISORDERS AGENTS

Nursing considerations/Cautions

- ophthalmological examination (slit lamp examination) is recommended before starting therapy
- liver function tests (including serum alpha fetoprotein levels) and liver imaging studies are recommended regularly during therapy. If liver nodules appear or serum alpha fetoprotein levels increase, the patient should be immediately assessed for liver malignancy
- WBC and platelet count should be monitored 6-monthly during therapy
- dose adjustment is dependent on urine succinylacetone levels, liver function tests and serum alpha fetoprotein levels, as well as any changes to body weight
- for patients weighing < 20 kg, the dose should be administered as 2 divided doses
- if the diet is not restricted in tyrosine and phenylalanine, plasma tyrosine levels increase leading to toxic effects in the eyes, skin and nervous system. Plasma tyrosine levels should be measured regularly
- (Suspension) contains sodium benzoate, which can cause bilirubin displacement from albumin, potentially causing jaundice (especially in neonates). Bilirubin levels should be measured before starting and regularly throughout therapy. If the bilirubin level is elevated in premature infants (with risk of acidosis and low albumin levels), treatment with capsule/tablet (rather than oral suspension) is recommended
- (Suspension) contains 0.7 mg sodium per mL suspension. Therapy with capsules should be considered if the sodium content is problematic
- (Suspension) contains 500 mg glycerol per mL suspension, which can cause headache, stomach upset and diarrhoea if 20 mL or more of suspension is administered. If the patient does not tolerate suspension (develops these adverse effects), therapy with capsules/tablets should be considered

Patient education

- advise the patient/carer to administer with food
- the patient/carer should be instructed to maintain dietary restriction of tyrosine and phenylalanine (to maintain plasma tyrosine levels below 500 micromol/L)
- advise the patient/carer to immediately report any eye pain, changes to vision, inflammation in cornea/eye/eyelid or sensitivity to light
- the patient/carer should be instructed in correct administration of the oral suspension, including:
  - the suspension should be administered directly into mouth using the syringe provided without any dilution
  - the oral suspension is supplied with 3 oral syringes (1 mL, 3 mL, 5 mL)
    - 1 mL syringe should be used for doses less than 1 mL. The syringe is marked from 0.1 to 1 mL, with graduations of 0.01 mL
    - 3 mL syringe should be used for doses from 1 to 3 mL and has 0.1 mL graduations
    - 5 mL syringe should be used for doses > 3 mL and has 0.2 mL graduations
  - new bottle:
    - a new bottle should be stored upright in refrigerator in its box
    - remove the bottle from refrigerator, label with the date the bottle was removed and opened
    - shake vigorously for at least 20 seconds to ensure the suspension is uniformly dispersed and mixed
    - remove the cap, place bottle upright on table and insert the plastic adapter firmly into the bottle neck (as far as it goes)
    - the cap can then be replaced
  - administering dose:
    - shake the bottle for at least 5 seconds
    - open the cap and syringe plunger into the top of the

adapter and carefully turn the bottle upside down (with syringe in place)
- pull the plunger slowly down until the top edge of the black ring is exactly level with the dose marking
- if air bubbles are present in the syringe, push the plunger back up until air bubble is expelled and slowly pull the plunger down to the dose level required
- turn the bottle upright and remove the syringe by gently twisting
- administer directly into the mouth slowly (rapid administration may cause choking)
- replace the cap and store the bottle in refrigerator or below 25°C
- discard 2 months after opening
- the syringe should be cleaned immediately with water, separating barrel and plunger and rinsing both. Allow to air dry

Available as an oral suspension. Tablet can be crushed, or the capsule opened and contents mixed with formula or a spoonful of yoghurt or oral suspension.

Not recommended during pregnancy unless benefits outweigh risks. Animal studies show adverse effects.

Avoid, as animal studies have shown adverse postnatal effects on offspring.

SAPROPTERIN

Trade name
Kuvan

Available forms
Tablets (soluble): 100 mg;
Powder for oral solution (sachet): 100 mg, 500 mg

Action
- synthetic form of naturally occurring 6R-tetrahydrobiopterin (BH_4) (co-factor for hydroxylases for phenylalanine, tyrosine and tryptophan)
- enhances activity of defective phenylalanine hydroxylase enzyme, increasing/restoring phenylalanine metabolism, preventing (or decreasing) accumulation in the blood
- sustained phenylalanine levels in those with phenylketonuria or tetrahydrobiopterin deficiency can result in neurological damage including severe mental retardation, microcephaly, delayed speech, seizures and behavioural abnormalities
- half-life is 6—7 hours

Use
- treatment of hyperphenylalaninaemia in those with phenylketonuria (PKU) or BH_4 deficiency

Dose
- (Phenylketonuria) initially 10 mg/kg orally once daily with food, adjusting dose according to blood levels (recommended range 5—20 mg/kg/day) **OR**
- (BH_4 deficiency) initially 2—5 mg/kg orally daily with food in 2—3 divided doses, adjusting dose according to blood levels (recommended range 2—20 mg/kg/day in 2—3 divided doses)

Adverse effects
- headache
- fever
- rash
- rhinorrhoea, pharyngolaryngeal pain, cough, nasal stuffiness, upper respiratory tract infection
- diarrhoea, vomiting, abdominal pain
- hypophenylalaninaemia
- (Rare) seizures, hypersensitivity reaction, gastritis, oesophagitis

Interaction
- caution if used with levodopa because of the risk of increased excitability and irritability
- caution if used with glyceryl trinitrate, isosorbide dinitrate, sodium nitroprusside, minoxidil and phosphodiesterase

METABOLIC DISORDERS AGENTS

type 5 (PDE5) inhibitors (e.g. sildenafil) that are nitric oxide donors
- caution if used with methotrexate, trimethoprim or other dihydrofolate reductase inhibitors

Nursing considerations/Cautions

- therapy should be initiated as early as possible to prevent non-reversible neurological disorders in children and cognitive deficits and psychiatric disorders in adults
- phenylalanine blood levels should be measured before and then 1 week after starting therapy. If blood level is not sufficiently reduced, the dose can be increased to 20 mg/kg/day maximum and blood levels monitored weekly for 4 weeks with dietary restrictions being maintained. A reduction of 30% or more in blood phenylalanine level is considered satisfactory. If this is not achieved after 4 weeks of therapy, the patient is considered a non-responder and therapy should be stopped
- (PKU) blood levels of phenylalanine should reduce within 24 hours of single dose, although about 4 weeks is needed for the maximum effect to occur
- phenylalanine blood levels should also be measured 1–2 weeks after any dose adjustment, especially in children
- blood phenylalanine levels may increase above pretreatment levels if therapy is suddenly stopped
- not recommended in children under 4 years
- caution if used in those with a history of seizures, kidney or liver impairment, or those over 50 years

Patient education

- the patient/carer should be instructed to maintain a strict phenylalanine diet and have regular clinical assessment, including serum phenylalanine and tyrosine levels, nutrient intake and psychomotor development
- advise the patient/carer to take with food (preferably high-fat, high-calorie meal) at the same time each day for maximum effect
- the patient/carer should be warned not to stop therapy suddenly
- instruct the patient/carer to seek medical advice if illness occurs, as this may cause phenylalanine levels to rise
- an adult patient should be instructed to dissolve tablets or sachets in 120–240 mL of water or apple juice and drink within 15–20 minutes. For children, doses above 100 mg should be dissolved in 120 mL or less of water. For doses less than 100 mg, 1 tablet (100 mg) should be dissolved in 100 mL of water and the required amount given
- advise the patient/carer that tablets will dissolve faster if they are crushed
- female patients should be counselled that strict control of maternal serum phenylalanine levels is recommended before and during pregnancy because of potential risks to mother and fetus (e.g. high incidence of neurological, cardiac, facial dysmorphism and growth abnormalities). Therapy is recommended only if strict dietary management is inadequate to control serum phenylalanine levels
- the patient/carer should be advised to seek medical advice if any of the following occur:
  - abdominal pain, belching, heartburn, nausea, vomiting, loss of appetite, indigestion (symptoms of gastritis)
  - difficulty swallowing, pain on swallowing, sore throat, hoarse voice, heartburn, acid reflux, nausea, chest

pain which is worse on swallowing (symptoms of oesophagitis)

Tablets can be crushed and dissolved in water or apple juice, or mixed with soft foods (e.g. yoghurt, mashed banana).

Human data are limited. Use during pregnancy only if strict dietary management does not sufficiently control blood phenylalanine levels, as uncontrolled levels may lead to fetal harm.

Excretion in human milk is unknown. Due to potential risks, avoid use while breastfeeding.

SEBELIPASE ALFA
Trade name
Kanuma

Available form
Vial: 2 mg/mL

Action
- lysosomal acid lipase deficiency is a rare autosomal recessive lysosomal storage disorder characterised by a decrease or loss of lysosomal acid lipase activity, resulting in accumulation of cholesteryl esters and triglycerides in liver, spleen, intestine and blood vessel walls. This can result in hepatomegaly, progressive liver disease, cirrhosis and end-stage liver disease; splenomegaly, anaemia and thrombocytopenia; malabsorption in the intestine and growth retardation; dyslipidaemia and increased risk of cardiovascular disease and atherosclerosis

Use
- long-term enzyme replacement therapy in patients with lysosomal acid lipase deficiency

Dose
- (Infants < 6 months) initially 1 mg/kg by IV infusion once weekly, increasing dose to 3 mg/kg weekly if required **OR**
- (Children and adults) 1 mg/kg by IV infusion every second week

Adverse effects
- diarrhoea, vomiting, nausea, constipation
- headache, asthenia
- fever
- rhinitis, cough, nasopharyngitis, oropharyngeal pain
- anaemia
- urticaria
- transient hyperlipidaemia (occurring within first 2—4 weeks and improving by week 8)
- development of anti-drug antibodies
- anaphylaxis, hypersensitivity reactions

Nursing considerations/Cautions
- patient should be assessed for any egg allergy before starting therapy
- the patient should be closely monitored for any anaphylaxis (e.g. fever, chills, abdominal pain, rash, nausea, vomiting, diarrhoea, laryngeal oedema), which can occur during or within 4 hours of infusion. Anaphylaxis can occur within 6 infusions or as late as 1 year after starting therapy
- medical personnel and emergency equipment should be readily available during administration and postinfusion
- if reaction occurs, infusion may be stopped or rate reduced and antihistamines, antipyretic and corticosteroid agents administered depending on severity of reaction
- allow the vial to come to room temperature before administration
- do not shake the vial
- dilute with sodium chloride 0.9% (10—250 mL depending on weight) and mix gently
- administer using a low-protein binding infusion set with an inline 0.2 micron filter
- contraindicated in those with life-threatening hypersensitivity to egg

Patient education
- the patient should be instructed that anaphylaxis can occur within 4 hours of infusion completion and to seek medical advice immediately if any signs or symptoms occur

METABOLIC DISORDERS AGENTS

Not recommended during pregnancy owing to lack of human data.

Not recommended during breastfeeding unless benefits outweigh risks.

SODIUM PHENYLBUTYRATE
Trade name
Pheburane

Available form
Granules: 483 mg/174 g

Action
- nitrogen scavenger
- prodrug, converted to phenylacetate
- reduces raised plasma ammonia and glutamine levels in patients with urea cycle disorders
- phenylbutyrate peak concentration in 1 hour, elimination half-life 0.8 hours
- phenylacetate peak concentration 3.55 hours, elimination half-life 1.3 hours

Use
- hyperammonaemia management associated with urea cycle disorders (with dietary protein restriction +/− dietary supplements)

Dose
- (Infants and children < 20 kg) up to 600 mg/kg per day orally in divided doses with meals **OR**
- (Children > 20 kg, adolescents, adults) up to 13 g/m^2 per day orally in divided doses with meals

Adverse effects
- anaemia, thrombocytopenia, leucopenia, leucocytosis, thrombocytosis
- metabolic acidosis, alkalosis
- decreased appetite, abdominal pain, vomiting, nausea, constipation, change in taste, increased weight
- rash, abnormal skin odour
- depression, irritability, headache
- syncope
- oedema
- renal tubular acidosis, increased liver enzymes, bilirubin, uric acid, chloride and sodium, decreased potassium, albumin, total protein and phosphate
- amenorrhoea, irregular menstruation
- neurotoxicity (somnolence, fatigue, lightheadedness, headache, disorientation, impaired memory, lack or change in taste, partial loss of hearing)

Interactions
- excretion may be inhibited by probenecid
- corticosteroids may cause breakdown of protein increasing plasma ammonia levels
- increased risk of hepatotoxicity if used with rifampicin
- increased risk of hyperammonaemia if given with haloperidol, sodium valproate, carbamazepine, phenobarbital (phenobarbitone) or topiramate

Nursing considerations/Cautions
- therapy should be started and managed by a practitioner with expertise in urea cycle disorder management
- urinalysis and plasma levels of ammonia, arginine, essential amino acids (especially branched chain amino acids), carnitine and serum proteins should be monitored during therapy. If needed, levels of phenylbutyrate (and metabolites) should be measured. The dose should be adjusted according to levels
- serum potassium should be monitored during therapy, as there may be increased potassium excretion
- a calibrated dosing spoon dispenses up to 3 g in 250 mg increments
- may be given via nasogastric or gastrostomy tube if needed
- contains 124 mg sodium/g sodium phenylbutyrate; therefore should be used with great caution (if at all) in those with congestive heart failure or severe kidney insufficiency, or with care in those on a sodium-controlled diet or where there is sodium retention with oedema

- contains sucrose (768 mg/g); therefore is not recommended in those with rare hereditary problems of fructose intolerance, glucose—galactose malabsorption or sucrase—isomaltase insufficiency, and should be taken into consideration by those with diabetes mellitus
- caution if used in those with liver or kidney impairment
- not recommended for management of acute hyperammonaemia, which is life threatening and requires a rapid response

Patient education

- the patient/carer should be instructed to use only the dosing spoon provided to measure the dose (no other measuring spoons should be used). Instructions include:
  - the lines on the spoon indicate the amount in grams
  - pour the granules into the spoon
  - tap the spoon on table to give a horizontal level and add more if needed
  - if more than 3 g is needed (the maximum amount held by the spoon), instructions should be repeated to give the total dose
- advise the patient/carer that granules can be taken directly with a drink (water, fruit juice, protein-free infant formula) or sprinkled on a spoonful of solid food (mashed potato or apple puree/sauce), but should be eaten or drunk straight away
- the patient/carer should be aware of need for dietary protein restriction and, if needed, essential amino acid and carnitine supplementation
- if dose is missed, the patient/carer should be instructed to take the dose as soon as possible with the next meal but there should be at least 3 hours between doses
- those with diabetes mellitus should be warned of the sucrose content and need to monitor blood glucose levels
- instruct the patient/carer to discard the bottle after 45 days of opening
- the patient should be advised to seek medical attention if any of the following occur:
  - nausea, vomiting, somnolence, fatigue, lightheadedness, headache, disorientation, impaired memory, lack or change in taste, partial loss of hearing
- women of childbearing potential should be counselled to use effective contraception during therapy to avoid pregnancy occurring

 Granules should not be crushed or chewed. They are designed for direct swallowing or mixing with a small amount of food (such as mashed potato or apple sauce) and should be taken immediately.

 Contraindicated during pregnancy because of the lack of safety data in humans and animal studies showing potential neurotoxicity effects on the fetus. Women of childbearing potential should use effective contraception while taking this medication.

 Contraindicated during breastfeeding.

 Reduced renal function: use with caution in patients with renal impairment (CrCl or eGFR < 60 mL/min), as sodium phenylbutyrate and its metabolites are excreted primarily by the kidneys, which may require dose adjustment and close monitoring.

TALIGLUCERASE ALFA (RPC)

Trade name
Elelyso

Available form
Vial: 200 U

Action
- recombinant form of human beta glucocerebrosidase

METABOLIC DISORDERS AGENTS

- a deficiency of glucocerebrosidase results in an accumulation of glucocerebroside in tissue macrophages, which become swollen (Gaucher cells)
- Gaucher cells are commonly found in the liver, spleen and bone marrow, as well as the lung, kidney and intestine
- consequences include anaemia, thrombocytopenia, hepatosplenomegaly and debilitating skeletal complications such as osteonecrosis, osteopenia with secondary pathological fractures, remodelling failure, osteosclerosis and bone crisis

Use
- type 1 Gaucher disease associated with splenomegaly, hepatomegaly, anaemia or thrombocytopenia

Dose
- 30—60 U/kg once every 2 weeks via IV infusion over 60—120 minutes

Adverse effects
- infusion-related reactions
- headache, dizziness, fatigue
- flushing, pruritus, rash, erythema
- eye swelling and pruritus, increased lacrimation
- sneezing, runny nose, throat irritation
- vomiting, abdominal pain, nausea, weight increase
- arthralgia, pain in extremity, bone pain, back pain
- peripheral oedema
- hypersensitivity
- infusion site pain
- (Rare) development of antibodies, pulmonary hypertension

Nursing considerations/Cautions
- any pulmonary hypertension should be evaluated regularly during therapy
- infusion-related reactions usually occur within 24 hours of infusion
- if infusion-related reactions occur, the rate should be slowed or stopped, then resumed at a reduced rate
- pretreatment with antihistamines and/or corticosteroids may be used to prevent subsequent reactions
- hypersensitivity reactions commonly occur in first 12 weeks of therapy
- can be switched from imiglucerase using the same dose
- reconstitute using 5.1 mL water for injections and mix the vial gently (do not shake)
- withdraw 5 mL of reconstituted solution and dilute with 100—200 mL sodium chloride 0.9% and administer by IV infusion
- an inline low protein binding 0.2 micron filter is recommended
- contains sodium and is administered in sodium chloride, which may need to be considered if the patient has sodium restriction
- caution if used in those with an allergy to carrots (as the agent has been developed in carrot plant)
- not recommended in those with type 2 Gaucher disease
- contraindicated in those with known allergy to similar glucocerebrosidase enzymes

Patient education
- warn the patient to avoid driving or operating machinery if dizziness occurs

 Should be used during pregnancy only if benefits outweigh risks.

 Should be used during breastfeeding only if benefits outweigh risks.

VELAGLUCERASE ALFA (GHU)
Trade name
VPRIV

Available form
Vial: 400 U

Action
- glycoprotein produced by gene activation technology
- recombinant macrophage (variant of human beta glucocerebrosidase) that

- catalyses hydrolysis of glucocerebroside (derived from haemopoietic cell turnover) to glucose and ceramide
- a deficiency of glucocerebrosidase results in an accumulation of glucocerebroside in tissue macrophages, which become swollen (Gaucher cells)
- Gaucher cells are commonly found in the liver, spleen and bone marrow, as well as the lung, kidney and intestine
- consequences include anaemia, thrombocytopenia, hepatosplenomegaly and debilitating skeletal complications such as osteonecrosis, osteopenia with secondary pathological fractures, remodelling failure, osteosclerosis and bone crisis

Use
- long-term enzyme replacement for those with type 1 Gaucher disease (with anaemia, thrombocytopenia or hepatosplenomegaly)

Dose
- 60 U/kg every 2 weeks by IV infusion over 60 minutes

Adverse effects
- (IV site) discomfort, pruritus, burning, swelling, sterile abscess
- infusion-related reactions (headache, dizziness, hypotension, hypertension, nausea, fatigue, asthenia, fever)
- nasopharyngitis, rhinitis, bronchitis, dyspnoea
- cystitis, urinary tract infection
- headache, dizziness
- paraesthesia
- cough, epistaxis
- abdominal pain, diarrhoea, vomiting, nausea
- urticaria, pruritus, rash, flushing
- chest discomfort, hypertension, hypotension, tachycardia
- arthralgia, bone/back pain, muscle spasm, myalgia, neck pain
- fever, flu-like illness
- peripheral oedema
- development of IgG antibodies, prolonged activated partial thromboplastin time (aPTT)
- (Rare) hypersensitivity, anaphylactoid reaction, allergic dermatitis

Nursing considerations/Cautions
- infusion-related reactions occur most commonly in the first 6 months of therapy for patients previously untreated with enzyme replacement therapy
- if the patient experiences infusion-related reaction, decreasing the rate and/or pretreatment with antihistamines and/or corticosteroids is recommended for next infusion
- if the patient has a severe infusion-related reaction or lack/loss of response, antibody testing is recommended
- reconstitute using 4.3 mL water for injections
- do not shake, as this will denature protein
- dilute further with 100 mL sodium chloride 0.9%, rotating gently to ensure even distribution before administration
- an inline low protein binding filter (0.2 micron) should be used
- the diluted solution should be administered over 60 minutes
- infusion in the home environment by a health professional may be considered if the patient has received at least 3 infusions in the hospital environment and has tolerated them well (infusion-related reaction free). The health professional must be adequately trained in cardiopulmonary resuscitative measures, have ready access to emergency services and be trained to recognise and manage serious infusion-related reactions, hypersensitivity reactions and medical emergencies
- not recommended in the management of type 2 or type 3 Gaucher disease
- caution if used in those with kidney or liver impairment

METABOLIC DISORDERS AGENTS

- caution if used in those with previous hypersensitivity reactions to other enzyme replacement therapies

Patient education

- warn the patient to avoid driving or operating machinery if dizziness occurs

Use during pregnancy only if the benefits outweigh the risks.

Caution if used during breastfeeding.

MOVEMENT DISORDER AGENTS

In this section, we are focusing on drugs that are used to manage and treat movement disorders such as multiple sclerosis (MS) and motor neurone disease (MND), which includes primary lateral sclerosis, primary muscular atrophy, and progressive bulbar palsy and amyotrophic lateral sclerosis (Cree & Hauser 2019).

MULTIPLE SCLEROSIS

Multiple sclerosis (MS) is an autoimmune disease affecting the central nervous system (CNS), characterised by chronic inflammation, demyelination, scarring or plaques and neuronal loss, with brain lesions developing over time in various areas of the brain (Cree & Hauser 2019). MS is more prevalent in women, with risk factors including vitamin D deficiency, smoking and Epstein—Barr virus exposure in later childhood. However, the exact cause remains unknown. MS affects approximately 2.3 million people globally, with over 33,000 Australians currently living with the condition — a number that has risen significantly over recent years. This increase is evident in the latest data released by MS Australia in 2023, showing a 30% rise in prevalence since 2017 (Cree & Hauser 2019; MS Australia 2023). Interestingly, the prevalence of MS increases the farther one lives from the equator, with particularly high rates in areas such as islands off Scotland. In Australia, for example, Tasmania has twice the prevalence rate compared with Queensland (Cree & Hauser 2019; MS Australia 2023).

In Australia, MS typically has an onset age between 20 and 40 years, with an average onset age around 30 years (Lane et al 2022). The symptoms of MS are highly variable and often depend on the specific areas of the central nervous system that are affected. Early symptoms may include visual disturbances, such as optic neuritis, motor weakness, sensory abnormalities and coordination issues. As MS progresses, individuals may experience more disabling symptoms like significant muscle weakness, spasticity, cognitive impairment, fatigue, and bladder or bowel dysfunction. Symptom presentation often varies, with relapses and remissions being common in the early stages, particularly for the relapsing remitting form of MS, which is the most common type initially diagnosed in Australian patients (Lane et al 2022).

- *relapsing remitting MS*, which accounts for about 85% of cases and is characterised by attacks that evolve over days to weeks, followed by recovery, with patients neurologically stable between attacks. However, as attacks continue, recovery may be less evident
- *secondary progressive MS*, which begins as relapsing remitting MS, but the

patient then experiences a steady deterioration in function not connected to acute attacks
- *primary progressive MS*, which accounts for about 10% of cases, with patients experiencing a steady functional decline from the onset (but no acute attacks) (Cree & Hauser 2019)
- *relapsing remitting MS*, which accounts for about 85% of cases and is characterised by attacks that evolve over days to weeks, followed by recovery, with patients neurologically stable between attacks. However, as attacks continue, recovery may be less evident
- *secondary progressive MS*, which begins as relapsing remitting MS, but the patient then experiences a steady deterioration in function not connected to acute attacks
- *primary progressive MS*, which accounts for about 10% of cases, with patients experiencing a steady functional decline from the onset (but no acute attacks) (Cree & Hauser 2019)

Management of MS involves a multifaceted approach to address both acute and long-term symptoms. Treatment of acute attacks typically involves corticosteroids, which help to control inflammation during initial attacks or acute exacerbations. For relapsing forms of MS, various pharmacological agents, such as disease-modifying therapies (DMTs), aim to reduce the frequency and severity of relapses, slow disease progression and potentially minimise the development of new lesions. Symptomatic therapies are essential to enhance quality of life and include treatments for common symptoms such as ataxia, tremor, spasticity, muscle spasms, weakness, pain, bladder dysfunction and depression. Supportive lifestyle changes are also encouraged, such as maintaining a balanced diet, engaging in regular exercise as tolerated and managing stress. These lifestyle measures may complement pharmacological treatments and support overall well-being in individuals with MS.

ALEMTUZUMAB
Trade names
Lemtrada, MabCampath

Available forms
Vial: 12 mg/1.2 mL (Lemtrada), 30 mg/mL (MabCampath)

Action
- anti-CD52 antibody (CD52 is a surface antigen on T and B lymphocytes, killer cells, monocytes and macrophages)
- multiple sclerosis (MS) activity is thought to be related to alteration in number, proportion and properties of some lymphocytes post-treatment

Use
- relapsing/remitting MS (in those with active disease) (Lemtrada)
- B-cell chronic lymphocytic leukaemia (MabCampath) (see Antineoplastic agents, p. 746)

Dose
- initially 12 mg daily by IV infusion over 4 hours for 5 consecutive days (60 mg total), followed by second course 12 mg daily by IV infusion over 4 hours for 3 consecutive days (36 mg total) after 12 months. Third and fourth courses (same as second course) can be given at 12-month intervals if needed

Adverse effects
- infusion-related reaction (headache, rash, fever, nausea, urticaria, pruritus, insomnia, chills, flushing, fatigue, dyspnoea, taste alteration, chest discomfort, tachycardia, dyspepsia, dizziness, pain)
- flushing, fever, chills, fatigue
- rash, urticaria, pruritus, erythema
- peripheral oedema, tachycardia
- back pain, pain in extremities, arthralgia, muscle weakness, myalgia, muscle spasm
- nausea, diarrhoea, vomiting, abdominal pain, dyspepsia, altered taste
- depression (new or worsened), anxiety, confusion, insomnia
- cough, dyspnoea, oropharyngeal pain, flu-like illness, pneumonitis

- paraesthesia, dizziness, hypoaesthesia, headache
- neutropenia, haemolytic anaemia, pancytopenia, leucopenia
- elevated serum creatinine, haematuria, proteinuria
- infection (nasopharyngitis, urinary tract infection, upper respiratory tract infection, sinusitis, oral herpes, influenza, bronchitis, *Listeria monocytogenes*, cervical infection)
- elevated liver enzymes, liver dysfunction, acute liver failure
- stroke, cervicocephalic arterial dissection
- superficial fungal infections (oral and vaginal candidiasis)
- hyper/hypothyroidism
- autobody development
- immune thrombocytopenic purpura (ITP)
- malignancy (thyroid cancer, breast cancer, basal cell carcinoma)
- (Rare) Graves' disease, reactivation of tuberculosis, haemophagocytic lymphohistiocytosis, acute acalculous cholecystitis

Interactions

- not recommended with live or live attenuated vaccines
- 28-day interval should be allowed between stopping interferons or glatiramer acetate and starting therapy

Nursing considerations/Cautions

- all patients should be carefully screened for history of tuberculosis (TB), hepatitis B and C or active infection and therapy delayed if treatment is required
- FBC (with differential), thyroid function tests, serum creatinine and urinalysis (with cell count) is recommended before starting therapy and then at monthly intervals (thyroid function tests 3-monthly) during therapy and continuing for 4 years after last infusion
- premedication with corticosteroid (1 g methylprednisolone), antihistamine and/or antipyretic is recommended just before infusion on first 3 days of any course
- the patient should be observed during and for 2 hours after infusion
- prophylactic oral antiherpes agent (e.g. 200 mg aciclovir twice daily) should be started on first day of therapy and continued for at least 4 weeks after each course
- immunisation should be up to date and completed at least 6 weeks before starting therapy
- the patient's immunity to varicella zoster virus (chicken pox, herpes zoster (shingles)) should be assessed (including serological testing) before starting therapy because the response to the virus may be severe if exposed and unprotected
- female patients should be screened for human papilloma virus (HPV) on a yearly basis
- administer alone
- dilute with 100 mL sodium chloride 0.9% or glucose 5% and administer IV over 4 hours
- caution if used in those with a cardiac history, as infusion-related reactions can include cardiac symptoms
- caution if used in those who are hepatitis B or C carriers because of increased risk of liver damage due to reactivation of virus
- caution if used in those with pre-existing or ongoing malignancy
- not recommended in those with stable or inactive MS
- contraindicated in those with murine protein hypersensitivity or HIV

Patient education

- the patient should be advised to carry a Patient Wallet Guide during and for 4 years post-therapy in case the person develops a severe infection or autoimmune condition that requires medical treatment
- advise the patient not to drive or operate machinery if dizziness occurs
- ensure that the patient understands the importance of the blood and urine tests

MOVEMENT DISORDER AGENTS

taken before starting and monthly for up to 4 years after stopping treatment
- warn the patient that infusion-related reactions commonly occur within 24 hours and that they will need to be monitored during and for 2 hours after the infusion. The patient should be given medication before the infusion to try and minimise any reactions
- the patient should be instructed regarding avoidance of foods that may increase the risk of L. monocytogenes infections (e.g. salads from salad bars, soft and semi-soft cheeses, soft serve ice cream, unpasteurised dairy products, ready-to-eat meals, raw shellfish and seafood)
- advise the patient to seek medical advice immediately if any of the following occur:
  - bruising or bleeding that is hard to stop or if the skin develops any small, scattered, red, pink or purple spots
  - signs of infection, including fever, chills, aching muscles or joints, swollen glands
  - shortness of breath, cough, wheezing, chest pain or tightness, cough, blood-stained sputum
  - abdominal pain and tenderness, fever, nausea and vomiting
  - nausea, vomiting, abdominal pain, fatigue, anorexia, dark urine, yellow skin or whites of the eyes
  - sudden numbness or weakness of face, arm or leg (especially one side of the body), confusion, difficulty speaking or slurring, loss of balance or coordination, dizziness
  - headache, neck pain
- women of childbearing potential should be advised to use effective contraception during and for 16 weeks after stopping therapy

 Avoid: women of childbearing potential should use effective contraception during and for 4 months after treatment.

 Avoid: excretion in human breastmilk unknown. Breastfeeding should be avoided during treatment and for 4 months after.

CLADRIBINE
Trade names
Leustatin, Litak, Mavenclad

Available forms
Vial: 10 mg/5 mL, 10 mg/10 mL (Leustatin, Litak);
Tablets: 10 mg (Mavenclad)

Action
- antimetabolite (purine nucleoside analogue)
- prodrug
- also known as chlorodeoxyadenosine, CdA or 2-CdA.

Use
- hairy cell leukaemia, Waldenstrom's macroglobulinaemia (after failure of alkylating agents), B-cell chronic lymphocytic leukaemia (CLL) (after failure of alkylating agents) (Leustatin, Litak) (see Antineoplastic agents, p. 622)
- treatment of relapsing remitting multiple sclerosis (MS) to decrease frequency of clinical relapses and delay physical disability progression (Mavenclad)

Dose
- (Mavenclad) relapsing remitting MS 20—30 mg orally daily for 4—5 days (week 1, month 1, year 1), repeated at the start of month 2. Regimen is repeated for year 2 (recommended cumulative dose 3.5 mg/kg over 2 years)

Adverse effects
- infections (nasopharyngitis, upper respiratory tract infection, urinary tract infection, influenza, oral herpes, herpes zoster)
- nausea, diarrhoea
- rash, alopecia
- headache

- lymphopenia, leucopenia
- back pain, arthralgia, pain in extremities
- fatigue, flu-like symptoms
- pharyngolaryngeal pain
- depression, insomnia
- vertigo
- (Rare) progressive multifocal leukoencephalopathy (PML), increased risk of malignancies

Interactions

- contraindicated with immunosuppressive or myelosuppressive agents (except corticosteroids)
- may increase lymphocyte count reduction if given with beta interferon
- not recommended within 3 hours of other oral medications
- not recommended with or within 6 weeks of live or live attenuated vaccines
- not recommended with any other MS-modifying treatment
- not recommended with dipyridamole, nifedipine, nimodipine or eltrombopag during 4–5 days of cladribine therapy
- caution if given with carbamazepine or non-steroidal anti-inflammatory drugs (NSAIDs) because of the additive haematological adverse effects
- decreased serum levels may occur if given with corticosteroids, rifampicin or St John's wort

Nursing considerations/Cautions

- the patient should not receive any more than 2 treatment courses over 2 consecutive years
- before starting therapy, the patient should be screened for any active tuberculosis, HIV and/or hepatitis B and C and any infection treated
- any active infection should be treated before starting therapy
- the patient's immunity to varicella zoster virus (chicken pox, herpes zoster (shingles)) should be assessed (including serological testing) before starting therapy because the response to the virus may be severe if exposed and unprotected. If the patient is antibody negative, vaccination is recommended 4–6 weeks before starting therapy
- lymphocyte count should be measured before each course and at 2 and 6 months after each course of treatment. A second course should not be started unless the count is at least 800 cells/mm^3. If the lymphocyte count does not recover within 6 months, a second course of therapy should not be given. Additionally, red blood cell, neutrophil and platelet counts, haemoglobin and haematocrit should also be measured
- if the patient is switching from another MS medication that has a risk of PML, baseline magnetic resonance imaging (MRI) is recommended
- pregnancy must be excluded before starting therapy in year 1 and year 2
- if the patient requires a blood transfusion, irradiation of cellular blood components is recommended to decrease risk of transfusion-related graft versus host disease
- tablets contain 64 mg sorbitol/tablet and are not recommended in those with fructose intolerance
- not recommended in those over 65 years or under 18 years
- not recommended in patients with active malignancy
- contraindicated in those with HIV infection, active chronic infections (tuberculosis, hepatitis) or who are immunosuppressed (including taking immunosuppressive agents) or with moderate-to-severe kidney impairment

Patient education

- instruct the patient to swallow tablets whole without chewing. They should be taken at the same time every day and can be taken with or without food
- advise the patient to handle tablets with dry hands and wash hands thoroughly after administration
- the patient should be instructed to separate cladribine administration from any other oral medications by at least 3 hours

MOVEMENT DISORDER AGENTS

- the patient should be advised to conduct regular self-examinations for any new or changing skin lesions, have an annual examination by a dermatologist, seek medical advice if any new or changing skin lesions occur, avoid direct sun exposure and use skin protection (including clothing and sunscreen)
- female patients of childbearing potential should be counselled to use adequate and reliable contraception to prevent pregnancy occurring during and for 6 months after last dose of therapy. If using hormonal contraceptive, an additional barrier method is recommended
- male patients should be counselled to take precautions to avoid pregnancy of their partner occurring during therapy and for at least 6 months after last dose

Tablets should be swallowed whole to prevent exposure to the drug's cytotoxic components. Do not crush or split.

Contraindicated in pregnancy because of its potential to cause congenital malformations by interfering with DNA synthesis. Women of childbearing potential must use reliable contraception during and for at least 6 months.

Contraindicated during breastfeeding and for 1 week after the last dose because of the potential adverse effects on nursing infants.

Reduced renal function: contraindicated in patients with moderate-to-severe renal impairment (CrCl < 60 mL/min) because of decreased clearance and potential toxicity. No dosage adjustment is required for mild renal impairment, but caution is advised.

Reduced hepatic function: not recommended in patients with moderate-to-severe hepatic impairment (Child–Pugh score > 6) because of lack of safety data in this population.

DIMETHYL FUMARATE
Trade names
APO-Dimethyl Fumarate, Dimethyl Fumarate MSN, Dimethyl Fumarate Sandoz, Pharmacor Dimethyl Fumaratea, Tecfidera, Trazent

Available forms
Capsules (enteric-coated): 120 mg, 240 mg

Action
- activates nuclear factor (erythroid-derived 2)-like 2 transcriptional pathway
- anti-inflammatory and immunomodulatory properties reduce release of pro-inflammatory cytokines
- active metabolite (monomethyl fumarate) whose half-life is about 1 hour

Use
- relapsing remitting multiple sclerosis (MS) (to reduce frequency of relapses and delay disease progress)

Dose
- initially 120 mg orally twice daily for 7 days, then increasing to 240 mg orally twice daily

Adverse effects
- flushing, burning sensation, feeling hot
- diarrhoea, nausea, abdominal pain, vomiting, dyspepsia, gastritis
- rash, pruritus, erythema
- gastroenteritis
- lymphopenia, leucopenia
- proteinuria, microalbuminuria, urine albumin present, elevated liver enzymes
- (Rare) prolonged lymphopenia, progressive multifocal leukoencephalopathy (PML), anaphylaxis, herpes zoster infections (including disseminated, ophthalmicus, meningoencephalitis, meningomyelitis)

Interactions
- not recommended with live or live attenuated vaccines
- caution if used with nephrotoxic agents such as aminoglycosides, diuretics,

non-steroidal anti-inflammatory drugs (NSAIDs) and lithium
- not recommended with other topical or systemic fumaric acid derivatives

Nursing considerations/Cautions

- complete blood count (including lymphocytes) and urinalysis are recommended before starting therapy (within 6 months) and then every 6–12 months
- if lymphocyte count falls below $0.5 \times 10^9/L$ for more than 6 months, interrupting therapy is recommended
- therapy should be interrupted if severe infection occurs
- dose can be decreased to 120 mg twice daily temporarily if flushing and gastrointestinal adverse effects are severe
- caution if used in those under 18 and over 65 years or if patient has pre-existing low lymphocyte count

Patient education

- warn the patient that flushing and gastrointestinal adverse effects (nausea, vomiting, diarrhoea, abdominal pain, dyspepsia) are common in first month and decrease with use. Taking capsules with food may decrease adverse effects
- advise the patient that taking 325 mg aspirin before therapy may decrease flushing
- instruct the patient to swallow capsules whole and not to crush, divide or dissolve them
- ensure the patient understands the importance of completing the urine test before starting therapy and then once per year
- the patient should be advised to wear a MedicAlert bracelet outlining the risks of PML
- the patient and carer/partner should be advised to immediately report any unusual, worse or prolonged neurological symptoms, including difficulty performing mental tasks, unusual behaviour, confusion or personality changes (may be signs of PML or progression of MS)
- advise the patient to seek medical advice immediately if any of the following occur:
  - any signs of infection including fever, chills, swollen glands, feeling unwell
  - skin rash, itching, hives, swelling of lips/throat/tongue, wheezing, difficulty breathing, dizziness, nausea, vomiting, feeling of dread (signs of anaphylaxis)
  - any signs of herpes zoster infection which can vary depending on location but could include headache, one-sided stabbing pain, fever, chills, headache, tingling/burning/itching or stinging sensation before rash appears

 Advise the patient to swallow capsules whole and not to crush, divide or dissolve them.

 Recommended during pregnancy only if benefits are thought to outweigh risks.

 Excretion in breastmilk is unknown; therefore should be used during breastfeeding only if benefits outweigh risks.

FAMPRIDINE

Trade name
Fampyra

Available form
Tablets (modified-release): 10 mg

Action
- non-selective potassium channel blocker that blocks potassium channels in demyelinated nerves, reducing current leakage from axons and restoring neuronal conduction and action potential formation
- readily crosses blood–brain barrier
- elimination half-life about 6 hours

Use
- symptomatic improvement of walking ability in adults with multiple sclerosis (MS)

MOVEMENT DISORDER AGENTS

Dose
- 10 mg orally twice daily (12 hours apart)

Adverse effects
- insomnia, anxiety, dizziness, headache, tremor, paraesthesia, asthenia
- pharyngolaryngeal pain
- nausea, vomiting, constipation, dyspepsia
- dyspnoea
- back pain
- balance disorder
- urinary tract infection
- nasopharyngitis
- seizures
- exacerbation of pre-existing trigeminal neuralgia

Interactions
- contraindicated with any form of fampridine/4-aminopyridine
- caution if given with agents which lower seizure threshold
- caution if given with agents which are renally excreted

Nursing considerations/Cautions
- before starting therapy, the patient should be assessed for any history of or predisposing factors for seizures or which may lower seizure threshold
- therapy should be re-evaluated after 8 weeks and continued only if a walk test shows a positive response
- caution if used in those with mild kidney impairment (creatinine clearance 50–80 mL/min) (monitoring renal function regularly is recommended)
- contraindicated in those with moderate-to-severe kidney impairment (creatinine clearance < 50 mL/min) or a history of seizures

Patient education
- instruct the patient that tablets should be swallowed whole (not broken, crushed or divided)
- advise the patient that walking will be assessed after 8 weeks and therapy stopped if no improvement has occurred
- warn the patient against driving or operating machinery if dizziness, balance problems or tremor occurs
- the patient should be advised to immediately report any seizures (fitting)

Do not crush, split, dissolve, suck, or chew. Formulated as modified-release tablets, which must be swallowed whole to ensure proper absorption and effectiveness.

Use during pregnancy should be considered only if the potential benefit justifies the risk to the fetus, as there are no adequate and well-controlled studies in pregnant women.

Avoid, as there are limited human data. Excretion in human breastmilk is unknown.

Reduced renal function: primarily excreted unchanged by the kidney. Contraindicated in patients with moderate-to-severe renal impairment (CrCl < 50 mL/min or eGFR < 59 mL/min/1.73m^2) because of an increased risk of adverse effects, particularly neurological ones. Caution and monitoring of renal function are advised for patients with mild renal impairment (CrCl 50–80 mL/min or eGFR 60–89 mL/min/1.73m^2).

FINGOLIMOD
Trade names
Fingolis, Fingolimod, Filosir, Fingolimod Dr. Reddy's, Fingolimod Sandoz, Fingolimod Sun, Fingolimod-Teva, Fynod, Gilenya, Pharmacor Fingolimod

Available forms
Capsules: 0.25 mg, 0.5 mg

Action
- sphingosine 1-phosphate receptor modulator that is metabolised to active metabolite fingolimod phosphate
- binds to specific receptors on lymphocytes leading to a redistribution rather

than depletion of lymphocytes, reducing the infiltration into the CNS (and associated nerve inflammation and tissue damage)
- readily crosses blood—brain barrier

Use
- relapsing/remitting and secondary progressive multiple sclerosis (MS) (to delay disability and/or reduce number of relapses)

Dose
- 0.5 mg orally daily

Adverse effects
- headache, dizziness, migraine, paraesthesia, asthenia
- eczema, alopecia, pruritus, decreased weight
- diarrhoea
- cough, dyspnoea
- infection (influenza, sinusitis, bronchitis, herpes zoster, tinea)
- depression
- eye pain, blurred vision, decreased visual acuity, macular oedema
- back pain
- bradycardia, hypertension
- leucopenia, lymphopenia
- abnormal liver tests, increased liver enzymes, increased triglycerides
- (Rare) posterior reversible encephalopathy syndrome (PRES), progressive multifocal leukoencephalopathy (PML), lymphomas, skin cancers, seizures

Interactions
- contraindicated with Class Ia or Class III (amiodarone, sotalol) antiarrhythmic agents
- not recommended with digoxin, ivabradine, calcium-channel blockers (that lower heart rate) or beta adrenoreceptor blocking agents because of the risk of increased bradycardia
- caution if given with antineoplastic or immunosuppressive therapy (including corticosteroids) because of additive effects on immune system
- decreased serum levels may occur if given with carbamazepine
- not recommended with or within 2 months of live or live attenuated vaccines
- not recommended with citalopram, chlorpromazine, haloperidol, methadone or erythromycin because of an increased risk of QT prolongation and torsades de pointes
- not recommended with phototherapy with UV-B radiation or PUVA (psoralen and UVA) photochemotherapy

Nursing considerations/Cautions
- patient's immunity to varicella zoster virus (chicken pox, herpes zoster (shingles)) should be assessed (including serological testing) before starting therapy because the response to the virus may be severe if exposed and unprotected
- vaccination against human papilloma virus (HPV) is recommended before starting therapy
- any infection should be excluded or treated before starting therapy
- complete blood count and ophthalmologic examination (including visual acuity and fundus examination) should be performed before starting therapy. Ophthalmologic examination should be repeated after 3—4 months of therapy (especially in those with diabetes mellitus or a history of uveitis)
- an ECG is recommended before starting therapy (especially in those with pre-existing slow or irregular heartbeat, cardiac risk factors or taking medications with antiarrhythmic actions)
- (First-dose procedure) monitoring heart rate and BP hourly for 6 hours after initial dose is recommended, along with an ECG at the completion of the monitoring time. If the postprocedure ECG shows QTc interval prolongation (> 470 msec in female patients, > 450 msec in male patients), the patient should be monitored overnight in hospital setting
- after 6 hours, extra observation is required if the patient's heart rate < 45

MOVEMENT DISORDER AGENTS

- beats/min or if the ECG shows any new-onset second-degree or higher AV block
- first-dose procedure (as above) will need to be repeated if therapy is discontinued or interrupted for:
  - more than 2 weeks after first 4 weeks, or
  - 1 day or more in first 2 weeks, or
  - 7 days during weeks 3 and 4
- because of the very long half-life, the patient should be monitored for adverse effects (such as infection) for up to 8 weeks after stopping therapy
- if switching from other immunomodifying agents, the half-life and mode of action should be considered before starting therapy to avoid additive immunosuppression
- can be started immediately after interferons, glatiramer acetate or dimethyl fumerate are stopped
- not recommended after alemtuzumab
- allow an interval of 2–3 months after natalizumab
- accelerated elimination of teriflunomide is recommended (see p. 1387)
- if therapy is discontinued, patient should be closely monitored, as severe exacerbation of disease may occur within 12 weeks of stopping
- caution if used in those > 65 years or < 10 years
- caution if used in those with history of uveitis or diabetes mellitus because of the increased risk of macular oedema
- caution if used in those with a history of recurrent syncope, symptomatic bradycardia or QT prolongation (QTc > 470 msec (females), > 450 msec (males)) (cardiology advice is recommended before starting therapy)
- caution if used in those with severe liver disease
- not recommended in those with risk factors for QT prolongation, such as hypokalaemia, hypomagnesaemia or congenital QT prolongation
- not recommended in patients with ischaemic heart disease, a history of myocardial infarction or cardiac arrest, congestive heart failure, uncontrolled hypertension, cerebrovascular disease or untreated sleep apnoea
- contraindicated in those with SA block, second-degree AV block or higher, sick sinus syndrome (unless the patient has a pacemaker) or with QTc interval prolongation ($\geq$ 500 msec)
- contraindicated in those who, in the last 6 months, have experienced myocardial infarction, unstable angina, stroke, transient ischaemic attacks (TIAs), decompensated heart failure or Class III/IV heart failure requiring hospitalisation

Patient education

- the patient should be advised after first-dose procedure involving hourly heart rate and blood pressure monitoring for 6 hours with ECG at the end. This will need to be repeated if there is a break in therapy for any length of time
- warn the patient that their heart rate may slow down during therapy
- the patient should be advised not to drive or operate machinery if dizziness or visual disturbances occur
- caution the patient to avoid exposure to sunlight without protection and to have regular skin examinations during therapy
- advise the patient to seek medical advice immediately if any of the following occur:
  - changes to vision (e.g. centre of vision is blurry or has shadows, blindspot, difficulty seeing colour or fine details), especially in first 4 months of therapy
  - nausea, vomiting, abdominal pain, fatigue, loss of appetite, yellowing of skin or eyes, dark urine
  - sudden severe headache, nausea, vomiting, visual disturbances, fitting or altered mental state
  - any signs of infections including flu-like symptoms, fever, chills, sore throat, joint or aching muscles,

- cough (up to 8 weeks after stopping therapy)
- any new or changed skin lesions
- the patient and carer/partner should be advised to immediately report any unusual, worse or prolonged neurological symptoms, including difficulty performing mental tasks, unusual behaviour, confusion or personality changes (may be signs of PML or progression of MS)
- female patients of childbearing potential should be counselled to use effective contraception during and for at least 8 weeks after stopping therapy. If pregnancy occurs the patient should be advised to immediately seek medical advice. If the patient plans to become pregnant, therapy should be stopped for at least 8 weeks before conception
- live vaccines should be avoided during and up to two months after discontinuation

Capsules should not be crushed or opened; capsules should be swallowed whole to ensure proper dosing and maintain the drug's effectiveness.

Contraindicated; use effective contraception during treatment and for two months post-treatment because of potential fetal risks.

Excretion in breastmilk is unknown; therefore not recommended during breastfeeding.

Reduced hepatic function: monitor for liver enzyme elevations. Discontinue if significant liver injury is confirmed.

Caution if used in those over 65 years.

GLATIRAMER ACETATE
Trade names
Copaxone Pen, Copaxone Prefilled syringe, Glatira, Glatiramer Acetate-Teva

Available forms
Pen: 40 mg/mL;
Prefilled syringe: 20 mg/mL, 40 mg/mL

Action
- immunomodulator thought to modify the immune process responsible for pathogenesis of multiple sclerosis (MS)

Use
- relapsing remitting MS (to reduce frequency of relapses and delay progression)
- treatment of patients with a single clinical event and at least 2 silent brain lesions (confirmed on MRI) suggestive of MS

Dose
- 20 mg SC daily **OR**
- 40 mg SC 3 times weekly

Adverse effects
- mild injection site reactions (erythema, pain, inflammation, pruritus, oedema, mass)
- (Postinjection reaction) flushing, chest pain, palpitations, anxiety, dyspnoea, throat constriction, urticaria
- vasodilation
- tachycardia, palpitations, transient chest pain, hypertension
- visual field defects, diplopia
- infection (influenza, rhinitis, bronchitis, gastroenteritis, vaginal or oral candidiasis, herpes zoster)
- back pain
- syncope
- nausea, vomiting, dysphagia, increase in weight, enlarged salivary glands, tooth caries, bowel urgency, ulcerative stomatitis

MOVEMENT DISORDER AGENTS

- anxiety, tremor, asthenia, nervousness, migraine, abnormal dreams, emotional lability, stupor
- dyspnoea, cough, hyperventilation
- fever, chills
- pruritus, urticaria, rash, sweating, eczema
- lymphadenopathy
- peripheral oedema, facial oedema
- urinary urgency, impotence
- menorrhagia, amenorrhoea, haematuria, vaginal haemorrhage
- autobody development
- skin neoplasm (benign)
- (Rare) hypersensitivity, seizures, allergic reactions
- (Injection site, rare) lipoatrophy, necrosis

Nursing considerations/Cautions

- should not be given IV or IM
- for injection site management, rotate sites to minimise irritation and the risk of lipoatrophy
- should be discontinued only under medical supervision
- caution if used in those with a history of asthma, previous anaphylactoid reaction or kidney impairment
- contraindicated in those with known hypersensitivity to mannitol

Patient education

- instruct the patient/family member/carer in correct administration, including:
  - remove the pen or prefilled syringe from the refrigerator 20 minutes before injection and allow to come to room temperature before use (this reduces pain)
  - wash hands before administration
  - check the pen or prefilled syringe for any signs of particles or cloudiness (and do not use if these are present) and expiry date
  - the importance of rotating administration sites (abdomen (avoiding area 5 cm around navel), thighs (front, avoiding area 5 cm above knees and below groin), arms (fleshy area at back) and upper hips (below waist area)), and do not use the same site more than once per week
  - injection technique into fatty layer under skin (not into muscle); hold the syringe in dominant hand, similar to holding a pencil; pinch skin between thumb and index finger (about 5 cm fold); insert the needle and release skin fold; inject medication by pushing the plunger down until none remains; pull the syringe straight out; using a cotton wad, press down on the injection site but do not massage
  - (40 mg/mL) given 3 times per week with at least 48 hours between injections
  - dispose of the used syringe in an appropriate container, such as a hard-walled detergent container that has a lid and can be stored out of reach of children; when full, seek advice from doctor or pharmacist regarding correct disposal
  - prefilled syringes should only be used once
  - unused syringes should be stored in fridge, but not frozen
- advise the patient that postinjection reaction (reddening of face and/or neck, chest tightness, rapid heartbeat, anxiety and/or difficulty breathing) is transient, will pass quickly, generally does not require treatment and usually occurs several months after start of therapy

Caution: animal studies show no harm to fetal development. However, limited human data mean glatiramer acetate should be used in pregnancy only if benefits outweigh potential risks.

Excretion in human milk is unknown. Its low oral absorption suggests minimal exposure to the infant, but caution is advised. Consider the benefits of breastfeeding alongside potential risks.

Reduced hepatic function: cases of severe liver injury, including hepatitis and liver failure, have been reported. Pretreatment liver function tests are recommended, with periodic monitoring. Discontinue use if signs of liver injury appear.

NATALIZUMAB
Trade name
Tysabri

Available form
Ampoules: 300 mg/15 mL;
Prefilled syringe: 150 mg/mL

Action
- IgG$_4$ humanised monoclonal antibody that binds to alpha4 integrin found on leucocyte (except neutrophil) cell surface, preventing migration of leucocytes into inflamed parenchymal tissue

Use
- relapsing remitting multiple sclerosis (MS) (to reduce frequency of relapses and delay progression)

Dose
- 300 mg SC every 4 weeks (given as two SC injections, administered no more than 30 minutes apart) **OR**
- 300 mg by IV infusion over 1 hour every 4 weeks

Adverse effects
- headache, fatigue, depression, somnolence, vertigo, dizziness
- arthralgia, muscle cramp, joint swelling, pain in extremities
- rigors, fever
- diarrhoea, abdominal pain/discomfort, nausea, vomiting, weight increase or decrease
- rash, dermatitis, pruritus, night sweating, urticaria
- irregular menstruation, dysmenorrhoea, amenorrhoea, ovarian cyst
- chest discomfort
- infection (urinary tract infection, lower respiratory tract infection, tonsillitis, gastroenteritis, vaginitis, tooth infection, herpes encephalitis, herpes meningitis, acute retinal necrosis)
- development of antibodies (transient or persistent)
- increased liver enzymes, elevated bilirubin, liver injury
- nasopharyngitis
- infusion-related reaction (headache, dizziness, fatigue, rigors, localised or generalised hypersensitivity reaction)
- (SC) injection site pain, reaction
- progressive multifocal leukoencephalopathy (PML) (an opportunistic viral brain infection which may lead to death or disability), immune reconstitution inflammatory syndrome (IRIS) if therapy is stopped due to PML, John Cunningham virus (JCV) granule cell neuronopathy

Interactions
- contraindicated with beta interferons, glatiramer acetate or other antineoplastic or immunosuppressive agents because of the increased risk of opportunistic infection and PML

Nursing considerations/Cautions
- therapy should be started in centre with MRI facilities and under the supervision of a neurologist
- antibody testing for JCV is recommended before starting therapy (using a JCV antibody assay) and repeated 6-monthly in negative patients or in positive patients with lower index values
- a recent (within 3 months) MRI scan is required before starting therapy, and then repeated yearly. The scan would assist in differentiating between PML symptoms and MS. More frequent MRI is recommended in those at higher risk of PML (i.e. having all 3 risk factors; having anti-JVC antibody index > 1.5 without prior immunosuppression and > 2 years on therapy)
- therapy should be interrupted if PML is suspected. A new MRI scan may be necessary to compare pre- and post-therapy. Other tests include

MOVEMENT DISORDER AGENTS

- neurological assessment and testing the CSF for John Cunningham viral DNA
- therapy must not be resumed if the patient has PML or develops an opportunistic infection
- FBC and liver function tests are recommended in those with active or a history of liver disease
- natalizumab remains in the blood for up to 12 weeks after the last dose
- the patient should be re-evaluated by a neurologist 3 months after the first infusion, 6 months after the first infusion and then at 6-month intervals
- testing for persistent antibodies is recommended if the patient has had a long interruption (12 weeks or more) to therapy and has had antibodies detected twice, 6 weeks apart. Persistent antibodies are related to a decrease in treatment effectiveness
- if plasma exchange procedure is performed, an interval of 14 days should be allowed before serum anti-JVC antibody testing
- (SC) administration sites include thigh, abdomen or posterior side of upper arm, avoiding any areas that are bruised, irritated scarred or infection. Second SC injection should be at least 2.5 cm from first site
- patient should be monitored during and for 1 hour after infusion for any signs of infusion-related reaction or SC administration
- dilute in 100 mL sodium chloride 0.9%, invert gently (do not shake) and infuse over 1 hour
- not recommended by IV bolus or IV push
- administer alone
- risk of hypersensitivity is increased early in therapy and if the patient is re-exposed to therapy after being stopped (short course e.g. 3 infusions) and a long period (over 12 weeks) without treatment
- caution if used in those with liver disease. If used, liver function should be closely monitored during therapy
- contraindicated in those with or who have had PML, with a murine hypersensitivity or at high risk of opportunistic infection, HIV, organ transplant or active malignancy, or who are immunocompromised

Patient education

- before starting therapy, the patient should be advised of the importance of continuing therapy uninterrupted, especially at the start. The neurologist is required to obtain individual, written, fully informed consent from the patient or legal guardian to the use of natalizumab and the possible adverse effects (PML, opportunistic infection)
- warn the patient not to drive or operate machinery if dizziness or vertigo occurs
- the patient should be advised to wear a MedicAlert bracelet and carry a Patient Alert Card outlining the risks of PML
- the patient and carer/partner should be advised to seek medical advice immediately if any of the following occur:
  - unusual, worse or prolonged neurological symptoms, including difficulty performing mental tasks, unusual behaviour, confusion and personality changes
  - severe or prolonged symptoms of infection, including prolonged dizziness, unexplained fever, severe diarrhoea, headache, stiff neck, weight loss or listlessness
  - decreased visual acuity, eye redness, painful eye

Avoid natalizumab crosses the placenta and may affect the fetus's blood cells. Monitoring for blood abnormalities is recommended in newborns exposed to natalizumab in utero.

Natalizumab is excreted in human milk. Due to the potential for serious adverse reactions in infants, breastfeeding is not recommended.

OCRELIZUMAB
Trade name
Ocrevus

Available form
Vial: 300 mg/10 mL

Action
* recombinant humanised monoclonal antibody
* selectively targets CD-20 expressing B cells, reducing their number and function
* terminal half-life 26 days

Use
* treatment of patients with relapsing multiple sclerosis (MS) to delay progression of physical disability and reduce frequency of relapses
* treatment of primary progressive MS to delay progression of physical disability

Dose
* 600 mg IV every 6 months, given as:
  * (initial dose) initially, 300 mg IV given at 30 mL/hour, then 2 weeks later, 300 mg IV starting at 30 mL/hour and increasing rate every 30 minutes by 30 mL/hour to a maximum of 180 mL/hour, then
  * (subsequent doses) 600 mg IV starting at 40 mL/hour, then increasing every 30 minutes by 40 mL/hour to a maximum of 200 mL/hour

Adverse effects
* infusion-related reactions
* infections (upper respiratory tract infection, nasopharyngitis, sinusitis, bronchitis, influenza, gastroenteritis, oral herpes, viral infection, herpes zoster, conjunctivitis, cellulitis)
* cough, increased sputum
* neutropenia
* (Rare) increased risk of malignancy, progressive multifocal leukoencephalopathy (PML)

Interactions
* not recommended with immunosuppressive agents (except corticosteroids) because of the increased risk of serious infections
* not recommended with other disease-modifying MS therapies
* not recommended with live or live attenuated vaccines

Nursing considerations/Cautions
* any active infection should be treated before starting therapy
* the patient should be screened for hepatitis B virus (HBV), as reactivation can occur during therapy. If the patient has active HBV, therapy should not be started. If the patient has positive serology (negative for hepatitis B surface antigen, positive for HB core antibody and carriers of HBV), they should consult a liver disease expert before starting therapy and be monitored closely if therapy occurs
* immunisation should be complete and up to date 6 weeks before starting therapy
* because hypotension can occur as part of infusion-related reactions, consideration should be given to withholding any antihypertension medication 12 hours before each infusion
* the patient should be premedicated with 100 mg IV methylprednisolone (or equivalent) about 30 minutes before infusion, along with antihistamine (given 30—60 minutes before infusion). An antipyretic may also be administered with antihistamine
* not given as IV push or bolus
* initial infusions given over about 2.5 hours; subsequent infusions administered over 3.5 hours
* initial infusions (300 mg) diluted in 250 mL sodium chloride 0.9% and subsequent infusions (600 mg) diluted in 500 mL sodium chloride 0.9%
* observe the patient for at least 1 hour after infusion is completed for any symptoms of infusion-related reactions (which can occur within 24 hours of infusion but more commonly during first infusion):

MOVEMENT DISORDER AGENTS

- if a life-threatening (e.g. bronchospasm, asthma exacerbation) reaction occurs, the infusion should be stopped and the patient treated using supportive therapies. Therapy should be discontinued permanently
- if a serious reaction (e.g. flushing, fever, throat pain) occurs, the infusion should be stopped and the patient receive symptomatic treatment. The infusion can be restarted when symptoms have totally resolved at a rate half the infusion rate when the reaction occurred
- if a mild-to-moderate reaction (e.g. headache) occurs, the infusion rate should be reduced to half that at onset of symptom and this rate maintained for at least 30 minutes. If tolerated, the infusion rate can be increased according to the patient's original infusion schedule

Patient education

- the patient should be warned that infusion-related reactions (e.g. rash, pruritus, flushing, throat irritation, oropharyngeal pain, shortness of breath, flushing, fever, fatigue, dizziness, headache) can occur within 24 hours of infusion they should seek medical attention immediately if any reaction occurs
- the patient and carer/partner should be advised to seek medical advice immediately if any of the following occur:
  - unusual, worse or prolonged neurological symptoms, including difficulty performing mental tasks, unusual behaviour, confusion, personality changes (signs of PML or worsening MS)
  - any signs of infection including fever, chills, swollen glands and fatigue
- women of childbearing potential should be counselled to use effective contraception during therapy and for 6 months after the last infusion

 Avoid during pregnancy unless the benefits outweigh the risks. Effective contraception is recommended during treatment and for 6 months postinfusion.

 Avoid, as unknown whether excreted in human breastmilk.

OFATUMUMAB
Trade name
Kesimpta

Available forms
Pre-filled syringe/pen: 20 mg/0.4 mL

Action
- recombinant human anti-CD20 monoclonal antibody (IgG$_1$)

Use
- relapsing forms of multiple sclerosis (to reduce frequency of relapse and delay progression of physical disability)

Dose
- 20 mg SC weekly for 3 weeks, then 20 mg SC monthly

Adverse effects
- (Injection-related reactions) fever, chills, headache, myalgia, fatigue, rash, urticaria, dyspnoea, angioedema
- (Injection site) redness, pain, itching, swelling
- nasopharyngitis, flu-like illness
- urinary tract infection
- back pain, muscle weakness
- constipation
- fever
- anxiety
- (Rare) progressive multifocal leukoencephalopathy, reactivation of hepatitis B, hypersensitivity

Interactions
- immunisation with live or live attenuated vaccines should be completed at least 4 weeks before starting therapy

- immunisation with inactivated vaccines should be completed at least 2 weeks before starting therapy
- not recommended with other immunosuppressants except corticosteroids for symptomatic management of relapses

Nursing considerations/Cautions

- the patient can be taught self-administration, with the first injection administered under medical supervision
- screening for hepatitis B virus (HBV) is recommended before starting therapy
- not recommended if the patient is severely immunocompromised or has an active malignancy, or if active infection is present

Patient education

- warn the patient that injection-related reactions commonly occur with the first injection
- the patient can be taught to self administer including:
  - when injections are due
  - injection technique under skin
  - importance of rotation of SC injection sites
  - correct storage and safe disposal of pen/syringe
- females of childbearing potential should be counselled to use effective contraception during and for 4 months after stopping therapy
- counsel the patient that, if pregnancy occurs during therapy, the infant should not receive live or live attenuated vaccines until B-cell counts have reached the lower limit of normal, as there is an increased risk of receiving these vaccines. The child can receive inactivated vaccines

Not recommended during pregnancy unless benefits to the mother outweigh risks to the fetus. Transient peripheral B-cell depletion and lymphocytopenia has been observed in infants born to mothers exposed to anti-CD20 antibodies during pregnancy.

Unknown whether ofatumumab is transferred to breastmilk.

OZANIMOD

Trade names
Zeposia, Zeposia – Initiation Pack

Available forms
Capsule: 230 microgram, 460 microgram, 920 microgram

Action
- sphingosine 1-phosphate (S1P) receptor modulators
- modulates S1P receptors 1 and 5, causing lymphocyte retention in lymph nodes
- reduces peripheral lymphocyte count, limiting migration to CNS and intestines, reducing inflammation and demyelination

Use
- treatment of adult patients with relapsing multiple sclerosis (MS)
- treatment of adult patients with moderately to severely active ulcerative colitis

Dose
- initial dose escalation over 7 days, starting at 230 micrograms daily and reaching 920 micrograms on day 8, followed by 920 micrograms once daily

Adverse effects
- headache
- nasopharyngitis
- hypertension
- back pain
- lymphopenia
- increased liver enzymes (alanine aminotransferase (ALT), gamma glutamyltransferase (GGT))
- risk of infections (e.g. herpes, respiratory tract infection; may be serious)
- macular oedema
- bradycardia on initiation
- basal cell carcinoma
- slight reduction in lung function tests

Interactions
- increased risk of immunosuppression when combined with immunomodulatory or antineoplastic agents
- avoid strong CYP2C8 inducers (e.g. rifampicin); caution with CYP2C8 inhibitors (e.g. gemfibrozil)

Nursing considerations/Cautions
- monitor liver function and CBC, including lymphocytes, before initiation and regularly during treatment
- consider cardiac monitoring in those with pre-existing heart conditions
- use with caution in patients with hepatic impairment; contraindicated in severe hepatic impairment
- has active metabolites; effects may last for 3 months after stopping treatment

Patient education
- advise against live vaccines during and up to 3 months post-treatment
- report symptoms of infections or liver dysfunction (e.g. jaundice, fatigue)
- if a dose is missed, do not take two doses on the same day. Resume with the next scheduled dose
- limit sun exposure and use sunscreen, as basal cell carcinoma is a possible risk
- patients with diabetes or uveitis should report any vision changes; an eye exam may be recommended

Take capsule whole with or without food; do not crush or open.

Women of childbearing age should use effective contraception and avoid pregnancy during and for 3 months post-treatment because of the potential fetal risk.

Not recommended in breastfeeding because of risks to the infant.

Reduced hepatic function: Ozanimod may be used with caution in cases of mild-to-moderate hepatic impairment (Child—Pugh class A or B). These patients should follow a modified dosing regimen, completing the 7-day dose escalation but taking the maintenance dose of 920 micrograms every other day instead of daily. Additionally, close monitoring of liver function is recommended. It is not recommended for patients with severe hepatic impairment (Child—Pugh class C) because of the lack of safety data and potential risks associated with impaired metabolism and clearance.

SIPONIMOD
Trade name
Mayzent

Available forms
Tablets: 0.25 mg, 1 mg, 2 mg

Action
- selective immunosuppressant
- sphingosine 1-phosphate receptor modulator that is metabolised to the active metabolite fingolimod phosphate
- binds to specific receptors on lymphocytes, leading to a redistribution rather than depletion of lymphocytes, reducing the infiltration into the CNS (and associated nerve inflammation and tissue damage)
- readily crosses blood—brain barrier
- reduces lymphocyte migration into CNS to limit inflammation

Use
- treatment of secondary progressive multiple sclerosis (SPMS)

Dose
- (Titration) start at 0.25 mg once daily, increasing over 5 days to 2 mg daily maintenance dose
  - adjust to 1 mg daily for patients with CYP2C923 or 13 genotype
- (Maintenance) 2 mg once daily or 1 mg once daily based on genotype

Adverse effects
- (Common) headache, hypertension, liver enzyme elevation, bradycardia, AV block, macular oedema, lymphopenia
- dizziness, asthenia, tremor, seizures

- diarrhoea, nausea
- change in lung function
- infection (herpes zoster)
- eye pain, blurred vision, decreased visual acuity
- pain in extremity
- (Serious) progressive multifocal leukoencephalopathy (PML), cryptococcal meningitis, herpes viral infections
- (Rare) posterior reversible encephalopathy syndrome (PRES), lymphomas, skin cancers

Interactions

- avoid with Class Ia and III antiarrhythmic drugs, QT-prolonging drugs, CYP2C9/CYP3A4 inducers and inhibitors
- caution with beta blockers, drugs that lower heart rate and immunosuppressants
- caution if given with antineoplastic or immunosuppressive therapy (including corticosteroids) owing to additive effects on immune system
- not recommended with or within 1 month of live or live attenuated vaccines
- not recommended after therapy with alemtuzumab (unless benefits clearly outweigh risks)

Nursing considerations/Cautions

- check liver function before starting; monitor liver enzymes periodically
- before starting therapy, the patient's CYP2C9 genotype should be determined
- an ECG is recommended before starting therapy (especially in those with pre-existing slow or irregular heartbeat, cardiac risk factors or taking medications with antiarrhythmic actions)
- monitor for infection signs
- avoid live vaccines during treatment
- screen for varicella immunity and complete vaccination prior if not immune
- perform ophthalmic evaluations for patients with a history of diabetes or uveitis
- (First-dose procedure for those with sinus bradycardia, AV block or history of myocardial infarction or heart failure) monitoring heart rate and BP hourly for 6 hours after initial dose is recommended, along with an ECG at the completion of the monitoring time
- if one dose is missed during the titration period (days 1 to 6) or if therapy is interrupted for 4 or more days, the titration regimen needs to be restarted
- if switching from other immunomodifying agents, half-life and mode of action should be considered before starting therapy to avoid additive immunosuppression. Remains in blood for up to 10 days
- if therapy is discontinued, the patient should be closely monitored, as severe exacerbation of disease may occur
- caution if used in those with a history of recurrent syncope or symptomatic bradycardia
- caution if used in those with asthma
- not recommended in those with risk factors for QT prolongation such as hypokalaemia, hypomagnesaemia or congenital QT prolongation
- not recommended in patients with a history of myocardial infarction or cardiac arrest, congestive heart failure, uncontrolled hypertension, cerebrovascular disease or untreated sleep apnoea
- not recommended in those with SA block, second-degree AV block or higher, sick sinus syndrome (unless the patient has a pacemaker) or with QTc interval prolongation (≥ 500 msec)

Patient education

- increases skin cancer risk: advise the patient to avoid excessive sunlight, use high-SPF sunscreen, wear protective clothing and monitor skin for changes in skin lesions, reporting concerns promptly
- advise the patient not to stop medicine abruptly, but taper as directed to avoid disease rebound

MOVEMENT DISORDER AGENTS

- advise the patient they can take with or without food
- advise the patient that after-first-dose procedure involves hourly heart rate and blood pressure monitoring for 6 hours with ECG at the end
- warn the patient that their heart rate may slow down during therapy
- the patient should be advised not to drive or operate machinery if dizziness or visual disturbances occur
- advise the patient to seek medical advice immediately if any of the following occur:
  - changes to vision (e.g. centre of vision is blurry or has shadows, blindspot, difficulty seeing colour or fine details), especially in first 4 months of therapy
  - nausea, vomiting, abdominal pain, fatigue, loss of appetite, yellowing of skin or eyes, dark urine
  - sudden severe headache, nausea, vomiting, visual disturbances, fitting or altered mental state
  - any signs of infections including flu-like symptoms, fever, chills, sore throat, joint or aching muscles, cough (up to 8 weeks after stopping therapy)
- the patient and carer/partner should be advised to immediately report any unusual, worse or prolonged neurological symptoms, including difficulty performing mental tasks, unusual behaviour, confusion or personality changes (may be signs of PML or progression of MS)
- female patients of childbearing potential should be counselled to use effective contraception during and for at least 10 days after stopping therapy. If pregnancy occurs the patient should be advised to immediately seek medical advice

Do not crush or split tablets. Tablets must be swallowed whole with water to ensure proper dosing and efficacy.

Contraindicated, as may harm the fetus. Advise effective contraception for women of childbearing potential during and for 10 days after discontinuing treatment. Use in pregnancy only if potential benefits justify potential risks.

Avoid, as excretion in human milk is unknown.

TERIFLUNOMIDE

Trade names
APO-Teriflunomide, Pharmacor Teriflunomide, Teriflagio, Teriflunomide Dr. Reddy's, Teriflunomide GH, Teriflunomide Sandoz, Terimide

Available form
Tablets: 14 mg

Action
- immunomodulator that selectively and reversibly inhibits dihydroorotate dehydrogenase needed for pyrimidine synthesis, thereby blocking the activation and proliferation of stimulated lymphocytes. This is thought to reduce the number of activated lymphocytes which can migrate into the CNS
- long terminal half-life (about 19 days)

Use
- relapsing remitting multiple sclerosis (MS) (to reduce frequency of relapses and delay progression)

Dose
- 14 mg orally daily

Adverse effects
- nausea, vomiting, diarrhoea, upper abdominal pain, toothache
- paraesthesia
- palpitations, hypertension
- alopecia, rash
- musculoskeletal pain, myalgia, arthralgia
- menorrhagia
- elevated liver enzymes, elevated creatine phosphokinase
- neutropenia

- influenza, sinusitis
- (Rare) severe liver injury, thrombocytopenia, interstitial lung disease, peripheral neuropathy, pancreatitis, severe skin reactions, hypersensitivity

Interactions

- caution if switching from one immuno-modifying agent to another, as added haemotoxicity may occur
- not recommended with or within 6 months of live or live attenuated vaccines
- serum levels may be reduced if given with carbamazepine, phenobarbital (phenobarbitone), rifampicin, phenytoin or St John's wort, and should therefore be given with caution
- may increase serum levels of paclitaxel, pioglitazone, repaglinide, rosiglitazone, rosuvastatin, methotrexate, topotecan, sulfasalazine, daunorubicin, doxorubicin, atorvastatin, simvastatin, pravastatin or rifampicin
- caution if used with cefaclor, penicillin G, ciprofloxacin, indometacin, ketoprofen, furosemide (frusemide), methotrexate or zidovudine
- may decrease serum levels of caffeine, duloxetine, ondansetron, theophylline or agomelatine
- may decrease INR if given with warfarin; therefore careful monitoring is recommended
- caution if given with NSAIDs because of added hepatotoxicity

Nursing considerations/Cautions

- FBC (including differential WBC count and platelets) and liver function tests (alanine aminotransferase (ALT), aspartate aminotransferase (AST) and bilirubin) should be measured before starting therapy, then monthly for 6 months, then 6–8-weekly if stable
- if liver enzyme levels are more than 3 times normal, therapy should be stopped and colestyramine or activated charcoal administered to reduce levels rapidly. If levels are mildly or moderately elevated 2–4-weekly monitoring is recommended
- blood pressure should be measured before starting therapy and then regularly during therapy
- all patients should be carefully screened for history or symptoms of acute or chronic infection (including pneumonia, urinary tract infection), tuberculosis (TB) or hepatitis, including detailed medical history and possible previous exposure to TB. Before starting therapy, any infection should be treated
- if switching from another MS medication to teriflunomide, the following are recommended:
  - interferon beta or glatiramer acetate: no waiting period is required
  - fingolimod: a 6-week interval should be allowed between discontinuing fingolimod for clearance and 4–8 weeks for lymphocyte recovery before starting teriflunomide
  - natalizumab: caution if switching as natalizumab has a very long half-life and will cause added effects on the immune system for 2–3 months if natalizumab is discontinued and teriflunomide started immediately
- pregnancy must be excluded before starting therapy. Therapy should be started only if effective contraception is being used in females of childbearing potential
- (Accelerated elimination procedure) if rapid elimination is required, an 11-day program of either colestyramine (4 g 3 times a day or 8 g 3 times a day) or activated charcoal (50 g twice daily) is recommended, with colestyramine being faster to reduce levels. The choice between the three procedures is dependent on patient tolerability. The 11 days do not need to be consecutive unless rapid elimination is needed. Plasma levels should be measured and verified on two separate tests 14 days apart and be ≤ 0.02 mg/L to reduce risk

MOVEMENT DISORDER AGENTS

- caution if used in those with history of interstitial lung disease or kidney impairment
- not recommended in those under 18 or over 65 years
- contraindicated in those with hypersensitivity to leflunomide
- contraindicated in those with severe immunodeficiency (e.g. AIDS), significant bone marrow impairment, significant anaemia, leucopenia or thrombocytopenia, severe uncontrolled infections, severe hypoproteinaemia or severe liver function impairment
- contraindicated in those who have (or have had) Stevens—Johnson syndrome, toxic epidermal necrolysis or erythema multiforme

Patient education

- the patient should be advised to seek medical advice immediately if any of the following occur:
  - unexplained nausea and vomiting, abdominal pain, fatigue, loss of appetite, yellowing of eyes or skin, dark urine
  - any signs of infection including unexplained fever, chills, aching muscles or joints, cough
  - any skin or mucosal reactions
  - bilateral numbness or tingling of hands or feet
  - cough, shortness of breath, with/without fever
- warn the patient that, if accelerated elimination procedure is used, disease activity may potentially return
- women of childbearing potential should be counselled to use effective contraception during therapy and notify the doctor immediately if pregnancy is suspected. If pregnancy occurs, an accelerated elimination procedure should be performed to lower plasma levels to $\leq$ 0.02 mg/L

 Teriflunomide tablets are film coated and should not be crushed, as altering the tablet may affect drug release and absorption.

Tablets should not be crushed by pregnant staff. If crushing the tablet, gloves and eye protection must be worn and closed pill crusher used.

 Teriflunomide is contraindicated in pregnancy because of the teratogenic effects. It must not be used in women who are pregnant or planning to conceive without ensuring a safe washout period or using reliable contraception until the drug is fully cleared from the body.

Women planning pregnancy should ensure teriflunomide plasma levels are below 0.02 mg/L or undergo a washout procedure with cholestyramine or activated charcoal to accelerate elimination.

 Contraindicated: teriflunomide is excreted into animal milk and poses potential serious adverse reactions in infants.

 Reduced hepatic function: mild-to-moderate hepatic impairment requires no dose adjustment. Contraindicated in patients with severe hepatic impairment because of the risk of life-threatening hepatotoxicity.

INTERFERONS

General Actions of interferons

- naturally occurring, small protein molecules produced and secreted by cells in response to viral infections or to various synthetic and biological inducers
- bind to specific cell surface receptors that are linked to inner cell networks that control enzyme activity, cell proliferation and immune activity enhancement (e.g. inhibit viral replication in virus-infected cells, enhance activity of macrophages and lymphocytes)
- there are three main forms of interferons: interferon alpha (IFN-α) and interferon beta (IFN-β), classified as type I interferons, which are primarily involved in antiviral defence and modulation of the immune response.

Interferon gamma (IFN-γ), classified as a type II interferon, plays a critical role in immune regulation and activation of macrophages, enhancing the body's defence against various pathogens.
- produced by recombinant DNA technology

General Adverse effects of interferons
- flu-like symptoms (including fever, malaise, chills, sweating, fatigue, myalgia, loss of appetite, headache)
- malaise, fatigue, asthenia, insomnia, dizziness, depression, confusion, vertigo
- fever, chills
- headache, migraine
- nausea, vomiting, anorexia, diarrhoea, abdominal pain, constipation, weight change
- sinusitis, dyspnoea, rhinitis, cough, upper respiratory tract infection, bronchitis, nasopharyngitis
- anaemia, leucopenia, thrombocytopenia, neutropenia
- elevated liver enzymes, hypertriglyceridaemia
- transient mild skin rash, reversible alopecia, sweating/flushing
- arthralgia, myalgia, back pain, musculoskeletal weakness, pain and/or stiffness, pain in extremities, muscle spasm
- palpitations, chest pain, oedema
- menorrhagia, metrorrhagia
- cystitis, urinary frequency, urinary tract infection
- (Uncommon) serum neutralising antibodies
- (Rare) hypersensitivity reaction (including bronchospasm, urticaria, anaphylaxis, angioedema), suicidal ideation, liver injury, seizures, thyroid dysfunction, nephrotic syndrome, thrombotic microangiopathy (thrombotic thrombocytopenia purpura, haemolytic anaemia)
- (Injection site) pain, swelling, redness, pruritus, haematoma
- (Rare) injection site necrosis

General Interactions of interferons
- caution if given with agents with narrow therapeutic index
- caution if given with another myelosuppressive agent
- caution if used with other agents that are hepatotoxic including alcohol
- not recommended with other immuno-modifying agents

General Nursing considerations/Cautions for interferons
- treatment should be started and supervised by a neurologist experienced in management of multiple sclerosis (MS)
- monitor blood cell counts (with WBC differential, platelet count), thyroid and liver function before starting therapy, then at monthly or appropriate intervals during treatment
- paracetamol 0.5—1 g can be taken orally 30 minutes before administration of interferon to alleviate symptoms of fever and headache, then up to 1 g 4 times daily
- chest X-ray is recommended if the patient develops a cough, dyspnoea or other respiratory symptoms
- any persistent fever should be investigated thoroughly
- all patients should be monitored for any signs of depression or suicidal ideation
- the patient should be monitored for any signs of nephrotic syndrome, including proteinuria, oedema and changes in kidney function
- if the patient develops seizures, therapy should be stopped and aetiology of seizures established
- at the discretion of the doctor, the patient may be educated to self-administer medication
- first self-administered injection should be done under supervision
- when reconstituting solution, care should be taken to avoid foaming or shaking the solution when dissolving
- administer alone

MOVEMENT DISORDER AGENTS

- caution if used in those with severe bone marrow suppression because of the increased risk of infection and/or bleeding
- caution if used in those with a history of seizures (especially if not well controlled), or of liver disease or active liver disease
- caution if used in those with kidney impairment (kidney function should be monitored regularly)
- caution if used in those with cardiac disorders such as angina, congestive cardiac failure or arrhythmias (cardiac function should be closely monitored)
- contraindicated in those with severe depression and/or suicidal ideation
- contraindicated in those with hypersensitivity to interferons (natural or recombinant), autoimmune disease

General Patient education for interferons

- patients should be advised not to drive or operate machinery if adverse effects such as dizziness, confusion, somnolence, visual disturbance or fatigue occur
- advise the patient that flu-like syndrome usually occurs within hours to days of injection
- the patient should be advised to report any skin breaks, swelling, pain, fluid drainage or multiple sores at the injection sites, as this may require a temporary stopping of therapy until the skin heals. Therapy may continue if a single sore exists and skin cell death (necrosis) is small
- instruct the patient/family member/carer in correct administration, including:
  - self-administration instructions including importance of aseptic technique
  - ensure the patient/family member/carer is clear about the route (SC or IM)
  - importance of rotation of SC injection sites (abdomen, thigh, upper outer arm) and not using areas that show any signs of redness, scarring
  - if the vial of powder and diluent (water for injections) are required to be mixed, this must be done carefully and according to instructions, especially not shaking the solution to mix it
  - not mixing anything else in the same syringe with the interferon
- advise the patient to seek medical advice immediately if any of the following occur:
  - nausea, vomiting, abdominal pain, itchiness, yellowing of eyes or skin, dark urine
  - feelings of sadness, anxiety, nervousness or hopelessness, getting upset easily, or having thoughts of hurting yourself or suicide
  - skin reactions, including any swelling or drainage at injection site
  - swelling of feet or legs, shortness of breath, irregular heartbeat
  - signs of frequent infections such as fever, sore throat, unusual bleeding or bruising
- women of childbearing potential should be counselled to use adequate and effective contraception to avoid pregnancy during therapy

 Avoid, as excretion in human breastmilk unknown.

INTERFERON BETA-1a
Trade name
Avonex

Available form
Prefilled syringe: 30 microgram (6 million IU)/0.5 mL

Action
- interferon beta-1a
- see also General Actions of interferons (p. 1389)

Use

- relapsing/remitting multiple sclerosis (MS)
- single demyelinating event at risk of progression to clinical MS (based on MRI)
- secondary progressive MS with continuous relapse, or relapse in last 12 months

Dose

- (Relapsing/remitting MS, single demyelinating event) initially 1.5 million (7.5 micrograms) IU IM weekly (week 1), then 3.0 million (15 micrograms) IU IM (week 2), 4.5 million (22.5 micrograms) IU IM (week 3), then 6 million (30 micrograms) IU IM (week 4) and thereafter **OR**
- (Secondary progressive MS with recent or continuing relapse) 12 million (60 micrograms) IU IM weekly

Adverse effects/Interactions

- see General Adverse effects and Interactions of interferons (p. 1390)

Nursing considerations/Cautions

- (Secondary progressive MS) not recommended unless relapse is continuous or has occurred in last 12 months
- (Avonex) not recommended SC
- not recommended in those under 12 or over 65 years
- contraindicated in those with hypersensitivity to any interferon beta (natural or recombinant) or albumin
- see also General Nursing considerations/Cautions for interferons (p. 1390)

Patient education

- see General Patient education for interferons (p. 1391), along with some extra information regarding the specific injection devices:
  - allow syringes to come to room temperature for at least 30 minutes before administration to reduce pain
  - Avonex is available as a prefilled syringe with needle that needs to be attached before administration IM (either thigh or arm)

Avoid, as potential abortifacient effects observed in animal studies. Women of childbearing potential should use appropriate contraceptive measures.

Avoid, as excretion in human breastmilk unknown.

Reduced renal function: caution is advised in patients with severe renal impairment, as clearance of the drug may be impacted. Regular monitoring of renal function is recommended during therapy.

Reduced hepatic function: use with caution. Liver function tests are recommended before and during treatment, and discontinuation should be considered if hepatic enzyme levels significantly increase.

Elderly patients may require closer monitoring, particularly for adverse effects like flu-like symptoms, liver function changes, or worsening of pre-existing conditions.

INTERFERON BETA-1b

Trade name
Betaferon

Available form
Vial: 8 million IU (0.3 mg)

Action

- interferon beta-1b
- see also General Actions of interferons (p. 1389)

Use

- treatment of single event suggestive of multiple sclerosis (MS) (with 2 lesions proven on magnetic resonance imaging (MRI))
- relapsing remitting MS (2 attacks in 2 years with recovery intervals)
- reduction in frequency and severity of relapses in those with secondary progressive MS

Dose

- (Single event suggestive of MS) initially 2 million IU SC every second day for 3 doses (days 1, 3, 5), 4 million IU SC for 3

MOVEMENT DISORDER AGENTS

doses (days 7, 9, 11), 6 million IU SC for 3 doses (days 13, 15, 17) then 8 million IU every second day **OR**
- (Relapsing MS, secondary progressive MS) 8 million IU SC every second day

Adverse effects
- hypertension
- dysmenorrhoea, intermenstrual bleeding
- conjunctivitis, abnormal vision
- (Rare) systemic capillary leak syndrome (with shock-like symptoms and fatal outcomes), pancreatitis
- see also General Adverse effects of interferons (p. 1390)

Interactions
- see General Interactions of interferons (p. 1390)

Nursing considerations/Cautions

- to reconstitute, connect the vial adapter to the vial with attached needle, then connect the prefilled syringe containing diluent and inject 1.2 mL into the vial and dissolve powder gently without shaking. Resultant solution should be clear to light yellow. Withdraw 1 mL of reconstituted solution
- contains human plasma; therefore theoretical risk exists for transmission of Creutzfeldt–Jakob disease (CJD) and viral diseases
- caution if used in those with pre-existing monoclonal gammopathy because of the increased risk of systemic capillary leak syndrome
- not recommended in those under 18 years
- contraindicated in those with hypersensitivity to any interferon (natural or recombinant), mannitol or albumin
- see also General Nursing considerations/Cautions for interferons (p. 1390)

Patient education
- see General Patient education for interferons (p. 1391) with modification to syringe preparation for SC administration

Avoid, as potential abortifacient effects observed in animal studies. Women of childbearing potential should use appropriate contraceptive measures.

Avoid, as excretion in human breastmilk unknown.

Reduced renal function: caution is advised in patients with severe renal impairment, as clearance of the drug may be impacted. Regular monitoring of renal function is recommended during therapy.

Reduced hepatic function: use with caution. Liver function tests are recommended before and during treatment, and discontinuation should be considered if hepatic enzyme levels significantly increase.

Elderly patients may require closer monitoring, particularly for adverse effects like flu-like symptoms, liver function changes or worsening of pre-existing conditions.

PEGINTERFERON BETA-1a
Trade name
Plegridy

Available forms
Prefilled pen: 63 microgram/0.5 mL, 94 microgram/0.5 mL, 125 microgram/0.5 mL

Action
- combination (termed pegylated) of recombinant interferon beta-1a and monomethoxy polyethylene glycol (PEG reagent)
- prolonged half-life compared with non-pegylated interferon beta-1a

Use
- treatment of remitting relapsing multiple sclerosis (MS)

Dose
- initially 63 micrograms SC, then 94 micrograms SC 2 weeks later, followed by 125 micrograms SC after a further 2 weeks, then continued at 125 micrograms SC every 2 weeks

Adverse effects/Interactions
- see General Adverse effects and Interactions of interferons (p. 1390)

Nursing considerations/Cautions
- contraindicated in those with hypersensitivity to natural or recombinant interferon beta or peg interferon
- liver function tests are recommended before initiation and periodically during treatment because of the risk of hepatic injury, and caution is advised when used in patients with severe hepatic impairment or with hepatotoxic agents
- see also General Nursing considerations/Cautions for interferons (p. 1390)

Patient education
- see General Patient education for interferons (p. 1391)

Contraindicated: initiation during pregnancy is contraindicated owing to potential abortifacient activity observed in animal studies with interferon beta. Women of childbearing potential should use effective contraception and, if pregnancy occurs, treatment should continue only if benefits outweigh risks.

Avoid, as excretion in human breastmilk unknown. Due to the potential for adverse reactions in infants, a decision should be made to discontinue breastfeeding or cease therapy, weighing the benefits for the mother and child.

CANNABIDIOL, TETRAHYDROCANNABINOL, NABIXIMOLS

Trade name
Sativex

Available form
Oromucosal spray:

Action
- there are at least two types of cannabinoid (CB) receptors in the brain, with CB1 found mainly in nerve terminals in the CNS, where it modulates neurotransmitter release. CB2 receptors are found mainly in cells within the immune system
- tetrahydrocannabinol (THC) is the main psychotropic constituent of cannabis and acts as a partial agonist at both CB1 and CB2 receptors
- in animal models of multiple sclerosis (MS), CB receptor agonists have been shown to improve both limb stiffness and motor function
- cannabidiol (CBD) has little activity at CB receptors, but has neuroprotective properties thought to be due to an ability to modulate intracellular calcium, as well as inhibiting microglial activity and T-cell proliferation

Use
- symptom improvement in patients with moderate-to-severe spasticity due to MS who have not responded adequately to other antispasticity medication and who have shown clinical improvement in spasticity-related symptoms during an initial trial

Dose
- (Titration period) initially 1 spray in the evening (days 1 and 2), then 2 sprays in the evening (days 3 and 4), then 1 spray in the morning and 2 sprays in the evening (day 5), then 1 spray in the morning and 3 sprays in the evening (day 6), then 1 spray in the morning and 4 sprays in the evening (day 7), then 2 sprays in the morning and 4 sprays in the evening (day 8), then 2 sprays in the morning and 5 sprays in the evening (day 9), then 3 sprays in the morning and 5 sprays in the evening (day 10), then 3 sprays in the morning and 6 sprays in the evening (day 11), then 4 sprays in the morning and 6 sprays in the evening (day 12), then 4 sprays in the morning and 7 sprays in the evening (day 13) and then 5 sprays in the morning and 7 sprays in the evening (day 14)

MOVEMENT DISORDER AGENTS

Adverse effects
- mild-to-moderate dizziness, disorientation, euphoric mood, dissociation, insomnia
- tachycardia, hypertension
- vertigo, dizziness, somnolence, headache, disturbed attention, lethargy, memory impairment, amnesia, tremor, paraesthesia
- blurred vision
- nausea, dry mouth, diarrhoea, vomiting, constipation, dyspepsia, abdominal pain, altered taste, anorexia or increased appetite
- fatigue, asthenia, feeling drunk or abnormal, pain, malaise
- infections (urinary tract, nasopharyngitis, pharyngitis, viral, respiratory tract)
- muscle spasm, back pain, pain in extremities, muscle weakness, arthralgia, balance disorder
- cough, pharyngolaryngeal pain
- (Application site) stinging, pain, discomfort, altered taste, mouth ulceration, glossodynia
- (High doses) psychosis, hallucinations, delusions, homicidal and suicidal ideation

Interactions
- may reduce effectiveness of hormonal contraceptive
- may increase metabolism of warfarin, statins, beta adrenergic blocking agents or corticosteroids
- caution if itraconazole, ritonavir or clarithromycin is started or stopped with therapy
- decreased serum levels may occur if given with rifampicin, carbamazepine, phenytoin, phenobarbital (phenobarbitone) or St John's wort
- caution if used with hypnotics, sedatives or other agents with sedating properties, as increased sedation may occur
- caution if used with alcohol, as coordination, concentration and reflexes may all be affected

Nursing considerations/Cautions
- the patient should be assessed by neurologist or rehabilitation physician for suitability, and should then be reassessed after 4 weeks of therapy for clinical improvement (defined as 20% improvement in spasticity-related symptoms on a 0–10 patient reported numeric rating scale). If there is no significant clinical improvement, therapy should be discontinued
- therapy should be given in addition to the patient's current antispasticity medication
- if adverse effects occur, depending on their seriousness or intensity, the dose may be continued, reduced or interrupted temporarily
- a titration period is required to achieve the optimal dose (number and timing of sprays will vary between patients). Caution during titration, as there may be alterations in pulse rate or blood pressure
- an afternoon/evening dose can be given any time between 4 pm and bedtime. A morning dose can be taken any time between rising and midday
- there should be at least 15 minutes between sprays
- the maximum number of consecutive sprays should not exceed 7 within a 3-hour period
- once the optimum dose is achieved, the patient can spread doses out during the day according to response and tolerance
- the dose may require retitration upwards or downwards if there are any changes in severity of the patient's condition
- doses should not exceed 12 sprays in any 24-hour period
- contains 50% v/v ethanol, with each spray containing 0.04 g ethanol; therefore caution if used in patients with severe alcohol use disorder

- caution if used in those with moderate-to-severe liver impairment
- caution if used in those with a history of epilepsy or recurrent seizures
- caution if used in those with a history of depression. If used, the patient should be closely monitored and therapy stopped if there is significant worsening of depression
- caution if used in those with history of substance abuse, as there is an increased risk of abuse
- caution if used in those > 65 years, as there is increased risk of CNS adverse effects
- not recommended in those under 18 years
- not recommended in those with serious cardiovascular disease
- contraindicated in those with hypersensitivity to cannabinoids, known or suspected history or a family history of schizophrenia or other psychotic illness, history of severe personality disorder or other significant psychiatric disorder (other than depression associated with MS)

Patient education

- advise the patient that it might take 2 weeks to find optimal dose
- warn the patient that side-effects can occur during this time, especially dizziness, but these are usually mild and resolve within a few days
- the patient should be warned not to exceed the maximum dose
- advise the patient to avoid alcohol during therapy
- caution the patient that there is an increased risk of falls when spasticity is reduced if they have insufficient muscle strength to maintain posture or gait
- advise the patient not to drive, operate machinery or participate in activities that are potentially dangerous (e.g. cooking, handling hot foods or liquids) if adverse effects such as dizziness, vertigo, blurred vision or disorientation occur
- the patient should be instructed in use of spray, including:
  - prime the container before first use and if not used for 21 days shake the container gently, removing the cap and pressing the actuator 2–3 times into a tissue until a fine spray appears
  - (After first use) shake the container gently before use and direct spray at different sites on the oromucosal surface, changing site each time the product is used
  - spray should not be applied to areas that are sore or inflamed
  - mouth should be inspected regularly
  - if mouth lesions occur or persist, therapy should be interrupted until the area resolves
  - the unopened container can be stored upright in a refrigerator
  - the open container does not need to be refrigerated, but should be stored below 25°C and discarded 42 days after opening
- female patients of childbearing potential should be counselled to use effective contraception during and for 12 weeks after discontinuing therapy. A barrier method should be used in addition to hormonal contraception

Avoid: should not be used during pregnancy unless the potential risks to the fetus are outweighed by the benefit of treatment, as there is insufficient experience in humans.

Contraindicated in breastfeeding mothers because high levels of cannabinoids are likely in maternal breastmilk, with potential adverse developmental effects in infants.

Reduced hepatic function: can be used in patients with mild hepatic impairment without dose adjustment but should be used cautiously in moderate-to-severe hepatic impairment because of the potential for exaggerated or prolonged effects. Frequent clinical evaluation is recommended.

MOVEMENT DISORDER AGENTS

Elderly patients may be more prone to CNS adverse reactions, including dizziness and fatigue. Care should be taken in activities requiring alertness, such as handling hot food or drinks, as these patients are at an increased risk of falls.

MOTOR NEURONE DISEASE (MND)

Motor neurone disease (MND), also known as amyotrophic lateral sclerosis (ALS) or Lou Gehrig's disease, is a progressive neurological condition affecting nerve cells responsible for muscle control. In Australia, the prevalence of MND has been increasing over recent years. The prevalence is estimated at 8.7 per 100,000 Australians. It is estimated that there are currently about 2318 Australians living with MND (MND Australia 2024).

Although the onset of MND may only involve loss of upper or lower motor neurone function, it eventually progresses to involve both. Clinical manifestations include asymmetric weakness (usually distal in one limb), cramping (especially in early hours of the morning while stretching in bed), weakness with progressive muscle wasting and atrophy and twitching/fasciculation. If facial muscles are involved, problems chewing and swallowing are experienced, along with movement issues of the tongue and face (Brown 2019). No one muscle group is known to be the first one to show signs; however, with time, as the disease progresses, more muscle groups become involved until there is a symmetrical distribution with both upper and lower motor neurone involvement. Unfortunately, the disease is relentlessly progressive, ending in death due to respiratory paralysis with a 3–5-year median survival time from diagnosis (Brown 2019). The cause of MND is unknown, with a small number of cases being inherited. Currently, there is no treatment for MND that prevents the disease's progress, with only one drug available that lengthens survival time (Brown 2019).

RILUZOLE
Trade names
Pharmacor Riluzole, Rilutek, Riluzole Sandoz, Teglutik

Available forms
Tablets: 50 mg;
Oral suspension: 5 mg/mL

Action
- glutamate antagonist (hypothesis suggests that vulnerable motor neurones are injured by glutamate)
- inactivates voltage-dependent sodium channels and impairs glutamatergic neurotransmission
- crosses blood–brain barrier
- decreases cerebral glucose metabolism
- neuroprotective
- myorelaxant, sedative and antiepileptic properties at high doses
- elimination half-life is approximately 9–15 hours

Use
- motor neurone disease (MND) (amyotrophic lateral sclerosis)

Dose
- 50 mg orally twice daily

Adverse effects
- anorexia, nausea, abdominal pain, vomiting, flatulence, constipation, diarrhoea, dysphagia, dry mouth, dyspepsia, weight loss
- asthenia, pain, back pain, stiffness, arthralgia, myalgia
- increased or abnormal liver enzymes (alanine aminotransferase (ALT), aspartate aminotransferase (AST))
- headache, dizziness, somnolence, insomnia, paraesthesia, nervousness, anxiety
- decreased lung function, apnoea, rhinitis, increased sputum, aspiration pneumonia, cough, dyspnoea
- tachycardia, peripheral oedema, hypertension
- infection (bronchitis, pneumonia, pharyngitis)
- eczema, pruritus, sweating

- urinary frequency
- (Rare) neutropenia, interstitial lung disease

Interactions
- absorption decreased by fat-containing meals
- increased serum levels may occur if given with quinolone antibacterial agents, diazepam, diclofenac, caffeine, clomipramine, imipramine, fluvoxamine, theophylline or amitryptyline
- decreased serum levels may occur if given with rifampicin, omeprazole or the patient cigarette smoking

Nursing considerations/Cautions

- serum transaminases should be measured before starting therapy, monthly for 3 months, then 3-monthly for the first year and regularly thereafter
- chest X-ray is recommended if the patient develops a dry cough and/or dyspnoea
- (Oral suspension) contains sorbitol, which may have laxative effect or cause diarrhoea in some people and is not recommended in those with rare hereditary problems of fructose intolerance
- caution if given to those with kidney dysfunction, abnormal liver function or neutropenia
- contraindicated in those with liver disease/impairment (transaminase level three times greater than normal)

Patient education

- instruct the patient to swallow the tablet whole
- the patient should be advised not to take medication with meals containing fat, because this will reduce absorption
- the patient should be instructed in correct administration of oral suspension, including:
  - shake the bottle gently for at least 30 seconds before use
  - after opening the bottle, insert the syringe into the bottle neck adapter and turn the bottle upside down
  - pull the plunger down slightly to allow suspension to enter the syringe, then push the plunger upwards again to remove any air bubbles
  - pull the plunger down to the graduation mark that corresponds with prescribed dose
  - turn the bottle upright and remove syringe
  - administer suspension directly into the mouth (no dilution is needed)
  - recap bottle
  - take the syringe apart and wash barrel and plunger separately with water and allow to air dry
  - discard the oral suspension 15 days after opening (bottle should be dated on opening)
  - store in a cool place below 25°C
- advise the patient to seek medical advice immediately if any of the following occur:
  - frequent infections, including fever, chills, mouth ulcers and sore throat
  - dry cough, shortness of breath, difficulty breathing
  - irregular or rapid heart rate
  - swelling of feet, legs or hands
  - itchy or yellow skin, yellow whites of the eyes, severe abdominal pain, nausea and vomiting, fatigue
- warn the patient against driving or operating machinery if dizziness, vertigo or somnolence occurs
- female patients of childbearing potential should be counselled to use adequate contraception during therapy to avoid pregnancy occurring

An oral suspension is available. Riluzole tablets are film coated and should not be crushed, as altering the tablet may affect drug stability and absorption.

Contraindicated: a risk of fetal harm was observed in animal studies, where fetal growth and development were slightly affected.

Riluzole and its metabolites are excreted in animal milk at higher levels than in maternal plasma and may cause harm to a nursing infant. Women should not

MOVEMENT DISORDER AGENTS

breastfeed while undergoing treatment with riluzole.

 Reduced hepatic function: contraindicated in patients with hepatic impairment or liver disease, particularly with baseline transaminases more than three times the upper limit of normal, owing to potential hepatotoxicity.

OTHER MOVEMENT DISORDERS

TETRABENAZINE
Trade names
Tetrabenazine, Tetrabenazine Sun

Available form
Tablets: 25 mg

Action
- depletes amines (such as dopamine) in the CNS
- inhibits monoamine transportation into presynaptic neuronal vesicles
- active metabolite thought to be responsible for therapeutic effects

Use
- management of movement disorders such as chorea, tardive and buccolingual dyskinesia and some dystonic syndromes

Dose
- initially 25 mg orally twice daily, increasing by 25 mg every 3—4 days (to a maximum of 200 mg daily or until therapeutic control is achieved)

Adverse effects
- drowsiness, Parkinsonism (at higher doses)
- postural hypotension, small prolongation of QT interval
- dysphagia, choking attacks
- agitation, insomnia, confusion, depression, anxiety
- (Rare) neuroleptic malignant syndrome, suicidal ideation, bronchopneumonia (resulting from dysphagia and choking)

Interactions
- contraindicated with or within 14 days of monoamine oxidase inhibitors (MAOIs)
- blocks action of levodopa; therefore therapies should be separated by at least 1 day and are contraindicated together
- extreme caution if given with other agents known to prolong QT interval
- increased dopamine depletion may occur if given with haloperidol, chlorpromazine or metoclopramide, resulting in Parkinsonism and, rarely, neuroleptic malignant syndrome
- sedative effects may be additive if given with alcohol or other CNS depressants
- may potentiate hypotensive action of antihypertensive agents
- increased serum levels may occur if given with fluoxetine, paroxetine, duloxetine, sertraline or amiodarone

Nursing considerations/Cautions
- check supine and standing BP regularly for postural hypotension
- if no improvement in symptoms is seen after 7—10 days of therapy at maximum dose, therapy should be re-evaluated
- dose reduction may be required in those with kidney or liver impairment or the elderly
- caution if used in those with history of depression or previous suicidal ideation or attempts
- caution if used in those with congenital QT prolongation or history of cardiac arrhythmias
- contains lactose; therefore not recommended in those with galactose intolerance, Lapp lactase deficiency or glucose—galactose malabsorption
- contraindicated in those with depression or Parkinsonism, as conditions may be worsened

Patient education
- advise the patient to avoid postural hypotension by moving gradually to a

- sitting or standing position, especially after sleep
- warn the patient to avoid alcohol during therapy
- the patient should be warned not to drive or operate machinery if drowsiness occurs
- the patient should be carefully observed during meals if dysphagia and choking attacks are problems, especially early in therapy
- advise the patient to seek medical attention if any of the following occur:
  - sweating, uncontrolled movements of legs, arms, hands or head or stiffness/tightness in arms or legs
  - feelings of depression, sadness or thoughts of self-harm or suicide
  - difficulty swallowing or choking attacks

Tablets can be crushed and mixed with a spoonful of yoghurt or apple puree.

Not recommended, as there are inadequate safety data and an unknown potential risk to humans. Animal studies showed increased stillbirths and neonatal mortality at higher doses.

Contraindicated during breastfeeding, as it is excreted in milk and may harm the infant.

Reduced hepatic function: dosage adjustments are needed, as tetrabenazine and its metabolites rely on hepatic metabolism. It should be used cautiously in patients with hepatic impairment.

ZILUCOPLAN

Trade name
Zilbrysq

Available forms
Pre-filled syringe: 16.6 mg, 23 mg, 32.4 mg

Action
- in those with generalised myasthenia gravis, binding of anti-acetylcholine receptor (AChR) autoantibodies (IgG_1, IgG_3) to AChR results in uncontrolled and inappropriate activation of the classical complement pathway, specifically C1 component. leading to enzymatic cleavage steps finally to C5 cleavage to C5a and C5b and deposition of a cytolytic membrane attack complex (C5b-9, MAC) on the postsynaptic membrane of the neuromuscular junction, injuring the end-plate and resulting in failed neuromuscular transmission
- zilucoplan inhibits C5 effects by binding to the C5 complement protein (preventing the subsequent steps described above), as well as binding to C5b, preventing binding to C6 and any assembly of MAC
- half-life 172 hours (7—8 days)

Use
- as add-on to standard therapy for treatment of generalised myasthenia gravis who are AChR antibody positive

Dose
- (Body weight $\geq$ 43 to $<$ 56 kg) 16.6 mg SC daily
- (Body weight $\geq$ 56 to $<$ 77 kg) 23 mg SC daily
- (Body weight $\geq$ 77 to $<$ 150 kg) 32.4 mg SC daily

Adverse effects
- (Injection site) bruising, haematoma, pain, rash, bleeding
- nasopharyngitis, sinusitis, tonsillitis, upper respiratory tract infection
- diarrhoea
- confusion
- increase in pancreatic enzymes (lipase, amylase)
- transient increase in eosinophils
- morphoea/scleroderma
- increased risk of *Neisseria* infection, other infections

Interactions
- not recommended with immunosuppressants because of additive immunosuppression

MOVEMENT DISORDER AGENTS

Nursing considerations/Cautions

- before starting therapy, all patients must be vaccinated against *Neisseria meningitidis* at least 2 weeks before the first dose unless the risks of delaying therapy outweigh the risks of developing meningococcal infection
- if therapy is started less than 2 weeks after meningococcal vaccination, the patient must receive prophylactic antibiotics until 2 weeks after vaccination
- the patient/carer can be instructed in administration technique
- contraindicated in those who have not been currently vaccinated against *N. meningitidis* unless receiving appropriate antibiotics until 2 weeks after first vaccination dose or in those with unresolved *N. meningitidis* infection

Patient education

- the patient should be made aware that vaccination with meningococcal vaccine dose not totally eliminate the risk of developing the infection; therefore they should seek medical advice if they develop any symptoms including:
    - headache with stiff neck or back, nausea, vomiting
    - fever (with or without rash)
    - eyes become sensitive to light
    - drowsiness or confusion
    - muscle pain with flu-like symptoms
- the patient should be aware that they are susceptible to other infections, including other *Neisseria* species infections (e.g. gonorrhoea) and seek medical advice if any symptoms develop
- the patient/carer can be instructed in administration technique including:
    - the importance of rotating injection sites (thighs, abdomen, back of upper arm) and not injecting into an area that is red, inflamed, infected, bruised, indurated or has scars or stretch marks
    - the daily dose should be given at about the same time every day. If a dose is missed, it should be given as soon as possible on the same day (but only one dose should be given per day)
    - the prefilled syringe should be removed from refrigerator 30—45 minutes before administration
    - do not warm the prefilled syringe in any way, including placing in a microwave, hot water or direct sunlight
    - check the expiry date and ensure the syringe is intact before use
    - wash and dry hands thoroughly
    - clean the injection site with alcohol swab and allow area to dry for 10 seconds
    - remove the needle cap and avoid allowing it to touch anything before injection
    - pinch the skin at injection site and hold firmly and insert the entire needle into pinched skin at a 45 to 90 degree angle; holding the needle in place, release pinched skin
    - push the plunger down holding on to the finger grip to inject medication
    - release the plunger by lifting the thumb. The needle guard will cover the needle automatically and a click may be heard
    - do not rub the injection site; however, a cotton ball or gauze can be used to press the injection site for 10 seconds; an adhesive strip (e.g. Bandaid) can be applied if needed
    - dispose of the used syringe into a sharps container
    - discard after the expiry date or 3 months after being removed from the refrigerator

 Not recommended during pregnancy or in women of childbearing potential not using contraception. Animal studies indicate an increased risk of embryofetal death at all tested doses.

 Unknown whether excreted in breastmilk.

MUSCLE RELAXANTS

Spasticity, as seen in neurological disorders like cerebral palsy, spinal injury, multiple sclerosis and stroke, often requires a multimodal treatment approach involving both muscle relaxants (spasmolytic drugs) and physiotherapy. Spasticity is an involuntary, often intermittent or sustained, contraction of skeletal muscles, resulting in stiffness. Depending on which muscles are involved, muscle stiffness can hinder mobility, impair coordination, and affect speech (Kruidering-Hall & Campbell 2018).

Muscle relaxants act by modifying the stretch or directly interfering with the skeletal muscle. Although currently available agents relieve painful spasms, they are typically limited in their ability to enhance functional outcomes like mobility (Kruidering-Hall & Campbell 2018).

BACLOFEN
Trade names
APO-Baclofen, Bacthecal, Clofen, Lioresal, Lioresal Intrathecal, Sintetica Baclofen Intrathecal, Stelax

Available forms
Tablets: 10 mg, 25 mg;
Ampoules: 0.05 mg/mL (for screening), 10 mg/5 mL, 10 mg/20 mL, 40 mg/20 mL

Action
- derivative of gamma aminobutyric acid (GABA)
- selective agonist at presynaptic GABA-B receptors
- inhibits adenylyl cyclase, blocking calcium channels and release of transmitter
- antispasticity activity via spinal cord, inhibiting motor neuron activation
- thought to reduce pain threshold associated with spasticity by inhibiting substance P in the spinal cord
- does not affect neuromuscular transmission
- does not reduce overall muscle strength as much as dantrolene
- stimulates gastric acid secretion
- (Intrathecal bolus) onset of action 30—60 minutes, peak response about 4 hours, duration of action 4—8 hours, half-life 1—5 hours
- (Intrathecal — continuous) response seen in 6—8 hours, maximum efficacy 24—48 hours
- (Oral) onset of action is variable (hours to weeks), half-life 2.5—6 hours

Use
- (Oral) skeletal muscle spasm in multiple sclerosis (MS) and spinal cord injuries
- (Intrathecal) used when there is no response to oral therapy and/or adverse effects are unacceptable

MUSCLE RELAXANTS

Dose
- initially 5 mg orally 3 times daily with food, then increasing at 3-day intervals by 5 mg/dose until desired response is achieved (optimal daily range 30—75 mg) **OR**
- initially 25—50 micrograms intrathecally (via spinal catheter or lumbar puncture), increasing by 25 micrograms daily until response lasts for 4—8 hours (screening dose). Screening dose is then doubled and given over 24 hours via intrathecal pump. Dose may be further adjusted to maintain muscle tone as normal as possible and reduce frequency and severity of muscle spasm without intolerable adverse effects

Adverse effects
- decreased appetite, nausea, retching, vomiting, diarrhoea, dry mouth, constipation, increased salivation
- muscle weakness/hypotonia, ataxia, myalgia, disturbed gait, paraesthesia
- headache, insomnia, somnolence, nightmares, drowsiness, dizziness, sedation, tremor, fatigue, asthenia
- confusion, hallucination, depression, disorientation, abnormal thinking, agitation, anxiety, concentration difficulty
- seizures
- tinnitus, vertigo
- double or blurred visual disturbance, nystagmus
- slurred speech
- rash, pruritus, urticaria, hyperhidrosis
- dysuria, enuresis, urinary retention, daytime urinary frequency, urinary incontinence
- sexual dysfunction
- pain, fever, chills
- facial and peripheral oedema
- respiratory depression, dyspnoea, chest tightness, pneumonia
- hypotension, decreased cardiac output, hypertension
- tolerance (may occur after several months)
- (Intrathecal) inflammatory mass at catheter tip, infection, dislodgement
- (Rare) scoliosis or worsening of pre-existing scoliosis
- (Withdrawal syndrome) initially high fever, altered mental state, aggravation of spasticity, muscle rigidity, seizures, coagulopathy, rhabdomyolysis, organ failure, death
- (Overdose symptoms) excessive muscular hypotonia, drowsiness, light-headedness, dizziness, somnolence, seizures, loss of consciousness, hypothermia, increased salivation, nausea and vomiting, respiratory depression, bradycardia, apnoea, coma

Interactions
- increased sedation and respiratory depression may occur if given with CNS depressants and alcohol
- may lower seizure threshold
- may increase confusion, hallucinations, agitation, nausea and headaches in patients with Parkinson's disease if given with levodopa—carbidopa
- may be potentiated by tricyclic antidepressants (TCAs), resulting in pronounced muscular hypotonia
- may potentiate hypotensive effect of antihypertensive agents
- caution if given with monoamine oxidase inhibitors (MAOIs), as increased CNS effects and hypotension may occur
- (Oral) may aggravate hyperkinesia if given with lithium and therefore should be given with caution
- may increase blood glucose, requiring a dose adjustment of insulin and/or oral hypoglycaemic agents
- increased risk of sedation and respiratory depression if given with opioid analgesics
- (Intrathecal) increased risk of seizures and cardiac disturbances if given with propofol or fentanyl
- caution if used with other agents that impact on kidney function. If used together, kidney function should be closely monitored

Nursing considerations/Cautions

- initiation of therapy should be done in a hospital setting for close patient monitoring to reduce spasticity to an acceptable level where muscle tone is sufficient for independence and adverse effects are minimal
- (Spasticity due to head injury) symptoms of spasticity should be stable and at least 1 year postinjury before intrathecal therapy is started
- (Post-traumatic spasticity) myelography of subarachnoid space is recommended before starting therapy and not commenced if any signs of arachnoiditis is evident (see Glossary)
- intrathecal route is recommended only when the patient has been unresponsive to other treatment, including oral baclofen
- the patient should be gradually withdrawn from oral antispasmodic agent (including baclofen) to decrease the risk of adverse effects (rebound spasticity and CNS disturbances)
- clinical effect is usually noticeable in 6–8 weeks
- liver enzymes should be monitored in those with liver impairment or diabetes mellitus
- resuscitation equipment should be readily available during initial intrathecal administration
- (Intrathecal) no dose increase should occur in first 24 hours of therapy
- (Intrathecal) incompatible with glucose 5%
- intrathecal bolus test dose of 100 micrograms should not be exceeded
- intrathecal pump should not be implanted until the patient response to the test dose (intrathecal bolus) and dose titration has been adequately evaluated and it is advisable that the patient is free of infection before pump insertion, as systemic infection can complicate dose adjustments
- monitor respiratory and cardiovascular function closely (especially in those with cardiopulmonary disease or respiratory muscle weakness)
- a patient with an intrathecal implant should be very carefully monitored whenever dosage is increased
- (Intrathecal) the patient should be carefully monitored for any signs that the intrathecal catheter tip may be occluded by a mass, which may include any decrease in response when previously well controlled, withdrawal symptoms, poor response to increasing doses, pain or neurological dysfunction
- only experienced staff should fill the intrathecal pump reservoir and the refill schedule should be calculated in a manner to prevent sudden stopping of therapy, which may induce withdrawal syndrome
- for a programmable pump, dose increase should be limited to once per 24 hours. If using a non-programmable pump (76 cm catheter delivering 1 mL/ 24 hours), dose increase should be once every 48 hours to evaluate response. Pump function and catheter patency should be checked if there is no clinical effect after substantial dose increase
- once the patient is stabilised on therapy, the regimen may be tailored to individual circumstances, such as the patient who experiences increased spasm at night. In this case the infusion rate may be increased overnight, but this should be done only under medical advice. Altered flow rate should be programmed to occur 2 hours before the time of desired clinical effect
- for patients with spasticity of spinal origin, dose increments should be limited to 10–30%. For patients with spasticity of cerebral origin, dose increments should be no greater than 5–15% to decrease the risk of overdose
- if withdrawal syndrome occurs, therapy should be restarted and withdrawn over a longer timeframe. Those receiving intrathecal therapy are at increased risk of withdrawal syndrome

MUSCLE RELAXANTS

- with chronic therapy, there is usually an increased dose requirement with time and some patients develop tolerance. In some cases, tolerance can be overcome by stopping therapy gradually and restarting after a 2—3-day break at the initial continuous infusion dose, followed by titration as previously
- if overdose occurs, the solution should be removed as soon as possible from the pump and emergency medical advice sought. The patient should be intubated and ventilated in the event of respiratory depression occurring, and IV diazepam administered for seizures. Cardiovascular function should be closely monitored and supported until the patient recovers
- adverse effects are more common and severe in the elderly and those with psychiatric illness, stroke or cortical/organic brain disorders
- (Intrathecal) caution if used in those with abnormal CSF flow, as response may be suboptimal
- caution if the patient uses spasticity to maintain an upright position or balance when moving, as use of baclofen may decrease independence
- caution if used in those with pre-existing bladder sphincter hypertonia, as urine retention may occur
- caution if used in those with schizophrenia, confusion, psychosis, depression or mania (as these may be exacerbated), or those with epilepsy, significant EEG abnormalities, brain damage, peptic ulcers, cerebrovascular disease, respiratory, liver or kidney failure/impairment, hypertension, porphyria, alcoholism or diabetes mellitus
- extreme caution if used in children under 6 years
- not recommended in those with Parkinson's disease, or if spasticity is caused by cerebral palsy, stroke or rheumatoid disorders
- (Intrathecal) contraindicated IV, IM, SC or via epidural, or in those with epilepsy that is refractory to therapy

Patient education

- instruct the patient to take tablets with food to decrease the gastrointestinal side-effects
- advise patients with diabetes mellitus to monitor blood glucose levels more frequently
- warn the patient against driving a vehicle or operating machinery if drowsy, dizzy or experiencing double or blurred vision
- instruct the patient not to stop therapy abruptly. Withdrawal should be gradual and over 1—2 weeks
- warn the patient to avoid alcohol during therapy because of increased sedation
- (Intrathecal) everyone caring for the patient should receive adequate instruction in caring for the insertion site and pump, as well as being aware of signs and symptoms of overdose and knowledge of what to do if this occurs, as this is an emergency situation. It is also important that everyone understands withdrawal symptoms may occur if the pump is allowed to run out of medication, the catheter becomes blocked or dislodged, the battery on the pump runs out or the pump malfunctions. This is an emergency situation which could be potentially fatal
  - overdose symptoms include unusual muscle weakness, sleepiness, dizziness, lightheadedness, nausea and vomiting, excessive saliva, breathing problems, fainting and fitting
  - withdrawal symptoms include uncontrolled spasms, difficulty with muscle movement, dizziness, lightheadedness, severe itching, numbness/tingling of hands/feet, anxiety, high fever, agitation, confusion, hallucinations and abnormal thinking

 Tablet can be dispersed in water, or crushed and mixed with a spoonful of yoghurt or apple puree.

HAVARD'S NURSING GUIDE TO DRUGS

Crosses the placental barrier. Use only if the expected benefit justifies the potential risk to the fetus. Withdrawal reactions, including postnatal convulsions, have been reported in neonates following intrauterine exposure. In cases where baclofen is necessary, monitor for neonatal convulsions and potential withdrawal symptoms.

Excreted in breastmilk in very small amounts. Adverse effects in the infant are unlikely at low levels; however, caution is advised.

Reduced renal function: to avoid drug accumulation, dose reduction is advised for patients with renal impairment. In patients with end-stage renal disease, baclofen should be used only if the benefit outweighs the risk. Close monitoring for toxicity signs (e.g. somnolence and confusion) is recommended.

Elderly patients are more likely to experience side-effects, particularly due to potential renal impairment and CNS effects. Monitor for adverse effects.

BOTULINUM TOXIN TYPE A
Trade names
Botox, Dysport

Available forms
Vial: 50 U, 100 U, 200 U;
Ipsen units: 125, 300, 500

Action
* purified neurotoxin from *Clostridium botulinum* (toxin type A) that blocks neuromuscular conduction by binding to motor nerve terminals
* enters nerve terminals and inhibits the release of acetylcholine
* when given IM, it causes localised chemical denervation, flaccid muscle paralysis, including decreased muscle tone and contractility, leading to muscle atrophy
* when given intradermally, it causes localised chemical denervation of sweat gland, decreasing sweating in that local area

Use
* blepharospasm associated with dystonia including hemifacial spasm associated with nerve VII disorder and benign blepharospasm (in those over 12 years)
* strabismus (children and adults)
* spasmodic dysphonia
* cervical dystonia (spasmodic torticollis)
* focal spasticity of upper and lower limbs including dynamic equinus foot deformity due to juvenile cerebral palsy (over 2 years)
* focal spasticity (adults)
* severe primary hyperhidrosis of axillae
* chronic migraine (where person has headaches at least 15 days per month, 8 of which are migraine)
* overactive bladder (with symptoms of incontinence, frequency and urgency where adult patient is intolerant or response has been inadequate to anticholinergics)
* neurogenic detrusor overactivity (due to multiple sclerosis or spinal cord injury, not controlled by anticholinergics)
* (Cosmetic use) glabellar lines, crow's feet, forehead lines

Dose
* dependent on site (see manufacturer's instructions)

Adverse effects
General
* generalised weakness, headache, fatigue, flu-like symptoms
* (Injection site) pain, inflammation, erythema, oedema/swelling, bleeding, bruising, tenderness, paraesthesia, hypoaesthesia, localised infection
* development of antibodies that reduce the effectiveness of subsequent injections requiring an increase in dosage
* (Rare) allergic reaction, spread of toxin effect (adverse effects away from injection site)

As well as general adverse effects (listed above), specific adverse effects for conditions include:

MUSCLE RELAXANTS

Blepharospasm
- diplopia, ptosis, dry eyes, photophobia, inability to close eyelids completely, entropion, ectropion
- facial muscle weakness

Strabismus
- partial ptosis, vertical deviation, diplopia
- (Infrequent) cycloplegia, ocular vertigo, corneal irritation
- (Rare) retrobulbar haemorrhage, sclera perforation, spatial disorientation, past pointing

Spasmodic dysphonia
- breathy dysphonia (paralytic dysphonia), dysphagia, aspiration, persistent cough

Cervical dystonia (spasmodic torticollis)
- dysphagia (lasting up to 3 weeks), dry mouth, nausea
- neck pain, asthenia, dizziness, general muscle weakness or stiffness, myalgia, facial paresis, hypertonia, hyperaesthesia
- upper respiratory tract infection, flu-like illness, rhinitis
- malaise, somnolence
- dysphonia

Nerve VII disorder (hemifacial spasm)
- blurred vision, facial droop, dizziness, tiredness (plus adverse effects for strabismus)

Focal spasticity (adult, upper and lower limb, post-stroke)
- (Upper limb) arm pain, hypertonia, muscle weakness, arthralgia, musculoskeletal pain, pain in extremities
- (Lower limb) falls, injury, lack of coordination, paraesthesia, hypertonia, asthenia, headache, hyperkinesia, peripheral oedema, arthralgia
- fever, flu-like illness
- ecchymosis

Focal spasticity (children)
- local and general weakness, clumsiness, falling, hypokinesia, paraesthesia, muscle spasm, leg/knee/ankle pain, leg cramps, myalgia, abnormal gait, joint dislocation, trigger finger
- vomiting
- lethargy, somnolence
- fever
- nasopharyngitis, flu-like illness, pneumonia, viral infection, ear infection
- rash
- increased micturition, urinary incontinence
- seizures

Hyperhidrosis
- increased non-axillary sweating, pain, hot flushes, transient arm weakness
- headache, asthenia, paraesthesia
- nausea
- pruritus

Chronic migraine
- worsening migraine/headache
- facial paresis, eyelid ptosis
- neck pain, myalgia, muscle spasm/tightness/weakness/stiffness
- pruritus, rash
- (Uncommon) dysphagia, jaw pain, skin pain

Overactive bladder/neurogenic detrusor overactivity
- urinary tract infection, bacteriuria, dysuria, urinary retention, increase in residual urine volume, frequent urination
- fatigue, insomnia

Glabellar lines
- headache, blepharoptosis, eyelid oedema, face pain, local muscle weakness, skin tightness, nausea, paraesthesia, ecchymosis

Crow's feet
- headache, flu-like symptoms, temporary lower lid droop

Forehead lines
- headache, eyebrow ptosis, eyelid swelling, aching/itching forehead, nausea, tension, flu-like symptoms

Interactions
- effects may be potentiated if given

1407

with aminoglycosides, colistimethate (polymyxin), tetracyclines, lincomycin, penicillamine, muscle relaxants or other agents that interfere with neuromuscular transmission and acetylcholine release, and should therefore be given with caution

Nursing considerations/Cautions

- administration should be performed only by a suitably qualified and experienced clinician (e.g. intradetrusor administration for bladder dysfunction should be done only by a urologist or urogynaecologist)
- dosage is kept as low as possible
- increasing frequency of treatment may result in tolerance developing. More than one ineffective treatment course should occur before a patient is classified as a non-responder
- neutralising antibodies are more likely to develop if dose is high, there is a short interval (< 3 months) between treatments and/or booster injections are given within 4 weeks of treatment
- denatured by violent agitation; therefore instil the diluent and swirl gently to dissolve powder
- reconstitute using sodium chloride 0.9% (1—10 mL) for a concentration of 1.25—40 U/0.1 mL (Botox) or sodium chloride 0.9% (0.6—2.5 mL) for a concentration of 20—50 units/0.1 mL (Dysport). Manufacturer's instructions should be followed for dilution
- use within 24 hours of reconstitution if refrigerated
- avoid contact with eyes and skin, and wash area thoroughly with water if contact occurs
- wear gloves and eye protection when reconstituting solution
- given IM generally; however, it can be injected SC (blepharospasm) or intradermally (hyperhidrosis)
- preparations from different manufacturers may not be equipotent; therefore do not substitute brands
- (Bladder dysfunction) urinary tract infection should not be present at time of administration
- (Bladder dysfunction) any antiplatelet therapy should be discontinued 3 days before injection
- (Bladder dysfunction) prophylactic antibiotics (not aminoglycosides) are recommended for 1—3 days before and 1—3 days after injection
- (Overactive bladder) clinical improvement may be seen within 2 weeks, duration about 24 weeks. Further injection not within 3 months
- (Overactive bladder) the patient should be observed for at least 30 minutes postinjection or until a spontaneous void has occurred
- (Overactive bladder) clinical trials showed response to therapy was far greater in females when compared with male patients, who, in many cases, either had no response or the condition was worsened
- (Overactive bladder) urinary tract infection (as an adverse effect) occurs more commonly in patients with diabetes mellitus than those without
- (Neurogenic detrusor overactivity) clinical improvement may be seen within 2 weeks. Fixed interval retreatment is not recommended and reinjection should occur when there is a reduced clinical effect, but no sooner than 3 months
- (Bladder dysfunction) postvoid residual urine volume should be measured 2 weeks post-treatment and regularly for 12 weeks
- (Primary hyperhidrosis of the axillae) before starting therapy, any underlying causes for the hyperhidrosis (e.g. hyperthyroidism, pheochromocytoma) should be investigated first
- (Primary hyperhidrosis of the axillae) repeat injections at less than 16-week intervals are not recommended
- (Spasmodic dysphonia) diagnosis using a laryngoscope (preferably a nasendoscope) should be made to

MUSCLE RELAXANTS

- rule out any other structural disorder of the larynx
- (Chronic migraine) retreatment schedule is every 12 weeks; however, if no response is seen after 2 treatment cycles, therapy should be discontinued
- (Blepharospasm) ecchymosis of soft eyelid tissue can be decreased by applying light pressure to the site immediately after injection
- (Blepharospasm) after the first injection, effect is seen within 3 days, peaking at 1—2 weeks and lasting about 12 weeks. Dose may be increased if subsequent injections do not last longer than 8 weeks. Cumulative dose in 8 weeks should be greater than 200 U
- (Strabismus) several drops of anaesthetic eye drops and an ocular decongestant should be applied prior to the injection
- (Strabismus) paralysis occurs within 1—2 days, increasing in intensity during first week, lasting 2—6 weeks and gradually resolving over 2—6 weeks
- (Nerve VII disorders/hemifacial spasm) cumulative dose over 2 months should not exceed 200 U
- (Cervical dystonia) clinical improvement is usually seen in 1—2 weeks, peak effect about 6 weeks, duration 12—16 weeks. Retreatment in less than 8 weeks is not recommended. Total dose of 360 U every 8 weeks should not be exceeded
- (Focal spasticity, children) clinical improvement is usually seen in 1—2 weeks, therapy repeated when clinical effects diminish but not more frequently than every 12 weeks
- (Focal spasticity, adults) maximum treatment dose of 360 U (upper limbs) or 400 U (lower limbs) divided between muscles. Clinical improvement occurs within 2 weeks, peaking 4—6 weeks after treatment
- (Glabellar lines) improvement seen in 1 week, lasting up to 16 weeks
- any leftover solution should be inactivated using dilute hypochlorite (0.5—1%) solution for 5 minutes and then disposed of as medical waste
- (Blepharospasm) caution if used in those at risk of acute angle closure glaucoma
- contains albumin; therefore there is a theoretical risk for transmission of viral or prion diseases
- caution if used in those predisposed to seizures
- caution if given to those with prolonged bleeding time because of increased risk of bleeding and bruising at injection site(s)
- caution if used in those with pre-existing swallowing or breathing problems, or any defective neuromuscular transmission
- caution if administered in lung region (especially lung apex) due to risk of pneumothorax
- (Spasmodic dysphonia) not recommended in those due to have elective surgery with general anaesthetic because of increased risk of aspiration due to relaxed vocal cords
- not recommended in those with motor neuron disease or motor neuropathy
- (Overactive bladder) not recommended in men with overactive bladder and signs of urinary obstruction
- (Focal spasticity, adults) not recommended for treatment of lower limb spasticity in adult post-stroke patients if reduced muscle tone is not expected to improve function (e.g. gait) or symptoms (e.g. pain) or to facilitate care
- contraindicated in those with myasthenia gravis or Lambert-— Eaton syndrome, or if any infection is present at the injection site
- (Bladder dysfunction) contraindicated in those with acute urinary tract infection or acute retention who do not routinely or are not willing to self-catheterise post-treatment (if required)

Patient education

- warn the patient to resume activity gradually to prevent falls and accidental injury if previously sedentary
- all patients should be advised that headache, flu-like symptoms and injection site reactions occur commonly postinjection
- instruct the patient to seek medical advice if any drooping of upper eyelid, double or blurred vision, difficulty speaking or swallowing, generalised or local muscle weakness or numbness occurs
- (Cervical dystonia) the patient should be warned of the possibility of difficulty swallowing and breathing. A soft diet may be recommended until swallowing returns to normal. However, if swallowing, speaking or breathing difficulties occur after administration, the patient should seek medical advice immediately
- (Chronic migraine) warn the patient that there may be initial worsening of headache/migraine in the first month after injection
- (Bladder dysfunction) the patient should be warned that there may be some blood in the urine after injection
- (Bladder dysfunction) ensure that the patient is aware that they will need to see doctor again about 2 weeks after injection to measure the amount of urine that is left in the bladder using ultrasound. This test needs to be done a number of times in the following 12 weeks
- (Bladder dysfunction) instruct the patient to seek medical advice immediately if they experience difficulties passing urine, as catheterisation (passing a small plastic tube into the bladder) may be required
- (Bladder dysfunction) the patient should be alerted to the signs of urinary tract infection (increase in frequency, difficulty passing urine, stinging/burning sensation) and the need to seek medical advice if they occur
- (Bladder dysfunction) female patients should be advised to pass urine after sexual intercourse in order to avoid urinary tract infection
- (Strabismus) if the patient experiences any spatial disorientation, double vision or past point after therapy, covering the affected eye with a patch may alleviate these symptoms

 Not recommended unless benefits outweigh risks.

 Not recommended unless benefits outweigh risks.

DANTROLENE
Trade names
Dantrium Capsules, Dantrium Powder for Injection

Available forms
Capsules: 25 mg, 50 mg;
Vial: 20 mg

Action
- hydantoin derivative (related to phenytoin) that interferes with release of calcium ions from skeletal muscle sarcoplasmic reticulum, thus producing muscle relaxation. However, cardiac and smooth muscle are minimally depressed
- no effect on neuromuscular transmission
- half-life 5 hours (IV) or about 8.7 hours (oral)

Use
- relieves long-standing spasticity associated with multiple sclerosis, stroke and spinal cord injury
- malignant hyperthermia (with supportive measures) (IV)

Dose
- (Muscle relaxation) initially 25 mg orally daily, increasing to 25 mg 2, 3 or 4 times daily, then by increments of 25 mg up to 50 mg orally 2, 3 or 4 times daily (daily maximum 200 mg) **OR**

MUSCLE RELAXANTS

- (Malignant hyperthermia) initially 1 mg/kg by IV push, up to a total dose of 10 mg/kg or until symptoms subside; may be repeated

Adverse effects
- drowsiness, dizziness, arm/leg weakness, fatigue, malaise
- loss of appetite, diarrhoea, nausea, vomiting, abdominal cramps, altered taste, swallowing difficulties, constipation
- disturbed speech
- chills, fever
- depression, confusion, nervousness
- increased liver enzymes, hepatitis, hepatotoxicity
- photosensitivity, abnormal hair growth, acne-like rash, pruritus, urticaria, sweating
- headache, insomnia
- visual disturbance, diplopia, excessive tearing
- pleural effusion, pericarditis
- seizures
- myalgia, backache
- tachycardia, erratic blood pressure
- haematuria, increased urinary frequency, crystalluria, nocturia, urinary retention, difficult urination
- difficult erection
- (IV) thrombophlebitis, erythema, urticaria, anaphylaxis, loss of grip strength, leg weakness, drowsiness, dizziness
- (IV, rare) malignant hyperthermia crisis

Interactions
- (IV) not recommended with calcium-channel blockers
- caution if given with oestrogen therapy (especially in women over 35 years) because of increased risk of hepatotoxicity
- may potentiate neuromuscular blockade of non-depolarising muscle relaxants such as vecuronium
- effects may be potentiated by alcohol and CNS depressants

Nursing considerations/Cautions
- baseline liver function tests are recommended before starting and then regularly during therapy (especially in females and those over 35) because of risk of hepatotoxicity
- the patient should be observed during meals because swallowing difficulties may lead to choking
- (Oral) dose should not exceed 400 mg
- (Oral) when establishing dose by titration, each dose level should be maintained for up to 7 days to determine response
- usually not continued for more than 45 days if there is no response
- (Capsules) should not be used for management of neuroleptic malignant syndrome
- (IV) prevent extravasation, as solution has a high pH and will cause tissue necrosis
- reconstitute the vial for IV use with 60 mL water for injections, shaking the solution until clear
- (Malignant hyperthermia) the dose is dependent on the patient's susceptibility, amount and time of exposure to triggering agent, and time between symptoms occurring and treatment
- (Malignant hyperthermia) supportive measures include oxygen, managing metabolic acidosis and electrolyte imbalance, cooling the patient (if needed) and ensuring adequate urinary output
- caution if used in those with pre-existing liver disease/dysfunction, or pulmonary, kidney or cardiac impairment
- not recommended for spasticity related to electroconvulsive treatment (ECT) or rheumatic disorders
- contraindicated in those with active hepatitis, active cirrhosis or those where spasticity to maintain upright position or balance when moving as use with baclofen may decrease independence

HAVARD'S NURSING GUIDE TO DRUGS

Patient education

- warn the patient against driving a vehicle or operating machinery if drowsy, dizzy or fatigued or within 48 hours of IV treatment
- the patient (and family members/carers) should be instructed that muscle strength may diminish, resulting in a risk of swallowing difficulties and choking at mealtime and therefore the patient should be closely observed
- the patient should be advised to avoid prolonged exposure to sunlight and to wear protective clothing, hat, sunglasses and sunscreen (SPF 30+ or greater) if going outdoors
- instruct the patient to immediately seek medical advice if any of the following occur:
  - yellowing of eyes or skin, dark urine, nausea, vomiting or loss of appetite, fever, itching or general feeling of being unwell (signs of liver impairment)
  - severe diarrhoea
  - fitting
  - crystal or blood in urine, difficulty passing urine
- counsel the patient to avoid alcohol or any medications that reduce anxiety during therapy to avoid enhancement of dizziness and drowsiness

Capsule can be opened and mixed with water or orange juice until the suspension is even and then drunk. Contents can be mixed with a spoonful of yoghurt or apple puree.

Crosses the placenta; should be used only if benefits outweigh risks.

Caution, as excreted in human breast-milk.

Can cause hepatotoxicity, with fatal hepatic failure reported, especially with prolonged or high-dose oral use. It should only be used when necessary, and liver function should be monitored frequently. Hepatic injury risk is higher in females, patients over 35 years of age, and those taking other medications alongside dantrolene.

INCOBOTULINUMTOXIN A

Trade name
Xeomin

Available forms
Vial: 50 LD50 U, 100 LD50 U

Action
- purified neurotoxin synthesised from *Clostridium botulinum* type A which has had complexing proteins removed making it low molecular weight
- blocks acetylcholine transmission at the neuromuscular junction

Use
- cervical dystonia (adults)
- blepharospasm (adults)
- spasticity of upper limb (adults)
- upper facial lines (glabellar frown lines, horizontal forehead lines, crow's feet) (adults)

Dose
- (Cervical dystonia) 0.1—0.5 mL/injection site, not exceeding 200 U/treatment session or 50 U/injection site during first course of treatment, repeated no more frequently than 6-weekly. For second and subsequent treatment, 300 U/treatment session **OR**
- (Blepharospasm) 1.25—2.5 U (0.05—0.1 mL)/injection site, not exceeding 25 U per eye. Total dose should not exceed 100 U/treatment session, repeated no more frequently than 6-weekly **OR**

1412

MUSCLE RELAXANTS

- (Post-stroke spasticity) initially 10—80 U/injection site, then 5—200 U/injection site (1—4 injection sites per muscle). Maximum dose 400 U/treatment session, repeated no more frequently than 3-monthly. No more than 250 U in shoulder muscles **OR**
- (Glabellar frown lines) 4 U (0.1 mL) into each of 5 injection sites (2 into each corrugator muscle, 1 into procerus muscle). Standard dose is 20 U, increasing to 30 U if needed. Injection interval ≥ 3 months **OR**
- (Crow's feet) 4 U bilaterally into 3 injection sites (1 injection 1 cm lateral from bony orbital rim, 2 injections approximately 1 cm above and 1 cm below first injection site). Total dose 24 units (12 per side) **OR**
- (Crow's feet) 3 U bilaterally into 4 injection sites (first 2 injections 0.5 cm above and below point that is 1 cm lateral from bony orbital rim; second 2 injections 1 cm above and below this point). Total dose 24 units (12 per side) **OR**
- (Horizontal forehead lines) 10—20 U into frontalis muscles at 5 injection sites at least 2 cm above bony orbital rim

Adverse effects

General
- general or local weakness
- (Injection site) pain, burning, stinging, erythema, oedema/swelling, ecchymosis, bruising, rash, paraesthesia
- development of antibodies that reduce the effectiveness of subsequent injections requiring an increase in dosage
- (Rare) hypersensitivity, flu-like symptoms
- (Very rare) toxin spread (resulting in adverse effects spreading to sites away from injection site), exaggerated muscle weakness, dysphagia, dysphonia, aspiration pneumonia, breathing difficulties

As well as general adverse effects (listed above), specific adverse effects for conditions include:

Blepharospasm
- dry eye, ptosis, blurred vision, visual disturbance, increased tearing
- dry mouth, diarrhoea, dysphagia, lip disorder, gastroenteritis
- nasopharyngitis, respiratory tract infection
- urinary tract infection
- asthenia, headache
- dyspnoea
- muscle strain
- hypertension
- tooth infection

Cervical dystonia (spasmodic torticollis)
- neck pain, muscle spasm/pain/stiffness/weakness
- dysphagia, nausea
- headache, dizziness, lightheadedness
- sinusitis, asthma, upper respiratory tract infection
- oropharyngeal pain
- sweating

Spasticity (upper limb, post-stroke)
- headache
- diarrhoea, dry mouth
- seizures (new onset or recurrent)

Glabellar lines
- headache
- bronchitis, sinusitis, nasopharyngitis, flu-like illness
- eye disorders
- gastrointestinal disorders
- outer end of eyebrow located above inner end (Mephisto sign)

Crow's feet
- viral infection
- eyelid oedema, dry eye

Horizontal forehead lines
- eyelid ptosis, dry eye, brow ptosis, outer end of eyebrow located above inner end (Mephisto sign)
- headache
- hypoaesthesia

Interactions
- caution if given with aminoglycosides, colistimethate, tetracyclines, lincomycin, penicillamine, tubocurarine-like muscle relaxants or other agents that interfere with neuromuscular transmission

Nursing considerations/Cautions

- recommended doses and frequency of administration should be adhered to in order to decrease the risk of adverse effects occurring away from the site of the injection owing to spread of the toxin
- optimal dose and frequency should be individualised for each patient by physician
- if areas to be injected are marked with pen, these areas should not be injected through, as permanent tattooing may result
- (Post-stroke spasticity) initial and maintenance dose is dependent on the muscle group being treated (e.g. biceps muscle (flexed elbow) requires 80 U initially, followed by 75–200 U spread over 1–4 injection sites/muscle)
- (Cervical dystonia) onset of effect within 7 days of injection, lasting 3–4 months
- (Blepharospasm) onset of effect within 4 days of injection, lasting 3–4 months
- (Blepharospasm) immediate gentle pressure at injection site will limit ecchymosis
- (Blepharospasm) corneal sensation testing is recommended
- (Post-stroke spasticity) onset of effect within 4 days of injection, maximum improvement within 4 weeks, lasting 12 weeks
- (Glabellar frown lines) onset of effect within 2–3 days of injection, maximum effect on day 30, lasting up to 4 months
- (Crow's feet) duration up to 12 weeks
- (Crow's feet) injection close to zygomaticus major muscle should be avoided to prevent lip ptosis
- (Horizontal forehead lines) duration up to 16 weeks
- (Horizontal forehead lines) avoid injecting near orbit rim to decrease risk of brow ptosis
- increasing frequency of treatment may result in tolerance developing
- neutralising antibodies are more likely to develop if dose is high or there is a short interval between injections
- botulinum toxin products are not interchangeable
- denatured by violent agitation; therefore instil diluent and swirl gently to dissolve the powder
- avoid contact with eyes and skin and wash the area thoroughly with water if contact occurs
- wear gloves and eye protection when reconstituting solution
- reconstitute using sodium chloride 0.9% according to the manufacturer's recommendations. If vacuum does not pull diluent into the vial, it should be discarded
- reconstituted solution should be clear, colourless and free of particles
- any leftover solution should be inactivated using diluted sodium hypochlorite (at least 1%) solution, diluted sodium hydroxide solution, 70% ethanol or 50% isopropanol for 5 minutes and then disposed of as medical waste
- any reconstituted solution spill should be wiped up using dry absorbent material or absorbent material impregnated with one of the solutions listed in the above point if the powder is spilt
- contains albumin; therefore there is a theoretical risk for transmission of viral or prion diseases
- caution if used in those with bleeding disorders or taking anticoagulants
- caution if used in those with motor neurone disease, peripheral neuromuscular dysfunction or if targeted muscles show pronounced weakness or atrophy
- extreme caution if used for neurological indications in those with a history of dysphagia or aspiration because of an increased risk of excessive muscle weakness
- (Cervical dystonia) caution if used in those with respiratory disorders who are dependent on accessory muscles.

MUSCLE RELAXANTS

- Caution in those with smaller neck muscles or who require bilateral injections into sternocleidomastoid muscles because of an increased risk of dysphagia
- (Blepharospasm) caution if used in those who at risk of developing narrow-angle glaucoma
- (Glabellar frown lines, crow's feet, horizontal forehead lines) not recommended in those with history of dysphagia or aspiration
- contraindicated in those with myasthenia gravis, Lambert–Eaton syndrome or other muscle activity disorders, if there is inflammation or infection at the injection site or if the person has a sensitivity to botulinum toxin or albumin

Patient education

- (Cervical dystonia) the patient should be warned of the possibility of difficulty swallowing (dysphagia) and difficulty breathing (dyspnoea). A soft diet may be recommended until swallowing returns to normal. However, if swallowing, speaking or breathing difficulties occur after administration, the patient should seek medical advice immediately
- instruct the patient to seek medical advice immediately if any of the following occur:
  - drooping of upper eyelid, double or blurred vision
  - difficulty breathing, speaking or swallowing
  - generalised or local muscle weakness (can occur within hours to weeks of injection)
- the patient should be warned to avoid driving, operating machinery or engaging in hazardous activities if muscle weakness, blurred vision, tiredness, dizziness or drooping eyelids occur

 Not recommended. Use only if clearly necessary, as studies in animals have shown reproductive toxicity, though the significance to humans is uncertain.

 Not recommended. Excretion in human breastmilk unknown.

ORPHENADRINE
Trade name
Norflex

Available form
Tablets: 100 mg

Action
- skeletal muscle relaxant

Use
- painful muscle spasm associated with strains, sprains, fibrositis, whiplash injuries, torticollis or prolapsed intervertebral disc
- tension headache, persistent hiccups

Dose
- 100 mg orally twice daily (may be increased to 300 mg/24 hours in severe cases)

Adverse effects
- nausea, dry mouth
- blurred or double vision
- (Rare) rash, drowsiness

Interaction
- caution if used with other agents with anticholinergic action

Nursing considerations/Cautions

- adverse effects related to anticholinergic activity
- if used long term, monitoring of liver function, blood counts and urine testing are recommended
- caution if used in those with tachycardia, arrhythmias, coronary insufficiency or coronary decompensation

- contraindicated in patients with glaucoma, myasthenia gravis, urinary retention or obstruction of bladder neck, or prostatic hypertrophy because of anticholinergic properties

Patient education

- patient should be advised against driving or operating machinery if blurred vision or drowsiness occurs
- if dry mouth is an ongoing problem, instruct patient to suck sweets, sugarless gum or ice, or use saliva substitute. However, if this continues for more than 2 weeks a dentist should be consulted because the patient is at risk of tooth decay, gum disease and fungal infection

Tablet can be crushed and mixed with water or a spoonful of yoghurt or apple puree.

The safety of orphenadrine during pregnancy has not been established, so it should be used only when the potential benefits outweigh the risks.

Avoid, as no human data.

Available in combination with

- orphenadrine 35 mg + paracetamol 450 mg (Norgesic)

PRABOTULINUMTOXIN A

Trade name
Nuceiva

Available form
Vial: 100 units

Action

- purified neurotoxin synthesised from *Clostridium botulinum* type A
- blocks acetylcholine transmission at neuromuscular junction
- recovery takes about 12 weeks after IM injection

Use

- temporary improvement in appearance of moderate-to-severe glabellar lines in adults

Dose

- 4 units (0.1 mL of reconstituted solution) IM into 5 sites (inferomedial and superior middle of each corrugator and one in the midline of the procerus muscle) (total dose 20 units in 0.5 mL)

Adverse effects

- (Injection site) pain, infection, inflammation, tenderness, swelling, redness, pruritus, paraesthesia, bleeding, bruising
- (Uncommon) dizziness, headache, migraine
- (Uncommon) muscle weakness
- (Uncommon) blepharospasm, brow ptosis, eyelid oedema, eye swelling, blurred or double vision, dry eye
- (Repeated administration) muscle atrophy
- development of antibodies that may reduce effectiveness of subsequent injections
- (Rare) hypersensitivity (anaphylaxis, serum sickness, urticaria, oedema, dyspnoea)
- (Very rare) toxin effect spread (resulting in adverse effects spreading to sites away from injection site) (e.g. asthenia, generalised muscle weakness, diplopia, ptosis, dysphagia, dysphonia, dysarthria, urinary incontinence, blurred vision, breathing difficulty)

Interactions

- caution if used with other neuromuscular transmission effects such as aminoglycosides, anticholinergics, muscle relaxants and other botulinum neurotoxin products

Nursing considerations/Cautions

- botulinum toxin units are not interchangeable between products
- administration should be performed only by a suitably qualified and experienced clinician

MUSCLE RELAXANTS

- before administration, the patient should be examined for any excessive weakness or atrophy of muscles to be injected, any facial asymmetry, ptosis, excessive dermatochalasis (loose and redundant eyelid skin), deep dermal scarring or thick sebaceous skin
- reconstituted using 2.5 mL sodium chloride 0.9%, resulting in a concentration of 4 units per 0.1 mL
- should be administered within 24 hours of reconstitution
- to reduce risk of eyelid ptosis, physical manipulation (e.g. rubbing) of injection site should be avoided post administration; lateral corrugator injections should be at least 1 cm above supraorbital ridge
- recommended dose and frequency of administration should not be exceeded
- if there is a lack of response (no improvement of glabellar lines at maximum frown) one month after the first course of treatment, the cause may be inappropriate injection technique, incorrect muscles injected and/or formation of botulinum toxin-neutralising antibodies
- retreatment should be no more frequently than every 12 weeks. If other botulinum toxin products have been used, a cumulative dose should be considered
- referral to an ophthalmologist should be considered if the patient has persistent eye problems
- approved only for treatment of glabellar lines
- the product contains albumin; therefore it carries an extremely remote risk of viral illness transmission including variant Creutzfeldt–Jacob disease
- caution if used in those with swallowing or breathing difficulties because of the increased risk of complications related to muscles that control breathing and swallowing
- caution if used in those with cardiovascular disease
- caution if used in those with bleeding disorders, as IM injection can lead to bruising
- contraindicated in those with hypersensitivity to any botulinum toxin preparations, in the presence of infection or inflammation at injection sites or with generalised muscle activity disorders (e.g. myasthenia gravis, Lambert–Eaton syndrome, amylotrophic lateral sclerosis/motor neuron disease)

Patient education

- the patient/carer should be instructed to seek medical advice immediately if they experience any:
  - difficulty with speech (e.g. hoarseness, change or loss of voice), swallowing or breathing
  - blurred or double vision, decreased blinking, dry eyes (including irritation or photophobia)
  - loss of bladder control
  - loss of body strength generally
- warn the patient/carer that swallowing, speech or breathing problems may occur within hours or weeks after injection
- women of childbearing potential should be counselled to use adequate contraception during therapy

Not recommended in pregnancy or women of childbearing potential not using contraception. Animal studies have shown adverse embryofetal development effects.

Not recommended during breastfeeding; lack of human data.

ROPINIROLE

Trade names
Appese, Repreve

Available forms
Tablets: 0.25 mg, 0.5 mg, 2 mg

Action
- non-ergot dopamine receptor (D2/D3) agonist
- half-life 6 hours

Use
- primary restless leg syndrome

Dose
- initially 0.25 mg orally daily at bedtime for 2 days, increased to 0.5 mg daily if tolerated for remainder of week 1, then increasing to 1 mg daily (week 2), 1.5 mg daily (week 3), 2 mg daily (week 4), 2.5 mg daily (week 5), 3 mg daily (week 6) and 4 mg daily (week 7) until optimal therapeutic response is reached

Adverse effects
- nausea, vomiting, abdominal pain, diarrhoea, dry mouth
- headache, migraine, dizziness, drowsiness, somnolence, fatigue, vertigo, syncope, sudden sleep onset, paradoxical worsening of restless leg syndrome (earlier onset, increased intensity, spread of symptoms to other limbs, symptoms recurring in early morning)
- nervousness
- arthralgia, myalgia
- paraesthesia
- increased sweating
- coughing, rhinitis, sinusitis, upper respiratory tract infection
- (Rare) impulse control disorder, aggression, hypersensitivity, fibrotic complications (e.g. retroperitoneal fibrosis, pericarditis, cardiac valvulopathy)

Interactions
- not recommended with antipsychotic (neuroleptic) agents or centrally active dopamine antagonists (e.g. metoclopramide) because effects of ropinirole may be decreased
- increased serum levels may occur if given with ciprofloxacin or fluvoxamine
- not recommended with alcohol
- increased drug clearance may occur in those who smoke cigarettes. Dose adjustment may be necessary if patient starts or stops smoking cigarettes during therapy with ropinirole
- caution if used with CNS depressants, such as benzodiazepines, antipsychotics and antidepressants because of added sedative actions
- dose adjustment may be required if hormone replacement therapy (HRT) is stopped or started during therapy

Nursing considerations/Cautions
- before starting therapy, the patient should be assessed for the presence of any sleep disorders or use of sedating medications
- if therapy is interrupted for more than a few days, it should be restarted using the titration method described in the dose section until optimal effects are seen
- caution if used in those with severe cardiovascular diseases, Parkinson's disease or major psychotic disorders
- not recommended in those under 18 years
- not recommended for treatment of neuroleptic-induced akathisia (muscular quivering, urge to constantly move and inability to sit still) or in those with liver impairment or kidney impairment (creatinine clearance < 30 mL/min)

Patient education
- the patient should be warned that sudden onset of sleep may occur without prior warning or daytime sleepiness. If significant daytime sleepiness or episodes of falling asleep occur, the patient should be advised to avoid operating heavy machinery, driving or performing any other hazardous task(s)
- instruct the patient that a bedtime dose can be taken up to 2 hours before retiring
- the patient should be advised to avoid alcohol during therapy
- the patient should be warned to advise doctor if smoking cigarettes is started or stopped, because dose adjustment may be needed
- the patient (and family member/carer) should be advised to seek medical advice immediately if:

MUSCLE RELAXANTS

- symptoms worsen (e.g. start earlier, are more intense, move to other limbs, recur early in the morning) or
- if the patient suddenly develops compulsive behaviours such as an urge to gamble or increased sexual urges or behaviours
- female patients of childbearing years should be counselled to use adequate contraception to avoid pregnancy occurring

Tablets can be crushed (tablet can be dispersed in 10–20 mL of water, or crushed and mixed with water or a spoonful of yoghurt or apple puree).

Not recommended for use during pregnancy owing to a lack of established safety and adverse findings in animal studies.

Not recommended for breastfeeding mothers, as ropinirole may inhibit lactation and there is no established safety for infants.

Reduced renal function: no dose adjustment is required for mild-to-moderate renal impairment. However, in patients with end-stage renal disease on dialysis, the maximum recommended dose is 3 mg/day. It is not recommended for severe renal impairment without dialysis.

NEUROMUSCULAR BLOCKING AGENTS

The neuromuscular junction is a narrow gap between the motor neurone and skeletal muscle cell. The nerve's action potential depolarises its terminal causing an influx of calcium ions into nerve cytoplasm, causing storage vesicles to release their contents (acetylcholine). The acetylcholine molecules diffuse across the gap (synaptic cleft) and bind to receptors (nicotinic cholinergic receptors) on the postsynaptic muscle cell membrane. For muscle contraction to occur, it requires activation of these receptors. The acetylcholine is rapidly hydrolysed to acetate and choline by the enzyme acetylcholinesterase. This allows the muscle end-plate to repolarise and the muscle cell to relax (Kruidering-Hall & Campbell 2024).

Neuromuscular blocking agents are drugs that act on the neuromuscular junction. There are two classes of agents:
- *non-depolarising agents* compete at the receptor site with acetylcholine, thereby reducing the response at the postsynaptic receptor site (or end-plate)
- *depolarising agents* act at the motor end-plate and maintain depolarisation, resulting in the receptor sites being unable to respond to any other stimulation, causing paralysis.

NON-DEPOLARISING BLOCKING AGENTS

General Actions of non-depolarising blocking agents
- antagonise acetylcholine by competing at the cholinergic receptor sites at motor end-plate, producing a rapid blockade, causing motor weakness that progresses to total flaccid paralysis
- small muscles are the first to be affected (e.g. eyelids), followed by limbs, neck and trunk, then diaphragm and intercostal muscles. Recovery is the opposite, with the respiratory muscles recovering first
- action blocked by anticholinesterase agents (e.g. neostigmine), increasing the amount of acetylcholine available to compete at the receptor site
- have no effect on consciousness, pain threshold or cerebration; therefore care should be taken to ensure the patient is asleep before administration

General Uses of non-depolarising blocking agents
- as an adjunct to general anaesthesia
- facilitate endotracheal intubation

- relax skeletal muscles during surgery or mechanical ventilation
- facilitate mechanical ventilation in the ICU

General Adverse effects of non-depolarising blocking agents

- mild transient hypotension, hypertension
- tachycardia, bradycardia
- erythema, pruritus, rash, urticaria, localised skin reaction
- skin flushing on the neck and upper chest
- bronchospasm, wheezing, increase in bronchial secretions, hypoxia, dyspnoea, laryngospasm
- pain and reaction at injection site, phlebitis
- (Rare) malignant hyperthermia (signs include muscle rigidity, tachycardia, tachypnoea, increased oxygen requirements, increased carbon dioxide production, increased temperature and metabolic acidosis), anaphylactoid reaction, anaphylactic reaction, muscle weakness, myopathy

General Interactions of non-depolarising blocking agents

- inhalation anaesthetics (e.g. isoflurane) increase the blockade and duration of non-depolarising neuromuscular blocking agents
- potentiated by some antibiotics, including some of the aminoglycosides, tetracyclines, polymyxin (colistimethate), clindamycin, lincomycin, metronidazole and vancomycin
- potentiated by magnesium sulfate heptahydrate
- effects are reversed by calcium salts
- intensity is increased and duration prolonged by acetazolamide, alpha adrenoceptor blocking agents, calcium-channel blockers, furosemide (frusemide), glucocorticoids, ketamine, lidocaine (lignocaine) (IV, high dose), lithium salts, possibly mannitol, monoamine oxidase inhibitors (MAOIs), oral contraceptives, organophosphates, phenytoin, propranolol, protamine, quinine, selective serotonin reuptake inhibitors (SSRIs) and thiazide diuretics
- onset of action may be lengthened and duration of blockade shortened by chronic use of antiepileptic agents (e.g. phenytoin)
- effects are variable if given with muscle relaxants
- prior administration of suxamethonium hastens onset and increases depth of blockade if given as part of the same procedure
- evidence of spontaneous recovery from suxamethonium should be evident before administration of non-depolarising neuromuscular blocking agents
- suxamethonium should not be used to extend the blockade of non-depolarising blocking agents because the prolonged blockade may be difficult to reverse
- activity is decreased (duration shortened) by a corticosteroid (high dose), phenytoin, adrenaline (epinephrine), carbamazepine, azathioprine, theophylline (high dose), potassium chloride, sodium chloride or calcium chloride dihydrate and anticholinesterases (e.g. donepezil)
- hypokalaemia can potentiate neuromuscular blockade; therefore agents that cause hypokalaemia (e.g. amphotericin B (amphotericin), cisplatin, thiazide or loop diuretics, corticosteroids) should be given with caution
- (ICU) increased risk of myopathy if given long term with corticosteroids
- some agents (some antibiotics, propranolol, hydroxychloroquine, D-penicillamine) may aggravate or unmask latent myasthenia gravis, increasing the person's sensitivity to non-depolarising neuromuscular blocking agents

General Nursing considerations/Cautions for non-depolarising blocking agents

- a small number of people have an atypical cholinesterase gene, which results in the person being very sensitive to neuromuscular blocking agents
- generally administered in the operating theatre or ICU by an anaesthetist or experienced doctor with resuscitation equipment and anticholinesterase reversal agents readily available
- any dehydration, altered blood pH or electrolyte imbalance should be corrected before administering a non-depolarising blocking agent; otherwise the neuromuscular blocking effect will be increased
- an appropriate neuromuscular monitoring technique should be used to monitor blockage and recovery
- if given as IV infusion, the degree of blockade should be monitored continually
- non-depolarising neuromuscular blocking agents may cause some histamine release locally and systemically, leading to adverse effects including hypersensitivity or anaphylactic reaction. Resuscitation equipment should be readily available
- each agent should be adequately flushed through the IV cannula using sodium chloride 0.9% before the introduction of the next drug
- reversed by neostigmine or pyridostigmine with an anticholinergic (e.g. atropine)
- treatment for malignant hyperthermia includes stopping the anaesthetic agent and neuromuscular agent, administration of oxygen, lowering temperature, restoring fluid and electrolyte balance, maintaining urine output, reversing any acidosis and administration of IV dantrolene
- (ICU) prolonged ($>$ 48 hours) administration with corticosteroids should be avoided
- should not be mixed with alkaline solutions (e.g. barbiturates) because a precipitate may occur
- caution if used in severely obese patients (weight $>$ 30% ideal body weight), as dose estimation should be based on lean body weight, not actual weight, to prevent overdosage and prolonged blockade
- caution if used in those with conditions which may lead to electrolyte imbalance, such as adrenal insufficiency
- caution if used in those with pulmonary disease, asthma, cardiovascular diseases, history of anaphylactic reaction or a family history of malignant hyperthermia
- caution if used in those with known hypersensitivity to a non-depolarising blocking agent, as cross-sensitivity between agents may exist
- caution if used in those with neuromuscular disease/disorders (e.g. polio, Eaton—Lambert syndrome, myasthenia gravis), as effects may be potentiated when given normal doses of neuromuscular blocking agents
- patients with burns may have a resistance to non-depolarising blocking agents; the dose will be dependent on the extent of the burns and the time elapsed since the burns occurred
- prolonged use over several days for maintenance of intubation and muscle paralysis is contraindicated
- contraindicated in patients known to be homozygous for atypical plasma cholinesterase gene because of increased sensitivity to blocking effects

General Patient education for non-depolarising blocking agents

- the patient should be advised not to drive or operate machinery within 12—24 hours of treatment with a non-depolarising blocking agent

NEUROMUSCULAR BLOCKING AGENTS

Should not be used during pregnancy unless benefits outweigh potential risks. Respiratory depression may occur in the newborn if used during delivery via caesarean section. If the patient has received magnesium sulfate heptahydrate for toxaemia during pregnancy, the dose of non-depolarising neuromuscular blocking agent should be reduced.

Caution if used during breastfeeding.

ATRACURIUM BESYLATE

Trade names
Atracurium Besylate Medsurge Injection, DBL Atracurium Besylate Injection, Tracrium Injection

Available forms
Vial: 25 mg/2.5 mL, 50 mg/5 mL

Action
- onset within 2—6 minutes, duration 30—60 minutes, half-life about 20 minutes
- recovery time is 25—45 minutes (depending on the type of anaesthesia used)
- causes histamine release from mast cells at higher clinical doses
- see also General Actions of non-depolarising blocking agents (p. 1420)

Dose
- initially 0.3—0.6 mg/kg by IV bolus, then 0.08—0.10 mg/kg (maintenance) 20—45 minutes later, then at 15—25-minute intervals if needed

Adverse effects
- flushing, rash, hypotension, bronchospasm
- (Rare) seizures
- see also General Adverse effects of non-depolarising blocking agents (p. 1421)

Use/Interactions
- see General Uses/Interactions of non-depolarising blocking agents (p. 1420)

Nursing considerations/Cautions/Patient education
- should not be given IM
- should not be administered in the same IV line as blood transfusion
- if body temperature is reduced, the dose also needs to be reduced
- if the patient has hypovolaemia, administration should be over 60 seconds
- causes histamine release; therefore should be used with caution in those who have increased sensitivity to histamine release (e.g. previous severe anaphylactoid reaction) or those with significant respiratory or cardiovascular disease
- contraindicated on a long-term basis (continuous over a period of days) because of accumulation of laudanosine (metabolite), which has CNS activating properties
- contraindicated in those with hypersensitivity to cisatracurium or benzenesulfonic acid
- see also General Nursing considerations/Cautions/Patient education for non-depolarising blocking agents (p. 1422)

In pregnancy the physician should determine whether the potential benefit outweighs any potential risk to the fetus.

Caution should be exercised when atracurium besilate is administered to a nursing woman, as many drugs are excreted in breastmilk.

It is recommended that in elderly patients the initial dose be at the lower end of the range and that it be administered slowly.

CISATRACURIUM

Trade names
Cisatracurium Accord, Cisatracurium Juno, Cisatracurium Medsurge, Cisatracurium-AFT, Nimbex

Available forms
Vial: 5 mg/mL, 5 mg/2.5 mL, 10 mg/5 mL, 150 mg/30 mL

Action
- stereoisomer of atracurium but more potent
- onset within 2—7 minutes, duration 10—35 minutes, half-life 22—29 minutes
- less likely to cause histamine release than atracurium (therefore less flushing, hypotension and/or bronchospasm)
- see also General Actions of non-depolarising blocking agents (p. 1420)

Dose
- initially 0.15 mg/kg by IV bolus, then 0.03 mg/kg (maintenance) at 20-minute intervals (if needed) **OR**
- initially 0.18 mg/kg/hour by IV infusion, then reduced to 0.06—0.12 mg/kg/hour (maintenance)

Use/Adverse effects/Interactions
- see General Uses/Adverse effects/Interactions of non-depolarising blocking agents (p. 1420)

Nursing considerations/Cautions
- incompatible with Ringer's solution, propofol and ketorolac
- should not be given with alkaline solutions (e.g. thiopentone)
- should not be administered in the same IV line as blood transfusions
- solution is pale yellow or greenish in colour
- contraindicated in those with hypersensitivity to atracurium or benzenesulfonic acid
- see also General Nursing considerations/Cautions for non-depolarising blocking agents (p. 1422)

MIVACURIUM CHLORIDE
Trade name
Mivacron

Available form
Ampoules: 2 mg/1 mL

Action
- effective within 1—4 minutes, duration of 15—30 minutes, half-life 1.5—3 minutes
- causes histamine release from mast cells
- see also General Actions of non-depolarising blocking agents (p. 1420)

Dose
- (Tracheal intubation) 0.2 mg/kg by IV bolus over 30 seconds **OR**
- 0.5—0.6 mg/kg/hour by IV infusion following bolus dose (above)

Use/Adverse effects/Interactions/Nursing considerations/Cautions/Patient education
- IV infusion rate should be maintained for 3 minutes before altering rate
- solution is pale yellow in colour
- caution if used in those with TB, severe or chronic infection, malnutrition, chronic anaemia, malignancy, myxoedema, collagen disease, peptic ulcer, end-stage liver failure or acute/chronic/end-stage kidney failure
- see also General Uses/Adverse effects/Interactions/Nursing considerations/Cautions/Patient education for non-depolarising blocking agents (p. 1420)

 Mivacron should not be used during pregnancy unless the expected clinical benefit to the mother outweighs any potential risk to the fetus.

 Mivacron should not be used during breastfeeding unless the expected clinical benefit to the mother outweighs any potential risk to the fetus.

 Reduced dosage and/or dosage monitoring in those with reduced renal or hepatic function.

 Reduced dosage and/or dosage monitoring in elderly patients.

ROCURONIUM BROMIDE
Trade names
DBL Rocuronium Bromide Injection, Rocuronium Bromide Medsurge, Rocuronium-hameln Solution

Available form
Vial: 50 mg/5 mL

NEUROMUSCULAR BLOCKING AGENTS

Action
- analogue of vecuronium with faster onset of action
- onset of action within 1–3 minutes IV, duration 30–40 minutes, half-life 66–80 minutes
- see also General Actions of non-depolarising blocking agents (p. 1420)

Dose
- 0.6 mg/kg (loading dose) IV, then 0.15 mg/kg (maintenance) **OR**
- 0.6 mg/kg IV, then 0.3–0.6 mg/kg/hour by IV infusion

Use/Adverse effects
- see General Uses/Adverse effects of non-depolarising blocking agents (p. 1420)

Interactions
- increases the onset of action of lidocaine (lignocaine)
- see also General Interactions of non-depolarising blocking agents (p. 1421)

Nursing considerations/Cautions/Patient education
- incompatible with amoxicillin, amphotericin B (amphotericin), azathioprine, cefazolin, dexamethasone, diazepam, erythromycin, famotidine, furosemide (frusemide), hydrocortisone, insulin, intralipid, methylprednisolone, prednisolone, propofol, thiopentone, trimethoprim and vancomycin
- ensure IV line is adequately flushed with sodium chloride 0.9% before and after administration
- solution is clear to pale yellow in colour
- should not be returned to refrigerator after being used at room temperature
- contraindicated in those with hypersensitivity to bromide
- see also General Nursing considerations/Cautions/Patient education for non-depolarising blocking agents (p. 1422)

VECURONIUM BROMIDE
Trade names
Vercure, Vecuronium Sun

Available form
Vial: 10 mg

Action
- effective within 2–4 minutes IV, duration 20–40 minutes, half-life 36–117 minutes
- see also General Actions of non-depolarising blocking agents (p. 1420)

Dose
- initially 0.10 mg/kg IV, then 0.02–0.04 mg/kg at 20–40-minute intervals **OR**
- 0.8–1.4 microgram/kg/min by IV infusion

Interactions
- may increase the onset of action of lidocaine (lignocaine)
- blockade increased and duration increased if used during surgery under hypothermia
- see also General Interactions of non-depolarising blocking agents (p. 1421)

Use/Adverse effects/Nursing considerations/Cautions/Patient education
- reconstitute using 5 mL water for injections
- incompatible with thiopentone
- contraindicated in those with hypersensitivity to bromide or pancuronium (as cross-sensitivity exists)
- see also General Uses/Adverse effects/ Nursing considerations/Cautions/Patient education for non-depolarising blocking agents (p. 1420)

 Should be used with caution in patients with clinically significant hepatic and/or biliary diseases and/or renal failure.

DEPOLARISING BLOCKING AGENTS

Suxamethonium is the only current depolarising blocking agent in clinical use.

SUXAMETHONIUM CHLORIDE
Trade names
Suxamethonium Juno (Suxamethonium Medsurge)

Available form
Ampoules: 100 mg/2 mL

Action
- also known as succinylcholine
- consists of two acetylcholine molecules that are joined at the acetyl ends
- binds to cholinergic receptors, resulting in persistent stimulation while maintaining depolarisation at motor endplate; therefore the receptor site is unable to respond to any other stimuli
- rapidly hydrolysed by cholinesterase (pseudocholinesterase) in liver and plasma
- onset of action within 30—60 seconds (IV) or 2—3 minutes (IM), duration 4—6 minutes (IV) or 10—30 minutes (IM), rapid half-life 2—4 minutes
- duration of action prolonged in those with low plasma cholinesterase levels
- muscle relaxation may be preceded by painful muscular fasciculations
- has no effect on consciousness, pain threshold or cerebration
- action not reversed by anticholinesterase

Use
- procedures requiring brief but profound relaxation, such as endotracheal intubation, electroconvulsive therapy (ECT), endoscopic examination or orthopaedic manipulations

Dose
- (Short procedures) 0.6 mg/kg IV over 10—30 seconds **OR**
- (Prolonged surgical procedures) 1—2 mg/mL solution given by IV infusion at a rate of 2.5—4.3 mg/min **OR**
- up to 2.5 mg/kg IM (maximum 150 mg) (if IV not possible)

Adverse effects
- postoperative muscle pain (particularly chest, abdominal and shoulder girdle muscles), muscle fasciculations, hypertonia
- myoglobinuria, myoglobinaemia, rhabdomyolysis, increased creatine phosphokinase (CPK)
- trismus
- apnoea, prolongs respiratory depression, bronchospasm
- transient rise in intraocular pressure
- increase in intracranial pressure
- excessive salivation, increased gastric secretions and bowel movements, increased bronchial secretions
- hyperkalaemia, arrhythmias, hypotension, hypertension, bradycardia, tachycardia, cardiac arrest
- (Rare) malignant hyperthermia (signs include muscle rigidity, tachycardia, tachypnoea, increased oxygen requirements, increased carbon dioxide production, increased temperature and metabolic acidosis), porphyria, hypersensitivity

Interactions
- may increase risk of apnoea, malignant hyperthermia and arrhythmias when given with inhalation anaesthetics, including nitrous oxide
- increased risk of bradycardia and asystole if given with fentanyl or propofol
- decreased dose required in those with hypocalcaemia or hypokalaemia
- effects may increase when given with amphotericin B (amphotericin) and thiazide diuretics because of risk of electrolyte imbalance
- causes immediate increase in serum potassium, which may be prolonged

- and is increased by beta adrenoceptor blocking agents, leading to an increased risk of cardiac arrest
- intensity and duration may be altered when given before or with non-depolarising muscle relaxants
- effect may be prolonged or enhanced when given with some non-penicillin antibiotics, aprotinin, azathioprine, beta adrenoceptor blocking agents, carbamazepine, hydroxychloroquine, high-dose corticosteroids, cyclophosphamide, lidocaine (lignocaine), lithium, magnesium salts, oral contraceptives, oxytocin, phenytoin, procaine, quinine, selective serotonin reuptake inhibitors (SSRIs), thiotepa or terbutaline
- increased risk of arrhythmias when given with digoxin or verapamil, or in those with digoxin toxicity
- prolonged depolarisation may occur if given with cholinesterase inhibitors (e.g. donepezil, metoclopramide, neostigmine, pyridostigmine, rivastigmine)
- duration may be decreased by atracurium or diazepam
- caution if exposed to neurotoxic insecticides and weed killers, antimalarial agents, antineoplastic agents, monoamine oxidase inhibitors (MAOIs), oral contraceptives, pancuronium, chlorpromazine or neostigmine, as these may decrease levels of pseudocholinesterase

Nursing considerations/Cautions

- should be given only by experienced medical staff with immediate access to resuscitation equipment
- any known hyperkalaemia or electrolyte imbalance should be corrected before administration of suxamethonium if possible
- should not be given to a conscious patient, as respiratory muscles become paralysed
- administer alone
- initial test dose of 0.1 mg/kg IV may be given to test response
- for IV infusion, should be diluted using glucose 5% or sodium chloride 0.9% to a concentration of 1–2 mg/mL
- may be given IM if vein is not accessible
- if prolonged apnoea occurs after administration, neostigmine should not be used as a reversal agent, as it may intensify blockade
- repeated administration is not recommended, as prolonged respiratory depression and apnoea may occur
- treatment for malignant hyperthermia includes stopping the anaesthetic agent and neuromuscular agent, administration of oxygen, lowering temperature, restoring fluid and electrolyte balance, maintaining urine output, reversing any acidosis and administration of IV dantrolene
- caution if used in those with bone fractures, as muscle contractions will occur before relaxation phase, causing increased pain
- caution if used in those with burns or trauma, as abnormal response to suxamethonium may persist for up to 2 years post-injury, with the greatest risk being between 10 and 90 days post-injury, but may also be prolonged if there is infection or prolonged healing (see contraindication below)
- caution if used in those with hypoxia, cardiovascular, liver, kidney, metabolic or lung disease or myasthenia gravis
- caution if used in those with pre-existing hyperkalaemia or electrolyte imbalance, uraemia, hemiplegia, paraplegia, head injury, encephalitis, ruptured cerebral aneurysm, tetanus, acute anterior horn disease, extensive denervation of skeletal muscle or degenerative neuromuscular disease (especially between 3 weeks and 6 months of onset), as hyperkalaemia increases the risk of cardiac arrest
- caution if used in those with decreased serum levels of pseudocholinesterase (cancer, severe dehydration, malnutrition, severe hepatic disease, severe anaemia, myxoedema, burns, pregnancy, abnormal body temperature, collagen

HAVARD'S NURSING GUIDE TO DRUGS

- diseases, severe infection, myocardial infarction or kidney impairment
- not recommended in those with phaeochromocytoma or during intraocular surgery in those with glaucoma
- not recommended in those with severe sepsis of greater than 7-day duration. Infection must be cleared before administering suxamethonium because of the risk of hyperkalaemia
- not recommended in patients with myotonias because of unpredictable effects
- contraindicated in those who have had malignant hyperthermia or have a family history of malignant hyperthermia, a penetrating eye injury or acute narrow-angle glaucoma, myopathies associated with increased CPK, Duchenne's muscular dystrophy or genetic disorders of pseudocholinesterases
- contraindicated after multiple trauma, severe burns (acute phase), extensive muscle degeneration (e.g. recent paraplegia), severe hyperkalaemia, kidney impairment or severe long-lasting sepsis because there is an increased risk of cardiac arrhythmias and arrest owing to severe hyperkalaemia resulting from administration of suxamethonium

Patient education

- the patient should be advised not to drive or operate machinery if there are any residual adverse effects
- advise the patient to seek medical advice immediately if any of the following occur:
  - change in heart rate or palpitations
  - eye pain
  - muscle stiffness

Used during pregnancy only if benefits outweigh risks. Plasma pseudocholinesterase levels are decreased during pregnancy and remain low for several days after delivery.

Use with caution in patients who have renal and hepatic disorders.

OPIOID ANALGESICS

Pain can be described as 'an unpleasant sensory and emotional experience associated with actual or potential tissue damage, or described in terms of such damage' (International Association for the Study of Pain (IASP) 2017). Pain is a subjective experience affected by a person's individual biological, psychological (including previous experience with pain) and cultural makeup, which means that ideally a person's pain management is individually tailored to their needs.

Pain may be *acute* (usually related to tissue damage and sharp in nature, also termed nociceptive), *chronic* (lasting longer than the original injury and for more than 6 months and variable in nature) or *neuropathic* (resulting from damage to nerves and presenting as burning, tingling or electric shock-type quality) (Rathmell & Fields 2018). Each of these pain types requires a different management strategy. For example, neuropathic pain may not respond to Opioid Treatment Program traditional NSAIDs or opioid analgesics and requires adjunct medications, such as tricyclic antidepressants (TCAs) or anticonvulsant medications (Knights et al 2023).

The opioid analgesics, as they are known today (also termed narcotic analgesics because of their sedation-producing properties), is a group of both natural and synthetic agonist drugs that have morphine-like properties and interact with specific opioid receptors (mu, delta and kappa, but predominantly the mu receptors) in the brain to lessen or remove the sensation of pain. Mu receptor activation is also responsive for other effects, including euphoria, sedation, respiratory depression, constipation and pupillary constriction. Opioid receptors are also located in other tissues, including the gastrointestinal tract and cardiovascular and immune systems (Rathmell & Fields 2018).

Drug tolerance, particularly with opioids, means that over time the body becomes less responsive to the drug, requiring higher doses to achieve the same effect (Knights et al 2023). Tolerance may develop not only to the analgesic effects but also to sedation, nausea and vomiting. However, patients do not become tolerant to other adverse effects, such as constipation, confusion and hallucinations, which only worsen with increasing doses to overcome the tolerance (Knights et al 2023). Fear of physical and psychological dependence on analgesics often leads to poor pain management (especially in the elderly), and is of little consequence in palliative or terminal care. Other reasons for poor pain management and unrelieved pain include nurses' inadequate knowledge and misconceptions about pain and its assessment (including nurses not believing it is a patient's right to expect total pain relief); poor, infrequent or unsystematic pain assessment; inadequate time to assess and manage a patient's pain (i.e. workload), irregular reassessment for pain relief (i.e. assessing the effectiveness of the analgesia); and nurses not accepting patients' report of pain (Knights et al 2023).

A 'good' pain management plan is one that incorporates treatment of the cause of the pain (if possible) rather than treating the symptoms. Accurate and ongoing pain assessment using a validated tool is essential in establishing pain levels and the efficacy of the management plan (including analgesics) (e.g. has the analgesic reduced pain levels so the patient is comfortable and able to function?). Analgesics should be administered at regular intervals (rather than PRN) in order to prevent pain from occurring. Opioids such as the ones discussed in this section are prescribed for moderate-to-severe pain, where NSAIDs (see p. 10) are used for mild pain. Known adverse effects (such as constipation, nausea and vomiting) should be prevented by use of appropriate agents administered concurrently with the opioid (Knights et al 2023).

Consideration should also be given to complementary medicine as an adjunct to traditional pain management strategies. There is strong evidence that acupuncture is effective in the management of chronic pain, resulting in a decreased usage of opioids. The evidence for other therapies, such as yoga, relaxation, tai chi and massage, is positive but weak (Lin et al 2017). The pain management plan should also consider non-pharmacological therapies, such as patient education, psychological therapies, exercise program, sleep hygiene and looking at activities that precipitate pain, and pacing or management of these activities in order to reduce the pain (e.g. timing, postural components, aids). Multidisciplinary input will often be required to facilitate these plans and includes clinicians such as psychologists, physiotherapists, occupational therapists and exercise physiologists (Faculty of Pain Medicine (FPM) & Australian and New Zealand College of Anaesthetists (ANZCA) 2015).

General Actions of opioids
- main actions are on CNS and smooth muscle
- analgesic action is caused by binding with specific opioid receptors (mu, delta and kappa) both pre- and post-synaptically, decreasing pain transmission in the spinal cord and modulating descending inhibitory pathways from the brain
- depresses respiratory centre (brainstem), decreasing the response to carbon dioxide
- suppresses cough centre (medulla)
- stimulates vomiting centre (chemoreceptor trigger zone (CTZ))
- stimulates the vagus nerve

OPIOID ANALGESICS

- produces miosis
- increases smooth muscle tone in the GI tract (especially the sphincters)
- reduces peristalsis and secretions
- relieves anxiety
- may produce euphoria or dysphoria, sedation and raised intracranial pressure
- causes histamine release, resulting in bronchospasm and itching
- tolerance and dependence may occur
- generally not well absorbed after oral administration owing to extensive first-pass metabolism in the liver

General Adverse effects of opioids
- nausea, anorexia, constipation, vomiting, dry mouth, dyspepsia
- respiratory depression, apnoea, dyspnoea, cyanosis
- urinary retention
- increased intracranial pressure
- ureteric or biliary spasm, increased intracholedochal pressure
- blurred vision, diplopia, miosis, visual disturbances
- cough suppression
- drowsiness, euphoria or dysphoria, headache, dizziness, confusion, vertigo, sedation, somnolence, mood change, slurred speech, hallucinations, delirium, tremor
- bradycardia, orthostatic hypotension (in ambulant patients), hypotension, tachycardia
- facial flushing, pruritus, urticaria
- sweating, hypothermia, chills
- muscle rigidity (including thoracic muscles), myoclonic movements
- prolongation of labour (reduction of strength, duration and frequency of contractions) or shortening of labour (increased rate of cervical dilation)
- seizures (high doses)
- tolerance and dependence (physical and/or psychological) may develop
- withdrawal symptoms (usually on rapid discontinuation)
- allergy, hypersensitivity, including rash, hives, pruritus, bronchospasm

General Interactions of opioids
- not recommended or contraindicated with alcohol, antihistamines, barbiturates, benzodiazepines, general anaesthetics, phenothiazines, sedative/hypnotics, other opioids or TCAs because CNS and respiratory depressant effects may be enhanced
- contraindicated with or within 2 weeks of monoamine oxidase inhibitors (MAOIs) because significant respiratory depression, hypotension and hyperpyrexia may occur
- actions may be antagonised by naloxone and naltrexone
- increased risk of respiratory depression if given with neuromuscular blocking agent or benzodiazepines
- miosis may be counteracted by atropine and atropine-like agents
- use with anticholinergic agents, tricyclic antidepressants (with anticholinergic effects), anti-Parkinson's agents and antihistamines (with anticholinergic effects) may increase the risk of severe constipation, urinary retention and/or paralytic ileus
- caution if used with other agents that depress respiratory function
- increased risk of severe constipation if given with antidiarrhoeal or antiperistaltic agents (e.g. loperamide, kaolin)
- may increase hypotensive effects if given with antihypertensive agents, diuretics or other agents with hypotensive effects

- if buprenorphine is given before other opioids, therapeutic effects of opioids may be reduced
- respiratory and cardiovascular depressant effects may be potentiated by halogenated inhalation anaesthetic agents
- metabolism may be inhibited by amiodarone, clarithromycin, diltiazem, erythromycin, fluconazole, itraconazole, ritonavir, verapamil and voriconazole, increasing risk of prolonged respiratory depression because of increased serum levels of opioid
- caution if an oral opioid is used with metoclopramide because gastric emptying and absorption may be increased, potentiating the CNS effects of the opioid
- delays gastric emptying and absorption; therefore all concurrent oral medication may be affected
- caution if given with rifampicin as opioid serum levels and effects may be decreased
- may interfere with gastric emptying studies and hepatobiliary imaging

General Nursing considerations/Cautions for opioids

- administration and storage precautions are as per state and territory Acts and Regulations for controlled drugs
- an opioid-tolerant patient is considered to be one who takes at least 60 mg morphine daily
- patient should be assessed for any known allergy to opioids (it is important to have the patient describe the allergy because some will describe the adverse effects (especially nausea and vomiting) as 'allergy')
- adverse effects are more common and severe in ambulant patients
- analgesia is more effective if given before onset of intense pain. Plan to give patient analgesia 15–30 minutes before undertaking any procedure that will cause pain or discomfort
- patient should be closely monitored for any signs of respiratory depression and drug withheld, and doctor informed if the respiratory rate shows marked decline (especially if 8 breaths/minute or less). Respiratory depression can occur at any time during therapy (not just initially) and special care should be taken with opioids with long half-life (e.g. fentanyl) as respiratory depression can occur after agent has been discontinued
- any hypovolaemia should be corrected before starting therapy to reduce risk of hypotension
- even if initial dose causes vomiting, subsequent doses depress the vomiting centre
- antiemetic should be given at the same time if vomiting is likely to be a problem; laxatives should also be commenced concurrently to prevent severe constipation from developing
- urinary output, presence of bowel sounds and bowel pattern should be monitored
- if opioid is used intraoperatively, patients should be closely observed postoperatively for any signs of delayed respiratory depression
- opioid-induced hyperalgesia should be considered if there is insufficient pain control in response to increased dose
- tolerance may develop in 24–48 hours, with larger doses being required to produce the same effect
- both physical and psychological dependence may occur. If opioid is

OPIOID ANALGESICS

- withheld, withdrawal syndrome (aggression, irritability, runny nose, body aches, yawning, fever, sweating, pupil dilation, nausea, vomiting, diarrhoea, stomach cramps, insomnia, nervousness, restlessness, tachycardia, tremor and goosebumps) may be seen
- naloxone and resuscitation equipment should be readily available to reverse respiratory depression
- ensure that the correct strength of syrup, ampoules/vials or correct tablet type (immediate release versus sustained release) is selected, as some opioids have multiple formulations
- caution if used in those with myasthenia gravis or phaeochromocytoma
- caution if used in those with hypothyroidism, adrenocortical insufficiency (e.g. Addison's disease), shock or myxoedema as symptoms may be exacerbated and/or there may be increased risk of respiratory and/or CNS depression
- caution if used in those with pulmonary disease, decreased respiratory reserve, alcoholism or impaired liver or kidney function
- caution if used in those with hypovolaemia or shock as hypotension may occur
- caution if used in those with acute abdominal conditions (including GI obstruction or obstructive bowel disorder) or postoperatively after abdominal surgery as intestinal mobility is decreased by opioids
- caution if using opioids in the elderly as they may have reduced liver or kidney function, reduced protein binding and reduced cardiac output, which may lead to accumulation of opioid and possible toxicity
- caution if used in those with diabetes as hyperglycaemia may occur
- caution if used in those with epilepsy or at risk of seizures (e.g. head injury, metabolic disorders, alcohol or drug withdrawal) because of the increased risk of seizures
- caution if used in those with prostatic obstruction/hypertrophy, urethral stricture or recent urinary tract surgery because of the risk of urinary retention
- caution if prescribed to those with a known history of drug/alcohol abuse/dependence, emotional instability or suicidal ideation/attempts
- not recommended/contraindicated in those with head injury, increased intracranial pressure, impaired consciousness, brain tumour or coma as carbon dioxide retention may further increase intracranial pressure (which may obscure clinical course in those with head injury)
- contraindicated in those with biliary or renal tract spasm or after biliary tract surgery
- contraindicated in those with diarrhoea caused by pseudomembranous colitis, poisoning or other toxic organisms because the slowing of the GI tract by opioids will prolong the diarrhoea
- contraindicated in those with respiratory depression, a low respiratory reserve, acute bronchial asthma, cardiac arrhythmias, CNS depression, heart failure (secondary to chronic pulmonary disease), acute alcoholism, delirium tremens, severe liver/kidney disease, hepatic encephalopathy, diabetic acidosis with danger of coma, or convulsive disorders (including status epilepticus, pre-eclampsia or eclampsia)

General Patient education for opioids

- advise patient not to drive or operate machinery if dizziness, drowsiness, sedation or confusion occur
- warn patient to take care when going from lying to standing position as dizziness may occur because of hypotension
- patient should be warned to avoid alcohol during therapy with opioid analgesics
- instruct patient to deep breathe, cough and move frequently (if permitted) postoperatively
- encourage patient to practise good dental hygiene as opioids can cause dry mouth, increasing the risk of dental caries
- advise patients with diabetes to monitor blood glucose levels closely during therapy

> Contraindicated during pregnancy as it may cause respiratory depression in newborn infants; therefore naloxone should be readily available. May cause withdrawal symptoms in newborn if there has been prolonged maternal use during pregnancy.

> Not recommended during or within 24 hours of breastfeeding. If used, baby should be observed for signs of sedation and other adverse effects.

> Opioids are banned in sport.

ALFENTANIL
Trade name
Alfentanil GH, Alfentanil-hameln, Medsurge Alfentanil, Rapifen

Available forms
Ampoule: 1 mg/2 mL, 5 mg/10 mL

Action
- potent short-acting synthetic opioid analgesic with mu receptor activity that is related to fentanyl (with more rapid onset)
- onset of analgesia and respiratory depression is 1—2 minutes, short duration of action (dose-related), elimination half-life is 90—110 minutes
- see also General Actions of opioids (p. 1430)

Use
- anaesthetic induction
- analgesic supplement

Dose
- generally given by specialist anaesthetist

Adverse effects
- laryngospasm
- muscle rigidity
- see also General Adverse effects of opioids (p. 1431)

Interactions
- may increase serum levels of propofol
- increased serum levels may occur if given with propofol
- metabolism may be decreased leading to increased serum levels by diltiazem, erythromycin, voriconazole and fluconazole
- increased risk of serotonin syndrome if given with selective serotonin reuptake inhibitors (SSRIs) or monoamine oxidase inhibitors (MAOIs)
- see also General Interactions of opioids (p. 1431)

Nursing considerations/Cautions
- oxygen, resuscitation and intubation equipment should be readily available
- if analgesia > 60 minutes is required, IV infusion is recommended
- the patient should be monitored for at least 2 hours postoperatively for any signs of respiratory depression
- muscle rigidity can be avoided by slow IV administration (especially at high doses), premedication with benzodiazepines or use of muscle relaxants

OPIOID ANALGESICS

- staff should be advised to wear gloves during administration. If contact with skin occurs, area should be thoroughly washed with water only
- not recommended in the last 10 minutes before the completion of surgery
- caution if used in those who are obese or have uncontrolled hypothyroidism as clearance may be reduced (requiring a lower dose)
- contraindicated as postoperative pain management
- see also General Nursing considerations/Cautions for opioids (p. 1432)

Patient education

- the patient should be advised to wait 3–6 hours (for 0.5–1.5 mg) or 12–24 hours (for higher doses) before driving or operating machinery because of possible delayed respiratory depression
- see also General Patient education for opioids (p. 1434)

BUPRENORPHINE

Trade name
B-Patch, Bupredermal, Buprenorphine Sandoz, Buvidal Monthly, Buvidal Weekly, Norspan, Sublocade, Subutex, Temgesic

Available forms
Sublingual tablets: 200 microgram, 400 microgram, 2 mg, 8 mg;
Transdermal patches: 5 mg, 10 mg, 15 mg, 20 mg, 25 mg, 30 mg, 40 mg;
Ampoules: 300 microgram/mL;
Modified-release solution (prefilled syringe): 8 mg/0.16 mL, 16 mg/0.32 mL, 24 mg/0.48 mL, 32 mg/0.64 mL, 64 mg/0.18 mL, 96 mg/0.27 mL, 100 mg/0.5 mL, 128 mg/0.36 mL, 160 mg/0.45 mL, 300 mg/1 mL, 300 mg/1.5 mL

Action
- synthetic opioid that has both opioid agonist (mu receptors) and antagonist (delta and kappa receptors) properties
- more potent than morphine and longer acting
- active metabolite (norbuprenorphine)
- see also General Actions of opioids (p. 1430)

Use
- moderate-to-severe pain (short-term management) (transdermal patches, IV or IM)
- opioid dependence (detoxification or maintenance) (sublingual tablets, modified-release solution)

Dose
- (Pain) 0.3–0.6 mg IM or slow IV injection (over at least 2 minutes) 6–8-hourly **OR**
- (Pain) 0.2–0.4 mg sublingually 6–8-hourly **OR**
- (Pain) initially 5 mg patch (releasing 5 micrograms/hour), applied to skin weekly, increasing at 3–7-day interval until satisfactory analgesia is achieved (maximum 40 mg) **OR**
- (Opioid dependence) initially 4–8 mg sublingually with additional 4 mg if needed (day 1, target 8–12 mg), then gradually increasing in increments of 2–8 mg according to response (daily maximum 32 mg). Dose frequency may be reduced once patient is stable **OR**
- (Opioid dependence, modified-release solution) 8–32 mg slow SC weekly **OR**
- (Opioid dependence, modified-release solution) 64–128 mg slow SC monthly **OR**
- (Opioid dependence, modified-release solution, adults stabilised on transmucosal buprenorphine for ≥ 7 days) 300 mg SC monthly for 2 months, then 100 mg SC monthly (maintenance); however, maintenance dose can be increased to 300 mg monthly if no satisfactory response after second maintenance dose (Sublocade)

Adverse effects
- miosis more marked than for morphine and lasting > 24 hours
- (IM, IV) injection site reaction
- (SC, injection site) pain, pruritus, erythema, induration, swelling, bruising, ulceration

- (Transdermal patch) erythema, oedema, rash, pruritus
- (Transdermal patch, high dose) prolongation of QT interval
- liver injury (including elevated liver enzymes, hepatitis, liver failure, liver necrosis, encephalopathy) (especially in those with previous liver damage, such as hepatitis B or C, alcoholism)
- see also General Adverse effects of opioids (p. 1431)

Interactions
- caution if given with rifampicin, phenytoin or carbamazepine as metabolism may be increased, decreasing serum levels
- caution if given with protease inhibitors, azole antifungals or macrolide antibiotics as serum levels may be increased
- caution if given with other hepatotoxic agents
- if given with warfarin, may increase INR; therefore this should be carefully monitored
- if buprenorphine is given before other opioids, therapeutic effects of opioids may be reduced
- elimination may be reduced if given with general anaesthetics or other agents that reduce liver blood flow
- (IV) not recommended with IV benzodiazepines
- (Transdermal patch) not recommended with other agents known to prolong QT interval or cause electrolyte imbalances, especially hypokalaemia or hypomagnesaemia
- see also General Interactions of opioids (p. 1431)

Nursing considerations/Cautions
- liver function test monitoring is recommended before starting and regularly throughout therapy
- may cause withdrawal symptoms if used in patients who are dependent on other opioid analgesics, because of its antagonistic properties
- not fully reversed by naloxone; therefore if respiratory depression occurs, ensure patient is adequately ventilated
- (Opioid dependence) should be part of a coordinated treatment program (medical and psychosocial), not a standalone therapy
- (Opioid dependence) part of Opioid Treatment Program requiring special authority
- (Opioid dependence) first dose may produce mild withdrawal symptoms in those being detoxified (i.e. with a dependence on opioids) if given too soon after opioid
- (Opioid dependence) methadone dose should be reduced to 30 mg daily before starting therapy
- (Opioid dependence) if transferring from methadone, a 24-hour gap should be left before starting therapy because of the long half-life of methadone. If transferring from short-acting opiates (including street heroin), there should be at least a 6-hour gap and signs of withdrawal before starting therapy
- (Opioid dependence) drug should not be stopped abruptly, but gradually over 3 weeks
- (Opioid dependence, SC) patient should be stabilised on sublingual therapy for at least 7 days before starting SC therapy, which can be commenced the day after last sublingual dose was administered
- (Opioid dependence, SC) patient may receive an additional 8 mg SC during dosing period if required (maximum dose 128 mg)
- (Opioid dependence, SC) if transitioning from sublingual tablets to weekly or monthly SC injections, the following is recommended:
    - 2–6 mg sublingual = 8 mg SC weekly
    - 8–10 mg sublingual = 16 mg SC weekly = 64 mg SC monthly
    - 12–16 mg sublingual = 24 mg SC weekly = 96 mg SC monthly
    - 18–24 mg sublingual = 32 mg SC weekly = 128 mg SC monthly

OPIOID ANALGESICS

- (Opioid dependence) if transitioning from SC monthly to daily sublingual, dose should be administered one month after last monthly SC injection was given
- (Opioid dependence) SC injections must only be administered by health professionals
- (Opioid dependence, SC) SC sites include buttock, thigh and upper arm and should be rotated
- (Transdermal patch) not suitable as an 'as needed (PRN)' analgesic because of delayed onset of action, including as pain relief immediately postsurgery
- (Transdermal patch) if adequate analgesia cannot be achieved using 40 mg patch, therapy should be discontinued and a stronger opioid used
- (Transdermal patch) patient with severe febrile illness should be closely monitored as increased skin blood flow may increase drug absorption
- (Transdermal patch) during titration of dose, dose should not be increased at less than 3-day intervals. Patch can be removed and a stronger strength patch applied, or a second patch can be added. However, no more than 2 patches should be applied to any one site and dose should not be greater than 40 mg
- (Transdermal patch) when discontinuing therapy, dose should be tapered downwards at 7-day intervals
- (Transdermal patch) when therapy is stopped, another opioid should not be given within 24 hours
- IV/IM route should be used only when sublingual route is not available
- (Prefilled syringes) needle cap may contain rubber latex, which may cause hypersensitivity reaction in sensitive individuals
- risk of abuse/misuse is present
- (Transdermal patches or IV/IM administration) not recommended for opioid dependence/withdrawal management
- (SC, modified-release solution) must not be administered IV or intradermally. Gel depot will form on contact with body fluids causing occlusion, local tissue necrosis and/or thromboembolic events
- (Modified-release solution) contraindicated in those with history of hypersensitivity reactions
- see also General Nursing considerations/Cautions for opioids (p. 1432)

Patient education

Sublingual tablets
- advise the patient that tablets should be kept under the tongue for at least 10 minutes before swallowing and they should have nothing else to eat or drink until tablet is completely dissolved. Warn the patient that tablets are less effective if chewed or swallowed

Transdermal patch
- the patient should be instructed to stop any other opioid analgesics when starting therapy with transdermal patches. However, the patient should be encouraged to take analgesics until transdermal patch takes effect
- if the patient develops a fever, they should be advised to monitor for any opioid adverse effects, because heat increases the release of the drug from the buprenorphine transdermal patch (increasing the risk of overdose and respiratory depression)
- advise the patient to continue swimming, bathing or showering as normal as these have no effect on transdermal patches
- the patient should be advised that transdermal patches should:
    - not be cut or damaged
    - be applied to skin on upper outer arms, upper chest or back or side of chest. Application area should not be red, irritated, burnt, scarred or damaged in any way. Application sites should be rotated and not reused within 3 weeks
    - be applied to cleaned (using water only) skin, with area completely dried before application. Hair can be

- clipped (not shaved) for application if necessary
- be removed from pouch, then silver backing foil removed and patch applied to skin with pressure from the palm for 30 seconds, taking care not to touch sticky section. If the edges of the patch start to peel, they can be taped to the skin
- be changed weekly
- be replaced by a new patch if old one falls off accidentally
- not be exposed to external heat source(s) (e.g. electric blanket, hot water bottle, saunas, spas, sunbathing), because heat increases release of buprenorphine, increasing risk of overdose and respiratory depression
- be carefully/safely disposed of (used patches should be folded (with adhesive sides sticking together), wrapped and disposed of carefully to prevent any misuse of product by non-patients)
* wash hands after applying patch
* ensure that the patient understands which patch or combination of patches should be applied to skin, including no more than 2 patches being applied to same site
* the patient should be instructed to rotate application sites to prevent irritation to area and patch not reapplied to same area within 3—4 weeks
* instruct the patient to seek medical advice immediately if any of the following occur:
  - severe skin reaction after applying transdermal patch, including severe reddening, blistering or burning sensation
  - sudden fainting for no reason or after exercise/emotional excitement, rapid or erratic heartbeat
* warn the patient against stopping therapy suddenly
* see also General Patient education for opioids (p. 1434)

 Sublingual tablet can be dissolved under tongue or in cheek, but must not be chewed or swallowed.

 Caution if used in those with severe liver impairment, as accumulation may occur.

Available in combination with
* buprenorphine 2 mg + naloxone 500 microgram (Suboxone 2 mg/0.5 mg Film)
* buprenorphine 8 mg + naloxone 2 mg (Suboxone 8 mg/2 mg Film)

CODEINE PHOSPHATE HEMIHYDRATE
Trade names
Actacode Linctus, Aspen Codeine Tablets, Codeine Tablets

Available forms
Linctus: 5 mg/mL;
Tablets: 30 mg

Action
* structurally similar to morphine and oxycodone
* one-sixth of the analgesic action of morphine
* metabolised in the liver to morphine and norcodeine
* antitussive action occurs as a result of suppression directly on cough centre in medulla; dries respiratory tract mucus and increases viscosity of bronchial secretions
* onset of analgesic action 15—30 minutes, duration 4—6 hours
* onset of antitussive action 1—2 hours, duration up to 4 hours
* half-life 2—4 hours
* withdrawal symptoms occur more slowly than with morphine
* less euphoria or sedation than with morphine

Use
* antitussive for unproductive dry and intractable cough
* relieves mild-to-moderate pain

OPIOID ANALGESICS

Dose
- (Pain relief) 30—60 mg orally 4—6-hourly
OR
- (Antitussive) 5 mL (25 mg) linctus orally 4—6-hourly

Adverse effects
- may increase plasma levels of amylase and/or lipase
- see also General Adverse effects of opioids (p. 1431)

Interactions
- see General Interactions of opioids (p. 1431)

Nursing considerations/Cautions
- analgesic effect is variable between patients
- no benefit is gained by exceeding 60 mg per dose
- naloxone blocks the effects of codeine phosphate hemihydrate
- not recommended for chronic pain
- contraindicated in those under 12 years, or 12—18 years if respiratory function is compromised (e.g. post tonsillectomy and/or adenoidectomy)
- contraindicated in those with hypersensitivity to morphine or oxycodone
- contraindicated in patients with acute respiratory depression with cyanosis and excessive bronchial secretions as these may be exacerbated
- see also General Nursing considerations/Cautions/Patient education for opioids (p. 1432)

Opioids can cause urinary retention and should therefore be used with caution in those with prostatic hypertrophy/obstruction, urethral stricture or recent urinary tract surgery.
Use with caution in patients with hepatic disease, as metabolism occurs in the liver.

Available in combination with
- codeine phosphate hemihydrate 8 mg + aspirin 300 mg (Aspalgin)
- codeine phosphate hemihydrate + paracetamol tablets (see Paracetamol p. 33)
- codeine phosphate hemihydrate + ibuprofen (see Ibuprofen p. 25)

FENTANYL CITRATE
Trade names
Abstral, Actiq, APO-Fentanyl, B.Braun Fentanyl Solution, DBL Fentanyl, Denpax, Durogesic, Dutran, Fentanyl GH, Fentanyl Juno, Fentanyl Medsurge, Fentanyl Sandoz, Fentanyl-hameln, Fentora, Sublimaze

Available forms
Transdermal patches: 12 microgram/hour, 25 microgram/hour, 50 microgram/hour, 75 microgram/hour, 100 microgram/hour;
Ampoules: 100 microgram/2 mL, 500 microgram/10 mL;
Lozenges: 200 microgram, 400 microgram, 600 microgram, 800 microgram;
Sublingual tablets: 100 microgram, 200 microgram, 300 microgram, 400 microgram, 600 microgram, 800 microgram;
Orally disintegrating tablets: 100 microgram, 200 microgram, 400 microgram, 600 microgram, 800 microgram

Action
- potent opioid analgesic that acts on mu receptors (brain, spinal cord, smooth muscle)
- more potent analgesic effect than morphine
- peak respiratory depression seen in 15—30 minutes after administration and lasts for several hours (longer than analgesic effects)
- duration of action 0.5—2 hours (SC, IM, IV, IT), 6—8 hours (oral) or 3 days (transdermal patch)
- half-life 3—12 hours (IV), 22—25 hours (transdermal patch, after 72-hour application) and 7 hours (oral)
- clearance is reduced and half-life increased in the elderly
- rarely produces histamine release and related adverse effects
- 157 micrograms fentanyl citrate = 100 micrograms fentanyl

Use
- premedication
- induction and maintenance of anaesthesia
- adjunct to general/regional anaesthesia
- postoperatively (in recovery room)
- chronic pain, including breakthrough pain

Dose
- (Premedication) 50—100 micrograms IM 30—60 minutes before surgery **OR**
- (Adjunct to general anaesthesia) 50—100 micrograms IV, repeated at 2—3-minute intervals until desired effect is achieved, then 25—50 micrograms IV or IM (maintenance) **OR**
- (Adjunct to regional anaesthesia) 50—100 micrograms IM or slow IV if additional anaesthesia is required during procedure **OR**
- (Postoperatively) 50—100 micrograms IM repeated 1—2-hourly as necessary **OR**
- (Transdermal patches) initially 25 micrograms/hour patch replaced 72-hourly, then titrate up or down by 12—25 micrograms/hour patch every 3 days **OR**
- (Breakthrough pain (sublingual tablets)) initially 100 micrograms orally sublingually, if adequate pain relief is achieved after 30 minutes; this dose should be used for further episodes of breakthrough pain. If adequate pain relief is not achieved after 30 minutes, a second 100-microgram dose may be given (no more than 2 tablets/episode of breakthrough) pain. If this does not relieve pain, next dose should be higher (daily maximum 800 micrograms) **OR**
- (Breakthrough pain (lozenge)) initially 200-microgram lozenge orally over 15 minutes; after waiting 15 minutes, if analgesia is inadequate, a second 200-microgram lozenge may be consumed. This dose (200 or 400 micrograms) may then be used for several episodes of breakthrough pain, but if still inadequate the dose may be increased (maximum daily dose 4 lozenges (4 episodes of breakthrough pain))

Adverse effects
- (IV) bradycardia, myoclonic movements, muscle rigidity
- (Patches) skin irritation, rash, pustules, redness, oedema, itching
- (Lozenge) gum bleeding, irritation, pain, ulcer, dental caries, gingivitis
- see also General Adverse effects of opioids (p. 1431)

Interactions
- increased risk of respiratory depression and hypotension (and sometimes hypertension) if given with droperidol; therefore blood pressure should be closely monitored during concurrent therapy
- (IV) increased risk of severe bradycardia, hypotension and sinus arrest if given with amiodarone
- increased risk of serotonin syndrome if given with selective serotonin reuptake inhibitors (SSRIs), serotonin and noradrenaline (norepinephrine) reuptake inhibitors (SNRIs) and other serotoninergic agents
- cardiovascular depression may occur if given in high doses with nitrous oxide
- (IV) increased risk of severe hypotension if given with calcium-channel blockers or beta adrenoceptor blocking agents
- sublingual, orally disintegrating and lozenges are not interchangeable
- see also General Interactions of opioids (p. 1431)

Nursing considerations/Cautions
- (Transdermal patch) an opioid-naive patient should be initially managed using immediate-release opioid to establish dose before commencing transdermal patch
- background persistent pain should be controlled with other opioid analgesics before starting therapy with lozenges for breakthrough pain. If the patient experiences more than 4 episodes of breakthrough pain per day, a dose of background (long-acting) opioid analgesic will need adjusting. If this occurs,

OPIOID ANALGESICS

- fentanyl lozenge dose may also require adjusting
- patients experiencing adverse effects should be monitored for at least 24 hours after discontinuation because of the long half-life
- lozenges and sublingual tablets are recommended only in those who have been previously treated with opioid analgesics (not opioid-naive patients)
- (Sublingual tablets) no more than 2 sublingual tablets and an interval of at least 2 hours is recommended per episode of breakthrough pain
- to convert from oral formulations to transdermal patches, calculate the previous 24-hour analgesic amount, then convert to equianalgesic oral morphine dose using the manufacturer's instructions (e.g. 45 mg morphine orally daily is roughly equivalent to 12-micrograms/hour patch) (equianalgesic dose refers to dose of one analgesic that is equivalent in pain-relieving effect to that of another analgesic)
- switching from one brand of transdermal patch to another should be done cautiously because of different properties and should be carried out under medical supervision
- respiratory depression may occur within 15—30 minutes of administration and persist for several hours in non-tolerant (opioid-naive — no previous exposure to opioids) patients. Risk of respiratory depression is less in those who have developed tolerance to opioids
- (Lozenge) if respiratory depression occurs, the lozenge should be removed immediately
- (Lozenge) contains almost 2 g glucose per lozenge, which may be important in blood glucose level management in those with diabetes
- (Sublingual tablets) caution if used in those with mouth ulcers or mucositis
- (IV) patient should be closely monitored during therapy for any signs of respiratory depression. Resuscitation equipment should be readily available
- (IV) when fentanyl and a neuroleptic agent (e.g. droperidol) are given in combination, adverse effects that may be observed include chills, shivering, restlessness, postoperative hallucinations (sometimes with transient mental depression) and extrapyramidal symptoms (up to 24 hours postoperatively)
- (IV) incompatible with thiopentone
- (Transdermal patches, lozenges) not recommended for use in those who are non-tolerant (opioid naive) with non-cancer pain
- caution if used in those with liver or kidney impairment or in the elderly (because of reduced clearance and prolonged half-life)
- (Transdermal patch) contraindicated for acute or postoperative pain where dose cannot be titrated, where pain can be managed by non-opioid agent, where PRN analgesia/starting dose > 25 micrograms/hour, or in those with acute respiratory disease and respiratory depression
- (IV) contraindicated in those with myasthenia gravis
- see also General Nursing considerations/Cautions for opioids (p. 1432)

Patient education

- advise the patient to take extra care in storage and disposal of lozenges/patches if children are in the household, as dose can be fatal in children
- see also General Patient education for opioids (p. 1434)

Lozenge

- advise the patient that lozenges should be sucked, not chewed, moved around inside cheek (using applicator provided) to maximise surface area exposure and held for 15 minutes
- instruct the patient that the lozenge should be used before or after food, but not with food or drink
- advise the patient to moisten mouth with water before using lozenge if dry mouth is a problem
- lozenges contain glucose (1.89 g/dose) and it is therefore important to instruct

- patient to brush teeth regularly during therapy to prevent dental caries
- patients with diabetes should be warned about glucose content (1.89 g/dose) of lozenge
- instruct the patient to tell doctor if lozenge is required more than 4 times per day

Sublingual tablets

- instruct the patient that sublingual tablets should be:
  - removed carefully from foil container so as not to damage tablet
  - placed under the tongue as far back as possible and allowed to dissolve, not sucked, chewed or swallowed
  - not taken with food or drink
- advise the patient to moisten the mouth with water before using sublingual tablet if dry mouth is a problem
- the patient should be instructed not to take more than 2 tablets per episode of breakthrough pain and to wait at least 2 hours before taking more tablets
- instruct the patient to tell the doctor if sublingual tablets are required more than 4 times per day for 4 consecutive days

Transdermal patches

- the patient should be advised that patches should:
  - not be cut or damaged
  - be applied to non-irritated, non-scarred and non-irradiated skin (torso or upper arms)
  - be changed every 72 hours
  - be worn only one at a time
  - be dated to remind patient when next patch is due
  - not be exposed to external heat source(s) (e.g. electric blanket, hot water bottle, saunas, spas, sunbathing), because heat increases release of fentanyl, increasing risk of overdose and respiratory depression
  - be carefully/safely disposed of (used patches should be folded with adhesive sides sticking together), wrapped and disposed of carefully to prevent any misuse of product by non-patients)
- the patient should be instructed to rotate application sites to prevent irritation to area
- advise the patient that hair can be clipped (not shaved) for application if necessary. Skin should be cleaned (using water only) and area completely dried before application
- instruct the patient to remove patch from pouch, and apply to skin with pressure from the palm for 30 seconds, avoiding contact with the adhesive
- if gel contacts the skin of the carer or health care worker, it should be washed with copious amounts of water only
- instruct the patient to wash hands after applying patch
- advise the patient to wait until patch has been in situ (in place) for at least 24 hours and other analgesic doses have been titrated accordingly before making initial evaluation of effectiveness of patch
- if removed because of adverse effects, continue to monitor the patient for at least 24 hours
- if the patient develops a fever, they should be advised to monitor for any opioid adverse effects, because heat increases the release of fentanyl from the transdermal patch (increasing risk of overdose and respiratory depression)

Sublingual tablets can be placed under the tongue and allowed to dissolve. Lozenge should be allowed to dissolve over 15 minutes.

Tablets should not be dispersed, crushed or chewed.

Use of patches in childbirth is contraindicated.

OPIOID ANALGESICS

Caution if used in those with kidney dysfunction. Monitor closely for signs of fentanyl toxicity.
Monitor patients with hepatic impairment for toxicity because of the potential delay in elimination. Consider reducing dose.

HYDROMORPHONE
Trade names
Dilaudid, HYDROmorphone hydrochloride 1 mg/mL oral solution, Hydromorphone Juno, Hydromorphone June-HP, Hydromorphone June-XHP, Hydromorphone-hameln, Hydromorphone-hameln-HP, Hydromorphone Medsurge, Hydromorphone Medsurge HP

Available forms
Tablets: 2 mg, 4 mg, 8 mg;
Oral liquid: 1 mg/mL;
Ampoules: 2 mg/mL, 10 mg/mL, 50 mg/5 mL, 50 mg/mL

Action
- opioid mu receptor agonist that is related to morphine, but 5–8 times more potent
- duration of action 2–4 hours (orally) or 4–5 hours (IM, SC or IV)
- half-life is approximately 2.6 hours

Use
- moderate-to-severe pain in opioid tolerant patients

Dose
Non-tolerant (opioid-naive) patients
- 4–8 mg orally daily, titrating dose upwards/downwards by 4–8 mg increments every 4 days if needed (modified-release tablets) **OR**
- 2–4 mg orally 4-hourly **OR**
- 1–2 mg IM or SC 4–6-hourly **OR**
- 0.5–1 mg by slow IV over 2–3 minutes **OR**
- 0.3 mg/hour by IV infusion **OR**
- (Patient-controlled analgesia) 0.1 mg/hour IV (background infusion) plus patient-administered bolus 0.2 mg at 5-minute intervals (1.2 mg/hour maximum)

Patients currently receiving opioids
- starting dose is based on previous day's opioid dose (converted using manufacturer's instructions)

Adverse effects
- (IV) injection site irritation
- see also General Adverse effects of opioids (p. 1431)

Interactions
- see General Interactions of opioids (p. 1431)

Nursing considerations/Cautions
- (IV) Dilaudid-HP is a high-potency preparation and is recommended for use only in opioid-tolerant patients; therefore use caution when selecting correct formulation
- (IV) incompatible with soluble barbiturates
- oral solution contains hydrobenzoate, which may cause allergic reaction in sensitive patients
- caution if used pre- or intraoperatively or within 24 hours postoperatively
- not recommended within 24 hours of chordotomy or other pain-relieving procedures
- see also General Nursing considerations/Cautions for opioids (p. 1432)

Patient education
- the patient to be advised to swallow modified-release tablets whole, not crushed, chewed or divided
- see also General Patient education for opioids (p. 1434)

Oral liquid available. Plain tablet can be crushed and mixed with water.

Caution if used in those with kidney or liver impairment.

Reduction of initial dose is recommended in those over 65 years.

METHADONE HYDROCHLORIDE
Trade names
Aspen Methadone Syrup, Biodone Forte, Methadone-AFT, Physeptone

Available forms
Oral liquid: 5 mg/mL;
Tablets: 10 mg;
Ampoules: 10 mg/mL

Action
- synthetic opioid with properties similar to morphine, but less hypnotic
- duration of action 4—24 hours (oral, IM or IV)
- long half-life of 15 hours in non-tolerant (opioid-naive) people, increasing to 22 hours with chronic use (with variation of 15—60 hours being reported)

Use
- severe pain (especially visceral)
- substitution therapy in the treatment of opioid dependence (Biodone Forte)

Dose
- (Analgesia) initially 5—10 mg orally, SC or IM 6—8-hourly **OR**
- (Opioid dependence) initially 10—20 mg orally, increasing by 5—10 mg daily, then 30—50 mg as maintenance (daily maximum 80 mg)

Adverse effects
- (Injection site) pain, induration, local irritation
- (Rare, high dose) prolongation of QT interval
- (Prolonged use) gynaecomastia
- see also General Adverse effects of opioids (p. 1431)

Interactions
- contraindicated with other agents that prolong QT interval or cause electrolyte disturbance, especially hypokalaemia or hypomagnesaemia
- phenytoin, rifampicin, St John's wort, protease inhibitors, efavirenz, nevirapine and carbamazepine may increase metabolism of methadone, lowering the serum level and increasing the risk of withdrawal symptoms
- metabolism may be decreased by fluconazole and some SSRIs (particularly fluvoxamine)
- may increase serum levels of fluconazole, desipramine and zidovudine
- may decrease serum levels of abacavir
- may cause false positive urine test (using Gravindex test)
- see also General Interactions of opioids (p. 1431)

Nursing considerations/Cautions
- (Opioid dependence) dose increases should not be greater than 5—10 mg daily or 30 mg in a 7-day period
- (Opioid dependence) part of the Opioid Treatment Program requiring special authority
- addition of non-opioid analgesic to methadone improves analgesia
- because of long half-life, repeated doses should be given with caution
- IV infusion of naloxone is recommended if overdose occurs, because of ongoing risk of respiratory depression associated with methadone's long half-life. Patient should be observed for at least 48 hours after recovery in case of relapse
- caution if used in those with phaeochromocytoma
- (Syrup) contraindicated in those with hypersensitivity to permicol red
- contraindicated in those with congenital long QT syndrome or at risk of long QT syndrome (e.g. cardiac hypertrophy), hypokalaemia or hypomagnesaemia
- see also General Nursing considerations/Cautions for opioids (p. 1432)

Patient education
- advise the patient to seek medical advice immediately if sudden fainting for no reason or after exercise/emotional excitement, rapid or erratic heartbeat occurs

- see also General Patient education for opioids (p. 1434)

Oral liquid available. Tablet can be dispersed in water, or crushed and mixed with spoonful of yoghurt or apple puree.

Should be used only if benefit outweighs the risk.

Caution if used in those with liver impairment where methadone metabolism is slowed. Reduced doses are recommended.
Caution if used in those with renal impairment. If GFR is < 10 mL/min, dosing interval should be a minimum of 12-hourly. If GFR is 10–50 mL/min, dosing interval should be a minimum of 8-hourly.

MORPHINE HYDROCHLORIDE TRIHYDRATE (MORPHINE HYDROCHLORIDE)

MORPHINE SULFATE PENTAHYDRATE
Trade names
Anamorph, DBL Morphine Sulfate Injection BP, Kapanol, Morphine Sulfate Medsurge, Morphine Sulfate Oral Solution, MS Contin

Available forms
Oral solution: 2 mg/1 mL, 10 mg/5 mL;
Tablets: 30 mg;
Capsules: 10 mg, 20 mg, 50 mg, 100 mg, 120 mg;
Capsules (controlled-release): 10 mg, 20 mg, 30 mg, 50 mg, 60 mg, 90 mg, 100 mg, 120 mg;
Tablets (controlled-release): 5 mg, 10 mg, 15 mg, 30 mg, 60 mg, 100 mg, 200 mg;
Ampoules: 5 mg/mL, 10 mg/mL, 15 mg/mL, 30 mg/mL

Action
- opioid analgesic derived from opium with high affinity for mu receptors
- poor oral availability; undergoes extensive first-pass metabolism and has multiple active metabolites
- morphine-induced analgesia increases both pain threshold and pain tolerance
- alters response where patient is still aware of pain but not distressed by it
- peak effect 30–60 minutes (IM), 50–90 minutes (SC), 20 minutes (IV)
- duration of action varies with formulation (2–4 hours (oral solution, tablets), 12–24 hours (sustained-release preparations), 4–6 hours (IV, IM or SC))
- half-life is 1.5–2 hours

Use
- moderate-to-severe pain
- premedication (with atropine or hyoscine)
- supplementary analgesia during general anaesthesia
- chronic breathlessness

Dose
- 10–30 mg orally 4–6-hourly (immediate-release tablets) **OR**
- 5–20 mg orally 4-hourly (oral solution) **OR**
- initially 30 mg orally 12-hourly, then adjusted at 48-hour intervals according to breakthrough pain (sustained-release tablets) **OR**
- initially 20 mg orally 12-hourly or 40 mg orally daily, increasing the dose at 24-hour intervals minimum as needed (sustained-release capsules) **OR**
- initially 60 mg orally daily, increasing dose at 3-day intervals if needed (controlled-release capsules) **OR**
- (Chronic breathlessness) 10 mg orally daily, increasing dose after 7 days if needed (maximum daily dose 30 mg) (sustained-release capsules) **OR**
- 5–20 mg SC or IM 4–6-hourly **OR**
- 2.5–15 mg by slow IV injection (over 4–5 minutes) diluted to at least 5 mL with water for injections **OR**
- 0.5–2 mg/hour by continuous IV infusion **OR**
- (Patient-controlled analgesia (PCA)) 1 mg/hour background infusion, with 0.5–1.5 mg bolus doses via PCA pump, with lock-out interval of 6–10 minutes

Adverse effects
- (Injection site) pain, induration, irritation
- (Rare) supraventricular tachycardia
- see also General Adverse effects of opioids (p. 1431)

Interactions
- increased risk of severe hypotension and CNS depression if given with diazepam
- may decrease efficacy of diuretics by increasing release of antidiuretic hormone
- may potentiate effects of warfarin; therefore INR should be closely monitored, especially when starting or stopping therapy
- not recommended with zidovudine
- decreased serum levels may occur if given with ritonavir or rifampicin
- if given with dexamfetamine, analgesic effect may be enhanced with reduced sedation
- may interfere with hepatobiliary imaging
- see also General Interactions of opioids (p. 1431)

Nursing considerations/Cautions
- shorter-acting opioid should be tried before starting therapy with sustained-release preparation
- sustained-release preparation should not be used for onset of acute pain management
- first dose of sustained-release preparation can be taken with last dose of immediate-release preparation
- (Cancer pain) should be given around the clock (including waking patient at night to prevent morning pain)
- (Sustained-release preparations) if breakthrough pain occurs at the end of the time interval, the dose should be increased, NOT the frequency of administration
- (Chronic breathlessness) breathlessness should be reviewed weekly using a validated tool to determine clinical effectiveness
- ensure that correct strength of tablets, syrup and controlled-release capsules and granules is selected, as they are available in varying strengths
- formulations are not bioequivalent
- 200 mg sustained-release preparation is suitable only for opioid-tolerant patients
- for patients using PCA, adequate assessment and education should be conducted before surgery to ascertain the patient's suitability. Only staff who have completed the required in-service sessions and associated assessment should care for patients with PCA, according to individual institution policy
- conversion from/to other opioid analgesics or other formulations of morphine should be done according to manufacturer's recommendations (e.g. 10 mg morphine IM = 30 mg oral morphine). There may not be bioequivalence between different brands of the same formulation (e.g. sustained-release capsules/tablets)
- (IM, SC) rotate injection sites to decrease pain and induration
- (IM, SC, IV) once analgesia is achieved, parenteral route should be changed to oral
- (IM, SC, IV) increases in dose should be made at no less than 24-hour intervals
- (IM, SC, IV) not normally mixed in the same syringe with other drugs, but is compatible with chlorpromazine, metoclopramide or prochlorperazine, as long as the resultant solution is used within 15 minutes and there is no precipitation
- (IV) incompatible with thiopentone, promethazine, barbiturates, pethidine and phenytoin
- have naloxone and resuscitation equipment readily available to reverse respiratory depression
- those over 50 years usually require lower doses
- (MS Contin) tablets contain lactose and are therefore not recommended in those with galactose intolerance, Lapp lactase deficiency or glucose—galactose malabsorption
- (Chronic breathlessness, sustained-release preparations) not recommended

OPIOID ANALGESICS

- for acute or acute-on-chronic breathlessness
- (Sustained-release preparations) not recommended within 24 hours of cordotomy or other procedures that interrupt pain transmission pathway
- (SC, IM) caution if used in those with shock, especially if repeated doses are given, as overdose may occur when circulation is restored
- caution if used in those with kidney impairment because of the risk of accumulation of active metabolite which may cause respiratory and CNS depression
- caution if used in those with atrial flutter or other supraventricular tachycardias
- (IV) continuous IV infusion is contraindicated in those with liver or kidney disease
- contraindicated in those with cardiac arrhythmias
- see also General Nursing considerations/Cautions for opioids (p. 1432)

Patient education

- advise the patient to swallow sustained-release tablets whole, not chewed, crushed or broken/divided
- the patient should be advised that sustained-release capsules should be swallowed whole, not chewed, crushed or broken. If swallowing is difficult, capsules may be opened and pellets sprinkled into 30 mL liquid (water, orange juice or milk) or soft food (yoghurt, custard, ice-cream, jam, apple sauce) and consumed within 30 minutes, taking care not to chew pellets. Another 30 mL of water should be used to rinse container to ensure entire dose has been taken. Pellets may also be sprinkled into water and administered via gastrostomy tube (not nasogastric tube), ensuring tube is flushed well before and after administration
- advise the patient to use measuring cup or oral syringe to measure correct oral solution/syrup dose
- instruct the patient to date bottle and discard oral solution/syrup 6 months after opening
- see also General Patient education for opioids (p. 1434)

Oral liquid is available. Plain (immediate-release) tablet can be crushed and mixed with water, or a spoonful of yoghurt or apple puree.

Sustained/modified/controlled-release tablets/capsules should not be crushed, broken or chewed. Pellets should not be chewed.

Caution if used in those with liver or kidney impairment, as there may be a prolonged duration and cumulative effects resulting in adverse effects. Reduced dosage is recommended.

OXYCODONE HYDROCHLORIDE
Trade names
Endone, Mayne Pharma Oxycodone IR<OxyContin, Oxyndone, Oxycodone BNM, Oxycodone HCl Medsurge Solution, Oxycodone Juno. Oxycodone Juno, Oxycodone Sandoz, Oxycodone Viatris, Oxycodone Wockhardt, Oxycodone-hameln, OxyNorm, Proladone

Available forms
Tablets: 5 mg;
Tablets (controlled-release): 5 mg, 10 mg, 15 mg, 20 mg, 30 mg, 40 mg, 80 mg;
Capsules: 5 mg, 10 mg, 20 mg;
Ampoules: 10 mg/mL, 20 mg/2 mL, 50 mg/mL;
Suppositories: 30 mg

Action
- semisynthetic opioid analgesic with actions similar to morphine
- (Oral) onset of action 10–15 minutes, peak effect 30–60 minutes, duration of action 3–6 hours
- duration of action 4–6 hours (SC, IV) or 6–8 hours (rectal)
- half-life is about 2–4 hours

- see also General Actions of opioids (p. 1430)

Use
- moderate-to-severe pain

Dose
- initially 5 mg orally after food 4—6-hourly, increasing dose as required (daily maximum 400 mg) (immediate-release tablet, oral solution) **OR**
- initially 5—10 mg orally 12-hourly, increasing dose as required (controlled-release tablets) **OR**
- 1 rectal suppository (30 mg) 6—8-hourly **OR**
- (10 mg/mL, 20 mg/mL) 1—5 mg IV bolus over 1—2 minutes, further doses may be given at 5—10-minute intervals if needed while monitoring patient, then 4-hourly (maintenance) **OR**
- 2 mg/hour by IV infusion **OR**
- (10 mg/mL) initially 5—10 mg SC, repeated 4-hourly as needed **OR**
- (Patient-controlled analgesia (PCA)) 0.03 mg/kg IV bolus (patient lock-out 5 minutes) **OR**
- (50 mg/mL, opioid-tolerant patient in palliative care setting) initially 2 mg/hour IV infusion, then increasing dose as needed

Adverse effects
- injection site pain and hypersensitivity
- see also General Adverse effects of opioids (p. 1431)

Interactions
- may increase effects of warfarin; therefore INR should be carefully monitored especially when starting or stopping therapy
- see also General Interactions of opioids (p. 1431)

Nursing considerations/Cautions
- not recommended as first-line management for non-malignant pain; however, it can be used if patient assessment shows other analgesics to be ineffective, pain continues impacting on quality of life and there is no history of drug abuse or drug-seeking behaviour
- shorter-acting opioid should be trialled before using controlled-release preparation
- if the patient was previously on morphine, 1 mg IV oxycodone = 1 mg IV morphine; 2 mg oral oxycodone = 1 mg parenteral oxycodone
- if the patient was previously on transdermal fentanyl, 10 mg oxycodone oral (controlled-release) = 25 microgram fentanyl/hour (transdermal patch)
- IV bolus doses 5—15 mg are not recommended because of the risk of sedation and respiratory depression
- IV solution should be diluted to 1 mg/mL with sodium chloride 0.9%, glucose 5% or water for injections before administering as IV bolus, infusion or patient-controlled analgesia
- antagonised by acidifying agents and potentiated by alkalising agents
- incompatible with prochlorperazine and fluorouracil (5FU)
- 10 mg/mL and 20 mg/mL formulations are recommended via IV/SC injection or IV/SC infusion; 50 mg/mL formulation is recommended as IV/SC infusion, in palliative care setting
- (50 mg/mL) is not recommended for more than 28 days consecutively
- 80 mg controlled-release tablets are recommended for opioid-tolerant patients only
- (Controlled-release tablets) not recommended preoperatively or 24 hours postoperatively
- see also General Nursing considerations/Cautions for opioids (p. 1432)

Patient education
- the patient should be advised to take controlled-release tablet whole, not crushed, broken or divided, as this may result in rapid release, overdose and respiratory depression
- advise the patient to take tablets (immediate-release) whole with milk or food to reduce gastric upset
- instruct the adult patient in the correct technique for suppository insertion, including:

OPIOID ANALGESICS

- the need to empty bowel if possible before suppository insertion
- wash hands with soap and water
- if suppository feels soft, place it (unwrapped) in the fridge or hold it under cold water to firm it up
- put on disposable glove if wanted
- remove wrapper from suppository and moisten slightly by dipping in cool water
- lie on side with knees raised to chest
- push suppository (blunt end first) gently into rectum taking care not to break suppository
- remain lying down for a few minutes to allow suppository to dissolve
- wash hands thoroughly after insertion
- advise the patient not to use bowels for at least 1 hour (if possible) after suppository insertion
- see also General Patient education for opioids (p. 1434)

For those with liver impairment or renal impairment (CrCl < 60 mL/min), dose should be reduced by one-third to a half and any dose titration cautiously managed.

Available in combination with

- oxycodone hydrochloride 10 mg + naloxone 5 mg tablets (ARX-Oxydodone/Naloxone 10/5, Targin 10/5)
- oxycodone hydrochloride 15 mg + naloxone 7.5 mg tablets (ARX-Oxydodone/Naloxone 15/7.5, Targin 15/7.5)
- oxycodone hydrochloride 2.5 mg + naloxone 1.25 mg tablets (ARX-Oxydodone/Naloxone 2.5/1.25, Targin 2.5/1.25)
- oxycodone hydrochloride 20 mg + naloxone 10 mg tablets (ARX-Oxydodone/Naloxone 20/10, Targin 20/10)
- oxycodone hydrochloride 30 mg + naloxone 15 mg tablets (ARX-Oxydodone/Naloxone 30/15, Targin 30/15)
- oxycodone hydrochloride 40 mg + naloxone 20 mg tablets (ARX-Oxydodone/Naloxone 40/20, Targin 40/20)
- oxycodone hydrochloride 5 mg + naloxone 2.5 mg tablets (ARX-Oxydodone/Naloxone 5/2.5, Targin 5/2.5)
- oxycodone hydrochloride 60 mg + naloxone 30 mg tablets (ARX-Oxydodone/Naloxone 60/30, Targin 60/30)
- oxycodone hydrochloride 80 mg + naloxone 40 mg tablets (ARX-Oxydodone/Naloxone 80/40, Targin 80/40)

PETHIDINE HYDROCHLORIDE

Trade names
DBL Pethidine Hydrochloride Solution, Pethidine Juno

Available forms
Ampoules: 50 mg/mL, 100 mg/2 mL

Action
- synthetic opioid analgesic that acts on mu receptors with similar properties to morphine (not as effective in management of cough or diarrhoea)
- pethidine 75–100 mg = 10 mg morphine = 120 mg codeine = 200 micrograms fentanyl = 8–10 mg methadone
- analgesia onset 10–15 minutes (IM, SC), 1 minute (IV), duration 3–5 hours (IM, IV, SC) (non-tolerant (opioid-naive) patients)
- active metabolite, norpethidine (half the analgesic properties, but twice the convulsant properties of pethidine)
- half-life 3.5 hours (pethidine) and 8–21 hours (norpethidine); therefore the risk of accumulation and associated adverse effects is high (especially in those with liver impairment)

Use
- moderate-to-severe pain (short-term (24–36 hours) management)
- obstetric analgesia
- premedication

- adjunct to general anaesthesia

Dose
- (Analgesia) 25—100 mg SC or IM 3—4-hourly, up to 150 mg for severe pain **OR**
- 25—50 mg 3—4-hourly by slow IV injection or infusion (diluted to at least 5 mL with sodium chloride 0.9%) (up to 200 mg daily) **OR**
- 0.3 mg/kg/hour as IV infusion **OR**
- (Premedication) 50—100 mg IM or SC 30—90 minutes before start of anaesthesia **OR**
- (Obstetric analgesia) 50—100 mg IM or SC when labour becomes regular; may be repeated 1—3-hourly (maximum daily dose 400 mg) **OR**
- (Adjunct to analgesia) repeated slow IV injection of 10 mg/mL solution, not exceeding 25—50 mg **OR**
- (Patient-controlled analgesia (PCA)) 5—20 mg bolus dose with 6—20-minute lock-out period (with or without background infusion) (not exceeding 800 mg/day)

Adverse effects
- see General Adverse effects of opioids (p. 1431), but has less constipation and urinary retention effects than morphine
- transient increase in BP and systemic vascular resistance
- (Large dose, rapid administration) rapid respiratory depression, apnoea, hypotension, peripheral circulatory collapse, bradycardia, cardiac arrest
- pethidine-associated neurotoxicity (related to the long-acting metabolite norpethidine with symptoms including irritability, agitation, hypomania, tremor, paranoia, delirium, vertigo, headache, sweating, cold/clammy skin, pallor, hallucinations, seizures, respiratory depression)
- (IM) irritation, induration, fibrosis (with repeated injections)

Interactions
- contraindicated with anticoagulants
- phenobarbital (phenobarbitone) and phenytoin may increase metabolism and generation of norpethidine and increase risk of pethidine-associated neurotoxicity
- may cause recurrence of seizures if given with phenothiazines if the two are used in eclampsia
- see also General Interactions of opioids (p. 1431)

Nursing considerations/Cautions
- IM is the preferred route of administration
- avoid intra-arterial route as this may result in necrosis and gangrene
- should be given slowly IV to prevent respiratory depression, hypotension, apnoea and bradycardia
- (IV) opioid antagonist and resuscitation equipment should be readily available
- (PCA) adequate assessment and education should be conducted before surgery to ascertain the patient's suitability. Only staff who have completed the required in-service sessions and associated assessment should care for patients with PCA, according to individual institution policy
- compatible with chlorpromazine, metoclopramide, prochlorperazine or promethazine when mixed in the same syringe, as long as the resultant solution is used within 15 minutes and there is no precipitation
- physically or chemically incompatible with aciclovir, aminophylline, doxorubicin, furosemide (frusemide), heparin, idarubicin, imipenem, iodine, morphine, phenobarbital (phenobarbitone), phenytoin, sodium bicarbonate, sodium iodide, thiopental, alkali, iodine and iodide solutions
- therapy should be limited to 24—36 hours to prevent pethidine-associated neurotoxicity due to accumulation of metabolite (norpethidine)
- (PCA) if dose is > 800 mg/day, the patient should be closely monitored for signs of

OPIOID ANALGESICS

- pethidine-associated neurotoxicity (initial signs include anxiety and twitching)
- it is recommended that intraocular pressure is monitored if used in patients with glaucoma
- not recommended for pain associated with myocardial infarction
- contraindicated as IV infusion or patient-controlled analgesia in those with kidney impairment
- (PCA) contraindicated in patients with poor cognitive function
- contraindicated in patients with supraventricular tachycardia or cor pulmonale owing to vagolytic action
- contraindicated during eclampsia or pre-eclampsia, during convulsive conditions (e.g. tetanus, strychnine poisoning, status epilepticus), during diabetic acidosis (with coma) or if the patient has a low platelet count or coagulation disorder
- see also General Nursing considerations/Cautions for opioids (p. 1432)

Patient education
- see General Patient education for opioids (p. 1434)

Continuous pethidine IV infusion or PCA is contraindicated in patients with kidney impairment.
Pethidine is metabolised in the liver and excreted via the kidneys; therefore caution and close monitoring are recommended if used in those with liver or kidney impairment.

REMIFENTANIL
Trade names
Remifentanil-AFT, Remifentanil Viatris

Available forms
Vial: 1 mg, 2 mg, 5 mg

Action
- potent opioid analgesic
- selective mu opioid receptor agonist with rapid onset and very short duration of action and with similar properties to fentanyl
- does not produce histamine release
- opioid and analgesic effects disappear within 5—10 minutes of stopping or reversal
- elimination half-life 3—10 minutes
- clearance is decreased during hypothermic cardiopulmonary bypass (decrease is about 3% per degree Celsius)
- see also General Actions of opioids (p. 1430)

Use
- opioid adjunct during induction and/or maintenance of general anaesthesia
- analgesia and sedation in mechanically ventilated patients or in immediate postoperative period

Dose
- generally given by specialist anaesthetist

Adverse effects
- skeletal muscle rigidity, shivering
- hypotension, bradycardia, hypertension, tachycardia
- postoperative nausea, vomiting
- respiratory depression, apnoea, hypoxia
- pruritus
- (Infusion site) erythema, pruritus, rash
- (Postprocedure) fever, dizziness, headache, visual disturbances

Interactions
- increased sedation may occur if given with other CNS depressants
- may decrease dose requirements of inhaled or IV anaesthetics, hypnotics and/or benzodiazepines
- increased hypotension and bradycardia may occur if given with beta adrenoceptor blocking agents or calcium-channel blocking agents

Nursing considerations/Cautions
- respiratory depression can occur for up to 30 minutes after administration; therefore it is important that the patient is fully conscious and spontaneously breathing before discharge from recovery area

1451

HAVARD'S NURSING GUIDE TO DRUGS

- bolus dose should be given slowly (over at least 60 seconds) to prevent muscle rigidity (especially chest wall)
- depending on severity, muscle rigidity can be treated by decreasing rate or stopping remifentanil, using antagonist (naloxone), neuromuscular blocking agent and/or additional hypnotic. The patient may require intubation and ventilation
- reconstitute using water for injections, glucose 5% or sodium chloride 0.9%, and then further dilute before administration
- if possible, should be administered via a dedicated line which is removed after administration. If this is not possible, should be administered into fast-flowing IV close to venous cannula to prevent a bolus dose being given if IV line is flushed
- incompatible with lactated Ringer's solution or propofol (in same infusion bag) or blood or blood products
- abrupt stopping is not recommended after prolonged administration
- caution if used in those with known sensitivity to opioids
- not recommended during labour or Caesarean section
- not recommended as sole agent during general anaesthesia, spontaneous ventilation anaesthesia or as analgesic in postoperative period
- contraindicated in those with hypersensitivity to fentanyl analogues or for epidural or intrathecal use
- see also General Nursing considerations/Cautions for opioids (p. 1432)

Patient education

- see General Patient education for opioids (p. 1434)

Caution if used in those with severe liver impairment, as they may be more sensitive to respiratory depressant effects and should be closely monitored.

If used for general anaesthesia, the dose should be halved and carefully titrated in those over 65 years.

TRAMADOL
Trade names
APO-Tramadol, APO-Tramadol SR, Tramadol AN, Tramadol Sandoz, Tramadol SR Generichealth, Tramadol-WGR, Tramal, Tramal SR, Tramedo, Tramedo SR, Zydol, Zydol SR

Available forms
Capsules: 50 mg;
Controlled release Tablets: 50 mg, 100 mg, 150 mg, 200 mg;
Ampoules: 100 mg/2 mL;
Oral drops: 100 mg/mL

Action
- centrally acting synthetic analgesic with opioid-like properties without being chemically related to the opioids
- binds to mu opioid receptors
- blocks reuptake of noradrenaline (norepinephrine) and serotonin
- does not cause histamine release
- produces less respiratory depression than morphine
- little evidence to suggest drug abuse and dependence occurs
- active metabolite (desmethyltramadol) has a greater affinity for mu receptors and is more potent than tramadol. Elimination half-life of metabolite is 6–8 hours
- duration of action is 3–6 hours (oral) or 5–6 hours (IM)
- half-life is 5–7 hours
- half-life of both tramadol and its active metabolite are both increased in those with liver or kidney impairment

Use
- moderate-to-severe pain

Dose
- (Postoperative) initially 100 mg IM or IV over 2–3 minutes, then 50–100 mg

OPIOID ANALGESICS

4—6-hourly (maximum daily dose 600 mg) **OR**
- (Less severe pain) 50—100 mg IM or IV over 2—3 minutes 4—6-hourly (maximum daily dose 400 mg) **OR**
- (Moderate pain) 50—100 mg orally 2—3 times daily **OR**
- (Moderate-to-severe pain) initially 100 mg orally, then 50—100 mg 4—6-hourly (maximum daily dose 400 mg) **OR**
- (SR preparations) 100—200 mg orally 1—2 times daily (depending on daily or twice daily preparations), increasing in 100 mg increments if needed (maximum daily dose 400 mg)

Adverse effects
- (Rare) anaphylactoid reaction (sometimes after first dose), seizures
- see also General Adverse effects of opioids (p. 1431), but with less respiratory depression

Interactions
- contraindicated with linezolid
- contraindicated with or within 14 days of monoamine oxidase inhibitors (MAOIs)
- metabolism may be increased, lowering the serum level, if given with carbamazepine
- increased risk of convulsions if given with selective serotonin reuptake inhibitors (SSRIs), serotonin and noradrenaline (norepinephrine) reuptake inhibitors (SNRIs), tricyclic antidepressants (TCAs), antipsychotics or other agents that lower the seizure threshold
- caution if used with CNS depressants (alcohol, opioids, anaesthetics, phenothiazines, tranquillisers, sedatives/hypnotics)
- analgesic effect may be reduced by ondansetron
- increased risk of serotonin syndrome if given with SSRIs, SNRIs, TCAs, mirtazapine and other serotoninergic agents
- caution if used with warfarin; INR should be closely monitored, especially when starting or stopping therapy
- increased serum levels may occur if given with phenothiazine or antipsychotic agents, increasing risk of adverse effects
- not recommended with buprenorphine, as analgesic action will be reduced
- not recommended with very light anaesthetics

Nursing considerations/Cautions
- IV injection should be given over at least 2—3 minutes
- (IV) incompatible with diclofenac, indometacin (indomethacin), diazepam, flunitrazepam, midazolam or glyceryl trinitrate
- naloxone reverses respiratory depression but not other symptoms of overdose
- caution if used for pain relief after throat surgery, tonsillectomy and/or adenoidectomy as patients are more susceptible to toxicity or overdose and should be carefully monitored
- (Tramal) SR tablets contain galactose; therefore should be used with caution in those with galactose intolerance, Lapp lactase deficiency or glucose–galactose intolerance
- (Tramal oral drops) contain sucrose and are therefore not recommended in those with rare hereditary problems of fructose intolerance, glucose–galactose intolerance or sucrase–isomaltase insufficiency
- not recommended for opioid withdrawal treatment
- contraindicated in those with acute alcohol intoxication
- contraindicated in all children under 12 years, and in postoperative management of children under 18 years after tonsillectomy and/or adenoidectomy
- controlled-release tablets for acute pain are not recommend because of the slow onset.
- see also General Nursing considerations/Cautions for opioids (p. 1432)

Patient education
- advise the patient to take controlled-release preparations whole, not chew, crush, divide or break tablets

- see also General Patient education for opioids (p. 1434)

Oral drops are available. Capsules can be opened and contents dispersed in water, or mixed with yoghurt or apple puree.

If patient has advanced cirrhosis, the dose should be reduced or dosing interval increased.
For renal impairment, dosing interval increase is recommended. If renal insufficiency is severe, prolonged/extended-release tablets are not recommended.

For those aged 75 years and over, the dose should not exceed 300 mg daily.

Available in combination with
- Tramadol 37.5 mg + paracetamol 325 mg tablets (Zaldair)

TAPENTADOL
Trade names
Palexia IR, Palexia SR

Available forms
Tablets (sustained release): 50 mg, 100 mg, 150 mg, 200 mg, 250 mg;
Tablets (immediate release): 50 mg

Action
- centrally acting synthetic analgesic with opioid and non-opioid activity
- binding affinity to mu receptors is much less than with morphine; however, it has only slightly less analgesic action
- noradrenaline (norepinephrine) re-uptake inhibiting activity
- antagonised by naloxone
- no active metabolite
- elimination half-life 5–6 hours
- see also General Actions of opioids (p. 1430)

Use
- moderate-to-severe pain (unresponsive to non-opioid analgesia)

Dose
- initially 50 mg orally twice daily, increasing by 50 mg at 3-day intervals if needed (daily maximum 500 mg) (sustained-release tablets) **OR**
- initially 50 mg orally every 4–6 hours (daily maximum 700 mg), increasing to 50–100 mg every 4–6 hours (to maintain adequate analgesia) (daily maximum 600 mg) (immediate-release tablets)

Adverse effects
- (Rare) suicidal ideation
- see also General Adverse effects of opioids (p. 1431)

Interactions
- increased risk of serotonin syndrome if given with serotoninergic agents such as SSNIs, SNRIs, TCAs, MAOIs or triptans
- see also General Interactions of opioids (p. 1431)

Nursing considerations/Cautions
- in those already taking opioids, the dose should be initiated taking into account type, dose and frequency of previous opioid
- (Immediate-release tablet) on first day; if pain control is not achieved within 1 hour, a second dose may be given
- withdrawal should be gradual to avoid withdrawal symptoms
- not recommended in those under 18 years
- contraindicated in those with or suspected of having paralytic ileus or intoxication with alcohol, hypnotics, centrally acting analgesics or psychotropic agents
- see also General Nursing considerations/Cautions for opioids (p. 1432)

Patient education
- advise the patient that sustained-release tablets should be swallowed whole, not chewed, broken or divided

OPIOID ANALGESICS

- warn the patient that the shell of sustained-release tablet may not be totally digested and appear in bowel motion
- see also General Patient education for opioids (p. 1434)

Plain (immediate-release) tablet can be crushed and mixed with water, or spoonful of yoghurt or apple puree.

Sustained-release tablets should be swallowed whole, not chewed, broken or divided.

Due to limited data available in humans, should be used only if benefit outweighs the risk.

Contraindicated because of the limited data available in breastfeeding mothers.

PREGNANCY, CHILDBIRTH AND BREASTFEEDING

The agents discussed in this section are those commonly used to treat infertility, to prevent premature labour or preeclampsia, or are used during labour, or to suppress lactation.

Most medications cross the placental and therefore have the potential to cause problems to the developing fetus. The severity of the impact can be related to where in the pregnancy the medication is taken (e.g. first trimester versus late pregnancy).

In Australia, drugs are classified according to whether they cause birth defects (e.g. cleft palate), possible problems (reversible or irreversible) at birth (e.g. sedation) or later in life. The classification system is Category A, B1, B2, B3, C, D and X. The risk of birth defects is dependent on facts such as systemic exposure and exposure to the fetus, which is determined by dose, route of administration and/or the dosing regimen. However, this classification is not hierarchical (e.g. category B is not necessarily safer than category C) except for category X medications, which are at high risk of causing permanent fetal damage and should not be used during pregnancy or in women who are planning to become pregnant (Australian Government, Department of Health (TGA) 2024).

AGENTS USED TO TREAT INFERTILITY

During the follicular stage, luteinising hormone (LH) stimulates ovarian theca cells to produce androgens, which are then used by ovarian granulosa cells to make estradiol (oestradiol), which supports the induction of follicle development by follicle-stimulating hormone (FSH). At mid-cycle, when LH levels are high, ovulation and subsequent corpus luteum formation are triggered, after which LH stimulates the production of progesterone by the corpus luteum. If fertilisation occurs, the progesterone level remains high, sustaining the endometrium and maintaining the pregnancy. However, if fertilisation does not occur, the production of progesterone by the corpus luteum decreases.

Worldwide, infertility is thought to affect as many as one in six people of reproductive age during their lifetime (WHO 2024e). Infertility is defined as 'the inability to conceive after 12 months of unprotected sexual intercourse or after 6 months in women aged 35 years and over' (WHO 2024e). Infertility may be due to male factors (e.g. sperm transport problems, abnormal sperm function and quality, hormonal disorders, testicular disease, genetic disorders), female factors (e.g. endocrine hormonal disorders (insufficient LH, FSH or progesterone); tubal defects (e.g. blocked fallopian tubes); uterine disorders (e.g. endometriosis) or ovarian disorders (e.g. polycystic ovary syndrome)), both male and female factors including lifestyle factors (e.g. smoking, obesity, excessive alcohol intake, exposure to pollutants) and, in some cases, it may be unexplained (WHO 2024e).

- discussion should take place about timing of intercourse and any modifiable factors, such as smoking, alcohol, caffeine and obesity (however, both high and low BMI can be associated with female infertility, as well as increased morbidity during pregnancy)
- the couple should have their infertility thoroughly investigated, and this may include:
  - confirmation of ovulation and tubal patency
  - identification of any menstrual cycle disorder or abnormal vaginal bleeding
  - evaluation of sperm quality and quantity via semen analysis
  - identification of any issues, such as ovarian failure, malformation of sexual organs or uterine fibroid tumours, that would be incompatible with pregnancy; otherwise LH preparations will be ineffective
  - identification and treatment of hypothyroidism, adrenocortical deficiency, hyperprolactinaemia, or pituitary or hypothalamic tumours.
- any systemic disease which may worsen with pregnancy should be identified, and
- any contraindications to pregnancy should be identified (Hall 2018).

Infertility treatment may involve stimulation of ovulation with agents such as clomifene (clomiphene), intrauterine insemination, use of gonadotrophins, in vitro fertilisation (IVF), or other assisted reproductive technologies. Success of infertility treatment is dependent on the age of the woman and the cause of the infertility. Because infertility, infertility treatment and its consequences can be extremely stressful, counselling and stress management should also be instigated early on as part of a holistic management plan (Hall 2018).

- ultrasound monitoring (fluid in cul-de-sac, ovarian stigmata, collapsed follicle and secretory endometrium) and estradiol (oestradiol) measurement are recommended to minimise the risk of ovarian hyperstimulation syndrome and multiple pregnancy, and
- treatment should be individualised according to follicle size (determined by ultrasound) and oestrogen response.

General Adverse effects of infertility agents

- ovarian hyperstimulation syndrome (OHSS), results from an excessive response to ovarian stimulation with FSH resulting in multiple ovarian follicles (> 17). Human chorionic gonadotrophin (hCG) or gonadotrophin-releasing hormone (GnRH) agonist is given to trigger follicle release and this is followed by the ovaries producing growth factors and cytokines, which induce vascularisation of multiple corpus lutea, increasing blood vessel permeability leakage into extravascular tissue and resulting in complications (e.g. oedema, ascites, plural/pericardial effusions) and decreased circulating vascular volume (haemoconcentration, thrombosis, decreased renal perfusion and oliguria). OHSS can be classified as mild, moderate, severe or critical. Management is aimed at the prevention of complication. Generally mild-to-moderate OHSS is managed on an outpatient basis with severe and critical cases requiring hospitalisation. OHSS resolves spontaneously with the onset of menses; therefore the patient should refrain from intercourse or use barrier contraceptive methods for at least 4 days. Risk factors for OHSS include polycystic ovaries,

previous episodes of OHSS, young age, low BMI, high doses of FSH, many follicles (> 17) and a rapid or high level of estradiol (oestradiol). If the woman has polycystic ovaries, it is recommended that the ovaries are monitored by ultrasound before and during stimulation to prevent OHSS
- increased risk of multiple pregnancies and births (related to number of embryos transferred)
- higher rate of miscarriage and congenital malformations (compared with the normal population)
- ectopic pregnancy
- thromboembolism
- headache, dizziness, fatigue
- breast tenderness/discomfort
- (Uncommon) mood swings, depression
- rash
- nausea, vomiting, abdominal pain
- ovarian disorder (including ovarian torsion), ovarian cysts, ovarian enlargement (with/without abdominal pain/distension), intermenstrual bleeding
- (Injection site reaction) pain, redness, swelling, irritation, bruising, itching
- (Rare) hypersensitivity, benign or malignant reproductive system neoplasms

General Nursing considerations/ Cautions for infertility agents

- pregnancy should be excluded before the start of therapy
- (Ovulation induction) treatment regimen is highly individualised and requires clinical, biochemical (e.g. oestrogen levels) and ultrasonic monitoring
- the first dose should be administered under supervision
- rotate SC injection sites
- caution if used in those with risk of thromboembolism or polycystic ovarian syndrome
- caution if used in those with porphyria, as gonadotrophins can increase the risk of acute attack
- caution in those who have shown previous sensitivity to gonadotrophin preparations (without FSH) because cross-sensitivity may occur. If given, the patient should be closely observed after first injection
- contraindicated in those who have had prior hypersensitivity reaction to hCG or FSH preparations, primary ovarian failure, uncontrolled thyroid or adrenal dysfunction, uncontrolled hypothalamic or pituitary tumours, ovarian enlargement or cyst (not caused by polycystic ovarian disease), hormone-dependent tumours of the reproductive tract and accessory organs (including ovarian, breast and uterine cancer), uterine fibroid tumours (incompatible with pregnancy), are postmenopausal, or had an ectopic pregnancy (previous 3 months), active thromboembolic disorders or gynaecological haemorrhage (of unknown cause)

General Patient education for infertility agents

- before starting therapy, the patient and partner should receive counselling regarding the potential risk of multiple birth occurring
- the patient should be advised to immediately seek medical advice if any of the following occur:
    - nausea, vomiting, diarrhoea, pelvic or abdominal pain, discomfort or distension (which may be early symptoms of OHSS)
    - swelling, redness, warmth or tingling in legs/arms, severe headache or shortness of breath (possible sign of blood clot)
- the patient should receive adequate education in the correct use of the equipment, correct injection technique, importance of rotating sites, storage information and safe disposal of used equipment before self-administration can begin; the first injection should be under medical supervision
- warn the patient against driving or operating machinery if dizziness occurs

PREGNANCY, CHILDBIRTH AND BREASTFEEDING

CETRORELIX ACETATE

Trade name
Cetrotide

Available form
Vial: 250 microgram

Action
- luteinising hormone-releasing hormone (LHRH) antagonist, which controls the secretion of LH and follicle-stimulating hormone (FSH) by the pituitary gland (also referred to as gonadotrophin-releasing hormone (GnRH) antagonist)

Use
- prevention of premature luteinisation and ovulation in women undergoing controlled ovarian stimulation (followed by oocyte pick-up and assisted reproductive techniques)

Dose
- 250 micrograms SC daily at 24-hour intervals (if given in the morning, should be started on day 5 or 6 of ovarian stimulation with FSH preparation, including day of ovulation induction with human chorionic gonadotrophin (hCG), or, if given in the evening, should be started on day 5 of ovarian stimulation with FSH preparation and continued until the evening before ovulation induction)

Adverse effects
- see General Adverse effects of infertility agents (p. 1457)

Nursing considerations/Cautions
- the patient should be closely monitored for 30 minutes after the first injection for any signs of allergic reaction
- the cycle should be repeated only after risk—benefit has been evaluated
- reconstitute with water for injections, and avoid vigorous shaking because it will denature product
- caution if used in those with any hypersensitivity to other GnRH products or any allergic predisposition
- contraindicated in those who have a hypersensitivity to extrinsic peptide hormone or mannitol, or those with moderate or severe kidney/liver impairment
- see also General Nursing considerations/Cautions for infertility agents (p. 1458)

Patient education
- see General Patient education for infertility agents (p. 1458)

 Contraindicated during pregnancy.

 Contraindicated during breastfeeding.

 Contraindicated in those with moderate-to-severe kidney or liver impairment.

CHORIOGONADOTROPHIN ALFA

Trade name
Ovidrel Pen

Available form
Prefilled syringe/pen: 250 microgram /0.5 mL

Action
- recombinant human chorionic gonadotrophin (hCG) that stimulates late follicular maturation, resumption of oocyte meiosis and initiates rupture of preovulatory ovarian follicle
- 250 micrograms choriogonadotrophin alfa are equivalent to urinary-derived hCG 5000—10,000 IU in terms of the number of oocytes retrieved

Use
- women undergoing superovulation prior to assisted reproductive techniques, such as in vitro fertilisation (IVF)
- anovulatory or oligo-ovulatory women

Dose
- (Women undergoing superovulation) 250 micrograms SC 24—48 hours after last dose of follicle-stimulating hormone (FSH) preparation **OR**
- (Anovulatory or oligo-ovulatory women) 250 micrograms SC 24—48 hours after optimal follicular growth stimulation has been achieved

Adverse effects
- see General Adverse effects of infertility agents (p. 1457)

Interactions
- may interfere with immunological determination of serum/urinary hCG for up to 10 days, resulting in a false positive pregnancy test

Nursing considerations/Cautions
- if ovaries are abnormally large after FSH therapy, chorigonatrophin alfa should be withheld because of an increased risk of OHSS
- see also General Nursing considerations/Cautions for infertility agents (p. 1458)

Patient education
- (Anovulatory or oligo-ovulatory women) the patient is advised to have intercourse on the day of and the day following administration
- see also General Patient education for infertility agents (p. 1458)

 Not recommended during pregnancy.

 Not recommended during breastfeeding.

 Permitted in sport for females only.

CLOMIFENE (CLOMIPHENE) CITRATE
Trade name
Clomid

Available form
Tablets: 50 mg

Action
- acts by stimulating output of pituitary gonadotrophins, stimulating maturation of ovarian follicle and then development and function of corpus luteum

Use
- stimulate ovulation in infertile women with ovarian dysfunction

Dose
- initially 50 mg orally daily for 5 days starting on the 5th day of the menstrual cycle (any time if there is amenorrhoea). If ovulation occurs but is not followed by pregnancy, this regimen can continue for 6 cycles **OR**
- dose increased to 100 mg for subsequent cycles if ovulation does not occur, repeated for 3 cycles (if ovulation does not occur) or 6 cycles (if ovulation occurs but is not followed by pregnancy)

Adverse effects
- hot flushes
- insomnia, anxiety, nervousness, light-headedness
- visual blurring, visual spots/flashes, 'after' images
- enlargement of existing uterine fibroids
- endometriosis or exacerbation of pre-existing endometriosis
- increased risk of ovarian cancer
- hypertriglyceridaemia, pancreatitis
- see also General Adverse effects of infertility agents (p. 1457)

Nursing considerations/Cautions
- pelvic examination is recommended before each cycle of treatment (to assess for ovarian cyst, ovarian cancer or pregnancy)
- therapy should be stopped if no ovulation occurs after 3 consecutive courses of therapy. Diagnosis should be re-evaluated
- record the weight and basal temperature to determine the day of ovulation
- liver function and serum triglycerides should be assessed before starting therapy
- ophthalmic examination is recommended if visual disturbances occur
- caution if used in women with known uterine fibroids, as they may enlarge during therapy

PREGNANCY, CHILDBIRTH AND BREASTFEEDING

- caution if used in those with a family history of or pre-existing hyperlipidaemia (especially in those undergoing prolonged therapy)
- contraindicated in those women with liver dysfunction or disease, or visual disorders related to prior use of clomifene
- see also General Nursing considerations/Cautions for infertility agents (p. 1458)

Patient education

- the patient should be advised to report any blurred vision or other visual symptoms (e.g. spots or flashes or loss of vision) immediately and to stop therapy if they occur. Visual disturbances may be worse in brightly lit environments
- warn the patient not to drive or operate machinery if visual blurring, lightheadedness, dizziness or headache occurs
- see also General Patient education for infertility agents (p. 1458)

 Tablet can be crushed and mixed with spoonful of yoghurt or apple puree.

 Contraindicated during pregnancy.

 Contraindicated during breastfeeding.

 Pregnant staff should not crush tablets.

 Banned in sport.

CORIFOLLITROPIN ALFA

Trade name
Elonva

Available forms
Prefilled syringe: 100 microgram/0.5 mL, 150 microgram/0.5 mL

Action
- gonadotrophin with sustained follicle-stimulating properties allowing once-weekly administration

Use
- controlled ovarian stimulation for follicle development and pregnancy in women undergoing assisted reproductive techniques

Dose
- (Body weight ≤ 60 kg and ≤ 36 years) 100 micrograms SC on day 1, followed by gonadotrophin-releasing hormone (GnRH) antagonist on day 5 or 6 depending on ovarian response (e.g. number/size of follicles and/or serum estradiol (oestradiol)), then on day 8, daily 150 IU follicle-stimulating hormone (FSH) until there are 3 follicles ≥ 17 mm, followed by 5000–10,000 IU hCG (to induce final maturation) **OR**
- (Body weight > 60 kg (regardless of age) or body weight > 50 kg and > 36 years) 150 micrograms SC on day 1, then as above

Adverse effects
- see General Adverse effects of infertility agents (p. 1457)

Interaction
- not recommended with GnRH agonist

Nursing considerations/Cautions

- only one SC injection is recommended per cycle
- no FSH is recommended in first 7 days after SC administration
- not recommended in those with kidney impairment
- contraindicated in those with previous controlled ovarian stimulation resulting in > 30 follicles ≥ 11 mm (on ultrasound) or basal antral follicle count > 20
- see also General Nursing considerations/Cautions for infertility agents (p. 1458)

Patient education

- see General Patient education for infertility agents (p. 1458)

 Contraindicated during pregnancy.

 Contraindicated during breastfeeding.

FOLLITROPIN ALFA

Trade names
Afolia, Bemfola, Gonal-f Pen, Ovaleap

Available forms
Prefilled Pen: 75 IU/0.125 mL, 150 IU/0.25 mL, 225 IU/0.375 mL, 300 IU/0.5 mL, 450 IU/0.75 mL, 900 IU/1.5 mL

Action
- recombinant human follicle-stimulating hormone (FSH) that stimulates development of mature follicles (in females) and spermatogenesis (in males)

Use
- infertility in women (where clomifene (clomiphene) has failed or is contraindicated)
- controlled ovarian hyperstimulation (assisted reproductive technology)
- hypogonadotrophic hypogonadism (HH) (where human chorionic gonadotrophin (hCG) alone is ineffective)

Dose
- (Anovulatory infertility) starting in first 7 days of menstrual cycle, initially 75–150 IU SC daily, increasing if necessary by 37.5–75 IU at 7- or 14-day intervals until an adequate response is achieved, followed by hCG preparation 24–48 hours after the last injection (to induce follicular maturation) **OR**
- (Controlled ovarian hyperstimulation) initially 150–225 IU SC daily, starting on day 2 or 3 of the cycle and continued until adequate follicle development has occurred, followed by hCG preparation 24–48 hours after the last injection (to induce follicular maturation). The dose should be adjusted according to response (daily maximum 450 IU) **OR**
- (HH) (males) 150 IU SC 3 times weekly with hCG preparation for at least 4 months

Adverse effects
- (Males) gynaecomastia, acne, weight gain
- see also General Adverse effects of infertility agents (p. 1457)

Nursing considerations/Cautions
- (Males) pretreatment with hCG alone should be started to achieve a testosterone level > 9–10 nanomol/L for up to 6 months, increasing the dose if this is not achieved
- (Males) serum should be analysed to determine clinical response
- (Males) therapy can be continued for up to 24 months to achieve spermatogenesis
- (Anovulatory infertility) if response is inadequate in 5 weeks, treatment should be stopped
- reconstitute with water for injections, and avoid vigorous shaking because it will denature product
- caution if used in those with porphyria, as acute crisis may be triggered
- (Males) contraindicated in men with primary testicular failure (elevated gonadotrophin levels) or infertility (from causes other than HH) or tumours of the hypothalamus or pituitary gland
- see also General Nursing considerations/Cautions for infertility agents (p. 1458)

Patient education
- (Anovulatory infertility) the patient should be advised to have intercourse on day of and day following administration of hCG preparation
- advise male patients to seek medical advice if any breast swelling or tenderness occurs

- see also General Patient education for infertility agents (p. 1458)

 Contraindicated during pregnancy.

 Contraindicated during breastfeeding.

Available in combination with
- follitropin alfa 900 IU and lutropin alfa 450 IU (Pergoveris)

FOLLITROPIN BETA
Trade name
Puregon

Available forms
Multidose cartridges: 300 IU/0.36 mL, 600 IU/0.72 mL, 900 IU/1.08 mL

Action
- recombinant human follicle-stimulating hormone (FSH)

Use
- (Females) anovulatory infertility; controlled ovarian hyperstimulation
- (Males) hypogonadotrophic hypogonadism (HH)

Dose
- (Anovulatory infertility) initially 50—150 IU SC daily for 5—7 days, increasing dose if needed to achieve a rise in oestrogen level (40—100% increase is considered optimal), daily dose is maintained to achieve preovulatory conditions estradiol (oestradiol) level 300—900 picogram/mL or total urinary estradiol (oestradiol) excretion 75—200 microgram/day and/or follicle $\geq$ 18 mm is present), followed by 5000—10,000 IU human chorionic gonadotrophin (hCG). hCG (1000—3000 IU) may be repeated up to 3 times in the following 9 days to support the luteal phase **OR**
- (Controlled ovarian hyperstimulation) 75—300 IU SC daily (alone, with clomifene (clomiphene) citrate or gonadotrophin-releasing hormone (GnRH) agonist), continued until adequate follicle development has occurred ($\geq$ 3 follicles 16—20 mm), followed by hCG 5000—10,000 IU preparation 30—40 hours after last injection and oocytes retrieved 34—35 hours later. hCG (1000—3000 IU) may be repeated up to 3 times in the following 9 days to support the luteal phase after embryo transfer **OR**
- (HH) 75 IU SC daily or 2—3 times weekly (with 1000—2000 IU hCG preparation 2—3 times weekly) and continued for at least 12 weeks

Adverse effects
- (Males) gynaecomastia, acne
- (Rare) atelectasis, acute respiratory distress
- see also General Adverse effects of infertility agents (p. 1457)

Interactions
- enhanced follicular response may be seen if given with clomifene (clomiphene)
- higher dose may be required following treatment with GnRH agonists

Nursing considerations/Cautions
- if oestrogen levels rise too fast (i.e. doubling daily for 2—3 days), dose should be decreased
- (Males) testosterone should be stopped before starting therapy
- (Males) semen analysis should be conducted 4—6 months after starting therapy
- (Males) contraindicated in those with primary testicular failure
- see also General Nursing considerations/Cautions for infertility agents (p. 1458)

Patient education
- advise male patients to seek medical advice if any breast swelling or tenderness occurs
- see also General Patient education for infertility agents (p. 1458)

Contraindicated during pregnancy.

 Contraindicated during breastfeeding.

FOLLITROPIN DELTA
Trade name
Rekovelle

Available forms
Prefilled pen: 12 microgram/0.36 mL, 36 microgram/1.08 mL, 72 microgram/2.16 mL

Action
* recombinant follicle-stimulating hormone (FSH) produced by recombinant DNA technology

Use
* controlled ovarian stimulation for the development of multiple follicles in women undergoing assisted reproductive technologies (e.g. IVF, intracytoplasmic sperm injection)

Dose
* (First treatment) dose is calculated based on anti-Mullerian hormone (AMH) concentration and body weight
  * (AMH < 15 picomol/L, regardless of body weight) 12 micrograms SC daily
  * (AMH > 15 picomol/L) daily dose decreases from 0.19 to 0.10 microgram/kg (daily maximum for first treatment cycle 12 micrograms)
* therapy should be started day 2 or 3 after menstrual bleeding starts, and continue until follicular development is adequate (determined by ultrasound and serum estradiol (oestradiol) levels), followed by 250 micrograms of recombinant human chorionic gonadotropin (hCG) or 5000 IU to induce follicular maturation
* (Subsequent cycles) daily dose should be maintained or modified according to response to previous cycle (daily maximum dose 24 micrograms)
  * (No ovarian hyperstimulation syndrome (OHSS) development) same daily dose
  * (Ovarian hyporesponse) daily dose should be increased by 25% or 50% depending on response
  * (Ovarian hyperresponse) daily dose should be decreased by 20% or 33% depending on response
  * (OHSS developed/risk of OHSS) daily dose should be decreased by 33%

Adverse effects
* see General Adverse effects of Infertility agents (p. 1457)

Nursing considerations/Cautions
* AMH is a biomarker of ovarian response to gonadotrophins. The dose should be based on a recent (within the last 12 months) determination of AMH levels using a specific diagnostic test such as Access AMH Advanced Immunoassay or Elecsys AMH Plus Immunoassay
* bodyweight should be measured without shoes and overcoat
* individual daily dose should be maintained during stimulation period
* AMH levels should be expressed as picomol/L and rounded off to nearest integer. If the concentration is expressed as nanogram/mL, it should be converted to picomol/L by multiplying by 7.14 (nanogram/mL × 7.14 = picomol/L)
* adequate follicular development (3 or more follicles 17 mm or larger) is achieved on average by the 9th day (range 5–20 days)
* if the woman is at risk of OHSS, a gonadotrophin-releasing hormone (GnRH) agonist should be considered in place of hCG to lower the risk
* if the woman experiences excessive ovarian response and produces > 35 follicles with a diameter of 12 mm or greater, final follicular maturation should not be triggered and the cycle cancelled
* see also General Nursing considerations/Cautions for Infertility agents (p. 1458)

PREGNANCY, CHILDBIRTH AND BREASTFEEDING

Patient education
- the patient should receive adequate education in the correct use of equipment, correct injection technique, importance of rotating injection sites, storage information and safe disposal of used equipment before self-administration can begin; the first injection should be under medical supervision
- see also General Patient education for Infertility agents (p. 1458)

Contraindicated during pregnancy.

Contraindicated during breastfeeding.

GANIRELIX ACETATE
Trade names
ARX Ganirelix, Ganirelix Lupin, Ganirelix Sun, Ganirelix Theramex, Orgalutran

Available form
Prefilled syringes: 250 microgram/0.5 mL

Action
- gonadotrophin-releasing hormone (GnRH) antagonist that binds to GnRH receptors in the pituitary gland
- inhibitory effect is greater for luteinising hormone (LH) release than for follicle-stimulating hormone (FSH)
- pituitary recovers within 2 days of stopping therapy

Use
- prevention of premature luteinisation and ovulation in women undergoing controlled ovarian stimulation (followed by oocyte pick-up and assisted reproductive techniques)

Dose
- 250 micrograms SC daily starting on day 5 or 6 of FSH therapy (depending on level of ovarian response) and continued until there are sufficient follicles of adequate size, followed by human chorionic gonadotrophin (hCG) to induce maturation and ovulation

Adverse effects
- headache, malaise
- nausea
- (Rare) hypersensitivity (rash, shortness of breath, facial swelling, urticaria)
- (Injection site) redness (with or without swelling)
- (Rare) OHSS, ectopic pregnancy, pelvic pain, abdominal distension

Nursing considerations/Cautions
- should not be mixed in the same syringe with FSH, but should be administered at the same time
- the time between last ganirelix and hCG administration should not exceed 30 hours
- contraindicated in those with allergy to latex rubber
- contraindicated in those with hypersensitivity to GnRH or GnRH analogues, or with moderate-to-severe kidney or liver impairment
- see also General Nursing considerations/Cautions for infertility agents (p. 1458)

Patient education
- see General Patient education for infertility agents (p. 1458)

Contraindicated during pregnancy.

Contraindicated during breastfeeding.

LUTROPIN ALFA
Trade name
Luveris

Available form
Vial: 75 IU

Action
- recombinant human luteinising hormone (LH)

- binds to receptor shared with human chorionic gonadotrophin (hCG)

Use
- stimulation of follicular development in women with severe LH and follicle-stimulating hormone (FSH) deficiency (usually with FSH preparation)

Dose
- 75 IU SC daily (with FSH preparation 75–150 IU) followed by hCG (5000–10,000 IU) when adequate response is obtained

Adverse effects
- see General Adverse effects of infertility agents (p. 1457)

Nursing considerations/Cautions
- if there is no response in 3 weeks, therapy should be stopped and restarted at a higher dose
- should not be mixed in same syringe with any other products except follitropin alfa
- treatment should be stopped if excessive response occurs and FSH levels may be decreased for next cycle
- contraindicated in those with hypersensitivity to gonadotrophins
- see also General Nursing considerations/Cautions for infertility agents (p. 1458)

Patient education
- patient should be advised to have intercourse on the day of and day following hCG administration. Alternatively, intrauterine (artificial) insemination may be performed at this time
- see also General Patient education for infertility agents (p. 1458)

 Contraindicated during pregnancy.

 Contraindicated during breastfeeding.

 Permitted in sport for females only.

Available in combination with
- lutropin alfa 450 IU and follitropin alfa 900 IU (Pergoveris)

MENOPAUSAL GONADOTROPHIN (HUMAN)
Trade name
Menopur

Available forms
Vial: 600 IU, 1200 IU

Action
- gonadotrophin that induces ovarian follicular growth and development and gonadal steroid production in women without primary ovarian failure

Use
- anovulatory infertility (including polycystic ovarian disease) in women unresponsive to clomifene (clomiphene) citrate
- controlled ovarian hyperstimulation to induce multiple follicle stimulation for assisted reproductive technologies

Dose
- (Anovulatory infertility) initially 75–150 IU SC daily for at least 7 days, with subsequent doses depending on clinical monitoring and patient response. Dose may be increased by 37.5 IU at intervals not less than 7 days (daily maximum 225 IU). When an optimal response is achieved, 5000–10,000 IU human chorionic gonadotrophin (hCG) should be given 1 day after last SC injection **OR**
- (Controlled ovarian hyperstimulation) initially 150–225 IU SC daily for at least 5 days of therapy, with subsequent dose depending on clinical monitoring and patient response. Dose may be increased by not more than 150 IU per adjustment (daily maximum 450 IU)

Adverse effects
- see General Adverse effects of infertility agents (p. 1457)

PREGNANCY, CHILDBIRTH AND BREASTFEEDING

Interactions
- enhanced follicular response may be seen if given with clomifene (clomiphene)
- higher dose may be required following treatment with gonadotrophin-releasing hormone (GnRH) agonists

Nursing considerations/Cautions
- may be used alone or with a gonadotrophin-releasing hormone (GnRH) agonist or antagonist
- (Anovulatory infertility) therapy should be started within 7 days of menstrual cycle
- (Anovulatory infertility) if no response after 4 weeks of therapy, the cycle should be stopped and restarted at a higher starting dose than the abandoned cycle
- (Controlled ovarian hyperstimulation) should be started 2 weeks after the start of agonist treatment (protocol using downregulation with a GnRH agonist), or on day 2 or 3 of menstrual cycle (protocol using downregulation with GnRH antagonist)
- (Controlled ovarian hyperstimulation) therapy > 20 days is not recommended
- to reconstitute, use one prefilled syringe of solvent (provided) for 600 IU vial and two prefilled syringes for 1200 IU vials
- roll the vial between the hands to dissolve any remaining powder after solvent has been added but avoid shaking
- extracted from human urine; therefore there may be a risk of pathogen transmission
- see also General Nursing considerations/Cautions for infertility agents (p. 1458)

Patient education
- (Anovulatory infertility) the patient should be advised to have sexual intercourse on the day of and the day following hCG administration (or artificial insemination may be performed)
- see also General Patient education for infertility agents (p. 1458)

 Contraindicated during pregnancy.

 Not recommended during breastfeeding.

 Permitted in sport for females only.

NAFARELIN ACETATE
Trade name
Synarel

Available form
Metered-dose nasal spray: 200 microgram/dose

Action
- gonadotrophin-releasing hormone (GnRH) analogue
- suppression of pituitary-gonadal system is restored 4—8 weeks after stopping treatment

Use
- endometriosis (visually proven) management (e.g. pain relief, to reduce lesions)
- controlled ovarian stimulation program

Dose
- (Endometriosis) initially 200 micrograms to one nostril in the morning, then 200 micrograms to the other nostril at night (total daily dose 400 micrograms), starting on days 2—4 of the menstrual cycle, increasing to 400 micrograms (given as 200 micrograms to each nostril morning and night) (total daily dose 800 micrograms) if symptoms of endometriosis are not controlled, for up to 6 months **OR**
- (Controlled ovarian stimulation) 400 micrograms twice daily given as 1 spray (200 micrograms) to each nostril, morning and night, starting either day 2 or day 21 of the menstrual cycle. Once downregulation is achieved,

gonadotrophin is commenced and nafarelin continued until human chorionic gonadotrophin (hCG) is given for follicular maturation (8–12 days)

Adverse effects

- hot flushes, headache, mood swings, insomnia
- changes in libido, vaginal dryness, decreased breast size
- acne, hirsutism, oily skin
- change in weight
- oedema
- myalgia
- irritation to nasal mucosa
- decreased bone density
- transient ovarian cysts
- increased cholesterol levels
- (Rare) hypersensitivity, ovarian hyperstimulation syndrome (OHSS), multiple pregnancy

Interaction

- diagnostic tests for pituitary–gonadal function may be inaccurate/misleading if conducted during or within 4 to 8 weeks of stopping therapy

Nursing considerations/Cautions

- (Endometriosis) bone density should be measured if symptoms recur and retreatment is necessary. A 2-year interval between treatment cycles is recommended
- (Controlled ovarian stimulation) should be stopped for 3 days before embryo transfer
- Controlled ovarian stimulation) if downregulation does not occur in 12 weeks, therapy should be stopped
- (Controlled ovarian stimulation) caution if used in those with polycystic ovarian syndrome because of an increased risk of excessive follicle development
- caution if used in women who are at risk of reduced bone mass (e.g. menstrual disturbances due to low weight or weight loss, athletic or other forms of hypothalamic amenorrhoea, immobilisation, glucocorticoid use or strong family history of osteoporosis). Baseline bone density should be measured before starting therapy in these at-risk women
- not recommended in women < 18 years
- contraindicated in women with undiagnosed abnormal vaginal bleeding or with hypersensitivity to GnRH or GnRH analogues

Patient education

- if the patient has rhinitis (runny nose), absorption of nafarelin may be decreased and may require use of nasal decongestant
- the patient should be advised to allow at least 30 minutes between using nasal decongestant and nafarelin
- the patient should be instructed regarding the correct use of the nasal pump, including:
  - priming pump with 5–10 sprays to obtain an even spray before first use
  - blowing nose before administration of the nasal spray
  - correct technique
  - cleaning and storage requirements
- warn the patient that symptoms of endometriosis may be exacerbated during the first few weeks of treatment
- the patient should be advised to immediately contact the doctor if one or more doses are missed, as there is a potential for breakthrough ovulation to occur. A pregnancy test may be recommended in this situation
- the patient should be counselled to use barrier methods of contraception during therapy and pregnancy should be excluded before starting therapy

 Contraindicated during pregnancy owing to the risk of abortion or fetal abnormality.

 Contraindicated during breastfeeding.

 Permitted in sport for females only.

PREGNANCY, CHILDBIRTH AND BREASTFEEDING

PROGESTERONE

Trade names
Crinone 8%, Cyclogest, Endometrin, Oripro, ProFeme Cream, Prolutex, Prometrium, Utrogestan

Available forms
Vaginal gel (prolonged release): 90 mg/applicator;
Vaginal pessaries: 100 mg, 200 mg, 300 mg, 400 mg;
Cream: 100 mg/mL;
Capsules: 100 mg;
Vial: 25 mg/1.112 mL

Action
- naturally occurring female sex hormone secreted from the ovary, placenta and adrenal gland
- if fertilisation occurs, progesterone levels remain high and this sustains the endometrium and maintains pregnancy
- rapidly absorbed from vagina

Use
- assisted reproductive technology in infertile women with progesterone deficiency (requiring supplementation to support embryo implantation and maintenance of pregnancy)
- preterm birth prevention with singleton pregnancy (in women with short cervix ≤ 25 mm)
- progesterone-deficient conditions (e.g. natural or surgical menopause)
- menstrual irregularities
- hormone replacement therapy (HRT) (with oestrogen product)

Dose
- (Pessary) 100 mg intravaginally 1—2 times daily, starting within several days of ovulation and continued until approximately 11 weeks gestation (daily maximum 400 mg twice daily) (Oripro) **OR**
- (Pessary) 100 mg intravaginally 3 times daily, starting at oocyte retrieval and continuing for 10 weeks (Endometrin) **OR**
- (Pessary) 200 mg intravaginally 3 times daily from embryo transfer until at least 7th week of pregnancy (and no later than 12th week) (Utrogestan) **OR**
- (Pessary) 400 mg intravaginally twice daily (morning, night) starting at oocyte retrieval and continuing for 38 days from start of therapy or up to 12 weeks of pregnancy (Cyclogest) **OR**
- (Prevention of preterm labour) 200 mg intravaginally nightly, from 16—24 weeks gestation and continued to 36 weeks or until delivery (Oripro, Utrogestan) **OR**
- (Threatened miscarriage) 200—400 mg intravaginally daily as 2 divided doses until week 12 (Utrogestan) **OR**
- (Gel) 90 mg (one application) intravaginally 1—2 times daily, starting 2 days after hCG administration, and continuing for 10—12 weeks if pregnancy occurs **OR**
- (HRT, intact uterus) 200 mg orally at night, from day 15—26, withdrawal bleeding following next week (with oestrogen) **OR**
- (HRT, intact uterus) 100 mg orally at night, from day 1—25, withdrawal bleeding following next week (with oestrogen) **OR**
- (Secondary amenorrhoea) 400 mg orally nightly for 10 days **OR**
- (Menstrual irregularities due to ovulation disorder, anovulation) 200—300 mg orally daily as single or divided dose (200 mg orally nightly, 100 mg morning (if needed)) for days 17—26 of the menstrual cycle **OR**
- (Menopause) 0.3 mL (30 mg) (10% cream) daily or in divided doses for either 25 days per calendar month or 3 weeks on and 1 week off (Profeme 10%) **OR**
- (Perimenopause) 0.3 mL (30 mg) (10% cream) daily or in divided doses for days 12—26 of menstrual cycle (if menstrual cycle begins before day 26) (Profeme 10%) **OR**
- (Premenstrual syndrome) 0.3 mL (30 mg) (10% cream) daily or in divided doses for days 12—26 of menstrual cycle (Profeme 10%) **OR**

1469

- (Premenstrual dysphoric disorder) 0.5—1 mL (50—100 mg) daily or in divided doses for days 12—26 (Profeme 10%) **OR**
- (Endometriosis, menorrhagia, postpartum depression) 1—2 mL (100—200 mg) daily or in divided doses (depending on condition severity), can be started days 12—26, but frequency can be increased to 3 weeks in 4 if symptoms recur after stopping therapy (Profeme 10%) **OR**
- (Infertility) 1 mL (100 mg) daily or in divided doses for days 12—26 until pregnancy is confirmed and then continued at 1—2 mL until at least week 13 or full term (Profeme 10%) **OR**
- (Repeated first-term miscarriage) 0.3 mL (30 mg) daily or in divided doses for days 12—26 until pregnancy is confirmed. If spotting occurs at week 6 or 7, 1—2 mL (100—200 mg) 2—3 times daily can be used until full term (Profeme 10%) **OR**
- (Infertility) 25 mg SC or IM daily from day of oocyte retrieval for up to 12 weeks where pregnancy is confirmed (Prolutex)

Adverse effects

- amenorrhoea, abnormal breakthrough bleeding, metromenorrhagia, spotting, genital itchiness, dyspareunia, perineal pain, uterine spasm, vaginal discomfort/burning/dryness, vaginal discharge
- abdominal cramping/distension/pain, bloating, weight gain
- breast pain/tenderness, breast swelling/enlargement, galactorrhoea
- fluid retention
- papillary oedema, retinal haemorrhage
- rash, pruritus
- arthralgia
- nocturia
- headache, dizziness, drowsiness
- depression, decreased libido, nervousness, somnolence, insomnia
- nausea, vomiting, diarrhoea
- hyperglycaemia, hyperlipidaemia
- ovarian enlargement, ovarian cyst formation
- (SC) pain, pruritus, haematoma, irritation
- (Rare) thromboembolism
- (Abrupt discontinuation) anxiety, moodiness, seizures

Interactions

- effects may be decreased if given with carbamazepine, phenobarbital (phenobarbitone), phenytoin, rifabutin, rifampicin or St John's wort
- may decrease serum levels of ciclosporin
- effects may be increased by itraconazole
- may potentiate levothyroxine levels, potentially leading to hyperthyroidism
- glucose tolerance test and coagulation test results may be affected
- liver, thyroid and endocrine function tests may be affected
- metyrapone test may show lower response than usual
- not recommended with other vaginal products

Nursing considerations/Cautions

- before starting therapy, breast, abdominal and pelvic organ examination is recommended, as well as a Papanicolaou (Pap) smear
- SC/IM administration is recommended for women who are unable to use or tolerate vaginal preparations
- (Prolutex) IM administration by medical practitioner, SC self-administration by the patient after adequate education
- (Cream) symptoms generally diminish 8—12 weeks after starting therapy
- (Secondary amenorrhoea) causes of secondary amenorrhoea, such as outflow obstruction, prolactinoma, thyroid disorders, pituitary and hypothalamic disorders, should be excluded before starting therapy
- (Endometrin) in women under 35 years with adequate ovarian reserve, twice daily application is appropriate; in women over 35 years with decreased ovarian reserve, 3 times daily application is necessary

PREGNANCY, CHILDBIRTH AND BREASTFEEDING

- caution if used in women with a history of depression
- caution if used in women with diabetes mellitus, as glucose tolerance may be altered during therapy
- caution if used in those women whose conditions would be aggravated by fluid retention (e.g. asthma, cardiac, migraine, renal dysfunction), or with a history of depression, diabetes mellitus or hyperlipidaemia
- caution if used in those with myocardial infarction, cardiovascular disorders, retinal thrombosis or mild-to-moderate liver dysfunction
- caution if used in those > 35 years, smokers or with risk factors for atherosclerosis because of the risk of risk of retinal vascular lesions
- contraindicated in women with a hypersensitivity to hard fat or with porphyria, vaginal or urinary tract bleeding (of unknown origin), liver impairment, deep vein thrombosis, pulmonary embolism, previous hormone-associated thrombophlebitis or thromboembolism, seizure disorder, missed abortion or ectopic pregnancy, or cancer (ovary, breast or uterine)
- contraindicated in pregnancy during assisted reproductive technology when normal progesterone levels are present

Patient education

- instruct the patient that the pessary should be inserted deep into the vagina while squatting or lying on back or side, and that no other intravaginal preparations should be used at the same time
- advise the patient that, if the pessary is used once daily, preferably administer in the evening
- the patient should be instructed to seek medical advice immediately if any sudden severe headache and/or visual disturbances occur
- if the patient has diabetes, she should be advised to monitor blood glucose levels closely during therapy
- (Prolutex) the patient should receive adequate education in the correct use of equipment, correct injection technique, importance of rotating injection sites, storage information and safe disposal of used equipment before self-administration can begin; the first injection should be under medical supervision
- (Vaginal gel) instruct the patient to shake down the gel applicator, holding on to the thick end without removing the cap. When gel is in the thin end, twist off the tab, insert applicator deep into the vagina and press the thick end to deposit prolonged-release gel. Remove applicator and discard appropriately
- warn the patient not to drive or operate machinery if dizziness or drowsiness occurs
- instruct the patient that capsules should be taken at bedtime without food
- ensure the patient has the following information regarding application of cream:
  - maximum absorption occurs when applied over a large skin area (e.g. inner aspects of arms, upper thighs, abdomen, upper chest and neck)
  - cream should be massaged until completely absorbed
  - perimenopausal women with irregular menstrual cycles should be warned that menses may return
  - for perimenopausal women, therapy should be synchronised with normal progesterone production (days 12–26 menstrual cycle). If menstruation occurs after 5–10 days, cream should be stopped and restarted 12 days later

 Contraindicated during pregnancy in which progesterone levels are normal.

 Not recommended during breastfeeding.

1471

AGENTS USED TO TREAT PRE-ECLAMPSIA AND ECLAMPSIA

Pre-eclampsia is a serious pregnancy complication, with mild pre-eclampsia occurring in 5—10% of all pregnancy and severe pre-eclampsia accounting for 1—2% of pregnancies. Pre-eclampsia and related complications are responsible for 15% of direct maternal deaths in Australia, as well as 10% of perinatal mortality. Rates of pre-eclampsia are higher in Aboriginal women, those from the Torres Strait Islands and Pacific Island women, while they are lower in Asian women (Australian Action on Pre-eclampsia n.d.; Fasanya et al 2021).

The exact cause of pre-eclampsia is still unknown, although it is thought that placental dysfunction may start the systemic vasospasm, ischaemia and thrombosis that ultimately results in damage to maternal organs. Risk factors for developing pre-eclampsia include a previous history or family history of pre-eclampsia, previous gestational hypertension, chronic hypertension, pre-existing diabetes, autoimmune disease such as systemic lupus erythematosus (SLE) or antiphospholipid syndrome. Other possible risk factors include nulliparity, first pregnancy, multiple birth pregnancy, advanced maternal age, assisted reproduction, BMI > 30, pre-existing kidney disease and increasing maternal glucose levels (Karrer, Martingano & Hong 2024). However, any pregnant woman is at risk.

Commonly, pre-eclampsia occurs after 20 weeks gestation and frequently near term. Symptoms include high BP, proteinuria (resulting from kidney dysfunction) and swelling of the hands, feet and face. If severe, dizziness, headache and visual problems occur, and, when left untreated, progress to eclampsia and convulsions which are life threatening for both the mother and the baby (Australian Action on Pre-eclampsia n.d.). While management includes BP and convulsion control, delivery of the fetus is needed.

MAGNESIUM SULFATE HEPTAHYDRATE (MAGNESIUM SULFATE)

Trade names
DBL Magnesium Sulfate Concentrated Injection, Medsurge Magnesium Sulfate Heptahydrate 50%, Phebra Magnesium Sulfate Heptahydrate 50% Injection

Available forms
Ampoules: 2.465 g/5 mL, 2.5 g/5 mL, 5 g/10 mL

Action
* second most abundant intracellular cation that is essential in more than 300 enzymatic processes, glycolysis, Krebs' cycle, protein and nucleic acid synthesis
* neuroprotective mechanism of action is unclear, but thought to be related to blockade of glutamate receptors preventing post-hypoxic brain injury decreasing perinatal death and risk of cerebral palsy
* anticonvulsant effects
* (IV) onset of action 30 minutes

Use
* prevent and treat hypomagnesaemia (see Vitamins, minerals and electrolytes, p. 1659)
* prevent and treat seizures associated with toxemias of pregnancy (pre-eclampsia and eclampsia)

Dose
* initially 4 g IV over 10—15 minutes (loading dose), followed by IV infusion of 1—2 g/hour **OR**
* initially 4 g IV over 5—10 minutes (loading dose), followed by 4—5 g IM into each buttock, then 4—5 g IM into alternate buttocks 4-hourly if needed
* (Neuroprotection of fetus) initially 4 g IV over 20—30 minutes, followed by 1 g per hour by IV infusion for 24 hours or birth (whichever comes first)

Adverse effects
- flushing (hands, face, neck), sensation of warmth
- nausea, vomiting
- (Uncommon) headache, dizziness
- (IM) pain, irritation at injection site
- (Excess, hypermagnesaemia) thirst, nausea, vomiting, flushing, hypotension, bradycardia, slurred speech, muscle weakness and paralysis, blurred/double vision, loss of deep tendon reflexes, respiratory and CNS depression, cardiac arrest, coma

Interactions
- caution if given with cardiac glycosides
- increased CNS depression may result if given with CNS depressants
- increased neuromuscular blockade may occur if given with neuromuscular blocking agents
- increased hypotension and neuromuscular blockade may occur if given with nifedipine

Nursing considerations/Cautions
- pulse, BP, respiratory rate, patellar reflexes and urine output should be checked before loading dose is given (as baseline), 10 minutes after loading dose has started and at the end of the loading dose (or according to hospital/facility protocol). Respiratory rate should be at least 16 breaths/min before start of infusion. During maintenance infusion, pulse, BP, respiratory rate, patellar reflexes and urinary output should be checked at least 4-hourly and infusion stopped if the respiratory rate is less than 12 breaths/min, patellar reflexes are absent, if hypotension occurs or urine output is less than 100 mL/4 hours
- serum magnesium should be measured regularly to ensure normal serum levels are not exceeded
- calcium salt (e.g. calcium gluconate monohydrate) should be available when IV magnesium sulfate heptahydrate is given (to treat hypermagnesaemia)
- IV doses should be diluted to a concentration of 20% or less
- total daily dose should not exceed 30—40 g
- incompatible with calcium salts and will precipitate if mixed in the same IV infusion. Also incompatible with alkali carbonates, bicarbonates and soluble phosphates
- caution if given to those with myasthenia gravis because it may precipitate an acute crisis
- caution if used in those with impaired kidney function
- contraindicated in those with heart block, kidney failure (creatinine clearance < 20 mL/min) or within 2 hours of delivery (unless it is the only therapy available)

May cause hypermagnesaemia and depressed breathing in the newborn, as it readily crosses the placenta and fetal serum levels are similar to the maternal levels. If given parenterally for a prolonged time (5—7 days), neonate may have bony abnormalities and congenital rickets.

Caution if given during breastfeeding because the concentration in breastmilk may reach twice the maternal serum levels. Cleared from breastmilk within 24 hours of stopping therapy.

Caution if used in those with impaired kidney function and contraindicated in those with kidney failure (CrCl < 20 mL/min)

AGENTS USED TO MANAGE PREMATURE LABOUR

An estimated 13.4 million babies were born preterm worldwide in 2020, with preterm birth complications being the major cause of death in children under 5 years, as well being the cause of lifetime disabilities including learning difficulties and visual or hearing problems (WHO 2023a). Preterm is considered to be delivery before 37 completed weeks of gestation, with 32—37 weeks as being defined as moderate-to-late preterm, 28—32 weeks as very preterm, and before 28 weeks considered as extremely preterm (WHO 2023a).

Tocolytic agents are used to inhibit preterm labour in order to allow time for co-interventions (such as transferring to a facility with neonatal intensive care services and the administration of corticosteroids) in order to improve neonatal outcomes; however, these are not recommended if pregnancy prolongation is dangerous for either mother or fetus. Generally, because preterm neonates born after 34 weeks gestation do well, tocolytic agents are not recommended after 33 weeks gestation (Cunningham et al 2022).

Corticosteroids (e.g. betamethasone or dexamethasone) may be given to women at 24–34 weeks gestation who are at risk of preterm delivery within 7 days. The aim is to accelerate fetal lung maturity, reducing the risk of neonatal death, respiratory distress syndrome and cerebroventricular haemorrhage (Cunningham et al 2022).

NIFEDIPINE
Trade names
Adalat, APO-Nifedipine XR

Available forms
Tablets: 10 mg, 20 mg;
Tablets (extended-release): 30 mg, 60 mg

Action
- calcium-channel blocker that relaxes smooth muscle via blockade of calcium channels
- evidence suggests that it appears to be more effective than salbutamol (with fewer births within 7 days of treatment), fewer maternal adverse effects and decreased neonatal morbidity
- half-life 6–12 hours

Use
- threatened or established preterm labour (< 34 weeks gestation)

Dose
- initially 20 mg orally, then dose repeated after 30 and 60 minutes if contractions continue. If maternal BP remains stable, 20 mg orally every 6 hours for 48 hours, unless contractions cease or labour is established (daily maximum dose 160 mg)

Adverse effects
- hypotension and possible fetal hypoxia
- headache, fatigue, dizziness
- flushing
- tachycardia, palpitations
- nausea, heartburn, constipation
- peripheral oedema (secondary to arteriolar vasodilation)
- transient risk in liver function tests

Interactions
- caution if given with magnesium sulfate heptahydrate, as significant hypotension and neuromuscular weakness may occur
- caution if used with IV salbutamol or glyceryl trinitrate (GTN)

Nursing considerations/Cautions
- maternal BP, temperature, pulse and respiratory rate and fetal heart rate should be measured before starting therapy, then maternal BP, temperature and heart rate should be measured hourly for 4 hours. BP should be measured before administration of nifedipine (regularity of observations can be tapered according to clinical situation and/or hospital protocol)
- cardiotocograph (CTG) monitoring should be continuous during contractions and if there is regular abdominal pain/tenderness, change in the amount/colour of liquor or antepartum haemorrhage occurs
- tablets may be crushed or chewed to increase absorption
- extended-release formulation should not be used
- if given with magnesium sulfate heptahydrate, BP, deep tendon reflexes and respiratory function should be closely monitored
- therapy should be stopped if there is marked hypotension (< 90 mmHg) or significant dyspnoea

- caution if there is suspected intrauterine infection, fetal growth restriction, multiple pregnancy, preterm labour with placenta praevia or undiagnosed significant vaginal bleeding
- (Fetal) contraindicated if there is proven intrauterine infection, fetal compromise during delivery, placental abruption or insufficiency, severe growth restriction, lethal fetal anomalies or intrauterine fetal death
- (Maternal) contraindicated if woman has hypotension (BP < 90 mmHg) or cardiac disease, if any condition exists that would make prolongation of pregnancy dangerous, advanced cervical dilation or liver dysfunction

Note
- Extended-release tablets (APO-Nifedipine XR) are commercially available for management of hypertension (see p. 939)
- Immediate-release formulation must be accessed through the Special Access Scheme (SAS)

SALBUTAMOL SULFATE (known as albuterol in the USA)
Trade names
Ventolin Obstetric Injection

Available form
Ampoules: 1 mg/mL

Action
- direct-acting sympathomimetic agent related to adrenaline (epinephrine), noradrenaline (norepinephrine) and isoprenaline, with a longer duration of action
- causes bronchodilation
- relaxes uterine smooth muscle via effect on uterine beta2 adrenoreceptors
- (IV) half-life 4—6 hours
- crosses the placenta, increasing fetal heart rate

Use
- relief of reversible bronchospasm in asthma, chronic bronchitis and emphysema (see Antiasthma agents, bronchodilators and respiratory agents, p. 104)
- management of threatened or established uncomplicated premature labour (24—33 weeks gestation)

Dose
- initially 10 microgram/min by IV infusion, increasing at 10-minute intervals until there is a decrease in strength, frequency or duration of contraction, then increasing infusion slowly until contractions have ceased. Infusion is then maintained for 1 hour at the same rate as when contractions ceased, then reducing rate by 50% 6-hourly

Adverse effects (for obstetric use)
- fine skeletal muscle tremor, especially in the hands
- nervousness, restlessness, anxiety
- dyspnoea
- oliguria
- maternal sinus tachycardia, palpitations, peripheral vasodilation, increased maternal pulse pressure and cardiac output, conduction disturbance (at high doses), hypotension
- nausea, vomiting
- headache, dizziness, flushing
- hypokalaemia, ketosis, disturbed carbohydrate metabolism, hyperglycaemia, exacerbation of diabetes
- (Uncommon) maternal pulmonary oedema, myocardial ischaemia
- (Neonatal) fetal tachycardia, and rarely hypoglycaemia, ileus
- (Rare) hypersensitivity, muscle cramps, maternal ileus

Interactions
- caution in patients who have already received therapy with high doses of other sympathomimetic agents
- may potentiate effects of chlorpromazine
- increased risk of hypokalaemia if given with xanthines, corticosteroids or diuretics

Nursing considerations/Cautions

- cardiovascular status should be assessed before starting therapy
- infusion should be started as soon as possible after diagnosis of premature labour
- hydration status (including fluid balance) should be closely monitored to prevent overhydration and maternal pulmonary oedema
- patient should lie on side during infusion to prevent aortocaval compression and hypotension
- electrolytes (especially serum potassium), glucose (especially in women with diabetes mellitus) and lactate should be monitored throughout therapy. If the patient has diabetes, she should be closely monitored for any signs of ketoacidosis
- monitor vital signs (HR, BP and ECG) throughout therapy (initially every 15 minutes), noting that an elevation of heart rate may be a side-effect and a reduced heart rate a sign of improvement. Maternal pulse rate should be monitored throughout therapy and adjusted to prevent an increase over 120 beats/min. The effect on diastolic BP is usually greater than on systolic
- fetal heart rate should be monitored continuously throughout therapy. If fetal distress occurs, the acid—base balance and oxygen saturation should be closely monitored to prevent fetal acidosis and hypoxia
- if fetal distress is present, monitoring for fetal acidosis is recommended. If acid—base balance continues to decrease, therapy should be stopped and labour allowed to proceed. Similarly, if fetal hypoxia does not improve, therapy should be stopped and labour allowed to proceed
- symptoms of overdose are eased by rest and reassurance
- note and report any cardiac arrhythmias, especially in patients receiving digoxin, because these may result from salbutamol-induced hypokalaemia
- for patients with diabetes, IV fluids containing glucose should be avoided
- infusion should be given via infusion pump and administered alone
- infusion is not recommended for more than 48 hours
- if membranes rupture or the cervix dilates to greater than 4 cm, salbutamol effectiveness is reduced and is not recommended
- therapy is generally stopped if strong contractions occur and labour progresses
- caution if used in those women with angina, hypertension or heart disease (especially tachyarrhythmias), coronary artery disease, congestive heart failure, acute severe asthma or thyrotoxicosis
- caution if used in those with impaired liver or kidney function; dose reduction is recommended
- contraindicated in women with sensitivity to salbutamol and related amines, if gestational age is < 24 weeks, or in those with diabetes mellitus, asthma, pre-existing (or with risk factors for) ischaemic heart disease, pulmonary hypertension, uncontrolled hypertension, ileus, is unconscious, has uncompensated potassium depletion, hypercalcaemia, hyperthyroidism, glaucoma, paroxysmal tachycardia, or has any condition where prolonged pregnancy could be dangerous for mother or fetus (e.g. severe pre-eclampsia, active uterine bleeding, premature rupture of membranes (with chorioamnionitis), cervical dilation > 4 cm, compression of umbilical cord, intrauterine fetal oedema, fetal acidosis or hypoxia, fetal distress, fetal death, known congenital or chromosomal malformations) or kidney insufficiency

Patient education

- warn the patient that tremor and palpitation may be experienced

PREGNANCY, CHILDBIRTH AND BREASTFEEDING

 Dose reduction may be needed in women with impaired kidney or liver function.

 Banned in sport.

Note
- salbutamol is available as Airomir Autohaler and Inhaler, Asmol CFC-free Inhaler, Salbutamol Cipla Inhalation, Ventolin preparations and Zempreon CFC-Free Inhaler, for management of asthma

AGENTS USED TO INDUCE LABOUR

DINOPROSTONE (prostaglandin E_2)

Trade names
Cervidil, Prostin E_2 Vaginal Gel

Available forms
Vaginal pessaries: 10 mg;
Vaginal gel: 1 mg/2.5 mL, 2 mg/2.5 mL

Action
- releases prostaglandin E_2 into cervical tissue, which promotes softening and effacement (ripening) of the cervix (relaxation of cervical smooth muscle) to allow passage of fetus through the birth canal

Use
- induction of labour (single pregnancy with vertex presentation) at or near term

Dose
- 1 mg intravaginally, with 1—2 mg after 6 hours if necessary (not exceeding 3 mg/6 hours) **OR**
- 10 mg pessary inserted high into posterior vaginal fornix (leaving sufficient withdrawal tape for easy removal)

Adverse effects
- fetal distress
- uterine hypertonus, hypercontractility, arrested labour
- headache
- fever
- (Rare) postpartum haemorrhage, amniotic fluid embolism, uterine rupture, disseminated intravascular coagulation (DIC), infection

Interactions
- not recommended with or within 30 minutes of other IV oxytocic agents, as effects are potentiated
- NSAIDs (including aspirin) should be stopped before using dinoprostone

Nursing considerations/Cautions
- the patient should be assessed before administration and have a cervical score (Bishop) of 8 or more
- should be administered only in facilities where continuous fetal and uterine monitoring is available
- (Pessary) only a small amount of water-based lubricant should be applied before insertion
- (Pessary) remove from freezer just before use and can be used without warming
- (Pessary) should not be inserted if retrieval tape is not in place
- (Gel) warm to room temperature for at least 30 minutes before administration
- (Gel, pessary) insert transversely high into the posterior fornix, avoiding the cervical canal. With the pessary, sufficient tape should remain outside the vagina for easy removal (not tucked inside). If the pessary is not correctly inserted, it will not make sufficient contact to be effective
- (Gel, pessary) the patient should remain recumbent for at least 30 minutes after insertion
- monitor the patient (uterine activity, progression of cervical dilation and effacement, fetal condition) closely after insertion
- (Pessary) the pessary should be removed immediately (by applying gentle traction on retrieval tape) if labour (painful uterine activity) commences (regardless of cervical state) before membranes rupture, if there are

- any adverse effects (maternal or fetal) or if there is insufficient cervical ripening in 12 hours or prior to amniotomy
- (Pessary) if oxytocin is to be used, a 30-minute interval should be allowed to elapse after removal of the pessary
- (Pessary) effective over 12 hours
- (Pessary) a second dose is not recommended
- caution if used in women aged 35 years or more, or with gestational diabetes, arterial hypotension, hypothyroidism, gestation greater than 40 weeks, compromised cardiovascular function, previous uterine hypertony, asthma, glaucoma or epilepsy, or who have had > 3 full-term deliveries
- caution if used in those with a cervical Bishop score ≥ 8 (i.e. greater chance of having a vaginal delivery)
- contraindicated in women with multiple pregnancy who have had five or more deliveries, previous uterine or cervical surgery, cervical rupture or current pelvic inflammatory disease (untreated), unexplained vaginal bleeding during pregnancy, if labour has started, membranes are ruptured or after amniotomy, if oxytocin will be given IV within 30 minutes, if the fetus is distressed, compromised or malpresented (non-vertex), if vaginal delivery is inappropriate (e.g. placenta praevia, active genital herpes), if strong prolonged contractions are inappropriate, or if there is cephalopelvic disproportion, uterine hyperstimulation or hypertonic uterine contractions
- (Gel) contraindicated in women with hypersensitivity to dinoprostone, triacetin or colloidal anhydrous silica

Not recommended for any other stage of pregnancy.

Not recommended for breastfeeding.

OXYTOCIC AGENTS

CARBETOCIN
Trade names
Carbetocin Interpharma, Duratocin

Available form
Ampoules: 100 microgram/mL

Action
- long-acting synthetic oxytocin analogue that stimulates uterine muscle contraction
- properties similar to oxytocin with less potent but more prolonged action
- contractions established within 2 minutes of IV duration of action about 1 hour (IV)
- may be given as IM for vaginal delivery (Duratocin only)

Use
- prevention of uterine atony and excessive bleeding after elective delivery via caesarean section (under spinal or epidural anaesthesia) or vaginal delivery

Dose
- (Caesarean section) 100 micrograms slowly IV over 1 minute as a single dose after delivery of infant (before or after delivery of placenta) **OR**
- (Vaginal delivery) 100 micrograms IM or slowly IV over 1 minute as a single dose after delivery of infant (before or after delivery of placenta) (Duratocin)

Adverse effects
- nausea, vomiting, abdominal pain, metallic taste
- pruritus
- flushing, feeling of warmth, sweating, fever, chills
- hypotension, tachycardia, chest pain
- headache, dizziness
- tremor, anxiety
- dyspnoea
- anaemia
- back pain

PREGNANCY, CHILDBIRTH AND BREASTFEEDING

Interaction
- may cause severe hypertension if given within 3—4 hours of vasoconstricting agent with caudal block anaesthesia

Nursing considerations/Cautions
- if bleeding persists, the patient should be closely examined for retained placental fragments, coagulopathy or genital tract trauma
- repeat administration is not recommended if uterine contraction post-delivery is not adequate. Other uterotonic agents such as oxytocin or ergometrine should be used
- (Vaginal delivery) may be given IM (Duratocin)
- caution if used in women with eclampsia or pre-eclampsia, as BP should be closely monitored
- not recommended post-emergency delivery via caesarean section or after vaginal delivery
- caution if used in those with epilepsy, migraine or asthma, or if rapid addition of extracellular water may be problematic
- contraindicated in those with known hypersensitivity to oxytocin, before delivery of infant or in those with cardiovascular disease (especially coronary artery disease), valvular heart disease, heart failure or cardiomyopathy

 Contraindicated during pregnancy.

ERGOMETRINE MALEATE
Trade name
DBL Ergometrine Injection

Available form
Ampoules: 500 microgram/mL

Action
- ergot alkaloid that stimulates contraction of uterine and vascular smooth muscle
- increases amplitude and frequency of uterine contractions and tone, impeding uterine blood flow, producing haemostasis
- increases strength and frequency of cervical contractions
- produces some arterial vasoconstriction by stimulating alpha adrenergic and serotonin receptors
- may decrease prolactin level post-delivery
- (IV) onset of action less than 1 minute, lasting for up to 45 minutes
- (IM) onset of action 2—5 minutes, lasting 3 hours

Use
- prevention and treatment of postpartum haemorrhage following delivery of placenta

Dose
- (Prophylaxis of postpartum haemorrhage) 200 micrograms IM after delivery is complete (after exclusion of second twin) **OR**
- (Treatment of postpartum haemorrhage) 200 micrograms IM **OR**
- (Emergency) 200 micrograms slowly IV over 1 minute

Adverse effects
- headache, dizziness, hallucination
- tinnitus, vertigo
- sweating
- nausea, vomiting, unpleasant taste, diarrhoea, abdominal pain, oesophageal spasm
- dyspnoea, nasal congestion, pulmonary oedema
- leg cramps
- bradycardia, palpitations, arrhythmias, chest pain (transient), hypotension, thrombophlebitis, peripheral vasospasm
- water intoxication
- haematuria
- (Rapid or undiluted IV infusion) hypertension (sometimes sudden and/or severe)

- (Prolonged therapy) gangrene, numbness/tingling of extremities
- (Rare) allergy, uterine rupture, amniotic fluid embolism

Interactions
- may precipitate angina and reduce effects of antianginal agents
- may cause additive peripheral vasoconstriction if given with beta adrenoceptor blocking agents, general anaesthetics, some local anaesthetics, sympathomimetic agents or vasoconstricting agents
- may cause hypertension, stroke, seizures or myocardial infarction if given with bromocriptine
- vasoconstriction may increase if given with nicotine (heavy smokers)
- effectiveness is reduced in calcium deficiency states
- not recommended with sumatriptan owing to an increased risk of coronary vasoconstriction
- increased risk of ergotism if given with erythromycin or doxycycline
- increased risk of hypertension, peripheral ischaemia and gangrene if given with dopamine; therefore not recommended together

Nursing considerations/Cautions
- the uterus should be inspected before administration for any retained placenta or second fetus. If administered before delivery, the infant may develop hypoxia and/or intracranial haemorrhage
- response may not be seen if hypocalcaemia is present
- IV route should be restricted to emergency situations, because the risk of adverse effects is increased
- if IV route is used, should be given slowly or diluted with 5 mL sodium chloride 0.9% before administration and given slowly over 1 minute to avoid hypertension
- prolactin level may be decreased in the postpartum period if multiple doses are given
- should be administered alone because of incompatibilities with many agents including adrenaline (epinephrine), ampicillin, cefalotin, chloramphenicol, heparin, metaraminol, sulfadiazine, thiopentone, vitamin B complex with C and warfarin
- should not be given for prolonged period, because ergotism and/or gangrene may result
- caution if used in those with porphyria because exacerbation may occur
- caution if used in those with Raynaud's phenomenon
- great caution if used in those with coronary artery disease, including mitral valve stenosis or venoatrial shunts
- caution if used in those with eclampsia or hypertension, as hypertensive effects may be exaggerated
- contraindicated in those with hypersensitivity to ergot alkaloids, during induction of labour or in the first or second stage of labour, if there is any suspicion of retained placenta, during eclampsia, pre-eclampsia or threatened spontaneous abortion, severe or persistent sepsis, peripheral vascular disease, heart disease, hypertension (existing or a history of), or liver or kidney impairment

Contraindicated during pregnancy (if given before delivery, may result in fetal hypoxia or intracranial haemorrhage).

Contraindicated during breastfeeding (secretion in breastmilk may result in fetal ergotism, although a single dose to prevent haemorrhage should not prevent women from breastfeeding).

Available in combination with
- ergometrine 0.5 mg + oxytocin 5 IU (Syntometrine)

OXYTOCIN

Trade names
Oxytocin APX, Oxytocin GH, Syntocinon, Viatocinon

Available forms
Ampoules: 5 IU/mL, 10 IU/mL

Action
- synthetic oxytocin with similar actions to endogenous oxytocin, but with little vasopressin (antidiuretic) activity
- stimulates uterine contraction and lactating breast to eject milk

Use
- induction and maintenance of labour (third stage)
- controlling postpartum bleeding

Dose
- (Induction of labour) initially 1–4 milliunits/min (0.1–0.4 mL/min) by IV infusion, increasing at intervals of at least 20 minutes and increments of 1–2 milliunits/min (to a maximum of 20 milliunits/min) until contractions are similar to normal labour, then reducing infusion rate **OR**
- (Management of the third stage of labour or postpartum haemorrhage) 5–10 IU IM or 5 IU slowly IV after delivery of shoulder **OR**
- (Caesarean section) 5 IU by slow IV injection, or IV infusion after delivery of the fetus

Adverse effects
- nausea, vomiting
- headache
- (Large doses) violent uterine contractions, leading to uterine rupture, fetal distress, asphyxia and death
- (Rapid infusion) severe hypotension, flushing and reflex tachycardia
- tachycardia, bradycardia and rarely ECG changes, QT prolongation
- (High dose, prolonged infusion) water intoxication, maternal hyponatraemia
- (Rare) hypertension, cardiovascular collapse, amniotic fluid embolism, disseminated intravascular coagulation (DIC), rash, anaphylaxis
- (Fetal) neonatal hyponatraemia, fetal distress, asphyxia, death

Interactions
- contraindicated within 6 hours of vaginal prostaglandins
- uterotonic effects potentiated if given with prostaglandins or their analogues. Careful patient monitoring is recommended if given together
- some inhalation anaesthetics (e.g. isoflurane) may reduce the action of oxytocin as well as potentiating hypotensive action and causing arrhythmias
- caution if used with other agents known to prolong QT interval
- oxytocin may potentiate pressor action of sympathomimetic vasoconstrictors if given during or after caudal block
- may enhance vasopressor effects of sympathomimetic or vasoconstricting agents (including if included in local anaesthetics)

Nursing considerations/Cautions
- 1000 milliunits = 1 unit (IU)
- not recommended SC, IM or by IV bolus
- multiple pregnancy should be excluded and maturity of the fetus should be established before starting infusion
- notify the doctor if contractions become prolonged and unduly strong, and be ready to reduce rate or stop infusion
- induction of labour should be stopped if infusion of 5 IU does not establish contractions
- during infusion, monitor maternal heart rate (HR), blood pressure (BP), strength, duration and frequency of uterine contractions, as well as fetal heart rate and rhythm
- infusion volume should be kept to a minimum if the woman has cardiovascular problems
- (High dose or prolonged administration) oral fluid restriction and strict fluid balance chart are recommended. Serum electrolytes should be measured 8–12-hourly to prevent water intoxication. If water intoxication occurs, oxytocin

should be stopped, fluids restricted, any electrolyte imbalance corrected, diuresis promoted and any seizures treated. Signs of water intoxication include headache, anorexia, nausea, vomiting, abdominal pain, lethargy, drowsiness, seizures, unconsciousness, hyponatraemia and acute pulmonary oedema (without hyponatraemia)
- a burette and infusion pump should be used to deliver the solution to prevent inadvertent overdose. This also avoids rapid administration, decreasing the risk of cardiovascular effects
- the solution should be prepared using glucose 4% with sodium chloride 0.18% and made to a solution strength of 10 IU/L. Glucose 5% is not recommended
- not compatible with solutions containing metasulfites or bisulfites
- gently rotate the IV container to distribute oxytocin evenly in admixture
- administer alone
- prolonged administration is not recommended in those with oxytocin-resistant uterine inertia, cardiovascular disorders or severe pre-eclampsia
- an increased risk of amniotic fluid embolism in women with fetal death in utero and/or meconium-stained amniotic fluid
- caution if used in those with borderline cephalopelvic disproportion, secondary uterine inertia, mild—moderate pregnancy-induced hypertension, cardiovascular disease (especially if affected by changes in HR or BP), over 35 years or with known QT syndrome or history of lower segment caesarean section
- caution if patient has latex allergy or intolerance, as there is an increased risk of anaphylaxis
- caution if used in women with predisposing factors for myocardial infarction (e.g. hypertrophic cardiomyopathy, valvular heart disease, ischaemic heart disease). If given, significant changes in HR and BP should be avoided
- caution if used in women with kidney impairment, as there is increased risk of water retention and oxytocin accumulation
- contraindicated if there is fetal distress, abnormal presentation, cephalopelvic disproportion, elderly multiparae, excessive distension of uterus, parity greater than four, multiple pregnancy, polyhydramnios, previous uterine surgery (including caesarean section), severe toxaemia, placenta praevia or prolapse, hypertonic contractions or predisposition to amniotic fluid embolism (e.g. fetal death in utero, presence of meconium-stained amniotic fluid)

Available in combination with
- oxytocin 5 IU and ergometrine 0.5 mg (Syntometrine)

AGENTS USED IN TERMINATION OF PREGNANCY

MIFEPRISTONE
Trade name
Mifepristone Linepharma

Available form
Tablets: 200 mg

Action
- synthetic steroid with antiprogestogen activity
- antagonises progesterone effect on endometrium and myometrium
- when used in first trimester of pregnancy, enables dilation and opening of the cervix
- when combined with a prostaglandin analogue after mifepristone, there is an increase in success rate and hastens the expulsion of the fetus
- also binds to the glucocorticoid receptor
- some antiandrogenic activity

Use
- medical termination of intrauterine pregnancy (in sequential combination

PREGNANCY, CHILDBIRTH AND BREASTFEEDING

with oral prostaglandin analogue) up to 49 days of gestation

Dose
- 200 mg orally either 2 hours before or 2 hours after food, followed 36—48 hours later with oral prostaglandin analogue (e.g. misoprostol)

Adverse effects
- nausea, vomiting, diarrhoea, gastric discomfort, abdominal pain
- dizziness, headache
- vaginal bleeding, uterine spasm, prolonged post-abortion bleeding, spotting, severe haemorrhage, endometritis, heavy bleeding
- breast tenderness
- fatigue, chills, fever
- fainting
- (Uncommon) rash, pruritus, hot flush, infection, haemorrhagic shock, hypotension
- (Rare) myocardial infarction, uterine rupture, toxic shock syndrome, seizures, severe skin reaction

Interactions
- may decrease efficacy of corticosteroids (including inhaled) for 3—4 days after administration, which may require dose adjustment in those receiving long-term therapy
- increased serum levels may occur if given with itraconazole, erythromycin and grapefruit juice
- decreased serum levels may occur if given with dexamethasone, St John's wort, phenytoin, phenobarbital (phenobarbitone) or carbamazepine
- caution if used with agents with a narrow therapeutic index

Nursing considerations/Cautions
- ectopic pregnancy should be excluded and gestation age confirmed before administration
- rhesus (Rh) factor should be determined before procedure to prevent rhesus alloimmunisation
- women undergoing medical termination must be fully counselled regarding the need for combination therapy with oral prostaglandin, follow-up therapy within 14—21 days to confirm complete abortion, risk of procedure failure, bleeding, infection and effects on fertility
- not recommended in those with anaemia, kidney failure, liver impairment or failure or if malnourished
- not recommended if there is an intrauterine contraception device (IUD) in place. The IUD must be removed first
- caution if used in those with asthma using long-term corticosteroid therapy (including inhaled), as efficacy may be reduced for 3—4 days after administration
- caution if used in women with cardiovascular disease because of an increased risk of cardiovascular events
- caution if used in women ≥ 35 years who are smokers
- contraindicated if pregnancy is not confirmed on ultrasound or biological test (e.g. urine, serum human chorionic gonadotrophin (hCG))
- contraindicated if there is any uncertainty about pregnancy age or suspected ectopic pregnancy, or in those with chronic adrenal failure, severe disease requiring exogenous glucocorticoid administration, known or suspected hypocoagulation diseases, or treatment with anticoagulants or hypersensitivity to prostaglandin analogue which will be given sequentially with mifepristone, or if there is lack of access to emergency care until complete expulsion has occurred

Patient education
- patients with asthma receiving long-term corticosteroid treatment (including inhaled) should be warned that corticosteroid effectiveness may be

reduced for 3—4 days after administration of mifepristone
- the patient should be instructed to seek medical advice if any severe skin reaction such as blistering occurs
- warn the patient to avoid grapefruit juice during therapy
- advise the patient to take mifepristone either 2 hours before or 2 hours after food
- ensure the patient fully understands all of the following:
  - oral prostaglandin (misoprostol) needs to be taken 36—48 hours after mifepristone
  - in a small number of cases, the fetus is expelled before taking the prostaglandin
  - the importance of attending the follow-up appointment 14—21 days after taking mifepristone to ensure abortion is complete (even if the fetus was expelled before taking prostaglandin). This follow-up may involve clinical examination, ultrasound or beta hCG measurement
  - risk of failure (if treatment does not work, a termination can be arranged using a different method. If treatment does not work and the patient decides to continue with the pregnancy, she should be counselled regarding possible risks to the fetus and needs to be carefully monitored for the pregnancy)
  - if patient is Rh negative, the doctor will need to take extra measures to prevent Rh factor sensitisation occurring
  - vaginal bleeding usually starts 1—2 days after taking mifepristone. Bleeding may be prolonged (10—16 days) and heavy. If the patient is concerned, she should contact the doctor or clinic
  - advise the patient not to travel away from home during the time that bleeding is occurring in case there is a need to visit or contact the doctor/clinic immediately (the patient should be provided with precise instructions with whom to contact (24-hour helpline) and where to go if prolonged heavy bleeding, pain or high temperature occurs)
  - the patient should be given a letter outlining information about the procedure to allow another practitioner to deal effectively with the case if the need arises
  - the importance of seeking medical advice immediately if the patient develops any fever, abdominal pain or discomfort, pelvic tenderness, general malaise, weakness, nausea, vomiting or diarrhoea more than 24 hours after taking prostaglandin
  - counsel the patient regarding the need to avoid pregnancy in the next menstrual cycle; reliable contraceptive precautions should start as soon as possible after mifepristone administration

Tablet can be crushed and mixed with water or a spoonful of yoghurt or apple puree.

Should be avoided during breastfeeding.

Pregnant staff should not crush the tablet.

Available in combination with
- misoprostol 200 microgram and mifepristone 200 mg (MS-2 Step (combination pack))

MISOPROSTOL
Trade names
Angusta, Cytotec, GyMiso

Available forms
Tablets: 25 microgram, 200 microgram

Action
- prostaglandin E1 analogue that induces contraction of myometrial smooth muscle and relaxation of uterine cervix
- facilitates cervical opening and evacuation of intrauterine contents
- when given sequentially with mifepristone, there is an increased success rate and hastened expulsion of the fetus (GyMiso, Augusta)

Use
- medical termination of developing intrauterine pregnancy ($\leq$ 49 days gestation) (with mifepristone 200 mg) (GyMiso)
- induction of labour (Angusta)
- prevention of gastric ulcers associated with NSAIDs or postsurgical stress (see Antiulcer agents, p. 883) (Cytotec)

Dose
- (Medical termination) 800 micrograms orally 2 hours before or 2 hours after food, as single or in 2 divided doses, 36–48 hours after mifepristone. May be repeated after 1–7 days if abortion has not occurred (GyMiso)
- (Labour induction) 25 micrograms every 2 hours or 50 micrograms every 4 hours; maximum dose 200 microgram/24 hours (Angusta)

Adverse effects
- transient and mild nausea, vomiting, diarrhoea, abdominal pain, gastric discomfort
- headache, dizziness
- vaginal bleeding, uterine contraction/spasm, prolonged post-abortion bleeding, spotting, severe haemorrhage, endometritis, heavy bleeding
- fainting
- breast tenderness
- fatigue, chills, fever
- (Rare) uterine rupture, infection, septic shock
- myocardial infarction, seizures, bronchospasm

Nursing considerations/Cautions
- ectopic pregnancy should be excluded and gestation confirmed before use
- should not be given if intrauterine contraceptive device (IUD) is in place. If present, the IUD should be removed before therapy is given
- if given as a divided dose, should be given as 400 micrograms, then second 400 micrograms 2 hours later
- may be administered buccally (kept between the cheek and gum for 30 minutes and any remainder swallowed with water)
- caution if used in those women with or with risk factors for cardiovascular disease, asthma or epilepsy
- not recommended in those women with viable pregnancy who intend to carry pregnancy to term
- contraindicated in those with known or suspected hypocoagulation diseases, treatment with anticoagulants, uncertainty about pregnancy age, suspected ectopic pregnancy or any hypersensitivity to mifepristone (which is administered first) or any prostaglandin

Patient education
- advise the patient that tablets should be taken either 2 hours before or 2 hours after food. Tablets may be placed between the cheek and gum for 30 minutes and any remainder swallowed with water
- if the patient prefers, tablets can be taken as 2 doses (400 micrograms each) 2 hours apart
- see also Patient education for mifepristone (p. 1483)

Tablet can be given buccally (between the cheek and gum for 30 minutes and remaining fragments swallowed with water).

Not recommended during breastfeeding, as may cause diarrhoea in the infant.

Available in combination with
- misoprostol 200 micrograms + mifepristone 200 mg (MS-2 Step (combination pack))

LACTATION INHIBITORS

BROMOCRIPTINE MESILATE (MESYLATE)
Trade name
Parlodel

Available form
Tablets: 2.5 mg

Action
- ergot derivative with no uterotonic and little vasoconstrictor activity
- stimulates dopaminergic receptors
- inhibits release of prolactin
- increases release of growth hormone for several hours after administration
- decreases size and growth of prolactin-secreting pituitary tumours (prolactinomas)

Use
- preventing onset of lactation (for clearly defined medical reasons, as routine use of dopaminergic agents for lactation suppression is not recommended)
- hyperprolactinaemia (where surgery/radiotherapy are ineffective or inappropriate)
- prolactinoma (conservative treatment before surgery to reduce size, and post-surgery if prolactin levels remain high)
- adjunctive therapy in acromegaly, Parkinson's disease (see Anti-Parkinson's agents, p. 802)

Dose
- (Inhibition of physiological lactation) 2.5 mg orally twice daily with food for 14 days (starting more than 4 hours after delivery) **OR**
- (Hyperprolactinaemia) initially 1.25 mg orally 2–3 times daily with food, increasing to 2.5 mg 2–3 times daily if needed **OR**
- (Prolactinoma) initially 1.25 mg orally twice daily with food, gradually increasing doses up to 15 mg daily in divided doses if needed to reduce prolactin levels

Adverse effects
- nausea, vomiting, constipation
- dizziness, headache (transient), somnolence
- postural hypotension, syncope
- nasal congestion
- (Uncommon) confusion, hallucinations, dyskinesias
- (Rare) gastrointestinal bleeding and ulceration, diabetic retinopathy, psychiatric disturbances, blurred vision, visual disturbances, impulse control disorders
- (Long-term, high dose) retroperitoneal fibrosis, pleural/pericardial effusions, pleural/pulmonary fibrosis
- (Very rare) sudden sleep onset, neuroleptic malignant syndrome (abrupt withdrawal), reversible pallor of toes/fingers on exposure to cold

Interactions
- tolerability may be decreased by alcohol
- hypotensive effect may be enhanced by antihypertensive agents
- increased plasma levels may result if given with erythromycin, octreotide or macrolide antibiotics
- effects may be antagonised by phenothiazines, butyrophenones, metoclopramide, methyldopa sesquihydrate, tricyclic antidepressants (TCAs), domperidone, oestrogens or thyrotropin-releasing factor
- effects may be increased if given with levodopa or clonidine
- increased risk of headache, nausea and vomiting if given with ergometrine

PREGNANCY, CHILDBIRTH AND BREASTFEEDING

- increased risk of hypertension and severe headache if given with sympathomimetic agents
- increased risk of vasospastic reaction if given with sumatriptan

Nursing considerations/Cautions

- hypoprolactinaemia should be thoroughly investigated before starting therapy to ensure cause is not severe hypothyroidism
- BP should be monitored during first week of therapy (hypotension is most common in first weeks of therapy) and then supine and standing BP checked regularly for postural hypotension
- gastric irritation is reduced if bromocriptine is taken with or immediately after food
- dosage increases are made gradually, usually over several days, to reduce the incidence of adverse effects
- (Prolactin-secreting adenomas) visual fields should be monitored throughout therapy
- (Prolactinoma) dosage is sufficient when serum prolactin level falls and tumour reduces in size
- when used for inhibiting physiological lactation, bromocriptine should not be used within 4 hours of delivery and only after vital signs have stabilised (especially BP). Therapy should be continued for 14 days to prevent rebound lactation. If secretion recurs, therapy may be restarted for another week at the same dose
- when given for hyperprolactinaemia associated with galactorrhoea or amenorrhoea, treatment is continued until breast secretions have ceased or the menstrual cycle has recommenced. May be continued over several menstrual cycles to prevent relapse if needed
- when given for hyperprolactinaemia, return of ovulation postpartum may be hastened; therefore adequate contraceptive methods should be used if pregnancy is not wanted
- (Long-term therapy) female patients should have regular gynaecological examination and all patients should have a regular chest X-ray (to monitor for pulmonary fibrosis)
- caution if used in those with suspected/known peptic ulceration, impaired liver function, diabetes mellitus or Raynaud's phenomenon
- not recommended in those with galactose intolerance, severe lactase deficiency or glucose–galactose malabsorption
- contraindicated in those with sensitivity to ergot alkaloids, uncontrolled hypertension, toxaemia, hypertensive disorders associated with pregnancy (including postpartum), coronary artery disease, severe cardiovascular conditions or serious psychiatric disorders (or history)

Patient education

- warn the patient that alcohol should be avoided during therapy
- advise the patient to take initial doses at bedtime, to reduce the incidence of hypotension and loss of consciousness
- warn the patient against driving a vehicle or operating machinery if drowsy, dizzy or experiencing daytime somnolence
- advise the patient to avoid postural hypotension by moving gradually to a sitting or standing position, especially after sleep; otherwise lightheadedness and fainting may occur
- the patient should be warned that milk secretion may recur 2–3 days after stopping treatment, which may necessitate restarting treatment at the same dosage for a further 7 days
- the patient should be advised to seek medical advice immediately if any of the following occur:
  - any shortness of breath, persistent cough or chest pain (signs of pulmonary fibrosis)
  - loin/flank pain, lower limb swelling or abdominal tenderness (signs of retroperitoneal fibrosis)

- family/carers should be asked to observe for any sudden sleep onset, as patients are often unaware that this occurs and it may be dangerous if the person drives or operates machinery
- women of childbearing years not wishing to become pregnant should be advised to use adequate contraception during therapy
- pregnancy must be avoided if a significant or expanding pituitary adenoma is diagnosed, and therefore woman should be counselled regarding the use of adequate contraception

Tablet can be dispersed in water, or crushed and mixed with a spoonful of yoghurt or apple puree.

Therapy should be discontinued if pregnancy occurs, unless there is a medical reason to continue. Close monitoring throughout pregnancy is recommended, especially for any signs such as headache or visual field deterioration.

Not recommended during breastfeeding (if mother wishes to breastfeed).

CABERGOLINE
Trade names
Cabaser, Dostamine, Dostinex

Available forms
Tablets: 500 microgram, 1 mg, 2 mg

Action
- ergot derivative that stimulates D_2 dopamine receptors, inhibiting prolactin secretion
- central dopaminergic effect

Use
- Parkinson's disease (Cabaser) (see Anti-Parkinson's agents, p. 804)
- inhibiting physiological lactation (for clearly defined medical reasons, as routine use of dopaminergic agents for lactation suppression is not recommended) (Dostamine, Dostinex)
- hyperprolactinaemia (Dostamine, Dostinex)

Dose
- (Preventing onset of physiological lactation) 1 mg orally with food as a once-only dose first day after delivery **OR**
- (Hyperprolactinaemia) initially 0.25 mg orally with food twice weekly (e.g. Monday and Thursday), increasing gradually by 0.5 mg weekly at 1-month intervals until a therapeutic response is achieved

Adverse effects
- nausea, vomiting, abdominal pain, constipation, dyspepsia, epigastric pain
- headache, dizziness, vertigo
- depression, somnolence, fatigue, asthenia
- paraesthesia
- breast pain
- hot flushes
- hypotension
- (Rare) pleural/pulmonary fibrosis, pleural effusions, palpitations, transient hemianopia, leg cramps, digital vasospasm, impulse control disorder, sudden sleep disorder, hypotension

Interactions
- not recommended with other ergometrine
- not recommended with agents that antagonise dopamine receptors (e.g. metoclopramide, phenothiazines, butyrophenones, thioxanthines)
- not recommended with macrolide antibacterial agents (e.g. erythromycin), as bioavailability may be increased

Nursing considerations/Cautions
- (Hyperprolactinaemia) before starting therapy, the patient should have a cardiovascular assessment (including ECG/echocardiogram), ESR, lung function test, chest X-ray and renal function
- (Hyperprolactinaemia) ECG/echocardiogram should be monitored within

- 3–6 months of starting therapy, then 6–12-monthly
- (Hyperprolactinaemia) chest X-ray and ESR are recommended if the patient develops any pulmonary symptoms
- (Hyperprolactinaemia) evaluation of pituitary function is recommended before starting therapy
- (Hyperprolactinaemia) serum prolactin levels should be measured monthly
- BP should be monitored regularly
- administration with food may lessen GI disturbances
- weekly doses may be given as single or divided doses, although doses over 1 mg/week should be divided to decrease GI disturbances
- caution if used in those with cardiovascular disease, Raynaud's syndrome, liver/renal disease, peptic ulcer, GI bleeding, pre-eclampsia, postpartum hypertension or psychiatric disorders
- contraindicated in those with a history of pulmonary, pericardial or retroperitoneal fibrotic disease, anatomical evidence of cardiac valvulopathy or hypersensitivity to other ergot alkaloids

Patient education

- advise the patient that adverse effects usually disappear with continued therapy
- the patient should be advised not to drive or operate machinery during the first days of therapy, or if vertigo, dizziness or somnolence are ongoing problems
- (Inhibition/suppression of lactation) if the patient experiences chest pain, or severe headache that is progressive and/or unremitting (especially with visual disturbance), medical treatment should be sought immediately
- the patient should be advised to immediately report:
  - any shortness of breath, persistent cough or chest pain (signs of pulmonary fibrosis)
  - loin/flank pain, lower limb swelling or abdominal tenderness (signs of retroperitoneal fibrosis)
- family/carers should be asked to observe for any:
  - sudden sleep onset, as patients are often unaware that this occurs and it may be dangerous if the person drives or operates machinery, or
  - persistent/recurring gambling, increased libido, hypersexuality, binge eating, compulsive buying or spending, or repetitive behaviours with no purpose (punding)
- women of childbearing years not wishing to become pregnant should be advised to use adequate contraception during therapy

 Tablet can be crushed and mixed with water or a spoonful of yoghurt or apple puree.

 Pregnancy should be excluded before starting and for 1 month after stopping therapy. A pregnancy test is recommended every 4 weeks or if the menstrual period is overdue by more than 3 days.

 Not recommended during breastfeeding (if mother wishes to breastfeed).

 Pregnant staff should not disperse or crush tablets.

PULMONARY HYPERTENSION AGENTS

Pulmonary hypertension is defined as being an elevated pulmonary arterial pressure (> 22 mmHg) or an estimated systolic pulmonary arterial pressure > 36 mmHg (Waxman & Loscalzo 2019). In the past, those with pulmonary hypertension often died owing to misdiagnosis and/or lack of appropriate management.

Early symptoms are non-specific (dyspnoea, fatigue); advanced symptoms include oedema, chest pain, pre-syncope and syncope. Diagnosis is based on clinical symptoms and tests such as echocardiogram, lung function tests and chest imaging (e.g. chest X-ray, CT and CT angiogram) (Waxman & Loscalzo 2019).

While medical treatments have improved the quality of life and survival rates for patients with pulmonary hypertension, there is currently no cure (Waxman & Loscalzo 2019). The agents discussed in this section are used in the management of pulmonary arterial hypertension (PAH) and include prostacyclin analogues (epoprostenol, iloprost), prostacyclin agonist (selexipag), endothelin receptor antagonists (ambrisentan, bosentan and macitentan) and phosphodiesterase-5 (PDE5) inhibitors (sildenafil and tadalafil; see Erectile dysfunction agents, p. 1120) (Waxman & Loscalzo 2019).

AMBRISENTAN
Trade names
Ambrisentan Viatris, Cipla Ambrisentan, Pulmoris, Volibris

Available forms
Tablets: 5 mg, 10 mg

Action
- endothelin receptor (type A) antagonist that inhibits the potent vasoconstrictor endothelin-1, which is increased in those with pulmonary arterial hypertension
- half-life 13.6–16.5 hours

Use
- familial pulmonary arterial hypertension (PAH), PAH associated with connective tissue disease or in patients with functional WHO Class II, III or IV symptoms

Dose
- initially 5 mg orally daily, increasing to 10 mg if needed

Adverse effects
- hypotension, peripheral oedema, fluid retention, heart failure, palpitations, chest pain
- headache, dizziness, fatigue

PULMONARY HYPERTENSION AGENTS

- nasal congestion, sinusitis, nasopharyngitis, epistaxis
- dyspnoea, cough, bronchitis
- elevated liver enzymes, hepatitis
- flushing
- anaemia
- constipation, abdominal pain, nausea
- (Rare) rash, hypersensitivity

Interactions

- caution if given with other hepatotoxic agents
- caution if given with ciclosporin. If given together, dose of ambrisentan should be limited to 5 mg daily
- increased risk of anaemia if given with tadalafil
- transient increase in serum levels may occur if given with rifampicin

Nursing considerations/Cautions

- liver function tests (serum liver enzymes and bilirubin) should be measured before starting and then monthly during therapy
- haemoglobin should be measured before starting therapy, after 1 month and then regularly
- BP should be monitored during therapy (especially in those with pre-existing hypotension)
- patient should be monitored for any signs of fluid retention and pulmonary oedema (especially if patient has severe systolic dysfunction in addition to PAH)
- pregnancy must be excluded before starting therapy
- caution if used in those with pre-existing hypotension or kidney impairment (especially if severe)
- caution if used in those with right heart failure, pre-existing liver disease, previous medication-induced elevation of liver enzymes or currently taking medications which may elevate liver enzymes
- not recommended in those with functional Class I symptoms
- contraindicated in those with severe liver impairment (with or without cirrhosis), elevated liver enzymes (3 times above normal) or idiopathic pulmonary fibrosis (with or without pulmonary hypertension)

Patient education

- patient should be advised to seek medical advice immediately if any of the following occur:
  - loss of appetite, nausea, upper abdominal pain, unusual tiredness, yellowing of eyes or skin, dark urine or pale stools
  - tiredness, weakness, shortness of breath, feeling unwell
  - swollen ankles or legs
- warn patient not to drive or operate heavy machinery if dizziness or fatigue occur
- women of childbearing potential should be counselled regarding the high risk of birth defects if conception occurs while taking therapy and be willing to perform monthly pregnancy tests and use two forms of reliable contraception if sexually active (oral contraceptive may not be reliable). Pregnancy must be avoided for 3 months after stopping therapy

 Disperse the tablet in water (administer within 3 minutes) OR tablet can be crushed and mixed with water or spoonful of yoghurt or apple puree.

 Contraindicated during pregnancy. Monthly pregnancy tests are recommended. Pregnancy must be avoided for 3 months after stopping therapy.

 Not recommended during breastfeeding.

 Teratogen. Pregnant staff must not crush or disperse tablets.

BOSENTAN
Trade names
Bosentan, APO, Bosentan Dr. Reddy's, Bosentan GH, Bosentan RBX, Bosentan Viatris

Available forms
Tablets: 62.5 mg, 125 mg

Action
- endothelin antagonist
- inhibits the potent vasoconstrictor endothelin-1 (ET-1), which is increased in those with pulmonary arterial hypertension
- slightly higher affinity for ETA receptors than for ETB

Use
- idiopathic or familial pulmonary arterial hypertension (PAH), PAH associated with connective tissue disease or in patients with functional WHO Class II, III or IV symptoms, PAH associated with congenital systematic to pulmonary shunt (including Eisenmenger's physiology)

Dose
- (Adult, child > 40 kg): start with 62.5 mg orally twice daily for the first 4 weeks. After 4 weeks, increase to 125 mg twice daily for maintenance
- children (based on weight):
    - 10—20 kg: start with 31.25 mg once daily. Increase to 31.25 mg twice daily after 4 weeks
    - > 20—40 kg: start with 31.25 mg twice daily. Increase to 62.5 mg twice daily after 4 weeks

Adverse effects
- joint swelling, arthralgia
- fever
- flushing, headache
- elevated liver enzymes and bilirubin
- anaemia
- peripheral oedema, fluid retention
- palpitations, chest pain, syncope, hypotension
- upper and lower respiratory tract infections, nasopharyngitis, sinusitis, nasal congestion, rhinitis, epistaxis
- pruritus, rash
- diarrhoea
- (Uncommon) thrombocytopenia
- (Rare) liver cirrhosis, liver failure

Interactions
- contraindicated with ciclosporin and glibenclamide
- not recommended with epoprostenol, fluconazole, itraconazole, voriconazole or ritonavir
- caution if given with other hepatotoxic agents including antiretroviral agents
- caution if given with tacrolimus or sirolimus
- increased serum levels may occur if given with itraconazole, voriconazole, ritonavir, sildenafil or rifampicin
- may decrease serum levels of digoxin, nimodipine, sildenafil, tacrolimus, sirolimus and simvastatin (and its active metabolite)
- may decrease efficacy of hormonal contraceptives (oral, injectable, transdermal, implantable)
- increased INR monitoring is recommended if given with warfarin
- caution if used with enzyme inducers: carbamazepine, phenobarbital (phenobarbitone), phenytoin and St John's wort

Nursing considerations/Cautions
- liver function tests (serum liver enzymes and bilirubin) should be measured before starting and then monthly during therapy
- haemoglobin should be measured after 1 and 3 months and then 3-monthly
- patient should be monitored for any signs of fluid retention (especially if patient has severe systolic dysfunction in addition to PAH)
- oxygen saturation monitoring is recommended in those with coronary heart disease
- discontinuation should be gradual over 3—7 days at a reduced dose
- caution if used in those with pre-existing anaemia or hypotension or with mild liver impairment
- contraindicated in those with moderate-to-severe liver impairment

Patient education
- patient should be advised to seek medical advice immediately if any of the following occur:

PULMONARY HYPERTENSION AGENTS

- nausea, vomiting, fever, lethargy, fatigue, abdominal pain, dark urine, pale stools (bowel motions) or yellowing of eyes or skin
- swelling of ankles or legs
- advise patient not to stop therapy abruptly
- women of childbearing potential should be counselled regarding the high risk of birth defects if conception occurs while taking bosentan and be willing to perform monthly pregnancy tests and use two reliable types of contraception if sexually active (oral contraceptive may not be reliable). Pregnancy must be avoided for 3 months after stopping therapy

Tablets can be crushed and mixed with water, yogurt, or apple puree. Compounding pharmacies can prepare a suspension from crushed tablets.

Contraindicated during pregnancy. Monthly pregnancy tests are recommended. Pregnancy must be avoided for 3 months after stopping therapy.

No clinical data. Not recommended during breastfeeding.

Contraindicated in moderate-to-severe liver impairment.

Pregnant staff must not crush or disperse tablets.

EPOPROSTENOL

Trade name
Veletri

Available forms
Vial: 500 microgram, 1.5 mg

Action
- prostacyclin
- direct vasodilation of pulmonary and systemic arterial vascular beds
- inhibits platelet aggregation
- elimination half-life less than 6 minutes

Use
- idiopathic or familial pulmonary arterial hypertension (PAH) (WHO functional Class III or IV) or PAH associated with connective tissue disease

Dose
- (Short-term (acute) dose, used to determine long-term infusion rate) initially 2 nanogram/kg/min by IV infusion, increasing by 2 nanogram/kg/min at 15-minute intervals until dose-limiting effects or maximum haemodynamic benefit is reached **OR**
- (Long term) initially 4 nanogram/kg/min less than the maximum dose achieved with acute dose. If acute dose was less than 5 nanogram/kg/min, then dose should be started at 1 nanogram/kg/min

Adverse effects
- general effects: flushing, headache, dizziness, fatigue, fever
- gastrointestinal: anorexia, nausea, vomiting, abdominal pain, diarrhoea
- cardiovascular: hypotension, bradycardia, tachycardia, syncope
- neurological/psychological: anxiety, nervousness, agitation, hypoaesthesia, paraesthesia
- musculoskeletal: arthralgia, myalgia, jaw pain, back pain, neck pain
- respiratory: dyspnoea
- dermatological: skin ulcer, rash, pruritus
- injection site reactions: pain, local reaction

Interactions
- may increase vasodilatory effects if given with other vasodilators
- may decrease the clearance of digoxin, leading to increased serum levels and a higher risk of toxicity, particularly in the early weeks of therapy

HAVARD'S NURSING GUIDE TO DRUGS

- may reduce the efficacy of tissue plasminogen activator by increasing its clearance
- increased risk of bleeding when used with NSAIDs or antiplatelet agents

Nursing considerations/Cautions

- for short-term dose-ranging procedures, administer via peripheral or central venous access in a controlled hospital environment
- reconstitute using sodium chloride 0.9% or water for injections
- ensure the IV administration set includes a 0.20–0.22 micron filter. Administer epoprostenol alone to prevent interactions
- avoid extravasation, as it may cause tissue damage. This is important to prevent local injury
- continuously monitor BP (supine and erect) and heart rate, especially when altering the infusion rate. Observe for signs of pulmonary oedema. If severe hypotension, sudden bradycardia, nausea, sweating or hypotension occur, reduce or stop the infusion
- cardiovascular effects generally disappear within 30 minutes of stopping the infusion. If severe hypotension occurs, adjust the infusion rate accordingly to manage potential overdose symptoms
- avoid abrupt cessation of chronic infusion, as it may cause rapid clinical deterioration, which can be potentially fatal. Sudden large reductions in infusion rate should also be avoided. Maintaining infusion continuity is vital for patient stability
- (Long term therapy) any dose adjustment should be based on recurrence or worsening or symptoms, or occurrence of adverse effects
- if no response is seen after 12 weeks, consider alternative treatment options
- anticoagulant therapy may be considered to reduce the risk of pulmonary thromboembolism or systemic embolism
- ensure proper training for handling and administering continuous IV infusions. Use appropriate equipment for haemodynamic monitoring and emergency care, especially for acute dose-ranging procedures in a hospital setting
- contraindicated in patients with congestive heart failure due to severe left ventricular dysfunction or those who develop pulmonary oedema during therapy. This is critical to prevent life-threatening complications

Patient education

- warn the patient not to stop therapy suddenly. Sudden discontinuation can lead to rapid clinical deterioration, dizziness, weakness and difficulty breathing. This is critical to prevent potentially life-threatening complications
- instruct patient to seek medical advice immediately if any of the following occur: This helps ensure timely intervention if serious side effects develop:
  - shortness of breath
  - jaw, muscle, or back pain
  - sweating, chest pain, or tightness
  - tingling or numbness in feet or hands
  - headaches, dizziness (especially on standing)
  - fever, fatigue
  - facial flushing
  - chills or flu-like symptoms
  - change in skin sensitivity (e.g. more sensitive, less sensitive)
  - redness or pain at the infusion site
- the patient should be advised not to drive or operate machinery if adverse effects occur

PULMONARY HYPERTENSION AGENTS

Should be used during pregnancy only if the potential benefits to the mother outweigh the possible risks to the fetus.

It is not known whether epoprostenol is excreted in human milk. A decision to continue breastfeeding or epoprostenol therapy should weigh the benefits to the child and the mother. A risk to the breastfeeding child cannot be excluded.

ILOPROST
Trade name
Ventavis

Available form
Nebuliser solution: 10 microgram/mL

Action
* synthetic prostaglandin analogue
* direct vasodilation of pulmonary arterial bed, improving pulmonary artery pressure, pulmonary vascular resistance and cardiac output
* duration 1–2 hours, biphasic half-life (3–5 minutes, 15–30 minutes)

Use
* moderate-to-severe idiopathic pulmonary hypertension (PH), PH secondary to drugs or connective tissue disease
* chronic pulmonary thromboembolism (where surgery is not possible)

Dose
* adults and children > 8 years: initially 2.5 microgram via nebulisation over 4–10 minutes 6–9 times daily, increasing to 5.0 microgram if needed and tolerated

Adverse effects
* vasodilation, hypotension, syncope, dizziness, tachycardia, palpitations
* cough, dyspnoea
* pharyngolaryngeal pain
* epistaxis, haemoptysis, bleeding
* headache, dizziness
* trismus/jaw pain, back pain, chest pain
* peripheral oedema
* rash
* nausea, vomiting, diarrhoea, irritation of mouth/tongue/throat
* (Rare) bronchospasm

Interactions
* may increase antihypertensive or vasodilatory effects of vasodilators or antihypertensive agents
* increased risk of bleeding if given with anticoagulants, antiplatelet agents, nitrates (such as glyceryl trinitrate), phosphodiesterase (PDE-5) inhibitors (e.g. sildenafil), aspirin or NSAIDs

Nursing considerations/Cautions
* administered via a nebuliser
* avoid sudden discontinuation as it can lead to rapid clinical deterioration. Patients should be monitored for rebound effects if therapy is interrupted or stopped
* when starting therapy, vital signs should be closely monitored to assess the patient's response and adjust treatment as needed
* use with caution in liver or kidney dysfunction. Not recommended for patients under 18 years, those with unstable pulmonary hypertension and advanced right heart failure, or with hypotension (systolic BP < 85 mmHg)
* close monitoring for any bronchial hyperreactivity is recommended if the patient has a concurrent lung infection, severe asthma or chronic obstructive pulmonary disease
* prevent contact with skin and eyes to avoid irritation or adverse effects
* contraindicated in those with an increased risk of haemorrhage (e.g. active peptic ulcer), unstable angina, myocardial infarction within the past 6 months, severe cardiac failure (not managed), severe arrhythmias, pulmonary congestion, stroke or transient ischaemic attack (TIA) within the past 3 months, pulmonary hypertension

due to venous occlusive disease, and congenital/acquired valvular defects with myocardial function disorder not related to pulmonary hypertension

Patient education
- avoid contact with eyes and skin; do not take orally
- use the nebuliser with a mouthpiece only, not a face mask (which would increase contact with eyes and skin)
- discard any unused solution after nebulisation
- if prone to syncope, avoid strain; take the first dose in bed if needed
- avoid driving or operating machinery if dizziness or fainting occurs

Not recommended during pregnancy.

Not recommended during breastfeeding because of the lack of human safety data.

Patients with hepatic dysfunction or renal failure (requiring dialysis) may have reduced elimination of iloprost, suggesting a possible need for dose reduction. It is recommended to use cautious initial dose titration with 3—4-hour dosing intervals.

MACITENTAN
Trade name
Opsumit

Available form
Tablets: 10 mg

Action
- endothelin (ET)-1 and its receptors (ETA, ETB) trigger vasoconstriction, fibrosis, proliferation, hypertrophy and inflammation. In pulmonary arterial hypertension, ET is upregulated and is involved in vascular hypertrophy and organ damage
- endothelin receptor (ETA, ETB) antagonist that binds to ET receptors in human pulmonary arterial smooth muscle cells and prefers penetration into lung tissue (particularly if diseased)
- maximum plasma concentration is reached in about 8 hours after administration
- active metabolite
- half-life about 18 hours (48 hours for metabolite)

Use
- idiopathic and heritable pulmonary arterial hypertension (PAH), PAH associated with connective tissue disease, or in patients with PAH associated with congenital heart disease with repaired shunt, with functional WHO Class II, III or IV symptoms (monotherapy or with phosphodiesterase-5 inhibitors or inhaled prostanoids)

Dose
- adult, child > 12 years and > 40 kg, oral 10 mg orally once daily

Adverse effects
- anaemia, thrombocytopenia
- hypotension
- headache, insomnia, depression
- pruritus, urticaria, flushing, skin ulceration
- bronchitis, nasopharyngitis, pharyngitis, influenza, nasal congestion, upper respiratory tract infection, rhinitis
- arthralgia, myalgia
- peripheral oedema, fluid retention
- diarrhoea, abdominal pain, gastroenteritis
- increased liver enzymes, hypokalaemia
- fever

Interactions
- caution if given with other hepatotoxic agents
- increased serum levels may occur if given with itraconazole, voriconazole, clarithromycin or ritonavir
- serum levels may be decreased if given with rifampicin, St John's wort, carbamazepine or phenytoin

PULMONARY HYPERTENSION AGENTS

Nursing considerations/Cautions

- liver function tests and full blood count (FBC) are recommended before starting and monthly during therapy
- BP and haemoglobin monitoring are recommended in those with kidney impairment or pre-existing hypotension because of the increased risk of anaemia and hypotension
- pregnancy must be excluded before starting therapy
- caution if used in those with pre-existing hypotension
- not recommended in those with significant anaemia, on dialysis or with severe kidney impairment
- not recommended in those under 12 years
- contraindicated in those with severe liver impairment (with or without cirrhosis) or clinically significant elevated liver aminotransferases (> than 3 times upper limit of normal)

Patient education

- instruct the patient to seek medical advice immediately if any if the following occur:
  - nausea, vomiting, fever, abdominal pain, yellowing eyes or skin, itching skin, dark urine, tiredness, exhaustion
  - flu-like syndrome, including chills, fever, joint and muscle pain
  - weight gain, swelling of feet or legs
- women of childbearing potential should be counselled regarding the high risk of birth defects if conception occurs during therapy, be willing to perform monthly pregnancy tests and use two reliable types of contraception if sexually active (oral contraceptives may not be reliable). Pregnancy must be avoided for 3 months after stopping therapy

 Tablet can be crushed and mixed with water or a spoonful of yoghurt or apple puree.

 Contraindicated during pregnancy. Monthly pregnancy tests are recommended. Pregnancy must be avoided for 3 months after stopping therapy.

 Not recommended during breastfeeding.

 Severe renal impairment: use with caution, as renal impairment may increase the risk of adverse reactions, particularly fluid retention.

Reduced hepatic function: perform liver function tests and an FBC before starting therapy and then monthly during treatment. Macitentan is contraindicated in patients with severe liver impairment or if liver enzyme levels are more than three times the normal limit.

 Pregnant staff must not crush or disperse tablets.

Available in combination with
- macitentan 10 mg + tadalafil 40 mg tablets (Opsynvi 10/40)

RIOCIGUAT
Trade name
Adempas

Available forms
Tablet: 0.5 mg, 1 mg, 1.5 mg, 2 mg, 2.5 mg

Action
- stimulates soluble guanylate cyclase (sGC) (enzyme found in most tissue and receptor for nitric oxide (NO)). When sGC binds to NO, cyclic guanosine monophosphate (cGMP) is synthesised. cGMP regulates processes that influence vascular tone, proliferation, fibrosis and inflammation
- pulmonary hypertension is associated with endothelial dysfunction, impaired NO synthesis and insufficient NO-sGC-cGMP pathway stimulation
- active metabolite
- half-life 7 hours (healthy patients) and 13 hours (patients with PAH)

Use
- idiopathic or heritable pulmonary arterial hypertension (PAH), PAH associated with connective tissue diseases, PAH associated with congenital heart disease in adults with WHO functional class II, III or IV symptoms
- chronic thromboembolic pulmonary hypertension (CTEPH) after surgical treatment, or inoperable CTEPH

Dose
- initially 1 mg orally 3 times daily (doses 6—8 hours apart) for 2 weeks, increasing at 2-week intervals by 0.5 mg increments (maximum 2.5 mg 3 times daily if patient has no signs or symptoms of hypotension and systolic BP ≥ 95 mmHg)

Adverse effects
- hypotension, palpitations, chest pain or discomfort
- headache, dizziness, fatigue
- dyspepsia, nausea, diarrhoea, vomiting gastro-oesophageal reflux disease (GORD), abdominal pain, constipation, gastritis, abdominal distension
- peripheral oedema
- nasopharyngitis, dyspnoea, cough, nasal congestion, epistaxis, haemoptysis
- anaemia
- pain in extremity
- (Uncommon) pulmonary oedema, pulmonary haemorrhage

Interactions
- contraindicated with nitrates or nitric oxide donor
- contraindicated with avanafil, sildenafil, tadalafil, dipyridamole or theophylline
- increased risk of respiratory tract bleeding if patient is taking anticoagulants
- not recommended with azole antifungal agents (e.g. itraconazole) or HIV protease inhibitors (e.g. ritonavir)
- caution if used with ciclosporin, erlotinib and gefitinib
- plasma levels are reduced by smoking
- plasma levels may be reduced if given with antacids, phenytoin, carbamazepine, phenobarbital (phenobarbitone) or St John's wort

Nursing considerations/Cautions
- therapy should be initiated in hospital setting with equipment for haemodynamic monitoring and emergency care readily available
- BP should be measured before starting therapy
- pregnancy should be ruled out before starting therapy
- if patient is thought not to be able to tolerate hypotensive action, dose should be started at 0.5 mg 3 times daily
- during titration:
  - if systolic BP ≥ 95 mmHg and patient has signs and symptoms of hypotension, dose should be reduced by 0.5 mg 3 times daily
  - if systolic BP < 95 mmHg and patient has no signs or symptoms of hypotension, dose should be maintained
  - if systolic BP < 95 mmHg and patient has signs and symptoms of hypotension, dose should be reduced by 0.5 mg 3 times daily
- if patient develops signs and symptoms of hypotension at any time during therapy, dose should be reduced by 0.5 mg 3 times daily
- if therapy is interrupted for 3 or more days, treatment should be restarted at 1 mg 3 times daily for 2 weeks, and titration continued as previously
- if patient was previously taking sildenafil, it should be stopped for at least 24 hours before starting riociguat and patient closely monitored for any signs of hypotension
- if patient was previously taking tadalafil, it should be stopped for at least 48 hours before starting riociguat and patient closely monitored for any signs of hypotension
- if patient is transitioning from riociguat to sildenafil or tadalafil, riociguat should

PULMONARY HYPERTENSION AGENTS

be stopped for at least 24 hours before starting sildenafil or tadalafil, and patient closely monitored for any signs of hypotension
- caution if used in those ≥ 65 years; increased risk of hypotension; start with the lowest dose and monitor BP, especially during dose titration
- not recommended in patients who have had recent episodes of serious haemoptysis or bronchial arterial embolisation owing to increased risk of respiratory tract bleeding
- contraindicated in those with pulmonary hypertension associated with idiopathic interstitial pneumonias

Patient education

- advise patient against driving or operating heavy machinery if dizziness, palpitations or hypotension occurs
- patient should be advised to stop smoking. However, if they do not, patient should be advised to let doctor know if there is any change to smoking habit as this will affect blood levels of riociguat
- if patient requires antacid, recommend that it is taken at least 1 hour after riociguat
- instruct patient to seek medical advice immediately if any of the following occur:
  - shortness of breath with activity or lying down, cough, pink frothy sputum, anxiety or sense of apprehension, feeling of drowning when lying down
- women of childbearing potential should be counselled regarding the high risk of birth defects if conception occurs during therapy, be willing to perform monthly pregnancy tests and use two reliable types of contraception if sexually active (oral contraceptives may not be reliable). Pregnancy must be avoided for 4 weeks after stopping therapy

Tablet can be crushed and mixed with water, yogurt, or apple puree.

Pregnant staff should not crush or disperse tablets.

Contraindicated during pregnancy. Monthly pregnancy tests are recommended. Pregnancy must be avoided for 4 weeks after stopping therapy.

Contraindicated during breastfeeding.

Caution if used in those with mild-to-moderate kidney impairment. If used, kidney function should be monitored regularly during therapy. Not recommended in those with severe liver or kidney impairment.

SELEXIPAG

Trade name
Uptravi

Available forms
Tablet: 200 microgram, 400 microgram, 600 microgram, 800 microgram, 1000 microgram, 1200 microgram, 1400 microgram, 1600 microgram

Actions
- selective prostacyclin receptor agonist
- it is a prodrug and is converted to the active form, ACT-333679, by hydrolysis
- it is not an analogue of prostacyclin. It has a different chemical structure and is classified as a non-prostanoid
- targets the same prostacyclin receptors but does so through a structurally different molecule
- has high selectivity for the prostacyclin receptor, which leads to vasodilation of the pulmonary arterial bed. By mimicking the effects of prostacyclin, selexipag reduces pulmonary vascular resistance, inhibits platelet aggregation, and exerts antiproliferative, anti-inflammatory and antithrombotic effects

- these actions collectively improve haemodynamics (blood flow) and exercise capacity in patients with pulmonary arterial hypertension

Use
- treatment of pulmonary arterial hypertension to delay disease progression and improve exercise capacity

Dose
- (Adults) start with 200 microgram twice daily. Based on response and tolerability, increase by 200 microgram twice daily at weekly intervals up to a maximum of 1600 microgram twice daily **OR**
- (Moderate hepatic impairment or use with moderate CYP2C8 inhibitors (e.g. clopidogrel)) start with 200 microgram once daily. Increase by 200 microgram daily at weekly intervals, up to 1600 microgram once daily

Adverse effects
- headache, flushing, dizziness, hypotension, tachycardia
- jaw pain, nausea, vomiting, diarrhoea, abdominal pain
- myalgia, anaemia, hyperthyroidism, eye pain

Interactions
- CYP2C8 inhibitors (e.g. gemfibrozil): co-administration with CYP2C8 inhibitors leads to a two-fold increase in selexipag exposure and an 11-fold increase in its active metabolite. Strong CYP2C8 inhibitors (like gemfibrozil) are contraindicated owing to the risk of significantly increased drug levels and potential toxicity
- moderate CYP2C8 inhibitors (e.g. clopidogrel, deferasirox, teriflunomide): increased exposure to the active metabolite; dosing of selexipag should be reduced to once daily during co-administration (i.e. halving the total daily dose). Note: while clopidogrel is typically considered a strong CYP2C8 inhibitor, the manufacturer treats it as a moderate inhibitor in this context
- UGT1A3 and UGT2B7 inhibitors (valproic acid): caution is recommended owing to potential increased exposure
- lopinavir/ritonavir: increases exposure to selexipag but not its active metabolite
- rifampicin: no change in selexipag exposure, but reduced active metabolite exposure
- co-administration with diuretics, antihypertensive agents, or other vasodilators may cause reductions in BP; careful monitoring is required

Nursing considerations/Cautions
- (Titration) a slower dose titration may minimise adverse effects, particularly in patients with severe renal impairment. If treatment is interrupted for 3 days or more, restart at a lower dose and re-titrate
- prostacyclins inhibit platelet aggregation, which may increase the risk of bleeding. Selexipag is an inhibitor of platelet aggregation in vitro. Monitor patients closely, particularly if they take other medicines that increase bleeding risk, such as anticoagulants
- contraindicated in patients with pulmonary veno-occlusive disease (PVOD), severe hepatic impairment (Child—Pugh class C), severe coronary heart disease or unstable angina, recent myocardial infarction (within the last 6 months), decompensated cardiac failure if not closely supervised, severe arrhythmias, recent cerebrovascular events, such as a transient ischaemic attack or stroke (within the last 3 months), significant congenital or acquired valvular defects with myocardial function disorders unrelated to pulmonary hypertension, concurrent use of potent CYP2C8 inhibitors (e.g. gemfibrozil)

PULMONARY HYPERTENSION AGENTS

Patient education

- when starting this medicine or when the dose is increased, take the first dose in the evening
- should be taken consistently with or without food, but they are better tolerated with food

 Tablets should be swallowed whole and not crushed or chewed.

 Not recommended during pregnancy.

 Breastfeeding is not recommended.

 Renal: titrate dose cautiously if eGFR < 30 mL/min/1.73 m^2; no clinical data or experience in patients with eGFR less than 15 mL/min/1.73 m^2.

Hepatic: adjust the dose for moderate impairment (Child–Pugh class B); contraindicated in severe impairment (Child–Pugh class C).

SEDATIVES AND HYPNOTICS

Insomnia is one of a number of sleep disorders that also include sleep apnoea, obstructive sleep apnoea and restless leg syndrome. Sleep disorders contribute to both motor vehicle and workplace accidents and are thought to cost the national economy about $51 billion in direct or indirect costs (AIHW 2021).

Insomnia is defined as occurring when there is difficulty initiating and/or maintaining sleep (e.g. frequent awakenings or inability to return to sleep after awakening) and/or early morning awakening with inability to return to sleep. This causes significant disturbance or impairment to the person (e.g. social or occupational functioning) and occurs at least 3 nights per week. It is usually not attributable to or adequately explained by other co-existing medical or mental disorders (Ng & Cunningham 2021). Insomnia can be subdivided into acute and chronic.

Acute insomnia generally has symptoms lasting less than 12 weeks, while chronic insomnia is a longer-term condition that can prolong, exacerbate or exist with other comorbidities. Acute insomnia can be caused by physiological factors (e.g. stress, being 'on-call', caring for a sick relative, being in an unknown environment such as a hospital), pharmacological factors (including prescribed medications (e.g. new diuretic causing nocturia, angiotensin converting enzyme (ACE) inhibitors, phenytoin, xanthines) and non-prescribed agents (e.g. caffeine, alcohol, heavy smoking, over-the-counter cold remedies), physical factors (e.g. coughing, noise, temperature) or disruption to circadian rhythm (e.g. jet lag). While the factors contributing to chronic insomnia are similar, they are longer term (e.g. depression, anxiety, dementia, substance abuse, ongoing medical conditions (e.g. pain, movement disorders, thyroid, respiratory or cardiac disorders), working shiftwork, caffeine, heavy smoking (> one pack/day) and alcohol use) (Raj et al 2024).

Treating insomnia is not always straightforward, but it is important to treat any underlying conditions (such as pain, anxiety, medical conditions or depression), as well as the patient receiving counselling regarding sleep hygiene and stimulus control. This education can include adequate exercise during the day (and avoiding vigorous exercise before bed), relaxation exercises, avoiding daytime napping, going to bed and getting up at the same time (routine), removal of computers, telephone, televisions and pets from the bedroom, and reducing caffeine, heavy smoking and alcohol intake before retiring. Alcohol can cause insomnia, as well as being responsible for sleep disturbances and sedation (Ng & Cunningham 2021; Raj et al 2024).

Pharmacological agents should be used as adjuncts to the counselling described above and used in the short term (less than 4 weeks) to return a person's sleep pattern to normal and then ceased. Agents used to treat the short-term symptoms of insomnia are generally sedatives and hypnotics, with there being little distinction between them. Hypnotics produce drowsiness and help the onset of sleep, whereas sedatives are calming, decreasing activity and curbing excitement. Often the same drug can produce both effects, depending on the dosage. Benzodiazepines are commonly prescribed for insomnia because they promote sleep by increasing the total sleep time, decrease sleep latency (how long it takes to fall asleep) and decrease nocturnal awaking (Raj et al 2024).

Short-acting benzodiazepines (e.g. temazepam, alprazolam, oxazepam, zolpidem, zopiclone) are often used in the management of insomnia, because they do not have active metabolites or 'hangover' symptoms, but the risk of abuse, dependence and tolerance means they should be used only for short-term management. Withdrawal should be gradual, because an increase in sleep disturbance may occur if withdrawal is abrupt (Raj et al 2024).

General Adverse effects of sedatives and hypnotics

- withdrawal reaction (prolonged use and abrupt withdrawal)
- tolerance, dependence, abuse
- memory impairment (transient)
- slurred speech, hangover, tiredness, drowsiness, dizziness, vertigo, headache, unusual or unpleasant dreams, fatigue, lethargy, difficulty concentrating, decreased alertness
- anxiety, nervousness, confusion, excitation, numbed emotions
- double vision
- hypotension
- falls, ataxia, muscle weakness, decreased physical performance, tremor
- nausea, vomiting, diarrhoea, flatulence, abdominal distension, dry mouth
- (Uncommon) rash, sweating
- (Rare) blood dyscrasias, elevated liver enzymes, paradoxical reactions (rage, excitement, stimulation), angioedema, complex sleep-related behaviours (e.g. sleep walking, sleep driving, preparing and eating food, making phone calls, having sex), rebound phenomenon (increase in insomnia or anxiety above pre-treatment level when therapy is stopped), angioedema, unmasking pre-existing depression, suicidal ideation

General Interactions of sedatives and hypnotics

- may potentiate anticholinergic effects of atropine and related drugs, antihistamines and antidepressants
- may have additive CNS-depressant effects if given with alcohol, barbiturates, sedatives, antidepressants, monoamine oxidase inhibitors (MAOIs), phenothiazines, antipsychotics, antiepileptics, hypnotics, muscle relaxants, antihistamines, tricyclic antidepressants (TCAs), opioid analgesics or anaesthetic agents

- caution if given with antiepileptic agents because levels of both antiepileptic and benzodiazepine may be altered; therefore monitoring of antiepileptic serum levels is recommended
- increased euphoria may occur if given with opioid analgesics
- abrupt withdrawal may increase frequency and severity of seizures in those with epilepsy
- serum levels may increase if given with erythromycin, clarithromycin, diltiazem, ritonavir, azole antifungals, fluoxetine, omeprazole, atorvastatin, verapamil or disulfiram
- sedative effects may be reduced if given with xanthines (e.g. aminophylline, theophylline, caffeine)
- metabolism can be increased by carbamazepine, phenytoin, rifampicin and St John's wort, reducing serum levels
- benzodiazepines have an unpredictable effect on phenytoin levels and these should be closely monitored during therapy
- may cause delirium in the elderly (especially if given with anticholinergic agents)

General Nursing considerations/Cautions for sedatives and hypnotics

- FBC, liver and renal function should be monitored regularly during therapy with benzodiazepines
- if there is no improvement to sleep in 7–10 days, underlying causes for insomnia should be investigated
- prolonged use is not recommended
- withdrawal should be gradual; if stopped suddenly, sleep disturbance may occur
- tolerance and dependence may occur
- agent should be stopped if paradoxical reaction (acute rage, stimulation, excitation) occurs
- may increase depression in some patients or cause deterioration in severely disturbed patients with schizophrenia
- lower doses are usually required for older people
- transient amnesia may occur, especially with parenteral administration of benzodiazepines
- patients with cardiac or cerebral disease should be monitored closely if hypotension is likely to cause complications
- caution if used in the elderly or those where a fall in blood pressure may lead to cardiac or cerebral complications
- caution if used in those with depression, psychosis, schizophrenia, suicidal tendencies or drug/alcohol abuse
- caution if used in those with epilepsy, as abrupt withdrawal may lead to an increase in frequency or severity of seizures and there are also interactions with some antiepileptic agents (see Interactions)
- caution if used in those with blood dyscrasias, liver or kidney impairment, or respiratory insufficiency
- contraindicated in those with myasthenia gravis, severe liver insufficiency, sleep apnoea, chronic obstructive airways disease (with insipient respiratory failure) or in those with hypersensitivity to any benzodiazepine
- benzodiazepines are contraindicated in those with acute narrow-angle glaucoma (but can be used in those with open-angle glaucoma that is being treated)

SEDATIVES AND HYPNOTICS

General Patient education for sedatives and hypnotics

- caution the patient against increasing the dose or abruptly stopping medication without first seeking medical advice
- advise the patient to seek medical advice immediately if any swelling of the tongue, glottis or larynx occurs
- warn the patient against driving a vehicle or operating machinery if drowsy or experiencing decreased alertness
- the patient should be warned about the reduced tolerance to alcohol and other CNS depressants
- counsel the patient about reliance on sleeping pills and rebound insomnia that may occur on the first and second nights after stopping medication
- the patient should be warned about ataxia (clumsy movements affecting walking and balance) and muscle weakness, which increases the risk of falls (especially in the elderly)
- advise the patient that some sleep medication can cause short-term memory loss
- instruct the patient in ways to improve sleep hygiene, including:
    - using the bed only for sleep and sex
    - removing all computers, laptops, tablets, televisions, radios, videogames and smartphones from the bedroom
    - if sleep doesn't occur within 20 minutes, get out of bed and read or do something relaxing (e.g. listening to relaxing music) in dim light before returning to bed
    - avoid napping in the afternoon or early evening
    - go to bed and get up at the same times every day
    - ensure the environment is restful (comfortable bed, quiet, temperature not too hot or cold, dark)
    - prepare for sleep with 20—30 minutes of relaxation (e.g. warm bath, reading, listening to music, meditation, yoga)
    - avoid alcohol, caffeine, smoking, vigorous exercise or heavy eating 2—3 hours before bedtime
    - when trying to fall asleep, avoid problem solving, reviewing the day or thinking about life issues
- the patient/carer/partner should be advised to immediately report any unusual activities such as sleep walking, sleep driving, preparing and eating food, making phone calls or having sex without any memory of the event (especially with zolpidem and zopiclone)
- women of childbearing potential should be counselled to use adequate contraception during therapy to avoid pregnancy. If pregnancy occurs, the woman should seek medical advice immediately

Benzodiazepines cross the placental barrier and may cause hypotonia, decreased respiratory function and hypothermia in the newborn. Withdrawal symptoms in the newborn may also occur if there has been prolonged maternal use during pregnancy.

Not recommended during breastfeeding.

Use with caution in those with kidney or liver impairment. Dose reduction is recommended. Regular liver function tests are recommended in those with liver impairment.

Use in the elderly should be with great caution (if at all) because of the risk of

> interaction with other medications, as well as the risk of delayed elimination leading to accumulation and potential side-effects, such as prolonged sedation, ataxia (and falls) and confusion. Therefore, the safest agents to use in the elderly are those with a short half-life and no active metabolites that might accumulate and cause adverse effects.

CHLORAL HYDRATE

Trade name
Orion Chloral Hydrate Mixture

Available form
Syrup: 1 g/10 mL

Action
- sedative, hypnotic
- action similar to other barbiturates
- active metabolite (trichloroethanol) appears to be responsible for CNS depression and has a half-life of 4—12 hours. Metabolite inhibits alcohol metabolism, prolonging its actions
- effective within 30 minutes, duration 4—8 hours
- has been superseded by more effective and less toxic agents

Use
- insomnia (short term)
- preoperative sedation

Dose
- (Hypnotic) 0.5—1 g orally nocte 15—30 minutes before bedtime (daily maximum 2 g) **OR**
- (Preoperatively) 0.5—1 g orally 30 minutes before surgery (daily maximum 2 g)

Adverse effects
- nausea, vomiting, diarrhoea, flatulence, unpleasant taste, abdominal distension
- residual sedation, hangover
- (Uncommon) leucopenia, eosinophilia, disorientation, tolerance, dependence
- (Prolonged therapy) gastritis, skin eruptions, kidney damage
- (Rare) rash, urticaria, pruritus, angioedema, ketonuria, paradoxical reactions

Interactions
- CNS-depressant effects are increased by other CNS depressants, including alcohol, benzodiazepines, barbiturates, antihistamines, tricyclic antidepressants (TCAs), sedatives, hypnotics, opioids or antipsychotics
- caution if given with warfarin, as there may be a transient increase in serum levels; therefore INR should be monitored closely, especially when starting or stopping therapy
- hypermetabolic state (sweating, flushing, labile BP, sense of unease) may result if IV furosemide (frusemide) is given after chloral hydrate
- an increased risk of vasodilation reaction (tachycardia, palpitations, facial flushing, dysphoria) if given with alcohol
- an increased risk of delirium if given with psychotropic or anticholinergic agents (especially in the elderly)
- may interfere with some laboratory tests (including urinary glucose using Clinitest)

Nursing considerations/Cautions
- contraindicated in children with obstructive sleep apnoea
- contraindicated in those with liver or kidney impairment, severe cardiac disease, gastritis, oesophagitis, gastric or duodenal ulcers or porphyria
- see also General Nursing considerations/Cautions for sedatives and hypnotics (p. 1504)

Patient education
- advise the patient that gastric irritation may be minimised by taking the mixture immediately after food, or diluting with a full glass of water, fruit juice or ginger ale
- see also General Patient education for sedatives and hypnotics (p. 1505)

SEDATIVES AND HYPNOTICS

 Not recommended during pregnancy, as it may cause sedation in newborn.

 Not recommended during breastfeeding, as it may cause sedation in the breastfed infant.

 Dose reduction is recommended in those with kidney or liver impairment.

 Dose reduction is recommended in the elderly. May lead to delirium if given in combination with cholinergic or psychotropic agents.

DEXMEDETOMIDINE
Trade names
Dexdor, Dexmedetomidine Accord, Dexmedetomidine Ever Pharma, Dexmedetomidine Medsurge, Dexmedetomidine Sandoz, Dexmedetomidine Viatris, Precedex, Precedex Ready to Use

Available forms
Ampoules: 200 microgram/2 mL, 400 microgram/4 mL;
Vials: 200 microgram/2 mL, 400 microgram/4 mL, 1000 microgram/10 mL;
Infusion: 200 microgram/50 mL, 400 microgram/100 mL

Action
- selective alpha2 adrenoreceptor antagonist with sedative and analgesic actions but no amnesic properties
- half-life is approximately 2 hours

Use
- ICU sedation (intubated patients)
- procedural sedation (non-intubated patients)

Dose
- initially 1 microgram/kg IV over 10—20 minutes (loading dose), followed by 0.2—1.0 microgram/kg/hour (maintenance) (titrating maintenance dose according to response)

Adverse effects
- hypotension, transient hypertension, bradycardia, tachycardia, atrial fibrillation, sinus arrest
- fever, rigors
- agitation, confusion
- hypoxia, respiratory depression
- dry mouth, nausea, vomiting, thirst
- decreased lacrimation, corneal dryness
- oliguria
- hyper- or hypoglycaemia
- anaemia

Interactions
- increased effects may occur if given with anaesthetics, sedatives, hypnotics or opioid analgesics
- bradycardia and/or hypotension may be potentiated if given with propofol or midazolam

Nursing considerations/Cautions
- should be administered only by an anaesthetist or in an ICU setting
- ECG, BP and oxygen saturation should be monitored throughout infusion. Transient hypertension (due to initial vasoconstriction) may occur with loading dose
- any hypovolaemia should be corrected before starting therapy
- lubrication of the eyes is recommended to prevent corneal dryness and damage
- if amnesia is also required, an amnesic agent should also be administered
- onset of sedation is 10—15 minutes after start of infusion
- patients receiving dexmedetomidine are easily rousable and alert when stimulated. However, this does not indicate a lack of drug efficacy
- IV therapy should continue for 24 hours only
- a loading dose may not be required if other sedative agents have been used previously
- use of a loading dose has been associated with increased risk of adverse effects

- therapy does not need to be ceased for extubation
- not recommended as bolus or rapid IV administration because of the increased risk of bradycardia and sinus arrest
- use a controlled infusion device
- 2 mL of solution is added to 48 mL of sodium chloride 0.9% and gently shaken to make up IV solution (100 microgram/mL concentrate solution)
- not recommended with blood or blood products
- incompatible with amphotericin B and diazepam
- not recommended in those under 18 years
- caution if used in those with pre-existing bradycardia, heart block or ventricular dysfunction, > 65 years or those with diabetes
- caution if used in those with severe cardiac disease or chronic hypertension
- see also General Nursing considerations/Cautions for sedatives and hypnotics (p. 1504)

Safety has not been established during pregnancy. Crosses the placental barrier and is recommended during pregnancy only if benefits to the mother outweigh risks to the fetus.

Is excreted in breastmilk. Breastmilk should be discarded for 24 hours after administration to decrease potential effects on the newborn.

Dose reduction for both loading and maintenance doses is recommended in those over 65 years.

FLUNITRAZEPAM
Trade name
Hypnodorm

Available form
Tablets: 1 mg

Action
- long-acting benzodiazepine related to nitrazepam and clonazepam, with marked hypnotic and sedative properties, as well as anxiolytic and muscle-relaxant properties
- rapid onset of action, half-life 20—30 hours
- two active metabolites, but less active than parent but have half-lives ranging from 10 to 33 hours

Use
- severe insomnia (short-term management)

Dose
- (Adult) 1—2 mg orally nocte, immediately before going to bed **OR**
- (Elderly) 0.5—1 mg orally nocte, immediately before going to bed

Adverse effects/Interactions/Nursing considerations/Cautions/Patient education
- contraindicated in children
- see also General Adverse effects/Interactions/Nursing considerations/Cautions/Patient education for sedatives and hypnotics (p. 1503)

Tablet can be dispersed in water, or crushed and mixed with a spoonful of yoghurt or apple puree.

Recommended dose for elderly (> 65 years) is 0.5—1 mg orally nocte, immediately before going to bed.

LEMBOREXANT
Trade name
Dayvigo

Available forms
Tablet: 5 mg, 10 mg

Action
- competitive antagonist of both orexin (OX1R, OX2R) receptors, with high affinity for OX2R (orexin is a neuropeptide that promotes wakefulness)
- metabolite has a low level of activity
- half-life 17—19 hours

SEDATIVES AND HYPNOTICS

- time to sleep onset is delayed if taken with food

Use
- treatment of insomnia

Dose
- 5—10 mg orally at bedtime

Adverse effects
- somnolence, abnormal dreams, nightmares, sleep paralysis
- headache
- (Uncommon) complex sleep behaviours

Interactions
- not recommended with other sedatives, hypnotics or other CNS depressants including benzodiazepines, tricyclic antidepressants (TCAs) or opioids
- not recommended with clarithromycin and azole antifungal agents
- dose should be limited to 5 mg if given with fluoxetine
- not recommended with carbamazepine, phenytoin, rifampicin, dexamethasone, efavirenz, rifabutin or St John's wort, as serum levels may be reduced
- not recommended with alcohol

Nursing considerations/Cautions
- not recommended in those under 18 years
- not recommended in those with severe liver impairment
- contraindicated in those with narcolepsy
- contraindicated in those with hypersensitivity to other orexin receptor antagonists
- see also General Nursing considerations for sedatives and hypnotics (p. 1504)

Patient education
- warn the patient that sleep onset will be delayed if taken with or soon after a meal
- the patient should take the dose at bedtime, 7 hours or more before the planned awakening time
- see also General Patient education for sedatives and hypnotics (p. 1505)

 Tablets can be crushed and mixed with water or a spoonful of yoghurt or apple puree.

 Safety has not been established; therefore not recommended during pregnancy unless benefits outweigh risks to the fetus.

 Excreted in breastmilk; therefore not recommended during breastfeeding.

 Maximum recommended dose in those with moderate liver impairment is 5 mg.

MELATONIN
Trade names
APO Health Melatonin Sleep Aid, Chemists Own Melatonin Sleep Aid, Circadin, Melatonin ARX, Melatonin MR Teva, Melatonin Sandoz Sleep Aid, Melatonin Viatris, Melotin MR, Slenyto, Somnicare, Voquily, Wagner Health Melatonin

Available forms
Tablets (prolonged release): 1 mg, 2 mg, 3 mg, 5 mg;
Oral solution: 1 mg/mL

Action
- naturally occurring hormone produced by pineal gland
- related to serotonin
- naturally secreted soon after onset of darkness, peaks between 2 am and 4 am, diminishing during second half of night
- associated with circadian rhythm control, hypnotic effect and increased sleep tendency
- acts at melatonin receptors (MT1-inhibit neuron firing, MT2-phase shifting response) in the hypothalamus
- inactive metabolite
- half-life 3.5—4 hours
- melatonin metabolism declines with age

Use
- insomnia (short-term management) in those aged 55 years and over
- jet lag

- sleep disorders in children (6 to 18 years) with neurodevelopmental disorders (e.g. autism, attention deficit hyperactivity disorder (ADHD))

Dose
- (Insomnia) 2 mg orally 1—2 hours before bedtime and after food **OR**
- (Jet lag) 2 mg orally at the preferred local sleep time, up to 5 mg if needed **OR**
- (Sleep disorder associated with neurodevelopmental disorders) 2 mg orally 30—60 minutes before bedtime, up to 5 mg daily if needed

Adverse effects
- headache, asthenia, dizziness, migraine, drowsiness, nightmares, irritability
- anxiety
- nasopharyngitis, influenza, upper and lower respiratory tract infection, rhinitis, cough, nasopharyngeal pain
- urinary tract infection
- back ache, arthralgia, muscle cramp, neck pain, pain in extremity
- abdominal pain, constipation, diarrhoea, nausea, vomiting

Interactions
- not recommended with alcohol
- may enhance sedative properties of other sedatives and hypnotics
- increased sensation of fuzzy-headedness when given with imipramine
- serum levels may be reduced by carbamazepine, rifampicin or smoking
- increased serum levels may occur if given with fluoroquinolone antibiotics or oestrogen-containing agents (e.g. oral contraceptives, hormone replacement therapy)
- not recommended with fluvoxamine
- caution if given with warfarin; INR should be closely monitored if given together
- serum levels may be decreased in those who smoke

Nursing considerations/Cautions
- (Sleep disorder associated with neurodevelopment disorders) evaluation of therapy is recommended after 12 weeks to determine clinical effectiveness
- (Voquily) should be taken on an empty stomach, and food not eaten an hour before or after administration
- (Voquily oral solution) oral solution contains sorbitol and is therefore not recommended in those with hereditary fructose intolerance
- tablets contain lactose: therefore are not recommended in those with rare hereditary problems of galactose intolerance, Lapp lactase deficiency or glucose—galactose malabsorption
- not recommended in those under 18 years (not Voquily, which is used for sleep disorders in children (6 to 18 years) with neurodevelopmental disorders)
- not recommended in those with autoimmune diseases or liver impairment

Patient education
- advise the patient that tablets should be swallowed whole, not chewed or split
- (Voquily) instruct the patient/carer that therapy should be taken on an empty stomach and food not consumed an hour before or after therapy
- (Oral solution) advise the patient that the solution should be stored below 25°C and discarded 2 months after opening.
- see also General Patient education for sedatives and hypnotics (p. 1505)

 Tablet should not be divided, crushed or chewed.

 Safety has not been established in pregnancy; therefore not recommended.

 Not recommended during breastfeeding.

 Not recommended in those with kidney or liver impairment.

SEDATIVES AND HYPNOTICS

MIDAZOLAM HYDROCHLORIDE

Trade names
B.Braun Midazolam Solution, Hypnovel, Midazolam Accord Solution, Midazolam Apotex Solution, Midazolam Solution, Midazolam Viatris Solution, Midazolam Baxter Solution, Zyamis Oromucosal Solution

Available forms
Ampoules: 5 mg/5 mL, 5 mg/mL, 15 mg/3 mL, 50 mg/10 mL;
Prefilled oral syringe: 2.5 mg/0.25 mL, 5 mg/0.5 mL, 7.5 mg/0.75 mL, 10 mg/1 mL

Action
- very short-acting benzodiazepine with rapid onset
- induces sedation, hypnosis, amnesia, anaesthesia, muscle relaxation
- induces sedation in 15 minutes (IM), peak effect 30–60 minutes, half-life 1.4–2.4 hours
- induces anaesthesia (IV), onset of action is 1.5–2.5 minutes (depending on dose and/or opioid premedication)
- approximately 2 hours are required for full recovery after anaesthesia (time dependent on dose and usage of other drugs)
- active metabolite (half-life 1–3 hours)
- half-life is prolonged in the elderly, obese, critically ill and those with congestive heart failure

Use
- preoperative sedation, relief of anxiety and to impair memory of perioperative events (IM)
- conscious sedation before endoscopy (lung, stomach, bladder), coronary angiography and cardiac catheterisation (IV) (alone or with opioid)
- induction of anaesthesia before anaesthetic agent (IV)
- sedation in intensive care unit (ICU) (IV)
- generalised convulsive status epilepticus (GCSE) (in those > 6 months) (Zyamis Oromucosal Solution)

Dose
- (Preoperative sedation) 0.07–0.08 mg/kg IM 1 hour before surgery **OR**
- (Endoscopic/cardiovascular procedures) initially 1 mg by slow IV injection (starting with lowest dose and titrating dose to desired sedation at 2–3-minute intervals) **OR**
- (Induction of anaesthesia) 0.15–0.2 mg/kg by slow IV at a rate of 2.5 mg/10 seconds. A further dose may be given if needed (to a total of 0.35 mg/kg) **OR**
- (Sedation in ICU) 0.03–0.2 mg/kg/hour by IV infusion **OR**
- GCSE (administered into buccal cavity)
  - (adult) 10 mg
  (> 6 months to < 12 months: 7 kg to < 12 kg) 2.5 mg
  (12 months to < 5 years: 12 kg to < 21 kg) 5 mg
  (5 years to < 10 years: 21 kg to < 29 kg) 7.5 mg
  (10 years and above: > 29 kg) 10 mg

Adverse effects
- (IV) hiccups, acid taste, coughing, phlebitis
- (IV, IM injection site) induration, redness, pain, muscle stiffness, headache, tenderness
- (Surgical procedures) respiratory depression, apnoea, variation in heart rate and BP
- see also General Adverse effects of sedatives and hypnotics (p. 1503)

Interactions
- thiopental sodium induction dose requirement may be reduced when IM midazolam is used as premedication
- erythromycin, other macrolide antibiotics and cimetidine inhibit metabolism of midazolam, prolonging duration of sedation
- increased effect if given with sodium valproate
- not recommended with St John's wort

Nursing considerations/Cautions

- half-life decreased if given with echinacea
- half-life may be increased if given with aprepitant
- see also General Interactions of sedatives and hypnotics (p. 1503)
- continuous cardiorespiratory function monitoring is recommended during IV administration
- any fluid or electrolyte imbalance should be corrected before administration or dose reduced
- extravasation and intra-arterial administration should be avoided
- not recommended as IV bolus or by rapid IV administration
- vital signs should be monitored carefully during administration and recovery period
- for conscious sedation, the dose should be titrated until the patient slurs speech, then wait for 2–3 minutes to establish effect and give a further dose if needed
- the patient should not be discharged until at least 3 hours post-procedure and any information given immediately post-procedure repeated on discharge, as anterograde amnesia may last longer than sedation; therefore the patient may not remember what was said to them in the immediate post-procedure period
- may be mixed in the same syringe with morphine, pethidine, atropine or hyoscine
- contraindicated in those in shock or coma, or with acute alcohol intoxication with depressed vital signs
- (GCSE) oromucosal solution should be used only in patients who have had a diagnosis of epilepsy
- (GCSE) carers should be carefully instructed in the correct administration of oromucosal solution to prevent choking occurring
- (GCSE) second or repeat doses are not recommended unless under medical advice including the patient's individual written care plan for seizure management
- (Oromucosal solution) the solution contains mannitol and should be used in those with rare hereditary problems of fructose intolerance only if benefits outweigh the risks
- see also General Nursing considerations/Cautions for sedatives and hypnotics (p. 1504)

Patient education

- the patient should be advised to avoid alcohol for at least 12 hours after administration, because mutual potentiation can cause unpredictable reactions
- instruct the patient/carer/parent in the correct administration of the oromucosal solution including;
  - the patient should be carefully monitored during and after a seizure (fit) ensuring they are in the recovery position on their side and safe
  - check expiry date and solution before use. Do not use if the solution is cloudy or is past the expiry date
  - do not attach a needle to the syringe and administer the solution by any other route than the mouth
  - remove the syringe from the plastic container
  - holding the syringe by the finger grips, unscrew the amber sheath cap in an anticlockwise direction and remove the amber sheath cap
  - using finger and thumb, gently pinch and pull back on the patient's cheek to open their lips and insert the syringe into the space between the cheek and lower gum (buccal cavity)
  - slowly administer about half the syringe into the buccal cavity and the remaining amount on the other side, pressing the syringe plunger until it stops
  - if it is too hard to administer into one buccal cavity, administer the whole dose over 4–5 seconds into the other buccal cavity

SEDATIVES AND HYPNOTICS

- dispose of the used syringe and cap safely
- observe the patient closely, taking note of the time the seizure started and finished
- the oromucosal solution must be administered into the buccal cavity only and not into the mouth or throat to prevent choking
- if the patient's condition does not improve quickly after administration, an ambulance should be called immediately
- if patient's condition improves, but has another seizure (fit), an ambulance should be called immediately
- a second dose should not be administered unless medical advice is given to do so
- the prefilled oral syringe should be stored in original packaging to protect from light at below 25°C but not frozen or refrigerated
- the prefilled oral syringe is single use only
- see also General Patient education for sedatives and hypnotics (p. 1505)

 The half-life may be prolonged up to 4 times in the elderly.

NITRAZEPAM
Trade names
Alodorm, Mogadon

Available form
Tablets: 5 mg

Action
- long-acting benzodiazepine with no active metabolites
- sedative, anxiolytic, antiepileptic and muscle-relaxing properties
- facilitates action of gamma aminobutyric acid (GABA) in the brain
- effective as a hypnotic within 30—60 minutes, duration 6—8 hours, long half-life (average 27 hours)

Use
- insomnia (short-term management)

Dose
- (Adult) 5—10 mg orally nocte, 20—30 minutes before bedtime **OR**
- (Elderly) 2.5—5 mg orally nocte, 20—30 minutes before bedtime

Adverse effects/Interactions/Nursing considerations/Cautions
- (Infants, children, debilitated elderly) bronchial hypersecretion and excessive salivation (can lead to aspiration pneumonia)
- dose may be increased to 20 mg in hospitalised patients if needed
- contains lactose and is therefore not recommended in those with rare hereditary galactose intolerance, total lactase deficiency or glucose—galactose malabsorption
- see also General Adverse effects/Interactions/Nursing considerations/Cautions for sedatives and hypnotics (p. 1503)

 Tablet can be dispersed in water, or crushed and mixed with a spoonful of yoghurt or apple puree.

 Recommended dose for those > 65 years is 2.5—5 mg orally nocte, 20—30 minutes before bedtime.

SUVOREXANT
Trade name
Belsomra

Available forms
Tablets: 15 mg, 30 mg

Action
- highly selective dual orexin receptor antagonist (OX1R, OX2R) (orexin A and orexin B are neuropeptides are central promotors of wakefulness)
- non-active metabolite
- increases REM sleep
- does not appear to produce dependence

- half-life 12 hours

Use
- treatment of insomnia

Dose
- (Adult ≥ 65 years) 15 mg orally nocte 30 minutes before bedtime **OR**
- (Adult < 65 years) 20 mg orally nocte 30 minutes before bedtime

Adverse effects
- fatigue, somnolence, dizziness, headache
- abnormal dreaming, nightmares
- anxiety
- nausea, dry mouth, diarrhoea
- palpitations, tachycardia
- (Rare) complex behaviours, worsening of depression, suicidal ideation, sleep paralysis (inability to walk or talk for several minutes during sleep—wake transition), mild catalepsy (e.g. mild leg weakness not associated with normal triggering event such as laughter or surprise), hypnagogic/hypnopompic hallucinations (vivid and sometimes disturbing sleep hallucinations that occur at sleep—wake transition)

Interactions
- CNS depression increased if given with other CNS depressants, including alcohol, benzodiazepines, tricyclic antidepressants (TCAs) and opioid analgesics
- not recommended with other hypnotic or sedative agents
- not recommended with aprepitant, diltiazem, ciprofloxacin, erythromycin, azole antifungal agents or HIV protease inhibitors (e.g. ritonavir), imatinib, grapefruit juice or verapamil
- efficacy may be reduced if given with rifampicin, carbamazepine or phenytoin
- may increase digoxin levels slightly; therefore blood levels should be monitored especially when starting or stopping therapy

Nursing considerations/Cautions
- if medication is not effective in improving insomnia in 7—10 days, other causes (e.g. medical or psychiatric illness) should be investigated
- caution if used in those with compromised respiratory function (e.g. sleep apnoea, chronic obstructive pulmonary disease)
- caution in those with a history of drug abuse if given for a long period
- not recommended in those with severe liver impairment
- contraindicated in those with narcolepsy

Patient education
- the patient should be instructed to take medication 30 minutes before retiring when they will get a full night's sleep (at least 7 hours) before needing to be awake
- warn the patient that daytime wakefulness can be impaired, and this may persist for several days after discontinuing therapy
- the patient should be instructed against driving or operating machinery if drowsy or experiencing decreased alertness
- advise the patient to avoid alcohol and grapefruit juice during therapy
- the patient should be warned against increasing the dose
- instruct the patient in ways to improve sleep hygiene (see General Patient education for sedatives and hypnotics, p. 1505)
- the patient/carer/partner should be advised to immediately report any of the following:
  - unusual activities, such as sleep walking, sleep driving, preparing and eating food or making phone calls without any memory of the activity
  - depression (new or worsening) or thoughts of self-harm

SEDATIVES AND HYPNOTICS

- temporary inability to walk or talk for minutes when falling asleep or waking up
- abnormal thoughts or behaviours, including being aggressive or more outgoing than normal, confusion, agitation or experiencing hallucinations, which may be vivid and disturbing
- sudden leg weakness or collapse

Tablet can be crushed and mixed with water or a spoonful of yoghurt or apple puree.

Not recommended during pregnancy unless benefits outweigh risks.

Caution if used during breastfeeding.

Dose for adults over 65 years is 15 mg orally nocte 30 minutes before bedtime.

TEMAZEPAM
Trade names
APO-Temazepam, Normison, Temaze, Temazepam-WGR, Temtabs

Available form
Tablets: 10 mg

Action
- short-acting benzodiazepine with no long-acting active metabolite; tends not to accumulate with long-term therapy
- metabolised to oxazepam
- half-life is 5–15 hours (average 10 hours)

Use
- insomnia (short-term management)

Dose
- (Adult) 10–30 mg orally nocte, 20–30 minutes before retiring **OR**
- (Elderly) 2.5–5 mg orally nocte, 20–30 minutes before bedtime

Adverse effects/Interactions/Nursing considerations/Cautions/Patient education
- not recommended in those under 16 years
- see also General Adverse effects/Interactions/Nursing considerations/Cautions/Patient education for sedatives and hypnotics (p. 1503

Tablet can be dispersed in water, or crushed and mixed with a spoonful of yoghurt or apple puree.

Recommended dose for those > 65 years is 2.5–5 mg orally nocte, 20–30 minutes before bedtime.

ZOLPIDEM TARTRATE
Trade names
APO-Zolpidem, Pharmcor Zolpidem, Somidem, Stildem, Stilnox, Stilnox CR, Zolpibell, Zolpidem Dr Reddy's, Zolpidem Sandoz Pharma, ZolpiMist

Available forms
Tablets: 10 mg;
Tablets (controlled/modified release): 6.25 mg, 12.5 mg;
Oral mucosal spray: 5 mg/actuation

Action
- imidazopyridine unrelated to other hypnotic agents
- selectively binds to benzodiazepine-1 subtype receptors (omega-1 subtype), whereas benzodiazepines bind non-selectively to all three omega receptor subtypes
- no active metabolite
- rapid onset, duration 6 hours, half-life 2 hours

Use
- insomnia (short-term management)

Dose
- (Adult) 10 mg orally at night 20—30 minutes immediately before bedtime (immediate-release tablets) **OR**
- (Elderly) 5 mg orally at night 20—30 minutes immediately before bedtime (immediate-release tablets) **OR**
- (Adult) 12.5 mg orally at night immediately before bedtime (modified-release tablets) **OR**
- (Elderly) 6.25 mg orally at night immediately before bedtime (modified-release tablets) **OR**
- (Oral mucosal spray) 5 mg (1 actuation) (women) or 5—10 mg (1—2 actuations) (men) immediately before bedtime

Adverse effects
- dizziness, daytime drowsiness, headache, memory impairment, drugged feeling, abnormal dreams, fatigue, somnolence, disorientation
- nausea, vomiting, diarrhoea, abdominal pain, dry mouth
- palpitations
- myalgia, back pain
- flu-like symptoms
- visual disturbances
- (Uncommon) complex sleep-related behaviours (e.g. sleep walking, sleep driving, preparing and eating food, making phone calls, having sex), rebound insomnia
- (Rare) angioedema

Interactions
- additive CNS-depressant effects may occur if given with other CNS-depressant drugs including barbiturates, benzodiazepines, sedatives, hypnotics, antianxiety agents, tricyclic antidepressants (TCAs), monoamine oxidase inhibitors (MAOIs), muscle relaxants, phenothiazines, antipsychotics, antihistamines, antiepileptics or anaesthetics
- caution if given with opioid analgesics because of increased CNS sedation and a risk of respiratory depression and coma
- serum levels may be decreased if given with rifampicin and St John's wort
- not recommended with ciprofloxacin or fluvoxamine
- contraindicated with alcohol because of an increased risk of complex sleep-related behaviours
- increased sedation may occur if given with imipramine or chlorpromazine

Nursing considerations/Cautions
- therapy should be limited to 4 weeks maximum under close medical supervision
- caution if used in those with long QT syndrome
- contraindicated in those who have experienced complex sleep behaviours when taking zolpidem
- see also General Nursing considerations/Cautions for sedatives and hypnotics (p. 1504)

Patient education
- advise the patient that modified-release tablets should be swallowed whole and not crushed or chewed
- warn the patient not to take tablets or use the spray with or immediately after food for maximum effect
- the patient should be warned about the serious effects of drinking alcohol during therapy
- (Oral mucosal spray) advise the patient that:
    - the pump needs to be primed with 7 sprays before first use, or 1 spray if not used for 14 days or more
    - spray directly into the mouth over the tongue while sitting or standing (not lying down)
    - if 2 doses (10 mg) are required, allow the pump to return to start position before the second actuation
    - should not be administered with or just after food
    - should not be used more than once per evening

SEDATIVES AND HYPNOTICS

- keep spray away from eyes and do not inhale it
- store in a cool dry place and keep out of reach of children
- the pump contains 28 actuations (after initial 7 priming actuations)
- see also General Patient education for sedatives and hypnotics (p. 1505)

Controlled-release (CR) tablets must not be crushed or chewed. Other tablets (10 mg) can be dispersed in water, or crushed and mixed with a spoonful of yoghurt or apple puree.

Safety in pregnancy has not been established; therefore not recommended during pregnancy.

A small amount is secreted in breastmilk; therefore not recommended during breastfeeding.

Recommended dose in those with liver impairment is 5 mg orally nocte.
Not recommended in those with severe liver impairment.

Recommended dose in those > 65 years is 5 mg orally nocte to decrease the risk of CNS adverse effects.

ZOPICLONE

Trade names
APO-Zopiclone, Imoclone, Imovane, Imrest, Pharmcor Zopiclone, Zopiclone GH

Available form
Tablets: 7.5 mg

Action
- cyclopyrrolone with sedative, anxiolytic, muscle relaxant, antiepileptic and amnesic properties
- one metabolite has weak activity
- half-life about 5.3 hours (extended in the elderly and those with liver impairment)

Use
- insomnia (short-term treatment)

Dose
- 3.75—7.5 mg orally nocte, 20—30 minutes before bedtime

Adverse effects
- bitter taste, dry mouth, anorexia, nausea, vomiting, diarrhoea/constipation, bad breath, coated tongue, heartburn, dyspepsia, epigastric pain
- drowsiness, headache, fatigue
- blurred vision
- urticaria, tingling, pruritus, rash
- impotence, ejaculation problems, libido disorder
- palpitations (elderly)
- withdrawal syndrome
- (Less commonly) impaired memory, confusion, dizziness, somnolence, euphoria, hypotonia, depression, asthenia, weakness, anxiety, agitation, euphoria, rebound insomnia, lack of coordination, complex sleep-related behaviours (e.g. sleep walking, sleep driving, preparing and eating food, making phone calls, having sex), rebound insomnia
- (Rare) altered micturition, altered liver enzymes, angioedema, muscle weakness

Interactions
- additive CNS-depressant effects may occur if given with other CNS-depressant drugs including barbiturates, benzodiazepines, sedatives, hypnotics, antianxiety agents, tricyclic antidepressants (TCAs), monoamine oxidase inhibitors (MAOIs), muscle relaxants, phenothiazines, antipsychotics, antihistamines, antiepileptics and anaesthetics
- not recommended with opioid analgesics owing to increased CNS sedation and a risk of respiratory depression and coma, and also a risk of dependence as euphoria may occur when given together
- increased serum level may occur if given with erythromycin, clarithromycin, ritonavir or itraconazole. increasing the risk of adverse effects
- decreased serum levels may occur if given with rifampicin, carbamazepine, phenobarbital (phenobarbitone), phenytoin or St John's wort

- contraindicated with alcohol because of the increased risk of complex sleep-related behaviours

Nursing considerations/Cautions

- therapy for greater than 4 weeks is not recommended
- not recommended in those with thyroid dysfunction or hormonal imbalance
- contraindicated in those with acute cerebrovascular accident (CVA) and in children
- contraindicated in those who have previously experienced complex sleep behaviours after taking zopiclone
- see also General Nursing considerations/Cautions for sedatives and hypnotics (p. 1504)

Patient education

- the patient should be warned about the serious effects of drinking alcohol during therapy
- advise the patient that the tablet has a bitter taste
- see also General Patient education for sedatives and hypnotics (p. 1505)

Tablet can be dispersed in water, or crushed and mixed with a spoonful of yoghurt or apple puree. The tablet has a bitter taste.

Not recommended during pregnancy.

Drug and metabolites are excreted in breastmilk; therefore not recommended during breastfeeding.

Recommended dose is 3.75 mg in those with kidney or liver impairment.

Caution in increasing dose above 3.75 mg in the elderly, as CNS adverse effects are more likely at higher dose.

SEX HORMONES

Steroid (sex) hormones (oestrogens and androgens) are produced mainly in the ovaries and testes, but also in the adrenal cortex and the placenta. Production is controlled by gonadotrophic hormones (follicle-stimulating hormone (FSH), luteinising hormone (LH)), released by the anterior pituitary gland (which is in turn controlled by the hypothalamus and circulating levels). They are generally synthesised and secreted (rather than being stored) and are lipid soluble and derived from cholesterol. The sex hormones have a role in the development and maintenance of the sex organs, as well as regulation of reproduction (Knights et al 2023).

Other agents described in this section are the sex hormone antagonists, oral contraceptive agents and agents that do not fit into any of these categories but still have an effect on the sex hormones.

ANDROGENS AND ANABOLIC STEROIDS

General Actions of androgens and anabolic steroids

- testosterone is the main androgen produced from within the Leydig (interstitial) cells in the testes, from precursors (dehydroepiandrosterone (DHEA) and androstenedione) produced in the adrenal glands
- some testosterone acts on seminiferous tubules to produce sperm; the remainder is secreted into the bloodstream and travels to target tissue
- (Before birth) androgens are responsible for masculinisation of reproductive tract and external genitalia and descent of the testes into the scrotum
- (Reproduction-related effects) growth and sexual maturation at puberty, as well as spermatogenesis, maintenance of reproductive tract and feedback control of gonadotrophin secretion
- development of male secondary sex characteristics (e.g. deepening of voice, male pattern hair growth, muscle growth, male body shape) and behaviours. Androgens are also responsible for male accessory sex organs (e.g. prostate gland, seminal vesicles, penis and bulbourethral glands)
- non-reproductive functions of androgens include anabolic effects on bone and skeletal muscle (i.e. resulting in increased skeletal weight, increased bone mass and growth), neuroprotective effect in central and peripheral nervous system, bone protection (due to decreased calcium excretion) and stimulation of vascular cell adhesion molecules in endothelial cells

General Uses of androgens and anabolic steroids
- replacement therapy in men with hypogonadism or eunuchoidism, and for the male climacteric (andropause)
- diseases in which there is protein and bone wasting (e.g. osteoporosis), and for which oestrogen therapy is contraindicated
- acute and chronic renal failure (including anaemia of chronic renal failure)
- inoperable breast carcinoma
- aplastic anaemia
- long-term corticosteroid therapy

General Adverse effects of androgens and anabolic steroids
- acne, rash, skin flushing, oily skin, greasy hair
- weight gain
- (Females) virilisation (e.g. acne, hirsutism, clitoral enlargement, menstrual irregularities (e.g. oligomenorrhoea, amenorrhoea), libido changes, voice changes, increased growth of pubic hair)
- (Males) increased frequency or persistence of erections, priapism
- (Prepubertal male) precocious sexual development, increased frequency of penile erection, phallic enlargement, premature epiphyseal closure
- excessive sexual stimulation, increase in libido
- gynaecomastia
- abdominal pain, nausea, gastrointestinal bleeding
- altered glucose tolerance
- hyperlipidaemia, decreased serum high-density lipoprotein (HDL) cholesterol
- headache (common), insomnia, anxiety, depression, excitation, aggression, emotional lability, mania, hypomania
- (Metastatic cancer) exacerbation of hypercalcaemia/hypercalciuria
- (Prolonged therapy) oligospermia, decreased ejaculatory volume, decreased sperm count, inhibition of spermatogenesis
- salt and water retention, hypertension, oedema
- (Rare) bladder irritability, decreased urine flow, impotence, testicular atrophy, prostate hyperplasia
- (Rare) leucocytosis, polycythaemia, hyperlipidaemia
- (Rare, long term) benign or malignant liver or prostate tumours, peliosis hepatis
- (Rare) liver function test abnormalities, cholestatic hepatitis, jaundice

General Interactions of androgens and anabolic steroids
- may increase the effects of warfarin; therefore INR should be closely monitored, especially when starting, stopping or altering dose
- androgens may improve glucose tolerance, thereby altering requirements for insulin and/or oral hypoglycaemic agents
- may potentiate effects and also the risk of nephrotoxicity if given with ciclosporin
- caution if given with levothyroxine
- increased risk of oedema if given with adrenocorticotrophic hormone (ACTH) or corticosteroids
- may alter results of some laboratory tests including glucose tolerance test, metyrapone test (pituitary test), thyroxine and iodine studies, suppression of clotting factors

General Nursing considerations/Cautions for androgens and anabolic steroids
- digital rectal (prostate) examinations and measuring prostate-specific antigen (PSA) level should be carried out before starting therapy (to rule out presence of prostate cancer) and then regularly throughout
- (Hypogonadism) diagnosis (e.g. clinical and physical assessment, serum testosterone, luteinising hormone (LH) and follicle-stimulating hormone (FSH) levels) should be confirmed before starting therapy

SEX HORMONES

- liver function, serum cholesterol and BP should be monitored regularly throughout therapy
- haemoglobin and haematocrit should be checked before starting therapy to rule out polycythaemia
- the dose should be decreased if frequent or persistent erections occur
- females should be closely monitored for any signs of virilisation and therapy stopped to reverse changes
- should not be used to enhance muscle development or increase physical ability in healthy individuals because of serious health risks. Furthermore, most androgens and anabolic steroids are banned in sport
- caution if used in those with bony (skeletal) metastases, as hypercalcaemia/hypercalciuria may develop or be aggravated
- caution if used in those with benign prostatic hypertrophy, as urinary obstruction may occur
- caution if used in those with psychological disturbances, as depression may be aggravated
- caution if used in those whose growth is incomplete, because high doses may cause premature closure of epiphyseal plates
- caution if given to those with cardiac or renal failure/impairment, hypertension, epilepsy or migraine where fluid retention/overload may aggravate conditions
- caution if given to those with a history of myocardial infarction or chronic artery disease, thrombophilia or liver dysfunction
- caution if given to those with diabetes mellitus, androgen-sensitive polycythaemia, sleep apnoea or porphyria
- contraindicated in those with hypercalcaemia, liver tumours (current or history), prostate cancer or breast cancer (males), cardiac failure, liver disease (with impaired bilirubin excretion), nephrosis or the nephrotic phase of nephritis

General Patient education for androgens and anabolic steroids

- females should be advised to report any changes, such as hoarseness or voice changes, that might be suggestive of virilisation
- instruct male patients to seek medical advice immediately if any of the following occur:
    - frequent or prolonged erection (this can become a medical emergency)
    - breast enlargement or tenderness
- patients with diabetes mellitus should be instructed to closely monitor blood glucose levels during therapy, as androgens may improve glucose tolerance, decreasing requirement for insulin and/or oral hypoglycaemics
- the patient (or carer) should be advised to seek medical advice immediately if any of the following occur:
    - thoughts/talk about self-harm, harm to others, suicide or death or recent attempts at self-harm or increase in aggression or hostility
    - change in mood
    - worsening of depression

 Contraindicated during breastfeeding.

 Banned in sport.

NANDROLONE DECANOATE
Trade names
Deca-Durabolin Solution

Available form
Ampoule: 50 mg/mL

Action/Use
- anabolic agent with greater anabolic but less androgenic activity than testosterone
- duration of action about 3 weeks

- acute renal failure, chronic renal insufficiency and anaemia of chronic renal failure
- for the palliative treatment of inoperable mammary carcinoma
- osteoporosis (where oestrogen therapy is contraindicated)
- aplastic anaemia
- patients on long-term treatment with corticosteroids
- see also General Actions/Uses of androgens and anabolic steroids (p. 1519)

Dose
- (Renal conditions) 25—50 mg deep IM every 2—3 weeks (initially 50 mg weekly may be required) **OR**
- (Inoperable breast carcinoma, osteoporosis, long-term corticosteroid therapy) 50 mg deep IM every 2—3 weeks **OR**
- (Aplastic anaemia) 50—150 mg deep IM weekly **OR**
- (Anaemia of chronic renal failure) 200 mg IM weekly (males) or 100 mg IM weekly (females) until haemoglobin returns to normal and then therapy is gradually withdrawn

Adverse effects
- urticaria at injection site
- see also General Adverse effects of androgens and anabolic steroids (p. 1520)

Interactions
- not recommended with heparin
- if given with recombinant erythropoietin (especially in females) may enhance effects, requiring a decrease in dosage of erythropoietin
- see also General Interactions of androgens and anabolic steroids (p. 1520)

Nursing considerations/Cautions/Patient education
- for optimal effects, the patient should be advised to ensure their diet is rich in protein, vitamins and minerals
- contains benzyl alcohol and is not recommended in children < 3 years because of the increased risk of toxicity and anaphylaxis
- contraindicated in those with peanut or soya allergy
- see also General Nursing considerations/Cautions/Patient education for androgens and anabolic steroids (p. 1520)

 Contraindicated during pregnancy.

TESTOSTERONE
Trade names
AndroFeme 1, AndroForte 2, AndroForte 5, Testavan, Testogel

TESTOSTERONE DECANOATE
Trade name
Sustanon 250

TESTOSTERONE ENANTATE (ENANTHATE)
Trade name
Primoteston Depot

TESTOSTERONE UNDECANOATE
Trade names
Gonadron, Reandron 1000, Rejunon 1000, Testosterone ADVZ

Available forms
Ampoules (depot solution): 250 mg/mL, 1000 mg/4 mL;
Prefilled syringes (depot): 250 mg/mL;
Cream (testosterone): 10 mg/mL, 50mg/mL;
Transdermal gel (testosterone): 1%, 2%

Action
- androgen and anabolic
- female requirement is 10—20 times less than male
- (Undecanoate) maximum levels achieved after 7—14 days, then declines; half-life about 53 days
- see also General Actions of androgens and anabolic steroids (p. 1519)

SEX HORMONES

Use
- testosterone deficiency in females (AndroFem 1)
- see also General Uses of androgens and anabolic steroids (p. 1519)

Dose
- 250 mg IM every 3 weeks (Sustanon 250) **OR**
- 250 mg IM every 2–3 weeks then 250 mg IM every 3–6 weeks as maintenance (Primoteston Depot) **OR**
- 1000 mg IM every 10–14 weeks (Reandron 1000) **OR**
- (Transdermal gel) 50 mg testosterone (5 g gel (4 actuations)) applied in the morning, not exceeding 10 g of gel per day. The adjustment of dosage should be achieved by 2.5 g of gel steps. then dose adjusted by 2.5 g increments if needed after 3 days, according to serum testosterone levels (Testogel) **OR**
- (Transdermal gel) 23 mg (1 actuation) applied in the morning, adjusting dose by 23 mg increments according to serum testosterone levels; daily maximum 69 mg (3 actuations) (Testavan) **OR**
- (Females, cream) initially 5 mg (0.5 mL) via applicator applied daily to upper outer thigh or lower torso (AndroFem 1) **OR**
- (Male, cream) (0.5 mL/25 mg of testosterone) applied daily to scrotum with dose adjusted according to clinical response (AndroForte 5). The daily dose should be adjusted by the doctor depending on the clinical and/or laboratory response in individual patients, not exceeding 1 mL of cream per day. The adjustment of dosage should be achieved by 0.25 mL increments

Adverse effects
- (Injection site) pain, redness, irritation, itching, haematoma
- (Depot) urge to cough, coughing, respiratory distress, chest pain
- (Cream) mild skin irritation, rash, redness, itching, dermatitis, dryness
- (Depot, rare) pulmonary microembolism
- see also General Adverse effects of androgens and anabolic steroids (p. 1520)

Interactions
- see General Interactions of androgens and anabolic steroids (p. 1520)

Nursing considerations/Cautions
- (Depot) should be injected IM slowly to prevent coughing and respiratory distress. Oxygen may be administered to relieve any respiratory symptoms
- (Depot) injection intervals may be varied for maintenance
- (Transdermal patch/gel) serum testosterone should be measured (morning after application) before adjusting dose
- (Cream) may take 3–4 weeks before clinical response is apparent
- (Females, cream) serum testosterone levels should be measured 3 weeks after starting therapy and dose maintained at upper normal therapeutic range for females and then titrated. Follow-up is recommended at 4 and 12 weeks
- (Testavan) contains propylene glycol, which may cause skin irritation
- (Cream) contains almond oil and is therefore contraindicated if any allergy exists
- (Cream) contraindicated in females with normal reproductive function
- (Depot) some preparations contain arachis (peanut) oil, which is contraindicated in those with a peanut allergy. Should also be avoided in those with soya allergy because of the relationship between peanut and soya allergies
- see also General Nursing considerations/Cautions for androgens and anabolic steroids (p. 1520)

Patient education
- the patient should be advised to swallow capsules whole without chewing, and if an uneven number of tablets is taken the greater number should be taken in the morning
- see also General Patient education for androgens and anabolic steroids (p. 1521)

Transdermal gel
- gel is available in sachets or metered dose pump
- advise the patient to shower if skin-to-skin contact is anticipated to avoid transfer
- the patient should be advised to:
  - spread the gel on skin (clean, dry, healthy) and allow to dry for 3–5 minutes
  - cover the area with clothing after the gel has dried. This is especially important before contact with children or during sexual intercourse (the patient can shower and remove gel before sexual intercourse)
  - apply gel to shoulders, arms or abdomen, but not genital area
  - avoid bathing, swimming or showering for 6 hours after application
  - thoroughly wash hands with water and soap after application
  - if using gel from a metered dose pump:
    - the pump should be primed before first use by depressing the actuator 3–4 times and discarding any gel in these actuations
    - if using an application device, the applicator head should be placed under the pump and then the applicator used to spread gel evenly on required sites. The applicator should be cleaned with tissue and protective cap replaced
    - (Testogel pump) 50 mg = 4 actuations, 75 mg = 6 actuations, 100 mg = 8 actuations once daily

Transdermal cream
- instruct the patient to:
  - use the measuring applicator to ensure correct dosage
  - apply the cream to clean, dry, unbroken skin on the upper outer thigh or lower torso in areas of minimal hair and body fat
  - not apply cream to genitalia or perineum (unless otherwise directed)
  - (AndroForte 5) apply cream to clean, dry scrotal skin (unshaved)
  - massage cream into skin until absorbed
  - cover the area with clothing once the cream is absorbed
  - wash hands well with soap and water after application
  - avoid swimming or bathing for 1 hour after application
  - avoid contact with children or partner for 1 hour after application
  - rinse the applicator after use
  - (AndroFeme 1) do not apply perfume, deodorant or moisturiser to the same area

Contraindicated during pregnancy. Pregnant women should avoid contact with the application area (e.g. gel, cream, solution).

Contraindicated during breastfeeding. Testosterone suppresses prolactin in lactating females and may cause adverse effects in the infant.

OESTROGENS

General Actions of oestrogens
- secreted primarily by the ovarian follicles (from menarche to menopause) at a daily rate of about 70–500 micrograms of estradiol (oestradiol) (depending on the phase of the menstrual cycle). Estradiol (oestradiol) is converted to oestrone and small amounts of estriol (oestriol). After menopause, oestrogen is produced from the adrenal cortex (androstenedione) and converted to oestrone in peripheral tissues
- estradiol (oestradiol) is more potent than oestrone or estriol (oestriol) at receptor sites. Oestrogen receptors are found in the uterus, hypothalamus, pituitary, vagina, urethra, breast, liver and osteoblasts
- control ovulation and menstrual cycle and maintain pregnancy
- important for development and maintenance of accessory sex organs

(e.g. breasts, uterus, vagina) and secondary sex characteristics (e.g. differences in skeletal and muscle size, body fat and hair distribution)
- oestrogen production in ovaries decreases during menopause, resulting in vasomotor symptoms (sweating, hot flushes and atrophic vaginitis)
- decreased rate of bone absorption

General Adverse effects of oestrogens
- menstrual disorders (bleeding or spotting, dysmenorrhoea), reactivation of endometriosis, endometrial hyperplasia, pelvic pain, changes to cervical secretions, increase in size of uterine fibroids, uterine spasm/disorder
- breast tenderness/discomfort/tension, enlargement, pain and discharge
- change to corneal curvature, intolerance of contact lenses, visual disturbances, double vision and, rarely, retinal vascular thrombosis
- muscle cramps, back pain, arthralgia
- nausea, vomiting, abdominal pain/cramps, bloating, diarrhoea
- changes in libido
- hypertension
- headache, migraine, mood swings, nervousness, anxiety, depression, fatigue, dizziness
- acne, pruritus, rash, hirsutism, alopecia
- fluid retention/oedema
- body weight changes
- glucose intolerance
- increased serum triglycerides and, rarely, pancreatitis, gallbladder disease, cholestatic jaundice
- venous and arterial thromboembolic events (pulmonary embolism, deep vein thrombosis (DVT), stroke, myocardial infarction)
- (Rare/very rare) breast, ovarian or endometrial cancer, fibrocystic breast changes, dementia

General Interactions of oestrogens
- serum levels may be decreased by carbamazepine, phenobarbital (phenobarbitone), primidone, some antiviral agents, phenytoin, rifampicin, rifabutin, topiramate or St John's wort
- serum levels may be increased if given with erythromycin, clarithromycin, ciclosporin, itraconazole, ritonavir, paracetamol or grapefruit juice
- hot flushes and vaginal bleeding may occur if taken with St John's wort
- may affect serum levels and therefore the actions of antihypertensive agents theophylline, phenothiazines, diazepam, caffeine and tricyclic antidepressants (TCAs). For this reason, serum levels should be closely monitored and the dose adjusted accordingly
- may require an increased dose of thyroid hormones if given with oestrogens
- may affect a number of laboratory tests, including serum folate level, serum triglycerides and phospholipid, response to metyrapone test, glucose tolerance, gonadotrophin, plasma cortisol, thyroid function test, prothrombin and coagulation time. It is therefore recommended that the test(s) be repeated when the person has been oestrogen free for 1–2 months

General Nursing considerations/Cautions for oestrogens
- the patient should have a thorough examination (including personal and family history, breast, pelvic and abdominal examination and cervical cytology) before starting therapy and at 6- to 12-monthly intervals
- BP should be monitored regularly during therapy
- prolactinoma should be ruled out before starting therapy
- any persistent or recurring abnormal bleeding should be investigated to rule out malignancy before starting therapy
- if prolonged immobilisation is foreseen (e.g. elective surgery, especially of the lower limbs), therapy should be stopped for 4–6 weeks before surgery because of the risk of thromboembolic events

- if the patient is being treated for secondary amenorrhoea, the presence of a pituitary tumour should be excluded before starting therapy
- breast discomfort, breakthrough bleeding, water retention or bloating lasting for more than 6 weeks may indicate that the dose should be reduced
- continual therapy with oestrogen preparations (e.g. hormone replacement therapy) is thought to increase the risk of endometrial cancer and may also mask a predisposition to oestrogen-dependent breast cancer. Women with an intact uterus should also have progestogen daily for 10—14 days of each month added to oestrogen therapy. However, therapy should be at the lowest dose and for the shortest duration to produce effective results
- if possible, oestrogens should be stopped for 4—6 weeks before surgery or other lengthy periods of immobility
- thyroid function should be monitored regularly in those treated with thyroid hormone replacement therapy
- oestrogen treatment may increase the risk of gallbladder disease
- may lead to hypercalcaemia in patients with breast cancer and bone metastases
- not recommended for prevention of cardiovascular disease and dementia
- caution if used in those with cardiac or renal dysfunction, as fluid retention may exacerbate conditions
- caution if used in those with asthma, endometriosis, uterine fibroids, otosclerosis, migraine or severe headache, epilepsy, hereditary angioedema or hepatic haemangiomas, as conditions may be exacerbated
- caution if used in women with risk factors for arterial vascular disease (e.g. hypertension, diabetes mellitus, tobacco use, hypercholesterolaemia, obesity) and/or venous thromboembolism (e.g. a personal or family history of venous thromboembolism, obesity, systemic lupus erythematosus (SLE))
- caution if used in those with hypertriglyceridaemia, hypocalcaemia, hypothyroidism, impaired liver function, hepatic cholestasis, cholelithiasis, severe pruritus, cholestatic jaundice or a history of pregnancy-induced jaundice
- caution if used in those with a history of oestrogen-dependent tumours, endometriosis (or any endometrial hyperplasia) or fibrocystic disease of the breast
- contraindicated in those with undiagnosed genital bleeding; a confirmed venous thromboembolic event; recurrent venous or arterial thromboembolism; known thrombophilic disease (not receiving anticoagulants), thrombophlebitis; known, suspected or history of breast cancer; undiagnosed breast pathology; a suspected or known oestrogen-dependent tumour; endometrial hyperplasia (untreated); porphyria; hyperlipoproteinaemia; pregnancy-related problems (jaundice, severe pruritus, otosclerosis, herpes gestationis); severe uncontrolled hypertension; sickle cell anaemia; severe diabetes with vascular changes; endometriosis; acute liver disease or a history of liver disease (with abnormal liver function)
- contraindicated in non-hysterectomised women (unless progestogen therapy is given concurrently)

General Patient education for oestrogens

- the patient should be warned of possible weight gain
- advise the patient not to smoke while having oestrogen therapy, because it increases the risk of cardiovascular effects
- instruct the patient to avoid grapefruit juice during therapy
- the patient should be advised to seek medical advice if any of the following occur:
  - any shortness of breath or sudden chest pain, cough, lightheadedness, dizziness, rapid heart rate

SEX HORMONES

- sudden painful or tender leg swelling, increased limb warmth, skin discolouration
- any loss of vision, double vision, bulging eyes
- new or worsening migraine or headache
- any yellowing of skin or eyes, loss of appetite, nausea, itching, upper abdominal pain, dark urine or pale stools
- vaginal bleeding
* instruct patients with diabetes to closely monitor blood glucose levels, because glucose tolerance may be affected
* the patient should be advised that hormone replacement therapy (HRT) is recommended only for menopausal symptoms and is not meant for long-term therapy, so should be reviewed after 6 months
* warn the patient that slight spotting is normal but that heavier or persistent bleeding should be reported
* advise the patient to avoid driving or operating machinery if dizziness occurs
* women should be aware of an increased risk of heart disease and stroke associated with taking an oestrogen/progestogen combination
* if the patient wears contact lenses, she should be warned that intolerance to lenses may occur
* woman should be counselled to perform monthly breast self-examinations

 Not recommended during breastfeeding.

ESTRADIOL (OESTRADIOL)
Trade names
Estraderm MX, Estradot, Estramon, Estrofem, Estrogel, Estro-Pess, Progynova, Sandrena, Vagifem Low, Zumenon

Available forms
Tablets: 1 mg, 2 mg;
Transdermal patches: 25 microgram/24 hours, 37.5 microgram/24 hours, 50 microgram/24 hours, 75 microgram/24 hours, 100 microgram/24 hours;
Gel: 1 mg/g 1.25 g (actuation), 0.75 mg/g;
Vaginal tablet/pessary (modified-release): 10 microgram

Action
* (Transdermal patches) constant serum oestrogen levels produced while avoiding gastrointestinal adverse effects
* see also General Actions of oestrogens (p. 1524)

Use
* oestrogen deficiency due to natural or surgically induced menopause
* prevention of postmenopausal bone mineral density loss in women at high risk of osteoporosis and fractures

Dose
* (Menopausal symptoms) 1–2 mg orally daily, with a drug-free interval every 6 months to establish whether symptoms are still present **OR**
* (Menopausal symptoms) 0.75–1.5 mg (1–2 actuations) once daily, increasing the dose after 4 weeks if needed (gel) (Estrogel) **OR**
* (Menopausal symptoms) initially 0.5 mg daily, applied to the lower trunk or thigh, increasing the dose to 1.5 mg if needed (gel) (Sandrena) **OR**
* (Atrophic vaginitis) initially 10 micrograms PV daily for 14 days, then 10 micrograms twice weekly (vaginal tablet) **OR**
* (Oestrogen deficiency due to menopause) initially 50 microgram/24-hour patch applied every 3–7 days, then dose adjusted according to symptoms (transdermal patch) **OR**
* (Prevention of bone mineral density loss) initially 50–100 microgram/24-hour patch applied every 3–7 days, then dose adjusted according to symptoms (transdermal patch) **OR**
* (Prevention of bone mineral density loss) 1.5 mg (2 actuations) once daily (gel) (Estrogel)

Adverse effects
- (Transdermal patches) skin redness, itching, stinging, vesicle formation
- (Gel) skin irritation, itching, erythema
- see also General Adverse effects of oestrogens (p. 1525)

Interactions
- (Gel) not recommended with other medications that alter skin production
- see also General Interactions of oestrogens (p. 1525)

Nursing considerations/Cautions
- (Oral therapy, no uterus) therapy can be started on any day
- (Oral therapy, oligomenorrhoea) therapy should start on day 5 of bleeding
- Estraderm MX 25 transdermal patch is not recommended for prevention of bone mineral density loss in postmenopausal women
- in women not taking oral oestrogen currently, therapy with transdermal patch can be started immediately. If taking oral oestrogens, therapy can be started 5–7 days after stopping therapy
- (Postmenopausal bone mineral density loss) if the patient has established bone mineral loss, therapy should be started using 100 microgram/24 hour-transdermal patch
- (Women with intact uterus) progestogen should be taken for 10 days to avoid overstimulation of endometrial tissue
- if hot flushes have ceased, consideration should be given to changing to local vaginal therapy
- see also General Nursing considerations/Cautions for oestrogens (p. 1525)

Patient education
- see General Patient education for oestrogens (p. 1526)

Transdermal patch
- patches are available in different strengths that may have different application intervals (e.g. Estraderm is applied twice weekly)
- instruct the patient on the correct application technique, including:
    - rotation of application sites (e.g. upper buttock, lower part of the back or abdomen), allowing a 7-day interval before reusing the same site
    - applying the patch to a clean, dry area of the lower trunk or buttocks that will be covered by clothing (not waistline or skin folds where the patch may be easily rubbed loose)
    - pressing the patch firmly and holding it in place for 10 seconds
    - if the the patch falls off, it should be replaced for the remaining time
    - the patch should not be applied to breasts or broken skin
    - the patch should not be cut or torn
    - the patch should not be exposed to sunlight or solariums
    - the patient can bathe or shower as normal if the patch is correctly applied; however, it may fall off if exposed to a hot bath or sauna
- transdermal patches should be kept out of reach of children before and after use, because used patches still contain active hormone

Gel
- (Sandrena) gel should be applied and spread over an area 2–3 times the size of the hand
- advise the patient to wash hands well after application of gel and avoid applying to breasts, face, vulval area or any broken or irritated skin
- the patient should be instructed to vary application sites to avoid skin irritation
- instruct the patient that other skin products should not be applied within 1 hour of gel application
- gel should be allowed to dry for at least 5 minutes
- skin contact with others (e.g. partner, children) should be avoided for at least 1 hour after gel application. If contact is made, the person should wash the area well with soap and water

SEX HORMONES

- instruct the patient to avoid use of strong skin cleansers or detergents, products with high alcohol content or keratolytics
- advise the patient if the dose is forgotten (≤ 12 hours) it may be applied as soon as possible; if > 12 hours, apply gel the next day as per routine. Warn the patient not to apply a double dose
- if using a pump, the patient should be instructed to:
  - prime pump before first use and discard gel from this actuation
  - apply to intact skin (e.g. arms, shoulder, inner thighs)

Intravaginal tablets
- the patient should be instructed in the correct technique for application and insertion of intravaginal tablets, including correct care of the applicator

Tablet can be crushed and mixed with water or a spoonful of yoghurt or apple puree. Occupational hazard. Mask and gloves must be worn and a closed tablet crusher used.

Contraindicated during pregnancy.

Pregnant staff must not disperse or crush tablets.

Available in combination with
- estradiol 1.0 mg, drospirenone 2.0 mg. (Angeliq 1/2)
- estradiol 50 microgram (Estalis Sequi Week 1 and 2) (release/day));
- estradiol 50 microgram, norethisterone acetate 140 microgram (Estalis Sequi 50/140 Week 3 and 4 (release/day))
- estradiol (as hemihydrate) 0.75 mg (Estrogel gel); Progesterone (micronised) 100 mg (Prometrium capsules) (Estrogel Pro)
- estradiol (as hemihydrate) norethisterone acetate 1 mg (Kliogest)
- estradiol (as hemihydrate) 1 mg, norethisterone acetate 0.5 mg (Kliovance)
- estradiol valerate 3 mg (2 dark yellow tabs); estradiol valerate 2 mg, dienogest 2 mg (5 medium red tabs); estradiol valerate 2 mg, dienogest 3 mg (17 light yellow tabs); estradiol valerate 1 mg (2 dark red tabs), placebo (2 white tabs); lactose monohydrate (placebo) (Qlaira)
- estradiol 2 mg; estradiol 2 mg, norethisterone 1 mg (Trisequens)
- estradiol 1.0 mg, nomegestrol acetate 2.5 (Zoely)

ESTRIOL (OESTRIOL)
Trade names
Ovestin Cream, Ovestin Ovula Pessaries, Ovestin Tablets

Available forms
Tablets: 1 mg;
Pessaries: 0.5 mg;
Vaginal cream: 1 mg/g

Action
- short-acting
- particularly effective in managing urogenital symptoms
- increases urogenital epithelial cell resistance to infection and inflammation, reducing vaginal complaints
- half-life 5—7 hours
- see also General Actions of oestrogens (p. 1524)

Use
- vulvo-vaginal complaints due to oestrogen deficiency (e.g. atrophic vaginitis, pruritus vulvae, dyspareunia due to vulvovaginal atrophy)
- adjunct to vaginal infection treatment
- pre-vulvovaginal surgery
- suspect cytological smear

Dose
- initially up to 4 mg orally daily for the first 5—7 days, then reduced to 1—2 mg daily during the next 1—3 weeks as required **OR**
- (Vulvovaginal symptoms associated with menopause) initially 0.5 mg vaginal cream or pessary daily PV for 2—3 weeks, then 1—2 weekly for 2—3 months.

1529

Discontinued for 4 weeks every 2—3 months to assess necessity for further treatment **OR**
- (Before vulvovaginal surgery) 0.5 mg vaginal cream or pessary daily PV, starting 2 weeks preoperatively **OR**
- (Suspect cytological smear) 0.5 mg vaginal cream or pessary daily PV for 7 days before re-evaluation of smear

Adverse effects
- flu-like symptoms
- (Cream, pessary) local irritation, pruritus
- see also General Adverse effects of oestrogens (p. 1525)

Interactions
- may increase effects of corticosteroids, theophylline and succinylcholine
- see also General Interactions of oestrogens (p. 1525)

Nursing considerations/Cautions
- 1 applicatorful = 0.5 mg cream
- if switching from cyclic hormone replacement therapy (HRT), therapy should be started 7 days after completion of HRT cycle
- (Oral) may be given continuously or intermittently (tablet-free 5—7 days may be started after 3 weeks of treatment)
- tablets are contraindicated in those with hereditary galactose intolerance, Lapp lactase deficiency or glucose—galactose malabsorption
- see also General Nursing considerations/Cautions for oestrogens (p. 1525)

Patient education
- advise the patient that cream and pessaries should be used at night for optimal effect
- the patient should be instructed in the correct insertion technique for vaginal cream or pessaries
- after use, the applicator should be taken apart and washed in warm (not hot) soapy water
- (Oral) the patient should be advised that, if a dose is missed (> 12 hours), the dose should be taken when next scheduled. Warn the patient not to double the dose
- see also General Patient education for oestrogens (p. 1526)

Tablet cannot be crushed.

Contraindicated during pregnancy.

Caution with use in patients with a history of thromboembolic disorders.

Occupational hazard. Pregnant staff must not disperse or crush tablets.

OESTROGENS (CONJUGATED)
Trade name
Premarin

Available forms
Tablets: 0.3 mg, 0.625 mg

Action
- similar effects to endogenous oestrogens
- conjugated oestrogens are a mixture of natural oestrogens (of equine origin)
- see also General Actions of oestrogens (p. 1524)

Use
- natural or surgically induced menopause symptoms (moderate-to-severe vasomotor symptoms and atrophic vaginitis)
- hypoestrogenic states (e.g. female hypogonadism, primary ovarian failure, female castration)
- prevention of postmenopausal osteoporosis

Dose
- (Menopausal symptoms) 0.3—1.25 mg orally daily **OR**
- (Female hypogonadism) 2.5—7.5 mg orally daily in divided doses for 20 days, rest for 10 days. If no bleeding has occurred, dose is repeated **OR**

SEX HORMONES

- (Prevention of postmenopausal osteoporosis) 0.3—0.625 mg orally daily **OR**
- (Female castration, primary ovarian failure) initially 0.3—1.25 mg orally daily, then dose adjusted according to response

Adverse effects/Interactions
- see General Adverse effects/Interactions of oestrogens (p. 1525)

Nursing considerations/Cautions
- if used for atrophic vaginitis only, topical vaginal products should be considered first
- (Female hypogonadism) the number of courses needed to produce bleeding varies between women. If bleeding occurs before the end of the 10-day period, a 20-day combined oestrogen—progestogen regimen is suggested (with 2.5—7.5 mg daily in divided doses, with progestogen added in the last 5 days)
- should be used for postmenopausal osteoporosis only in women who are at high risk of osteoporosis and fractures where non-oestrogen therapies were contraindicated or the patient was intolerant of them
- an increased risk of stroke and deep vein thrombosis has been reported
- see also General Nursing considerations/Cautions for oestrogens (p. 1525)

Patient education
- advise the patient to swallow tablets whole, not chewed, crushed, divided or dissolved
- (Postmenopausal osteoporosis) women should be encouraged to maintain weight-bearing exercise and an adequate intake of calcium and vitamin D (with supplements if required)
- see also General Patient education for oestrogens (p. 1526)

 Tablets should not be divided, chewed, crushed or dispersed.

 Contraindicated during pregnancy.

 Not recommended during breastfeeding.

 Occupational hazard. Pregnant staff must not disperse or crush tablets.

Available in combination with
- conjugated oestrogens 0.45 mg, bazedoxifene 20 mg (Duavive)

PROGESTOGENS

General Actions of progestogens
- convert the endometrial proliferative phase to the secretory phase in preparation for the fertilised ovum
- progestogens are synthetic derivatives of progesterone
- suppress uterine motility
- alter cervical mucus hindering passage of sperm and/or ova
- promote breast development
- raise core body temperature (thermogenic)
- affect glucose tolerance and insulin resistance
- prevent further ovulation

General Uses of progestogens
- alone or with oestrogen in menstrual disorders (e.g. primary or secondary amenorrhoea, uterine bleeding caused by hormonal imbalance, primary dysmenorrhoea)
- endometriosis
- oral contraception (either alone or combined with an orally active oestrogen)
- postcoital emergency contraception
- adjunct to oestrogen replacement therapy (to prevent endometrial hyperplasia)
- recurrent and/or metastatic breast or renal cell cancer, inoperable recurrent or metastatic endometrial carcinoma

General Adverse effects of progestogens
- dizziness, depression, fatigue, malaise, emotional lability, headache, migraine,

- insomnia, somnolence, nervousness, tremor
- breast pain, tension, tenderness, enlargement, galactorrhoea
- hirsutism, acne, sweating, alopecia, oily hair, hot flushes, urticaria, rash, pruritus, eczema, melasma (chloasma) (blotchy brown pigmentation)
- menstrual changes (frequent, longer and/or irregular bleeding), spotting, breakthrough bleeding, amenorrhoea, dysmenorrhoea, changes in cervical secretions, vulvovaginitis, (low dose) benign ovarian cysts
- muscle cramps
- dyspnoea
- increased triglyceride levels
- hypertension
- visual disorders (including loss of vision (partial or complete), diplopia, retinal vascular lesions, optic neuritis) and, rarely, retinal vascular thrombosis
- weight gain, fluid retention, oedema
- nausea, constipation, diarrhoea, dry mouth, abdominal pain/cramp, bloating, flatulence, weight changes
- decreased glucose tolerance, exacerbation of diabetes mellitus, glycosuria
- arterial or venous thromboembolic disease, thrombophlebitis
- (Cancer treatment) Cushingoid symptoms
- (Rare) cholestatic jaundice, changes in liver function, liver tumours (benign or malignant), gallbladder disease, hypercalcaemia, ectopic pregnancy, exacerbation of porphyria
- (Rare) anaphylactoid-like reaction, anaphylaxis, angioedema

General Interactions of progestogens

- decreased serum levels may occur if given with phenytoin, barbiturates, primidone, carbamazepine, rifampicin, oxcarbazepine, rifabutin, griseofulvin, topiramate, bosentan or St John's wort
- increased serum levels may occur if given with itraconazole, fluconazole, voriconazole, erythromycin, clarithromycin, diltiazem, verapamil or grapefruit juice
- caution if given with HIV protease (e.g. ritonavir) and non-nucleoside transcript inhibitors (e.g. efavirenz) because of variable effects
- may increase serum levels of ciclosporin, increasing the risk of toxicity
- may interfere with a number of laboratory tests, including plasma testosterone level (males), plasma progestogen and oestrogen levels (females), gonadotrophin level, cortisol level, glucose tolerance, metyrapone test, sex hormone binding globulin level and coagulation test values for prothrombin and factors VII, VIII, IX and X

General Nursing considerations/ Cautions for progestogens

- the patient should have a thorough examination (including personal and family history, BP, breast, pelvic and abdominal examination and cervical cytology) before starting therapy and at 6- to 12-monthly intervals
- pregnancy should be excluded before starting therapy
- therapy should be stopped if there is a constantly elevated BP or if raised BP does not respond to antihypertensive therapy
- fluid retention occurs frequently, therefore some patients, including those with cardiac and renal disorders, asthma, epilepsy or migraine, may require closer than usual monitoring, especially in the initial phases of the therapy
- patients with an intact uterus should be given a progestogen daily for 10—14 days of each month of oestrogen therapy
- therapy should be stopped 4 weeks before planned surgery and restarted 2 weeks after complete mobilisation
- prolactin-producing tumour should be excluded before starting therapy for amenorrhoea

SEX HORMONES

- caution if used in those with liver impairment, as progestogens may be poorly metabolised
- caution if used in women with a previous history of extrauterine pregnancy or impaired tube function because of an increased risk of ectopic pregnancy
- caution if used in women with hyperlipidaemia, as some progestogens may increase low-density lipoprotein (LDL) levels and increase risk of pancreatitis
- caution if used in patients with pre-existing depression
- caution if used in patients with pre-existing diabetes mellitus, because glucose tolerance may be affected by progestogens
- caution if used in women with history of chloasma gravidarum
- caution if used in women with endometriosis, because of an increased risk of breakthrough bleeding
- the risk of thromboembolic events increases with age, obesity, positive family history, prolonged immobilisation, major surgery or trauma, leg surgery, smoking (especially in women > 35 years), valvular heart disease, migraine, atrial fibrillation and dyslipoproteinaemia
- contraindicated in those with history of or active severe liver disease or dysfunction (where liver function tests have not returned to normal), Dubin—Johnson syndrome, Rotor syndrome, active venous or arterial thromboembolic disorders, thrombophlebitis, severe hypertension, sickle cell anaemia, migraine (with focal neurological symptoms), diabetes mellitus (with nephropathy, retinopathy, neuropathy or vascular disease), undiagnosed abnormal vaginal or urinary tract bleeding, cervical dysplasia, cerebrovascular or coronary artery disease, carcinoma of breast or genital organ, benign or malignant liver tumours or hormone-dependent tumour

General Patient education for progestogens

- women treated for endometriosis should be warned that breakthrough bleeding may occur
- the patient should be advised to seek medical advice immediately if any of the following occur:
  - migraine headache for the first time or an increase in frequency or severity of headache
  - dizziness, weakness, numbness (especially if marked and one-sided), slurred speech or difficulty speaking
  - disturbed vision, including asymmetrical vision loss or double vision
  - pain/tenderness or swelling in leg, increased limb warmth, discolouration
  - pain/tightness in the chest (especially if radiating down the left arm), unexplained cough, breathlessness or difficulty breathing
  - depression, sadness, change in appetite, loss of interest in previously pleasurable activities, social withdrawal
  - yellowing of skin or eyes or itching of skin
- the patient should be warned about increase in weight and changes to menstrual bleeding pattern (frequency, duration and/or heaviness)
- advise the patient to avoid driving or operating machinery if dizziness occurs
- instruct the patient to avoid grapefruit juice during therapy
- instruct the patient with diabetes mellitus to monitor blood glucose levels more frequently
- if the patient has a tendency to melasma (chloasma) (blotchy brown pigmentation), she should be advised to avoid excessive sunlight or UV exposure during therapy
- the patient should be warned that withdrawal bleeding usually occurs on discontinuation of treatment

- women should be advised that oral contraceptives do not protect against HIV infection, AIDS and other sexually transmitted diseases
- barrier method contraception is recommended during combined therapy and for 28 days after stopping some medication such as rifampicin

ETONOGESTREL

Trade name
Implanon NXT

Available form
Implants: 68 mg

Action
- biologically active metabolite of desogestrel that inhibits ovulation
- effects reversible on removal of implant
- see also General Actions of progestogens (p. 1531)

Use
- long-term contraception

Dose
- implants (68 mg) are inserted under the skin (inner side of upper arm) after area is locally anaesthetised; replaced every 3 years

Adverse effects
- (Insertion site) pain, redness, swelling, bruising, irritation, itching, fibrosis, abscess, scar
- expulsion (if insert not correctly inserted) or migration (if inserted too deeply)
- see also General Adverse effects of progestogens (p. 1531)

Interactions
- see General Interactions of progestogens (p. 1532)

- plasma levels are inversely related to woman's weight; therefore some consideration should be given to replacing insert earlier in women with heavier body weight, as implant may be less effective by the third year
- if no hormonal contraceptive was taken during the preceding month, the implant should be inserted on day 1 to 5 of menstrual cycle (day 1 = first day of bleeding)
- if changing from a combination oral contraceptive, vaginal ring or transdermal patch, the implant should be inserted on next day after last day of active tablet of combination contraceptive, day of removal or when application was due
- if changing from progestogen-only contraceptive, the implant should be inserted immediately, with no break from progestogen-only tablets
- if changing from non-oral progestogen-only contraception (i.e. injection or implant), the implant should be inserted on removal of different implant or when next injection was due
- if following first-trimester abortion/miscarriage, the implant should be inserted immediately
- if following second-trimester abortion/miscarriage, the implant should be inserted on day 21 to 28 after abortion/miscarriage
- if postpartum and not breastfeeding, the implant should be inserted on day 21 to 28 after delivery
- if postpartum and breastfeeding, the implant should be inserted after the 4th postpartum week
- see also General Nursing considerations/Cautions for progestogens (p. 1532)

Nursing considerations/Cautions
- inserted subdermally into non-dominant arm
- medical review is recommended 3 months after insertion to monitor BP and any side-effects

Patient education
- women should be given a user card which records batch number and date of insertions
- until the presence and effect of the implant has been confirmed, it is

SEX HORMONES

- recommended that barrier contraception is used
- barrier method contraception is recommended for first 7 days if avoiding pregnancy when changing from another method to an etonogestrel implant
- warn the patient that bleeding pattern during first 3 months after implant insertion is likely to be the future pattern of bleeding
- advise the patient that she should be able to feel implant under skin
- warn the patient that effects wear off quickly after implant is removed
- see also General Patient education for progestogens (p. 1533)

 Contraindicated during pregnancy; the implant should be removed if pregnancy occurs.

Available in combination with
- etonogestrol 11.7 mg, ethinyloestradiol 2.7 mg (NuvaRing).

LEVONORGESTREL
Trade names
Kyleena, Levonelle-1, Levonorgestrel-1, Microlut, Mirena, NorLevo-1, Novella-1, Postella-1, Postinor-1, Postrelle-1

Available forms
Tablets: 30 microgram, 1.5 mg;
Intrauterine device (IUD): 19.5 mg, 52 mg

Action
- inhibits ovulation
- may also cause endometrial changes that prevent implantation
- (Postcoital emergency contraception) efficacy decreases with time after intercourse (95% efficacy if used within 24 hours, reduces to 58% between 48 and 72 hours)
- (IUD) low-dose release directly into uterine cavity
- no antiandrogenic or glucocorticoid properties but some partial androgenic activity
- see also General Actions of progestogens (p. 1531)

Use
- postcoital emergency contraception (within 72 hours) (Levonelle-1, NorLevo-1, Postella-1, Postinor-1, Postrelle-1)
- see also General Uses of progestogens (p. 1531)

Dose
- (Long-term contraception) 52 mg device inserted into uterine cavity (IUD) (Mirena) **OR**
- (Long-term contraception) 19.5 mg device inserted into uterine cavity (IUD) (Kyleena) **OR**
- (Oral contraception) 30 micrograms orally daily **OR**
- (Postcoital emergency contraception within 72 hours) 1.5 mg orally as soon as possible after unprotected sexual intercourse and within 72 hours

Adverse effects
- (IUD) expulsion, bleeding, pain and, rarely, infection, perforation or penetration of uterus or cervix, ectopic pregnancy
- (High dose) nausea, vomiting, vaginal bleeding, headache, breast pain
- see also General Adverse effects of progestogens (p. 1531)

Interactions
- see General Interactions of progestogens (p. 1532)

Nursing considerations/Cautions
- (Contraception) pregnancy should be excluded before starting therapy
- (IUD) any genital infection should be treated before insertion of an IUD
- (IUD) the patient should be assessed for any pelvic infection risk factors (e.g. previous history of pelvic infection, sexually transmitted disease, multiple sexual partners)

- (Postcoital contraception) BP should be measured before therapy is given
- (Postcoital contraception) efficacy may be impaired if the patient has severe diarrhoea, vomiting or malabsorption such as Crohn's disease
- (Postcoital emergency contraception only) can be taken at any time during menstrual cycle
- for oral contraception:
  - if no hormonal contraceptive was taken during preceding month, oral therapy should be started on the first day of the menstrual cycle
  - if changing from a combination oral contraceptive, oral therapy should be started on the next day after the last day of active tablet of combination contraceptive and omit a pill-free interval
  - if changing from a progestogen-only contraceptive, oral therapy can be started immediately with no break from progestogen-only tablets
  - if changing from non-oral progestogen-only contraception, oral therapy can be started on the day of implant removal or when the next injection was due. Barrier method contraception is recommended for the first 7 days if avoiding pregnancy
  - if following abortion, oral therapy can be started immediately
  - if following delivery, oral therapy can be started 4 weeks after delivery if not breastfeeding. Barrier method contraception is recommended for the first 7 days if avoiding pregnancy
- (IUD) levonorgestrel is slowly released and contains sufficient quantities to be effective for up to 5 years
- IUD should be inserted within 7 days of onset of menstruation or immediately after first-trimester abortion
- postpartum IUD insertion should be postponed for at least 6 weeks after delivery or longer until the uterus is fully involuted
- for those with amenorrhoea, IUD insertion can be at any time or the last day of menstruation or withdrawal bleeding
- insertion/removal of IUD is associated with pain and bleeding, and this may precipitate a vasovagal reaction (or seizure if the patient has epilepsy)
- (IUD) the patient should be examined after 4–12 weeks post-insertion and then yearly (or more frequently if needed)
- (IUD) infection may occur within 4 weeks of insertion. If infection recurs, is severe or does not respond to antibiotics, the IUD should be removed
- (IUD) should be removed after 5 years and a new system re-inserted if the patient wants to continue with IUD therapy
- (IUD) should not be first-line treatment for nulligravid women or postmenopausal women with advanced uterine atrophy (making insertion difficult)
- (IUD) caution if used in those with a history of ectopic pregnancy, congenital heart disease or valvular heart disease at risk of infectious endocarditis. Antibiotic prophylaxis is required when inserting or removing the IUD
- (IUD) caution if used in women with migraine, focal migraine with asymmetrical visual loss (or other symptoms of transient cerebral ischaemia), severe headache, jaundice, increased BP, stroke or myocardial infarction. If any of these occur for the first time, consideration should be given to removing the IUD
- (IUD) contraindicated in women with pelvic inflammatory disease (current or recurrent history), lower genital tract infection, postpartum endometriosis, infected abortion in the last 3 months, cervicitis, cervical dysplasia, uterine or cervical neoplasm, confirmed or suspected hormone-dependent tumour, undiagnosed abnormal uterine bleeding, congenital or acquired uterine anomaly, predisposition to infection or active liver disease or tumour

SEX HORMONES

- see also General Nursing considerations/Cautions for progestogens (p. 1532)

Patient education

- see General Patient education for progestogens (p. 1533)

Postcoital emergency contraception

- if the patient presents multiple times for postcoital contraception, she should be counselled to consider long-term contraception
- if the patient vomits within 2 hours, she should be advised to return to the doctor, pharmacy or clinic

Oral contraception

- the patient should be advised to take oral medication at same time every day
- barrier method contraception is recommended until onset of the next period
- if vomiting or diarrhoea occurs within 4 hours of oral administration, advise the patient to replace it using the last tablet from pack
- if the tablet is forgotten (more than 27-hour interval between doses), it should be taken when remembered regardless of timing, and barrier method contraception used during sexual intercourse for the next 7 days if avoiding pregnancy
- warn women that ectopic pregnancy may occur if pregnancy occurs during treatment

IUD

- the patient should be instructed to feel for two threads at the end of the device after each menstrual period
- the patient should be warned that irregular bleeding or spotting (in addition to normal menstrual bleeding) is common with an IUD for the first 3–6 months after insertion
- the patient should be advised that re-examination should occur 4–12 weeks after insertion and then yearly until removed after 5 years
- advise the patient that if an IUD is removed mid-cycle and they have sexual intercourse, there is an increased risk of pregnancy occurring
- the patient should be advised to seek medical advice immediately if any of the following occur:
  - length of removal threads increases or stem of IUD becomes visible in the cervix (expulsion may be imminent)
  - there is a noticeable increase in menstrual flow
  - removal threads cannot be felt
  - there is persistent lower abdominal pain, fever, abnormal bleeding or discharge and/or pain during sexual intercourse (especially in first 4 weeks after IUD insertion, as it may indicate infection)

 Crushing tablets is not recommended as the dose may be altered.

 (IUD) not recommended during pregnancy. If pregnancy occurs, the IUD should be removed.

(Oral contraception) contraindicated during pregnancy.

(Postcoital emergency contraception) not recommended during pregnancy.

Available in combination with

- ethinyloestradiol 30 microgram, levonorgestrel 150 microgram (Eleanor, Evelyn, Femme-Tab ED 30/150, Lenest, Levlen ED, Microgynon 30 ED, Monofeme)
- ethinyloestradiol 20 microgram, levonorgestrel 100 microgram (Femme-Tab ED 20/100, Louette, Microgynon 20 ED)
- levonorgestrel 150 microgram, ethinylestradiol 30 microgram (pink tablet); ethinylestradiol 10 microgram (white tablet) (Seasonique)
- levonorgestrel 50 microgram (brown tablet); ethinylestradiol 40 microgram, levonorgestrel 75 microgram (white tablet); ethinylestradiol 30 microgram,

levonorgestrel 125 microgram (ochre/yellow tablet) (Trifeme, Triquilar ED)

MEDROXYPROGESTERONE ACETATE

Trade names
Depo-Provera, Depo-Ralovera, Provera, Ralovera

Available forms
Vial: 150 mg/mL;
Prefilled syringe: 150 mg/mL;
Tablets: 2.5 mg, 5 mg, 10 mg, 100 mg, 200 mg, 250 mg, 500 mg

Action
- more potent than progesterone
- has anabolic effects with little to no androgenic or oestrogenic activity
- see also General Actions of progestogens (p. 1532)

Use
- see General Uses of progestogens (p. 1531)

Dose
- (Inoperable, recurrent metastatic endometrial and renal carcinoma) 600–1200 mg IM weekly, then 450–600 mg every 1–4 weeks (maintenance) **OR**
- (Breast cancer) 500 mg IM daily for 4 weeks, then 500–1000 mg at weekly intervals (maintenance) **OR**
- (Endometriosis) 50 mg IM weekly or 100 mg IM 2-weekly for at least 6 months **OR**
- (Endometrial or renal cell carcinoma) 200–400 mg orally daily **OR**
- (Breast cancer) 500 mg orally daily until progression of disease **OR**
- (Endometriosis) 10 mg orally 3 times daily for 90 consecutive days, starting day 1 of the menstrual cycle **OR**
- (Secondary amenorrhoea) 2.5–10 mg orally daily for 5–10 days beginning with day 16–21 of cycle and repeated for 3 consecutive cycles **OR**
- (Abnormal uterine bleeding) 2.5–10 mg orally daily for 5–10 days, beginning day 16–21 of the cycle and repeated for 3 consecutive cycles **OR**
- (Adjunct to oestrogen therapy) 10–20 mg orally daily for at least 10 days of the cycle **OR**
- (Adjunct to oestrogen therapy) 5 mg orally daily for 28 days of the cycle **OR**
- (Contraception) 150 mg IM every 3 months

Adverse effects
- (IM) gluteal infiltration, abscess formation
- decreased bone mineral density
- see also General Adverse effects of progestogens (p. 1531)

Interactions
- see General Interactions of progestogens (p. 1532)

Nursing considerations/Cautions
- (IM, contraception) if the interval between IM injections is > 14 weeks, pregnancy should be excluded
- (IM, contraception) the first injection should be given during the first 5 days of onset of normal menstrual period, within 5 days postpartum (if not breastfeeding), or if breastfeeding at sixth week postpartum (after pregnancy has been excluded)
- volumes of 2.5 mL or greater should be given IM in divided doses to prevent gluteal infiltration and abscess formation
- vial should be well shaken before use
- administration should be by deep IM injection into the gluteal muscle
- bone mineral density should be measured regularly if prolonged therapy is indicated
- (Endometriosis, contraception) should be used long term (> 2 years) only if other methods are inadequate
- (Depo-Provera/Depo-Ralovera) not recommended for secondary amenorrhoea or dysfunctional uterine bleeding
- (Endometriosis, contraception) caution if used in those with chronic alcohol and/or tobacco use, a strong family history of osteoporosis, or chronic use of agents that decrease bone mass (e.g. antiepileptic agents, corticosteroids) because of the increased risk of osteoporosis
- see also General Nursing considerations/Cautions for progestogens (p. 1532)

SEX HORMONES

Patient education

- women with endometriosis should be advised that breakthrough bleeding is likely to occur
- women should be warned that therapy may result in prolonged contraception. Median time to conceive was 10 months (range 4—31 months) after last injection and was not related to duration of use
- (Oral) advise patient to swallow tablets whole and not crush or chew
- (Prolonged therapy) all patients should be advised to have sufficient calcium and vitamin D in their diets
- see also General Patient education for progestogens (p. 1533)

Tablets can be dispersed in water. May be crushed and given with yoghurt or apple puree. Occupational hazard. Mask and gloves must be worn and closed tablet crusher used.

Contraindicated during pregnancy.

Pregnant staff must not disperse or crush tablets (crush if enteral feeding tube).

NORETHISTERONE

Trade names
Noriday 28, Primolut N

Available forms
Tablets: 350 microgram, 5 mg

Action
- little androgenic effect
- thermogenic, altering basal body temperature
- partly metabolised to ethinylestradiol
- see also General Actions of progestogens (p. 1531)

Use
- see General Uses of progestogens (p. 1531)

Dose
- (Dysfunctional bleeding) 5 mg orally 3 times daily for 10 days (Primolut N) **OR**
- (Prevention of recurrence of dysfunctional bleeding) 5 mg orally 1—2 times daily from day 16 to day 25 of menstrual cycle (Primolut N) **OR**
- (Primary or secondary amenorrhoea) endometrial priming with oestrogen product for 14 days, then 5 mg norethisterone orally 1—2 times daily for 10 days and continued for 2—3 cycles (Primolut N) **OR**
- (Premenstrual syndrome) 5 mg orally 1—3 times daily from day 19 to day 26 of the menstrual cycle (Primolut N) **OR**
- (Endometriosis) 5 mg orally twice daily starting between day 1 and day 5 of menstrual cycle for 4—6 months. If spotting occurs, dose can be increased to 10 mg twice daily, then decrease dose when bleeding has decreased (Primolut N) **OR**
- (Tming of menstruation) 5 mg orally 2—3 times daily for 10—14 days, starting 3 days before expected menstruation. Bleeding should occur in 2—3 days after stopping medication (Primolut N) **OR**
- (Contraception) 350 micrograms orally daily, starting on first day of menstrual cycle (Noriday 28)

Adverse effects
- see General Adverse effects of progestogens (p. 1531)

Interactions
- see General Interactions of progestogens (p. 1532)

Nursing considerations/Cautions

- (Dysfunctional bleeding) bleeding usually stops in 1—3 days; however, if it does not stop, an organic or extragenital cause should be investigated
- see also General Nursing considerations/Cautions for progestogens (p. 1532)

Patient education

- (Contraception) if the tablet is forgotten (more than 27-hour interval between doses), the patient should be instructed to take it when remembered, regardless

of timing, and barrier method contraception used for the next 7 days if avoiding pregnancy
- see also General Patient education for progestogens (p. 1533)

Crushing may pose an unacceptable level of risk to those preparing or giving medicine.

Contraindicated during pregnancy, as progestogens can cause masculinisation of a female fetus.

Occupational hazard. Pregnant staff must not disperse or crush tablets.

Available in combination with
- estradiol 50 microgram + norethisterone acetate 140 microgram release/day (Estalis Continuous 50/140 Transdermal patches)
- estradiol 50 microgram + norethisterone acetate 250 microgram release/day (Estalis Continuous 50/250 Transdermal patches)
- estradiol 50 microgram (Estalis Sequi Week 1 and 2) (release/day)); estradiol 50 microgram, norethisterone acetate 140 microgram (Estalis Sequi 50/140 Week 3 and 4 (release/day))
- estradiol 50 microgram (Estalis Sequi Week 1 and 2) (release/day)); estradiol 50 microgram, norethisterone acetate 250 microgram (Estalis Sequi 50/250 Week 3 and 4 (release/day))
- estradiol (as hemihydrate) 2 mg, norethisterone acetate 1 mg (Kliogest)
- estradiol (as hemihydrate) 1 mg, norethisterone acetate 0.5 mg (Kliovance)
- ethinyloestradiol 35 microgram, norethisterone 1mg (Norimin-1)
- ethinyloestradiol 35 microgram, norethisterone 500 microgram (Norimin)
- mestranol 50 microgram, norethisterone 1 mg (Norinyl-1)
- relugolix 40 mg, estradiol (as hemihydrate) 1 mg, norethisterone acetate 0.5 mg (Ryeqo)
- estradiol 2 mg; estradiol 2 mg, norethisterone 1 mg (Trisequens)

OTHER AGENTS

CYPROTERONE ACETATE
Trade names
Androcur, Anterone, Cyrotone, Cyproterone Sandoz

Available forms
Tablets: 50 mg, 100 mg

Action
- antiandrogenic agent with progestogenic and antigonadotrophic properties

Use
- (Women) moderate-to-severe signs of androgenisation (hirsutism, androgenic alopecia, acne and/or seborrhoea)
- (Men) reduce drive for men with sexual deviations, inoperable prostatic carcinoma (with a luteinising hormone-releasing hormone (LHRH) agonist)

Dose

Women
- (Hirsutism secondary to androgenisation in premenopausal women) 50 mg orally daily for 10 days from days 1—10 of the menstrual cycle until there is a satisfactory response, then reduce dose **OR**
- (Signs of androgenisation in premenopausal women) 100 mg orally at the same time each day with some liquid after a meal from days 1—10 of the menstrual cycle, reducing to 10—50 mg with clinical improvement (with progestogen/oestrogen contraceptive starting on day 1 of cycle) **OR**
- (Androgenisation in postmenopausal/hysterectomised women) 25—50 mg orally daily for 21 days followed by 7 days drug free, continuing for several months

Men
- (Reduction of sexual drive) initially 50 mg orally twice daily, then increasing dose to 100 mg 2—3 times daily to achieve a satisfactory response; the dose

SEX HORMONES

may then be gradually reduced to 25—50 mg (maintenance) **OR**
- (Prostate cancer: to decrease 'flare' associated with LHRH agonists) initially 100 mg orally twice daily for 5—7 days, then 100 mg twice daily for 3—4 weeks with LHRH agonists **OR**
- (Prostate cancer, advanced without orchiectomy) 100 mg orally 2—3 times daily **OR**
- (Prostate cancer, treatment for hot flushes associated with LHRH agonists or in those who have had orchiectomy) 50 mg orally 1—3 times daily, increasing gradually to 100 mg 3 times daily if needed

Adverse effects
- tiredness, headache, depression, fatigue, restlessness
- GI disturbances, nausea
- increased or decreased weight
- reduced libido
- hot flushes, sweating
- anaemia
- (High dose) shortness of breath
- (Women) inhibited ovulation, menstrual cycle irregularity, spotting, breast pain, breast tension
- (Men) impaired spermatogenesis, gynaecomastia, breast tenderness, osteoporosis, erectile dysfunction
- arterial or venous thromboembolic events
- (Rare) benign or malignant liver tumours, liver toxicity, rash, meningioma

Interactions
- may alter requirements for insulin or oral hypoglycaemic agents
- increased risk of myopathy and/or rhabdomyolysis if given with 3-hydroxy-3-methylglutaryl coenzyme A (HMG-CoA) inhibitors (statins)
- metabolism may be inhibited by itraconazole, ritonavir and clotrimazole increasing serum levels
- increased metabolism may occur if given with rifampicin, phenytoin or St John's wort, decreasing serum levels

Nursing considerations/Cautions
- (Female) complete medical examination, including cervical cytological smear and breast examination, should be completed before the start and regularly throughout therapy. Other causes of androgenisation (e.g. adrenal or ovarian cancer) should be ruled out before starting therapy
- pregnancy should be excluded before starting therapy
- baseline liver function tests, blood counts, blood clotting, thyroid function, adrenal function, blood glucose and agglutination should be measured before starting therapy and regularly throughout
- in premenopausal women (of childbearing potential) an oestrogen/progestogen combination should be added to ensure contraception and stabilise the cycle
- (Women) treatment should start on the first day of the menstrual cycle (first day of bleeding). Women with amenorrhoea or an irregular menstrual cycle can start therapy immediately
- (Men) one control spermatogram is made before the start of treatment; spermatogenesis may take 3—20 months to return to normal after discontinuing treatment
- tablets contain lactose and are not recommended in those with rare hereditary problems of galactose intolerance, Lapp lactase deficiency or glucose—galactose malabsorption
- caution when used to treat prostate cancer, because there is an increased risk of liver toxicity
- caution if used in those with diabetes mellitus
- not recommended before conclusion of puberty
- contraindicated in those with liver disease (including jaundice and pruritus associated with pregnancy), previous or current

liver tumours, a history of herpes in pregnancy, wasting diseases (not prostate cancer), severe chronic depression, predisposition to thromboembolic events, severe diabetes mellitus (with vascular changes), sickle cell anaemia, present or a history of meningioma, Dubin–Johnson syndrome or Rotor syndrome

Patient education

- the patient should be advised to avoid driving or operating machinery if tiredness or inability to concentrate occurs
- instruct women to seek medical attention if any persistent or recurrent bleeding occurs at irregular intervals
- women should be warned that hirsutism and alopecia may recur when therapy is stopped
- the patient should be advised to report any unusual tiredness, dark urine, persistent loss of appetite, yellowing of skin or eyes, upper abdominal pain or unexplained flu-like symptoms
- women should be instructed to take medication at the same time every day
- if tablets are missed, contraceptive effectiveness may be reduced and the patient should be advised to use barrier contraceptive methods, and continue to take tablets according to the normal regimen
- instruct female patients that tablet taking should not be interrupted if unscheduled bleeding occurs during the 3-week cycle in which the tablets are being taken

 Tablet can be dispersed in water or crushed and mixed with yoghurt or apple puree if necessary. Occupational hazard. Mask and gloves must be worn and closed tablet crusher used.

 Pregnancy must be excluded at the start of treatment and ethinylestradiol taken as well to ensure contraception. If taken during pregnancy, may lead to feminisation of male fetus; therefore it is contraindicated.

 Contraindicated during breastfeeding.

 Pregnant staff must not disperse or crush tablets.

Available in combination with
- ethinylestradiol 35 microgram, cyproterone acetate 2 mg (Brenda-35 ED, Diane-35 ED, Estelle-35 ED, Jene-35 ED, Juliet-35 ED)

FLUTAMIDE
Trade name
Flutamin

Available form
Tablets: 250 mg

Action
- non-steroidal antiandrogen with specific effects on the prostate

Use
- advanced prostatic carcinoma (with luteinising hormone-releasing hormone (LHRH) agonist) in previously untreated patients
- prophylaxis of disease 'flare' associated with LHRH agonist

Dose
- 250 mg orally 3 times daily, at 8-hour intervals, starting 24 hours before taking LHRH agonist

Adverse effects
- anorexia, constipation, diarrhoea
- insomnia, tiredness, headache, dizziness, malaise, drowsiness, depression, confusion
- peripheral oedema
- urine colour change (amber to yellow-green)
- blood dyscrasias, anaemia
- gynaecomastia, breast tenderness, galactorrhoea
- elevated liver enzymes and blood urea nitrogen (BUN)
- decreased glucose tolerance

SEX HORMONES

- cholestatic jaundice, hepatic encephalopathy, hepatic necrosis
- (With LHRH agonist) hot flushes, decreased libido, impotence, nausea, vomiting, diarrhoea, decreased bone density
- (Rare) prolongation of QT interval, increased risk of cardiovascular disease

Interactions

- may increase prothrombin time if given with warfarin; therefore should be monitored carefully, especially when starting or stopping therapy
- caution if given with paracetamol, NSAIDs or opioids
- caution if used with agents known to prolong QT interval
- may increase serum levels of theophylline

Nursing considerations/Cautions

- only for use in males
- before starting therapy, cardiovascular and osteoporosis risk factors should be evaluated
- haemoglobin should be monitored regularly during therapy
- liver function tests are recommended before starting, monthly for 4 months and throughout therapy. If serum transaminases are 2–3 times normal, therapy should not be started
- blood glucose levels and/or glycated haemoglobin (HbA1c) should be monitored if combined with LHRH analogues
- caution if used in men at risk of cardiovascular disease or with congenital QT interval, electrolyte imbalance or congestive cardiac failure
- caution if used in those with chronic alcohol and/or tobacco use, a strong family history of osteoporosis or chronic use of agents that decrease bone mass (e.g. antiepileptic agents, corticosteroids)
- contraindicated in those with severe liver impairment

Patient education

- the patient should be advised to seek medical advice if any unusual tiredness, itching, dark urine, persistent loss of appetite, yellowing of eyes or skin, upper abdominal pain or unexplained flu-like symptoms occur
- warn the patient that urine colour change (amber to yellow-green) is harmless
- advise the patient to avoid driving or operating machinery if dizziness, drowsiness or confusion occurs
- the patient should be warned that he may experience an increase in breast size, breasts may become tender and sometimes secrete fluid

 Tablets can be dispersed in water, or crushed and mixed with a spoonful of yoghurt or apple puree. Occupational hazard: mask and gloves must be worn and a closed tablet crusher used.

 No studies have been conducted in pregnant women; therefore consider the possibility of harm to the fetus.

 No studies have been conducted in lactating women; therefore consider the possibility of harm from the drug entering breastmilk.

 Caution in hepatic impairment: hospitalisation and, rarely, death due to liver failure in patients taking flutamide. Evidence of hepatic injury included elevated serum transaminase levels, jaundice, hepatic necrosis and hepatic encephalopathy,

 Pregnant staff must not open capsules.

PRASTERONE

Trade name
Intrarosa

Available form
Pessary: 6.5 mg

Action
- biochemically and biologically identical to endogenous human dehydroepiandrosterone (DHEA)
- steroid precursor with little or no activity, but is converted into oestrogens and androgens (metabolites), which then activate both oestrogen and androgen receptors

Use
- treatment of vulvar and vaginal atrophy in postmenopausal women experiencing moderate-to-severe symptoms

Dose
- 6.5 mg (one pessary) intravaginally nocte

Adverse effects
- vaginal discharge
- abnormal Pap smear
- weight fluctuation
- urinary tract infection
- (Uncommon) breast mass (benign), cervical/uterine polyps
- (Rare) increased risk of breast cancer, ovarian cancer, venous thromboembolism, coronary artery disease, ischaemic stroke

Interactions
- not recommended with systemic hormone replacement therapy or vaginal oestrogens
- caution if used in women on chronic anticoagulant therapy

Nursing considerations/Cautions
- any vaginal infection should be treated before starting therapy
- therapy should be started in women only where symptoms are negatively impacting on quality of life
- re-evaluation (including check-ups, blood pressure monitoring, Pap smears) should occur every 6 months and therapy continued only while benefits of therapy outweigh risks
- before starting therapy, a complete personal and family history should be taken, including physical (pelvic, breast) examination to identify any contraindications
- if the woman has pre-existing hypertriglyceridaemia, triglyceride monitoring during therapy is recommended
- if the patient is to undergo surgery and prolonged immobilisation is anticipated, therapy should be stopped 4 to 6 weeks before surgery and not restarted until the woman is completely mobile
- may cause fluid retention; therefore should be used with caution in those with cardiac or kidney dysfunction
- caution if used in women who have undergone hysterectomy because of endometriosis, as residual endometriosis may be present and become stimulated by oestrogen
- caution and close supervision is recommended if the woman has had endometriosis, uterine fibroids, risk factors for thromboembolic disorders or oestrogen-dependent tumours (e.g. first-degree hereditary for breast cancer), hypertension, liver disorders, diabetes mellitus (with or without vascular involvement), cholelithiasis, migraine or severe headache, systemic lupus erythematosus, a history of endometrial hyperplasia, epilepsy, asthma or otosclerosis
- contraindicated in women with undiagnosed genital bleeding, breast cancer (past, known or suspected), known or suspected oestrogen-dependent malignant tumours (e.g. endometrial cancer), untreated endometrial hyperplasia, acute liver disease, history of liver disease (if liver function tests have not returned to normal), previous/current venous thromboembolism, known thrombophilic disorders (e.g. protein C, protein S, antithrombin deficiency), active or recent arterial thromboembolic disease (e.g. angina, myocardial infarction) or porphyria

SEX HORMONES

Patient education

- the woman should be advised to seek medical advice immediately if any of the following occurs:
    - new onset of migraine-type headache
    - yellowing of skin or whites of the eyes, nausea, upper abdominal pain, fever, chills, dark coloured urine, pale bowel motions
    - painful swelling or redness in legs, sudden chest pain, difficulty breathing
    - any changes to breasts (women should be encouraged to regularly examine breasts)
    - any vaginal bleeding or spotting
- advise the patient that if dose is forgotten it should be used when she remembers unless the next dose is due in less than 8 hours, in which case the dose should be skipped
- the woman should be warned to expect an increase in vaginal discharge that is due to vaginal secretion increase resulting from therapy as well as melting of the hard fat used in the pessary
- instruct the patient is correct insertion technique including:
    - wash hands before and after insertion of pessary
    - if using fingers, the pessary should be inserted into vagina as far as is comfortable (without force)
    - if using the applicator
        - activate the applicator by pulling the plunger back
        - place the flat end of pessary into the open end of activated applicator
        - insert the applicator into the vagina as far as is comfortable (without force)
        - press the plunger to release pessary
        - withdraw the applicator
        - disassemble the applicator and rinse the two pieces for 30 seconds under running water, then dry with a paper towel and then reassemble
    - the washed applicator should be stored in a clean place (separate from unused applicators)
    - a used applicator should be discarded after 7 days of use
    - pessaries should be stored in a cool (below 30°C) place, away from sunlight, moisture or heat
- women should be warned that therapy can weaken condoms, diaphragms or cervical caps made of latex

 Contraindicated during pregnancy, as the formation of oestradiol and testosterone may pose potential risks to fetal development.

 Not recommended during breastfeeding. Lack of data regarding excretion in human milk and potential effects on the breastfed infant.

 Banned in sport.

TIBOLONE
Trade names
APO Tibolone, Livial, Livilan, Xyvion

Available form
Tablets: 2.5 mg

Action
- related to naturally occurring steroids with progestogenic and androgenic properties
- three active metabolites (two with oestrogenic properties and one with progestogenic/androgenic properties)
- oestrogenic effects on vagina, bone and thermoregulatory centre
- androgenic effect on some metabolic and haematological factors
- improves vaginal dryness and atrophy, as well as mood and libido

Use
- relief of symptoms of natural or surgical menopause (short term)
- second-line treatment in prevention of postmenopausal bone mineral density

loss (in those at high risk of fractures where other treatment is contraindicated or not appropriate)

Dose
- (Natural or surgical menopause, prevention of postmenopausal bone mineral density loss) 2.5 mg orally daily

Adverse effects
- fluid retention, oedema, weight gain
- headache, dizziness, depression
- lower abdominal pain
- breast tenderness
- cervical dysplasia, vulvo-vaginitis, vaginal bleeding/discharge, genital pruritus/discharge, pelvic pain, endometrial wall thickening
- hypertension
- abnormal hair growth
- altered high-density lipoprotein (HDL) cholesterol, total triglycerides and lipoprotein (a)
- rash, pruritus, acne
- blurred vision
- arthralgia, myalgia
- (Long-term use > 3 years, uncommon) endometrial, ovarian or breast cancer, venous or arterial thromboembolism, stroke
- (Rare) jaundice, impaired liver function

Interactions
- anticoagulant effect of warfarin may be increased; therefore INR should be carefully monitored especially when starting or stopping therapy
- decreased serum levels may occur if given with phenobarbital (phenobarbitone), carbamazepine, phenytoin, rifampicin or St John's wort

Nursing considerations/Cautions
- patients should have a thorough medical examination, including breast, abdominal and pelvic examination, to rule out presence of carcinoma before starting therapy. Assessment should also include personal and family history. Yearly breast and pelvic examinations are recommended while on therapy
- BP should be monitored regularly during therapy
- serum cholesterol and triglycerides should be monitored regularly if patient has pre-existing hypertriglyceridaemia
- therapy should be stopped immediately if there is any decrease in liver function, jaundice, increase in blood pressure or new onset of migraine-type headache
- treatment duration should be as short as possible and reviewed after 6 months. Symptoms usually improve after first few weeks of therapy but may take up to 12 weeks to be optimal
- (Menopause) started within 12 months after last natural bleed, or immediately after surgically induced menopause
- if switching from oestrogen-only therapy, a withdrawal bleed should be induced before starting therapy
- if switching from continuous hormone replacement therapy (HRT), therapy can be started at any time
- if switching from sequential HRT preparations, therapy should be started after progestogen phase
- tablets contain lactose and are therefore not recommended in those with galactose intolerance, Lapp lactase deficiency or glucose–galactose malabsorption
- caution and increased monitoring in those with uterine fibroids or endometriosis, risk factors for thromboembolic disorders or oestrogen-dependent tumours (e.g. first-degree relative with breast cancer), hypertension, liver disorders, diabetes mellitus (with or without vascular involvement), cholelithiasis, migraine or severe headache, systemic lupus erythematosus (SLE), epilepsy, asthma, otosclerosis or history of endometrial hyperplasia
- caution if used in those with cardiac or renal failure that may be aggravated by fluid retention
- caution if used in those with pre-existing hypertriglyceridaemia
- contraindicated in those with a history of (or suspicion of) breast cancer,

SEX HORMONES

oestrogen-dependent malignant tumours, undiagnosed genital bleeding, endometrial hyperplasia (untreated), idiopathic/current venous thromboembolism, arterial thromboembolic disease, known thrombophilic disorders, acute liver disease or history of liver disease (with abnormal liver function) or porphyria

Patient education

- advise the patient to avoid driving or operating machinery if blurred vision or dizziness occurs
- the patient should be advised to seek medical advice immediately if any of the following occur:
  - loss of appetite, nausea, vomiting, abdominal pain, unusual tiredness, dark urine or yellowing of skin or eyes
  - new or worsening headache/migraine
  - painful leg swelling
  - sudden onset of chest pain or difficulty breathing
  - any vaginal bleeding is present 6 months after starting therapy, starts after 6 months of therapy or continues after therapy has been stopped
- warn the patient that vaginal bleeding or spotting may occur when starting therapy
- the patient should be instructed that if missed dose is noticed within 12 hours, it should be taken; if > 12 hours has elapsed, the patient should wait until the next dose. The patient should be aware that there will be an increased risk of breakthrough bleeding and spotting

Tablets can be crushed and mixed with water, or a spoonful of yoghurt or apple puree. Occupational hazard: mask and gloves must be worn and a closed tablet crusher used.

Contraindicated during pregnancy.

Contraindicated during breastfeeding.

Pregnant staff must not crush tablets.

Banned in sport.

COMBINED ORAL CONTRACEPTIVES (COC)

Available form
Tablets

General Actions of oral contraceptives

- oral contraceptives are a combination of oestrogens (e.g. ethinylestradiol, mestranol) and progestogens (e.g. norethisterone, levonorgestrel, cyproterone, drospirenone, desogestrel)
- oestrogens inhibit the secretion of follicle-stimulating hormone (FSH), preventing follicular development and release of luteinising hormone (LH)
- progestogens, in combination, appear to inhibit the preovulatory rise of LH
- combination preparations decrease the likelihood of conception and implantation by causing changes in both the cervical mucus and the endometrium
- most widely used form of hormonal contraception
- progestogen-only preparations alter the cervical mucus and endometrium without influencing ovulation and are used when oestrogen is not wanted (e.g. during breastfeeding). Levonorgestrel is the most androgenic, with third-generation progestogens (desogestrel, gestodene, drospirenone) less androgenic
- available in three formulations: fixed-dose oestrogen—progestogen combination, phasic oestrogen—progestogen combination and progestogen only

- menstrual cycle becomes regular, less painful and bleeding lighter

General Uses of oral contraceptives
- oral contraception (regular or emergency)
- androgenisation in women (e.g. treatment of severe acne (with inflammation, nodularity and/or at risk of scarring) where prolonged oral antibiotics or local treatment have been unsuccessful; mild-to-moderate hirsutism)
- menstrual disorders, endometriosis

General Adverse effects of oral contraceptives
- nausea, abdominal pain or bloating, weight gain and, uncommonly, vomiting, diarrhoea
- mental depression, altered mood, nervousness, dizziness
- headache and, uncommonly, migraine
- oedema and, uncommonly, fluid retention
- acne, rash, pruritus, urticaria
- spotting, breakthrough bleeding, abnormal withdrawal bleeding, pelvic pain
- leucorrhoea, vaginal candidiasis, vaginitis
- breast tenderness, pain or engorgement
- changes to libido
- (Uncommon) hypertension
- (Rare) increased risk of cervical, endometrial, ovarian, liver or breast cancer
- (Rare) venous or arterial thromboembolic or thrombotic disorders, ocular lesions, dry eyes, intolerance to contact lenses (changed corneal curvature), chloasma (blotchy dark pigmentation), cholestatic jaundice, benign hepatic adenomas, gallbladder disease

General Interactions of oral contraceptives
- efficacy may be reduced by some broad-spectrum antibiotics; therefore additional contraception is recommended
- may increase serum levels of benzodiazepines, tacrolimus or ciclosporin, increasing the risk of toxicity
- may decrease serum levels of lamotrigine
- decreased serum levels, pregnancy or menstrual irregularities may occur if given with barbiturates, carbamazepine, griseofulvin, phenobarbital (phenobarbitone), phenytoin, primidone, rifabutin, rifampicin, St John's wort or topiramate. A different or additional form of contraception is recommended during therapy with these agents
- if used with rifampicin, a barrier method should be used during therapy and for 28 days after stopping
- increased serum levels may occur if given with azole antifungals, verapamil, diltiazem, macrolide antibiotics, atorvastatin or grapefruit juice
- HIV protease and non-nucleoside transcriptase inhibitors may have a variable (increase or decrease) effect on serum levels of oral contraceptives and should therefore be given with caution
- may affect a number of laboratory tests, including serum folate, triglycerides and phospholipid, response to metyrapone test, glucose tolerance, thyroid, renal, adrenal and liver function tests, prothrombin and coagulation time. It is therefore recommended that the test(s) be repeated when the person has been oestrogen free for 1–2 months

General Nursing considerations/Cautions for oral contraceptives
- complete medical examination (including family history, BP and examination of breasts, pelvis and abdomen, cervical cytology and urinalysis) should occur before starting oral contraceptives. Clotting tests should be performed on any women with a family history of thromboembolic disease
- pregnancy should be excluded before starting therapy
- (Androgenisation of women) an androgen-producing tumour or adrenal enzyme defect should be excluded before starting therapy (especially if

hirsutism has only recently appeared or intensified)
- increase in frequency or severity of migraine, loss of vision, double vision, slurred speech, aphasia, weakness or marked numbness on one side, or collapse (with or without focal seizures) could also be a sign of imminent stroke
- the patient should be monitored for signs of depression, especially if pre-existing depression
- therapy should be discontinued for at least 4 weeks before elective surgery and restarted 2 weeks after complete mobilisation. Other causes of immobilisation that require stopping therapy include long-haul flights, major trauma or emergency surgery
- many oral contraceptives contain lactose and are therefore not recommended in those with rare hereditary problems of galactose intolerance, Lapp lactase deficiency or glucose—galactose malabsorption
- caution if used in women with porphyria, systemic lupus erythematosus (SLE), haemolytic uraemic syndrome, Crohn's disease, ulcerative colitis, cholestasis, gallstones or otosclerotic-related hearing loss
- caution if used in women with hypertension
- caution if used in women with diabetes mellitus because of decreased glucose tolerance
- caution if used in women with hereditary angioedema, as condition may be exacerbated
- caution if used in women post-bariatric surgery because of the possibility of malabsorption
- caution if used in women with hypertriglyceridaemia because of the increased risk of pancreatitis
- caution if used in women who may be affected by fluid retention (e.g. cardiac or renal disease, asthma, migraine)
- the risk of venous or arterial thrombotic, thromboembolic or cerebrovascular accidents increases with age, smoking (further risk increase if over 35 and heavy smoker), a family history of venous/arterial thromboembolism (especially at an early age), obesity or overweight, hypertension, migraine, dyslipoproteinaemia, valvular heart disease, atrial fibrillation, prolonged immobilisation (including post-surgery or after any leg surgery), recent delivery or second-trimester abortion, or temporary immobilisation (e.g. air travel > 4 hours)
- contraindicated in those with or who have a history of thrombophlebitis or thromboembolic disorder, predisposition to thromboembolism (including acquired or hereditary disorders such as antithrombin III deficiency or protein C deficiency), a past history of deep vein thrombosis (DVT), cerebrovascular or coronary artery disease, a history of migraine with focal neurological symptoms, known/suspected breast/uterine/vaginal or cervical cancer, known/suspected/previous oestrogen-dependent tumour, undiagnosed abnormal vaginal bleeding, liver disease (if liver function has not returned to normal), cholestatic jaundice, pruritus in pregnancy or with contraceptive use, Dubin—Johnson or Rotor syndrome, benign or malignant liver tumour, otosclerosis (which deteriorated during pregnancy), herpes in pregnancy, abnormal lipid metabolism or hypertriglyceridaemia, pancreatitis or history of pancreatitis with severe hypertriglycidaemia, severe hypertension or severe diabetes mellitus (with or without vascular changes)

General Patient education for oral contraceptives

- instruct the patient in the importance of telling health professionals that oral contraceptive is being used when being questioned during routine medical examination

- recommend a routine of taking oral contraceptive pill at the same time each day so that it is taken regularly, including when to start (i.e. day 1 is the first day of menstrual bleeding), following the arrows on the packet. The patient should also be advised on what to do if a dose is missed or if vomiting or diarrhoea occurs
- advise the patient to keep follow-up appointments so that BP can be checked and breasts may be examined (and a cytology smear taken if needed)
- teach the patient how to examine her own breasts immediately after each menstrual period
- advise the patient to seek medical advice immediately if any of the following occur:
  - any sudden leg/foot pain, tenderness or swelling, increased warmth and/or discolouration of the leg/foot (these may be signs of DVT)
  - sudden chest pain, sudden breathlessness or unexplained sudden cough, lightheadedness, dizziness, rapid heart rate (these may be signs of pulmonary embolism)
  - loss of appetite, nausea, unusual tiredness, upper abdominal pain, yellowing of skin or eyes, dark urine or whole-body itching (signs of jaundice)
  - blurred or double vision, loss of vision
  - any changes in migraine/headache frequency and/or severity
  - any change in mood, or worsening of depression
  - sudden numbness/weakness of the face/arm/leg (especially if one-sided), dizziness, loss of balance or coordination, trouble walking, prolonged or severe headache, loss of consciousness
- a patient who is a heavy smoker (>15 cigarettes/day) and taking oral contraceptives should be advised that she runs a higher risk of developing DVT than those who do not smoke
- women who wear contact lenses should be warned that intolerance to lenses sometimes occurs
- women should be advised that oral contraceptive efficacy may be reduced if a dose is missed, during severe vomiting or diarrhoea, or with some concurrent medications (including some OTC, antibiotic or herbal preparations)
- advise the woman that not all women experience withdrawal bleeding during the placebo/no tablet period
- women should be warned that slight spotting is common; however, persistent or heavy bleeding should be reported to her doctor
- advise the patient to contact her doctor if she has missed a dose or if, despite following the prescribed dose pattern, she has missed two consecutive 'periods'
- women should be advised that oral contraceptives do not protect against HIV infection, AIDS and other sexually transmitted diseases

 Tablets should not be crushed.

 Contraindicated during pregnancy.

 Contraindicated during breastfeeding.

STIMULANTS

The main groups of drugs used as central nervous stimulants are the amphetamines and methylxanthines (e.g. caffeine). The amphetamines are mainly used in the management of narcolepsy and some hyperkinetic states in children (e.g. attention deficit hyperactivity disorder (ADHD), previously known as attention deficit disorder (Knights et al 2023). Amphetamine-like substances such as phentermine are utilised as appetite suppressants.

ADHD in childhood is characterised by persistent symptoms of inattention, impulsive behaviour and hyperactivity, resulting in a child who may be irritable and moody, have low self-esteem and experience learning difficulties. Management of ADHD involves family therapy and support, educational programs and directed activities, and speech and occupational therapy, with pharmacological therapy being an adjunct if needed. It should be noted that a number of patients with ADHD will either not respond or be intolerant to a stimulant and another therapy may need to be trialled (Knights et al 2023).

Narcolepsy is an incurable neurological condition in which the person experiences excessive drowsiness and uncontrollable 'sleep attacks' that can occur at any time, including during everyday activities such as eating, working and driving. Patients may also experience sleep paralysis (inability to move that occurs when just falling asleep or waking up), cataplexy (stress-induced, generalised muscle weakness) and vivid auditory or visual dreams when falling asleep (Knights et al 2023).

General Adverse effects of stimulants
- palpitations, increase in BP, tachycardia
- depression, agitation, irritability, nervousness, restlessness, hostility, aggression (or worsening of aggression or hostility)
- headache, migraine, dizziness, somnolence, insomnia, sedation
- fatigue, asthenia
- loss of appetite, anorexia, nausea,
- vomiting, abdominal pain, dry mouth or unpleasant taste, thirst, weight loss, dyspepsia, constipation, diarrhoea
- (Children) retarded growth (height and weight)
- fever
- sweating, flushing

- pharyngitis, upper respiratory tract infection, cough, dyspnoea, flu-like illness
- erectile dysfunction, decreased libido, impotence, menstrual irregularities
- pruritus, dermatitis, rash, urticaria
- (Rare) angioedema, anaphylactic reactions
- (Rare) seizures
- (Rare) suicidal ideation, emergence of new psychotic or manic symptoms (e.g. hallucinations, delusional thinking, mania), onset/exacerbation of motor or vocal tics
- (Rare) peripheral vasculopathy, including Raynaud's phenomenon

General Nursing considerations/Cautions for stimulants

- before starting therapy, the patient should have a thorough assessment to identify any pre-existing or underlying cardiovascular (e.g. hypertension, cardiac abnormalities, sudden death) or psychiatric history (e.g. history of depression, bipolar disorder, suicide attempts)
- blood pressure, heart rate and psychiatric status should be regularly reviewed throughout therapy
- children should have their height and weight monitored regularly throughout therapy. Growth and weight will return to normal when medication is stopped, and some specialists recommend drug-free periods to minimise these complications
- if therapy is stopped for more than 1 week, it should be restarted at the initial dose
- (Narcolepsy) evaluation of excessive sleepiness and diagnosis of narcolepsy, obstructive sleep apnoea/hypopnea syndrome (OSAHS) and chronic shiftwork sleep disorder (SWSD) should be made according to diagnostic criteria, including history and physical examination, and may also be supplemented by laboratory testing (e.g. sleep studies)
- patients should be closely monitored for any suicidal thoughts or behaviours during therapy
- (ADHD) caution if used in those with ADHD and co-morbid bipolar disorder, as mixed/mania episodes may be induced
- caution if used in those who partake in strenuous exercise, use stimulants and/or have a family history of sudden/cardiac death, because of an increased risk of sudden/cardiac death
- caution if used in those with pre-existing depression, mania, psychosis, hyperthyroidism, epilepsy, mild hypertension, tachycardia, ventricular arrhythmias, recent myocardial infarction, cardiovascular disease (including unstable angina and significant cardiac abnormalities), liver or kidney dysfunction or a family history of cardiac arrest or sudden death (including congenital or acquired QT syndrome), or conditions that could be worsened by increasing blood pressure and/or heart rate
- contraindicated in those with moderate-to-severe hypertension, severe cardiovascular disease, atrial fibrillation/flutter, ventricular tachycardia, ventricular fibrillation/flutter, advanced atherosclerosis, pheochromocytoma or uncontrolled hyperthyroidism, arteriosclerosis, glaucoma, severe anxiety, tension or agitation, motor tics, Tourette's syndrome, severe depression, anorexia nervosa, psychotic or

STIMULANTS

suicidal tendencies, hypersensitivity to sympathomimetic amines or a history of drug or alcohol abuse

General Patient education for stimulants

- the patient (or carer) should be advised to report any:
  - dark urine, itching, yellowing of eyes or skin, right upper abdominal pain or tenderness, nausea, loss of appetite or flu-like illness
  - thoughts/talk about self-harm, harm to others, suicide or death, or recent attempts at self-harm
  - increase in aggression, agitation, irritability, panic attacks or hostility
  - occurrence of fitting, confusion or hallucinations
  - exertional chest pain, unexplained fainting
  - discolouration of toes and/or fingers on exposure to temperature change (cold or heat), or emotional events accompanied by numbness in the same area
- adult patients should be advised not to drive or operate machinery if dizziness, drowsiness, tiredness or visual disturbances occur
- warn the patient to take care getting out of bed or suddenly standing up, as dizziness, lightheadedness and/or fainting may occur
- adult patients should be advised to avoid (or reduce) alcohol intake during therapy
- (ADHD) the parent/carer should regularly monitor the child's growth (height and weight) and discuss any concerns with the doctor, as therapy may need to be temporarily interrupted
- warn the patient/carer not to suddenly stop therapy, as unwanted side-effects will occur. Any interruption or stopping of therapy should be gradual and under medical supervision
- counsel the adult patient that there may be changes to sexual function during therapy

Not recommended.

Not recommended.

ARMODAFINIL

Trade name
Nuvigil

Available forms
Tablets: 50 mg, 150 mg, 250 mg

Action
- non-amphetamine that promotes wakefulness by an unknown action that is different to that of the sympathomimetic amines, but thought to involve orexinergic and histaminergic systems
- chemically related to modafinil (R-enantiomer) with similar properties
- indirect dopamine receptor agonist
- half-life about 15 hours

Use
- narcolepsy
- obstructive sleep apnoea/hypopnoea syndrome (OSAHS) with continuous positive airway pressure (CPAP) (adjunct)
- treatment of excessive sleepiness associated with moderate-to-severe chronic shiftwork sleep disorder (SWSD) (where non-pharmacological interventions were ineffective or inappropriate)

Dose
- (Narcolepsy) 150 mg or 250 mg orally daily (in the morning) 1 hour before or 2 hours after food **OR**
- (OSAHS) 150 mg or 250 mg orally daily (in the morning) 1 hour before or 2 hours after food (with CPAP) **OR**
- (SWSD) initially 150 mg orally daily 1 hour before or 2 hours after food, 1 hour before starting shiftwork

Adverse effects
- abuse, dependence
- (Rare, high dose) serious skin reactions, angioedema, multi-organ hypersensitivity reaction
- see also General Adverse effects of stimulants (p. 1551)

Interactions
- decreased serum levels may occur if given with carbamazepine, oxcarbazepine, phenytoin, rifabutin, phenobarbital (phenobarbitone), rifampicin or St John's wort
- increased serum levels may occur if given with ritonavir, indinavir, saquinavir, nelfinavir, chloramphenicol, clarithromycin, erythromycin, itraconazole, diltiazem or verapamil
- may increase serum level of diazepam, phenytoin, propranolol, omeprazole, esomeprazole and clomipramine
- caution if used with monoamine oxidase inhibitors (MAOIs)
- increased monitoring of INR is recommended if given with warfarin, especially when starting or stopping therapy
- may decrease serum level of oral contraceptives, midazolam, ciclosporin, quetiapine and carbamazepine

Nursing considerations/Cautions
- patients with sleep apnoea should be fully investigated by an experienced doctor with access to sleep laboratory diagnostic facilities before starting therapy
- armodafinil and modafinil are not bioequivalent or interchangeable
- patient with persistent sleepiness should have their levels assessed frequently to determine the effectiveness of the medication
- therapy should not be started unless negative pregnancy test is confirmed at least 1 week before starting therapy
- not recommended in those under 18 years
- caution if used in those with a psychiatric history (including anxiety), history of drug/stimulant abuse or liver dysfunction
- caution if used in the elderly, as lower dosage may be required
- not recommended in those with history of left ventricular hypertrophy or mitral valve prolapse who have history of CNS stimulant-induced valve prolapse
- contraindicated in those with hypersensitivity to modafinil
- see also General Nursing considerations/Cautions for stimulants (p. 1552)

Patient education
- ensure patient has an understanding of good sleep hygiene principles, such as limiting alcohol and caffeine intake before bedtime, regular bed and waking time and comfortable sleeping environment (no TV or electronics, cool room temperature)
- patient should be advised to seek medical attention immediately if any of the following occur:
  - rash or mouth blistering, fever or hives, abnormal physical weakness or lack of energy
  - swelling of face, eyes, lips, tongue or throat, hoarseness, difficulty swallowing
  - chest pain or unusual heartbeat
- if patient has abnormal levels of sleepiness, advise that medication may not return wakefulness to normal levels
- women of childbearing potential who use oral contraceptives should be warned that their effectiveness may be impaired, and therefore an additional

STIMULANTS

form of contraception is recommended to prevent pregnancy occurring. Contraception should be continued for 4 weeks after discontinuing therapy
- see also General Patient education for stimulants (p. 1553)

Tablets can be crushed and mixed with water, or spoonful of yoghurt or apple puree. Crushed tablets have a very bitter taste.

Contraindicated during pregnancy.

Not recommended during breastfeeding.

The dose of armodafinil should be reduced in patients with severe hepatic impairment, with or without cirrhosis.

Elimination of armodafinil and its metabolites may be reduced as a consequence of ageing. Therefore consideration should be given to the use of lower doses and close monitoring.

There is inadequate information to determine safety and efficacy of armodafinil dosing in patients with renal impairment, mild, moderate or severe.

Banned in sport.

ATOMOXETINE
Trade names
APO-Atomoxetine, Atomoxetine Sandoz

Available forms
Capsules: 10 mg, 18 mg, 25 mg, 40 mg, 60 mg, 80 mg, 100 mg

Action
- sympathomimetic agent that inhibits noradrenaline (norepinephrine) uptake, serotonin (5HT) uptake and (weakly) dopamine
- non-stimulant
- has an active equipotent metabolite
- half-life 5—22 hours
- considered second-line treatment
- does not cause dependence

Use
- attention deficit hyperactivity disorder (ADHD) (in those aged 6 years and over) as part of total treatment program

Dose
- ($\leq$ 70 kg) initially 0.5 mg/kg orally daily for at least 3 days, then increasing to 1.2 mg/kg as a single or divided dose (morning and late afternoon or early evening), increasing to a maximum 1.4 mg/kg or 100 mg after a further 2—4 weeks if optimal results have not been achieved **OR**
- (> 70 kg) initially 40 mg orally daily for at least 3 days, then increasing to 80 mg as a single or divided dose, increasing to a maximum 100 mg after a further 2—4 weeks if optimal results have not been achieved

Adverse effects
- urinary retention, urinary hesitancy
- sexual dysfunction
- chest pain
- (Rare) liver injury, seizures, stroke, myocardial infarction
- see also General Adverse effects of stimulants (p. 1551)

Interactions
- contraindicated with or within 2 weeks of stopping/starting MAOIs
- may increase serum levels of diazepam, paroxetine and phenytoin
- caution if used with salbutamol or other beta adrenoceptor agonists, because cardiovascular effects (e.g. palpitations) may be potentiated
- additive effect may occur if given with alpha1 agonist or noradrenaline (norepinephrine) uptake inhibitors
- increased serum level may occur if given with fluoxetine or paroxetine
- not recommended with tricyclic antidepressants (TCAs) because of increased risk of cardiovascular adverse effects

1555

- not recommended with other agents that prolong QT interval or cause electrolyte imbalance
- caution if given with antihypertensive or pressor agents

Nursing considerations/Cautions

- may be discontinued without tapering dose
- caution if used in males with enlarged prostate or have a history of urinary retention
- caution if used in those with history of seizures
- should be discontinued if evidence of liver injury or jaundice
- see also General Nursing considerations/Cautions for stimulants (p. 1552)

Patient education

- advise patient (or carer) to take divided dose in the morning and late afternoon/early evening for best effect
- patient (or carer) should be advised not to open capsules as powder is irritating to the eyes. Eyes should be immediately flushed with water if contact occurs
- see also General Patient education for stimulants (p. 1553)

Gloves and safety glasses must be worn when opening capsules or dispersing in water. Capsules can be opened and contents dispersed in water, or mixed with spoonful of yoghurt or apple puree.

No adequate and well-controlled studies have been conducted in pregnant women; it should not be used during pregnancy unless the potential benefit justifies the potential risk to the fetus.

It is not known whether atomoxetine is excreted in human milk; caution when administering to a nursing woman.

The safety and efficacy of atomoxetine in elderly patients (over 65) have not been established.

CAFFEINE
Trade name
No Doz Awakeners

Available form
Tablets: 100 mg

Action
- methylxanthine, related to theophylline
- stimulant effect on CNS, producing wakefulness and increased mental activity
- antagonises adenosine receptors, leading to contraction of cardiac muscle and relaxation of airway smooth muscle
- may indirectly stimulate dopamine activity
- weak vasodilator and weak diuretic effect

Use
- relieves mental fatigue and drowsiness and increases alertness
- adjunct to enhance analgesic actions
- respiratory stimulant in premature infants (see Antiasthma agents, bronchodilators and respiratory agents, p. 120)

Dose
- 100 mg orally, may be repeated after 3–4 hours (daily maximum 400 mg)

Adverse effects
- insomnia, anxiety, tremor, palpitations, increased BP, nervousness, withdrawal syndrome (including headache, irritability, weakness)
- gastric irritation, nausea, dyspepsia

Interactions
- may antagonise effects of dipyridamole when used during cardiac stress testing
- antagonises adenosine
- may increase CNS stimulation if given with other CNS-stimulating agents or other caffeine-containing products

Nursing considerations/Cautions
- a standard cup of coffee contains 50–150 mg caffeine, with espresso coffee containing 145 mg/50 mL; therefore intake of chocolate or beverages that

STIMULANTS

- contain caffeine, including coffee, tea, energy drinks, cola and cocoa, or any products containing guarana, may require a reduction in dose
- caution if used in those with insomnia, nervousness or tachycardia
- not recommended in those with severe anxiety, severe cardiac disease, liver impairment or hypertension
- contraindicated in children under 12 years or those with caffeine/xanthine sensitivity

Patient education
- instruct patient that dose should not be repeated within 3 hours

Available in combination with:
- Dimenhydrinate 50 mg, hyoscine hydrobromide 200 mcg, caffeine 20 mg (Travacalm Original). Also contained in Endura Sports Energy Gels, No Doz Plus, Panadol Extra, Travacalm Original (as well as commercial products such as energy drinks)

DEXAMFETAMINE (DEXAMPHETAMINE) SULFATE

Trade name
Dexamfetamine Tablets

Available form
Tablets: 5 mg

Action
- centrally acting sympathomimetic agent with alpha and beta adrenergic activity
- CNS stimulation, especially of the cerebral cortex, respiratory and vasomotor centres, causing increased motor activity, mental alertness and wakefulness, and producing euphoria. Peripheral actions include elevation of systolic and diastolic BP and some weak bronchodilator and respiratory activity
- excretion half-life is about 16—31 hours in urine with a pH of more than 7.5 and falls to 6—8 hours when the urinary pH is 5.0 or less

Use
- attention deficit hyperactivity disorder (ADHD) (in children 3 years or over) as part of total treatment program
- narcolepsy

Dose
Narcolepsy
- (Adult) 5—60 mg orally daily in divided doses **OR**
- (6—12 years) initially 5 mg orally daily, increasing by 5 mg at weekly intervals if needed **OR**
- (12 years and over) initially 10 mg orally daily, increasing by 10 mg at weekly intervals if needed

ADHD (over 3 years)
- initially 2.5 mg orally daily, increasing at weekly intervals by 2.5 mg until satisfactory response is achieved (maximum daily dose 40 mg in 2 divided doses)

Adverse effects
- tolerance, dependence, abuse potential
- (High dose, abrupt withdrawal) extreme fatigue, depression, changes on sleep EEG
- see also General Adverse effects of stimulants (p. 1551)

Interactions
- contraindicated with, or within 2 weeks of stopping, monoamine oxidase inhibitors (MAOIs)
- urinary excretion may be increased by urinary acidifiers
- urinary excretion may be decreased by acetazolamide, sodium bicarbonate and some thiazide diuretics
- absorption may be lowered by GI acidifying agents, including fruit juices, decreasing serum levels
- may enhance activity of tricyclic antidepressants (TCAs) (including cardiovascular effects), sympathomimetic agents and other CNS-stimulating agents; therefore combined use is not recommended
- may decrease the sedative effect of antihistamines

- may antagonise the hypotensive action of antihypertensive agents
- CNS-stimulant effects may be antagonised by haloperidol, chlorpromazine and lithium
- may slow absorption of ethosuximide
- may potentiate the analgesic effect of pethidine
- may enhance the effects of adrenaline (epinephrine) and noradrenaline (norepinephrine)
- may delay the absorption of phenobarbital (phenobarbitone) and phenytoin and may also produce a synergistic antiepileptic effect
- may cause elevation in serum corticosteroid levels (especially in the evenings) and therefore interfere with urinary steroid test

Nursing considerations/Cautions

- under same control as drugs of addiction (S8) (Drugs, Poisons and Controlled Substances Regulations)
- limited, by law, to the above uses in most Australian states and territories. Requires special authority
- (ADHD) a drug-free interval is suggested to determine whether there are changes in behavioural patterns. If therapy is stopped for more than a week, it should be restarted at the initial dose
- any withdrawal should be gradual
- caution if used in those with mild hypertension. If used, BP should be closely monitored throughout therapy
- not recommended in those with lactose allergy
- possibility for abuse and dependence exists, especially in those with a history of drug or alcohol abuse; therefore contraindicated
- see also General Nursing considerations/Cautions for stimulants (p. 1552)

Patient education

- to avoid sleep disturbances, doses should not be given in the evening
- (ADHD) first dose should be given on awakening, second dose should then be given 4–6 hours later
- female patients of childbearing potential should be counselled to use adequate and reliable contraception during therapy to avoid pregnancy occurring
- see also General Patient education for stimulants (p. 1553)

 Tablet can be crushed and mixed with water, or spoonful of yoghurt or apple puree.

 Not recommended during pregnancy. If used, there is an increased risk of premature delivery and low birthweight, and infants may experience withdrawal symptoms after birth including agitation and lassitude

 Not recommended during breastfeeding unless benefits outweigh risks.

 Banned in sport.

GUANFACINE

Trade name
Intuniv

Available forms
Tablets (modified-release): 1 mg, 2 mg, 3 mg, 4 mg

Action
- selective alpha2A adrenergic receptor agonist
- not a CNS stimulant
- modulates signalling in prefrontal cortex and basal ganglia through direct modification of synaptic noradrenaline (norepinephrine) transmission acting at the alpha2 adrenergic receptors
- elimination about 18 hours

Use
- attention deficit hyperactivity disorder (ADHD) in children and adolescents 6–17 years, as monotherapy (when

STIMULANTS

stimulants or atomoxetine are not suitable, not tolerated or have been ineffective), or as adjunctive therapy (with psychostimulants where the response has been suboptimal) (as part of total treatment program)

Dose
- initially 1 mg orally daily, increasing by increments of 1 mg at weekly intervals (daily maximum 4 mg if given with psychostimulants or 4–7 mg as monotherapy)

Adverse effects
- syncope, hypotension, orthostatic hypotension, bradycardia
- somnolence, sedation, nightmares
- enuresis
- (Abrupt discontinuation) rebound effects (increased blood pressure and heart rate)
- see also General Adverse effects of stimulants (p. 1551)

Interactions
- caution if used with antihypertensive agents or other agents that lower blood pressure or heart rate
- caution if used with alcohol, sedatives, hypnotics, antipsychotics, phenothiazines, barbiturates or benzodiazepines, as additive sedation may occur
- decreased serum levels may occur if given with rifampicin
- may increase serum levels of sodium valproate
- not recommended with grapefruit juice

Nursing considerations/Cautions
- before starting therapy, heart rate and blood pressure should be measured and repeated during dose increases and then regularly throughout therapy
- height, weight and BMI should be measured before starting, every 3 months for first 12 months, then 6-monthly (or more frequently during dose adjustment)
- therapy should be re-evaluated regularly to determine long-term usefulness
- if two or more consecutive doses are missed, retitration starting at initial dose is recommended
- abrupt discontinuation is not recommended because of rebound effects including increased blood pressure and heart rate
- if discontinuation is required, daily dose should be tapered downwards in increments of 1 mg every 3–7 days to minimise risk of blood pressure increasing when therapy is stopped altogether. Blood pressure and pulse should be monitored when reducing or stopping therapy
- dose reduction may be required in those with liver or kidney impairment
- caution if used in those with history of hypotension, heart block, bradycardia or other cardiac conditions including arrhythmia, sick sinus syndrome, ischaemic heart disease, congestive heart failure or congenital long QT syndrome
- caution if used in those with a history of syncope or a condition which might predispose to syncope (e.g. hypotension, orthostatic hypotension, dehydration)
- caution if used in those with gastrointestinal illnesses that lead to vomiting because inability to take medication may result in rebound effects
- not recommended in those under 6 years
- see also General Nursing considerations/Cautions for stimulants (p. 1552)

Patient education
- advise patient/parent/carer that medication should not be given with high-fat meal, nor tablets chewed, crushed or broken
- patient/parent/carer should be advised to avoid becoming dehydrated or overheated
- warn the patient/parent/carer against abrupt discontinuation of medication to avoid rebound effect
- advise patient/parent/carer to avoid grapefruit juice during therapy

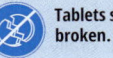 **Tablets should not be chewed, crushed or broken.**

Not recommended during pregnancy unless benefits outweigh risks.

Should be used during breastfeeding only if benefits outweigh risks.

Dose reduction may be required in patients with different degrees of hepatic impairment.

Dose reduction may be required in patients with severe renal impairment (GFR 29–15 mL/min) and an end-stage renal disease (GFR < 15 mL/min) or requiring dialysis.

Should not be used in adults and elderly with ADHD, as the safety and efficacy of guanfacine has not been established.

LISDEXAMFETAMINE DIMESILATE
Trade name
Vyvanse

Available forms
Capsules: 20 mg, 30 mg, 40 mg, 50 mg, 60 mg, 70 mg

Action
- inactive prodrug
- rapidly absorbed and hydrolysed in the blood to dexamfetamine (dexamphetamine)
- non-catecholamine sympathomimetic amine with CNS-stimulant activity thought to be due to blocking noradrenaline (norepinephrine) and dopamine reuptake
- short half-life (less than 1 hour)

Use
- treatment of attention deficit hyperactivity disorder (ADHD) as part of total treatment program
- treatment of binge eating disorder (BED) where non-pharmacological therapy is unavailable or unsuccessful

Dose
- (ADHD) initially 30 mg orally in the morning, increasing by 20 mg at weekly intervals if needed (daily maximum 70 mg) **OR**
- (BED) initially 30 mg orally in the morning, increasing to 50–70 mg

Adverse effects
- blurred vision, accommodation difficulty
- teeth grinding at night (bruxism)
- fever
- abuse, dependence
- see also General Adverse effects of stimulants (p. 1551)

Interactions
- contraindicated with or within 14 days of monoamine oxidase inhibitors (MAOIs)
- stimulant effects may be blocked by haloperidol, lithium and chlorpromazine
- may potentiate analgesic actions of opioid analgesics
- urinary acidifiers (e.g. ascorbic acid) increase excretion, decreasing serum levels
- urinary alkalinisers (e.g. sodium bicarbonate) decrease excretion, increasing serum levels
- may increase serum levels of guanfacine
- may decrease effect of antihypertensive agents
- caution if used with selective serotonin reuptake inhibitors (SSRIs), serotonin and noradrenaline (norepinephrine) reuptake inhibitors (SNRIs) or other serotonergic agents because of the risk of serotonin syndrome
- may interfere with estimation of urinary steroid test

Nursing considerations/Cautions
- (ADHD) therapy should be reviewed on a yearly basis
- (BED) should be prescribed for shortest amount of time and reassessed for effectiveness after 12 weeks
- under same control as drugs of addiction (S8) (Drugs, Poisons and Controlled Substances Regulations)
- limited, by law, to the above uses in most Australian states and territories; requires special authority

STIMULANTS

- not recommended in children under 6 years or adults over 55 years
- caution if used in those with kidney insufficiency. Maximum daily dose should not exceed 50 mg if glomerular filtration rate is between 15 and 30 mL/min
- contraindicated in those with severe depression, anorexia nervosa, psychotic symptoms or suicidal tendencies
- see also General Nursing considerations/Cautions for stimulants (p. 1552)

Patient education

- advise patient/carer that capsule should be swallowed whole, or can be opened and contents mixed in a glass of water. The mixture should be stirred to ensure mixing and drunk immediately (not stored)
- female patients of childbearing potential should be counselled to use effective and reliable contraception during therapy
- see also General Patient education for stimulants (p. 1553)

Capsule can be opened and given with a spoonful of yoghurt or apple puree.

Not recommended during pregnancy. If used, there is an increased risk of premature delivery and low birthweight, and infants may experience withdrawal symptoms after birth including agitation and lassitude.

Not recommended during breastfeeding.

Caution if used in those with kidney insufficiency.

Safety and efficacy has not been established in adult patients over the age of 55 years.

Banned in sport.

METHYLPHENIDATE HYDROCHLORIDE

Trade names
Artige, Concerta Extended-Release Tablets, Methylphenidate Orifarm, Methylphenidate Sandoz XR, Methylphenidate-Teva XR, Ritalin 10, Ritalin LA, Rubifen LA

Available forms
Tablets: 10 mg;
Tablets (extended release): 18 mg, 27 mg, 36 mg, 54 mg;
Capsules (modified release): 10 mg, 20 mg, 30 mg, 40 mg, 60 mg

Action
- sympathomimetic agent that stimulates the CNS by inhibiting dopamine and noradrenaline (norepinephrine) uptake, elevating mood and improving the powers of judgement and concentration
- half-life 3.5 hours

Use
- attention deficit hyperactivity disorder (ADHD) as part of total treatment program
- narcolepsy

Dose
- (ADHD, children > 6 years, adolescents) initially 5 mg orally daily 1–2 times daily (breakfast and lunch) increasing at 5–10 mg increments at weekly intervals if needed (daily maximum 60 mg) (immediate-release tablets) **OR**
- (ADHD, children > 6 years, adolescents) initially 18 mg orally daily, then increasing at 9 mg increments at weekly intervals to 36 mg, then increasing at 18 mg increments at weekly intervals if needed (daily maximum 54 mg) (extended-release tablets) **OR**
- (ADHD, children > 6 years, adolescents) initially 10 mg orally daily, increasing at 10 mg increments at weekly intervals if needed (daily maximum 60 mg) (modified-release capsules) **OR**
- (ADHD, adults) 10–60 mg orally daily in 2–3 divided doses (immediate-release tablets) **OR**
- (ADHD, adults) initially 18–36 mg orally daily, increasing at 18 mg increments at

weekly intervals if needed (daily maximum 72 mg) (extended-release tablets) **OR**
- (ADHD, adults) initially 20 mg orally daily, increasing at 20 mg increments at weekly intervals if needed (daily maximum 80 mg) (modified-release capsules) **OR**
- (Narcolepsy, adults) 20–60 mg orally daily in 2–3 divided doses (daily maximum 60 mg) (immediate-release tablets)

Adverse effects
- fever
- vertigo
- arthralgia, muscle twitching, myalgia
- tachycardia, palpitations
- teeth grinding at night (bruxism)
- dyskinesia, paraesthesia, tremor
- (Rare) priapism
- tolerance, dependence, potential for abuse
- (Rare) leucopenia, thrombocytopenia, anaemia
- see also General Adverse effects of stimulants (p. 1551)

Interactions
- contraindicated with, or within 2 weeks of, monoamine oxidase inhibitors (MAOIs)
- not recommended on same day as halogenated anaesthetics because of the sudden increase in blood pressure
- may decrease effects of antihypertensive agents
- may enhance effects of phenytoin, primidone, phenobarbital (phenobarbitone) and tricyclic antidepressants (TCAs)
- may enhance effects of warfarin; therefore INR should be closely monitored, especially when starting and stopping therapy
- not recommended with selective serotonin reuptake inhibitors (SSRIs), serotonin and noradrenaline (norepinephrine) reuptake inhibitors (SNRIs) or other serotonergic agents because of the risk of serotonin syndrome
- not recommended with antipsychotic agents
- alcohol may increase CNS effects and is therefore not recommended
- not recommended with clonidine or other alpha agonists
- may cause false positive on laboratory test for amphetamine, particularly immunoassay screening tests

Nursing considerations/Cautions
- FBC, differential and platelet counts should be monitored regularly during prolonged therapy
- has possibility for abuse, tolerance and habit formation
- under same control as drugs of addiction (S8) (Drugs, Poisons and Controlled Substances Regulations)
- limited, by law, to the listed uses in most Australian states and territories; Requires special authority
- drug should be discontinued if there is no improvement after 1 month of stable dosage
- single doses > 20 mg should be avoided because of adverse effects
- should be stopped on day of surgery
- (Modified-release capsules) contain both immediate-release and extended/delayed-release beads
- when patient is converting from immediate-release formulation to extended- or modified-release formulation, follow manufacturer's conversion table
- (Extended-release tablets) not recommended in those with pre-existing GI narrowing, dysphagia or significant swallowing difficulties
- not recommended in children under 6 years of age
- not recommended for prevention or treatment of normal fatigue states
- contraindicated in those with severe depression, anorexia nervosa, psychotic symptoms or suicidal tendencies
- see also General Nursing considerations/Cautions for stimulants (p. 1552)

STIMULANTS

Patient education

- if using 10 mg tablets and sleeplessness is a problem, patient should be advised to take last dose before 6 pm
- advise patient that extended-release tablets should be swallowed whole, not chewed, crushed or divided. Patient should also be warned that tablet shell may appear in their stools
- patient should be advised that modified-release capsules should be swallowed whole. However, contents may be sprinkled on cold soft food (e.g. apple sauce) and eaten unchewed. Uneaten food containing capsule contents should not be stored
- instruct male patient/carer to immediately seek medical attention if prolonged and painful erection occurs as this is a medical emergency
- see also General Patient education for stimulants (p. 1553)

Plain tablet (10 mg) can be dispersed in water, or crushed and mixed with spoonful of yoghurt or apple puree. Ritalin LA capsules can be opened and beads mixed with cold apple puree. Beads must not be chewed or mixed with warm food.

Not recommended during pregnancy unless benefits outweigh risks.

Not recommended during breastfeeding unless benefits outweigh risks.

Banned in sport.

MODAFINIL

Trade names
Modafin, Modavigil, APO-Modafinil, Modafinil GH, Modafinil Sandoz, Modafinil Viatris, Modafinil-WGR

Available form
Tablets: 100 mg

Action
- non-amphetamine that promotes wakefulness by an unknown action that is different to that of the sympathomimetic amines but thought to involve histaminergic systems
- no effect on appetite, behaviour, nocturnal sleep or autonomic nervous system
- half-life 10—12 hours
- clearance delayed in the elderly

Use
- narcolepsy
- obstructive sleep apnoea/hypopnoea syndrome (OSAHS) with continuous positive airway pressure (CPAP) (adjunct)
- treatment of excessive sleepiness associated with moderate-to-severe chronic shiftwork sleep disorder (SWSD)

Dose
- (Narcolepsy) 200—400 mg orally daily as single dose (morning) or divided doses (morning and noon) **OR**
- (OSAHS) 200—400 mg orally daily as single dose (morning) or divided doses (morning and noon) (with CPAP) **OR**
- (SWSD) initially 200 mg daily, 1 hour before starting shiftwork

Adverse effects
- neck rigidity
- dependence, euphoria, abuse potential
- (Rare) paraesthesia
- (Rare, high dose) serious skin reactions, multi-organ hypersensitivity reaction, serious rash
- see also General Adverse effects of stimulants (p. 1551)

Interactions
- absorption may be delayed if given with methylphenidate
- caution if used with monoamine oxidase inhibitors (MAOIs)
- caution if used with carbamazepine, phenobarbital (phenobarbitone), rifampicin or itraconazole, as decreased serum modafinil levels may occur

- may increase serum level of diazepam, phenytoin, propranolol, tricyclic antidepressants (TCAs) and selective serotonin reuptake inhibitors (SSRIs)
- may decrease serum level of oral contraceptives, triazolam, ciclosporin and theophylline
- INR should be closely monitored if given with warfarin, especially when starting or stopping therapy or if adjusting dose
- if given with phenytoin, serum level of phenytoin should be closely monitored to prevent toxicity

Nursing considerations/Cautions

- patients with obstructive sleep apnoea should be fully investigated by an experienced doctor with access to sleep laboratory diagnostic facilities before starting therapy
- ECG monitoring is recommended before starting therapy
- not recommended in those under 18 years
- caution if used in those with a psychiatric history (including anxiety), history of drug/stimulant abuse or liver dysfunction
- armodafanil and modafanil are not bioequivalent or interchangeable.
- see also General Nursing considerations/Cautions for stimulants (p. 1552)

Patient education

- ensure patient has an understanding of good sleep hygiene principles, such as limiting alcohol and caffeine intake before bedtime, regular bed and waking time and comfortable sleeping environment (no TV or electronics, cool room temperature)
- patient should be advised to report any rash, skin blistering, fever or hives immediately
- instruct patient to swallow tablets whole with glass of water
- women of childbearing potential who use oral contraceptives should be warned that their effectiveness may be impaired, and therefore an additional form of contraception is recommended to prevent pregnancy from occurring. Contraception should be continued for 4 weeks after discontinuing therapy
- see also General Patient education for stimulants (p. 1553)

 Tablet can be crushed and mixed with water, or spoonful of yoghurt or apple puree

 Contraindicated during pregnancy.

 Not recommended during breastfeeding.

 Caution in severe hepatic failure.

 No satisfactory data on the safety and efficacy in patients ≥ 65 years of age. The clearance of modafinil may be reduced in the elderly.

 Banned in sport.

SYMPATHOMIMETIC AGENTS

The autonomic nervous system (ANS) consists of two main divisions: the sympathetic and the parasympathetic nervous system. Each manages specific physiological responses to help the body adapt to various situations. The sympathetic nervous system (SNS), often called the 'fight or flight' system, prepares the body to respond to stress. When activated, the SNS increases heart rate and the force of cardiac contractions, ensuring that oxygen-rich blood reaches the muscles more efficiently. It also dilates the airways in the lungs to enhance oxygen intake, dilates the pupils to improve vision, and raises blood glucose levels to provide a quick energy source. Additionally, it suppresses digestive activity to redirect blood flow to muscles and essential organs for immediate action.

The main transmitter substance of the sympathetic nervous system is noradrenaline (norepinephrine); however, adrenaline (epinephrine) is also released from the adrenal cortex in times of stress and produces the same effects. Noradrenaline (norepinephrine) acts on postsynaptic receptors (adrenoceptors), which can be divided into alpha (α) and beta (β). Alpha adrenoceptors can be further subdivided into α1A, α1B, α1D, α2A, α2B and α2C, while beta adrenoceptors are subdivided into β1 (found in the heart), β2 (found predominantly in smooth muscle of bronchioles, arteries and skeletal muscle blood vessels) and β3 (found in the plasma membrane of adipocytes and mediate lipolysis; also found in the brain, heart, prostate, urinary bladder detrusor and GI tract) (Knights et al 2023).

Sympathomimetic (adrenergic) agents include naturally occurring catecholamines (adrenaline (epinephrine), noradrenaline (norepinephrine) and dopamine) and drugs that mimic the effects of sympathetic nerve stimulation. Direct-acting agents stimulate the adrenergic receptors, whereas indirect-acting agents release stored noradrenaline (norepinephrine) from nerve endings, block its uptake from nerve terminals or block monoamine oxidase (MAO) or catechol-*O*-methyltransferase (COMT) enzymes, which metabolise the catecholamines (Knights et al 2023).

General Interactions of sympathomimetic agents

- contraindicated with halogenated general anaesthetics because they may provoke ventricular arrhythmias

- not recommended with agents that sensitise the heart to arrhythmias, such as digoxin. If given together, ECG monitoring is recommended
- not recommended with monoamine oxidase inhibitors (MAOIs), tricyclic antidepressants (TCAs), some antihistamines, thyroid hormones or cocaine, as sudden hypertension, tachycardia, arrhythmias and/or hyperpyrexia may occur because of potentiated effect
- additive effect may occur if given with other sympathomimetic agents and therefore are not recommended together
- actions may be antagonised if given with rapidly acting vasodilating agents
- increased serum levels may occur if given with entacapone, increasing the risk of arrhythmias
- severe hypertension may occur if given with oxytocin
- hypotension and cardiac acceleration may occur if given with alpha adrenoceptor blocking agents (e.g. prazosin)
- severe hypertension and reflex bradycardia (and possibly heart block) may occur if given with non-specific beta adrenoceptor blocking agents (e.g. propranolol)
- increased hypokalaemia may occur if given with other agents known to deplete potassium (e.g. diuretics, corticosteroids, aminophylline, theophylline)
- may affect control of blood glucose levels in those with diabetes managed with hypoglycaemic agents, so careful monitoring is required
- caution if used with antihypertensive agents, as severe hypertension may occur

General Nursing considerations/Cautions for sympathomimetic agents

- any hypovolaemia, hypercapnia, hypoxia or acidosis should be corrected before starting therapy or at the same time
- frequently monitor BP, arterial blood gases, heart rate and rhythm (ECG), arterial pressure, cardiac output, central venous pressure (CVP) or pulmonary wedge pressure, mental status, skin temperature and urinary output
- serum potassium should be monitored frequently throughout therapy
- if there is a disproportionate increase in diastolic BP, the infusion rate should be slowed or infusion stopped and the patient carefully observed (unless this is the desired effect)
- shock state may continue if vasopressor amines are given for a prolonged period, because resultant vasoconstriction may prevent adequate expansion of circulating volume
- a burette, infusion pump or drip regulator should be used to deliver the solution
- monitor infusion for rate and free flow to avoid extravasation
- should be given into large blood vessels and, if infiltration or thrombosis occurs at IV site, infusion should be stopped immediately
- administer alone
- reduce rate gradually before discontinuing infusion to avoid rebound hypotension
- contraindicated in those with sulfite/metasulfite allergy, which may

SYMPATHOMIMETIC AGENTS

evoke allergic reaction in susceptible individuals, including those with asthma (adrenaline (epinephrine), dobutamine, dopamine, isoprenaline, metaraminol, phenylephrine)

ADRENALINE (EPINEPHRINE)
Trade names
Adrenaline Jr Viatri, Adrenaline Juno, Adrenaline Viatris, Adrenaline—Link Injection BP, Anapen, Aspen Adrenaline, Emerade, Epipen, Epipen Jr

Available forms
Autoinjector: 150 microgram/0.3 mL, 300 microgram/0.3 mL;
Ampoules: 0.1 mg/mL, 1 mg/mL, 1 mg/10 mL;
Prefilled syringe: 0.1 mg/mL, 1 mg/10 mL

Action
- direct-acting sympathomimetic agent that stimulates both alpha and beta adrenoceptors
- cardiac stimulant causing increased heart rate, output, myocardial contractility and BP
- relaxes bronchial smooth muscle, causing bronchodilation
- constricts blood vessels in skin and mucous membranes
- relaxes gastrointestinal smooth muscle
- increases secretion of renin
- stimulates lipolysis, increasing free fatty acids in blood
- inhibits insulin secretion, increases glycogenolysis, resulting in hyperglycaemia
- inhibits uterine contraction
- decreases desire to void, which can lead to urinary retention
- crosses placenta but not blood—brain barrier
- rapid onset (IV)
- half-life about 2 minutes

Use
- adjunct in treatment of cardiac arrest
- emergency management of severe anaphylactic reactions and severe acute reactions to allergens (first-line management)
- relief of respiratory distress due to bronchospasm, angioedema, croup, mucosa and upper airway obstruction (e.g. laryngeal oedema)
- provides inotropic support in acute chronic heart failure and septic shock
- adjunct to local anaesthetic, prolonging action by delaying absorption
- as a haemostatic agent, applied topically to control superficial bleeding from arterioles and capillaries in skin, mucous membranes and other tissue
- in ocular surgery to control bleeding, relieve mucosal and conjunctival congestion, decrease intraocular pressure and produce mydriasis

Dose
anaphylaxis
- 100—500 micrograms (0.1—0.5 mL of 1:1000 solution) SC or IM (SC dose may be repeated at 20-minute to 4-hour intervals if required) **OR**
- (Severe anaphylaxis) 100—250 micrograms (1—2.5 mL of 1:10,000 solution) IV slowly over 10 minutes **OR**
- 500 micrograms SC or IM initially, then 25—50 micrograms (0.25—0.5 mL of 1:10,000 solution) IV every 5—15 minutes until relief **OR**
- 150—300 micrograms IM, which may be repeated at 5—15-minute intervals if symptoms have not subsided or recur (autoinjector)

cardiopulmonary resuscitation (in absence of ventricular fibrillation)
- 1 mg (10 mL of 1:10,000 solution) IV, repeated every 3—5 minutes during cardiopulmonary resuscitation. Line should be flushed with 20 mL of sodium chloride 0.9% to ensure that patient receives the full dose

Adverse effects
- tachycardia, palpitations, ectopic beats, ventricular fibrillation, arrhythmias, severe hypertension, anginal pain, non-specific chest pain, vasodilation

- with hypotension, hypertension with reflex bradycardia
- anxiety, fear, restlessness, irritability, impaired memory, psychosis, hallucinations, confusion, nervousness, disorientation, exacerbation of psychiatric disorders
- pallor, sweating, flushing of face and skin
- headache, weakness, dizziness, insomnia
- nausea, vomiting, anorexia, hypersalivation
- peripheral vasoconstriction, coldness of extremities, gangrene of the feet if there is pre-existing peripheral vascular disease
- muscle tremor
- hypokalaemia, hyperglycaemia
- difficulty with micturition, urinary retention
- increased rigidity and tremor (if given to those with Parkinson's disease)
- (Children) syncope
- (High doses) ventricular arrhythmias, severe hypertension, cerebral haemorrhage, pulmonary oedema
- (Repeated injections) skin necrosis
- (Accidental IV injection) convulsions, metabolic acidosis, renal failure with anuria
- (Prolonged use, overdose) severe metabolic acidosis

Interactions
- see General Interactions of sympathomimetic agents (p. 1565)

Nursing considerations/Cautions

- select correct type of solution and note concentration, dose and route carefully
- 1:1000 solution means 1 g in 1000 mL or 1 mg in 1 mL
- 1:10,000 solution means 1 g in 10,000 mL or 0.1 mg in 1 mL
- discard any discoloured (brown) or precipitated solutions
- if given SC, aspirate to ensure needle is not in a vein and inject very slowly. If SC formulation is given IV, hypertension may occur
- if giving injection IM, do NOT give into the buttocks
- SC route is not recommended because of variable absorption
- intracardiac administration is no longer recommended
- rotate injection sites to avoid local ischaemic necrosis
- if given IV, monitor cardiac rate and BP, especially in the first 5 minutes
- avoid interarterial administration, as gangrene may occur from vasoconstriction of vessel
- adrenaline (epinephrine) is incompatible with alkaline solutions (e.g. sodium bicarbonate), metals (e.g. copper, iron, zinc, silver) and a large number of drugs, and is therefore best infused alone
- (Autoinjector) junior formulation is recommended in children weighing 15–30 kg
- contains sodium metabisulfite, which may cause allergic reactions in those with hypersensitivity
- extreme caution if used in the elderly, or those with cardiovascular disease, hypertension, cerebrovascular insufficiency, circulatory collapse (induced by phenothiazines), chronic lung disease, angina, prostatic hypertrophy, urinary retention, Parkinson's disease, asthma/emphysema (with degenerative heart disease) or psychoneurosis
- contraindicated with local anaesthetics for use in infiltration injection for digits, ears, nose, penis or scrotum, owing to risk of ischaemic tissue necrosis
- contraindicated in those with hypersensitivity to other sympathomimetic agents, shock (except anaphylaxis), hypertension, ischaemic heart disease, arrhythmias, cardiac dilation, coronary insufficiency, cerebral arteriosclerosis, narrow-angle glaucoma, diabetes mellitus, organic brain damage, hyperthyroidism, pheochromocytoma or thyrotoxicosis, or in obstetrics (where maternal BP > 130/80 mmHg)

- see also General Nursing considerations/Cautions for sympathomimetic agents (p. 1566)

Patient education
- warn the patient against driving or operating machinery because of dizziness, weakness and tremor
- ensure the patient/family member has been instructed in correct use of auto-injector, including:
  - carry autoinjector at all times
  - it is important to seek medical emergency care/assistance immediately
  - check expiry date and colour of solution before use (cloudy or brown solutions should not be used)
  - injection technique into outer thigh only (through clothing if necessary) (training autoinjector is available to assist with education, demonstration and practising technique)
  - record time injection was given
  - once-only use per autoinjector (however, more than one injection may be required)
  - storage conditions (not in fridge, protect from light and heat)
  - safe disposal
  - if accidental injection of other sites (e.g. hands, feet, nose, ears, genitalia) occurs, seek medical treatment immediately because of potential loss of blood supply to the area
- those with diabetes mellitus should be advised to monitor blood glucose levels carefully after adrenaline (epinephrine) use, as hyperglycaemia may occur

Safe. There is no evidence of harm to the fetus when used in a large number of pregnant women. However, it should be avoided during labour as it may delay contractions and prolong labour. There are no absolute contraindications to adrenaline (epinephrine) in anaphylactic reactions. As a life-saving medication, use it if required.

No human data available.

Banned in sport.

Available in combination with
- Adrenaline (epinephrine) + lidocaine (lignocaine) or articaine or bupivacaine or mepivacaine (see Local anaesthetics p. 1326)

DOBUTAMINE
Trade names
DBL Dobutamine Hydrochloride Injection, Dobutamine-Claris

Available form
Ampoules: 250 mg/20 mL

Action
- synthetic catecholamine that acts directly on beta1 adrenoceptors, resulting in potent inotropic effects and mild vasodilatory effects
- little increase in heart rate or peripheral resistance (and therefore BP)
- does not cause release of noradrenaline (norepinephrine)
- no effect on dopamine receptors
- does not cause renal vasodilation
- onset 1–2 minutes, peak effect within 10 minutes, duration of action up to 10 minutes, plasma half-life < 3 minutes

Use
- short-term treatment of cardiac failure secondary to acute myocardial infarction or cardiac surgery

Dose
- 2.5–10 microgram/kg/min IV infusion (rate and duration of therapy adjusted according to patient response)

Adverse effects
- marked increased heart rate, increased systolic BP, ventricular ectopic beats,

- hypotension (occasionally), angina, palpitations, chest pain (non-specific)
- shortness of breath
- nausea
- headache
- mild decrease in serum potassium and, rarely, hypokalaemia
- (Hypersensitivity) rash, bronchospasm, fever, eosinophilia
- (IV site) phlebitis, necrosis (rare)
- (Rare) cardiac rupture (during dobutamine stress testing)

Interactions
- when given with sodium nitroprusside or glyceryl trinitrate, may increase cardiac output and lower pulmonary wedge pressure
- contraindicated with halogenated general anaesthetics because they may provoke ventricular arrhythmias

Nursing considerations/Cautions
- loading dose/bolus not recommended
- available as a powder or solution
- solution should be diluted to 50 mL with either glucose 5% or sodium chloride 0.9% before IV administration
- reconstitute powder with 10 mL water for injections (add another 10 mL if not completely dissolved) then add to at least 50 mL glucose 5%, Ringer's solution or sodium lactate. Sodium chloride 0.9% should not be used to reconstitute powder
- incompatible with sodium bicarbonate or any other strongly alkaline solution
- pink discolouration does not indicate loss of potency
- if the patient has atrial fibrillation with rapid ventricular response, digitalisation is recommended before starting therapy
- solution contains sodium metabisulfite, which may cause allergic reactions in those with hypersensitivity
- caution if used in those with pre-existing hypertension, atrial flutter/fibrillation, ventricular ectopics or with any risk factors for cardiac rupture (e.g. within 4–12 days of myocardial infarction)
- contraindicated in those with idiopathic hypertrophic subaortic stenosis
- see also General Nursing considerations/Cautions for sympathomimetic agents (p. 1566)

 Not used during pregnancy unless expected benefit outweighs any potential risk.

 Excretion in human breastmilk unknown. Not used during breastfeeding unless expected benefit outweighs any potential risk.

 Banned in sport.

DOPAMINE
Trade names
DBL Sterile Dopamine Concentrate, Dopamine Juno

Available form
Ampoules: 200 mg/5 mL

Action
- both direct and indirect sympathomimetic effects
- stimulates alpha and beta adrenergic and dopamine receptors (depending on dose)
  - (0.5–2 microgram/kg/min) dopaminergic (D_1) receptors are selectively activated, leading to renal and mesenteric vasodilation resulting in increased renal blood flow and urine output
  - (2–10 microgram/kg/min) β1-receptors are activated, increasing cardiac output and systolic BP
  - (> 10 microgram/kg/min) α receptors are activated, resulting in peripheral vasoconstriction, increases in both systolic and diastolic BP and decreased urine flow (because of decreased renal blood flow)
- inotropic effect on the heart increases cardiac output and systolic BP
- physiological precursor of noradrenaline (norepinephrine) and adrenaline (epinephrine)

SYMPATHOMIMETIC AGENTS

- physiological neurotransmitter, mainly in the brain; however, does not cross blood—brain barrier when given systemically
- rapid onset of action (within 5 minutes), duration 5—10 minutes, half-life 2 minutes

Use
- correction of haemodynamic imbalance in acute hypotension/shock (e.g. acute myocardial infarction, endotoxic shock, trauma, renal failure)
- adjunct after open-heart surgery (when there is persistent hypotension despite correction of hypovolaemia)
- chronic cardiac decompensation in severely refractory congestive cardiac failure (short-term management)

Dose
- initially 2—5 microgram/kg/min IV, increasing by 5—10 microgram/kg/min increments, up to 50 microgram/kg/min as required **OR**
- (Severe refractory cardiac failure) 0.5—2 microgram/kg/min IV, increasing to 1—3 microgram/kg/min as urine flow increases (maintenance) as required. Rate should be decreased if diastolic BP or HR increases

Adverse effects
- tachycardia, palpitations, ectopic beats, angina, hypotension, vasoconstriction
- nausea, vomiting
- headache
- dyspnoea
- gangrene of feet (in pre-existing peripheral vascular disease or high doses)
- (Rare) ventricular arrhythmias
- (IV site extravasation) skin/tissue necrosis

Interactions
- bradycardia, hypotension and possible cardiac arrest may occur if given with phenytoin (IV)
- hypotension may occur if given with calcium-channel blockers, nitroprusside or glyceryl trinitrate
- if given with or within 3 weeks of monoamine oxidase inhibitors (MAOIs), dopamine dose should be reduced to 1/10th normal dose
- may interfere with urine tests for amino acids, catecholamines, uric acid or urobilinogen
- see also General Interactions of sympathomimetic agents (p. 1565)

Nursing considerations/Cautions
- frequently check conscious state and nail bed capillary filling
- note changes in temperature or colour of extremities if there is pre-existing peripheral vascular disease
- urine output should be carefully monitored during therapy; if it decreases without any associated hypotension, dose reduction is recommended
- must be diluted before administration: 200 mg may be added to 250 mL of the recommended infusion solution to make a concentration of 800 microgram/mL, or to 500 mL for a concentration of 400 microgram/mL
- to avoid tissue necrosis, administer into a large vein high up in a limb, preferably the arm
- incompatible with amphotericin B (amphotericin) and ampicillin and alkaline solutions such as sodium bicarbonate
- hypotension may occur when weaning from dopamine and this may require an increase in blood volume or changing to another pressor agent while slowly decreasing dose
- have phentolamine available as antidote for peripheral ischaemia resulting from extravasation (phentolamine 5—10 mg in sodium chloride 0.9%; infiltrate area with 10—15 mL)
- contains sodium metabisulfite, which can cause allergic reactions in those with hypersensitivity
- caution if used in those with pulmonary hypertension, as condition may be worsened with therapy
- caution if given to those with cardiac ischaemia or pre-existing peripheral vascular disease (including

atherosclerosis, frostbite and Raynaud's disease), as these people may be at greater risk of peripheral ischaemia and gangrene
- contraindicated in those with pheochromocytoma, atrial/ventricular arrhythmias or hyperthyroidism
- see also General Nursing considerations/Cautions for sympathomimetic agents (p. 1566)

Not used during pregnancy unless expected benefit outweighs any potential risk.

Not used during breastfeeding unless expected benefit outweighs any potential risk.

Elderly patients may be more susceptible to dopamine's effects, including fluctuations in blood pressure, urine output and peripheral perfusion. Close monitoring is recommended.

Banned in sport.

EPHEDRINE HYDROCHLORIDE
Trade names
Ephedrine Hydrochloride Juno, Ephedrine Interpharma, Ephedrine-hameln

EPHEDRINE SULFATE
Trade name
DBL Ephedrine Sulfate Injection

Available form
Ampoules: 30 mg/mL, 30 mg/10 mL

Action
- direct and indirect sympathomimetic effects on both alpha and beta adrenoceptors
- more prolonged, but less potent than adrenaline (epinephrine)
- CNS and respiratory centre stimulant
- increases cardiac output and peripheral vasoconstriction, increasing systolic and diastolic BP
- causes bronchodilation
- reduces intestinal tone and motility
- relaxes bladder wall, contracts sphincter muscle and relaxes detrusor muscle
- usually reduces activity of the uterus
- onset 10–20 minutes (IM) or 3–5 minutes (IV), duration 1 hour (IM) or 10–15 minutes (IV)
- half-life 3–6 hours (increased in acidic urine)

Use
- hypotension associated with spinal anaesthesia
- shock unresponsive to fluid replacement
- treatment of bronchospasm in asthma (although more selective agents are now available)

Dose
- (Hypotension secondary to spinal anaesthetic) 3–7.5 mg by slow IV, repeated if needed every 3–4 minutes (maximum 30 mg) (Ephedrine Hydrochloride) **OR**
- (Pressor) 10–50 mg IM or SC, or 10–25 mg slow IV, repeated 5–10 minutes until desired response (maximum daily dose 150 mg) (Ephedrine Sulfate) **OR**
- (Bronchospasm) 12.5–25 mg IM, SC or slow IV, then determined by response (maximum daily dose 150 mg) (Ephedrine Sulfate)

Adverse effects
- pallor, fever, sweating
- headache, insomnia
- angina, palpitations, bradycardia, tachycardia, hypertension, hypotension, chest pain
- nausea, vomiting, epigastric distress, increased salivation
- shortness of breath, dyspnoea
- dry mouth, nose, throat
- urinary retention, dysuria
- nervousness, anxiety, restlessness, fear, mood changes, irritability, trembling
- hyperglycaemia, hypokalaemia

SYMPATHOMIMETIC AGENTS

- (High dose) dizziness, lightheadedness, vertigo, confusion, delirium, euphoria
- (Long-term use) physical addiction
- (IV) necrosis (if extravasation occurs)

Interactions
- contraindicated with, or within 2 weeks of, monoamine oxidase inhibitors (MAOIs)
- contraindicated with linezolid
- increased risk of paroxysmal hypertension and arrhythmia if given with venlafaxine or sibutramine
- cardiac and bronchodilator effects may be reduced if given with beta adrenergic blocking agents
- may increase serum levels of phenytoin, primidone and phenobarbital (phenobarbitone) if given together
- increased risk of headache, palpitations and hypertension if given with moclobemide
- decreased vasopressor effects may occur if given with methyldopa sesquihydrate
- increased effect may occur if pretreated with clonidine
- elimination may be reduced if given with urinary alkalinisers (e.g. acetazolamide, sodium bicarbonate and sodium citrate)
- increased risk of adverse effects of both agents if given with theophylline
- vasopressor effects may be increased by atropine sulfate monohydrate, oxytocin and ergot alkaloids
- increased risk of peripheral vascular ischaemia and gangrene if given with oxytocin or ergot alkaloids
- see also General Interactions of sympathomimetic agents (p. 1565)

Nursing considerations/Cautions
- any hypoxia, hypercapnia and acidosis should be corrected before starting therapy
- IV route is recommended for those in shock to ensure adequate absorption
- avoid extravasation
- 3 mg/mL solution requires dilution before use
- (IV, ephedrine hydrochloride 3 mg/mL) dilute 1 mL with 10 mL sodium chloride to give a concentration of 3.5 mg/mL
- (IV, ephedrine hydrochloride) if maximum dose of 30 mg does not produce required effect, another therapeutic agent should be considered
- incompatible with phenobarbital (phenobarbitone), thiopentone and hydrocortisone
- caution if used in those with prostatic hypertrophy, diabetes mellitus, cardiovascular disease (e.g. angina, arrhythmias or cardiac insufficiency) or myocardial infarction (as ischaemia may be increased)
- extreme caution (if given at all) to those with hyperthyroidism or hypertension because of the increased risk of adverse effects
- contraindicated in those with closed-angle glaucoma, pheochromocytoma, asymmetric septal hypertrophy, tachyarrhythmias, ventricular fibrillation or psychoneurosis
- see also General Nursing considerations/Cautions for sympathomimetic agents (p. 1566)

Patient education
- patients with diabetes mellitus should be warned that blood glucose levels may become unstable during therapy

If used during delivery, it may increase the fetal heart rate. It is not recommended if the maternal blood pressure is greater than 130/80 mmHg.

Not recommended. Excreted in breast-milk and may cause adverse effects in nursing infants.

Elderly patients, particularly men with prostatic hypertrophy, are at increased risk of urinary retention when using ephedrine. Caution and close monitoring are recommended.

Banned in some sports, while permitted in other sports subject to restrictions.

ISOPRENALINE HYDROCHLORIDE (ISOPROTERENOL)

Trade names
Cipla Isoprenaline, Isoprenaline Macure, Isoprenaline Medsurge

Available forms
Ampoules: 200 microgram/mL, 1000 microgram/5 mL

Action
- non-selective synthetic catecholamine structurally related to adrenaline (epinephrine), but acts almost exclusively on beta adrenergic receptors
- increased cardiac output because of positive inotropic and chronotropic actions, increases venous return
- increased peripheral vasodilation resulting in lower diastolic BP in normal individuals
- relaxes bronchial smooth muscle causing bronchodilation, as well as relaxation of skeletal muscle, GI tract and splanchnic bed
- stimulates insulin release
- metabolite has weak beta adrenergic blocking activity
- half-life 2–3 minutes (IV) or up to 2 hours (SC)

Use
- mild or transient heart block (not requiring electric shock or pacemaker)
- cardiac arrest (until electric shock or pacemaker is available)
- serious heart block or Stokes–Adams attack (unless caused by ventricular tachycardia or fibrillation)
- bronchospasm during anaesthesia
- adjunct in management of cardiogenic, hypovolaemic and septic shock or congestive heart failure

Dose
- (Bronchospasm during anaesthesia) 0.01–0.02 mg by IV bolus (diluted solution 0.2 mg in 10 mL of sodium chloride 0.9% or glucose 5%), repeated as necessary **OR**
- (Shock, hypoperfusion) 1 mg (5 mL) in 500 mL glucose 5% by IV infusion at a rate of 0.5–5 microgram/min **OR**
- (Heart block, cardiac arrest, Stokes–Adams attack) initially 0.2 mg IM or SC, then 0.02–1 mg IM or 0.15–0.2 mg SC (undiluted solution) **OR**
- (Heart block, cardiac arrest, Stokes–Adams attack) initially 0.02–0.06 mg by IV bolus, then 0.01–0.2 mg (diluted solution 0.2 mg in 10 mL of sodium chloride 0.9% or glucose 5%) **OR**
- (Heart block, cardiac arrest, Stokes–Adams attack) 5 microgram/min by IV infusion (diluted solution 2 mg in 500 mL glucose 5%) **OR**
- (Heart block, cardiac arrest, Stokes–Adams attack) 0.02 mg by intracardiac injection (undiluted solution)

Adverse effects
- tachycardia, palpitations, angina, hypertension, hypotension, ventricular arrhythmias, Stokes–Adams attack, pulmonary oedema
- hot flushes, skin flushing, sweating
- mild tremor, weakness
- nervousness, restlessness, fear, tension
- headache, dizziness
- (Rare) tinnitus, asthenia, lightheadedness, nausea, vomiting

Interactions
- increased risk of cardiotoxicity if given with IV corticosteroids or IV aminophylline
- not recommended with chlorpromazine or monoamine oxidase inhibitors (MAOIs)
- not recommended with adrenaline (epinephrine) or digoxin because of the increased risk of cardiac arrhythmias (although may be given separately with adequate time interval separating agents)

Nursing considerations/Cautions
- if time is not an essential factor, IM or SC administration is preferred
- if the patient has pre-existing asthma, oxygen should be administered at the same time as IV infusion

SYMPATHOMIMETIC AGENTS

- infusion rate is adjusted according to the heart rate, ECG, central venous pressure (CVP), systemic BP, arterial blood gases and urine output (reduce infusion rate if adult heart rate exceeds 110 beats/min or ventricular hyperexcitability is apparent on ECG). Cardiac enzyme (CPK MB) should be measured if ECG shows any signs of myocardial ischaemia
- caution if given to the elderly or those with coronary insufficiency, ischaemic heart disease, cardiogenic shock (due to coronary arterial occlusion or myocardial infarction), hypertension, diabetes mellitus or hyperthyroidism or if sensitive to other sympathomimetic agents
- contraindicated in those with digitalis-induced tachycardia/heart block, tachyarrhythmias, ventricular arrhythmias (requiring inotropes), recent myocardial infarction or angina
- see also General Nursing considerations/Cautions for sympathomimetic agents (p. 1566)

Not used during pregnancy unless the expected benefit outweighs any potential risk.

Caution: excretion in human breastmilk unknown.

Banned in sport.

METARAMINOL

Trade names
Aramine, Metaraminol ARX, Metaraminol GH Pharma, Metaraminol Juno, Metaraminol MYX, Metaraminol Phebra, Metaraminol Torbay

Available forms
Ampoules: 2.5 mg/5 mL, 3 mg/6 mL, 5 mg/10 mL, 10 mg/mL

Action
- direct and indirect sympathomimetic effects on both alpha and beta adrenoreceptors
- mainly alpha adrenergic stimulant effects, with some beta effects, resulting in potent effects that increase systolic and diastolic BP and peripheral vasoconstriction
- increases coronary blood flow, slows heart rate
- less potent than noradrenaline (norepinephrine)
- effective within 1–2 minutes (IV), lasting 20–60 minutes

Use
- prevention or treatment of acute hypotension following spinal anaesthesia
- adjunct to treatment of hypotension associated with haemorrhage, septicaemia, reaction to medications, surgical complications or cardiogenic shock

Dose
- (Adjunctive treatment of hypotension) 15–100 mg diluted in 500 mL of sodium chloride 0.9% or glucose 5% regulated by burette or microdrip with IV infusion rate adjusted to maintain BP at desired level **OR**
- (Emergency treatment of severe shock) 0.5–5 mg IV bolus, followed by infusion as above

Adverse effects
- tachycardia, arrhythmias
- (IV site, rare) abscess formation, tissue necrosis, sloughing

Interactions
- contraindicated with halogenated hydrocarbon anaesthetics
- caution if used with digoxin as ectopic arrhythmias may occur
- effects may be potentiated by monoamine oxidase inhibitors (MAOIs) and tricyclic antidepressants (TCAs) and therefore not recommended together

Nursing considerations/Cautions

- monitor heart rate and systemic BP every 5 minutes until stabilised, then every 15 minutes during and for several hours after infusion is completed
- avoid excessive BP response
- allow at least 10 minutes to elapse between altering dosage
- IV bolus should be used only as life-saving measure
- response may be poor in those with shock and acidosis
- not used regularly in routine clinical practice
- caution if used in those with cirrhosis, heart or thyroid disease, hypertension or diabetes mellitus
- contains sodium metabisulfite; therefore it is contraindicated in those with sulfite hypersensitivity
- see also General Nursing considerations/Cautions for sympathomimetic agents (p. 1566)

May cause fetal hypoxia by constricting uterine vessels and limiting placental perfusion. Use during pregnancy only if the potential benefit justifies the potential risk.

Caution: excretion in human breastmilk unknown.

Banned in sport.

NORADRENALINE (NOREPINEPHRINE)
Trade names
Noradrenaline BNM, Noradrenaline Juno, Noradrenaline Medsurge, Noralin

Available forms
Ampoules: 2 mg/2 mL, 4 mg/4 mL, 3 mg/50 mL, 6 mg/50 mL

Action
- direct-acting sympathomimetic agent with action on alpha and beta adrenoceptors
- dilates coronary arteries, increasing blood flow
- peripheral vasoconstriction resulting in increase in both systolic and diastolic BP
- no changes in heart rate or cardiac output
- physiological neurotransmitter released from postganglionic adrenergic nerve fibres when stimulated
- rapid onset of action, half-life 30 seconds to 3 minutes

Use
- treatment of acute hypotensive states when blood volume is adequate
- adjunct to cardiac arrest treatment (to restore and maintain adequate BP after effective cardiac arrest management measures)

Dose
- initially 8—12 microgram/min IV, then adjusted to maintain the BP at the desired level, then 2—4 microgram/min (maintenance)

Adverse effects
- arrhythmias, palpitations, reflex bradycardia, hypotension
- anxiety, transient headache
- respiratory distress
- (IV site) necrosis (if extravasation occurs)
- (Rare) gangrene of extremities
- (Overdose or in those who are hypersensitive) severe hypertension, violent headache, photophobia, stabbing retrosternal pain, pallor, intense sweating, vomiting

Interactions
- prolonged hypertension may result if given with monoamine oxidase inhibitors (MAOIs) or tricyclic antidepressants (TCAs) and should be given with extreme caution, if at all

SYMPATHOMIMETIC AGENTS

- contraindicated with halogenated hydrocarbon general anaesthetics

Nursing considerations/Cautions

- monitor conscious state, temperature and colour of extremities, urinary output and infusion site every 15 minutes (for any signs of blanching; IV should be resited if this occurs)
- monitor heart rate and BP every 2 minutes until stabilised at desired level, then every 5 minutes. Patient should not be left unattended
- preferably given via central venous catheter (CVC) to decrease risk of extravasation and necrosis
- must be diluted before use. Add 2 mg to 500 mL or 4 mg to 1000 mL of glucose 5% to make a concentration of 4 microgram/mL
- therapy should be continued until adequate BP and tissue perfusion can be maintained, then rate reduced gradually, avoiding abrupt withdrawal
- noradrenaline (norepinephrine) should not be added to whole blood, plasma or saline solutions
- should not be used if solution is brown
- incompatible with alkalis, barbiturates, chlorpheniramine, iron salts, nitrofurantoin, phenytoin, sodium bicarbonate or sodium iodide
- have phentolamine (5–10 mg in 10–15 mL of sodium chloride 0.9%) available if extravasation occurs
- increased risk of hypersensitivity reaction in those with hyperthyroidism
- contains sodium metabisulfite, which may cause allergic reaction in hypersensitivity individuals; therefore is not recommended
- not recommended for infusion via leg veins in those > 65 years
- contraindicated in those with hypotension (because of hypovolaemia) or mesenteric or peripheral vascular thrombosis (because of the increased risk of ischaemia)

- see also General Nursing considerations/Cautions for sympathomimetic agents (p. 1566)

Not recommended during pregnancy unless the benefits outweigh the risks. Animal studies indicate that noradrenaline (norepinephrine) may reduce placental perfusion and cause fetal bradycardia, potentially resulting in fetal asphyxia in late pregnancy.

Caution: excretion in human breastmilk unknown.

Use with caution. Start at a lower dose because of likely reduced hepatic, renal or cardiac function and other conditions or drug interactions. Avoid leg vein infusions to reduce ischaemia risk.

Banned in sport.

PHENYLEPHRINE

Trade names
Neo-Synephrine, Phenylephrine Baxter, Phenylephrine BNM

Available forms
Ampoules: 0.5 mg/5 mL (0.01%), 10 mg/mL (1%)

Action
- synthetic sympathomimetic structurally related to adrenaline (epinephrine) and ephedrine
- vasoconstrictor, pressor
- slows heart rate and increases stroke output with no effect on rhythm
- main actions are on postsynaptic alpha receptors
- little effects on coronary beta receptors
- increases systolic and diastolic BP, marked reflex bradycardia
- constricts vascular beds, but coronary blood flow is increased
- constricts pulmonary vessels, increasing pulmonary arterial pressure

- more sustained action than adrenaline (epinephrine) (20 minutes (IV) or 50 minutes (SC))

Use
- maintains BP during spinal and inhalation anaesthesia
- vascular failure in shock, shock-like states or drug-induced hypotension
- overcomes paroxysmal supraventricular tachycardia
- prolongs spinal anaesthesia
- vasoconstrictor in regional anaesthesia
- mydriatic (see Eye, Ear, Nose and Throat agents, p. 1132)

Dose
- (Mild/moderate hypotension) 2–5 mg SC or IM (initial dose not greater than 5 mg) **OR**
- (Mild/moderate hypotension) 0.1–0.5 mg IV (initial dose not greater than 0.5 mg) increasing dose at 15-minute intervals if needed **OR**
- (Severe hypotension and shock) 100–180 microgram/min by IV infusion (10 mg (of 1% solution) diluted in 500 mL glucose 5% or sodium chloride 0.9%) until BP is stabilised, then reduced to 40–60 microgram/min **OR**
- (Spinal anaesthesia – hypotension) 2–3 mg IM or SC given 3–4 minutes before spinal anaesthetic **OR**
- (Hypotensive emergency during spinal anaesthesia) initially 0.2 mg IV, increasing dose by 0.1–0.2 mg if needed (maximum single dose 0.5 mg) **OR**
- (Prolong spinal anaesthesia) 2–5 mg added to anaesthetic solution **OR**
- (Vasoconstrictor for regional anaesthesia) optimal strength is 1:20,000 (add 1 mg (1% solution) phenylephrine to 20 mL local anaesthetic) **OR**
- (Paroxysmal supraventricular tachycardia) initially up to 0.5 mg rapid IV, then increasing dose by not more than 0.1–0.2 mg of initial dose (depending on BP) (maximum dose 1 mg)

Adverse effects
- headache, excitability, restlessness
- reflex bradycardia
- (Rare) arrhythmias

Interactions
- see General Interactions of sympathomimetic agents (p. 1565)

Nursing considerations/Cautions
- can be given SC, IM, IV injection or IV infusion
- (Phenylephrine BNM) not recommended SC or IM
- (Spinal anaesthesia prolongation) phenylephrine hydrochloride prolongs duration of motor block by up to 50% with no increase in adverse effects
- 5 mg IM will produce increased BP for 1–2 hours, while 0.5 mg IV will produce an increase for 15 minutes
- extreme caution if used in the elderly or those with hyperthyroidism, bradycardia, partial heart block, myocardial disease or severe arteriosclerosis
- contraindicated in those with severe hypertension or ventricular tachycardia
- see also General Nursing considerations/Cautions for sympathomimetic agents (p. 1566)

Use in pregnancy only if the potential benefits outweigh the risks. May cause persistent hypertension if given with some oxytocic agents, which may result in cerebral vessel rupture postdelivery.

Caution: excretion in human breastmilk unknown.

Caution: start at the lower end of dosing, as elderly patients are more likely to have reduced hepatic, renal or cardiac function and concurrent conditions. Avoid infusion in leg veins to reduce ischaemia risk.

Note
- Phenylephrine is combined with a number of other agents (see Eye, ear, nose and throat agents p. 1132)

THYROID AND ANTITHYROID AGENTS

The thyroid gland is a highly vascular organ consisting of two connected lobes which have small parathyroid glands on the posterior surface. The thyroid gland produces two hormones, thyroxine sodium (T4) (precursor) and liothyronine (T3) (active hormone), which influence growth, development and metabolic processes (Jameson, Mandel & Weetman 2022c). Iodine is needed for the synthesis of both hormones and is generally acquired via the diet, with an adult requiring approximately 1 mg/week. Iodine can be found in foods such as dairy products, seafood, kelp, eggs, bread (since 2009, all breads made in Australia are made with iodised salt, except for organic bread), some vegetables (if grown in iodine-rich soil) and iodised salt (Food Standards, Australia & New Zealand 2019). Over the past few decades, iodine intake levels have dropped and reasons are thought to include the increased consumption of processed food (manufacturers generally do not use iodised salt), less iodine in milk (treatment methods have changed), a reduction in iodine in soil, and less use of salt in cooking and eating (particularly iodised salt; sea salt and 'boutique' salts do not contain iodine) (Food Standards, Australia & New Zealand 2023).

Control of thyroid hormone secretion is via a complex feedback system that involves both the hypothalamus and the pituitary gland. Decreased blood concentrations of thyroid hormone are detected by receptors in the hypothalamus, leading to the release of thyrotrophin (thyrotropin)-releasing hormone (TRH). TRH stimulates the anterior pituitary gland to release thyroid-stimulating hormone (TSH), which in turn stimulates the thyroid gland to release T3 and T4. T4 is de-iodinated in the liver to T3, further increasing the concentration of T3 (active) in the blood. This then feeds back to the hypothalamus and pituitary gland to stop production (negative feedback) (Jameson, Mandel & Weetman 2022c). It should be noted that goitrogenic foods, such as cruciferous vegetables (e.g. cabbage, broccoli, Brussels sprouts, cauliflower, kale, bok choy (pak choi)), interfere with thyroid hormone synthesis by impairing the binding of iodine to thyroglobulin (Food Standards, Australia & New Zealand 2023).

Thyroid hormones are needed for normal growth and development and to maintain metabolic rate. Effects of thyroid hormones include activation of osteoclast and osteoblast activities in the bones; increase in cardiac output and blood volume and decrease in systemic vascular resistance; regulation of lipolysis; regulation of triglyceride and cholesterol metabolism; regulation of pituitary hormone synthesis, inhibition of TSH and stimulation of production of growth hormone; and stimulation of axonal growth and development in the brain (Jameson, Mandel & Weetman 2022c).

Thyroid gland dysfunction can manifest as hypo- or hyperthyroidism.

Hypothyroidism is the most common thyroid dysfunction, affecting about 1 in 33 Australians (Hormones Australia 2023). It is a decrease in thyroid gland activity from a range of causes, including congenital, autoimmune disease (e.g. Hashimoto's disease), surgery, iodine deficiency or excess intake, some medications and radioactive iodine ingestion. Symptoms include tiredness, weakness, weight gain with poor appetite, constipation, intolerance to heat, feeling cold, cool peripheries, decreased libido, dry and coarse skin, brittle nails, hoarse/husky voice, bradycardia, difficulty concentrating and poor memory (Jameson, Mandel & Weetman 2022b). Hypothyroidism is treated using thyroid hormone replacement therapy. The term myxoedema refers to those patients with thyroid hormone deficiency of such severity that profound hypothermia, hypoventilation, hypotension and central nervous system signs are evident on physical examination and can be life threatening.

Thyroid dysfunction occurs commonly in women of childbearing years, second only to diabetes mellitus, with the incidence of hyperthyroidism in pregnancy ranging from 0.1 to 0.4%. It is important to note that overt hypothyroidism and hyperthyroidism have been associated with some adverse obstetric outcomes, including pre-eclampsia, miscarriage and low birthweight babies, and subclinical hypothyroidism associated with pre-eclampsia and perinatal mortality. If a woman with pre-existing thyroid disease becomes pregnant, thyroid hormone levels should be closely monitored and medications adjusted accordingly to maintain a euthyroid state (Pregnancy, Birth & Baby 2023).

Hyperthyroidism is caused by an overfunctioning thyroid gland (e.g. Graves' disease), toxic adenoma, toxic multinodular goitre or excessive intake of thyroid agents or iodine. Symptoms include palpitations, tachycardia, palpably enlarged thyroid gland, ophthalmopathy, nervousness, irritability, labile emotions, heat intolerance and sweating, weight loss (in spite of increased food intake), loose stools/diarrhoea, decreased or absent menstrual flow, decreased libido, muscle weakness, warm, moist skin, fine hair, diffuse alopecia, fine tremor and excessive sweating (Jameson, Mandel & Weetman 2022a). Hyperthyroidism treatment is aimed at reducing thyroid hormone production and blocking the peripheral effects of excessive thyroxine sodium, such as tachycardia, tremor and sweating. Treatment may include surgery (subtotal resection of thyroid gland), radioactive iodine therapy or medical management using antithyroid agents (Jameson, Mandel & Weetman 2022a).

Thyrotoxicosis is defined as the state of thyroid hormone excess and is not synonymous with *hyperthyroidism*, which is the result of excessive thyroid function (Jameson, Mandel & Weetman 2022a).

Antithyroid agents inhibit the synthesis of thyroid hormones, but do not affect the thyroid hormones that are already stored or circulating in the blood. Antithyroid agents are usually given in high doses for 3–4 months until thyroid function returns to normal (euthyroid), and the dose is then reduced to the minimum dose required to maintain the euthyroid state. Treatment is sometimes a combination of antithyroid agents and thyroid hormones. Antithyroid compounds (also termed thyrostatic compounds) can be subdivided into thioureas (also called thionamides) (e.g. carbimazole, propylthiouracil) and anion inhibitors (e.g. iodine, potassium perchlorate).

THYROID AGENTS

LEVOTHYROXINE SODIUM
Trade names
APO-Levothyroxine, Eltroxin, Eutroxsig, Oroxine, Levothox, Levoxine, Levothyroxine Lup, Levothyroxine Sandoz, Thyrox

Available forms
Tablets: 25 microgram, 50 microgram, 75 microgram, 100 microgram, 125 microgram, 150 microgram, 200 microgram

Action
- also called L-thyroxine sodium
- converted to more active T3 form
- slow onset of action (3–4 weeks)
- long duration of action 7–21 days (even when thyroxine sodium is stopped)
- elimination half-life 6–7 days (euthyroid patient), 9–10 days (hypothyroidism) or 3–4 days (hyperthyroidism)

Use
- thyroid hormone deficiencies
- thyroid-stimulating hormone (TSH)-responsive thyroid tumours

Dose
- (Adult $\geq$ 70 kg) initially 50–100 micrograms orally daily 30–60 minutes before food, increasing by 25–50 micrograms and at least 4-weekly intervals to 100–200 micrograms daily as maintenance **OR**
- (Adult > 60 years or with ischaemic heart disease) initially 25–50 micrograms orally daily 30–60 minutes before food, then increasing to 75–125 micrograms orally daily as maintenance

Adverse effects
- usually associated with overdosage and consists of the following:
  - nervousness, tremor, restlessness, anxiety, irritability, fatigue
  - sweating, flushing, intolerance to heat, fever
  - headache, insomnia, sleep disturbance, poor concentration, emotional lability
  - mania, psychosis, psychotic depression
  - seizures
  - tachypnoea, shortness of breath
  - tachycardia, palpitations, cardiac arrhythmias, angina pectoris, chest pain
  - myopathy, muscle cramps and weakness
  - eyelid lag
  - diarrhoea, nausea, vomiting, abdominal pain, weight loss, malabsorption
  - alopecia, hyperpigmentation
  - amenorrhoea, menstrual irregularities, decreased libido, gynaecomastia (males)
  - decreased glucose tolerance

Interactions
- may enhance the clinical effects of warfarin, requiring close monitoring of INR especially when starting therapy
- may reduce the effect of digoxin

- use with ketamine may result in marked hypertension and tachycardia
- effect may be reduced by colestyramine (cholestyramine), colestipol, soya flour, soy-containing foods, high-fibre diet, sucralfate, aluminium hydroxide, calcium carbonate, magnesium hydroxide, ferrous sulfate heptahydrate and proton pump inhibitors
- coronary insufficiency may occur if given with sympathomimetic agents
- increased dosage of oral hypoglycaemics and insulin may be needed. Blood glucose levels should be carefully monitored, especially when starting, stopping or changing doses of levothyroxine sodium
- effect may be reduced by beta adrenoceptor blocking agents and amiodarone, because peripheral conversion of thyroxine sodium to T3 is decreased
- increase in therapeutic and toxic effects of levothyroxine sodium and tricyclic antidepressants (TCAs) may occur if given together
- absorption may be decreased if given with ciprofloxacin; a 6-hour interval is recommended if the two are given together
- an increase in dose of levothyroxine sodium may be required if given with oestrogen (in those with a non-functioning thyroid gland)
- dose adjustment of corticosteroids may be required if given with levothyroxine sodium
- decreased plasma levels may result if given with phenytoin, carbamazepine, barbiturates, rifampicin, proguanil or ritonavir
- effects may be reduced if given with sertraline or other selective serotonin reuptake inhibitors (SSRIs)
- caution if given with lithium, as hypothyroidism may result
- decreased dose may be required if given with androgens
- absorption may be decreased by orlistat and should be separated by a 4-hour interval if given together
- thyroid function tests can be modified by NSAIDs, salicylates, diazepam and heparin

Nursing considerations/Cautions

- formulations are not interchangeable (e.g. Eltroxin versus Oroxine/Eutroxsig). If the patient is switched between formulations, careful TSH monitoring is required and dose adjustment may be necessary
- where possible, the patient should be administered whole tablets
- monitor heart rate, reporting if it is more than 100 beats/min or if there is any marked change in rate or rhythm
- signs of overdose may take 3–6 days to be manifested
- T4, T3, TSH and response to thyrotrophin-releasing hormone (TRH) should be monitored regularly throughout therapy
- blood sampling times should be related to ingestion time
- if the patient has hypopituitarism or adrenal insufficiency, corticosteroid replacement therapy should be started before thyroxine sodium to prevent Addisonian crisis
- therapy should be started at a low dose (25–50 microgram/day) and increased gradually. If the patient has cardiac disease or is elderly, the starting dose should be 12.5–25 microgram/day and increased in increments of not more than 25 micrograms, at intervals of not less than 14 days. If not tolerated because of angina, increments should be reduced and/or angina controlled with beta adrenoceptor blocking agents
- caution if used in postmenopausal women, as a decrease in bone mineral density may occur
- caution if used in those with diabetes insipidus or diabetes mellitus, as an adjustment to insulin or oral antidiabetic medication may be required

THYROID AND ANTITHYROID AGENTS

- caution if used in those with a history of hyperthyroidism or thyrotoxicosis, long-standing hypothyroidism or myxoedema or cardiac disease
- caution if given to those with malabsorption syndromes, as absorption may be reduced
- not recommended for treatment of obesity or weight loss
- contraindicated in those with untreated hyperthyroidism, thyrotoxicosis, uncorrected adrenal insufficiency, acute myocarditis, acute pancreatitis or acute myocardial infarction uncomplicated by hypothyroidism

Patient education

- the patient should be warned that it may take a few weeks for therapy to be effective and changes in symptoms to occur
- instruct the patient to take as a single daily dose 30–60 minutes before breakfast (on an empty stomach)
- advise the patient that the replacement therapy is lifelong and that follow-up appointments need to be kept. The importance of regular blood tests should also be emphasised
- the patient should be warned that therapy interacts with a number of other medications, including over-the-counter (OTC) preparations such as antacids, calcium and iron supplements, and it is therefore important to discuss dosing schedule in relation to these. The patient should also be instructed to allow a 6-hour interval if prescribed ciprofloxacin or a 5-hour interval if prescribed colestyramine (cholestryramine) or colestipol with thyroxine sodium
- the patient should be directed to report palpitations, difficulty in breathing (dyspnoea) or chest pain
- if the patient has diabetes mellitus, it is important to remind them that insulin and/or oral hypoglycaemic agent requirements will increase with therapy and blood glucose levels should be monitored frequently, especially when starting therapy
- (Oroxine/Eutroxsig) instruct the patient to store tablets in refrigerator (2–8°C); however, a single blister strip can be stored at up 25°C for up to 2 weeks and then any remaining tablets should be discarded

If tablet is crushed and dispersed in water, it should be taken immediately as the dispersion settles quickly and is sensitive to light.

Increased dose may be required if used during pregnancy. Serum thyroxine sodium and TSH levels should be monitored 3–4-weekly during pregnancy, as an increase in dosage requirements is usually required. Requirements then decrease postpartum. If possible, thyroxine sodium therapy should be optimised before conception.

Breastfeeding should be continued during therapy.

Therapy should be initiated at a low dose.

LIOTHYRONINE SODIUM

Trade names
Tertroxin

Available form
Tablets: 20 microgram

Action
- also called L-triiodothyronine
- similar to that of thyroxine sodium, but much more potent and rapid in onset (within a few hours of administration), with briefer duration of action and disappears within 24–48 hours of stopping therapy
- half-life 1–2 days (in euthyroid patient), prolonged in hypothyroidism, reduced in hyperthyroidism

Use
- severe and acute hypothyroid states
- myxoedema coma
- thyrotoxicosis (as an adjunct to carbimazole to prevent subclinical hypothyroidism)

Dose
- (Myxoedema) 10—20 micrograms orally 8-hourly, increasing gradually to a total of 60 micrograms daily in 2—3 divided doses **OR**
- (Myxoedema coma) 60 micrograms via stomach tube, then 20 micrograms 8-hourly **OR**
- (Thyrotoxicosis) 20 micrograms orally 8-hourly (with carbimazole)

Adverse effects
- headache, restlessness, flushing, sweating, excitability
- diarrhoea, excessive weight loss
- palpitations, anginal pain, tachycardia, cardiac arrhythmias
- skeletal muscle cramps and/or weakness

Interactions
- may enhance activity of oral anticoagulants; therefore prothrombin times should be closely monitored when therapy with liothyronine is started or the dose altered
- absorption may decrease if given with colestyramine (cholestryramine)
- may increase plasma levels of phenytoin, increasing the risk of toxicity
- metabolism may be increased by phenytoin and carbamazepine
- increased risk of cardiac arrhythmias if given with TCAs
- may require adjustment to dose of digoxin (as liothyronine may potentiate digitalis toxicity)
- decreased serum levels may result if given with oral contraceptives
- ketamine may cause hypertension and tachycardia when given with thyroid replacement therapy
- increased oral hypoglycaemics and insulin may be needed. Blood glucose levels should be carefully monitored

Nursing considerations/Cautions
- regular thyroid function tests are recommended
- adverse effects are uncommon
- adrenal deficiency should be corrected with adrenocorticotrophic hormones before starting therapy
- if treating myxoedema coma, ECG monitoring, assisted ventilation and corticosteroids are also required
- caution if used in elderly patients, who may be more sensitive to thyroid replacement therapy
- caution if used in those with endocrine disorders (e.g. diabetes mellitus, adrenocortical insufficiency)
- contraindicated in those with angina, cardiovascular disorders, untreated adrenal cortical insufficiency or untreated hyperthyroidism

Patient education
- the patient should be advised of the importance of continuing therapy, keeping follow-up appointments and having regular blood tests
- warn the patient to report any chest pain or palpitations, excessive sweating or weight loss immediately
- if the patient has diabetes mellitus, it is important to remind them that insulin and/or oral hypoglycaemic agent requirements will increase with therapy and blood glucose levels should be monitored frequently, especially when starting therapy
- if the patient is taking anticoagulant medication (e.g. warfarin), blood test for prothrombin should be monitored frequently when starting therapy

THYROID AND ANTITHYROID AGENTS

Tablet may be crushed and mixed with water (does not disperse well), or a spoonful of yoghurt or apple puree.

Excreted in breastmilk.

Initial dose in elderly patients should be 5 micrograms daily, as they may show increased sensitivity to the thyroid replacement therapy.

ANTITHYROID AGENTS

CARBIMAZOLE
Trade names
Neo-Mercazole, Thirazol, WP Carbimazole

Available form
Tablets: 5 mg

Action
- depresses thyroid hormone synthesis by inhibiting the binding of iodine to tyrosine
- clinical response does not occur until circulating and stored thyroid hormone has been used
- has no effect on iodine uptake by thyroid gland
- active metabolite (methimazole) is responsible for antithyroid activity, half-life 3–6 hours

Use
- hyperthyroidism (induction of remission in either primary or secondary thyrotoxicosis)
- preparation for thyroidectomy
- pre- and post-radioactive iodine treatment

Dose
- (Hyperthyroidism, mild cases) initially 15–20 mg orally daily in divided doses; (moderate cases) 30 mg orally daily in divided doses; (severe cases) 40–45 mg orally daily in divided doses (up to 60 mg) until euthyroid, then 10–15 mg daily as maintenance for 1–2 years **OR**
- (Changeover from thiouracils) 5 mg of carbimazole is equivalent to 50 mg of propylthiouracil **OR**
- (Preparation for thyroidectomy) preoperatively carbimazole is prescribed in doses that will make the patient euthyroid and continued until surgery, with iodide being added in the last 2 weeks

Adverse effects
- nausea, mild gastric disturbances, loss of taste
- headache, neuritis
- mild rash, pruritus, urticaria, hair loss
- arthralgia
- bone marrow depression, agranulocytosis
- jaundice, hepatitis, abnormal liver function tests
- (Rare) aplastic anaemia, myopathy, vasculitis, severe hypersensitivity reaction

Interactions
- may increase serum levels of theophylline, increasing the risk of toxicity
- caution if given with other agranulocytosis-inducing agents
- may increase effects of anticoagulants; therefore prothrombin time/INR should be carefully monitored especially when starting or stopping therapy or if a surgical procedure is planned
- may increase clearance of prednisolone
- may decrease clearance of erythromycin
- may increase digoxin and beta adrenergic blocking agent levels when hyperthyroid patients become euthyroid

Nursing considerations/Cautions
- treatment should not be commenced if patient is not able to be regularly monitored or is unlikely to be concordant with therapy
- dosage is titrated to thyroid function until patient is euthyroid and maintenance dose continued for 12–24 months
- patient monitoring should be monthly for the first year, then 3–6-monthly to

- prevent overtreatment resulting in hypothyroidism
- adverse reactions usually occur within 8 weeks of starting therapy
- if patient complains of myalgia, creatine phosphokinase (CPK) levels should be monitored
- therapy is usually stopped when radioactive iodine is administered
- response to carbimazole may be delayed (weeks to months) if there are large amounts of thyroid hormones present (e.g. nodular goitre), whereas response in thyrotoxicosis is seen in 3—4 days
- caution if given to those with memory loss or confusion, as they may not be able to report symptoms of adverse effects. Regular monitoring of full blood counts is recommended
- caution if used in those with mild-to-moderate liver impairment
- caution if used in those with tracheal obstruction, as high doses may lead to thyroid enlargement, which in turn may exacerbate symptoms of obstruction
- not recommended in those with galactose intolerance, Lapp lactase deficiency or glucose—galactose malabsorption
- contraindicated in those with a retrosternal goitre
- contraindicated in those with severe liver impairment or pre-existing blood disorders
- contraindicated in those with previous acute pancreatitis due to carbimazole/active metabolite
- contraindicated in those with hypersensitivity to thiamazoles or propylthiouracil, as cross-allergy may exist

Patient education

- advise the patient to keep appointments throughout therapy, including the need for blood tests
- warn the patient to immediately report any of the following:
  - rash, fever, mouth ulcers, malaise, sore throat, bruising or bleeding immediately (early signs of bone marrow depression)
  - muscle pain (possible myopathy)
  - yellow eyes or skin, itchiness, upper abdominal pain, nausea, vomiting or loss of appetite, loss of weight, fever or dark urine (signs of liver dysfunction)
- women of childbearing potential should be advised to use effective contraception during therapy

Tablet does not disperse easily in water. Tablet can be crushed and mixed with water (does not disperse easily) or mixed with spoonful of yoghurt or apple puree.

Crosses the placental barrier. Should be given during pregnancy only if benefits (mother's needs) outweigh risk to the fetus, and if propylthiouracil is unsuitable. Dose may need to be adjusted during pregnancy, because of the increase in basal metabolic rate (BMR). Dose should not exceed 15 mg twice daily during last trimester. Administration should stop 3—4 weeks before delivery date because carbimazole may inhibit thyroid hormone synthesis in the fetus, leading to congenital goitre, and substituted with iodine. If used during pregnancy, close maternal and fetal monitoring is recommended, and the neonate monitored for any signs of hypothyroidism.

Carbimazole is concentrated in breastmilk and therefore breastfeeding is contraindicated.

Pregnant staff must not crush or disperse tablet. Gloves, mask and closed tablet crusher should be used.

THYROID AND ANTITHYROID AGENTS

PROPYLTHIOURACIL
Trade name
PTU

Available form
Tablets: 50 mg

Action
- depresses thyroid hormone synthesis by inhibiting the binding of iodine to tyrosine
- clinical response does not occur until circulating and stored thyroid hormone has been used
- has no effect on iodine uptake by thyroid gland
- does not interfere with release or action of exogenous thyroid hormone
- half-life about 2 hours
- may become euthyroid in 4–6 weeks

Use
- hyperthyroidism (induction of remission in either primary or secondary thyrotoxicosis)
- preparation for thyroidectomy
- pre- and post-radioactive iodine treatment

Dose
- initially 200–400 mg orally daily in 3–4 divided doses until euthyroid, then 50–800 mg daily in 2–4 divided doses
OR
- (Thyrotoxic crisis) 800–1200 mg daily in divided doses (orally or via nasogastric tube) together with other agents such as iodine, and general supportive measures

Adverse effects
- itching
- dizziness
- joint pain
- loss of taste, nausea, vomiting, stomach pain
- agranulocytosis, mild leucopenia. granulocytosis, thrombocytopenia
- (Rare) cholestatic jaundice, hepatotoxicity, ototoxicity, lymphadenopathy, hypoprothrombinaemia, nephritis, vasculitis, peripheral neuropathy, severe hypersensitivity reaction
- (Rare) hyperplasia of thyroid gland

Interactions
- patients receiving heparin or oral anticoagulants require close monitoring of prothrombin time, because propylthiouracil can cause hypoprothrombinaemia
- risk of agranulocytosis is increased if propylthiouracil is taken with another agranulocytosis-inducing agent

Nursing considerations/Cautions
- those with severe hyperthyroidism may require up to 1200 mg daily
- regular thyroid function tests are recommended before starting therapy, monthly during stabilisation and then 2–3-monthly. Liver function tests and full blood count monitoring are also recommended
- women under 30 should be closely monitored, as they are at greater risk of hepatotoxicity (especially in first 3 months of therapy). Liver function tests monthly for first 6 months of therapy are recommended
- iodine is given with propylthiouracil in preparation for surgery to decrease friability and vascularity of thyroid gland
- caution if used in those with asthma
- contraindicated in those with hypersensitivity to thioamide derivatives

Patient education
- advise the patient to keep appointments during initial therapy
- the patient should be warned not to drive or operate machinery if dizziness occurs
- the patient should be instructed to seek medical advice immediately if any of the following occur:
  - rash, fever, chills, headache, malaise, mouth ulcers, sore throat, bleeding or bruising (signs of agranulocytosis)
  - upper abdominal discomfort, fever, nausea, vomiting, weight loss, yellowing of eyes or skin, dark urine (signs of hepatotoxicity)

- diarrhoea, fever, vomiting, rapid heartbeat, irritability, weakness, listlessness (signs of excess thyroid hormone)
- tiredness, lethargy, muscle weakness/cramping, slow heartbeat, feeling cold, dry/flaky skin, hair loss, deep/husky voice, weight gain, change in menstrual cycle, headache (signs of hypothyroidism)
- signs of hepatotoxicity should be emphasised in women under 30 because of their increased risk
- the patient should be informed to keep dosing intervals equal (e.g. 6- or 8-hour intervals)

May be dispersed in water, or crushed tablet mixed with yoghurt or apple puree.

May cause damage to fetal thyroid, causing fetal hypothyroidism and neonatal goitre, or congenital abnormalities; therefore should be avoided during pregnancy unless the benefits to the mother outweigh risks to the fetus. If used, dose should be as low as possible to provide therapeutic effects and discontinued if patient shows any signs of hypothyroidism.

Excreted in breastmilk. Breastfeeding should be stopped before starting therapy with propylthiouracil.

If crushing tablets, mask, gloves and closed tablet crusher should be used. Pregnant staff should not crush or disperse tablet.

SODIUM IODIDE (^{131}I)

Trade names
ANSTO Health Sodium Iodide (^{131}I) Injection, ANSTO Health Sodium Iodide (^{131}I) Therapy Capsules, ANSTO Health Sodium Iodide (^{131}I) Therapy Solution Oral liquid

Available forms
Capsule (contained in a glass vial and lead container): 50—6000 MBq;
Oral solution (contained in a glass vial and lead container): 50—16 000 MBq;
Injection (contained in 10 mL glass vial): 200—1600 MBq;
MBq (megabecquerel) is a measure of radiation

Action
- radioactive iodide that concentrates in thyroid tissue. Therapeutic effect is due to beta radiation
- mostly excreted via kidneys but also via sweat and saliva

Use
- hyperthyroidism in patients who have a poor surgical risk or have not responded well to therapy
- detection and ablation of residual thyroid tissue (thyroid cancer)

Dose
- (Thyrotoxicosis) 150—600 MBq orally (capsules, oral solution) **OR**
- (Thyroid ablation) 800—2000 MBq orally (capsules, oral solution) **OR**
- (Thyroid carcinoma) 2000—6000 MBq in 2 capsules orally **OR**
- (Hyperthyroidism, wt $\geq$ 70 kg) 148—370 MBq IV **OR**
- (Thyroid imaging) 0.185—3.7 MBq IV

Adverse effects
- vomiting, nausea
- tachycardia
- rash, pruritus
- (Elderly patient with total thyroidectomy) hyponatraemia
- (Rare, high dose) radiation-induced thyroiditis, inflamed salivary glands, transient worsening of hyperthyroidism
- (Potential) radiation sickness, bone marrow depression, acute leukaemia, anaemia, pulmonary fibrosis, acute thyroid crisis

Interactions
- uptake may be affected by intake of stable iodine within last 4 weeks (e.g. seafood, radiographic contrast media, antithyroid drugs, thyroxine sodium)

THYROID AND ANTITHYROID AGENTS

- contraindicated with thyroid hormones or antithyroid agents

Nursing considerations/Cautions

- the patient should be well hydrated before and during therapy to promote excretion
- the patient should be encouraged to urinate as often as possible for 4—6 hours after administration to reduce exposure of bladder, kidney and stomach to radiation
- antithyroid drugs should be stopped for 3—4 days before treatment and withheld for 7—14 days after administration of radioactive iodide
- levothyroxine sodium should be withheld for 4 weeks before treatment with radioactive iodide
- the patient should be screened for any recent intake of stable iodine (e.g. seafood, radiographic contrast media, antithyroid drugs, thyroxine sodium). Patient should also be screened for any risk of hyponatraemia, including age, being female, use of thiazide diuretics and previous thyroidectomy
- women of childbearing age should have pregnancy test before administration
- the patient should be managed in a single room (according to hospital protocol) to prevent unwanted radiation exposure to others. Isolation precautions are recommended for those receiving greater than 600 MBq
- only a doctor qualified and licensed to handle radioisotopes should administer dosage
- staff exposure should be minimised
- disposable gloves (for staff and patient); disposal cup with water and tissues should be prepared before removal of vial from lead container
- handling and disposal of radioactive waste (including disposable gloves, paper cup, empty vial, stopper and cap) is according to hospital policy and NHMRC 'Code of Practice for the disposal of radioactive wastes by the user' (1985, 1990)
- the patient will require lifelong follow-up
- capsules and IV solution have a 14-day expiry from the day of calibration and should not be administered if expired
- iodine allergy IS NOT a contraindication to the use of sodium iodide, as there is only a very small amount of iodine in the capsule (3 micrograms in a 500 MBq capsule)
- not recommended in those with renal insufficiency or under 18 years
- caution if given to those with nephrosis or decreased kidney function, or who eat goitrogenic foods (see p. 1579), as these interfere with accumulation of iodine by thyroid
- contraindicated in those currently undergoing treatment with thyroid or antithyroid agents, or if the person is vomiting or has diarrhoea

Patient education

- the patient should be advised to swallow capsule whole (not chewed)
- the patient should be encouraged to drink copious amounts of fluid before and after treatment to reduce dose (radioactivity) to kidney, bladder and stomach
- secreted in saliva; therefore kissing is discouraged for at least 10 days after therapeutic dose (especially children)
- double flushing of toilet and careful washing of hands should be encouraged strongly
- urine, stool and vomit are radioactive and should be disposed of carefully, avoiding contact with others
- the patient should be instructed that they will require lifelong follow-up
- close contact with children and pregnant women should be avoided for a week after administration, as well as lengthy duration with others closer than 1 metre

- encourage daily showering to remove excess perspiration (radioactive iodide is excreted in sweat) for a week after administration
- both males and females should be counselled regarding the need for effective contraception after administration of radioactive iodide for 6 months (those with benign thyroid conditions) or 12 months (thyroid cancer)
- males should be counselled regarding sperm banking if they have extensive disease necessitating high dosage

Contraindicated during pregnancy.

Breastfeeding must be stopped at least 8 weeks before administration and should not be restarted.

Increased risk of hyponatraemia in elderly patients who have undergone total thyroidectomy. Regular serum electrolyte monitoring is recommended.

VACCINES AND IMMUNOGLOBULINS

A vaccine is a biological preparation that contains antigens (or ANTIbody GENerating substances) that are derived from a disease-causing microorganism. When introduced into the body, a vaccine confers acquired immunity to a specific disease (Knights et al 2023). *Vaccination* is the administration of a vaccine and *immunisation* is the development of protective levels of antibodies (confirmed by serological testing). Immunological agents are used for both active and passive immunity. Active immunity results when the body itself responds to an antigenic agent, producing antibodies. This may happen naturally as a result of an infection or artificially after immunisation.

Not all vaccines use the same technology to stimulate an immune response, hence there are different types of vaccines. Conventional vaccine types include live attenuated vaccines, inactivated (killed whole antigen) vaccines and subunit (purified antigen) vaccines. Over recent decades, a better understanding of the genomes of pathogens, coupled with enhanced laboratory and computer technologies, has led to new types of vaccines. New vaccine types include nucleic acid vaccines (e.g. mRNA) and viral vector vaccines. The COVID-19 global pandemic, and the urgent need for the widespread use of an effective vaccine, resulted in the novel vaccine types being used extensively in humans for the first time (Iwasaki & Omer 2020).

Passive immunisation is immunity given as already formed antibodies. These antibodies may be of animal origin (antivenom, also known as antisera) or of human origin (immunoglobulins) and provide temporary protection.

VACCINES

General Actions of vaccines
- vaccines are ANTIbody GENerating (antigenic) materials that, when introduced into the body, induce active artificial immunity to a specific infectious disease
- subsequent doses of vaccine (booster doses) provide protection by increasing declining antibody levels
- live attenuated vaccines include oral typhoid, oral rotavirus, BCG, yellow fever, Japanese encephalitis, varicella, zoster, measles—mumps—rubella (MMR) and varicella (chickenpox) vaccines

General Uses of vaccines
- a vaccine provides complete or partial protection for months or years to specific infectious diseases

- the primary immunisation schedule starts early in life and is lifelong (see National Immunisation Program Schedule, below)

General Interactions of vaccines

- if live vaccines are not administered simultaneously (i.e. on the same day at the same visit), they should be separated by at least 4 weeks
- people who have received immunoglobulins or blood products (e.g. blood transfusion) may need to wait 3—11 months before vaccination; the presence of naturally occurring circulating antibodies in the blood products may result in vaccine failure
- revaccination may be required if an immunoglobulin is given within 2 weeks of vaccine
- not recommended within 14 days of high-dose corticosteroid therapy
- live vaccines are often contraindicated during corticosteroid or immunosuppressive therapy, including radiation, as they may result in an extensive vaccine-related rash or disseminated disease
- live vaccines are often contraindicated or used with caution in people with HIV/AIDS or other immunocompromised states, depending on the individual's immune function
- may temporarily depress tuberculin skin sensitivity for 4—6 weeks, giving a possible false negative response

Nursing considerations/Cautions

- assess the patient's medical history, including allergies, immunocompromised status, pregnancy, recent immunoglobulin or blood product administration and current medications (especially immunosuppressants)
- be aware of contraindications and temporary precautions, such as recent illness, moderate/severe acute illness or pregnancy, in the case of live vaccines
- ensure patients understand the purpose of the vaccine, potential side-effects and any contraindications before administering vaccines
- valid consent should be obtained before each vaccination. A parent or legal guardian can consent for a child. However, if a child/adolescent refuses a vaccination that has been consented to by a parent or legal guardian, their wishes should be respected and the parent or legal guardian informed. Consent may be written or verbal (depending on the protocols of the health facility). It should be obtained after the person has been given information (verbal and/or written) about the vaccine, its use, risks and benefits and any possible adverse effects
- ensure appropriate needle length and gauge based on the patient's age, size and injection route (IM or SC). For instance, a 23- to 25-gauge, 1-inch (25 mm) needle is typically recommended for most adult IM injections
- be sure to landmark properly to avoid surrounding structures and minimise the risk of shoulder injury related to vaccine administration (SIRVA)
- different sites can be used (e.g. one injection into each deltoid muscle). If the same muscle (muscle mass needs to be sufficiently large) is used for multiple injections, at least 2.5 cm should be allowed between sites
- in paediatric patients, non-pharmacological methods such as distraction techniques (e.g. toys, blowing bubbles or singing) may help alleviate anxiety and discomfort during vaccination
- post-vaccine, nurses should monitor patients for 15 minutes for immediate reactions, including anaphylaxis. Adrenaline (epinephrine) should be readily available for emergency use
- vasovagal episodes (fainting) occur commonly in adolescents and adults post-vaccination but not in infants or children. If an infant or child loses consciousness, an anaphylactic reaction

VACCINES AND IMMUNOGLOBULINS

should be presumed if a strong central (carotid) pulse is not present. Vasovagal episodes tend to occur within minutes of vaccination, whereas anaphylactic reaction usually occurs within 15 minutes, although it can be delayed
- to maintain vaccine efficacy, nurses must follow protocols for proper vaccine storage (e.g. refrigeration or freezing, depending on the vaccine)
- accurately document vaccine administration, including the vaccine name, lot number, expiration date, site of injection and any adverse reactions
- guide patients on catch-up schedules if they missed doses of vaccines or have incomplete vaccine histories
- report serious adverse events following immunisation (AEFI) to appropriate health authorities (relevant state and territory health department or Therapeutic Goods Administration)
- ensure you upload data to the Australian Immunisation Register (AIR): full name, date of birth, Medicare number or AIR identification number and vaccine details (brand, dose number, batch number, date administered, injection site)
- if using a multidose vial, ensure the vial is used within the manufacturer's specified time frame (e.g. 28 days) once opened, to avoid contamination and preserve vaccine efficacy
- premature infants should be immunised as per the normal schedule (not adjusted for prematurity), although some (depending on gestation or birthweight) may require extra doses of some vaccines, as preterm infants may be at increased risk of vaccine-preventable diseases (e.g. pneumococcal disease) and may not develop sufficient antibodies after some vaccinations (e.g. hepatitis B)

General Patient education for vaccines

- (Prevaccination) advise individuals to wear loose, comfortable clothing that makes it easy to access the injection site (usually the deltoid muscle of the upper arm)
- educate patients/parents/carers on the signs of an allergic reaction (e.g. difficulty breathing, swelling of the face or throat, hives) and advise them to seek immediate medical attention if any of these symptoms occur
- patient/parent/carer should be advised that vaccination may not confer 100% protection (e.g. immunised children may still develop chicken pox after exposure, but the number of vesicles and duration of illness is reduced)
- patient/parent/carer should be warned that vaccination often results in soreness, itching, swelling or burning at injection site, which lasts for 1—2 days
- adult patients should be warned not to drive or operate machinery after vaccination if drowsiness or dizziness occurs
- advise the patient to avoid vigorous exercise and excessive alcohol consumption for several hours after vaccination
- explain that some vaccines (e.g. tetanus, diphtheria, pertussis, hepatitis B) may require booster doses to maintain immunity over time

Notes

Overseas travel and vaccination
- the individual's doctor will decide on the type, dosage and timing of vaccination in consultation with the patient (or parents in the case of a child), and this decision is generally made according to such factors as length of stay overseas, risk of exposure, age of the patient and how endemic the disease is in the country to be visited

Health care workers and vaccination
- health care workers may be exposed to a range of vaccine-preventable diseases
- it is recommended that all health care workers (including students) involved in direct patient care or who come into

contact with human tissue (e.g. laboratory staff, mortuary staff) are vaccinated against hepatitis B, influenza, pertussis, MMR (if non-immune) and varicella (if seronegative). In addition, those working with remote Aboriginal and Torres Strait Islander communities in the Northern Territory, Western Australia, Queensland and South Australia should also be vaccinated against hepatitis A. Staff who may be at high risk of exposure to drug-resistant tuberculosis should also receive BCG. There are also recommendations for people who work with animals
- health care workers should consider that vaccination may not only protect themselves from developing diseases and requiring time away from the workplace, but also protect the patients they care for from the potential spread of illness (e.g. influenza, COVID-19), which may be potentially life threatening in some groups of particularly vulnerable patients (e.g. the elderly, immunocompromised, after transplantation, after radiation or chemotherapy)
- some workplaces have immunisation requirements and comprehensive occupational vaccination programs in place. This may include the management of vaccine refusal by the health care worker (e.g. reducing the risk of the health care worker transmitting a disease to vulnerable individuals)
- BCG vaccination is recommended in staff at high risk of TB (e.g. staff working in chest clinics, infectious diseases wards, physiotherapists, diagnostic laboratory staff, autopsy room staff, and medical and nursing staff in public hospitals)

National Immunisation Program Schedule

Age	Disease
Birth (preferably within 24 hours for the greatest benefit, but within 7 days of birth)	Hepatitis B
2 months (can be given from 6 weeks)	Hepatitis B, diphtheria, tetanus, pertussis (whooping cough), *Haemophilus influenzae* type b, poliomyelitis, pneumococcal, rotavirus
Aboriginal and Torres Strait Island children	Meningococcal B
4 months	Hepatitis B, diphtheria, tetanus, pertussis (whooping cough), *H. influenzae* type b, poliomyelitis, pneumococcal, rotavirus
Aboriginal and Torres Strait Island children	Meningococcal B
6 months	Hepatitis B, diphtheria, tetanus, pertussis (whooping cough),

(Continued)

VACCINES AND IMMUNOGLOBULINS

— cont'd

Age	Disease
	H. influenzae type b, poliomyelitis,
Additional dose for children with specified medical risk conditions and Aboriginal and Torres Strait Island children from WA, SA, NT and Queensland	Pneumococcal
Additional dose for children with specified medical risk conditions (Aboriginal and Torres Strait Island children)	Meningococcal B
6 months to 5 years (annually)	Influenza
12 months	Measles, mumps and rubella, meningococcal ACWY (MenACWY), pneumococcal
Aboriginal and Torres Strait Island children	Meningococcal B
18 months	Diphtheria, tetanus, pertussis (whooping cough), measles, mumps, rubella and varicella (chickenpox), *H. influenzae* type b (Hib)
Additional vaccine for Aboriginal and Torres Strait Island children in WA, NT, SA and Queensland	Hepatitis A
4 years	Diphtheria, tetanus, pertussis (whooping cough), poliomyelitis
Additional dose for children with specified medical risk conditions, and Aboriginal and Torres Strait Island	Pneumococcal

(Continued)

— cont'd

Age	Disease
children in WA, NT, SA and Queensland	
Additional vaccine for Aboriginal and Torres Strait Island children in WA, NT, SA and Queensland	Hepatitis A
≥ 5 years (annually) Children with specified medical risk conditions, Aboriginal and Torres Strait Islander children	Influenza
12—13 years	Human papillomavirus Diphtheria, tetanus, pertussis (whooping cough)
14—16 years	MenACWY
50 years and over (Aboriginal and Torres Strait Island adults)	Pneumococcal, shingles
65 years and over	Influenza (annually) (non-Aboriginal and Torres Strait Islander adults), shingles (herpes zoster) (non-Aboriginal and Torres Strait Islander adults)
70 years and over	Pneumococcal (non-Aboriginal and Torres Strait Islander adults)
Pregnant women (ideally between 20—32 weeks, but may be given up to delivery)	Influenza, pertussis (whooping cough)

National Immunisation Program Schedule © 2024 Commonwealth of Australia as represented by the Department of Health and Aged Care

VACCINES AND IMMUNOGLOBULINS

BACILLUS CALMETTE-GUERIN (BCG) VACCINE
Trade names
BCG S11 Vaccine, BCG Vaccine AJV

Action
- prepared from attenuated strain of *Mycobacterium bovis*

Use
- Aboriginal and Torres Strait Islander children under 5 in certain high-risk areas
- health care workers with high exposure to tuberculosis
- young children travelling to tuberculosis endemic regions
- children born to parents from countries with high tuberculosis incidence
- children in contact with household members who have leprosy

Dose
- 0.1 mL intradermally

Adverse effects
- local reaction of a small indurated red papule occurs in 1–3 weeks, which softens then ulcerates and heals over several weeks, leaving superficial scar, lymphadenopathy
- (Rare) keloid scarring, local or generalised infection, anaphylactoid reaction

Interactions
- response may be inhibited if given within 4–6 weeks of measles-containing vaccine or measles infection

Nursing considerations/Cautions
- tuberculin test (Mantoux test) is recommended before vaccination (unless under 6 months old) and vaccine given if induration is less than 5 mm with test dose of 10 units
- given intradermally using specialised tuberculin syringe
- those with latent or previous TB infection will have accelerated response to BCG
- does not prevent TB if patient is already infected, but reduces mortality
- not used in TB treatment
- revaccination is not recommended
- contains polysorbate 80 and is not recommended in those with known hypersensitivity to these
- contraindicated in people who have an immunodeficiency disorder or have had TB or a positive tuberculin reaction > 5 mm
- see also General Nursing considerations/Cautions for vaccines (p. 1592)

Patient education
- patient should be advised that small red lump will form, will ulcerate in about 2–3 weeks after vaccination and will heal with a small scar. Swelling and tenderness under the arm also commonly occur
- see also General Patient education for vaccines (p. 1593)

 Live vaccine not recommended during pregnancy.

 Safe in breastfeeding.

CHOLERA VACCINE
Trade names
Dukoral, Vaxchora

Action
- cholera is an acute diarrhoeal disease that can kill a person within hours if untreated with oral rehydration salts
- (Vaxchora) live, attenuated oral cholera vaccine containing a weakened strain of *Vibrio cholerae* O1. Protection lasts for about 3–6 months
- (Dukoral) inactivated (killed) oral cholera vaccine. It contains killed *Vibrio cholerae* bacteria and a non-toxic component of cholera toxin. Provides protection against cholera (serogroup O1 *Vibrio cholerae*), which is one of the virulent strains of the disease; not active against other species of cholera; confers 85%

protection for 4—6 months in all age groups

Use
- travellers to high-risk areas where cholera is endemic or the person is at high risk (e.g. immunocompromised)

Dose
- Dukoral
  - (adults, children > 6 years) 2 doses orally, at least 1 week apart **OR**
  - (children 2—6 years) 3 doses orally, at least 1 week apart
  - dissolve the effervescent powder in 150 mL of water.
  - add the vaccine suspension to the water and drink it within 2 hours
  - (children 2—6 years) discard half of the effervescent solution (75 mL) and add the vaccine to the remaining half
- Vaxchora
  - (adults, children > 2 years) oral, single dose
  - dissolve the buffer powder in 100 mL of bottled water
  - add the contents of the vaccine sachet to the water and drink it within 15 minutes
  - (children 2—6 years) discard half of the buffer solution, then add the vaccine sachet to the remaining half

Adverse effects
- Dukoral (common): diarrhoea, abdominal pain/cramps/discomfort, gas; (rare) nausea, vomiting
- Vaxchora (common): abdominal pain, nausea, vomiting, diarrhoea

Interactions
- should be separated by at least 8 hours from oral typhoid vaccine
- see also General Interactions of vaccines (p. 1592)

Nursing considerations/Cautions
- not recommended for children under 2 years
- administration should be delayed if person has acute gastrointestinal illness
- avoid food and drink for 1 hour before and after taking the vaccine
- should be started at least 2 weeks before arrival at destination
- if more than 6 weeks elapse between doses, immunisation should be restarted
- (Dukoral) offers protection for about 6 months after vaccination. Booster dose is recommended after 2 years for repeated travel or ongoing risk
- (Dukoral) contains 1.2 g sodium/dose, which may need to be considered if patient requires sodium-/salt-restricted diet
- (Dukoral) contraindicated in those with hypersensitivity to formaldehyde
- (Vaxchora) treatment with antibacterial or antimalarial agents may inactivate Vaxchora vaccine. Wait at least 14 days after completing antibacterial or antimalarial treatment before administering the vaccine. Avoid starting antibacterial or antimalarial therapy for at least 10 days after the vaccine is given to ensure its effectiveness
- (Vaxchora) immunosuppression— Vaxchora is contraindicated
- see also General Nursing considerations/Cautions for vaccines (p. 1592)

Patient education
- take on an empty stomach at least 1 hour before or after food
- avoid eating or drinking anything for at least 60 minutes after taking the vaccine
- patient should be warned to take care with selection of food and water while travelling in endemic areas
- see also General Patient education for vaccines (p. 1593)

Vaxchora is a live attenuated vaccine — contraindicated in pregnancy.

It is unknown whether the Vaxchora vaccine is excreted in human milk; a risk to the breastfed child cannot be ruled out.

Dukoral is considered safe in breastfeeding.

VACCINES AND IMMUNOGLOBULINS

COVID-19 VACCINE
Trade names
Comirnaty, Comirnaty Omicron XBB.1.5, Comirnaty JN.1, Spikevax, Spikevax JN.1, Nuvaxovid

Action
- Comirnaty (tozinameran and famtozinameran) — single-stranded messenger RNA (mRNA) encoding the viral spike (S) protein of severe acute respiratory syndrome coronavirus 2 (SARS-CoV-2)
- Comirnaty JN.1 (bretovameran) — single-stranded messenger RNA (mRNA) encoding the viral spike (S) protein of severe acute respiratory syndrome coronavirus 2 (SARS-CoV-2) (JN.1)
- Comirnaty Omicron XBB.1.5 (raxtozinmeran) — single-stranded messenger RNA (mRNA) encoding the viral spike (S) protein of severe acute respiratory syndrome coronavirus 2 (SARS-CoV-2) (Omicron XBB.1.5)
- Spikevax (elasomeran/imelasomeran) — single-stranded messenger RNA (mRNA) encoding the viral spike (S) protein of severe acute respiratory syndrome coronavirus 2 (SARS-CoV-2)
- Spikevax JN.1 (SARS-CoV-2 JN.) — single-stranded messenger RNA (mRNA) encoding the viral spike (S) protein of SARS-CoV-2 JN.1
- Nuvaxovid (SARS-CoV-2 rS (NVX-CoV2373)) COVID-19 vaccine — severe acute respiratory syndrome coronavirus 2 (SARS-CoV-2) recombinant spike protein (rS) with Matrix M adjuvant to boost the immune response. This vaccine introduces proteins that prompt the body's immune system to respond without using live viruses

Use
- active immunisation to prevent coronavirus disease 2019 (COVID-19) caused by SARS-CoV-2

Dose
Primary
- Nuvaxovid: given IM in two 0.5 mL doses, with second dose recommended 3 weeks after first
- Comirnaty: given IM in two 0.3 mL doses, with second dose recommended 3 weeks after first
- Spikevax: given IM in two 0.5 mL doses, with second dose recommended 4 weeks after first
- Spikevax JN.1: given IM in two 0.5 mL doses, with second dose recommended 28 days after first
- Comirnaty JN.1, Comirnaty Omicron XBB.1.5:
  - (3 microgram/dose: patient age 6 months to under 5 years) given IM in three 0.2—0.3 mL. Doses 1 and 2 at least 3 weeks apart, third dose at least 8 weeks after 2 dose
  - (10 microgram/dose: patient age 5 to under 12 years) given IM in two 0.2—0.3 mL doses, with second dose recommended 3 weeks after first
  - (30 microgram/dose: patient age 12 years and older) given IM in two 0.3 mL doses, with second dose recommended 3 weeks after first

Booster
- ($\geq$ 75 years): every 6 months
- (65—74 years & 18—64 years with severe immunocompromise): every 12 months; consider 6 months based on risk
- (All other adults 18—64 years): consider every 12 months based on risk
- (Children 5 to under 18 years with severe immunocompromise): consider every 12 months based on risk

Adverse effects
- headache, fatigue, malaise
- fever, chills
- nausea
- myalgia, arthralgia
- (Injection site) tenderness, warmth, pain, swelling, redness
- (Rare) hypersensitivity, anaphylaxis
- (Rare) myocarditis, pericarditis (commonly after second dose and more frequently in adolescents or young men)

Nursing considerations/Cautions
- administered IM, with preferred vaccination site the deltoid muscle

- COVID-19 vaccines can be co-administered with an influenza vaccine
- name and batch number should be recorded to assist traceability of vaccine
- use of same brand of vaccine for first 2 doses (primary series) is preferred
- medical recommendations regarding preferred vaccine according to patient's age should be considered before vaccination
- allow to thaw for 30 minutes at room temperature before use
- (Comirnaty Omicron XBB.1.5, Comirnaty JN.1) available as suspension for injection or prefilled syringes not requiring dilution, or as a concentrate that requires dilution with sodium chloride 0.9% (see manufacturer's information for dilution instructions)
- mRNA vaccines (Comirnaty, Comirnaty JN.1, Comirnaty Omicron, Spikevax, Spikevax JN.1) must be stored frozen. Comirnaty is stored at −90°C to −60°C and Spikevax at −50°C to −15°C. Once thawed, both can be refrigerated at +2°C to +8°C for up to 30—31 days, depending on the vaccine. After dilution or puncture, must be used within 6—12 hours and not refrozen
- see also General Nursing considerations/Cautions for vaccines (p. 1592)

Patient education

- the patient should be instructed to seek medical advice immediately if they experience any of the following, which may be signs of myocarditis or pericarditis:
    - acute and persisting chest pain, shortness of breath and/or rapid heart rate
    - fatigue, nausea, vomiting, abdominal pain, dizziness, fainting
- see also General Patient education for vaccines (p. 1593)

DIPHTHERIA—TETANUS VACCINE
Trade name
ADT Booster

Action
- (Diphtheria) protects against *Corynebacterium diphtheriae*, which produces a toxin that can lead to severe throat and respiratory problems. The toxin can also cause life-threatening heart failure and paralysis
- (Diphtheria) the vaccine contains diphtheria toxoid, a chemically inactivated form of the toxin
- (Tetanus) protects against *Clostridium tetani*, a bacterium that produces a toxin that affects the nervous system and leads to painful muscle contractions
- (Tetanus) the vaccine contains tetanus toxoid, the inactivated form of the toxin produced by the bacterium

Use
- revaccination of adults and children over 5 who have received at least 3 doses of vaccine for immunisation against diphtheria and tetanus
- tetanus prophylaxis after injury (see Tetanus-prone wounds p. 1629)

Adverse effects
- (Injection site) redness, swelling
- headache, fever, lethargy, malaise, myalgia
- (Rare) urticaria, peripheral neuropathy, anaphylaxis

Interactions/Nursing considerations/Cautions/Patient education
- intramuscular (IM) injection
- not recommended as primary immunisation
- laboratory workers should have serology tests for diphtheria antibody levels every 10 years and booster given if diphtheria antitoxin < 0.1 IU/mL
- caution if used in those with formaldehyde sensitivity

- see also General Nursing considerations/Cautions/Patient education for vaccines (p. 1592)

Safe to use. Inactivated vaccine.

Safe to use. Tetanus and diphtheria toxoid vaccines are safe for breastfeeding women as they are inactivated and pose no risk of infection to the infant.

DIPHTHERIA–TETANUS–PERTUSSIS VACCINE

Trade names
Adacel, Boostrix, Infanrix, Tripacel

Action
- active immunisation against diphtheria, tetanus and pertussis (whooping cough)
- (Diphtheria) the vaccine contains diphtheria toxoid, a chemically inactivated form of the toxin. Protects against *Corynebacterium diphtheriae*, which produces a toxin that can lead to severe throat and respiratory problems. The toxin can also cause life-threatening heart failure and paralysis
- (Tetanus) the vaccine contains tetanus toxoid, the inactivated form of the toxin produced by the bacterium. It protects against *Clostridium tetani*, a bacterium that produces a toxin that affects the nervous system and leads to painful muscle contractions
- (Pertussis) the vaccine contains inactivated acellular components of the pertussis bacterium. It protects against *Bordetella pertussis*, a bacterium that causes severe coughing fits, difficulty breathing and the characteristic 'whooping' sound. It can lead to serious complications, especially in infants, such as pneumonia, seizures, brain damage, and death (1 in 200 infants)
- effect of diphtheria and tetanus vaccines is enhanced when administered with pertussis vaccine
- adult formulations provide lower diphtheria and pertussis antigens (dTpa) than formulations for children (DTP)

Use
- as primary immunisation in infants aged 2–12 months (Infanrix, Tripacel)
- recommended in those over 10 years as a booster after primary immunisation (Adacel)

Adverse effects
- (Injection site) pain, swelling, redness
- (Children) crying, irritability, somnolence, extensive limb swelling, loss of appetite, diarrhoea, vomiting, headache
- fever, chills, body aches
- headache, lethargy, malaise
- nausea, diarrhoea
- myalgia
- (Children, rare) febrile convulsion, hypotonic–hyporesponsive episodes (child becomes pale, limp and unresponsive)
- (Rare) limb/joint swelling

Interactions
- see General Interactions of vaccines (p. 1592)

Nursing considerations/Cautions
- intramuscular (IM) injection
- any reaction is likely to be caused by pertussis component and any further diphtheria–tetanus–pertussis or pertussis-only vaccines should be avoided
- diphtheria and tetanus toxoid-containing vaccines should be avoided within 5 years of previous booster dose to avoid risk of local adverse reactions
- it is not recommended to give paracetamol before vaccination as a preventive measure. Studies suggest it might slightly reduce the immune response to the vaccine (except for children aged < 2 years receiving meningococcal B vaccine)
- (Boostrix, Adacel) not to be used as primary immunisation for those with no or incomplete primary immunisation
- not recommended if encephalopathy occurred after prior immunisation with

pertussis-containing vaccine or neurological complications after diphtheria—tetanus—pertussis combination or in those with progressive or unstable neurological disorders, uncontrolled epilepsy or progressive encephalopathy until condition has stabilised
- contraindicated in those with allergy to formaldehyde or glutaral (glutaraldehyde)
- see also General Nursing considerations/Cautions for vaccines (p. 1592)

Patient education

- parent should be advised that limb swelling occurs commonly in children, especially after fourth dose. Swelling can be extensive, as well as redness and pain, and usually occurs within 48 hours of vaccination and may last for 1—7 days
- see also General Patient education for vaccines (p. 1593)

Safe to use. dTpa vaccine is funded through the National Immunisation Program for all pregnant women.

Safe to use. Tetanus and diphtheria toxoid vaccines and pertussis vaccines are safe for breastfeeding women as they are inactivated and pose no risk of infection to the infant.

Available in combination with

- contained in Infanrix Hexa with hepatitis B vaccine, poliomyelitis and *Haemophilus influenza* type B vaccine
- contained in Adacel Polio, Boostrix-IPV, Infanrix-IPV and Quadacel with poliomyelitis vaccine

HAEMOPHILUS INFLUENZAE TYPE B VACCINE

Trade names
Act-HIB, Hiberix

Action/Use

- immunisation against *Haemophilus influenzae* type b (Hib) in infants and children between 2 months and 5 years
- *H. influenzae* type b (Hib): protects against infections caused by Hib, which can lead to serious diseases such as meningitis, pneumonia, epiglottitis and sepsis, particularly in young children
- Hib vaccine: the vaccine contains Hib polysaccharide, a sugar derived from the bacteria's capsule, conjugated to a protein carrier (like tetanus toxoid) to enhance the immune response, providing protection against Hib

Dose

- infants and children are recommended to receive an Hib-containing vaccine at 2, 4, 6 and 18 months of age as part of the routine immunisation schedule
- Dose: reconstitute with diluent supplied; admin 0.5 mL immediately by IMI or SCI in anterolateral thigh (< 2 yrs), anterolateral thigh or deltoid (greater than or equal to 2 yrs). Infants 2—6 mths: 3 injections at 1 or 2 mth intervals; 7—11 mths: 2 injections at 1 or 2 mth intervals; booster dose at 18 mths. Children > 12 mths: single injection (Act-Hib)
- Dose: reconstitute with diluent supplied (add entire contents of prefilled syringe to vial), shake well until powder completely dissolved, use promptly or refrigerate and use within 24 hrs. Admin 0.5 mL IMI at age 2, 4 and 6 mths; booster dose at age 12 mths. Children < 12 mths: admin into anterolateral thigh; > 12 mths: deltoid region or anterolateral thigh (Hiberix)

Adverse effects

- (Injection site reaction) pain, swelling
- vomiting, prolonged crying, irritability, unusual tiredness, runny nose, cough, otitis media, conjunctivitis, fever, rash, loss of appetite, diarrhoea

Interactions/Nursing considerations/ Cautions/Patient education

- intramuscular (IM) injection or SCI in anterolateral thigh (Act-Hib)
- does not protect against all strains of *Haemophilus*

VACCINES AND IMMUNOGLOBULINS

- see also General Interactions/Nursing considerations/Cautions/Patient education for vaccines (p. 1592)

Available in combination with
- Hexaxim, Infanrix Hexa, Vaxelis: combines vaccines for diphtheria, tetanus, pertussis, hepatitis B, poliomyelitis and Hib

HEPATITIS A VACCINE
Trade names
Avaxim, Havrix 1440, Havrix Junior, VAQTA Adult Formulation, VAQTA Paediatric/adolescent Formulation Suspension

Action
- inactivated (killed) vaccine. It contains inactivated hepatitis A virus (HAV), which stimulates the immune system to provide protection without causing infection
- HAV is a highly contagious disease that is generally spread via a faecal–oral route through contact with contaminated food and/or water or direct contact with an infectious person

Use
- for use in susceptible people over the age of 2 years at risk of exposure to HAV (e.g. travellers to endemic areas, occupational risk, lifestyle risk factors, medical risk factors, Aboriginal and Torres Strait Island children)

Dose
- usually given as a single dose IM

Adverse effects
- (Local reaction) pain, redness, swelling, induration, haematoma
- headache, malaise, fatigue, fever, asthenia
- diarrhoea, loss of appetite, nausea, vomiting
- (Uncommon) rash, myalgia, arthralgia

Interactions/Nursing considerations/Cautions/Patient education
- intramuscular (IM) injection
- can be given at the same time as other vaccines required for overseas travel
- if the person has had previous hepatitis or unexplained jaundice, was born before 1950 or lived childhood in endemic area, vaccination may not be required. Screening is recommended
- should be given 2 weeks before expected exposure
- immunity occurs after about 4 weeks and persists for up to 12 months, and may be reinforced by booster dose given 6–36 months after initial vaccination
- does not protect against other strains of hepatitis
- (Avaxim) caution if used in those with hypersensitivity to neomycin or formaldehyde
- (Havrix) caution if used in those with hypersensitivity to neomycin
- (Havrix, VAQTA) available in both an adult ($\geq$ 16 years) and a paediatric (2–15 years) formulation
- see also General Interactions/Nursing considerations/Cautions/Patient education for vaccines (p. 1592)

 Safe to use.

Available in combination with
- Twinrix, Twinrix Junior: combines vaccines for HAV and hepatitis B (HBV)

HEPATITIS B VACCINE
Trade names
Engerix-B, H-B-Vax II

Action
- recombinant vaccine. It contains hepatitis B virus (HBV) surface antigen (HBsAg), which is a protein produced through recombinant DNA technology, triggering an immune response to protect against HBV infection
- causes seroconversion in 97–99% of normal adults
- will not protect against other hepatitis viruses such as A, C or E

Use
- recommended in those with chronic liver impairment or transplantation, hepatitis C, post-exposure prophylaxis or other susceptible groups (including high-risk occupational groups, infants born to HBV-positive mothers, susceptible sexual contacts, injecting drug users)

Dose
- (Adult) 3 doses IM at 0, 1- and 6-month intervals **OR**
- (Infants) 4 doses IM at birth, and 2, 4 and 6 months **OR**
- (Dosage for infants born of HBsAg-positive mothers) one 0.5 mL dose of hepatitis B immunoglobulin at birth and three 5 microgram (0.5 mL) doses of H-B-Vax II, the first dose given within one week after birth, second dose 0.5 mL at one month and third dose 0.5 mL at 6 months of age.

Adverse effects
- (Injection site) redness, swelling, pain
- fever, headache, drowsiness, irritability, fatigue
- loss of appetite, nausea, vomiting, diarrhoea, abdominal pain
- (Uncommon) myalgia
- (Rare) lymphadenopathy

Interactions/Nursing considerations/ Cautions/Patient education
- neonates should be vaccinated within 24 hours of birth (and no later than 7 days)
- if neonate is born of HBV-positive mother, HBV immunoglobulin should also be given within 12 hours of birth as efficacy decreases if given after 48 hours
- will not prevent disease if infection was already present when vaccination occurred (long incubation period) or if protective antibody titres are not achieved
- available in both adult and paediatric formulations. Paediatric formulation can be used in young adults ≤ 20 years (Energix-B)
- antibody titres should be measured after primary course in those at high occupational risk, at high risk of serious disease, household contacts or where response is expected to be poor
- reduced response may occur in those > 40 years, male, smokers or those who are obese
- if more rapid protection is required (e.g. travel to endemic area within 4 weeks), vaccination may be given at 0, 7 and 21 days (adult)
- low birthweight (< 2000 g) and preterm infants (< 32 weeks regardless of weight) doses as per infants (above) plus booster at 12 months **OR** surface antigen measured at 7 months and booster given if level is < 10 mIU/mL
- booster doses are recommended in immunocompromised people (especially if HIV positive) or dialysis dependent. Antibody levels should be measured every 6–12 months
- for post-exposure prophylaxis, vaccine should be given within 7 days of exposure and then course completed as usual. HBV immunoglobulin should be given within 72 hours of exposure (and in different limb if administered at the same time)
- larger doses may be required in those with renal failure owing to impaired immune response
- HIV infection is not a contraindication to vaccine
- see also General Interactions/Nursing considerations/Cautions/Patient education for vaccines (p. 1593)

 Safe to use.

Available in combination with
- Infanrix Hexa, Hexaxim: combines vaccines for diphtheria, tetanus, pertussis (whooping cough), hepatitis B, poliomyelitis and *Haemophilus influenzae* type b (Hib)
- Twinrix, Twinrix Junior: combines vaccines for hepatitis A (HAV) and HBV

HUMAN PAPILLOMAVIRUS (HPV) VACCINE

Trade name
Gardasil 9

Action
- persistent infection with HPV appears to be primary cause of cervical cancer and most precursor lesions with HPV types 16 and 18 are responsible for about 70% of cervical cancers worldwide
- contains recombinant virus-like particles which are not capable of causing infection as they are not viruses and not able to reproduce

Use
- (Females, 9—45 years) prophylactic vaccine against several strains (HPV types 6, 11, 16, 18, 31, 33, 45, 52, 58 of HPV thought to be responsible for persistent infection, premalignant lesions, genital warts, and cervical, vaginal, vulval and anal cancers
- (Males, 9—45 years) prevention of anal cancer, premalignant or dysplastic lesions, external genital lesions caused by HPV types 6, 11, 16, 18, 31, 33, 45, 52, 58

Dose
- 3 doses given IM at 0, 2- and 6-month intervals (Gardisil-9 i.e. 9vHPV) **OR**
- (9—14 years) 2 doses given IM at 0 and 5—13 months (if second dose is given earlier than 5 months, a third dose should be given)

Adverse effects
- (Injection site reaction) pain, redness, swelling, bruising
- arthralgia, myalgia
- fatigue, headache, dizziness
- nausea, vomiting, abdominal pain, diarrhoea
- rash, urticaria, pruritus
- fever

Interactions/Nursing considerations/ Cautions/Patient education
- intramuscular (IM) injection
- most effective if given before sexually active
- regular cytological screening (every 5 years for women aged 25—70 years) is still recommended as vaccine does not protect against cancer
- will not protect against diseases not caused by HPV, nor if established lesions are present
- vaccine is not recommended for treatment of active genital lesions, or cervical, vulval, vaginal or anal cancers
- see also General Interactions/Nursing considerations/Cautions/Patient education for vaccines (p. 1592)

 Women who are pregnant or trying to become pregnant should postpone vaccination.

INFLUENZA VACCINE

Trade names
Afluria Quad, Fluad Quad, Fluarix Tetra, Flucelvax Quad, Fluquadri, Fluzone High-Dose Quadrivalent, Influvac Tetra, Vaxigrip Tetra

Action
- prevents influenza caused by influenza virus types A and B
- vaccine is composed of two current influenza A subtypes and influenza B, representing recently circulating viruses (in Australia, these tend to be those circulating in the European winter season), with composition being revised annually
- protection occurs within 2—3 weeks and lasts for 6—12 months

Use
- prevention of influenza type A and B
- recommended for everyone aged over 6 months, but particularly those aged $\geq$ 65 years, all Aboriginal and Torres Strait Islander people, children aged 6 months to 5 years, pregnant or breastfeeding women, people with medical conditions increasing their risk of influenza (e.g. being immunocompromised, chronic medical conditions, chronic liver or kidney failure, chronic alcohol misuse,

obesity), occupational groups (e.g. health care workers, carers, staff, volunteers and visitors to long-term or aged care facilities, essential services providers), residents of long-term or aged care facilities, those travelling during influenza season and homeless people

Dose
- 1 dose annually **OR**
- (Children under 9 years and over 6 months receiving first influenza vaccine, first influenza vaccine after solid organ or stem cell transplant) 2 doses annually 4 weeks apart

Adverse effects
- (Injection site reaction) pain, redness, swelling, induration
- fever, malaise, fatigue, headache, sweating, shivering
- myalgia, arthralgia
- (Rare) allergic reaction

Interactions
- may cause false positive serological test for hepatitis C
- see also General Interactions of vaccines (p. 1591)

Nursing considerations/Cautions
- administered (IM) intramuscularly
- vaccination usually recommended from autumn before the start of the influenza season
- (Afluria Quad, Fluarix Tetra, Flucelvax Quad, Fluad Quad, Fluquadri, Fluzone High-Dose Quadrivalent, Influvac Tetra, Vaxigrip Tetra) provide protection against 4 strains (two A subtypes and two B subtypes)
- (Vaxigrip Tetra) caution if used in those with hypersensitivity to neomycin or formaldehyde
- (Fluzone High-Dose Quadrivalent) recommended for patients aged 60 years and over
- not recommended in those who developed Guillain–Barre syndrome within 6 weeks of previous influenza vaccination
- (Afluria Quad) contraindicated in children under 5 years
- (Influvac Tetra) contraindicated in those with hypersensitivity to formaldehyde, gentamicin, cetrimonium or polysorbate 80
- see also General Nursing considerations/Cautions for vaccines (p. 1592)

Patient/staff education
- all health care workers who have direct patient contact should be vaccinated against influenza every year. This is not just to protect the health care worker against influenza but also to prevent transmission of influenza to patients, particularly those who are elderly or immunosuppressed, for whom influenza can be fatal, as was seen in the influenza pandemic of 1918 when almost 23 million people died worldwide (more than died as a result of the First World War, which had just finished)
- unfortunately, many myths surround the influenza vaccine and influenza itself and people (health care workers among them) often confuse the 'common cold' with true influenza
- influenza vaccine cannot give anyone the 'flu'. It may give the person a sore arm, mild fever or muscle ache, but it does not give anyone the flu or a cold
- influenza vaccine does not protect against coughs, colds or any other viral diseases, nor from influenza caused by strains not contained in the vaccine. The person is also not protected if they are incubating influenza at the time of immunisation
- influenza vaccine is effective only for that year, because each year a new vaccine is developed from the most common influenza strains from the previous winter (e.g. in Australia the vaccine contains the most common influenza strains from the previous northern hemisphere winter)
- influenza is not just the common cold, is highly contagious and is spread by direct contact with respiratory secretions or respiratory aerosol droplets (i.e. coughing and sneezing)

VACCINES AND IMMUNOGLOBULINS

- influenza incubation period is usually 1–3 days
- influenza symptoms vary between mild and severe illness lasting for 7–10 days, high fever, loss of appetite, malaise, chills and shivering, muscle pains, need for bed rest, dry sensation in the nose and throat initially, severe headache and dry cough that may become moist; pneumonia may be a secondary bacterial complication
- common cold symptoms include symptoms that last for 1–2 days generally, mild fever (if at all), no muscle pain, runny nose and sneezing, mild headache, which is generally because of congested sinuses, cough with mild or no complications
- management of influenza includes bed rest until temperature has returned to normal, drinking plenty of fluids and using paracetamol to control fever, aches and pains. If cough worsens or phlegm becomes green/yellow or breathing becomes difficult, a doctor should be consulted
- influenza vaccine effectiveness tends to range between 40% and 60%, depending on the match between the vaccine and circulating strains

JAPANESE ENCEPHALITIS VIRUS (JEV) VACCINE
Trade names
Imojev, Jespect

Action
- (Imojev) live attenuated virus vaccine
- (Jespect) adsorbed inactivated virus vaccine
- does not protect against other forms of encephalitis

Use
- Japanese encephalitis (JE) is caused by infection with the mosquito-borne Japanese encephalitis virus (JEV). The disease primarily affects the central nervous system, leading to inflammation of the brain (encephalitis). While many infections are asymptomatic or mild, severe cases can result in serious neurological complications, such as seizures, paralysis and, in some cases, death
- it is most common in rural and agricultural areas of Asia and the Western Pacific, where mosquitoes breed in rice paddies and stagnant water
- the vaccine provides protection against JE
- vaccine is usually administered to
  - people who plan to live in or travel to areas where JE is endemic or epidemic during the transmission season (e.g. workers who work in the outer Torres Strait Islands for a total of 30 days or more during the wet season)
  - laboratory workers with potential exposure to infected material

Dose
- (Jespect) 2 doses given IM 28 days apart
OR
- (Imojev) single SC dose

Adverse effects
- (Injection site) redness, swelling, bruising, pruritus, pain
- diarrhoea, nausea, vomiting, abdominal pain
- dyspnoea, runny nose, cough, wheezing, nasal congestion, pharyngeal pain
- fatigue, malaise, headache, dizziness, feeling hot, chills
- myalgia, arthralgia

Interactions/Nursing considerations/Cautions
- should be given at least 14 days before exposure (adults) or 28 days (children) (Imojev) or 7 days (Jespect)
- (Imojev) booster given at 12–24 months (if under 18 years) or 5 years (if > 18 years) if risk is ongoing
- immunity last for at least 5 years (adults) or 3 years (children) (Imojev) or 12 months (Jespect)
- see also General Nursing considerations/Cautions for vaccines (p. 1592)

Patient education

- the patient should be advised to avoid mosquito bites while travelling in endemic areas by using insect repellent, protective clothing and mosquito netting, and also avoiding outdoor activities during twilight or in the evening
- female patients of childbearing age should be advised to avoid pregnancy for 28 days after vaccination (Imojev)
- see also General Patient education for vaccines (p. 1593)

> Imojev is contraindicated during pregnancy and breastfeeding (live vaccine).
>
> JE infection in early pregnancy can lead to miscarriage, but no adverse pregnancy outcomes have been linked to Jespect. Jespect can be used in pregnant or breastfeeding women at risk of JE infection.

> Imojev is contraindicated during breastfeeding owing to being a live vaccine.
>
> Jespect has limited human data but can be used for breastfeeding women at increased risk of JE.

MEASLES–MUMPS–RUBELLA (MMR) VACCINE
Trade names
MMRII, Priorix

Action
- live attenuated virus

Use
- active immunisation against measles, mumps and rubella

Dose
- (Child) dose SC or IM at 2 doses at least 1 month apart (usually given at age 12 months and 18 months; the second dose can be given as MMRV) **OR**
- (Adult with no immunity) 1 dose IM or SC

Adverse effects
- (Injection site) redness, pain, swelling
- headache, fever, rash
- pharyngitis, bronchitis, rhinitis, cough, otitis media, upper respiratory tract infection
- vomiting, diarrhoea
- (Uncommon) parotid swelling
- (Rare) febrile seizures, arthralgia, lymphadenopathy

Interactions
- measles virus inhibits tuberculin skin response. Mantoux test may be unreliable for 4–6 weeks after vaccination
- see also General Interactions of vaccines (p. 1592)

Nursing considerations/Cautions

- limited protection if vaccination is given within 72 hours of contact with measles (and no protection against contact with mumps or rubella in this timeframe)
- may be given to asymptomatic HIV-infected people (however, it should be noted that immunisation is less effective in this group)
- caution if used in those with a history of convulsions or cerebral injury where fever should be avoided
- contraindicated if used in those with untreated TB, as condition may be exacerbated
- contraindicated in those with hypersensitivity to eggs and chicken feathers, history of allergic diseases or neomycin (but not contact dermatitis due to neomycin)
- see also General Nursing considerations/Cautions for vaccines (p. 1592)

Patient education

- parents should be warned that children may experience fever 5–12 days after vaccination, which may be accompanied by non-infectious rash and/or a general feeling of being unwell
- female patients of childbearing age should be advised to avoid pregnancy for a month after vaccination

> Women of childbearing potential should be tested for rubella antibodies before pregnancy and, if negative and not pregnant, should be offered rubella vaccine and instructed to avoid pregnancy

for 3 months. Contraindicated during pregnancy, and pregnancy should be avoided for at least 1 month after vaccination.

 The MMR vaccine is generally considered safe for breastfeeding women. There is no evidence that the vaccine poses a risk to the breastfeeding infant.

Available in combination with
- contained in Priorix-Tetra and ProQuad with varicella zoster virus vaccine

MENINGOCOCCAL VACCINE
Trade names
Bexsero, MenQuadfi, Menveo, NeisVac-C, Nimenrix

Action
- meningococcal disease is caused by *Neisseria meningitidis* (meningococcus), with serogroups A, B, C, W135 and Y the most likely cause of disease (Serogroup B causes most of the cases in Australia)
- meningococcal ACWY (MenACWY) vaccine: conjugate vaccine against groups A, C, W135 and Y *N. meningitidis* (meningococcus) (MenQuadfi, Menveo, Nimenrix)
- MenC vaccine: conjugate vaccine against group C *N. meningitidis* (meningococcus) (NeisVac-C)
- MenB vaccine: recombinant vaccine against group B *N. meningitidis* (meningococcus) (Bexsero)

Use
- infants, children, adolescents and young adults (especially smokers and those who live in close contact with each other (e.g. student accommodation, new military recruits), travellers where disease is endemic, laboratory workers frequently handling specimens, those with medical risk factors increasing risk of invasive meningococcal disease
- inherited disease of properdin or factor H or D deficiency, HIV, stem cell transplantation, asplenia (functional or anatomical), treatment with eculizumab, Aboriginal and Torres Strait Islander people
- controlling epidemic caused by *N. meningitides* in confined communities

Dose
- MenACWY (MenACWY vaccine for infants and children under 2 years: the schedule depends on the brand and age, with 1, 2 or 3 doses required based on when the child starts the series)
  - Menveo:
    - age 6 weeks — 6 months: 3 doses IM 0.5 mL at 2, 4 and 12 months. Consider 4 doses if travelling to meningococcal A endemic areas
    - age 6—12 months: 2 doses IM 0.5 mL, second dose at 12 months or at least 8 weeks after the first
    - age 12—24 months: 2 doses IM 0.5 mL, at least 8 weeks apart. Age > 2 years: 1 dose IM 0.5 mL
  - Nimenrix:
    - age 6 weeks — 6 months: 3 doses IM 0.5 mL at 2, 4 and 12 months
    - age 6—12 months: 2 doses IM 0.5 mL, second dose at 12 months or at least 8 weeks after the first
    - age > 12 months: 1 dose IM 0.5 mL
- MenACWY vaccine booster dose (if ongoing risk):
  - age < 7 years: give the first booster after 3 years, then every 5 years
  - age ≥ 7 years: give every 5 years
- Men B vaccine:
  - infants aged 6 weeks — 6 months are recommended to receive:
    - standard 3-dose schedule: 3 doses IM at 6—8 weeks, 4 months and 12 months
    - medically at increased risk: 4 doses IM at 6—8 weeks, 4 months, 6 months and 12 months
  - Infants aged 6—12 months:
    - 3 doses IM: 2 doses given at least 8 weeks apart, followed by a third dose at 12 months (or at least 8 weeks after the primary course)
  - Individuals aged 12 months — 50 years

- 2 doses IM at least 8 weeks apart
- MenB vaccine booster dose (if ongoing risk):
  - age < 7 years: give a single dose 3 years after the primary series
  - age ≥ 7 years: give a single dose 5 years after the primary series

Adverse effects
- (Injection site) tenderness, redness, pain, swelling
- fever, chills, sleepiness, irritability, malaise, fatigue, headache, unusual crying
- nausea, vomiting, changes in appetite
- rash
- myalgia, arthralgia
- (Bexsero) fever (highest 6 hours after vaccination, decreasing by day 2)

Nursing considerations/Cautions
- intramuscular (IM) injection
- store at +2°C to +8°C. Do not freeze. Protect from light
- (Bexsero) supplied as a 1.0 mL suspension in a pre-filled syringe. A fine off-white deposit may form after storage. Shake well before use
- (Menveo) it must be reconstituted. Mix the liquid MenCWY with the lyophilised MenA and shake until dissolved. Use promptly or store at +2°C to +8°C for up to 24 hours
- (Nimenrix) it must be reconstituted. Reconstitute by adding the solvent to the vial. Shake until dissolved. Use promptly or store up to 30°C for 8 hours
- (Menveo) contraindicated in those with latex hypersensitivity or diphtheria-containing vaccines
- (NeisVac-C) contraindicated in those with known hypersensitivity to tetanus toxoid
- see also General Nursing considerations/Cautions for vaccines (p. 1592)

Patient education
- (Bexsero) parents should be advised that children under 2 can be given paracetamol (15 mg/kg) prophylactically with each dose of vaccine, either 30 minutes before or as soon as practicable after injection. Two more doses of paracetamol can be given 6 hours apart
- the effectiveness of the meningococcal vaccine may decrease over time, and it does not protect against all strains of meningococcal infections or other types of meningitis. If you notice any symptoms of these infections, seek medical attention immediately

Meningococcal vaccines are generally not recommended in pregnancy, except in rare cases where thers is a significant risk of exposure or special circumstances.

Meningococcal vaccines are generally not recommended for breastfeeding mothers, except in rare cases with a significant risk of exposure or special circumstances.

PNEUMOCOCCAL VACCINE
Trade names
Prevenar 13, Prevenar 20, Vaxneuvance, Pneumovax 23

Action
- 13vPCV (Prevenar 13): pneumococcal conjugate vaccine, protecting against 13 strains of *Streptococcus pneumoniae*
- 20vPCV (Prevenar 20): pneumococcal conjugate vaccine, protecting against 20 strains of *Streptococcus pneumoniae*
- 15vPCV (Vaxneuvance): pneumococcal conjugate vaccine, protecting against 15 strains of *Streptococcus pneumoniae*
- 23vPPV (Pneumovax 23): pneumococcal polysaccharide vaccine, protecting against 23 strains of *Streptococcus pneumoniae*

Use
- active immunisation in adults and children over 6 weeks for prevention of pneumococcal disease (Prevenar 13, Prevenar 20, Vaxneuvance)

VACCINES AND IMMUNOGLOBULINS

- prevention of pneumococcal disease in those aged over 65 years, immunocompromised, Aboriginal and Torres Islander people over 50 years, people > 2 yrs with asplenia including sickle cell disease, CSF leak, or at risk from pneumococcal disease complications (e.g. diabetes, alcohol dependence, heart, kidney and lung disease, smokers) (Pneumovax 23)

Dose
- 13vPCV, 15vPCV:
  - adults and children > over 6 weeks old: IM 0.5 mL. The primary course is 3 doses (at 2, 4 and 12 months)
  - a 4-dose schedule is recommended for high-risk individuals, with an extra dose at 6 months
  - for catch-up doses, refer to the *Australian Immunisation Handbook*
- 23vPPV:
  - adults and children > 2 years at increased risk: IM 0.5 mL, 2 doses 5–10 years apart
- booster doses:
  - Aboriginal and Torres Strait Islander children in high-risk areas: extra 13vPCV/15vPCV dose at 6 months (primary course), plus 2 doses of 23vPPV. First 23vPPV at 4–5 years or 2–12 months after the last 13vPCV/15vPCV
  - medically at-risk individuals: extra 13vPCV/15vPCV dose at 6 months (or at diagnosis if > 12 months), plus 2 doses of 23vPPV. First 23vPPV at 4–5 years or 2–12 months after the last 13vPCV/15vPCV

Adverse effects
- (Injection site) redness, swelling, pain/tenderness, induration
- fever, chills, drowsiness, irritability, headache, fatigue
- rash
- diarrhoea, vomiting, loss of appetite
- (Premature infants ≤ 30 weeks gestation) sleep apnoea

Interactions
- not recommended with zoster vaccine (Zostavax) as it may decrease responsiveness of zoster vaccine (Pneumovax 23)
- see also General Interactions of vaccines (p. 1592)

Nursing considerations/Cautions/Patient education
- Prevenar 13 (13vPCV) IM injection
- Vaxneuvance (15vPCV) IM injection
- Pneumovax 23 (23vPPV): IM injection or subcutaneous (SC) injection
- protection lasts for 5–10 years
- 13vPCV, 15vPCV: recommended for all unvaccinated individuals aged > 70 years (Aboriginal and Torres Strait Islander people aged > 50 years). Can usually be given with routine vaccinations. However, co-administration with the influenza vaccine may increase the risk of fever in children. If concerned, give the vaccines at least 3 days apart
- does not prevent diseases caused by other capsular types of *Pneumococcus*
- should be given 2 weeks before splenectomy or immunosuppressant therapy (including bone marrow transplantation) or as soon as possible after diagnosis of HIV
- (Premature infants ≤ 30 weeks gestation) infants should be closely monitored for 48–72 hours after vaccination
- (Pneumovax 23) caution if used in those with severely compromised cardiac and/or respiratory function
- see also General Nursing considerations/Cautions/Patient education for vaccines (p. 1592)

Pneumococcal vaccines are not routinely recommended for pregnant women. Women of childbearing age who have a risk condition(s) for pneumococcal disease are normally recommended to receive pneumococcal vaccine either before a planned pregnancy, or as soon as practicable after delivery.

Appears safe. Breastfeeding women can receive 13vPCV, 15vPCV and 23vPPV.

POLIOMYELITIS VACCINE

Trade name
Ipol

Action
- inactivated polio virus (IPV)
- vaccine against the three types of polio virus
- oral polio vaccine is no longer used in Australia
- Australia was declared polio-free in 2000; however, wild polio virus can be imported from countries where it is still endemic

Use
- all infants, unimmunised children and adolescents not previously vaccinated or those where oral polio vaccine was refused or contraindicated
- travellers to countries where poliomyelitis is epidemic or endemic
- health care workers (who may come into contact with those who might be excreting poliovirus) or laboratory workers (who may handle specimens)

Dose
- (Child > 6 weeks) SC 0.5 mL for 4 doses at 2, 4 and 6 months, with a booster at 4 years (or from 3.5 years) **OR**
- (Adult unvaccinated): SC 0.5 mL for 3 doses at 2-month intervals **OR**
- (Booster doses) not recommended for adults unless at special risk, such as travelling to polio-endemic areas. In these cases, give a booster every 10 years

Adverse effects
- (Injection site) redness, pain, induration
- fever, irritability, drowsiness
- diarrhoea, vomiting

Interactions/Nursing considerations/Cautions/Patient education
- booster dose not required in adults unless at high risk (e.g. travelling to endemic area, laboratory workers, healthcare workers)
- contraindicated in those with hypersensitivity to formaldehyde, neomycin, streptomycin or polymyxin B
- see also General Interactions/Nursing considerations/Cautions/Patient education for vaccines (p. 1592)

> IPV vaccines are not routinely recommended for pregnant women but can be given if necessary.

> IPV vaccines are not routinely recommended for breastfeeding women, but can be given if needed.

Available in combination with
- (Adacel Polio, Boostrix-IPV, Infanrix-IPV, Quadracel) includes vaccines for diphtheria, tetanus, pertussis and inactivated poliovirus
- (Infanrix Hexa, Hexaxim, Vaxelis) includes vaccines for diphtheria, tetanus, pertussis, inactivated poliovirus, hepatitis B and *Haemophilus influenzae* type b

Q FEVER (*COXIELLA BURNETII*) VACCINE

Trade name
Q-Vax

Available forms
Prefilled syringe: 25 microgram/0.5 mL (vaccine);
Prefilled vial: 2.5 microgram/mL (skin test)

Action
- killed *Coxiella burnetii*
- protects against infection by *C. burnetii*, which causes Q fever
- transmitted from both wild and domesticated animals, including sheep, cattle, goats, kangaroos, feral camels and cats
- infection is via inhalation of infected aerosol or dust
- vaccination during incubation period does not prevent onset of disease

Use
- recommended for those susceptible to Q fever (e.g. abattoir workers, veterinarians, veterinary nurses, veterinary students, laboratory workers, goat, cattle, sheep and dairy farmers, shearers,

livestock transporters or sale yard workers, professional cat and dog breeders, agricultural college staff and students, wildlife and zoo workers working with high-risk animals, animal refuge workers)
- after negative skin and serology tests (skin test for previous sensitisation to Q fever antigens)

Dose
- the Q fever vaccine is given as a single dose. Booster doses are not recommended
  - adults and children > 15 years: SC 0.5 mL, single dose

Adverse effects
- (Local reaction) redness, tenderness, induration
- headache, fever, chills, minor sweating
- delayed skin reaction (up to 6 months after vaccination at either test or injection site)
- (Uncommon) nausea, vomiting, diarrhoea

Interactions/Nursing considerations/Cautions/Patient education
- Q fever vaccine contraindications: immunity to Q fever (positive serology or skin test result), history of Q fever or prior Q fever vaccination. Anaphylaxis to eggs
- before vaccination, the patient should be questioned regarding any prior possible exposure to Q fever and duration of any such illness or egg allergy
- serum antibody levels and a skin test are recommended before vaccination to prevent serious hypersensitivity reactions from occurring
- (Skin test) skin testing and interpretation should be done only by immunisation providers who are trained to administer Q fever skin testing. The site is read after 7 days and any induration is considered positive and the vaccine should therefore not be given
- risk of Q fever is greatest in first year of exposure; therefore vaccination should be given as soon as possible after starting employment in high-risk settings
- revaccination is not recommended because of risk of severe hypersensitivity reaction
- see also General Interactions/Nursing considerations/Cautions/Patient education for vaccines (p. 1592)

 No data. Vaccination should be deferred.

 No human data. Avoid use.

RABIES VACCINE
Trade names
Verorab, Rabipur

Action
- rabies is a zoonotic disease transmitted through saliva or neural tissue from an infected animal. Humans can be exposed through bites, scratches that break the skin or contact with mucous membranes (nose, eyes or mouth). Rabies is almost always fatal
- inactivated rabies vaccine protects against zoonotic disease

Use
- post-exposure to the rabies virus
- prophylaxis for those who work with animals (e.g. veterinarians, veterinary students or veterinary nurses — depending on animals they come in contact with) or those who come into regular contact with bats (both 'flying foxes' and microbats), bat handlers, bat scientists, wildlife officers and zoo curators, as well as laboratory personnel who handle bat tissues or lyssaviruses
- prophylaxis for travellers to rabies-enzootic regions based on risk assessment

Dose
- dosage — rabies vaccine (pre-exposure)
  - adults and children:
    - IM 1 mL (Rabipur) or 0.5 mL (Verorab) on day 0, day 7, and a third dose between days 21 and 28
    - for immunocompromised individuals, give a fourth dose if rabies virus antibody levels are low 2–4 weeks after the third dose **OR**
- dosage — rabies vaccine (post-exposure)
  - non-immune adults and children:
    - IM 1 mL or 0.5 mL on days 0, 3, 7, 14 and 28.
    - give rabies immunoglobulin with the first vaccine dose (or within 7 days) if high-risk exposure (e.g. non-immune or immunocompromised)
  - immune adults and children (previously vaccinated or with adequate antibody levels):
    - IM 1 mL or 0.5 mL on days 0 and 3
  - for severely immunocompromised, administer doses on days 0, 3, 7, 14 and 28.
    - for immunocompromised adults and children, check antibody response 2–4 weeks after the last dose, as further doses may be required

Adverse effects
- (Local reaction) redness, swelling, tenderness, induration, pruritus, bruising
- fever, headache, dizziness, fatigue, malaise
- arthralgia, myalgia
- rash
- nausea, abdominal pain, decreased appetite
- (Rare) angioedema

Interactions
- anti-rabies immunoglobulin may decrease response to vaccine
- see also General Interactions of vaccines (p. 1592)

Nursing considerations/Cautions
- immediate first aid treatment should include cleaning area with soap and copious amounts of water and then applying 70% alcohol or iodine-containing antiseptic/disinfectant
- suturing bite(s) is not recommended
- deltoid should be used rather than buttock (as vaccine failure has been reported using this site)
- tetanus prophylaxis is also recommended post-exposure
- vaccination should be stopped if animal remains healthy for 10 days or the animal is euthanised humanely and found to be negative for rabies
- booster is recommended in those with ongoing risk (e.g. veterinarians, wildlife workers) if antibody level falls below 0.5 IU/mL
- antibody levels should be tested 6-monthly for those where risk remains high (e.g. laboratory workers) or every 2 years in those who are at continuing risk of exposure (e.g. veterinarians, wildlife workers)
- (Rabipur) (as pre-exposure prophylaxis) contraindicated in those with hypersensitivity to neomycin or bovine gelatin, egg or chicken proteins, chlortetracycline and amphotericin B (amphotericin)
- see also General Nursing considerations/Cautions for vaccines (p. 1592)

Patient education
- travellers should be given advice about avoiding contact with bats, wild and domestic animals (including feeding and patting monkeys at tourist spots such as temples). Travellers should also be discouraged from carrying food and they should be aware of immediate first aid measures if contact or injury occurs. Parents travelling with children should be given advice about the increased risk in children of facial injuries because of their height and the importance of discouraging children to pat or touch animals

VACCINES AND IMMUNOGLOBULINS

Pregnant women are recommended to receive the rabies vaccine and human rabies immunoglobulin, if needed, after potential exposure to rabies virus or lyssaviruses — that is, if the benefit outweighs the risk.

Breastfeeding women are recommended to receive the rabies vaccine and human rabies immunoglobulin, if needed, after potential exposure to rabies virus or lyssaviruses — that is, if the benefit outweighs the risk.

ROTAVIRUS VACCINE
Trade name
Rotarix Oral Liquid

Action
- live attenuated virus vaccine
- rotavirus infection commonly occurs in children under 5 years, especially between 6 and 24 months, causing sudden vomiting and diarrhoea

Use
- prevention of rotavirus gastroenteritis, which can lead to dehydration and hospitalisation in infants < 6 months

Dose
- oral: 1.5 mL for 2 doses
  - first dose: at 6—14 weeks of age
  - second dose: before 25 weeks of age
- minimum of 4 weeks between doses
- repeat the dose if most of it is spat out or vomited within minutes of administration

Adverse effects
- vomiting, loss of appetite, diarrhoea
- fever, irritability
- cough, runny nose
- (Rare) intussusception

Interactions
- see General Interactions of vaccines (p. 1592)

Nursing considerations/Cautions
- administer orally by squeezing the entire contents of the tube directly into the inside of the infant's cheek, with no dilution needed
- vaccination should be postponed if infant has moderate-to-severe vomiting or diarrhoea
- does not protect against gastroenteritis due to other pathogens
- not recommended in infants > 24 weeks
- contraindicated in those with chronic gastrointestinal history, including uncorrected gastrointestinal congenital malformation that might lead to intussusception or combined immunodeficiency disorder
- see also General Nursing considerations/Cautions for vaccines (p. 1592)

Parent education
- parent/carer should be advised to immediately report if child experiences any abdominal pain or distress, persistent vomiting, blood in stools (bowel motions), high fever and/or bloated stomach
- see also General Patient education for vaccines (p. 1593)

TYPHOID (*SALMONELLA TYPHI*) VACCINE
Trade names
Typhim Vi, Vivotif (Oral)

Action
- oral: live, attenuated *Salmonella typhi*
- IM: Vi polysaccharide.

Use
- typhoid fever is spread via faecally contaminated food and water
- vaccine provides immunisation against typhoid fever caused by *S. typhi* and recommended for military personnel, travellers (≥ 2 years) going to typhoid-endemic areas and laboratory workers routinely working with *S. typhi*

Dose
- oral vaccine: 1 capsule on days 1, 3 and 5
  OR
- IM vaccine: 25 micrograms IM, single dose

1615

Adverse effects
- (IM) (common) local site reaction (tenderness/pain, redness, induration) headache, nausea, malaise, fever
- (Oral) (uncommon) diarrhoea, constipation, nausea, vomiting, loss of appetite, abdominal cramps, fever, headache, rash
- (Rare) allergic reaction

Interactions
- (Oral) not recommended with antimalarials or sulfonamides that may be active against *Salmonella* spp. A 3-day gap should be allowed between vaccination and the administration of these agents
- (Oral) should be given at least 8 hours apart from oral cholera vaccine
- see also General Interactions of vaccines (p. 1592)

Nursing considerations/Cautions
- IM dose should be given at least 2 weeks before, and oral vaccine at least 1 week before potential *S. typhi* exposure
- repeat vaccination is recommended 2—3-yearly in those who have continued or repeated exposure
- (Typhim Vi) contains traces of formaldehyde; therefore should be given with caution in anyone with a formaldehyde sensitivity
- see also General Nursing considerations/Cautions for vaccines (p. 1592)

Patient education
- advise patient to swallow capsules whole, not chewed or crushed, and take 1 hour before meals with cold or lukewarm (not hot) drink or food
- see also General Patient education for vaccines (p. 1593)

The oral vaccine is contraindicated during pregnancy and pregnancy should be avoided for 12 weeks after oral vaccination.

The Vi polysaccharide vaccine is not routinely recommended for pregnant women. Still, it may be given if travelling to areas with poor water quality and sanitation, where the benefits outweigh the risks.

No human data for the oral vaccine.

The Vi polysaccharide vaccine is not routinely recommended for breastfeeding women but may be given if travelling to areas with poor water quality and sanitation, where the benefits outweigh the risks.

Available in combination with
- (Vivaxim) combined vaccine that provides protection against both typhoid (Vi polysaccharide) and hepatitis A (inactivated virus)

VARICELLA VACCINE
Trade names
Varilrix, Varivax Refrigerated

Action
- live attenuated vaccine given as active immunisation against varicella virus (chickenpox)

Use
- children aged ≥12 months to < 14 years
- adolescents aged ≥ 14 years and adults who are non-immune, particularly health care workers, childhood educators and carers, and people working in long-term care facilities

Dose
- Adult, child >1 year: administer 2 doses of 0.5 mL SC at least 4 weeks apart
- The National Immunisation Program currently includes only 1 dose of varicella vaccine (given as MMRV at 18 months of age). A second dose for children < 14 years will boost immunity; check with your local state or territory public health unit for specific guidelines

VACCINES AND IMMUNOGLOBULINS

Adverse effects
- (Injection site) pain, swelling, redness, swelling, pruritus, induration, haematoma
- a mild papular-vesicular rash (small, raised bumps and fluid-filled blisters) within 5–26 days of vaccination, fever, rash, pruritus

Interactions
- people vaccinated with a varicella-containing vaccine should avoid immunoglobulin-containing products for 3 weeks unless the benefits outweigh the vaccine. If immunoglobulin is given within 3 weeks of vaccination, the person should be revaccinated at the appropriate time
- antiviral medication may interfere with vaccine; therefore it should be stopped for at least 24 hours before vaccination and withheld for at least 14 days after
- see also General Interactions of vaccines (p. 1592)

Nursing considerations/Cautions
- contraindicated in people who are significantly immunocompromised or receiving high-dose immunosuppressive therapy, such as chemotherapy, radiation or corticosteroids
- individuals with possible IFNAR1 deficiency, a rare inherited condition in some Western Polynesian people (Tongan, Samoan, Niuean), may experience severe illness from viral infections and live vaccines like MMR, yellow fever or varicella. Healthcare providers should monitor children of Western Polynesian heritage who become very unwell 1–2 weeks after MMRV or varicella vaccination for possible immune deficiency and report any adverse events. Family members of those with severe reactions to live vaccines or known IFNAR1 deficiency should see an immunologist before vaccination
- varicella vaccine and zoster vaccine (p. 1619) are not interchangeable
- varicella vaccine can be given at the same time as other vaccines
- it can prevent infection if administered within 5 days after exposure (ideally within 3 days). May also require zoster immunoglobulin (p. 1630)
- vaccination is strongly recommended for household contacts of immunosuppressed individuals, people in high-risk occupations (e.g. health care workers, child educators) and non-immune women prior to pregnancy
- rarely, the vaccine virus may be transmitted from the recipient to seronegative contacts, so recipients should avoid contact with immunosuppressed individuals if a vaccine-associated rash occurs
- vaccinating individuals who are already immune poses no issues
- see also General considerations/Cautions for vaccines (p. 1592)

Patient education
- female patients of childbearing age should be counselled to avoid pregnancy for 4 weeks after vaccination
- see also General Patient education for vaccines (p. 1593)

Contraindicated during pregnancy (live, attenuated vaccine) and pregnancy should be avoided for at least 4 weeks after vaccination.

Inadvertent varicella vaccination during pregnancy has not been shown to cause harm to the fetus and is not a reason to terminate the pregnancy.

Breastfeeding women can safely receive the varicella vaccine. Most live vaccines are not passed into breastmilk. There is no evidence of the virus in breastmilk, and no effects on breastfed infants have been reported.

Available in combination with
- contained in Priorix-Tetra and ProQuad with measles, mumps and rubella

YELLOW FEVER VACCINE
Trade name
Stamaril

Action
- live attenuated virus vaccine for active immunisation against yellow fever
- immunity appears 10 days after vaccination and lasts for at least 10 years

Use
- prevention of yellow fever in those living in or travelling through endemic areas, or laboratory workers handling infected material

Dose
- adults and children > 9 months: SC/IM 0.5 mL single dose

Adverse effects
- (Injection site reaction) pain, tenderness, redness, induration, swelling, haematoma
- fever, headache, asthenia
- myalgia
- nausea, vomiting
- rash
- (Very rare occurring within 10 days of vaccination) yellow fever vaccine-associated viscerotropic disease (fever, fatigue, myalgia, headache, hypotension, metabolic acidosis, muscle and liver cytolysis, lymphocytopenia, thrombocytopenia, renal failure, respiratory failure). May be fatal
- (Very rare occurring within 30 days of vaccination) yellow fever vaccine-associated neurotropic disease (high fever, headache, confusion, encephalopathy, meningitis and seizures). May be fatal

Interactions
- not recommended within 4 weeks of cholera or typhoid vaccines (unless given at the same time into different sites)
- can cause false positive results for other flaviviruses (e.g. dengue, Japanese encephalitis)
- may be given to adults at same time as Japanese encephalitis vaccine (Imojev) in separate sites
- see also General Interactions of vaccines (p. 1592)

Nursing considerations/Cautions
- given SC or IM
- immunity appears in 10 days after vaccination and lasts for at least 10 years (may be lifelong)
- must be given by approved vaccination centre and registered on international certificate, which is valid for 10 years
- reconstituted using sodium chloride 0.4%
- caution if used in those > 60 years or with thymus disease, as there is an increased risk of yellow fever-associated viscerotropic disease
- contains lactose and sorbitol and therefore contraindicated in those with fructose intolerance
- contraindicated in infants under 9 months owing to risk of encephalitis
- contraindicated in those who have an allergy to egg or egg proteins, or with thymus disorders (e.g. myasthenia gravis)
- see also General Nursing considerations/Cautions for vaccines (p. 1592)

Patient education
- instruct the patient to seek medical advice immediately if any of the following occur:
  - fever, fatigue, myalgia or headache within 10 days of vaccination
  - high fever, headache, confusion, stiff neck, fitting (seizures) within 30 days of vaccination
- mosquitoes transmit yellow fever; therefore, patients should be encouraged to use insect spray, protective clothing and mosquito nets while sleeping to avoid mosquito bites while in endemic areas

VACCINES AND IMMUNOGLOBULINS

- see also General Patient education for vaccines (p. 1593)

Live viral vaccines are typically contraindicated during pregnancy unless necessary. Pregnant women should avoid the yellow fever vaccine unless there is a significant risk of exposure. If travel to a high-risk area is unavoidable, vaccination may be considered.

Women breastfeeding infants under 9 months should avoid yellow fever vaccination. There have been rare cases of the vaccine strain being transmitted through breastmilk, leading to probable vaccine-associated neurotropic disease in infants. This adverse event is extremely rare, and affected infants showed normal neurological development upon follow-up.

ZOSTER VACCINE
Trade name
Shingrix

Action
- adjuvanted recombinant varicella-zoster virus (VZV) glycoprotein E (gE) subunit vaccine is a non-live vaccine used to prevent shingles (herpes zoster)
- it stimulates the immune system using the gE protein from the virus, combined with an adjuvant to enhance the immune response
- shingles is a reactivation of the varicella–zoster virus, the same virus that causes chicken pox. Shingles is not contagious; however, a person who has never had chicken pox or had the chicken pox (varicella) vaccine can get chicken pox if they come into contact with someone who has shingles

Use
- prevention of herpes zoster (shingles) and postherpetic neuralgia (PHN) in those > 50 years and for those over 18 years who are at increased risk of developing herpes zoster

Dose
- (Adults > 50 years) IM 0.5 mL for 2 doses, given 2–6 months apart
- (Immunocompromised patients > 18 years) IM 0.5 mL for 2 doses, given 1–2 months apart (this accelerated schedule may be used if rapid protection is needed, such as before starting immunosuppressive treatment)

Adverse effects
- headache, fatigue, gastrointestinal symptoms (such as nausea, vomiting, diarrhoea, abdominal pain), shivering, muscle pain (myalgia)
- increased risk of Guillian–Barre disease development

Interactions
- Shingrix is not a live vaccine, so it can be administered to individuals on immunosuppressive therapy. However, the immune response may be reduced in those on high doses of immunosuppressive drugs (e.g. corticosteroids, chemotherapy)

Nursing considerations/Cautions
- ensure proper storage: Shingrix must be stored in the refrigerator (not frozen) between 2°C and 8°C
- Shingrix can be administered simultaneously with other vaccines, such as influenza
- need for booster dose has not been established
- vaccination of household contacts aged >50 years of unvaccinated immunocompromised individuals is recommended to help protect the immunocompromised person from exposure to shingles to prevent the possibility of catching varicella (chicken pox) (see Action for discussion of the link between shingles and chickenpox)
- not recommended for prevention of varicella (chicken pox) or treatment of herpes zoster (shingles) or PHN
- see also General Nursing considerations/Cautions for vaccines (p. 1592)

Patient education
- reduces the incidence of PHN by approximately 90%

- ensure the patient schedules the second dose 2–6 months after the first dose to complete the series for optimal protection
- educate the patient that Shingrix offers long-term protection (for at least 10 years)

No current data available for vaccine use during pregnancy.

No current information available on use of vaccine during breastfeeding.

IMMUNOGLOBULINS

General Actions of immunoglobulins
- immunoglobulins provide acquired passive immunity as they contain high titres of antibodies
- these antibodies target specific antigens (in the case of specific immunoglobulins) or are pooled from multiple donors, offering a broader range of antibody protection (pooled immunoglobulins)
- protection using immunoglobulins is immediate but lasts for only 3–4 weeks

General Uses of immunoglobulins
- individuals who are unable to produce antibodies
- prevention of disease when time does not permit active immunity (post-exposure)
- treatment of some diseases that are normally prevented by immunisation
- treatment of conditions where active immunisation is not available or is impractical

General Adverse effects of immunoglobulins
- (IM site) redness, stiffness, tenderness, induration, pain, irritation, bruising
- (IV site, high dose, prolonged administration) thrombophlebitis
- headache, malaise, drowsiness
- chest tightness
- fever
- facial flushing or pallor, feeling hot, chills, sweating
- abdominal pain, nausea, vomiting
- dyspnoea
- rash, pruritus
- hypotension (transient)
- (Delayed reaction, within 24 hours) nausea, vomiting, chest pain, chills or shivering, dizziness, aching legs
- (Infrequently, high dose) aseptic meningitis syndrome occurring from several hours up to 2 days after administration and consisting of headache, nuchal rigidity, drowsiness, fever, photophobia, painful eye movement, nausea and vomiting
- (Rare) renal dysfunction, acute renal failure, haemolysis, haemolytic anaemia, thrombotic events, abscess
- (Very rare) anaphylactic reaction, transfusion-related acute lung injury
- any human serum carries the risk of transmitting blood-borne viral or prion diseases

General Interactions of immunoglobulins
- caution if immunoglobulins are given with nephrotoxic agents because of increased risk of renal dysfunction and acute renal failure
- immunoglobulins should not be given within 14 days of vaccination (if possible), as they can reduce the effectiveness of vaccines by neutralising the vaccine antigen. This may necessitate revaccination once the immunoglobulin effects have diminished
- vaccination with live attenuated vaccines (e.g. measles, mumps, rubella, varicella, yellow fever) should not be given within 3 months of immunoglobulin
- may produce misleading positive (false positive) results on serological testing
- some immunoglobulins contain maltose or glucose, which may interfere with measurements of blood glucose levels

General Nursing considerations/ Cautions for immunoglobulins
- ensure the patient is well hydrated before administration to help reduce the risk of renal dysfunction

VACCINES AND IMMUNOGLOBULINS

- check and record blood pressure, heart rate, respiratory rate and temperature (vital signs) before starting immunoglobulin therapy. Continue to monitor vital signs after the infusion to detect any delayed reactions
- transfusion-related acute lung injury occurs 1–6 hours after administration and patient should be monitored for any signs of respiratory distress or fever
- infusion rate should commence slowly and be gradually increased after 15–30 minutes if tolerated by the patient
- if the patient is at risk of thromboembolic events, therapy should be administered at minimal dose infused at a slow rate while observing patient closely. Consideration should be given to evaluation of blood viscosity
- if adverse reactions occur, infusion should be stopped for 5–10 minutes and restarted at a slower rate, monitoring the patient carefully
- batch number of product should be recorded each time it is administered to enable linking between the patient and product if an untoward event occurs
- if given IM, no more than 5 mL should be given per site
- reconstituted solutions should not be shaken as this denatures the protein
- monitor for signs of hypersensitivity reactions, including hives, rash, difficulty breathing and anaphylaxis, particularly during the first infusion. Have readily available adrenaline (epinephrine) 1 in 1000 (drawn up), antihistamines, IV corticosteroid, oxygen, suction and resuscitation equipment in the event of anaphylaxis occurring
- allow the preparation to reach room temperature before injection/infusion
- turbid-looking preparation should not be administered and should be returned to manufacturer (Australian Red Cross)
- immunoglobulin should not be used if it has been frozen
- administer alone
- if container breaks and/or spillage occurs, it should be cleaned with sodium hypochlorite 1% for 15 minutes, avoiding inhalation or any contact with spill. Standard precautions should be strictly applied
- produced from human plasma; therefore there is a potential risk of disease transmission (e.g. viruses, Creutzfeldt–Jacob disease)
- caution if immunoglobulins are used in those with pre-existing renal impairment, diabetes mellitus, volume depletion, sepsis or paraproteinaemia, or who are older than 65 years, because of increased risk of renal dysfunction and possible acute renal failure
- caution if used in those with increased risk of thrombotic events (e.g. immobile, elderly, with cardiovascular risk factors (e.g. impaired cardiac output, atherosclerosis), hypertriglyceridaemia, monoclonal gammopathies, previous history of thrombotic event, severe hypovolaemia, hyperviscosity, oestrogen use, acquired/inherited hypercoagulation states) or if the person has an indwelling vascular catheter
- caution if used in those with non-O blood group, with underlying associated inflammatory conditions or receiving high cumulative doses of immunoglobulins over several days because of increased risk of haemolysis
- IM administration is contraindicated in those with severe thrombocytopenia or coagulation disorders
- immunoglobulins are contraindicated in those who have had a previous anaphylactic reaction following administration of immunoglobulins or in those with IgA deficiency (unless tested and found to be negative for anti-IgA antibodies)

General Patient education for immunoglobulins

- warn the patient that nausea, vomiting, chills or shivering, chest pain, dizziness and/or aching legs may occur with 24 hours of immunoglobulin administration

- the patient should be advised to seek medical advice immediately if any of the following occur:
  - headache, nausea, vomiting, drowsiness, fever, stiff neck, painful eye movement or inability to tolerate bright light (especially within 2 days of immunoglobulin administration) (may be signs of aseptic meningitis syndrome)
  - fatigue, fever, pallor, confusion, dizziness, lightheadedness and weakness/inability to complete any physical activity (signs of haemolysis)
  - fever or any signs of respiratory difficulty (signs of transfusion-related acute lung injury)
- inform the patient that any product prepared from human blood or plasma has the potential for transmission of blood-borne viral or prion diseases (e.g. Creutzfeldt–Jakob disease), although stringent procedures now exist for careful selection of blood donors and removal and inactivation of known enveloped viruses from blood products (e.g. HIV, hepatitis B and C) and non-enveloped viruses (e.g. hepatitis A)
- if the patient has diabetes mellitus, it is important to instruct them to seek advice from doctor regarding the possibility that maltose/glucose contained in some immunoglobulins may interfere with the estimation of blood glucose levels

CYTOMEGALOVIRUS (CMV) IMMUNOGLOBULIN

Trade name
CSL CMV Immunoglobulin-VF

Available form
Vial: 1.5×10^6 U

Action
- trace of IgA present
- half-life about 3 weeks (but less if patient is immunocompromised)
- see also General Actions of immunoglobulins (p. 1620)

Use
- prevention of CMV infection in those with bone marrow or kidney transplantation when the donor is CMV positive and the recipient is CMV negative
- (Adjunct) treatment of established CMV infection (e.g. CMV pneumonitis)

Dose
- (Prophylaxis) 25,000 U/kg IV given on days −4, −2, day of transplant (intraoperatively) and then weekly for 8 weeks **OR**
- (Therapy) 50,000 U/kg IV, repeated after 4–5 days and then every 10–14 days until clinical improvement is seen

Adverse effects/Interactions/Nursing considerations/Cautions/Patient education
- may be given undiluted or diluted with glucose 5% or sodium chloride 0.9%. Infusion rate should start at 1 mL/min for 15 minutes, then increased gradually to 3–4 mL/min if patient's vital signs remain stable
- administer alone
- only given IV
- contains maltose
- see also General Adverse effects/Interactions/Nursing considerations/ Cautions/Patient education for immunoglobulins (p. 1620)

HEPATITIS B IMMUNOGLOBULIN (HBIG)

Trade name
CSL Hepatitis B Immunoglobulin-VF

Available forms
Vial: 100 IU, 400 IU

Action
- contains specific neutralising antibodies against hepatitis B surface antigen (HBsAg)
- see also General Actions of immunoglobulins (p. 1620)

Use
- post-exposure prophylaxis (PEP) in those never previously vaccinated, with

VACCINES AND IMMUNOGLOBULINS

- incomplete vaccination or whose HBsAg antibody level is inadequate (< 10 IU/L) who have been exposed to HBsAg-positive or suspected HBsAg-positive material
- prophylaxis in infants born to HBsAg-positive mothers

Dose
- (Prophylaxis in infants born to HBsAg-positive mother) 100 IU IM at birth and hepatitis B vaccination started at same time (in different limbs) **OR**
- (Confirmed exposure to HBsAg, person has no/incomplete immunisation) 400 IU IM stat within 72 hours of exposure, start hepatitis B vaccination at same time (in different limbs) **OR**
- (Confirmed exposure to HBsAg, person has complete immunisation) antibody level should be measured and if inadequate (< 10 IU/L), 400 IU IM stat and hepatitis B vaccine booster dose (in different limbs) **OR**
- (High risk for HBsAg but not confirmed, person has no/incomplete immunisation) start hepatitis B vaccination regimen, test potential source of infection; if positive, give 400 IU IM stat **OR**
- (High risk for HBsAg but not confirmed, person has complete immunisation) antibody level should be measured and if inadequate (< 10 IU/L), source tested and, if positive, 400 IU IM stat and hepatitis B vaccine booster dose (in different limbs) **OR**
- (Uncertain or low risk of exposure, person has no/incomplete immunisation) start hepatitis B vaccination regimen **OR**
- (Uncertain or low risk of exposure, person has complete immunisation) no treatment required

Adverse effects/Interactions
- see General Adverse effects/Interactions of immunoglobulins (p. 1620)

Nursing considerations/Cautions
- HBIG is administered via IM injection
- post-exposure prophylaxis should be considered after percutaneous or permucosal exposure to HBsAg-positive or suspected positive material (e.g. needlestick, sexual exposure, oral ingestion)
- if given with hepatitis B vaccine, different limbs should be used
- immunoglobulin is not necessary if hepatitis B antibodies are present in adequate levels
- contraindicated in those who are HBsAg positive or have adequate hepatitis B antibodies ($\geq$ 10 IU/L)
- see also General Nursing considerations/Cautions for immunoglobulins (p. 1620)

Patient education
- warn patient that local reaction (pain, redness, tenderness, induration) is normal and may persist for some hours after IM administration
- see also General Patient education for immunoglobulins (p. 1621)

NORMAL (HUMAN) IMMUNOGLOBULIN
Trade names
CSL Normal Immunoglobulin-VF, Cuvitru, Flebogamma 5% DIF, Flebogamma 10% DIF, Gammanorm, Gamunex, Hizentra, Hyqvia, Kiovig, Octagam, Privigen

Available forms
Solution for Infusion: 320 mg/2 mL, 1 g/5 mL, 0.8 g/10 mL, 1 g/10 mL, 1.6 g/2 mL, 2 g/10 mL, 1 g/20 mL, 2 g/20 mL, 3.3 g/20 mL, 4 g/20 mL, 2.5 g/25 mL, 2.5 g/50 mL, 5 g/50 mL, 10 g/50 mL, 5 g/100 mL, 10 g/100 mL, 10 g/200 mL, 20 g/200 mL, 40 g/400 mL, 0.16 g/mL, 165 mg/mL;
Prefilled syringe: 1 g/5 mL, 2 g/10 mL

Action
- contains a range of IgG antibodies collected from pooled plasma from at least 1000 donors

Use
- replacement therapy in primary immunodeficiency (e.g. severe combined immunodeficiency, congenital agammaglobinaemia and hypogammaglobinaemia, common variable immunodeficiency)
- replacement therapy in secondary immunodeficiency (e.g. myeloma, children with AIDS, allogenic bone marrow transplantation)
- immunomodulation (e.g. Guillain—Barre syndrome, Kawasaki disease, idiopathic thrombocytopenic purpura at high risk of bleeding or before surgery, susceptible contacts of hepatitis A, measles and poliomyelitis)

Dose
- (Primary immunodeficiency replacement) initially 0.4—0.8 g/kg IV every 2—4 weeks, then 0.2—0.8 g/kg IV every 2—4 weeks, to achieve IgG trough level of ≥ 4—6 g/L (Flebogamma, Kiovig, Octagam 5% or 10%, Privigen) **OR**
- (Primary immunodeficiency replacement) 300—600 mg/kg by SC infusion weekly (first week), second dose after 2 weeks, third dose after 3 weeks, fourth dose after 4 weeks, then every 3—4 weeks. Therapy should start 1 week after treatment with previous immunoglobulin (with infusion of vorhyaluronidase alfa) (Hyqvia) **OR**
- (Primary immunodeficiency replacement) ≥ 0.2—0.5 g/kg by SC infusion, divided over several days (loading dose), then repeated to achieve 0.3—1 g/kg cumulative monthly dose (Cuvitru) **OR**
- (Primary immunodeficiency replacement in children) initially 0.2—0.5 g/kg SC to achieve steady-state IgG levels, then repeated to achieve 0.4—0.8 g/kg cumulative monthly dose (Gammanorm) **OR**
- (Primary immunodeficiency replacement) 300—600 mg/kg IV or SC every 3—4 weeks to reach IgG trough level of ≥ 5 g/L (Gamunex) **OR**
- (Primary immunodeficiency replacement or hypogammaglobinaemia in children) 0.2—0.5 g/kg SC divided over several days until steady-state IgG trough level is achieved, maintenance doses administered to achieve 0.4—0.8 g/kg cumulative monthly dose (Hizentra) **OR**
- (Primary immunodeficiency replacement in children) 100 mg (0.6 mL)/kg weekly via syringe driver at 10 mL/hour. Rate may be increased by 1 mL/hour/pump every 3—4 weeks (maximum dose 40 mL/hour using 2 pumps) (Gammanorm) **OR**
- (Secondary immunodeficiency replacement, symptomatic hypogammaglobinaemia) 0.2—0.4 g/kg IV every 3—4 weeks to achieve IgG trough level of ≥ 4—6 g/L (Flebogamma, Gamunex, Kiovig, Octagam 5% or 10%, Privigen) **OR**
- (Allogenic bone marrow transplantation (infection, graft vs host disease)) 0.5 g/kg/week IV, starting 7 days pretransplant up to 12 weeks post-transplant (Octagam 5% or 10%) **OR**
- (Allogenic bone marrow transplantation (persistent lack of antibody production)) 0.5 g/kg IV monthly until antibody levels return to normal (Octagam 5% or 10%) **OR**
- (Kawasaki disease) 1.6—2.0 g/kg IV as a single dose or in divided doses over 2—5 days with aspirin (Gamunex, Octagam 5% or 10%, Privigen, Flebogamma) **OR**
- (Kawasaki disease) 2 g/kg IV as a single dose with aspirin (Flebogamma, Kiovig, Octagam 10%, Privigen) **OR**
- (Idiopathic thrombocytopenic purpura) 0.8—1 g/kg IV, repeated once in next 3 days if needed (Flebogamma, Kiovig, Octagam 5% or 10%, Privigen) **OR**
- (Idiopathic thrombocytopenic purpura) 2 g/kg IV as single dose, 1 g/kg over 2 consecutive days or 0.4 g/kg over 5 consecutive days (Gamunex) **OR**

VACCINES AND IMMUNOGLOBULINS

- (Idiopathic thrombocytopenic purpura) 0.4 g/kg/day IV for 2—5 days (Flebogamma, Kiovig, Octagam 5% or 10%, Privigen) **OR**
- (Guillain—Barre syndrome) 0.4 g/kg/day IV for 3—7 days starting within 14 days of symptom onset (Gamunex, Flebogamma, Kiovig, Octagam 5% or 10%, Privigen) **OR**
- (Children with AIDS and recurrent infection) 0.2—0.4 g/kg IV every 3—4 weeks (Flebogamma, Octagam 5% or 10%) **OR**
- (Hepatitis A household contact/institutional contact/staff in institution where hepatitis A is endemic) 0.06 mL/kg deep IM 5—6-monthly (or until active immunity develops or risk no longer exists (long-term protection) (CSL Normal Immunoglobulin-VF) **OR**
- (Hepatitis A household contact) 0.03 mL/kg deep IM (short-term protection) (CSL Normal Immunoglobulin-VF) **OR**
- (Measles) 0.2 mL/kg deep IM (CSL Normal Immunoglobulin-VF) **OR**
- (Poliomyelitis) 0.3 mL/kg deep IM (CSL Normal Immunoglobulin-VF) **OR**
- (Hypogammaglobinaemia) 0.6 mL/kg at monthly intervals (with an extra dose during first month) (CSL Normal Immunoglobulin-VF) **OR**
- (Chronic inflammatory demyelinating polyneuropathy) initially 2 g/kg in divided doses over 2—4 consecutive days (loading dose), then 1 g/kg over 1 day or 500 mg/kg over 2 consecutive days, every 3 weeks (Gamunex, Privigen) **OR**
- (Multifocal motor neuropathy (MMN)) initially 2 g/kg in divided doses over 2—5 days, then 0.4—2 g/kg every 2—6 weeks for 3—6 months (Kiovig, Privigen) **OR**
- (Myasthenic gravis exacerbation (e.g. before surgery, during myasthenic crisis) initially 1—2 g/kg IV in divided doses over 2—5 days, then 0.4—1 g/kg every 4—6 weeks (maintenance) (Privigen) **OR**
- (Lambert—Eaton myasthenic syndrome) initially 2 g/kg IV in divided doses over 2—5 days, then 0.4—1 g/kg every 2—6 weeks (maintenance) (Privigen) **OR**
- (Stiff person syndrome) initially 2 g/kg IV in divided doses over 2—5 days, then 1—2 g/kg every 4—6 weeks (maintenance) (Privigen)

Adverse effects/Interactions
- see General Adverse effects/Interactions of immunoglobulins (p. 1620)

Nursing considerations/Cautions
- higher doses may be required at the start of therapy to provide rapid protection
- IgG trough levels should be measured before next infusion. It may take 3—6 months for IgG trough levels to equilibrate
- the patient should be closely monitored if new to immunoglobulin therapy, if there has been a large time interval between administrations or if changing from one formulation to another
- (SC) the patient and/or carer/family member may be taught SC administration technique
- (Hyqvia) only given SC
- (Hyqvia) infusion of vorhyaluronidase alfa (160 U/mL) is administered first at 1—2 mL/min, followed within 10 minutes by infusion of immunoglobulin through same needle. Vorhyaluronidase alfa acts increases permeability of subcutaneous tissue allowing better absorption of immunoglobulin
- (Hyqvia) if using two sites, doses of both should be divided and contralateral sites used
- (Flebogamma) initial infusion rate should be 0.01—0.02 mL/kg/min for first 30 minutes, then increasing gradually to maximum of 0.08—0.1 mL/kg/min if tolerated
- (Flebogamma) contains sorbitol and is not recommended in those with fructose intolerance

- (Gammanorm) SC infusion site should be changed after 5—15 mL has been administered. Multiple sites can be used simultaneously (as long as they are at least 5 cm apart)
- (Gammanorm) SC is preferred route, but IM may be used for small doses or if SC route is not applicable
- (Cuvitru) administered by SC infusion at 10 mL/hour/site initially, increasing by ≥ 10-minute intervals if well tolerated, to 20 mL/hour/site. More than one pump can be used at same time
- (Kiovig) SC route is recommended only for primary immunodeficiency replacement therapy. Initial recommended infusion rate is 0.5 mL/kg/hour increasing to < 6 mL/kg/hour if tolerated
- (Kiovig, MMN) therapy should continue for 3—6 months to establish patient response. Six months may be required if significant axonal degeneration has occurred. Regular review by neurologist is also recommended
- (Gamunex) may be diluted with glucose 5% (not sodium chloride 0.9%) and infused IV at an initial rate of 1 mg/kg/min for 30 minutes, then increasing gradually to 8 mg/kg/min if tolerated
- (Gamunex) high-dose regimen (1 g/kg over 1—2 days) for idiopathic thrombocytopenic purpura is not recommended if there is any concern about patient's fluid volume
- (Gamunex — idiopathic thrombocytopenic purpura) after first dose (of 2 consecutive day regimen), platelet count should be measured and if adequate, second dose not given. This also applies to 0.4 g/kg regimen
- (Hizentra) only given SC
- (Hizentra) doses greater than 50 mL should be administered over multiple sites, at least 5 cm apart
- (Hizentra) infusion rate ≤ 20 mL/hour/site, gradually increasing to 35 mL/hour/site if tolerated
- (Octagam 10%) infusion rate 0.6—1.2 mL/kg/hour for first 30 minutes, increasing gradually to 7.2 mL/kg/hour if tolerated
- (Octagam 5%) infusion rate 1 mL/kg/hour for first 30 minutes, increasing gradually to 5 mL/kg/hour if tolerated
- (Octagam 5% or 10%) contain maltose
- (Privigen) not given with sodium chloride 0.9%
- (Privigen — primary immunodeficiency replacement) infusion rate 0.3 mL/kg/hour, increasing gradually to 4.8 mL/kg/hour, and finally to 7.2 mL/kg/hour if very well tolerated
- (Privigen, Hizentra) contraindicated in those with hypoprolinaemia type I or II
- (Kiovig, CSL Normal Immunoglobin-VF) contain glycine and are therefore contraindicated if glycine hypersensitivity exists
- (Hyqvia) contraindicated in those with hypersensitivity to vorhyaluronidase or hyaluronidase (as this is given as infusion before immunoglobulin)
- see also General Nursing considerations/Cautions for immunoglobulins (p. 1620)

Patient education

- instruct the patient in SC administration technique, including importance of:
    - allowing solution to come to room temperature before use (usually 20—60 minutes)
    - not shaking vial
    - collecting all equipment before starting procedure (e.g. infusion pump, administration tubing, SC needle or catheter set, Y-connector, alcohol swab, syringe, vial adapter, gauze or transparent dressing, tape, sharps disposal container, treatment diary (if used))
    - checking expiry date and solution for any turbidity or sediment (not used if out of date, turbid or contains sediment)
    - washing hands with soap and water before starting
    - drawing up of solution technique and preparation of infusion tubing

- insertion of SC needle (including choice of sites and technique and use of multiple sites, e.g. at least 5 cm apart if multiple sites are administered at same time)
- starting infusion at correct infusion rate
- use of syringe driver or other infusion pumps (if used)
- correct disposal of used equipment
- recording treatment (including recording label information or removing label and putting this in diary/log book)
* see also General Patient education for immunoglobulins (p. 1621)

RABIES IMMUNOGLOBULIN
Trade name
KamRAB

Available form
Vial: 300 IU/2 mL

Action
- rabies virus is transmitted via saliva of infected mammals
- see also General Actions of immunoglobulins (p. 1620)

Use
- given immediately after exposure to virus (single or multiple bites or scratches or if contamination with mucous membrane (e.g. licks)) occurs (unless the person already has adequate antibody levels from previous vaccination)

Dose
- 20 IU/kg with largest portion infiltrated around wound(s) (if possible) and remainder IM at a site distant to vaccination site (at time of first vaccine dose)

Adverse effects/Nursing considerations/Cautions/Patient education
- administered IM
- bites/scratches should be washed with copious amount of water and detergent, and then treated with disinfectant. Tetanus prophylaxis is also recommended
- may be given up to 7 days (168 hours) after initial dose of rabies vaccine
  - should not be given in same syringe or at same anatomical site as rabies vaccine
- repeated doses of immunoglobulin should not be given once vaccination schedule has started
- not given IV because of risk of shock
- may be diluted with sodium chloride 0.9% before administration
- should be given with rabies vaccine (p. 1613) (different limb)
- see also General Adverse effects/Nursing considerations/Cautions/Patient education for immunoglobulins (p. 1620)

RHESUS (Rh(D)) IMMUNOGLOBULIN
Trade names
CSL Rh(D) Immunoglobulin-VF, Rhophylac

Available forms
Vial (solution): 250 IU;
Vial (powder): 625 IU;
Prefilled syringe: 1500 IU/2 mL

Action
- when mother is Rh(D)-negative and fetus is Rh(D)-positive, mother can become immunised to Rh(D) antigen producing anti-Rh(D) antibodies, which may cross the placenta and cause haemolytic anaemia in the newborn

Use
- prevention of Rh sensitisation in Rh(D)-negative female (at or below childbearing age). Sensitising events include antepartum haemorrhage, maternal abdominal trauma (likely to cause bleeding to both mother and fetus (feto—maternal haemorrhage)), external cephalic version, cordocentesis, amniocentesis or chorionic villi sampling,

normal delivery, miscarriage, pregnancy termination and ectopic pregnancy
- treatment of Rh(D)-negative person after incompatible transfusion of Rh(D)-positive blood or other products containing red blood cells (RBC)

Dose
- (Sensitising event in pregnancy unless fetus is confirmed Rh(D)-negative) 250 IU IM (in first trimester) or 625 IU IM (in second or third trimester or if multiple pregnancy) (CSL Rh(D) Immunoglobulin-VF) **OR**
- (Gestational age is unknown but possibly ≥ 13 weeks) 625 IU IM (CSL Rh(D) Immunoglobulin-VF) **OR**
- (Abdominal trauma causing haemorrhage > 6 mL) 100 IU/mL IM of Rh(D)-positive RBC (CSL Rh(D) Immunoglobulin-VF) **OR**
- (Abdominal trauma causing haemorrhage ≤ 6 mL) 625 IU IM (CSL Rh(D) Immunoglobulin-VF) **OR**
- (Transfusion of Rh(D)-positive blood) 100 IU/mL IM of Rh(D)-positive RBC (CSL Rh(D) Immunoglobulin-VF) **OR**
- (Antepartum prophylaxis, 28–30-week gestation) 1500 IU IM or IV (Rhophylac) **OR**
- (Postpartum prophylaxis if newborn is Rh(D) positive) 1500 IU IM or IV within 72 hours of delivery (Rhophylac) **OR**
- (Prophylaxis after pregnancy complication or invasive procedure) 1500 IU IM or IV within 72 hours of event (Rhophylac) **OR**
- (Large haemorrhage > 15 mL) 1500 IU IM or IV within 72 hours of haemorrhage plus 100 IU/mL fetal RBC > 15 mL (Rhophylac) **OR**
- (Incompatible blood transfusion) 100 IU per 2 mL of transfused Rh(D)-positive blood or 1 mL erythrocyte concentrate IV (maximum dose 15,000 IU) (Rhophylac)

Adverse effects/Interactions/Nursing considerations/Cautions/Patient education
- dose should be given within 72 hours of sensitising event
- (IM administration) slow deep intramuscular injection; local anaesthetic may be added to lessen pain
- if > 5 mL is required IM, dose should be divided and given into different sites
- if patient body mass index (BMI) ≥ 30, IV route is recommended as IM administration may be ineffective
- contraindicated in those who are Rh(D) positive or Rh(D) negative and have been immunised, or in Rh(D)-positive postpartum babies
- see also General Adverse effects/Interactions/Nursing considerations/Cautions/Patient education for immunoglobulins (p. 1620)

TETANUS IMMUNOGLOBULIN
Trade names
CSL Tetanus Immunoglobulin-VF (For Intramuscular Use), Tetanus Immunoglobulin-VF (For Intravenous Use)

Available forms
Vial: (for IM use) 250 IU, (for IV use) 4000 IU

Action
- see General Actions of immunoglobulins (p. 1620)

Use
- passive protection in those with a tetanus-prone wound (see Tetanus-prone wounds below) with no or doubtful tetanus immunity or greater than 10 years since last booster dose
- treatment of clinical tetanus

Dose
- 250 IU IM or 500 IU IM if wound is grossly contaminated or 24 hours has elapsed before seeking medical advice (CSL Tetanus Immunoglobulin-VF (for IM use)) **OR**
- (Clinical tetanus) 4000 IU by IV infusion starting at 1 mL/min for 15 minutes, then increasing rate to 3—4 mL/min if tolerated (Tetanus Immunoglobulin-VF (for IV use))

VACCINES AND IMMUNOGLOBULINS

Adverse effects/Nursing considerations/Cautions/Patient education
- may be diluted using sodium chloride 0.9% or glucose 5%, or may be given undiluted IV (IV preparation) or by IM injection (IM preparation)
- local anaesthetic can be added to IM to lessen pain
- IV formulation contains maltose
- administer IV alone
- IV preparation should not be given IM
- IM preparation should not be given IV
- see also General Adverse effects/Nursing considerations/Cautions/Patient education for immunoglobulins (p. 1620)

Tetanus-prone wounds
- *Clostridium tetani* is a Gram-positive organism responsible for tetanus. It forms spores which can easily enter a wound where they can then grow anaerobically and produce a toxin that contains both a neurotoxin and haemolysin. The neurotoxin acts on the CNS, producing muscle rigidity and painful spasms. Incubation period is 3—21 days, the median being 10 days after injury (or less with heavily contaminated wounds). Early signs of tetanus include trismus (lockjaw), dysphagia and pain or stiffness in the neck, back or shoulder muscles. Violent, painful generalised muscle spasms may also occur. The person may or may not be febrile and mental status is generally not impaired. Death usually results from respiratory failure, hyper/hypotension or cardiac arrhythmias
- most deaths occur in those > 70 years and is often associated with apparently minor injuries (e.g. prick with a rose thorn while gardening) in those who may never have been vaccinated or vaccinated > 10 years ago
- all wounds (except clean minor cuts) should be considered tetanus prone
- growth of *C. tetani* is favoured in compound fractures, bite wounds, deep penetrating wounds, wounds complicated by extensive tissue damage (such as burns), pyogenic infection or with foreign bodies (particularly wood splinters) or superficial wounds contaminated with soil, dust or horse manure that have remained untreated for 4 hours. Reimplantation of an avulsed tooth is considered a tetanus-prone event as washing and cleaning is often minimised to improve implantation of the tooth. Depot injections (SC or intradermal) in those who inject drugs may also cause tetanus-prone wounds
- wound should be thoroughly cleaned and any foreign or necrotic material removed
- regardless of the patient's immune status, local disinfection and, if needed, surgical treatment should be included as part of the overall management plan. Antibiotic prophylaxis is usually not required; however, may be needed if bacterial infection is present
- booster doses are recommended for adults > 50 years who have not received a booster dose in previous 10 years (with pertussis), in those ≥ 65 years (if not received in previous 10 years) or in travellers to countries where health services may be difficult to access (if more than 10 years has elapsed since last dose of tetanus-containing vaccine)
- when tetanus vaccine and immunoglobulin are administered at the same time, each is given into a different limb and a separate syringe is used
- tetanus prophylaxis is dependent on the person's history of active immunisation, time since last dose of tetanus-containing vaccine and the type of wound. The following table shows the current recommendations

Recommendations for tetanus prophylaxis in wound management

History of tetanus vaccination	Time since last dose	Type of wound	Tetanus vaccine	Tetanus immunoglobulin
≥ 3 doses	< 5 years	Clean minor wound	NO	NO
≥ 3 doses	< 5 years	All other wounds	NO	NO (unless person is immunodeficient)
≥ 3 doses	5–10 years	Clean minor wound	NO	NO
≥ 3 doses	5–10 years	All other wounds	YES	NO (unless person is immunodeficient)
≥ 3 doses	> 10 years	Clean minor wound	YES	NO
≥ 3 doses	> 10 years	All other wounds	YES	NO (unless person is immunodeficient)
< 3 doses	Uncertain	Clean minor wound	YES	NO
< 3 doses	Uncertain	All other wounds	YES	YES

Immunodeficient: those who have humoral immune deficiency or with HIV (regardless of CD4+ count) if tetanus-prone wound has occurred regardless of when last dose of tetanus-containing vaccine was administered
Australian Technical Advisory Group on Immunisation (ATAGI). The Australian Immunisation Handbook (2023). Available from: https://immunisationhandbook.health.gov.au/resources/handbook-tables/table-guide-to-tetanus-prophylaxis-in-wound-management © Commonwealth of Australia as represented by the Department of Health

ZOSTER IMMUNOGLOBULIN

Trade name
CSL Zoster Immunoglobulin-VF

Available form
Vial: 200 IU

Action
- most effective if given within 96 hours of exposure
- see also General Actions of immunoglobulins (p. 1620)

Use
- prevention of varicella in susceptible high-risk patients (e.g. leukaemia, lymphoma, congenital or acquired immunodeficiency (e.g. AIDS), corticosteroid or antineoplastic therapy), after exposure to chicken pox or shingles, with

VACCINES AND IMMUNOGLOBULINS

no/unknown history of prior exposure to chicken pox

Dose
- (Patient weight > 40 kg) 600 IU IM **OR**
- (Patient weight 30.1–40 kg) 500 IU IM **OR**
- (Patient weight 20.1–30 kg) 375 IU IM **OR**
- (Patient weight 10.1–20 kg) 250 IU IM **OR**
- (Patient weight 0–10 kg) 125 IU IM

Nursing considerations/Cautions

- administered by IM injection
- should be administered within 96 hours of exposure
- not recommended prophylactically in those who are immunodeficient
- if greater than 5 mL is required, dose should be administered over several sites
- local anaesthetic can be added to lessen pain
- see also General Nursing considerations/Cautions for immunoglobulins (p. 1620)

VASODILATORS

The vasodilators are a heterogeneous (diverse) group of agents that act either directly or indirectly, resulting in vasodilation and improved circulation. Directly acting vasodilators include those that affect the smooth muscle within blood vessels, such as the nitrates (e.g. glyceryl trinitrate; see Antianginal agents, p. 59); calcium-channel blockers, which act by inhibiting the cellular influx of calcium ions into vascular smooth muscle, thereby reducing contractile ability (e.g. diltiazem; see Antihypertensive agents, p. 536); and potassium-channel activators (e.g. nicorandil; see Antianginal agents, p. 66). Indirectly acting vasodilators include centrally acting agents (e.g. clonidine; see Antihypertensive agents, p. 543), ACE inhibitors (e.g. captopril; see Antihypertensive agents, p. 506) and angiotensin II receptor antagonists (e.g. losartan; see Antihypertensive agents, p. 516).

Other vasodilators that do not fall into these categories are included in this chapter.

ALPROSTADIL (PROSTAGLANDIN E1)
Trade names
Caverject Impulse, Neupedix, Prostin VR

Available forms
Ampoules: 500 microgram/mL;
Vial: 10 microgram, 20 microgram

Action
- prostaglandin
- vasodilator, prevents platelet aggregation
- relaxes ductus arteriosus, supporting patency
- elevates body temperature
- most effective if used within 96 hours of birth (ductus arteriosus)
- (IV) half-life 5–10 minutes

Use
- maintain patency of the ductus arteriosus in neonates with congenital heart failure until surgery is possible (Prostin VR, Neupedix)
- erectile dysfunction in adult men (see Erectile dysfunction agents, p. 1116) (Caverject impulse)

Dose
- (Ductus arteriosus) 0.1 microgram/kg/min IV until effective, then dose is decreased

VASODILATORS

Adverse effects
- (IV) apnoea, fever, flushing, hypotension, bradycardia, tachycardia, seizures, diarrhoea, oedema, cardiac arrest, hypokalaemia, disseminated intravascular coagulation (DIC), sepsis
- (Long term) reversible cortical proliferation of long bones

Nursing considerations/Cautions
- use is recommended only in facilities where intubation and ventilatory support can be accessed immediately in the event of an emergency
- babies (especially those weighing < 2 kg) should be closely monitored for apnoea (especially during the first 60 minutes of infusion)
- arterial pressure should be monitored during therapy and the infusion rate decreased if there is a significant fall
- if therapy > 120 hours, babies should be monitored for antral hyperplasia and gastric outlet obstruction
- solution should be replaced every 24 hours
- should be given into a large blood vessel or via umbilical artery catheter
- dilute with sodium chloride 0.9%
- the infusion rate is calculated using dosage, neonate's weight and final concentration to be used
- administer using an infusion pump
- avoid Prostin VR (undiluted) coming into contact with a plastic container, because a hazy solution will result, which should be discarded
- caution if used in neonates with a history of bleeding because of the risk of DIC
- not recommended in neonates with respiratory distress syndrome or for more than 2–3 days continuously
- contraindicated in neonates with persistent fetal circulation (with cyanosis), with total anomalous pulmonary venous return (below the diaphragm), or with asplenia or polysplenia in whom pulmonary atresia is combined with anomalous pulmonary venous return that may be obstructed

BETAHISTINE DIHYDROCHLORIDE
Trade names
Betahistine GH, Betahistine Lupin, Betahistine Sandoz, Betahistine Viatris, Betasert, Serc, Setear

Available forms
Tablets: 16 mg, 24 mg

Action
- histamine-like drug that increases blood flow in the microcirculation in the inner ear
- half-life about 3.5 hours

Use
- Ménière's syndrome (symptoms include vertigo with nausea and/or vomiting, tinnitus and hearing loss)

Dose
- initially 8–16 mg orally 3 times daily (maximum daily dose 48 mg) **OR**
- 24 mg twice daily (maximum daily dose 48 mg)

Adverse effects
- headache
- nausea, dyspepsia
- (Rare) dizziness, malaise, tiredness, mild skin or GI disturbances, hypersensitivity

Interactions
- may antagonise antihistamines
- caution if used with monoamine oxidase inhibitors (MAOIs) inhibitors (including MAO-B selective), as betahistine metabolism may be inhibited

Nursing considerations/Cautions
- monitoring is required if patient has asthma
- caution if used in those receiving antihistamines or who have asthma
- contraindicated in those with a history of or current active peptic ulcer or pheochromocytoma or under 18 years

Patient education

- advise the patient that improvement in the condition should be seen within a few days of starting therapy
- warn the patient not to drive or operate machinery if dizziness or tiredness occurs
- the patient should be advised to take with meals if GI disturbances occur
- female patients should be counselled to use adequate contraception to prevent pregnancy occurring

Tablet can be crushed and mixed with water or a spoonful of yoghurt or apple puree.

Contraindicated during pregnancy.

Contraindicated during breastfeeding.

PENTOXIFYLLINE (OXPENTIFYLLINE)
Trade name
Trental 400

Available form
Tablets (controlled release): 400 mg

Action
- xanthine derivative thought to improve blood flow in the affected microcirculation by reducing blood viscosity, platelet adhesion and aggregation and increasing tissue oxygenation
- half-life 0.4–0.8 hours
- active metabolites (elimination half-lives 1–1.6 hours)

Use
- intermittent claudication in peripheral arterial disease of limbs

Dose
- 400 mg orally 3 times daily with or after food

Adverse effects
- nausea, dyspepsia, vomiting, bloating, flatulence, belching, abdominal pain, diarrhoea
- dizziness, headache, tremor, insomnia, sleep disturbances
- pruritus, rash, urticaria
- (Uncommon) angina/chest pain
- (Rare) jaundice, cholestasis

Interactions
- combined use with other xanthine derivatives or with sympathomimetics may cause excessive CNS stimulation
- may increase serum levels of theophylline and the risk of adverse effects
- may increase the effects of hypoglycaemic agents, requiring a dose adjustment to prevent hypoglycaemia occurring in patients with diabetes
- may cause bleeding if given with oral anticoagulants or antiplatelet agents. Those on warfarin should have the INR time monitored more frequently than normal
- effects of antihypertensive agents may be enhanced
- serum levels may increase if given with ciprofloxacin
- may cause false positive result on urinary assay for pregnanediol

Nursing considerations/Cautions
- blood pressure (BP) should be measured regularly during therapy, especially in those with pre-existing low or labile BP
- observe for improvement of skin colour, temperature and peripheral pulses
- note if the patient can walk further without pain after treatment
- treatment is recommended for at least 8 weeks to assess effectiveness
- caution if used in elderly patients, those with low/labile blood pressure, at risk of bleeding, severe coronary heart disease, or stenosis of cerebral blood vessels
- not recommended in those with severe liver or kidney impairment
- contraindicated in those with or history of peptic ulceration or myocardial

VASODILATORS

infarction, or who have recently experienced a severe haemorrhage or have an intolerance to other methylxanthines (e.g. caffeine, theophylline)

Patient education

- advise the patient to avoid smoking and alcohol
- instruct the patient that a controlled-release tablet is swallowed whole (not broken, chewed or crushed) with a glass of water
- suggest taking with food to reduce stomach disturbances if they occur
- advise the patient against driving or operating heavy machinery if dizziness or tremor occurs
- those with diabetes should be instructed to monitor blood glucose levels regularly during therapy, as adjustment to the hypoglycaemic agent (insulin or oral medication) may be required
- prevent ulceration of affected lower extremities by advising good skin care, close attention to toenails, properly fitting shoes and hosiery and by avoiding garters, hot water bottles and any trauma

Tablet should not be crushed, broken or chewed.

Not used in pregnancy unless the expected benefit outweighs potential risk.

Not used in breastfeeding unless the expected benefit outweighs potential risk.

Dose adjustment and monitoring is recommended in those with impaired kidney function (creatinine clearance < 30 mL/min).

Not recommended in those with severe liver or kidney impairment.

Caution if used in elderly patients.

VITAMINS, MINERALS AND ELECTROLYTES

Vitamins are organic substances the body requires in small amounts for various metabolic processes. Minerals are inorganic nutrients or trace elements, also required in small quantities, which act as essential co-factors in various enzyme systems. Deficiency states are rare in people who have an adequate diet. However, oral vitamin and mineral supplements may be necessary in cases of restricted diet, malabsorption syndrome and where there are increased requirements, such as in pregnancy, lactation, fever, hyperthyroidism, burn injuries, large wounds and wasting diseases. They may also be added to parenteral and enteral nutrition solutions.

Vitamins are categorised based on their solubility: the B-group vitamins and vitamin C are water soluble, whereas vitamins A, D, E and K are fat soluble. Numerous multivitamin preparations containing vitamins A, B-group, C, D and E are available, some of which also include minerals. For individuals with a well-balanced diet, prolonged use of high-dose multivitamins offers little benefit and can have serious consequences, particularly because of the excessive intake of fat-soluble vitamins A and D.

VITAMINS

VITAMIN A (also known as Retinol)
Trade names
Bio-Logical Vitamin A, Blackmores Vitamin A 5000

Available forms
Capsules: 5000 IU;
Oral solution: 2.75 mg/0.2 mL (5000 IU)

Action
- fat-soluble vitamin necessary for normal formation and function of epithelial and mucosal cells, normal bone growth, embryonic development (particularly spinal cord, vertebrae, limbs, eyes, ears and heart) and immune function
- necessary for formation and regeneration of rhodopsin (visual purple), which is needed for vision, particularly in dim light
- available in a number of forms (retinol, retinal, retinoic acid, retinyl ester)
- preformed vitamin A is available only in animal-derived foods; oils, fruits and vegetables contain provitamin A carotenoid (precursor of retinol)

VITAMINS, MINERALS AND ELECTROLYTES

Deficiency
- night blindness; later, xerophthalmia
- dry rough skin (follicular hyperkeratosis)
- infection due to immune dysfunction

Use
- deficiency states, night blindness
- some skin diseases (e.g. dermatitis, skin ulcers), chronic infection (e.g. acne)
- premenstrual tension
- prophylaxis against respiratory infection
- replacement in decreased intestinal absorption conditions (e.g. steatorrhoea, biliary obstruction, coeliac disease)
- xerophthalmia

Optimal daily requirements
- 700 micrograms (women), 900 micrograms (men)

Dose
- 5000 IU orally daily with food **OR**
- (Severe deficiency) 50,000 IU orally twice daily for 3 days, then daily for 14 days

Adverse effects

Acute toxicity (very high doses)
- drowsiness, sedation, dizziness, irritability, severe headache (because of increased intracranial pressure), papilloedema
- nausea, vomiting, hepatomegaly
- erythema, pruritus, desquamation
- (Infants) vomiting, bulging fontanelles

Chronic toxicity (excessive amounts over prolonged period)
- anorexia, weight loss
- irritability, headache, fatigue
- cracking and bleeding lips
- dry itching, peeling skin, dermatitis, disturbed hair growth
- bone pain, hyperostosis
- papilloedema
- haemorrhage

Nursing considerations/Cautions
- contraindicated in those with hypervitaminosis A

Patient education
- (Oral solution) advise patient that oral solution can be mixed in water or juice

Vitamin A capsules should not be opened. Available as an oral solution.

Not recommended. High doses of Vitamin A are teratogenic and can cause serious birth defects, particularly if taken during the first trimester.

Breastfeeding women should aim for the recommended daily intake of vitamin A without exceeding the upper limit. Excessive supplementation should be avoided as it may lead to high levels in breastmilk, which could pose a risk to the infant.

VITAMIN B

THIAMINE HYDROCHLORIDE (Vitamin B$_1$)

Trade names
Betavit, Biologicals Therapies Thiamine Hydrochloride Solution

Available forms
Tablets: 100 mg;
Vial: 100 mg/mL

Action
- member of the water-soluble vitamin B group necessary for carbohydrate metabolism, including detoxification of oestrogen in the liver
- not stored in any significant amounts (about 30 g); therefore any excess is excreted in the liver
- found predominantly in cereal foods; thiamine-enrichment of baking flour exists in Australia (but not New Zealand)

Deficiency
- dietary deficiency (e.g. beriberi, chronic alcoholism (as alcohol metabolism requires thiamine), anorexia)

- (Chronic) peripheral neuropathy, Wernicke's encephalopathy, Korsakoff's syndrome, psychosis, cardiac failure
- (Acute) weakness, fatigue, nausea, anorexia, hypotension, decreased reflexes and sensation, paralysis

Use
- thiamine deficiency due to restricted diet (including those receiving total parenteral nutrition), extensive burns, diabetes, impaired kidney or liver function, hyperthyroidism, alcoholism, benign breast dysplasia

Optimal daily requirements
- 0.9—1.1 mg (male), 0.7—0.8 mg (female), 1.2 mg (during pregnancy)

Dose
- 50—100 mg orally daily as a single dose or 2 divided doses, **OR**
- (Critically ill thiamine-deficient adult, malabsorption syndrome) 5–100 mg IM or IV over 10 minutes, three times daily, **OR**
- (Wernecke's encephalophy) initially 100 mg IV over 30 minutes, then 50–100 mg daily IM or IV until patient resumes normal diet, **OR**
- (Alcohol withdrawal) initially 100 mg IM or IV, followed by 100 mg orally, IM or IV daily for up to 5 days

Nursing considerations/Cautions
- parenteral thiamine should be used only when an oral route is not available because of the risk of anaphylaxis
- consideration should be given to administering other water-soluble vitamins with thiamine, as simple thiamine deficiency is rare
- (IV) administration should be over at least 10 minutes
- high-carbohydrate diet or glucose infusion may worsen thiamine deficiency symptoms. If patient requires glucose-containing IV solution, it should be administered after thiamine
- (100 mg/mL) contraindicated in children under 2 years due to benzyl alcohol content

Tablets can be crushed and mixed with water or spoonful of yoghurt or apple puree.

Safe.

Women who are breastfeeding require 1.2 mg of thiamine delay to compensate for 100–200 mg that is distributed daily into breastmilk; however, over-supplementation should be avoided.

Available in combination with
- contained in Biological Therapies B-Dose 2 mL injection and Biological Therapies B-Dose Forte 2 mL injection with other B vitamins cyanocobalamin (B_{12}), (nicotinamide (B_3), pyridoxine (B_6), riboflavine (B_2) and dexpanthenol (B_5)) for treatment of beriberi, Wernicke's encephalopathy (Forte formulation), pellagra (as patients often have other vitamin B deficiencies), peripheral neuritis, pernicious anaemia and chronic alcoholism
- contained in multivitamin preparations

NICOTINAMIDE (also known as Vitamin B_3, Nicotinic acid and Niacin)

Trade names
Blackmores InSolar, Caruso's Vitamin B3

Available form
Tablets: 500 mg

Action
- member of the water-soluble vitamin B group
- peripheral vasodilator
- hypolipidaemic, hypotriglyceridaemic and hypocholesterolaemic
- forms co-enzymes important in tissue respiration

VITAMINS, MINERALS AND ELECTROLYTES

- available in a wide range of foods, including beef, pork, wholegrain cereals, eggs and cow's milk

Deficiency
- pellagra (glossitis, dermatitis, diarrhoea and, in severe cases, dementia or delirium)

Use
- pellagra
- skin health
- hypercholesterolaemia, hypertriglyceridaemia, hyperlipoproteinaemia (most types) (see also Lipid-regulating agents (p. 1318))

Optimal daily requirements
- 16 mg (males), 14 mg (females), 18 mg (pregnancy), 17 mg (breastfeeding)

Dose
- (Pellagra) 250 mg orally twice daily after meals **OR**
- 500 mg orally daily **OR**
- (Solar damaged skin, prevention recurrence of skin cancers) 500 mg orally twice daily

Adverse effects/Interactions/Nursing considerations/Cautions/Patient education
- it is important to differentiate between nicotinic acid (niacin) and nicotinamide (niacinamide, e.g. Insolar). Nicotinic acid is used for treating hyperlipidaemia; nicotinamide is used for treating solar-damaged skin. These uses are not interchangeable; however, either can be used for treating B₃ deficiency
- not recommended in those < 18 years
- see also general points for Thiamine hydrochloride (p. 1637)

High doses are not recommended.

High doses should be avoided while breastfeeding because of the potential for side effects in both the mother and infant, including skin flushing or gastrointestinal discomfort.

PYRIDOXINE (VITAMIN B₆)
Trade names
Blackmores Vitamin B6, Pyridox

Available forms
Tablets: 25 mg, 100 mg;
Tablets (sustained-release): 240 mg

Action
- member of the water-soluble vitamin B group, important in carbohydrate, lipid and protein metabolism
- assists in formation of haemoglobin
- made up of 6 compounds (pyridoxal, pyridoxine, pyridoxamine and their phosphates)
- found in a wide range of foods (e.g. organ meats, muscle meats, breakfast cereals, vegetables, fruits)

Deficiency
- irritability, convulsions, depression, confusion
- hypochromic (microcytic) anaemia
- seborrhoeic dermatitis

Use
- some types of anaemia
- nausea and vomiting in pregnancy
- radiation sickness
- symptoms associated with premenstrual tension
- acute alcoholism
- homocystinuria

Optimal daily requirements
- 1.3–1.7 mg (males), 1.3–1.5 mg (females), 1.9 mg (pregnancy), 2.0 mg (breastfeeding)

Dose
- 25–100 mg orally daily or as prescribed **OR**
- 240 mg orally daily (sustained-release)

Adverse effects
- gastrointestinal upset, headache
- (High dose, prolonged therapy) peripheral neuropathy, nervousness, tremors, abnormal ECG

Interactions
- may reduce effects of levodopa (not if a dopa decarboxylase inhibitor is also given)

Nursing considerations/Cautions
- contraindicated if there is inadequate dietary protein intake to avoid undesirable increase in amino acid catabolism
- see also general points for Thiamine hydrochloride (p. 1637)

Patient education
- (Premenstrual tension) patient should be advised to take pyridoxine daily for the number of days the symptoms occur before the onset of menstruation
- advise the patient to seek medical advice if any tingling, burning, prickling or tightening sensation of hands or feet occurs

 Plain tablets can be dispersed in water, or crushed and mixed with spoonful of yoghurt or apple puree.

 Sustained-release tablets should not be chewed, broken or crushed.

CYANOCOBALAMIN (VITAMIN B$_{12}$)

Trade names
B12 Liquid, Biological Therapies Cyanocobalamin 1 mg in 1 mL Injection, Biological Therapies Cyanocobalamin 20 mg in 2 mL Injection, Blackmores B12, Eagle Sublingual B12, Methylcobalamin 10 mg in 2 mL injection, Methyl B12 Chewable, NanoCelle B12

Available forms
Tablets: 100 microgram;
Tablets (sublingual): 1 mg;
Ampoules: 1 mg/mL, 10 mg/2 mL, 20 mg/2 mL;
Sublingual spray: 500 microgram/spray

Action
- member of the water-soluble vitamin B group, essential for normal cell growth, production of epithelial cells, haemopoiesis and maintenance of myelin throughout the nervous system
- acts as a coenzyme in nucleic acid synthesis
- dietary sources include red meats, milk and milk products

Deficiency
- megaloblastic anaemia (macrocytosis) (similar to folate deficiency)
- neurological damage (e.g. sensory disturbance of feet and hands, motor disturbance, cognitive changes, visual disturbance)
- GI disturbance

Use
- pernicious anaemia
- prophylaxis and treatment of other macrocytic anaemias associated with vitamin B$_{12}$ deficiency (unable to be corrected orally)
- peripheral neuropathy, diabetic polyneuropathy (adjunct)
- diet supplement for vegan and vegetarian diets

Optimal daily requirements
- 2.4 micrograms; (pregnancy) 2.6 micrograms; (breastfeeding) 2.8 micrograms

Dose
- 20 mg slow IM stat **OR**
- 5 mg slow IM daily for 5 days **OR**
- 10 mg slow IM, repeated as needed **OR**
- 1 mg slow IM, repeated as needed **OR**
- 1 mg daily orally (dissolved under tongue) (sublingual tablets) **OR**
- 100 micrograms orally twice daily with food or as prescribed **OR**
- 500–1000 micrograms sublingually 1–2 times daily after meals (or as prescribed) (sublingual spray)

Adverse effects
- diarrhoea, prolonged nausea or vomiting, abdominal pain
- IM pain, redness, induration
- (Rare) hypersensitivity reaction, anaphylaxis, pulmonary oedema, congestive cardiac failure, hypokalaemia, cardiac arrest

VITAMINS, MINERALS AND ELECTROLYTES

Interactions
* malabsorption may occur if given with colchicine or heavy alcohol use (> 2 weeks)
* serum levels by decreased by combined oral contraceptives or folic acid (high dose, prolonged use)
* response may be decreased if given with methotrexate

Nursing considerations/Cautions
* diagnosis of pernicious anaemia should be made before starting therapy
* before starting therapy, haematocrit, reticulocyte count, vitamin B_{12}, folate and iron levels should be checked. Haematocrit and reticulocyte count should also be checked daily from day 5 to 7 of therapy, then regularly depending on haematocrit. If reticulocyte count does not increase or reticulocyte count remains elevated with haematocrit < 35%, therapy should be re-evaluated
* serum potassium levels should be monitored during therapy, especially initially, and any hypokalaemia corrected immediately
* FBC and serum vitamin B_{12} should be monitored 6–12-monthly (if the patient is well), or more frequently if the patient has some condition that may increase the need for vitamin B_{12}. Monitoring of levels should continue for life
* oral administration may be insufficient to treat pernicious anaemia, malabsorption disorders, gastrectomy and gastrointestinal pathologies
* if the patient has an allergic disposition to B vitamins, this can be checked giving a dermal dose
* antihistamines, corticosteroids and adrenaline (epinephrine) (1:1000) should be readily available in the event of anaphylaxis
* not given IV
* solution should be warmed before use to reduce pain
* solution is a crimson–red colour
* not recommended in children < 12 years
* caution if used in those with liver disease, myeloproliferative disorders or Leber's disease
* contraindicated in those with hypersensitivity to cobalt, hypervitaminosis or megaloblastic anaemia of pregnancy

Patient education
* the patient should be advised to allow sublingual tablets to dissolve under the tongue
* advise the patient with pernicious anaemia that therapy is for life to prevent nerve damage to the spinal cord

 Available as chewable or sublingual tablets.

HYDROXOCOBALAMIN (VITAMIN B_{12})
Trade names
Cobal-B12, Hydroxo-B12, Neo-B12 Injection, Pure Liposome Vitamin B12 Liquid, Vita B12

Available forms
Ampoule: 1000 microgram/mL; Liquid: 500 microgram/0.5 mL

Action
* as for cyanocobalamin (p. 1640), but produces a higher and more prolonged vitamin B_{12} level when given IM at the same dose
* excreted slowly via bile and urine

Use
* prevention and treatment of pernicious anaemia and other macrocytic anaemias associated with vitamin B_{12} deficiency
* treat optic neuropathies (e.g. tobacco amblyopia, Leber's disease, optic atrophy)

Dose
* (Pernicious anaemia, macrocytic anaemias without neurological involvement) initially 250–1000 micrograms IM alternate days for 1–2 weeks, then 250

micrograms IM weekly until RBC count is normal, then 1000 micrograms every 2–3 months for life (maintenance) **OR**
- (Pernicious anaemia, macrocytic anaemia with neurological involvement) initially 1000 micrograms IM on alternate days for 1–2 weeks, then 1000 micrograms every 2 months for life (maintenance) **OR**
- (Optic neuropathies) initially 1000 micrograms IM daily for 2 weeks, then twice weekly for 4 weeks, then monthly for life (maintenance) **OR**
- (Prevention of macrocytic anaemia and associated B_{12} deficiency) 1000 micrograms IM every 2–3 months, **OR** 0.5–2.0 mL orally daily

Adverse effects
- itching, sensation of hot and cold, urticaria, eczema, acne, folliculitis
- nausea, vomiting, diarrhoea
- headache, dizziness, malaise
- chest pain/discomfort, hypokalaemia, arrhythmias (secondary to hypokalaemia), cardiac arrest
- feeling of body swelling
- development of antibodies
- peripheral vascular thrombosis
- IM site reaction
- (Rare) anaphylaxis, pulmonary oedema, congestive cardiac failure

Interactions
- poor response if given with chloramphenicol or other agents with bone marrow depressing properties
- serum levels may be decreased by oral contraceptives
- vitamin B_{12} levels may be lowered by large, continuous doses of folic acid, as well as potentiating neurological complications
- vitamin B_{12} blood assay may be invalidated by antibacterial agents

Nursing considerations/Cautions
- diagnosis of pernicious anaemia should be made before starting therapy
- intradermal test is recommended in those with sensitivity to cobalamins
- not given IV
- serum potassium should be monitored during therapy, especially initially, and any hypokalaemia should be corrected immediately
- serum vitamin B_{12} should be monitored regularly during therapy
- therapy may unmask polycythaemia vera
- solution is dark red in colour
- iron and folic acid supplements may also be necessary if there is severe anaemia
- caution if used in those with iron or folate deficiency, uraemia or a concurrent infection because the therapeutic effect may be decreased
- contraindicated in those with hypersensitivity to cobalt or with megaloblastic anaemia of pregnancy

Patient education
- the patient should be advised to seek medical advice if any of the following occur:
  - breathlessness that worsens on lying down
  - changes in heart rate
  - chest tightness or pain

FOLIC ACID (FOLATE)
Trade names
Biological Therapies Folic Acid 15 mg in 1 mL, Biological Therapies Folic Acid 5 mg in 1 mL, Blackmores Folate, Foltabs, Megafol

Available forms
Vial: 5 mg/mL, 15 mg/mL;
Tablets: 500 microgram

Action
- member of the water-soluble vitamin B group, required for the maturation of RBC and necessary for DNA synthesis and mitosis, and hence growth
- available in different forms in foods; dietary sources include cereals, cereal products, vegetables, fruits and legumes

VITAMINS, MINERALS AND ELECTROLYTES

- stored in the liver and excreted in the urine (4–5 microgram/day)
- folate utilisation is increased in pregnancy and lactation, haemolytic anaemia, hyperthyroidism, exfoliative dermatitis and chronic infection

Deficiency
- megaloblastic anaemia

Use
- to prevent or treat megaloblastic anaemia caused by folic acid deficiency
- prevention of deficiency during pregnancy and breastfeeding
- decreases risk of spina bifida (neural tube defect in fetus) if taken 4 weeks before conception and during pregnancy

Optimal daily requirements
- 400 micrograms (males and females), 600 micrograms (pregnancy), 500 micrograms (breastfeeding)

Dose
- (Prevention during pregnancy and breastfeeding) 0.5 mg orally daily **OR**
- (Treatment of megaloblastic anaemia) 1–5 mg orally, IV or IM adjusted according to severity of anaemia **OR**
- (Prevention of spina bifida) 0.5 mg orally daily starting 4 weeks before conception

Adverse effects
- (Uncommon) nausea, flatulence, diarrhoea
- (Uncommon) sleep disturbance, irritability
- (Uncommon) rash, bronchospasm
- (IV) seizures, EEG changes
- (Rare) anaphylaxis

Interactions
- absorption decreased by chronic alcohol intake and sulfasalazine
- metabolism may be inhibited by methotrexate, trimethoprim and pyrimethamine
- may decrease serum levels of phenytoin and phenobarbital (phenobarbitone) leading to possible loss of seizure control

Nursing considerations/Cautions
- vitamin B_{12} deficiency should be excluded before starting therapy
- folic acid does not correct folate deficiency due to methotrexate; folinic acid should be used
- (Parenteral) usually given IM, but may be given IV or SC
- (Parenteral) may be diluted with 49 mL of 5 mg/mL sodium chloride 0.9% or glucose 5% for IV administration
- (Parenteral, 15 mg/mL) for IV use, should be diluted with 149 mL of sodium chloride 0.9% or glucose 5%
- contains 34.5 mg of sodium/mL
- caution if used in those with folate-dependent tumours
- contraindicated for treatment of megaloblastic anaemia caused by vitamin B_{12} deficiency

Patient education
- advise the patient to avoid alcohol during therapy

 Tablets can be dispersed in water, or crushed and mixed with spoonful of yoghurt or apple puree.

VITAMIN C

ASCORBIC ACID (VITAMIN C)
Trade names
Biological Therapies Sodium Ascorbate Solution, Blackmores Vitamin C, Cenovis MegaC 1000 mg Chewable Tablets, Cenovis Sugarless C 500 mg Chewable Tablets

Available forms
Tablets: 250 mg, 500 mg, 1 g;
Tablets (chewable): 250 mg, 500 mg, 1 g;
Vial: 90 mg/mL, 150 mg/mL, 300 mg/mL (as calcium ascorbate)

Action
- water-soluble agent essential for synthesis of collagen and intercellular material
- necessary for wound healing and resistance to infection
- necessary for the conversion of folic acid to folinic acid, carbohydrate and iron metabolism, lipid and protein synthesis
- necessary for maintenance of teeth, bone matrix and capillary walls
- antioxidant properties
- facilitates absorption of iron and copper
- necessary for RBC production
- dietary sources include fruit (e.g. blackcurrants, guava, citrus, kiwi fruit) and vegetables (e.g. broccoli and sprouts)

Deficiency
- scurvy (petechiae, coiled hairs, inflamed and bleeding gums, joint effusion, fatigue, poor wound healing, lesions, pain in extremities, haemorrhage, oedema)

Use
- prevention of ascorbic acid (vitamin C) deficiency
- as a supplement when on a restricted diet
- treatment of scurvy
- promotion of healing of wounds and fractures at times of increased requirement that cannot be met by normal dietary intake (e.g. burns, trauma, postoperatively, thyrotoxicosis)
- adjunct in the treatment of idiopathic methaemoglobinaemia

Optimal daily requirements
- 45 mg (males, females), 60 mg (pregnancy), 85 mg (breastfeeding)

Dose
- (Dietary supplement) 1–3 tablets orally daily or as prescribed **OR**
- (IV when oral treatment is not feasible) 100–500 mg IV as bolus or IV infusion **OR**
- (Antioxidant) 500 mg orally 1–2 times daily or as prescribed

Adverse effects
- headache, dizziness
- (Large doses) diarrhoea, renal calculi
- (Doses > 600 mg) diuretic action
- stomach cramps, nausea, vomiting
- (High dose) may precipitate gout or sickle cell crisis
- (IV) pain, thrombophlebitis, dehydration
- (IV, rapid infusion) temporary dizziness or faintness

Interactions
- may increase absorption of aluminium hydroxide from gut and therefore not recommended together in those with renal failure
- increased urinary excretion may occur if given with aspirin, primidone or barbiturates
- may decrease excretion of aspirin increasing serum levels
- caution if given with warfarin
- (Oral) may increase bioavailability of ethinyloesterol
- (Oral) may increase absorption of iron
- increases excretion of desferrioxamine when given together. Vitamin C should be given 1–2 hours after desferrioxamine infusion has started
- decreases chronotropic effect of isoprenaline
- decreased serum levels may occur if given with alcohol
- (Chronic/high dose) may interfere with disulfiram
- may decrease effects of phenothiazines
- may interfere with some laboratory tests including theophylline serum levels and occult blood

Nursing considerations/Cautions/Patient education
- (IV) ensure patient is adequately hydrated during therapy
- (IV) large vein should be used
- (IV) pain at infusion site can be minimised by decreasing infusion rate or diluting infusion (50:50) with water for injections or warming solution to body temperature before administration
- (IV) avoid extravasation
- caution if used in those with iron overload (e.g. haemochromotosis,

thalassaemia, polycythaemia, sideroblastic anaemia), G6PD deficiency, sickle cell anaemia (high dose), diabetes mellitus, gout, active peptic ulcer, advanced cancer, congestive cardiac failure, severely impaired kidney function, hypernatraemia, hyperoxaluria or prone to kidney stones

Chewable, dispersible and effervescent formulations are available.

High doses should not be used during pregnancy or breastfeeding.

VITAMIN D

General Actions of vitamin D
- endogenous vitamin D is obtained from sunlight's action on the skin, and is then activated in the liver and kidneys (D_3 or colecalciferol (cholecalciferol)); also found in some foods (D_2 or ergocalciferol)
- group of closely related fat-soluble sterol compounds involved in the regulation of calcium and phosphate homeostasis and bone mineralisation
- enhances calcium absorption from the small intestine
- immune function

Optimal daily requirements
- 5 micrograms (males, females, pregnancy, breastfeeding)
- 10 micrograms (males, females 51–70 years)
- 15 micrograms (males, females over 70 years of age)

Deficiency
- osteomalacia (adults), bone softening, leading to bone pain and muscle weakness
- rickets (children)
- studies have found deficiencies in elderly people with restricted access to sunlight, many of whom live in residential care

COLECALCIFEROL (CHOLECALCIFEROL) (VITAMIN D_3)

Trade names
Bio-Logical Vitamin D3 Solution, Blackmores Vitamin D3, Caltrate Vitamin D 1000 IU, D3 Capsules and Drops Forte, Caruso's Vitamin D3, Eagle Vitamin D3, Ethical Nutrients Daily D, NanoCelle D3 Oromucosal spray, Ostelin Vitamin D, OsteVit-D, OsteVit-D Vitamin D3 Oral Drops for Children, OsteVit-D One-A-Week, Phyta D

Available forms
Tablets: 25 microgram (1000 IU), 175 microgram (7000 IU);
Capsules: 25 microgram (1000 IU);
Drops: 5 microgram (200 IU), 25 microgram (1000 IU);
Oral spray: 25 microgram/spray (1000 IU);
Oral solution: 25 microgram/0.5 mL

Use
- treatment and prevention of vitamin D deficiency states, including those associated with malabsorption, hypocalcaemia, hypophosphataemic rickets, hypoparathyroidism and metabolic disorders
- osteoporosis
- prevention of osteoporosis associated with corticosteroids

Dose
- 25 micrograms (1000 IU) orally daily with food or as prescribed **OR**
- 175 micrograms (7000 IU) orally with food once per week **OR**
- 1 spray (25 micrograms (1000 IU)) once daily **OR**
- (Adult) 1 drop (25 micrograms (1000 IU)) once daily (Forte drops)

Adverse effects
- nausea, abdominal pain
- headache, drowsiness, weakness
- hypercalcaemia, hypercalciuria
- (High dose, prolonged therapy) vitamin D intoxication
- severe dehydration

- (Uncommon) ectopic calcification, nephrocalcinosis, proteinuria, casts in urine
- (Uncommon) diarrhoea, constipation, rash, pruritus, urticaria
- (Children, high dose, rare) retarded growth

Interactions

- not recommended with other vitamin D-containing preparations because of the risk of vitamin D intoxication
- phenobarbital (phenobarbitone), phenytoin, and primidone may increase metabolism and decrease effects
- caution if used with calcitonin, gallium nitrate, pamidronate, calcium-containing preparations or thiazide diuretics because of the risk of hypercalcaemia
- mineral oil, orlistat or lipid-lowering agents (e.g. colestipol or colestyramine (cholestyramine)) may decrease absorption of fat-soluble vitamins including vitamin D
- hypermagnesaemia may develop if calcitriol is used concurrently with magnesium-containing antacids
- may increase aluminium levels and risk of toxicity if given with aluminium-containing antacids (if used as phosphate binders in hyperphosphataemia)
- caution if vitamin D and digoxin are given together as this may precipitate cardiac arrhythmias
- may decrease the effectiveness of calcium-channel blockers

Nursing considerations/Cautions

- monitor serum calcium and phosphate levels regularly (twice weekly when starting therapy) then 2–3-monthly. Magnesium, alkaline phosphatase and urinary calcium and phosphorus (24-hour) should also be monitored
- if possible, bloods should be drawn without using a tourniquet to minimise local calcium effects
- parathyroid hormone (PTH) levels should be monitored regularly during therapy
- patients who are immobile (e.g. post-surgery) are at increased risk of hypercalcaemia
- vitamin D-resistant state may exist in uraemic patient owing to failure of kidneys to convert precursor to active component
- caution if used in those with hyperphosphataemia because of the risk of ectopic calcifications occurring
- caution if used in those with impaired renal function or renal calculi, history of raised urinary oxalates, sarcoidosis or granulomas
- caution if used in those with arteriosclerosis or cardiac function impairment
- contraindicated in those with vitamin D toxicity, hypercalcaemia or renal osteodystrophy with hyperphosphataemia

Patient education

- advise the patient to take 1 hour before or 4–6 hours after colestyramine (cholestyramine) or orlistat
- the patient should be instructed to seek medical advice immediately if any of the following occur:
    - loss of appetite, nausea, vomiting, diarrhoea
    - profuse sweating, excessive thirst or urination
    - headache, muscle weakness or bone pain
- instruct the patient/parent/carer that drops should be dispensed using graduated dropper; can be taken directly or added to water or juice
- the patient should be advised to avoid magnesium or aluminium-containing antacids during therapy
- inform the patient that daily dietary calcium intake should not exceed 1000 mg (calcitriol therapy) and that calcium supplements are not required unless diet is clearly inadequate
- advise the patient that vitamin D supplements are not required if they receive a sufficient daily sunlight exposure (20 minutes daily)

VITAMINS, MINERALS AND ELECTROLYTES

- instruct the patient to shake the spray or oral solution well before use

 Oral solution is available. Tablets can be crushed and mixed with spoonful of yoghurt or apple puree.

 Not recommended during breastfeeding.

Note
- Calcitriol (1,25-dihydroxycholecalciferol) is discussed in Bone and calcium regulating agents (p. 966)

VITAMIN E

VITAMIN E (ALPHA TOCOPHERYL)
Trade names
Blackmores Natural E, Eagle Natural Vitamin E 500 IU, E-Prime

Available forms
Capsules: 100 IU, 200 IU, 250 IU, 500 IU, 1000 IU

Action
- water-soluble vitamin consisting of several tocopherols that function as antioxidants
- doses of vitamin E, no matter which tocopherol, should be expressed as d-alpha tocopherol equivalents
- 10 mg of d-alpha tocopherol is ~15 IU (= 14.9)
- main dietary sources are fats and oils

Deficiency (very uncommon)
- peripheral neuropathy, ataxia, skeletal muscle atrophy, retinopathy (symptoms include hyporeflexia, gait disturbances, reduced sensitivity to vibration and proprioception, ophthalmoplegia) (this is due to genetic abnormalities rather than dietary deficiency)

Use
- impairment of fat-soluble vitamin absorption (cystic fibrosis, chronic cholestasis, A-beta lipoproteinaemia)
- antioxidant

Optimal daily requirements
- 10 mg (males), 7 mg (females), 7 mg (pregnancy), 11 mg (breastfeeding)

Dose
- 100 IU orally with food 1–3 times daily or as prescribed **OR**
- 200 IU orally with food twice daily or as prescribed **OR**
- 250 IU orally with food 1–3 times daily or as prescribed **OR**
- 500 IU orally with food 1–2 times daily or as prescribed **OR**
- 1000 IU orally daily with food or as prescribed

Adverse effects
- (High dose) nausea, diarrhoea, abdominal pain, fatigue and weakness

Interactions
- may antagonise effects of vitamin K, leading to increased blood clotting time
- caution if used with warfarin; INR should be monitored
- caution if given with ciclosporin, as ciclosporin levels may decrease or increase. Serum levels should be monitored if given together

Nursing considerations/Cautions/Patient education
- should be taken with food

VITAMIN K

General Actions of vitamin K
- a group of fat-soluble compounds that promote the hepatic biosynthesis of prothrombin (factor II) and coagulation factors VII, IX and X and anticoagulant proteins C and S

- antagonises the effects of indirect-acting oral anticoagulants
- dietary sources include leafy green vegetables (e.g. spinach, salad greens, broccoli, cabbage, brussels sprouts) and some plant oils (e.g. soybean and canola oils and products derived from them)

General Uses of vitamin K
- prothrombin deficiency
- prevention and therapy of vitamin D deficiency bleeding of the newborn
- haemorrhage (or threatened haemorrhage) resulting from hypoprothrombinaemia
- hypovitaminosis K
- to reverse the effects of oral anticoagulants (as an adjunct to blood transfusion)

Deficiency
- hypoprothrombinaemia, bleeding
- haemorrhagic disease of the newborn (neonates)

Optimal daily requirements
- 70 micrograms (males), 60 micrograms (females, pregnancy, breastfeeding)

PHYTOMENADIONE (VITAMIN K$_1$)
Trade names
Konakion MM Adult, Konakion MM Paediatric

Available forms
Ampoule (adult): 10 mg/mL;
Ampoule (newborn): 2 mg/0.2 mL

Dose
- (Adult, asymptomatic high INR with/without mild haemorrhage) (INR 5—9) 0.5—1.0 mg IV **OR**
- (Adult, asymptomatic high INR with/without mild haemorrhage) (INR > 9) 1.0 mg IV **OR**
- (Adult, major haemorrhage) 5—10 mg slowly IV with fresh frozen plasma (FFP) and prothrombin complex concentrate (PCC) **OR**
- (Adult, life-threatening haemorrhage) 10 mg slowly IV with fresh frozen plasma (FFP) and prothrombin complex concentrate (PCC) **OR**
- (Prophylaxis, neonate) 1 mg IM at birth (Konakion MM Paediatric) **OR**
- (Prophylaxis, neonate) 2 mg orally at birth, then at 3—5 days old and at 4 weeks (Konakion MM Paediatric) **OR**
- (Prophylaxis, neonate weight < 1.5 kg) 0.5 mg IM at birth (Konakion MM Paediatric) **OR**
- (Bleeding, neonate) 1 mg IV, repeated if needed (Konakion MM Paediatric)

Adverse effects
- unusual taste, facial flushing, sweating
- (Adult, IV injection site) phlebitis
- (Neonate, IM) (rare) injection site reaction
- (Rare) anaphylactoid reaction

Interactions
- antagonises warfarin
- action may be impaired by phenobarbital (phenobarbitone), phenytoin, rifampicin and isoniazid
- effects may be decreased by cephalosporins, aspirin and salicylates

Nursing considerations/Cautions/Patient education
- ineffective in heparin overdose
- IV rate not more than 1 mg/min
- (IV) administer alone and should not be diluted
- (Adult, major or life-threatening haemorrhage) prothrombin time should be measured after 3 hours and dose repeated if needed
- (Adult) if patient has severe liver impairment, INR should be closely monitored after administration
- (Adult) should be discontinued if ineffective after 1—2 days in those with severe liver disease
- (Neonate, oral) dispenser is supplied with ampoule. Open ampoule and place dispenser in it vertically. Withdraw solution to 2 mL mark on dispenser.

VITAMINS, MINERALS AND ELECTROLYTES

- Contents can be given directly into infant's mouth. If infant spits it out or vomits, dose can be readministered
- important to check expiry date, as impurities may develop over time
- (Adult) caution as risk of thromboembolism will return if given to reverse anticoagulant action in those being treated for thromboembolism
- (Neonate) increased risk of kernicterus if given to premature infants weighing < 2.5 kg
- (Adult) contraindicated IM because of variable absorption (may act as a depot) and also increased risk of haematoma if given to those receiving anticoagulant therapy
- (Adult) contraindicated in those with severe allergic predisposition
- see also general points for Vitamin K (p. 1647)

Contraindicated during pregnancy.

Use only if clearly indicated and the benefits outweigh the potential risks. Vitamin K$_1$ is poorly excreted in breastmilk.

Reduced hepatic function: use with caution in severe liver impairment; monitor INR closely after administration, as response may vary with liver function.

Elderly patients may have increased sensitivity to vitamin K$_1$'s effects; lower doses are generally effective in this population for reversing anticoagulation.

MINERAL SUPPLEMENTS

CALCIUM

General Actions of calcium
- essential for the functioning of muscular, skeletal and nervous systems and cardiac function
- involved as a co-factor in blood coagulation and transmission of nerve impulses, contraction of cardiac, smooth and skeletal muscle, renal function and respiration
- storage and release of hormones and neurotransmitters
- regulates intracellular signaling pathways important for various cellular processes
- important for the activation of certain enzymes necessary for metabolic functions
- absorbed from small intestine
- absorption of vitamin B$_{12}$
- bone has 99% of body's calcium stores
- main dietary sources are milk and milk products, with smaller amounts in bony fish, legumes, some nuts, fortified soy products and breakfast cereals

Optimal daily requirements
- 1000—1300 mg (males, females, pregnancy, breastfeeding)

CALCIUM CARBONATE
Trade names
CAL-500 Tablets, CAL-600 Tablets, Cal-Care, Calci-Tab 600, Cal-Sup Chewable

Available forms
Tablets: 500 mg, 600 mg (of elemental calcium)

Action
- see General Actions of calcium left

Use
- antacid (see Antacids, p. 887)
- calcium supplement in prevention and treatment of calcium deficiency (e.g. osteoporosis)
- supplement in pregnancy
- phosphate binder in chronic renal failure

Dose
- 1—2 tablets orally daily after food or as prescribed

Adverse effects
- GI irritation, nausea, vomiting, diarrhoea, abdominal pain and distension, flatulence, constipation

Interactions
- may interfere with absorption of oral iron
- forms a complex when given with tetracyclines; therefore should not be given together

Nursing considerations/Cautions
- contraindicated in those with hypercalcaemia, hypercalciuria or severe renal failure

Patient education
- advise patient that chewable tablets can be chewed, sucked or swallowed whole (Cal-Sup Chewable)
- advise patient to take oral calcium at least 2 hours apart from oral iron compounds and oral tetracyclines

 Chewable tablets are available. Tablets are difficult to crush.

CALCIUM GLUCONATE
Trade name
Phebra Calcium Gluconate 953 mg/10 mL Injection

Available form
Ampoules: 100 mg/mL (contains 8.9 mg (or 0.44 mEq) elemental calcium/mL)

Action
- see General Actions of calcium (p. 1649)

Use
- prevention and treatment of hypocalcaemia
- acute hypocalcaemia
- hypocalcaemic tetany
- severe hyperkalaemia
- cardiac resuscitation
- magnesium sulphate toxicity
- acute renal, biliary or intestinal colic

Dose
- (Hypocalcaemia) 7—14 mEq IV repeated every 1—3 days if needed **OR**
- (Hypocalcaemic tetany) 4.5—16 mEq IV until response occurs (daily maximum 15 g calcium gluconate (calcium ion 67.5 mEq)) **OR**
- (Hypermagnesaemia) initially 7 mEq IV, may be repeated if necessary **OR**
- (Severe hyperkalaemia) 4.5—9.0 mEq IV, as an adjunct (with ECG monitoring)

Adverse effects
- (High dose) hypercalcaemia (anorexia, nausea, vomiting, constipation, abdominal pain, muscle weakness, polydipsia, polyuria, mental disturbances, bone pain, renal calculi, cardiac arrhythmias, coma, cardiac arrest), nephrolithiasis
- (IV) sweating, hypotension, irregular heart rate, hot flushed sensation, tingling, 'chalky' taste, feeling of oppression, dizziness, nausea, vomiting, sweating
- (Rapid IV) peripheral vasodilation, hot flushes, bradycardia, arrhythmias, hypotension, syncope, cardiac arrest, skin necrosis
- transient increase in BP (elderly or hypertensive patient)
- (IV) burning, redness, rash, pain
- (IM/SC) sloughing, necrosis, burning, cellulitis
- (Extravasation) skin redness, rash, pain, burning, soft tissue calcification

Interactions
- (Parenteral) contraindicated with digoxin owing to calcium's effects on the heart and increased risk of digoxin toxicity
- may interfere with absorption of oral iron
- may reduce response to verapamil and other calcium-channel blockers
- increased risk of calcium deposition in soft tissue if given with potassium and/or sodium phosphate
- forms a complex when given with tetracyclines; therefore should not be given together
- increased risk of hypercalcaemia and hypermagnesaemia if given with other calcium-containing agents or magnesium-containing agents

VITAMINS, MINERALS AND ELECTROLYTES

- (especially in those with impaired renal function)
- increased risk of hypercalcaemia if given with high doses of vitamin A (as vitamin A stimulates bone loss of calcium)
- vitamin D increases absorption of calcium from the diet; therefore high doses of vitamin D should be avoided during therapy
- may reverse actions of non-depolarising neuromuscular blocking agents
- may antagonise effects of calcitonin (if used to treat hypercalcaemia)
- increased risk of hypercalcaemia if given with thiazide diuretics
- increased calcium serum levels (but not risk of toxicity) if calcium is given to patients who have recently received citrated blood transfusions

Nursing considerations/Cautions

- any hyperphosphataemia should be corrected before treating hypocalcaemia in patients who have both conditions
- any fluid or electrolyte imbalance should be corrected before starting IV therapy, including adequate hydration to prevent formation of renal calculi
- ECG monitoring is recommended during IV injection to detect bradycardia (especially if given to treat hyperkalaemia), and therapy discontinued if significant bradycardia occurs
- the patient should remain recumbent during IV therapy to prevent dizziness and should be cautioned to move slowly when first standing
- serum levels of calcium and kidney function should be measured regularly throughout therapy, especially if large doses are given
- solution should be warmed to body temperature (if possible) before IV administration
- do not dilute if using any phosphate-containing solutions as precipitate may form
- do not use if a precipitate is present

- vitamin D analogues may be given concurrently with calcium, especially when hypocalcaemia is caused by vitamin D deficiency; however, high vitamin D intake should be avoided
- solution should be injected very slowly into a large vein. IV infusion rate should not exceed 2 mL/min (or calcium ion 0.9 mEq/min). May also be given by direct IV injection at a rate of 1.5–3 mL/min
- calcium gluconate injection should be administered via slow IV infusion. Avoid intramuscular or subcutaneous injection because of the risk of severe tissue irritation and necrosis
- incompatible with 10% IV fat emulsions, cephalosporins, dobutamine, methylprednisolone, prochlorperazine, metoclopramide, indometacin (indomethacin), soluble carbonates, sulphates and phosphates
- caution if used in those with sarcoidosis or other diseases associated with elevated vitamin D levels, mild hypercalcaemia, impaired renal function, cardiac disease or history of calcium-containing renal calculi
- contraindicated in galactosaemic patients
- contraindicated in those with hypercalcaemia, hypercalciuria, severe renal failure, severe cardiac disease, severe calcium loss due to immobilisation or calcium level above normal (4.2–5.2 mEq/L)

Patient education

- the patient should be advised to immediately report any loss of appetite, nausea, vomiting, increased thirst and urination, constipation, confusion, muscle or joint pain, or general weakness (early signs of hypercalcaemia)

 Crosses the placenta and may reach higher levels in fetal than in maternal blood. Use during pregnancy should balance the potential benefits to the mother against possible risks to the fetus.

HAVARD'S NURSING GUIDE TO DRUGS

Excreted in breastmilk, though no adverse effects have been documented in breastfeeding infants. Weigh potential benefits for the mother against possible risks to the infant.

Use with caution in reduced renal function, as there is increased risk of calcium accumulation. Serum calcium levels should be monitored regularly.

Elderly patients may be at higher risk of experiencing adverse effects, such as hypercalcemia, from calcium gluconate administration. Monitor serum calcium levels closely.

IRON AND IRON COMPOUNDS

General Actions of iron and iron compounds

- approximately 15–20 g of iron is absorbed from the diet, with the main site of absorption being the duodenum and jejunum, and this iron more than adequately replaces the small amount that is lost in the faeces, urine, skin and sweat
- rate of absorption is dependent on acid secretion from the stomach, as well as the amount of iron already stored within the body. The actual amount needed depends on such factors as loss through menstruation, whether a child/adolescent is growing or whether a woman is pregnant or breastfeeding
- approximately 4 g of the iron is present in the body in the form of haemoglobin or stored as ferritin, haemosiderin or myoglobin, as well as small amounts in the plasma (bound to transferrin) and in haem-containing enzymes
- only very small amounts of iron are excreted, hence the risk of iron overload
- main dietary sources of iron include meat, fish and poultry and some leafy vegetables, wholegrain cereals and legumes; however, iron from plant sources is less bioavailable. Phytates (found in legumes, rice and other grains), calcium and zinc can inhibit absorption of iron
- iron (as oxide or hydroxide) is used as a colouring agent

General Uses of iron and iron compounds

- iron deficiency anaemia
- iron deficiency
- (IV) when oral therapy is contraindicated or impractical or if patient is non-adherent with oral therapy

Optimal daily requirements

- 8 mg (males), 8–18 mg (females), 27 mg (pregnancy), 9 mg (breastfeeding)
- requirements increase during periods of rapid growth such as early childhood and adolescence

General Adverse effects of iron and iron compounds

- metallic taste, GI irritation, nausea, vomiting, constipation, dark/discoloured stools, diarrhoea, abdominal pain
- (Oral) teeth or skin staining
- generalised lymph node enlargement
- rash, urticaria, pruritus, angioedema
- bronchospasm, dyspnoea
- transient hypophosphataemia
- sensation of stiffness in arms, legs and/or face, joint and muscle pain, muscle spasm, arthralgia
- headache, dizziness, faintness
- tachycardia, faintness, syncope, hypotension, hypertension
- elevated liver enzymes
- (Parenteral) flushing, sweating, chills, fever, chest and back pain, fatigue
- (IV) hypersensitivity, anaphylactoid reaction, anaphylaxis, phlebitis, thrombophlebitis
- (IM) pain, bruising, burning, irritation, lower quadrant abdominal pain, local inflammation, sterile abscess formation, enlarged inguinal lymph nodes, permanent skin discolouration, pain (if incorrectly administered)

VITAMINS, MINERALS AND ELECTROLYTES

General Interactions of iron and iron compounds
- vitamin C can enhance non-haem iron absorption
- (Oral) absorption may be reduced by antacids, colestipol, colestyramine (cholestryramine) and tetracyclines
- (Oral) absorption of oral tetracyclines, quinolones, penicillamine, levodopa and methyldopa sesquihydrate may be reduced by oral iron compounds
- parenteral iron is not recommended with oral iron, because the absorption of oral iron is decreased
- oral iron should not be given within 7 days of parenteral iron
- increased risk of erythema, abdominal cramps, nausea, vomiting and hypotension if given with ACE inhibitors
- parenteral iron interferes with a number of laboratory tests (and continues for up to 3 weeks post-administration), including serum bilirubin (falsely elevated) and serum calcium (falsely decreased). Scanning using gallium or technetium (Tc-99m) may be affected. Blood samples appear brown colour within hours of administration. Darkened stools may mask GI bleeding; however, this darkening does not affect haemoccult test

General Nursing considerations/ Cautions for iron and iron compounds
- the type of anaemia should be investigated to determine the cause before starting treatment with iron
- regular monitoring of haemoglobin, haematocrit, serum ferritin and transferrin saturation is recommended to prevent iron overload as excretion is limited
- observe the patient carefully for any breathing difficulties, tachycardia or hypotension (frequently reported in haemodialysis patients) during the initial stages of IV injection or infusion in case of anaphylactoid reaction. Patient should be observed for at least 30 minutes post infusion for any reaction
- IM injection should not be given into arm or exposed area
- give IM injection by drawing subcutaneous tissue to one side before inserting needle (5—6 cm long) (Z-track technique) to promote absorption and prevent skin staining and pain. Pressure should be applied to injection site for 1 minute. Consult manufacturer's instructions for recommended injection sites
- extravasation should be avoided as it may result in brown discolouration of the skin
- administer alone
- have available adrenaline (epinephrine), IV corticosteroids, oxygen and resuscitation equipment; antihistamines may be used for minor allergic reactions
- overdose is very serious in young children, because the gut lining may be destroyed and should be treated urgently by emptying the stomach and giving milk to form an iron-protein complex (first aid) and then the iron-chelating agent, desferrioxamine (see p. 1644)
- caution if used in those with rheumatoid arthritis and other inflammatory disease because there is increased risk of delayed reaction, including fever and exacerbation or reactivation of joint pain
- caution if used in those with asthma or history of allergic disorders (e.g. eczema, atopic allergies), low iron-binding capacity or folic acid deficiency, because they are at increased risk of allergy or anaphylactoid reaction
- (IM/IV) caution if used in those with acute or chronic infection and should be discontinued if any bacteraemia occurs
- caution if used in those with severe liver or kidney inflammation as iron accumulates in inflamed tissue
- caution if used in those with GI disease resulting from the gastrointestinal

irritation because oral iron may exacerbate mucosal irritation
- not recommended in those with liver dysfunction related to iron overload such as porphyria cutanea tarda
- not recommended in those who have had previous reactions to parenteral iron
- contraindicated in those with anaemia not caused by simple iron deficiency, iron overload, chronic polyarthritis, asthma, uncontrolled hyperparathyroidism, acute kidney infection, infectious hepatitis, haemosiderosis, haemochromatosis or thalassaemia

General Patient education for iron and iron compounds

- warn patient not to drive or operate machinery until any dizziness or faintness subsides
- advise patient to keep iron preparations out of the reach of children as they are particularly sensitive to high doses
- inform the patient that gastrointestinal irritation can be reduced if oral iron preparations are taken with or immediately after food (although iron is absorbed better if taken between meals)
- instruct the patient that oral iron, tetracyclines, zinc salts and aluminium salts are each given at least 2 hours apart to allow adequate absorption
- instruct the patient that iron mixtures should be taken in milk or through a straw to avoid temporary staining of teeth, and teeth staining may be minimised by brushing teeth with baking soda
- warn patient that faeces become darker/discoloured during treatment
- if patient was receiving oral iron before receiving parenteral iron, advise patient not to restart oral therapy until at least 5 days post-infusion/injection

 (Parenteral) contraindicated in first trimester of pregnancy. Use during second or third trimester only if benefits outweigh potential risks. May cause transient fetal bradycardia. Unborn child should be monitored if pregnant mother is given IV iron during second or third trimester.

 Caution if used during breastfeeding.

FERRIC CARBOXYMALTOSE
Trade name
Ferinject

Available forms
Ampoules: 100 mg/2 mL, 500 mg/10 mL, 1 g/20 mL (as elemental iron)

Use
- parenteral administration is recommended when oral route is not available or is impractical

Dose
- cumulative dose calculated according to following formula (Ganzoni):

cumulative iron dose = body weight kg × (target Hb − actual Hb g/L) × 0.24 + iron stores mg

Adverse effects/Interactions
- see General Adverse effects/Interactions for iron and iron compounds (p. 1652)

Nursing considerations/Cautions/Patient education
- maximum weekly dose 1 g
- if patient is overweight, normal body weight and blood volume relation should be assumed when calculating iron requirements
- target Hb = 130 g/L if < 35 kg or 150 g/L if ≥ 35 kg
- iron stores (depot) = 15 mg/kg if < 35 kg or 500 mg if ≥ 35 kg
- for patient ≤ 66 kg, calculated cumulative dose should be rounded down to nearest 100 mg
- for patient > 66 kg, calculated cumulative dose should be rounded up to nearest 100 mg
- 1 mL (undiluted) contains up to 5.5 mg (0.24 mmol) sodium, which may need to be considered if patient has sodium restriction
- not for IM or SC use

VITAMINS, MINERALS AND ELECTROLYTES

- administer alone
- IV dilution with sodium chloride 0.9% only as follows: 100–200 mg iron diluted in 50 mL and given over 3 minutes; > 200–500 mg iron diluted in 100 mL and given over 6 minutes; > 500 mg–1 g iron diluted in 250 mL and given over 15 minutes
- may be given as IV bolus injection to a daily maximum of 200 mg (4 mL) and not repeated more than 3 times per week
- may be given at IV infusion (not greater than 20 mg/kg or maximum 1 g (20 mL)), should only be given weekly
- may be given during haemodialysis undiluted via venous limb of dialyser
- contains 5.5 mg (0.24 mmol) sodium/mL, which should be considered if person has sodium restriction
- see also General Nursing considerations/Cautions/Patient education for iron and iron compounds (p. 1653)

FERROUS FUMARATE
Trade names
APOHealth Iron tablets, Ferro-tab

Available form
Tablets: 200 mg (= elemental iron 65.7 mg)

Dose
- (Prophylaxis) 1 tablet orally daily **OR**
- (Treatment) 1 tablet orally 2–3 times daily

Use/Adverse effects/Interactions/Nursing considerations/Cautions
- see general points for iron and iron compounds (p. 1652)

Patient education
- advise the patient that tablets may be taken with or without water. However, if taken between meals, the patient should take them with at least 240 mL water and avoid lying down for ≥ 30 minutes
- see also General Patient education for iron and iron compounds (p. 1654)

Tablets can be crushed and mixed with water or spoonful of yoghurt or apple puree.

Available in combination with
- ferrous fumarate 310 mg (providing 100 mg of elemental iron) + folic acid 350 microgram (Ferro-F-Tab) — prevents and treats iron and folic acid deficiencies, including during pregnancy

FERROUS SULFATE
Trade names
Ferrogen Ferrous Sulfate, Ferro-Grad, Ferro-Liquid

Available forms
Oral solution: 150 mg (= 30 mg elemental iron)/5 mL;
Tablets (slow-release): 325 mg (= 105 mg elemental iron)

Dose
- 325 mg orally daily before food or as prescribed **OR**
- 450–900 mg (15–30 mL) orally daily or as prescribed (oral liquid)

Use/Adverse effects/Interactions
- see General Uses/Adverse effects/Interactions of iron and iron compounds (p. 1652)

Nursing considerations/Cautions/Patient education
- advise patient that tablets should be swallowed whole (not crushed or chewed) and, if gastric irritation occurs, may be taken with food
- (Oral solution) contains sorbitol and bisulfite, and may cause diarrhoea and allergic reaction in susceptible individuals
- tablets contain lactose
- prolonged administration > 12 months is not recommended
- see also General Nursing considerations/Patient education for iron and iron compounds (p. 1653)

Oral solution available. Slow-release tablets should not be chewed, broken or crushed.

Can be used during pregnancy when iron deficiency anaemia is diagnosed, as adequate iron levels are essential for both maternal health and fetal development.

IRON POLYMALTOSE COMPLEX

Trade names
Ferrosig Injection, Maltofer

Available forms
Ampoule: 100 mg/2 mL (as elemental iron); Tablets: 370 mg (= 100 mg elemental iron); Syrup: 185 mg/5 mL (= 50 mg elemental iron/5 mL)

Action
- (IM) evokes local inflammatory response and is transported to regional lymph nodes without being broken down. Then enters blood reaching maximum concentration in 24 hours
- half-life 22.4 hours
- see also General Actions of iron and iron compounds (p. 1652)

Dose
- (Treatment) 100–200 mg orally daily with food or as prescribed **OR**
- (Prophylaxis) 100 mg orally daily with food or as prescribed **OR**
- 100 mg of iron IM every second day until total dose is achieved **OR**
- 200 mg IM at intervals longer than 2 days until total dose is achieved **AND**
- (IM) total dose is calculated using the Ganzoni formula:

iron dose (mg) = body weight (kg) × target Hb − actual Hb (in g/L) × 0.24 + iron depot

Adverse effects/Interactions
- see General Adverse effects and Interactions of iron and iron compounds (p. 1652)

Nursing considerations/Cautions
- 100 mg = 1 tablet = 10 mL syrup. If dose is less than 100 mg, syrup should be used
- (IV) administer alone
- (Ferrosig) for IV use, dilute in 500 mL of sodium chloride 0.9% and infuse first 50 mL at a rate of 5–10 drops/min, then carefully observe the patient. If tolerated, continue infusion at 30 drops/min
- for body weight > 34 kg, target Hb = 150 g/L and iron depot = 500 mg; for body weight < 34 kg, target Hb = 130 g/L and iron depot 15 mg/kg
- for adult > 45 kg; daily maximum is 200 mg
- test dose of 25 mg may be given before first therapeutic dose
- dose given by IM injection is 2 mL (100 mg) on alternate days until total dose is attained, or 4 mL (200 mg) at longer intervals
- monitor treatment by regular determination of haemoglobin
- adverse effects may occur up to 1–2 days after administration
- IV route can be used if IM is impractical or unacceptable and when bone marrow stores show no iron
- (Oral solution) contains hydroxybenzoates, which may cause allergic reactions in sensitive individuals
- (Oral solution) contains a small amount of alcohol (3.25 mg/mL)
- (Oral solution) contains sorbitol and sucrose and is therefore not recommended in those with rare hereditary problems of fructose intolerance, glucose–galactose malabsorption or sucrase–isomaltase insufficiency
- contraindicated in those with any hypersensitivity to iron (III) hydroxide polymaltose complex
- see also General Nursing considerations/Cautions for iron and iron compounds (p. 1653)

Patient education
- advise patient to swallow tablets whole, not chewed or crushed
- instruct the patient that oral solution can be mixed with fruit or vegetable juice. This may show a slight discolouration, but is fine to ingest
- see also General Patient education for iron and iron compounds (p. 1654)

VITAMINS, MINERALS AND ELECTROLYTES

Swallow tablets whole, not chewed or crushed; oral solution available.

Avoid during the first trimester. In the second and third trimesters, use only if the benefits outweigh potential risks. Fetal bradycardia may occur because of hypersensitivity reactions in the mother.

Caution: no human data available.

IRON SUCROSE
Trade name
Venofer

Available form
Ampoule: 100 mg/5 mL (as elemental iron)

Use
- treatment of iron deficiency anaemia in patients receiving chronic haemodialysis and supplemental erythropoietin therapy

Dose
- 100 mg by IV infusion or slow IV injection into venous limb of dialysis line during dialysis session, no more than 3 times weekly until haemoglobin, haematocrit and laboratory parameters of iron storage are within acceptable limits

Action/Adverse effects/Interactions/Patient education
- see General Actions/Adverse effects/Interactions/Patient education for iron and iron compounds (p. 1652)

Nursing considerations/Cautions
- most patients require a cumulative dose of 1 g over 10 sequential dialysis sessions
- dilute with 100 mL sodium chloride 0.9% just before IV infusion and administer over at least 15 minutes
- slow IV injection should be at least 5 minutes into venous line of dialysis machine
- not given IM or SC because of strong alkaline nature
- administer alone
- if not effective in 1–2 weeks, original diagnosis should be reconsidered
- see also General Nursing considerations/Cautions for iron and iron compounds (p. 1653)

MAGNESIUM

General Actions of magnesium
- second most abundant cation
- essential for more than 300 enzyme processes
- necessary for glycolysis, the Krebs cycle, and protein and nucleic acid synthesis
- neurochemical transmission
- anticonvulsant effect
- role in calcium homeostasis and bone mineralisation
- 90% stored in bone, muscle and soft tissue
- dietary sources include most green vegetables, legumes, peas, beans and nuts, some shellfish and spices, unrefined cereals

Optimal daily requirements
- 400–420 mg (males), 310–320 mg (females), 350–360 mg (pregnancy), 310–320 mg (breastfeeding)

General Adverse effects of magnesium
- hypermagnesaemia (nausea, vomiting, flushing, hypotension, muscle weakness and paralysis, blurred or double vision, loss of reflexes and CNS depression; more severe: respiratory depression/paralysis, renal failure, coma, arrhythmias, cardiac arrest)
- hypocalcaemia with tetany (secondary to hypermagnesaemia)
- (IM injection site) irritation and pain

General Interactions of magnesium
- increased CNS depression may occur if given with CNS depressant drugs
- not recommended with other agents containing magnesium, including antacids, because of increased risk of magnesium toxicity
- excessive neuromuscular blockade may occur if given with neuromuscular blocking agents or aminoglycosides
- caution if used with digoxin, as heart block may occur
- increased hypotension can occur if given with nifedipine and other antihypertensive agents

General Nursing considerations/Cautions for magnesium
- patient should be adequately hydrated before starting therapy and urine output should be at least 100 mL for the preceding 4 hours before the infusion is started
- serum magnesium levels and renal function should be monitored frequently during therapy
- patellar reflexes should be assessed before repeating doses, because decreased reflexes are indicative of toxicity
- respiratory rate should be monitored throughout infusion (maintained at a rate of at least 16 breaths/min)
- have IV calcium salts (e.g. calcium gluconate) readily available to treat any toxicity when parenteral magnesium chloride is administered
- incompatible with carbonates, bicarbonates, phosphates and calcium salts
- may precipitate myasthenic crisis
- caution if used in those with renal or liver impairment because of risk of hypermagnesaemia
- contraindicated in those with heart block or renal failure (creatinine clearance < 20 mL/min)
- contraindicated in those with hypermagnesaemia

(Parenteral) should not be given within 2 hours of delivery, because respiratory depression may occur in the newborn (unless there are no other options in treatment of eclamptic seizures). Readily crosses the placenta and fetal serum levels are similar to maternal; bony abnormalities and congenital rickets may occur in neonates if given for prolonged periods (4–13 weeks) during pregnancy.

Not recommended during breastfeeding, as concentration in breastmilk is twice maternal serum levels. Cleared from breastmilk within 24 hours of stopping IV therapy.

MAGNESIUM ASPARTATE
Trade names
Mag-A, Magmin, Mag-Sup, Pharmacy Care Magnesium

Available form
Tablets: 500 mg (= elemental magnesium 37.4 mg)

Use
- magnesium deficiency
- symptom relief of muscle cramps and spasm

Dose
- 1–3 g daily orally with meals or as prescribed

Action/Adverse effects/Nursing considerations/Cautions
- see Action/Adverse effects/Nursing considerations/Cautions for magnesium (p. 1657)

Tablets can be crushed and mixed with water or spoonful of yoghurt or apple puree.

VITAMINS, MINERALS AND ELECTROLYTES

MAGNESIUM CHLORIDE
Trade names
DBL Magnesium Chloride Concentrated Injection

Available form
Ampoule: 480 mg/5 mL

Use
- acute hypomagnesaemia
- prevention of hypomagnesaemia in those receiving total parenteral nutrition (TPN)

Dose
- (Acute hypomagnesaemia) initially 3.3—7.2 g (70—150 mEq) by slow IV infusion (day 1), then reduced to 2.4 g (50 mEq) daily until hypomagnesaemia has been corrected (maximum daily dose 18.7 g) **OR**
- (Prevention of hypomagnesaemia in those receiving TPN) 0.2—1.2 g (4—24 mEq) by slow IV infusion daily

Action/Adverse effects/Interactions/Nursing considerations/Cautions
- administer alone
- IV dose should be diluted with glucose 5%
- 1 mL = 1 mmol = 2 mEq magnesium ions
- use cautiously with cardiac glycosides; magnesium toxicity may necessitate calcium administration, risking heart block
- avoid use with neuromuscular blocking agents, as it can lead to excessive neuromuscular blockade if used together
- caution when using magnesium with antihypertensives (e.g. nifedipine), as it may result in exaggerated hypotensive effects
- see also Action/Adverse effects/Interactions/Nursing considerations/Cautions for magnesium (p. 1657)

Available in combination with
- sodium: 110 mmol + chloride: 160 mmol + potassium: 16 mmol + magnesium: 16 mmol + calcium: 1.2 mmol (Cardioplegia Solution A [Baxter], DBL Sterile Cardioplegia Concentrate) used in cardiac surgery to induce cardiac arrest

MAGNESIUM SULFATE
Trade names
DBL Magnesium Sulfate Concentrated Injection, Magnesium Sulfate Heptahydrate Concentrated 50% Injection

Available forms
Ampoules: 2.465 g/5 mL;
Vial: 2.5 g/5 mL, 5 g/10 mL

Use
- acute hypomagnesaemia
- prevention of hypomagnesaemia in those receiving total parenteral nutrition (TPN)
- seizures associated with pre-eclampsia and eclampsia (see Pregnancy, p. 1472)
- cardiac arrhythmias

Dose
- (Severe hypomagnesaemia) 0.25 g/kg IM over 4 hours **OR**
- (Severe hypomagnesaemia) 5 g by slow IV infusion over 3 hours **OR**
- (Mild hypomagnesaemia) 1 g (8 mEq) IM 6-hourly for 4 doses **OR**
- (Arrhythmias) 2 g (8.2 mmol) by slow IV infusion over 20 minutes **OR**
- (Prevention of hypomagnesaemia in those receiving TPN) 0.5—3.0 g daily IV or IM

Action/Adverse effects/ Interactions/Nursing considerations/Cautions/Patient education
- total daily dose should not exceed 30—40 g
- given IV or IM only
- IV dose should be diluted to 20% before administration
- IM administration may be given diluted or undiluted
- 2 mL = 1 g = 4 mmol = 8 mEq magnesium ions
- drug interactions: CNS depressants, neuromuscular blocking agents (risk of excessive neuromuscular blockade),

nifedipine (may cause an exaggerated hypotensive response). aminoglycosides, amphotericin B and diuretics (risk of renal magnesium loss when co-administered).
- see also General Nursing considerations/Cautions for magnesium (p. 1658)

Magnesium sulfate may be used in pregnancy to prevent seizures in pre-eclampsia and eclampsia, but it crosses the placenta and can cause fetal hypermagnesaemia, respiratory depression and musculoskeletal abnormalities if given within 2 hours of delivery. Use cautiously in pregnancy and avoid near delivery unless absolutely necessary.

Magnesium is excreted into breastmilk at concentrations approximately double that of maternal serum. Use with caution in lactating women, as it clears from breastmilk within 24 hours after the infusion ends.

Reduced renal function: use with caution in patients with impaired renal function because of an increased risk of hypermagnesaemia. Avoid if CrCl < 20 mL/min.

OTHER MINERALS

PHOSPHORUS/PHOSPHATE
Trade names
DBL Potassium Dihydrogen Phosphate Concentrated Injection, DBL Potassium Phosphate — Monobasic and Potassium Phosphate — Dibasic Concentrated Injection, Phosphate Phebra Tablets, Potassium Dihydrogen Phosphate 13.6% Concentrated Injection, Sodium Phosphate and Potassium Phosphate Concentrated Injection

Available forms
Tablets (effervescent): 500 mg;
IV solution: contains phosphate, potassium and sodium ions

Action
- most of the body's phosphate is found in bones, giving rigidity, and some is also in soft tissue
- main anion of intracellular fluid
- involved in metabolic and enzymatic pathways
- involved in energy storage and transfer, utilisation of vitamin B, buffering and renal excretion of hydrogen ions
- excretion controlled by parathyroid gland
- mainly (85%) stored in bone, the rest in soft tissue
- inverse relationship with serum calcium (i.e. increased phosphate level leads to decreased calcium level)
- normal serum concentration 0.8—1.5 mmol/L
- widely distributed in foods; plant seeds (e.g. beans, peas, cereals, nuts) have phosphate stored in a form (phytic acid) that is not bioavailable to mammals

Use
- hypercalcaemia associated with hyperparathyroidism, metastatic bone disease
- hypophosphataemia associated with vitamin D-resistant rickets
- hypophosphataemia (serum level < 0.3 mmol/L)

Optimal daily requirement
- 1000 mg

Dose
- (Hypercalcaemia) up to 3 g orally daily **OR**
- (Vitamin D-resistant rickets) 2—3 g orally daily **OR**
- (Hypophosphataemia) up to 10 mmol by slow IV infusion over 12 hours, may be repeated until serum level > 0.3 mmol/L

Adverse effects
- (Oral) diarrhoea, nausea, vomiting, abdominal pain
- (IV) hypotension, fluid retention, weight gain
- (IV) hyperkalaemia (confusion, weakness, irregular or slow heartbeat, numbness/tingling of lips, hands or feet, anxiety, difficulty breathing or shortness of breath, heaviness of legs)
- (IV) hypernatraemia (confusion, tiredness, weakness, convulsions, oliguria,

VITAMINS, MINERALS AND ELECTROLYTES

- tachycardia, headache, dizziness, increased thirst)
- (IV) hyperphosphataemia, hypocalcaemia or hypomagnesaemia (convulsions, muscle cramps, numbness, tingling, pain or weakness of feet or hands, shortness of breath, tremor)
- (IV) soft tissue calcification, nephrocalcinosis
- (Rare) myocardial infarction, acute renal failure

Interactions
- hyperkalaemia may occur if given with ACE inhibitors, potassium-sparing diuretics, NSAIDs, potassium-containing agents, or in patients with heart block who are taking cardiac glycosides (digoxin) or with renal impairment
- increased risk of calcium deposition in soft tissue if given with calcium or phosphate-containing agents (including supplements)
- oedema may occur if given with corticosteroids that have mineralocorticoid actions
- may increase serum salicylate levels leading to toxicity
- hypernatraemia may occur if given with sodium-containing agents
- hyperphosphataemia may occur if given with phosphate-containing products or vitamin D
- (Oral) efficacy decreased if given with aluminium-, calcium- or magnesium-containing antacids
- increased urinary excretion may occur if given with parathyroid hormone
- may interfere with some bone imaging studies

Nursing considerations/Cautions
- cause of hypophosphataemia should be investigated and treated
- serum sodium, potassium, phosphate and calcium levels and renal function should be monitored 12—24-hourly during therapy
- parenteral therapy should be replaced with oral therapy as soon as possible
- tablets contain sodium (469 mg or 20.4 mEq) and potassium (123 mg or 3.1 mEq) in addition to phosphate
- IV solution should be diluted with sodium chloride 0.9% or glucose 5% and given by slow IV infusion to prevent toxicity
- incompatible with iron-, aluminium-, calcium- or magnesium-containing solutions as precipitates may occur
- caution if given to those with myotonia congenita or heart disease
- caution in those with potentially high phosphate levels (e.g. rhabdomyolysis, hypoparathyroidism, chronic renal disease), low calcium levels (e.g. osteomalacia, hypoparathyroidism, rickets, acute pancreatitis), high potassium level (e.g. acute dehydration, pancreatitis, rhabdomyolysis, severe burns or other extensive tissue damage) or high sodium levels (e.g. toxaemia of pregnancy, hypertension, congestive cardiac failure, electrolyte imbalance, peripheral oedema, liver cirrhosis, pulmonary oedema, severe liver disease)
- contraindicated in those with severe renal impairment ($< 30\%$ of normal), hyperphosphataemia, hypocalcaemia, hyperkalaemia, hypernatraemia, Addison's disease or urolithiasis

Patient education
- the patient should be advised to dissolve effervescent tablets in half a glass of water
- advise the patient to avoid aluminium-, calcium- or magnesium-containing antacids within 2 hours of phosphate
- instruct the patient to seek medical advice immediately if any of the following occur:
  - swelling of feet or lower legs, weight gain
  - increased thirst
  - muscle weakness, weakness or heaviness in hands or feet, muscle cramps
  - irregular heart rate

- unexpected anxiety
- tiredness
- confusion
- seizures
- pain or numbness
- breathing difficulties
- tingling, prickling or burning sensation

Effervescent tablets are available.

Not recommended.

Not recommended. It is unclear whether phosphates are excreted in human milk.

Reduced renal function: caution due to the risk of hyperphosphatemia. Use is contraindicated in severe renal impairment (less than 30% of normal function).

POTASSIUM

General Actions of potassium
- main intracellular ion
- involved in maintaining intracellular tonicity, nerve—muscle transmission, muscle contraction and normal renal function
- best dietary sources of potassium include leafy green vegetables, vine fruit (e.g. tomatoes, zucchini (courgettes), cucumbers, pumpkin, eggplant (aubergine)) and root vegetables. Other sources include beans, peas, tree fruit (e.g. apples, bananas, oranges), milk, yoghurt and meats
- normal serum concentration 3.5–5 mmol/L

General Uses of potassium
- hypokalaemia
- potassium replacement therapy after long-term use or high doses of potassium-depleting diuretics, especially if the patient is also receiving digoxin
- long-term or high-dose corticosteroid therapy, ACTH or benzylpenicillin
- low-salt, low-potassium diet
- poor absorption or loss from GI tract after excessive vomiting or diarrhoea, fistula or enterostomy drainage, or use of laxatives
- metabolic alkalosis (including hypochloraemic alkalosis)
- hyperaldosteronism
- renal disease associated with increased potassium excretion
- liver cirrhosis with diuretic therapy
- electrolyte supplement with TPN

Optimal daily requirements
- 3800 mg (males), 2800 mg (females, pregnancy), 3200 mg (breastfeeding)

General Adverse effects of potassium
- (IV) nausea, vomiting, diarrhoea, abdominal discomfort, fall in BP, arrhythmias, heart block, cardiac depression, ECG abnormalities
- (IV site) pain, phlebitis
- hyperkalaemia (lethargy, listlessness, confusion, weakness and heaviness of legs, flaccid paralysis, cold skin, grey pallor, paraesthesia of extremities, hypotension, heart block, cardiac arrhythmias, ECG abnormalities, cardiac arrest) (potentially fatal hyperkalaemia can develop rapidly and be asymptomatic)

General Interactions of potassium
- contraindicated with potassium-sparing diuretics (amiloride, spironolactone or triamterene) owing to risk of hyperkalaemia
- caution if given with ACE inhibitors (such as captopril and enalapril) and angiotensin II receptor antagonists owing to risk of hyperkalaemia
- hyperkalaemia may result if given with NSAIDs or heparin
- caution if used with other potassium-sparing agents such as renin inhibitors or proton pump inhibitors owing to risk of hyperkalaemia
- not recommended in those taking digoxin for heart block (severe or complete)

VITAMINS, MINERALS AND ELECTROLYTES

- caution if given with beta adrenoceptor blocking agents as serum potassium levels may increase, as well as increasing time to return to basal levels
- serum potassium levels may decrease if used with insulin, sodium bicarbonate, ciclosporin or tacrolimus

General Nursing considerations/Cautions for potassium

- potassium replacement should be undertaken cautiously and include monitoring acid—base balance, serum electrolytes, ECG and urine output
- serum potassium level should be closely monitored during therapy
- any dehydration should be corrected before treating potassium imbalance
- any hypomagnesaemia should be treated at same time as potassium deficiency, as magnesium deficiency prevents restoration of intracellular potassium deficit
- IV administration is usually given via a large vein to minimise vein irritation
- prevent extravasation
- must be diluted before using and should be diluted with sodium chloride 0.9% rather than glucose 5%, because the glucose may decrease the serum potassium concentration
- IV potassium must be given as a thoroughly mixed dilute solution of uniform concentration. This avoids a sudden increase in plasma potassium concentration, which may lead to cardiac arrest and death. If potassium chloride is to be added to a hanging IV solution, ensure that there is sufficient solution to make the correct dilution, then, after adding the potassium, invert the container several times to guarantee complete and even mixing
- ensure container is labelled carefully
- monitor IV infusion rate by using a burette or infusion pump or syringe pump
- potassium should not be added to a burette or injection port
- IV rate should be not greater than 20 mmol/hour

- (Metabolic acidosis) hypokalaemia should be treated with potassium salt (with alkalinising anion e.g. potassium bicarbonate), not potassium chloride
- administer alone
- (IV) incompatible with mannitol and fat emulsions containing soya oil or lecithin
- (Oral) caution if used in those with oesophageal stasis, a history of peptic ulcer, delayed intestinal transit, intestinal ischaemia or GI tract obstruction
- caution if used in those with chronic renal disease or liver impairment because of increased risk of hyperkalaemia
- caution if used in those with heart block, as degree of block may be increased
- caution if used in those on low salt diet because of risk of hypokalaemic hypochloraemic alkalosis occurring
- contraindicated in those with hypersensitivity to potassium or potassium administration (e.g. congenital paramyotonia), renal impairment with oliguria or azotaemia, severe tissue damage (including severe burns), severe renal failure, untreated Addison's disease, acute dehydration, hyperkalaemia, hyperchoraemia, uncontrolled diabetes mellitus, severe or prolonged diarrhoea, slowed or obstructed GI disease, heat cramps, hyperadrenalism associated with adrenogenital syndrome, metabolic or respiratory acidosis, ventricular fibrillation or atrioventricular/intraventricular heart block

General Patient education for potassium

- advise the patient to seek medical advice immediately if any confusion, weakness, irregular or slow heartbeat, numbness/tingling of lips, hands or feet, anxiety, shortness of breath or heaviness of legs occurs

 Serum potassium levels should be closely monitored if used during pregnancy. Potassium needs in pregnancy can often be met through a balanced diet rather than supplements. Natural sources (e.g. fruits such as bananas, oranges and leafy greens) provide potassium in a controlled amount and minimise the risk of overdose.

 Excessive potassium supplementation should be avoided as it could lead to hyperkalaemia (elevated potassium levels), which might indirectly affect milk composition.

POTASSIUM ACETATE
Trade name
DBL Potassium Acetate Concentrated Injection

Available form
Ampoule: 5 mEq/mL

Dose
- (IV) dose and rate are dependent on individual patient's condition, with maximum concentration of 40 mmol/L

Action/Use/Adverse effects/ Interactions/Patient education
- see General Action/Use/Adverse effects/Interactions/Patient education for potassium (p. 1662)

Nursing considerations/Cautions
- must be diluted before IV use
- total dose should not exceed > 150 mEq/24 hours
- if potassium level > 2.5 mEq/L (2.5 mmol/L), infusion rate < 10 mEq/hour (10 mmol/hour)
- see also General Nursing considerations/Cautions for potassium (p. 1663)

POTASSIUM CHLORIDE
Trade names
Bridgewest Sterile Potassium Chloride Concentrate, Chlorvescent, Phebra Potassium Chloride 22.3% Concentrated Injection, Potassium Chloride Aborns Concentrate, Span-K

Available forms
Tablets (slow-release): 600 mg;
Effervescent tablets: 548 mg (14 mmol);
Vials: 2.23 g/10 mL;
Ampoules: 75 mg/mL, 150 mg/mL, 10 mmol (0.75 g)/10 mL, 13.4 mmol (1 g)/10 mL, 20 mmol (1.5 g)/10 mL, 13.4 mmol (1 g)/4 mL, 26.8 mmol (2 g)/8 mL

Action/Use
- see General Actions and Uses of potassium (p. 1662)

Dose
- (With potassium-losing diuretic) 600 mg—1.2 g orally daily with or after food (slow-release tablets) **OR**
- (Potassium deficiency) 600 mg—1.2 g orally daily 2—3 times daily with or after food (slow-release tablets) **OR**
- (Potassium deficiency) 1—2 tablets orally daily 2—3 times daily with or after food (effervescent tablets) **OR**
- (IV) dose and rate are dependent on individual patient's condition, with maximum concentration of 40 mmol/L

Adverse effects
- (Slow-release tablets) nausea, vomiting, diarrhoea, abdominal pain, flatulence, gastrointestinal bleeding and, rarely, stricture, ulceration or perforation of bowel
- (Effervescent tablets) nausea, vomiting, diarrhoea, abdominal pain
- see also General Adverse effects of potassium (p. 1662)

Interactions
- (Oral, slow-release) caution if given with anticholinergic agents that reduce intestinal motility because of increased risk of gastrointestinal ulceration and haemorrhage
- see also General Interactions of potassium (p. 1662)

Nursing considerations/Cautions
- dilute well before IV use
- if serum potassium > 2.5 mmol/L, rate should not exceed 10 mmol/hour and daily dose maximum 150—200 mmol
- if serum potassium < 2 mmol/L with ECG changes or paralysis, rate can be

VITAMINS, MINERALS AND ELECTROLYTES

- increased to 40 mmol/hour and daily dose maximum 400 mmol
- (IV) incompatible with amikacin, amphotericin B, amoxicillin, benzylpenicillin, diazepam, dobutamine, etoposide with mannitol and cisplatin, methylprednisolone, phenytoin, promethazine or sodium nitroprusside
- see also General Nursing considerations/Cautions for potassium (p. 1663)

Patient education

- advise the patient to stop medication and seek medical advice immediately if there are any GI symptoms, including marked nausea, vomiting, flatulence, abdominal pain, diarrhoea with black or blood-stained stools
- advise the patient to swallow slow-release tablets whole (not chewed, crushed or broken) with water and not to allow to dissolve in the mouth
- warn the patient that, if taking slow-release preparations, potassium is released gradually from an insoluble wax core or matrix, which is excreted (and may be seen) in the faeces
- (Oral) warn the patient against using potassium salt substitutes during therapy
- (Effervescent tablets) instruct the patient to dissolve tablets in 120—240 mL cold water and take with or after food
- see also General Patient education for potassium (p. 1663)

Slow-release tablet should not be chewed, crushed or broken. Effervescent tablets can be dissolved in 5 mL water and then added to 120 mL thickened fluids.

Not recommended.

Not recommended: potassium is excreted into breastmilk.

Monitor serum potassium levels closely because of a generally increased risk of adverse effects in elderly patients.

(IV) this product is permitted in some sports and prohibited in others.

BICARBONATE

SODIUM BICARBONATE
Trade names
Sodibic, Sodium Bicarbonate Injection, Sodium Bicarbonate Injection 8.4%

Available forms
Capsules: 840 mg;
Prefilled syringe (Min-I-Jet): 1 mmol/mL;
Vial: 84 mg/mL (1 mmol/mL)

Actions
- bicarbonate is a normal constituent of body fluids
- part of the buffering system that maintains the acid—base balance in the body
- can cause redistribution of potassium ions into cells
- increases urinary pH
- normal plasma concentration 24—31 mmol/L

Uses
- renal tubular acidosis
- alkaliniser used in treatment of metabolic acidosis (e.g. cardiac arrest, shock, severe dehydration, diabetes mellitus)
- urinary alkaliniser to increase solubility of some weak acids (e.g. cysteine, uric acid, sulfonamides)
- forced alkaline diuresis in acute poisoning from weakly acidic drugs (e.g. salicylates, methanol, phenobarbital (phenobarbitone)), resulting in decreased renal absorption of the drug

Dose
- (Renal tubular acidosis) 840 mg orally daily **OR**

- (Cardiac arrest) initially 1 mmol/kg IV, followed by 0.5 mmol/kg at 10-minute intervals during arrest (depending on arterial blood gases) **OR**
- (Non-urgent metabolic acidosis) 2–5 mmol/kg by IV infusion over 4–8 hours

Adverse effects
- (Oral) anorexia, nausea
- (IV) alkalosis, hypokalaemia, sodium and water retention, oedema, congestive heart failure, hypernatraemia, hyperosmolality, hyperirritability, tetany, cerebral oedema and, rarely, intracranial haemorrhage
- hypercapnia (if patient is on fixed ventilation)
- (IV, extravasation) vascular irritation, chemical cellulitis, tissue necrosis, ulceration

Interactions
- caution if used in those taking corticosteroids or corticotrophin (corticotropin)
- urinary alkalinisation will increase clearance of tetracyclines (especially doxycycline)
- urinary alkalinisation will increase half-life and action of amphetamines, ephedrine and pseudoephedrine
- if used with thiazide diuretics, furosemide (frusemide) or hypochloraemic alkalosis may occur
- may enhance or prolong action of flecainide because of decreased excretion due to alkalinisation of urine
- may decrease effects of aspirin and other salicylates, barbiturates or lithium because of increased excretion owing to alkalinisation of urine
- may produce false positive on urine protein test

Nursing considerations/Cautions
- any hypokalaemia or hypocalcaemia should be corrected before starting therapy
- arterial blood gases (especially carbon dioxide and arterial/venous blood pH) and serum electrolytes should be monitored before starting and during therapy to prevent alkalosis
- levels should be monitored frequently to avoid excessively elevated plasma sodium levels occurring, which can lead to brain dehydration, confusion, somnolence, convulsions and coma
- therapy should be carried out in a slow step-wise manner to prevent alkalosis
- if patient has respiratory acidosis and metabolic acidosis, pulmonary ventilation and perfusion should be supported to ensure carbon dioxide is removed
- avoid extravasation. However, if it occurs, treat extravasation by elevating and warming the limb and giving a local injection of lidocaine (lignocaine) or hyaluronidase
- excessive sodium-containing solution may cause fluid overload, electrolyte dilution and pulmonary oedema
- see manufacturer's instructions for dilution and compatibility with solutions and other drugs as there are a large number of incompatibilities
- ensure IV is flushed with sodium chloride 0.9% before and after administration
- may be diluted with sodium chloride 0.9% or glucose 5%
- not recommended with IV calcium-containing solutions as precipitation will occur
- caution if used in those with cirrhosis
- caution if used in those with tissue hypoxia (type A lactic acidosis) as increased lactate production will occur, worsening acidosis
- extreme caution if used in those predisposed to sodium retention and oedema or those with congestive heart failure or renal insufficiency because of the sodium content (12 mEq/g)
- not recommended for diabetic ketoacidosis with pH between 6.9 and 7.1
- contraindicated in those with renal failure, metabolic/respiratory alkalosis, hypertension, oedema, congestive heart failure, hypoventilation, chloride depletion, hypernatraemia, hypocalcaemia,

VITAMINS, MINERALS AND ELECTROLYTES

co-existing potassium depletion, history of urinary calculi, eclampsia or aldosteronism

Capsules can be opened and mixed with water or a spoonful of yoghurt or jam.

Permitted in some sports but prohibited in others.

Also available in combination with
- contained in Citravescent and Ural for the treatment of cystitis
- contained in antacids and laxatives and multi-electrolyte preparations

SODIUM

General Actions of sodium
- sodium is a key electrolyte in the body
- a major cation that plays a central role in maintaining extracellular volume and serum osmolality
- 95% is found in extracellular fluid, maintained with sodium/potassium–ATPase pumps
- sodium is essential for maintaining cell membrane potential
- absorbed in the small intestine along with chloride
- found in most foods in a variety of forms
- primarily excreted through urine and sweat

Recommended daily intake
- 460–920 mg (20–40 mmol) (males, females, pregnancy, breastfeeding)
- daily intake should not exceed 2300 mg (100 mmol)

SODIUM CHLORIDE
Trade names
Sodium Chloride 0.9% (Normal Saline) Sterile Injection, Sodium Chloride (0.9%) for Irrigation Solution BP, Saltabs, Toppin Salt Tablets

Available forms
Tablets: 600 mg;
IV solution: 0.45%, 0.9%;
Ampoule: 0.9%;
Vial: 0.9%

Action
- source of sodium and chloride ions
- sodium is a principal electrolyte

Use
- prevention and/or correction of fluid and electrolyte deficits or imbalance
- diluent for drugs and vehicle for drug admixtures
- prevention or treatment of sodium chloride loss in sweat when heavy work is being done in a hot environment
- replacement of urinary sodium chloride loss in Addison's disease (adrenocortical atrophy)
- dialysis fluid
- priming fluid for haemodialysis procedures
- eye lotion, mouthwash and irrigating solution

Dose
- mainly given by IV infusion as sodium chloride 0.9% (isotonic saline) **OR**
- (Prophylaxis during light work) 2.4–3.6 g (4–6 tablets) orally daily or as prescribed **OR**
- (Prophylaxis during heavy work) 7.2–9 g (12–15 tablets) orally daily

Adverse effects
- electrolyte imbalance, fluid overload, acid–base imbalance
- (IV site) phlebitis, burning sensation, itching

Interactions
- caution if given with lithium, as clearance may be increased, reducing serum levels
- caution if given with corticosteroids or corticotrophin (corticotropin) because of potential sodium and fluid retention
- increased risk of hyponatraemia if given with antiepileptic agents, antipsychotics, selective serotonin reuptake inhibitors (SSRIs), NSAIDs, opioids, cyclophosphamide, vincristine or clofibrate

1667

Nursing considerations/Cautions

- select the correct concentration of sodium chloride: isotonic (0.9%), hypotonic (less concentrated) or hypertonic (more concentrated), noting also that sodium chloride is often combined with glucose
- monitor heart rate, BP, fluid intake and output and serum electrolytes, especially throughout prolonged IV therapy
- rapid correction of hyponatraemia or hypernatraemia is potentially dangerous
- (IV) not recommended with blood products
- caution if used in the elderly or those with cardiac failure, hypertension, kidney impairment, oedema (peripheral, pulmonary, cerebral), cirrhosis or pre-eclampsia
- caution if used in children or the elderly, women or postoperatively because of the risk of hyponatraemia
- caution if used in those at risk of hypernatraemia, hyperchloraemia or hypervolaemia
- contraindicated in those for whom salt retention may be undesirable (e.g. heart disease, oedema, renal impairment, primary/secondary aldosteronism)

Patient education

- the patient should be advised to maintain an adequate water intake with oral preparations to prevent high salt levels, especially during hot weather, fever, diarrhoea, exercise or heavy manual labour
- advise the patient to seek medical advice immediately if any of the following occur:
  - swelling in arms or legs, difficulty breathing or frothy pink sputum, or
  - thirst, swollen tongue, decreased saliva, dry eyes, flushing, fever, rapid breathing, rapid heart rate, weakness, dizziness, decreased urination and/or headache

 Tablets can be dispersed in water, or crushed and mixed with spoonful of yoghurt or apple puree.

Available in combination with

- nasal spray or drops, eye drops
- also available as part of multi-ingredient intravenous solutions (e.g. sodium chloride and glucose; sodium chloride, glucose and potassium chloride; sodium chloride, sodium lactate, potassium chloride and calcium chloride), multi-ingredient peritoneal dialysis solutions or oral electrolyte replacement solutions (e.g. Hydralyte)

ZINC

General Actions of zinc

- zinc acts as a co-factor in numerous biochemical pathways.
- involved in wound healing and protein, DNA and collagen synthesis
- essential for enzyme reactions critical to healthy skin gland function
- mobilisation of vitamin A
- essential for immune function
- involved in normal prostate function
- aids in maintenance of taste and smell
- present with insulin in the pancreas
- normal serum levels 0.7—1.5 mg/L

General Uses of zinc

- zinc deficiency (growth deterioration, skin lesions, alopecia, delayed wound healing, impaired prostate gland development and function)

Optimal daily requirements

- 14 mg (males), 8 mg (females), 11 mg (pregnancy), 12 mg (breastfeeding)

ZINC CHLORIDE

Trade names
DBL Zinc Chloride Injection, Zinc Chloride Concentrated Injection

Available forms
Ampoules: 5.1 mg/2 mL, 10.6 mg/2 mL

Action/Use
- see General Actions/General Uses of zinc above

Dose
- 2.5—4 mg daily by IV infusion over 8—24 hours, with additional 2 mg daily for acute catabolic states

VITAMINS, MINERALS AND ELECTROLYTES

Adverse effects
- (Prolonged therapy) copper deficiency, anaemia
- increased serum amylase, lipase and alkaline phosphatase

Interactions
- if given without copper, may cause decrease in serum copper levels

Nursing considerations/Cautions
- direct intravenous or intramuscular injection is contraindicated owing to tissue irritation risk. Zinc chloride injection should be diluted and administered as a slow intravenous infusion, avoiding undiluted direct injection into a vein to reduce phlebitis risk. Ensure careful handling, avoiding contact with eyes and skin, and wash thoroughly with water if contact occurs.
- for IV use, dilute in 1000 mL of glucose 5% or sodium chloride 0.9% and infuse over 8–24 hours
- serum copper and zinc levels should be regularly monitored
- increased amount is required in those on a vegetarian diet as there is lower zinc absorption
- further zinc supplementation may also be required in situations of acute catabolism (2 mg per day) or for fluid loss from small intestine (12.2 mg/L of fluid lost or 17.1 mg/kg of stool/ileostomy output)
- (IV solution) avoid contact with eyes and skin. If contact occurs, wash area immediately with copious amounts of water
- caution if given to those with renal impairment as zinc may accumulate
- contraindicated by IM or IV bolus injection

 Not recommended: no human data. Zinc chloride injection should be used in pregnancy only if clearly indicated, as no animal reproduction studies have been conducted to evaluate potential risks to the fetus.

 Zinc is excreted in breastmilk, and excessive zinc intake may risk causing copper deficiency in the infant. The potential benefits to the mother must be weighed against the risks to the infant.

 Reduced renal function: caution when administering zinc chloride injection to patients with renal impairment because of the potential for zinc accumulation.

ZINC SULFATE
Trade name
Zincaps

Available form
Capsules: 50 mg

Action/Use
- see General Actions/General Uses of zinc (p. 1668)

Dose
- 50 mg orally daily with food

Adverse effects
- nausea, mild epigastric discomfort

Interactions/Nursing considerations/Cautions
- administer on an empty stomach to maximise absorption, particularly for patients with Wilson's disease. If gastrointestinal side-effects occur, consider giving with food
- see also Interactions/Nursing considerations/Cautions of zinc chloride (p. 1668)

Patient education
- advise the patient that capsules may be taken with food to overcome gastric irritation

 Capsules can be opened and contents dispersed in water or mixed with spoonful of yoghurt or apple puree.

# AMINO ACIDS

ARGININE
Trade names
Arginine Hydrochloride 60% Concentrated Injection

Available form
Vial: 15 g/25 mL

Action
- essential amino acid
- absorbed from GI tract and processed by liver
- important part of urea cycle enabling body to safely store and excrete ammonia

Use
- stimulates the release of growth hormone and may be used instead of, or in addition to, other tests to evaluate growth disorders
- acidifying agent in severe metabolic alkalosis
- severe deficiency of ornithine carbamoyl transferase or carbamoyl phosphate synthetase where respiratory alkalosis is present

Dose
- 30 g by IV infusion over 30 minutes

Adverse effects
- nausea, vomiting
- flushing
- headache, numbness
- (Rare) hypotension, anaphylaxis, allergic reactions, severe hyperkalaemia
- (IV site) irritation (if infused too rapidly)

Interactions
- caution if given with spironolactone

Nursing considerations/Cautions
- BP should be monitored during and for 24 hours after IV infusion because of the risk of hypotension
- antihistamines should be readily available in the event of allergic reaction
- a single test should not be used as an evaluation for growth disorders as false positive and false negative results are common
- should be diluted with sodium chloride 0.9% or glucose 5% before IV administration
- caution if used in those with electrolyte disturbance because of the risk of hyperchloraemic acidosis
- caution if used in those with severe liver disease or moderate kidney insufficiency
- caution if used in those with uraemia, anuria or kidney disease because of the risk of elevated potassium levels
- contraindicated in those who are highly allergic or with hypersensitivity to arginine, severe acidosis, hypotension or any disease/defect related to nitric oxide production

 Limited use in humans. Use only if clearly necessary.

 Caution: passes into breastmilk, but adverse effects on nursing infants are not expected.

 Reduced renal or hepatic function: use with caution in patients with moderate renal insufficiency or severe liver disease. Risk of elevated plasma potassium levels in uraemic patients; monitor closely.

MISCELLANEOUS AGENTS

The agents included in this section are a heterogeneous group of drugs which do not fit into any of the other more clearly defined chapters.

FEZOLINETANT

Trade name
Veoza

Available form
Tablet: 45 mg

Action
- non-hormonal selective neurokinin-3 (NK3) receptor antagonist that blocks neurokinin B (NKB) (the thermoregulatory centre in the hypothalamus is inhibited by oestrogen and stimulated by NKB); during menopause, with declining oestrogen levels, the balance of oestrogen and NKB becomes disrupted, with increased NKB activity resulting in vasomotor symptoms including hot flushes and night sweats)
- metabolite has less activity than parent
- half-life is less than 15 hours

Use
- moderate-to-severe vasomotor symptoms associated with menopause

Dose
- 45 mg orally daily

Adverse effects
- headache, fatigue, insomnia
- diarrhoea, nausea, abdominal pain
- increased liver enzymes
- nasopharyngitis, upper respiratory tract infection
- arthralgia, back pain

Interactions
- contraindicated with fluvoxamine, ciprofloxacin, mexiletine, ethinyl oestradiol-containing contraceptives, imipramine, bortezomib
- not recommended with hormonal replacement therapy (except topical vaginal preparations)

Nursing considerations/Cautions
- a baseline liver function test is recommended before started therapy and then monthly for the first 3 months
- caution if used in women with a current or past history of oestrogen-dependent breast or other tumour, or currently being treated with antioestrogen therapy. Benefit—risk assessment should be undertaken before starting therapy
- contraindicated in those with moderate-to-severe liver impairment or severe kidney impairment or end-stage liver disease

Patient education
- advise the patient to take the tablet at the same time of day and swallowed whole (not crushed, cut or chewed)

- if the patient misses a dose, they should take the tablet as soon as possible unless it is 12 hours or less until next dose
- instruct patient to seek medical advice if they develop any new-onset fatigue, decreased appetite, nausea, vomiting, pruritus, dark urine, pale stools, abdominal pain or yellowing of eyes or skin
- perimenopausal women of childbearing potential should be instructed to use a non-hormonal contraceptive method during therapy

Tablet should not be crushed.

Not recommended during pregnancy.

Not recommended during breastfeeding.

Contraindicated in those with chronic liver impairment (Pugh-Child Class B or C), or severe or end-stage renal impairment (eGFR< 30 mL/min)

HYALURONIC ACID

Trade name
Durolane

Available form
Glass syringe: 20 mg/mL

Action
- hyaluronic acid is a normal part of synovial fluid, acting as a lubricant for cartilage and ligaments, as well as a shock absorber
- in joints affected by osteoarthritis (OA), synovial fluid has a lower viscosity and elasticity; therefore hyaluronic acid is used to restore viscosity and elasticity, reducing pain and improving mobility
- half-life is about 4 weeks

Use
- symptomatic treatment of mild-to-moderate OA

Dose
- 60 mg (3 mL) intra-articular injection into knee

Adverse effects
- transient knee pain, swelling or stiffness
- joint infection

Interactions
- not recommended with other intra-articular injections

Nursing considerations/Cautions

- current evidence suggests that joint injections with hyaluronic acid may not be effective, and potential risks (pain, swelling, infection) outweigh benefits
- any joint effusion should be removed before intra-articular injection
- same needle can be used for both removal of effusion and intra-articular injection
- if both limbs are being treated, a separate syringe should be used for each limb
- re-injection in less than 6 months is not recommended
- caution if used in those with venous or lymphatic stasis of the limb
- caution if used in those with pre-existing chondrocalcinosis, as administration may lead to acute attack
- not recommended if there is any infection or severe inflammation of the knee joint or skin infection/disease at or near the injection site
- not recommended IV, extra-articularly or in synovial tissue or capsule
- not recommended in those with known hypersensitivity to hyaluronic acid

Patient education

- patient should be instructed to avoid strenuous exercise (e.g. tennis, jogging, long walks) for 48 hours after injection
- warn patient that there may be some transient mild-to-moderate pain, swelling or stiffness during the first week after injection. If these symptoms persist for more than 1 week,

patient should be advised to seek medical advice

Limited data; use only if benefits justify risks.

Not recommended. Unknown whether excreted in human breastmilk.

LAUROMACROGOL 400
Trade name
Aethoxysklerol

Available forms
Ampoule: 10 mg/2 mL, 20 mg/2 mL, 60 mg/2 mL

Action
- irritates vein wall intima, causing thrombus, which permanently occludes vessel by causing fibrosis when compression is applied

Use
- treatment of varicose veins (up to 6 mm) in lower limbs (with compression therapy)

Dose
- injected slowly into lumen of affected vein (daily maximum 2 mg/kg)

Adverse effects
- (Immediate) pain, inflammation, swelling, haematoma, local allergic reaction
- (Delayed) hyperpigmentation, vein thrombosis, ecchymosis, neovascularisation
- (Rare) allergic reaction, angioedema, anaphylactoid reaction

Interaction
- may intensify effects of anaesthetics, especially cardiac effects

Nursing considerations/Cautions
- avoid intra-arterial injection as it can cause severe necrosis, potentially requiring amputation
- before injection, ensure valvular competence and deep vein patency
- before injection, leg should be elevated 30—45 degrees above the horizontal
- if patient has a history of hypersensitivities or allergies, only 1 injection should be given initially under careful observation
- amount injected is dependent on size of vessel (e.g. spider veins 0.1—0.2 mL of 0.5% solution, whereas medium-sized varices require 0.5—1 mL of 2—3% solution)
- once injections are complete and sites covered, a firm compression bandage is applied and patient should walk under observation for at least 30 minutes
- bandage should remain in situ for 2—3 days (spider veins), 3—7 days (small varices) or 4—6 weeks (medium-to-large sized varices)
- repeat treatments at 1—2-week intervals may be necessary depending on size and extent of varices
- contains alcohol, which may need to be considered in patients with alcoholism
- oxygen, adrenaline (epinephrine), IV corticosteroids and resuscitation equipment should be available in the event of anaphylaxis
- caution if injecting into malleolus area. Small quantities of low concentration solution should be used
- contraindicated intra-arterially
- caution or contraindicated (depending on severity) in those with leg oedema (that can't be compressed), symptoms of microangiopathy or neuropathy, hypercoagulability, spider veins, inflammatory skin reaction at injection site, acute severe cardiac disease, febrile states or advanced age (with impaired mobility or very poor general condition) or right-to-left shunt (asymptomatic)
- contraindicated in those who are bedridden or unable to walk or those with arterial occlusive disease, acute superficial thrombophlebitis, thromboembolic disorders or high risk of thromboembolic disorders, significant valvular or deep vein incompetence,

huge superficial veins that communicate to deeper veins, acute cellulitis or infections, phlebitis migrans, varicosities caused by abdominal/pelvic tumours (unless tumour has been removed), uncontrolled systemic disease (e.g. diabetes mellitus, hypertension), tuberculosis, toxic hyperthyroidism, asthma, blood dyscrasias, acute respiratory or skin disease or strong predisposition to allergies

Not recommended. Lauromacrogol 400 has shown embryo-fetal toxicity and malformations in animal studies at high doses. It crosses the placenta and is associated with an increased risk of fetal malformations. It should not be used during pregnancy unless the potential benefit justifies the risk.

Caution. Excretion into human breast-milk unknown.

METYRAPONE
Trade name
Metopirone

Available form
Capsules: 250 mg

Action
* reversibly inhibits production of cortisol, corticosterone and aldosterone by the adrenal cortex
* if pituitary feedback control system is intact, causes a compensatory increase in adrenocorticotrophic hormone (ACTH), resulting in increased cortisol precursor production
* rapidly absorbed orally
* elimination half-life is 20—26 minutes
* active metabolite

Use
* diagnostic agent for assessing anterior pituitary and adrenocortical function
* differential diagnosis of adrenal hyperfunction in Cushing's syndrome

Dose
Short single-dose test (ambulant patient)
* 1—2 g (based on 30 mg/kg) orally at approximately midnight with yoghurt or milk; 8 hours later, take blood for estimation of ACTH and/or 11-deoxycortisol, then give cortisone acetate 50 mg prophylactically

Multiple-dose test (in hospital setting)
* obtain urine samples in the 24 hours preceding the test (for control values of urinary steroid excretion)
* 500—750 mg orally 4-hourly for 6 doses after food or with milk (total 3.0—4.5 g/24 hours)
* collect all urine for the next 24 hours and store at $-10°C$ until analysis

Adverse effects
* nausea, vomiting
* headache, dizziness, sedation
* hypotension
* (Rare) skin reactions

Interactions
* may potentiate paracetamol, increasing risk of toxicity
* test results may be influenced by phenytoin, barbiturates, amitriptyline, chlorpromazine, alprazolam, hormone preparations, corticosteroids, cyproheptadine and antithyroid agents

Nursing considerations/Cautions
* requires some functioning of the adrenal cortex for satisfactory results; otherwise acute adrenal insufficiency may be induced
* drugs affecting pituitary or adrenocortical function (e.g. antiepileptics, psychoactive drugs, hormone preparations, corticosteroids, antithyroid drugs) must be withdrawn before the test
* if adrenocortical insufficiency is suspected, patient should be observed overnight in hospital if a carer/supervision is not available

MISCELLANEOUS AGENTS

- caution if used in those with ectopic Cushing's syndrome because of the risk of opportunistic infection
- caution if used in those with liver damage (response may be delayed) or thyroid hypofunction (urinary steroid excretion may not increase at all or very slowly)
- contraindicated in those with adrenocortical insufficiency

Patient education
- patient should be advised against driving or operating machinery if dizziness or sedation occurs

Contents of capsule can be squeezed into water or spoonful of yoghurt; however, content is very thick and dose may not be correct. Mask, gloves and safety glasses should be worn if opening capsule.

Not recommended during pregnancy unless the benefits outweigh the risks.

Not recommended. Breastfeeding should be discontinued during treatment, because of the potential risks to the infant.

Paediatric warning: Use in children requires a reduced dosage, and administration should be carefully monitored in hospital settings, especially when evaluating adrenal function, owing to the potential to provoke transient adrenocortical insufficiency.

PATISIRAN
Trade name
Onpattro

Available form
Vial: 10 mg

Action
- double-stranded small interfering ribonucleic acid (siRNA)
- in those with hereditary transthyretin (TTR)-mediated amyloidosis, TTR proteins are abnormal and clump together in deposits (amyloid) which can build up around nerves, the heart and other areas of the body, leading to symptoms
- formulated as lipid nanoparticles that deliver the siRNA to hepatocytes where there is degradation of TTR mRNA reducing serum TTR protein
- reduction of serum TTR protein can lead to decreased vitamin A (retinol) levels

Use
- treatment of hereditary TTR-mediated amyloidosis in adults with stage 1 or stage 2 polyneuropathy

Dose
- 300 micrograms/kg by IV infusion once every 3 weeks **OR**
- (Patient weight > 100 kg) 30 mg by IV infusion once every 3 weeks

Adverse effects
- (Infusion-related reactions) flushing, back pain, nausea, abdominal pain, dyspnoea, headache, hypotension, syncope
- vitamin A deficiency (night blindness, reduced night vision, persistent dry eyes, eye inflammation, corneal inflammation or ulceration, corneal thickening or perforation)
- bronchitis, sinusitis, rhinitis, dyspnoea
- vertigo
- peripheral oedema
- muscle spasms
- dyspepsia
- skin redness
- (Uncommon) extravasation

Nursing considerations/Cautions
- serum vitamin A levels should be measured before starting therapy and any deficiency corrected
- pregnancy should be excluded before starting therapy
- infusion-related reactions (IRR) most commonly occur within the first 2 infusions

- all patients should receive premedication at least 60 minutes before infusion to decrease the risk of IRR. Premedication should include:
  - IV corticosteroid (e.g. 10 mg dexamethasone or equivalent)
  - oral paracetamol 500 mg
  - IV H1 blocker (e.g. diphenhydramine 50 mg or equivalent)
  - IV H2 blocker (e.g. famotidine 20 mg or equivalent)
- if IV premedication is not available, the oral equivalent may be given
- the patient should be monitored during infusion for any signs of IRR
- if the patient has 3 consecutive IV infusions of patisiran without IRR, consideration can be given to tapering corticosteroid dose by 2.5 mg increments to 5 mg
- vial should be removed from fridge before use but not shaken and not used if frozen
- the required volume of patisiran (calculated on patient weight) should be withdrawn from the vial through a sterile 0.45 micron polyethersulfone (PES) syringe filter into a sterile container. The required volume is then withdrawn from the sterile container into an infusion bag of sodium chloride 0.9% to a total volume of 250 mL
- the infusion set and lines should be free of di-(2-ethylhexyl)phthalate (DEHP)
- the infusion bag should be gently inverted to mix solution (not shaken)
- infuse alone using a 1.2 micron PES inline infusion filter
- the initial infusion rate should be 1 mL/min for first 15 minutes, then increasing to 3 mL/min for the remainder of the infusion (approximately 80 minutes — can be extended if IRR occur)
- the infusion site should be monitored regularly for any signs of extravasation
- the infusion line should be flushed with sodium chloride 0.9% at completion of the infusion
- if the patient has tolerated 3 infusions of patisiran, consideration should be given to home administration by a health professional (e.g. a community nurse)

- not recommended in those with moderate-to-severe liver impairment, severe kidney impairment or end-stage kidney disease

Patient education

- advise the patient to take vitamin A supplement (2500 IU) daily to prevent vitamin A deficiency
- during the infusion, ensure the patient understands the importance of immediately reporting any IRR including:
  - nausea, abdominal pain
  - shortness of breath, difficulty breathing, cough
  - body aches or pains
  - skin flushing, feeling of warmth, rash, itching
  - feeling faint
  - pain, redness, swelling, burning at infusion site
- women of childbearing potential should be counselled to use effective contraception during therapy to prevent pregnancy, as vitamin A levels (too high or too low) can lead to fetal malformation. If the patient plans to become pregnant, patisiran and vitamin A supplementation should both be stopped and serum vitamin A levels monitored until normal before becoming pregnant is attempted

 Not recommended during pregnancy. If unplanned pregnancy occurs, the fetus should be closely monitored especially during first trimester.

 Not recommended in those with moderate or severe liver impairment, severe renal impairment or end-stage renal disease. Should be used only if clinical benefit outweighs potential risk

PHENOL
Trade name
Haemorol

Available form
Ampoule: 250 mg/5 mL

MISCELLANEOUS AGENTS

Action
- sclerosing agent

Use
- first- to second-degree symptomatic haemorrhoids (unresponsive to conservative treatment such as dietary manipulation)

Dose
- 100–250 mg (2–5 mL) into submucosal space above each of the 3 main haemorrhoids (maximum per treatment 500 mg (10 mL))

Adverse effects
- pain, discomfort
- dizziness
- local ulceration, sterile abscess
- (Rare) necrotising fasciitis

Interactions
- incompatible with alkaline salts and non-ionic surfactants
- interferes with a number of laboratory tests, including plasma estimation for adrenaline (epinephrine) and noradrenaline (norepinephrine), ferric chloride test for urinary ketones or salicylates, serum calcium, serum sulfonamides and Benedict's test for glycosuria

Nursing considerations/Cautions
- for submucosal injection only. It must not be injected intrathecally, into a blood vessel or into deep tissues. Misplacement may result in serious complications, such as prostatic abscess or sterile abscess formation
- not recommended over large areas of skin owing to absorption and toxicity
- glass syringes are recommended; however, plastic syringes with plastic hubs can be used if administered immediately
- contraindicated in those with hypersensitivity to phenol or almond oil, or over large areas
- contraindicated for use in neonates and children, as significant phenol absorption can occur, leading to potential toxic effects

Patient education
- warn patient to avoid driving or operating machinery if dizziness occurs

Not recommended. Phenol has shown evidence of fetal damage in animal studies, including fetal resorptions and malformations at doses not toxic to the mother.

Limited human data. Given the lack of established safety in neonates and children, it should not be used during lactation.

POVIDONE–IODINE
Trade names
Betadine Preparations, Difflam Sore Throat Gargle with Iodine Concentrate, Herron Riodine Concentrated Gargle, Inadine Dressing, Inadine, Microshield PVP

Available forms
Surgical body wash solution: 7.5%;
Cream: 5%;
Ointment: 10%;
Cold sore ointment: 10%;
Spray: 5%;
Liquid throat gargle: 1%, 7.5%;
Solution: 7.5%, 10%;
Dressing

Action
- rapidly effective against bacteria, viruses and fungal spores
- low-concentration solutions provide kill rate equal to or greater than concentrated solutions

Use
- broad-spectrum antiseptic and disinfectant

Dose
- (Sore throat) dilute 7.5% solution according to instructions (1 in 20) and gargle for greater than 30 seconds, then expel. Repeat 3–4-hourly (some

solutions (1%) do not need to be diluted) **OR**
- (Presurgical body wash) wet body and hair, apply solution and work into a lather (paying particular attention to hair, groin and axilla) for at least 2 minutes, rinse thoroughly with running water and dry. Should be repeated at least twice before surgery **OR**
- (Minor burns, wounds, cuts, abrasions) apply to affected area according to the manufacturer's instructions and cover with dressing, if required **OR**
- (Surgical hand scrub) apply 3.5 mL (1 pump) to 5 mL to wet hands and arms and wash for at least 2 minutes, scrub nails with nail brush, rinse, then repeat, and dry with sterile towel **OR**
- (Surgical skin preparation) paint operative field with skin preparation (10%) and allow to dry before starting procedure **OR**
- (Cold sore ointment) ointment applied to cold sore at least 4 times per day **OR**
- (Dressing) apply dressing to cleansed wound and leave intact until colour fades (usually up to 72 hours)

Adverse effects
- irritation, redness, swelling

Nursing considerations/Cautions
- (Skin preparation) 10% solution contains alcohol and may be hazardous if allowed to pool on surgical drapes or under patient before diathermy
- (Dressing) dressing should be changed when colour fades. For highly exuding or infected wounds, dressing may require changing twice daily, with frequency reducing as healing occurs. A secondary dressing is required
- multiple preparations and strengths are available; therefore care should be taken to select the correct preparation and strength
- (Solution) avoid contact with mucous membranes, eyes or ears
- (Dressing) caution if used in deep ulcers or burns, or over large areas
- prolonged (> 14 days) or extensive use (> 10% total body surface) should be avoided
- not recommended or used on premature newborns, and caution if used on full-term infants, because of the risk of transient hypothyroidism if used for extended time or over large area of body
- contraindicated if used in those with thyroid disorders or within 4 weeks of thyroid cancer treatment
- contraindicated in those with known iodine sensitivity

Patient education
- (Cold sore ointment) warn patient not to apply close to eyes, ears or mucous membranes
- (Gargle solution) advise patient not to swallow solution
- (Sore throat) instruct patient that, if symptoms persist for > 2 days, medical advice should be sought

SODIUM TETRADECYL SULFATE
Trade name
Fibrovein

Available forms
Solution: 0.2%, 0.5%, 1%, 3%

Action
- sclerosing agent that irritates the intima of the vein wall so that when compressed the vein is permanently occluded because of vein fibrosis

Use
- compression sclerotherapy of varicose veins

Dose
- 0.5–1.0 mL IV into lumen of emptied, isolated segment of superficial vein, followed by immediate compression (maximum 4 sites (4 mL) per treatment) (3% solution) **OR**
- 0.25–1.0 mL IV into lumen of emptied, isolated segment of superficial vein, followed by immediate compression

MISCELLANEOUS AGENTS

(maximum 10 sites (10 mL) per treatment) (1% solution) **OR**
- 0.25—1.0 mL IV into lumen of emptied, isolated segment of superficial vein (medium venules), followed by immediate compression (maximum 10 sites (10 mL) per treatment) (0.5% solution) **OR**
- 0.1—1.0 mL IV into lumen of emptied, isolated segment of superficial vein (minor venules, spider veins), followed by immediate compression (maximum 10 sites (10 mL) per treatment) (0.2% solution)

Adverse effects
- superficial thrombophlebitis
- (Local) pain, burning sensation, skin pigmentation, necrosis, ulceration (superficial extravasation)
- (Rare) anaphylaxis, allergy, deep vein thrombosis, pulmonary embolism

Interactions
- contraindicated in those taking oral contraceptives or hormone replacement therapy

Nursing considerations/Cautions
- pre-injection assessment for valvular competence and deep vein patency must be carried out. Allergy history should also be taken from patient before administration, including any previous treatment with sodium tetradecyl sulfate, because there is an increased risk of allergic reaction with repeated treatments
- strength of solution used is dependent on size of vein to be sclerosed
- avoid extravasation, as it may cause local tissue damage, including necrosis. Use care in injection technique, and consider immediate compression at the injection site
- not given intra-arterially because of the risk of tissue necrosis and ischaemia
- caution if used in those with history of allergy/anaphylaxis. If deemed necessary, a test dose (0.25—0.5 mL) can be given 24 hours before treatment
- because the possibility of anaphylaxis exists (although rare), it is necessary to have ready availability of adrenaline (epinephrine), aminophylline, hydrocortisone, an antihistamine and equipment for mucous extraction and endotracheal intubation in the event of a reaction occurring
- class 1 compression stocking can be applied over bandages for retention and compression
- (Fibrovein 1%) bandages can be replaced by class 2 or 3 compression stockings at an early stage but must be worn for at least 6 weeks
- available in four strengths; therefore ensure that correct solution is selected
- patient should walk for 30—60 minutes immediately postprocedure
- extreme caution if used in those with arterial disease including peripheral atherosclerosis and thromboangiitis obliterans
- contraindicated in those who are bedridden or unable to walk 5 km/day, or those with arterial occlusive disease, acute superficial thrombophlebitis, thromboembolic disorders or high risk of thromboembolic disorders, significant valvular or deep vein incompetence, high superficial veins that communicate to deeper veins, acute cellulitis or infections, phlebitis migrans, varicosities caused by abdominal/pelvic tumours (unless tumour has been removed), uncontrolled systemic disease (e.g. diabetes mellitus, hypertension), tuberculosis, toxic hyperthyroidism, asthma, blood dyscrasias, recent surgery, acute respiratory or skin disease, or strong predisposition to allergies

Patient education
- patient should be advised to seek medical attention immediately if any of the following occur:
  - sudden shortness of breath, sudden chest pain which worsens on deep

breathing or coughing, coughing up pinky frothy sputum, rapid heart rate and/or breathing, anxiety, fainting, sweating
* pain in calf, foot or leg, swelling of extremity (usually one side), tenderness, warmth
* after procedure, patient should be given the following instructions:
  * bandages/stockings must not be removed for at least 6 weeks after injection, and then removed only after doctor has specified this can occur
  * bandages/stockings should be kept dry during bathing or showering
  * daily exercise (walking) for at least 1 hour or 5 km is recommended from day of injection and should be continued after removal of bandages/stockings
  * standing still for any period of time is not recommended

 Not recommended.

 Not recommended. Excretion in human breastmilk unknown.

THYROTROPHIN ALFA (RCH)
Trade name
Thyrogen

Available form
Vial: 0.9 mg/mL

Action
* human thyroid-stimulating hormone (TSH) produced by recombinant DNA technology
* similar to human pituitary TSH
* binds to TSH receptors on normal thyroid epithelial cell or well-differentiated thyroid cancer cells, stimulating iodine uptake, organification, synthesis of thyroglobulin (Tg), triiodothyronine (T3) and thyroxine (T4)

Use
* use with serum thyroglobulin (Tg) testing (with or without radioactive iodine imaging) to detect thyroid remnants or well-differentiated thyroid cancer in post-thyroidectomy patients on hormone suppression therapy
* combined with radioactive iodine in the ablation of thyroid remnant tissue post-thyroidectomy on hormone suppression therapy

Dose
* 0.9 mg IM, followed by 0.9 mg after 24 hours

Adverse effects
* nausea, vomiting, diarrhoea
* headache, fatigue, dizziness, asthenia, paraesthesia
* transient flu-like symptoms (including fever ($> 38°C$), chills, shivering, myalgia, arthralgia, fatigue, malaise, headache)
* elevated (short-term) TSH levels, which may stimulate tumour or metastatic growth (where thyroid hormones have been withdrawn for diagnostic purpose)
* (Rare) hypersensitivity

Nursing considerations/Cautions
* use should be restricted to patients who are at low risk of disease recurrence
* Tg levels are generally lower and do not correlate with Tg levels after thyroid hormone withdrawal. If a detectable Tg level appears or rises after administration, or there is a high index of suspicion of metastatic disease, further evaluation is recommended immediately
* in clinical trials, undetectable thyrotrophin alfa-stimulated Tg levels (< 2.5 nanogram/mL) suggested the absence of clinically significant disease
* whole-body scanning with thyroglobulin testing after administration increased detection rate of remnant cancer when compared with either method alone

MISCELLANEOUS AGENTS

- reconstitute with 1.2 mL water for injections
- administer by deep IM into buttocks
- radioactive imaging or treatment: radioactive administration is recommended 24 hours after second IM injection
- diagnostic scanning should be performed 48 hours after radioactive administration (72 hours after last IM injection)
- for serum Tg testing, serum sample should be collected 72 hours after final IM injection
- thyroglobulin antibodies will interfere with Tg assay, leading to uninterpretable results. If this occurs, a thyroid hormone withdrawal scan is recommended to determine the site and extent of thyroid cancer
- administer alone
- caution if used in those who have previously experienced hypersensitivity reaction to bovine TSH
- caution if used in those with history of heart disease with residual thyroid tissue, as a rise in thyroid hormone levels may lead to thyrotrophin alfa-induced hyperthyroidism
- caution if used in those with thyroid cancer with metastases in confined spaces (e.g. brain, spinal cord, orbit, neck infiltration), as elevated TSH levels after administration may result in symptoms such as acute hemiplegia, hemiparesis, pain or swallowing difficulties. Pretreatment with corticosteroids may prevent this from occurring

Patient education

- warn patient to avoid driving or operating machinery if dizziness or fatigue are ongoing
- patient should be warned that flu-like symptoms may occur for up to 48 hours after procedure

 Not recommended. To be used during pregnancy only if the potential benefits outweigh possible risks.

 Not recommended. Excretion in human breastmilk unknown.

 Reduced renal function: In patients with end-stage renal disease (ESRD) who are dialysis-dependent, clearance is significantly reduced, resulting in prolonged elevation of TSH levels for up to two weeks. Increased risk of headache and nausea may occur. Use with caution and monitor closely in patients with renal impairment.

 In patients over 65 years, a careful risk—benefit assessment is recommended, especially those with heart disease or high-risk thyroid tumours.

APPENDIX 1: POISONING AND ITS TREATMENT

A poison can be defined as 'a substance (other than an infectious substance) that is harmful if ingested, inhaled, injected or absorbed through the skin' (Australian Resuscitation Guidelines (ARC) 2021). It should be noted, however, that any substance can be poisonous if the dose is large enough.

Poisons can include:
- prescription, over-the-counter (OTC) medications or other readily available substances taken in doses that are higher than recommended (e.g. alcohol, paracetamol, aspirin)
- illegal drug overdoses (e.g. heroin, morphine, ecstasy)
- gases (e.g. carbon monoxide from gas appliances or car emissions, bromine or chlorine gas)
- household products (e.g. cleaning products, furniture polish)
- pesticides
- plants (including mushrooms)
- metals (e.g. lead, mercury).

It is essential to prevent poisoning by:
- surveying home or workplace to identify any poisonous substances present
- minimising the amount of poisonous substances stored in the house
- correctly disposing of unwanted and out-of-date medicines by returning them to the local pharmacy (and not disposing in domestic waste or flushing down the toilet)
- leaving medicines and chemicals in the original containers (and not decanted into other containers such as soft drink bottles)
- ensuring medicines and chemicals are stored safely out of reach of children in locked or child-proof cupboards
- never leaving medicines unattended or within reach of children
- storing medicines separately from household products
- not referring to medicines as 'lollies'
- not taking other people's medicine
- checking with a pharmacist or doctor if uncertain about when or how to take medicines
- using appropriate protection (personal protective equipment) and ensuring adequate ventilation when using toxic or caustic chemicals (e.g. over-cleaning, spraying pesticides, painting) (ARC 2021).

Diagnosis of poisoning is usually made from the history and circumstantial evidence. Signs and symptoms of poisoning may include:
- burns or redness around the mouth and/or lips
- breath that smells like chemicals
- burns, stains and/or odour on the person or his/her clothing, furniture, floor or other surrounding area
- empty container(s), medication bottles or scattered pills
- person unexpectedly vomiting, becoming sleepy, restless or agitated, confused or having breathing difficulty, having either pinpoint or dilated pupils, unusual heart rate (slow or fast depending on the poisoning agent), having a seizure or becoming unconscious.

APPENDIX 1: POISONING AND ITS TREATMENT

- some poisons have delayed symptoms (hours, days or even months), which may make it difficult to connect the signs and symptoms with the offending agent(s) (e.g. paracetamol, lead, sustained/modified-release preparations).

Aims
The aims in treating poisoning are to:
- assess the severity of the poisoning
- identify the poison or poisons, if possible
- prevent poisoning of the rescuer
- remove or neutralise the poison before absorption or corrosion occurs
- apply first aid treatment.

Action
When treating poisoning, the Australian Resuscitation Council (2021) makes the following recommendations:
- If the person has collapsed, ring for an ambulance NOT the Poisons Information Centre.
- Do not put yourself in any danger (e.g. poorly ventilated room, contact with chemicals on the person's skin).
- Ensure that the person's airway, breathing and circulation are maintained. Commence cardiopulmonary resuscitation (CPR) if necessary and if the environment is safe to do so.
- Protect the spine, especially in an unconscious patient.
- If possible, obtain a history to ascertain the name of the product (and manufacturer), the type of contact with the poison (ingestion, inhalation, skin contamination), the amount ingested, the length of time elapsed since contact, any existing illnesses or allergies, current medications, any symptoms since contact and the weight of the person (especially if a child is involved). However, if the person is unconscious and the event was unwitnessed, this information may be difficult, if not impossible, to obtain. At times, some of this information may be obtained by counting missing tablets or questioning partners, carers or family members regarding what was available and/or quantities.
- Observe level of consciousness (e.g. conscious, unconscious, drowsy, responding to questions and commands), any seizure activity, colour (flushed, pallor, cyanotic), heart rate (is pulse present? rapid, slow, strong and bounding, weak and thready), peripheral perfusion, breathing (including any increased or decreased respiratory rate, breathing is laboured, wheezing or stridor present), difficulty swallowing, voice alteration, temperature (increased or decreased), hydration status and urine output.
- Collect evidence (e.g. medication containers, spilled pills) and samples of gastric contents, urine and blood, if required, possible and appropriate.

Swallowed poison
- Do not try and make the person vomit. Adsorbing with activated charcoal lowers blood concentrations more effectively than inducing vomiting. Vomiting is not recommended in all cases as severe damage to the oesophagus may occur if the substance taken is corrosive. Activated charcoal is not recommended in ALL cases of poisoning, so it is important to seek advice before taking any action.

- A sip of water may be used to wash out mouth.
- If the ingested poison is a button battery, it is time critical that an X-ray of neck, chest and abdomen is conducted. Endoscopic removal of the battery may be needed urgently.
- Seek advice from the Poisons Information Centre (see Appendix 2, p. 1687).

Inhaled poison
- Move patient into fresh air or admit fresh air to the area, if safe to do so. Avoid breathing in fumes.
- Check for any stridor or hoarse voice.
- Call for ambulance.

Poison in contact with skin
- Remove contaminated clothing and shoes and socks, avoiding contact with the poison/chemical.
- Drench contaminated area with tepid running water for at least 15—20 minutes, then wash area gently with soap and water and rinse well, taking care to wash behind ears, under nails and in skin folds.
- Use soap or shampoo if the poison was oily.
- Call for ambulance.

Poison in contact with eyes
- Timing is important as the corneal surface can be damaged rapidly and permanently scarred.
- Contact lenses should be removed if present.
- Holding eyelids apart, wash eyes thoroughly with copious amounts of water or saline for 15—20 minutes.
- Evert the lids to ensure adequate removal of the agent.
- Cover the eye(s) and transport patient for medical assessment.

Hospital management
- After the person has been transferred to hospital, Murray and collegues (2015) outline the following as being priorities of care:
  - airway, breathing and circulation
- assessment and correction of any:
  - seizure activity (generally managed with IV benzodiazepines; phenytoin is contraindicated in seizure management due to acute poisoning)
  - hypoglycaemia (may be associated with poisoning/overdose due to insulin, oral hypoglycaemic agents, chloroquine, salicylates, beta-adrenoceptor blocking agents and sodium valproate)
  - hypo- or hyperthermia (temperature $> 39.5°C$ is life threatening and requires immediate management to prevent organ damage or failure; severe hypothermia $< 29°C$ can imitate or cause cardiac arrest)
- administration of antidote — this is not always part of the resuscitation phase of poisoning management; however, it is dependent on the agent used (e.g. naloxone for opioid overdose; atropine for organophosphate poisoning)
- risk assessment is the next element of hospital management and involves identifying potential problems and making decisions about subsequent care (Murray et al 2015), involving steps identified earlier (identifying agent(s), amount ingested, time since ingestion, clinical features and progress, as well as patient-specific factors such as weight and co-morbidities)

APPENDIX 1: POISONING AND ITS TREATMENT

- initial hospital investigations should include:
  - 12-lead ECG (assessing rate, rhythm, PR interval, QRS interval, QT interval)
  - serum paracetamol level (normally done if 4 hours has elapsed and is implicated in overdose; however, non-detectable paracetamol levels more than 1 hour after ingestion excludes significant ingestion). Alanine amino-transferase (ALT) should also be measured in all patients along with serum paracetamol levels (Toxicology and Toxinology Expert Group 2020)
  - other investigations may include arterial blood gases, urine blood screen, baseline blood count, electrolytes, renal function, blood sugar, creatine kinase, troponins (especially if cocaine was used), and, if indicated, coagulation studies, liver function tests, and/or specific drug tests
- the patient should be closely and continuously monitored, including the circulation (pulse, blood pressure, peripheral perfusion), urine output, temperature, hydration, respiration (airway protective reflexes, respiratory rate, air entry, breath sounds, pulse oximetry) and neurological status (including conscious state) (Glasgow Coma Scale, seizure activity)
- duration of observation is dependent on agent(s) ingested, formulation (e.g. immediate-release tablets or sustained release) and potential complications
- determine the time of poison ingestion (if possible), because there is little benefit in emptying the stomach if more than 3 hours have elapsed since ingestion
- stomach should not be emptied if the airway cannot be protected or if a petroleum distillate or corrosive substance has been ingested
- specific antidotes may be given for a limited number of drugs (e.g. naloxone for opiates, acetylcysteine for paracetamol, fresh frozen plasma and vitamin K for warfarin, chelating agents for heavy metals, flumazenil for benzodiazepines, hyperbaric oxygen for carbon monoxide, glucagon, isoprenaline and pacing for beta-adrenergic blocking agents) (see Antidotes, antagonists and chelating agents, p. 334)
- the patient may also need fluid therapy and oxygen
- enhanced removal techniques may be used to remove some agents. These include repeat doses of activated charcoal, forced diuresis, alkalinisation of the urine, peritoneal or haemodialyis or haemoperfusion
- admission to ICU may be required if haemodialysis, prolonged or invasive haemodynamic monitoring is required and/or the patient is ventilated
- formal psychiatric and social work assessments may be necessary before discharge, with the patient given access to social work, counselling and other resources (e.g. drug and alcohol counselling) if the poisoning was a deliberate attempt at self-harm.

TREATMENT WITH ACTIVATED CHARCOAL (CARBOSORB X)

Action and use

- absorbs most inorganic and organic compounds in the alimentary tract, so reducing or preventing systemic

absorption. Drugs that are well absorbed include aspirin, amphetamines, barbiturates, cocaine, digoxin, morphine and phenothiazines. Drugs that are poorly bound to activated charcoal include corrosive acids or alkalis, metals (e.g. lithium, iron, potassium, lead, arsenic and mercury), alcohols and hydrocarbons
- may be given after emptying stomach contents by emesis or washout (gastric lavage), although activated charcoal is increasingly being used in emergency departments as first-line management of ingested poisoning. The earlier the charcoal is given, the more effective it is likely to be. Emesis should not be used if the person is drowsy, unconscious, fitting or likely to become drowsy within 30 minutes of taking an emetic.

Adult dose
- 1 g/kg orally or via nasogastric/orogastric tube as soon as possible after ingestion or suspected ingestion of the potential poison or after induced emesis or stomach washout (may be repeated 2—6-hourly until first black stool has been passed (maximum dose 50 g)).

Paediatric dose
- 1 g/kg orally or via nasogastric tube.

Nursing considerations/Cautions
- if antidote to a specific drug is available, it should be used as first-line treatment. Specific antidotes should not be given with activated charcoal as they may be adsorbed
- risk versus harm should be assessed before administration
- activated charcoal should be administered as soon as possible after poison ingestion or up to 2 hours after immediate-release or 4 hours after sustained-release preparations
- any concurrent medication should preferably be given parenterally
- bowel sounds should be assessed before any dose (or repeat dose) of activated charcoal
- colours faeces black
- caution if given to patients with diabetes as Carbosorb X contains 0.46 g sucrose/mL
- contraindicated in poisoning due to strong acids and alkalis and where adsorptive capacity is too low to treat poisoning (e.g. iron salts, ferrous sulfate, cyanides, other sulfonylureas, malathion, lithium, ethanol, methanol, ethylene glycol and hydrocarbons)
- contraindicated if airway is not protected, corrosive agent was ingested or the gastrointestinal tract is not intact
- see also Antidotes, antagonists and chelating agents (p. 334)

Note
- contained in Carbosorb XS with sorbitol.

APPENDIX 2: POISONS INFORMATION CENTRES

When contacting the Poisons Information Centre, it is useful to provide the following information if possible or available:

- name of toxin or drug (with exact name and spelling, if possible)
- patient details (age, weight, sex, medical history, medication history)
- whether the poisoning was deliberate, intentional or accidental
- exposure details (e.g. time since exposure, route, dose)
- any immediate first aid action taken
- basic observations if possible (including heart rate, respiratory rate, temperature, consciousness level) and
- any clinical symptoms (Toxicology and Toxinology Expert Group 2020).

Australia

Please call: 13 11 26
(24-hour line, Australia-wide) (cost of a local call excluding mobile phones) for information and advice on emergency treatment of poisoning, bites and stings in all Australian states and territories.

New Zealand

In New Zealand call: 0800 764 766 (0800 POISON)

APPENDIX 3: CHANGES TO DRUG NAMES

From April 2016, drug ingredient names are being updated to bring Australia in line with the rest of the world. The goal of this is to ensure international conformity in order to promote patient safety by eliminating major name differences between Australia and other countries. It is expected that these changes will be completed by 2023, with products displaying dual labelling until that time. The table below outlines these changes.

Previous term	Current term
Adrenaline and noradrenaline	
adrenaline	adrenaline (epinephrine)
noradrenaline	noradrenaline (norepinephrine)
Other significant changes	
diclofenac diethylammonium	diclofenac diethylamine
hexamine hippurate	methenamine hippurate
insulin — human	insulin
tetrahydrozoline hydrochloride	tetryzoline hydrochloride
thyroxine sodium	levothyroxine sodium
Minor spelling changes	
amoxycillin	amoxicillin
amoxycillin sodium	amoxicillin sodium
amoxycillin trihydrate	amoxicillin trihydrate
atracurium besylate	atracurium besilate
beclomethasone	beclometasone (beclomethasone)
beclomethasone dipropionate	beclometasone dipropionate
benztropine mesylate	benztropine mesilate

Previous term	Current term
bromocriptine mesylate	bromocriptine mesilate
cephalexin	cefalexin monohydrate
cephalothin sodium	cefalotin sodium
cephazolin	cefazolin
cephazolin sodium	cefazolin sodium
chlorthalidone	chlortalidone
cholecalciferol	colecalciferol
cholestyramine	colestyramine
clomiphene citrate	clomifene citrate
cyclosporin	ciclosporin
dexamphetamine sulfate	dexamfetamine sulfate
dextropropoxyphene napsylate	dextropropoxyphene napsilate
dolasetron mesylate	dolasetron mesilate monohydrate
ethacrynic acid	etacrynic acid
ethinyloestradiol	ethinylestradiol
flumethasone	flumetasone
flupenthixol decanoate	flupentixol decanoate
glutaraldehyde	glutaral

APPENDIX 3: CHANGES TO DRUG NAMES

Previous term	Current term
heparinoid	heparinoids
indomethacin	indometacin
lapatinib ditosylate monohydrate	lapatinib ditosilate monohydrate
oestradiol	estradiol
oestradiol valerate	estradiol valerate
oestriol	estriol
oestrogens — conjugated	conjugated estrogens
pentamidine isethionate	pentamidine isetionate
pericyazine	periciazaine
sorafenib tosylate	sorafenib tosilate
testosterone enanthate	testosterone enantate
thioguanine	tioguanine
Additional minor changes	
disodium pamidronate	pamidronate disodium
pramipexole hydrochloride	pramipexole dihydrochloride
samarium	samarium (153Sm)

Previous term	Current term
Dual labelling required till 2023	
actinomycin D	dactinomycin (actinomycin D)
amethocaine hydrochloride	tetracaine (amethocaine) hydrochloride
amphotericin	amphotericin B (amphotericin)
Bacillus Calmette and Guerin	Mycobacterium bovis (Bacillus Calmette and Guerin (BCG) strain)
benzhexol hydrochloride	trihexyphenidyl (benzhexol) hydrochloride

Previous term	Current term
colaspase	asparaginase (colaspase)
cysteamine bitartrate	mercaptamine (cysteamine) bitartrate
dothiepin hydrochloride	dosulepin (dothiepin) hydrochloride
doxycycline hydrochloride	doxycycline hyclate (hydrochloride)
eformoterol fumarate	formoterol (eformoterol) fumarate
eformoterol fumarate dihydrate	formoterol (eformoterol) fumarate dihydrate
frusemide	furosemide (frusemide)
glycopyrrolate	glycopyrronium bromide (glycopyrrolate)
hydroxyurea	hydroxycarbamide (hydroxyurea)
lignocaine	lidocaine (lignocaine)
lignocaine hydrochloride	lidocaine (lignocaine) hydrochloride monohydrate
oxpentifylline	pentoxifylline (oxpentifylline)
phenobarbitone	phenobarbital (phenobarbitone)
procaine penicillin	procaine benzylpenicillin (procaine penicillin)
salcatonin	calcitonin salmon (salcatonin)
tetracosactrin	tetracosactide (tetracosactrin)
trimeprazine tartrate	alimemazine (trimeprazine) tartrate

Source: Therapeutic Goods Administration (TGA) (2020). Updating medicine ingredient names — list of affected ingredients. Therapeutic Goods Administration, Department of Health, Australian Government, www.tga.gov.au/updating-medicine-ingredient-names-list-affected-ingredients

BIBLIOGRAPHY

Advanced Pharmacy Australia (2025). Don't rush to crush. https://app.emims.plus/Drtc#beforeyoucrush

Alzheimer's Research Australia (2024). What is Alzheimer's? https://alzheimersresearch.org.au/alzheimers/what-is-alzheimers/

Anderson, I. (2013). How to ... Ten top tips on compliance, concordance and adherence. Wounds International 4(2), 9–12.

Andrews, G., Bell, C., Boyce, P. et al (2018). Royal Australian and New Zealand College of Psychiatrists clinical practice guidelines for the treatment of panic disorder, social anxiety disorder and generalised anxiety disorder. Australian and New Zealand Journal of Psychiatry 52(12), 1109–1172.

Antman, E. & Loscalzo, J. (2019). Ch. 267. Ischaemic heart disease. In: J.L. Jameson, A.S. Fauci, D.L. Kasper et al (eds). Harrison's principles of internal medicine, 20th edn. McGraw-Hill (Online edition).

Appleton, L., Gill, T., Lang, C. et al (2018). Prevalence and comorbidity of sleep conditions in Australian adults: 2016 Sleep Health Foundation national survey. Sleep Health 4, 13–19.

Arruda, V. & High, K. (2018). Ch. 112. Coagulation disorders. In: J.L. Jameson, A.S. Fauci, D.L. Kasper et al (eds). Harrison's principles of internal medicine, 20th edn. McGraw-Hill. (Online edition).

Arthritis Australia (2024). Rheumatoid arthritis. https://arthritisaustralia.com.au/types-of-arthritis/rheumatoid-arthritis/

Aruanno, M., Glampedakis, E., & Lamoth, F. (2019). Echinocandins for the treatment of invasive Aspegillosis: From laboratory to bedside. Antimicrob Agents Chemother. 25;63(8):e00399-19. https://doi.org/10.1128/AAC.00399-19

Atik, A. (2013). Adherence to the Australian National Inpatient Medication Chart: the efficacy of a uniform national drug chart on improving prescription error. Journal of Evaluation in Clinical Practice 19(5), 769–772.

Australian Action on Pre-Eclampsia (N.D.) What is pre-eclampsia? https://www.aapec.org.au/what-is-preeclampsia/

BIBLIOGRAPHY

Australian Bureau of Statistics (ABS) (2023). National study of mental health and well being. https://www.abs.gov.au/statistics/health/mental-health/national-study-mental-health-and-wellbeing/latest-release

Australian Bureau of Statistics (ABSB) (2023B). Hypertension and high measured blood pressure. https://www.abs.gov.au/statistics/health/health-conditions-and-risks/hypertension-and-high-measured-blood-pressure/latest-release

Australian Bureau of Statistics (ABS) (2022). Waist circumference and BMI. ABS. https://www.abs.gov.au/statistics/health/health-conditions-and-risks/waist-circumference-and-bmi/latest-release.

Australian Bureau of Statistics (ABS) (2019). Australian Health Survey: first results, 2017–2018. Cat. no. 4364.0.55.001. Online. Available: www.abs.gov.au/ausstats/abs.

Australian Commission on Safety and Quality in Health Care (ACSQHC) (2024) Delirium clinical standard 2021. https://www.safetyandquality.gov.au/standards/clinical-care-standards/delirium-clinical-care-standard

Australian Commission on Safety and Quality in Health Care (ACSQHC) (2025). Electronic medication chart. https://www.safetyandquality.gov.au/our-work/medicines-safety-and-quality/electronic-medication-charts

Australian Commission on Safety and Quality in Health Care (ACSQHC) (2019). National inpatient medication chart – development and background. Online. Available: www.safetyandquality.gov.au/our-work/medication-safety/medication-charts/background-and-development-medication-charts/national-inpatient-medication-chartdevelopment-and-background.

Australian Commission on Safety and Quality in Health Care (ACSQHC) (2021). National standard medication charts. Online. Available:. https://www.safetyandquality.gov.au/our-work/medicines-safety-and-quality/medication-charts

Australian Commission on Safety and Quality in Health Care (ACSQHC) (2016a). National recommendations for user-applied labelling of injectable medicines, fluids and lines. Online. Available: www.safetyandquality.gov.au/our-work/medication-safety/safer-naming-labelling-and-packaging-medicines/recommendations-terminologyabbreviations-and-symbols-used-medicines-documentation.

Australian Commission on Safety and Quality in Health Care (ACSQHC) (2016b). Recommendations for terminology, abbreviations and symbols used in the prescribing and administration of medicines. Online. Available: www.safetyandquality.gov.au/sites/default/files/migrated/Recommendations-for-terminology-abbreviations-and-symbolsused-in-medicines-documentation-Summary-sheet-December-2016.pdf.

Australian Commission on Safety and Quality in Health Care (ACSQHC) (2002). Second national report on patient safety: improving medication safety. Australian Department of Health and Ageing, Canberra.

Australian Government, Department of Health (2020). National Immunisation Program. Online. Available: https://www.health.gov.au/health-topics/immunisation/immunisationthrough
out-life/national-immunisation-program-schedule.

Australian Government, Department of Health (2019). Clinical practice guidelines: pregnancy care. Online. Available: https://www.health.gov.au/resources/pregnancy-careguidelines.

Australian Government, Department of Health and Aged Care. (2023). Australian categorization system for prescribing drugs in pregnancy. Online. Available: https://www.tga.gov.au/australian-categorisation-system-prescribing-medicines-pregnancy.

Australian Government, Department of Health, Disability and Aging (2023). National return and disposal of unwanted medication program (NatRUM). Available https://www.health.gov.au/our-work/national-return-and-disposal-of-unwanted-medicines-program-natrum?language=en

Australian Government, Department of Health (2024a). Chronic respiratory conditions: Asthma - Australian Institute of Health and Welfare, Available https://www.aihw.gov.au/reports/chronic-respiratory-conditions/asthma

Australian Government, Department of Health (2024b). Diabetes. https://www.aihw.gov.au/reports-data/health-conditions-disability-deaths/diabetes/overview

Australian Government, Department of Health (2024c). Mental health. https://www.aihw.gov.au/mental-health

Australian Government, Department of Health (2024d). Dementia. https://www.aihw.gov.au/reports-data/health-conditions-disability-deaths/dementia/overview

Australian Institute of Health and Welfare (AIHW) (2024e). Chronic musculoskeletal conditions. Online. Available: https://www.aihw.gov.au/reports-data/health-conditions-disability-deaths/chronic-musculoskeletal-conditions/overview.

Australian Institute of Health and Welfare (AIHW)(2024). Chronic musculoskeletal conditions. https://www.aihw.gov.au/reports/chronic-musculoskeletal-conditions/musculoskeletal-conditions/contents/arthritis

BIBLIOGRAPHY

Australian Government, Department of Health and Welfare (2024). Chronic musculoskeletal conditions: Gout. https://www.aihw.gov.au/reports/chronic-musculoskeletal-conditions/gout

Australian Government, Department of Health (2022). Epilepsy in Australia. https://www.aihw.gov.au/reports/chronic-disease/epilepsy-in-australia/contents/about

Australian Government, Department of Health (2021). Sleep problems as a risk factor for chronic conditions. Online. Available: https://www.aihw.gov.au/reports/risk-factors/sleep-problems-as-a-risk-factor/summary

Australian Institute of Health and Welfare (AIHW) (2020). Australia's health – causes of death. Online. Available: https://www.aihw.gov.au/reports/australias-health/causes-of-death.

Australian Institute of Health and Welfare (AIHW) (2019a). Arthritis. Cat. no. PHE 234. AIHW, Canberra. Online. Available: https://www.aihw.gov.au/reports/chronic-musculoskeletalconditions/arthritis.

Australian Institute of Health and Welfare (AIHW) (2019b). Asthma. AIHW, Canberra. Online. Available: https://www.aihw.gov.au/reports/chronic-respiratory-conditions/asthma/contents/asthma.

Australian Institute of Health and Welfare (AIHW) (2019c). Dementia. Online. Available: https://www.aihw.gov.au/reports-data/health-conditions-disability-deaths/dementia/overview.

Australian Institute of Health and Welfare (AIHW) (2019d). Diabetes. AIHW, Canberra. Online. Available: https://www.aihw.gov.au/reports/diabetes/diabetes/contents/what-is-diabetes.

Australian Institute of Health and Welfare (AIHW) (2019e). Incidence of gestational diabetes in Australia. AIHW, Canberra. Online. Available: https://www.aihw.gov.au/reports/diabetes/incidence-of-gestational-diabetes-in-australia/contents/what-is-gestational-diabetes.

Australian Institute of Health and Welfare (AIHW) (2019f). Osteoporosis. Cat. no. PHE 178. AIHW, Canberra. Online. Available: https://www.aihw.gov.au/reports/chronic-musculoskeletal-conditions/osteoporosis/contents/what-is-osteoporosis.

Australian Institute of Health and Welfare (AIHW) (2019g). Rheumatoid arthritis. Cat. no. PHE 252. AIHW, Canberra. Online. Available: https://www.aihw.gov.au/reports/chronicmusculoskeletal-conditions/rheumatoid-arthritis.

Australian Institute of Health and Welfare (AIHW) (2017). Gout. AIHW, Canberra. Online. Available: www.aihw.gov.au/.

Australian Resuscitation Council (ARC) (2011). Guideline 9.4.8. Envenomation – pressure immobilization technique. Online. Available: resus.org.au/?wpfb_dl=44.

Australian Resuscitation Council (ARC) (2011, amended 2021). Guideline 9.5.1. Emergency management of a patient who has been poisoned. Online. Available: resus.org.au/guidelines/.

Australian Technical Advisory Group on Immunisation (ATAGI) (2018). Australian immunisation handbook. Australian Government Department of Health, Canberra. Online. Available: immunisationhandbook.health.gov.au.

Austroads (2022). Assessing fitness to drive – seizures and epilepsy. https://austroads.gov.au/publications/assessing-fitness-to-drive/ap-g56/neurological-conditions/seizures-and-epilepsy.

Banga, S. & Chalfoun, N.T. (2018). Ch. 9. Arrhythmias and antiarrhythmic drugs. In: A. Elmoselhi (ed). Cardiology: an integrated approach. McGraw-Hill. (Online edition).

Barbieri, R. & Repke, J. (2018). Ch. 466. Medical disorders during pregnancy. In: J.L. Jameson, A.S. Fauci, D.L. Kasper et al (eds). Harrison's principles of internal medicine, 20th edn. McGraw-Hill. (Online edition).

Brenner, G. & Stevens, C. (2017). Brenner & Stevens' pharmacology, 5th edn. Elsevier, Philadelphia.

Bringhurst F, Kronenberg H.M., & Liu E.S. (2022). Ch 409. Bone and mineral metabolism in health and disease. Loscalzo J, & Fauci A, & Kasper D, & Hauser S, & Longo D, & Jameson J(Eds.), *Harrison's Principles of Internal Medicine, 21e.* McGraw-Hill Education

Bringhurst, F.R., Demay, M. & Kronenberg, H. (2019). Ch. 402. Bone and mineral metabolism in health and disease. In: J.L. Jameson, A.S. Fauci, D.L. Kasper et al (eds). Harrison's principles of internal medicine, 20th edn. McGraw-Hill. (Online edition).

Brown, R.H. (2019). Ch. 429. Amyotrophic lateral sclerosis and other motor neuron diseases. In: J.L. Jameson, A.S. Fauci, D.L. Kasper et al (eds). Harrison's principles of internal medicine, 20th edn. McGraw-Hill. (Online edition).

Bryant, B., Knights, K., Darroch, S. et al (2019). Pharmacology for health professionals, 5th edn. Elsevier, Chatswood.

Butterworth, J., Mackey, D. & Wasnick, J. (2018). Morgan & Mikhail's clinical anesthesiology, 6th edn. McGraw-Hill. (Online edition).

BIBLIOGRAPHY

Camilleri, M., & Murray, J.A. (2026). Diarrhea and constipation. In: Longo, D, & Fauci, A, & Kasper, D, & Hauser, S, & Jameson, J, & Loscalzo J, & Holland, S, & Langford, C (Eds.), *Harrison's Principles of Internal Medicine, 22nd Edition*. McGrawHill. https://accessmedicine.mhmedical.com/content.aspx?bookid=3541&sectionid=293067526

Capuano V, Marchese F, Capuano R, et al. Hyperuricemia as an independent risk factor for major cardiovascular events: a 10-year cohort study from Southern Italy. J Cardiovasc Med (Hagerstown). 2017 Mar;18(3):159-164. https://doi.org/10.2459/JCM.0000000000000347.

Carruthers, A., Naughton, K. & Mallarkey, G. (2008). Accuracy of packaging of dose administration aids in regional aged care facilities in the Hunter area of New South Wales. Medical Journal of Australia 188(5), 280–282.

Centers for Disease Control & Prevention (CDC) (2016). About parasites. Online. Available: https://www.cdc.gov/parasites/about.html.

Cheeley, J.T., & Lawley, L.P. (2026). Eczema, psoriasis, cutaneous infections, acne, and other common skin disorders. In: Longo, D., Fauci, A., Kasper, D., Hauser, S., Jameson, J., Loscalzo, J., Holland, S., & Langford, C. (Eds.), *Harrison's Principles of Internal Medicine, 22nd Edition*. McGraw Hill. https://accessmedicine.mhmedical.com/content.aspx?bookid=3541&sectionid=293068042

Cree, B. & Hauser, S. (2019). Multiple sclerosis. In: J.L. Jameson, A.S. Fauci, D.L. Kasper et al (eds). Harrison's principles of internal medicine, 20th edn. McGraw-Hill. (Online edition).

Preterm birth. In Cunningham F, Leveno K.J., Dashe J.S., Hoffman B.L., Spong C.Y., Casey B.M. (Eds.), *Williams Obstetrics, 26e*. McGraw Hill. https://accessmedicine.mhmedical.com/content.aspx?bookid=2977&sectionid=263821201

Del Valle J. Peptic Ulcer Disease and Related Disorders. In: Longo D, Fauci A, Kasper D, Hauser S, Jameson J, Loscalzo J, Holland S, Langford C. eds. *Harrison's Principles of Internal Medicine, 22nd Edition*. McGraw Hill; 2026. Accessed October 02, 2025. https://accesspharmacy.mhmedical.com/content.aspx?bookid=3541&sectionid=296167454

Del Valle, J. (2018). Ch. 317. Peptic ulcer disease and related disorders. In: J.L. Jameson, A.S. Fauci, D.L. Kasper et al (eds). Harrison's principles of internal medicine, 20th edn. McGraw-Hill. (Online edition).

Del Valle J. (2026). Peptic Ulcer Disease and Related Disorders. In: Longo D, Fauci A, Kasper D, Hauser S, Jameson J, Loscalzo J, Holland S, Langford C. eds. Harrison's Principles of Internal Medicine, 22nd Edition. McGraw Hill; 2026. (Online edition).

Deloitte Access Economics (2019). The cost of pain in Australia. Online. Available: www.deloitte.com/au/en/pages/economics/articles/cost-pain-australia.html.

Deloitte Access Economics (2018). Migraine in Australia Whitepaper. Online. Available: www.painaustralia.org.au/static/uploads/files/deloitte-au-economics-migraine-australiawhitepaper-101018-wfsydysdysky.pdf.

Department For Health & Ageing, Government Of South Australia (2018). Perinatal practice guidelines – Ovarian Hyperstimulation Syndrome. https://www.sahealth.sa.gov.au/wps/wcm/connect/9b61ed004ee5348da663afd150ce4f37/Ovarian+Hyperstimulation+Syndrome_PPG_v3_0.pdf?MOD=AJPERES&CACHEID=ROOTWORKSPACE-9b61ed004ee5348da663afd150ce4f37-p4choud

Derry, S., Wiffen, P., Kalso, E. et al (2019). Topical analgesics for acute and chronic pain in adults – an overview of Cochrane reviews. Cochrane Database of Systematic Reviews 2017, 5, CD008609; CD008609.pub2 (updated).

Douglas V.C. & Aminoff M.J. (2025). Movement disorders. Papadakis M.A., & Rabow M.W., & McQuaid K.R., & Gandhi M(Eds.), *Current Medical Diagnosis & Treatment 2025*. McGraw-Hill Education. https://accessmedicine.mhmedical.com/content.aspx?bookid=3495&sectionid=288492928

Eatforhealth.gov.au. (n.d.). Nutrient reference values for Australia and New Zealand – iodine https://www.eatforhealth.gov.au/search?search=iodine

Edwards, J.E. (2018). Ch. 206. Diagnois and treatment of fungal infections. In: J.L. Jameson, A.S. Fauci, D.L. Kasper et al (eds). Harrison's principles of internal medicine, 20th edn. McGraw-Hill. (Online edition).

Eilers H, & Yost S (2024). Ch 25. General anesthetics. In: Vanderah T.W. (Ed.), Katzung's basic & clinical pharmacology, 16th edn. McGraw-Hill. (Online edition).

Elliott, R. (2014). Appropriate use of dose administration aids. Australian Prescriber, 37, 46–50.

Faculty of Pain Medicine (FPM), Australian and New Zealand College of Anaesthetists (ANZCA) (2015). Recommendations regarding the use of opioid analgesics in patients with chronic non-cancer pain. Online. Available: http://fpm.anzca.edu.au/documents/pm1-2010.

Fantry G.T. (2024). Ch 62. Drugs used in the treatment of gastrointestinal diseases. In: Vanderah T.W. (Ed.), Katzung's basic & clinical pharmacology, 16th edn. McGraw-Hill. (Online edition).

Fasanya, H., Hsiao, C., Armstrong-Sylvester, K. & Beal, S. *Journal of Applied Laboratory Medicine*, Volume 6, Issue 1, January 2021, Pages 247–256, https://doi.org/10.1093/jalm/jfaa149

Favus, M. & Vokes, T. (2019). Ch. 405. Paget's disease and other dysplagias of bone. In: J.L. Jameson, A.S. Fauci, D.L. Kasper et al (eds). Harrison's principles of internal medicine, 20th edn. McGraw-Hill. (Online edition).

Flenady, V., Wojcieszek, A.M., Papatsonis, D.N.M. et al (2014). Calcium channel blockers for inhibiting preterm labour and birth. Cochrane Database of Systematic Reviews 6, CD002255.

Food Standards, Australia & New Zealand (2023). Iodine fortification. Online. Available: https://www.foodstandards.gov.au/consumer/food-fortification/iodine-fortification.

Food Standards, Australia & New Zealand (2023). Iodine fortification. Online. Available: https://www.foodstandards.gov.au/consumer/food-fortification/iodine-fortification

Gao, K. (2024). Mood disorders. Ebert M.H., & Martin P.R., & McVoy M, & Ronis R.J., & Weissman S.H.(Eds.), *Current Diagnosis & Treatment: Psychiatry, 4th Edition*. McGraw Hill. https://accessmedicine.mhmedical.com/content.aspx?bookid=3507&sectionid=289853568

Gelber, R.H. (2018). Ch. 203. Leprosy. In: J.L. Jameson, A.S. Fauci, D.L. Kasper et al (eds). Harrison's principles of internal medicine, 20th edn. McGraw-Hill. (Online edition).

Gilmartin, J.F-M., Marriott, J.L. & Hussainy, S.Y. (2016). Improving Australian care home medicine supply services: evaluation of quality improvement intervention. Australian Journal of Ageing 35(2), E1–6.

Goadsby, P.J. (2021). Headache research in 2020: disrupting and improving practice. *Lancet Neurology*, 20(1), 7-8. https://dx.doi.org/10.1016/S1474-4422(20)30457-9

Migraine & Headache Australia (2024). Migraine. https://headacheaustralia.org.au/migraine/

Goel, H., Lusher, A. & Boneh, A. (2010). Pediatric mortality due to inborn errors of metabolism in Victoria, Australia: a population-based study. JAMA. 2010;304(10):1070–1072. https://doi.org/10.1001/jama.2010.1259

Gowan, J. & Roller, L. (2010). Crushing medications: dose delivery challenges for people with impaired swallowing. Australian Journal of Pharmacy 91, 50–54.

Grosser, T., Smyth, E. & FitzGerald, G. (2018). Ch. 38. Pharmacotherapy of inflammation, fever, pain and gout. In: L. Brunton, R. Hilal-Dandan & B.C. Knollman (eds). Goodman and Gilman's: the pharmacological basis of therapeutics, 13th edn. (Online edition).

Gunning, K., Pippitt, K., Kiraly, B. et al (2012). Lice and scabies: treatment update. American Family Physician 99(10), 635–642.

Hall, J. (2018). Ch. 389. Infertility and contraception. In: J.L. Jameson, A.S. Fauci, D.L. Kasper et al (eds). Harrison's principles of internal medicine, 20th edn. McGraw-Hill. (Online edition).

Harris, B.R. & Cooper, A.J. (2017). Modern management of acne. Medical Journal of Australia 206(1), 41–45.

Hasler W.L. (2022). Ch 45. Nausea, vomiting, and indigestion. In: J. Loscalzo, A. Fauci, D. Kasper, S. Hauser, D. Longo, & J. Jameson (eds.), Harrison's Principles of Internal Medicine, 21st edn. Mcgraw-Hill. (Online edition).

Hasler, W. (2018). Ch. 41. Nausea, vomiting and indigestion. In: J.L. Jameson, A.S. Fauci, D.L. Kasper et al (eds). Harrison's principles of internal medicine, 20th edn. McGraw-Hill. (Online edition).

Heart Foundation (2023). Hypertension clinical information and guidelines. Online. Available: https://www.heartfoundation.org.au/for-professionals/hypertension

Hempenstall, A., Smith, S. & Hanson, J. (2019). Leprosy in Far North Queensland: almost gone, but not to be forgotten. Medical Journal of Australia 211(4), 182–183.

Hendrick, L. (2017). Ch. 16. The structure and function of the haematological system. In: J. Craft & C. Gordon (eds). Understanding pathophysiology, 3rd edn. Elsevier, Chatswood.

Hogg, K. & Weitz, J. (2018). Ch. 32. Blood coagulation, anticoagulant, fibrinolytic and antiplatelet drugs. In: L. Brunton, R. Hilal-Dandan & B.C. Knollman (eds). Goodman and Gilman's: the pharmacological basis of therapeutics, 13th edn. (Online edition).

Holland, S. (2018). Ch. 175. Nontuberculous mycobacterial infections. In: J.L. Jameson, A.S. Fauci, D.L. Kasper et al (eds). Harrison's principles of internal medicine, 20th edn. McGraw-Hill. (Online edition).

Hopkins, R. & Grabowski, G. (2019). Ch. 411. Lysosomal storage diseases. In: J.L. Jameson, A.S. Fauci, D.L. Kasper et al (eds). Harrison's principles of internal medicine, 20th edn. McGraw-Hill. (Online edition).

Hormones Australia (2023). The thyroid gland. Online. Available: https://www.hormones-australia.org.au/the-endocrine-system/thyroid/

Hotham, N. & Hotham, E. (2015). Drugs in breastfeeding. Australian Prescriber 38(5), 156–160.

International Association for the Study of Pain (IASP) (2017). IASP terminology. Online. Available: www.iasp-pain.org/Education/Content.aspx?ItemNumber=1698#Pain.

BIBLIOGRAPHY

International Diabetes Federation (IDF) (2021). Facts and figures. https://idf.org/about-diabetes/diabetes-facts-figures/

International Headache Society (2019). The international classification of headache disorders, 3rd edn. Online. Available: https://ichd-3.org/.

Iwasaki, A. & Omer, S.B. (2020). Why and how vaccines work. Cell. 2020 Oct 15;183(2):290-295. https://doi.org/10.1016/j.cell.2020.09.040. PMID: 33064982; PMCID: PMC7560117.

Jain R.K. & Vokes T.J. (2022). Ch 412 Paget's disease and other dysplasias of bone. In: J. Loscalzo, A. Fauci, D. Kasper, S. Hauser, D. Longo, & J. Jameson (eds.), Harrison's principles of internal medicine, 21st edn. McGraw-Hill Education. (Online edn).

Jameson, J.L., Fauci, A.S., Kasper D.L. et al (eds). (2020). Ch. 123. Chronic stable angina. In: J.L. Jameson, A.S. Fauci, D.L. Kasper (eds). Harrison's manual of medicine, 20th edn. McGraw-Hill. (Online edition).

Jameson, J.L., Mandel, S. & Weetman, A. (2022a). Hyperthyroidism. In: Loscalzo, J., Fauci A., Kasper, D., Hauser, S., Longo, D. & Jameson, J. (eds). Harrison's principles of internal medicine, 21st edn. McGraw-Hill Education. https://accessmedicine.mhmedical.com/content.aspx?bookid=3095&sectionid=265439848

Jameson, J.L., Mandel, S. & Weetman, A. (2022b). Hypothyroidism. In: Loscalzo, J., Fauci A., Kasper, D., Hauser, S., Longo, D. & Jameson, J. (eds). Harrison's principles of internal medicine, 21st edn. McGraw-Hill Education. https://accessmedicine.mhmedical.com/content.aspx?bookid=3095&sectionid=265439848

Jameson, J.L., Mandel, S. & Weetman, A. (2022c). Thyroid gland physiology and testing. In: Loscalzo, J., Fauci A., Kasper, D., Hauser, S., Longo, D. & Jameson, J. (eds). Harrison's principles of internal medicine, 21st edn. McGraw-Hill. (Online edition).

Jokanovic, N., Ferrah, N., Lovell, J. et al (2019). A review of coronial investigations into medication-related deaths in residential care. Research in Social and Administrative Pharmacy 15, 410–416.

Karrer, S., Martingano, D. & Hong, P. (2024). Pre-eclampsia. https://www.ncbi.nlm.nih.gov/books/NBK570611/

Karsan, N., Bose, P. & Goadsby, P. (2018). The migraine premonitory phase. Continuum: Lifelong Learning in Neurology 24(4), 996–1008.

Katzung, B. (2018). Ch. 12. Vasodilators and the treatment of angina pectoris. In: B. Katzung (ed). Basic and clinical pharmacology, 14th edn. (Online edition).

Keiser, J., McCarthy, J. & Hotez P.J. (2018). Chemotherapy of helminth infections. In: L. Brunton, R. Hilal-Dandan & B.C. Knollman (eds). Goodman and Gilman's: the pharmacological basis of therapeutics, 13th edn. (Online edition).

Khosla, S. (2019). Ch. 50. Hypercalcemia and hypocalcemia. In: J.L. Jameson, A.S. Fauci, D.L. Kasper et al (eds). Harrison's principles of internal medicine, 20th edn. McGraw-Hill. (Online edition).

Knights, K., Darroch, S., Rowland, A. & Bushell, M. (2023). Pharmacology for health professionals (6th ed.). Elsevier Australia. https://www.google.com.au/books/edition/Pharmacology_for_Health_Professionals/I5iZEAAAQBAJ?hl=en&gbpv=1&printsec=frontcove

Konkie, B. (2018). Ch. 111. Disorders of platelets and vessel wall. In: J.L. Jameson, A.S. Fauci, D.L. Kasper et al (eds). Harrison's principles of internal medicine, 20th edn. McGraw-Hill. (Online edition).

Kruidering-Hall M, & Campbell L.J. (2024). Ch 27. Skeletal muscle relaxants. In: T.W. Vanderah (ed.), Katzung's basic & clinical pharmacology, 16th edn. Mcgraw-Hill. (Online edn).

Kushner, R.F. (2022). Evaluation and management of obesity. Loscalzo J, & Fauci A, & Kasper D, & Hauser S, & Longo D, & Jameson J (Eds.), Harrison's Principles of Internal Medicine, 21e. McGraw-Hill Education. https://accessmedicine.mhmedical.com/content.aspx?bookid=3095&sectionid=265445754

Lander, C. (2008). Antepileptic drugs in pregnancy and lactation. Australian Prescriber 31(3), 70–72.

Lawley, L., McCall, C. & Lawley, T. (2025). Ch. 53. Eczema, psoriasis, cutaneous infections, acne and other common skin infections. In: Longo, D., Fauci, A., Kasper, D., Hauser, S., Jameson, J., Loscalzo, J., Holland, S., & Langford, C. (Eds.), *Harrison's Principles of Internal Medicine, 22nd Edition*. McGraw Hill. https://accessmedicine.mhmedical.com/content.aspx?bookid=3541&sectionid=293068042

Levison, W. (2014). Review of medical microbiology and immunology, 13th edn. McGraw-Hill. (Online edition).

Lin, Y.C., Wan, L. & Jamison, R. (2017). Using integrative medicine in pain management: an evaluation of current practice. Anesthesia and Analgesia 125(6), 2081–2093.

Lindsay, R. & Cosman, F. (2019). Ch. 404. Osteoporosis. In: J.L. Jameson, A.S. Fauci, D.L. Kasper et al (eds). Harrison's principles of internal medicine, 20th edn. McGraw-Hill. (Online edition).

Lindsay, R. & Samuels, B. (2022). Ch 411. Osteoporosis. In: J. Loscalzo, A. Fauci, D. Kasper, S. Hauser, D. Longo, & J. Jameson (eds). Harrison's principles of internal medicine, 21st edn. McGraw-Hill Education. (Online edition).

Loosen, P. & Shelton, R. (2019). Ch. 17. Mood disorders. In: M. Ebert, J. Leckman & I. Petrakis (eds). Current diagnosis and treatment: psychiatry, 3rd edn. McGraw-Hill. (Online edition).

Lowenstein, D. (2019). Ch. 418. Seizures and epilepsy. In: J.L. Jameson, A.S. Fauci, D.L. Kasper et al (eds). Harrison's principles of internal medicine, 20th edn. McGraw-Hill. (Online edition).

MacNaughton, W.K., & Sharkey, K.A. (2023). Pharmacotherapy of inflammatory bowel disease. In: L.L. Brunton & B.C. Knollmann (eds.), Goodman & Gilman's: The pharmacological basis of therapeutics, 14th edn. McGraw-Hill Education. (Online edition).

Malhi, G.S., Bell, E., Bassett, D., et al. (2021). The 2020 Royal Australian and New Zealand College of Psychiatrists clinical practice guidelines for mood disorders *Australian and New Zealand Journal of Psychiatry*, 55(1), 7-117. https://doi.org/10.1177/0004867420979353.

Mahli, G., Outhred, T., Hamilton, A. et al (2018). Royal Australian and New Zealand College of Psychiatrists clinical practice guidelines for mood disorders: major depression summary. Medical Journal of Australia 208(4), 175–180.

McQuaid, K. (2018). Ch. 62. Drugs used in the treatment of gastrointestinal diseases. In: B.G. Katzung (ed.). Basic and clinical pharmacology, 14th edn. (Online edition).

Migraine & Headache Australia (2021). Migraine. Online. Available: https://headacheaustralia.org.au/migraine/

MIMS Australia. MIMS Online. Available: www.mims.com.au.

MND Australia (n.d.). What is MND? Facts and figures. Online. Available: www.mndaust.asn.au/Get-informed/What-is-MND/Facts-and-figures.aspx.

MS Australia (2019). Key facts and figures about multiple sclerosis. Online. Available: www.msaustralia.org.au.

Murray, L., Little, M., Pascu, O. et al (2015). Toxicology handbook, 3rd edn. Elsevier, Chatswood.

National Asthma Council Australia (2022). Australian asthma handbook (Version 2.2). Online. Available: www.nationalasthma.org.au/health-professionals/australian-asthmahandbook.

National Heart Foundation of Australia (2016). Guidelines for the diagnosis and management of hypertension in adults. Online. Available: www.heartfoundation.org.au.

National Health & Medical Research Council (NHMRC), New Zealand Ministry of Health (NZ MoH) (2017). Sodium. Online. Available: www.nrv.gov.au/nutrients/sodium.

National Vascular Disease Prevention Alliance (2012). Guidelines for the management of absolute cardiovascular disease risk. Online. Available: www.cvdcheck.org.au/pdf/Absolute_CVD_Risk_Full_Guidelines.pdf.

Newman-Casey, P. & Myers, J. (2019). Preliminary steps to address glaucoma medication adherence beginning to tackle the elephant in the room. JAMA Ophthalmology 137(3), 246–247.

Ng, L. & Cunningham, D. (2021). Management of insomnia in primary care. *Australian Prescriber*, 44, 124-128.

Nursing and Midwifery Board of Australia (NMBA), Australian Health Practitioner Regulation Agency (AHPRA) (2023). Fact sheet: enrolled nurses and medication administration. Online. Available: https://www.nursingmidwiferyboard.gov.au/Codes-Guidelines-Statements/FAQ/Enrolled-nurses-and-medicine-administration.aspx

Nursing and Midwifery Board of Australia (NMBA), Australian Health Practitioner Regulation Agency (AHPRA) (2020a). Fact sheet: endorsement for scheduled medicines for midwives. Online. Available: www.nursingmidwiferyboard.gov.au/codes-guidelinesstatements/faq/fact-sheet-endorsement-for-scheduled-medicines-for-midwives.aspx.

Nursing and Midwifery Board of Australia (NMBA), Australian Health Practitioner Regulation Agency (AHPRA) (2020b). Fact sheet: endorsement for scheduled medicines for midwives. Online. Available: www.nursingmidwiferyboard.gov.au/codes-guidelinesstatements/faq/fact-sheet-endorsement-for-scheduled-medicines-for-midwives.aspx.

Nursing and Midwifery Board of Australia (NMBA), Australian Health Practitioner Regulation Agency (AHPRA) (2025a). Endorsement for scheduled medicines designated RN prescriber. Online. Available: https://www.nursingmidwiferyboard.gov.au/Registration-Standards/Endorsement-for-scheduled-medicines-designated-RN-prescriber.aspx

Nursing and Midwifery Board of Australia (NMBA), Australian Health Practitioner Regulation Agency (AHPRA) (2020b). Fact sheet: enrolled nurses and medication administration. Online. Available: www.nursingmidwiferyboard.gov.au/Codes-Guidelines-Statements/FAQ/Enrolled-nurses-and-medicine-administration.aspx.

BIBLIOGRAPHY

Nursing and Midwifery Board of Australia (NMBA) (2017). Guidelines: for midwives applying for endorsement for scheduled medication. Online. Available: https://www.nursingmidwiferyboard.gov.au/Codes-Guidelines-Statements/Codes-Guidelines/Guidelines-for-Midwives-applying-for-endorsement-for-scheduled-medicines.aspx

Olanow, C.W., Klein, C. & Schapira, A. (2019). Ch. 427. Parkinson's disease and other movement disorders. In: J.L. Jameson, A.S. Fauci, D.L. Kasper et al (eds). Harrison's principles of internal medicine, 20th edn. McGraw-Hill. (Online edition).

Powers, A. (2019). Ch. 417. Diabetes mellitus. In: J.L. Jameson, A.S. Fauci, D.L. Kasper et al (eds). Harrison's principles of internal medicine, 20th edn. McGraw-Hill. (Online edition).

Powers A.C., Fowler M.J. & Rickels M.R. (2022a). Diabetes mellitus: management and therapies. Loscalzo J, & Fauci A, & Kasper D, & Hauser S, & Longo D, & Jameson J(Eds.), *Harrison's Principles of Internal Medicine, 21e.* McGraw-Hill Education. https://accessmedicine.mhmedical.com/content.aspx?bookid=3095&sectionid=265445871

Powers, A.C. Niswender, K.D. & Evans-Mollina, C. (2022). Diabetes mellitus: diagnosis, classification, and pathophysiology. Loscalzo, J., Fauci, A., Kasper, D., Hauser, S., Longo, D., & Jameson, J. (Eds.), *Harrison's Principles of Internal Medicine, 21e.* McGraw-Hill Education. https://accessmedicine.mhmedical.com/content.aspx?bookid=3095&sectionid=265445787

The Poisons Standard (the SUSMP). Online. Available: https://www.tga.gov.au/how-we-regulate/ingredients-and-scheduling-medicines-and-chemicals/poisons-standard-and-scheduling-medicines-and-chemicals/poisons-standard-susmp. or update reference to legal instrument: https://www.legislation.gov.au/Details/F2023L01294

Pregnancy, Birth & Baby (2023). Pre-eclampsia. https://www.pregnancybirthbaby.org.au/pre-eclampsia

Pretorius, A., Searle, J. & Marshall, B. (2015). Barriers and enablers to emergency department nurses' management of patients' pain. Pain Management Nursing 16(3), 372–379.

Psychotropic Expert Group (2021). Therapeutic guidelines: Psychotropic. eTG.

Rabinovici G.D., Seeley W.W. & Miller B.L. (2022). Alzheimer's disease. Loscalzo J, & Fauci A, & Kasper D, & Hauser S, & Longo D, & Jameson J(Eds.), *Harrison's Principles of Internal Medicine, 21e.* McGraw-Hill Education. https://accessmedicine.mhmedical.com/content.aspx?bookid=3095&sectionid=262997915

Radhakrishnan, R., Ganesh, S., Meltzer, H.Y., et al (Eds.), *Current Diagnosis & Treatment: Psychiatry, 4th Edition.* McGraw Hill. https://accessmedicine.mhmedical.com/content.aspx?bookid=3507&sectionid=289853094

Raj, K.S., Williams, N.R., Debattista, C. & Johnson, M.D. (2025). Sleep-wake disorders. Papadakis M.A., & Rabow M.W., & McQuaid K.R., & Gandhi M(Eds.), *Current Medical Diagnosis & Treatment 2025*. McGraw-Hill Education. https://accessmedicine.mhmedical.com/content.aspx?bookid=3495&sectionid=288494036

Ramasamy, S., Baysari, M., Lehnbom, E. et al (2013) Evidence briefings on intervention to improve medication safety: double checking medication administration. Online. Available: www.safetyandquality.gov.au/wp-content/uploads/2013/12/Evidence-briefings-on-interventions-to-improve-medication-safety-Double-checking-medicationadministration-PDF-888KB.pdf.

Rao, V.R. & Lowenstein, D.H. (2022). Seizures and epilepsy. Loscalzo J, & Fauci A, & Kasper D, & Hauser S, & Longo D, & Jameson J(Eds.), *Harrison's Principles of Internal Medicine, 21e*. McGraw-Hill Education. https://accessmedicine.mhmedical.com/content.aspx?bookid=3095&sectionid=265447874

Rathmell, J. & Fields, A. (2018). Ch. 10. Pain: pathophysiology and management. In: J.L. Jameson, A.S. Fauci, D.L. Kasper et al (eds). Harrison's principles of internal medicine, 20th edn. McGraw-Hill. (Online edition).

Raviglione, M. (2018). Ch. 173. Tuberculosis. In: J.L. Jameson, A.S. Fauci, D.L. Kasper et al (eds). Harrison's principles of internal medicine, 20th edn. McGraw-Hill. (Online edition).

Reddy, D. & O'Donnell, M. (2018). Ch 176. Antimycobacterial agents. In: J.L. Jameson, A.S. Fauci, D.L. Kasper et al (eds). Harrison's principles of internal medicine, 20th edn. McGraw-Hill. (Online edition).

Roach, S. (2005). Pharmacology for health professionals. Lippincott Williams & Wilkins, Philadelphia.

Roberson, E. (2018). Ch. 18. Treatment of central nervous system degenerative disorders. In: L. Brunton, R. Hilal-Dandan & B.C. Knollman (eds). Goodman & Gilman's: the pharmacological basis of therapeutics, 13th edn. (Online edition).

Robinson, P. & Stamp, L. (2016). The management of gout: much has changed. Australian Family Physician 45(5), 299–302.

Rogers, V. & Worley, K. Ch. 19.12. Preeclampsia-eclampsia. In: M. Papadakis, S. McPhee, & M. Rabow (eds) (2021). Current medical diagnosis and treatment. McGraw-Hill. (Online edition).

Roman-Rodriguez, M., Metting, E., Gacia-Pardo, M., et al. `(2019). Wrong inhalation technique is associated to poor asthma clinical outcomes. Is there room for improvement? Current Opinion in Pulmonary Medicine 25(1), 18–26.

Ropper A.H., Samuels M.A., Klein J.P. & Prasad S. (2023). Epilepsy and other seizure disorders. Ropper A.H., & Samuels M.A., & Klein J.P., & Prasad S. (Eds.), *Adams and Victor's Principles of Neurology, 12e*. McGraw-Hill Education. https://accessmedicine.mhmedical.com/content.aspx?bookid=3313&sectionid=27673232

Royal Australian College of General Practitioners (RACGP) (2015). Prescribing drugs of dependence in general practice, Part B: Benzodiazepines. RACGP, Melbourne. Online. Available: www.racgp.org.au/clinical-resources/clinical-guidelines/key-racgp-guidelines/view-all-racgp-guidelines/prescribing-drugs-of-dependence/prescribing-drugs-ofdependence-part-b/evidence-based-guidance-for-benzodiazepines/insomnia.

Salmon, J. (2018). Ch. 11. Glaucoma. In: P. Riordan-Eva & J. Augsburger (eds). Vaughan & Asbury's general ophthalmology, 19th edn. McGraw-Hill. (Online edition).

Schumacher, H.R. & Chen, L.X. (2018). Ch. 365. Gout and other crystal-associated arthropathies. In: J.L. Jameson, A.S. Fauci, D.L. Kasper et al (eds). Harrison's principles of internal medicine, 20th edn. McGraw-Hill. (Online edition).

Schwedt, T. (2018). Preventive therapy of migraine. Continuum: Lifelong Learning in Neurology 24(4), 1052–1065.

Seifter J.L. (2022). Urinary tract obstruction. In: Loscalzo J, & Fauci A, & Kasper D, & Hauser S, & Longo D, & Jameson J (Eds.), *Harrison's Principles of Internal Medicine, 21e*. McGraw-Hill Education. https://accessmedicine.mhmedical.com/content.aspx?bookid=3095&sectionid=263550254

Seeley, W. & Miller, B. (2018). Ch. 423. Alzheimer's disease. In: J.L. Jameson, A.S. Fauci, D.L. Kasper et al (eds). Harrison's principles of internal medicine, 20th edn. McGraw-Hill. (Online edition).

Shakir, S. M., Shakir, F. A., & Couturier, M. R. (2023). Updates to the Diagnosis and Clinical Management of Helicobacter pylori Infections. *Clinical Chemistry, 69*(8), 869–880. https://doi.org/10.1093/clinchem/hvad081

Sharkey, K.A. & Wallace, J.L. (2018). Ch. 50. Gastrointestinal motility and water flux, emesis, and biliary and pancreatic disease. In: L. Brunton, R. Hilal-Dandan & B.C. Knollman (eds). Goodman and Gilman's: the Pharmacological basis of therapeutics, 13th edn. (Online edition).

Shelton R.C. & Anand A. (2024). Anxiety disorders. In Ebert M.H., & Martin P.R., & McVoy M, & Ronis R.J., & Weissman S.H.(Eds.), *Current Diagnosis & Treatment: Psychiatry, 4th Edition*. McGraw Hill. https://accessmedicine.mhmedical.com/content.aspx?bookid=3507&sectionid=289854116

Skidgel, R. (2018). Ch. 39. Histamine, bradykinin and their antagonists. In: L. Brunton, R. Hilal-Dandan & B.C. Knollman (eds). Goodman and Gilman's: the pharmacological basis of therapeutics, 13th edn. McGraw-Hill. (Online edition).

Sly, B. & Taylor, J. (2023). Blood glucose monitoring devices: Current considerations. *Australian Prescriber*, 45, 54-59 https://doi.org/10.18773/austprescr.2023.013

Snyder, B. (2014). Revisiting old friends: update on opioid pharmacology. Australian Prescriber 17(2), 56–60.

Society of Hospital Pharmacists of Australia (SHPA) (2018). Don't rush to crush. SHPA.

Sorense,n M., Hehemann, M.C. & Haider, M.A. (2025). Male sexual dysfunction & erectile dysfunction. Papadakis M.A., & Rabow M.W., & McQuaid K.R., & Gandhi M(Eds.), *Current Medical Diagnosis & Treatment 2025*. McGraw-Hill Education. https://accessmedicine.mhmedical.com/content.aspx?bookid=3495&sectionid=288492213

Urinary incontinence. In South-Paul J.E., & Matheny S.C., & Lewis E.L.(Eds.), *CURRENT Diagnosis & Treatment: Family Medicine, 5e*. McGraw Hill. https://accessmedicine.mhmedical.com/content.aspx?bookid=2934&sectionid=247402461

The National Return & Disposal of Unwanted Medicines Ltd. (2020). Return Unwanted Medicines. Online. Available: https://returnmed.com.au/about-us/.

Therapeutic Goods Administration (TGA) (2023). Scheduling basics of medicines and chemicals in Australia. Online. Available: https://www.tga.gov.au/how-we-regulate/ingredients-and-scheduling-medicines-and-chemicals/scheduling-basics-medicines-and-chemicals-australia

Therapeutic Goods Administration (TGA) (2020). No. 31 Poisons Standard October 2020. Australian Government, Department of Health. Online. Available: www.legislation.gov.au/Details/F2020L01255.

Therapeutic Goods Administration (TGA) (2018). Current list of up-scheduled codeine containing products. Australian Government, Department of Health. Online. Available: www.tga.gov.au/node/770507.

Therapeutic Guidelines (2024). Rheumatology. December 2024 updates. Online. Available: https://www.tg.org.au/products/therapeutic-guidelines/updates/rheumatology/.

Thomas, J., Van Hove, J., Larson, A. et al (2020). Ch. 36. Inborn errors of metabolism. In: W. Hay, M. Levin, M. Abzug & M. Bunik (eds). Current diagnosis and treatment: pediatrics, 25th edn. McGraw-Hill. (Online edition).

Tortora, G. & Derrickson, B. (2021). Principles of anatomy and physiology, 16th edn. Wiley.

Toxicology and Toxinology Expert Group (2020). Therapeutic guidelines: toxicology and toxinology. Online. Available: https://tgldcdp.tg.org.au/guideLine?guidelinePage=Toxicology+and+Toxinology&frompage=etgcomplete

Traver, J. & Cheng, A. (2016). Multidrug-resistant tuberculosis in Australia and our region. Medical Journal of Australia 204(7), 251–252.

Vargas, B. (2018). Acute treatment of migraine. Continuum: Lifelong Learning in Neurology 24(4), 1032–1051.

Victorian Government (2017) (authorised version with amendments November 2025). Drugs, Poisons and Controlled Substances Regulations. Statutory Rule No. 29/2017 version 020. Online. Available: https://content.legislation.vic.gov.au/sites/default/files/2025-11/17-29sra020-authorised.pdf.

Waxman, A. & Loscalzo, J. (2019). Ch. 277. Pulmonary hypertension. In: J.L. Jameson, A.S. Fauci, D.L. Kasper et al (eds). Harrison's principles of internal medicine, 20th edn. McGraw-Hill. (Online edition).

Westbrook, J., Li, L., Lehnbom, E., et al (2015). What are incident reports telling us? A comparative study at two Australian hospitals of medication errors identified at audit, detected by staff and reported to an incident system. International Journal for Quality in Health Care 27(11), 1–9.

White, N.J. & Ashley, E.A. (2026). Ch. 231. Malaria. In: J.L. Jameson, A.S. Fauci, D.L. Kasper et al (eds). Harrison's principles of internal medicine, 22th edn. McGraw-Hill. (Online edition).

World Anti-Doping Agency (WADA) (2025). Prohibited list. Online. Available: https://www.wada-ama.org/en/prohibited-list

World Anti-Doping Agency (WADA) (2025). Therapeutic use exemptions (TUE). Online. Available: https://www.wada-ama.org/en/athletes-support-personnel/therapeutic-use-exemptions-tues

World Health Organization (WHO)(2025). Malaria. Online. Available: https://www.who.int/news-room/fact-sheets/detail/malaria

World Health Organization (Who) (2024). Infertility. https://www.who.int/news-room/fact-sheets/detail/infertility

World Health Organization (Who) (2024b). Leprosy. https://www.who.int/news-room/fact-sheets/detail/leprosy

World Health Organisation (WHO)(2025). Malaria. https://www.who.int/news-room/fact-sheets/detail/malaria

World Health Organization (Who) (2023). Preterm birth. https://www.who.int/news-room/fact-sheets/detail/preterm-birth#:~:text=Preterm%20is%20defined%20as%20babies,(32%20to%2037%20weeks).

World Health Organization (WHO) (2023). Global tuberculosis programme. https://www.who.int/teams/global-tuberculosis-programme/tb-reports/global-tuberculosis-report-2023

World Health Organisation (WHO) (2023c) Mental health – anxiety disorders https://www.who.int/news-room/fact-sheets/detail/anxiety-disorders

World Health Organization (WHO) (2019a). Leishmaniasis. Online. Available: www.who.int/mediacentre/factsheets/fs375/en/.

World Health Organization (WHO) (2019b). Soil transmitted helminth infection. Online. Available: www.who.int/news-room/fact-sheets/detail/soil-transmitted-helminthinfections.

Wright, E.K., Ding, N.S. & Niewiadomski, O. (2018). Management of inflammatory bowel disease. Medical Journal of Australia 209(7), 318–323.

Zaenglein, A.L., Pathy, A.L., Schlosser, B.J. et al (2016). Guidelines of care for the management of acne vulgaris. Journal of the American Academy of Dermatology 74(5), 945–973. Updated: *Friday, February 2, 2024 @ 2:37 PM*

GLOSSARY

Anaphylactoid reactions (pseudoallergic reactions): thought to be caused by direct release of histamine provoked by unclear non-immune mechanisms. Unlike anaphylactic reactions, there may be no prior exposure or triggering factors with anaphylactoid reactions, which may be seen with the first dose of a drug

Anaphylaxis: manifestation of immediate hypersensitivity (also called type 1 hypersensitivity). The sensitised individual (i.e. the person who has had prior exposure or contact with the drug or substance) is exposed to a specific antigen or hapten, resulting in urticaria, pruritus and angio-oedema, which may progress to vascular collapse, shock and respiratory distress and require immediate treatment

Angio-oedema: a vascular reaction involving the deep dermis or subcutaneous or submucosal tissue, leading to localised oedema and wheals. Hereditary angio-oedema (dominant trait) may be mediated by minor trauma, sudden increases or decreases in environmental temperature or sudden emotional stress, and the result is visceral lesions

Anhidrosis: absence of sweating

Arachnoiditis: signs and symptoms include tingling, numbness or weakness of legs, leg sensation (e.g. insects crawling, water running over limb), severe shooting pain, muscle cramps and spasms, uncontrollable twitches, bladder, bowel and sexual problems

Aseptic meningitis syndrome: occurs from several hours up to 2 days after administration of IV human immunoglobulin (high dose: 2 g/kg) and consists of headache, nuchal rigidity, drowsiness, fever, photophobia, painful eye movement, nausea and vomiting

Asthenia: loss of strength and energy, weakness

Bier's block: anaesthetic technique for surgical procedures on the extremities where a local anaesthetic is injected intravenously

Blepharitis: inflammation of eyelid glands and lash follicles

Charcot-type arthropathy: progressive degeneration of weight-bearing joint characterised by bony destruction, bone resorption and eventual deformity

'Cheese reaction': a combination of tyramine-containing food and MAOIs which can result in headache, severe hypertension and subarachnoid haemorrhage, even up to 2 weeks after discontinuation of the MAOI. Tyramine-containing foods include: products that have been aged, pickled, fermented or smoked; some types of red wines (especially those of the Chianti and Alicante types) and beer (or large quantities of beer or wine); caviar; pickled herrings; chicken liver; vegetable, yeast and meat extracts (e.g. Vegemite, Promite, Bovril, Bonox, Marmite); mature cheeses; sour cream; yoghurt; liver; dry sausage (e.g. salami); aged meats; sauerkraut; excessive amounts of coffee or chocolate; coffee substitutes; avocados; broad-bean pods; stock cubes; packet or canned soup; and dehydrated foods

Cheilitis: lip inflammation

Cryptorchism (cryptorchidism): failure of one or both testes to descend into the scrotum; may be treated with surgery (usually when the child is 5–7 years old) or with gonadotrophic hormones

Disulfiram–alcohol reaction: characterised by intense flushing of the face and neck accompanied by heat and sweating, feeling of constriction and irritation of throat and trachea, chest pains, restlessness, headache, tachycardia, palpitation, dyspnoea, hypertension initially, then hypotension; later, pallor, weakness, vertigo, nausea, vomiting, abdominal cramps, thirst, dizziness, blurred vision, numbness of hands and feet, insomnia and, finally, in severe reactions, cardiopulmonary arrest. Disulfiram reaction is managed by giving the patient 1 g ascorbic acid IV, chlorpromazine 5–100 mg IM and resuscitation measures as necessary

Dubin–Johnson syndrome: hereditary, chronic non-haemolytic jaundice

Eaton–Lambert syndrome: limb muscle weakness similar to myasthenia gravis, but not involving ocular or bulbar muscles

Embryotoxic: causing injury to the embryo, resulting in death, growth retardation or abnormal development in a part that may affect either its structure or its function

Erythema nodosum leprosum (ENL) (lepromatous reaction) (type 2 reaction): which occurs within the first 2 years of treatment. Symptoms include high fever and raised, tender erythematous skin nodules (which may become pustular and/or ulcerate), and may also include malaise, neuritis, orchitis, albuminuria, joint swelling, iritis, epistaxis, acute vasculitis and depression. Usual treatment consists of corticosteroids, analgesics and/or other agents that suppress the reaction

Erythrasma: superficial skin infection caused by *Corynebacterium minutissimum*, resulting in brown, scaly skin patches, affecting the skin in the armpits, groin and between the toes. It may co-exist or be mistaken for tinea or *Candida* fungal infection. It may also be more generalised and found on the trunk of the body, under the breasts or in the umbilicus

Extrapyramidal reactions or syndromes: may include some or all of the following symptoms and may occur after a single dose, especially in children and young adults:
- Parkinsonian symptoms: akinesia, rigidity, tremor at rest
- akathisia: motor and mental restlessness
- acute dystonic reaction: facial grimacing, torticollis, oculogyric crisis
- tardive dyskinesia: exaggerated and persistent chewing movements, tongue protrusion.

Drugs that may be used to reverse the extrapyramidal reaction include benztropine and diphenhydramine

Fanconi syndrome: syndrome of inadequate reabsorption in the proximal renal tubules which can be caused by congenital or acquired diseases, toxicity or adverse drug reactions

Glossodynia (also known as burning mouth syndrome): burning sensation, discomfort, pain, irritation or rawness of tongue, lips or oral cavity

Goodpasture's syndrome: syndrome characterised by cough, production of frothy mucus containing bright red blood, nausea, pruritus, constipation and decreased urination

Hyperostosis: excessive growth of bony tissue

Hypersensitivity: altered reactivity in which the body reacts with an exaggerated immune response to a foreign substance. It may be subdivided into immediate (type 'I'), cytotoxic (type II), immune complex (type III) or delayed (type IV) reactions. Immediate (type 'I') reactions are antibody mediated and occur within minutes of the sensitised person being exposed to an antigen; they may result in anaphylaxis or atopic allergy (allergic rhinitis, asthma, dermatitis, urticaria and/or angio-oedema). Cytotoxic (type II) reactions occur when an antigen combines with an antibody resulting in a complement-mediated lysis (e.g. transfusion reaction). Immune complex (type III) reactions result in a complement being activated when antigen–antibody immune complexes are deposited into tissues. Polymorphonuclear cells are then attracted to the site, resulting in the release of lysosomal enzymes and tissue damage. Delayed (type IV) reactions take 12–48 hours to develop and are produced by natural infection, vaccination with live attenuated virus vaccines or by injection of antigens and are mediated through T lymphocytes

Lepra reaction, reversal reaction (type 1): usually seen early in therapy and thought to be due to a decrease in antigens where the immune system mounts a response to the remaining infection. It consists of swelling of any skin and nerve lesions and is generally treated using corticosteroids (especially if neuritis is present), analgesics or surgical decompression, if necessary. Non-treatment may result in irreversible nerve damage

Livedo reticularis: mottled discolouration of skin appearing net-like, reddish-blue in colour with surrounding pale areas, occurring mainly on arms, legs and trunk, worse in cold weather

Lymphopenia: low level of lymphocytes in the blood

Lypodystrophy syndrome: redistribution/accumulation of body fat, peripheral and facial wasting, breast enlargement, central obesity, dorsocervical fat enlargement ('buffalo hump'), elevated serum lipids and blood glucose concentration

Malignant hyperthermia (also called malignant hyperpyrexia): rare but potentially fatal condition associated mainly with halogenated general anaesthetic agents. It occurs more commonly in males and is genetically determined. There appears to be a skeletal hypermetabolic state caused by a sudden increase in calcium concentration in the muscle cytoplasm, leading to high oxygen demand. Symptoms include muscle rigidity, acidosis, hyperkalaemia, tachycardia, arrhythmias, tachypnoea, cyanosis, sweating and unstable blood pressure. The body temperature rises at a rate of at least $2°C$ per hour, but sometimes this is a late sign. Late complications may include renal failure, intravascular coagulopathy and pulmonary oedema. The reaction is thought to be induced by preoperative exercise, muscle trauma, fever or anxiety, or induction by inhalation anaesthetics, suxamethonium or prolonged anaesthesia

Melasma (also called chloasma): facial hyperpigmentation consisting of sharply demarcated blotchy brown macules that are symmetrically spread over cheeks and forehead and, sometimes, upper lip and neck.

Metrorrhagia: abnormal uterine bleeding

Neuroleptic malignant syndrome: a potentially fatal reaction to antipsychotic drugs. Symptoms include hyperthermia and severe extrapyramidal symptoms (muscle rigidity, altered consciousness, tachycardia, labile blood pressure, profuse sweating and dyspnoea). Skeletal muscle damage may occur as a consequence. Predisposing factors include dehydration, pre-existing organic brain disease and AIDS. Infants and the elderly are particularly susceptible. It is usually managed by discontinuing antipsychotic drugs and monitoring and treating symptoms

Oligohidrosis: decreased sweating

Paracervical block: anaesthetic procedure used in obstetrics and gynaecology where the anaesthetic is injected into between two and six sites at a depth of 3–7 mm alongside the vaginal portion of the cervix in the vaginal fornices

Peliosis hepatitis: liver, and sometimes splenic, tissue replaced by blood-filled cysts; may be associated with liver failure and life-threatening intra-abdominal haemorrhage

Phaeochromocytoma: catecholamine-producing tumour of the adrenal medulla, resulting in the excessive production of adrenaline and noradrenaline (norepinephrine) and associated symptoms, including palpitations, weight loss, sweating and high blood pressure

Porphyria: porphyrins usually combine with haem to produce haemoproteins, including haemoglobin, and the process involves multiple enzymes. Abnormal enzymes result in a build-up and excretion of porphyrin. Porphyria are inherited disorders affecting either the skin (e.g. on exposure to sun, the skin develops blisters, itching and swelling) or the nervous system (resulting in pain in the chest, abdomen, limbs or back, muscle numbness, tingling, paralysis or cramping; vomiting, constipation and personality disorders). Attacks of porphyria may be triggered by a number of agents, including some medications (e.g. sedatives, oral contraceptives, barbiturates and tranquillisers), chemicals, smoking, alcohol, infection, sun exposure, menstrual hormones and emotional or physical stress

Pulmonary wedge pressure: indirect measure of left atrial pressure, measured by placing a catheter (Swanz Ganz) into the pulmonary artery and attaching it to a pressure transducer

Prader–Willi syndrome: genetic disorder of chromosome 15, resulting in hypotonia (e.g. floppiness and weakened/absent suck reflex in babies); poor large muscle strength, sometimes with poor coordination and balance; hypogonadism (immature development of sexual organs and sexual characteristics); hyperphagia (excessive appetite and overeating, resulting in obesity if food intake is not controlled); CNS and endocrine gland dysfunction (resulting in learning disabilities, short stature, hyperphagia, somnolence and poor emotional and social development)

Priapism: abnormal erection of penis, accompanied by pain and tenderness

Proptosis: bulging eyes

Pseudomembranous colitis: severe acute inflammation of the bowel mucosa, commonly associated with antibiotic therapy. Pseudomembranous plaques (yellow–green) in the bowel are common, and symptoms include watery diarrhoea, fever and abdominal cramps

Pyrosis: burning sensation in the stomach and oesophagus with belching (sour taste)

'Purple toe' syndrome: characterised by toes becoming dark, purple or mottled in appearance, usually within 3–10 weeks of starting therapy with warfarin or related drugs. Other symptoms include purple colour of the plantar surfaces and sides of toes. The colour blanches when moderate pressure is applied and fades when legs are elevated. Toes may also become painful and tender. In some cases, purple toes may progress to gangrene or necrosis requiring debridement or amputation

Radical cure: aims to eliminate dormant schizonts from the liver during malaria

Raynaud's disease/syndrome: a disease characterised by spasm of the arteries in the extremities (especially fingers) and brought on by cold or vibration, resulting in pallor, pain, numbness and, in severe cases, and gangrene

'Red man' syndrome: flushing of upper body, hypotension, angio-oedema, pruritus

Reye's syndrome: rare but fatal disease that may occur as a sequel to varicella or viral upper respiratory infection, and which has been associated with the taking of aspirin by children under 12 years for febrile, viral illnesses. Symptoms include recurrent vomiting, liver and visceral changes, deteriorating to encephalopathy with acute brain swelling, disturbance in consciousness and seizures

Rotor syndrome: rare, idiopathic form of hyperbilirubinaemia

Serotonin syndrome: a triad of altered mental status, autonomic dysfunction and neuromuscular abnormalities associated with the use of 'serotonergic' antidepressants or antidepressant combination. Symptoms include agitation, coma, confusion, delirium, hallucinations, mania, mutism, fluctuating blood pressure, sweating, diarrhoea, hyperthermia, lacrimation, mydriasis, shivering, tachycardia, restlessness, hyperreflexia, clonus, myoclonus, nystagmus, oculogyric crisis, tetanic body arching, tremor, rigidity and rhabdomyolysis

Stevens–Johnson syndrome: a form of erythema multiforme that is sometimes fatal. It may be preceded by influenza-like symptoms and is characterised by systemic and more severe mucocutaneous lesions. It usually involves oronasal and anogenital mucous membranes, with characteristic grey–white pseudomembranes, and haemorrhagic crusts on the lips. Ocular lesions (iritis, uveitis, corneal vesicles, erosions and perforations) may lead to corneal opacities and blindness. There may also be pulmonary, gastrointestinal, cardiac and renal involvement

Stokes–Adams syndrome: condition caused by heart block and characterised by sudden attacks of unconsciousness with or without convulsions

Superinfection: overgrowth of non-susceptible organisms with prolonged or repeated treatment

Suppressive cure: if a suppressive drug is continued for long enough after a patient has left a malarial area, the liver cycle of the plasmodium is no longer maintained by re-infection, resulting in a cure

Suppressive prophylaxis: suppression of the erythrocyte cycle of malaria, preventing acute attacks

Teratogen: any substance that can cause a disturbance in growth and development of embryo or fetus or may cause a stop to the pregnancy altogether. Teratogens can include drugs, chemicals, radiation and maternal infection

Teratogenic: able to disturb the growth and development of the embryo or fetus

Torsades de pointes: atypical, rapid ventricular tachycardia with periodic waxing and waning of the amplitude of the QRS complex on ECG. It may be self-limiting or progress to ventricular fibrillation

Vasomotor reaction (nitritoid reaction): vasodilation, facial flushing, loss of consciousness, hypotension, syncope, nausea, vomiting and cerebrovascular accident. May occur immediately after taking ACE inhibitor or months later. Is most common when ACE inhibitor is given with systemic gold preparation, but can also occur with oral gold

Vitiligo: skin condition in which melanocytes are destroyed, resulting in patches of de-pigmented areas, often surrounded by hyperpigmentation

Water intoxication: increased water intake causes decreased sodium concentration (hyponatraemia) and the excess water is absorbed into the blood, accumulating in the brain and lungs, leading to symptoms of breathlessness and nausea

Wernicke's encephalopathy: associated with thiamine deficiency and generally related to chronic alcohol abuse, although other conditions can cause it. Symptoms include paralysis of eye muscles, diplopia, nystagmus, ataxia and mental changes

Wolff–Parkinson–White syndrome: an extra electrical pathway exists in the heart leading to the electrical signal reaching the ventricles prematurely. Symptoms include tachycardia, dizziness, chest palpitations, fainting and, rarely, cardiac arrest

Xerostomia: dry mouth associated with dysfunction of the salivary glands

Xerophthalmia: abnormal dryness and thickening of conjunctiva and cornea

Zollinger–Ellison syndrome: rare disorder causing pancreatic and duodenal tumours, as well as gastric and duodenal ulcers. The tumour secretes gastrin, which causes the stomach to produce acid and in turn causes gastric and duodenal ulcers that are less responsive than ordinary ulcers to treatment

Drug administration

Oral preparations

Capsule: gelatin container, swallowed whole, containing a drug that is to be released or has an unpleasant taste; the drug is released when the capsule is dissolved in the stomach or intestine

Elixir: flavoured, sweetened alcoholic solution of a potent or unpleasant-tasting drug in a small dose volume

Emulsion: mixture of oil and water, the oil remaining dispersed by an emulsifying agent; the container needs to be shaken before use

Extract: concentrated preparation of a drug that may remain in fluid form or be evaporated and the solid sediment incorporated into a tablet or capsule

Granule: small pellet of the active substance

Linctus: drug prepared as a sweet syrup, given in doses of small volume to be swallowed slowly without the addition of water, usually for the relief of cough

Lozenge: solid drug form that acts by slow disintegration in the mouth and is used when a local drug action in the mouth or throat is required

Mixture: contains several drugs dissolved or suspended in an aqueous vehicle

Powder: usually a mixture of two or more powdered drugs intended for internal use

Suspension: solid insoluble particles of a drug dispersed in a liquid; must be shaken well before use

Syrup: drug contained in a concentrated sugar solution

Tablet: dried, powdered drug mixed with a binding base and compressed into a variety of shapes; may be swallowed whole or crushed if required

Tablet – enteric-coated: coated tablet containing a drug that is a gastric irritant or is broken down by gastric acid; the tablet is swallowed whole

Tablet – slow-release: the tablet, swallowed whole, contains a drug that is released over a prolonged period

Tincture: drug contained in an alcoholic solution

Injections

Intra-arterial: mainly cytotoxic (antineoplastic) agents delivered directly to an organ or tissue via the feeding artery

Intra-articular: injected into a joint cavity

Intracardiac: drug is delivered directly into the ventricle or myocardium for an immediate cardiac response

Intradermal: drug is given into the superficial skin layers, mainly in skin testing

Intramuscular: delivered into muscle (e.g. oily solutions, suspensions or potentially irritant substances) or if rapid absorption is required; the site is not massaged if the Z-track technique is used

Intraperitoneal: drugs have direct contact with intraperitoneal organs during peritoneal dialysis

Intrathecal: for drugs that do not penetrate the blood–brain barrier; they may be delivered to the cerebrospinal fluid in the subarachnoid space, usually after lumbar puncture

Intravenous: if a very rapid effect is required or if the preparation is too irritating to the tissues

Subcutaneous: used if relatively slower absorption is required

Topical applications

Cream: semi-solid emulsion that may be aqueous or oily

Drops: for the eye, ear and nose; avoid touching eye, ear or nose with the dropper and return the dropper to the bottle without washing (eye drops are sterile and may be supplied with a dropper or administered directly from the container)

Dusting powder: usually a mixture of two or more substances in fine powder; should not be applied to open wounds or large areas of raw surface

Gel: aqueous preparation used to apply water-soluble medicament to body surfaces for longer retention than with an aqueous solution

Inhalation: liquid preparation containing volatile substances, which, on vaporisation, are inhaled to produce a local or systemic effect via the respiratory tract (e.g. steam inhalation, nebuliser, atomiser or aerosol spray)

Insufflation: powder intended for introduction into the ear, nose, throat, body cavities or wounds

Irrigation: washing of a body cavity or wound by a stream of water or other solution

Liniment: thin cream or oily preparation applied to the intact skin by rubbing; may contain substances possessing analgesic, rubefacient, soothing or stimulating properties

Lotion: agent contained in an aqueous, alcoholic or emulsified vehicle, applied to the skin without friction, having an astringent, emollient or other therapeutic action

Ointment: semi-solid preparation in a greasy base

Paint: liquid preparation for application in limited amounts to the skin or mucous membranes

Paste: semi-solid preparation containing a high proportion of drug that is not intended to be absorbed

Pessary: solid preparation shaped suitably for vaginal administration and containing an agent intended to act locally

Suppository: solid preparation shaped suitably for rectal administration and containing an agent intended for local or systemic medication

INDEX

A

abacavir, 920—922
abatacept, 1068—1070
abdominal distension, ganirelix acetate and, 1465
Abilify, 839—841
Abilify Maintena, 839—841
abiraterone acetate, 600
Abisart, 515—516
Abraxane, 663—665
absence seizures, 395
absolute neutrophil count (ANC), 1245
absorption, aspirin and, 817
abstinence
    acamprosate calcium for, 1102
    from opioids, naltrexone hydrochloride for, 1108
Abstral, 1439—1442
abuse, drug, 1102
Abyraz, 839—841
acamprosate calcium, 1102—1103
acarbose, 314—315
Acetadote Concentrated Injection, 334—336
acetazolamide, 388, 462
Acetec, 508
acetylcholine, 984
    non-depolarising agents, 1420
acetylcholine chloride, 1134—1136
acetylcholinesterase, 944
acetylcysteine, 334—336
    action of, 334
    adverse effects of, 334—335
    dose of, 334
    interactions of, 335
    nursing points/cautions for, 335—336
    use of, 334
aciclovir, 898—899
Aciclovir Intravenous Infusion, 898—899
aciclovir-resistant herpes simplex virus infection, foscarnet sodium for, 903
acid alfa-glucosidase deficiency, alglucosidase alfa (RHU) for, 1338—1340
Acimax, 880—881
Acinetobacter spp., infections due to, colistimethate sodium for, 199
acitretin, 4—5
Aclasta, 964—965
acne treatment, 1—9
    topical agents for, 6

acne vulgaris
    clindamycin phosphate for, 207
    erythromycin lactobionate for, 204
    genetic factors and, 1
    management of, 1—2
    types of lesions in, 1
acquired immune deficiency syndrome (AIDS), 898
acromegaly
    bromocriptine mesilate for, 804, 1487
    lanreotide acetate for, 1222
    octreotide for, 1223
    pasireotide for, 1224
    pegvisomant for, 1226
ACS. *See* acute coronary syndrome
Actacode Linctus, 1438—1439
Actemra, 1073—1075
ACTH. *See* adrenocorticotropic hormone
Act-HIB, 1602
Actilax, 1289—1290
Actilyse, 1153
actinic keratoses
    methyl aminolevulinate hydrochloride for, 657
    mild-to-moderate, aminolevulinic acid for, 668
Actinomycin D, 627—628
actinomycotic mycetoma, dapsone for, 586
Actiq, 1439—1442
activated carbon (AC) chamber, of methoxyflurane, 1179
activated charcoal, 337
    leflunomide and, 1047
activated factor Xa, 237
activated partial thromboplastin time (aPTT), 237
active immunity, 1591
Actonel, 963—964
Actonel 150 mg Once-A-Month, 963—964
Actonel EC 35 mg Once-a-Week, 963—964
Actos, 315—317
Actrapid, 303
Acular Eye Drops, 27—28
acute angina, isosorbide mononitrate for, 63
acute attack, glyceryl trinitrate for, 59
acute bacterial sinusitis, cefaclor monohydrate for, 168
acute/chronic bronchitis, cefuroxime axetil for, 177
acute coronary syndrome (ACS), bivalirudin for, 255

1716

INDEX

acute cystitis
  aztreonam for, 180
  fosfomycin for, 22
acute deep vein thrombosis (DVT)
  dalteparin sodium for, 241
  fondaparinux sodium for, 253
acute diarrhoea, 330
acute dystonia, 835
acute febrile respiratory illness, idursulfase for, 1351
acute function psychosis, chlorpromazine hydrochloride for, 844
acute herpes zoster, famciclovir for, 902
acute hypotension
  dopamine hydrochloride for, 1572
  metaraminol tartrate for, 1575
acute inflammatory large bowel disease, mesalazine for, 1163
acute influenza, peramivir for, 911
acute insomnia, 1502
acute left ventricular failure, isosorbide mononitrate for, 63
acute lung exacerbation, tobramycin sulfate for, 191
acute lymphoblastic leukaemia
  dasatinib for, 708
  daunorubicin for, 629
  imatinib for, 715
  inotuzumab ozogamicin for, 763
  methotrexate for, 1051
  ponatinib for, 729
acute lymphocytic leukaemia
  blinatumomab for, 750
  clofarabine for, 623
  cytarabine for, 625
acute myeloblastic leukaemia
  daunorubicin for, 629
  etoposide for, 639
  tioguanine for, 678
acute myelogenous leukaemia, mercaptopurine monohydrate for, 654
acute myeloid leukaemia
  azacitidine for, 604
  cytarabine for, 626
acute myocardial infarction
  alteplase for, 1095
acute pain, 1429
  management of, 1429
acute pelvic inflammatory disease, erythromycin lactobionate for, 204
acute postoperative urinary retention, bethanechol chloride for, 944
acute promyelocytic leukaemia arsenic trioxide for, 604
acute pulmonary oedema, furosemide for, 1086

acute renal colic, calcium gluconate monohydrate for, 1650
acute shock, dopamine hydrochloride for, 1572
acute sinusitis, moxifloxacin hydrochloride for, 218
acute ST segment elevation myocardial infarction (STEMI), enoxaparin sodium for, 244
acute stress, 70
AD. *See* Alzheimer's disease
Adacel, 1601—1602
Adacel Polio, 1602, 1612
Adalat, 1474—1475
adalimumab, 1060—1062
adapalene, 6—7
Adcetris, 751
Adcirca, 1124—1125
addiction, drugs, 1102
Addison's disease
  cortisone acetate for, 1003
adefovir dipivoxil, 915—916
Adempas, 8—10
Adenocor, 90—92
adenohypophysis, 1216
Adenoscan, 90—92
adenosine, 90—92
  action of, 90—91
  adverse effects of, 91
  dose of, 91
  interactions of, 91
  nursing points/cautions for, 91
  patient teaching and advice for, 92
  use of, 91
Adenosine Juno Solution, 90—92
Adenuric, 479
Adesan, 515
ADH. *See* antidiuretic hormone
ADHD. *See* attention deficit hyperactivity disorder
ADP, 817
adrenal cortex, 991, 1519
adrenaline (epinephrine), 1321, 1519, 1567—1569
  effect, droperidol and, 849
  promethazine and, 496
Adrenaline-Link Injection BP, 1567—1569
adrenergic agents, 1565
adrenoceptors, 1565
  alpha, 1565
  beta, 1565
adrenocorticosteroids, 991
adrenocorticotropic hormone (ACTH), 991, 1216
Adriamycin, 633—635
ADT Booster, 1600—1601
Advagraf XL, 1275—1278
advanced atherosclerosis, stimulants and, 1552—1553

1717

advanced liver cirrhosis, high-ceiling (loop) diuretics and, 1028
advanced symptomatic HIV disease, 899
Advantan, 1011
Advate, 1203
Advil preparations, 24
Adynovate, 1203—1205
Aerius, 490
Aerrane, 1175—1177
Aethoxysklerol, 1673—1674
afatinib, 693—694
Afinitor, 1251—1254
aflibercept, 1139
Afluria Quad, 1605—1607
agalsidase alfa (GHU), 1336—1337
agalsidase beta (RCH), 1337—1338
Agarol, 1294—1295
age-related bone loss, 958
age-related macular degeneration
   aflibercept for, 1139
   ranibizumab for, 1140
Aggrastat, 823—824
aggression, droperidol for, 849
aggressive systemic mastocytosis
   imatinib for, 715
agitated states, 833
agitation
   chlorpromazine hydrochloride for, 844
   severe, droperidol for, 849
   stimulants and, 1551—1552
agomelatine, 288—289
agranulocytosis, propylthiouracil and, 1585
Agrylin, 601—602
aHUS. See atypical haemolytic uraemic syndrome
AIDS. See acquired immune deficiency syndrome
Aimovig, 573—574
Airomir Autohaler and Inhaler, 104—108
Ajovy, 574—575
Akamin, 197—198
akathisia, 834
Alacare, 1028—1029
Albalon, 1136—1137
albendazole, 43—45
   action of, 43
   adverse effects of, 44
   dose of, 43—44
   interactions of, 44
   nursing points/cautions for, 44—45
   patient teaching and advice for, 45, 45b
   use of, 43
albuterol, 104—108, 1475—1477
Alcaine Eye Drops 0.5%, 1334
alcohol
   antiepileptic agents and, 385
   cyclizine lactate and, 382
   griseofulvin and, 440

alcohol (*Continued*)
   methotrexate and, 1042
alcohol dependence
   acamprosate calcium for, 1102
   naltrexone hydrochloride for, 1108
alcohol withdrawal, haloperidol decanoate for, 852
alcoholism
   chronic, disulfiram for, 1106
   erectile dysfunction and, 1116
Aldactone, 1096—1098
Aldara, 1033—1034
Aldiq, 1033—1034
Aldomet, 545—547
Aldurazyme, 1353—1354
alemtuzumab, 746—747, 1369—1371
alendronate sodium, 961
alendronic acid, 961
Alepam, 77
Aleve, 30—31
Alfentanil GH, 1434—1435
alglucosidase alfa (RHU), 1338—1340
   action of, 1338
   adverse effects of, 1339
   dose of, 1339
   nursing points/cautions of, 1339
   patient teaching and advice of, 1340
   use of, 1339
Alimta, 667—668
alirocumab, 1315
Alkeran, 653
alkylating agents, 595—596
Allegron, 273—276
Allereze, 494—495
allergic conjunctivitis
   lodoxamide trometamol, 1136
allergic disorders, cortisone acetate for, 1003
allergic reactions, in retinoids, 3
allergic rhinitis
   budesonide for
      patient teaching and advice for, 127
      prophylaxis of, 125
   ciclesonide for, 129
   fexofenadine hydrochloride for, 493
   fluticasone furoate for, 130
   montelukast sodium for, 142
allergic states, betamethasone valerate for, 1000
allergy
   cyproheptadine hydrochloride sesquihydrate for, 484
   monitoring for, rasburicase rys and, 482
   promethazine hydrochloride for, 496
   tendency, 1255
Allersoothe, 496
Allmercap, 654
allogeneic haemotopoietic stem cell transplant, letermovir, 908

INDEX

allograft transplantation, 1237
Allopurinol-WGR, 475—476
Allosig, 475—476
Alodorm, 1513
alogliptin, 318
alopecia androgenetica, 1034
Aloxi, 372—373
alpha-1 adrenoreceptor antagonist, alfuzosin hydrochloride in, 943
alpha-1 receptors, 943
alpha 1A (a_{1A}) adrenoceptor antagonist, silodosin in, 943
alpha-1-proteinase inhibitor, 1340—1341
alpha-2A-adrenergic receptor agonist, 1558
alpha adrenergic receptor, 68
  asenapine maleate and, 841
  chlorpromazine hydrochloride and, 844
  paliperidone and, 860
  quetiapine and, 863
  risperidone and, 865
  ziprasidone and, 80
alpha-adrenoceptor blocking agents, 500, 501, 931
alpha adrenoceptors, 1565
5-alpha dihydrotestosterone (DHT), 946
alpha-galactosidase A enzyme
  in agalsidase alfa (GHU), 1365
alpha glucosidase inhibitors, 304, 314—315
alpha-L-iduronidase deficiency, laronidase (RCH) for, 1353
alpha tocopheryl, 1647
AlphaClav Duo Viatris, 156
AlphaClav Duo Forte Viatris, 156—158
Alphagan Eye Drops, 466—467
Alphagan P, 466—467
Alphamox, 154—155
Alphapress, 549—550
Alprax, 73—74
alprazolam, 73—74
Alprim, 233—235
Alprolix, 1213—1214
alprostadil, 1118—1119, 1632—1633
alteplase, 1153—1155
aluminium hydroxide, 886—887
  sodium polystyrene sulfonate hydrogen with, 362
aluminium hydroxide hydrate, 886—887
aluminium levels, plasma, with desferrioxamine mesylate, 345
Alunbrig, 699—700
Alu-Tab, 886—887
Alvesco, 128—130
Alzene, 488—489
Alzheimer's disease (AD), 50
A&M Fintab-1, 947—948
amantadine hydrochloride, 799—800
Amaryl, 309—310
AmBisome, 429—432

ambrisentan, 1490—1491
ambulant patient, metyrapone in, 1674
Amdarone, 86—88
amenorrhoea
  progesterone and, 1471
  secondary
    medroxyprogesterone for, 1539
    norethisterone for, 1540
amethocaine hydrochloride, (*See* tetracaine (amethocaine) hydrochloride)
Amgevita, 1060—1062
amide-like local anaesthetics, 1321
amifostine, 781
amikacin, 188—189
Amiloxyn, 154—156
amino acids, 1670
  arginine, 1670
aminoglycosides, 186—188
  actions of, 186—187
  adverse effects of, 187
  interactions of, 187
  nursing points/cautions for, 187—188
  patient teaching and advice for, 188
  uses of, 187
aminolevulinic acid hydrochloride, 1028
aminophylline, 118—119
aminoquinoline, hydroxychloroquine sulfate, 1045
aminosalicylic acid-based agents, 1159
amiodarone, methotrexate and, 1052
amiodarone, 86—88
  action of, 86
  adverse effects of, 86
  dose of, 86
  interactions of, 86—87
  nursing points/cautions for, 87—88
  patient teaching and advice for, 88
  use of, 86
Amira, 277—278
amisulpride, 839
amitriptyline hydrochloride, 270
Amlo, 534—535
amlodipine, 534—535
ammonium chloride, 1019—1020
amoebae, 825
amoebiasis, metronidazole for, 827
amorolfine, 428—429
amoxicillin sodium, 154
amoxicillin, 154—155
  action of, 154
  adverse effects of, 155
  dose of, 154—155
  interactions of, 155
  nursing points/cautions for, 155
  patient teaching and advice for, 155
  use of, 154

HAVARD'S NURSING GUIDE TO DRUGS

amoxicillin trihydrate with clavulanic acid, 156—158
Amoxiclav, 156
Amoxil, 154—156
Amoxycillin Generichealth, 154—156
AmoxyClav, 156
amphetamines, 1551
   decreased absorption, 407
amphotericin B (amphotericin), 429—431
   suxamethonium chloride and, 1426
ampicillin sodium, 158
Ampicyn, 158
amyotrophic lateral sclerosis, riluzole and, 1397
anaemia
   of chronic renal failure, nandrolone decanoate for, 1520
   epoetin alfa for, 1189
   epoetin beta for, 1190
   imiglucerase (RCH) for, 1352
   macitentan and, 1095
   megaloblastic, overdose, calcium folinate for, 336
   in non-myeloid malignancy, 1185
   pyridoxine for, 1634
transfusion-dependent, treatment of, 1259
anaerobic infections,
   metronidazole for, 827
anaerobic organisms, severe,
   metronidazole for, 826
anaesthetics
   general, 1172—1174
      adverse effects of, 1173
      dose of, 1127
      interactions of, 1173
      nitrous oxide, 1180
      nursing points/cautions for, 1174
      patient teaching and advice for, 1174
      procedure, 1172
   induction of, 1172
      alfentanil hydrochloride for, 1434
      fentanyl citrate for, 1439
      remifentanil for, 1451
   inhalation, 1172—1173
   intravenous, 1173
   local, 1321—1335
Anafranil, 270—271
Anagraine, metoclopramide hydrochloride monohydrate and, 379
anagrelide, 601—602
anakinra, 1070—1071
anal cancer, human papillomavirus (HPV) vaccine for, 1606
analgesics, 10—34
   opioid, 1429—1670
   supplement, 1107
      alfentanil hydrochloride and, 1434
      morphine sulfate pentahydrate and, 1445
Anamorph, 1445—1447

anaphylactic reactions, adrenaline for, 1567
anaphylaxis
   adrenaline and, 1568
   antivenom and, 1592
Anaprox, 30—31
anastrozole, 602
ANC. See absolute neutrophil count
Androcur, 1540—1542
AndroFeme, 1, 1522
AndroForte, 2, 1522
AndroForte, 5, 1522
androgen, 1519—1520
   non-reproductive functions of, 1519
androgenisation
   oral contraceptives for, 1548, 1549
   in post-menopausal/hysterectomised women, cyproterone acetate for, 1540
   in pre-menopausal women, cyproterone acetate for, 1540
androgens, 991
   anabolic steroids and, 1519—1521
      actions of, 1519
      adverse effects of, 1520
      interactions of, 1520
      nandrolone decanoate, 1521—1522
      nursing points/cautions for, 1520—1521
      patient teaching and advice for, 1521
      testosterone, 1522
      testosterone decanoate, 1522
      testosterone enantate, 1522
      testosterone undecanoate, 1522—1524
      use of, 1520
androgen-sensitive polycythaemia, androgens and anabolic steroids and, 1521
Anexate, 348
angina
   amlodipine for, 534
   diltiazem hydrochloride for, 536
   verapamil hydrochloride for, 541
angina pectoris, 63
   atenolol for, 524
   isosorbide mononitrate for, 63
   metoprolol tartrate for, 528
   propranolol hydrochloride for, 531
angio-oedema
   from agalsidase alfa (GHU), 1337
   from alglucosidase alfa (RHU), 339
   human C1 esterase inhibitor for, 1255
   icatibant for, 1256
angioneurotic oedema, cortisone acetate for, 1003
angiotensin-converting enzyme (ACE) inhibitors, 500, 504
   actions of, 504
   adverse effects of, 504
   interactions of, 504—505
   nursing points/cautions for, 505—506

INDEX

angiotensin-converting enzyme (ACE) inhibitors (*Continued*)
    patient teaching and advice for, 506
angiotensin-converting enzyme (ACE) inhibitors blockers, 312
angiotensin II receptor antagonists, 500, 513
    actions of, 513
    adverse effects of, 513
    interactions of, 513—514
    nursing points/cautions for, 514
    patient teaching and advice for, 514
anidulafungin, 432
anion inhibitors, 1581
ankylosing spondylitis
    adalimumab for, 1039
    certolizumab pegol for, 1062
    etanercept for, 1063
    golimumab for, 1064
    infliximab for, 1065
anogenital warts, podophyllotoxin for, 1037
Anopheles mosquito, 555
anorectics, 35—41
    use of, 36
anovulatory infertility
    choriogonadotropin alfa for, 1460
    follitropin beta for, 1464
    menopausal gonadotropin and, 1466
anovulatory sterility, chorionic gonadotropin (human), 1459
Anpec, 541—543
Antabuse, 1106—1107
antacids, 806, 886
    aluminium hydroxide hydrate, 886—887
    bisphosphonates and, 887
    calcium carbonate, 887
    domperidone and, 376
    magnesium hydroxide, 887
antagonists, 334
Antenex, 75—77
anterior pituitary gland, 922, 1216—1217
anterior pituitary hormones, 1216—1217
    adrenocorticotropic hormone, 1216
    gonadotrophins, 1216
    growth hormone, 1216, 1221
Anterone, 1540—1542
Anthel, 49
anthelmintics, 42—49
anti-Alzheimer's agents, 50—53
    actions of, 51
    adverse effects of, 51
    interactions of, 51—52
    nursing points/cautions for, 52
    patient/carer teaching and advice for, 52—53
antianginal agents, 58—69
    patient teaching and advice for, 73
antianxiety agents, 70—80
    actions of, 71

antianxiety agents (*Continued*)
    adverse effects of, 71
    interactions of, 71—72
    nursing points/cautions for, 72—73
    patient teaching and advice for, 73
antiarrhythmic agents, 79—96
    atypical, 90—92
    class I, 79
    class IA, 80—82
    class IB, 82—84
    class IC, 84—85
    class II, 85
    class III, 85—90
    class IV, 90—96
    terbinafine hydrochloride and, 454
antiasthma agents, bronchodilators, and respiratory agents, 97—146
    patient teaching and advice for, 98—100
        aerolizer, 100
        nebuliser, 99—100
        spacer device, 99
    symptom controllers, 98
    symptom preventers, 98—100
    symptom relievers, 98
antibacterial agents, 147—235
    antidiarrhoeal agents and, 330
    nursing points/cautions for, 149—150
    patient teaching and advice for, 150—151
antibiotic-induced pseudomembranous colitis, vancomycin hydrochloride for, 185
antibiotics
    cephalosporin, with vitamin K, 366
    non-depolarising blocking agents and, 1411
anticholinergic (antimuscarinic) agents, 110—111
    actions of, 791
    adverse effects of, 110, 791
    atropine sulfate monohydrate, 986
    domperidone and, 376
    glycopyrronium bromide, 987—988
    hyoscine butylbromide, 988—989
    hyoscine hydrobromide, 988
    interactions of, 985
    nursing points/cautions for, 110—111, 893—894
    patient teaching and advice for, 111, 986
    propantheline bromide, 990
anticholinergic anti-Parkinson's agents, 791—793
    actions of, 791
    adverse effects of, 791—792
    benzatropine mesilate, 793—794
    interactions of, 792
    nursing points/cautions for, 792
    patient teaching and advice for, 792—793
    trihexyphenidyl (benzhexol) hydrochloride, 794—795
    uses of, 791
anticholinergic effects, antipsychotics, 835, 836

1721

anticholinesterases. *See also* anti-Alzheimer's agents
  agents, 981
anticoagulants
  antithrombotic agents and, 236–263
  patient teaching and advice for, 237
  coumarin-type, vitamin K, 366
  liothyronine sodium and, 1584
  propylthiouracil and, 1587
anticonvulsants, 385
antidepressants, 264–295
  nursing points/cautions for, 266
  patient teaching and advice for, 266–267
antidiabetic agents, 296–329
  glucagon-like peptide-1 (GLP-1) analogues, 321–322
  insulins, 298–304
  oral hypoglycaemic agents, 304–306
  sodium-glucose cotransporter 2 inhibitors (SGLT2 inhibitors), 324–325
antidiarrhoeal agents, 330–331
  nursing points/cautions for, 331
  patient teaching and advice for, 331
antidiuretic hormone (ADH), 1217, 1231–1236
antidotes, 334–367
antiemetic agents, 368–383, 596
  dopamine antagonists, 376–377
  neurokinin-$_1$ (NK$_1$) receptor antagonists, 374–375
antiepileptic agents, with vitamin K, 367
antiepileptic therapy, 385
antiepileptics, 384–427
  acetazolamide, 388
  adverse effects of, 385–386
  brivaracetam, 389–390, 390b
  carbamazepine, 385, 392–385, 394b
  clonazepam, 395–396
  ethosuximide, 397, 397b
  gabapentin, 397–399
  lacosamide, 399–400
  lamotrigine, 400–402
  levetiracetam, 402–403
  non-adherence to, 384
  nursing points/cautions for, 386
  oxcarbazepine, 403–405
  patient teaching and advice for, 386–388, 388b
  perampanel, 405–406
  phenobarbital, 406–409, 409b
  phenytoin sodium, 385, 409–412
  pregabalin, 412–414
  primidone, 414–415
  rufinamide, 415–416
  selection of, 385
  sodium valproate, 385, 416–419
  stiripentol, 419–421
  sulthiame, 421–422, 422b

antiepileptics (*Continued*)
  tiagabine hydrochloride, 422
  topiramate, 422–424
  vigabatrin, 424, 425b
  zonisamide, 425–427, 427b
antifolate, pyrimethamine and, 831
antifungal agents, 428–459
antiglaucoma agents, 460–462
  actions of, 461
  nursing points/cautions for, 461
  ocular adverse effects of, 461
  patient teaching and advice for, 461–462
antigout agents, 473–483
antihistamines, 484–486
  actions of, 484
  adverse effects of, 484–485
  interactions of, 485
  nursing points/cautions for, 485
  patient teaching and advice for, 485–486
    eye drop instillation, 486
    nasal spray instillation, 485–486
antihypertensive agents, 499–554
  alpha-adrenoceptor blocking agents, 500, 501
  angiotensin II receptor antagonists, 500, 513
    actions of, 513
    adverse effects of, 513
    interactions of, 513–514
    nursing points/cautions for, 514
    patient teaching and advice for, 514
  angiotensin-converting enzyme (ACE) inhibitors, 500, 504
    actions of, 504
    adverse effects of, 504
    interactions of, 504–505
    nursing points/cautions for, 505–506
    patient teaching and advice for, 506
  beta-adrenoceptor blocking agents, 500, 521–524
    actions of, 521
    adverse effects of, 521–522
    interactions of, 522
    nursing points/cautions for, 522–523
    patient teaching and advice for, 523–524
  calcium-channel blockers, 500, 532–534
  centrally acting agents, 500, 543
  direct acting vasodilators, 500, 548–549
  hypotensive effects of, antipsychotics and, 836
  thiazide diuretics, 500
anti-infective agents, for oropharynx, 1149
antimalarial agents, 555–568
antimetabolites, 595
antimigraine agents, 569–583
antimuscarinic agents, 949
antimycobacterial agents, 584–594
  dapsone, 586–587

INDEX

antimycobacterial agents (*Continued*)
  ethambutol, 587—588
  isoniazid, 588—590
  rifabutin, 590—591
  rifampicin, 592—594
  thalidomide, 585
antineoplastic agents, 595—779
  adverse effects of, 596
  interactions of, 596
  nursing points/cautions for, 596—598
  patient teaching and advice for, 598—599
antineoplastic chemotherapy, methotrexate for, 1050
antineoplastic support agents, 780—781
  granulocyte colony stimulating factor (G-CSF), 784
anti-Parkinson's agents, 790—816
  anticholinergic, 791—793
    actions of, 791
    adverse effects of, 791—792
    benzatropine mesilate, 793—794
    interactions of, 792
    nursing points/cautions for, 792
    patient teaching and advice for, 792—793
    trihexyphenidyl (benzhexol) hydrochloride, 794—795
    uses of, 791
  catechol-o-methyl transferase (COMT) inhibitors, 795—796
    entacapone, 795—796
    opicapone, 796—797
  dopamine agonists, 798—799
    adverse effects of, 798
    amantadine hydrochloride, 799—800
    apomorphine hydrochloride hemihydrate, 800—802
    benserazide hydrochloride, 802
    bromocriptine mesilate, 802—804
    cabergoline, 804—805
    carbidopa monohydrate, 805
    interactions of, 798
    levodopa, 805—809
    nursing points/cautions for, 798
    patient teaching and advice for, 798—799
    pramipexole dihydrochloride monohydrate, 809—810
    rotigotine, 810—812
  monoamine oxidase type B enzyme (MAO-B) inhibitors, 812
    patient teaching and advice for, 812
    rasagiline, 812—813
    safinamide, 813—814
    selegiline hydrochloride, 814—816
antiplatelet agents, 817—824
antiplatelet therapy, aspirin and, 818
antiprotozoal agents, 825—832

antipsychotic agents, 833—838
  adverse effects of, 834—835
  anticholinergic effects, 835, 836
  atypical, 833
  dopamine antagonism and, 836
  interactions of, 835—836
  nursing points/cautions for, 836—837
  patient teaching and advice for, 837—838
  typical, 833
antiretroviral agents, 918—920
  adverse effects of, 918—919
  entry inhibitors, 898, 936—939
    bulevirtide, 936—937
    maraviroc, 937—938
    nirsevimab, 938—939
  integrase inhibitors, 898, 939—941
    dolutegravir, 939—940
    raltegravir, 940—941
  interactions of, 919
  non-nucleoside reverse transcriptase inhibitors, 897—898, 927—931
    efavirenz, 927—929
    etravirine, 929—930
    rilpivirine hydrochloride, 930—931
  nucleoside/nucleotide reverse transcriptase inhibitors (NRTIs), 823, 920—927
    abacavir, 920—922
    emtricitabine, 922—923
    lamivudine, 923—924
    tenofovir alafenamide, 924
    tenofovir disoproxil fumarate, 924—925
    zidovudine, 925—927
  nursing points/cautions for, 919—920
  patient teaching and advice for, 920
  protease inhibitors, 897, 931—936
    atazanavir, 931—933
    darunavir, 933—934
    ritonavir, 935—936
    tipranavir, 935
antirheumatic drugs, 1038—1078
  conventional, 1039
  cytokine modulators, 1067—1068
  tumour necrosis factor alpha (TNF-α) antagonists, 1057—1060
antisecretory drugs, domperidone and, 376
antisera, 1591
antithrombin III-dependent anticoagulants, 253—255
antithymocyte globulin (equine), 1238
antithymocyte globulin (rabbit), 1238—1240
  action of, 1238
  adverse effects of, 1239
  dose of, 1238—1239
  interactions of, 1239
  nursing points/cautions for, 1239—1240
  patient teaching and advice for, 1240

antithymocyte globulin (rabbit) (*Continued*)
   use of, 1238
antithyroid agents, 1579—1590
   carbimazole, 1585—1586
   propylthiouracil, 1587—1588
   sodium iodide (^{131}I), 1588—1590
antithyroid compounds, 1579—1590
antiulcer agents, 871—888
   antacids, 886
   cytoprotective agents, 883
   histamine H$_2$-receptor antagonists, 872—873
   proton pump inhibitors, 875
anti-vascular endothelial growth factor (VEGF), brolucizumab, 1140
antivenoms, 889—896
   actions of, 889
   adverse effects of, 889
   black snake, 892
   box jellyfish, 892
   brown snake, 892—893
   death adder, 893
   funnel-web spider, 893
   monovalent snake, 889
   nursing points/cautions for, 889—890
   patient teaching and advice for, 891
   polyvalent snake, 893—894
   pressure immobilisation first aid technique, 891
   red back spider, 894
   sea snake, 894
   spider, 889
   stone fish, 895
   taipan, 895
   tiger snake, 895
   uses of, 889
antiviral agents, 897—941
   abacavir, 920—922
   aciclovir, 898—900
   adefovir dipivoxil, 915—916
   atazanavir, 931—933
   cidofovir, 900—902
   darunavir, 933—934
   dolutegravir, 939—940
   efavirenz, 927—929
   emtricitabine, 922—923
   entecavir monohydrate, 916
   etravirine, 929—930
   famciclovir, 902—903
   fosamprenavir, 842
   foscarnet, 903—905
   ganciclovir, 905—907
   lamivudine, 923—924
   letermovir, 907—908
   maraviroc, 935
   oseltamivir, 910—911
   peramivir, 911—912
   raltegravir, 940—941

antiviral agents (*Continued*)
   ribavirin, 917—918
   rilpivirine, 930—931
   ritonavir, 934—936
   sofosbuvir, 913—914
   tenofoviralafenamide, 924
   tenofovir disoproxilfumarate, 924—925
   valaciclovir, 908—909
   valganciclovir, 909—910
   zanamivir, 912—913
   zidovudine, 925—927
Antizol Concentrated Injection, 349—350
Antroquoril, 1000—1001
anxiety, 70
   erectile dysfunction and, 1116
   quetiapine for, 863
   severe, periciazine for, 863
   stimulants and, 1552—1553
anxiety disorders, 70
Anzatax Injection, 663—665
Anzole, 602
apalutamide, 603—604
aperients, 1285
aphakia, latanoprost and, 469
Apidra, 303
apixaban, 259—260
aplastic anaemia, nandrolone decanoate for, 1522
Aplidin, 668—669
apnoea, suxamethonium chloride and, 1426
APO-Adefovir, 915—916
APO-Azathioprine, 1243—1245
APOHealth Anti-Inflammatory Pain Relief Rapid 25, 22
APOHealth Cardio Aspirin, 15—17
APO-Isotretinoin, 5—6
APOC-5FU Cream, 642—643
apolipoproteins, 1300
Apomine, 800—802
apomorphine hydrochloride, 800—802
apomorphine hydrochloride hemihydrate, 800—802
Aporyl, 428—429
Appese, 1417—1419
appetite suppression, mode of action in, 36
apraclonidine, 463—464
apremilast, 1240—1241
aprepitant, 374—375
Apresoline, 549—550
aprotinin, 1427
aPTT. *See* activated partial thromboplastin time
arachis, 1523
Aramine, 1575—1576
Aranesp, 1187—1188
Aratac, 86—88
Arava, 1047—1050
Arazil, 53

INDEX

Arcoxia, 22—23
Ardix Gliclazide MR, 309
arginine, 1670
Arginine Hydrochloride 60% Concentrated Injection, 1670
argipressin, 1670
Arianna, 602
Aricept, 53
Aridol, 137
Aridon APN, 53
Arimidex, 602
aripiprazole, 839—841
Aristocort, 1017
Arixtra, 253—255
armodafinil, 1553—1555
Arnuity Ellipta, 130—133
Aromasin, 640
Aropax, 282—283
arrhythmias
 antipsychotics and, 835
 idursulfase and, 1351
 suxamethonium chloride and, 1426
 verapamil hydrochloride for, 541
arsenic trioxide, 604—605
Artane, 794—795
artemether and lumefantrine, 557—559
 action of, 557—558
 adverse effects of, 558
 dose of, 558
 interactions of, 558
 nursing points/cautions for, 558—559
 patient teaching and advice for, 559
 use of, 558
arterial thrombi, 236, 1151
arterial thromboembolic events, antipsychotics and, 837
arteriosclerosis, stimulants and, 1552—1553
arthralgia, progesterone and, 1470
Arthrexin, 26—27
arthritis, 970
articaine hydrochloride, 1324—1325
Artige, 1561—1563
Artiss, 1198
Asacol, 1163—1165
ascorbic acid (vitamin C), 1643—1645
 desferrioxamine mesylate and, 342
asenapine maleate, 841—842
aseptic meningitis syndrome, 1620
asfotase alfa, 1341—1342
Asmol CFC-free Inhaler, 104—108
aspartame, ondansetron and, 372
Aspecillin VK, 163—164
Aspen Ciprofloxacin Injection for Intravenous Infusion, 216—218
Aspen Methadone Syrup, 1107, 1444
aspergillosis, itraconazole for, 443

Aspergillus, 428
aspiration pneumonia, antipsychotics and, 837
aspirin, 15—17, 817—818
 action of, 15
 adverse effects of, 16
 dose of, 16
 interactions of, 16
 nursing points/cautions for, 16—17
 patient teaching and advice for, 17
 use of, 15—16
asplenia, meningococcal vaccine for, 1609
Aspro Clear, 15—17
Aspro Clear Extra Strength, 15—17, 817—818
Aspro preparations, 817—818
asthenia
 from agalsidase beta (RCH), 1338
 from carglumic acid, 1343
asthma, 97
 budesonide for, 1002
  patient teaching and advice for, 127
 dupilumab for, 1248
 mannitol for, 137
 sodium cromoglycate for, 98
asthma action plan, 98
asthma prophylaxis
 budesonide, 1002
 ciclesonide for, 128
 fluticasone furoate for, 130
 montelukast sodium for, 142
 sodium cromoglycate, 98
Astrix, 100, 817—818
Astrix Tablets, 817—818
asystole, suxamethonium chloride and, 1426
Atacand, 515
Ataris, 1047—1049
atazanavir, 931—932
atenolol, 524
Atgam, 1238
Atgam skin testing, antithymocyte globulin and, 1239
atherosclerosis, 1299
atherothrombotic events, ticagrelor for, 822
Ativan, 77
atomoxetine, 1555—1556
atonic seizures, 384
atopic dermatitis
 ciclosporin for, 1041
 dupilumab for, 1248
 mild-to-moderate, crisaborole for, 1031
 pimecrolimus for, 1036
Atorvachol, 1302—1303
atorvastatin, 1302—1303
atovaquone, 559—561, 825—826
 action of, 559—560
 adverse effects of, 560
 dose of, 560

1725

HAVARD'S NURSING GUIDE TO DRUGS

atovaquone (*Continued*)
  interactions of, 560
  nursing points/cautions for, 560
  patient teaching and advice for, 560—561
  use of, 560
atracurium besylate, 1423
Atrax robustus, 893
atrial fibrillation
  apixaban for, 259
  dabigatran etexilate for, 256
  digoxin for, 980
  rivaroxaban for, 260
  stimulants and, 1552—1553
atrial flutter, stimulants and, 1552—1553
atrophic vaginitis, estradiol for, 1527
atropine, activated charcoal and, 337
Atropine Injection BP, 986—987
atropine sulfate, 1131—1132
atropine sulfate monohydrate, 949, 987, 1131, 1573
Atropt, 986—987, 1131—1132
Atrovent preparations, 113—114
attention deficit hyperactivity disorder (ADHD), 1551
  atomoxetine for, 1555
  dexamfetamine (dexamphetamine) sulfate for, 1557
  guanfacine for, 1558
  lisdexamfetamine dimesilate for, 1560
  methylphenidate hydrochloride for, 1561
atypical antidepressant agents, 288—295
atypical antipsychotic agents, 834
atypical haemolytic uraemic syndrome (aHUS), 1249
  eculizumab for, 1249
atypical pneumonia, roxithromycin for, 205
auranofin, 1039—1041
auranofin-induced diarrhoea, 1040
Aurorix, 277
Ausfam, 873—874
Ausgem, 1311—1312
Australian Immunisation Register, 1593
Austrapen, 158—159
autoimmune diseases, DMARDs and, 1038
autologous pre-donation, 1185
  epoetin alfa for, 1189
  epoetin beta for, 1190
  epoetin lambda for, 1191
autonomic nervous system, 981, 1565
Avamys, 130—133
avanafil, 1121—1122
Avanza, 293—294
Avapro, 515—516
Avapro HCT, 516
Avaxim, 1603
Avelox, 218—219

avelumab, 748
Avodart, 946—947
Avonex, 1391—1392
Avsartan, 515—516
axicabtagene ciloleucel, 605—607
Axit, 293—294
axitinib, 695—696
Axotide, 130
azacitidine, 607—608
Azactam, 179—180
Azadine, 607—608
Azapin, 1243—1245
azathioprine, 1243—1245
  action of, 1243
  adverse effects of, 1243
  dose of, 1243
  interactions of, 1243—1244
  nursing points/cautions of, 1244
  patient teaching and advice of, 1244
  sulfasalazine and, 1167
  use of, 1243
Azathioprine Sandoz, 1243—1245
Azathioprine-WGR, 1243—1245
Azclear Medicated Lotion, 7—8
Azelaic acid, 7—8
Azelastine, 486—487
Azep Nasal Spray, 486—487
Azilect, 812—813
Azith, 201—202
azithromycin, 201—202
azole antifungal agents, amphotericin B and, 430
Azonaire Hayfever & Allergy Prevention Nasal Spray, 1013—1014
Azopt Eye Drops 1%, 467
aztreonam, 179—180

B

B lymphocyte stimulator, belimumab, 1247
B lymphocytes, rituximab, 1071
B12 Liquid, 1640—1641
Bacillus Calmette-Guerin (BCG) vaccine, 1597
baclofen, 1402—1406
  action of, 1402
  adverse effects of, 1403
  dose of, 1403
  interactions of, 1403
  nursing points/cautions of, 1404—1405
  patient teaching and advice of, 1405—1406
  use of, 1402
bacteraemia
  daptomycin for, 225
  teicoplanin for, 184
bacterial cell membrane, disrupting, 147
bacterial conjunctivitis
  chloramphenicol for, 209
  ciprofloxacin lactate for, 217

INDEX

bacterial conjunctivitis (*Continued*)
framycetin sulfate for, 189
gentamicin sulfate for, 190
ofloxacin for, 220
bacterial endocarditis, amoxicillin trihydrate for, 154
bacterial keratitis
ciprofloxacin lactate for, 217
framycetin sulfate for, 189
bacterial meningitis
ampicillin sodium for, 158
chloramphenicol for, 209
bacterial protein synthesis, other miscellaneous inhibitors of, 209—211
bacterial septicaemia, amoxicillin trihydrate for, 154
bacterial vaginosis
clindamycin phosphate for, 207
metronidazole for, 827
bactericidal drugs, 147
bacteriostatic drugs, 147
Bacthecal, 1402—1405
Bactrim DS, 222—225
Bactroban, 214
Bactroban Nasal Ointment, 214
balsalazide sodium, 1160
barbiturates, 414
non-depolarising blocking agents and, 1422
bariatric surgery, 35—36
baricitinib, 1245
barrier method contraception, 1536
basal cell carcinoma
methyl aminolevulinate hydrochloride for, 658
vismodegib for, 742
basiliximab, 1246—1247
Bavencio, 748
B-cell chronic lymphocytic leukaemia, alemtuzumab for, 746, 1369
BCG (non-vaccine), 608—619
BCG Vaccine, 1597
beclometasone (beclomethasone) dipropionate, 124, 1000
Beconase Allergy & Hayfever 12 hour, 123—124
behaviour, changes in, and clonazepam, 396
behavioural disturbances, chlorpromazine hydrochloride for, 844
Bekunis Senna Tablets, 1294
belimumab, 1247—1248
Belkyra, 1031—1033
belladonna alkaloid, 1131
Belsomra, 1513—1515
Bemfola, 1462—1463
bendamustine hydrochloride, 609—610
BeneFIX, 1211—1212
benign prostatic hyperplasia
alfuzosin hydrochloride for, 943

benign prostatic hyperplasia (*Continued*)
finasteride for, 947
prazosin hydrochloride for, 503
silodosin for, 952
tadalafil for, 1124
benign prostatic hypertrophy
androgens and anabolic steroids and, 1521
tamsulosin hydrochloride for, 954
Benlysta, 1247—1248
BenPen, 160—161
benralizumab, 133
benserazide hydrochloride, 802
Benzac, 8—9
Benzac AC Wash, 8—9
benzalkonium chloride, 461
olopatadine hydrochloride and, 495
Benzathine Benzylpenicillin, 159—160
benzatropine mesilate, 793—794
benzodiazepines
first trimester, 73b
short-acting, 1511
benzoyl peroxide, 8—9
Benztrop, 793—794
benztropine mesylate, 793—794
benzydamine, 17—18
benzyl alcohol, 1202
clonazepam and, 396
nandrolone decanoate and, 1522
benzyl benzoate, 1026
Benzylpenicillin, 160—161
Beovu, 1140
beractant, 133—134
Berinert, 1255
Besponsa, 763—764
beta-adrenoceptor blocking agents, 500, 521—524
actions of, 521
adverse effects of, 521—522
interactions of, 522
nursing points/cautions for, 522—523
patient teaching and advice for, 523—524
beta adrenoceptors, 1427
beta-glucocerebrosidase
in imiglucerase (RCH), 1352
in velaglucerase alfa (GHU), 1366
beta-lactam resistant Gram-positive organisms, vancomycin hydrochloride for, 185
beta-lactams, probenecid co-therapy with, 480
beta3 adrenergic agonist, 948
Betadine Preparations, 1677
Betadine Sore Throat Gargle, 1150
Betadine Sore Throat Gargle - Ready To Use, 1150
Betaferon, 1392—1393
betahistine dihydrochloride, 1633—1634
betaine, 1342—1343
Betaloc, 528
betamethasone, 999

betamethasone acetate, 999
betamethasone dipropionate, 1000
betamethasone sodium phosphate, 999
betamethasone valerate, 1000–1001
Betavit, 1637–1638
betaxolol, 464–465
bethanechol chloride, 944
Betmiga, 948–949
Betnovate preparations, 1000–1001
Betoptic, 464–465
Betoquin, 464–465
bevacizumab, 748–750
   action of, 748
   adverse effects of, 749
   dose of, 748–749
   interactions of, 749
   nursing points/cautions for, 749–750
   patient teaching and advice for, 750
   use of, 748
Bexsero, 1609–1610
Bicalox, 610–611
bicalutamide, 610–611
bicarbonate, 1665–1667
   serum levels of, zonisamide and, 426
   sodium bicarbonate, 1665–1667
Bicard, 524–525
Bicillin LA, 159–160
BiCNU, 618–619
Bicor, 524–525
Bier's block, 1321
bifonazole, 433
biguanides, 304, 310–313
bile acid binding agents, 1307
   actions of, 1307
   adverse effects of, 1307–1308
   interactions of, 1308
   nursing points/cautions for, 1308
   patient teaching and advice for, 1308
   uses of, 1307
biliary atresia, lanthanum, 353
biliary surgery prophylaxis, cefotaxime sodium for, 171
Biltricide, 48–49
bimatoprost, 465–466
Bimprozt, 465–466
binge eating disorder (BED), lisdexamfetamine dimesilate for, 1560
Biodone Forte, 1107, 1444
Biological Therapies Sodium Ascorbate Solution, 1643–1645
Bio-Logical Vitamin A, 1636–1637
Bio-Logical Vitamin D3 Solution, 1645–1647
biopsy, golimumab, 1065
Biostate, 1205–1206
biphasic anaphylactic reaction, idursulfase for, 1351

bipolar disorders, 833
   carbamazepine for, 843
bipolar I disorder
   aripiprazole for, 840
   asenapine maleate for, 841
   haloperidol decanoate and, 852
   olanzapine pamoate monohydrate for, 858
   quetiapine for, 863
birth defects, due to thalidomide, 675
bisacodyl, 1293
Bisalax, 1293
Bisolvon Chesty Forte Oral Liquid, 1020
Bisolvon Chesty Forte Tablets, 1020
Bisolvon Chesty Oral Liquid, 1020
Bisolvon Dry (Oral Liquid), 1021–1022
Bisolvon Dry Pastilles, 1021–1022
bisphosphonates, 958–960
   actions of, 958
   adverse effects of, 959
   alendronic acid, 961
   ibandronate, 961–962
   interactions of, 959
   nitrogen-containing, 958
   nursing points/cautions for, 959–960
   pamidronate disodium, 962–963
   patient teaching and advice for, 960
   risedronate sodium, 963–964
   uses of, 958
   zoledronic acid, 964–965
Bispro, 524–525
bivalirudin, 255–256
black snake antivenom, 892
Blackmores B12, 1640–1641
Blackmores Folate, 1642–1643
Blackmores InSolar, 1638–1639
Blackmores Natural E, 1647
Blackmores Vitamin A, 5000, 1636–1637
Blackmores Vitamin B6, 1639–1640
Blackmores Vitamin C, 1643–1645
Blackmores Vitamin D3, 1645–1647
bladder, 942
bladder cancer
   BCG (non-vaccine) for, 608
   cisplatin for, 621
   doxorubicin hydrochloride for, 633–634
   epirubicin hydrochloride for, 636–637
   fluorouracil for, 642
   gemcitabine for, 646
   surgery, erectile dysfunction and, 1116
bladder function disorder
   causes of, 942
   cholinergic agents for, 942–943
   sympathomimetic agents for, 943
bladder function disorder agents, 942–956
bleeding
   adrenaline for, 1567

INDEX

bleeding (*Continued*)
  coagulation factor deficiencies and, 1201
  control of, factor VIII inhibitor bypassing fraction (Feiba-NF) for, 1207
  dysfunctional, norethisterone for, 1539
  oestrogens and, 1530–1532
  during pregnancy rifabutin, 591b
    rifampicin, 594
    risk, prasugrel with, 821
  as side-effect of anticoagulants, 236–237
bleomycin sulfate, 611–613
  action of, 611–612
  adverse effects of, 612
  dose of, 612
  nursing points/caution for, 612–613
  patient teaching and advice for, 613
  use of, 612
blepharitic corneal abrasions and burns, framycetin sulfate for, 189
blepharospasm
  botulinum toxin type A for, 1406
  incobotulinumtoxinA for, 1412
blinatumomab, 750–751
Blincyto, 750–751
Blistex Antiviral Cold Sore Cream, 898–900
blood counts, antipsychotics and, 836
blood dyscrasias, TNF-α antagonists and, 1058
blood glucose levels (BGLs), 296
  monitoring of, probenecid and, 481
blood levels, monitoring of, for antiepileptic agents, 386
blood lipids, retinoids and, 3
blood phenylalanine levels, sapropterin for, 1361
blood pressure (BP)
  factors affecting, 499
  monitoring
    epoprostenol and, 1495
    macitentan and, 1498
    riociguat and, 1499
  pentoxifylline and, 1635
blood stasis, 1151
blurred vision
  mercaptamine bitartrate for, 1355
  olopatadine hydrochloride and, 495
BMI. *See* body mass index
body louse, 1024
body mass, 1024
  benzyl benzoate for, 1026
body mass index (BMI), 35
body weight, changes in, antipsychotics and, 835
Bondronat, 961–962
bone, 957
bone and calcium regulating agents, 957–978
  bisphosphonates, 958–960
  other, 965–966
bone fractures, suxamethonium chloride and, 1427

bone infection, gentamicin sulfate for, 191
bone loss, age-related, 958
bone marrow depression
  allopurinol and, 475
  methotrexate and, 656
bone marrow transplant, G-CSF for, 784
bone mass, 957
bone remodelling, 957
Bonjela Mouth Ulcer Gel, 19–20
Bonjela Teething Gel, 19–20
bony (skeletal) metastases, androgens and anabolic steroids and, 1521
Boostrix, 1601–1602
Boostrix-IPV, 1602
bortezomib, 698–699
bosentan, 1491–1493
Botox, 1406–1410
botulinum toxin type A, 1406–1410
  action of, 1406
  adverse effects of, 1406–1408
  dose of, 1406
  interactions of, 1407–1408
  nursing points/cautions for, 1408–1409
  patient teaching and advice of, 1410
  use of, 1406
Bowen's disease, fluorouracil for, 642
bowing
  femur or tibia, 957
  in Paget's disease, 957
box jellyfish antivenom, 892
bradycardia
  dexmedetomidine and, 1507
  suxamethonium chloride and, 1426
brain tumours
  lomustine for, 651
  temozolomide for, 674
Braltus, 114–116
branch retinal vein occlusion (BRVO), aflibercept for, 1139
breast cancer
  anastrozole for, 602
  androgens and anabolic steroids and, 1520
  bevacizumab for, 748
  capecitabine for, 616
  chlorambucil for, 619
  cyclophosphamide for, 624
  docetaxel for, 632
  doxorubicin hydrochloride for, 633
  epirubicin hydrochloride for, 636–637
  eribulin mesilate for, 638
  everolimus for, 1251
  exemestane for, 640
  fluorouracil for, 642
  fulvestrant for, 644
  gemcitabine for, 646
  goserelin acetate for, 1217

1729

breast cancer (*Continued*)
  ifosfamide for, 648
  invasive, raloxifene hydrochloride for, 973
  lapatinib ditosylate monohydrate for, 718
  letrozole for, 651
  medroxyprogesterone acetate for, 1538
  melphalan for, 653
  methotrexate for, 655
  mitozantrone for, 660
  olaparib for, 727
  paclitaxel for, 663
  pertuzumab for, 771
  tamoxifen for, 672
  toremifene for, 682
  trastuzumab for, 777
  vinblastine sulfate for, 686
  vincristine sulfate for, 687
  vinorelbine for, 688
breastfeeding
  alpha-adrenoceptor blocking agents and, 501b
  angiotensin-converting enzyme (ACE) inhibitors and, 514b
  angiotensin II receptor antagonists and, 514b
  apremilast and, 1241b
  artemether and lumefantrine and, 559b
  azathioprine and, 1245b
  baclofen and, 1406
  baricitinib and, 1246b
  basiliximab and, 1247b
  belimumab and, 1248b
  botulinum toxin type A and, 1406
  calcium-channel blockers and, 532b
  carbimazole and, 1586
  clonidine hydrochloride and, 545b
  dantrolene sodium hemiheptahydrate and, 1412
  desmopressin and, 1235b
  dupilumab and, 1249b
  eculizumab and, 1251b
  everolimus and, 1254
  goserelin acetate and, 1217
  guselkumab and, 1255
  human C1 esterase inhibitor and, 1256
  hydralazine hydrochloride and, 549
  icatibant and, 1257
  incobotulinumtoxinA and, 1415
  ixekizumab (RCH) and, 1258
  lanreotide and, 1222
  leuprorelin acetate and, 1220
  methyldopa sesquihydrate and, 547b
  minoxidil and, 552b
  moxonidine and, 548b
  mycophenolate mofetil and, 1263
  octreotide and, 1224
  pasireotide and, 1226
  pegvisomant and, 1227b

breastfeeding (*Continued*)
  pirfenidone and, 1267
  plerixafor and, 1268
  propylthiouracil and, 1588
  rifabutin and, 591
  rifampicin and, 594
  risankizumab and, 1271
  ropinirole hydrochloride and, 1419
  secukinumab and, 1272
  sirolimus and, 1274
  sodium iodide (^{131}I) and, 1590
  sodium nitroprusside and, 554b
  tacrolimus and, 1278
  terlipressin and, 1236
  tetracosactide and, 835
  thalidomide and, 678
  tildrakizumab and, 1279
  ustekinumab and, 1280
brentuximab vedotin, 751
Brenzys, 1063–1064
Bretaris Genuair, 111–112
Brevibloc, 526–527
brexpiprazole, 842
brigatinib, 699–700
bright lights, seizure triggers, 386
Brilinta, 822–823
brimonidine, 466–467, 1029–1030
brimonidine tartrate, 467
Brineura, 1344–1346
Brintellix, 294–295
brinzolamide, 467–468
BrinzoQuin Eye Drops 1%, 467–468
Brivact, 389–390
brivaracetam, 389–390
brolucizumab, 1140
bromazepam, 74
Bromhexine, 1020–1021
bromocriptine mesilate (mesylate), 802–804, 1486–1488
  action of, 1486
  adverse effects of, 1486
  dose of, 1486
  interactions of, 1486–1487
  nursing points/cautions for, 1487
  patient teaching and advice for, 1487–1488
  use of, 1486
bromocriptine mesylate, 802–804
bronchial hyperresponsiveness, mannitol for, 138
bronchiectasis, 584
bronchitis, cefaclor monohydrate for, 168
Bronchitol, 137
bronchodilators (beta-2 adrenoceptor agonists), 100–101
  adverse effects of, 100
  interactions of, 101
bronchogenic carcinoma, methotrexate for, 656

INDEX

bronchospasm
 ephedrine sulfate for, 1572
 idursulfase and, 1351
brown snake antivenom, 892–893
Brufen, 24
BRVO. *See* branch retinal vein occlusion
buccolingual dyskinesia, tetrabenazine for, 1399
Budamax, 124–128, 1001–1002
Budenofalk, 124–128, 1001–1002
Budenofalk Foam Enema, 124–128, 1001–1002
budesonide, 124–128, 1001–1002
 action of, 124–125
 adverse effects of, 125–126
 dose of, 125
 interactions of, 126
 nursing points/cautions for, 126–127
 patient teaching and advice for, 127–128
 use of, 125
Bugesic Oral Suspension, 24
bulbar conjunctival inflammation, fluorometholone acetate for, 1008
bulk-forming laxatives, 1285, 1287
bumetanide, 1084–1085
bupivacaine hydrochloride monohydrate, 1325
Bupivacaine Hydrochloride Injection BP, 1325
Bupivacaine Spinal Heavy BNM, 1325
Bupredermal, 1103, 1435–1438
buprenorphine, 1103–1104, 1435–1438
 action of, 1435
 adverse effects of, 1435–1436
 dose of, 1435
 interactions of, 1436
 nursing points/cautions for, 1436–1437
 patient teaching and advice for, 1437–1438
 sublingual tablets, 1103
 transdermal patches, 1103
 use of, 1435
bupropion hydrochloride, 36–38
Burinex, 1084–1085
Burkitt's lymphoma, methotrexate for, 655
burns
 silver sulfadiazine for, 232
 suxamethonium chloride and, 1427
bursitis, betamethasone valerate for, 1000
Buscopan, 988–989
busulfan, 613–615
 action of, 613
 adverse effects of, 614
 dose of, 613–614
 interactions of, 614
 nursing points/cautions for, 614–615
 patient teaching and advice for, 615
 uses of, 613
Busulfex, 613–615
Buvidal Monthly, 1103–1104, 1435–1438
Buvidal Weekly, 1103–1104, 1435–1438

C

C. difficile, confirmed infection with, fidaxomicin for, 227
Cabaser, 804, 1488–1489
cabazitaxel, 615–616
cabergoline, 804–805, 1488–1489
CAD. *See* coronary artery disease
Caelyx, 633–635
caesarean section prophylaxis
 cefoxitin sodium for, 171
 cefotaxime sodium for, 172
caffeine, 1556–1557
caffeine citrate, 120–121
Cafnea, 120–121
CAL-500 Tablets, 1649–1650
CAL-600 Tablets, 1649–1650
Cal-Care, 1649–1650
calcimimetic agents, 958
calcipotriol, 1001
Calcipotriol/Betamethasone 50/500, 1030–1031
Calci-Tab 600, 1649–1650
calcitonin, 957
calcitonin salmon (salcatonin), 965–966
calcitriol, 966–968, 1647
Calcitrol, 966–968
calcium, 1649–1652
 calcium carbonate, 1650–1650
 calcium gluconate monohydrate, 1473
calcium carbonate, 887, 1649–1650
calcium-channel blockers, 311, 1632
 as antihypertensives, 500, 533
calcium chloride, 968–969
calcium chloride dihydrate, 968–969
Calcium Chloride Injection, 968–969
calcium-dependent intracellular signals, 1272
calcium folinate, 336–337
calcium gluconate, 1650–1652
Calcium Gluconate 953 mg/10 mL Injection, 1650–1652
calcium gluconate monohydrate, 1473
calcium-independent intracellular signals, 1272
calcium polystyrene sulfonate hydrogen, 363
calcium regulating agents, 957–978
Calcium Resonium, 363
calcium supplements, bisphosphonates, 959
Caldolor, 24–25
Calindamin, 207–209
Cal-Sup Chewable, 1649–1650
Caltrate Vitamin D 1000 IU, 1645–1647
Calutex, 610–611
Campral, 1102–1103
candesartan cilexetil, 515
Candida, 428
candidiasis
 amphotericin B dosages for, 430
 cutaneous

candidiasis (*Continued*)
    clotrimazole for, 435
    nystatin for, 450
  intestinal, nystatin for, 450
  invasive, micafungin for, 447
  itraconazole for, 444
  micafungin for, prophylaxis of, 448
    itraconazole for, 443
    micafungin for, 447
  oral
    itraconazole for, 443
    nystatin for, 450
    posaconazole for, 452
  oropharyngeal, fluconazole for, 438
  vaginal
    clotrimazole for, 435–436
    miconazole nitrate for, 449
    nystatin for, 450
  vulvovaginal
    clotrimazole for, 435
    itraconazole for, 444
Canesoral, 438–440
Canesten Once Daily Bifonazole Cream 1%, 433
cannabidiol, 1394–1397
capecitabine, 616–617
capillariasis, albendazole for, 44
captopril, 506–508
Carafate, 884–885
carbachol, 1135
Carbaglu, 1343–1344
carbamazepine, 392, 842–843
  ondansetron with, 371
  tiagabine hydrochloride and, 422
carbamazepine epoxide, brivaracetam and, 389
carbamazepine toxicity, use with lamotrigine, 393
carbamide peroxide, 1144
carbamoyl phosphate synthetase 1 (CPS 1), in carglumic acid, 1343
carbetocin, 1478–1479
Carbidopa, 805
carbidopa monohydrate, 805
carbonic anhydrase, 1081
carbonic anhydrase inhibitors, 1081–1082
  acetazolamide, 388
  zonisamide and, 425
carboplatin, 617–618
Carboplatin Solution for Infusion, 617–618
Carbosorb X, 337–338
carcinoid tumour, lanreotide acetate for, 1221
carcinoma, renal cell, 700
Cardasa, 15–17, 817–818
cardiac arrest
  adrenaline for, 1567
  isoprenaline hydrochloride for, 1574
  sodium bicarbonate for, 1665
  stimulants and, 1552

cardiac arrhythmias
  atenolol for, 524
  metoprolol tartrate for, 529
  propranolol hydrochloride for, 531
cardiac disease, betaxolol and, 465
cardiac dysfunction, oestrogens and, 1526
cardiac failure/impairment
  androgens and anabolic steroids and, 1521
  dobutamine hydrochloride for, 1569
cardiac glycosides, 92–96, 979–980
cardiac ischaemia, tirofiban hydrochloride for, 823
cardiac monitoring, for ketamine hydrochloride, 1178
cardiac oedema, acetazolamide for, 1081
cardiac resuscitation
  calcium chloride dihydrate for, 968
  calcium gluconate monohydrate for, 1650
cardiac surgery
  milrinone lactate for, 980
  tranexamic acid for, 1200
cardiopulmonary resuscitation
  adrenaline and, 1567
cardiovascular death, eplerenone for, 1095
cardiovascular disease
  antipsychotics and, 834
  apraclonidine hydrochloride and, 464
  stimulants and, 1552
Cardiprin, 100, 15–17, 817–818
Cardizem, 536–537
Cardizem CD, 536–537
Cardol, 88–90
Cardol 80 mg, 88–90
carglumic acid, 1343–1344
carmustine, 618–619
Cartia, 15–17, 817–818
carvedilol, 525–526
Carvidol, 525–526
Caspofungin, 434–435
cataplexy associated with narcolepsy, clomipramine hydrochloride for, 271
Catapres, 543–545
cataract formation, in desferrioxamine mesylate, 343
catecholamines, 1565
catechol-o-methyl transferase (COMT)
  inhibitors, 795–796
  entacapone, 795–796
  opicapone, 796–797
cathartics, 1285
catridecacog, 1214–1215
Caverject Impulse, 1118–1119, 1632–1633
Cavstat, 1305–1306
Ceclor, 168–169
Ceclor CD, 168–169
CeeNU, 651

INDEX

Cefaclor, 168—169
Cefalexin, 169
cefazolin (cephazolin) sodium, 170
Cefepime, 170—171
Cefepime-AFT, 170—171
Cefepime Kabi, 170—171
Cefotaxime Sodium for Injection, 171—172
Cefotaxime, 171—172
Cefoxitin Juno Powder for Injection, 172—173
cefoxitin sodium, 480
ceftaroline fosamil, 173
ceftazidime, 173—174
Ceftazidime Powder for Injection, 173—174
ceftazidime with avibactam, 174—175
ceftolozane with tazobactam, 175—176
Ceftriaxone Powder for Injection, 176—177
cefuroxime axetil, 177—178
Celapram, 280
Celaxib, 18—19
Celebrex, 18—19
celecoxib, 18—19
Celecoxib GH, 18—19
Celebrex Relief, 18—19
Celecoxib Sandoz, 18—19
Celecoxib-WGR, 18—19
Celestone Chronodose, 999
Celestone M Cream and Ointment, 1000
Celexi, 18—19
cell replication, methotrexate on, 1050
CellCept, 1263
Cellplant, 1263
Celsentri, 937—938
Cenovis MegaC 1000 mg Chewable Tablets, 1643—1645
Cenovis Sugarless C 500 mg Chewable Tablets, 1643—1645
central nervous system, 981
central retinal vein occlusion, aflibercept for, 1139
centrally acting agents, 543
Cepacol Solution, 1149
Cephalex, 169
Cephalexin, 169
cephalosporins, 166—168
    actions of, 166
    adverse effects of, 166
    interactions of, 166—167
    nursing points/cautions for, 167—168
    patient teaching and advice for, 168
    uses of, 166
    with vitamin K, 167
Ceprotin, 262—263
Ceptolate, 1263—1265
Cerdelga, 1346—1347
cerebral oedema, furosemide for, 1086
cerebrovascular disease, antipsychotics and, 836
Cerezyme, 1352—1353

cerliponase alfa, 1344—1346
    action of, 1344
    adverse effects of, 1344
    dose of, 1344
    nursing points/cautions of, 1344—1346
    patient teaching and advice of, 1346
    use of, 1344
Certican, 1251—1254
certolizumab pegol, 1062—1063
cervical cancer
    bevacizumab for, 748
    fluorouracil for, 642
    human papillomavirus (HPV) vaccine for, 1605
    ifosfamide for, 647
    topotecan hydrochloride for, 681
    vincristine sulfate for, 687
cervical dystonia
    botulinum toxin type A for, 1406
    incobotulinumtoxinA for, 1412
Cervidil, 1477—1478
cestodes, 42
cetirizine, 488—489
cetrorelix acetate, 1459
Cetrotide, 1459
cetuximab (RMC), 752—753
cetylpyridinium chloride, 1149
CF. *See* cystic fibrosis
CFlox, 216
CFTR gene mutation, ivacaftor for, 135
charcoal, activated, 337—338
    leflunomide and, 1048
Charcocaps, 338
Charcotabs, 338
chelating agents, 334—367
chemoreceptor trigger zone (CTZ), 368, 1431
chemotherapy
    pegfilgrastim for, 788
chest X-ray
    immunomodifiers and, 1237
    interferons and, 1281
chewing gum, nicotine as, 1109
children, helminth infestations in, 42
Children's Claratyne Chewable Tablets, 494—495
Children's Claratyne Syrup, 494—495
Chirocaine, 1325—1326
Chironex fleckeri, 892
chlamydial infection
    azithromycin for, 201
    erythromycin lactobionate for, 204
chloasma, 1532
chloasma gravidarum, progestogens and, 1533
chloral hydrate, 1506—1507
Chloral Hydrate Mixture, 1506—1507
chlorambucil, 619—620
chloramphenicol, 209—211
chlorhexidine gluconate, 1149

1733

Chloromycetin Succinate, 209—211
chlorpromazine, zolpidem tartrate and, 1516
chlorpromazine hydrochloride, 844—846
Chlorsig, 209—211
chlortalidone, 1088—1089
Chlorvescent, 1664—1665
cholecalciferol, 1645—1647
cholera vaccine, 1597—1598
cholesterol, 1299
cholestyramine, 1318
choline salicylate, 19—20
cholinergic agents, 981—990
    actions of, 981
    adverse effects of, 981—982
    for bladder function disorder, 942—943
    neostigmine methylsulfate, 982
    pyridostigmine bromide, 983
cholinergic agonists, 981
cholinesterase gene, atypical, non-depolarising blocking agents and, 1420
cholinomimetics, 987
Cholstat, 1304
chorea
    phenoxymethylpenicillin potassium for, 163
    tetrabenazine for, 1399
choriocarcinoma
    bleomycin sulfate for, 612
    methotrexate for, 655
    vinblastine sulfate for, 686
chorionic gonadotropin (human), 1457—1460
choroidal neovascularisation
    ranibizumab for, 1140
'Christmas disease', 1194
    factor IX for, 1210
    nonacog alfa for, 1211
    nonacog gamma for, 1212
chronic alcoholism, disulfiram for, 1106
chronic artery disease, androgens and anabolic steroids and, 1521
chronic autoimmune diseases, 1243
chronic bronchitis
    ampicillin sodium for, 158
    moxifloxacin hydrochloride for, 219
chronic cardiac decompensation, dopamine hydrochloride for, 1571
chronic cholestatic liver disease, ursodeoxycholic acid for, 1158
chronic diarrhoea, 331
chronic granulocytic leukaemia
    busulfan for, 613
    mercaptopurine monohydrate for, 654
    tioguanine for, 678
chronic granulomatous disease, interferon gamma 1b for, 1282
chronic heart failure
    adrenaline for, 1567

chronic heart failure (*Continued*)
    digoxin and, 980
    eplerenone for, 1095
chronic kidney disease, methoxy polyethylene glycol epoetin beta for, 1193
chronic left ventricular failure, isosorbide mononitrate for, 63
chronic liver impairment, hepatitis B vaccine for, 1604
chronic liver transplantation, hepatitis B vaccine for, 1604
chronic lymphocytic leukaemia
    alemtuzumab for, 746
    bendamustine hydrochloride for, 609
    chlorambucil for, 619
    cladribine for, 622
    cytarabine for, 625
    fludarabine phosphate for, 641
    ibrutinib for, 713
    idelalisib for, 714—715
    obinutuzumab for, 767
    rituximab for, 773
chronic migraine, botulinum toxin type A for, 1406
chronic myelocytic leukaemia
    azacitidine for, 607
    hydroxycarbamide for, 645
chronic myelogenous leukaemia, mitozantrone for, 660
chronic myeloid leukaemia
    cytarabine for, 625
    dasatinib for, 708
    imatinib for, 716
    nilotinib for, 725
    ponatinib for, 729
chronic neuronopathic type 3, imiglucerase (RCH) for, 1352
chronic neutropenia
    filgrastim for, 786
    G-CSF for, 784
chronic obstructive pulmonary disease (COPD), 584
    TNF-α antagonists and, 1059
chronic pain, 1429
    fentanyl citrate for, 1440
chronic plaque psoriasis, moderate-to-severe, etanercept for, 1063
chronic recurrent urinary tract infection, norfloxacin for, 219
chronic renal failure
    darbepoetin alfa for, 1187
    epoetin alfa for, 1189
    epoetin beta for, 1190
    epoetin lambda for, 1191
    haemopoietic agents and, 1184, 1185
chronic renal insufficiency, somatropin (somatotrophin/somatotropin) for, 1228

INDEX

chronic respiratory disorders, antipsychotics and, 837
chronic shiftwork sleep disorder
  armodafinil for, 1553
  modafinil for, 1563
chronic stable angina, 58
  nifedipine for, 539
chronic stable congestive heart failure, chlortalidone for, 1088
chronic stable plaque psoriasis, calcipotriol for, 1030
chronic suppurative otitis media
  ciprofloxacin lactate for, 217
chylomicrons, 1299
Cialis, 1124—1125
ciclesonide, 128—130
ciclopirox, 435
ciclosporin, 1041—1045
  allopurinol and, 475
  amphotericin B and, 430
  caspofungin acetate and, 434
  tacrolimus and, 1277
Cidala, 1124—1125
cidofovir, 900—902
cilia, 825
ciliate, 825
Cilicaine Syringe, 165—166
Cilicaine V, 163
Cilicaine VK, 163
Cilopam-S, 280—281
CiloQuin, 216
Ciloxan, 216
Ciloxan Ear Drops, 216
cimetidine, 926
Cimzia PEGOL, 1062—1063
cinacalcet, 969—971
cinchonism, 565
Cinryze, 1255—1256
Cipramil, 280
ciprofloxacin
  sevelamer hydrochloride and, 360
  zolpidem tartrate and, 1516
ciprofloxacin hydrochloride, 216
ciprofloxacin lactate, 216—218
Ciprol, 216
Ciproxin HC Ear Drops, 218
Circadin, 1509—1510
cisatracurium, 1423—1424
cisplatin, 621—622
citalopram, 280
Citanest, 1330—1331
Citanest Dental with Octapressin, 3%, 1331
cladribine, 622—623, 1371—1373
Claratyne, 494—495
Claratyne Reditabs, 494—495
Clarithro, 202—204

clarithromycin, 202—204
'classic' haemophilia, 1194
claudication, intermittent, pentoxifylline for, 1634
Clear Eyes, murine, 1136—1137
clevidipine, 535—536
Cleviprex, 535—536
Clexane, 244—246
Clexane Forte, 244—246
clindamycin hydrochloride, 207
clindamycin phosphate, 207—209
Clindamyk, 207
ClindaTech, 207
clobazam, 74—75
Clobemix, 277
Clobetasol, 1002
Clobetasone, 1003
Clobex, 1002
clofarabine, 623—624
Clofen, 1402—1406
Clomid, 1460—1461
clomifene (clomiphene) citrate, 1460—1461
clomipramine hydrochloride, 270—271
Clonac, 20—22
clonazepam, 395—396
Clonea, 435—437
Clonea Clotrimazole Thrush Treatment 3 Day cream, 435—437
Clonea Clotrimazole Thrush Treatment 6 Day cream, 435—437
clonic seizures, 381
clonidine hydrochloride, 543—545
clonus, serotonin syndrome and, 265
clopidogrel, 818—819
Clopine, 847—849
Clopixol, 869
Clopixol Acuphase, 869
Clopixol Depot, 869—870
clostridial infection, benzylpenicillin sodium for, 160
Clostridium tetani, 1600—1601
clotrimazole, 435—437
clotting, prevention during haemodialysis, nadroparin calcium for, 247
Clovix, 818—819
clozapine, 847—849
Clozaril, 847—849
Clozole Topical Cream, 435—437
Clozole Vaginal Cream 10 mg/g & 20 mg/g, 435—437
cluster headaches
  pizotifen maleate for, 577
  sumatriptan for, 581
CMV. *See* cytomegalovirus
CMV Immunoglobulin-VF, 1622
CMV pneumonitis, ganciclovir for, 905

CMV retinitis
  in AIDS, ganciclovir for, 905
  cidofovir for, 900
  foscarnet sodium for, 903
  valganciclovir for, 909
CNS disease, TNF-α antagonists and, 1059
coagulation factor deficiencies, 1194
coagulation factors, 1201
  factor VII, 1201
  factor VIII, 1203
    inhibitor bypassing fraction (Feiba-NF), 1206—1208
    inhibitors to, eptacog alfa for, 1201
  factor IX, 1209
    inhibitors to, eptacog alfa for, 1201
  factor XIII, 1214
coagulopathies, tranexamic acid for, 1200—1201
Cobal-B, 12, 1641—1642
cobimetinib, 705—706
Codeine Linctus, 1438—1439
codeine phosphate hemihydrate, 1438—1439
Codeine Phosphate Tablets, 1438—1439
Co-Diovan, 521
Colazide, 1160
colchicine, 477—479
cold sores
  famciclovir for, 902
  valaciclovir for, 909
colecalciferol, 1645—1647
Colese, 1156
colestyramine, 1308
  leflunomide and, 1048
Colgout, 477—478
colistimethate sodium, 221—222
Colistin, 221—222
collagen diseases, betamethasone valerate for, 1000
Colofac, 1156—1157
colon cancer
  capecitabine for, 616
  fluorouracil for, 642
  irinotecan hydrochloride for, 649
  oxaliplatin for, 662
colon electrolyte lavage, 1288—1289
ColonLYTELY, 1288—1289
colonoscopy, golimumab, 1065
colorectal cancer
  bevacizumab for, 748
  capecitabine for, 616
  cetuximab for, 752
  oxaliplatin for, 662
  panitumumab for, 769
  pembrolizumab for, 770
  raltitrexed for, 670
Coloxyl Tablets, 1294
Combantrin Chocolate Squares, 49

Combantrin-1 with Mebendazole, 47—48
Combantrin-1 with Mebendazole Chocolate Square, 47—48
combined oral contraceptive pills, 1270
comedones, 1
Comirnaty, 1599—1600
common cold
  ammonium chloride for, 1019
  bromhexine hydrochloride for, 1020
community-acquired pneumonia
  azithromycin dihydrate for, 201
  linezolid for, 212
  moxifloxacin hydrochloride for, 219
Comtan, 795—796
Concerta Extended-Release Tablets, 1561—1563
Condyline Paint, 1037
congenital factor VII deficiency, eptacog alfa for, 1202
congenital fibrinogen deficiency, fibrinogen for, 1197
congestive heart failure
  captopril for, 507
  carvedilol for, 526
  digoxin for, 92
  fosinopril sodium for, 509
  lisinopril dihydrate for, 509
  milrinone lactate for, 980
  perindopril erbumine for, 510
  prazosin hydrochloride for, 503
conjugate vaccines, 1609
conjunctivitis
  due to *Chlamydia trachomatis*, azithromycin dihydrate for, 201
conscious sedation, midazolam hydrochloride and, 1511
consent, vaccination and, 1592
constipation, 1285
  antipsychotics and, 838
contact lenses
  antiglaucoma agents and, 461
  oral contraceptives and, 1548
contraception
  griseofulvin and, 441
  itraconazole and, 446
  long-term, etonogestrel for, 1534
  medroxyprogesterone and, 1538
  post-coital emergency, levonorgestrel as, 1535, 1537
  travoprost and, 472
Contrave 8/90, 36—38
controlled ovarian hyperstimulation
  follitropin alpha for, 1462
  follitropin beta for, 1463
  menopausal gonadotropin and, 1466
controlled ovarian stimulation, nafarelin acetate for, 1467

INDEX

conventional DMARDs, 1039, 971
    auranofin, 1039–1041
    ciclosporin, 1041–1045
    hydroxychloroquine, 1045–1047
    leflunomide, 1047–1049
    methotrexate, 1050–1054
    penicillamine, 1054–1056
    sulfasalazine, 1056–1057
Copaxone Prefilled Syringe, 1378–1380
COPD. *See* chronic obstructive pulmonary disease
copper-releasing intrauterine devices, 1262, 1270
Coralan, 65
Cordarone X, 86–88
Cordilox SR, 541–543
corifollitropin alfa, 1461–1462
corneal ulcers
    ciprofloxacin lactate for, 217
    infected, ciprofloxacin lactate for, 217
    ofloxacin for, 220
coronary artery disease (CAD), 58
    dalteparin sodium for, 241
    rivaroxaban for, 260
coronary occlusion, warfarin sodium for, 249
coronary vasodilator activity, dipyridamole and, 819
coronavirus disease 2019 (COVID-19), COVID-19 Vaccine for, 1599
Cortate, 1003–1004
Cortic DS, 1009
corticosteroid eye drops, 997
corticosteroids, 123–133, 991–1018, 1406
    actions of, 991–992
    adverse effects of, 992–993
    for Crohn's disease, 1096–1097
    eye drop instillation, 999
    interactions of, 993–994
    intra-articular, 995
    nasal spray instillation, 999
    nursing points/cautions for, 994–998
    ocular, 992
    ophthalmic, 997–998
    patient teaching and advice for, 998–999
    therapy, vaccination and, 1592
    topical, 996–997, 999
    uses of, 992
    withdrawal, 998
corticotrophin-releasing factor (CRF), 991
corticotropin-releasing hormone (CRH), 1216
Cortiment, 124–128, 1001–1002
cortisol, 991
cortisone acetate, 1003–1004
Cortival, 1000–1001
Cosamide, 610–611
Cosentyx, 1271–1272
Cosmegen, 627–628
Cosudex 50, 610–611

Cotellic, 705–706
co-trimoxazole, 222–225
    action of, 222
    adverse effects of, 222–223
    dose of, 222
    interactions of, 223
    nursing points/cautions for, 223–224
    patient teaching and advice for, 224–225
    use of, 222
cough
    ammonium chloride for, 1019
    dextromethorphan hydrobromide monohydrate for, 1021
    dihydrocodeine tartrate for, 1022
    guaifenesin for, 1023
cough suppressants, 1019–1023
Coumadin, 249–253
coumarin-induced skin necrosis, protein C for, 262
coumarin-type anticoagulants, vitamin K, 366
Coversyl, 510
Coversyl Plus, 511
COVID-19 Vaccine, 1599–1600
COX. *See* cyclo-oxygenase
COX platelet activity, aspirin and, 817
COX-2. *See* cyclo-oxygenase 2
Coxiella burnetii, 1612–1613
Cozaar, 516–517
Cozavan, 516–517
crab louse, 1024
craniosynostosis, from asfotase alfa, 1341
Cream and Ointment, 30
creatine kinase, pregabalin and, 413
creatinine, serum, deferasirox and, 339
Creon Capsules, 1170–1171
Creon Micro, 1170–1171
Cresemba, 442–443
Crestor, 1305–1306
CRF. *See* corticotrophin-releasing factor
CRH. *See* corticotropin-releasing hormone
Crinone 8%, 1469–1471
crisaborole, 1031–1032
crizotinib, 706
Crohn's disease, 1159
    adalimumab for, 1060
    antidiarrhoeal agents and, 331
    budesonide for, 125, 1002
    patient teaching and advice for, 127
    DMARDs and, 1038
    infliximab for, 1066
    lanthanum and, 353
    mild-to-moderate, budesonide for, 1002
    sulfasalazine for, 1056
    vedolizumab (rch) for, 1168
Crosuva, 1305–1306
crotamiton, 1027

1737

crow's feet
  botulinum toxin type A for, 1406
  incobotulinumtoxinA for, 1412
crusted scabies, ivermectin for, 45
cryptococcal meningitis, fluconazole for, 438
cryptococcosis, disseminated, HIV-associated, amphotericin B for, 430
Cryptococcus, 428
Crysanal, 30–31
crystalline penicillin, 160–161
CSL Zoster Immunoglobulin-VF, 1630–1631
CTZ. *See* chemoreceptor trigger zone
cumulative iron deficit, 1654
Curam preparations, 156
Curosurf, 145–146
Cushing syndrome
  metyrapone for, 1674
  pasireotide for, 1224
cutaneous larva migrans, albendazole for, 43
cutaneous T cell lymphoma, 620
Cuvitru, 1623–1627
cyanide
  poisoning, sodium nitrite, 361
  sodium thiosulfate pentahydrate with, 363
cyanocobalamin, 1640–1641
Cyanocobalamin 1 mg in 1 mL Injection, 1640–1641
Cyanocobalamin 20 mg in 2 mL Injection, 1640–1641
cyanosis, from idursulfase, 1351
cyclizine hydrochloride, 382
cyclizine lactate, 382–383
Cyclogyl, 1132
Cyclonex, 624–625
cyclo-oxygenase (COX), 10
cyclo-oxygenase 2 (COX-2), 10
cyclopentolate hydrochloride, 1132
cyclophosphamide, 624–625
cycloplegia
  atropine sulfate monohydrate for, 1131
  cyclopentolate hydrochloride for, 1132
cycloplegic and mydriatic drops, 1130
  actions of, 1130
  adverse effects of, 1130
  atropine sulfate as, 1131
  cyclopentolate hydrocholoride as, 1132
  interactions of, 1130
  nursing points/cautions for, 1130–1131
  patient teaching and advice for, 1131
  phenylephrine as, 1132–1133
  tropicamide as, 1133–1134
cyclosporin, 1041–1045
Cyklokapron, 1200–1201
Cymbalta, 286–287
Cymevene, 905–907
cyproheptadine, 489

cyproterone acetate, 1540–1542
Cyramza, 770–773
Cyrotone, 1540–1542
Cystadane, 1342–1343
Cystagon, 1354–1355
cysteamine bitartrate. *See* mercaptamine (cysteamine) bitartrate
cystic fibrosis (CF)
  colonisation and lung infection due to *P. aeruginosa* in those with, colistimethate sodium for, 221
  dornase alfa for, 135
  mannitol for, 138
  pancreatic enzyme replacement therapy for, 1170
  tobramycin sulfate for, 191
  ursodeoxycholic acid for, 1158
cystinosis, mercaptamine bitartrate for, 1354–1355
cystinuria, penicillamine for, 1055
cysts, 1
cytarabine, 625–626
cytokine modulators, 1067–1068
  abatacept, 1068–1070
  adverse effects of, 1067
  anakinra, 1070–1071
  interactions of, 1067
  nursing points/cautions for, 1067–1068
  patient teaching and advice for, 1068
  rituximab, 1071–1072
  tocilizumab, 1073–1075
  tofacitinib, 1075–1077
  upadacitinib, 1077–1078
cytological smear, estriol and, 1529
cytomegalovirus (CMV), 898, 919
cytomegalovirus (CMV) disease, ganciclovir for, 905
cytomegalovirus (CMV) immunoglobulin, 1622
cytomegalovirus (CMV) infection
  cytomegalovirus immunoglobulin for, 1622
  letermovir for, 907
  valganciclovir for, 909
cytoprotective agents, 883
  misoprostol, 883–884
  sucralfate, 884–885
Cytotec, 883–884, 1484–1485
cytotoxic antibiotics, 595–596
cytotoxic therapy, prevention of nausea and vomiting induced by, 373

D

D Penamine, 1054–1056
D3 Capsules and Drops Forte, 1645–1647
dabigatran, idarucizumab and, 352
dabigatran etexilate, 256–258
dabrafenib, 706–708
dacarbazine, 626–627

INDEX

dactinomycin, 627—628
Daivobet 50/500, 1030—1031
Daivobet 50/500 Ointment, 1030—1031
DaktaGOLD Cream, 446—447
Daktarin Oral Gel, 448—450
Daktarin Tincture, 448—450
Dalacin C Capsules, 207
Dalacin C Phosphate Injection, 207—209
Dalacin T Topical Lotion, 207—209
Dalacin V Cream 2%, 207—209
Dalteparin, 241—243
   action of, 241
   adverse effects of, 242
   dose of, 241—242
      acute DVT treatment, 241
      anticoagulation for haemodialysis, 241
      thromboprophylaxis (general surgery associated with high thrombosis risk), 241
      thromboprophylaxis (orthopaedic surgery e.g. hip replacement), 241
      thromboprophylaxis (surgery), 241
      treatment of symptomatic VTE in those with solid tumour cancers, 241
      unstable CAD, 242
   interactions of, 242
   nursing points/cautions for, 242—243
   patient teaching and advice for, 243
   use of, 241
danaparoid, 243—244
Dantrium Capsules, 1410—1412
Dantrium Powder for Injection, 1410—1412
dantrolene, 1410—1412
   adverse effects of, 1411
   dose of, 1410—1411
   interactions of, 1411
   nursing points/cautions of, 1411
   patient teaching and advice of, 1412
   use of, 1410
Daonil, 308—309
dapagliflozin, 325—326
DapaTabs, 1090—1091
Dapoxetine, 1125—1127
dapsone, 586—587
daptomycin, 225—226
Daraprim, 831—832
darbepoetin alfa, 1187—1188, 1193
darifenacin hydrobromide, 945—946
darolutamide, 628—629
darunavir, 933—934
dasatinib, 708—709
daunorubicin, 629—630
   leflunomide and, 1048
Daunorubicin Injection, 629—630
DBL Acetylcysteine Injection Concentrate, 334—336
DBL Amikacin Injection, 188—189
DBL Aminophylline Injection, 118—119
DBL Atracurium Besylate Injection, 1423
DBL Bleomycin Sulfate for Injection, 611—613
DBL Carboplatin Solution for Infusion, 617—618
DBL Cisplatin Solution for Infusion, 621—622
DBL Dacarbazine for Injection, 626—627
DBL Desferrioxamine Mesylate for Injection BP, 342—345
DBL Dexamethasone Sodium Phosphate Injection, 1005—1007
DBL Dobutamine Hydrochloride Injection, 1569—1570
DBL Ephedrine Sulfate Injection, 1572—1573
DBL Ergometrine Injection, 1479—1480
DBL Fentanyl Injection, 1439—1442
Flopen, 162
DBL Fluorouracil Solution, 642—643
DBL Gemcitabine Solution, 646
DBL Glyceryl Trinitrate Concentrate injection, 59—62
DBL Heparin Sodium Injection, 237—240
DBL Magnesium Chloride Concentrated Injection, 1659
DBL Magnesium Sulfate Concentrated Injection, 1472—1473, 1659
DBL Methotrexate Injection, 655—657
DBL Morphine Sulfate Injection, 1445—1447
DBL Oxaliplatin Concentrate, 662—663
DBL Papaverine Hydrochloride Injection, 1119—1120
DBL Pemetrexed, 667—668
DBL Pentamidine Isethionate, 829—831
DBL Pethidine Hydrochloride Solution, 1449—1451
DBL Phenytoin Injection BP, 409—412
DBL Potassium Acetate Concentrated Injection, 1664
DBL Potassium Dihydrogen Phosphate Concentrated Injection, 1660—1662
DBL Potassium Phosphate - Monobasic and Potassium Phosphate - Dibasic Concentrated Injection, 1660—1662
DBL Promethazine Hydrochloride Injection, 496
DBL Rocuronium Bromide Injection, 1424—1425
DBL Sodium Nitroprusside Concentrated Injection, 552—554
DBL Sodium Thiosulfate Injection, 363—364
DBL Sterile Dopamine Concentrate, 1570—1572
DBL Vinblastine Injection, 686—687
DBL Zinc Chloride Injection, 1668—1669
death adder antivenom, 893
debilitating skeletal complications, imiglucerase (RCH) for, 1352—1353
Deca-Durabolin Solution, 1521—1522

HAVARD'S NURSING GUIDE TO DRUGS

decongestants, 948
Decozol Oral Gel, 448–450
deep vein thrombosis (DVT)
   apixaban for, prophylaxis of, 259
   dabigatran etexilate for, 256
   rivaroxaban for, 260
deferasirox, 338–340
   action of, 338
   adverse effects of, 339
   dose of, 338–339
   interactions of, 339
   nursing points/cautions for, 339–340
   patient teaching and advice for, 340
   use of, 338
deferiprone, 341–342
deficiency states, 1636
   vitamin A for, 1636–1637
degarelix, 631–632
dehydration
   antidiarrhoeal agents and, 330
   diuretics and, 1079
delay organ rejection, ciclosporin for, 1041
delirium, chloral hydrate and, 1506
Delucon, 863–865
dementia, 50
Dencorub Anti-Inflammatory Gel, 20–22
denosumab, 670, 755–759
Denpax, 1439
dental work, delay in, and colchicine, 475
deoxycholic acid, 1032–1033
dependence
   drug, 1102–1115
      acamprosate calcium for, 1102–1103
      buprenorphine for, 1103–1104
      bupropion for, 1104–1106
      disulfiram for, 1106–1107
      methadone for, 1107
      naltrexone hydrochloride for, 1108–1109
      nicotine for, 1109–1114
      varenicline, 1114–1115
   physical, on drugs, 1102
depolarising agents, 1420
depolarising blocking agents, 1426
Depo-Medrol, 1011–1012
Depo-Nisolone, 1011–1012
Depo-Provera, 1538–1539
Depo-Ralovera, 1538–1539
depression, 264
   agomelatine for, 288
   amitriptyline hydrochloride for, 270
   chlorpromazine hydrochloride for, 844
   citalopram for, 280
   clomipramine hydrochloride for, 270
   desvenlafaxine for, 286
   dosulepin (dothiepin) hydrochloride for, 271
   doxepin for, 272

depression (*Continued*)
   duloxetine for, 286
   erectile dysfunction and, 1117
   escitalopram for, 281
   fluoxetine for, 281
   fluvoxamine maleate for, 282
   imipramine hydrochloride for, 272
   mercaptamine bitartrate for, 1355
   mianserin hydrochloride for, 292
   mirtazapine for, 293
   moclobemide for, 277
   nortriptyline for, 273
   oral contraceptives and, 1548
   paroxetine for, 283
   phenelzine for, 276
   progestogens and, 1531
   reboxetine for, 287
   sertraline for, 283
   stimulants and, 1551–1552
   tranylcypromine for, 276
   venlafaxine hydrochloride for, 287
   vortioxetine for, 294
Depreta, 286–287
Deptran, 272
Deralin, 531–532
DermAid products, 1009
Dermatane, 5–6
dermatitis, clobetasone butyrate for, 1003
dermatitis herpetiformis, dapsone for, 586
dermatofibrosarcoma protuberans (DFSP),
     imatinib for, 716
dermatological agents, 1024–1037
   absorption of, 1024
   goals of therapy for, 1024
   other dermatological preparations, 1028
   topical ectoparasitical agents, 1024
dermatomycosis, itraconazole for, 443
dermatophytes, in cutaneous candidiasis,
     clotrimazole for, 435
dermatoses, desonide for, 1004
Desfax, 285–286
desferrioxamine mesylate, 342–345
   action of, 342
   adverse effects of, 343
   dose of, 343
   interactions of, 343
   nursing points/cautions for, 343–345
   patient teaching and advice for, 345
   use of, 342
desflurane, 1175
desloratadine, 490
desmopressin, 1232
desmopressin acetate, 1232–1235
desonide, 1004
Desowen, 1004
desvenlafaxine, 285–286

INDEX

Desvenlafaxine GH XR, 285–286
Detrusitol, 955
detrusor overactivity
   darifenacin hydrobromide for, 945
   oxybutynin for, 949–950
   solifenacin succinate for, 953
   tolterodine tartrate for, 955
DeWorm Chewable Tablets, 47–48
dexamethasone, 1005
   ondansetron and, 372
Dexamethasone Medsurge, 1005–1007
dexamethasone phosphate, 1005–1007
Dexamethasone Sodium Phosphate Injection, DBL, 1005–1007
dexamfetamine (dexamphetamine) sulfate, 1557–1558
Dexamfetamine Tablets, 1557–1558
dexchlorpheniramine maleate, 484
dexmedetomidine, 1507–1508
Dexmethsone, 1005
Dextromethorphan, 1021–1022
Deztron, 964–965
DFSP. *See* dermatofibrosarcoma protuberans
diabetes
   antipsychotics and, 837, 838
   fluconazole and, 439
   probenecid and, 481
   sympathomimetic agents and, 1566
diabetes mellitus, 296
   androgens and anabolic steroids and, 1521
   betaxolol and, 465
   diuretics and, 1080
   erectile dysfunction and, 1116
   immunoglobulins and, 1622
   levothyroxine sodium and, 1582
   liothyronine sodium and, 1584
   oral contraceptives and, 1549
   progestogens and, 1532
   thiazide and, 1092
   timolol maleate and, 471
diabetic control, metoclopramide hydrochloride monohydrate and, 378
diabetic foot infections, ertapenem for, 180
diabetic gastroparesis, 376
   domperidone and, 376
diabetic macular oedema (DME)
   aflibercept for, 1139
   dexamethasone phosphate for, 1005
   ranibizumab for, 1140
diabetic nephropathy, captopril for, 507
diabetic neuropathic pain, duloxetine for, 286
diabetic polyneuropathy, cyanocobalamin for, 1639
Diabex, 310–313
Diabex XR, 310–313
Diacomit, 419–420

Diaformin Alphapharrm XR, 310–313
Diaformin Viatrix, 310–313
dialysis
   allopurinol and, 476
   amphotericin B and, 431
Diamicron 60 mg MR, 309
Diamox, 388, 462–463, 1081–1082
diarrhoea, 330
   from alglucosidase alfa (RHU), 1339
   diphenoxylate hydrochloride for, 332
   loperamide hydrochloride for, 333
diazepam, 75–77
   action of, 75
   adverse effects of, 76
   dose of, 76
   interactions of, 76
   nursing points/cautions of, 76–77
   patient teaching and advice for, 77
   use of, 75–76
Diazepam Elixir, 75–77
Diazepam Solution for Injection, 75–77
diazoxide, 548–549
Diazoxide Injection BP, 548–549
Dibenyline, 501–502
Dicarz, 525–526
diclofenac diethylamine, 22
diclofenac diethylammonium, 22
diclofenac potassium, 22
diclofenac sodium, 20–22
Dicloxacillin, 161
diet, iodine in, 1579
diethyltoluamide, 557
Differin Topical Cream, 6–7
Differin Topical Gel, 6–7
Difflam Anti-inflammatory Gel, 17–18
Difflam Sore Throat Gargle and Mouth Solution, 17–18
Difflam Sore Throat Gargle with Iodine Concentrate, 1150, 1677
Difflam Sore Throat Spray, 17–18
Difflam Sore Throat Spray Forte, 17–18
diffuse large B-cell lymphoma
   axicabtagene ciloleucel for, 605
   polatuzumab vedotin for, 772
   tisagenlecleucel for, 679
Dificid, 226–227
Diflucan, 438–440
Diflucan One, 438–440
DigiFab, 345–346
Digitalis, 979
digitalis toxicity, amphotericin B and, 430
digoxin, 979
   sodium polystyrene sulfonate hydrogen with, 362
   sympathomimetic agents and, 1567
   topiramate and, 423
   toxicity, 93

1741

digoxin specific immune antigen binding fragment, 95, 345
Dihydrocodeine, 1022
Dilantin, 409—412
Dilart, 519—521
Dilatrend, 525—526
Dilaudid, 1443
Diltiazem, 536—537
Dimetapp 12 Hour Nasal Spray, 1147
Dimetapp preparations, 1022
dimethyl fumarate, 1373—1374
dimorphic fungus, 428
dinoprostone, 1477—1478
Diovan, 519—521
Dipentum, 1165—1166
dipeptidyl peptidase-4 (DPP-4) inhibitors, 317—319
Diphenhydramine, 491—492
diphenoxylate hydrochloride, 332
diphtheria-tetanus vaccine, 1600—1601
diphtheria-tetanus-pertussis (DTP) vaccine, 1601—1602
Diprivan, 1180—1181
Diprosone, 1000—1001
Diprosone OV, 1000—1001
dipyridamole, 819—820
direct-acting agents, 1565
direct acting vasodilators, 500, 548—554
direct factor Xa inhibitors, 259
  action of, 259
direct thrombin inhibitors, 255—259
directly acting vasodilators, 1632
discoid lupus erythematosus, hydroxychloroquine sulfate for, 1045
disease-modifying antirheumatic drugs (DMARDs), 1038—1078
  conventional, 1038, 1039
  cytokine modulators, 1067
  tumour necrosis factor alpha (TNF-α) antagonists, 1039, 1057
disodium edetate, 346—348
  action of, 346—347
  adverse effects of, 347
  dose of, 347
  interactions of, 347
  nursing points/cautions for, 347—348
  use of, 347
Disodium Edetate 3 g + Sodium Ascorbate 5 g in 50 mL Solution, 348
disodium pamidronate, 962—963
disopyramide, 80
  action of, 80
  adverse effects of, 80
  dose of, 80
  interactions of, 80—81
  nursing points/cautions for, 81

disopyramide (*Continued*)
  patient teaching and advice for, 81
  use of, 80
Disprin preparations, 15—17, 817—818
disrupted ability, antipsychotics and, 835
disseminated intravascular coagulation
  dinoprostone and, 1477
  oxytocin and, 1481
disseminated lupus erythematosus, cortisone acetate for, 1003
disseminated *Mycobacterium avium* complex (MAC), azithromycin dihydrate for, 201
disseminated neuroblastoma, daunorubicin for, 629
Distaph, 161—162
disulfiram, 1106—1107
Dithiazide, 1088—1090
Ditropan, 949—950
diuresis, mannitol for, 1100
diuretic-induced hypokalaemia, spironolactone for, 1096
diuretics, 1079—1101
  carbonic anhydrase inhibitors, 1081—1091
  classifications of, 1079
  high-ceiling (loop), 1082
  induced hypokalaemia, spironolactone for, 1096
  nursing points/cautions for, 1079—1080
  osmotic, 1079, 1098
  patient teaching and advice for, 1080
  potassium-sparing, 1080, 1093, 1661
  thiazide, 500, 1079, 1088
  uses of, 1079
Dizole, 438—440
Dizole One, 438—440
dizziness, mercaptamine bitartrate for, 1355
DMARDs. *See* disease-modifying antirheumatic drugs
DME. *See* diabetic macular oedema
DNA polymerase inhibitors, 897, 898—913
  aciclovir, 898—900
  cidofovir, 900—902
  famciclovir, 902—903
  foscarnet sodium, 903—905
  ganciclovir, 905—907
  letermovir, 907—908
  valaciclovir, 908—909
  valganciclovir, 909—910
  oseltamivir, 910—911
  peramivir, 911—912
  zanamivir, 912—913
DNA synthesis, inhibitors of, 214—216
dobutamine hydrochloride injection, 1569—1570
docetaxel, 632—633
Docetaxel Concentrated Injection, 632—633
docosahexaenoic acid ethyl ester, 1316—1317
docusate sodium, 1144, 1294

INDEX

Dolapril, 512
dolutegravir, 939—940
Domion, 288—289
domperidone, 376—377
Donepezil-GH, 53
donepezil hydrochloride, 53
Donnatab, 987
dopamine (D_2), 1565
   lithium carbonate and, 854
   paliperidone and, 860
dopamine agonists, 798—799
   adverse effects of, 798
   amantadine hydrochloride, 799—800
   apomorphine hydrochloride hemihydrate, 800—802
   benserazide hydrochloride, 802
   bromocriptine mesilate, 802—804
   cabergoline, 804—805
   carbidopa monohydrate, 805
   interactions of, 798
   levodopa, 805—809
   nursing points/cautions for, 798
   patient teaching and advice for, 798—799
   pramipexole dihydrochloride monohydrate, 809—810
   rotigotine, 810—812
dopamine (D_2) antagonists, 376—383
   domperidone, 376—377
   haloperidol decanoate and, 832—854
   lurasidone hydrochloride and, 857
   metoclopramide hydrochloride monohydrate, 377—379
   olanzapine pamoate monohydrate and, 858
   prochlorperazine maleate, 380
   risperidone and, 865
   ziprasidone and, 868
dopamine receptors
   amisulpride, 839
   clozapine and, 847
   quetiapine and, 863
dornase alfa, 134—135
Dostinex, 804, 1488—1489
dosulepin (dothiepin) hydrochloride, 271
Dothep, 271
double vision, mercaptamine bitartrate for, 1355
Down syndrome, diphenoxylate hydrochloride and, 332
doxepin, 272
doxorubicin, leflunomide and, 1048
doxorubicin hydrochloride, 633—635
   action of, 633
   adverse effects of, 633—634
   dose of, 633
   interactions of, 634

doxorubicin hydrochloride (*Continued*)
   liposomal, 634—635
   nursing points/cautions for, 634—635
   patient teaching and advice for, 635
   use of, 633
Doxorubicin Hydrochloride, 633
Doxsig, 195—196
doxycycline hyclate (hydrochloride), 196
doxycycline monohydrate, 196
doxylamine succinate, 492—493
Doxylin, 195
Dozile, 492—493
driver's licence, and seizures, 387
driving, antiglaucoma agents and, 461
Drixine Decongestant Nasal Spray, 1147
Drixine No Drip Formula, 1147
droperidol, 849—850
drowsiness, 1503—1505
   antipsychotics and, 1543
   caffeine for, 1556
   entacapone and, 677
drug abuse, 1102
drug dependence, 1102—1115
   acamprosate calcium for, 1102—1103
buprenorphine for, 1103—1104
   bupropion for, 1104—1106
   disulfiram for, 1106—1107
   methadone for, 1107
   naltrexone for, 1108—1109
   nicotine for, 1109—1114
   varenicline, 1114—1115
drug-induced extrapyramidal reactions, amantadine hydrochloride for, 799
drug-induced oedema, acetazolamide for, 1081
drug-induced Parkinsonism
   benzatropine mesilate for, 793
   trihexyphenidyl (benzhexol) hydrochloride for, 794
drug misuse, 1102
drug sensitisation, cortisone acetate for, 1003
drug tolerance, definition of, 1429—1430
ductus arteriosus, alprostadil for, 1632
Dukoral, 1597—1598
dulaglutide, 322
Dulcolax, 1293
Dulcolax SP Drops, 1295—1296
Dulose, 1289—1290
Duloxecor, 286—287
duloxetine, 286—287
duodenal ulcers, 871
dupilumab, 1248—1249
Dupixent, 1248—1249
Duratocin, 1478—1479
Duride, 63—65
Durogesic, 1439—1443
Durolane, 1672—1673

1743

Duromine, 40—41
DuroTuss Chesty Cough Liquid Double Strength (1.6 mg/mL), 1020—1021
DuroTuss Chesty Cough Liquid Regular, 1020—1021
durvalumab, 759—760
dutasteride, 946—947
Dutran, 1439—1443
DVT. See deep vein thrombosis
Dymadon suspension, 31—34
dyskinesia, tardive, 835
dyslipidaemias, 1300
dyspareunia, progesterone and, 1470
dysphonia, spasmodic, botulinum toxin type A for, 1406
dysplastic lesions, human papillomavirus (HPV) vaccine for, 1605
dyspnoea
 abacavir and, 921
 agalsidase beta (RCH) and, 1338
 carbetocin and, 1478
 salbutamol sulfate and, 1475
Dysport, 1406—1410
dystonia
 acute, 835
 cervical botulinum toxin type A for, 1406
 incobotulinumtoxinA for, 1412
dysuria, topiramate and, 423
Dytrex, 286—287

E

E. coli, certolizumab pegol and, 1062
Eagle Sublingual B12, 1640
ear, 1143—1145
 agents for, 1128—1150
 instillation of ear drops in, 1143
 nursing points and caution for, 1143
 teaching and advice for, 1144
 wax softeners for, 1144
Ear Clear for Ear Wax Removal, 1144
ear drops, instillation of, 1143
Early Bird Chocolate Squares, 49
Ebixa, 54
eclampsia, 1472
 agents for, 1472
Econazole, 437
Ectoparasites, 1024
ectoparasitical agents, topical, 1024
 benzyl alcohol, 1025
 benzyl benzoate, 1026
 crotamiton, 1027
 for pediculosis (lice infestation), 1024—1025
 permethrin, 1027—1028
ectopic pregnancy, ganirelix acetate and, 1465
eculizumab, 1249
 action of, 1249

eculizumab (Continued)
 adverse effects of, 1249—1250
 dose of, 1249
 nursing points/cautions of, 1250
 patient teaching and advice of, 1251
 use of, 1249
eczema
 mild, clobetasone butyrate for, 1003
 pimecrolimus for, 1036
Edronax, 287
EDTA. See ethylenediamine tetra-acetic acid
Edurant, 930—931
efavirenz, 927—929
efexor XR, 287—288
efmoroctocog alfa, 1203
Eformoterol (See formoterol (eformoterol)) fumerate
eftrenonacog alfa, 1213—1214
Efudix, 642—643
EGPA. See eosinophilic granulomatosis with polyangiitis
eicosapentaenoic acid ethyl ester, 1316—1317
Elaprase, 1351—1352
Elaxine SR, 287—288
Eldepryl, 814—816
elderly
 neuroleptic malignant syndrome in, 835
 thiazide and, 1092
elective surgery
 epoetin alfa for, 1189
 epoetin lambda for, 1191
electrolytes, 1636—1670
Elelyso, 1364—1365
eletriptan hydrobromide, 570—572
Eleuphrat, 1000—1001
Eleva, 283—284
Elidel, 1036—1037
Eligard, 1219—1220
eliglustat, 1346—1347
Eliquis, 259—260
Elmiron, 951—952
Elocon, 1013—1014
Eloctate, 1203—1205
Elonva, 1461—1462
elosulfase alfa (RCH), 1348—1349
 action of, 1348
 adverse effects of, 1348
 dose of, 1348
 nursing points/cautions of, 1348—1349
 patient teaching and advice of, 1349
 use of, 1348
Elovax One Dose, 902
eltrombopag olamine, 1195
 action of, 1195
 adverse effects of, 1195
 dose of, 1195

INDEX

eltrombopag olamine (*Continued*)
   interactions of, 1195
   nursing points/cautions for, 1195—1196
   patient teaching and advice for, 1196—1197
   use of, 1195
Eltroxin, 1581—1583
embolus, dipyridamole for, 820
embryonal testicular cancer, bleomycin sulfate for, 612
Emend IV, 375—376
Emerade, 1567—1569
emetic centre, 368
Emexlon, 377—379
Emgality, 575—576
emicizumab, 1208—1209
EMLA, 1331
emollient laxatives, 1285
emollients, retinoids and, 3
empagliflozin, 326
Empovir, 900—902
emtricitabine, 922—923
Emtriva, 922
Emycin Mayne Pharma Erythromycin, 204
Enablex, 945—946
Enalapril, 508
Enanthate, 1522
Enbrel, 1063—1064
Endep, 270
endocarditis prophylaxis
   erythromycin lactobionate for, 204
   vancomycin hydrochloride for, 185
endometrial cancer, pembrolizumab for, 770
endometrial carcinoma, recurrent metastatic, medroxyprogesterone for, 1538
Endometrin, 1469—1471
endometriosis
   medroxyprogesterone for, 1538
   nafarelin acetate for, 1467
   norethisterone for, 1539
Endone, 1447—1449
Endoxan, 624—625
Engerix-B, 1603—1604
Enidin, 466—467
Enlafax-XR, 287—288
Enoxaparin, 244—247
   action of, 244
   adverse effects of, 245
   dose of, 244—245
   interactions of, 245
   nursing points/cautions for, 245—246
   patient teaching and advice for, 246
   use of, 244
Enstilar Foam Spray, 1001
Entac, 916
entacapone, 795—796
entecavir monohydrate, 916

enteral feeds, phenytoin sodium and, 411
Enterobacteriaceae spp., infection due to, fosfomycin for, 227
enterococcal infections, linezolid for, 212
Enterococcus faecalis, infection due to, fosfomycin for, 227
Entocort, 124—128, 1001
Entrip, 270
entry inhibitors, 898, 936—939
   enfuvirtide, 936—937
   maraviroc, 937—938
   nirsevimab, 938—939
Entyvio, 1168—1170
enzalutamide, 635—636
envenomation, 890
enzyme replacement, 1170
   agalsidase alfa (GHU), 1336
   agalsidase beta (RCH), 1336
eosinophilic asthma benralizumab for, 133
   mepolizumab for, 140
eosinophilic granulomatosis with polyangiitis (EGPA), mepolizumab for, 140
ephedrine hydrochloride, 1572
Ephedrine HydrochlorideJuno, 1572
ephedrine sulfate, 1572—1573
epidermoid carcinoma, methotrexate for, 656
epilepsy, 381
   acetazolamide for, 1081
   androgens and anabolic steroids and, 1521
   antipsychotics and, 837
   carbamazepine for, 843
   sodium valproate for, 868
   stimulants and, 1552
Epilim, 416—419, 867—868
Epilim IV, 416—419, 867—868
epinephrine, 1567—1569
   beta, 1565
Epipen, 1567—1569
Epipen Jr, 1567—1569
Epiramax, 422—424
epirubicin hydrochloride, 636—638
eplerenone, 1095—1096
epoetin alfa, 1188—1190
epoetin beta, 1190—1191
epoetin lambda, 1191—1192
epoprostenol, 1493—1495
Eprex, 1188—1190
E-Prime, 1647
eptacog alfa, 1201—1203
Eraxis, 432—433
Erbitux, 752—753
erectile dysfunction, 1116
   alprostadil for, 1118
erectile dysfunction agents, 1116—1127
   alprostadil as, 1118
   intracavernosal administration of, 1117

1745

erectile dysfunction agents (*Continued*)
  other agents for, 1125—1127
  papaverine hydrochloride as, 1119
  phosphodiesterase type 5 (PDE5) inhibitors, 1120
  sildenafil as, 1122—1123
  tadalafil as, 1124
erenumab, 573—574
ergometrine maleate, 1479—1480
ergot alkaloids, posaconazole and, 452
eribulin mesilate, 638
Erivedge, 742
erlotinib hydrochloride, 711—712
Erlyand, 603—604
Ertapenem, 180—181
erythema, from alglucosidase alfa (RHU), 1339
erythema nodosum leprosum, thalidomide for, 675
Erythrocin IV, 204
erythrocytes, 556
erythromycin, 204
  midazolam hydrochloride and, 1511
erythromycin ethyl succinate, 204
erythromycin lactobionate, 204
erythropoiesis, 1184
erythropoiesis stimulating agent (ESA), 1192
erythropoietin
  human, 1042
    ciclosporin with, 1042
  recombinant, nandrolone decanoate and, 1522
ESA. *See* erythropoiesis stimulating agent
Esbriet, 1266—1267
Escherichia coli, infections due to, colistimethate sodium for, 221
escitalopram, 280—281
  oral solution, 281
Esipram, 280—281
Eskazole, 43—45
esmolol, 526—527
esomeprazole, 877—878
Esopreze, 877—878
Espler, 1095—1096
essential hypertension, spironolactone for, 1096
essential thrombocythaemia, busulfan for, 613
essential thrombocytopenia, anagrelide for, 601
essential tremor, propranolol hydrochloride for, 531
established DVT, enoxaparin sodium for, 244
Estraderm MX, 1527—1529
estradiol, 1456, 1524, 1527—1529
  gel, 1528—1529
  intravaginal tablets/cream, 1529
  transdermal patch, 1528
Estradot, 1527—1529
estriol, 1529—1530
Estrofem, 1527—1529
Estrogel, 1527—1529
etacrynic (ethacrynic) acid, 242

etanercept, 1063—1064
ethambutol, 587
ethanol, 1035
ethosuximide, 397
ethylenediamine tetra-acetic acid (EDTA), 346
etonogestrel, 1534—1535
Etopophos, 639—640
etoposide, 639—640
etoricoxib, 22—23
etravirine, 929—930
Eulactol Antifungal Spray, 448
Eumovate, 1003
Eurax, 1027
Eutroxsig, 1581—1583
evacuants, 1285
Everocan, 1251—1254
everolimus, 1251—1254
  action of, 1251
  adverse effects of, 1252
  dose of, 1251—1252
  interactions of, 1252—1253
  nursing points/cautions of, 1253
  patient teaching and advice of, 1253—1254
  use of, 1251
evolocumab, 1316
Evoltra, 623—624
Ewing's sarcoma
  dactinomycin for, 627
  vincristine sulfate for, 687
excessive sleepiness, mercaptamine bitartrate for, 1355
Exelon, 55—57
Exelon patch, 55—57
exemestane, 640
exenatide, 304
exercise-induced asthma, sodium cromoglycate for, 98
expectorants, 1019—1023
external genital lesions, human papillomavirus (HPV) vaccine for, 1605
external sphincter, 942
Extine, 282—283
extracorporeal circulation, heparin sodium for, 238
extrapulmonary TB, 584
extrapyramidal reactions or syndrome, 834
extreme drug resistant TB (XDR-TB), 585
eye, 1128—1143
  agents for, 1128—1150
  antiglaucoma agents, 460—462
  colour, change in
    travoprost and, 471—472
  cycloplegic and mydriatic drops for, 1130—1131
  eye drop instillation, 1128
  eye ointment insertion, 1129
  macular degeneration agents, 1138—1139

INDEX

eye (*Continued*)
  miotics and ocular decongestants, 1134—1138
  nursing points/cautions for, 1128—1129
  other agents for, 1141
  patient teaching and advice for, 1129—1130
eye drop instillation, 999
eye drops
  benzalkonium chloride, 487
  contact lenses and, 1129
  corticosteroid, 997
  instillation of, 1128
  local anaesthetics and, 1332
  NSAIDs, 14—15
eye infection, tobramycin sulfate for, 191, 192
eye movement, mercaptamine bitartrate for, 1355
eye ointment, insertion of, 1129
eye pain, mercaptamine bitartrate for, 1355
eyelash, changes in
  travoprost and, 472
Eyezep, 486—487
Eylea, 1139
Ezemichol, 1317—1318
ezetimibe, 1317—1318
Ezetrol, 1317—1318
Ezovir, 902—903
Ezovir Cold Sore Relief, 902—903

F

FAB, 345
FAB fragment-digoxin complex, 345
Fabrazyme, 1337—1338
Fabry disease
  agalsidase alfa (GHU) for, 1336—1337
  agalsidase beta (RCH) for, 1337—1338
  migalastat for, 1356
facial/flexure dermatitis, hydrocortisone sodium succinate for, 1009
factor VII, 1201
factor VIII, 1203, 1205—1206
  action of, 1205
  adverse effects of, 1205
  dose of, 1205
  inhibitors to, eptacog alfa for, 1202
  nursing points/cautions of, 1205—1206
  patient teaching and advice of, 1206
  use of, 1205
factor VIII inhibitor bypassing fraction (Feiba-NF), 1206—1208
  actions of, 1206—1207
  adverse effects of, 1207
  dose of, 1207
  interactions of, 1142
  nursing points/cautions for, 1207—1208
  patient teaching and advice for, 1208
  use of, 1207

factor IX, 1144
  deficiency of, 1128
factor XIII, 1214
factor D deficiency, meningococcal vaccine for, 1609
factor H deficiency, meningococcal vaccine for, 1609
faecal softeners, 1294
fallopian cancer, olaparib for, 727
Fallot's tetralogy, propranolol hydrochloride for, 531
famciclovir, 902
famotidine, 873—874
fampridine, 1374—1375
Fampyra, 1374—1375
Famvir, 902—903
Fareston, 682
Fasenra, 133
Fasturtec, 482
fat soluble vitamins, 1636
fatigue, from agalsidase beta (RCH), 1337
Faverin, 282
Favic, 902—903
Febridol, 31—32
febuxostat, 479
Feiba-NF, 1206—1208
Feldene D, 34
Feldene Gel, 34
Felodil XR, 537—538
felodipine, 537—538
Felodur ER, 537—538
female castration, oestrogens (conjugated) for, 1530—1531
female hirsutism, spironolactone for, 1096
Femara, 651
Femazole One, 438—440
Femolet, 651
Femrelief One, 438—440
femur, bowing, 957
Fenac, 22
Fenocol, 1310—1311
fenofibrate, 1310—1311
FenPaed, 24—25
fentanyl, 1439
fentanyl citrate, 1439—1443
  action of, 1439
  adverse effects of, 1440
  dose of, 1440
  interactions of, 1440
  lozenge, 1436
  nursing points/cautions for, 1440—1441
  patient teaching and advice for, 1441—1442
  sublingual tablets, 1439
  transdermal patches, 1439—1440
  use of, 1440
Fentora, 1439

Ferinject, 1654–1655
ferric carboxymaltose, 1654–1655
ferrioxamine, 342
Ferriprox, 341–342
ferritin
  deferasirox in, 339
  deferiprone and, 341
Ferro-Grad, 1655
Ferro-Liquid, 1655
Ferrosig Injection, 1656–1657
Ferro-tab, 1655
ferrous fumarate, 1655
ferrous sulfate, 1655
ferrous sulfate heptahydrate, 1167
fetal hypoxia, nifedipine and, 1474
fetus, neuroprotection of, magnesium sulfate heptahydrate for, 1472
Fexit, 493
fexofenadine, 493
Fexotabs, 493
fibrates, 1309, 1310
  actions of, 1309
  adverse effects of, 1309
  interactions of, 1309
  nursing points/cautions for, 1309–1310
  patient teaching and advice for, 1310
  uses of, 1309
fibrin, 1087
fibrin non-specific agents, 1151
fibrinogen, 1197–1198
fibrinolysis, 1200
fibrinolytic agents, 1153–1154
  adverse effects of, 1151
  alteplase as, 1153
    interactions of, 1151
    nursing points/cautions for, 1151–1153
    tenecteplase, 1155
fibrositis, betamethasone valerate for, 1000
Fibsol, 509–510
fidaxomicin, 226
'fight or flight' mechanism, 981
filariae, 42
filgrastim, 785–788
  action of, 785
  adverse effects of, 786
  dose of, 785
  interactions of, 786
  nursing points/cautions for, 786–787
  patient teaching and advice for, 787–788
  use of, 785
Finacea, 7–8
Finapen, 947–948
finasteride, 947–948
fingertip injuries, silver sulfadiazine for, 232
fingolimod, 1375–1378
  action of, 1375

fingolimod (Continued)
  adverse effects of, 1376
  dose of, 1376
  interactions of, 1376
  nursing points/cautions for, 1376–1377
  patient teaching and advice for, 1377–1378
  teriflunomide and, 1388
  use of, 1376
Finnacar, 947–948
Finpro, 947–948
Firazyr, 1256–1257
Firmagon, 631–632
Fisamox, 154
5-aminosalicylic acid, 1056–1057
$5HT_3$ receptor, 368–369
  adverse effects of, 369
  granisetron, 370
  interactions of, 369
  nursing points/cautions for, 369
  ondansetron, 371–372
  palonosetron hydrochloride, 372–373
  patient teaching and advice for, 369–370
  tropisetron, 373
Fixta 60, 973–974
flagellates, 825
flagellum, 825
Flagyl, 826–829
Flagyl S Suspension, 826–829
Flamazine, 232–233
Flarex, 1008
Flebogamma 5% DIF, 1623–1627
Flebogamma 10% DIF, 1623–1627
Flecainide Sandoz, 84–85
Flecatab, 84–85
Fleet Ready-to-Use-Enema, 1290–1292
Flixonase Allergy & Hayfever 24 hr, 130
Flixonase Nasule Drops, 130
Flixotide, 130
Flo Rapid Relief, 1148
Flomaxtra, 954
Florinef, 1007
Flosix, 954
Fluad Quad, 1605–1607
Fluanxol, 850–851
Fluarix Tetra, 1605–1607
Flubiclox, 162
Flucil, 162
flucloxacillin, 162–163
Flucon, 1008
fluconazole, 438–440
  tofacitinib and, 1076
Fluconazole Injection for Intravenous Infusion, 438–440
flucytosine, 431
Fludara, 641
fludarabine phosphate, 641

INDEX

Fludrocortisone, 1007
Flufeme, 438–440
fluid retention, progestogens and, 1532
flukes, 42
flumazenil, 348, 396
flunitrazepam, 1508
fluorometholone, 1008
fluorometholone acetate, 1008
fluoroquinolones, 214–216
   for tuberculosis, 584–585
fluorouracil, 642–643
   calcium folinate and, 336
Fluotex, 281–282
fluoxetine, 281–282
flupenthixol decanoate, 850–851
flupentixol decanoate, 850–851
FluQuadri, 1605–1607
flurbiprofen, 23
flutamide, 1542–1544
Flutamin, 1542–1543
fluticasone furoate, 130–133
   action of, 130
   adverse effects of, 130–131
   dose of, 130
   interactions of, 131
   nursing points/cautions for, 131
   patient teaching and advice for, 131–132
   use of, 130
fluticasone propionate, 130
fluvastatin, 1303–1304
fluvoxamine, zolpidem tartrate and, 1516
fluvoxamine maleate, 282
Fluzole, 438–440
FML, 1008
focal seizures, 384
focal spasticity, botulinum toxin type A for, 1407
folate, 1642–1643
folic acid, 1642–1643
   methotrexate, 1050
   phenobarbital and, 407
folinic acid, 336
folinic acid rescue, 336
follicle-stimulating hormone (FSH), 1216, 1456
follicular hyperkeratosis, 1637
follicular lymphoma
   idelalisib for, 715
   obinutuzumab for, 797
follitropin alfa, 1462–1463
follitropin beta, 1463–1464
foltabs, 1642–1643
fomepizole, 349–350
Fonat, 961
Fondaparinux, 253–255
Foradile, 101–102
forehead lines, botulinum toxin type A for, 1407
Formet, 310–313

formoterol (eformoterol), 101–102
Forteo, 977–978
Forxiga, 325
Fosamax, 961
Fosamax Plus Once Weekly, 961
fosamprenavir, 842
fosaprepitant, 375–376
foscarnet sodium, 903–905
Foscavir, 903–905
fosfomycin, 227–228
Fosinopril, 508–509
Fosrenol, 352–353
fotemustine, 643–644
foxglove, 979
fractures
   ascorbic acid for, 1644
   in Paget's disease, 957
Fragmin, 241–243
Framycetin, 189–190
Fraxiparine, 247–249
Fraxiparine Forte, 247–249
fremanezumab, 574–575
Fresofol 1% Injection, 1180–1181
Fresofol 1% MCT/LCT, 1180–1181
Frisium, 74–75
frusemide, 1085–1088
Frusemix, *See* furosemide (frusemide)
Frusemix-M, 1085–1088
FSH. *See* follicle-stimulating hormone
Fucidin, 211–212
Fucidin Topical, 211–212
fulvestrant, 644–645
Fumarate dihydrate, 102
fungal infections, 428
   systemic, amphotericin B dosages for, 430
   tumour necrosis factor alpha (TNF-α) antagonists and, 1058
fungal keratitis, itraconazole for, 443
Fungilin, 429–431
funnel-web spider antivenom, 893
furosemide (frusemide), 1085–1088
fusidic acid, sugammadex sodium with, 365
fusospirochaetosis of oropharynx, phenoxymethylpenicillin potassium for, 163
Fybogel, 1287
Fycompa, 405–406

G

G6PD deficiency
   dapsone and, 587
   methylene blue trihydrate and, 355
GA Tramadol Tramal, 1452–1454
Gabacor, 397–399
gabapentin, 397–398
Gabitril, 422
gait abnormalities, in Paget's disease, 957

Galafold, 1355
galantamine, 53
Galantamine MR, 53
Galantyl, 53
galcanezumab, 575
galsulfase, 1349
Galvus, 320
Gamine XR, 53
gamma-aminobutyric acid (GABA), sodium valproate and, 416
Gammanorm, 1623—1627
Gamunex, 1623—1627
ganciclovir, 905—907
ganirelix acetate, 1465
Gapentin, 397—398
Gardasil-9, 1605
Gastrex, 332—333
gastric acid secretion, reduction of, 872
gastric cancer
  epirubicin hydrochloride for, 636
  fluorouracil for, 642
gastric hyperacidity, aluminium hydroxide hydrate for, 886
gastric symptoms, probenecid and, 481
gastric ulcers, 871
gastrointestinal agents (miscellaneous), 1156—1171
  agents used in inflammatory bowel disease, 1159
    balsalazide sodium as, 1160
    mesalazine as, 1163—1165
    olsalazine sodium as, 1165—1166
    vedolizumab as, 1168—1170
  for enzyme replacement, 1170
  mebeverine hydrochloride as, 1156
  sulfasalazine as, 1166—1168
  teduglutide as, 1157—1158
  ursodeoxycholic acid as, 1158—1159
gastrointestinal stromal tumour
  imatinib for, 716
  sunitinib for, 737
gastro-oesophageal junction adenocarcinoma, ramucirumab for, 772
Gastro-Sooth, 988
Gastro-Stop, 332—333
Gaucher disease
  imiglucerase (RCH) for, 1352
  miglustat for, 1357
  velaglucerase alfa (GHU) for, 1366
Gazyva, 767
G-CSF. *See* granulocyte colony stimulating factor
gefitinib, 712—713
Gemaccord, 646
gemcitabine, 646
gemeprost, 27
gemfibrozil, 1311

general anaesthetics, 1172—1183
  adverse effects of, 1173
  dose of, 1173
  inhalation, 1172—1173
  interactions of, 1173
  intravenous, 1173
  nitrous oxide, 1176
  nursing points/cautions for, 1174
  patient teaching and advice for, 1174
  procedure, 1172
    induction, 1172
    maintenance, 1172
    premedication, 1172
    recovery, 1172
    reversal, 1172
generalised anxiety disorder, 70
  duloxetine for, 286
  escitalopram for, 281
  paroxetine for, 283
  sertraline for, 283
  venlafaxine hydrochloride for, 287
genital herpes
  aciclovir for, 898
  famciclovir for, 902
  valaciclovir for, 909
genital itchiness, progesterone and, 1470
genital tract infections, co-trimoxazole for, 222
genital warts
  human papillomavirus (HPV) vaccine for, 1605
  imiquimod for, 1033
genitourinary tract infection, amoxicillin trihydrate for, 154
Genotropin, 1228—1230
Genotropin GoQuick, 1228—1230
Genotropin MiniQuick, 1228—1230
Genox, 672—673
Gentamicin Injection BP, 190—191
  eye drops, 14—15
GEP endocrine tumour
  lanreotide acetate for, 1221
  octreotide for, 1222
germ cell carcinoma
  ifosfamide for, 648
  metastatic, cisplatin for, 621
gestational diabetes mellitus, 267
GH. *See* growth hormone
GHRH. *See* growth hormone-releasing hormone
GHRIF. *See* growth hormone release-inhibiting factor
GHRIH. *See* growth hormone release-inhibiting hormone
GI infections
  ampicillin sodium for, 158
  co-trimoxazole for, 222
giant cell arteritis, cortisone acetate for, 1003
giant cell tumour, denosumab for, 755, 971

INDEX

Gilenya, 1375—1378
Gilles de la Tourette syndrome
   haloperidol decanoate for, 852
   haloperidol for, 852
Gilmat, 715—717
gingival hyperplasia, ciclosporin, 1042
gingivitis, chlorhexidine gluconate, 1149
Giotrif, 693—694
GIP. *See* glucose-dependent insulinotropic polypeptide
GIT 1, 1288
glabellar lines
   botulinum toxin type A for, 1406
   incobotulinumtoxinA for, 1412
Glanzmann's thrombasthenia, eptacog alfa for, 1202
glatiramer acetate, 1378—1380
   teriflunomide and, 1388
glaucoma, 460
   acetazolamide for, 1081
   antipsychotics and, 835
   closed-angle, 460
   naphazoline hydrochloride for, 1137
   open-angle, 460
      acetazolamide for, 462
      bimatoprost for, 465
      dorzolamide for, 468
   secondary, 460
      acetazolamide for, 462
   stimulants and, 1552—1553
Glaumox Powder for Injection, 388, 462, 1081—1082
glibenclamide, 308—309
gliclazide, 309
glimepiride, 309—310
glioblastoma multiforme, temozolomide for, 674
glioma, bevacizumab for, 748
glipizide, 310
Glivec, 715—717
globotriaosylceramide (Gb3)
   in agalsidase alfa (GHU), 1336
   in agalsidase beta (RCH), 1337
glomerulonephritis prophylaxis, benzathine penicillin for, 159
GlucaGen HypoKit, 350—352
glucagon, 300
glucagon hydrochloride, 350—352
glucagon-like peptide 1 (GLP1), 304
glucagon-like peptide-1 (GLP-1) analogues, 321—322
   actions of, 321
   adverse effects of, 321
   interactions of, 321
   nursing points/cautions for, 321
   patient teaching and advice for, 321
   uses of, 321

glucagonoma, glucagon hydrochloride in, 351
Glucobete, 310
glucocerebrosidase deficiency, in imiglucerase (RCH), 1352
glucocorticoids, 991, 1216
gluconeogenesis, corticosteroids in, 991
glucose, 1098
   tolerance, androgens and, 1520, 1521
Glucose 50%, 1098
glucose-dependent insulinotropic polypeptide (GIP), 317
Glucovance, 309, 313
Glybosay, 314—315
glycated haemoglobin (HbA$_{1c}$), 297
glycerol, 1293
Glycerol Suppositories BP, 1293
glyceryl trinitrate, 59—62
   action of, 59—60
   adverse effects of, 60
   dose of, 60
   interactions of, 60—61
   nursing points/cautions of, 61—62
   patient teaching and advice for, 62
   use of, 60
glyceryl trinitrate concentrate injection, 59
glycopeptides, 183
   actions of, 183
   adverse effects of, 183
   nursing points/cautions for, 183—184
   patient teaching and advice for, 184
Glycoprep, 1288
Glycoprep-C, 1293
glycoprotein IIb/IIIa receptors
   tirofiban and, 823
glycopyrrolate, 112, 987—988
glycopyrronium (glycopyrrolate), 112—113
glycopyrronium bromide (glycopyrrolate), 987—988
glycosides, cardiac, 979—980
Glypressin Solution, 1235
GnRH. *See* gonadotropin-releasing hormone
golimumab, 1064—1065
Gonal-f Pen, 1462
gonadotrophins, 1216
gonadotropin-releasing hormone (GnRH), 1217—1219
gonorrhoea
   amoxicillin trihydrate for, 154
   aztreonam for, 180
   cefotaxime sodium for, 171
   cefoxitin sodium for, 172
   ceftriaxone sodium for, 176
   cefuroxime axetil for, 177
   probenecid for, 480, 481
   procaine benzylpenicillin for, 165
Gopten, 512

goserelin, 1217–1219
gout, 473
    allopurinol for, 475
    probenecid for, 480
gout flares, 477
GPA. *See* granulomatosis with polyangiitis
graft *versus* host disease, ciclosporin for, 1041
Gram-negative bacilli, penicillins and, 151
Gram-negative sepsis, gentamicin for, 190
Gram-positive organisms, serious infections due to, linezolid for, 212
grand mal seizures, 381
granisetron, 370–371
Granisetron-AFT, 370–371
Granisetron Kabi, 370–371
granulocyte colony stimulating factor (G-CSF), 784, 1267
    actions of, 784
    adverse effects of, 784–785
    interactions of, 785
    nursing points/cautions for, 785
    patient teaching and advice for, 785
    uses of, 784
granulomatosis with polyangiitis (GPA), rituximab for, 773
griseofulvin, 440–441
Grisovin, 440–441
growth, thyroid hormones on, 1216–1217
growth hormone (GH), 1216, 1227–1230
growth hormone release-inhibiting factor (GHRIF), 1221–1157
    adverse effects of, 1221
    interactions for, 1221
    lanreotide, 1221–1222
    octreotide, 1222–1224
    pasireotide, 1224
    patient teaching and advice for, 1221
    pegvisomant, 1226–1227
growth hormone release-inhibiting hormone (GHRIH), 1216
growth hormone-releasing hormone (GHRH), 1216
guaifenesin, 1023
guanfacine, 1558–1559
Guardium Acid Reflux Relief, 877–878
guselkumab, 1254
GyMiso, 883, 1484
Gynotril, 651–652

H

H. pylori eradication, clarithromycin for, 202
H_1 receptors, 368
H_1-receptor antagonists, 484–485
H_2 receptors, 453

Hadlima, 1060–1062
haematopoiesis, 957
haemodialysis
    with desferrioxamine mesylate, 343
    thrombotic complications of, dalteparin sodium for, 241
haemodynamic monitoring, sugammadex sodium, 365
haemoglobin
    methoxy polyethylene glycol epoetin beta and, 1192
    monitoring
        ambrisentan and, 1491
        bosentan monohydrate and, 1492
        macitentan and, 1497
    sodium nitrite, 361
haemophilia A, 1194
    factor VIII for, 1205
    moroctocog alfa for, 1203
haemophilia B, 1194
    factor IX, 1210
    nonacog alfa for, 1211
    nonacog gamma for, 1212
Haemophilus influenzae, 178
Haemophilus influenzae type B prophylaxis, rifampicin for, 592
Haemophilus influenzae type B vaccine, 1602
haemopoietic agents, 1184–1193
    actions of, 1184
    adverse effects of, 1184–1185
    nursing points/cautions for, 1185–1186
    patient teaching and advice for, 1186–1187
Haemorol, 1676–1677
haemorrhagic cystitis, mesna for, 780
haemorrhagic skin infarction, protein C for, 262
haemorrhoids, phenol for, 1677
haemosiderosis, transfusion, desferrioxamine mesylate, 342
haemostasis, 1194
haemostatics, 1194–1215
    coagulation factors, 1201
        factor VII, 1201
        factor VIII, 1203, 1205
        factor IX, 1209–1210
        factor XIII, 1214–1215
    eltrombopag olamine, 1195–1197
    fibrinogen, 1197–1198
    romiplostim, 1198–1199
    tranexamic acid, 1200–1201
haemotoxicity, auranofin and, 1040
Hair A-Gain, 551, 1034–1036
Hair Science Anti-Dandruff Shampoo, 446
hairy cell leukaemia
    cladribine for, 622, 1371
Halaven, 638

INDEX

Haldol Decanoate, 852–854
halogenated anaesthetics, sympathomimetic agents and, 1565
haloperidol, 852–857
haloperidol decanoate, 852–854
Hansen's disease, 584
Harmonise, 332–333
Havrix, 1440, 1603
Havrix Junior, 1603
H-B-Vax II, 1603–1604
HDLs. *See* high-density lipoproteins
HE. *See* hepatic encephalopathy
head injuries, flumazenil in, 349
head louse, 1024
    benzyl alcohol for, 1025
    crotamiton for, 1027
headache
    medication overuse, 570
    mercaptamine bitartrate for, 1355
    refractory, 570
healthcare workers, vaccination and, 1593–1594
hearing, deferasirox and, 339–340
heart block, isoprenaline hydrochloride for, 1574
heart disease, erectile dysfunction and, 1116
heart failure
    amiloride hydrochloride dihydrate for, 1093
    bisoprolol fumarate for, 525
    candesartan cilexetil for, 515
    chronic, digoxin and, 980
    congestive
        digoxin for, 980
        milrinone lactate for, 980
    eplerenone for, 1095
    metoprolol tartrate for, 529
    nebivolol for, 530
    TNF-α antagonists and, 1059
heart transplantation, 1276
    everolimus for, 1251
heartburn
    calcium carbonate for, 887
    magnesium hydroxide for, 887
Heartburn Relief, 880–881
heavy metals, penicillamine for, 1054
Helicobacter pylori, 871
helminth infestations, 42
    patient teaching and advice for, 43
helminths, 42
    subdivision of, 42
Hemlibra, 1208–1209
heparin
    disodium edetate, 347
    epoetin beta in, 1191
    protamine sulfate in, 359
heparin and low molecular weight heparins (LMWHs), 237–240

heparin sodium, 237–240
    action of, 237–238
    adverse effects of, 238
    dose of, 238
    interactions of, 238–239
    nursing points/cautions for, 239–240
    general, 239–240
    subcutaneous injection technique, 239
    patient teaching and advice for, 240
    use of, 238
Heparin Sodium Injection, 237–240
Heparinised Saline, 237–240
heparinoids, 243
hepatic cirrhosis, amiloride hydrochloride dihydrate for, 1093
hepatic encephalopathy (HE), rifaximin for, 231
hepatitis A vaccine, 1603
hepatitis A virus, hepatitis A vaccine for, 1603
hepatitis B
    chronic
        adefovir dipivoxil for, 915
        entecavir monohydrate, 916
        interferon alfa 2a for, 1283
        lamivudine for, 923
        peginterferon alfa 2a for, 1283
    vaccine, 1603–1604
hepatitis B immunoglobulin, 1622
Hepatitis B Immunoglobulin-VF, 1622
hepatitis C
    chronic
        peginterferon alfa 2a for, 1283
        sofosbuvir for, 913
        tenofovir disoproxil fumarate for, 924
    hepatitis B vaccine for, 1603
hepatitis C-associated thrombocytopenia, eltrombopag olamine for, 1195
hepatocellular carcinoma
    nivolumab for, 766
    sorafenib tosilate for, 735
hepatomas, doxorubicin hydrochloride for, 633
hepatosplenomegaly, imiglucerase (RCH) for, 1352
hepatotoxic agent, methotrexate on, 656
hepatotoxicity, leflunomide, 1048
Hequinel, 1045–1047
Herb-a-lax, 1288
Herceptin SC, 777
hereditary angio-oedema attack, symptomatic treatment of, 1256
hereditary angioneurotic oedema, tranexamic acid for, 1200
herpes labialis, 899
    famciclovir for, 902
    valaciclovir for, 909
herpes simplex encephalitis
    aciclovir for, 899

herpes simplex encephalitis (*Continued*)
  immunocompetent or immunocompromised, 899
herpes simplex infections
  aciclovir for, 898
  famciclovir for, 902
herpes simplex keratitis, aciclovir for, 898
herpes zoster (shingles)
  aciclovir for, 898
  valaciclovir for, 909
  varicella zoster vaccines for, 1161
Herron Nicaway Lozenges, 1109–1114
Herron Riodine Concentrated Gargle, 1677
Herzuma, 777
Hiberix, 1602
hidradenitis suppurativa, adalimumab for, 1060
high-ceiling (loop) diuretics, 1082, 1085
  actions of, 1082–1083
  adverse effects of, 1083
  bumetanide, 1084–1085
  furosemide, 1085–1088
  interactions of, 1083
  nursing points/cautions for, 1083–1084
  patient teaching and advice for, 1084
  uses of, 1083
high-density lipoproteins (HDLs), 1077
hip arthroplasty, total, tranexamic acid for, 1200
Hiprex, 228
hirsutism, cyproterone acetate for, 1540
histamine, non-depolarising blocking agents and, 1422
histamine H$_2$-receptor antagonists, 872–873
  famotidine, 873–874
  nizatidine, 874
  ranitidine hydrochloride, 875
histiocytosis X, vinblastine sulfate for, 686
histoplasmosis, itraconazole for, 443
HIV infection
  abacavir for, 921
  aciclovir for, 898
  efavirenz for, 927
  emtricitabine for, 922
  filgrastim for, 786
  lamivudine for, 923
  meningococcal vaccine for, 1609
  tenofovir disoproxil fumarate for, 924
  zidovudine for, 926
HIV-1 infection
  atazanavir for, 931
  darunavir for, 933
  dolutegravir for, 939
  etravirine for, 929
  maraviroc for, 937
  rilpivirine hydrochloride for, 930
  ritonavir for, 934
HIV testing, 915, 919

HIV-1 infection
  raltegravir potassium for, 940
Hizentra, 1623–1627
HMG-CoA reductase inhibitors (statins), 1300–1302
  actions of, 1300
  adverse effects of, 1301
  interactions of, 1301
  leflunomide and, 1048
  nursing points/cautions for, 1301
  patient teaching and advice for, 1301–1302
  uses of, 1300–1301
Hodgkin lymphoma
  bleomycin sulfate for, 612
  brentuximab vedotin for, 751
  carmustine for, 618
  chlorambucil for, 619
  doxorubicin hydrochloride for, 633
  etoposide for, 639
  lomustine for, 651
  nivolumab for, 766
  procarbazine for, 669
  vinblastine sulfate for, 686
  vincristine sulfate for, 687
Holoxan, 647–649
homozygous familial hypercholesterolaemia, alirocumab and, 1316
hookworms, 42
  albendazole for, 43
  mebendazole for, 47
horizontal forehead lines, incobotulinumtoxinA for, 1412
hormonal contraceptives, antiepileptics reacting with, 393
hormone replacement therapy (HRT), 1418
hormones, thyroid, 1579–1580
Horton's syndrome, pizotifen maleate for, 577
Hospira Levetiracetam concentrate for IV infusion, 402–403
hospital-acquired pneumonia, ceftazidime with avibactam for, 174
hospital setting, metyrapone in, 1674
HRT. *See* hormone replacement therapy
Humalog, 303
human C1 esterase inhibitor, 1255
human erythropoietin, 1184
  ciclosporin with, 1042
human IgG 1g monoclonal antibody, 1247
human papillomavirus (HPV) vaccine, 1605
Humatrope, 1230
Humira, 1060–1062
Humulin 30/70, 303
Humulin NPH, 303
Humulin R, 303
Hunter syndrome, idursulfase for, 1351
hyaluronic acid, 1672–1673
Hycamtin, 681

INDEX

hydatid disease, albendazole for, 43—45
Hydopa, 545—546
Hydralazine, 549—550
hydration, topiramate and, 424
Hydrea, 645
hydrochloric acids, 871
hydrochlorothiazide, 1089—1090
hydrocortisone, 1009
hydrocortisone acetate, 1009
hydrocortisone sodium succinate, 1009—1011
hydromorphone hydrochloride, 1443
Hydroxo-B12, 1641—1642
hydroxocobalamin, 1641—1642
hydroxybenzoates, and levetiracetam, 403
hydroxycarbamide (hydroxyurea), 645
hydroxychloroquine, 1045—1047
4-hydroxyphenylpyruvate dioxygenase inhibitor, nitisinone and, 1358
Hydrozole, 1010
Hygroton, 1088
hyoscine butylbromide, 988
Hyoscine Butylbromide SXP for Injection, 988
hyoscine hydrobromide, 988—989
hyperacidity, magnesium hydroxide for, 887
hyperactivity, in psychotic disorders, droperidol for, 849
hyperammonaemia
  carglumic acid for, 1343
  management, sodium phenylbutyrate for, 1363
  topiramate and, 423
hypercalcaemia, 958, 1650
  androgens and anabolic steroids and, 1520
  calcitonin salmon for, 965
  cinacalcet for, 969
  digoxin toxicity and, 93
  furosemide for, 1085
  of malignancy, 755
  denosumab for, 971
  sevelamer hydrochloride and, 360
  sodium phosphate for, 976
  tumour-induced, 755
hypercalciuria, androgens and anabolic steroids and, 1520
hypercholesterolaemia, 1299
  nicotinamide for, 1639
hypercontractility, dinoprostone and, 1477
hypereosinophilic syndrome, imatinib for, 716
hyperglycaemia
  carglumic acid and, 1343
  salbutamol sulfate and, 1475
hyperhidrosis, botulinum toxin type A for, 1406
hyperkalaemia, 1660, 1662
  calcium chloride dihydrate for, 968
  calcium gluconate monohydrate for, 1650
  ciclosporin and, 1042
hyperkinetic states, amphetamines for, 1551

hyperlactataemia, from abacavir, 921
hyperlipidaemia, 1300
  progestogens and, 1471
hyperlipoproteinaemia, nicotinamide for, 1639
hypermagnesaemia, 1657, 1658
  magnesium sulfate heptahydrate and, 1472
hypermetabolic state, chloral hydrate and, 1506
hyperphenylalaninaemia, sapropterin dihydrochloride for, 1360
hyperprolactinaemia
  bromocriptine mesilate for, 803, 1486
  cabergoline for, 804
  Dostinex for, 1488
hyperreflexia, serotonin syndrome and, 265
hypersensitivity
  allopurinol and, 475
  corticosteroids and, 996, 997
hypertension, 499
  amiloride hydrochloride dihydrate for, 1093
  amlodipine for, 534
  androgens and anabolic steroids and, 1520
  atenolol for, 524
  candesartan cilexetil for, 515
  captopril for, 507
  carvedilol for, 525
  chlortalidone for, 1088
  clevidipine for, 535
  clonidine hydrochloride for, 543
  diltiazem hydrochloride for, 536
  enalapril maleate for, 508
  erectile dysfunction and, 1116
  felodipine for, 537
  fosinopril sodium for, 509
  furosemide for, 1085
  hydralazine hydrochloride for, 549
  hydrochlorothiazide for, 1089
  indapamide hemihydrate for, 1090
  irbesartan for, 516
  labetalol hydrochloride for, 528
  lercanidipine hydrochloride for, 538
  lisinopril dihydrate for, 509
  losartan potassium for, 516
  methyldopa for, 545
  metoprolol tartrate for, 529
  minoxidil for, 551
  moxonidine for, 547
  nebivolol for, 530
  nifedipine for, 539
  olmesartan medoxomil for, 517
  perindopril erbumine for, 510
  phenoxybenzamine for, 502
  prazosin for, 503
  propranolol hydrochloride for, 531
  pulmonary, agents, 1490—1491
    ambrisentan as, 1490—1491

hypertension (*Continued*)
    bosentan as, 1491—1493
    epoprostenol as, 1493—1495
    iloprost as, 1495—1496
    macitentan as, 1496—1497
    riociguat as, 1497—1499
    ramipril for, 511
    stimulants and, 1552
    sympathomimetic agents and, 1566
    telmisartan for, 518
    trandolapril for, 512
    valsartan for, 519—520
hypertensive crisis
    clonidine hydrochloride for, 543
    diazoxide for, 548
hydralazine hydrochloride for, 549
hyperthermia
    dantrolene sodium hemiheptahydrate for, 1410
    malignant
    signs, 1421
    suxamethonium chloride and, 1426
    treatment for, 1422
hyperthyroidism, 1515
    antipsychotics and, 835
    carbimazole for, 1585
    propylthiouracil for, 1587
    stimulants and, 1552
hypertriglyceridaemia, nicotinamide for, 1639
hyperuricaemia
    allopurinol for, 475
    rasburicase rys for, 482
hyphaema, tranexamic acid for, 1200
Hypnodorm, 1508
Hypnovel, 1511—1513
hypoalbuminaemia, phenytoin sodium and, 411
hypocalcaemia, 192, 1666
    calcitriol for, 966
    calcium chloride dihydrate for, 968
hypocalcaemic tetany, 1650
hypoestrogenic states, oestrogens (conjugated) for, 1530
hypoglycaemia, 300
    glucose for, 1099
    symptoms of, 305
hypoglycaemic agents, oral, 304—306
    alpha glucosidase inhibitors, 314—315
    biguanides, 310
    dipeptidyl peptidase-4 (DPP-4) inhibitors, 317—317
    nursing points/cautions for, 305
    patient teaching and advice for, 305—306
    sulfonylureas, 306—308
    thiazolidinediones, 315
hypogonadism
    oestrogens (conjugated) for, 1530

hypogonadotropic hypogonadism
    follitropin alpha for, 1462
    follitropin beta for, 1463
hypokalaemia
    digoxin toxicity and, 93
    milrinone lactate and, 980
    non-depolarising blocking agents and, 1422
    sympathomimetic agents and, 1566
hypomagnesaemia
    acute, 1659
    digoxin toxicity and, 93
    magnesium sulfate heptahydrate for, 1472
    mild, 1660
    severe, 1660
hyponatraemia, diuretics and, 1081
hypophosphataemia, 1660
    sodium phosphate for, 976
hypophosphatasia, asfotase alfa for, 1341
hypophysis, 1216
hypopnoea syndrome armodafinil for, 1553
    modafinil for, 1563
hyposmia, 1145
hypotension
    ambrisentan and, 1490
    amifostine and, 530
    antipsychotics and, 835
    bosentan monohydrate and, 1492
    dexmedetomidine and, 1507
    ephedrine sulfate for, 1572
    epoprostenol and, 1493
    idursulfase and, 1351
    iloprost trometamol and, 1495
    macitentan and, 1496
    milrinone lactate and, 980
    nifedipine and, 1474
    riociguat and, 1498
    salbutamol sulfate and, 1475
hypothalamic hormones, 1216—1236
    gonadotrophin-releasing hormone, 1216, 1217—1227
    growth hormone release-inhibiting factor, 1216, 1221
hypothalamic-pituitary adrenal (HPA) axis suppression, 125
hypothalamus, 1216, 1579
hypothyroid states, liothyronine sodium for, 1584
hypothyroidism, 1580
    antipsychotics and, 838
hypovolaemia, diuretics and, 1080
hypoxia
    digoxin toxicity and, 93
    nitrous oxide, 1180
Hyqvia, 1623—1627
Hyrimoz, 1060—1062
Hysone, 1009

INDEX

I

ibandronate, 961–962
Ibavyr, 917–918
Ibiamox, 154
Ibilex, 169
Ibimycin, 158
ibrutinib, 713–714
ibuprofen, 24–25
ibuprofen lysine, 25
icatibant, 1256–1257
Iclusig, 729–730
ICU sedation, dexmedetomidine and, 1507
Idaprex, 510–511
idarubicin hydrochloride, 647
idarucizumab, 352
idelalisib, 714–715
idiopathic methaemoglobinaemia, ascorbic acid for, 1644
idiopathic Parkinson's disease, rasagiline of, 812
idiopathic pulmonary fibrosis
  nintedanib for, 726
  treatment of, 1266
idiopathic thrombocytopenic purpura (ITP)
  eltrombopag olamine for, 1195
  romiplostim for, 1198
IDL. See intermediate-density lipoprotein
iduronate-2-sulfatase, in idursulfase, 1351
idursulfase, 1351–1352
ifosfamide, 647–649
  action of, 647
  adverse effects of, 648
  dose of, 648
  interactions of, 648
  nursing points/cautions for, 648–649
  patient teaching and advice for, 649
  use of, 647–648
Ikotab, 66–67
Iloprost, 1495–1496
Ilumya, 1278–1279
imatinib, 715–717
Imazan, 1243–1244
Imbruvica, 713–714
Imdur, 63–65
Imfinzi, 759
imiglucerase (RCH), 1352–1353
Imigran, 580–582
Imigran FDT, 580–582
imipenem (with cilastatin sodium), 181–182
imipramine, zolpidem tartrate and, 1516
imipramine hydrochloride, 272–273
imiquimod, 1033
immunisation, 1591
  passive, 1591
immunity, active, 1591
immunocompetent patient, famciclovir for, 902

immunocompromised patient, famciclovir for, 902
immunoglobulins, 1591–1631
  actions of, 1620
  adverse effects of, 1620
  cytomegalovirus (CMV) immunoglobulin, 1622
  hepatitis B immunoglobulin, 1622
  interactions of, 1620
  normal immunoglobulin, 1623–1627
  nursing points/cautions for, 1620–1621
  patient teaching and advice for, 1621–1622
  rabies immunoglobulin, 1627
  Rhesus (Rh(D)) immunoglobulin, 1627–1628
  tetanus immunoglobulin, 1628–1630
  uses of, 1620
  zoster immunoglobulin, 1630–1631
immunological agents, 1591
immunomodifiers, 1237–1238
  adverse effects of, 1237
  interactions of, 1237–1238
  interferons, 1280
  nursing points/cautions for, 1237–1238
  patient teaching and advice for, 1238
immunomodulation, normal immunoglobulin and, 1623
immunosuppressants, 1038
Imoclone, 1517–1518
Imodium, 332–333
Imojev, 1607–1608
Imovane, 1517–1518
impetigo
  mupirocin calcium for, 214
Implanon NXT, 1534–1535
Imrest, 1517–1518
Imukin, 1282
Imuran, 1243–1244
Inadine, 1677
Inadine Dressing, 1677
Incobotulinumtoxin A, 1412–1415
  action of, 1412
  adverse effects of, 1413
  dose of, 1412
  interactions of, 1413
  nursing points/cautions of, 1414–1415
  patient teaching and advice of, 1415
  use of, 1412
incontinence
  darifenacin hydrobromide for, 945
  oxybutynin for, 949
  solifenacin succinate for, 953
  tolterodine tartrate for, 955
Incruse Ellipta, 117
indacaterol, 102–104
indapamide hemihydrate, 1090–1091
Inderal, 531–532

indigestion, calcium carbonate for, 887
indirect-acting agents, 1565
indirectly acting vasodilators, 1632
Indocid, 26—27
indomethacin, 26—27
  action of, 26
  adverse effects of, 26
  interactions of, 26
  nursing points/cautions for, 26
  patient teaching and advice for, 26
  use of, 26
Indosyl Mono, 510—511
induction, anaesthetic procedure, 1172
Infanrix, 1601
Infanrix Hexa, 1602
Infanrix-IPV, 1602
infants, neuroleptic malignant syndrome in, 834
infected corneal ulcer, framycetin sulfate for, 189
infected skin lesions, mupirocin calcium for, 214
infections
  protozoan, 825
  TNF-α antagonists and, 1058, 1059
infective endocarditis, daptomycin for, 225
infertility, 1456
  agents for, 1456
    adverse effects of, 1457—1458
    cetrorelix acetate as, 1460
    choriogonadotropin alfa as, 1459—1460
    clomifene citrate as, 1460—1461
    corifollitropin alfa as, 1461—1462
    follitropin alpha as, 1462—1463
    follitropin beta as, 1463—1464
    follitropin delta as, 1464—1465
    ganirelix acetate as, 1465
    lutropin alfa as, 1465—1466
    menopausal gonadotropin as, 1466—1467
    nafarelin acetate as, 1467—1468
    nursing points/cautions for, 1458
    patient teaching and advice for, 1458
    progesterone as, 1469—1471
infestation, of lice, 1024—1025
inflammation, of globe, fluorometholone acetate for, 1008
inflammatory bowel disease, agents for, 1159
  balsalazide sodium as, 1160
  etrasimod, 1161—1162
  mesalazine as, 1163—1165
  olsalazine sodium as, 1165—1166
  sulfasalazine, 1166—1168
  vedolizumab as, 1168—1170
inflammatory mass, baclofen and, 1403
inflammatory process, certolizumab pegol in, 1062
infliximab, 1065—1067
influenza
  bromhexine hydrochloride for, 1020

influenza (*Continued*)
  prophylaxis for, oseltamivir phosphate and, 910
influenza type A
  influenza vaccine for, 1605
  prophylaxis for, amantadine hydrochloride for, 799
  treatment of
    oseltamivir phosphate for, 910
    zanamivir for, 912
influenza type B
  influenza vaccine for, 1605
  treatment of
    oseltamivir phosphate for, 910
    zanamivir for, 912
influenza vaccine, 1605—1607
Influvac Tetra, 1605—1607
inhalation anaesthetics, 1172—1173
  non-depolarising blocking agents and, 1421
inhalator, nicotine, 1109, 1110
inhibitors of bacterial cell wall synthesis, 151
inhibitors of bacterial protein synthesis, 186—188
Inlyta, 695
inoperable breast carcinoma, nandrolone decanoate for, 1522
inotuzumab ozogamicin, 763—764
Inovelon, 415—416
Inpler, 1095—1096
insect repellent, 557
Insig, 1090
insomnia, 1502
  acute, 1502
  chloral hydrate for, 1506—1507
  dexmedetomidine, 1507—1508
  diphenhydramine hydrochloride for, 491
  doxylamine succinate, 492
  flunitrazepam for, 1508
  lemborexant, 1508—1509
  melatonin for, 1509—1510
  midazolam hydrochloride, 1511—1513
  nitrazepam for, 1513
  severe, flunitrazepam and, 1508
  suvorexant for, 1513—1515
  temazepam for, 1515
  treating, 1502
  zolpidem tartrate for, 1515—1517
  zopiclone for, 1517—1518
Inspra, 1095—1096
insulin(s), 298—304
  actions of, 298
  administration of, 301
  adverse effects of, 298—299
  characteristics of, 303
  classification of, 298
  correct storage for, 302
  dose of, 298

insulin(s) (*Continued*)
  functions of, 296
  interactions of, 299
  long-acting, 300
  nursing points/cautions for, 299—300
  patient teaching and advice for, 301—302
  preparation, 301
  short-acting, 300
  storage, 300
  use of, 298
insulin aspart, 303
insulin aspart + insulin aspart protamine, 303
insulin detemir, 303
insulin glargine, 303
insulin glulisine, 303
insulin lispro, 303
insulinoma, glucagon hydrochloride in, 351
integrase inhibitors, 898, 939—941
  dolutegravir, 939—940
  raltegravir, 940—941
Intelence, 929—930
intense itching, in scabies, 1025
interferon beta, teriflunomide and, 1388
interferon beta, 1a, 1391—1392
interferon beta, 1b, 1392—1393
interferon gamma, 1B, 1282—1283
interferons, 1280, 1389—1391
  actions of, 1280, 1389—1390
  adverse effects of, 1280—1281, 1390
  interactions of, 1390
  interferon beta, 1a, 1391—1392
  interferon beta, 1b, 1392—1393
  nursing points/cautions for, 1281—1282, 1390—1391
  patient teaching and advice for, 1282, 1391
  peginterferon beta-1a, 1393—1394
interleukin-1 receptor antagonist, non-glycosylated, anakinra, 1070—1071
interleukin, 6
  receptors, tocilizumab and, 1073
intermediate-density lipoprotein (IDL), 1299—1300
intermittent claudication, pentoxifylline for, 1634
internal sphincter, 942
interstitial cystitis, pentosan polysulfate sodium for, 951
intestinal colic, calcium gluconate monohydrate for, 1650
intestinal obstruction, charcoal, activated, 337
intra-abdominal infection
  ceftazidime with avibactam for, 174
  ceftolozane with tazobactam for, 175
intra-articular corticosteroids, 995
intracavernosal administration, 1117—1118
intracellular signals, calcium-independent, 1272
intracranial pressure (ICP), mannitol for, 1100

intractable hiccups, chlorpromazine hydrochloride for, 844
intractable nausea, haloperidol decanoate for, 852
intraocular infections, chloramphenicol for, 209
intraocular lens placement, acetylcholine chloride for, 1134
intraocular pressure, reducing, antiglaucoma agents for, 460
intrathecal mass, baclofen and, 1403
intrauterine devices (IUDs)
  copper-releasing, 1262, 1270
  levonorgestrel and, 1535
intravascular thrombosis, protein C for, 262
intravenous anaesthetics, 1173
intravenous regional anaesthesia, 1321
intrinsic factor, 871
Intuniv, 1558—1559
Invanz, 180—181
Invega, 860—862
Invega Sustenna, 860—862
Invega Trinza, 860—862
Inza, 30
iodine, 1579
  propylthiouracil and, 1587
Iopidine, 463—464
I-Pantoprazole, 881—882
ipecacuanha, 1019
ipilimumab, 764—765
Ipol, 1612
ipratropium bromide, 1148
Iptam, 580—582
irbesartan, 515—516
Iressa, 712—713
iridectomy, acetylcholine chloride for, 1134
irinotecan (liposomal), 649—651
irinotecan hydrochloride, 649—651
irinotecan hydrochloride trihydrate, 649
iron, sucroferric oxyhydroxide with, 364
iron and iron compounds, 1652—1657
  actions of, 1652
  adverse effects of, 1652
  ferric carboxymaltose, 1654—1655
  ferrous fumarate, 1655
  ferrous sulfate heptahydrate, 1655
  interactions of, 1652—1653
  iron polymaltose complex, 1656—1657
  iron sucrose, 1657
  nursing points/cautions for, 1653—1654
  optimal daily requirements for, 1652
  patient teaching and advice for, 1654
  uses of, 1652
iron overload, chronic
  deferasirox, 338
  deferiprone, 341

iron overload, chronic (*Continued*)
desferrioxamine mesylate, 342
iron poisoning, desferrioxamine mesylate, 343
iron polymaltose complex, 1656—1657
iron sucrose, 1657
iron supplementation, penicillamine and, 1055
Irprestan, 515—516
irritable bowel syndrome, mebeverine hydrochloride for, 1156
isavuconazole sulfate, 442
ischaemic stroke
alteplase for, 1153
dipyridamole for, 819
Iscover, 818
Isentress, 940—941
islets of Langerhans, 296
Isobide MR, 63—65
isoflurane, 1175—1176
isoniazid, 588—590
isophane insulin (with protamine), 303
isoprenaline hydrochloride, 1574—1575
isoproterenol, 1574
Isoptin, 541—543
Isoptin SR, 541—543
Isopto Carpine, 469
Isordil, 63
isosorbide dinitrate, 63
isosorbide mononitrate, 63—65
action of, 63
adverse effects of, 63
dose of, 63
interactions of, 63—64
nursing points/cautions of, 64
patient teaching and advice for, 64—65
use of, 63
isotretinoin, 5—6
Isotretinoin GX, 5—6
Isotretinoin Lupin, 5—6
Isotretinoin-WGR, 5—6
ispaghula, 1287
Istodax, 671
Itracap, 443—446
itraconazole, 443—446
triazolam and, 1447
Itranox, 443—446
IUDs. *See* intrauterine devices
ivabradine, 65
ivacaftor, 135—137
ivermectin, 45—47
ixekizumab (RCH), 1257—1258

J
Jadenu, 338—340
Jakavi, 731—733
Janus kinase (JAK1-3) inhibitor, 1075
Januvia, 319—320

Japanese encephalitis virus vaccine, 1607—1608
Jardiance, 326
jaw, osteonecrosis of, 959
Jespect, 1607
Jetrea, 1142
Jock Itch DermaGel, 448
Jorveza, 124, 1001
juvenile idiopathic arthritis, 1038

K
Kadcyla, 777—779
Kalexico, 202—204
Kalma, 73—74
Kalydeco, 135—137
Kanjinti, 777
Kanuma, 1362—1363
Kapanol, 1445—1447
Kaposi's sarcoma, 633, 635, 686
AIDS-related
doxorubicin hydrochloride for, 633
interferon alfa 2a for, 1283
vinblastine sulfate for, 686
Kaptan, 863—865
Karvea, 515—516
Karvezide, 516
Keflex, 169
Keflor, 168—169
Keflor CD, 168—169
Kefzol, 169—170
Kenacomb, 1018
Kenacomb Otic, 1018
Kenacort-A10, 1017—1018
Kenacort-Alignocaine, 40, 1017—1018
Kenalog in Orabase, 1017—1018
Keppra Oral, 402—403
keratin, ketoconazole and, 446
keratitis
ciprofloxacin lactate for, 217
Kerron, 402—403
Ketalar, 1177—1178
ketamine hydrochloride, 1177—1178
Ketamine solution for injection, 1177—1178
ketoconazole, 446—447
ketoprofen, 27
Ketorolac Solution for Injection, 27—28
ketorolac trometamol, 28
Kevtam, 402—403
Keytruda, 770
kidney impairment
antipsychotics and, 325
digoxin and, 92
kidney transplantation, 1276
Kineret, 1070—1071
Kiovig, 1623—1627
Klacid, 202—204

INDEX

Klebsiella spp. infections, colistimethate sodium for, 194
Kloxema, 1003
knee arthroplasty, total, tranexamic acid for, 1200
Kodatef, 567—568
Konakion, 366—367
Konakion MM Adult, 1648—1649
Konakion MM Paediatric, 366—367, 1648—1649
Kozenis, 567—568
Kuvan, 1360—1362
Kwells, 988
Kyleena, 1535—1538
Kymriah, 679—681
Kytril, 370—371

L

labetalol, 528
labour
    induction of, agents for, 1477—1478
    premature, 1456
        management of, agents for, 1473—1474
        salbutamol sulfate for, 104
lacosamide, 399—400
lactation inhibitors, 1486—1489
    bromocriptine mesilate (mesylate) and, 1486—1488
    cabergoline and, 1488—1489
lactic acidosis, 311
lactose
    deferasirox with, 340
    domperidone and, 376
    in oral contraceptives, 1549
    in pizotifen maleate, 578
lactulose, 1289—1290
Lamictal, 400—402
Lamisil Cream, 454—456
Lamisil Dermgel, 454—456
Lamisil Once, 454—456
Lamisil Spray, 454—456
Lamisil Tablets, 454—456
Lamitan, 400—402
lamivudine, 923—924
lamotrigine, 400—402
Lamotrust, 400—402
Lanoxin, 979
Lanreotide, 1221
lansoprazole, 879—880
lanthanum, 352—353
Lantus, 303
Lanvis, 678—679
Lanzopran, 879—880
Largactil, 844—846
Lariam, 561—562
laronidase (RCH), 1353—1354
laryngotracheobronchitis, budesonide for, 125
Lasix, 1085—1088

Lasix High Dose, 1085—1088
latanoprost, 468—469
latrodectism, 894
Latrodectus hasselti, 894
Latuda, 857
Lauromacrogol, 400, 1673—1674
Lax-Active, 1288
laxatives, 1285—1289
    adverse effects of, 1286
    bulk-forming, 1285, 1287—1288
    emollient, 1285
    faecal softeners, 1294—1296
    nursing points/cautions for, 1286
    osmotic, 1285, 1288—1292
    patient teaching and advice for, 1286
    stimulant, 1285, 1292—1294
    uses of, 1285—1286
Laxettes with Senna, 1294
Laxettes with Sennosides, 1294
Lax-Tab, 1293
lead poisoning, 346
leflunomide, 1047—1049
left ventricle impairment, eplerenone for, 1095
left ventricular systolic dysfunction, eplerenone for, 1095
leg ulcers, silver sulfadiazine for, 232
Legionnaire's disease
    clarithromycin for, 199
    erythromycin lactobionate for, 204
Leishmania aethiopica, pentamidine isetionate for, 829
leishmaniasis
    pentamidine isetionate for, 829
    visceral, amphotericin B for, 430
Lemsip Cold & Flu, 31—34
Lemsip Max, 31—34
Lemtrada, 746—747, 1369—1371
lenalidomide, 1258—1262
    action of, 1258
    adverse effects of, 1259—1260
    dose of, 1259
    interactions of, 1260
    nursing points/cautions for, 1260—1261
    patient teaching and advice for, 1261—1262
    use of, 1258—1259
Lengout, 477—478
leprosy, 567
    BCG Vaccine for, 1597
    dapsone for, 586
    rifampicin for, 592
    thalidomide, 675
leprosy reactional states, 585
Lercan, 538—539
lercanidipine, ciclosporin with, 1042
Lercanidipine, 538—539
Lescol XL, 1303—1304

HAVARD'S NURSING GUIDE TO DRUGS

letermovir, 907—908
lethargy, from agalsidase beta (RCH), 1338
letrozole, 651
Leucovorin Calcium Injection and Tablets, 336—337
leukaemia
  acute lymphoblastic
    dasatinib for, 708
    daunorubicin for, 629
    imatinib for, 716
    mercaptopurine monohydrate for, 654
    methotrexate for, 655
    ponatinib for, 729
  acute lymphocytic
    blinatumomab for, 750
    clofarabine for, 623
    cytarabine for, 625
  acute myeloblastic
    daunorubicin for, 629
    etoposide for, 639
    tioguanine for, 678
  acute myelogenous, mercaptopurine monohydrate for, 654
  acute myeloid
    azacitidine for, 607
    cytarabine for, 625
    idarubicin hydrochloride for, 647
  acute promyelocytic
    arsenic trioxide for, 604
    tretinoin for, 684
  chronic granulocytic
    busulfan for, 613
    mercaptopurine monohydrate for, 654
    tioguanine for, 678
  chronic lymphocytic
    alemtuzumab for, 746
    bendamustine hydrochloride for, 609
    chlorambucil for, 619
    cladribine for, 622
    cytarabine for, 625
    fludarabine phosphate for, 641
    ibrutinib for, 713
    idelalisib for, 714—715
    obinutuzumab for, 767
    rituximab for, 773
  chronic myelocytic, hydroxycarbamide for, 645
  chronic myeloid
    cytarabine for, 625
    dasatinib for, 708
    imatinib for, 716
    nilotinib for, 725
    ponatinib for, 729
  hairy cell
    cladribine for, 622
Leukeran, 619—620
leukotriene receptor antagonists, 139

Leuprorelin, 1219—1220
Leustatin, 622—623, 1371—1373
Levactam, 402—403
Levecetam, 402—403
Levemir, 303
levetiracetam, 402—403
  adjunct therapy with, 402
Levi, 402—403
Levitam, 402—403
levobupivacaine hydrochloride, 1325—1326
levocabastine, 493—494
levodopa, 805—809
  benserazide hydrochloride and, 802
  carbidopa monohydrate and, 805
  dose of, 795
Levonelle-1, 1535—1538
levonorgestrel, 1535—1538
  IUD, 1536—1537
  oral contraception, 1535, 1536
  post-coital emergency contraception, 1535, 1536
levothyroxine sodium, 1581—1583
Lexapro, 280—281
Lexotan, 74
lice infestation, 1024—1025
lidocaine (lignocaine), 82, 1326—1329
  action of, 1326—1327
  adverse effects of, 1327
  cream, 1328
  dose of, 1327
  interactions of, 1327—1328
  nursing points/cautions for, 1327
  ointment, 1328
  oral solution/spray, 1328
  patient teaching and advice for, 1328—1329
  transdermal patches, 1328—1329
  use of, 1327
lidocaine (lignocaine) hydrochloride, 82—84
  action of, 82
  adverse effects of, 82
  dose of, 82
  interactions of, 82—83
  nursing points/cautions for, 83
  use of, 82
life-threatening infections, vancomycin hydrochloride for, 185
lifitegrast, 1141—1142
lignocaine. *See* lidocaine (lignocaine)
Lignocaine Injection, 1326—1329
Lignospan Special, 1329
linagliptin, 318—319
Lincocin, 209
lincomycin, 209
lincomycin SXP, 209
lincosamides, 206—207
  actions of, 206

INDEX

lincosamides (*Continued*)
  adverse effects of, 206
  interactions of, 206
  nursing points/cautions for, 206
  patient teaching and advice for, 207
  uses of, 206
Linevox, 212—213
linezolid, 212—213
Lioresal, 1402—1406
Lioresal Intrathecal, 1402—1406
liothyronine (T₃), 1579
liothyronine sodium, 1583—1584
lipegfilgrastim, 788
Lipex, 1306
lipid regulating agents, 1299—1320
  bile acid binding agents, 1300, 1307
    actions of, 1307
    adverse effects of, 1307
    interactions of, 1307
    nursing points/cautions for, 1308
    patient teaching and advice for, 1308
    uses of, 1307
  fibrates, 1300, 1309
    actions of, 1309
    adverse effects of, 1309
    interactions of, 1309
    nursing points/cautions for, 1309—1310
    patient teaching and advice for, 1310
    uses of, 1309
  HMG-CoA reductase inhibitors (statins), 1300—1302
    actions of, 1300
    adverse effects of, 1301
    interactions of, 1301
    nursing points/cautions for, 1301
    patient teaching and advice for, 1301
    uses of, 1300—1301
  other lipid-lowering agents, 1300, 1316—1320
  PCSK9 inhibitors, 1314
Lipidil, 1310—1311
lipid-lowering agents, 1315
lipids, 1299
  retinoids and, 3
Lipigem, 1311—1312
Lipitor, 1302—1303
lipoprotein lipase, 951, 1299
lipoproteins, 1074
liposarcoma, eribulin mesilate for, 638
Liposomal Doxorubicin SUN, 633—635
Lipostat, 1304
liraglutide, 36
  actions of, 36
  uses of, 36
lisdexamfetamine dimesilate, 1560—1561
Litak, 622—623, 1371—1373
Lithicarb, 854—857

lithium carbonate, 854—857
live attenuated vaccines, 1591
liver cancer
  doxorubicin hydrochloride for, 633
  fluorouracil for, 642
liver disease
  androgens and anabolic steroids and, 1520
  progestogens and, 1526
liver dysfunction
  androgens and anabolic steroids and, 1521
  stimulants and, 1552
liver flukes, albendazole in, 43
liver function
  antipsychotics and, 835
  deferasirox and, 339
  lanthanum and, 353
  retinoids and, 3
liver function tests
  ambrisentan and, 1492
  bosentan monohydrate and, 1492
  gastrointestinal symptoms or jaundice and, 1156
  macitentan, 1497
  nitisinone, 1359
liver impairment antipsychotics and, 836
  progestogens and, 1533
liver transplantation
  amphotericin B for, 430
  everolimus for, 1251
  tacrolimus for, 1276
liver tumours, androgens and anabolic steroids and, 1520
Livial, 1545—1547
Livilan, 1545—1547
Livostin Eye Drops, 493—494
Livostin Nasal Spray, 493—494
LMX 4, 1326—1328
local anaesthetics, 1321—1324
  actions of, 1321—1322
  adverse effects of, 1322
  doses of, 1322
  infiltration anaesthesia, 1321
  interactions of, 1322—1323
  nerve block anaesthesia, 1322
  nursing points/cautions for, 1323—1324
  patient teaching and advice for, 1324
  spinal anaesthesia, 1322
  surface or topical anaesthesia, 1321
  uses of, 1322
Loceryl, 428—429
lodoxamide, 11326
Lofenoxal, 331—332
Logem, 400—401
Logicin Rapid Relief Nasal Spray, 1147
Lomide Eye Drops 0.1%, 1136
Lomotil, 331, 987
lomustine, 651—652

long-acting insulin, 300
long-term contraception, etonogestrel for, 1534
Loniten, 551–552
Lonquex, 788
loop diuretics, ciclosporin with, 1043
loperamide hydrochloride, 332–333
Lorano, 494–495
Lorapaed, 494–495
loratadine, 494–495
lorazepam, 77
lorlatinib, 722–723
Lorstat, 1302
Lorviqua, 722–723
losartan, 516–517
Losec, 880–881
loss of appetite, mercaptamine bitartrate for, 1355
low molecular weight heparins, 237–240
low-density lipoproteins (LDLs), 1299
lower respiratory tract infections
 amoxicillin trihydrate for, 154
lower urinary tract infection
 cefaclor monohydrate for, 168
 fosfomycin for, 227
lower urinary tract symptoms, silodosin for, 952
Loxalate, 280–281
Lozanoc, 443–445
lozenge, nicotine, 1109
LPV, 163–164
L-thyroxine sodium, 1581
L-triiodothyronine, 1583
Lucentis, 1140–1141
Lucrin, 1219–1220
Lucrin Depot, 1219–1220
Lukair, 142–143
lumefantrine, artemether and, 557–559
Lumigan Eye Drops, 465–466
Lumigan PF, 465–466
Lumin, 291–292
Lunava, 1047–1049
lung cancer
 cyclophosphamide for, 624
 doxorubicin hydrochloride for, 633
 ifosfamide for, 648
 non-small cell
  afatinib for, 726
  bevacizumab for, 748
  brigatinib for, 699
  crizotinib for, 706
  dabrafenib for, 707
  docetaxel for, 632
  durvalumab for, 759
  erlotinib hydrochloride for, 711
  gefitinib for, 713
  gemcitabine for, 646
  ipilimumab for, 764
  lorlatinib for, 722

lung cancer (*Continued*)
 nintedanib for, 726
 nivolumab for, 766
 paclitaxel for, 663
 pembrolizumab for, 770
 pemetrexed disodium for, 667
 trametinib for, 739
 vinorelbine for, 688
 small cell
  carboplatin for, 617
  epirubicin hydrochloride for, 636
  etoposide for, 639
  topotecan hydrochloride for, 681
 vincristine sulfate for, 687
lupus nephritis, mycophenolate mofetil for, 1263
lupus-like syndrome, TNF-α antagonists and, 1058
lurasidone hydrochloride, 857
luteinising hormone (LH), 1216, 1520
lutropin alfa, 1465–1466
Luveris 75 IU, 1465–1466
Luvox, 282
Lyclear, 1027
lymphocytic lymphoma
 small, ibrutinib for, 713
 vinblastine sulfate for, 686
lymphosarcoma
 methotrexate for, 655
 procarbazine for, 669
Lynparza, 727–728
Lyrica, 412–414
lysosomal acid lipase deficiency, sebelipase alfa for, 1362
lysosomal enzyme, alglucosidase alfa (RHU), 1338
lysosomes, 1349
lytic bone metastases, 962
Lyzalon, 412–413

M

MabCampath, 746–748, 1369–1371
MAC. See *Mycobacterium avium* complex
macitentan, 1496–1497
macrocytic anaemias, cyanocobalamin for, 1640
Macrodantin, 229–231
Macrogol, 1291
macrolide lactone, 1276
macrolides, 199–200
 actions of, 199
 adverse effects of, 199
 interactions of, 199–200
 nursing points/cautions for, 200
 patient teaching and advice for, 200–201
 for tuberculosis, 584
 uses of, 199
Macrovic Powder, 1288–1289
macular degeneration, agent for, 1138–1139

INDEX

macular degeneration, agent for (*Continued*)
adverse effects for, 1138
aflibercept as, 1139
brolucizumab as, 1140
nursing points/cautions for, 1138
patient teaching and advice for, 1138–1139
ranibizumab as, 1140–1141
macular oedema, latanoprost and, 468
Mag-A, 1658–1661
Magmin, 1658
magnesium, 1657–1658
magnesium aspartate, 1658–1661
magnesium chloride, 1659–1661
magnesium hydroxide, 887–888
sodium polystyrene sulfonate hydrogen, 362
magnesium sulfate heptahydrate, 1472–1473, 1659–1660
Magnesium Sulfate Heptahydrate 50% Injection, 1472–1473
Magnesium Sulfate Heptahydrate Concentrated 50% Injection, 1659
magnesium sulphate toxicity, calcium gluconate monohydrate for, 1650
magnesium toxicity, calcium chloride dihydrate for, 968–969
magnesium trisilicate, 887–888
Mag-Sup, 1658
maintenance, anaesthetic procedure, 1172
malabsorption, caused by pancreatic insufficiency, pancrelipase for, 1170
malabsorption syndrome, 1636
malaise, from agalsidase beta (RCH), 1337
malaria
diagnostic test for, 556
hydroxychloroquine sulfate for, 1045
initial symptoms of, 555
life cycle of, 555–557
patient teaching and advice for, 557
pregnancy and, 557
prevention of, 556–557
prophylaxis, doxycycline monohydrate for, 196
treatment of, 556
vectors, 555
Malarone, atovaquone and, 559
Malarone Junior Tablets 62.5/25, 559–560
Malarone Tablets 250/100, 559–561
maldigestion, pancreatic enzyme replacement therapy for, 1170
male pattern baldness, finasteride for, 947
Malean, 508
malignant glioma, carmustine for, 618
malignant hypertension, spironolactone for, 1096
malignant hyperthermia
signs, 1421
suxamethonium chloride and, 1426
treatment for, 1422, 1427

malignant lymphoma, cyclophosphamide for, 624
malignant melanoma
dacarbazine for, 626–627
fotemustine for, 643–644
pembrolizumab for, 770
temozolomide for, 674–675
vincristine sulfate for, 687–688
malignant pleural effusion, bleomycin sulfate for, 613
malignant syndrome, neuroleptic, 834
Maltofer, 1656–1657
mania, 836
acute
olanzapine pamoate monohydrate for, 858
quetiapine for, 863–865
risperidone for, 865–867
aripiprazole for, 839–841
carbamazepine for, 843
chlorpromazine hydrochloride for, 844–846
lithium carbonate and, 854–856
sodium valproate for, 416–418
stimulants and, 1553
manic depression, lithium carbonate for, 854
manic or mixed episodes, acute
asenapine maleate for, 841
olanzapine pamoate monohydrate for, 858
ziprasidone for, 868
mannitol, 137, 1099–1101
action of, 137
adverse effects of, 138
dose of, 138
interactions of, 138
nursing points/cautions for, 138–140
diagnostic procedure, 138–139
treatment, 139
patient teaching and advice for, 140
use of, 138
mantle cell lymphoma
bendamustine hydrochloride for, 609
bortezomib for, 698
ibrutinib for, 713
lenalidomide for, 1259
Mantoux test, 1597
MAOIs. *See* monoamine oxidase inhibitors
maraviroc, 898
Marcain, 1325
Marcain Epidural, 1325
Marcain Spinal 0.5%, 1325
Marcain Spinal 0.5% Heavy, 1325
Marcain with Adrenaline, 1325
Marevan, 249–253
Maroteaux-Lamy syndrome, galsulfase and, 1349
mast cell stabilisers, 98
maternal sinus tachycardia, salbutamol sulfate and, 1475

Mavenclad, 622—623, 1317—1373
Maxalt, 579—580
Maxamox, 154—155
Maxidex (Eye Drops), 1005
Maxolon, 377—379
Maxor, 880—881
Maxor Heartburn Relief, 880—881
Mayzent, 1385—1387
McGloin's Benzemul, 1026
measles-mumps-rubella vaccine, 1608—1609
mebendazole, 47—48
mebeverine hydrochloride, 1156
MedicAlert bracelet/pendant, 988
medication overuse, headaches and, 570
Meditab Irinotecan, 649—650
medroxyprogesterone acetate, 1538—1539
mefenamic acid, 28—29
mefloquine, 561
Megafol, 738—739
megaloblastic anaemia, folic acid for, 1643
Mekinist, 738—739
melanocyte-stimulating hormone, 1217
melanoma
  malignant
    dacarbazine for, 627
    fotemustine for, 643
    pembrolizumab for, 770
    temozolomide for, 674
    vincristine sulfate for, 687
  metastatic
    cobimetinib for, 705
    dabrafenib for, 706
    ipilimumab for, 764
    nivolumab for, 766
    trametinib for, 738
    vemurafenib for, 741
melasma, 1532
melatonin, 1509, 1510
Melobic, 29
Melotin MR, 1509—1510
Melox Capsules, 29
meloxibell, 29
meloxicam, 29
Melpha, 653
melphalan, 653
memantine hydrochloride, 54—55
Memanxa, 54
menarche, 653
Ménière's syndrome, betahistine dihydrochloride for, 1633
meningeal leukaemia
  cytarabine for, 626
  methotrexate for, 655
meningococcal disease
  meningococcal vaccine for, 1609
  rifampicin for, 592

meningococcal meningitis, benzylpenicillin sodium for, 160
meningococcal vaccine, 1609
menopausal flushing, clonidine hydrochloride for, 543
menopause
  oestrogen deficiency due to, estradiol for, 1527
  progesterone, 1469
  vulvovaginal symptoms associated with, estriol for, 1529
Menopur, 1466
menorrhagia, tranexamic acid for, 1200
Men's Regaine Extra Strength, 1034—1036
menstrual abnormalities, terbinafine hydrochloride and, 454
menstruation, timing of, norethisterone for, 1539
mental fatigue, caffeine for, 1556
Menveo, 1609
mepivacaine hydrochloride, 1329—1330
mepolizumab, 140
  action of, 140
  adverse effects of, 140—141
  dose of, 140
  nursing points/cautions for, 141
  patient teaching and advice for, 141—142
    pen instructions, 141—142
    syringe instructions, 142
  use of, 140
Mepreze, 877—878
mercaptamine (cysteamine) bitartrate, 1354—1355
mercaptopurine
  methotrexate and, 1052
  sulfasalazine and, 1167
mercaptopurine monohydrate, 654—655
Merkel cell carcinoma, avelumab for, 748
merozoites, 555—556
mesalazine, 1163—1165
Mesasal, 1163—1165
mesna, 780—781
mesterolone, 250
Mestinon, 983—984
Mestinon Timespan, 983—984
metabolic acidosis
  topiramate and, 423
  zonisamide and, 426
metabolic disorders agents, 1336—1367
  agalsidase alpha (GHU), 1336—1337
  agalsidase beta (RCH), 1337—1338
  alglucosidase alfa (RHU), 1338—1341
  asfotase alfa, 1341—1342
  carglumic acid, 1343
  elosulfase alfa (RCH), 1348—1349
  idursulfase, 1351—1352
  imiglucerase (RCH), 1352—1353
  laronidase (RCH), 1353—1354

INDEX

metabolic disorders agents (*Continued*)
  mercaptamine bitartrate, 1354—1355
  migalastat, 1355—1356
  miglustat, 1357—1358
  nitisinone, 1358—1360
  sapropterin, 1360—1362
  sebelipase, 1362—1363
  sodium phenylbutrate, 1363—1364
  taliglucerase alfa (RPC), 1364—1365
  velaglucerase alfa (GHU), 1365—1367
Metalyse, 1155
Metamucil, 1287—1288
Metaraminol, 1575—1576
metaraminol ARX, 1575—1576
Metaraminol GH, 1575—1576
Metaraminol Juno, 1575—1576
Metaraminol MYX, 1575—1576
Metaraminol Torbay, 1575—1576
metasulfite allergy, sympathomimetic agents and, 1566
Metermine, 40
Metex XR, 310
metformin hydrochloride, 310
  actions of, 310—311
  adverse effects of, 311
  dose of, 311
  interactions of, 311—312
  nursing points/cautions for, 312
  patient teaching and advice for, 312—313
  uses of, 311
methadone hydrochloride, 1444
methaemoglobin, 60
methaemoglobinaemia
  methylene blue trihydrate in, 354
  sodium nitrite, 361
methenamine (hexamine) hippurate, 228—229
methicillin-resistant *Staphylococcus aureus* (MRSA), 148—149
  mupirocin calcium for, 214
Methoblastin, 655—657, 1050—1054
methotrexate, 655—657, 666, 1050—1054
  action of, 655
  adalimumab and, 1060
  adverse effects of, 656
  dose of, 656
  interactions of, 656—657
  leflunomide and, 1048
  nursing points/cautions for, 657
  overdose, calcium folinate, 336
  patient teaching and advice for, 657
  probenecid and, 481
  use of, 655—656
Methotrexate Ebewe, 655—657
Methotrexate Injection, 655—657
methoxsalen, 781—783
  action of, 781

methoxsalen (*Continued*)
  adverse effects of, 782
  dose of, 781—782
  interactions of, 782
  nursing points/cautions for, 782—783
  patient teaching and advice for, 783
  use of, 781
methoxy polyethylene glycol epoetin beta, 1192—1193
methoxyflurane, 1178—1179
  increased risk of nephrotoxicity, 408
methyl aminolevulinate hydrochloride, 657—659
Methyl B12 Chewable, 1640—1641
methyl salicylate, 30
Methyl Salicylate Liniment, 30
Methylcobalamin 10 mg in 2 mL Injection, 1640—1641
methyldopa, 545—546
methyldopa sesquihydrate, 551
  with desferrioxamine mesylate, 343
Methylene Blue Injection, 354—355
methylene blue trihydrate, 354—355
methylnaltrexone, 1296—1297
methylphenidate hydrochloride, 1561—1563
methylprednisolone aceponate, 1011
methylprednisolone acetate, 1011
methylprednisolone sodium succinate, 1011—1012
methylxanthines, 1551
metoclopramide hydrochloride, 377—379
Metoclopramide Injection, 377—379
Metomax, metoclopramide hydrochloride monohydrate and, 379
Metopirone, 1674—1675
Metoprolol IV Viatris, 528
metoprolol succinate, 528—529
metoprolol tartrate, 528
Metrogyl, 826—829
Metrol, 528
Metrol-XL, 528
metromenorrhagia, progesterone and, 1470
metronidazole, 826—829
Metronidazole Intravenous Infusion, 826—829
Metronide, 826—829
Metvix, 657—659
metyrapone, 1674—1675
Mezavant, 1163—1165
Miacalcic, 965—966
mianserin hydrochloride, 291—293
micafungin, 447—448
Micardis, 518—519
Micardis Plus, 519
Micolette micro-enema, 1292
miconazole, 448
  oral administration of, 449
  oral gel, 450

1767

miconazole (*Continued*)
    spray powder, 450
    tincture, 450
    topical cream, 450
Microlax Enema, 1292
Microlut, 1535–1538
Microshield PVP, 1677
micturition frequency, increased, mirabegron for, 948
midazolam hydrochloride, 1511–1513
Midazolam Solution, 1511–1513
midostaurin, 659
mifepristone, 1482–1484
Mifepristone Linepharma, 1482–1484
migalastat, 1355–1356
miglustat, 1357–1358
migraine, 569
    androgens and anabolic steroids and, 1521
    chronic, botulinum toxin type A for, 1406
    eletriptan hydrobromide for, 571
    erenumab for, 573
    fremanezumab for, 574
    galcanezumab for, 575
    naratriptan hydrochloride for, 576
    pizotifen maleate for, 577
    premonitory phase (predrome) of, 569
    prophylaxis
        clonidine hydrochloride for, 544
        metoprolol tartrate for, 529
        propranolol hydrochloride for, 531
    rizatriptan benzoate for, 579
    sumatriptan for, 581
    zolmitriptan for, 582
Milrinone, 979–980
milrinone GH, 979
Milrinone-Baxter, 979–980
Minax, 528
Minax-XL, 528
mineral supplements, 1649–1652
    amino acids, 1670
    bicarbonate, 1665–1668
    calcium, 1649–1652
    iron and iron compounds, 1652–1654
    magnesium, 1658–1660
    other, 1660–1663
    phosphorus/phosphate, 1660–1662
    potassium, 1662–1665
    sodium, 1667–1669
    zinc, 1668–1669
mineralocorticoids, 991, 1216
minerals, 1636–1670
Minidiab, 310
Minims Amethocaine Eye Drops, 1334–1335
Minims Atropine Eye Drops, 986–987, 1131–1132
Minims Chloramphenicol 0.5% Eye Drops, 209–211

Minims Cyclopentolate Eye Drops, 1132
Minims Oxybuprocaine, 1333
Minims Phenylephrine Eye Drops, 1132–1133
    Pilocarpine, 469
Minims Prednisolone Eyedrops, 1014–1016
Minims Tropicamide, 1133–1134
Minipress, 503–504
Minirin Injection, 1232–1235
Minirin Melt, 1232
Minirin Nasal Spray or Drops, 1232–1235
Minirin Tablets, 1232
Minitran, 59–62
minocycline, 197
Minomycin, 167
minoxidil, 1034–1036
Miochol-E, 1134–1135
Miostat, 1135
miotics and ocular decongestants, 1134–1069
    acetylcholine chloride, 1134–1135
    carbachol, 1135
    lodoxamide, 1136
    naphazoline, 1136–1137
    tetryzoline (tetrahydrozoline), 1137
mirabegron, 948–949
Mircera, 1192–1193
Mirena, 1535–1538
Mirtanza, 293–294
mirtazapine, 293–294
Mirvaso, 1029–1030
misoprostol, 883–884, 1484–1486
misuse, drug, 1102
mite infestation, 1024
mitotic inhibitors, 595–596
mitozantrone, 660–661
Mitozantrone Ebewe, 660–661
Mivacron, 1424
mivacurium chloride, 1424
mixed drug overdose, flumazenil for, 348
mixed worm infestation
    albendazole for, 44
    mebendazole for, 47
Mixtard, 303
Mizart, 518–519
MMR II, 1608–1609
MND. *See* motor neurone disease
Mobic, 29
Mobilis, 34
Mobilis D, 34
moclobemide, 277–278
Modafin, 1563–1564
modafinil, 1563–1564
Modavigil, 1563–1564
Moduretic, 1093, 1094
Mogadon, 1513
moisturisers, retinoids and, 3
Molaxole, 1288–1289

INDEX

mometasone furoate, 1013—1014
monoamine oxidase (MAO), 273
monoamine oxidase inhibitors (MAOIs), 273—276
    actions of, 273
    adverse effects of, 274
    interactions of, 274
    nursing points/cautions for, 275
    patient teaching and advice for, 275—276
    uses of, 274
monoamine oxidase type B enzyme (MAO-B) inhibitors, 812
    patient teaching and advice for, 812
    rasagiline, 812—813
    safinamide, 813—814
    selegiline hydrochloride, 814—816
monobactams and carbapenems, 178—179
    adverse effects of, 178
    interactions for, 178
    nursing points/cautions for, 179
    patient teaching and advice for, 179
    uses of, 178
monoclonal antibody IgG$_{1kappa}$, 1271
Monodur, 63—65
MonoFIX-VF, 1210—1211
Monopril, 508—509
monovalent snake antivenom, 889
Montelair, 142—143
montelukast, 142—143
Monurol, 227—228
mood-stabilising agents, 833—870
moroctocog alfa, 1203
morphine hydrochloride, 1445
morphine hydrochloride trihydrate, 1445
morphine sulfate injection, 1445—1447
morphine sulfate pentahydrate, 1445—1447
    action of, 1445
    adverse effects of, 1446
    dose of, 1445
    interactions of, 1446
    nursing points/cautions for, 1446—1447
    patient teaching and advice for, 1447
    use of, 1445
Morquio A syndrome, elosulfase alfa (RCH) for, 1348
mosquito nets, 557
Motilium, 376—377
motion sickness
    hyoscine hydrobromide for, 988
    promethazine hydrochloride and, 496
motor neurone disease (MND), 1397
    cannabidiol for, 1394—1397
    riluzole for, 1397—1398
    tetrabenazine for, 1399—1400
    tetrahydrocannabinol for, 1394—1397
motor tics, stimulants and, 1552
moulds, 428

mouth, 1148
mouth hygiene, antipsychotics and, 838
mouth ulcer, chlorhexidine gluconate, 1149
Movapo, 800—802
movement disorder agents, 1368—1401
    interferons, 1389—1391
        actions of, 1389—1390
        adverse effects of, 1390
        interactions of, 1390
        interferon beta 1a, 1391—1392
        interferon beta 1b, 1392—1393
        nursing points/cautions for, 1390—1391
        patient teaching and advice for, 1391
        peginterferon beta-1a, 1393—1394
    motor neurone disease, 1397
        cannabidiol, 1394—1397
        riluzole, 1397—1399
        tetrabenazine for, 1399—1400
        tetrahydrocannabinol, 1394—1397
    multiple sclerosis, 1368—1369
        alemtuzumab, 1369—1371
        cladribine, 1371—1373
        dimethyl fumarate, 1373—1374
        fampridine, 1374—1375
        fingolimod, 1375—1378
        glatiramer acetate, 1378—1379
        natalizumab, 1380—1381
        ocrelizumab, 1382—1383
        ofatumumab, 1383—1384
        ozanimod, 1384—1385
        siponimod, 1385—1387
        teriflunomide, 1387—1389
        primary progressive, 1369
        relapsing/remitting, 1368
        secondary progressive, 1368
        teriflunomide, 1387—1389
Movicol preparations, 1288—1289
Moviprep, 1288
Movox, 282
Moxicam, 29
moxifloxacin, 218—219
moxonidine, 547—548
Moxotens, 547—548
Mozobil, 1267—1268
MRSA. See methicillin-resistant *Staphylococcus aureus*
MS Contin, 1445—1447
mucopolysaccharidosis II, idursulfase for, 1351
mucopolysaccharidosis type IVA, elosulfase alfa (RCH) for, 1348
mucopolysaccharidosis VI, galsulfase and, 1349
Mucosoothe, 1326—1329
multiple myeloma (MM), 887
    bortezomib for, 698
    carmustine for, 618
    cyclophosphamide for, 624

multiple myeloma (MM) (*Continued*)
    doxorubicin hydrochloride for, 633
    lenalidomide for, 1258
    melphalan for, 653
    plerixafor for, 1267
    plitidepsin for, 668
    thalidomide for, 675
multiple pregnancy, nafarelin acetate and, 1468
multiple sclerosis, 1237, 1368—1369
    alemtuzumab for, 1369—1371
    cladribine for, 622, 1371—1373
    dimethyl fumarate for, 1373—1374
    erectile dysfunction and, 1116
    fampridine for, 1374
    fingolimod for, 1375—1378
        action of, 1375—1376
        adverse effects of, 1376
        dose of, 1376
        interactions of, 1376
        nursing points/cautions for, 1376—1377
        patient teaching and advice for, 1377—1378
        use of, 1376
    glatiramer acetate for, 1378
    natalizumab for, 1382
        action of, 1380
        adverse effects of, 1380
        dose of, 1380
        interactions of, 1380
        nursing points/cautions for, 1380—1381
        patient teaching and advice for, 1381
        teriflunomide and, 1387
        use of, 1380
    ocrelizumab for, 1382
    primary progressive, 1368—1369
    relapsing, alemtuzumab for, 746
    relapsing/remitting, 1368—1369
    secondary progressive, 1368—1369
    teriflunomide for, 1387—1389
        action of, 1387
        adverse effects of, 1387—1388
        dose of, 1387
        interactions of, 1388
        nursing points/cautions for, 1388—1389
        patient teaching and advice for, 1389
        use of, 1387
Muphoran, 643—644
mupirocin, 214
Murelax, 77
Murine Clear Eyes, 1136—1137
Murine Sore Eyes, 1137
muscarinic M$_3$ antagonist, darifenacin hydrobromide in, 945
muscarinic receptor antagonist, 953, 955
muscarinic receptors, 955
muscle relaxants, 1402—1419
    baclofen, 1402—1405

muscle relaxants (*Continued*)
    botulinum toxin type A, 1406—1410
    dantrolene, 1410—1412
    incobotulinumtoxinA, 1412—1415
    orphenadrine, 1415—1416
    prabotulinumtoxin A, 1416—1417
    ropinirole hydrochloride, 1417—1419
muscle spasms
    baclofen for, 1402
    orphenadrine citrate for, 1415
muscle toxicity, ciclosporin and, 1042
myalgia, nafarelin acetate and, 1468
Myambutol, 587—588
myasthenia gravis
    neostigmine methylsulfate for, 982
    pyridostigmine bromide for, 983
Mycamine, 447—448
mycobacteria, 584
mycobacterial infection, clarithromycin for, 202
Mycobacterium avium complex (MAC), 590
Mycobacterium bovis, 608, 1597
Mycobacterium leprae, 586
Mycobacterium tuberculosis, 584
Mycobutin, 590—591
MycoNail, 428—429
mycophenolate mofetil, 1263
mycophenolate sodium, 1263—1265
mycoplasma infection, erythromycin lactobionate for, 204
mycoses, 428
mycosis fungoides
    bleomycin sulfate for, 612
    cyclophosphamide for, 624
    methotrexate for, 655
    vinblastine sulfate for, 686
    vincristine sulfate for, 687
Mycostatin Topical, 450—451
Mydriacyl, 1133—1134
mydriasis
    atropine sulfate monohydrate for, 1131
    cyclopentolate hydrochloride for, 1132
myelodysplastic syndrome (MDS), azacitidine for, 607
myelodysplastic/myeloproliferative disorder (MDS/MPD), imatinib for, 716
myelofibrosis
    busulfan for, 613
    ruxolitinib for, 731
myelomonocytic leukaemia, chronic, azacitidine for, 607
myelosuppressive therapy
    filgrastim for, 786
    G-CSF for, 784
Myfortic, 1263—1265
Mylan, 613—615
myocardial contraction, digoxin and, 92

myocardial infarction
    androgens and anabolic steroids and, 1522
    atenolol for, 524
    captopril for, 507
    metoprolol tartrate for, 529
    propranolol hydrochloride for, 531
    ramipril for, 511
    stimulants and, 1552
    trandolapril for, 512
    warfarin sodium for, 249
myocardial ischaemia, isosorbide mononitrate
        for, 63
myoclonic seizures, 384
myolysis, signs of, 890
myositis, betamethasone valerate for, 1000
Myozyme, 1338−1340
Mysoline, 414−415
myxoedema, 1183
myxoedema coma, liothyronine sodium for, 1584

N

nabiximols, 1394−1396
N-acetylgalactosamine 4-sulfatase deficiency,
        galsulfase and, 1349
N-acetylglutamate (NAG), in carglumic acid,
        1343
nadroparin calcium, 247−249
nafarelin acetate, 1467−1468
Naglazyme, 1349
naloxone (Narcan) challenge test, 1108
naloxone hydrochloride, 355−358
    action of, 355
    adverse effects of, 356
    dose of, 356
    interactions of, 356
    nursing points/cautions for, 356−357
    patient teaching and advice for, 357−358
    use of, 355−356
Naloxone Hydrochloride Injection, 355−358
Naltrexone GH, 1108−1109
naltrexone hydrochloride, 36−38
nandrolone decanoate, 1521−1522
NanoCelle B12, 1640
naphazoline, 1136−1137
Naphcon Forte, 1136−1137
nappy dermatitis, hydrocortisone sodium
        succinate for, 1009
Naprogesic, 30
Naprosyn, 30−31
Naprosyn SR, 30−31
naproxen, 30
naproxen sodium, 30−31
Naproxen Suspension, 30
Naramig, 576−577
naratriptan hydrochloride, 576−577
Narcan, 355−358

narcolepsy, 1551
    amphetamines for, 1551
    armodafinil for, 1553
    dexamfetamine (dexamphetamine) sulfate for,
        1557
    methylphenidate hydrochloride for, 1561
    modafinil for, 1563
narcotic analgesics, 1429
Naropin, 1331−1332
narrow therapeutic index, lithium carbonate and,
        854
nasal drops, instillation of, 1145
nasal polyps, fluticasone furoate for, 130
nasal spray instillation, 999
Nasonex Aqueous Nasal Spray, 1013−1014
nasopharyngitis, from carglumic acid, 1343
natalizumab, 1382
    action of, 1380
    adverse effects of, 1380
    dose of, 1380
    interactions of, 1380
    nursing points/cautions for, 1380−1381
    patient teaching and advice for, 1381
    teriflunomide and, 1388
    use of, 1380
National Immunisation Program Schedule,
        1594−1596t
Natrilix SR, 1090
Natulan, 669
nausea and vomiting
    from agalsidase alfa (GHU), 1337
    chemotherapy-induced, 374
    chlorpromazine hydrochloride for, 844
    management of, 368
    mercaptamine bitartrate for, 1355
    postoperative, 374
        prevention of, 374
    promethazine hydrochloride for, 496
    pyridoxine for, 1639
Nausetil, 380
Nausicalm, 382−383
Nausrelief, 380−382
Navelbine, 688−690
Navelbine Oral, 688−690
Nebilet, 530−531
nebivolol, 530
Neo-B12 Injection, 1641−1642
Neo-Mercazole, 1585−1587
Neoral, 1041−1045
NeoRecormon, 1190−1191
Neostigmine, 982−983
nedocromil sodium, 98
Neisseria meningitidis, 1609
NeisVac-C, 1609
nematocysts, 892
nematodes, 42

Neostigmine Juno, 982–983
Neo-Synephrine, 1577–1578
Neotigason, 4–5
nephritis, androgens and anabolic steroids and, 1521
nephrocalcinosis, from asfotase alfa, 1341
nephrolithiasis, topiramate and, 423
nephrosis, androgens and anabolic steroids and, 1521
nephrotic syndrome
　amiloride hydrochloride dihydrate for, 1093
　ciclosporin for, 1041
　spironolactone for, 1096
nephrotoxic drugs, ciclosporin with, 1042
nephrotoxicity
　auranofin and, 1039
　ciclosporin and, 1042
　signs of, 890
neratinib, 723–724
Nerlynx, 723–724
nerve block anaesthesia, 1322
nerve VII disorder, botulinum toxin type A for, 1407
Nervoderm, 1326–1329
nervous system, 981
Nesina, 318
Neulactil, 863
Neupro, 810–812
neuralgia, carbamazepine for, 843
neuraminidase inhibitors, 897, 912
　oseltamivir phosphate, 910
　peramivir, 911
　zanamivir, 912
neuroblastoma
　carboplatin for, 617
　cyclophosphamide for, 624
　doxorubicin hydrochloride for, 633
　vincristine sulfate for, 687
Neuroccord, 412
neurocysticercosis, albendazole for, 43
neuroendocrine tumours
　everolimus for, 1251
　octreotide for, 1223
neurogenic atony of urinary bladder, bethanechol chloride for, 944
neurogenic detrusor overactivity, botulinum toxin type A for, 1406
neurohypophysis, 1216
neurokinin-1 (NK1) receptor antagonists, 369
　aprepitant, 369
　fosaprepitant, 369
neuroleptanalgesia, haloperidol decanoate for, 852
neuroleptic malignant syndrome, 836
neurological diseases, erectile dysfunction and, 1116

neuromuscular blocking agents, 1420–1428
　depolarising blocking agents, 1426
　non-depolarising blocking agents, 1420–1423
neuromuscular disease/disorders, non-depolarising blocking agents and, 1420
neuromuscular junction, 1420
neuromyelitis optica spectrum disorder (NMOSD), eculizumab for, 1249
neurons, lithium carbonate and, 854
Neurontin, 397–398
neuropathic pain, 1429
neuropathy, peripheral, leflunomide, 1048
neurosyphilis, benzathine penicillin, 159
neutral (regular, soluble) insulin, 304
NeutraLice Advance, 1025
neutropenia
　deferiprone and, 341
　G-CSF for, 784
neutrophil count, deferiprone and, 341
neutrophils, G-CSF and, 784
Nexavar, 735–736
Nexium, 877–878
Nexole, 877–878
niacin, 1638–1639
Nicabate preparations, 1109–1114
nicorandil, 66–67
Nicorette preparations, 1109–1114
nicotinamide, 1638–1639
nicotine, 1109–1114
　chewing gum, 1112, 1113
　inhaler/inhalator, 1113
　lozenge, 1113
　oral spray, 1113, 1114
　transdermal patches, 1112
nicotine dependence
　bupropion hydrochloride for, 1104
　nicotine for, 1109
Nicotinell preparations, 1109–1114
nicotinic acid, 1318–1320, 1638–1639
Nidem, 309
Niemann-Pick type C disease, miglustat for, 1357
nifedipine, 539–540, 1474–1475
night blindness, vitamin A for, 1637
nilotinib, 724–726
　action of, 724
　adverse effects of, 725
　dose of, 725
　interactions of, 725
　nursing points/cautions for, 725
　patient teaching and advice for, 725–726
　uses of, 725
Nilstat Oral, 450–451
Nilstat Vaginal, 450–451
Nimbex, 1423–1424
Nimenrix, 1609

INDEX

nimodipine, 540—541
Nimotop, 540—541
nintedanib, 726—727
nitisinone, 1358—1360
　action of, 1358
　adverse effects of, 1358
　dose of, 1358
　interactions of, 1358
　nursing points/cautions of, 1359
　patient teaching and advice of, 1359—1360
　use of, 1358
nitrazepam, 1513
nitrofurantoin, 229—231
nitrogen-containing bisphosphonates, 958
Nitrolingual Pump Spray, 59—62
Nitrostat, 59—62
nitrous oxide, 1180
　methotrexate and, 656
Nityr, 1358—1360
Nivestim, 785—788
nivolumab, 766—767
Nizac, 874
nizatidine, 874
Nizoral Cream and Anti-Dandruff Shampoo, 446—447
NMDA receptors, ketamine hydrochloride and, 1177
NoDoz, 1556
Nocturnal, 1232
nocturnal enuresis
　amitriptyline hydrochloride for, 270
　imipramine hydrochloride for, 282
nodules, 1
Nolvadex-D, 672—673
nonacog alfa, 1211—1212
nonacog gamma, 1212—1213
non-barbiturate short-acting anaesthetic agent, 1177
non-competitive antagonist, ketamine hydrochloride and, 1177
non-depolarising blocking agents, 1420—1423
　actions of, 1420
　adverse effects of, 1421
　interactions of, 1421
　nursing points/cautions for, 1455
　patient teaching and advice for, 1422—1423
　uses of, 1420—1421
non-Hodgkin lymphoma
　bendamustine hydrochloride for, 609
　bleomycin sulfate for, 612
　carmustine for, 618
　chlorambucil for, 619
　cytarabine for, 625
　doxorubicin hydrochloride for, 633
　epirubicin hydrochloride for, 636
　etoposide for, 639

non-Hodgkin lymphoma (*Continued*)
　mitozantrone for, 660
　rituximab for, 773
　vincristine sulfate for, 687
non-mycobacterial infections, clarithromycin for, 202
non-myeloid malignancies
　darbepoetin alfa for, 1187—1188
　epoetin alfa in, 1189
　epoetin beta for, 1190
　epoetin lambda for, 1191
　haemopoietic agents and, 1185
non-nucleoside reverse transcriptase inhibitors (NNRTIs), 897—898, 927—931
　efavirenz, 927—929
　etravirine, 929—930
　rilpivirine hydrochloride, 930—931
non-Q wave myocardial infarction
　enoxaparin sodium for, 244
　tirofiban for, 823
non-radiographic axial spondyloarthritis
　etanercept for, 1063
　golimumab for, 1065
nonretrovirals, 898—918
　DNA polymerase inhibitors, 897, 898—918
　　aciclovir, 898—900
　　cidofovir, 900—902
　　famciclovir, 902—903
　　foscarnet, 903—905
　　ganciclovir, 905—907
　　letermovir, 907—908
　　valaciclovir, 908—909
　　valganciclovir, 909—910
　neuraminidase inhibitors, 897
　　oseltamivir phosphate, 910—911
　　peramivir, 911—912
　　zanamivir, 912—913
　NS3/4A protease inhibitors, 913
　NS5A inhibitors, 897
　NS5B RNA-dependent RNA protease inhibitors, 823, 913—914
　　sofosbuvir, 913—914
non-small cell lung cancer
　afatinib for, 694
　bevacizumab for, 748
　brigatinib for, 699
　crizotinib for, 706
　dabrafenib for, 707
　docetaxel for, 632
　durvalumab for, 759
　erlotinib hydrochloride for, 711
　gefitinib for, 713
　gemcitabine for, 646
　ipilimumab for, 764
　lorlatinib for, 722
　nintedanib for, 726

non-small cell lung cancer (*Continued*)
  nivolumab for, 766
  paclitaxel for, 663
  pembrolizumab for, 770
  pemetrexed disodium for, 667
  trametinib for, 739
  vinorelbine for, 688
non-ST-elevation myocardial infarction (NSTEMI)
  clopidogrel for, 818
  fondaparinux sodium for, 253—254
  ticagrelor for, 822
non-steroidal anti-inflammatory drugs (NSAIDs), 10—34, 570, 1038
  actions of, 11
  adverse effects of, 11
  interactions of, 11—15
  methotrexate and, 656
  nursing points/cautions for, 12—13
  patient teaching and advice for, 13—14
    eye drops, 14—15
    suppositories, 15
    topical gel, 14
non-surgical fat removal, deoxycholic acid for, 1032
noradrenaline, 1555, 1565
  haloperidol decanoate and, 852
  lithium carbonate and, 854
noradrenaline (norepinephrine) acid tartrate, 1576
Noralin, 1576—1577
Nordip, 534—535
Norditropin FlexPro, 1228—1230
norepinephrine, 1565, 1576
norethisterone, 1539—1540
Norflex, 1415—1416
norfloxacin, 219—220
Noriday, 28, 1539—1540
NorLevo-1, 1535—1537
normal blood pressure, 499
normal (human) immunoglobulin, 1623—1627
Normal Immunoglobulin-VF, 1623—1627
normal saline, 1667—1668
Normison, 1515
Norspan Transdermal Patch, 1103
nortriptyline, 273
NortriTABS, 273
Norvasc, 534—535
Norvir, 934—936
nose, 1145—1146
  agents for, 1128—1150
  instillation of nasal drops, 1145
  nursing points/cautions for, 1145
  patient teaching and advice for, 1145—1146
  sympathomimetic nasal decongestants, 1146

nosocomial pneumonia, linezolid for, 212
Noten, 524
Noumed Azathioprine, 1243—1245
Noumed Diazepam, 53, 75
Novasone, 1013—1014
Novicrit, 1191—1192
NovoMix, 303
NovoRapid, 303
NovoThirteen, 1214
Noxafil, 452—453
Noxicid Caps, 877—878
Nplate, 1198—1199
NRTIs. *See* nucleoside/nucleotide reverse transcriptase inhibitors
NS3/4A protease inhibitors, 913
NS5A inhibitors, 897
NS5B RNA-dependent RNA protease inhibitors, 897, 913—914
  sofosbuvir, 913—914
NSAIDs. *See* non-steroidal anti-inflammatory drugs
NSTEMI. *See* non-ST-elevation myocardial infarction
Nubeqa, 628—629
Nucala, 140
nuclear metabolism, pentamidine isetionate and, 829
nucleic acid atovaquone and, 825
  metronidazole and, 826
  pyrimethamine and, 831
  viral, methylene blue trihydrate, 354
nucleoside/nucleotide reverse transcriptase inhibitors (NRTIs), 897, 920—927
  abacavir, 920—922
  emtricitabine, 922—923
  lamivudine, 923—924
  tenofovir alafenamide, 924
  tenofovir disoproxil fumarate, 924—925
  zidovudine, 925—927
Nuelin SR, 121—123
Nuelin Syrup, 121—123
Nupentin, 397—399
Nurofen preparations, 24—25
Nurofen QuikZorb, 25
Nuvigil, 1553—1555
Nyal Antiviral Cold Sore Cream, 898—900
Nyal Bronchitis Cough Medicine, 1019—1020
nystatin, 450—452
Nyxoid, 355—358

O

obesity
  degree of, 35
  erectile dysfunction and, 1116
  management of, 35

INDEX

obesity (*Continued*)
  secondary causes of, 36
obinutuzumab, 767–769
obsessive-compulsive disorder (OCD), 70
  clomipramine hydrochloride for, 270–271
  escitalopram for, 281
  fluoxetine for, 281
  fluvoxamine maleate for, 282
  paroxetine for, 283
  sertraline for, 283
obstructive sleep apnoea
  armodafinil for, 1553
  modafinil for, 1563
occlusive dressings, topical corticosteroids and, 996
ocrelizumab, 1382–1383
Ocrevus, 1382–1383
ocriplasmin, 1142–1143
Octagam, 1623–1627
octocog alfa, 1203
Octostim Injection, 1232–1235
octreotide, 1222–1224
Octreotide Acetate Omega, 1222–1224
Octreotide GH, 1222–1224
Octreotide Sun, 1222–1224
Ocuflox, 220–221
ocular corticosteroids, 997
Odaplix SR, 1090–1091
oedema
  amiloride hydrochloride dihydrate for, 1093
  chlortalidone for, 1088
  dexamethasone phosphate for, 1005
  furosemide for, 1085
  mannitol for, 1100
  periorbital
    from alglucosidase alfa (RHU), 1339
  premenstrual tension (PMT) with, hydrochlorothiazide for, 1089
  spironolactone for, 1096
oesophagogastric cancer, capecitabine for, 616
Oestradiol, 1527–1529
Oestriol, 1529–1530
oestrogen deficiency, estradiol for, 1527
  vulvo-vaginal complaints due to, estriol for, 1529
oestrogens, 1519, 1524
  actions of, 1524
  adjunct, medroxyprogesterone for, 1538
  adverse effects of, 1525
  conjugated, 1527–1528
  contraindications to, 1526
  deficiency due to menopause, estradiol for, 1527
  estradiol, 1527–1529
  estriol, 1529–1530
  interactions of, 1525
  nursing points/cautions for, 1525–1526
  patient teaching and advice for, 1526–1527

oestrone, 1524
ofatumumab, 1383–1384
Ofev, 726–727
ofloxacin, 220–221
Ogivri, 777
OHSS. *See* ovarian hyperstimulation syndrome
olanzapine pamoate monohydrate, 858–860
olaparib, 727–728
olfaction receptors, 1145
oliguria, furosemide for, 1085
olmesartan medoxomil, 517–518
Olmetec, 517–518
Olmetec Plus, 517
Olopatadine, 495–496
olsalazine sodium, 1165–1166
Olumiant, 1245–1246
Omacor, 1316–1317
omalizumab (rch), 143–145
Omepral, 880–881
omeprazole, 880–881
Omnaris Nasal Spray, 128–130
Omnitrope, 1228–1230
Onbrez Breezhaler, 102–104
onchocerciasis, ivermectin for, 45–47
OncoTICE, 608–609
ondansetron, 371–372
Ondansetron Injection, 371–372
Onglyza, 319
Onivyde, 649–651
Onkotrone, 660–661
onychomycoses
  amorolfine for, 429
  itraconazole for, 443
Opdivo, 766–767
open-heart surgery, dopamine hydrochloride for, 1571
ophthalmic zoster, valaciclovir for, 909
opioid analgesics, 1429–1455
  actions of, 1430–1431
  adverse effects of, 1431
  alfentanil hydrochloride, 1434–1435
  buprenorphine, 1435–1438
  codeine phosphate, 1438–1439
  fentanyl, 1439–1443
  fentanyl citrate, 1439–1443
  hydromorphone, 1443
  interactions of, 1431–1432
  methadone hydrochloride, 1444–1445
  morphine hydrochloride trihydrate, 1445
  morphine sulfate pentahydrate, 1445–1447
  nursing points/cautions for, 1432–1433
  oxycodone, 1447
  oxycodone hydrochloride, 1447–1449
  patient teaching and advice for, 1434
  pethidine hydrochloride, 1449–1451
  remifentanil, 1451–1452

HAVARD'S NURSING GUIDE TO DRUGS

opioid analgesics (*Continued*)
   tapentadol hydrochloride, 1454—1455
   tramadol hydrochloride, 1452—1454
opioids
   abstinence from, naltrexone hydrochloride for, 36
   dependence
      Biodone Forte for, 1444
      buprenorphine for, 1435
      methadone hydrochloride for, 1107
      naltrexone hydrochloride for, 1108
      Subutex for, 1103, 1435
   naloxone hydrochloride dihydrate with, 355—358
Opsumit, 1496—1497
optic neuropathies, hydroxocobalamin for, 1641
Optrex Eye Drops, 1136—1137
oral contraceptive pills, combined, 1550
oral contraceptives, 1548
   actions of, 1547—1548
   adverse effects of, 1548
   etonogestrel and, 1534
   interactions of, 1548
   levonorgestrel as, 1535
   norethisterone for, 1539
   nursing points/cautions for, 1548—1549
   oxcarbazepine and, 404
   patient teaching and advice for, 1549—1550
   perampanel and, 405
   primidone and, 414
   terbinafine hydrochloride and, 454
   topiramate and, 423
   uses of, 1548
   voriconazole and, 458
oral glucose, 302
oral hypoglycaemic agents, 304—306
   alpha glucosidase inhibitors, 314—315
   biguanides, 311
   dipeptidyl peptidase-4 (DPP-4) inhibitors, 317
   nursing points/cautions for, 305
   patient teaching and advice for, 305—306
   sulfonylureas, 307
   thiazolidinediones, 315—317
oral spray, nicotine as, 1109, 1113
oral therapy, retinoids, 4
Oratane, 5—6
Orencia, 1068—1070
Orfadin, 1358—1360
Orgalutran, 1465
organ rejection
   everolimus for, 1251
   mycophenolate mofetil for, 1263
   sirolimus for, 1272
organ transplantation, azathioprine for, 1243
organophosphate poisoning, atropine sulfate monohydrate for, 986
Orgaran, 243—244

Oripro, 1469—1471
Orion Phenobarbital Elixir, 406—408
orlistat, 38—40
oropharynx, 1148
   anti-infective agents for, 1149
   nursing points/cautions for, 1148
   patient teaching and advice for, 1148
Oroxine, 1581—1583
Orphenadrine, 1415—1416
orthostatic hypotension, antipsychotics and, 835
Oruvail SR, 27
Oselltamivir, 910—911
Osmitrol Intravenous Infusion, 1099—1101
osmotic diuretics, 1098—1101
   glucose, 1098
osmotic laxatives, 1288
Ospolot, 421—422
osteitis deformans, 957
Ostelin Vitamin D, 1645—1647
osteoarthritis (OA), 1038
   hyaluronic acid for, 1672
osteoblasts, 957
osteoclasts, 657
osteogenic sarcoma, methotrexate for, 656
Osteomol, 31—34
osteomyelitis, teicoplanin for, 184—185
osteonecrosis, of jaw, 959
osteopenia, denosumab for, 755
osteoporosis, 957—958
   calcitriol for, 966
   colecalciferol for, 1645
   denosumab for, 971
   in post-menopausal women, denosumab for, 755
   raloxifene hydrochloride for, 973
   teriparatide for, 977
Osteovan, 964—965
OsteVit-D, 1645—1647
OsteVit-D One-A-Week, 1645—1647
OsteVit-D Vitamin D3 Oral Drops for Children, 1645—1647
Otezla, 1240—1241
otitis externa
   framycetin sulfate for, 189
otitis media, phenoxymethylpenicillin potassium for, 163
Otocomb Otic, 1018
Otodex, 1007
Otrivin Menthol Spray, 1148
Otrivin Nasal Drops Adult, 1148
Otrivin Nasal Drops Junior, 1148
Otrivin Nasal Spray Adult, 1148
Otrivin Nasal Spray Junior, 1148
ovarian adenocarcinoma
   chlorambucil for, 619
   cyclophosphamide for, 624
   melphalan for, 653

INDEX

ovarian cancer
  bevacizumab for, 748
  carboplatin for, 617
  cisplatin for, 621
  docetaxel for, 632
  doxorubicin hydrochloride for, 633
  epirubicin hydrochloride for, 636
  fluorouracil for, 642
  gemcitabine for, 646
  hydroxycarbamide for, 645
  ifosfamide for, 647
  olaparib for, 727
  paclitaxel for, 663
  topotecan hydrochloride for, 681
ovarian dysfunction, clomifene (clomiphene) citrate for, 1460
ovarian hyperstimulation, controlled
  follitropin alpha for, 1462
  follitropin beta for, 1463
  menopausal gonadotropin and, 1466
  ovarian hyperstimulation syndrome (OHSS), 1457–1458
  ganirelix acetate and, 1465
ovarian stimulation, controlled corifollitropin alfa, 1461
  nafarelin acetate for, 1467
overactive bladder
  botulinum toxin type A for, 1406
  mirabegron for, 948
overdose
  baclofen, 1403
  thyroxine sodium, 1582
overseas travel, vaccination and, 1593
overweight, 35
Ovestin Cream, 1529–1530
Ovestin Ovula Pessaries, 1529–1530
Ovestin Tablets, 1529–1530
Ovidrel Pen, 1459–1460
oxaliplatin, 662–663
oxazepam, 77–78
oxcarbazepine, 403–405
Oxis Turbuhaler, 101–102
oxpentifylline (*See* pentoxyfyline (oxypentifylline)) Oxy Cream, 8–9
Oxy Vanishing Cream, 8–9
oxybuprocaine hydrochloride, 1333–1334
oxybutynin, 949–951
oxycodone, 1439
oxycodone hydrochloride, 1447–1449
oxygen saturation, monitoring, bosentan monohydrate and, 1492
Oxymetazoline, 1147
OxyNorm, 1447–1449
oxytocic agents, 1478–1482
  carbetocin and, 1478
  ergometrine maleate and, 1479–1480

oxytocic agents (*Continued*)
  oxytocin and, 1481–1482
oxytocin, 1481–1482, 1573
Oxytrol Transdermal System, 949–951
Oxyuranus microlepidotus (fierce snake), 895
Oxyuranus scutellatus, 895
Ozidal, 865–867
Ozin, 858
Ozmep, 880–881
Ozole, 438–440
Ozole 150 mg, 438–440
Ozpan, 881–882
Ozurdex, 1005–1007

P

$P2Y_{12}$ receptor, 817, 819, 821, 822
paclitaxel, 663–665
  action of, 663
  adverse effects of, 664
  dose of, 663–664
  interactions of, 664
  nursing points/cautions for, 664–665
  patient teaching and advice for, 665
  use of, 663
Pacrolim, 1275–1278
paediatric cerebral tumour, carboplatin for, 617
Paget's disease, 957
  calcitonin salmon for, 965
PAH. *See* pulmonary arterial hypertension
pain, 1429
  acute, 1429
    management of, 1430
  buprenorphine for, 1103, 1435
  chronic, 1430
    fentanyl citrate for, 1440
  codeine phosphate hemihydrate for, 1439
  hydromorphone hydrochloride for, 1443
  methadone hydrochloride for, 1107, 1444
  neuropathic, 1429
  oxycodone hydrochloride for, 1448
  in Paget's disease, 957
  pethidine hydrochloride for, 1449
  tapentadol hydrochloride for, 1454
  tramadol hydrochloride for, 1452
  varicella zoster associated with, varicella zoster vaccines for, 1591
Paladopt, 495
Palexia IR, 1454–1455
Palexia SR, 1454–1455
paliperidone, 860–862
palivizumab, 1265–1266
palonosetron hydrochloride, 372–373
palpebral conjunctival inflammation, fluorometholone acetate for, 1008
pamidronate disodium, 962–963

Pamisol, 962—963
Panadol preparations, 31—34
Panafcort, 1016—1017
Panafcortelone, 1014—1016
Panamax, 31—34
pancreatic adenocarcinoma
    gemcitabine for, 649
    irinotecan hydrochloride for, 649
    paclitaxel for, 663
pancreatic cancer
    erlotinib hydrochloride for, 711
    fluorouracil for, 642
    gemcitabine for, 646
pancreatic enzyme replacement, 1170
pancreatic neuroendocrine tumour, sunitinib for, 737
pancreatic surgery, octreotide for, 1222
pancreatitis, chronic, pancrelipase for, 1105
pancrelipase, 1170—1171
panic disorder, 70
    sertraline for, 283
    venlafaxine hydrochloride for, 287
panitumumab, 769—770
Panthron, 881—882
pantoprazole, 881—882
Panzytrat 25000, 1170—1171
papaverine hydrochloride, 1119—1120
papillary cancer, epirubicin hydrochloride for, 637
papules, 1
paracetamol, 31—34, 570, 1281
    action of, 31
    adverse effects of, 32
    diphtheria-tetanus-pertussis (DTP) vaccine and, 1602
    dose of, 32
    interactions of, 32
    nursing points/cautions for, 32—33
    patient teaching and advice for, 33—34
    phenobarbital and, 407
    use of, 31
Paracetamol preparations, 31—34
Paracetamol Solution for Infusion, 31—34
Parachoc, 1294—1295
paraesthesia, from agalsidase beta (RCH), 1338
paraffin, liquid, 1294—1295
Paralgin, 31—34
paralytic ileus, antipsychotics and, 837
parasympathetic nervous system, 981, 1565
parasympathomimetics, 981—982
parathyroid hormone, 957
Parbezol, 882—883
parenteral beclomethasone, 1000
Pariet, 882—883
parietal cells, 871
Parkinson, James, 790
Parkinsonian symptoms, antipsychotics and, 834

Parkinsonism
    benserazide hydrochloride for, 802
    benztropine mesilate for, 793
    carbidopa monohydrate for, 805
    levodopa for, 806
    symptoms of, 790
    trihexyphenidyl (benzhexol) hydrochloride for, 794
Parkinson's disease, 790
    amantadine hydrochloride for, 799
    apomorphine hydrochloride hemihydrate for, 800
    benserazide hydrochloride for, 802
    bromocriptine mesilate for, 803, 1486
    cabergoline for, 804, 1488
    entacapone for, 795
    pramipexole dihydrochloride monohydrate for, 809
    rotigotine for, 810
    safinamide of, 813
    selegiline hydrochloride for, 815
Parlodel, 802—804, 1486—1488
Parnate, 276
paroxetine, 282—283
paroxysmal atrial tachycardia, digoxin for, 92
paroxysmal nocturnal haemoglobinuria (PNH), 1249
    eculizumab for, 1249
partial seizures, 384
pasireotide, 1224—1226
passive immunisation, 1591
Patanol, 495—496
patient education, tuberculosis and, 584—585
patiromer, 358—359
Paxam, 395—396
Paxtine, 282—283
pazopanib, 728—729
PBC. See primary biliary cholangitis
PCI. See percutaneous coronary intervention
PCP. See Pneumocystis carinii pneumonia
PCSK9 inhibitors, 1300, 1314
PDE5 inhibitors. See phosphodiesterase type 5 (PDE5) inhibitors
pediculicides, 1024
pediculosis, 1024—1025
Pegasys, 1283—1284
pegfilgrastim, 788—789
Peginterferon alfa, 2a, 1283—1284
    action of, 1283
    adverse effects of, 1283
    interactions of, 1283
    nursing points/cautions of, 1283—1284
    patient teaching and advice of, 1284
    use of, 1283
peginterferon beta-1a, 1393—1394
pegvisomant, 1226—1227

Pelgraz, 788—789
pellagra, 1319
pelvic abscess/cellulitis, metronidazole for, 827
pelvic pain, ganirelix acetate and, 1465
pembrolizumab, 770
pemetrexed disodium, 667—668
Pemzo, 880—881
penetrating keratoplasty, acetylcholine chloride for, 1134
penicillamine, 1054—1056
penicillin G, 160—161
penicillins, 151—154
  actions of, 151
  adverse effects of, 152
  interactions of, 152
  nursing points/cautions for, 152—153
  patient teaching and advice for, 153—154
  uses of, 151—152
penile desensitiser, lidocaine as, 1127
pentamidine isethionate, 829—831
Pentasa preparation, 1163—1165
Penthrox, 1178—1180
Penthrox inhaler, 1179
pentosan polysulfate sodium, 951—952
pentoxifylline (oxpentifylline), 1634—1635
peptic ulcers, 805
  aluminium hydroxide hydrate for, 886
perampanel, 405—406
percutaneous coronary intervention (PCI), bivalirudin for, 255
Pergoveris, 1463, 1466
Perhexiline, 68—69
Periactin, 489
perianal warts, imiquimod for, 1033
periarteritis nodosa, cortisone acetate for, 1003
periciazine, 863
pericyazine, 863
peri-menopause, progesterone, 1469
Perindo, 510—511
perindopril arginine, 510—511
perindopril erbumine, 510—511
peripheral arterial disease, rivaroxaban for, 260
peripheral blood progenitor cell (PBPC) mobilisation, G-CSF for, 784
peripheral demyelinating disease, TNF-α antagonists and, 1059
peripheral nervous system, 981
peripheral neuropathy
  cyanocobalamin for, 1640
  leflunomide, 1048
peritoneal cancer
  bevacizumab for, 748
  olaparib for, 727
Perjeta, 771
permethrin, 1027—1028
pernicious anaemia

pernicious anaemia (*Continued*)
  cyanocobalamin for, 1640
  hydroxocobalamin for, 1641
Persantin Ampoules, 819—820
pertuzumab, 771
pessary, progesterone, 1469
pethidine hydrochloride, 1449—1451
Petrus Bisacodyl Suppositories, 1293
Pevaryl Anti-fungal Cream, 437—438
Pevaryl Foaming Solution, 437—438
Pexsig, 68—69
phaeochromocytoma, glucagon hydrochloride in, 351
Pharmacy Action Diarrhoea Relief, 332—333
Pharmorubicin, 636—638
pharyngitis, from agalsidase alfa (GHU), 1337
Pheburane, 1363—1364
Phenasen, 604
phenelzine, 276
Phenergan, 496—498
Pheniramine 0.3%, 1137
Phenobarb, 406—409
phenobarbital (phenobarbitone), 406—409
  brivaracetam and, 389
  tiagabine hydrochloride and, 422
  tropisetron and, 373
Phenobarbital Injection, 406—408
phenobarbitone, 406—408
  tropisetron and, 373
phenol, 1676—1677
phenothiazines
  with desferrioxamine mesylate, 343
  metoclopramide hydrochloride monohydrate with, 378
Phenoxybenzamine, 501—502
Phenoxymethylpenicillin AFT, 163—164
phentermine, 40—41
phenylalanine
  epoetin beta in, 1191
  in rizatriptan benzoate, 580
  in zolmitriptan, 583
phenylalanine blood levels, sapropterin for, 1361
Phenylephrine BNM, 1577—1578
phenylephrine, 1132, 1577—1578
phenylketonuria, sapropterin dihydrochloride for, 1360
phenytoin
  brivaracetam and, 389
  ondansetron with, 371
  phenobarbital and, 407
  prochlorperazine maleate and, 380
  sulthiame and, 421
  tiagabine hydrochloride and, 422
phenytoin sodium, 409—412
phaeochromocytoma
  propranolol hydrochloride for, 531

1779

phaeochromocytoma (Continued)
  stimulants and, 1552
phobias, 70
  clomipramine hydrochloride for, 271
Phosphate Phebra, 976
Phosphate Phebra Tablets, 976—977
phosphodiesterase 3 (PDE$_3$) inhibitor, 979
phosphodiesterase 4 inhibitor, 1240
phosphodiesterase type 5 (PDE$_5$) inhibitors, 1120
  actions of, 1120
  interactions of, 1120—1121
  nursing points/cautions for, 1121
  patient teaching and advice for, 1121
phosphorus/phosphate, 1660—1662
Phospho-Soda, 1290—1292
Physeptone, 1107, 1444—1445
physical dependence, on drugs, 1102
Physiotens, 547—548
Phyta D, 1645—1647
phytomenadione, 366—367, 1648—1649
Piax, 818
Picolax, 1296
pilocarpine, 469—470
pimecrolimus, 1036—1037
pinworm, albendazole for, 43
pioglitazone, 315—317
Piperacillin with tazobactam, 164—165
piperazine antihistamine, 382
PiperTaz, 164
Piptaz, 164
pirfenidone, 1266—1267
piroxicam, 34
Pitressin, 1231
pituitary gland, 1216—1217
pituitary hormones, 1216—1236
  anterior pituitary hormones, 1216—1217
  posterior pituitary hormones, 1216—1217
pityriasis versicolor, itraconazole for, 443
pizotifen maleate, 577—578
placental barrier, rifampicin and, 594
Placil, 270—271
plaque, 1299
plaque psoriasis
  adalimumab for, 1060
  certolizumab pegol for, 1062
  etanercept for, 1063
  guselkumab for, 1254
  infliximab for, 1066
  ixekizumab for, 1257
Plaquenil, 1045—1047
plasma aluminium levels, with desferrioxamine mesylate, 345
plasma calcium, 957
plasma enzyme to p-aminobenzoic acid (PABA), 1321
plasmin, 1151

plasminogen, 1151
Plasmodium falciparum, 560, 564
  hydroxychloroquine sulfate for, 1045
Plasmodium malariae, 1045
  hydroxychloroquine sulfate for, 1045
Plasmodium parasites, 555
Plasmodium vivax, 555
  hydroxychloroquine sulfate for, 1045
platelet aggregation, 817
  clopidogrel and, 808
platelet-activating factor, 817
platelets, 817
Plavicor, 818—819
Plavix, 818—819
Plegridy, 1393—1394
Plendil ER, 537—538
Plenvu, 1288—1289
plerixafor, 1267—1268
pleural mesothelioma, pemetrexed disodium for, 667
Plidogrel, 818—819
plitidepsin, 668—669
pneumococcal disease, pneumococcal vaccine for, 1610—1611
pneumococcal infections,
  phenoxymethylpenicillin potassium for, 163
pneumococcal meningitis, benzylpenicillin sodium for, 160
pneumococcal vaccine, 1610—1010
Pneumocystis carinii pneumonia (PCP), 222
Pneumocystis jiroveci pneumonia, 674, 1011
pneumonia
  from alglucosidase alfa (RHU), 1339
  from carglumic acid, 1343
  cefaclor monohydrate for, 168
  Pneumocystis carinii
    atovaquone for, 825
    pentamidine isetionate for, 828
Pneumovax, 23, 1610—1611
podophyllotoxin, 1037
Polaramine, 490
polatuzumab vedotin, 771—772
poliomyelitis, poliomyelitis vaccine for, 1612
poliomyelitis vaccine, 1612
Polivy, 771—772
poloxalkol, 1295
poloxamer, 1295
polyarticular course juvenile chronic arthritis, etanercept for, 1063
polyarticular juvenile idiopathic arthritis
  abatacept for, 1068
  adalimumab for, 1060
  moderate-to-severe, adalimumab for, 1060
polycystic disease, acne and, 1
polycythaemia vera
  busulfan for, 613

INDEX

polycythaemia vera (*Continued*)
  melphalan for, 653
  ruxolitinib for, 731
Polymyxin B, 1612
polystyrene sulfonate, 362—363
polyvalent snake antivenom, 893, 894
pomalidomide, 1268—1271
  action of, 1268
  adverse effects of, 1268
  dose of, 1268
  interactions of, 1268
  nursing points/cautions for, 1269
  patient teaching and advice for, 12691271
  use of, 1268
Pomalyst, 1268—1271
ponatinib, 729—730
Ponstan, 28—29
poractant alfa, 145—146
porphyria
  androgens and anabolic steroids and, 1521
  hydroxychloroquine sulfate and, 1046
posaconazole, 452—453
post-coital emergency contraception, 1535, 1537
post-delivery sepsis, metronidazole for, 827
post-dose syndrome, zoledronic acid and, 964
Postella-1, 1535—1538
posterior pituitary gland, 1216—1217
posterior pituitary hormones, 1216—1217
  antidiuretic hormone, 1217, 1231—1236
  oxytocin, 1217
postherpetic neuralgia, varicella zoster vaccines for, 1619
Postinor-1, 1535—1538
post-menopausal bone mineral density loss, estradiol for, 1527
post-menopausal osteoporosis, oestrogens (conjugated) for, 1527
postoperative intestinal atony, neostigmine methylsulfate for, 982
postpartum haemorrhage dinoprostone and, 1477
  ergometrine maleate for, 1479
post-partum urinary retention, bethanechol chloride for, 944
Postrelle-1, 1535—1538
post-traumatic stress disorder (PTSD), 283
  paroxetine for, 283
postural hypotension, antipsychotics and, 835
potassium, 1662—1663
  actions of, 1662
  adverse effects of, 1662
  ciclosporin and, 1043
  deficiency, 1663
  interactions of, 1662—1663

potassium (*Continued*)
  levels, sodium polystyrene sulfonate hydrogen, 363
  nursing points/cautions for, 1663
  optimal daily requirements for, 1662
  patient teaching and advice for, 1662
  serum, suxamethonium chloride and, 1426
  uses of, 1662
potassium acetate, 1664
potassium chloride, 1664—1665
Potassium Chloride (2.23 g/10 mL) Injection, 1664—1665
Potassium Dihydrogen Phosphate 13.6% Concentrated Injection, 1660—1662
potassium-sparing diuretics, 500, 1080, 1662
  tacrolimus and, 1277
povidone-iodine, 1150, 1677
PPIX. *See* protoporphyrin IX
Pradaxa, 256—258
Prader-Willi syndrome, somatropin (somatotrophin/somatotropin) for, 1228
Praluent, 1315
Pramin, 377—379
pramipexole dihydrochloride monohydrate, 809—810
prasugrel, 821—822
Prasugrel Lupin, 821—822
Pravachol, 1304
Praxbind, 352
praziquantel, 48—49
prazosin, 503
Precedex, 1507—1508
Predmix Oral Solution, 1014
Prednefrin Forte, 1133
Prednefrin Forte (Eye Drops), 1016
prednisolone, 1014
prednisolone sodium phosphate, 1014
prednisone, 1016
Predsol Retention Enema and Suppositories, 1014
Predsolone, 1014
Predsone, 1016
pre-eclampsia, 1472
pregabalin, 412
pregnancy
  alpha-adrenoceptor blocking agents and, 501b
  ambrisentan and, 1491
  angiotensin II receptor antagonists and, 514b
  angiotensin-converting enzyme (ACE) inhibitors and, 506
  antiepileptic use during, 385
  apremilast and, 1241b
  artemether and lumefantrine and, 557
  azathioprine and, 1245
  baclofen and, 1402
  baricitinib and, 1246b
  basiliximab and, 1247b

pregnancy (*Continued*)
  belimumab and, 1248b
  beta-adrenoceptor blocking agents and, 523
  bleeding during rifabutin, 590
    rifampicin, 594
  bosentan monohydrate and, 1493
  botulinum toxin type A and, 1406
  calcium-channel blockers and, 534b
  carbimazole and, 1586b
  clonidine hydrochloride and, 545b
  dantrolene and, 1410
  dapsone and, 587
  desmopressin and, 1235b
  dupilumab and, 1249b
  eculizumab and, 1251b
  everolimus and, 1254
  goserelin acetate and, 1217
  guselkumab and, 1254
  human C1 esterase inhibitor and, 1256b
  icatibant and, 1257
  incobotulinumtoxinA and, 1412
  interferon alfa 2a and, 1284
  interferons, 1280
  isoniazid and, 590
  ixekizumab (RCH), 1258
  lanreotide acetate and, 1222
  leuprorelin and, 1220
  levothyroxine sodium for, 1583
  macitentan and, 1497
  malaria and, 557
  methyldopa sesquihydrate and, 546b
  minoxidil and, 552b
  moxonidine and, 548b
  mycophenolate mofetil and, 1264
  octreotide and, 1224
  orphenadrine citrate and, 1416b
  pasireotide and, 1226
  peginterferon alfa 2a, 1284b
  pegvisomant and, 1227
  pirfenidone and, 1267b
  plerixafor and, 1268
  propylthiouracil and, 1588b
  retinoids and, 4
  rifabutin and, 590
  rifampicin and, 594
  risankizumab and, 1271
  ropinirole hydrochloride and, 1419b
  secukinumab and, 1272b
  siponimod and, 1387b
  sirolimus and, 1274
  sodium iodide (^{131}I) and, 1589
  sodium nitroprusside and, 552b
  somatropin and, 1230b
  tacrolimus and, 1275
  terlipressin and, 1236b
  thalidomide and, 676

pregnancy (*Continued*)
  tildrakizumab and, 1279b
  ustekinumab and, 1280b
pregnancy, childbirth and breastfeeding, 1456–1489
  infertility treatment agents, 1456
    adverse effects of, 1457–1458
    cetrorelix acetate as, 1459
    choriogonadotropin alfa as, 1459–1460
    chorionic gonadotropin (human) as, 1457
    clomifene citrate as, 1460–1461
    corifollitropin alfa as, 1461–1462
    follitropin alpha as, 1462–1463
    follitropin beta as, 1463–1464
    ganirelix acetate as, 1465
    lutropin alfa as, 1465–1466
    menopausal gonadotropin as, 1466–1467
    nafarelin acetate as, 1467–1468
    nursing points/cautions for, 1458
    patient teaching and advice for, 1458
    progesterone as, 1469–1471
  labour induction agents, 1477–1478
  lactation inhibitors, 1486–1489
    bromocriptine mesilate (mesylate) and, 1486–1488
    cabergoline and, 1488–1489
  oxytocic agents and, 1478
    carbetocin as, 1478–1479
    ergometrine maleate and, 1479–1480
    oxytocin and, 1481–1482
  pre-eclampsia and eclampsia treatment agents, 1472
  pregnancy termination agents, 1482
    mifepristone in, 1482–1484
    misoprostol in, 1484–1486
  premature labour management, agents for, 1473–1474
    nifedipine, 1474–1475
    salbutamol sulfate, 1475–1477
pre-malignant lesions, human papillomavirus (HPV) vaccine for, 1605
Premarin, 1530–1531
premature ejaculation, dapoxetine for, 1125
premature infants
  caffeine for, 1556
  vaccination of, 1593
premature labour, 1473
  management of, agents for, 1473
  nifedipine, 1475
  salbutamol sulfate, 1475
premature luteinisation, prevention of
  cetrorelix acetate for, 1459
  ganirelix acetate for, 1465
premedication, anaesthetic procedure, 1172
premenstrual dysphoric disorder
  fluoxetine for, 281
  progesterone, 1469

INDEX

premenstrual dysphoric disorder (*Continued*)
    sertraline for, 283
premenstrual syndrome
    norethisterone for, 1539
progesterone, 1469
premenstrual tension
    with oedema, hydrochlorothiazide for, 1089
    pyridoxine for, 1639
    vitamin A for, 1637
Prenoxad, 355–358
preoperative sedation, midazolam hydrochloride and, 1511
Presolol, 528
pressure immobilisation first aid technique, for snake bite, 891
pressure injuries, silver sulfadiazine for, 232
preterm birth, 1469
Prevenar, 13, 1610
pre-vulvovaginal surgery, estriol for, 1529
Prevymis, 907–908
Prexum, 510–511
Prezista, 933
Prilace, 511–512
Priligy, 1125–1127
prilocaine hydrochloride, 1330–1331
Primacin, 563–564
primaquine, 563–564
    action of, 563
    adverse effects of, 563
    dose of, 563
    interactions of, 563
    nursing points/cautions for, 563–564
    patient teaching and advice for, 564
    use of, 563
primary adrenocortical insufficiency, corticosteroids for, 992
primary amenorrhoea, norethisterone for, 1539
primary biliary cholangitis (PBC), ursodeoxycholic acid for, 1158
primary hyperaldosteronism, spironolactone for, 1096
primary hypercholesterolaemia, alirocumab and, 1315
primary hyperhidrosis, botulinum toxin type A for, 1406
primary hyperlipidaemia, 1300
primary hyperparathyroidism, cinacalcet for, 969
primary immunisation schedule, 1592
primary immunodeficiency, 1624
primary ovarian failure, oestrogens (conjugated) for, 1530–1531
primary progressive multiple sclerosis, 1368–1369
primary sclerosing cholangitis (PSC), ursodeoxycholic acid for, 1158
Primaxin, 181

primidone, 414–415
    tiagabine hydrochloride and, 422
Primolut N, 1539
Primoteston Depot, 1522
Priorix, 1608
Pristiq, 285–286
Privigen, 1623–1627
Pro-Banthine, 990
probenecid, 480–482
Probitor, 880–881
procaine benzylpenicillin (procaine penicillin), 165–166
Procalm, 380
procarbazine, 669
    prochlorperazine mesilate and, 380
procedural sedation, dexmedetomidine and, 1507
prochlorperazine, 380
    with desferrioxamine mesylate, 343
prochlorperazine maleate, 380
prochlorperazine mesilate, 380–382
Pro-Cid, 480–482
ProFeme Cream, 1469–1471
progenitor (stem) cell, G-CSF in, 784
progesterone, 1469–1471
    action of, 1469
    adverse effects of, 1470
    deficiency, 1469
    dose of, 1469–1470
    interactions of, 1470
    nursing points/cautions for, 1470–1471
    patient teaching and advice for, 1471
    use of, 1469
progestogens, 1531
    actions of, 1531
    adverse effects of, 1531–1532
    etonogestrel, 1534
    interactions of, 1532
    levonorgestrel, 1535–1536
    medroxyprogesterone acetate, 1538–1539
    norethisterone, 1539
    nursing points/cautions for, 1532–1533
    patient teaching and advice for, 1533–1534
    uses of, 1531
Progout, 475–476
Prograf, 1275–1278
proguanil hydrochloride, 559–561
Progynova, 1527–1529
prolactin, 1216
    levels
        domperidone and, 376
        flupentixol decanoate and, 850
        olanzapine pamoate monohydrate and, 858
        raised, antipsychotics and, 835
        risperidone and, 865
    release

prolactin (*Continued*)
    chlorpromazine hydrochloride and, 844
    haloperidol decanoate and, 852
prolactin release-inhibiting factor (PRIH), 1216
prolactinoma
    bromocriptine mesilate (mesylate) for, 1486
    oestrogens and, 1525
Proladone, 1447
Prolastin C Solution for infusion, 1340—1341
Prolia, 755, 971—973
proliferative diabetic retinopathy (PDR), ranibizumab for, 1140
Prolistat, 38
promethazine hydrochloride, 496
Prometrium, 1469—1471
propantheline, 990
propecia, 947
    finasteride for, 947
properdin deficiency, meningococcal vaccine for, 1609
prophylactic and anti-inflammatory drugs, 98
propofol, 1180
    action of, 1180
    adverse effects of, 1180—1181
    interactions of, 1181
    nursing points/cautions of, 1181
    patient teaching and advice for, 1181
    use of, 1180
Propofol-Lipuro 1% and 2%, 1180
propranolol, prochlorperazine mesilate with, 380
propranolol, 531—532
propylthiouracil, 1587—1588
Proscar, 947—948
prostaglandin E$_1$, 1118, 1485, 1632
prostaglandin E$_2$, 1477—1478
prostaglandins, 992
prostate cancer
    abiraterone acetate for, 600
    androgens and anabolic steroids and, 1519
    apalutamide for, 603
    bicalutamide for, 611
    cabazitaxel for, 615
    cyproterone acetate for, 1541
    darolutamide for, 628
    degarelix for, 631
    docetaxel for, 632
    enzalutamide for, 635
    erectile dysfunction and, 1116
    goserelin acetate for, 1217
    leuprorelin acetate for, 1220
    radium (^{223}Ra) dichloride for, 689
prostate-specific antigen (PSA), 943
prostatic hypertrophy, antipsychotics and, 836
prosthetic heart valves, warfarin sodium for, 249
Prostin E$_2$ Vaginal Gel, 1477—1479
Prostin VR, 1118, 1632

protamine sulfate, 359—360
Protamine Sulphate Injection BP, 359—360
Protaphane, 303
protease inhibitors, 897, 931—936
    atazanavir, 931—933
    darunavir, 933—934
    ritonavir, 934—936
    tipranavir, 935
protein C, 262—263
prothrombin time (PT), 237
proton pump inhibitors, 875
    esomeprazole, 877—878
    lansoprazole, 879—880
    omeprazole, 880—881
    pantoprazole, 881—882
    rabeprazole sodium, 882—883
protoporphyrin IX (PPIX), 1028
protozoa, 825
protozoan infections, 825
Proveblue Solution for Injection, 354—355
Provera, 1538—1539
Provitamin A carotenoid, 1637
Provive 1%, 1180
Provive MCT/LCT 1%, 1180
Proxen SR, 30
proxymetacaine hydrochloride, 1334
Prozac, 281—282
prucalopride, 1297—1298
pruritus
    from aciclovir, 899
    from agalsidase alfa (GHU), 1337
    from alglucosidase beta (RHU), 1337
    crotamiton for, 1027
    cyproheptadine hydrochloride sesquihydrate for, 489
Pryzex, 858—860
Pryzex ODT, 858—860
PSC. *See* primary sclerosing cholangitis
pseudoaphakia, latanoprost and, 469
Pseudomonas aeruginosa infection, 148
    cephalosporins, 166
    cefepime, 170
    ceftriaxone, 176
    gentamicin, 190
    linezolid, 212
    tobramycin sulfate for, 191
pseudopodia, 825
psoriasis, 1237
    ciclosporin for, 1041
    hydrocortisone sodium succinate for, 1009
    hydroxychloroquine sulfate and, 1047
    methotrexate for, 1050
    tildrakizumab for, 1278
psoriatic arthritis, 1038
    abatacept for, 1068
    adalimumab for, 1060

INDEX

psoriatic arthritis (*Continued*)
  certolizumab pegol for, 1062
  DMARDs and, 1038
  etanercept for, 1063
  golimumab for, 1065
  infliximab for, 1066
  leflunomide for, 1047
  moderate-to-severe, adalimumab for, 1060
psychological disturbances, androgens and anabolic steroids and, 1521
psychosis, 791
  flupentixol decanoate for, 850
  haloperidol decanoate and, 852
  stimulants and, 1552
psychotic/suicidal tendencies, stimulants and, 1552—1553
psyllium, 1287—1288
PT. *See* prothrombin time
PTU, 1587—1588
pubic lice, 1027
  crotamiton for, 1027
Pulmicort, 124—128, 1001—1002
pulmonary arterial hypertension (PAH), 1490
  familial
    ambrisentan for, 1490
    bosentan monohydrate for, 1491—1493
    epoprostenol for, 1493—1495
    macitentan for, 1496
  idiopathic
    bosentan monohydrate for, 1491—1493
    epoprostenol for, 1493
    iloprost trometamol for, 1495—1496
    macitentan for, 1496—1497
    riociguat for, 1497—1499
    sildenafil for, 1122
    tadalafil for, 1124
pulmonary embolism
  alteplase for, 1153
  apixaban for, 259
  dabigatran etexilate for, 256
  fondaparinux sodium for, 253
  rivaroxaban for, 260
pulmonary hypertension, agents, 1490—1501
  ambrisentan as, 1490—1491
  bosentan monohydrate as, 1491—1493
  epoprostenol as, 1493—1495
  iloprost trometamol as, 1495—1496
  macitentan as, 1496—1497
  riociguat as, 1497—1499
pulmonary TB, 584
pulmonary thromboembolism
  epoprostenol and, 1494
  iloprost trometamol for, 1495
Pulmozyme, 134—135
pure red cell aplasia, 1185
Puregon, 1463

purgatives, 1285
Puri-Nethol, 654—655
purpura fulminans, protein C for, 262
PVC, clonazepam absorbed by, 395
pyelonephritis
  ceftazidime with avibactam for, 174
  ceftolozane with tazobactam for, 175
Pyralin EN, 1056—1057, 1166—1168
Pyrantel, 49
Pyridostigmine, 983—984
Pyridox, 1639—1640
pyridoxine, 1639—1640
pyrimethamine, 831
  overdose, calcium folinate, 336

Q

Q fever vaccine, 1612—1613
QT interval prolongation, antipsychotics and, 835
QT prolongation
  promethazine and, 496
  risk of, deferiprone and, 341
  voriconazole and, 457—458
Quadracel, 1612
Questran Lite, 1308—1309
Quetia, 863—865
Quetia XR, 863—865
Quilonum SR, 854—857
Quinate, 564—567
Quinbisul, 564
quinine bisulfate, 564
quinine dihydrochloride, 564
Quinine Dihydrochloride 6% Sterile Concentrate, 564
quinine sulfate, 564—567
  action of, 564
  adverse effects of, 565
  dose of, 565
  interactions of, 565
  nursing points/cautions for, 565—566
  patient teaching and advice for, 566
  use of, 564—565
quinolones, 214—216
  actions of, 214
  adverse effects of, 215
  interactions of, 215
  nursing points/cautions for, 215—216
  patient teaching and advice for, 216
  uses of, 215
QuitX preparations, 1109—1114
Qvar, 123—124
Q-vax, 1612

R

RA. *See* rheumatoid arthritis
rabeprazole sodium, 882—883
rabies immunoglobulin, 1627

rabies vaccine, 1613—1615
Rabipur, 1613—1615
radiation sickness, pyridoxine for, 1639
radiation therapy, erectile dysfunction and, 1116
Radium (^{223}Ra) dichloride, 669—670
Rafen, 24—25
Ralovera, 1538—1539
Ralovista, 973—975
raloxifene hydrochloride, 973—975
raltegravir, 940—941
raltitrexed, 670—671
Ramipril, 511—512
ramucirumab, 772—773
ranibizumab, 1140—1141
ranitidine hydrochloride, 875
Rapamune, 1272—1274
rapid miosis, acetylcholine chloride for, 1134
Rapifen, 1434—1435
Rapivab, 911—912
rasagiline, 812—813
rasburicase rys, 482—483
rash
  from alglucosidase alfa (RHU), 1339
  allopurinol for, 475
  mercaptamine bitartrate for, 1355
Raynaud's disease, prazosin for, 503
Raynaud's phenomenon, prazosin hydrochloride for, 503
Razit, 882—883
'rebound phenomena', 72
reboxetine, 287
recombinant monoclonal antibody (IgG1), 1057
recombinant tissue plasminogen activator (r-tPA)
  alteplase as, 1153
  tenecteplase as, 1155
recovery, anaesthetic procedure, 1172
recurrent brain tumours, temozolomide for, 674
recurrent glioblastoma multiforme, temozolomide for, 674
recurrent metastatic renal carcinoma, medroxyprogesterone for, 1538
recurrent unipolar depressive illness, lithium carbonate for, 854
red back spider antivenom, 894
red cell aplasia, pure, 1185
Redipred Solone, 1014—1016
Reedos, 400—402
refractory follicular lymphoma, idelalisib for, 715
refractory headaches, 570
refractory invasive fungal infection, posaconazole for, 452
Regaine, 551—552
Rejuvenail, 435
relapsing/remitting multiple sclerosis, 1371
  alemtuzumab, 746, 1369
  dimethyl fumarate, 1373

relapsing/remitting multiple sclerosis (*Continued*)
  fingolimod, 1376
  glatiramer acetate, 1378
  interferon beta, 1a, 1392
  interferon beta, 1b, 1392
  natalizumab, 1380
  peginterferon beta-1a, 1393
Relenza, 912—913
Relistor, 1296—1297
Remicade, 1065—1067
remifentanil, 1451—1452
Reminyl, 53—54
remodelling, bone, 957
Remsima, 1065—1067
Renagel, 360—361
renal angiomyolipoma, everolimus for, 1251
renal cancer, everolimus for, 1251
renal cell carcinoma
  axitinib for, 696
  bevacizumab for, 748
  ipilimumab for, 764
  nivolumab for, 766
  pazopanib for, 728
  pembrolizumab for, 770
  sorafenib tosilate for, 735
  sunitinib for, 737
renal dysfunction, oestrogens and, 1526
renal failure, chronic
  darbepoetin alfa for, 1187
  epoetin alfa for, 1189
  epoetin beta for, 1190
  epoetin lambda for, 1191
  haemopoietic agents for, 1184
renal stones, allopurinol for, 475
renal transplantation
  basiliximab for, 1246
  everolimus for, 1251
renal tubular acidosis, sodium bicarbonate for, 1665
Renflexis, 1065—1067
Renitec, 508
Renitec Plus 20/6, 508
renovascular hypertension, enalapril maleate for, 508
Repatha, 1316
Replagal, 1336—1337
Repreve, 1417—1419
Resolve Plus 1.0, Resolve Plus 0.5, 1010
Resonium A, 362—363
Resotrans, 1297—1298
respiratory agents, 133—146
respiratory depression
  diphenoxylate and, 332
  for ketamine hydrochloride, 1177
respiratory distress, adrenaline for, 1567
respiratory distress syndrome (RDS)

INDEX

respiratory distress syndrome (RDS) (*Continued*)
  beractant for, 133
  betamethasone valerate for, 1000
  poractant alfa for, 145
respiratory syncytial virus, palivizumab for, 1265
respiratory tract disease, prevention of, 1204
respiratory tract infection
  ampicillin sodium for, 157
  co-trimoxazole for, 221
  vitamin A for, 1575
Resprim, 222–225
Resprim Forte, 222–225
Restavit, 492–493
restless leg syndrome (RLS)
  pramipexole dihydrochloride monohydrate for, 809
  ropinirole hydrochloride for, 1418
  rotigotine for, 810
reteplase, 256
reticulosarcoma, procarbazine for, 669
retinal vein occlusion, ranibizumab for, 1140
retinoblastoma, cyclophosphamide for, 624
retinoids, 2–4
  actions of, 2
  adverse effects of, 2
  interactions of, 2
  nursing points/cautions for, 2
  patient teaching and advice for, 3–4
    oral therapy, 4
    topical therapy, 3–4
Retinol, 1636–1637
ReTrieve Cream, 6
Retrovir, 925–927
retroviruses, 897, 918
re-vaccination, 1620
Revatio, 1122–1124
reversible inhibitors of monoamine oxidase type A, 277–278
Revestive, 1157–1158
Revlimid, 1258–1262
Revolade, 1195–1197
Rexulti, 842
Reyataz, 931–933
rhabdomyosarcoma
  dactinomycin for, 627
  daunorubicin for, 629
  vincristine sulfate for, 687
Rhesus (Rh(D)) immunoglobulin, 1627–1628
rheumatic fever
  benzathine penicillin for, 159
  phenoxymethylpenicillin potassium for, 163
rheumatoid arthritis (RA), 970, 1237
  abatacept for, 1068
  adalimumab for, 1060
  adjunctive treatment for, 1039
  anakinra for, 1070

rheumatoid arthritis (RA) (*Continued*)
  auranofin for, 1039
  baricitinib for, 1245
  certolizumab pegol for, 1062
  ciclosporin for, 1041
  erectile dysfunction and, 1116
  etanercept for, 1063
  golimumab for, 1065
  hydroxychloroquine sulfate for, 1045
  infliximab for, 1066
  leflunomide for, 1047
  methotrexate for, 656, 1050
  penicillamine for, 1054
  rituximab for, 773
  sulfasalazine for, 1056
Rh(D) immunoglobulin, 1627–1628
Rh(D) Immunoglobulin-VF, 1627–1628
Rhinocort, 124–128, 1001–1002
Rhinocort Hayfever, 1001–1002
Rhinocort Hayfever & Allergy, 124–128
rhinorrhoea
  from agalsidase alfa (GHU), 1337
  from alglucosidase alfa (RHU), 1339
rhodopsin, 1636
Rhophylac, 1627–1628
Riamet, 557–559
RiaSTAP, 1197–1198
ribavirin, 917–918
riboflavine, 1638
Ribomustin, 609–610
rickettsial infections, chloramphenicol for, 209
Ridaura, 1039
rifabutin, 590–592
Rifadin, 592–594
rifampicin, 592–594
  action of, 592
  adverse effects of, 592
  dose of, 592
  interactions of, 592–593
  leflunomide and, 1048
  nursing points/cautions for, 593–594
  ondansetron with, 371
  patient teaching and advice for, 594
  tofacitinib and, 1076
  tropisetron and, 373
  use of, 592
  zolpidem tartrate and, 1516
rifaximin, 231–232
Rikodeine Oral Liquid, 1022
rilpivirine, 930–931
Rilutek, 1397–1399
riluzole, 1397–1399
Rimycin, 592–594
ringworm, tolnaftate, 456
Rinvoq, 1077–1078
riociguat, 1497–1499

Riodine Concentrated Gargle Solution, 1677
risankizumab, 1271
risedronate sodium, 963–964
Rispa, 865–867
Risperdal, 865–867
Risperdal Consta, 865–867
risperidone, 865–867
Rispernia, 865–867
Ritalin 10, 1561–1563
Ritalin LA, 1561–1563
ritonavir, 934–936
rituximab, 773–774, 1071–1072
Rivacol Chlorhexidine 0.2% Mouthwash, 1149
rivaroxaban, 260–261
rivastigmine, 55–57
Rivotril, 395–396
Rixadone, 865–867
Rixalt, 579–580
Riximyo, 773–774, 1071–1072
Rixubis, 1212–1213
rizatriptan benzoate, 579–580
Roaccutane, 5–6
Robinul, 987–988
Robitussin Chesty Cough Oral Liquid, 1023
Robitussin Dry Cough Forte, 1021–1022
Rocaltrol, 966–968
Rocta, 5–6
rocuronium, sugammadex for, 365
rocuronium bromide, 1424–1425
romidepsin, 671–672
romiplostim, 1198–1199
Ropibam, 1331–1332
Ropinirole, 1417–1419
Ropivacaine hydrochloride, 1331
rosacea
  brimonidine for, 1029
  ivermectin and, 45, 46
Rostor, 1305–1306
rosuvastatin, 1305–1306
Rotarix Oral Liquid, 1615
rotavirus gastroenteritis, rotavirus vaccine for, 1615
rotavirus vaccine, 1615
rotigotine, 810–812
roundworms, 42
  albendazole for, 43
  mebendazole for, 47
Roxar, 205–206
roxithromycin, 205–206
Roxtine 20, 282–283
Rozex Cream and Gel, 826–829
RSV infection, 917
rubella, measles-mumps-rubella vaccine for, 1608
rufinamide, 415–416
rurioctocog alfa pegol, 1203–1205
Rusquen, 1045–1047

ruxolitinib, 731–733
Rydapt, 659
Rythmodan, 80–82

S

Sabril, 424
safinamide, 813–814
Saizen, 1228–1230
Salazopyrin, 1056–1057, 1166–1168
Salazopyrin EN-Tabs, 1056–1057, 1166–1168
salbutamol sulfate, 1475–1477
  action of, 1475
  adverse effects of, 1475
  dose of, 1475
  interactions of, 1475
  nursing points/cautions for, 1476
  patient teaching and advice for, 1476–1477
    autohaler, 107–108
    metered dose aerosol inhaler, 106–107
    rotahaler, 107
  use of, 1475
salcatonin. *See* calcitonin salmon (salcatonin)
salicylates, varicella zoster vaccines and, 965
salicylic acid, aspirin and, 817
Salmeterol, 108–109
Salmonella typhi vaccine, 1615–1616
Salofalk preparations, 1163–1165
Salpraz, 881–882
Saltabs, 1667–1668
salt-losing adrenogenital syndrome, fludrocortisone acetate for, 1007
Sandimmun IV, 1041–1045
Sandomigran, 577–578
Sandostatin, 1222–1224
Sandostatin LAR, 1222–1224
Sandrena, 1527–1529
Saphris, 841–842
Sapropterin, 1360–1362
saquinavir, 1277
sarcoma botryoides, dactinomycin for, 627
sarcomas
  dacarbazine for, 627
  ifosfamide for, 648
  vincristine sulfate for, 687
Sativex, 1394–1396
Savacol Mouth & Throat Rinse, 1149
saxagliptin, 1319
Saxenda, 36–38, 322–324
scabicides, 1024
scabies, 1025–1026
  benzyl benzoate for, 1026
  crotamiton for, 1027
  ivermectin and, 45, 46
  permethrin for, 1027–1028
scalp psoriasis, moderate-to-severe, clobetasol propionate for, 1002

INDEX

Scandonest 2% Special, 1330
Scandonest 3%, 1329–1330
scarring, in acne, 1
schizoaffective disorder
  lithium carbonate for, 854
  paliperidone for, 860
schizonts, tissue, 555
schizophrenia, 835
  amisulpride for, 839–840
  aripiprazole for, 840–841
  asenapine maleate for, 841–842
  brexpiprazole for, 842
  carbramazepine, 842–843
  cariprazine, 843–844
  chlorpromazine hydrochloride for, 844–846
  clozapine for, 847–849
  droperidol, 849–850
  flupentixol decanoate for, 850–851
  haloperidol decanoate and, 852–854
  lithium carbonate for, 854–857
  lurasidone hydrochloride for, 857
  olanzapine pamoate monohydrate for, 858–860
  paliperidone for, 860–862
  periciazine, 863
  quetiapine for, 863–865
  risperidone for, 865–867
  sodium valproate, 867–868
  ziprasidone for, 868–869
SciTropin A, 1228–1230
scurvy, 1644
sea snake antivenom, 894
sebelipase alfa, 1362–1363
Sebizole Shampoo, 446–447
seborrhoeic dermatitis, ketoconazole for, 446
secondary adrenocortical insufficiency, corticosteroids for, 992
secondary amenorrhoea
  medroxyprogesterone for, 1538
  norethisterone for, 1539
  oestrogens and, 1531
  progesterone, 1469
secondary hyperparathyroidism, cinacalcet for, 969
secondary immunodeficiency, 1624
secondary progressive multiple sclerosis, 1376
  fingolimod, 1376
  interferon beta 1b, 1392
secukinumab, 1271–1272
Seda Lotion, 1326–1329
sedating action, periciazine and, 863
sedatives and hypnotics, 1502–1518
  adverse effects of, 1503
  chloral hydrate, 1506–1507
  dexmedetomidine, 1507–1508
  flunitrazepam, 1508

sedatives and hypnotics (*Continued*)
  interactions of, 1503–1504
  lemborexant, 1508–1509
  melatonin, 1509–1510
  midazolam hydrochloride, 1511–1513
  nitrazepam, 1513
  nursing points/cautions for, 1504
  patient teaching and advice for, 1505–1506
  suvorexant, 1513–1515
  temazepam, 1515
  zolpidem tartrate, 1515–1517
  zopiclone, 1517–1518
Seebri Breezhaler, 112
seizure, 384
  antipsychotics and, 835
  hydroxychloroquine sulfate and, 1046
  triggers for, avoidance of, 386
  unclassifiable, 384
selective alpha 1A (α_{1A}) adrenoceptor antagonist, silodosin in, 952–953
selective alpha-1 adrenoreceptor antagonist, alfuzosin hydrochloride in, 943
selective alpha-2A-adrenergic receptor agonist, 1558
selective (o)estrogen receptor modulator (SERM), 958
selective immunosuppressant agent, 1272
selective serotonin reuptake inhibitors (SSRIs), 278–280
  actions of, 278
  adverse effects of, 278–279
  interactions of, 279
  nursing points/cautions for, 279–280
  patient teaching and advice for, 280
Selegiline hydrochloride, 814–816
self-administer medication, 1069
semen, alprostadil and, 1119
semi-synthetic opioid, 1022
senna, 1294
Senna-Gen, 1294
sennosides A and B, 1294
Senokot, 1294
Sensease Nasal Allergy Relief Nasal Spray, 1013–1014
sensitising events, 1627
separation anxiety, 70
sepsis
  amikacin for, 189
  TNF-α antagonists and, 1059
Septanest—injection, 1324
septic arthritis, teicoplanin for, 184
septic shock, adrenaline for, 1567
septicaemia
  ampicillin sodium for, 158
  chloramphenicol for, 209
  co-trimoxazole for, 222

septicaemia (*Continued*)
   teicoplanin for, 184
Septrin Forte, 222—225
Septrin Sugar Free Oral Suspension, 222—225
Serc, 1633—1634
Serenace, 852—854
Serepax, 77—78
Serevent, 108—109
serial coagulation tests, 890
SERM. *See* selective (o)estrogen receptor modulator
Seroquel, 863—865
Seroquel XR, 863—865
serotonin (5HT), lithium carbonate and, 854
serotonin and noradrenaline reuptake inhibitors (SNRIs), 284—285
   actions of, 284
   adverse effects of, 284
   interactions of, 284—285
   nursing points/cautions for, 285
   patient teaching and advice for, 285
serotonin (5HT$_2$) antagonist
   risperidone and, 865
   ziprasidone and, 868
serotonin (5HT$_2$) receptors, quetiapine and, 863
serotonin (5HT$_{2A}$) receptors
   asenapine maleate and, 841
   lurasidone hydrochloride and, 857
   paliperidone and, 860
serotonin syndrome, 265
   methylene blue trihydrate and, 354
Sertra, 283—284
sertraline, 283—284
serum cholesterol, antipsychotics and, 836
serum sickness, 1239
   cortisone acetate for, 1003
Setear, 1633—1634
Setrona, 283—284
sevelamer, 360—361
sevoflurane, 1181—1182
Sevorane, 1181—1182
sex hormones, 1519—1550
   androgens and anabolic steroids, 1519—1521
   oestrogens, 1524—1527
   oral contraceptives, 1547—1550
   other agents, 1541—1547
   production of, 1519
   progestogens, 1531—1534
sex steroid, decreased, in osteoporosis, 957—958
sexual drive, reduced, cyproterone acetate for, 1540
sexual intercourse
   clotrimazole use and, 436
   nystatin use and, 451
SGLT2 inhibitors. *See* sodium-glucose cotransporter 2 inhibitors (SGLT2 inhibitors)

shigellosis, norfloxacin for, 220
Shilova, 908—909
shingles. *See* herpes zoster; herpes zoster (shingles)
shock, ephedrine sulfate for, 1572
short-acting benzodiazepines, 1503
short-acting insulin, 300
short-acting local anaesthetics, 1321
sho-saiko-to, Chinese herbal medicine, 1283
Sical, 966—968
Sifrol, 809—810
Sifrol ER, 809—810
Sigmacort, 1009
Sigmaxin, 979
Signifor, 1224—1226
Signifor LAR, 1224—1226
Siguent Hycor Eye Ointment, 1009
Silaran, 1122
Silcap, 1122—1124
Sildatio PHT, 1122—1124
sildenafil, 1122—1124
silodosin, 952—953
silver sulfadiazine, 232—233
Simipex, 809—810
Simipex XR, 809—810
Simponi, 1064—1065
Simpral, 809—810
Simulect, 1246—1247
Simvar, 1306—1307
simvastatin, 1306—1307
   tocilizumab and, 1074
Singulair, 142—143
Sintetica Baclofen Intrathecal, 1402—1406
siponimod, 1385—1387
   action of, 1385
   adverse effects of, 1385—1386
   dose of, 1385
   interactions of, 1386
   nursing points/cautions of, 1386
   patient teaching and advice of, 1386—1387
   use of, 1385
sirolimus, 1272—1274
   action of, 1272
   adverse effects of, 1273
   dose of, 1272—1273
   interactions of, 1273
   nursing points/cautions of, 1273—1274
   patient teaching and advice of, 1274
   use of, 1272
sitagliptin, 319—320
skin cancer, ciclosporin and, 1042
skin diseases, vitamin A for, 1637
skin health, nicotinamide for, 1639
skin infections
   amoxicillin for, 154
   cefaclor monohydrate for, 168

INDEX

skin infections (*Continued*)
    co-trimoxazole for, 222
    daptomycin for, 225
    linezolid for, 212
    moxifloxacin hydrochloride for, 219
skin irritation, hydrocortisone sodium succinate for, 1009
skin lesions
    mercaptamine bitartrate for, 1355
skin rash, lamotrigine and, 401
skin test
    Atgam, antithymocyte globulin and, 1238
    tuberculin (Mantoux), for immunomodifiers, 1237
skin ulceration, methotrexate, 1051
Skyrizi, 1271
SLE. *See* systemic lupus erythematosus
sleep apnoea, androgens and anabolic steroids and, 1521
sleep hygiene, 1430
sleepiness, armodafinil for, 1553
Slenyto, 1509–1510
small cell lung cancer
    carboplatin for, 617
    epirubicin hydrochloride for, 636
    etoposide for, 639
    topotecan hydrochloride for, 681
small lymphocytic lymphoma
    ibrutinib for, 713
    idelalisib for, 714–715
smoking
    cessation, varenicline tartrate for, 1114
    erectile dysfunction and, 1117
    oral contraceptives and, 1549
snake antivenom, 889
snake bite, pressure immobilisation first aid technique for, 891
snake venom detection kit, 891
SNRIs. *See* serotonin and noradrenaline reuptake inhibitors
Snuzaid Tabs, 491–492
social anxiety disorder, 70
    escitalopram for, 281
    paroxetine for, 283
    sertraline for, 283
    venlafaxine hydrochloride for, 287
Sodibic, 1665–1667
sodium, 1667–1668
    idarucizumab and, 352
    sodium chloride, 1667–1668
sodium ascorbate, disodium edetate, 346
sodium bicarbonate, 1665–1667
    topiramate and, 423
Sodium Bicarbonate Injection, 1665–1667
Sodium Bicarbonate Injection 8.4%, 1665–1667
sodium chloride, 1667–1668

Sodium Chloride 0.9%, 1667–1668
Sodium Chloride 0.9% (Normal Saline) Sterile Injection, 1667–1668
Sodium Chloride (0.9%) for Irrigation Solution BP, 1667–1668
sodium cromoglycate, 98
sodium fusidate, 211–212
sodium iodide (^{131}I), 1588–1590
Sodium Iodide (^{131}I) Capsules (Therapy), 1588–1590
Sodium Iodide (^{131}I) Injection, 1588–1590
sodium nitrite, 361–362
sodium nitroprusside, 552–554
sodium phenylbutyrate, 1363–1364
sodium phosphate, 976, 1290–1292
Sodium Phosphate and Potassium Phosphate Concentrated Injection, 1660–1662
sodium picosulfate, 1295–1296
sodium polystyrene sulfonate hydrogen, 362–363
sodium tetradecyl sulfate, 1678
sodium thiosulfate, 363–364
sodium thiosulfate pentahydrate, 553
sodium valproate, 416–419, 867–868
sodium-glucose cotransporter 2 inhibitors (SGLT2 inhibitors), 304, 324–325
    actions of, 324
    nursing points/cautions for, 324–325
    patient teaching and advice for, 325
    uses of, 324
sofosbuvir, 913–914
Soframycin Ear, 189
Soframycin Eye Drops, 189
soft tissue infection
    amoxicillin trihydrate for, 154
    gentamicin sulfate for, 191
soft tissue sarcoma
    carboplatin for, 617
    epirubicin hydrochloride for, 636
    pazopanib for, 728
solar (actinic) keratosis
    fluorouracil for, 642
    imiquimod for, 1033
Solaraze 3% Gel, 20–22
Solavert, 88–90
Solian, 839
Solicare, 953–954
solid allogeneic organ rejection, prevention of, 1263
solifenacin succinate, 953–954
Soliris, 1249
Solprin, 15–17, 817–818
SoluCortef, 1009–1011
Solu-Medrol, 1011–1013
SolvEasy Tinea Cream, Gel or Spray, 454–456
Somac, 881–882
Somac Injection, 881–882

1791

somatostatin, 1216
somatotropic hormones, 1228—1230
somatropin (somatrophin/somatotropin), 1228—1230
Somatuline Autogel, 1221—1222
Somavert, 1226—1227
Somidem, 1515—1517
Sone, 1016—1017
Soolantra, 45—47
sorafenib tosilate, 735—736
Sorbisol, 1292
sorbitol, 1292
  idarucizumab with, 352
  osmotic laxative, charcoal, activated, 338
sore throat, povidone-iodine for, 1677
Sotacor, 88—90
sotalol, 88—90
  action of, 88
  adverse effects of, 89
  dose of, 88—89
  interactions of, 89
  nursing points/cautions for, 89—90
  patient teaching and advice for, 90
  use of, 88
Sozol, 881—882
Span-K, 1664—1665
spasmodic dysphonia, botulinum toxin type A for, 1406
spasmodic torticollis
  botulinum toxin type A for, 1406
  incobotulinumtoxinA for, 1413
spasmolytic drugs, 1402
spasms, muscle
  baclofen for, 1402
  orphenadrine citrate, 1415
spasticity, 1402
  dantrolene sodium hemiheptahydrate for, 1410
  focal, botulinum toxin type A for, 1406
  incobotulinumtoxinA for, 1412
Spedra, 1121—1122
sphincters, 942
spider antivenom, 889
spider bites, 889
spina bifida, folic acid for, 1643
spinal anaesthesia, 1322
spinal cord injury, erectile dysfunction and, 1116
spinal cord lesions, 942
Spiractin, 1096—1098
Spiriva, 114—117
Spiriva Respimat, 114—117
spironolactone, 1096—1098
splenomegaly, ruxolitinib for, 732
spondyloarthropathies, 1038
sporotrichosis, itraconazole for, 443
sporozoans, 825
sporozoites, 555

sport
  beta-adrenoceptor blocking agents and, 524b
  desmopressin and, 1232b
  goserelin acetate and, 1219
  haemopoietic agents and, 1184
  leuprorelin acetate and, 1220
  somatropin and, 1230b
  terlipressin and, 1236b
Spray Tish, 1147
Spray Tish Menthol, 1147
Spren, 15—17, 817—818
Sprycel, 708—709
squamous cell carcinoma
  afatinib for, 694
  bleomycin sulfate for, 612
  cetuximab for, 752
  cisplatin for, 621
  docetaxel for, 632
  methyl aminolevulinate hydrochloride for, 658
  nivolumab for, 766
  pembrolizumab for, 770
SSRIs. See selective serotonin reuptake inhibitors
ST elevation myocardial infarction (STEMI)
  clopidogrel for, 818
  ticagrelor for, 822
St John's wort, phenobarbital and, 407
Stamaril, 1618—1619
Staphylex, 162—163
staphylococcal enterocolitis, vancomycin hydrochloride for, 185—186
staphylococcal infections
  amikacin for, 189
  teicoplanin for, 184
Staquis, 1031—1032
statins, 1300—1302
  actions of, 1300
  adverse effects of, 1301
  interactions of, 1301
  nursing points/cautions for, 1301
  patient teaching and advice for, 1301—1302
  uses of, 1300—1301
status asthmaticus, cortisone acetate for, 1003—1004
status epilepticus, 384
steatorrhoea, pancreatic enzyme replacement therapy for, 1170
Stelara, 1279—1280
Stelax, 1402—1406
stem cell transplantation
  busulfan for, 613
  meningococcal vaccine for, 1609
Stemetil Solution for Injection, 380—382
STEMI. See ST elevation myocardial infarction
steroid hormones, 1299
Stildem, 1515—1517
Stilnox, 1515—1517

INDEX

Stilnox CR, 1515—1517
stimulant laxatives, 1292—1293
stimulants, 1551—1553
   adverse effects of, 1551—1552
   nursing points/cautions for, 1552—1553
   patient teaching and advice for, 1553
stiripentol, 419—420
Stokes-Adams attack, isoprenaline hydrochloride for, 1574
stomach pain, mercaptamine bitartrate for, 1355
stone fish antivenom, 895
strabismus, botulinum toxin type A for, 1407
Strensiq, 1341—1342
strenuous exercise, stimulants and, 1552
Strepfen Intensive Lozenges, 23—24
Strepfen Throat Spray, 23—24
streptococcal infection
   phenoxymethylpenicillin potassium for, 163
   teicoplanin for, 184
streptococcal pharyngitis
   cefalexin monohydrate for, 169
streptococcal prophylaxis, erythromycin lactobionate for, 204
streptococcal (group A) upper respiratory tract infection, benzathine benzylpenicillin for, 159
stress
   erectile dysfunction and, 1116
   seizure triggers, 386
stridor, from agalsidase alfa (GHU), 1337
stroke
   apixaban for, 259
   dabigatran etexilate for, 256
   ischaemic, alteplase for, 1153
   rivaroxaban for, 260
Stromectol, 45—47
Strongyloides
   albendazole for, 43
   corticosteroids and, 996
strongyloidiasis, ivermectin for, 45
ST-segment elevation myocardial infarction (STEMI), fondaparinux sodium for, 253
Stud 100 Desensitising Spray for Men, 1127, 1326—1329
subependymal giant cell astrocytoma, everolimus for, 1251
Sublimaze, 1439—1442
Sublocade, 1103, 1435—1438
Suboxone, 1438
   naloxone hydrochloride dihydrate and, 357
substance P, 513
Subutex, 1103, 1435—1438
sucralfate, 884—885
sucroferric oxyhydroxide, 364
Sudafed Xylo Nasal Decongestant Nasal Spray, 1148

sudden death, stimulants and, 1552
sudden fainting, antipsychotics and, 838
sugammadex sodium, 365—366
suicidal thoughts, antiepileptics and, 386
suicide, 836
sulfapyridine, 1166—1167
sulfasalazine, 1056—1057, 1166—1168
   leflunomide and, 1048
sulfite allergy, sympathomimetic agents and, 1566
sulfonamides, hypersensitivity to, 577
sulfonylureas, 306—308
   actions of, 306
   adverse effects of, 306
   interactions of, 306—307
   nursing points/cautions for, 307
   patient teaching and advice for, 307—308
   uses of, 306
Sulprix, 869
sulthiame, 421
Sumatran, 580—582
sumatriptan, 580—582
sunitinib, 737—738
   action of, 737
   adverse effects of, 737
   dose of, 737
   interactions of, 737
   nursing points/cautions for, 737
   patient teaching and advice for, 737—738
   use of, 737
sunlight
   auranofin and, 1040
   skin exposure to
      griseofulvin and, 441
      voriconazole and, 459
superficial basal cell carcinoma, imiquimod for, 1033
suppositories, NSAIDs, 15
Suprane, 1175
surface (topical) anaesthesia, 1321
surgery prophylaxis
   benzylpenicillin sodium for, 160
   cefoxitin sodium for, 172
   ceftriaxone for, 176
Survanta, 133—134
Sustanon, 250, 1522
Sutent, 737—738
suvorexant, 1513—1515
suxamethonium
   metoclopramide hydrochloride monohydrate and, 378
   non-depolarising blocking agents and, 1421
suxamethonium chloride, 1426—1428
Suxamethonium Juno, 1426—1428
Symmetrel, 799—800
sympathetic nervous system, 1565
sympathomimetic agents, 1565—1578

sympathomimetic agents (*Continued*)
  for bladder function disorder, 942—943
  interactions of, 1565—1566
  nursing points/cautions for, 1566—1567
sympathomimetic nasal decongestants, 1146
symptomatic benign prostatic hyperplasia, dutasteride for, 946
symptomatic hypocalcaemia, 959
Synagis, 1265
Synanceia horrida, 895
Synanceia verrucosa, 895
Synarel, 1467
synthetic gold complex, auranofin, 1039
Syntocinon, 1481—1482
Syntometrine, 1480, 1482
syphilis
  benzathine benzylpenicillin for, 158
  erythromycin lactobionate for, 204
  procaine benzylpenicillin for, 165
Syquet, 863—865
Systane Red Eyes, 1136—1137
systemic embolism
  apixaban for, 259
  dabigatran etexilate for, 256
  epoprostenol and, 1494
  rivaroxaban for, 260
systemic inflammatory disease, erectile dysfunction and, 1116
systemic lupus erythematosus (SLE)
  belimumab for, 1247
  DMARDs and, 1038
  hydroxychloroquine for, 1045

T

T cell lymphoma
  brentuximab vedotin for, 751
  cutaneous, 781
  romidepsin for, 671
  vorinostat for, 690
TachoSil, 1198
tachyarrhythmias, verapamil for, 541
tachycardia
  from agalsidase alfa (GHU), 1337
  from idursulfase, 1351
  stimulants and, 1551
Tacidine, 874
Tacrograf, 1275—1278
tacrolimus, 1275—1278
  action of, 1276
  adverse effects of, 1276—1277
  ciclosporin with, 1042
  dose of, 1276
  interactions of, 1277
  nursing points/cautions for, 1277—1278
  patient teaching and advice for, 1278
  use of, 1276

Tadacip, 1124—1125
Tadalaccord, 1124—1125
tadalafil, 1124—1125
Tadalca, 1124—1125
Tadalis, 1124—1125
Tadim, 221—222
Tafenoquine, 567—568
taipan antivenom, 895
Talam, 280
taliglucerase alfa (RPC), 1364—1365
Taltz, 1257
Tamate, 422—424
Tambocor, 84—85
Tamiflu, 910—911
Tamosin, 672—673
tamoxifen, 672—673
Tamsil, 454—456
tamsulosin hydrochloride, 954—955
Tapentadol, 1454—1455
tapeworms, 42
  albendazole for, 43
tetrabenazine for, 1399
Targocid, 184
Tasigna, 724—726
taste receptors, 1148
Tazac, 874
Tazarotene, 8
Tazopip, 164—165
TB. *See* tuberculosis
TCAs. *See* tricyclic antidepressants
Tecfidera, 1373—1374
teduglutide, 1157—1158
Teglutik, 1397—1399
Tegretol, 392—394, 842—843
teicoplanin, 184—185
Teicoplanin Sandoz, 184—185
Telfast, 493
telmisartan, 518—519
telotristat ethyl, 783—784
Teltartan, 518—519
Temaze, 1515
temazepam, 1515
Temgesic, 1103—1104, 1435—1438
Temizole, 674—675
Temodal, 674—675
temozolomide, 674—675
temperature regulation, chlorpromazine hydrochloride and, 844
temsirolimus, 505
Temtabs, 1515
Tenaxil SR, 1090—1091
tenecteplase, 1155
tenofovir alafenamide, 924
tenofovir disoproxil fumarate, 924—925
Tenormin, 524

INDEX

Tensig, 524
tension
   periciazine for, 863
   stimulants and, 1552–1553
tension headache, orphenadrine citrate for, 1415–1416
teratogen, 585, 1217b
Terbinafine, 454–456
Terbutaline, 109–110
Teriflagio, 1387–1389
teriflunomide, 1387–1389
   action of, 1387
   adverse effects of, 1387–1388
   dose of, 1387
   interactions of, 1388
   nursing points/cautions for, 1388–1389
   patient teaching and advice for, 1389
   use of, 1387
Terimide, 1387–1389
teriparatide, 977–978
terlipressin, 1235–1236
Terlipressin Ever Pharma Solution for Injection, 1235–1236
termination of pregnancy, agents for, 1482
   mifepristone in, 1482–1484
   misoprostol in, 1484–1486
Tertroxin, 1583–1585
Testavan, 1522
testicular cancer
   carboplatin for, 617
   dactinomycin for, 627
   vinblastine sulfate for, 686
testicular tumour, etoposide for, 639
Testogel, 1522
testosterone, 1522
testosterone decanoate, 1522
testosterone deficiency, testosterone undecanoate for, 1523
testosterone enantate, 1522
testosterone undecanoate, 1522–1524
   correct application technique for, 1524
   transdermal cream, 1524
   transdermal gel, 1524
   transdermal patches, 1528
tetanus
   diphtheria-tetanus vaccine for, 1601
tetanus immunoglobulin, 1628–1630
Tetanus Immunoglobulin-VF (For Intramuscular Use), 1628–1630
Tetanus Immunoglobulin-VF (For Intravenous Use), 1628–1630
tetanus-prone wounds, 1600, 1629–1630t
tetrabenazine, 1399–1400
tetracaine (amethocaine) hydrochloride, 1334–1335
tetracosactide (tetracosactrin), 80

tetracyclines, 194–195
   actions of, 194
   adverse effects of, 194
   interactions of, 194
   nursing points/cautions for, 195
   patient teaching and advice for, 195
   uses of, 194
tetrahydrobiopterin (BH$_4$) deficiency, sapropterin dihydrochloride for, 1360
tetrahydrocannabinol, 1394–1397
Tetryzoline, 1137–1138
Tevatiapine XR, 863–865
thalassaemia syndrome
   deferasirox, 339
   desferrioxamine mesylate, 342
thalidomide, 585, 675–678
   action of, 675
   adverse effects of, 675–676
   dose of, 675
   interactions of, 676
   nursing points/cautions for, 676–677
   patient teaching and advice for, 677–678
   use of, 675
Thalomid, 675–678
theophylline, 121–123
   allopurinol and, 475
   febuxostat and, 479
   methotrexate and, 656
thiamine deficiency, thiamine hydrochloride for, 1637
thiamine hydrochloride, 1637–1638
thiazide diuretic-induced hypokalaemia, 1092
thiazide diuretics, 489, 1091, 1079
   actions of, 1091
   adverse effects of, 1091
   chlortalidone, 1088
   ciclosporin with, 1043
   hydrochlorothiazide for, 1089–1090
   indapamide hemihydrate for, 1090
   interactions of, 1092
   nursing points/cautions for, 1092–1093
   patient teaching and advice for, 1093
   prochlorperazine maleate and, 380
   suxamethonium chloride and, 1426
   uses of, 1091
thiazolidinediones, 299, 315–317
   actions of, 315
   adverse effects of, 315–316
   interactions of, 316
   nursing points/cautions for, 316
   patient teaching and advice for, 316–317
   uses of, 315
thiocyanate, 361
thioguanine, 678–679
thionamides, 1581
thiopentone, 1323

1795

Thioprine, 1243—1245
thioureas, 1581
threadworms, 42
  albendazole for, 43
  corticosteroids and, 993
  mebendazole for, 47
3TC, 923—924
throat, agents for, 1128—1150
thrombin, 817, 1214
thrombocytopenia
  imiglucerase (RCH) for, 1352
  for romiplostim, 1198
thromboembolic disorders, heparin sodium for, 238
thromboembolic events, progestogens and, 1532
thromboembolism
  in atrial fibrillation, warfarin sodium for, 249
  oral contraceptives and, 1548
  pulmonary
    chronic, iloprost trometamol for, 1495
    epoprostenol and, 1495
    iloprost trometamol for, 1495
thrombolysis, in myocardial infarction
  tenecteplase for, 1155
thrombolytic agents, 1151
thrombophilia, androgens and anabolic steroids and, 1521
thrombophlebitis, oral contraceptives and, 1549
thrombosis, 1151
  enoxaparin sodium for, 244
thrombotic agents, 262—263
thrombotic events, immunoglobulins and, 1621
thromboxane A_2, 817
thrombus, formation of, 817
Thymoglobuline, 1238—1240
Thyrogen, 1680—1681
thyroid agents, 1579—1585
  levothyroxine sodium, 1581—1583
  liothyronine sodium, 1583—1585
thyroid cancer
  dabrafenib for, 707
  doxorubicin hydrochloride for, 633—635
  sorafenib tosilate for, 735
  trametinib for, 739
thyroid function monitoring, lenalidomide and, 1260
thyroid function tests, propylthiouracil and, 1587
thyroid gland, 1579
  dysfunction, 1580
thyroid hormone deficiencies, levothyroxine sodium for, 1581
thyroid hormone secretion, control of, 1579
thyroid hormones, 1579—1580
thyroidectomy
  carbimazole for, 1585
  propylthiouracil for, 1587

thyroid-stimulating hormone (TSH), 1216, 1680
thyrostatic compounds, 1581
thyrotoxic crisis, propylthiouracil for, 1587—1588
thyrotoxicosis, 1580
  antipsychotics and, 837
  betaxolol and, 465
  liothyronine sodium for, 1584
thyrotrophin alfa, 1680—1681
thyrotropin, 1579
thyrotropin-releasing hormone (TRH), 1486, 1579
thyroxine sodium (T_4), 1579
tiagabine hydrochloride, 422
tibolone, 1545—1547
ticagrelor, 822—823
tigecycline, 198
tiger snake antivenom, 895—896
tildrakizumab, 1278—1279
Timoptol, 470—471
Timoptol XE, 470—471
Tinaderm Powder, 456
Tinasil, 454—456
Tinea spp., 428
tioguanine, 678—679
tiotropium bromide, 139
  HandiHaler, 115—116
  Zonda device, 116
tipranavir, 913
Tirofiban, 823
Tirofiban Juno Concentrate, 823
tisagenlecleucel, 679
  action of, 679
  adverse effects of, 679
  dose of, 679
  interactions of, 680
  nursing points/cautions for, 680—681
  patient teaching and advice for, 681
  use of, 679
tissue plasminogen activator (tPA), 1153
  tenecteplase as, 1155
tissue schizonts, 555—556
Tivicay, 939—940
Tixol, 286—287
TNF. *See* tumour necrosis factor
TNF-α antagonists. *See* tumour necrosis factor alpha (TNF-α) antagonists
Tobi, 191—194
Tobramycin Injection, 191—194
Tobramycin PF, 191—194
Tobramycin SUN, 191—194
tobramycin sulfate, 191—194
Tobrex, 191—194
tocilizumab, 1073—1075
tocolytic agents, 1474
tofacitinib, 1075—1077
Tofranil, 272

INDEX

tolnaftate, 456
tolterodine tartrate, 955–956
Tomudex, 670
tonic seizures, 384
tonic–clonic seizures, 385
tonsillitis, cefalexin for, 169
Topamax, 422–424
topical agents, for acne management, 6–7
topical anaesthesia, 1321
topical corticosteroids, 995–996, 999
topical ectoparasitical agents, 1024
    benzyl alcohol, 1025
    benzyl benzoate, 1026
    crotamiton, 1027
    for pediculosis (lice infestation), 1024–1025
    permethrin, 1027–1028
    scabies, 1025–1026
topical gel, NSAIDs, 14
topical therapy, retinoids, 3–4
topiramate, 422–424
    monotherapy with, 423
topotecan, leflunomide and, 1048
topotecan hydrochloride, 681
Toppin Salt Tablets, 1667–1668
Topra, 881–882
Toprol-XL, 528–529
Toradol, 27–28
toremifene, 682–683
    action of, 682
    adverse effects of, 682
    dose of, 682
    interactions of, 682
    nursing points/cautions for, 682
    patient teaching and advice for, 682
    sugammadex sodium with, 365
    use of, 682
Torlemo DT, 400–402
torticollis, spasmodic
    botulinum toxin type A for, 1406
    incobotulinumtoxinA for, 1413
Torvastat, 1302–1303
Torzole, 881–882
total hip arthroplasty, tranexamic acid for, 1200
total knee arthroplasty, tranexamic acid for, 1200
Toujeo, 301
Tourette's syndrome, stimulants and, 1552–1553
toxoplasmosis, pyrimethamine for, 825
Tracrium Injectable, 1423
Trajenta, 318–319
tramadol, ondansetron on, 371
Tramal SR, 1452–1454
tramazoline, 1147–1148
Tramedo, 1452–1454
Tramedo SR, 1452–1454
trametinib, 738–739
Tranalpha, 512–513

trandolapril, 512–513
tranexamic acid, 1200–1201
    action of, 1200
    adverse effects of, 1200
    dose of, 1200
    interactions of, 1200
    nursing points/cautions of, 1200–1201
    patient teaching and advice of, 1201
    use of, 1200
Tranexamic Acid Solution for Injection, 1200–1201
transdermal patches, nicotine, 1110
transfusion haemosiderosis, desferrioxamine mesylate, 342
transfusion-dependent anaemia, treatment of, 1259
Transiderm-Nitro, 59–62
transient ischaemic attack, dipyridamole for, 819
transient ovarian cysts, nafarelin acetate and, 1468
tranylcypromine, 276
trastuzumab, 777
trastuzumab emtansine, 777–779
    action of, 777
    adverse effects of, 778
    dose of, 777–778
    interactions of, 778
    nursing points/cautions for, 778
    patient teaching and advice for, 778–779
    use of, 777
Travacalm HO, 988–989
Travatan Eye Drops, 471–472
traveller's diarrhoea
    norfloxacin for, 220
travoprost, 471–472
Trazimera, 777–779
trematodes, 42
Tremfya, 1254
Trental 400, 1634
Tretinoin, 6
tretinoin, 6
Trexject, 655–657, 1050–1054
TRH. *See* thyrotropin-releasing hormone
triamcinolone acetonide, 1017
triamterene, 810
Tricortone, 1017
tricyclic antidepressants (TCAs), 267–269
    actions of, 267
    adverse effects of, 267
    interactions of, 267–268
    nursing points/cautions for, 268–269
    patient teaching and advice for, 269
triglycerides, 1299–1300
    antipsychotics and, 836
trihexyphenidyl (benzhexol) hydrochloride, 794–795
Trileptal, 403–405

1797

trimethoprim, 233—235
trimethoprim with sulfamethoxazole, 222—225
Tripacel, 1601—1602
Triprim, 233—235
triptans, 570
Tritace, 511—512
tropicamide, 1133—1134
tropisetron, 373
Tropisetron-AFT, 373
Tropisetron-MYX, 373
Trovas, 1302—1303
Trulicity, 322
Trusamide, 468
Trusopt, 468
Trust Fexit, 493
Trust Stomach Ease, 988—989
Truxima, 773—774, 1071—1073
trypanosomiasis, pentamidine isetionate for, 829
Tryzan, 511—512
TSH. *See* thyroid-stimulating hormone
TSH-responsive thyroid tumours, levothyroxine sodium for, 1581
tuberculin skin test (Mantoux), for immunomodifiers, 1237
tuberculin test, 1058
tuberculosis (TB), 584
   BCG Vaccine for, 1596
   ethambutol hydrochloride for, 587
   isoniazid, 588
   rifabutin for, 590
   rifampicin for, 592
tuberous sclerosis complex, everolimus for, 1251
tumour necrosis factor (TNF), 1067
tumour necrosis factor alpha (TNF-α) antagonists, 1057, 1060
   actions of, 1057
   adalimumab, 1060—1062
   adverse effects of, 1057—1058
   certolizumab, 1062—1063
   etanercept, 1063—1064
   golimumab, 1064—1065
   infliximab, 1065—1067
   interactions of, 1058
   nursing points of, 1058—1059
   patient teaching and advice for, 1059—1060
tumour-induced hypercalcaemia, 958, 959
turbuhaler, terbutaline sulfate, 109
Turner's syndrome, somatropin (somatotrophin/ somatotropin) for, 1228
Tygacil, 198
Tykerb, 718—719
type 1 diabetes mellitus, 296—298
type 2 diabetes mellitus, 297, 324
   metformin hydrochloride for, 311
type II 5 alpha reductase, 947
Typhim Vi, 1615—1616

typhoid fever
   chloramphenicol for, 209
   typhoid (*Salmonella typhi*) vaccine, 1615
typhoid (*Salmonella typhi*) vaccine, 1615—1616
typical antipsychotic agents, 833
tyrosinaemia type 1, nitisinone for, 1358
Tysabri, 1380—1381

U

ulceration, deferasirox and, 339
ulcerative colitis, 1159
   adalimumab for, 1060
   antidiarrhoeal agents and, 331
   balsalazide sodium for, 1160
   budesonide for, 125, 127
   golimumab for, 1065
   infliximab for, 1066
   lanthanum and, 353
   olsalazine sodium for, 1166
   sulfasalazine for, 1056
   vedolizumab (rch) for, 1168
ulcerative proctitis, mesalazine for, 1163
ulcerative proctosigmoiditis, mesalazine for, 1163
umeclidinium, 117—118
uncontrolled hyperthyroidism, stimulants and, 1552—1553
Unisom Sleepgels, 491—492
unstable angina, 60
   clopidogrel for, 818
   enoxaparin sodium for, 244
   fondaparinux sodium for, 253
   ticagrelor for, 822
   tirofiban hydrochloride for, 823
upadacitinib, 1077—1078
upper respiratory tract infections, amoxicillin trihydrate for, 154
urate turnover conditions, high, allopurinol for, 475
urea cycle disorders, sodium valproate and, 418
Uremide, 1085—1088
urethral pressure, alfuzosin hydrochloride in, 943
urethritis, amoxicillin trihydrate for, 154
Urex Forte, 1085—1088
urgency incontinence
   darifenacin hydrobromide for, 945
   mirabegron for, 948
   oxybutynin for, 949
   solifenacin succinate for, 953
   tolterodine tartrate for, 955
uric acid, 473
uricolytic agents, 473—483
urinary frequency
   darifenacin hydrobromide for, 945
   oxybutynin for, 949—950
   solifenacin succinate for, 953
   tolterodine tartrate for, 955

urinary retention
  antipsychotics and, 837
  neostigmine for, 982
  phenoxybenzamine hydrochloride for, 502
urinary tract infection
  amoxicillin trihydrate for, 154
  ampicillin sodium for, 158
  aztreonam for, 179
  cefalexin monohydrate for, 169
  cefalotin (cephalothin) sodium for, 170
  cefepime hydrochloride for, 170
  cefotaxime for, 171
  ceftazidime for, 174
  ceftazidime with avibactam for, 173
  ceftolozane with tazobactam for, 175
  co-trimoxazole for, 222
  fosfomycin for, 227
  methenamine (hexamine) hippurate for, 229
  nitrofurantoin for, 229
  norfloxacin for, 219
  trimethoprim for, 222
Urocarb, 944
urogenital trichomoniasis, metronidazole for, 827
Uromitexan, 780–781
Urorec, 952–953
urothelial cancer
  enfortumab vedotin, 760
  nivolumab for, 766
  pembrolizumab for, 770–761
ursodeoxycholic acid, 1158–1159
Ursodox GH, 1158–1159
Ursofalk, 1158–1159
Ursosan, 1158–1159
urticaria
  from aciclovir, 899
  from agalsidase alfa (GHU), 1337
  from alglucosidase alfa (RHU), 1339
  fexofenadine for, 493
ustekinumab, 1279–1280
uterine atony, prevention of, carbetocin for, 1478
uterine bleeding, abnormal,
    medroxyprogesterone for, 1538
uterine cancer
  dactinomycin for, 627
  fluorouracil for, 642
  vincristine sulfate for, 687
uterine fibroids, goserelin acetate for, 1217
uterine hypertonus, dinoprostone and, 1477
uterine spasm
  mifepristone and, 1483
  progesterone and, 1470
Utrogestan, 1469–1471
Uvadex, 781–783
uveitis
  adalimumab for, 1060

uveitis (*Continued*)
  cyclopentolate hydrochloride for, 1132

V

vaccination, 1591
  leflunomide and, 1048
vaccines, 1591–1598
  actions of, 1592
  BCG Vaccine, 1597
  cholera vaccine, 1597–1598
  conjugate, 1602
  COVID-19 Vaccine, 1600–1600
  diphtheria-tetanus vaccine, 1600–1601
  diphtheria-tetanus-pertussis (DTP) vaccine, 1601–1602
  Haemophilus influenzae type B vaccine, 1602–1603
  healthcare workers, 1594–1594
  hepatitis A vaccine, 1603
  hepatitis B vaccine, 1603–1604
  human papillomavirus (HPV) vaccine, 1605
  influenza vaccine, 1605–1607
  interactions of, 1592–1593
  Japanese encephalitis virus vaccine, 1607–1608
  live attenuated, 1592
  measles-mumps-rubella vaccine, 1608–1610
  meningococcal vaccine, 1609–1610
  National Immunisation Program Schedule, 1594–1596
  nursing points/cautions for, 1593–1593
  overseas travel, 1594
  patient teaching and advice for, 1593–1594
  pneumococcal vaccine, 1610–1611
  poliomyelitis vaccine, 1612
  Q fever vaccine, 1612–1613
  rabies vaccine, 1613–1615
  rotavirus vaccine, 1615
  typhoid (*Salmonella typhi*) vaccine, 1615–1616
  uses of, 1591–1592
  varicella zoster vaccines, 1616–1617
  yellow fever vaccine, 1618–1619
  zoster vaccine, 1619–1620
Vaclovir, 908–909
Vagifem Low, 1527–1529
vaginal cancer, human papillomavirus (HPV) vaccine for, 1605
vaginal dryness, nafarelin acetate and, 1468
vaginal infection, estriol for, 1529
valaciclovir, 908–909
Valcyte, 909–910
Valdoxan, 288–289
valganciclovir, 909–910
Valium, 75–77
Valoid, 382–383
Valpam, 75–77
Valpro EC, 416–419, 867–868

valsartan, 519—521
Valtrex, 908—909
Vancocin, 185—186
Vancocin CP, 185—186
Vancomycin Powder for Infusion, 185—186
vancomycin-resistant *Enterococcus faecium* (VRE), 148—149
VAQTA Adult Formula, 1603
vardenafil, 733
varenicline Lupin, 1114—1115
variant (Prinzmetal's or vasospastic) angina, 58
  nifedipine for, 539
varicella zoster vaccines, 1616—1617
varicose veins
  sodium tetradecyl sulfate for, 1678
Varilrix, 1616—1617
Varivax Refrigerated, 1616—1617
Vasafil, 1122—1124
Vascalace, 511—512
vascular ischaemia, clopidogrel for, 818
Vasocardol, 536—537
Vasocardol CD, 536—537
vasodilation reaction, chloral hydrate and, 1506
vasodilators, 1633—1635
vasopressin, 1217, 1232
vasovagal episodes, in post-vaccination, 1593
Vaxigrip Tetra, 1605—1607
Vectibix, 769—770
vectors, malaria, 556
vecuronium, sugammadex sodium for, 365
vecuronium bromide, 1425
Vedafil, 1122—1124
vedolizumab (rch), 1168—1170
velaglucerase alfa (GHU), 1365—1367
Velcade, 698—699
Veletri, 1493—1495
Velphoro, 364
Veltassa, 358—359
Vemlidy, 924
vemurafenib, 741—742
venereal disease, benzathine penicillin for, 159
venlafaxine hydrochloride, 287—288
Venofer, 1657
venous thrombi, 236
venous thromboembolism (VTE)
  antipsychotics and, 836
  apixaban for, 259
  dabigatran etexilate for, 256
  dalteparin sodium for, 241
  danaparoid sodium for, 243
  enoxaparin sodium for, 244
  fondaparinux sodium for, 253
  nadroparin calcium for, 247
  rivaroxaban for, 260
  warfarin sodium for, 249
Ventavis, 1495

ventilator-associated pneumonia, ceftazidime with avibactam for, 174
Ventolin Obstetric Injection, 104—108, 1475—1477
Ventolin preparations, 104—108
ventricular arrhythmias, stimulants and, 1553
ventricular fibrillation
  adrenaline and, 1568
  stimulants and, 1552—1553
ventricular flutter, stimulants and, 1552—1553
ventricular tachycardia, stimulants and, 1552—1553
Vepesid, 639—640
verapamil, activated charcoal and, 337
verapamil hydrochloride, 513
Vercure, 1425
Vermox, 47—48
vernal keratoconjunctivitis, lodoxamide trometamol, 1136
Versacloz, 847—849
Versatis, 1326—1329
very-low-density lipoproteins (VLDL), 1299
Vesanoid, 6, 684—685
Vesicare, 953—954
Vexazone, 315—317
Vfend, 457—459
Viagra, 1122—1124
Viatocinon, 1481—1482
Vibrio cholerae, serogroup O, 1, 1597
Vicks Cough Syrup for Chest Coughs, 1023
Vicks Sinex Nasal Spray, 1147
Viclofen, 20—22
Victoza, 36, 322—324
vigabatrin, 424
vildagliptin, 320—321
Vimizim, 1348—1349
Vimpat, 399—400
vinblastine sulfate, 686—687
vincristine sulfate, 687—688
Vincristine Sulfate, 687—688
vinegar, as first aid, 892
vinorelbine, 688—690
Viread, 924—925
viruses, 827
Visine Advanced, 1137—1138
Visine Clear, 1137—1138
vision
  blurred, olopatadine hydrochloride and, 495
  deferasirox and, 339—340
  loss of, mercaptamine bitartrate for, 1355
vismodegib, 742—743
visual disturbances, bisphosphonates and, 960
Vita B12, 1641—1642
vitamin A, 1636—1637
vitamin B, 1637—1638
  cyanocobalamin, 1640

INDEX

vitamin B (*Continued*)
  folic acid, 1642–1643
  hydroxocobalamin, 1641–1642
  nicotinamide, 1638–1639
  pyridoxine, 1639
  thiamine hydrochloride, 1637–1638
vitamin B$_1$, 1637–1638
vitamin B$_2$, 1638
vitamin B$_3$, 1638–1639
vitamin B$_6$, 1639–1640
vitamin B$_{12}$, 1640–1641, 1641–1642
vitamin C, 1643–1645
  ascorbic acid, 1643–1645
  colchicine and, 478
  desferrioxamine mesylate and, 343
vitamin D, 1645–1647
  colecalciferol, 1645–1647
  deficiency, calcitriol for, 966
  toxicity, 967
vitamin D$_3$, 1645–1647
vitamin E, 1647
vitamin K, 366–367, 1647–1648
  phytomenadione, 1648–1649
  rifabutin and, 590
  rifampicin and, 592
vitamin K antagonists, 249–253
vitamin K$_1$, 366–367, 1648–1649
vitamins, 1636–1670
  fat soluble, 1636
  folic acid, 1642–1643
  vitamin A, 1636–1637
  vitamin B, 1637–1642
  vitamin C, 1643–1645
  vitamin D, 1645–1647
  vitamin E, 1647
  vitamin K, 1647–1649
  water soluble, 1636
vitreomacular traction, ocriplasmin for, 1142
Vivaxim, 1616
Vivotif (Oral), 1615–1616
Vizo-PF Bimatoprost, 465–466
Volibris, 1–2
Volirop, 525–526
Voltaren, 20–22
Voltaren Emulgel, 22
Voltaren Ophta, 22
Voltaren Osteo Gel, 22
Voltaren Osteo Gel 12-hourly, 22
Voltaren Rapid, 22
Vomiting. *See also* nausea and vomiting
  from agalsidase alfa (GHU), 1337
  chlorpromazine hydrochloride for, 844
  haloperidol decanoate for, 852
  mercaptamine bitartrate for, 1355
  pyridoxine for, 1639
von Willebrand disease, 1194

von Willebrand disease (*Continued*)
  Biostate for, 1205
voriconazole, 457–459
vorinostat, 690
vortioxetine, 294–295
Votrient, 728–729
VPRIV, 1365–1367
VTE. *See* venous thromboembolism
Vttack, 457–459
vulval cancer, human papillomavirus (HPV) vaccine for, 1605
vulvovaginal surgery, estriol before, 1530
Vytorin, 1307
Vyvanse, 1560–1561

W

Wafesil, 1122–1124
waist circumference, 35
Waldenstrom's macroglobulinaemia
  chlorambucil for, 619
  cladribine for, 622
  ibrutinib for, 714
  zanubrutinib, 743
warfarin
  androgens and anabolic steroids and, 1520
  aprepitant with, 374
  itraconazole and, 445
  phenobarbital and, 407
  phenytoin sodium and, 410–411
  tibolone and, 1546
  vitamin K, 367
warfarin sodium, 249–253
  action of, 249
  adverse effects of, 249
  dose of, 249
  interactions of, 249–250
  nursing points/cautions for, 250–252
  patient teaching and advice for, 252–253
  use of, 249
washout procedure, leflunomide, 1049
water soluble vitamins, 1647
wax softeners, 1144
Waxsol, 1144, 1294
weight
  etonogestrel and, 1534
  gain, pregabalin and, 413
weight-loss agents, 35–41
Wellvone Suspension, 825–826
whipworms, 42
  albendazole for, 43
  mebendazole for, 47
Wilms' tumour
  dactinomycin for, 627
  doxorubicin for, 633
  vincristine sulfate for, 687

Wilson's disease, 1054
withdrawal syndrome, baclofen and, 1403
Women Regaine, 1034—1036
wound healing, ascorbic acid for, 1644

X

Xadago, 813—814
Xalaprost, 468—469
Xalatan, 468—469
Xalkori, 706
xanthine derivative, 1634
xanthine oxidase, 475
xanthines, 118—123
Xarelto, 260—262
Xatral SR, 943—944
Xelabine, 616—617
Xeljanz, 1075—1077
Xenical, 38—40
Xeomin, 1412—1415
Xergic, 493
Xermelo, 783—784
xerophthalmia, vitamin A for, 1637
Xgeva, 755, 971—973
Xiao-Chai-Hu, Chinese herbal medicine, 1283
Xifaxan, 231—232
Xiidra, 1141—1142
Xofigo, 669—670
Xogel Dental Gel, 1326—1329
Xolair, 143—145
X-rays, retinoids and, 3
Xtandi, 635
Xylocaine preparations, 1326—1329
Xylocard, 82—84, 1326—1329
xylometazoline hydrochloride, 1148
Xyntha, 1203
Xyvion, 1545—1547

Y

yeast, 428
yellow fever, 1618
  vaccine, 1618
Yervoy, 764—765
Yescarta, 605—607

Z

Zabep, 882
Zactin Tabs, 281
Zaldair, 33, 1454
Zamic, 1200—1201
zanamivir, 897, 912—913
Zanidip, 538—539
Zantac Concentrate for Injection, 875
Zantac Oral Liquid, 875
Zantac preparations, 875
Zarontin, 397
Zarzio, 785—788

Zatamil, 1013—1014
Zavedos, 647
Zavesca, 1357—1358
Zavicefta, 174—175
Zedace, 506—508
Zedd, 201—202
Zeffix, 923—924
Zelboraf, 741—742
Zeldox, 868—869
Zeldox IM, 868—869
Zelitrex, 908—909
Zentel, 43—45
Zerbaxa, 175—176
Zestril, 509—510
Zetin, 4—5
Zetlam, 923—924
Ziagel Dental gel, 1326—1329
Ziagen, 920—922
Zidoval Vaginal Gel, 826—829
zidovudine, 925—927
  amphotericin B and, 430
Zient, 1317—1318
Ziextenzo, 788—789
Zimstat, 1306—1307
zinc, 1668
  deficiency, 1668
zinc chloride, 1668—1669
Zinc Chloride Concentrated Injection, 1668—1669
zinc sulfate, 1669
ZinCaps, 1670
Zinforo, 173
Zinnat, 177—178
Zinnat Suspension, 177—178
Zinopril, 509—510
ziprasidone, 868—869
Ziprox, 868—869
Zircol, 538—539
Zithro, 201—202
Zithromax, 201—202
Zithromax IV, 201—202
Zocor, 1306—1307
Zofran, 371—372
Zoladex 3.6 mg Implant, 1217—1219
Zoladex 10.8 mg Implant, 1217—1219
zoledronic acid, 964—965
Zolinza, 690
zolmitriptan, 582—583
Zoloft, 283—284
Zolpibell, 1515—1517
zolpidem tartrate, 1515—1517
Zoltrip, 582—583
Zometa, 964—965
Zomig, 582—583
Zonegran, 425—427
zonisamide, 425—427

INDEX

zopiclone, 1517—1518
Zopral, 879—880
Zopral ODT, 879—880
Zostavax, 1611
zoster immunoglobulin, 1630—1631
Zoton FasTabs, 879
Zovirax Cold Sore Cream, 898—900
Zovirax Ophthalmic Ointment, 898—900
Zovirax Tablets, 898—900
zuclopenthixol, 869
zuclopenthixol acetate, 869
zuclopenthixol decanoate, 869—870
Zumenon, 1527—1529
Zyban SR, 1104—1106
Zydelig, 714—715
Zydol, 1452—1454
Zydol SR, 1452—1454
Zyloprim, 475—476
Zypine, 858—860
Zypine ODT, 858—860
Zyprexa, 858—860
Zyprexa IM, 858—860
Zyprexa Relprevv, 858—860
Zyprexa Zydis Wafers, 858—860
Zyrtec, 488—489
Zyrtec Eye Drops, 493—494
Zyrtec Nasal Spray, 493—494
Zytiga, 600
Zyvox, 212—213